INFECTIOUS DISEASES

For Elsevier

Commissioning Editor: *Sue Hodgson*
Development Editor: *Sven Pinczewski*
Editorial Assistant: *Poppy Garraway*
Project Manager: *Elouise Ball*
Copyeditor: *Isobel Black*
Design: *Charles Gray*
Illustration Manager: *Merlyn Harvey*
Illustrator: *Ethan Danielson*
Marketing Manager(s) (UK/USA): *Clara Toombs/Brenna Christiansen*

INFECTIOUS DISEASES

THIRD EDITION

Edited by

Jonathan Cohen
MB BS FRCP FRCPath FRCPE FMedSci
Professor of Infectious Diseases, and Dean
Brighton and Sussex Medical School
Honorary Consultant Physician, Royal Sussex
County Hospital
Brighton, UK

Steven M Opal
MD
Professor of Medicine Infectious Disease
Division, The Warren Alpert Medical School
of Brown University, Providence, RI, USA

William G Powderly
MD FRCPI
Professor of Medicine and Therapeutics
Head, UCD School of Medicine and
Medical Sciences, Health Sciences Centre
University College Dublin
Dublin, Ireland

Section editors

Thierry Calandra MD PhD
Professor of Medicine
Head, Infectious Diseases
Service, Department
of Internal Medicine
Centre Hospitalier
Universitaire Vaudois
Lausanne, Switzerland

Nathan Clumeck MD PhD
Professor of Infectious Diseases
Head, Department of
Infectious Diseases
St Pierre University Hospital
Brussels, Belgium

Jeremy Farrar FRCP FRCP
(Ed) FMedSci PhD OBE
Director
Oxford University Clinical
Research Unit
The Hospital for Tropical
Diseases
Ho Chi Minh City, Vietnam

Roger G Finch MB BS FRCP
FRCPath FRCPEd FFPM
Professor of Infectious
Diseases
School of Molecular Medical
Science
Division of Microbiology
and Infectious Disease
Nottingham University
Hospitals NHS Trust
Nottingham, UK

Scott M Hammer MD
Professor of Medicine
and Public Health
(Epidemiology)
Columbia University
Presbyterian Hospital
New York, NY, USA

Andy IM Hoepelman
MD PhD
Professor in Medicine,
Infectious Diseases Specialist
Head, Department of Internal
Medicine and Infectious
Diseases
University Medical Center
Utrecht, The Netherlands

Timothy E Kiehn PhD
Chief, Microbiology Service
Memorial Sloan-Kettering
Cancer Center
New York, NY, USA

Kieren A Marr MD
Director, Transplant and
Oncology
John Hopkins University
School of Medicine
Baltimore, MD, USA

Keith P W J McAdam MA
MB BChir FRCP FWACP
Emeritus Professor of Clinical
Tropical Medicine
London School of Hygiene
and Tropical Medicine
London, UK

Didier Raoult MD PhD
Professor, Faculté de
Médecine, Unité des
Rickettsies
WHO Collaborative Center
for Rickettsial Reference and
Research
Marseille, France

Robert T Schooley MD
Professor and Head
Division of Infectious Diseases
Academic Vice Chair
Department of Medicine
University of California
San Diego, La Jolla, CA

Jack D Sobel MD
Professor of Infectious
Diseases
Division Head, Infectious
Diseases
Wayne State University -
Medicine
Detroit, MI, USA

Jos WM van der Meer
MD PhD FRCP
Professor of Medicine
Department of General
Internal Medicine, Nijmegen
Institute for Infection,
Inflammation and Immunity
Radboud University Medical
Centre
Nijmegen, The Netherlands

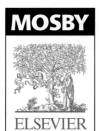

MOSBY

ELSEVIER

MOSBY is an imprint of Elsevier Limited.

© 2010, Elsevier Limited. All rights reserved.

First published 1999
Second edition 2004
Third edition 2010
Chapters 4, 13, PP37, 120, 121, 126, 182 and 184 are US Government works in the public domain and not subject to copyright.

The right of Jonathan Cohen, Steven M Opal, William G Powderly, Thierry Calandra, Nathan Clumeck, Jeremy Farrar, Roger G Finch, Scott M Hammer, Andy IM Hoepelman, Timothy E Kiehn, Kieren A Marr, Keith PWJ McAdam, Didier Raoult, Robert T Schooley, Jack D Sobel and Jos WM van der Meer to be identified as authors of this work has been asserted by them in accordance with the Copyright, Designs and Patents Act 1988.

ISBN: 978-0-323-04579-7

British Library Cataloguing in Publication Data
Infectious diseases.-3rd ed.
  1. Communicable diseases 2. Communicable diseases - Diagnosis 3. Communicable diseases - Treatment
I. Cohen, J. (Jon), 1949-
616.9
ISBN-13: 9780323045797

Infectious diseases.-3rd ed., Expert consult premium ed.
  1. Communicable diseases 2. Communicable diseases - Diagnosis 3. Communicable diseases - Treatment
I. Cohen, J. (Jon), 1949-
616.9
ISBN-13: 9780723435037

Library of Congress Cataloging in Publication Data
A catalog record for this book is available from the Library of Congress

Notice

Medical knowledge is constantly changing. Standard safety precautions must be followed, but as new research and clinical experience broaden our knowledge, changes in treatment and drug therapy may become necessary or appropriate. Readers are advised to check the most current product information provided by the manufacturer of each drug to be administered to verify the recommended dose, the method and duration of administration, and contraindications. It is the responsibility of the practitioner, relying on experience and knowledge of the patient, to determine dosages and the best treatment for each individual patient. Neither the Publisher nor the author assume any liability for any injury and/or damage to persons or property arising from this publication.

The Publisher

Printed in China
Last digit is the print number: 9 8 7 6 5 4 3 2 1

Contents

Contents

Section 3: Special Problems in Infectious Disease Practice

Contents

Section 4: Infections in the Immunocompromised Host

Thierry Calandra & Kieren A Marr

Volume 2

Section 5: HIV and AIDS

Nathan Clumeck & William G Powderly

PREVENTION

PATHOGENESIS

CLINICAL PRESENTATION

Section 6: International Medicine

Jeremy Farrar & Keith PWJ McAdam

MAJOR TROPICAL SYNDROMES: SKIN AND SOFT TISSUE

MAJOR TROPICAL SYNDROMES: THE CENTRAL NERVOUS SYSTEM

MAJOR TROPICAL SYNDROMES: THE GASTROINTESTINAL TRACT

Contents

Section 7: Anti-Infective Therapy

Roger G Finch & Scott M Hammer

Section 8:   Clinical Microbiology

Andy IM Hoepelman & Timothy E Kiehn

VIRUSES

BACTERIA

FUNGI

PARASITES

Preface to the Third Edition

These are extraordinary times in the fields of microbiology and infectious diseases. The genomes of essentially all the major bacterial and viral pathogens known to infect humankind have now been sequenced and are available on public databases. The human genome project is now complete and whole genome sequencing of the major malaria parasite *Plasmodium falciparum* and the common fungal pathogen *Candida albicans* are now available on line. We have learned an enormous amount of new information about the molecular mechanisms that underlie microbial pathogenesis and the host response to pathogens since the second edition of this book some five years ago. An expanding number of antiviral and antifungal agents are now available to clinicians, and new generations of vaccine constructs and adjuvants are now entering clinical practice.

Despite these advances, progress has been uneven with very little in the developmental pipeline for novel antibacterial agents, antituberculosis drugs, or chemotherapeutic agents against parasitic infection. We find ourselves increasingly on the defensive against a variety of newly emerging and remerging pathogens. The specter of progressive antimicrobial resistance now threatens the long-term viability of the very foundation of our primary treatment approach against bacterial pathogens, including extensively drug resistant tuberculosis (XDR-TB). Our collective vulnerability to airborne pathogens within our highly mobile and crowded global community has become poignantly evident with the H1N1 swine flu pandemic of 2009 and ongoing threats of human dissemination of H5N1 avian influenza strains. Environmental disruption and global warming largely attributable to our ever expanding human population is likely to have adverse health consequences; among them with be the spread of vector-borne, waterborne and airborne pathogens.

In preparing this third edition we have continued the themes that initially inspired the creation of this textbook of Infectious Diseases. The book maintains its tradition of well illustrated and tightly referenced chapters with an emphasis on clinical practicality along with a detailed review of disease pathogenesis and microbiology. Practice points are found throughout the text that highlight common, and not so common, clinical scenarios that require specific and targeted information to provide informed responses. The interactive website, complete with its frequently updated information sources and a downloadable set of illustrations, will continue to support the print version of the text and now includes a number of innovative new functions. The whole text has been carefully reviewed, many chapters have been totally re-written with new figures added, and new authors and editors have been commissioned to ensure that the material is fresh, up to date and relevant.

We are indebted to the superb group of section editors and the extensive collection of highly skilled, international, contributors for each chapter, without whom the third edition of this book would not have been possible. We would especially like to extend our sincere gratitude to Sue Hodgson, Sven Pinczewski, Poppy Garraway and the staff at Elsevier for their unflappable spirit and their attention to detail throughout this considerable undertaking. Finally, we thank the Section Editors from the second edition who have now stood down: Steven Holland, Dennis Maki, Ragnar Norrby, Allan Ronald, Claus Solberg and Jan Verhoef without whom we would never have been in the position of preparing a third edition. We trust that our readers will find the readily accessible knowledge distilled into these pages to have been well worth the effort in generating the Third Edition of Infectious Diseases.

Jon Cohen
William Powderly
Steven Opal

User Guide

Volumes, sections and color coding
Infectious Diseases is divided into two volumes. The book is divided into eight sections, which are color-coded as follows for reference:

Volume 1

Section 1   – Introduction to infectious diseases

Section 2   – Syndromes by body system

Section 3   – Special problems in infectious disease practice

Section 4   – Infections in the immunocompromised host

Volume 2

Section 5   – HIV and AIDS

Section 6   – International medicine

Section 7   – Anti-infective therapy

Section 8   – Clinical microbiology

Contributors

George J Alangaden MD
Professor of Medicine
Division of Infectious Diseases
Wayne State University School of
Medicine
Detroit, MI, USA

Michael J Aldape PhD
Affiliate Assistant Professor
Department of Microbiology
Molecular Biology and
Biochemistry
University of Idaho at Moscow
Assistant Research Scientist
Infectious Disease Section
Veterans Affairs Medical Center
Boise, ID, USA

**Jérôme Allardet-Servent
MD MSc**
Intensivist
Service de Réanimation
Fondation Hôpital Ambroise Paré
Marseille, France

**Upton D Allen MBBS MS
FAAP FRCPC**
Professor of Paediatrics
Consultant in Infectious Diseases
Division of Infectious Diseases
Hospital for Sick Children
Toronto, Ontario, Canada

Heidi SM Ammerlaan MD
PhD student/Resident in Internal
Medicine
Department of Medical
Microbiology
University Medical Centre
Utrecht, The Netherlands

**Emmanouil Angelakis PhD
MD**
Detection of Molecular
Mechanisms Resulting in Antibiotic
Resistance
Faculté de médecine
Urmite, UMR 6236, CNRS-IRD
Marseille, France

**Andrew Artenstein MD
FACP FIDSA**
Physician-in-Chief
Department of Medicine
Director, Center for Biodefense
and Emerging Pathogens Memorial
Hospital of Rhode Island,
Professor of Medicine and
Community Health
The Warren Alpert Medical School
of Brown University
Providence, RI, USA

**David Asboe MB ChB
Dip GUM FRCP**
Consultant Physician
Department of HIV and
Genitourinary Medicine
Chelsea and Westminster
Hospital Foundation Trust
London, UK

Kingsley B Asiedu MD
Medical Officer
Department of Control of
Neglected Tropical Diseases
World Health Organization
Geneva, Switzerland

John C Atherton MD FRCP
Professor of Gastroenterology;
Director
Nottingham Digestive Diseases
Centre
Biomedical Research Unit
Nottingham Digestive Diseases
Centre
University of Nottingham
Nottingham, UK

**Tar-Ching Aw MBBS PhD
FRCP FRCPC FFOM FFPHM**
Professor and Chair
Department of Community
Medicine
Faculty of Medicine and Health
Sciences
United Arab Emirates University
Al Ain, United Arab Emirates

**Seema Baid-Agrawal MD
FASN**
Attending Nephrologist
Department of Nephrology and
Medical Intensive Care
Campus Virchow-Klinikum
Berlin, Germany

**Robin Bailey BA BM DTMH
PhD FRCP**
Professor of Tropical Medicine
London School of Hygiene and
Tropical Medicine
London, UK

Christopher Bandel MD
Research Fellow
Department of Dermatology
University of Texas Southwestern
Medical School
Dallas, TX, USA

**Philip S Barie MD MBA
FCCM FACS**
Professor of Surgery and Public
Health
Department of Surgery
New York-Presbyterian Hospital
and Weill Medical College P713A
New York, NY, USA

David J Barillo MD FACS
Surgical Intensivist and Chief
Burn Flight Team and Special
Medical Augmentation Response
Team (Burn)
US Army Institute of Surgical
Research
Fort Sam Houston
San Antonio, TX, USA

Pierre-Alexandre Bart MD
Senior Scientist and Clinician
Division of Immunology and Allergy
University Hospital Center
Lausanne, Switzerland

**Roger Bayston MMedSci
PhD MSc FRCPath**
Associate Professor
Surgical Infection
Biomaterials-Related Infection
Group
School of Medical and Surgical
Sciences
University of Nottingham
Nottingham, UK

C. Ben Beard PhD
Chief
Bacterial Diseases Branch
Division of Vector-Borne Infectious
Diseases
US Centers for Disease Control and
Prevention
Fort Collins, CO, USA

**Nick J Beeching MA BM BCh
FRCP (Lond) FRACP FFTM
RCPS (Glasg) DCH DTM&H**
Senior Lecturer in Infectious Diseases
Clinical Group
Liverpool School of Tropical
Medicine
Liverpool, UK

Rodolfo E Bégué MD
Professor of Pediatrics
Chief Infectious Diseases
Department of Pediatrics
Health Sciences Center
Louisiana State University
New Orleans, LA, USA

Yves Benhamou MD PhD
Associate Professor
Service d'Hépato-Gastroentérologie
Hôpital Pitié-Salpêtrière
Paris, France

Constance A Benson MD
Professor of Medicine
Division of Infectious Diseases
University of California, San Diego
San Diego, CA, USA

Elie F Berbari MD
Assistant Professor of Medicine
Division of Infectious Diseases
Section of Orthopedic Infectious
Diseases
Department of Internal Medicine
Mayo Clinic College of Medicine
Rochester, MN, USA

**Anthony R Berendt BM BCh
MRCP(UK)**
Consultant Physician-in-Charge
Bone Infection Unit
Nuffield Orthopaedic Centre
Oxford, UK

Madhav P Bhatta MPH
Doctoral Candidate
Department of Epidemiology
University of Alabama at
Birmingham
Birmingham, AL, USA

Jacques Bille MD
Professor of Medical Microbiology
Institute of Microbiology
University of Lausanne and
University Hospital Centre
Lausanne, Switzerland

Ari Bitnun MD MSc FRCPC
Assistant Professor
University of Toronto
Staff Physician
Division of Infectious Diseases
Hospital for Sick Children
Toronto, Ontario, Canada

**Finn T Black MD DMSc
DTM&H**
Professor of Infectious Diseases and
Tropical Medicine
Department of Infectious Diseases
University Hospital of Aårhus
Aårhus, Denmark

Iain Blair MA MB BChir
Associate Professor
Department of Community Medicine
Faculty of Medicine and Health
Sciences
United Arab Emirates University
Al Ain, United Arab Emirates

Stéphane Blanche MD
Professor of Pediatrics
Hôpital Necker Enfant Malades
Paris, France

Thomas P Bleck MD FCCM
Professor of Neurological Sciences
Neurosurgery, Internal Medicine
(Pulmonary/Critical Care Medicine
and Infectious Diseases), and
Anesthesiology;
Assistant Dean, Rush Medical
College; and
Associate Chief Medical Officer
(Critical Care),
Rush University Medical Center
Chicago, IL, USA

**Chantal P Bleeker-Rovers
MD PhD**
Internist specialized in infectious
diseases
Department of Internal Medicine
Division of Infectious Diseases
Radboud University Nijmegen
Medical Center
Nijmegen, The Netherlands

Gijs Bleijenberg PhD
Professor of Clinical Psychology
Expert Centre Chronic Fatigue
University Medical Centre
Nijmegen
Nijmegen, The Netherlands

Karen C Bloch MD MPH
Assistant Professor of Medicine
(Infectious Disease) and Preventive
Medicine
Vanderbilt University Medical
Center
Nashville, TN, USA

Marc JM Bonten MD PhD
Professor of Molecular
Epidemiology of Infectious Diseases
Department of Medical
Microbiology
Julius Centre for Health Sciences
and Primary Care
Utrecht, The Netherlands

**Charles AB Boucher MD
PhD**
Clinical Virologist
Department of Virology
Erasmus Medical Center
Erasmus University
Rotterdam, The Netherlands

Rafik Bourayou MD
Specialist in Pediatrics
Department of Pediatrics
Pediatric Rheumatology and
Pediatric Emergency Medicine
Hôpital de Bicêtre
Le Kremlin-Bicêtre, France

Emilio S Bouza MD PhD
Head
Clinical Microbiology and Infectious
Diseases
Clinical Microbiology and Infectious
Diseases Department
Hospital General Universitario
Gregorio Marañón
Madrid, Spain

**William R Bowie MD
FRCPC**
Professor of Medicine
Division of Infectious Diseases
The University of British Columbia
Vancouver, BC, Canada

Barry D Brause MD
Clinical Professor of Medicine,
Weill-Cornell Medical College
Attending Physician
Hospital for Special Surgery and
New York Presbyterian Hospital
New York, NY, USA

Sylvain Brisse PhD
Researcher
Genotyping of Pathogens and
Public Health Institut Pasteur
Paris, France

**Warwick Britton PhD MB BS
BScMed FRACP FRCP FRCPA
DTM&H**
Bosch Professor of Medicine
and Professor of Immunology,
Centenary Institute and Disciplines
of Medicine
Infectious Diseases and Immunology
University of Sydney
Sydney, NSW, Australia

Itzhak Brook MD MSc
Professor of Pediatric Medicine
Department of Pediatrics
Georgetown University School of
Medicine
Washington, DC, USA

**David WG Brown MBBS
MSc FRCPath FFPH**
Director
Enteric and Respiratory Virus
Laboratory
London, UK

Christian Brun-Buisson MD
Service de Réanimation Médicale
C.H.U. Henri Mondor
University Paris Val-de-Marne
Assistance Publique-Hôpitaux de
Paris
Créteil, France

James CM Brust MD
Assistant Professor of Medicine
Divisions of General Internal
Medicine and Infectious Diseases
Montefiore Medical Center
and Albert Einstein College of
Medicine
Bronx, NY, USA

Amy E Bryant PhD
Affiliate Assistant Professor of
Medicine
University of Washington School of
Medicine
Seattle, WA
Research Scientist
Infectious Disease Section
Veterans Affairs Medical Center
Boise, ID, USA

André Bryskier MD
Consultant in Microbiology and
Infectious Diseases
Romainville
Le Mesnil Le Roi, France

R. Mark L Buller PhD
Professor of Molecular
Microbiology and Immunology
Department of Molecular
Microbiology and Immunology
St Louis University
St Louis, MO, USA

Karen Bush PhD
Adjunct Professor of Biology
Indiana University Bloomington
Bloomington, IN, USA

Thierry Calandra MD PhD
Professor of Medicine
Head, Infectious Diseases Service,
Department of Internal Medicine
Centre Hospitalier
Universitaire Vaudois
Lausanne, Switzerland

**D. William Cameron MD
FRCP FACP**
Professor of Medicine
Divisions of Infectious Diseases and
Respirology
University of Ottawa at The Ottawa
Hospital
Ottawa, ON, Canada

Michel Caraël PhD
Professor Emeritus of Medical
Sociology
Social Sciences Faculty
Free University Brussels
Brussels, Belgium

Michael J Carr BSc PhD
Clinical Scientist
National Virus Reference Laboratory
University College Dublin
Belfield, Dublin
Ireland

Inmaculada Casas PhD
Research Scientist
Alert and Emergency Unit
Virology Service
National Centre of Microbiology
Instituto de Salud Carlos III
Madrid, Spain

**Stephen T Chambers MD
ChB MSc FRACP**
Professor of Pathology,
Christchurch School of Medicine,
University of Otago
Clinical Director of Infectious
Diseases, Christchurch Hospital
Department of Infectious Diseases
Christchurch Hospital
Christchurch, New Zealand

**Katarina G Chiller MD
MPH&TM**
Assistant Clinical Professor of
Dermatology
Emory University School of
Medicine
Atlanta Skin Cancer
Specialists, PC
Atlanta, GA, USA

Tom M Chiller MD MPHTM
Deputy Chief, Mycotic Diseases
Branch
Division of Foodborne, Bacterial
and Mycotic Diseases
National Center for Zoonotic
Vector-Borne and Enteric
Diseases, Centers for Disease
Control and Prevention
Adjunct Assistant Professor of
Infectious Diseases
Emory University school of
Medicine
Atlanta, GA, USA

**Peter L Chiodini BSc MBBS
PhD MRCS FRCP FRCPath**
Consultant Parasitologist
Department of Clinical Parasitology
Hospital for Tropical Diseases
London, UK

**Ian Chopra BA MA PhD DSc
MD(honorary)**
Professor of Microbiology and
Director of the Antimicrobial
Research Centre
Institute of Molecular and Cellular
Biology
University of Leeds
Leeds, UK

Anthony C Chu FRCP
Consultant Dermatologist/Honorary
Senior Lecturer
Head of Dermatology, Unit of
Dermatology
Imperial College School of Medicine
London, UK

Kevin K Chung MD
Medical Intensivist
Medical Director
Burn ICU
US Army Institute of Surgical
Research
San Antonio, TX, USA

Benjamin M Clark MBChB MRCP (UK) DTM&H
Consultant in Infectious Diseases
Department of Infectious Diseases
Fremantle Hospital
Fremantle, WA, Australia

Nathan Clumeck MD PhD
Professor of Infectious Diseases
Head, Department of Infectious Diseases
St Pierre University Hospital
Brussels, Belgium

Clay J Cockerell MD
Professor of Dermatology and Pathology
Departments of Dermatology and Pathology
University of Texas
Dallas, TX, USA

Jonathan Cohen MB BS FRCP FRCPath FRCPE FmedSci
Professor of Infectious Diseases and Dean
Brighton and Sussex Medical School
Honorary Consultant Physician
Royal Sussex County Hospital
Brighton, UK

John Collinge MRCP MD FRCPath
Professor of Neurology
Head of Department
Department of Neurodegenerative Diseases/Director, MRC Prion Unit
Institute of Neurology
University College London
London, UK

Christopher P Conlon MA MD FRCP
Reader in Infectious Diseases and Tropical Medicine
University of Oxford Consultant in Infectious Diseases
Nuffield Department of Medicine
Oxford, UK

G. Ralph Corey MD
Gary Hock Professor of Global Health
Duke University Medical Center
Durham, NC, USA

Alan Cross MD
Professor of Medicine
Center for Vaccine Development and Department of Medicine
University of Maryland School of Medicine
Baltimore, MD, USA

John H Cross PhD
Professor
Tropical Public Health
Department of Preventive Medicine and Biometrics
Uniformed Services University of the Health Sciences
Bethesda, MD, USA

Judith Currier MD
Professor of Medicine
Division of Infectious Diseases
Center for Clinical AIDS Research and Education
David Geffen School of Medicine
University of California
Los Angeles, CA, USA

Carmel M Curtis PhD MRCP
Microbiology Specialist Registrar
Department of Parasitology
The Hospital for Tropical Diseases
London, UK

Gina Dallabetta MD
Director
Technical Support
HIV/AIDS Institute
Family Health International
Arlington, VA, USA

Robert N Davidson MD FRCP DTM&H
Consultant Physician
Hon. Senior Lecturer
Department of Infectious and Tropical Diseases
Northwick Park Hospital
Harrow, Middlesex, UK

Jane Davies MBBS MRCP DTM&H PGCTLCP
Specialist Registrar in Infectious Diseases and Tropical Medicine
Tropical and Infectious Disease Unit, Royal Liverpool University Hospital
Liverpool, UK

Jeremy Day MA MB BChir MRCP(London) DTM&H
Consultant in Infectious Diseases
Wellcome Trust Major Overseas Program
Oxford University Clinical Research Unit
Hospital for Tropical Diseases
Ho Chi Minh City, Vietnam

Nicholas PJ Day DM FRCP FMedSci
Professor of Tropical Medicine
Centre for Tropical Medicine
University of Oxford, UK
Director of the Mahidol Oxford Tropical Medicine Research Unit
Faculty of Tropical Medicine
Mahidol University
Bangkok, Thailand

Cillian F De Gascun MB MRCPI
Senior Registrar in Virology
National Virus Reference Laboratory
University College Dublin
Belfield, Dublin
Ireland

Stéphane de Wit MD PhD
Senior Physician
Division of Infectious Diseases
St Pierre University Hospital
Brussels, Belgium

Jean Delmont MD PhD
Physician, Professor of Infectious Diseases and Tropical Medicine
Infectious Diseases Department
Hôpital Nord, University Hospital of Marseille
Marseille, France

David T Dennis MD MPH DCMT
Medical Epidemiologist
Influenza Coordinator
Vietnam
Division of Influenza
Atlanta, GA, USA

David J Diemert MD FRCP(C) DTM&H
Assistant Professor
Department of Microbiology Immunology and Tropical Medicine
The George Washington School of Medicine
Director of Clinical Trials, Sabin Vaccine Institute
Washington DC, USA

Mehmet Doganay MD
Professor in Infectious Diseases
Department of Infectious Diseases
Faculty of Medicine
Erciyes University
Kayseri, Turkey

Tom Doherty MD FRCP DTM&H
Consultant Physician
Hospital for Tropical Diseases
London, UK

Christiane Dolecek MD
The Hospital for Tropical Diseases
Oxford University Clinical Research Unit
Ho Chi Minh City, Vietnam

Stéphane Y Donati MD
Intensivist
Medico-surgical ICU
Font Pré Hospital
Toulon, France

Arjen M Dondorp MD PhD
Infectious Diseases and Intensive Care Physician
Deputy Director
Mahidol-Oxford Tropical Medicine Research Unit (MORU)
Bangkok, Thailand

Barbara Doudier MD
Physician, Infectious Diseases Fellow
Assistant Professor, Infectious Diseases Department
Hôpital de la Conception
University Hospital of Marseille
Marseille, France

Michel Drancourt MD
Professor of Microbiology, Head of the Clinical Microbiology Laboratory
Unité de Recherche sur les Maladies Infectieuses et Tropicales Emergentes
Medical School, Méditerranée University
Marseille, France

Dimitri M Drekonja MD
Assistant Professor of Medicine
University of Minnesota
Infectious Diseases
VA Medical Center
Minneapolis, MN, USA

Richard H Drew PharmD MS BCPS
Professor, Campbell University
College of Pharmacy and Health Sciences
Associate Professor of Medicine (Infectious Diseases)
Duke University School of Medicine
Durham, NC, USA

Jay S Duker MD
Director
New England Eye Center
Professor and Chair of Ophthalmology
Tufts New England Medical Center
Tufts University School of Medicine
Boston, MA, USA

J. Stephen Dummer MD
Professor of Medicine
Division of Infectious Diseases
Vanderbilt University Medical Center
Nashville, TN, USA

Charles N Edwards FRCP FACP FACG
Associate Senior Lecturer
School of Clinical Medicine and Research
University of the West Indies
Barbados

Miquel B Ekkelenkamp MD
Clinical Microbiologist
University Medical Center Utrecht
Utrecht, The Netherlands

Mark C Enright PhD
Professor of Molecular Epidemiology
Department of Infectious Disease Epidemiology
Imperial College London
London, UK

Paul R Epstein MD MPH
Associate Director
Center for Health and the Global Environment
Harvard Medical School
Boston, MA, USA

Veronique Erard MD MSc
Division of Infectious Diseases
Centre Hospitalier University
Vadors Rue du Bugnon
Lausanne, Switzerland

Alice Chijioke Eziefula MBBS MA MRCP MRC Path
Department of Infection
Brighton and Sussex University Hospitals
Brighton, UK

Contributors

Mark B Feinberg MD PhD
Vice President
Policy, Public Health and Medical
Affairs
Merck & Co., Inc.
West Point, PA, USA

Florence Fenollar MD PhD
Associate Professor of Clinical
Microbiology
Unité des Rickettsies
Faculté de Médecine
Marseille, France

Alan Fenwick OBE
Professor of Tropical Parasitology
Director, Schistosomiasis Control
Initiative
Department of Infectious Disease
Epidemiology
Imperial College London
London, UK

Luis Fernandez MD FACS
Assistant Professor of Surgery
Department of Surgery
University of Wisconsin School of
Medicine and Public Health
Madison, WI, USA

Joshua Fierer MD
Michael and Marci Oxman Professor
of Medicine and Pathology
Chief, Infectious Diseases Section
VA San Diego Healthcare System
Director, Microbiology Laboratory
VA San Diego Healthcare System
San Diego, CA, USA

**Roger G Finch MB BS FRCP
FRCPath FRCPEd FFPM**
Professor of Infectious Diseases
School of Molecular Medical Science
Division of Microbiology and
Infectious Disease
Nottingham University Hospitals
NHS Trust
Nottingham, UK

Charles W Flexner MD
Professor of Medicine
Pharmacology and Molecular
Sciences and International Health
Johns Hopkins University
Baltimore, MD, USA

Ad C Fluit PhD
Associate Professor
Department of Medical Microbiology
University Medical Center Utrecht
Utrecht, The Netherlands

**Elizabeth Lee Ford-Jones
MD FRCPC**
Professor of Pediatrics
Division of Infectious Diseases
The Hospital for Sick Children
University of Toronto
Co-editor *Paediatrics and Child
Health*
Toronto, ON, Canada

**Pierre-Edouard Fournier
MD PhD**
Associate Professor
Unité des Rickettsies
Faculté dé Medecine, Université de
la Méditerranée
Marseille, France

Victoria Fraser MD
J William Campbell Professor of
Medicine and Co-Director
Infectious Diseases Division
Washington University School of
Medicine
St Louis, MO, USA

**Martyn A French MB
CRB MD FRCPath FRCP
FRACP**
Clinical Immunologist and
Winthrop Professor of Pathology
and Laboratory Medicine
Department of Clinical Immunology
Royal Perth Hospital and School of
Pathology and Laboratory Medicine
University of Western Australia
Perth, Australia

**Jon S Friedland MA PhD
FRCP FRCPE FMedSci**
Head, Department of Infectious
Diseases and Immunity
Imperial College London
Lead Clinician, Clinical Infection
Imperial College Healthcare
NHS Trust
London, UK

Joseph M Fritz MD
St Lukés Hospital
St Louis, MO, USA

E. Yoko Furuya MD MS
Assistant Professor of Clinical
Medicine
Division of Infectious Diseases
Columbia University
New York, NY, USA

Kenneth L Gage PhD
Chief, Flea-borne Disease Activity
Bacterial Diseases Branch
Division of Vector-Borne Infectious
Diseases
US Centers for Disease Control and
Prevention
Fort Collins, CO, USA

**Lynne S Garcia MS FAAM
MT(ASCP) CLS(NCA)
BLM(AAB)**
Director, LSG & Associates
Santa Monica, CA, USA

Arturo S Gastañaduy MD
Associate Professor of Pediatrics
Department of Pediatrics
Louisiana State University Health
Sciences Center
New Orleans, LA, USA

Khalil G Ghanem MD PhD
Assistant Professor of Medicine
Division of Infectious Diseases
Johns Hopkins University School of
Medicine
Assistant Professor Population
Family and Reproductive Health
Johns Hopkins University
Bloomberg School of Public Health
Baltimore, MD, USA

Maddalena Giannella MD
Research Assistant
Clinical Microbiology and Infectious
Diseases Department
Hospital General Universitario
Gregorio Marañón
Madrid, Spain

Carol A Glaser DVM MD
Chief, Viral and Rickettsial Disease
Laboratory Branch
California Department of Public
Health
Richmond, CA, USA

Marshall J Glesby MD PhD
Associate Professor of Medicine
and Public Health
Division of Infectious Diseases
Department of Medicine
Weill Cornell Medical College
New York, NY, USA

**Sarah Glover MBChB MRCP
FRCPath**
Specialist Registrar in Infectious
Diseases and Microbiology
Brighton and Sussex University
Hospitals NHS Trust
Brighton, UK

Youri Glupczynski MD
Professor of Microbiology
Laboratoire de Microbiologie
Cliniques universitaires UCL de
Mont-Godinne
Yvoir, Belgium

John W Gnann Jr MD
Professor of Medicine,
Pediatrics and Microbiology
Division of Infectious Diseases
University of Alabama at
Birmingham and Birmingham
Veterans Administration Medical
Center
Birmingham, AL, USA

**Andrew F Goddard MA MD
FRCP**
Consultant Gastroenterologist
Digestive Diseases Centre
Derby Hospitals NHS Foundation
Trust
Derby, UK

**Ellie JC Goldstein MD
FIDSA**
Director, RM Alden Research
Laboratory
Santa Monica, CA
Clinical Professor of Medicine
UCLA School of Medicine
Los Angeles, CA, USA

Iveth J González MD PhD
Scientific Officer
FIND Diagnostics
Geneva, Switzerland

Sherwood L Gorbach MD
Distinguished Professor
Departments of Public Health and
Medicine
Tufts University School of Medicine
Boston, MA, USA

**Bruno Gottstein PhD
AssEVPC CBA**
Professor and Director
Institute of Parasitology
Vetsuisse-Faculty and Faculty of
Medicine
University of Bern
Bern, Switzerland

**Ravi Gowda MBBS
MRCP(UK) DTM&H DCH
DRCOG MRCGP**
Consultant in Infectious Diseases
Department of Infection and
Tropical Medicine
University Hospitals Coventry and
Warwickshire
Coventry, UK

**John D Grabenstein RPh
PhD**
Senior Medical Director-Adult
Vaccines
Merck Vaccines & Infectious Diseases
Merck & Co., Inc.
West Point, PA, USA

**John M Grange MBBS
MSc MD**
Visiting Professor
Centre for Infectious Diseases and
International Heatlh
Windeyer Institute for Medical
Sciences
London, UK

Michael D Green MD MPH
Professor of Pediatrics and Surgery
University of Pittsburgh School of
Medicine
Division of Infectious Diseases
Children's Hospital of Pittsburgh
Pittsburgh, PA, USA

**Stephen T Green MD BSc
FRCP(Lond, Glas) FFTH
DTM&H**
Consultant Physician in Infectious
Disease and Tropical Medicine
Department of Infection and
Tropical Medicine
Royal Hallamshire Hospitals
Sheffield, UK

**Danielle T Greenblatt
MBChB MRCP**
Specialist Registrar
Department of Dermatology
Ealing Hospital NHS Trust
Southall, UK

Brian Greenwood MD
Professor of Tropical Medicine
Department of Infectious and
Tropical Diseases
London School of Hygiene and
Tropical Medicine
London, UK

Aric L Gregson MD
Assistant Clinical Professor of
Medicine
Department of Medicine
Division of Infectious Diseases
University of California
Los Angeles, CA, USA

Andreas H Groll MD
Infectious Disease Research Program
Center for Bone Marrow
Transplantation and Department of
Pediatric Hematology/Oncology
University Children's Hospital
Munster, Germany

**Aditya K Gupta MD PhD
MA(Cantab) CCI CCTI CCRP
DABD FAAD FRCPC**
Professor, Division of Dermatology
Department of Medicine
Sunnybrook and Women's Health
Science Center and the University
of Toronto
London, ON, Canada

**Kok-Ann Gwee MBBS
MMed MRCP FAMS PhD
FRCP**
Consultant Gastroenterologist
Gleneagles Hospital, Singapore
and Adjunct Associate Professor of
Medicine, Yong Loo Lin School of
Medicine
National University of Singapore
Singapore

**William Hall BSc PhD MD
DTMH**
Professor of Medical Microbiology
College of Life Sciences
School of Medicine & Medical
Science
Belfield, Dublin
Ireland

Scott M Hammer MD
Professor of Medicine and Public
Health (Epidemiology)
Columbia University
Presbyterian Hospital
New York, NY, USA

Sajeev Handa MD FMM
Director, Division of Hospital
Medicine
Rhode Island Hospital
Providence, RI, USA

Diane Hanfelt-Goade MD
Assistant Professor
Department of Medicine
The University of New Mexico
School of Medicine
Albuquerque, NM, USA

Alexandre Harari PhD
Project Leader
Service of Immunology and Allergy
Centre Hospitalier Universitaire
Vaudois
Lausanne, Switzerland

Marianne Harris MD CCFPC
Clinical Research Advisor
AIDS Research Program
Providence Health Care
Vancouver, BC, Canada

Barry J Hartman MD
Clinical Professor of Medicine
Department of International
Medicine and Infectious Diseases
Cornell University Medical College
New York
New York, NY, USA

**Roderick J Hay DM FRCP
FRCPath**
Honorary Professor, London School
of Hygiene and Tropical Medicine
Chairman
International Foundation for
Dermatology
London, UK

David K Henderson MD
Deputy Director for Clinical Care
Warren G Magnuson Clinical
Center
National Institutes of Health
Bethesda, MD, USA

Lisa E Hensley MD
Chief of Viral Therapeutics
Department of Viral Therapeutics
Virology Division
Fort Detrick, MD, USA

Luke Herbert FRCOphth
Consultant and Clinical Director
Department of Ophthalmology
The Queen Elizabeth II Hospital
Welwyn Garden City, UK

**David R Hill MD DTM&H
FRCP FFTM**
Honorary Professor, London
School of Hygiene and Tropical
Medicine
Director, National Travel Health
Network and Centre
Hospital for Tropical Diseases
London, UK

**Timothy J Hills
BPharm MRPharmS Dip
Clin Pharm**
Lead Pharmacist Antimicrobials and
Infection Control
Department of Pharmacy
Nottingham University Hospitals
NHS Trust
Nottingham, UK

John David Hinze DO
Pulmonary and Critical Care
Consultants of Austin
Austin, TX, USA

Hans H Hirsch MD MS
Professor of Clinical Virology
Division of Infectious Diseases
University Hospital Basel
Institute for Medical Microbiology
Basel, Switzerland

Bernard Hirschel MD
Division of Infectious Diseases
Unite VIH/SIDA Hôpital Universitaire
de Geneve
Geneva, Switzerland

**Andy IM Hoepelman
MD PhD**
Professor in Medicine, Infectious
Diseases Specialist
Head, Department of
Internal Medicine and Infectious
Diseases
University Medical Center
Utrecht, The Netherlands

Steven M Holland MD
Chief, Laboratory of Clinical
Infectious Diseases
National Institute of Allergy and
Infectious Disease
National Institutes of Health
Bethesda, MD, USA

Mary M Horgan MD FRCPI
Senior Lecturer in Medicine
University College Cork
Consultant in Infectious Diseases
Cork University Hospital
Cork, Ireland

**Robin Howe MA MBBS
FRCPath**
Consultant in Clinical Microbiology
Microbiology Cardiff (Velindre NHS
Trust),
University Hospital of Wales,
Heath Park, Cardiff, UK

James M Hughes MD
Professor of Medicine and Public
Health
Division of Infectious Diseases
Department of Medicine
Emory University School of Medicine
Atlanta, GA, USA

Mark W Hull MD FRCPC
Research Scientist
BC Centre for Excellence in
HIV/AIDS
Vancouver, BC, Canada

Clark B Inderlied PhD
Professor of Clinical Microbiology
Keck School of Medicine
University of Southern California
Los Angeles, CA, USA

Michael G Ison MD MS
Assistant Professor, Divisions of
Infectious Diseases and Organ
Transplantation
Medical Director, Transplant
& Immunocompromised Host
Infectious Diseases Service
Northwestern University Feinberg
School of Medicine
Chicago, IL, USA

**Peter J Jenks PhD MRCP
FRCPath**
Director of Infection Prevention and
Control/Consultant in Microbiology
Department of Microbiology
Plymouth Hospitals NHS Trust
Plymouth, UK

**James R Johnson MD FACP
FIDSA**
Professor of Medicine University of
Minnesota
Infectious Diseases
VA Medical Center
Minneapolis, MN, USA

Theodore Jones MD
Associate Professor
Wayne State University
Detroit, MI, USA

Mettassebia Kanno MD
Assistant Professor of Medicine
Division of Infectious
Diseases
Institute of Human Virology
University of Maryland
Baltimore, MD, USA

Carol Kauffman MD
Professor of Internal Medicine
University of Michigan
Chief, Infectious Diseases Section
VA Ann Arbor Healthcare System
Ann Arbor, MI, UK

Patrick Kelly BVSc PhD
Professor of Small Animal Medicine
Ross University School of Veterinary
Medicine
Basseterre
St Kitts, West Indies

Jason S Kendler MD
Clinical Associate Professor of
Medicine
Weill Cornell Medical College
New York, NY, USA

Yoav Keynan MD
Infectious Disease Fellow
Department of Internal Medicine
Laboratory of Viral Immunology
Department of Medical
Microbiology
Winnipeg, MB, Canada

Ali S Khan MD
Assistant Surgeon General and
Deputy Director
National Center for Zoonotic,
Vector-borne, and Enteric Diseases
Centers for Disease Control and
Prevention
Atlanta, GA, USA

Grace T Kho MD
Department of Dermatology and
Pathology
University of Texas Southwestern
Medical Center
Dallas, TX, USA

**George R Kinghorn MD
FRCP**
Clinical Director, Directorate of
Communicable Diseases
Royal Hallamshire Hospital
Sheffield, UK

Paul E Klapper PhD MRCPath
Consultant Clinical Scientist
Honorary Professor of Clinical
Virology,
University of Manchester
Clinical Virology Central
Manchester
University Hospitals
NHS Foundation Trust
Manchester, UK

Jan AJW Kluytmans MD PhD
Professor of Medical Microbiology
and Infection Control
VU University Medical Center
Laboratory for Microbiology and
Infection Control
Amsterdam, The Netherlands

Menno Kok PhD
Senior Staff Member
Medical Faculty
Erasmus MC
Rotterdam, The Netherlands

Isabelle Koné-Paut MD
Professor, Department of Pediatrics
Pediatric Rheumatology and
Pediatric Emergency Medicine
Hôpital de Bicêtre
Le Kremlin-Bicêtre, France

John N Krieger MD
Professor of Urology
Department of Urology
University of Washington and Chief
of Urology
VA Puget Sound Health Care System
Seattle, WA, USA

Aloys CM Kroes MD PhD
Professor of Medical Microbiology
and Clinical Virology
Department of Medical
Microbiology
Leiden University Medical Center
Leiden, The Netherlands

Frank P Kroon MD PhD
Department of Infectious Diseases
C5P
Leiden University Medical Center
Leiden, The Netherlands

Christine J Kubin PharmD BCPS
Clinical Pharmacy Manager
Infectious Diseases
Columbia University College of
Physicians and Surgeons
New York-Presbyterian Hospital
Columbia University Medical Centre
New York, NY, USA

Alberto M La Rosa MD
Director of Clinical Trials Unit
Asociacion Civil Impacta Salud Y
Educacion
Lima, Peru

Tahaniyat Lalani MBBS MHS
Assistant Professor, Division of
Infectious Diseases, Uniformed
Services
University of the Health Sciences
Naval Medical Center Portsmouth
Portsmouth, VA, USA

David G Lalloo MB BS MD FRCP
Professor of Tropical Medicine and
Head, Clinical Research Group
Liverpool School of Tropical Medicine
Liverpool, UK

Harold Lambert MD FRCP FRCPath
Emeritus Professor of Microbial
Diseases
St George's Hospital Medical School
London, UK

Luce Landraud MD PhD
Medical Doctor
Microbiology Department
Archet II-Hospital
Microbial Toxins in Host Pathogen
Interactions
Sophia Antipolis University
Nice, France

Stephen D Lawn BMedSci MBBS MRCP MD DTM&H Dip HIV Med
Reader in Infectious Diseases and
Tropical Medicine
Department of Infectious and
Tropical Diseases
London School of Hygiene and
Tropical Medicine, London, UK
Associate Professor of Infectious
Diseases and HIV Medicine
The Desmond Tutu HIV Centre
Institute for Infectious Disease and
Molecular Medicine
Faculty of Health Sciences
University of Cape Town
Cape Town, South Africa

Phillipe Lehours Pharm PhD
Associate Professor of Bacteriology
Université Victor Segalen
Bordeaux, France

Marc Leone MD PhD
Assistant Professor of Anesthesiology
and Critical Care Medicine
Service d'anesthésie et de
réanimation
Hôpital Nord
Marseille, France

Itzchak Levi MD
Infectious Diseases Unit
Sheba Medical Center
Tel Hashomer
Ramat Gan, Israel

Alexandra M Levitt PhD
Health Scientist
National Center for Preparedness,
Detection, and Control of
Infectious Diseases
Centers for Disease Control and
Prevention
Atlanta, GA, USA

H. D. Alan Lindquist PhD
Microbiologist
Water Infrastructure Protection
Division
National Homeland Security
Research Center
Office of Research and Development
US Environmental Protection Agency
Cincinnati, OH, USA

Graham Lloyd PhD MSc BSc FIBMS CMS
Health Protection Agency
Centre for Applied Microbiology
and Research
Salisbury, UK

David J Looney MD
Associate Professor of Medicine
of Residence
Director, UCSD Center for AIDS
Research Molecular Biology Core
University of California San Diego
San Diego, CA, USA

Franklin D Lowy MD
Professor of Medicine and Pathology
Division of Infectious Diseases
Columbia University
College of Physicians and Surgeons
New York, NY, USA

Benjamin J Luft MD
Edmund D Pellegrino
Professor Chairman,
Department of Medicine
State University of New York
at Stony Brook
Stony Brook, NY, USA

William A Lynn MD FRCP
Medical Director
Consultant in Infectious Diseases
Infection and Immunity Unit
Ealing Hospital
Southall, UK

Mark J Macielag PhD
Senior Research Fellow
Johnson & Johnson Pharmaceutical
Research / Development
Spring House PA, USA

Philip A Mackowiak MD MBA MACP
Director, Medical Care Clinical Center
Professor of Medicine and
Vice-Chairman, VA Maryland
Health Care System
Department of Medicine
University of Maryland School of
Medicine
Baltimore, MD, USA

Paul A MacPherson MD PhD FRCPC
Assistant Professor, University of
Ottawa
Specialist in Infectious Diseases
Ottawa Hospital
Scientist, Ottawa Hospital Research
Institute
Ottawa, ON, Canada

Valérie Maghraoui-Slim MD
Specialist in Pediatrics
Department of Pediatrics
Pediatric Rheumatology and
Pediatric Emergency Medicine
Hôpital de Bicêtre
Le Kremlin-Bicêtre, France

Janice Main FRCP(Ed, Lond)
Reader and Consultant Physician
in Infectious Diseases and General
Medicine
Department of Medicine
Imperial College
London, UK

Vincent Mallet MD PhD
Assistant Professor
Service d'Hepatologie
Université Paris Descartes
Assistance Publique Hôpitaux de
Paris, INSERM U.567
Paris, France

Julie E Mangino MD
Associate Professor of Internal
Medicine
Division of Infectious Diseases
Department of Internal Medicine
OSUMC Medical Director,
Department of Clinical
Epidemiology
The Ohio State University College
of Medicine
Columbus, OH, USA

Oriol Manuel MD
Attending in Transplant Infectious
Diseases
Service of Infectious Diseases
Transplantation Centre
University Hospital of Lausanne
(CHUV)
Lausanne, Switzerland

Oscar Marchetti MD
Privat Docent
Infectious Diseases Service
Department of Medicine
Centre Hospitalier Universitaire
Vaudois and University of Lausanne
Lausanne, Switzerland

Kristen Marks MD MS
Assistant Professor of Medicine
Division of Infectious Diseases
Department of Medicine
Weill Cornell Medical College
New York, NY, USA

Kieren A Marr MD
Director, Transplant and
Oncology
Johns Hopkins University School of
Medicine
Baltimore, MD, USA

Claude Martin MD
Professor of Anesthesiology and
Critical Care Medicine
Service d'anesthésie et de
réanimation
Hôpital Nord
Marseille, France

Pablo Martín-Rabadán MD DTMH
Consultant Physician
Servicio de Microbiologia y
Enjermedades Infecciosas
Hospital General Universitario
Gregorio Maranon
Madrid, Spain

Augusto Julio Martinez MD
(deceased)
Professor of Pathology
Department of Pathology
(Neuropathology)
University of Pittsburg School of
Medicine
Pittsburg, PA, USA

Ellen M Mascini MD PhD
Medical Microbiologist
Laboratory for Medical
Microbiology and Immunology
Alysis Zorggroep Arnhem,
The Netherlands

Kenneth H Mayer MD
Professor of Medicine and
Community Health
Brown University; Director of
Brown University
Infectious Diseases Division
The Miriam Hospital
Providence, RI, USA

Joseph B McCormick MD
Regional Dean and James H Steele
Professor
School of Public Health
University of Texas Houston Health
Science Center
Brownsville, TX, USA

Rose McGready MB BS PhD
Research Clinician
Obstetrics
Shoklo Malaria Research Unit
Tak Province, Thailand

**Michael W McKendrick
MB BS FRCP(Lond)
FRCP(Glasg)**
Lead Consultant Physician
Department of Infection and
Tropical Medicine
South Yorkshire Regional
Department of Infection and
Tropical Medicine
Sheffield, UK

Simon Mead MD
Honorary Consultant Neurologist
and Senior Lecturer
MRC Prion Unit
Institute of Neurology
University College London
London, UK

Francis Mégraud MD
Professor of Bacteriology
Université Victor Segalen
Bordeaux, France

André Z Meheus MD PhD
Professor Emeritus
Department of Epidemiology and
Social Medicine
Campus Drie Eiken
Antwerp, Belgium

**Graeme Meintjes MBChB
MRCP(UK) FCP(SA)
DipHIVMan(SA)**
Honorary Senior Lecturer
Division of Infectious Diseases and
HIV Medicine
Department of Medicine
University of Cape Town
Waterfront, South Africa

**Marian G Michaels
MD MPH**
Professor of Pediatrics and Surgery
University of Pittsburgh School of
Medicine
Division of Pediatric Infectious
Diseases
Pittsburgh, PA, USA

**Michael Miles MSc PhD DSc
FRCPath**
Professor of Medical Protozoology
London School of Hygiene and
Tropical Medicine
London, UK

**Alastair Miller MA FRCP
(Edin) DTM&H**
Consultant Physician
Tropical and Infectious Disease Unit
Royal Liverpool University Hospital
Honorary Fellow
Liverpool School of Tropical Medicine
Liverpool, UK

**Matthew J Mimiaga ScD
MPH**
Research Scientist
The Fenway Institute
Instructor in Psychiatry
Harvard Medical School
Boston, MA, USA

**Marie-Paule Mingeot-
Leclercq MSc PharmD PhD**
Professor of Pharmacology
Biochemistry and Biophysics
Unité de Pharmacologie cellulaire
et moléculaire & Louvain Drug
Research Institute
Université catholique de Louvain
Brussels, Belgium

Thomas G Mitchell PhD
Associate Professor
Department of Molecular Genetics
and Microbiology
Duke University Medical Center
Durham, NC, USA

Pamela A Moise PharmD
Clinical Scientific Director
Cubist Pharmaceuticals, Lexington
MA USA

Julio Montaner MD
Director, Infectious Disease Clinic
St Paul's Hospital
Vancouver, BC, Canada

Caroline B Moore PhD
Principle Clinical Mycologist
Regional Mycology Laboratory
University Hospital of South
Manchester (Wythenshawe
Hospital)
Manchester, UK

Philippe Moreillon MD PhD
Professor
Department of Fundamental
Microbiology
University of Lausanne
Lausanne, Switzerland

**Peter Morgan-Capner BSc
MBBS FRCPath FRCP Hon
FFPHM**
Honorary Professor of Clinical
Virology
Department of Microbiology
Royal Preston Hospital
Preston, UK

**Valentina Montessori MD
FRCPC**
Clinical Assistant Professor
Canadian HIV Trials Network
British Columbia Centre for
Excellence in HIV/AIDS
Division of Infectious Diseases
Vancouver, BC, Canada

Peter Moss MD FRCP DTMH
Consultant in Infectious Diseases
and Honorary Senior Lecturer in
Medicine
Director of Infection Prevention and
Control
Hull and East Yorkshire Hospitals
NHS Trust
East Riding of Yorkshire, UK

Patricia Muñoz MD PhD
Professor of Clinical Microbiology
and Infectious Diseases Department
Hospital General Universitario
Gregorio Marañón
Madrid, Spain

Kurt G Naber MD PhD
Associate Professor of Urology
Technical University Munich
Munich, Germany

Sammy Nakhla MD
State University of
New York at Stony Brook
Stony Brook, NY, USA

Jai P Narain MD
Director
Department of Communicable
Diseases
World Health Organization
New Delhi, India

**Dilip Nathwani MB
FRCP(Lond) FRCP(Edin)
FRCP(Glas) DTM&H**
Consultant Physician and Honorary
Professor of Infection
Infection Unit
Ninewells Hospital and Medical
School
Dundee, UK

Paul Newton MRCP
Reader in Tropical Medicine, Head
of the Laos Collaboration
Group Head/PI and Grant Holding
Senior Scientist
Wellcome Trust-Mahosot Hospital-
Oxford Tropical Medicine Research
Collaboration
Vientiane, Laos

Chinh Nguyen MD
Postdoctoral Fellow
Department of Infectious Diseases
University of Maryland School of
Medicine
Baltimore, MD, USA

**Lindsay E Nicolle BSc
BScMed MD FRCPC**
Professor of Internal Medicine and
Medical Microbiology
University of Manitoba
Winnipeg, MB, Canada

Michael S Niederman MD
Chairman
Department of Medicine
Winthrop-University Hospital
Professor of Medicine
Mineola, NY, USA

**Gary J Noel MD FIDSA
FAAP**
Clinical Professor of Pediatrics
Weill Cornell Medical College
Anti-Infectives Medical Leader
Johnson & Johnson Pharmaceutical
Research and Development
Raritan, NJ, USA

**S. Ragnar Norrby MD PhD
FRCP(Edin)**
Professor and Director General
The Swedish Institute for Infectious
Disease Control
Solna, Sweden

François Nosten MD
Professor
Shoklo Malaria Research Unit
Tak Province, Thailand

**Luigi Daniele Notarangelo
MD**
Professor of Pediatrics and
Pathology, Harvard Medical
School
Director of Research and Molecular
Diagnosis Program on Primary
Immunodeficiencies
Division of Immunology
Children's Hospital
Boston, MA, USA

Paul Nyirjesy MD
Professor
Departments of Obstetrics and
Gynecology and Medicine
Drexel University College of
Medicine
Philadelphia, PA, USA

**P. Ronan O'Connell MD
FRCSI FRCS(Glas)**
Head of Surgery and Surgical
Specialties
UCD School of Medicine and
Medical Fellow, Conway Institute
of Biomolecular and Biomedical
Research University College Dublin
Consultant Surgeon
St Vincent's University Hospital
Dublin, Ireland

Jon S Odorico MD FACS
Associate Professor of Surgery
Director of Pancreas and Islet
Transplantation
Division of Transplantation
University of Wisconsin-Madison
School of Medicine and Public
Health
Madison, WI, USA

Edmund LC Ong MBBS FRCP FRCPI MSC DTMH
Consultant Physician and Honorary Senior Lecturer
Department of Infection and Tropical Medicine
University of Newcastle Medical School
Newcastle upon Tyne, UK

Steven M Opal MD
Professor of Medicine,
Infectious Disease Division
The Warren Alpert Medical School of Brown University
Providence, RI, USA

L. Peter Ormerod BSc MBChB(Hons) MD DSc(Med) FRCP
Professor of Medicine
Chest Clinic
Blackburn Royal Infirmary
Blackburn, UK

Douglas R Osmon MD
Associate Professor of Medicine
Division of Infectious Diseases
Department of Internal Medicine
Mayo Clinic
Rochester, MN, USA

Eric A Ottesen MD
Director, Lymphatic Filariasis Support Center
Task Force for Global Health
Decatur, GA, USA
Technical Director, Neglected Tropical Disease Control Program
RTI International
Washington, DC, USA

Gustavo Palacios PhD
Assistant Professor
Center for Infection and Immunity
Mailman School of Public Health
Columbia University
New York, NY, USA

Giuseppe Pantaleo MD
Professor of Medicine
Division of Immunology and Allergy
Department of Medicine
Centre Hospitalier Universitaire
Vaudois (CHUV)
University of Lausanne
Lausanne, Switzerland

Laurent Papazian MD
Intensivist
Service de Réanimation Médicale
Hôpital Sainte Marguerite
Marseille, France

Philippe Parola MD PhD
Associate Professor
Unité de Recherche en Maladies Infectieuses et Tropicales Emergentes
Marseille, France

Manuel A Pascual MD
Professor and Chief
Transplantation Center
University of Lausanne
Lausanne, Switzerland

Eleni Patrozou MD
Clinical Instructor in Medicine
Alpert Medical School of Brown University
Providence, RI, USA
Internist-Infectious Diseases
Consultant, Hygeia Hospital
Athens, Greece Medical Director
The PROLEPSIS Institute
Athens, Greece

Carlos Paya MD PhD
Professor of Medicine, Consultant
Infectious Diseases
Division of Infectious Diseases and Transplant Center
Mayo Clinic
Rochester, MN, USA

Sharon J Peacock BM MSc FRCP FRCPath PhD
Professor of Clinical Microbiology
Department of Medicine
University of Cambridge
Addenbrooke's Hospital
Cambridge, UK

Jean-Claude Pechère MD
President, International Society of Chemotherapy
Universities of Geneva and Marrakech
Geneva, Switzerland

Mark D Perkins MD
Chief Scientific Officer
Foundation for Innovative New Diagnostics (FIND)
Cointrin, Switzerland

Barry Peters MBBS DFFP MD FRCP
Head of Academic Unit of HIV and STDs
Department of Infectious Diseases
Kings College London
London, UK

Gaby E Pfyffer PhD FAMH FAAM
Professor of Medical Microbiology
Head, Department of Medical Microbiology
Center for Laboratory Medicine
Luzerner Kantonsspital Luzern
Luzern, Switzerland

Paul A Pham PharmD BCPS
Research Associate
Johns Hopkins University School of Medicine
Division of Infectious Diseases
Baltimore, MD, USA

Peter Piot MD PhD FRCP
Director, Institute for Global Health at Imperial College
London, UK

Geraldine Placko-Parola MD
Physician, Radiology Fellow
Assistant Professor InfectRadiology
Department Hopital de la Conception
University Hôpital of Marseille
Marseille, France

Stainslas Pol MD PhD
Liver Unit Hôpital Cochin
Paris, France

Klara M Posfay-Barbe MD MS
Head of Pediatric Infectious Diseases
Department of Pediatrics
Children's Hospital of Geneva
University Hospitals of Geneva
Geneva, Switzerland

William G Powderly MD FRCPI
Professor of Medicine and Therapeutics
Head, UCD School of Medicine and Medical Sciences
Medical Professorial Unit
University College Dublin
Dublin, Ireland

Anton Pozniak MD FRCP
Consultant Physician and Director of HIV Services
Executive Director of HIV Research
Department of HIV and Genitourinary Medicine
Chelsea and Westminster Hospital
London, UK

Guy Prod'hom MD
Head of Bacteriology Unit
Institute of Microbiology
University of Lausanne and University Hospital Centre
Lausanne, Switzerland

Thomas C Quinn MD MSc
Associate Director for International Research,
Division of Intramural Research,
National Institute of Allergy and Infectious Diseases
Bethesda, MD, USA

Daniel W Rahn MD
President and Professor of Medicine
Medical College of Georgia
Augusta, GA, USA

Aadia I Rana MD
Fellow, Division of Infectious Diseases
Warren Alpert Medical School of Brown University
Providence, RI, USA

Didier Raoult MD PhD
Professor, Faculté de Médecine
Unité des Rickettsies
WHO Collaborative Center for Rickettsial Reference and Research
Marseille, France

Raul Raz MD
Director
Infectious Diseases Unit
Ha'Emek Medical Center
Afula, Israel

Raymund Razonable MD
Consultant, Division of Infectious Diseases
The William J von Liebig Transplant Center
Associate Professor of Medicine
Mayo Clinic College of Medicine
Rochester, MN, USA

Robert C Read MD FRCP FIDSA
Professor of Infectious Diseases
University of Sheffield Medical School
Sheffield, UK

Stephen J Reynolds PhD CIH
Staff Clinician
Division of Intramural Research
National Institute of Allergy and Infectious Diseases
Bethesda, MD, USA

Malcolm D Richardson PhD FIBiol FRCPath
Director
New England Eye Center
Boston, MA, USA

Christopher C Robinson MD
Director
New England Eye Center
Boston, MA, USA

Suzan HM Rooijakkers PhD
Post-Doctorate
Department of Medical Microbiology
University Medical Center Utrecht
Utrecht, The Netherlands

Daniel Rosenbluth MD
Professor of Medicine and Pediatrics
Medical Director, Jacqueline Maritz Lung Center
Fellowship Director
Division of Pulmonary and Critical Care Medicine
Washington University School of Medicine
St Louis, MO, USA

Sergio D Rosenzweig MD
Immunopathogenesis Unit
Clinical Pathophysiology Section
Laboratory of Host Defenses
National Institute of Allergy and Infectious Diseases
Bethesda, MD, USA

Clarisse Rovery MD
Specialist in Infectious Diseases
Infectious Disease Unit
Hôpital Nord
Marseille, France

Robert H Rubin MD FACP FCCP
Associate Director of Infectious Diseases
Brigham and Women's Hospital
Professor of Medicine, Harvard Medical School
Gordon and Marjorie Osborne Professor of Health Sciences and Technology
Director, Center for Experimental Pharmacology and Therapeutics
Co-Director, The Clinical Investigator Training Program Fellowship
Harvard–MIT Division of Health Sciences and Technology
Massachusetts Institute of Technology
Cambridge, MA, USA

Bina Rubinovitch MD
Sheba Medical Center
Tel Hashomer
Ramat Gan, Israel

Kathleen H Rubins PhD
Principal Investigator/Fellow
Rubins Lab
Whitehead Institute for Biomedical Research
Cambridge, MA, USA

Ethan Rubinstein MD Llb
Sellers Professor and Head
Section of Infectious Diseases
Faculty of Medicine
Winnipeg, Manitoba, Canada

Greg Ryan MB FRCOG FRCSC
Associate Professor
Department of Obstetrics and Gynecology
Division of Fetal and Maternal Medicine
University of Toronto
Toronto, ON, Canada

Stephen Ryder DM FRCP
Consultant Hepatologist
Division of Gastroenterology
Queen's Medical Centre
Nottingham University Hospital NHS Trust and Biomedical Research Unit
Nottingham, UK

Steven Safren PhD
Director of Behavioral Medicine
The Fenway Institute
Associate Professor in Psychology
Department of Psychiatry
Harvard Medical School
Boston, MA, USA

Vikrant V Sahasrabuddhe MBBS MPH DrPH
Assistant Professor
Department of Pediatrics and Institute for Global Health
Vanderbilt University School of Medicine
Nashville, TN, USA

Pekka AI Saikku MD PhD
Professor of Medical Microbiology
Department of Medical Microbiology
University of Oulu
Oulu, Finland

George Sakoulas MD
Assistant Professor
Department of Pediatrics
University of California
San Diego School of Medicine
La Jolla, CA

Juan Carlos Salazar MD MPH
Associate Professor of Pediatrics
Department of Pediatrics
University of Connecticut Health Center
Director, Division of Infectious Diseases
Connecticut Children's Medical Center
Hartford, CT, USA

Michelle R Salvaggio MD
Instructor of Medicine
Division of Infectious Diseases
University of Alabama at Birmingham and Birmingham Veterans Administration Medical Center
Birmingham, AL, USA

Kirsten Schaffer MD MRCPath
Consultant Microbiologist
Department of Medical Microbiology
St Vincent's University Hospital
Dublin, Ireland

Franz-Josef Schmitz MD PhD
Head, Institute for Laboratory Medicine, Microbiology, Hygiene and Transfusion Medicine Klinikum Minden,
Associate Professor of Medical Microbiology, Institute for Medical Microbiology and Virology
University of Düsseldorf
Düsseldorf, Germany

Robert T Schooley MD
Professor and Head
Division of Infectious Diseases
Academic Vice Chair
Department of Medicine
University of California, San Diego
La Jolla, CA, USA

Richard-Fabian Schumacher MD
Attending Physician, Children's Hospital
Clinica Pediatrica
Universita' degli Studi di Brescia
Brescia, Italy

Euan M Scrimgeour MD FRACP DTM&H FAFPHM
Clinical Associate Professor
Department of Immunology and Microbiology
School of Biomedical, Biomolecular and Clinical Sciences
Perth, Australia

James Seddon MBBS MA MRCPCH DTM&H
London School of Hygiene and Tropical Medicine
London, UK

Harald Seifert MD
Professor of Medical Microbiology and Hygiene
Institute for Medical Microbiology, Immunology and Hygiene
University of Cologne
Cologne, Germany

Graham R Serjeant CMG CD MD FRCP FRCPE
Sickle Cell Trust
Kingston, Jamaica

Beverly E Sha MD
Associate Professor of Medicine
Section of Infectious Diseases
Rush University Medical Center
Chicago, IL, USA

Keerti V Shah MD DrPH
Professor of Molecular Microbiology and Immunology
Johns Hopkins Bloombery School of Public Health
Baltimore, MD, USA

Daniel S Shapiro MD
Director, Clinical Microbiology Laboratory
Lahey Clinic
Burlington, MA
Adjunct Associate Professor of Medicine
Boston University School of Medicine
Boston, MA, USA

Gerard Sheehan MB FRCPI
Senior Lecturer
School of Medicine and Medical Sciences
University College Dublin
Consultant in Infectious Diseases
Mater Misericordiae University Hospital
Dublin, Ireland

Shmuel Shoham MD
Director of Transplant Infectious Diseases
Division of Infectious Diseases
Washington Hospital Center
Washington, DC
Immunocompromised Host Section
Pediatric Oncology Branch
National Cancer Institute
Bethesda, MD, USA

Cameron P Simmons BSc(Hons) PhD
Reader in Tropical Medicine
Oxford University Clinical Research Unit
Hospital for Tropical Diseases
Ho Chi Minh City, Vietnam

Kari A Simonsen MD
Assistant Professor of Pediatrics
Section of Pediatric Infectious Diseases
Nebraska Medical Center
Omaha, NE, USA

Neeraj Singh MBBS
Assistant Professor of Medicine
Division of Nephrology
The Ohio State University Medical Centre
Columbus, OH, USA

Mary PE Slack MAMBBChir FRCPath
Head of Haemophilus Influenzae Reference Unit
Respiratory and Systemic Infection Laboratory
Central Public Health Laboratory
London, UK

Jack D Sobel MD
Professor of Infectious Diseases
Division Head
Infectious Diseases
Wayne State University School of Medicine
Detroit, MI, USA

Madhuri M Sopirala MD MPH
Assistant Professor of Internal Medicine
Division of Infectious Diseases
Department of Internal Medicine
OSUMC
Assistant Medical Director, Clinical Epidemiology
The Ohio State University Medical Center
Columbus, OH, USA

Lisa A Spacek MD PhD
Assistant Professor
Division of Infectious Diseases
Department of Medicine
Johns Hopkins University
Baltimore, MD, USA

Shiranee Sriskandan PhD FRCP MA MBBChir
Professor of Infectious Diseases
Department of Infectious Diseases
Faculty of Medicine
Imperial College School of Medicine
London, UK

Samuel L Stanley Jr MD
President Stony Brook University
Stony Brook, NY, USA

James M Steckelberg MD
Professor of Medicine
Division of Infectious Disease
Department of Internal Medicine
Mayo Clinic
Rochester, MN, USA

Iain Stephenson FRCP MB MA (Cantab)
Senior Lecturer in Infectious Diseases
Infectious Diseases Unit
Leicester Royal Infirmary
Leicester, UK

Dennis L Stevens PhD MD
Professor of Medicine
University of Washington School of Medicine
Chief, Infectious Disease Section
Veterans Affairs Medical Center
Boise, ID, USA

Contributors

Walter L Straus MD MPH
Global Director for Scientific
Affairs-Vaccines
Merck Vaccines and Infectious
Diseases
Merck & Co., Inc.
West Point, PA, USA

Willem Sturm MD PhD
Professor of Medical Microbiology
Department of Medical
Microbiology
Nelson R Madela School of
Medicine
Congella, South Africa

Richard C Summerbell PhD
Senior Researcher
Centraalbureau voor
Schimmelcultures
Royal Netherlands Academy of
Sciences
Utrecht, The Netherlands

Joseph S Susa MD
Clinical Assistant Professor
Dermatology Department
University of Texas Southwestern
Medical Center
Dallas, TX, USA

**Sarah J Tabrizi BSc(Hons)
FRCP PhD**
Reader in Neurology and
Neurogenetics
Department of Neurodegenerative
Diseases/MRC Prion Unit
Institute of Neurology
London, UK

Marc A Tack MD
Infectious Diseases Consultant
Medical Associates of the Hudson
Valley P.C.
Kingston, NY, USA

Randy Taplitz MD
Associate Professor of Clinical
Medicine
Clinical Director
Division of Infectious Diseases
Associate Medical Director of UCSD
Infection Prevention and Clinical
Epidemiology
University of California at San Diego
San Diego, CA, USA

Pablo Tebas MD
Associate Professor of Medicine
Division of Infectious Diseases
University of Pennsylvania
Philadelphia, PA, USA

**Marleen Temmerman MD
MPH PhD**
Professor
Head of Department of Obstetrics
& Gynaecology
International Center for
Reproductive Health
WHO Collaborating Centre
for Research on Sexual and
Reproductive Health
Faculty of Medicine and Health
Sciences
Ghent University
Ghent, Belgium

Steven FT Thijsen MD PhD
Medical Microbiologist
Department of Medical
Microbiology
Diakonessenhuis
Utrecht, The Netherlands

Lora D Thomas MD MPH
Assistant Professor of Medicine
Division of Infectious Diseases
Vanderbilt University Medical Center
Nashville, TN, USA

**Gail Thomson MB ChB
MRCP & DTM&H**
Consultant in Infectious Diseases
North Manchester General Hospital
Manchester, UK

**Guy E Thwaites MA MBBS
MRCP MRCPath PhD**
Wellcome Trust Clinical Research
Fellow
Centre for Molecular Microbiology
and Infection
Imperial College London
London, UK

Umberto Tirelli MD
Director, Division of Medical Oncology
National Cancer Institute
Aviano, Italy

**Nina E Tolkoff-Rubin MD
FACP**
Director of Hemodialysis and CAPD
Units
Medical Director for Renal
Transplantation
Professor of Medicine
Harvard Medical School
Department of Medicine
Massachusetts General Hospital
Boston, MA, USA

Tone Tønjum MD PhD
Professor
Chief Physician
Institute of Microbiology, Centre for
Molecular Biology and Neuroscience
University of Oslo
Rikshospitalet
Oslo, Norway

Francesca J Torriani MD
Professor of Clinical Medicine
Medical Director of UCSD
Infection Prevention and Clinical
Epidemiology
Division of Infectious Diseases
University of California at San Diego
San Diego, CA, USA

Gregory C Townsend MD
Assistant Professor of Medicine
Division of Infectious Diseases
University of Virginia
Charlottesville, VA, USA

Gloria Trallero Masó BSc
Enterovirus Laboratory
Department of Virology
National Center for Microbiology
Instituto de Salud Carlos III
Madrid, Spain

Paul M Tulkens MD PhD
Professor of Pharmacology
Unité de Pharmacologie cellulaire
et moléculaire & Louvain Drug
Research Institute
Université catholique de Louvain
Brussels, Belgium

Allan R Tunkel MD PhD
Professor of Medicine
Drexel University College of Medicine
Chair, Department of Medicine
Monmouth Medical Center
Long Branch, NJ, USA

Emanuela Vaccher MD
Department of Medical Oncology
National Cancer Institute
Aviano, Italy

Anaïs Vallet-Pichard MD
Service d'Hepatologie
Hopital Necker
Paris, France

**Françoise Van Bambeke
PharmD PhD**
Senior Research Associate of
the Belgian Fonds National de la
Recherche Scientifique
Unité de Pharmacologie cellulaire
et moléculaire & Louvain Drug
Research Insitute
Université catholique de Louvain
Brussels, Belgium

**Diederik van de Beek MD
PhD**
Neurologist
Department of Neurology
Center of Infection and Immunity
Amsterdam (CINIMA)
Academic Medical Center
University of Amsterdam
Amsterdam, The Netherlands

**Jos WM van der Meer MD
PhD FRCP**
Professor of Medicine
Department of General Internal
Medicine
Nijmegen Institute for Infection
Inflammation and Immunity
Radboud University Medical Center
Nijmegen, The Netherlands

Anton M van Loon PhD
Director
Department of Virology
University Medical Centre Utrecht
Utrecht, The Netherlands

Jos van Putten MD PhD
Professor of Infection Biology
Infectious Diseases and
Immunology
Utrecht University
Utrecht, The Netherlands

Bernard P Vaudaux MD
Head, Unit of Pediatric Infectious
Diseases and Vaccinology
Department of Pediatrics
Centre Hospitalier Universitaire
Vaudois and Hôpital de l'Enfance
de Lausanne
Lausanne, Switzerland

Sten H Vermund MD PhD
Amos Christie Chair of Global Health
Vanderbilt University School of
Medicine
Nashville, TN, USA

**Hans Verstraelen MD MPH
PhD**
Research Fellow
Department of Obstetrics and
Gynaecology
Ghent University
Ghent, Belgium

Paul Verweij MD PhD
Professor of Medical Microbiology
Department of Medical
Microbiology
Radboud University Nijmegen
Medical Centre
Nijmegen Centre for Molecular Life
Sciences
Nijmegen, The Netherlands

Raphael P Viscidi MD
Professor of Pediatrics
Department of Pediatrics
Johns Hopkins University School of
Medicine
Baltimore, MD, USA

Kumar Visvanathan MD
Director, Innate Immunity
Laboratory and Infectious Diseases
Physician
Centre for Inflammatory Diseases
Department of Medicine (Monash
Medical Centre)
Monash University
Clayton, VIC, Australia

Govinda S Visvesvara PhD
Research Microbiologist
Division of Parasitic Diseases
National Center for Zoonotic,
Vector–Borne and Enteric Diseases
Centers for Disease Control
and Prevention
Atlanta, GA, USA

Lorenz von Seidlein MD PhD
Reader
London School of Hygiene and
Tropical Medicine
London, UK

**Florian ME Wagenlehner
MD PhD**
Consultant Urologist
Clinic for Urology and Pediatric
Urology
Justus-Liebig-University
Giessen, Germany

Victoria Wahl-Jensen MS PhD
Principal Investigator
Virology
United States Army Medical
Research Institute of Infectious
Disease (USAMRIID)
Fort Detrick, MD, USA

Thomas J Walsh MD
Head, Immunocompromised Host
Section
Pediatric Oncology Branch
National Cancer Institute
Bethesda, MD, USA

David C Warhurst BSc PhD DSc FRCPath
Emeritus Professor of Protozoan Chemotherapy
Department of Infections and Tropical Diseases
London School of Hygiene and Tropical Medicine
London, UK

David W Warnock BSc PhD FAAM FRCPath
Director
Division of Foodborne
Bacterial and Mycotic Diseases
National Center for Zoonotic, Vector-borne and Enteric Diseases
Centers for Disease Control and Prevention
Adjunct Professor of Pathology and Laboratory Medicine
Emory University School of Medicine
Atlanta, GA, USA

David A Warrell MA DM DSc FRCP FRCPE HonFCeylonCP FMedSci HonFZS FRGS
Emeritus Professor of Tropical Medicine
Nuffield Department of Clinical Medicine
University of Oxford
Oxford, UK

Mary J Warrell MBBS MRCP FRCPath
Oxford Vaccine Group University of Oxford
Centre for Clinical Vaccinology and Tropical Medicine
Oxford, UK

Adilia Warris MD PhD
Pediatric Infectious Diseases Specialist
Head of the Division of Pediatric Infectious Diseases and Immunology
Department of Pediatrics
Radboud University Nijmegen Medical Center
Nijmegen, The Netherlands

Rainer Weber MD DTMH(Lond)
Head of the Division of Infectious Diseases and Hospital Epidemiology
Division of Infectious Diseases and Hospital Epidemiology
Department of Internal Medicine
University Hospital Zurich
Zurich, Switzerland

Wolfgang Weidner MD
Professor of Urology
Head of Department of Urology
Clinic for Urology, Pediatric Urology and Andrology
Justus-Liebig University
Giessen, Germany

Vivienne C Weston MBBS MSc FRCPath FRCP(UK)
Consultant Medical Microbiologist
Department of Microbiology
Nottingham University Hospitals
NHS Trust
Nottingham, UK

Estella Whimbey MD
Associate Medical Director
University of Washington
Medicial Center
Seattle WA, USA

Michael Whitby MD BS DTM&H MPH FRACP FRCPA FRCPath FAFPHM
Director, Infection Management Services
Princess Alexandra Hospital
Brisbane, Australia

Peter J White PhD
Head
Modelling and Economics Unit
Health Protection Agency Centre for Infections, London;
MRC Centre for Outbreak Analysis and Modelling, Department of Infectious Disease Epidemiology
Imperial College London
London, UK

Christopher JM Whitty FRCP DTM&H
Consultant Physician
Hospital for Tropical Diseases
Professor of International Health
London School of Hygiene and Tropical Medicine
London, UK

Rob JL Willems PhD
Associate Professor
Medical Microbiology
University Medical Center Utrecht
Utrecht, The Netherlands

Emrys Williams MBBS MRCP DTM&H FRCPath
Consultant in Medical Microbiology
NPHS Microbiology Bangor
Ysbyty Gwynedd
Bangor, UK

Cara Wilson MD
Associate Professor
Infectious Diseases Division
University of Colorado School of Medicine
Denver, CO, USA

Mary E Wilson MD FACP FIDSA
Associate Clinical Professor of Medicine
Harvard Medical School
Associate Professor of Global Health and Population
Harvard School of Public Health
Washington DC, WA, USA

Richard E Winn MD
Division Director of Pulmonary Medicine and Infectious Diseases,
Scott and White Clinic
Professor of Internal Medicine
Texas A&M College of Medicine
Temple, TX, USA

Kevin L Winthrop MD MPH
Assistant Professor of Infectious Diseases, Ophthalmology, Public Health and Preventive Medicine
Oregon Health and Science University
Portland, OR, USA

Martin J Wiselka MD PhD FRCP
Consultant in Infectious Disease
Leicester Royal Infirmary
Leicester, UK

Hilmar Wisplinghoff MD
Physician
Institute for Medical Microbiology
Immunology and Hygiene
University of Cologne
Cologne, Germany

Cameron R Wolfe MD
Fellow
Department of Infectious Diseases and Internal Health
Duke University School of Medicine
Durham, NC, USA

Robin Wood BSc BM MMed DTM&H
Professor of Medicine
The Desmond Tutu HIV Centre
Institute of Infectious Disease and Molecular Medicine
Faculty of Health Sciences
University of Cape Town
Cape Town, South Africa

Natalie Wright BSc
University of Texas Health Science Center
Houston, TX, USA

James R Yankaskas MD MS BS
Professor of Medicine
Cystic Fibrosis/Pulmonary Research and Treatment Center
University of North Carolina
Chapel Hill, NC, USA

Najam A Zaidi MD
Assistant Professor of Medicine (Clinical)
Warren Alpert Medical School of Brown University
Providence, RI, USA

Jonathan M Zenilman MD
Professor of Medicine
Johns Hopkins University School of Medicine
Baltimore, MD, USA

Yaobi Zhang MD PhD
Field Programme Co-ordinator
Schistosomiasis Control Initiative
Department of Infectious Disease Epidemiology
Imperial College London
London, UK

Arie J Zuckerman MD DSc FRCP FRCPath FMedSci
Professor of Medical Microbiology in the University of London
Academic Centre for Travel Medicine and Vaccines
London, UK

Jane Nicola Zuckerman MD FRCP(Edin) FRCPath MRCGP FFPH FFPM FHEA
Senior Lecturer and Honorary Consultant
WHO Centre for Reference, Research and Training in Travel Medicine
Academic Centre for Travel Medicine and Vaccines
University College London Medical School
London, UK

Alimuddin Zumla BSc MBChB MSc PhD FRCP(Lond) FRCP(Edin)
Director, Centre for Infectious Diseases and International Health
Royal Free and University College London Medical School
Consultant Infectious Diseases Physician
University College London NHS Hospitals Trust
London, UK

Section | 5 |

Nathan Clumeck & William G Powderly

HIV and AIDS

Chapter | **84** | *Michel Caraël*
Peter Piot

Epidemiology of HIV infection

INTRODUCTION

This chapter describes the distribution and transmission patterns of HIV infections. Although the biology and modes of transmission are broadly the same in the developing world and in high-income countries, there are some large differences in the epidemiology, which are due to a variety of behavioral factors and socioeconomic conditions.

Twenty-five years after the recognition of the first AIDS cases, more than 25 million people have died because of this pandemic, one of the most significant health, social and security challenges facing the global community.[1] At the end of 2007, 33.2 million people (range 30.6–36.1 million) are living with HIV, including 2.5 million children.[2] The HIV epidemics are overwhelmingly affecting developing countries, where more than 90% of all people infected with HIV live, and there is an increasing proportion of adults living with HIV who are women (Fig. 84.1). In sub-Saharan Africa, almost 61% of adults living with HIV in 2007 were women and 42% in the Caribbean, while in the other regions the proportion of women has increased since 1990 as HIV is transmitted to the female partners of men who are likely to have been infected through intravenous drug use, during unprotected paid sex or sex with other men.

Despite a continuing increase in the number of people living with HIV, in a growing world population, in recent years, the adult HIV prevalence percentage has leveled off – 0.8% prevalence since 2001. In addition, the global number of new HIV infections has decreased. There were an estimated 2.5 million new infections in 2007, down from 3.2 million in 2001. The number of people dying of AIDS has declined in the last 2 years to 2.1 million. There are documented reductions in HIV prevalence in seven countries and a reduction in HIV-associated deaths, partly attributable to increased access to anti-retroviral treatment. Sub-Saharan Africa is still the most seriously affected region, where AIDS remains the leading cause of death. In the USA and Western Europe, despite the spectacular reduction in numbers of new AIDS cases due to advances in antiretroviral treatment, a constant number of new HIV infections persists every year, with evidence that in some settings high-risk behavior has increased, indicating failure in HIV prevention. The contribution of Asia to the HIV pandemic has considerably diminished.[2] Small variations in estimates of national adult HIV prevalence in India – from 0.9% to 0.4% – and also in China result in large differences in the number of people with HIV because of the population size of these two giant countries.

Trends suggest that HIV prevention efforts are having an impact in several of the most affected countries. Côte d'Ivoire, most East African

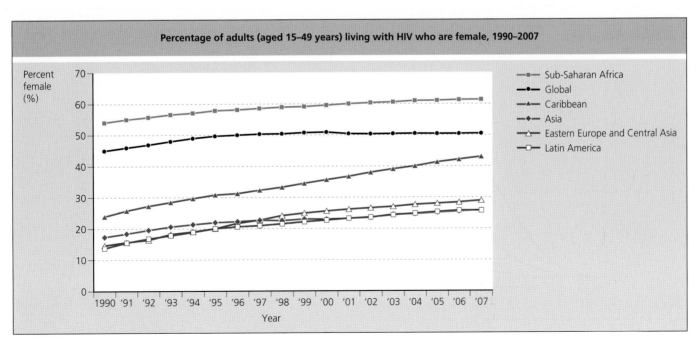

Fig. 84.1 Percentage of adults (aged 15–49 years) living with HIV who are female, 1990–2007. (From WHO: 2007 Aids Epidemic Update.)

countries and several Caribbean countries have all seen downward trends in their national prevalence percentages. HIV prevalence has also declined in South and South East Asia, notably in Cambodia, Myanmar and Southern India.

EXTENT OF HIV INFECTION

Shortly after the first reports of AIDS in the USA in 1981 among homosexual men and intravenous drug users, it became obvious that the disease was also present in Haitians living in North America and in Africans seen in Belgium for medical care at the end of 1983.[3,4] Subsequently, surveys in Haiti and Central Africa confirmed the occurrence of several epidemic foci of HIV in these areas.[5–7]

The identification of another variant, labeled HIV-2, among West African populations further increased the heterogeneity of what quickly emerged as a global pandemic. The routes of transmission and risk factors of HIV-2 and HIV-1 are similar, but it has become increasingly clear that the pathogenic effect of HIV-2 is lower than that of HIV-1.[8] In the rest of this chapter, HIV refers to HIV-1.

The exact magnitude of the HIV epidemic is still difficult to assess.[9] Indeed, despite the recognition that estimates of HIV are more accurate than for most other infectious diseases, the largely silent nature of this infection and the limited HIV surveillance systems in many countries make the tracking of HIV infection difficult. The selection of surveillance populations depends on the type of epidemic. In epidemics with at least 1% infection rates in the adult population, the recommended surveillance population are pregnant women attending antenatal clinics. In epidemics where HIV has not spread into the general population, the primary focus of the surveillance system is among high-risk populations. HIV surveillance systems have improved since 2000. In some countries, improvements have been through an increase of sentinel surveillance sites, both in number and in geographical coverage. For example in India the number of sites increased from 155 in 1998 to 1100 in 2006. In addition, 40 countries, mostly in Africa where heterosexual transmission of HIV is predominant, have conducted national representative population-based household surveys with HIV prevalence measurement. These surveys give a more precise picture of the HIV prevalence in men and women in rural areas, but clearly underestimate the extent of HIV infection among mobile populations and other vulnerable populations. As such, there is a need for several surveillance approaches to achieve the most accurate estimates.

Geographic distribution of HIV infection and AIDS

North America and Australia

In the USA, AIDS cases increased rapidly in the 1980s and peaked in 1992 with an estimated 78 000 cases diagnosed, before stabilizing in 1998; since then, approximately 40 000 AIDS cases have been diagnosed annually[10] (Fig. 84.2) but reaching around 60 000 in 2007. In 1992, during early prevention and treatment advances, the number of AIDS cases started to decrease in all demographic and transmission categories until around 1998 when the numbers started to increase again.

At the end of 2003, the most recent estimation, approximately 1 100 000 persons in the USA were living with HIV or AIDS, an estimated 25% of whom were unaware of their infection. Based on data from HIV reporting, men accounted for 74% of the HIV or AIDS diagnoses among adults and adolescents. More than half of all newly diagnosed HIV infections in 2005 were among men who have sex with men. Persons exposed to HIV through heterosexual intercourse with a nonregular partner accounted for just under one-third, while about 18% occurred among intravenous drug users.[11]

Racial and ethnic minorities continue to be disproportionately affected by the HIV epidemic. Although African-Americans represent about 13% of the population, they accounted for 51% of new HIV or AIDS diagnoses during 2001–2004. In 2004, estimated HIV and AIDS case rates for blacks and Hispanics were 8.5 and 3.3 times higher, respectively, than rates for whites. Among males and females, case rates among blacks were 7.0 and 21 times higher, respectively, than rates for whites. AIDS was the fourth leading cause of death among African-Americans aged 25–44 years in the United States in 2004.[12]

Between 1981 and 2004, more than half a million deaths among persons with AIDS were reported to the US Centers for Disease Control and Prevention (CDC). The most striking trend has been the decline in AIDS incidence and deaths that have occurred since 1995 when combination antiretroviral therapy first became available (see Fig. 84.2).

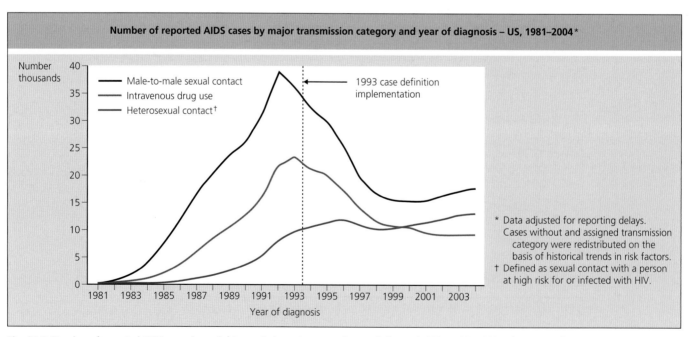

Number of reported AIDS cases by major transmission category and year of diagnosis – US, 1981–2004*

Number thousands (y-axis: 0, 5, 10, 15, 20, 25, 30, 35, 40)

- Male-to-male sexual contact
- Intravenous drug use
- Heterosexual contact†

1993 case definition implementation

Year of diagnosis (x-axis: 1981, 1983, 1985, 1987, 1989, 1991, 1993, 1995, 1997, 1999, 2001, 2003)

* Data adjusted for reporting delays. Cases without and assigned transmission category were redistributed on the basis of historical trends in risk factors.
† Defined as sexual contact with a person at high risk for or infected with HIV.

Fig. 84.2 Number of reported AIDS cases by major transmission category and year of diagnosis: USA, 1981–2004. (Courtesy of UN AIDS 2006 Report on the global AIDS epidemic.)

The proportion of individuals living at 2 years after AIDS diagnosis was 44% for 1981–1992, 64% for 1993–1995, 85% for 1996–2000 and 87% for 2000–2005.

After leveling off in the mid-1990s, the estimated total number of people living with HIV in Canada started to increase again in the late 1990s, mainly because of the life-prolonging effects of antiretroviral treatment to reach around 64 000. Women represented 17% of new HIV infections in 2006, as compared with 8.5% in 1995. The annual number of newly reported HIV infections stayed about the same during that period, at about 2500 per year.[13] Unprotected sex between men continues to account for nearly half of new HIV infections. An estimated 37% of new HIV infections in 2005 were attributed to unprotected heterosexual intercourse, with a substantial proportion among people born in countries with generalized HIV epidemic.

In Australia and New Zealand, just as in several countries of northern Europe and some parts of the USA and Canada, the vast majority of HIV infections have been acquired through sexual contacts between men. The annual number of HIV diagnoses in Australia peaked in 1987. There followed 12 years of decline, after which the rate of diagnoses grew again to reach nearly 1000 in 2006. The proportion of men having sex without a condom nearly doubled to 46% between 1997 and 2001, and the number of men who had unprotected sex with a casual partner climbed 10% to 26% over the same time period. Programs involving community members and allowing easy access to sterile injecting equipment and methadone treatment have permitted the prevalence in intravenous drug users to remain very low (<1%) in several major cities.[14]

Europe and Central Asia

This region had an estimated 2 360 000 persons living with HIV in 2007.[2] In Western Europe, the number of annual reported new HIV diagnoses almost tripled between 1999 and 2005 to reach nearly 20 000 but declined significantly thereafter.[15] Heterosexually acquired HIV infections, most of which were among immigrants and migrants, accounted for 42% of new HIV diagnoses in Western Europe in 2006. Of these newly diagnosed HIV infections, 29% were attributable to unsafe sex between men and only 6% (except in countries such as Spain and Italy) to intravenous drug use. More than half heterosexually transmitted HIV cases originate in countries with high HIV prevalence and, within that group, more than 50% of new HIV diagnoses are in women.[15]

Portugal has the highest HIV prevalence, estimated at around 0.3–0.5%. The annual number of newly diagnosed HIV infections has more than doubled in the UK, reaching about 9000 in 2006. This is mainly due to sustained levels of newly acquired infections among men who have sex with men, an increase in diagnoses among heterosexual men and women who acquired their infection in a high prevalence country, and improved reporting due to expanding HIV testing services. In central Europe, the number of newly diagnosed HIV infections in 2006 surpassed 100 only in Poland, Turkey and Romania. Elsewhere, the epidemics are comparatively small. Intravenous drug use is the most reported mode of HIV transmission in the three Baltic States where the epidemics appear to have stabilized.[16]

In Eastern Europe and Central Asia, the greatest majority of HIV cases in 2006 was from the two countries with the largest populations: the Russian Federation, with an estimated 1 million cases (three times the reported HIV cases) and to a lesser extent Ukraine, with around 380 000 persons living with HIV (four times the estimated number of reported cases) (Fig. 84.3). Nearly two-thirds were attributed to intravenous drug use and 37% were ascribed to unprotected sex. A large number of young and unemployed men inject and share drugs. Syringe exchange programs have recently increased but their coverage is too limited to make an impact on the HIV epidemic curve. As the Russian Federation's epidemics mature, AIDS mortality will contribute significantly to the demographic decline.

In addition to HIV, major epidemics of tuberculosis and syphilis have occurred in Central Asia against a background of political and economic instability, increased mobility, intravenous drug use and degradation of the public health infrastructure. In this region, the future course of the HIV epidemic is unpredictable.

Table 84.1 summarizes the levels of HIV prevalence in selected high-risk populations in Western, Central and Eastern Europe.

Sub-Saharan Africa

Sub-Saharan Africa is more heavily affected by AIDS than any other region of the world. An estimated 22.5 million people were living with HIV in the region in 2007, 61% of them women.[2] The region's epidemics vary significantly in scale, with national adult HIV prevalence ranging from less than 1% in some countries of the Sahel to around 15–20% in most of southern Africa. Southern Africa alone accounted for almost one-third of all new HIV infections and AIDS deaths

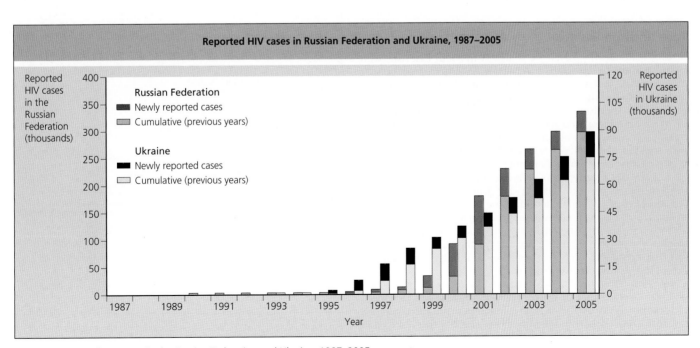

Fig. 84.3 Reported HIV cases in the Russian Federation and Ukraine, 1987–2005.

Table 84.1 HIV prevalence among high-risk populations by European regions

	Western Europe	Central Europe	Eastern Europe
Intravenous drug users	<5% in 11 countries >20% in Mediterranean countries	<2% in all countries except Poland (>20%)	5% in some countries Up to 60% in cities in Ukraine and Russia
Homosexual men	5–15%	3–10%	0–5%
Sex workers	Mostly <1%	<1%	Up to 15%
Patients with sexually transmitted disease	1–2%	<0.1%	0–2%
Adapted from EuroHIV.[15]			

globally in 2007. A total of 1.7 million people in sub-Saharan Africa became infected with HIV in the past year, of whom 500 000 were in South Africa, declining from 2.2 million new infections in 2001. AIDS continues to be the single largest cause of mortality in sub-Saharan Africa, before malaria and lower respiratory tract infections. There are an estimated 11.4 million orphans due to AIDS in this region.

HIV prevention efforts are having an impact in some countries[2] (Fig. 84.4). In Kenya, HIV prevalence among young pregnant women declined significantly by more than 25% in both urban and rural areas, while similar declines were observed in urban areas of Malawi and Zimbabwe. Less striking declines in HIV prevalence in young pregnant women have also occurred in numerous sub-Saharan countries. While there is evidence of a significant decline in the national HIV prevalence in Zimbabwe,[17] the epidemics in most of the rest of the South African region have either reached or are approaching a plateau, associated with significant changes in sexual behavior.

HIV-2 is primarily found in West Africa but has also been confirmed in other African countries. The highest prevalence of HIV-2 infection is found in Guinea-Bissau, with prevalence rates as high as 8.0% in 1987–88 but with a decline to 2.5% in 2004. In contrast to the increasing spread of HIV-1, the prevalence of HIV-2 has remained rather stable in West Africa and has declined in Guinea-Bissau and in the Gambia.[18] This is probably the result of the higher transmissibility of HIV-1 compared with that of HIV-2.[8]

Asia and the Pacific

In Asia, national HIV prevalence is highest in South East Asia, with wide variation in epidemic trends between different countries.[19] Overall in Asia, an estimated 4.9 million people were living with HIV in 2007, including the 440 000 people who became newly infected in the past year. Approximately 300 000 died from AIDS-related illnesses in 2007.[2] New, more accurate estimates of HIV indicate that approximately 2.5 million people in India were living with HIV in 2006, with a national adult HIV prevalence of around 0.4%. The epidemic is extremely heterogeneous; for example, in Mumbai, Pune and Tamil Nadu state, HIV prevalences of 24% have been reported in pregnant women, contrasting with Calcutta and Delhi where prevalence has remained below 1%. Intravenous drug use is the predominant mode of transmission in the north-eastern states near Myanmar, where prevalence among drug users exceeds 70%. In Manipur cities, many of the women who tested HIV positive are sexual partners of male drug injectors. HIV prevalence levels among intravenous drug users usually far exceed levels among sex workers (Fig. 84.5).

In China, HIV infection was first noted in Yunnan Province bordering the Golden Triangle where Myanmar, Thailand and Laos meet. Here the prevalence of HIV infection in intravenous drug users climbed rapidly to 70% or more in the early 1990s, and HIV first emerged in sex workers in this region. At least 650 000 persons were living with HIV in China in 2006, around half were intravenous drug users, while

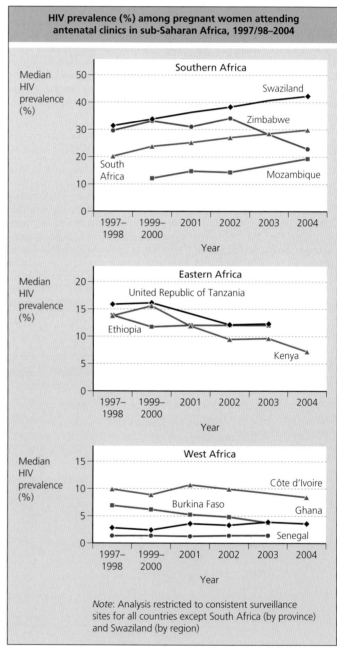

Fig. 84.4 HIV prevalence (%) among pregnant women attending antenatal clinics in sub-Saharan Africa, 1997/98–2004. (Courtesy of UN AIDS 2006 Report on the global AIDS epidemic.)

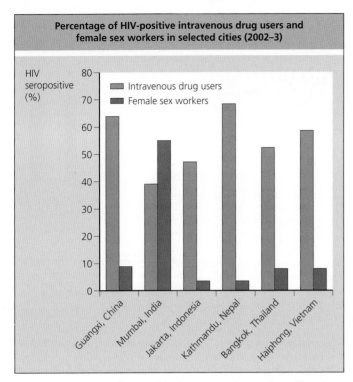

Fig. 84.5 Percentage of HIV-positive intravenous drug users and female sex workers in selected cities (2002–3).

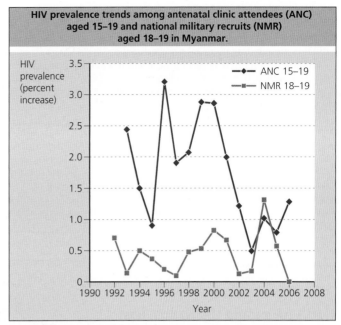

Fig. 84.6 HIV prevalence trends among antenatal clinic (ANC) attendees aged 15–19 and national military recruits (NMR) aged 18–19 in Myanmar.

the others became infected during unprotected paid sex. China has established more than 300 methadone clinics and needle exchange sites. In Sichuan Province these programs reduced the reuse of non-sterile needles by almost half. In 2000, serious HIV epidemics were documented in Henan Province in central China, where many thousands of rural villagers have become infected by selling their blood to illegal collecting centers.

The most heavily affected countries of South East Asia are Cambodia, Thailand and Myanmar, with intravenous drug use and commercial sex driving HIV transmission. In Thailand, the epidemic has spread in overlapping waves through intravenous drug users and sex workers, their clients and the female partners of clients. The prevalence among sex workers rose from 3% in 1989 to 30% in 1996, and that among sexually transmitted disease (STD) clinic patients rose from nearly zero to 9% over the same period before declining in the late 1990s. Risky behaviors were reduced following extensive programs to promote condom use in brothels and to discourage men from visiting them. The number of new annual HIV infections in Thailand continued to decline in 2008, although the decline in HIV prevalence has been slowing in recent years as more people are receiving antiretroviral therapy. HIV prevalence among intravenous drug users has remained high over the past 15 years, ranging between 30% and 50%.[20] Similarly, recent studies show increasing HIV prevalence among men who have sex with men in Bangkok from 17% in 2003 to 28% in 2007.[21]

The epidemic in Myanmar also shows signs of a decline, with HIV prevalence among pregnant women having dropped from 2.2% in 2000 to 1.5% in 2006, as well as in new military recruits (Fig. 84.6). The male to female ratio has changed from almost 8:1 in 1994 to 2.4:1 in 2006, showing a steady increase in the proportion of women being infected. While the epidemics in Cambodia also show declines in HIV prevalence, those in Vietnam and Indonesia (especially in the Papua Province) are growing. An HIV prevalence of more than 1% has been documented in Papua New Guinea, fueled mainly by heterosexual transmission. Risky behavior is widespread, with research showing high rates of unsafe sex with multiple partners and the frequent failure to use condoms.[22]

Recent sero-surveys conducted as part of national HIV surveillance in Asia show new HIV epidemics among men who have sex with men (MSM) in several countries, including India and China. Rates of HIV infection among MSM are as high as 14% in Phnom Penh, Cambodia; 16% in Andhra Pradesh, India, and 28% in Bangkok, Thailand. These data represent an alarming trend, since male–male sexual activity in the region is diverse, often completely hidden, and beyond the reach of current HIV prevention efforts. The increasing sex industry in parts of Asia is of concern, and male clients of sex workers and sex workers themselves are likely to be the most important group to target for prevention programs.[19]

Latin America and the Caribbean

With an estimated 100 000 people living with HIV in 2007, the HIV prevalence in Latin America remain generally stable, but HIV transmission continues to occur among populations at higher risk of exposure, including sex workers, their clients, intravenous drug users and MSM.[2] The epidemic in Latin America was initially similar to that in North America and Europe, with most cases among homosexual men and intravenous drug users. Systematic surveillance in the region is limited and the picture is complex, with MSM transmission predominating in some countries (Mexico, Chile, Ecuador and Peru, as well as in several Central American countries), while in others (Argentina and Brazil), intravenous drug use accounts for about half of all infections. However, in almost all countries there has been a rapid increase in cases attributed to heterosexual transmission, with a corresponding increase in the proportion of infections occurring among women. HIV rates in pregnant women are generally low, although there are estimates of prevalence higher than 1% in Honduras and Guatemala and in urban areas of Brazil and Argentina.

About one-third of all people living with HIV in Latin America reside in Brazil, where in 2005 an estimated 620 000 people were living with HIV. Although initially concentrated primarily among MSM, the epidemic subsequently spread to intravenous drug users and eventually into the general population, with increasing numbers of women becoming infected. It is estimated that a large proportion of infections among women can be attributed to the behavior of their male sexual partners. However, unprotected sex between men remains an important factor and is estimated to account for about half of all sexually transmitted HIV infections in Brazil. HIV prevalence among intravenous drug users in Brazil has declined in some cities as a result of harm-reduction programs, changing from injecting to inhaling drugs. Mortality among drug users has also declined.[23]

Of the Central American countries, Honduras and Guatemala have been especially widely affected by heterosexual transmission. Overall, however, HIV infection is highest among female sex workers and their clients and among MSM.

In the Caribbean, adult HIV prevalence is estimated at 1.0%. HIV prevalence is highest in the Dominican Republic and Haiti, which together account for nearly three-quarters of the 230 000 people living with HIV in the Caribbean.[2] HIV prevalence shows clear signs of decline in these two countries, but AIDS remains one of the leading causes of death among adults. Declining HIV is also documented in the Bahamas, Barbados and Cuba. The primary mode of HIV transmission in this region is sexual intercourse, with unprotected sex between sex workers and clients a significant factor in the transmission of HIV. Among female sex workers, HIV prevalence of 3.5% has been found in the Dominican Republic, 9% in Jamaica and 31% in Guyana. HIV infection rates remain relatively low in Jamaica but have risen in marginalized groups such as crack cocaine users and migrant laborers.

North Africa and the Middle East

Except for Sudan, the number of HIV infections in these countries is very low.[2] So far, the spread of the virus appears to be limited to paid sex, sex between men and intravenous drug use in large cities. About 75% of the AIDS cases have been reported from Morocco, Sudan, Saudi Arabia, Tunisia and Djibouti. HIV seroprevalence levels among the general population show seropositivity lower than 1%. Djibouti and South Sudan are the hardest hit countries in the region, with prevalence levels of up to 9% in pregnant women in Djibouti and 2–5% in cities in South Sudan. Iran has made needles and syringes available in pharmacies in an effort to cut the spread of HIV infection among an estimated 200 000 intravenous drug users.[24] Libya's epidemic has been growing, with almost 90% of the 6000–10 000 HIV infections in Tripoli attributed to intravenous drug use. Transmission through contaminated injecting equipment has been reported in Libya, Bahrain and Oman. Because of the illegal character of homosexuality, there is concern that HIV may spread undetected among MSM in the region.

Dynamics of the HIV epidemic

Under circumstances that are not yet fully understood, epidemics may suddenly explode, with rates of infection increasing several-fold within only a few years. For example, estimation of HIV seroprevalence among intravenous drug users seeking treatment in Bangkok increased from zero in 1985–6 to 16% in 1988 and 40–60% in 1992.

In Central and Eastern Europe, before 1995, the total number of HIV infections, with over 450 million inhabitants, was less than 30 000. In 2006, Russia estimated at around one million the number of people with HIV and AIDS. Between 1996 and 1998 alone, Russia experienced a 100-fold increase in new HIV infections, demonstrating the rapid onset of the epidemic among intravenous drug users. The epidemic has slowed through better knowledge of the risks of HIV transmission and a saturation effect. Outwith rapid HIV spread among intravenous drug users, contrasting situations have been found in the general population. Cambodia did not record its first diagnosis of HIV infection until 1991. By 1996, HIV prevalence among pregnant women was approaching 5% but was estimated to have declined to 1.6% at the end of 2005 through the implementation of 100% condom use in brothels.

In sub-Saharan Africa, most new HIV infections are occurring among young people and particularly among young girls (Fig. 84.7). There is often a doubling of the HIV rate between the 15–19 age group and the 20–24 age group. The pattern of higher HIV infection among girls than boys in sub-Saharan Africa is consistent regardless of the overall level of HIV prevalence, and regardless of whether the study is conducted in an urban or a rural area.

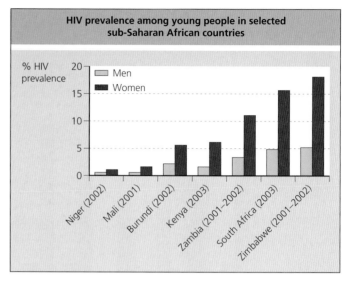

Fig. 84.7 HIV prevalence among 15–24-year-old men and women in selected sub-Saharan African countries, 2001–2003.

Sexual behavior patterns and sexual networks are believed to play a critical role due to an increased biologic susceptibility to HIV/STD associated with early age at first sexual intercourse[25,26] and because of new primary infections associated with a peak in infectiousness.[27] Age at first sex before 15 years is reported by around 15% of young women in selected countries (Fig. 84.8). In only five national surveys from 18 countries for which recent data are available, more men than women had had first sexual relations before age 15. Social factors increasing HIV exposure and susceptibility of young girls include gender inequality, older sexual partner, male sexual violence, standards of masculinity and low levels of access to information and services. The practical effect of these factors is a greater difficulty in refusing sex and/or negotiating protected sexual intercourse. Other factors increasing the efficiency of the transmission of HIV are the lack of male circumcision and the prevalence of other STDs. More attention is given now to the role of herpes simplex virus type 2 (HSV-2) as enhancing susceptibility to HIV.[28]

There is no evidence that different genetic subtypes of HIV-1 are associated with differences in the efficiency of spread of the virus in a population. The observation that some sex workers who had been repeatedly exposed to HIV infections remained HIV-antibody-negative raised the hypothesis that some people have less susceptibility to, or even immunity against, the virus or specific subtypes. Factors such as certain human leukocyte antigen (HLA) haplotypes and polymorphisms of the chemokine receptor gene CCR5, as well as genital HIV-neutralizing IgA and systemic HIV-specific proliferative responses, were associated with HIV nonacquisition.[29,30]

MODES OF TRANSMISSION

Sexual transmission

In contrast to the industrialized world, heterosexual intercourse accounts for more than 85% of cases of HIV infection in developing countries. Early epidemiologic studies showed that risk factors associated with HIV infection were unprotected sexual intercourse with multiple partners or an infected partner and the presence of STDs or a history of STDs.[31,32] More recent studies have highlighted sex differences in patterns of HIV transmission; for many monogamous women the main risk factor for HIV may be the heterosexual and homosexual behavior of their steady partner.[33] Although the probability of HIV transmission associated with unprotected vaginal sexual intercourse is not constant from one contact to another, estimates per episode – based on discordant couples – ranged from 0.0008 to 0.0015 in a study in Uganda.[34]

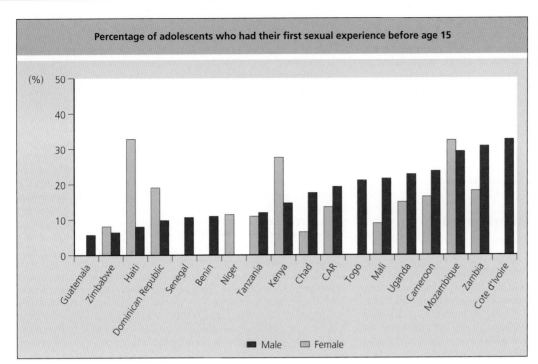

Fig. 84.8 Percentage of adolescents who had their first sexual experience before age 15 years.

A summary of biologic factors influencing the probabilities of HIV transmission from an infected person to a susceptible individual is given in Table 84.2. The presence of STDs suggests a marked risk of concurrent HIV infection, for at least two reasons:

- the modes of transmission of HIV and other STDs are similar; and
- the role of STD-induced genital ulcers, including genital herpes, chancroid and syphilis, as well as nonulcerative STD, facilitates transmission of HIV.

Early studies among female sex workers in Kinshasa and Nairobi found gonorrhea, chlamydial infections and trichomoniasis to be independent risk factors for HIV acquisition, with relative risks of 2.7–3.5.[35] HSV-2 infection may also enhance HIV acquisition and HSV-2 and HIV co-infection may facilitate HIV transmission and perhaps accelerate HIV disease progression.

A meta-analysis of prospective observational cohort studies showed that HSV-2 seropositive male and female patients had a threefold higher risk of acquiring HIV-1 compared with HSV-2 seronegative individuals.[36] More recently, in two cohorts studies in Uganda and Zimbabwe, hazard ratios for HIV-1 acquisition were 2.8% and 4.4% for prevalent HSV-2 infection, respectively, and 4.6% and 8.6% for incident HSV-2 infection, respectively.[37]

HSV-2 is now the leading cause of genital ulcer disease in both developing and developed countries. Several trials have been conducted or are currently in progress to measure the effect of aciclovir suppressive therapy in reducing HIV acquisition among HIV seronegatives, reducing HIV transmission from HIV and HSV-2 dually infected persons, and reducing HIV disease progression. Two recent trials reported no efficacy of HSV-2 suppressive therapy in reducing HIV acquisition, an unexpected outcome considering the extensive and consistent evidence for epidemiologic synergy between the two infections.[38,39]

Early diagnosis and treatment of STDs were shown to reduce the spread of HIV infection in two randomized trials in Mwanza, Tanzania and in Southern Uganda. In the intervention communities, a 42% decline in the rate of newly acquired HIV infections was observed[40,41] but later studies found no effect. Data from a randomized controlled trial undertaken in South Africa[42] and two others in Kenya and Uganda show that male circumcision reduces the risk of heterosexually acquired HIV infection in men by approximately 60%. This evidence supports the correlation between lower HIV prevalence and high rates of male circumcision in some countries in Africa. Lack of male circumcision is associated with the risk of acquiring other STDs, especially genital ulcer.[43]

The impact of male circumcision on HIV transmission to women is under study.

Perinatal transmission

As a result of heterosexual transmission in women, the number of infants born with HIV infection is growing dramatically. It is estimated that globally around 420 000 infants become infected with HIV-1 every year.[2] Nine out of 10 new infections in children occur in sub-Saharan Africa. Mother-to-child transmission of HIV can occur in utero, intrapartum or postnatally via breast-feeding. Out of these annual new pediatric infections, more than 200 000 are the result of breast milk transmission, almost exclusively in developing countries. Breast-feeding by HIV-positive mothers (in the absence of antiretroviral therapy for either mother or baby) can account for up to one-third of HIV infections among babies in sub-Saharan Africa. HIV transmission risk through breast-feeding is enhanced during primary maternal HIV infection acquired after the baby has been put to the breast.[44] The additional risk of postnatal transmission attributable to breast-feeding without a maternal primary HIV infection is estimated

Table 84.2 Biologic factors increasing the probability of sexual transmission of HIV

Confirmed	Lack of male circumcision Acute primary HIV infection Advanced clinical stage of HIV Viral load Sexually transmitted diseases Receptive anal intercourse Sex during menstruation
	HIV-1 versus HIV-2
Under study	First sex and traumatic sexual intercourse Cervical ectopy Genital trauma (use of vaginal products)
	Specific HIV-1 clades

at about 14%. Duration of breast-feeding, maternal plasma and breast milk viral load, cracked nipples, mastitis, breast abscess and infant thrush increase the risk for transmission of HIV-1. Exclusive breast-feeding is associated with a reduced risk of HIV-1 transmission as compared to mixed feeding.[45]

Most countries are making substantial progress towards preventing mother-to-child transmission of HIV, particularly in sub-Saharan Africa. In low- and middle-income countries, the proportion of HIV-positive pregnant women receiving antiretroviral prophylaxis to reduce the risk of transmission increased from 10% in 2004 to more than 30% at the end of 2007 (Fig. 84.9). Of note is the steady progress made in eastern and southern Africa, home to the majority of children who have been newly infected (see Chapters 97 and 98).

Blood products and contaminated equipment

Because of the rational use of blood, systematic HIV screening of blood donors and avoidance of donors self-reporting at higher risk, the risk of transmitting HIV infection through blood transfusion is estimated to be less than 1/100 000 units of blood. Although the situation of contaminated blood is improving and most countries have blood screening policies, implementation is still not universal. In some developing countries, however, a significant proportion of blood donations remain unscreened for HIV and an estimated 5% of HIV infections may still occur through blood transfusion, with women and children at greater risk because of frequent anemia. Clinical indications for appropriate blood transfusions are often not met outside of large cities in low-income countries.

Drug injecting is a strong driver of HIV infection in many regions. In 2003, there were estimated to be around 13 million intravenous drug users worldwide, the majority in Eastern and Central Europe and Asia (Fig. 84.10). Needle sharing with HIV-infected persons is one of the most effective ways of spreading HIV. In Russia, for example, it is estimated that 30–40% of intravenous drug users use nonsterile needles or share needles. In addition, a majority of intravenous drug users have sex not only with their female partners but also with sex workers. In 2007, 34% of countries with a concentrated epidemic implemented harm-reduction programs to reduce risk among intravenous drug users. Regionally, prevention coverage for intravenous drug users is highest in South and South East Asia, at 62%.

In many developing countries disposable needles and syringes are not available and sterilization practices are inadequate. The use of other skin piercing instruments, for instance for scarification and circumcision, also has some potential for HIV transmission. This results in potentially frequent parenteral exposure to HIV in populations where HIV prevalence is high, including among health-care workers.

The mean probability of HIV infection due to puncture by a contaminated needle was recently estimated to be 0.23% (0.00–2.38%).[46] The potential for HIV transmission by unsterilized needles in medical settings is probably weak, but localized outbreaks in the Russian Federation, Romania and Libya among infants and young children have shown that it can occur in special circumstances. In Romania, over 90% of cases have occurred in children living in public institutions as a result of the re-use of contaminated and inadequately sterilized injection equipment or repeated microtransfusions of contaminated blood from one child to another.

In 2001, it became widely known that in a number of Chinese provinces, but mostly in Henan in central China, paid blood donation had caused HIV infections, with estimates ranging from below 100 000 to several hundred thousand. Before 1996, poor rural farmers had been selling blood and plasma to commercial blood processing companies to supplement their small income. Blood from many

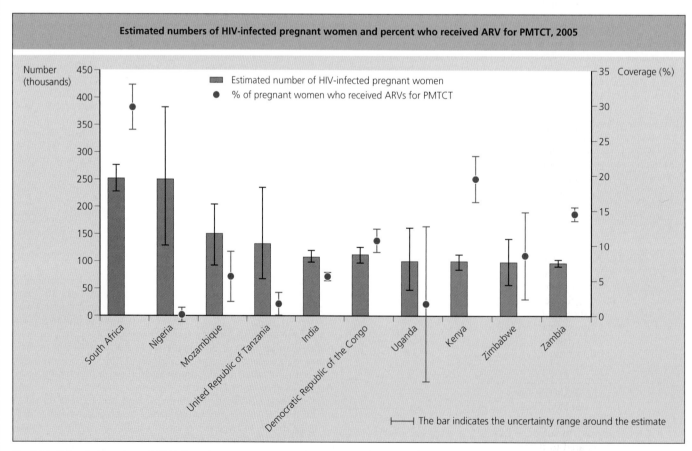

Fig. 84.9 Estimated numbers of HIV-infected pregnant women and percentage who received antiretrovirals (ARVs) for preventing mother-to-child transmission (PMTCT), 2005. Courtesy of WHO.

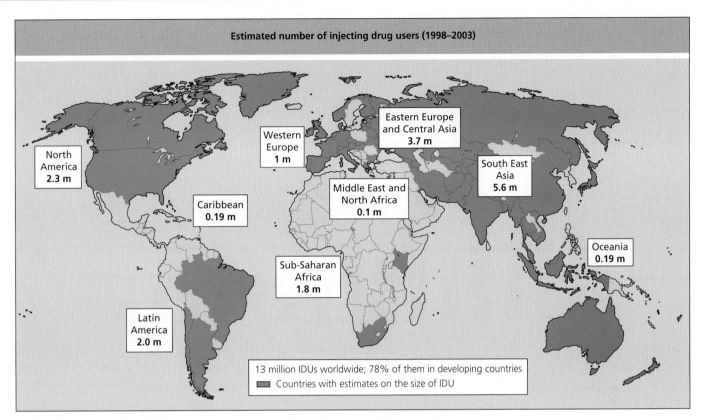

Fig. 84.10 Estimated number of intravenous drug users (IDUs) in 130 countries and territories, 1998–2003.

donors was collected and mixed. The red blood cells were separated from the pooled plasma and re-injected back into donors to reduce anemia. This unacceptable practice has been stopped.

NATURAL HISTORY

The natural history of HIV infection in many developing countries is similar to developed countries. Recently, the UNAIDS reference group estimated that the survival time from seroconversion to death in the absence of antiretroviral therapy (ART) is about 11 years (8 years latent period and 3 years from ART eligibility to death).

It is recognized that HIV-1 subtypes differ in biologic characteristics that affect pathogenicity. A recent study in Uganda found that HIV disease progression is affected by HIV-1 subtype. The median time to AIDS onset was shorter for persons with subtype D (6.5 years), recombinant subtypes (5.6 years) or multiple subtypes (5.8 years) compared with persons with subtype A (8.0 years).[47]

Pneumocystis jirovecii, pneumonia and Kaposi's sarcoma are less frequently associated with AIDS in developing countries than in high-income countries. There is evidence of pathologic interactions between HIV and malaria in dually infected patients. A transient elevation in HIV viral load occurs during febrile malaria episodes; in addition, susceptibility to malaria is enhanced in HIV-infected patients. Co-infection might also have facilitated the geographic expansion of malaria in areas where HIV prevalence is high. Hence, transient and repeated increases in HIV viral load resulting from recurrent co-infection with malaria may be a factor in promoting the spread of HIV in some part of sub-Saharan Africa.[48]

An unanticipated consequence of the AIDS epidemic has been a dramatic rise in the incidence of tuberculosis (TB). TB notification rates in Africa have doubled since the early 1980s, just after the start of the HIV epidemic, with the largest rise in countries most affected by the HIV epidemic. In sub-Saharan Africa, the relative risk of TB in those with, compared to those without, HIV infection has varied from four to more than 20.[49] In addition, among people who have HIV infection, TB is now the most common and deadly opportunistic infection, accounting for 40% of all adult death. In this population, extension of multiple resistance to anti-TB drugs is a major concern. The prevalence and consequences of multidrug-resistant and extensively drug-resistant (XDR) TB was assessed in a rural area in KwaZulu Natal, South Africa.[50] Of the 6% of patients who were diagnosed with XDR TB, all were co-infected with HIV. Of these patients, all except one died, with median survival of 16 days from the time of diagnosis.

This new situation has posed an unprecedented challenge to TB control programs in much of the developing world (see Chapter 93).[51] Only 31% of individuals living with HIV and TB co-infection received both antiretroviral and anti-TB drugs in 2007.

Health and social impact

Approximately 3 million people in low- and middle-income countries were receiving ART as of the end of 2007, compared to about 200 000 receiving ART in 2002. ART programs in Africa retain about 80% of patients 6 months after the initiation of treatment and 60% of patients at 2 years.[52] Antiretroviral therapy coverage has reached around 30% of those in need according to the most recent data but large variations can be seen (Fig. 84.11).

However, despite these achievements, the epidemic continues to outpace the response. With five new infections for every two people on treatment in 2007, it is obvious that HIV prevention efforts must be greatly intensified to stop this epidemic. AIDS remains the leading cause of death in Africa, before malaria and lower respiratory tract infection, with the biggest increase in mortality among adults aged 20–49. Demographic projections suggest that life expectancy in sub-Saharan countries most affected by HIV has been reduced by as much as 15 years when compared with projections without HIV (Fig. 84.12). The estimated impact of AIDS on juvenile mortality in these countries was extremely high between 2002 and 2005 (Fig. 84.13).

Outside of Africa, in regions with lower HIV prevalence, AIDS has slowed rather reversed gains in life expectancy. But for young adults aged between 20 and 35 years, even in Asia for example, AIDS deaths are among the leading cause of death as compared to other diseases (not accidents).[19]

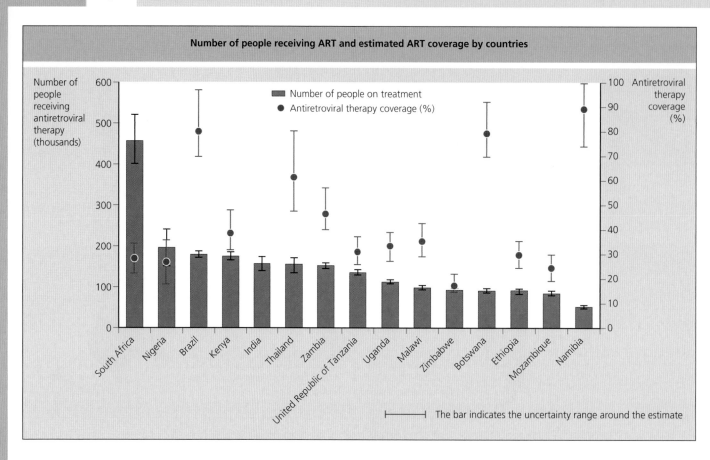

Fig. 84.11 Number of people receiving antiretroviral therapy (ART) and estimated ART coverage by country, 2007. (Courtesy of UN AIDS 2006 Report on the global AIDS epidemic.)

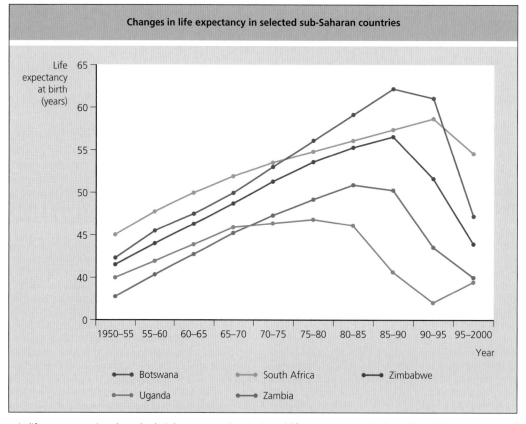

Fig. 84.12 Changes in life expectancy in selected sub-Saharan countries. Projected life expectancy at birth, 1950–2000.

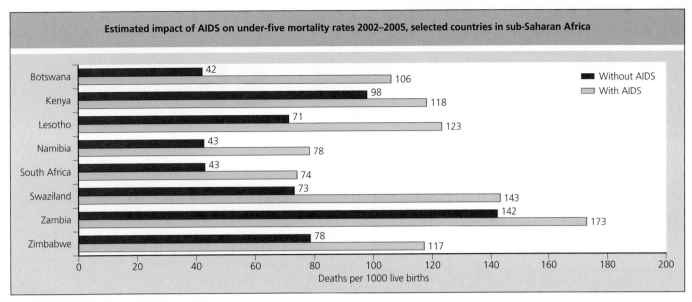

Fig. 84.13 Estimated impact of AIDS on under-five mortality rates, 2002–2005, in selected countries in sub-Saharan Africa. (Courtesy of UN AIDS 2006 Report on the global AIDS epidemic.)

In southern and eastern Africa, the economic impact of AIDS is felt not only on health-care costs but also on skilled labor forces, on certain economic sectors and on households, which in turn has a negative impact on many social indicators such as education and health.

AIDS has profoundly affected the health systems in high-income and developing countries alike. AIDS has illustrated the need to strengthen some of the weakest components of health services, such as access to appropriate care, counseling and prevention activities, and participation of persons living with HIV in treatment and medical decision making. Strong health systems are central to mitigating AIDS impact. The provision of widespread access to ART was central in bringing to light deficiencies in developing world public health systems, most of which are not equipped to manage chronic conditions on a large scale. In addition to severe shortages of basic infrastructure such as facilities and equipment, the countries where HIV is most widespread also face serious shortages of trained health-care providers, including doctors, nurses and support staff. According to the World Health Organization (WHO), 57 countries, mostly in sub-Saharan Africa but also including Bangladesh, India and Indonesia, face health workforce shortages: more than 4 million health workers are needed, including at least 2.4 million doctors, nurses and midwives. The epidemic itself is a leading cause of health worker attrition. Botswana, for example, lost nearly one-fifth of its health workforce to AIDS between 1999 and 2005.[53] Favorable task-shifting approaches, such as including community workers, have been documented by WHO. Most HIV prevention activities besides preventing mother-to-child transmission take place outside health services and many are implemented by nongovernmental organizations.

Recent evidence clearly indicates that at least in Africa, AIDS is a disease of inequality, often associated with economic transition, rather than a disease of poverty in itself.[54] Higher income groups usually living in urban settings have higher HIV prevalence than those living in rural areas. Among urban dwellers, those living in shanty towns and in poor slums also show higher risk behaviors and higher HIV prevalence than those with higher socioeconomic status. Unlike diseases such as TB, HIV is mostly transmitted through sex. This brings into play the economic perspective around reward and dependency, which influences the extent to which individuals are able to make and exercise choices about sexual behavior. Where women's economic and social safety is largely dependent on their partners' occupations and status, they have little choice in determining their own sexual safety. Gender inequality is one of many injustices fuelling the epidemic. The spread of HIV is disproportionately high among many groups that experience discrimination and suffer from a lack of human rights protection. This includes groups that have been marginalized socially, culturally and often economically, such as intravenous drug users, sex workers, migrants, internally displaced persons and MSM.

The HIV pandemic kills adults in their most productive years, when they are responsible for childcare. The epidemic is dramatically increasing the numbers of orphans, particularly in high-prevalence countries. More than 15 million children worldwide have lost their mothers or both parents because of AIDS, over 12 million of them in sub-Saharan Africa, overwhelming the capacity of social networks and traditional patterns of intergenerational dependency. According to recent surveys, an estimated 15% of orphans in 11 high-prevalence countries live in households receiving some form of assistance, including medical care, school assistance, financial support or psychosocial services. As a threat to development of many countries, the AIDS epidemic still requires large public funding, not only for ensuring universal access to HIV prevention, care and support programs, but also for research and development of new prevention tools, such as vaccines and microbicides.

REFERENCES

References for this chapter can be found online at http://www.expertconsult.com

Chapter | **85** |

Kenneth H Mayer
Matthew J Mimiaga
Steven Safren

Prevention of HIV transmission through behavioral change and sexual means

HIV TRANSMISSION DYNAMICS

HIV transmission is a high consequence, but low probability event with the majority of relevant exposures *not* resulting in new infections.[1] There are multiple co-factors that may affect HIV transmission, which is why there is a high level of variability around estimates of the relative risk of infection for specific exposures (Table 85.1).[2,3] HIV may be transmitted as cell-free or cell-associated virus, and different factors may affect expression of virus concentrations in different body fluids (i.e. blood, semen or cervicovaginal secretions). Although lower blood concentrations of HIV are associated with lower rates of HIV transmission,[4] antiretroviral drugs do not necessarily make HIV-infected people noninfectious or incapable of transmitting the virus. In fact, the sexual transmission of multidrug-resistant HIV has been well documented,[5,6] underscoring the need for providers to promote safer sex among the patients in their care, including those taking antiretroviral therapy.

BIOLOGIC ISSUES RELATED TO HIV TRANSMISSION

HIV is most often transmitted through intimate sexual contact by rapidly binding to cells that are present in the cervical, vaginal, penile, urethral and rectal mucosa.[7] The male foreskin contains abundant cells that can bind HIV; thus, being uncircumcised confers an additional risk for HIV seroconversion[8,9] (Table 85.2). All of the specific mechanisms responsible for the sexual transmission of HIV in humans are not fully understood, since HIV can be found either as cell-free or cell-associated virus in blood and genital secretions, and can bind multiple cell types.[10,11] The cells that can bind HIV in the genital tract include T-helper lymphocytes, monocyte/macrophage cells and Langerhans cells, as well as follicular dendritic cells. These latter cells may be particularly important because of their mobility, since they can bind HIV on their surface membranes and/or internalize it

Table 85.1 Estimates of per-contact risk of HIV infection

Type of contact	Risk
Needle sharing	6/1000 to 3/100
Occupational needlestick	1/300
Receptive anal	8/1000 to 3/100
Receptive vaginal	8/1000 to 2/1000
Insertive anal or vaginal	3/10,000 to 1/1000
Receptive oral	Case reports/no denominator

Table 85.2 Modifiers of the efficiency of HIV transmission

	Infectiousness	Susceptibility
Sexually transmitted diseases	↑	↑
Genital tract inflammation (e.g. traumatic sex, douching)	↑	↑
Circumcision	↓	↓
Cervical ectopy	?	↑
Genetics*	?	↓
HIV subtype†	↑	NA
Monocytotropic strain	↑	NA
Acute infection	↑	NA
Advanced infection	↑	NA
Antiretroviral therapy	↓?	NA

*CCR5 mutation.
†Subtype A or C compared to B.

and migrate via draining lymphatics to distal sites, where propagation in submucosal lymphoid tissue can occur, resulting in subsequent viral dissemination through the bloodstream.

Factors that are associated with increased HIV infectiousness include sexually transmitted infections[12] and noninfectious factors that can result in genital tract inflammation (e.g. douching), recruiting more white blood cells to genital mucosal surfaces.[13] Among the sexually transmitted diseases, ulcerative sexually transmitted infections such as syphilis, chancroid and genital herpes simplex virus infection afford additional portals of entry through mucosal ulcerations, but also recruit inflammatory cells that bind and propagate HIV infection.[14] Other local genital factors that are associated with increased inflammation include douching and traumatic sexual intercourse, particularly after sexual assault.

Different tissues in the genital tract have varying levels of susceptibility to being infected with HIV. The vaginal epithelium is stratified, and contains fewer cells with co-receptors that can bind HIV.[13] Thus, vaginal mucosa is less likely to become HIV infected than the endocervix, which has a thinner layer, is highly vascular and contains a much higher concentration of HIV-binding cells. Any physiologic event that results in ectropion (i.e. increased exposure of the endocervix), such as the use of hormonal contraceptives or occult *Chlamydia trachomatis* infection, will increase susceptibility to HIV.[15] The penile foreskin contains many cells that can readily bind and express HIV, resulting in increased HIV acquisition or transmission in uncircumcised males.[9] Three randomized trials of HIV-infected men in Africa have shown that adult male circumcision decreased HIV incidence by 50%.[16-18] The oropharynx contains many fewer cells that may bind HIV, which may partially explain the relative inefficiency of oral exposure to HIV as a means of transmission.[19] Moreover, salivary secretions contain several compounds that have been found to inhibit HIV transmission *in vitro*, most notably secretory leukocyte protease inhibitor (SLPI).[20] However, young rhesus macaques have been readily infected with simian immunodeficiency virus after oral challenge, with evidence of viral replication in tonsillar and adenoidal tissues.[21]

EPIDEMIOLOGIC ISSUES RELATED TO HIV TRANSMISSSION

Because of the multiple co-factors that may alter the amount of virus in the blood and genital tract, the calculation of the exact risk for infection for each type of HIV exposure is imprecise (see Tables 85.1, 85.2). Moreover, much of the data that have been obtained to generate per-contact risks have been based on cohort studies in which individuals recollect their level of risk during preceding time intervals (often every 3–6 months). Some of the participants in these studies may be worried that they have become newly infected or their sexual behavior may have been under the influence of drugs or alcohol, affecting precise recall. Thus, although many people want to have a precise calculation of risk associated with specific practices, it is very difficult to determine with any certainty the precise likelihood of transmission for each specific act. It is important when patients ask questions about the likelihood of risk after an exposure to reassure them that a single, one-time exposure to HIV is unlikely to result in transmission, but that the reason why the epidemic has become so widespread is because of individuals engaging in recurrent risk-taking behavior.

Having noted the limitations of how risk calculations have been obtained, certain key principles have emerged. Direct intravenous exposure to HIV (e.g. blood transfusions) is the most efficient way of transmitting the virus, while percutaneous needlestick injuries are much less efficient in transmitting HIV.[22] Individuals who share needles who pull back on the syringe and have substantial blood in the syringe when passing a syringe to their partner are more likely to transmit HIV than in a common health-care setting where an occupational needlestick injury occurs with a solid suture needle.[23] The range of risk for individuals who share intravenous drug paraphernalia ranges from 0.6% to 3% (see Table 85.1). This range overlaps with the level of risk for individuals who engage in unprotected receptive anal or unprotected receptive vaginal intercourse.[24] One study suggested that, on average, receptive anal intercourse was more than seven times as efficient in transmitting HIV as insertive anal intercourse.[25]

For each type of exposure, many contextual variables may alter the risk of transmission. For example, variations in the prevalence of HIV in different communities may mean that the same risk behavior has a different likelihood of resulting in an infection in two different communities. The amount of virus in the infected source plays a role in determining the risk of becoming HIV infected after a relevant contact. Co-factors, like a source with a high concentration of plasma HIV RNA[4,26] or concomitant sexually transmitted infection, can greatly increase the average per-contact risk.[27,28]

In the developed world, the epidemiologic data would suggest that men are more likely to transmit HIV to their female partners. However, in several studies of HIV serodiscordant couples in sub-Saharan Africa, the rates of male-to-female and female-to-male transmission were quite similar.[4] The reasons for the difference in the efficiency of female-to-male transmission in the developing world compared to the

developed world may be because of the decreased prevalence of male circumcision in the places where these studies were conducted, as well as the high co-prevalence of other sexually transmitted infections. For anal intercourse, the insertive partner is less likely to acquire HIV from an infected receptive partner than vice versa; however, there are sufficient cells in the distal male urethra and the male foreskin, and such an abundance of HIV-infected cells and mucus secretions containing virus in infected receptive partners, that an insertive partner still is at substantial risk of acquiring HIV from unprotected intercourse.

It is clear that receptive oral intercourse, either fellatio or cunnilingus, is a much less efficient way to acquire HIV, but case reports have been well documented showing that oral exposure to ejaculate may result in HIV transmission. The relative efficiency of oral exposure to HIV is below that of unprotected vaginal intercourse, thus it may be in the realm of less than 1 per 1000 contacts. However, animal studies have demonstrated that HIV can be readily transmitted orally, since there is lymphoid tissue in the oropharynx that may acquire HIV from genital secretions.[21] In counseling patients who have concerns about the risk of acquiring HIV through oral exposure, it is important to indicate that it is less efficient than unprotected anal or vaginal intercourse, but that transmission can still occur. Thus, if an individual wants a zero risk situation, it is preferable for them to avoid any oral exposure to semen or cervicovaginal secretions from a partner who is known to be HIV infected or at risk. However, if oral sex is a substitute for unprotected anal or vaginal sex, the patient can be told that this is less risky. Although HIV has been found in very small concentrations in pre-ejaculatory secretions, there are no reliable case reports of HIV transmission through exposure to pre-ejaculate without semen. Thus, it is important to counsel patients that being able to negotiate with their partners about limiting exposure to semen may be a helpful means for 'harm reduction'.

PREVENTION OF HIV TRANSMISSION

HIV transmission may be decreased by biologic or behavioral means (Fig. 85.1). Treating sexually transmitted infections can decrease genital tract HIV load in co-infected patients and can decrease susceptibility in at-risk persons.[20] Antiretroviral therapy can decrease genital, as well

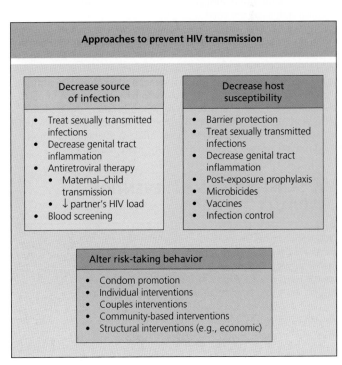

Approaches to prevent HIV transmission

Decrease source of infection
- Treat sexually transmitted infections
- Decrease genital tract inflammation
- Antiretroviral therapy
  - Maternal–child transmission
  - ↓ partner's HIV load
- Blood screening

Decrease host susceptibility
- Barrier protection
- Treat sexually transmitted infections
- Decrease genital tract inflammation
- Post-exposure prophylaxis
- Microbicides
- Vaccines
- Infection control

Alter risk-taking behavior
- Condom promotion
- Individual interventions
- Couples interventions
- Community-based interventions
- Structural interventions (e.g., economic)

Fig. 85.1 Approaches to preventing HIV transmission.

as plasma viral load, but the transmission of multidrug-resistant HIV suggests that these drugs may only have an impact on wider HIV transmission if coupled with programs that encourage safer sexual behavior and optimal drug therapy adherence. Antiretroviral drugs may be used to decrease the likelihood of mother-to-child transmission, or be used for postexposure prophylaxis. However, for any biologically plausible intervention to work, attention will need to be paid to the behavioral context in which the intervention will be undertaken. For example, a biologically effective microbicide may fail if the at-risk population refrains from lubricated sex. The next section will review interventions designed to decrease HIV through sexually transmitted infection treatment and behavioral interventions.

TREATING SEXUALLY TRANSMITTED INFECTIONS

As noted above, there are several different ways that HIV transmission may be minimized; aggressively diagnosing and treating sexually transmitted infections (STIs) is a biologically plausible way to alter HIV transmission dynamics, and remains cheaper than chronic antiretroviral therapy. There have been several studies conducted in sub-Saharan Africa to test this hypothesis with varying results. In a study in the Mwanza district of Uganda, specific syndromic management of STIs in an area where the epidemic was still in its early stages (i.e. 1% of the adult population were infected at the start of the study) resulted in decreasing HIV incidence in communities where the intervention was undertaken.[29] However, in a study in the Rakai district of Tanzania, periodic mass treatment of at-risk adults for STIs did not result in a decrease in HIV incidence.[27] In the latter study, the HIV epidemic was already much more advanced (i.e. 16% of the adult population were infected at the start of the study) and there was a high background rate of concomitant herpes simplex infection that was not treated in the course of the study.

Herpes simplex virus type 2 (HSV-2) seropositivity has been associated with increased risk for HIV transmission and acquisition.[30] Several studies have attempted to see whether chronic HSV-2 suppression with a thymidine kinase inhibitor (i.e. aciclovir or valaciclovir) could decrease susceptibility to HIV acquisition.[31,32] Unfortunately, these studies did not demonstrate a protective effect when anti-HSV-2 chemoprophylaxis was used.

Thus, the lessons from these studies of STI treatment to prevent HIV transmission are equivocal at best. For STI treatment to affect HIV spread, it should be specifically tailored to individual patients, focusing on aggressively diagnosing diseases that are common in specific communities, as opposed to using general algorithms. In addition, the benefit of STI control will be likely to have the greatest impact in areas of lower HIV prevalence. In communities where the epidemic is already more widespread, the likelihood of encountering a new partner who is HIV infected may be substantial, so the benefit of modifying a modest co-factor like an STI will be more limited.

HIV SCREENING AS A PREVENTION MODALITY

Other approaches to the prevention of HIV in the developed world are so well established that they seem routine (i.e. the routine screening of blood).[33] The use of more sensitive antibody screening and careful donor history have resulted in enhanced safety in the blood supply, such that the transmission of HIV via infected blood in the past two decades is exceedingly rare. In other parts of the world where the relative cost of blood screening is high, blood supplies may not be as safe.

Another routine practice that results in the prevention of HIV transmission is the guideline that pregnant women be universally offered HIV antibody testing before delivery.[34] Although compliance with this guideline is not 100%, the rate of new perinatally transmitted infections in the USA has decreased dramatically, with fewer than 100 new infections annually in recent years.

In the Fall of 2006, the US Centers for Disease Control and Prevention recommended that HIV be routinely screened for in most medical settings for patients aged 13–64 years old because more than a quarter of the more than 1 million HIV-infected Americans were unaware of their serostatus.[35] The net effect on the HIV/AIDS epidemic in the USA remains to be seen.

BEHAVIORAL APPROACHES – OVERVIEW

Despite increasing access to antiretroviral therapy, blood screening and treatment of STIs, the number of new HIV infections in the USA has increased to a plateau of approximately 56 000 new infections per year over most of this past decade.[36] The reason why people engage in HIV risk behavior are complex, and may involve issues related to early life events, such as childhood sexual abuse, low self-esteem, contextual issues in relationships and concomitant substance use, as well as addiction to specific forms of sexual pleasure.[37] Gender-related power dynamics (e.g. the role of women in many societies) may also limit the ability to promote safer sex.[38] Thus, no single behavioral approach will invariably lead to an adaptation of consistent safer sexual or drug-using practices. Much like dieting, regular exercise and smoking cessation, no single program of HIV risk reduction will work for all at-risk individuals. However, several studies have now indicated that the provision of either individual counseling and/or small group sessions can be helpful in assisting at-risk individuals in moderating their risk.[39–43]

Good elements of risk-reduction programs include the ability of the counselor to approach the patient in a nonjudgmental manner to elicit a realistic assessment of the person's pattern of risk-taking behavior. Given the slow progress in the development of cheap, safe and effective vaccines, microbicides and other biologic approaches to the prevention of HIV transmission, the role of the provider in patient education, discussion of risk-taking behavior, initiation of risk-reduction counseling and triage to appropriate prevention services is an essential part of stopping the epidemic's further spread.

PSYCHOSOCIAL MODELS OF RISK BEHAVIOR UNDERLYING PREVENTION INTERVENTIONS

Knowledge is one aspect of HIV prevention but ongoing risk taking is a function of many other complex psychosocial variables. The three most common models that have been employed to explain HIV risk taking are the health belief model, the theory of reasoned action and social cognitive theory (i.e. self-efficacy models).[44] Health beliefs models emphasize the role of perceived benefits and barriers to condom use and perceived severity and vulnerability to getting HIV.[45] In the theory of reasoned action, health behavior (e.g. condom use) is a function of intentions to use condoms and, in turn, intentions to use condoms are a function of variables such as attitudes and norms regarding HIV and condom use.[46] Social cognitive models (i.e. self-efficacy) explain condom use as a function of an individual's knowledge about HIV, expectation about the outcomes of using condoms (i.e. pleasure reduction versus disease prevention) and self-efficacy (i.e. that the individual will be able to use a condom in different sexual situations).[47,48] These psychosocial models of HIV prophylactic behavior have been tested in both cross-sectional and longitudinal studies in a variety of populations and are the basis for many of the behavioral interventions reviewed below.

Intervention models that address information, motivation and behavioral skills[49] typically take into account models of HIV risk prevention. One is the transtheoretical model of change[50] which posits that an intervention needs to be adaptable to an individual's current readiness to change. For example, people who are currently in a 'pre-contemplative' level of readiness to change do not see their behavior as problematic and do not see a reason to change; someone in a 'contemplative' level may be ambivalent about changing, and someone at a 'determination or preparation' level is ready to make a commitment. Additional levels of change include 'action', 'maintenance' and 'relapse prevention', each with different suggested strategies to assist an individual in a counseling situation. Interventions based on the transtheoretical model try to move individuals to a more serious, higher level of readiness to change than where they are initially. Accordingly, an individual at an earlier level may benefit most from information and education, whereas someone at a mid-level or higher might benefit from more intensive motivational support and skills training.

Many of the randomized controlled trials of interventions utilize aspects of the transtheoretical model of behavioral change, other information–motivation–behavior skills interventions, and/or variables related to self-efficacy, health beliefs and attitudes in the risk-reduction interventions. HIV prevention studies typically collect sexual risk-taking data on HIV-negative individuals, but STI or HIV incidence may also be used as end points. To address the overarching public health significance of HIV, community randomized designs employ more of a wider scale approach. These interventions are formulated to develop population-based HIV prevention approaches, and compare communities who receive the intervention to other similar communities who do not.

OUTCOME OF LARGE SCALE AND HIGH-IMPACT-FOR-HIV PREVENTION STUDIES IN THE UNITED STATES

Prevention trials delivered primarily to heterosexual individuals in STI and primary care clinics

Two different randomized controlled trials of HIV prevention interventions have examined the efficacy of risk-reduction counseling approaches in individuals at high risk for HIV infection, by studying heterosexual individuals attending STI or primary care clinics. The first study, the US National Institute of Mental Health's Multisite HIV Prevention Trial (Project Light), recruited 3706 individuals from 37 inner-city community-based clinics in seven sites across the USA.[51] The three risk groups were:

- men presenting in an STI clinic;
- women presenting in an STI clinic; and
- women presenting in health service organizations.

At screening, all participants reported engaging in unprotected vaginal or anal sex within 90 days. Approximately one-half were randomized to seven sessions of risk-reduction counseling in a group format, and the other half to watch a 1-hour AIDS video followed by a question-and-answer session. Those in the intervention group reported fewer unprotected sexual acts and were more likely to use condoms consistently over the follow-up period. The intervention group also reported higher overall levels of condom use. With respect to STIs, there were no overall differences in infection rates across intervention and control group; however, of the men who were recruited from STI clinics, there was a decreased incidence of gonorrhea.

The second large-scale study, Project RESPECT, recruited over 5787 heterosexual HIV-negative patients who presented for care at STI clinics across the USA.[52] Participants were randomized to a four-session ('enhanced counseling'), a two-session ('brief counseling') or a noninteractive ('didactic message') condition. Those assigned four-session and two-session interactive interventions had fewer new HIV infections at both 6- and 12-month intervals than those who received the noninteractive counseling. Additionally, self-reported 100% condom use was higher in both interactive counseling groups compared to the didactic message control.

Recently, Crepaz *et al.* evaluated the efficacy of a large number of HIV behavioral interventions in reducing unprotected sex and incident STI among African-American/Black and Latino/Hispanic STI clinic patients.[39] HIV behavioral interventions were found to significantly reduce unprotected sex (OR = 0.77; 95% CI 0.68–0.87; 14 trials; n = 11 590) and incident STIs (OR = 0.85; 95% CI 0.73–0.998; 13 trials; n = 16 172), providing evidence that HIV behavioral interventions provide an efficacious means of HIV/STI prevention for African-American/Black and Latino/Hispanic patients who attend STI clinics.

As HIV risk behavior is a necessary factor for HIV infection, these studies taken together reveal that HIV risk-reduction counseling can both increase condom use and decrease sexually transmitted infections.

Prevention trials for men who have sex with men (MSM)

Individually randomized controlled trials

One of the earlier individually randomized intervention trials[53] compared an integrated cognitive–behavioral intervention to a waiting list control among 104 gay men in a metropolitan area. The integrated intervention included AIDS risk information as well as cognitive–behavioral self-management training, sexual assertion training and strategies for increasing positive social supports/relationship skills. At the post-training assessment, the experimental group had fewer high-risk sexual practices and better behavioral skills for sexual coercive situations than the wait list control.

Project EXPLORE was a large-scale randomized HIV-prevention trial among MSM conducted in six US cities, with a total of 4295 participants.[37,54] Inclusion criteria for the EXPLORE study were men who were HIV uninfected, 16 years or older, had anal sex with another man during the past year, and had not been involved in a mutually monogamous relationship in the past 2 years with a male partner who was HIV uninfected. Men were randomized to receive a behavioral intervention versus standard risk-reduction counseling. Study results suggested a possible modest benefit of the intervention in reducing new HIV infections.[54] Further, the reporting of unprotected receptive anal sex with HIV-positive or unknown-status partners was significantly lower in the intervention group compared with the standard group.

Community randomized controlled trials

One of the first community randomized controlled trials, the Mpowerment Project, studied a peer-outreach program for young gay men (aged 18–29 years).[55] The intervention involved peer outreach (training peers to spread prevention messages and to recruit more individuals to participate), small groups which focused on misperceptions of safer sex, eroticizing safer sex, verbal and nonverbal safer sex strategies, informal outreach and a publicity campaign. To assess outcome, a cohort of 300 individuals from two communities were surveyed. In the intervention community, the proportion of participants who reported unprotected anal intercourse with nonprimary partners decreased, as did the proportion of participants who reported unprotected anal intercourse with their boyfriends. No significant changes occurred in the comparison community.

Another large-scale community randomized trial[56] involved delivering the intervention through opinion leaders (popular individuals) from the gay community in four US states. Each state randomly had both an intervention city and comparison city. In the intervention city, popular gay men were trained to spread behavior-change messages (to change norms), and in the comparison city pamphlets were placed at gay bars. The team identified 'popular' men with the assistance of bartenders in intervention city bars. Participants then completed surveys in the bars. Across all states, 1126 men completed baseline surveys and 1010 completed follow-up surveys. At 1-year follow-up, those in the intervention cities reported a significantly greater reduction in the frequency of unprotected anal sex during the previous 2 months, and a significantly greater increase in condom use for anal sex compared to comparison cities. Consistent with this finding, more condoms were taken from bars at the intervention cities than the comparison cities.

The community randomized trials among MSM validate the utility of providing HIV prevention, on a larger scale, to communities of MSM. From a public health perspective, raising awareness and changing norms regarding HIV prophylactic behavior can influence transmission rates at the community level. Although recruiting opinion leaders and/or providing an integrated prevention program involving peers, groups, workshops and outreach can be a complex undertaking, such efforts can be useful approaches to curtailing HIV risk taking, which, in turn, would curtail HIV transmission.

Meta-analyses of HIV behavioral intervention studies show that HIV behavioral interventions with adult MSM result in significant reductions in self-reported sexual risk behaviors.[41,42,57] A meta-analytic review by Herbst et al. synthesizing evidence and evaluating the effectiveness of HIV behavioral interventions found individual-level, group-level and community-level interventions to be effective in reducing the odds of unprotected anal intercourse (range 27% to 43% decrease) and increasing the odds of condom use for the group-level approach (by 81%).[40] Similarly, Johnson et al. found significant reductions in unprotected anal intercourse when comparing the effects of 38 HIV behavioral interventions to minimal or no HIV prevention interventions.[57] HIV behavioral interventions were shown to reduce the overall proportion of MSM reporting unprotected sex by 27% (95% CI 15–37%).[57] Interventions most successful in reducing risky sexual behavior are those based on theoretic models, including interpersonal skills training, incorporating several delivery methods, and being delivered over multiple sessions spanning a minimum of 3 weeks.

Prevention trials for women

Individually randomized controlled trials

Several large scale multisite studies have investigated risk-reduction counseling among low-income and/or minority women. Kelly et al. randomized 197 high-risk women from an urban primary health clinic to a cognitive–behavioral risk-reduction intervention or comparison.[58] Three months later, the intervention group evidenced better sexual communication and negotiation skills (assessed by role play and self-report), and less unprotected sexual intercourse. The comparison group had no changes on these measures.

A second study of HIV risk-reduction counseling among women[59] sought to adapt models of behavioral change to social and contextual variables relevant to 128 economically disadvantaged African-American women between the ages of 18 and 29 years. Accordingly, their intervention used the theory of gender and power as a guide, and was social-skills based. At the 3-month follow-up, women in the more intensive intervention showed increased consistent condom use, sexual self-control, sexual communication and sexual assertiveness, and partner's adoption of norms supporting consistent condom use than those in the delayed educational control.

A study of 206 pregnant inner-city women randomized participants to an AIDS prevention group or to one of two controls.[60] The AIDS prevention intervention consisted of four sessions, each delivered in group format, and included videos as well as group activities such as role play or discussions. After the intervention and after 6-month follow-up, the AIDS prevention group had increases in knowledge and safer sex behaviors in comparison with the two control groups.

Due to difficulties with retention and attrition of high-risk and hard-to-reach women in HIV prevention trials, Belcher et al. developed and tested the utility of a single session 2-hour one-on-one intervention using motivational interviewing and information–motivation–behavioral skills training.[61] No differences occurred in HIV knowledge, but the group that received skills training and motivational interviewing showed higher levels of HIV protective behaviors than the control group, including higher rates of condom use during vaginal intercourse, demonstrating the efficacy of a brief, minimal intervention.

Two randomized controlled trials of an HIV risk-reduction intervention using information, motivation enhancement and skills training intervention were developed for low-income, primarily African-American women.[62,63] In both studies, the intervention consisted of four 90-minute sessions, which included personalized feedback about their HIV knowledge, risk perceptions and sexual behavior. Women in the first study who received the intervention reported stronger intentions to practice safe sex and to communicate these intentions to partners, and less unprotected intercourse and substance use near the time of sexual activity; these gains were maintained at the 3-month follow-up. In the second study, 102 women comprising a new sample were randomized. Overall, the results of the second study were corroborated.

Taken together, the series of randomized controlled trials of HIV prevention counseling for high-risk women demonstrate both feasibility and efficacy of such approaches. While many of these approaches are useful, some may be difficult to disseminate. These interventions require special training and most require a significant amount of time for both the participants and the counselors. Future study of individually administered interventions should now focus on ways to implement and disseminate interventions to community-based settings.

Community randomized controlled trials

To attempt to address some of the limitations of clinic-based intervention approaches for women, two studies of community-randomized trials have been undertaken. The first used nine low-income housing developments[62] and nine demographically matched control developments. The community-level intervention included workshops and community HIV prevention events implemented by popular opinion leaders within each community. The women in the housing developments (n = 690) were surveyed at baseline and 1 year later. This revealed that women in the intervention communities showed better decreases in unprotected sex (past 2 months) and frequency of unprotected acts.

A second community-based randomized control trial targeted low-income, primarily African-American women in four urban settings.[63] Four communities in metropolitan areas were selected: two public housing communities, a low-income neighborhood and a group of inner-city neighborhoods. The intervention was specifically based on the transtheoretical model of change, attempting to reach women who would be at different levels of readiness to change. The intervention consisted of distribution of HIV prevention materials, developing a peer network of community organizers and businesses, and delivering prevention messages by outreach specialists, both individually and in groups. The intervention communities evidenced increases in talking with main partners about condoms and trying to get main partners to use condoms.

HIV behavioral interventions with women have been shown to be effective in reducing overall HIV risk.[38,64] Neumann et al. conducted a meta-analysis of HIV behavioral interventions among heterosexuals and found statistically significant effects in reducing sex-related risk (OR = 0.81, 95% CI 0.53–0.90) and decreased incidence of STIs (OR = 0.74, 95% CI 0.62–0.89). Four of the 10 studies (40%) included in the behavioral analyses were individual interventions and 6 out of 10 (60%) focused exclusively on women.[38]

HIV prevention interventions specific to intravenous drug users

A review of 42 studies between 1989 and 1999 suggested that the majority found that needle-exchange programs prevent HIV risk behavior and seroconversion among intravenous drug users.[65] Most other studies of HIV prevention interventions for drug users are observational or quasi-experimental evaluation studies; however, these studies do show significant within-participant reductions in HIV risk behavior.[66]

Semaan et al. examined the efficacy of 33 intervention studies with drug users (94% intravenous drug users, 21% crack users).[67] Relative to no HIV behavioral intervention, drug users in intervention conditions significantly reduced sexual risk behaviors (OR = 0.60, 95% CI 0.43–0.85). In other words, when extrapolating results to a population with a 72% prevalence of risk behaviors, the proportion of drug users who reduced their risk behaviors was 12.6% greater in the intervention groups than in the comparison groups.

Among the studies of prevention interventions for intravenous drug users, methodologies differ and, consequently, so do the results. Sexual behavior, as shown in previous sections, is a difficult and complex behavior to change. When co-morbid with drug dependence or addiction, its complexity grows; intensive multimodal interventions currently show the most utility in this population.

SUMMARY

Behavioral interventions to decrease HIV transmission have been successful in a wide array of settings and with diverse populations. However, in most situations, interventions were needed to sustain behavior change. Moreover, there is limited experience with these interventions in parts of the world where the epidemic is spreading most rapidly and where the social construction of reality (e.g. disempowerment of women, limited health-care infrastructure) may limit the effectiveness of programs developed in resource-rich settings. Clearly, additional work is needed to develop culturally specific behavioral interventions, while the development of more effective biologic prevention modalities (i.e. microbicides and vaccines) is underway.

REFERENCES

 References for this chapter can be found online at http://www.expertconsult.com

Joseph M Fritz
Victoria J Fraser
David K Henderson

Chapter | **86** |

Preventing occupational HIV infection in the health-care environment

This chapter addresses strategies designed to prevent the transmission of HIV in health-care settings.

EPIDEMIOLOGY

Occupational risks, including risks for physical injuries, chemical exposures and infectious diseases, have been well described in health-care settings. The introduction of HIV into the health-care workplace in the 1980s, however, focused the attention of health-care providers, perhaps for the first time, on the issue of occupational acquisition of HIV. Ironically, HIV infection is only one of the blood-borne pathogens that can be occupationally acquired in health-care settings. Hepatitis B virus (HBV), hepatitis C virus (HCV) and HIV can all be transmitted in health-care settings through needlestick injuries and other traumatic blood and body fluid exposures. Blood-borne pathogens have been identified as occupational risks for health-care workers (HCWs) since the epidemiology and routes of transmission of HBV were delineated in the 1960s. For reasons incompletely understood at present, occupational HIV infection remains relatively uncommon.

To date, the US Public Health Service's Centers for Disease Control and Prevention (CDC) had recorded only 57 instances of documented occupational HIV infections and 139 instances of probable or possible occupational HIV infections among HCWs in the USA.[1] For each of the documented 57 cases, the HCW sustained an occupational exposure to HIV, had a baseline serum sample drawn which was negative for HIV antibody and then, during follow-up, developed serologic evidence consistent with HIV infection. Fewer than 50 additional cases of documented occupational infections and approximately 60 instances of 'possible or probable' occupational infections have been reported from outside the USA. For the 139 'possible or probable' occupational infections reported to the CDC, the exposed HCWs were unaware of the occurrence of an occupational exposure, did not report the exposure and/or did not have baseline serologic studies performed to document that they were not HIV-infected prior to the occupational exposure.

A comparison of the demographics of the 'possible/probable' and definite occupational infection cases reveals substantial differences. When one compares the demographics of these categories of infection with those of all HCWs in the USA, the likelihood that some of the 'possible/probable' cases occurred as a result of traditional risk factors occurring outside the workplace (i.e. sexual behavior, intravenous drug use) seems quite high.[2]

A number of both general and specific factors determine an individual practitioner's risk for occupational infection with HIV.

- The prevalence of HIV infection among the population of patients served is a major determinant of the overall risk.
- The type of specialty practice (e.g. medical, emergency room, surgical) is associated with varying levels of risk for occupational exposure to blood-borne pathogens.

- The types and frequencies of procedures performed by the HCW, as well as the conditions under which the procedures are performed (i.e. emergent versus elective), also contribute to the risk equation.
- The extent to which the practitioner adheres to recommended infection control procedures and practices is also likely to be a determinant of risk for exposure and infection.
- The individual HCW's technique and attention to detail also contribute to the risk.

Several specific factors contribute to the risk for occupational HIV infection in the health-care workplace. Tables 86.1 and 86.2 list factors that have been demonstrated[3] or suggested in the literature to contribute to the risk for occupational HIV infection.

Many of the reported occupational HIV cases share several features in common. Most were due to percutaneous exposures and the majority of these were hollow-bore needlestick injuries. All of the clinical occupational HIV cases occurred following exposure to blood or grossly blood-stained bodily fluids from HIV-infected patients. As yet, no case of occupational HIV infection has been documented following a needlestick injury with a solid surgical needle.

Table 86.1 Factors contributing to the risk for occupational HIV infection

Exposure factors

1. Route of exposure (e.g. percutaneous,* mucous membrane, cutaneous)
2. Inoculum size
   - Size of the device producing injury
   - For needlestick exposures, type of needle (i.e. hollow-bore* vs solid)
   - Extent of contamination (e.g. visible blood on device,† whether or not device had been placed in an artery or vein†)
   - 'Depth/severity' of exposure*†
   - Type of contamination (e.g. blood,* pleural fluid, etc.)

Source/'donor' factors

1. Extent of viremia (e.g. by polymerase chain reaction or branch-chain DNA assay)
2. Stage of illness (as a presumed surrogate for extent of viremia†)
3. Circulating free (as opposed to cell-associated) virus
4. Antiretroviral chemotherapy (presumably reducing level of viremia)

*Features shared by many, if not most, of the occupational infections reported in the literature.
†Features identified as significantly associated with risk for occupational infection in the CDC case-control study.[3]

Table 86.2 Risk factors for occupational HIV infection identified in a retrospective case-control study conducted in the USA, UK and France[3]

The risk for occupational HIV infection was increased when:
- the occupational exposure was deep, as compared with superficial ($p<0.001$)
- blood was visible on the device causing the occupational exposure ($p=0.0014$)
- the device causing the exposure had been placed in a source-patient's vein or artery ($p=0.0028$)
- the source-patient died within 60 days of the exposure ($p=0.0011$)
- the exposed health-care worker did not take zidovudine postexposure chemoprophylaxis ($p=0.0026$).

Table 86.3 Occupational risks for HIV infection

	Percutaneous exposures	Mucous membrane exposures
Number of longitudinal studies	27	21
Number of exposures	6807	2768
Number of documented infections	21	0/1*
Infection rate per exposure	0.31%	0–0.11%†

*See text for discussion.
†Using rule of three.[10]

To attempt to identify specific factors associated with risk for occupational HIV infection, public health authorities from the USA, France and the UK conducted a retrospective case-control study, matching the known anecdotal case reports of occupational HIV infections with 'controls' from the public health surveillance studies of occupational exposures in each of these countries.[3] This study identified five specific risk factors for occupational infection; these five factors and the level of statistical significance assigned to each are listed in Table 86.2. The first four of these factors very likely relate directly to the inoculum effect. That an inoculum effect is present in this setting is supported by several pieces of information:

- transfusion of a unit of blood from an HIV-infected donor has been associated with virtually 100% risk for infection;[4]
- the depth of a percutaneous exposure has been shown to be an independent risk factor for occupational HIV infection;[3]
- the presence of visible blood on the device producing the injury has been independently associated with risk for infection;[3]
- instruments that had been placed in source-patients' vascular channels were more likely to result in occupational infection;[3] and
- the fact that all of the needlestick exposures to blood have been caused by hollow-bore needles (i.e. injection, as compared with suturing needles).

Both in the CDC study, as well as in the majority of the anecdotal case reports, the source-patients for the exposures that resulted in occupational HIV infections had advanced disease. This finding is likely to be a surrogate marker for either the level of the source-patient's viral load or the level of circulating free virus, or both. Finally, most occupational HIV infections have followed parenteral (as compared with mucosal or cutaneous) occupational exposures. These latter routes of exposure are associated with lower risks for occupational HIV infection.

Percutaneous exposure

It is estimated that nearly 400 000 percutaneous injuries occur annually among HCWs in the United States.[5] Several longitudinal studies have attempted to determine the magnitude of risk associated with different types of occupational exposure (summarized by Ippolito et al.[6] and Henderson[7]). Combining the data from the available studies, HCWs have sustained more than 6800 percutaneous exposures to sharp devices contaminated with blood or other blood-stained body fluids from patients known to be infected with HIV. Twenty-one occupational HIV infections have been documented in these studies, resulting in a risk of transmission per injury of 0.31% (Table 86.3). Thus, one in 324 parenteral exposures in these studies resulted in occupational HIV infection.

Although such a pooled risk estimate provides the best available data concerning the magnitude of risk for occupational HIV infection, this type of analysis has substantial limitations. For example, the longitudinal studies vary somewhat in experimental design and are therefore not directly comparable. Such an analysis implicitly assumes that all parenteral occupational exposures are associated with equal risk, an assumption that does not make intuitive sense and that has apparently been shown to be flawed by the CDC's case-control study cited above.[3] Similarly, all source-patients are also not likely to present the same level of risk for occupational infection. Patients with advanced disease and high viral loads are more likely to transmit HIV than patients with lower or undetectable viral loads (see Table 86.2). Because of the large number of factors that influence the risk for occupational infection, these summary data cannot address the risk associated with a specific, discrete exposure in an individual HCW.

Mucous membrane exposure

Occupational exposures other than parenteral exposures to blood present a lower level of risk for occupational HIV infection. Anecdotal reports document, in rare circumstances, that mucous membrane or cutaneous exposures may produce occupational HIV infections in HCWs.[8] Some of the longitudinal studies cited above have also addressed occupational risks associated with mucous membrane exposure to blood from HIV-infected patients. To date, with more than 2700 exposures followed prospectively, only one study has reported a seroconversion following a mucous membrane exposure.[9] Thus, as a maximum estimate (using the 'rule of three' as an approximation for a zero numerator),[10] the pooled risk estimate for infection associated with a mucous membrane exposure is 0.11% per exposure (see Table 86.3). Again, such a pooled risk estimate provides only a rough framework for considering the risks associated with a discrete exposure.

Occupational exposures other than percutaneous and mucous membrane exposures

Occupational exposures other than percutaneous and mucous membrane exposures are even less likely to result in infection. Prospective studies of nonpercutaneous and nonmucous membrane exposures, which include hundreds of person-years of follow-up, have not identified a single instance of HIV transmission.[11,12] Whereas exposures to other non-bloody fluids are likely to be associated with some occupational risk, this risk is below currently measurable levels.

When one evaluates the occupational exposures that have produced HIV infection, almost all of them result from exposure to blood from HIV-infected patients. Whereas other body fluids may ultimately be shown to represent a risk for occupational infection, the major risk in the health-care setting has come from occupational exposures to blood from HIV-infected patients.

PATHOGENESIS

Although the retrospective case-control study of risk factors for occupational HIV infection cited above[3] provided some insight into factors associated with risk for occupational HIV infection, the precise pathogenetic mechanisms of the occupational infection event are poorly understood. The major risk for occupational infection is associated with percutaneous injury with a hollow-bore needle or other sharp device that has been used on an HIV-infected patient. The risk is associated primarily with blood exposure. Precisely how the transmission event occurs in the skin, subcutaneous tissue or underlying muscle remains unclear. Current interest in the pathogenesis of HIV infection by this route focuses on the role of host defense and the role of the dendritic cell.

The role of host defense in protection against occupational infection is poorly understood. Scientists working at the National Cancer Institute have demonstrated that 75% of HCWs exposed to blood from HIV-infected patients who do not become infected with HIV develop HIV-specific T-helper activity.[13] In a subsequent study, these investigators demonstrated that 35% of uninfected HCWs who had sustained occupational exposure to blood from HIV-infected patients developed cytotoxic lymphocyte responses to HIV-related envelope antigens.[14] Among HCWs who had sustained occupational exposures to blood from patients who were not infected with HIV, none responded to HIV-associated envelope antigens. Whereas the precise role that cellular immunity plays in host defense against occupational HIV infection remains to be delineated, these data, when combined with results from animal studies, suggest that the role may be an important one. One recent case report also supports a significant role for cellular immunity in the defense against HIV infection.[15] In this case, an HCW who sustained an HIV needlestick exposure had HIV DNA detected by nucleic acid sequence-based amplification during a course of three-drug antiretroviral postexposure chemoprophylaxis. Despite the detection of proviral DNA, this individual ultimately remained uninfected (as assessed by serial nucleic acid tests and antibody determinations). The HCW did, however, develop a robust HIV-specific cellular immune response.

INTERVENTIONS DESIGNED TO DECREASE THE RISK FOR OCCUPATIONAL HIV INFECTION

Interventions designed to limit occupational exposures

Several approaches have been used to attempt to decrease risks for occupational exposure to (and therefore occupational infection with) blood-borne pathogens in the health-care setting (Table 86.4). Such interventions can be considered as primary prevention. Major categories of intervention include:
- education;
- work practice controls (e.g. adherence to infection control procedures designed to limit risk); and
- engineered controls.

Education and use of infection control procedures

Staff should be routinely informed about all occupational risks. Since the major risk for occupational HIV infection (and for infection with other blood-borne pathogens as well) is by parenteral inoculation, some critics of the recommendations to manage all patients as if they were potentially infected with blood-borne pathogens (e.g. universal precautions, body substance isolation, standard precautions; discussed below) have suggested that these precautions will have little

Table 86.4 Prevention strategies for health-care workers and institutions to decrease risks for occupational HIV infection[2]

1. Use of 'standard precautions' or other isolation procedures designed to place effective barriers between the health-care worker and blood or other body fluids.
2. Educating new staff and retraining existing staff regarding occupational risks for blood-borne pathogen infection in the context of other occupational risks present and prevalent in the health-care workplace; making sure staff are aware of these risks.
3. Including information about all occupational risks (including those associated with caring for patients who have blood-borne pathogen infections) in biomedical training schools' curricula.
4. Evaluating all procedures associated with occupational risk for exposure to blood-borne pathogens (particularly those presenting risks for transcutaneous exposures), with the intent of modifying the aspects of these procedures associated with risks for occupational exposures.
5. Aggressive use of newly developed engineered controls, including careful evaluation of 'safety devices' for safety, efficacy and cost-effectiveness; implementation of those devices that meet these tests.
6. Development of efficient, readily accessible, user-friendly institutional postexposure management systems, including the option for postexposure prophylaxis for documented occupational HIV exposures.

impact on the number of occupational infections. However, since these and later guidelines educate staff about the careful handling of needles and sharp objects, recommend against practices associated with needlestick injuries (e.g. needle recapping, needle bending or needle clipping) and stress appropriate disposal of needles and other sharp objects,[16,17] their implementation has been associated with a decreased parenteral exposure rate.

Two centers have documented a significant decrease in such exposures,[18,19] one in temporal association with training in, and implementation of, universal precautions.[18] Up to one-third of parenteral occupational exposures may be preventable by following guidelines designed to minimize occupational exposures.[20] The use of appropriate barriers also reduces occupational risk. The blood inoculum on needles is reduced by as much as 50% when penetrated through a latex glove.[21] Making HCWs aware of the presence of occupational risks also results in occupational behavior modification. In a survey of certified nurse-midwives, both knowledge of the routes of transmission of blood-borne pathogens and perception of risk for occupational infection were statistically associated with the appropriate use of precautions. However, risk perception and use of precautions were more closely linked, suggesting that knowledge, in itself, may be insufficient to produce behavior modification.[22]

Employers in the USA are governed by regulations issued by the Occupational Safety and Health Administration of the US Department of Labor in 1991. One regulation mandates that employers follow certain protocols when managing health-care workers who have sustained occupational exposures to blood-borne pathogens.[23] This 'final rule' requires mandatory education for HCWs at every health-care institution in the USA.

Work practice controls

In 1987, the CDC issued guidelines for the management of patients infected with blood-borne pathogens that have since provided the underpinnings for all subsequent guidelines in the USA.[16] These 'universal precautions' guidelines clearly set out the principle that HCWs should treat blood and blood-stained body fluids from all patients as potentially infectious, in order to prevent the transmission of blood-borne pathogens (in particular HIV) from patients to HCWs. Several years later, the CDC issued revised isolation guidelines, called 'standard precautions', which focus on the bidirectional spread of organisms to and from patients and health-care providers.[17] All of these sets of guidelines and precautions emphasize:

- that blood and other blood-containing body fluids represent risk to HCWs; and
- that HCWs should use barriers and take precautions to prevent occupational exposures to these materials.

Use of these kinds of precautions in health-care settings has resulted in decreased risk of occupational exposure to blood and decreased risk for occupational infections with blood-borne pathogens. Based on self-reports of occupational exposures to blood, Fahey and co-workers at the National Institutes of Health estimated that, in the year prior to training the staff in universal precautions, staff members experienced an average of 36 cutaneous exposures to blood.[24] Eighteen months after the staff were trained in universal precautions, this number decreased to 18. For all categories of employees and information analyzed, exposures to blood were reduced by approximately 50%. These results suggest that changes in behavior occurred between the two surveys, and, although a causal relationship with training cannot be proved, such a relationship can reasonably be inferred.

Initially, compliance with these precautions was problematic. Gerberding and co-workers identified substantial noncompliance at San Francisco General Hospital.[25] Although Fahey identified substantial improvement in her staff's compliance with universal precautions, the reduction in blood exposures was only 50% (implying that 50% of such exposures continued to occur, despite implementation of these precautions).[24]

Although data regarding procedure-specific adverse exposure rates are limited, certain procedures and devices seem intrinsically associated with increased risk for occupational exposures. To the extent that such modifications are possible, inherently risky procedures should be modified. In some instances, risk modification can be achieved by practitioners modifying the way the procedure is performed. In other circumstances, new devices or engineered controls (discussed below) have been developed and implemented. Some work practice interventions have been shown to reduce the risks for blood exposures. For example, the use of 'double-gloving' in surgery reduced the risk for skin exposure to blood significantly.[26,27]

Engineered controls

Whereas work practice controls can eliminate a substantial fraction of occupational exposures to blood-borne pathogens, modifying medical devices that, in their current formats, are intrinsically associated with exposure risks can reduce these risks further. Jagger and co-workers detailed the importance of medical devices designed to prevent occupational exposures to blood-borne pathogens.[28,29]

In the past several years, a number of engineered controls (i.e. 'safer' sharps and safety devices) have been introduced. Of these new safety devices, the following have been identified in at least one published study as being associated with decreased risks for cutaneous and/or percutaneous blood exposures:

- a surgical repair assist device
- blunt surgical needles;
- surgical finger guards and glove liners;
- phlebotomy equipment;
- needleless intravenous administration systems; and
- modified (e.g. self-capping) intravenous catheters.

At one center, the incidence of self-reported percutaneous injuries among HCWs was reduced by 58% after implementation of 'safety-engineered devices' allowing for needle-safe blood drawing, intravenous insertion, etc.[30] Despite implementation of safer devices, some exposures will still occur. Development of a process for the systematic, objective evaluation of these new devices is crucial to reduce the risk of sharps injuries in all health-care settings.[31]

Interventions designed to decrease the risk for occupational infection once exposure to HIV has occurred

Immediate postexposure management

Despite the emphasis on the prevention of occupational exposures, institutions should also develop strategies to effectively manage occupational exposures. Important constituents of a postexposure management program are listed in Table 86.5.

When an exposure occurs, first aid should be administered and the exposure site should be allowed to bleed freely. The wound should be cleansed and decontaminated as soon as patient safety permits. Wounds should be washed with soap and water and then irrigated with sterile saline, a disinfectant or other suitable solution. Mucosal exposures should be decontaminated by vigorously flushing with water. Eyes should be irrigated with clean water, saline or sterile eye irrigants.

HCWs must be educated about the importance of promptly reporting occupational exposures. Institutional reporting procedures should be simple, straightforward and widely publicized. A mechanism

---

Table 86.5 Components of postexposure management programs for health-care workers exposed to HIV

1. Institutions should develop thorough, thoughtful, aggressive, employee educational campaigns concerning the presence of occupational risks in the health-care setting, including the risks for blood-borne pathogen infection; these educational campaigns should emphasize risk prevalence, risk-reduction strategies, the importance of reporting adverse occupational exposures and postexposure management protocols.
2. Postexposure management systems must include mechanisms to facilitate both exposure reporting and the provision of follow-up care; these systems should be readily accessible, widely publicized, convenient and user friendly; occupational medicine personnel should be instructed to provide immediate 'first aid' for staff sustaining adverse exposures to blood and body fluids.
3. Institutions should develop a system for categorizing occupational exposures that require differing management strategies and different types of follow-up; protocols should address 'source-unknown' and 'source refuses serologic testing' exposures.
4. Postexposure management protocols should include appropriate serologic testing (mindful of state and local laws regarding consent) of both the source-patient as well as the employee sustaining the occupational exposure.
5. Occupational medicine staff should be thoroughly trained in the counseling of staff sustaining occupational exposures to HIV; all exposed staff should be given appropriate counseling regarding risks for infection and prevention of secondary transmission; all staff should have access to further counseling, if needed; all exposed staff should be given access to experts in the areas of occupational risks and HIV infection.
6. Exposed employees should be counseled to return for appropriate clinical and serologic follow-up and should be instructed to return if signs and/or symptoms of acute HIV infection develop.
7. Postexposure management protocols should offer postexposure prophylaxis, with appropriate follow-up, for health-care workers sustaining occupational exposure to HIV.
8. Counseling should include attention to the known/expected toxicities of the selected regimen. Pre-emptive therapy of these symptoms/side-effects (e.g. prescriptions to treat nausea, diarrhea, etc.) may increase regimen adherence.
9. Postexposure management protocols must, at all costs, maintain the exposed health-care worker's medical privacy and confidentiality.

to facilitate reporting and provide follow-up care should be readily accessible. Reporting systems should offer access to expert consultants. Institutional occupational medical systems must protect the confidentiality of the exposed worker.

At the time an exposure is reported, occupational medical personnel should draw baseline serology. For documented occupational exposures to HIV, follow-up should occur at 6 weeks, 3 months, and 6 months postexposure. The follow-up period should be prolonged to 1 year for HCWs who become infected with HCV after exposure to patients with HIV and HCV co-infection. Late seroconversion (i.e. more than 6 months following exposure) has been documented in case reports. However, routinely prolonging the duration of follow-up beyond 6 months for all exposed HCWs is generally not recommended unless a particular situation calls for such action. More aggressive diagnostic evaluation, such as the use of polymerase chain reaction analysis to detect viral or proviral nucleic acids, should be ordered if the HCW develops symptoms suggestive of acute HIV infection. Occupational medicine staff should counsel the exposed HCW about the signs and symptoms of acute HIV infection and should instruct the employee to return for evaluation should any illness consistent with this syndrome occur.

Institutions should have written policies and procedures regarding the testing of source-patients and employees that are consonant with local and state laws. If available, rapid HIV tests should be performed on source-patients as such testing allows faster determination of source-patients' HIV status with sensitivity and specificity that is similar to that of conventional serologic testing.[32,33] This approach has been shown to be cost-effective and can lead to reduced implementation of unnecessary postexposure prophylaxis (PEP), as well as reduce the stress and anxiety often seen with the exposed workers.[34-36]

Postexposure chemoprophylaxis with antiretroviral agents

The use of antiretroviral agents as PEP for occupational exposures was controversial in the mid-1980s.[37] Data accumulated over the past 20 years, however, provide a firmer foundation demonstrating the efficacy of PEP. Animal studies of PEP (most of which use substantially lower viral inocula) have been able to demonstrate efficacy. Another piece of scientific evidence that indirectly supports the use of PEP comes from the success of antiretroviral agents administered in pregnancy to reduce maternal–fetal transmission of HIV.[38,39] One of the factors identified in the collaborative retrospective case-control study of occupational HIV in HCWs as significantly associated with an increased risk for occupational HIV infection was 'not taking zidovudine chemoprophylaxis'.[3] In this study, administering zidovudine chemoprophylaxis to exposed HCWs was associated with an approximately 80% reduction in the risk for occupational infection following percutaneous exposures to HIV.[3]

The US Public Health Service (USPHS) updated its guidelines recommending the use of PEP in 2005.[40] For 'less severe' occupational exposures, the current recommendations (summarized in Table 86.6) advocate the use a basic two-drug regimen consisting of two nucleoside reverse transcriptase inhibitors (NRTIs) or one NRTI plus one nucleotide reverse transcriptase inhibitor (NtRTI). The most frequently used combinations are zidovudine and lamivudine (co-formulated as Combivir) or emtricitabine and tenofovir (co-formulated as Truvada). Other potential combinations include stavudine plus lamivudine or emtricitabine, and tenofovir plus lamivudine or emtricitabine. The combination of didanosine and stavudine is no longer recommended due to potential drug toxicity. Due to the risk of possible serious or life-threatening adverse drug events, abacavir, delavirdine, nevirapine, and zalcitabine are not routinely recommended for PEP.

For 'more severe' exposures, an expanded protease inhibitor-based three-drug (or possibly four-drug) chemoprophylaxis regimen

Table 86.6 Current US Public Health Service recommendations for chemoprophylaxis of occupational exposures to HIV[40]

HIV exposures with a recognized transmission risk	Preferred 'basic regimens': • Zidovudine (ZDV) + lamivudine (3TC) • Tenofovir (TDF) + emtricitabine (FTC) • ZDV + FTC • TDF + 3TC
	Alternate 'basic regimens': • 3TC + stavudine (d4T) • FTC + d4T • 3TC + didanosine† (ddI) • FTC + ddI
HIV exposures for which the nature of the exposure suggests an elevated transmission risk*	Basic regimen' plus one of the following agents: • Lopinavir–ritonavir (LPV–RTV) – preferred • Atazanavir (ATV) ± RTV • Fosamprenavir (FOSAPV) ± RTV • Saquinavir (SQV) + RTV • Indinavir† (IDV) ± RTV • Nelfinavir† (NFV) • Efavirenz† (EFV)

*Examples of elevated risk include deep puncture, injury with large-bore hollow needle, visible blood on the device, exposure to 'larger' volume of blood and/or blood from source-patient with high viral load.
†Agents not advisable for use in pregnancy and/or increasingly not recommended in practice.

is recommended. The preferred protease inhibitor (PI) is lopinavir–ritonavir (Kaletra), but others may be used as alternatives with certain exceptions (discussed below).

If the source-patient for an exposure is (or recently has been) receiving antiretroviral therapy, some authorities recommend the use of alternative regimens utilizing agents to which the source-patient's virus has not been exposed. Certain regimens may be inappropriate if the source-patient is known or suspected to harbor a resistant virus. This latter point underscores the importance of obtaining expert guidance from individuals knowledgeable about the use of antiretroviral agents to tailor a PEP regimen for HCWs. Clinicians who are skilled in providing care to HIV-infected patients are perhaps best suited to provide this kind of advice. If you cannot identify a local expert, the US Public Health Service sponsors a postexposure hotline that can provide this expertise (either over the telephone (1-888-448-4911) or at http://www.ucsf.edu/hivcntr/Hotlines/PEPline.html).

Another special circumstance worthy of additional consideration relates to PEP administration to a HCW who is (or thinks she may be) pregnant. Because of the extremely limited experience with the use of these agents in uninfected individuals, the risks associated with administering the drugs to pregnant women are essentially undefined. The only relevant clinical experience in humans comes from the administration of the drugs to HIV-infected pregnant women, a circumstance that is not exactly consonant with the postexposure prophylaxis setting. Based on the limited clinical data, as well as several relevant animal studies, general guidelines for this situation have been developed and are summarized in Table 86.7.[40-42]

Virtually all of the marketed antiretroviral agents have potential for carcinogenicity, teratogenicity and mutagenicity. Since publication of the USPHS guidelines, concern has been raised for potential teratogenicity associated with the use of nelfinavir in animals. Although no definite relationship has been established in humans, the use of this agent in PEP regimens for pregnant women or women of childbearing age is no longer recommended.[42] Efavirenz has been shown to be teratogenic in cynomolgus monkeys at drug levels similar to those used in humans. In addition, administration of the didanosine–stavudine combination in pregnancy has been associated with cases

Table 86.7 General principles for administering antiretroviral chemoprophylaxis to pregnant health-care workers[40-42]

1. A pregnant, exposed health-care worker is the only person who can decide whether to take chemoprophylaxis, and she must be empowered to make this decision. No one should attempt to make this decision for her.
2. The practitioner providing care to a pregnant, HIV-exposed woman must provide up-to-date and accurate information about what is known (and not known) concerning:
   - the magnitude of risk for infection associated with her exposure;
   - the efficacy of postexposure prophylaxis;
   - the safety of the treatment, including the potential for harm to the health-care worker and her fetus; and
   - the risk of the fetus becoming infected (and the possible interventions that could be taken to reduce this risk) should the health-care worker become infected from the exposure.
3. The practitioner should select a regimen appropriate for the exposure; i.e. pregnancy per se should not dictate the regimen, but consideration should be given to agents for which an experience base exists (e.g. zidovudine and lamivudine). Some agents/regimens with known toxicities in pregnancy should be avoided whenever possible (e.g. didanosine plus stavudine; indinavir, efavirenz, nelfinavir).
4. Pregnant workers electing to take postexposure prophylaxis must be followed closely for signs of toxicity (both maternal and fetal); pregnancy represents another circumstance in which expert consultative advice is essential.

of severe pancreatitis and severe lactic acidosis among HIV-infected women, and both maternal and fetal deaths have been recorded.[43] Other issues that may be relevant to the administration of chemoprophylaxis to pregnant HCWs include data from France suggesting a risk for severe mitochondrial toxicity in uninfected infants born to mothers who had taken nucleoside analogues[44] (an experience that has not been detected in the USA), as well as the potential for hepatotoxicity and nephrolithiasis associated with indinavir use.

Monitoring for PEP toxicity

If HCWs are prescribed PEP, chemistry (renal and hepatic function) and complete blood counts should be checked at baseline and 2 weeks into treatment. Additional monitoring may be necessary depending on the specific PEP regimen prescribed. Potential drug toxicity and interactions should be discussed with HCWs, as should the importance of adherence to treatment. Despite the encouraging data concerning the use and efficacy of PEP, legitimate concerns remain about the use of these agents in this setting. Antiretrovirals are not trivial agents in terms of potential toxicity. Virtually all studies of PEP for occupational HIV exposures in HCWs have demonstrated substantial side-effects, often limiting completion of the prescribed regimen.[45] Despite the availability of newer, more tolerable agents, recent data have shown that as many as 20% of HCWs stop PEP prematurely due to adverse events.[46,47] Finally, several cases of zidovudine chemoprophylaxis failure (eight of which have direct clinical relevance) have appeared in the literature.

The US Public Health Service last revised its guidelines concerning postexposure prophylaxis in 2005[40] and intends to revise the guidelines whenever new information becomes available concerning the risks or benefits of postexposure chemoprophylaxis. In spite of these considerations, all institutions need to have a policy on postexposure prophylaxis. Offering chemoprophylaxis is seen as 'empowering' by exposed workers. Workers who have had these frightening occupational exposures appreciate the fact that their institutions are willing to offer these drugs, ongoing support and prevention strategies to improve HCW safety.

REFERENCES

References for this chapter can be found online at http://www.expertconsult.com

HIV vaccines: past failures and future scientific challenges

INTRODUCTION: WHY WE NEED AN HIV VACCINE?

There are currently around 3 million deaths annually from HIV and AIDS, but this figure is projected to increase much further over the coming decades. By 2030, it is estimated that HIV will be one of the three major causes of death worldwide, alongside heart disease and stroke. Highly active antiretroviral therapy (HAART), which was introduced in the 1990s, will not prevent this outcome, because the majority of people worldwide do not have access to anti-HIV drugs. Even when HAART can be readily obtained, there are major problems associated with its use. These include adverse effects, drug interactions and the development of drug-resistant HIV strains. Measures that reduce or prevent transmission, such as condoms or male circumcision, are needed urgently. Of the various prevention measures, a prophylactic HIV vaccine is the only one likely to have a major impact on the global spread of HIV. There is, therefore, an urgent need for a safe, effective prophylactic HIV vaccine in order to improve global health. Unfortunately, as this chapter discusses, we are far from achieving this goal.

IT WAS NEVER GOING TO BE EASY

When HIV was discovered in 1983, there was initially hope that a vaccine might follow shortly afterwards. Expectations were further raised when experiments in nonhuman primates showed protection against a hybrid between the human and monkey AIDS virus SHIV (simian HIV). As we describe below, this proved to be a false dawn. Phase III efficacy trials in humans that had been predicated on such data failed completely to show any form of protection against HIV. The true magnitude of the challenge in designing an HIV vaccine became apparent as we gained a more thorough understanding of the complex molecular biology of HIV infection.

However, even a basic understanding of HIV and its evolution should enable us to anticipate major difficulties for HIV vaccine development. Ancestral retroviruses have been in existence for many tens of millennia and have had a head start on us in how to evade host immune responses. Combine this with the extraordinarily rapid rate of mutation during HIV replication and it is understandable that HIV has been able to evolve superlatively effective mechanisms against vaccination. These range from the 'hiding' of potential neutralizing domains from neutralizing antibodies to the development of restriction genes whose sole purpose is to defend HIV from the host. The enormity of the scientific challenge is now apparent to all those in the field (Table 87.1).

Table 87.1 Key difficulties in developing an HIV vaccine

- No natural sterilizing immunity to disease
- Huge difficulties in producing neutralizing antibodies
- No good animal models of HIV infection
- A pool of latently infected cells is formed early after infection
- No good correlates of T-cell vaccine efficacy have been identified

WHERE ARE WE WITH CURRENT CLINICAL TRIALS?

Thus far there have been three large efficacy studies, all of which have failed to show any benefit. The latest, the 'STEP trial' of an adenoviral vector HIV vaccine candidate[1] (described in more detail below), was halted prematurely in 2007. This candidate engendered hope as there was a strong T-cell recognition of HIV antigens as measured by enzyme-linked immunosorbent spot (ELISpot) assay responses. The dismal results of this study were a blow to the morale of HIV vaccine researchers.

These failures sent a clear message that we need to re-evaluate our approach to HIV vaccine development. As this chapter emphasizes, a 'quick fix' will not be achievable for HIV vaccines. The opposite is true, and a huge amount of basic scientific work is still required before we will have an HIV vaccine with any realistic chance of success. We will discuss a number of barriers that need to be overcome, including the difficulties in producing neutralizing antibodies to HIV, the problems in measuring and producing effective cytotoxic T-lymphocyte responses and the need to develop other approaches, including those that rely on innate immunity.

HOW WOULD WE DEFINE A 'SUCCESSFUL PROPHYLACTIC HIV VACCINE'?

There has also been a re-evaluation of what might be considered a 'successful prophylactic HIV vaccine' (PHV). An ideal PHV would be one that prevents infection in almost 100% of those vaccinated; it would be cheap, easily (self-) administered, stable in all commonly encountered environmental conditions (including those found in the tropics), be completely safe and have a lifelong effect. However, a PHV would still be valuable if it did not offer protection against infection, but instead mitigated the course of the disease after infection. This would reduce morbidity and mortality from HIV. Similarly, a vaccine that reduced the infectivity of the individual would reduce the spread of the HIV epidemic (Table 87.2).

Table 87.2 Definitions of a successful HIV vaccine

- Provides protection to 70–100% and markedly slows epidemic.
- Only provides protection in 30–70% but still has significant impact on HIV epidemic.
- Does *not* prevent infection at all, but reduces the viral load post infection, leading to:
  - slower disease progression in the individual;
  - reduced infectivity of the individual; and
  - slowing of the epidemic due to reduced transmission.

THE STARTING POINT: APPLYING APPROACHES THAT HAVE BEEN SUCCESSFUL FOR OTHER VACCINES

It is not a prerequisite to understand how the body protects against an infective agent to develop an effective vaccine against that organism. The first successful vaccine against a viral infection was developed by Edward Jenner without any knowledge of the causative infectious agent, the way the agent was transmitted or any knowledge of how the vaccine might mediate disease. Nonetheless, a vaccine against smallpox was developed.[2]

The three main types of vaccine that have been used successfully for the prevention of other viral illnesses are live attenuated, whole inactivated and recombinant proteins (Table 87.3). All of these vaccines protect by means of antibody responses, and hence it seemed only natural in HIV vaccine development to seek vaccines that might produce neutralizing antibodies. This would tie in with our knowledge of the immune response to HIV infection (Fig. 87.1). The choice of vaccine type, however, is limited by safety concerns. Live attenuated AIDS vaccines have protected against infection in the nonhuman primate model but are considered too dangerous for use in humans because of the possible reversion to a more pathogenic type of virus.[3] Whole inactivated viruses seemed to offer protection in nonhuman primate models. However, it transpired that this protection was mediated by neutralizing antibodies (NAbs) against human cellular proteins that had been incorporated into the vaccine during production in human cell lines.[4] Hence, for reasons of safety and efficacy, most HIV vaccine candidates are recombinant/subunit vaccines. The first such vaccine used a recombinant envelope protein of HIV, based on gp120 (Fig. 87.2).

There are many other instances of viral infections for which the 'neutralizing antibody' approach has not yielded a successful vaccine,

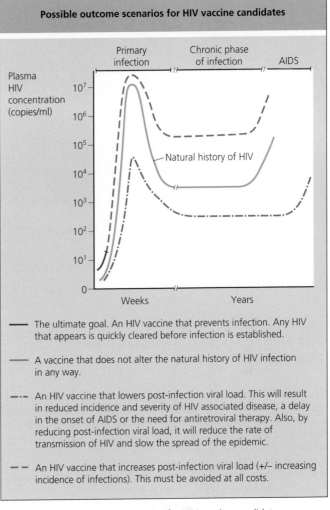

Possible outcome scenarios for HIV vaccine candidates

—— The ultimate goal. An HIV vaccine that prevents infection. Any HIV that appears is quickly cleared before infection is established.

—— A vaccine that does not alter the natural history of HIV infection in any way.

—·— An HIV vaccine that lowers post-infection viral load. This will result in reduced incidence and severity of HIV associated disease, a delay in the onset of AIDS or the need for antiretroviral therapy. Also, by reducing post-infection viral load, it will reduce the rate of transmission of HIV and slow the spread of the epidemic.

– – An HIV vaccine that increases post-infection viral load (+/– increasing incidence of infections). This must be avoided at all costs.

Fig. 87.1 Possible outcome scenarios for HIV vaccine candidates.

hepatitis C being one such example. There appear to be several reasons for this, including the rapid multiple mutations that occur, leading to evasion of a neutralizing antibody response. Also, it is not clear if hepatitis C even has a single principal neutralizing domain.

Table 87.3 Examples of vaccines used to prevent other viral illnesses

Vaccine type	Diseases	Correlate for protection	Safety issues for HIV vaccines
Live attenuated	Polio (oral) Measles Mumps Rubella Varicella Yellow fever Smallpox	Antibodies	Considered too unsafe to use in HIV because of possible reversion to virulent type
Whole inactivated	Inactivated polio Hepatitis A Influenza	Antibodies	Considered to be relatively safe, although some concerns exist
Recombinant proteins	Hepatitis B Human papillomavirus	Antibodies	Considered to be relatively safe, and is the main current approach, although some viral vectors might increase the risk of infection

Structure of HIV

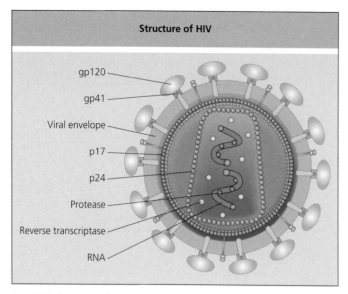

Labels: gp120, gp41, Viral envelope, p17, p24, Protease, Reverse transcriptase, RNA

Fig. 87.2 Structure of HIV.

THE NEUTRALIZING ANTIBODY APPROACH FOR HIV

Whereas HIV viruses cultured in the laboratory can be neutralized, primary isolates from HIV patients have so far been resistant to neutralization.[5] HIV does appear to have several neutralizing domains, but none of them is an easy target for potential vaccine-induced antibodies. There are several reasons for this (Table 87.4).

Firstly, the high mutation rate that occurs with HIV replication leads rapidly to escape mutations to most antibodies with neutralizing potential. Therefore, even though neutralizing antibodies against the HIV envelope do occur naturally after infection in humans, they almost immediately select for escape mutants.[6,7] It is sobering to realize that the degree of viral diversity that occurs amongst all influenza viruses in the world in a given year is far exceeded by the diversity of HIV within one newly infected person within the same time period. Hence any antibodies produced by such a vaccine would prove ineffective. Furthermore, 'natural infection' with HIV does not prevent the occurrence of superinfection with other viral clades.

The first phase III efficacy trial of a prophylactic HIV vaccine was based on the gp120 envelope protein and it is not surprising, therefore, that it proved completely ineffective. The study was conceived before the extent of escape mutants was clear, but the results of the study demonstrated the scale of this barrier to vaccine efficacy.

For neutralizing antibodies to be effective in HIV, they need to interfere with fusion of the virus. HIV fuses to target cells by using a trimeric

---

Table 87.4 Difficulties in producing neutralizing antibodies (NAbs)

- Exposed sequences on the envelope are highly variable, which rapidly leads to escape mutants
- Exposed sequences, e.g. gp120, do not lead to NAbs of great breadth or specificity
- The viral envelope exists as a trimer and immunogenic regions on the monomer are shielded (the envelope proteins are shielded by numerous *N*-linked glycans)
- The envelope protein undergoes structural changes when it binds to the CD4 receptor
- High levels of NAbs are probably required to prevent infection

---

envelope complex of gp120 and gp41 subunits, which attach to CD4+ receptors and a co-receptor (usually CCR5 or CXCR4). Neutralizing antibodies of primary isolates work in one of two ways: either they prevent receptor engagement by binding to the virus surface trimer or they inhibit fusion after viral attachment has occurred.[8]

HIV has evolved a number of mechanisms to evade this neutralization (Fig. 87.3).[9] The HIV envelope is heavily glycosylated. The glycans themselves are poorly immunogenic and they prevent access of antibodies to the peptides beneath them. The trimeric nature of the gp120–gp41 structure also shields the epitopes much more so than for the individual monomeric subunits. The reason for this is not completely clear, but is probably related to conformational changes that occur during trimerization. Hence any sites potentially vulnerable to neutralization are well shielded.

Finally, and partly as a result of the above features, those neutralizing antibodies that have been identified usually need very high levels to prevent infection, and the '2 log' or '100 times' rule has generally been observed to hold. This is where the titer of one of the known neutralizing antibodies required to neutralize the virus in vivo is around 100 times the levels required to neutralize the virus in sera.[10,11]

The potential for neutralizing antibodies against primary HIV *in vivo*

Despite all the forgoing reasons that neutralization of HIV *in vivo* is such a difficult prospect, there are reasons to expect progress in this area. Several naturally occurring neutralizing antibodies, with broadly neutralizing activity, have been identified in rare individuals.[12] Primary isolates from different HIV-1 subtypes can be neutralized by different broadly reactive human monoclonal antibodies which have been assigned the following labels: b12, 2G12, 2F5 and 4E10. These sera and monoclonal antibodies have been extensively studied and the way they neutralize HIV might provide some important insights for vaccine development.

It is instructive to look at an example of how one of these antibodies appears to achieve neutralization. B12 was the first broadly neutralizing antibody to be described and it acts by preventing attachment of HIV to the cell. It does this by occluding the CD4 binding site on gp120. There is a recess on the CD4 binding site that forms a contact site for an amino acid, Phe-43, that protrudes from a loop on CD4. This is a key interaction, for without it gp120 binds too weakly for fusion to occur. The b12 antibody acts by means of a long protruding CDR3 loop that 'spears' the center of the CD4 binding site. Although a large number of antibodies have been shown to act in a similar manner, it is only b12 that is able to neutralize primary isolates. The exact qualities of b12 that give it this specificity are yet to be determined, but if this can be established, we can attempt to induce neutralizing antibodies that act in the same way.

The other broadly neutralizing antibodies act in different ways; for example, 2F5 and 4E10 appear to act by inhibiting fusion, and 2G12 prevents virus entry by a different mechanism from b12. The ways that these antibodies neutralize have been the subject of considerable research and their mechanism of action has become much clearer over the past few years.[9]

Interestingly, the '2 log' rule described earlier does not seem to apply to one of the neutralizing antibodies, 2G12, where the relatively low levels required to achieve in-vitro neutralization are sufficient to achieve neutralization in vivo.[13] It might prove very instructive to find out why 2G12 'punches above its weight'.

Finally, some illuminating clinical studies have been performed in patients, whereby known human monoclonal antibodies have been infused into HIV-infected patients and have markedly reduced HIV viral load.[14] This will never constitute a practical form of therapy, because of the high levels of antibodies required, as well as the requirement for constant infusion. Nonetheless, these studies point to the potential efficacy of these neutralizing antibodies in humans and also provide a means of studying how best to deploy these approaches.

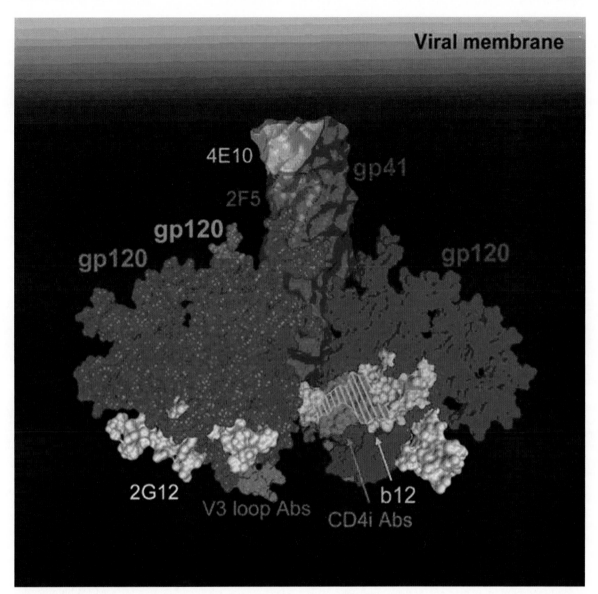

Fig. 87.3 HIV mechanisms of avoiding neutralization. From Burton *et al.*[9]

THE RATIONALE FOR T-CELL VACCINES AGAINST HIV

With the recognition that it will be some time, if ever, that a vaccine will be developed that produces a strong effective neutralizing antibody response, the field has turned to ways to elicit effective T-cell responses against HIV.

The basis of 'T-cell vaccines' is the ability of T cells to recognize peptide sequences of HIV. These sequences can be generated by proteolytic breakdown of the virus, and hence can include the internal, more conserved core proteins of HIV as well as the more variable Env proteins. CD8+ T cells recognize peptides that are 8–11 amino acids in length that are presented on the surface of cells by major histocompatibility complex (MHC) class I antigens; CD4+ T cells recognize peptides 10–18 amino acids in length that are presented on cells by MHC class II antigens. The MHC antigens of infected and of vaccinated individuals can recognize multiple CD4 and CD8 epitopes. This is promising for HIV vaccine development, because by targeting multiple epitopes,

there is less likelihood of the vaccine being selected against by escape mutation. This principle is similar to that applied successfully in combination anti-HIV drug therapy.

The disadvantage of T-cell vaccines compared to antibody vaccines is that they can only work once a cell has become infected. Thus T-cell vaccines do not prevent infection but are of potential value in controlling infections. Even with T-cell vaccines, however, there is the possibility of viral escape over time.[15]

There have been some key advances in our knowledge of the immunology of T-cell responses in recent years, and below is a brief summary of those most relevant to T-cell vaccine development.

For a vaccine to generate T cells, the antigens need to be presented by professional 'antigen presenting cells' or APCs. Usually, for an APC to be able to present class I antigens, proteins need to be produced within a cell. These do not have to be produced by the APC, as they could be produced by another cell and then the antigen is taken up by the APC, known as cross-presentation.[16] Class II presentation can occur whether the proteins are produced within the cell or are taken up from outside the cell. APCs need activating in order to initiate an immune response. This occurs by activating signals produced by pattern recognition receptors (PRRs),[17,18] to which Toll-like receptors belong. The PRRs recognize conserved patterns in the sequences of pathogen molecules and in turn stimulate the APCs to produce activation molecules and inflammatory cytokines. The APCs migrate to the lymph nodes where they present the foreign antigen to naive or memory T cells. The APCs stimulate T cells that recognize presented peptides to expand and differentiate into short-lived acute effector cells, long-lived effector memory cells and long-lived central memory cells.[19]

The vaccine antigen drives the acute effector T-cell response. It is only as the antigen is cleared that effector memory and central memory cells undergo differentiation. The effector memory cells provide an immediate response to a further antigen challenge, whereas the central memory cells traffic through the spleen and lymph nodes looking for their specific antigens. If found, central memory cells rapidly divide and differentiate to provide short-lived effector cells to fight the acute infection. During the clearance of the infection, the central memory cells change their profiles and replenish the effector and central memory cells in order to provide a long-term memory response.

Hence, the key aim of a T-cell vaccine is to present the antigen with the infective agent for which control is desired, such that they elicit both long-lived effector memory and central memory responses.

The problem is how best to generate these T-cell responses. Live attenuated viruses produce not only CD4+ T-lymphocyte responses, but also CD8+ responses, the latter as a result of MHC class processing of proteins that occurs during active replication of the viral vaccine *in vivo*. This approach is used with the current measles vaccine, for instance. Where live attenuated viruses are unsafe or impractical, such as hepatitis A, chemical treatment to remove replicative capacity has been used. However, as neither of these approaches is considered safe enough for HIV, the use of viral proteins that have been expressed by cells lines, such as with hepatitis B, appears to be the safest approach.

An approach that has been used for a recently developed papillomavirus vaccine is the administration of virus-like particles (VLPs). With this method, structural virus proteins are expressed that come together *in vitro* to form nonreplicating, noninfectious particles. These immunogens undergo MHC class II processing and hence are able to express antibodies and CD4+ T-lymphocyte responses. They cannot, however, induce CD8+ T-lymphocyte responses because they do not replicate *in vivo* and so cannot undergo MHC class I processing.

A number of approaches are being used in order to develop T-cell responses within an HIV vaccine. Those undergoing most development at present are the use of recombinant viral vectors, DNA delivery of antigenic material using adjuvant-supported proteins and peptides, and finally a combination of more than one of these approaches. For example, the 'prime-boost' approach uses DNA priming followed by boosting of the response by presenting the antigen by means of a delivery system such as a live or bacterial vector. It is beyond the scope of this chapter to give a detailed account of the advantages and disadvantages of DNA vaccination and the use of live viral vectors. Suffice it to say that the 'prime-boost' approach has been extensively developed and used in clinical trials because it appears the most effective means of eliciting good T-cell responses. Until recently, the two most favored boost approaches have used either the DNA priming adenovirus vectors or mammalian poxvirus vectors, with Adenovirus5 (Ad5) and modified vaccinia Ankara (MVA) being the best examples.

The prime boost approach using both of these vectors has delivered some impressive results in animal models, including nonhuman primates. However, none of these successes carried over into trials in humans. A recent MVA candidate vaccine was studied in two large phase II international studies in human volunteers; the results were very disappointing with no ELISpot responses in the majority of vaccines.[20] This has led to a complete halt of the clinical trial program that used this vaccine construct. Similar phase II studies with a construct delivered by Ad5 gave much stronger and sustained ELISpot responses. This gave the rationale for the investigation of this candidate in a much larger efficacy trial, the STEP trial. The results were eagerly awaited, but proved to be a major letdown – not only did the vaccine fail to afford any protection at all, there was also a slightly increased incidence of HIV infections in the vaccine arm compared to the placebo arm.[1] For this reason the use of this vector is being reconsidered.

Another efficacy study, the PAVE 100A trial (www.hivpave.org/about/pave100.html), using a different adenovirus vector and different immunogens, is still going ahead, but will be monitored very carefully for safety. PAVE 100A is designed to enroll several thousand volunteers in two studies focused on distinct populations in the Americas and Africa. The expectations for this study have been readjusted downwards in the light of the previous studies, and some question whether it should be going ahead at all. The rationale to perform such a large study is that we may still have much to learn in terms of breadth of immune responses. The argument against continuing with further studies until we have improved candidate PHV design is discussed later, but centers on the damage it might do to the standing of PHV trials in the future.

There are two key messages that have been reinforced by these two prime boost vaccine candidates:

- there are no good animal models from which results of HIV vaccine trials in humans can be extrapolated; and
- the current measures of immune responsiveness of potential HIV vaccines do not correlate with protection.

With the recognition of this, there are renewed efforts to try to improve these barriers to PHV development. For example, assays are being carried out to determine whether different states of differentiation of T cells can reveal any subset(s) that correlate with protection in nonhuman primates. It appears as if the central memory cells have a better correlation than other cells.

LESSONS FROM THE NATURAL HISTORY OF HIV PROGRESSION

The rates of progression of HIV in the complete absence of treatment, as measured by CD4+ cell count decline, can vary enormously between patients. At one extreme are the rare 'elite nonprogressors', alternatively termed 'HIV controllers', who maintain an undetectable HIV viral load in serum for long periods of time and have no discernable CD4+ count decline during these periods. Such control has been observed for long periods, up to 25 years so far in some patients. These controllers are much more likely to have certain genetic factors, specifically certain HLA class I alleles, and also CD8+ T-cell responses generated through these alleles.[21] They are also more likely to have virus-specific, strong CD4+ T-cell responses. However, no one feature is common to all HIV controllers. Clearly there might be much to learn from these patients with regard to HIV vaccines designed to prevent or treat HIV, and this population is being studied intensively for further clues.

MUCOSAL VACCINES AGAINST HIV

There is an extensive and growing knowledge base concerning mucosal immunity, and this is being applied to the development of HIV vaccine candidates. For successful vaccines for other infections given via the parenteral route, protection appears to be induced by systemic immune responses; the mucosal responses, although poorly studied, appear to be less robust. In nonhuman primate models, high doses of neutralizing antibodies given intravenously can reach mucosal sites and block mucosal transmission of SHIV.[13,22] Unfortunately, neutralizing antibodies of this concentration have not been induced by HIV vaccine candidates thus far.

Most HIV infections are acquired by the mucosal route, vaginally, rectally or, less commonly, orally. Once HIV has gained entry via mucosa, it is transmitted quickly throughout the body. After rhesus macaques were inoculated intravaginally with SIV, the virus was detected in Langerhans cells or dendritic cells under the vaginal epithelium within 4 hours, in the internal iliac lymph nodes within

48 hours and in the blood within 5 days.[23,24] SIV was found in distant lymph nodes and bone marrow at 12 days.[25] Once established in the lymphoid tissue, HIV undergoes massive replication in the largest mucosal-associated lymphoid tissue (MALT), the bowel, and this leads to a marked depletion of CD4+ cells in the intestinal tract.[26] A unique aspect of HIV, and a challenge for vaccine development, is that a pool of latently infected 'resting' CD4+ cells is established early in the course of the primary infection.[27] This pool seems resistant to clearance, even by prolonged antiretroviral therapy.[28]

Therefore, if early HIV infection is to be cleared before it becomes established, then HIV vaccines must induce effective immune responses at the point of entry within the first few days of exposure to the virus.[29] Certainly the effective induction of mucosal immunity is thought to be one of the most important requirements for an HIV vaccine. As such, it seems likely that the best defense against HIV would be vaccines that induce both systemic and mucosal responses against the virus. Mucosal vaccines might offer this more than immunization by other routes[30] because of the potential for enhancement of mucosal immunity, as well as being easier to deliver.

However, not all routes of mucosal vaccination are the same. Both the quality and the quantity of antigen-specific immune responses at a mucosal site appear to be highly dependent on the exact route of mucosal vaccination. As a rule of thumb, oral administration induces antigen–antibody-specific responses in the small intestine, colon, mammary and salivary glands, as well as systemically; however, although antigen–antibody responses in the large intestine and female genital tract are weak,[31-33] they do induce antigen-specific CD8+ cytotoxic T lymphocytes (CTLs) in the rectal mucosa.[34] Rectal administration has been poorly studied in humans, but mice models show that vaccines can induce strong antigen-specific mucosal IgA and CTL responses in the rectum and systemically.[33,35] Nasal administration in humans induces strong antigen-specific antibody responses in salivary glands, the respiratory tract, genital tract and systemically, but not in the intestine, although this route can induce strong antigen-specific IgA and CTLs in the female genital tract.[36,37] Thus, because HIV first infects the majority of people genitally, nasal vaccination is an attractive option for a mucosal HIV vaccine.[33,35] The vaginal and transcutaneous routes would also offer advantages as they have been shown to induce antigen-specific IgA and IgG in the human female genital tract.[33,38]

NOVEL HIV VACCINE STRATEGIES

The word 'novel' is often applied liberally to new HIV vaccine candidates even if they are merely an extension of existing approaches. There is a clear need to explore 'novel' approaches that are substantially, if not radically, different from anything that has preceded them. We are not going to attempt to list those approaches, but instead will briefly give a few examples. None of the examples given below are clear leaders in the race to find the best approach towards an effective HIV vaccine and they are not mutually exclusive. A broad agreement is emerging that a systematic examination of the most promising novel approaches needs to be carefully undertaken, and that those with the most valuable results should be given further accelerated support. This forms the basis of a number of current initiatives, including programs for innovative research from the Gates Foundation.

The following is a highly selective selection of some of the good new ideas that are being evaluated at present.

One example of innovative work is the induction of potent CD8+ T-cell responses by using novel biodegradable nanoparticles carrying: human immunodeficiency virus type 1 (HIV-1) gp120.[39] Another approach that is of promise is the use of passive immunization as a tool to identify protective HIV-1 Env epitopes that might be useful to incorporate in future HIV vaccines.[40] It seems that the adaptive immune response may emerge too slowly to prevent the spread of HIV after the initial inoculation. Hence alternative avenues of research are being directed to innate immune mechanisms that might be incorporated into novel vaccination strategies.

The strongest immune response in humans is the alloimmune response, mediated by presentation of foreign antigens by human leukocyte antigens. There is evidence that this immune response might play a significant role in natural protection against HIV.[41,42] This has encouraged current ongoing work in macaques to determine whether the protective potential of alloimmunity can be incorporated into effective vaccines against SIV and, if so, whether this might lead to studies in humans (T Lehner, personal communication, 2008).

THE FUTURE

It is highly unlikely that the current vaccine approaches that have entered human trials to date will prove successful by themselves. There is a broad consensus amongst the scientific community that we must call a halt to large trials of the efficacy of PHVs in humans unless they are with truly new candidates that offer some reasonable possibility of success. This consensus is not universal, however. The danger of continuing with studies of candidates with little chance of efficacy is the real possibility that volunteers and donors alike would withdraw support from future HIV vaccine trials. We are learning from behavioral studies just what it is that drives volunteers to participate or turn away from PHV trials[43] and more effort is required to keep abreast of this critical aspect of vaccine studies. Major advances are required before we will have a PHV candidate of true merit, one that we can reasonably hope will offer efficacy. At the present time our efforts should be directed towards building the foundations of HIV vaccine science.

So, how should we be directing our energies over the next few years? In the face of one of the greatest public health issues to face mankind, stopping work on HIV vaccines is not an option. The best tactic when facing a seemingly omnipotent 'enemy' is a tactical retreat in order to reconsider tactics.

This work has already begun in coordinating HIV vaccine efforts towards the 'big' questions that include:

- How do we identify and reproduce broadly neutralizing antibody responses in humans?
- How can we identify correlates of immunity in which to screen and select HIV vaccine candidates at an early stage?
- How can we improve animal models of HIV infection?
- How can we best identify those truly original vaccine concepts that deserve further evaluation?
- How can we maintain enthusiasm from volunteers and donors alike in the face of the lack of progress?

To this end a number of consortia are pooling efforts and identifying cohorts of patients to study, such as 'HIV controllers' and immunologic and virologic questions to tackle through groups such as 'neutralizing antibody consortia'.

When the next edition of this textbook is published, we hope that we can report some real progress with some of the 'big questions' of HIV vaccine development.

REFERENCES

References for this chapter can be found online at http://www.expertconsult.com

Alexandre Harari
Giuseppe Pantaleo

Chapter | **88** |

The immunopathogenesis of HIV-1 infection

This chapter examines the immunologic and virologic mechanisms involved in the pathogenesis of HIV-1 infection and the interaction between the virus and the host. The recent availability of highly active antiretroviral combination therapy (HAART) has significantly influenced the natural history of the infection, delaying the progression to overt AIDS and prolonging survival. At the same time, increasing knowledge of the pathogenic mechanisms and of the limitations of HAART has made it clear that eradication of the virus with the available conventional antiviral drugs is not feasible. Recent advances in our understanding of the correlates of protective immunity have drawn attention to the development of immune-based interventions in order to achieve long-term control of HIV-1 disease.

THE NATURAL HISTORY OF HIV INFECTION

The typical course of HIV-1 infection is defined by different phases that generally occur during a period of between 8 and 12 years. Although the pattern and the course of the infection are highly variable among HIV-1-infected patients, three distinct phases can be identified (Fig. 88.1):[1]

- primary HIV-1 infection;
- chronic asymptomatic phase; and
- overt AIDS.

Primary HIV-1 infection

Primary HIV-1 infection is a transient condition, often accompanied by a symptomatic illness of variable severity in 40–90% of patients, and is invariably accompanied by:

- an initial rapid rise in plasma viremia, often to levels in excess of 1 000 000 RNA copies/ml;
- a decrease in the blood CD4+ T cells and a massive decrease CD4+ T cells in tissues, particularly in the gut and lymph nodes; and
- a large increase in the blood CD8+ T-cell count.

The marked decline of plasma viremia generally coincides with resolution of the clinical syndrome.[2] The decrease in the viral load correlates with the appearance of virus-specific immune responses (see below), particularly HIV-1-specific cytotoxic T lymphocytes (CTLs), indicating that virus-specific immune responses certainly play a crucial role in the initial downregulation of virus replication.[3–6]

The signs and symptoms of primary HIV-1 infection generally appear 2–4 weeks after virus exposure (see Fig. 88.1). The duration of the clinical syndrome ranges between a few days and more than 10 weeks but generally lasts less than 14 days. The clinical presentation of the primary HIV-1 infection may mimic acute mononucleosis (see Chapter 89) as well as many other febrile acute illnesses, emphasizing the nonspecific nature of these symptoms and the difficulty of obtaining an accurate early diagnosis.

Because the acute clinical syndrome associated with primary infection is not specific for HIV-1, the diagnosis is based on laboratory tests. In this regard, it is important to underscore the fact that anti-HIV-1 antibodies are usually negative during the acute phase of illness, as well as the Western blot, which evaluates the generation of specific antibodies against different HIV-1 proteins. The Western blot is considered to be positive when there are at least three specific bands and/or two bands but with antibody reactivity against HIV-1 *env* and *gag*. Early diagnosis, therefore, relies on a history of exposure, a positive p24 antigen enzyme-linked immunosorbent assay (ELISA) or the detection of plasma viral RNA (almost always >50 000 copies/ml of plasma).[2]

The chronic asymptomatic phase

The primary HIV-1 infection is followed by a long phase of clinical latency (median time of 10 years), during which neither signs nor symptoms of illness are present. Relatively stable levels of virus replication and of CD4+ T-cell counts for a variable period of time characterize this phase of infection. This 'stability' of measures of disease activity is apparent in the blood only. Virus replication in the gut and the accumulation of extracellular virus trapped in the follicular dendritic cell network are particularly active in the lymphoid tissue, where a progressive anatomic and functional deterioration occurs, impairing the ability to maintain effective specific immune responses over time.[7,8] This is reflected by the rapid increase in the levels of viremia and by a drop in CD4+ T-cell counts, which can suddenly speed up the transition from this phase to the advanced stage of the disease.

The advanced stage of HIV-1 disease is marked by low CD4+ T-cell counts (<200 cells/ml) and by the appearance of constitutional symptoms. It may be complicated by the development of AIDS-defining opportunistic infections.[1]

Overt AIDS

Overt AIDS defines the end stage of HIV-1 infection. In the absence of antiretroviral therapy, this phase leads to death in 2–3 years. The risk for death and opportunistic infections significantly increases with CD4+ T-cell counts below 50 cells/ml. Fortunately, the recent advent of HAART, including at present as many as six different classes of antiretroviral drugs administered in different combinations, is significantly decreasing the rate of progression, morbidity and mortality of HIV-1 infection (see Chapter 100).

Clinical course of the infection

The clinical course of HIV-1 infection is variable. In the majority (60–70%) of HIV-1-infected patients, the median time between infection and development of AIDS, in the absence of therapy, is

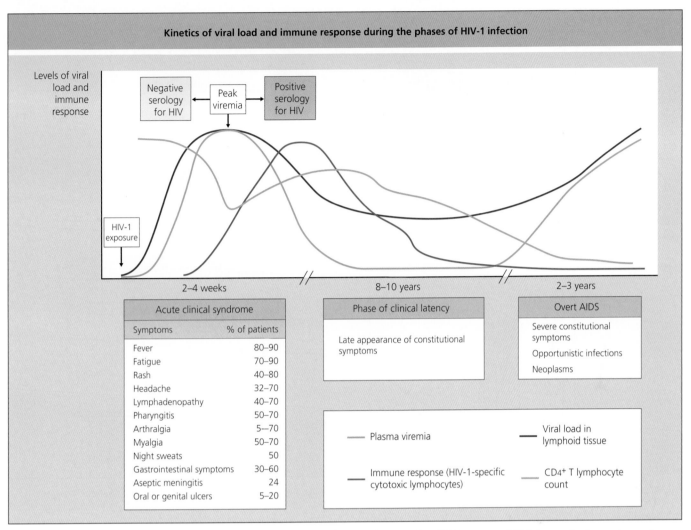

Fig. 88.1 Kinetics of viral load and immune response during the phases of HIV-1 infection. After HIV-1 exposure, initial virus replication and spread occur in the lymphoid organs, and systemic dissemination of HIV-1 is reflected by the peak of plasma viremia. A clinical syndrome of varying severity is associated with this phase of primary HIV-1 infection in up to 70% of HIV-1-infected persons. Downregulation of viremia during the transition from the primary to the early chronic phase coincides with the appearance of HIV-1-specific cytotoxic T cells and with the progressive resolution of the clinical syndrome. The long phase of clinical latency is associated with active virus replication, particularly in the lymphoid tissue. During the clinically latent period, CD4+ T-cell counts slowly decrease, as does the HIV-1-specific immune response. When CD4+ T-cell counts decrease below 200 cells/ml (i.e. when overt AIDS occurs), the clinical picture is characterized by severe constitutional symptoms and by the possible development of opportunistic infections and/or neoplasms.

10–11 years. These HIV-1-infected persons are defined as typical progressors (Fig. 88.2), and the clinical course of the infection that they generally experience is the one described above.

However, about 10–20% of subjects progress rapidly, developing AIDS in less than 5 years of infection, and they are therefore called rapid progressors (see Fig. 88.2). In these patients, after the primary HIV-1 infection, plasma virus levels are often >10⁵ copies of HIV-1 RNA/ml and, in particular, CD4+ T-cell counts start to decrease much earlier and more rapidly during the chronic asymptomatic phase, leading to the eventual development of AIDS. Furthermore, both humoral and cell-mediated HIV-1-specific immune responses are either never detected or rapidly lost after the transition from the acute to the chronic phase of infection.

At the other extreme, it is estimated that 5–15% of HIV-1-infected people will remain free of AIDS for more than 15 years; these people are termed slow progressors (see Fig. 88.2). In this situation, CD4+ T-cell counts remain stable and they are frequently >500 cells/ml, and plasma virus levels are usually <10 000 HIV-1 RNA copies/ml.

Slow progressors include a further subgroup of HIV-1-infected people, so-called long-term nonprogressors (see Fig. 88.2). About 1%

of HIV-1-infected subjects probably fall into this category. The definition of long-term nonprogressors should be limited to those who have had a documented infection for at least 8–10 years, are naive to antiretroviral therapy and have no signs of disease progression (e.g. constant high counts of CD4+ T cells and either low (500–1000 copies of RNA/ml) or very low (<50 copies/ml) plasma virus levels).[1,9] Recently, a subgroup of HIV-1 infected individuals with chronic infection and levels of viremia <50 copies/ml has been termed 'elite controllers'. The definition of elite controllers is independent of the length of the control of viremia.[10]

This wide variability of the natural course of the disease is evidenced by the presence of different driving forces – genetic, immunologic and virologic factors – that determine the evolutionary pattern of HIV-1 infection in the individual patient.[11] It is therefore important, first, to identify the different determinants of the rate of disease progression and, second, to elucidate how these driving forces work together. Furthermore, the potential ability of HAART to restore some determinants of long-term control of the virus must be evaluated in depth. These arguments are discussed in detail below.

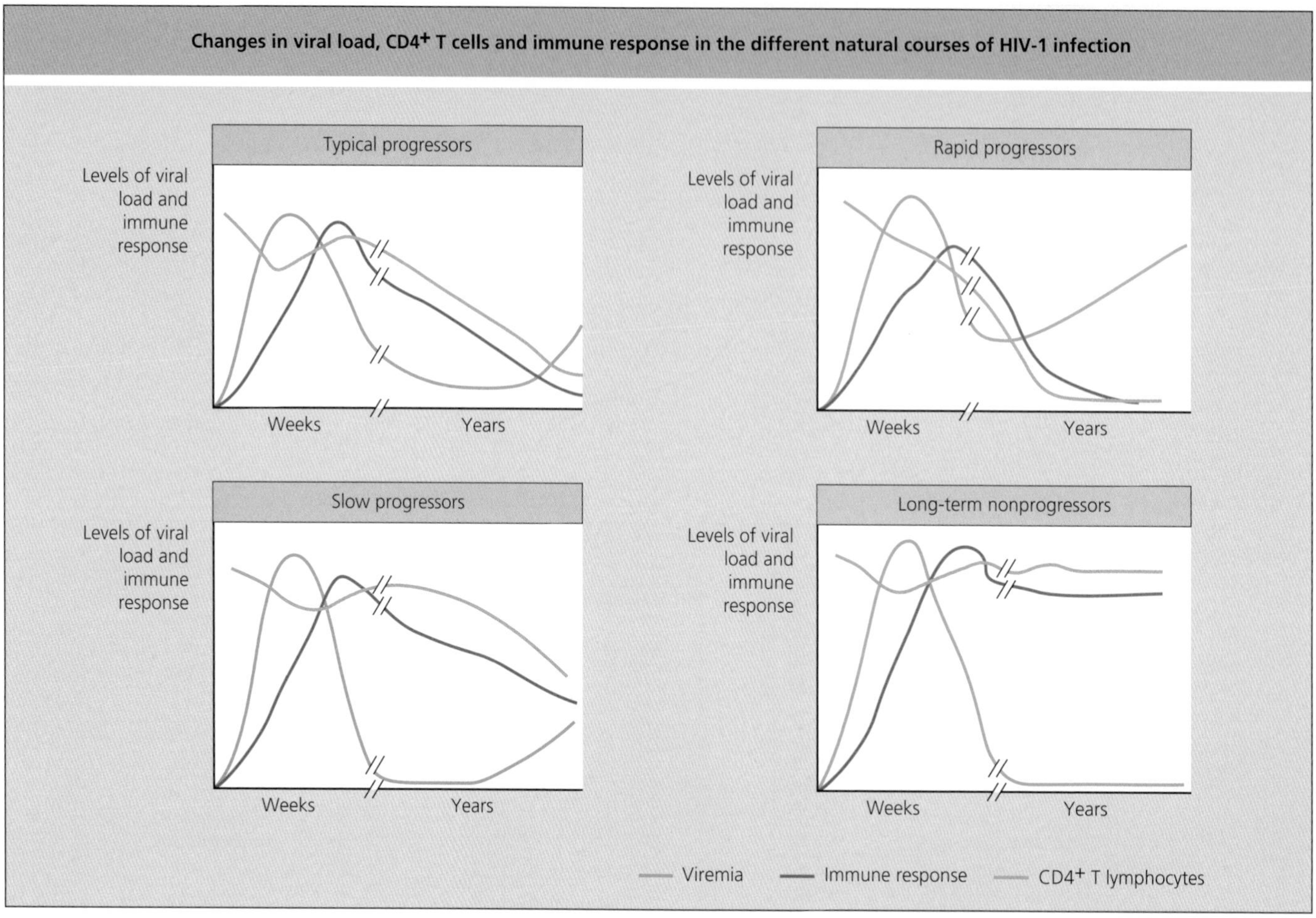

Changes in viral load, CD4+ T cells and immune response in the different natural courses of HIV-1 infection

Fig. 88.2 Changes in viral load, CD4+ T cells and immune response in the different natural courses of HIV-1 infection. Typical progressors represent 60–70% of the total HIV-1-infected population, rapid progressors represent 10–20%, slow progressors represent 5–15% and long-term nonprogressors represent 1%.

The variability of the natural course of HIV-1 infection also underlines the need for markers of disease progression that may identify as early as possible the patients who are at risk for a more rapid disease progression. This could warrant either the use of different, perhaps more aggressive, therapeutic strategies or the need to monitor these patients more closely, or both.

SEQUENCE OF PATHOGENIC EVENTS LEADING TO THE ESTABLISHMENT OF HIV-1 INFECTION

HIV-1 can be transmitted by different routes: by sexual contact, through either genital–genital or genital–oral sex; by blood–blood contamination, via either transfusion of blood and infected blood-derived products or needle sharing among intravenous drug users; and by maternal–fetal transmission. The most common route of infection is sexual transmission at the genital mucosa.[12]

Early pathogenic events after entry of HIV-1 into the body

The acute intravaginal infection of rhesus monkeys with the simian immunodeficiency virus (SIV) represents a very useful model for studying the sequence of cellular events that characterize the very early steps of infection after sexual transmission. In this model, tissue dendritic cells (i.e. Langerhans cells that reside in the lamina propria below the vaginal epithelium) are the first potential target cells of HIV-1 (Fig. 88.3).[13]

The dendritic cells constitute a complex and highly developed system of antigen-presenting cells that are able to prime naive T cells. Their potent antigen-presenting ability is associated with the high expression of major histocompatibility complex (MHC) class I and class II molecules and co-stimulatory molecules on the cell surface. The ability of dendritic cells to attract and prime naive T cells can be explained by the expression of a type II membrane protein with an external mannose binding, C-type lectin domain, named DC-SIGN (meaning dendritic cell-specific intercellular adhesion molecule (ICAM)-3 grabbing nonintegrin).[14,15] It has been suggested that interaction between DC-SIGN and ICAM-3 is responsible for the initial contact between dendritic cells and resting T cells, which represents a critical step for the initiation of the T-cell immune response. Furthermore, a major contribution to the ability of dendritic cells to initiate T-cell immunity is also provided by the fact that dendritic cells express high levels of specific chemokines that target naive rather than memory T cells.[16] Therefore, dendritic cells play a key role, both in priming the initial virus-specific immune response and in serving as a carrier for the transport of HIV-1 to the nearest lymphoid station.

It is important, however, to mention the differences that exist between the Langerhans cells (also called 'epidermal' or 'epithelial' dendritic cells) and the 'dermal' or 'subepithelial' dendritic cells.[15] Langerhans cells do not express DC-SIGN and, once they have

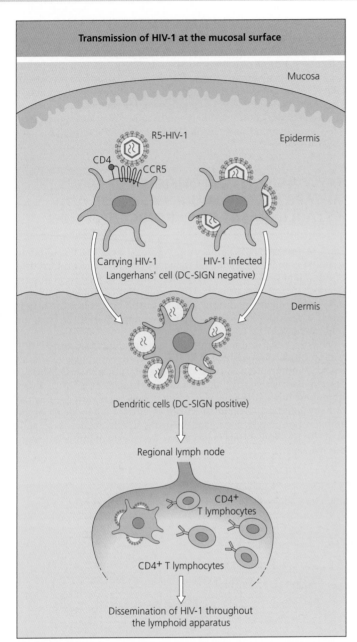

Transmission of HIV-1 at the mucosal surface

Mucosa

Epidermis

R5-HIV-1

CD4

CCR5

Carrying HIV-1
Langerhans' cell (DC-SIGN negative)

HIV-1 infected

Dermis

Dendritic cells (DC-SIGN positive)

Regional lymph node

CD4⁺ T lymphocytes

CD4⁺ T lymphocytes

Dissemination of HIV-1 throughout
the lymphoid apparatus

Fig. 88.3 Transmission of HIV-1 at the mucosal surface. After entry at the mucosal epithelium, Langerhans cells, also named epidermal dendritic cells, can either be infected by R5 (macrophage (M)-tropic) strains of HIV-1 or pick up HIV-1 virions. Epidermal, DC-SIGN-negative dendritic cells are thought to select for the M-tropic viruses that are the most frequently transmitted variants. The M-tropic HIV-1 carried by epidermal dendritic cells can bind to additional subepithelial DC-SIGN-positive dendritic cells. DC-SIGN can capture HIV-1 on the cell surface of dendritic cells without allowing viral entry. It is thought that DC-SIGN-positive dendritic cells play the major role in the delivery of virus to T cells, thus greatly amplifying HIV-1 infection.

encountered HIV-1 below the vaginal epithelium, they can either be infected or pick up HIV-1 virions. Epidermal, DC-SIGN-negative dendritic cells are thought to select for the macrophage (M)-tropic viruses that are the most frequently transmitted variants.[17,18] The M-tropic HIV-1 carried by epidermal dendritic cells can bind to additional subepithelial DC-SIGN-positive dendritic cells. DC-SIGN can capture HIV-1 on the cell surface of dendritic cells without allowing viral entry.[19] It is thought that DC-SIGN-positive dendritic cells

play the major role in the delivery of virus to T cells, thus greatly amplifying HIV-1 infection.[18] Subsequently, dendritic cells migrate to the internal iliac lymph nodes, where they target the T cell areas and then present the viral antigens to activated virus-specific T cells. Dendritic cells can support viral replication only in the presence of activated T cells.[16]

Recent advances in our understanding of the mechanisms that modulate the infectivity of HIV-1 can explain why 95% of viruses transmitted are M-tropic. For more than 10 years, it has been known that human CD4 is sufficient for binding HIV-1 gp120 to cells, but it is sufficient neither for fusion nor for penetration of the viral envelope into the host cell.[20-22] It is now clear that certain cell-surface receptors for chemokines function as co-receptors by co-operating with the CD4 molecule; moreover, different chemokine receptors, together with CD4, allow entry of HIV-1 strains with distinct cellular tropism. There are two major classes of chemokines: CC, if the first two cysteines are adjacent; and CXC, if they are separated by a single amino acid. The CC-chemokine receptor (CCR)5, a seven-transmembrane G-protein-coupled receptor, is the major co-receptor for M-tropic or R5 strains of HIV-1, whereas CXCR4 is the one for T-cell-tropic or X4 strains of HIV-1. Langerhans cells or epithelial dendritic cells express CCR5 but they may not express CXCR4, giving a reason for the preferential transmission of R5 HIV-1 strains.[23]

To this extent, it is worth noting that subepithelial dendritic cells are able to capture the virus through DC-SIGN,[19] a mechanism that is independent of CD4 and co-receptors. However, although both R5 and X4 strains of HIV-1 are carried by dendritic cells to the nearest lymphoid station, only R5 HIV-1 envelopes have the unique ability to mediate an activation signal into CD4⁺ T cells and to recruit them by chemotaxis.[24] Therefore, the combination of the two events (i.e. the differential expression of co-receptors on the initial target cells and the unique signaling ability of R5 envelopes of HIV-1) may explain why R5 HIV-1 variants are preferentially transmitted, ensuring the rapid recruitment of a large number of activated CD4⁺ T cells and spread of HIV-1 in the lymphoid organs. It is important to emphasize that rapid recruitment and spreading of target cells (i.e. activated CD4⁺ T cells) confers to HIV-1 a major advantage because these events occur before the appearance of effective virus-specific immune responses.

Within 2 days after infection, HIV-1 can be detected in the draining lymphoid tissue, and it rapidly disseminates throughout the lymphoid system. Afterwards, HIV-1 enters the bloodstream, where viral replication can be detected in plasma 5 days after infection (see Fig. 88.3). In humans, the time from mucosal infection and initial plasma viremia varies, ranging between 4 days and 11 days according to available estimates. It is of note that the risk of infection is increased by conditions that decrease the function of mucosal barriers, such as lesions caused by the presence of concomitant inflammatory or infectious diseases (e.g. cervicitis, urethritis, genital ulcers).

These same steps of infection can be described in the case of genital–oral HIV-1 transmission, because nasopharyngeal tonsils and adenoid tissue contain many cells of dendritic origin that can support viral replication more efficiently than Langerhans cells.[2]

The role of the gut and lymph nodes in primary HIV-1 infection

The study of virologic events occurring during primary infection with either HIV-1 or SIV emphasizes the key role of the gastrointestinal (GI) tract and lymphoid tissue in the establishment of infection. With regard to the role of the GI tract, it is important to mention that the majority of T cells, particularly CD4 T cells, are contained within the GI tract. Recent studies have demonstrated that memory CD4 T cells within the GI tract, which express the CCR5 HIV-1 co-receptor, are the earliest targets of HIV-1 during primary infection.[25] The monitoring of CD4 T-cell depletion following SIV infection has shown that initial decrease in CD4 T cells may vary between 60% and 80% in blood and lymph nodes while the loss of CD4 T cells is almost complete in the GI tract.[26] Studies performed in humans have also shown that, in addition to the greater depletion of CD4 T cells in the gut, the proportion of HIV-1 infected CD4 T cells resident in the gut is 10–100 fold higher compared to blood.[25]

With regard to the role of lymphoid tissues, longitudinal and cross-sectional analyses of HIV-1 or SIV distribution were performed on lymph node biopsies taken from rhesus monkeys or HIV-1-infected patients. In the SIV model of acute infection, virus can be detected in the lymph node as early as 5 days after infection. At this time, as shown by *in-situ* hybridization analysis for the detection of HIV-1/SIV RNA, virus is mostly present in the form of numerous individual cells expressing viral RNA, and the highest number of virus-expressing cells is observed 7 days after SIV inoculation. Interestingly, the occurrence of the peak number of virus-expressing cells in the lymph node occurs at the same time as the peak of plasma viremia, or shortly precedes it. The cross-sectional analysis of lymph nodes obtained from HIV-1-infected patients indicates that the kinetics of virus distribution in lymph nodes is consistent with those in the SIV model of acute infection.

Altogether, these findings indicate that the GI tract is the primary site for CD4 T-cell depletion caused by HIV-1 infection.[27] In addition, both gut and lymph nodes are primary anatomic sites of virus infection, replication and dissemination.[7,28]

During the transition from primary to chronic infection, a switch from individual virus-expressing cells to virus trapped by the follicular dendritic cell network of lymph node germinal centers occurs (Fig. 88.4). The trapped virus becomes the dominant form of virus present in lymph nodes, and this event is associated with a dramatic decrease in the number of individual cells expressing viral RNA.[7,28]

At least in part, this is the result of the emergence of virus-specific CTLs that can be detected very early during primary infection and may mediate the elimination of HIV-1-producing cells. Furthermore, the trapping of HIV-1 virions in the follicular dendritic cell network is itself the result of the HIV-1-specific humoral response. In fact, HIV-1 virions are complexed with immunoglobulins and complement, and the binding of these complexes on the extracellular surface of follicular dendritic cells occurs through complement receptors expressed on follicular dendritic cells. In both SIV and HIV-1 infection, the transition from primary to early chronic infection is marked by a decrease of viral RNA in plasma and the resolution of the acute clinical syndrome. Therefore, it is clear that virus-specific immune responses are not only present very early during primary infection but may also significantly affect virus distribution occurring in the early phase of both SIV and HIV-1 infection.[29]

MECHANISMS RESPONSIBLE FOR VIRUS ESCAPE FROM IMMUNE RESPONSE AND ESTABLISHMENT OF CHRONIC INFECTION

Early in primary HIV-1 infection, vigorous virus-specific immune responses can be detected, and they may contribute to both control of the initial peak of virus replication and the reduction in plasma viremia.[3–6] However, primary HIV-1 infection invariably results in the establishment of chronic disease in the host, inducing a progressive deterioration of the different components of the immune response.

HIV-1-specific immune responses lack the ability to control HIV-1 and to block the progression of the disease. Nevertheless, similar types of immune response are effective against other viruses, such as Epstein–Barr virus (EBV) and cytomegalovirus (CMV). HIV-1 differs from these other viruses by being able to target very early (during the primary infection) a broad spectrum of effector components of the antiviral immune response and in being able to render these antiviral effector mechanisms ineffective or reshape them into self-defense mechanisms.[30]

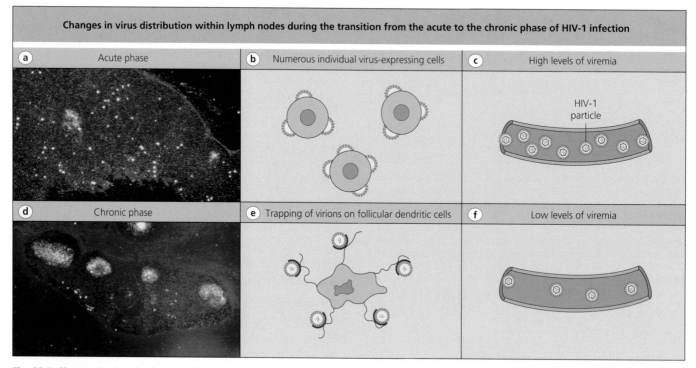

Fig. 88.4 Changes in virus distribution within lymph nodes during the transition from the acute to the chronic phase of HIV-1 infection. (a) During the initial weeks of primary HIV-1 infection, the virus is detected in lymphoid tissue as individual virus-expressing cells. This is shown by *in-situ* hybridization for the detection of HIV-1 RNA (white dots indicate HIV-1 RNA-positive cells). (b) Numerous individual virus-expressing cells seen in the acute phase. (c) Elevated virion levels are found in the circulation in the acute phase. (d) After transition to the chronic phase of the disease, virions trapped in the follicular dendritic cell network become the dominant form of HIV-1, as shown by *in-situ* hybridization for the detection of HIV-1 RNA (diffuse white areas indicate virus trapped within follicular dendritic cells). (e) Binding of virions on the extracellular surface of follicular dendritic cells in the chronic phase. (f) The number of circulating virions is dramatically reduced in the chronic phase.

Virologic mechanisms of HIV-1 escape from the immune response

HIV-1 possesses the ability to put in motion several mechanisms as the result of the interaction with the host. Some of these virologic mechanisms can be identified:

- formation of a stable pool of latently HIV-1-infected CD4+ T cells containing virus that is capable of replicating;[31–35]
- the genetic variability of HIV-1;[36] and
- trapping of infectious virions on the surface of follicular dendritic cells.[37]

The rapid formation of a pool of latently HIV-1-infected CD4+ T cells is a key event in the immunopathogenesis of HIV-1 infection for several reasons. First, this event occurs very early and most probably before the appearance of the host's virus-specific immune responses. Second, the pool of latently infected CD4+ T cells contains replication-competent HIV-1 proviral DNA. The proviral DNA can be detected even in compliant HIV-1-infected persons who have been receiving HAART for a long time (i.e. for more than 2 years); moreover, the virus is wild type with respect to known drug-induced mutations in the genome. This emphasizes the fact that this pool of cells is a stable reservoir in which HIV-1 remains sheltered from the effects of host immune responses and HAART.[31–35] Furthermore, it is worth noting that initiation of HAART very early during primary HIV-1 infection does not appear to have a significant impact on the size of this pool of CD4+ T cells, indicating that this pool is created very rapidly after infection. Third, the decay of this pool of infected CD4+ T lymphocytes is very slow, and the rate of decay is not much influenced by the effective suppression of virus replication obtained by HAART. This clearly represents a major obstacle to the goal of HIV-1 eradication (see below) and long-term control of virus replication.[33–35]

The high genetic variability of the virus is another efficient mechanism by which it escapes the host immune response.[36,38] HIV-1 possesses the intrinsic ability to mutate very rapidly. Both during primary and established chronic infection, rapid mutations in the epitopes recognized by HIV-1-specific CTLs may occur. As a consequence, both humoral and cell-mediated virus-specific immune responses quickly lose their ability to control the virus efficiently.

An additional way by which HIV-1 is able to reshape antiviral mechanisms is the trapping of the virus on the surface of follicular dendritic cells in lymphoid tissue germinal centers. As already described, HIV-1 is trapped by the follicular dendritic cell network during the transition from primary to chronic infection and this becomes the dominant form of virus in lymphoid tissue in the chronic phase. Formation of immune complexes and their attachment to the follicular dendritic cell network are physiologic mechanisms that are generally devoted to the clearance of the pathogen and to the generation and maintenance of effective immune responses. In HIV-1 infection, however, these mechanisms lead to the formation of a stable reservoir of infectious virions, representing a continuous source for the infection of CD4+ T cells, and to a chronic inflammatory reaction that ultimately results in the destruction of the lymphoid tissue.[7,8]

Immunologic mechanisms of HIV-1 escape from the immune response

In addition to the virologic mechanisms described above, through which HIV-1 escapes and reshapes the host immune response, there are some immunologic mechanisms that can be identified:

- deletion of HIV-specific CD4+ T-cell clones;[39]
- deletion/exhaustion of HIV-specific cytotoxic CD8+ T-cell clones;[40–43]
- generation of virus escape mutants mediated by CTLs;[30]
- impairment of the function of antigen-presenting cells;[30] and
- interference with humoral neutralizing response.[30]

In the majority of HIV-1-infected patients who have established chronic infection, HIV-1-specific CD4+ helper T-cell responses, particularly the ability of virus-specific CD4 T cells to proliferate after antigen-specific stimulation, cannot be detected, although it is possible to find evidence of such HIV-1-specific CD4+ T-cell responses in long-term nonprogressors.[39,44] In contrast, HIV-1-specific effector CD4+ T-cell responses, i.e. virus-specific CD4 T cells secreting interferon gamma (IFN-γ) and tumor necrosis factor (TNF), are consistently detected in patients who have chronic infection.[45] The persistence of the CD4+ helper T-cell response may represent one of the determinants of the course of the disease in long-term nonprogressors. In contrast, typical progressors do lose CD4+ helper T-cell responses very early in the natural history of the disease (during the primary HIV-1 infection) as a result of direct or indirect virus-induced cytopathology, particularly within the GI tract and lymph nodes.[39,46] Furthermore, initiation of HAART during chronic infection and even during early HIV-1 infection is associated with the restoration of the HIV-1-specific CD4+ helper T-cell responses only in a subset (about 30–40%) of patients after prolonged treatment.[47] It is, however, possible to preserve HIV-1-specific CD4+ T-cell responses if HAART is initiated at the time of the peak of plasma viral RNA (i.e. very early during primary HIV-1-infection).[39,46]

It is also worth noting that T helper (Th)1 cells, the CD4 T cells mounting the immune responses against HIV-1, preferentially express CCR5 on the membrane surface, suggesting that HIV-1 R5 strains may preferentially and selectively infect Th1 cells during primary HIV infection, when R5 quasispecies predominate. In this regard, a series of studies have demonstrated that the initial expansion of HIV-1-specific CD4+ T cells with effector function is aborted during primary infection.[48] In contrast, the expansion of CMV-specific CD4+ T cells in patients who experienced primary HIV-1 and CMV co-infection was not suppressed. These studies indicate a preferential infection of HIV-1-specific CD4+ T cells. Furthermore, they provide evidence that HIV-1-specific CD4+ T-cell clones may be rapidly deleted very early during primary HIV-1 infection and that the possibility of rescuing these responses is strictly dependent upon the time of initiation of HAART.[39,48]

Furthermore, the lack of HIV-1-specific CD4+ helper T-cell responses has two other important consequences. First, it can significantly affect the induction and persistence of HIV-1-specific CD8+ CTL responses, because the latter require continuous cognate Th function provided by antigen-specific CD4+ T cells. Therefore, generation and maintenance of vigorous virus-specific responses by CTLs can be compromised over time. Second, it can considerably affect the development of HIV-1-specific antibody responses, because the development of humoral responses is strictly dependent on CD4+ antigen-specific Th cells.[30]

A rapid deletion of certain HIV-1-specific cytotoxic CD8+ T-cell clones also occurs during primary HIV-1 infection, in a manner that is analogous to the HIV-1-specific responses mediated by CD4+ helper T cells.[41] These CD8+ T-cell clones undergo massive clonal expansion and may be deleted by a mechanism analogous to the clonal exhaustion that is observed in mice during acute lymphocytic choriomeningitis virus infection. This clonal exhaustion of HIV-1-specific CD8+ CTLs causes the early impairment of the virus-specific responses by CTLs. In this regard, recent studies suggest that during primary infection deletion of CD8 T cells equipped with high avidity T-cell receptors may occur.[49] The extent of this phenomenon may determine the varying ability to control virus replication efficiently and therefore it may significantly affect the rate of disease progression. In fact, it is now clear that the appearance of virus-specific responses by CTLs correlates with the decrease in plasma viremia.[5,50] Furthermore, the higher the relative frequency of HIV-1-specific CTLs, the lower the levels of circulating viral RNA, and higher levels of CTL activity correlate with slower rates of disease progression.[5,50,51] However, the clonal exhaustion of virus-specific CTLs does not necessarily result in a complete loss of HIV-1-specific CTL activity, although it does provide additional evidence of how HIV-1 is able to target and impair host immune responses early in the course of the infection.

The detection of CTL-escape variants is common during the course of chronic HIV-1 infection; however, there is increasing evidence that this phenomenon consistently occurs during primary HIV-1 infection.[52]

This event provides further evidence of the ability of HIV-1 to reshape some antiviral mechanisms of the immune response into self-defense mechanisms. In fact, although HIV-specific CTLs contribute to the control of both plasma viremia and disease progression,[5,50,51] the pressure exerted by CTLs can, at the same time, facilitate the selection of virus mutants that are able to escape the host immune response.[30,41]

In addition to CD4+ and CD8+ HIV-1-specific T cells, HIV-1 may interfere with the function of antigen-presenting cells. These cells play a central role in the generation of an effective host immune response. Cells of the monocyte–macrophage line and dendritic cells can function as specialized antigen-presenting cells and induce both humoral and cell-mediated immune responses. The effect of HIV-1 on these components of the immune system is produced by a quantitative depletion through direct cytopathogenesis or by interference with the formation of MHC-antigenic peptide complexes. To this extent, the expression of MHC class I molecules on antigen-presenting cells can be downregulated by HIV-1 Nef protein, thus affecting both generation of antigen-specific immune responses and recognition of virus-infected target cells by CTLs.[53]

Humoral response against HIV-1 can be detected early during primary HIV-1 infection. This response, however, comprises low-avidity Env-specific IgG that possesses little or no neutralizing activity. Although the reasons for the delay in the appearance of the neutralizing antibody response are poorly understood, such a response is detectable only either after the transition from primary HIV-1 infection to established early chronic HIV-1 infection, or even much later. The virologic and immunologic mechanisms described above significantly affect the global host immune response, within which the CD4+ Th cell function and the interactions between T cells and B cells are profoundly altered. These events may ultimately interfere with circulating titers, avidity maturation and neutralizing activity of HIV-1-specific antibodies.

HOST AND VIROLOGIC FACTORS THAT INFLUENCE THE COURSE OF HIV-1 INFECTION

The events that result in the establishment of chronic HIV-1 infection emphasize the ability of the virus to target the host's antiviral immune response and reshape it into a self-defense mechanism. In this context, the mutual interactions between the virus and the host are major determinants of disease progression. Primary HIV-1 infection is a key phase in the immunopathogenesis of the infection, because all of the events that occur at this stage can determine both the pattern and rate of progression of the disease. In the transition from primary to early chronic HIV-1 infection, levels of plasma viral RNA tend to reach a virologic set-point that is predictive of the rate of disease progression (see below).[54,55] The virologic set-point varies among HIV-1-infected patients and tends to remain stable in the same person during the chronic phase. The virologic set-point that a person attains is determined both by the mechanisms involved in the establishment of chronic infection and by host factors that can modulate the course of HIV-1 disease.

Several factors play an important role in modulating both the antiviral host immune response and the susceptibility to HIV-1, and these factors can thus result in a slower rate of disease progression. These factors are mainly genetic, immunologic and virologic (Table 88.1).[11,30]

Genetic host factors

Patients infected with HIV-1 who experience a nonprogressive disease are more likely to possess certain human leukocyte antigen (HLA) class I haplotypes than other members of the general population. These haplotypes are more efficient than others at binding peptides that correspond to epitopes recognized by virus-specific CTLs. This suggests that persons who have inherited these clusters of haplotypes could generate HIV-1-specific CTL responses against multiple epitopes, thus

Table 88.1 Host factors and virologic factors in HIV-1 infection

Genetic host factors	Immunologic host factors	Virologic factors
HLA class I haplotype Mutations in chemokine receptor or ligand genes: Ø32 in CCR5 m303 in CCR5 V641 in CCR2b G801A in SDF Levels of β-chemokines (RANTES, MIP-1α and MIP-1β)	Qualitative differences in the primary immune response Clonal deletion of HIV-1-specific cytotoxic T cells Persistence of HIV-1-specific CD4+ T-cell responses Chronic immune activation	Extent of HIV-1 replication Viral phenotype (syncytium-inducing or nonsyncytium-inducing strains of HIV-1) Trapping of virions in follicular dendritic cell network Viral latency Size of inoculum

resulting in a more efficient antiviral response, as a consequence of their HLA genetic background.[51] A panel of HLA class I haplotypes has been clearly shown to be associated with different rates of HIV disease progression.[56] HLA*B5701 and HLA*B5703 are strongly associated with delayed progression of disease.[57–59] Similar protective effects has also been observed with HLA*B27.[56] Other HLA haplotypes, including HLA*B5801, B1503, B13, Bw4 and B51, have also been found to be associated with control of virus replication and disease progression.[60] The interaction between HLA*Bw4 and the corresponding KIR3SD1 receptor expressed on natural killer cells has also been associated with slower disease progression.[61] Finally, recent observations have also shown a beneficial effect of HLA C on disease progression.[56]

The recent identification and study of the function of several α- and β-chemokine receptors that can serve as HIV-1 co-receptors have provided evidence of varying chemokine receptor genetic polymorphisms that can influence susceptibility to HIV-1 infection and are associated with different rates of disease progression. CXC or α-chemokine and CC or β-chemokine receptor molecules are part of the vast and functionally diverse family of seven-transmembrane G protein-coupled receptors. CXCR4, the first identified co-receptor, mediates T-cell-tropic viral fusion and entry (X4 HIV-1 strains), but it does not function as a co-receptor for the M-tropic HIV-1 envelope. The major co-receptor for M-tropic HIV-1 strains is CCR5; other CC chemokine receptors, such as CCR2b, CCR3 and CCR8, can serve as co-receptors for R5 or dual-tropic (i.e. primary HIV-1 isolates) HIV-1 strains.[62–67]

Some HIV-1-negative persons, despite being at high risk of exposure, appear to have an innate ability to 'resist' HIV-1 infection. Mapping of the CCR5 structural gene on the human chromosome 3p21 allowed the identification of a 32 base-pair deletion allele (Δ32CCR5) that encodes a truncated and nonfunctional molecule that fails to reach the cell surface. As a result, cells susceptible to HIV-1 are highly resistant to infection by R5 strains. Available prevalence estimates indicate that between 15% and 20% of Caucasians are heterozygous for the mutation, whereas 1% or fewer are homozygous.[68] The study of large cohorts of HIV-1-negative persons, including those who have had multiple exposures to HIV-1, and HIV-1-infected patients has provided evidence that the homozygous genotype for the mutation (i.e. Δ32CCR5–Δ32CCR5) confers high resistance to infection by HIV-1,[68] although a few HIV-1-infected patients possess the Δ32CCR5–Δ32CCR5 homozygous genotype. However, the heterozygous genotype (CCR5–Δ32CCR5) does not prevent HIV-1 from infecting susceptible cells but is significantly associated with a slower rate of disease progression in HIV-1-infected patients and is found more commonly in long-term nonprogressors.[69] In heterozygotes there is a decreased expression of the CCR5 receptor, which can be explained by a transdominant inhibition of wild-type CCR5 receptor function owing to the concomitant intracellular presence of both normal and defective gene products withheld in the endoplasmic reticulum.[70] Another mutation (m303) in the CCR5 gene prevents the expression of the receptor on the cell surface by introducing a premature stop codon. This mutation, when in *trans* with the Δ32CCR5 defective gene, confers resistance because no expression of CCR5 receptor occurs.[71] Studies centered on the investigation of the CCR5 promoter have shown a certain degree of CCR5 polymorphism and certain variants are associated with different rates of HIV disease progression.[72–74]

Furthermore, other genetic variants do not prevent infection but rather delay the progression of HIV-1 disease. However, their protective effect has not been confirmed in all studies, emphasizing the need to evaluate their role in larger cohorts. These genetic variants include a mutant CCR2b allele (V64I), which encodes a base mutation that replaces valine with isoleucine at position 64 in the transmembrane domain I of the CCR2b receptor,[75–79] and a guanosine-to-adenosine transition at position 801 (G801A) in the 3′ untranslated region of the reference sequence in the gene of the stromal-derived factor (SDF)-1,[80,81] which is the ligand for CXCR4.

Epidemiologically, the inheritance of the CCR2b mutant is less beneficial than the inheritance of the Δ32CCR5 mutant in terms of reducing the risk of progression to AIDS; however, as in the case of CCR5–Δ32CCR5 heterozygosity, the V64I mutant is more commonly found in long-term nonprogressors.[77] Biologically, it is not clear how the V64I allele could interfere with the co-receptor function, because valine and isoleucine are chemically very similar. It is possible that the V64I allele is in linkage disequilibrium with other mutations,[75,78,79] as it has been described with a point mutation in the CCR5 regulatory region.[75]

As far as the SDF-1 G801A mutant allele is concerned, available data are somewhat puzzling. On the one hand, the status of homozygosity for the mutation has been associated with a lower risk of progression to AIDS.[81] A possible explanation for such a protective effect is that the presence of mutant alleles induces a higher than usual release of SDF-1, which inhibits X4 HIV-1 strains. X4 strains tend to emerge during the late phase of the disease and their appearance is generally associated with a more rapid progression. The SDF-1 at high levels could therefore interfere with the spreading of X4 HIV-1 strains, thus reducing the rate of disease progression. Homozygosity for the SDF-1 mutant has been linked to a higher risk of death, although the potential explanation is unclear.[80] Recent analyses performed on different cohorts highly question the interpretation of the original observations.[82,83]

Different haplotypes of the chemokine receptor CX3CR1, a minor HIV-1 co-receptor, have been associated with different rates of HIV disease progression.[84] The CX3CR1–I249/M280 haplotype with more rapid progression to AIDS and the CX3CR1–I249/T280 haplotype have been more frequently found in long-term nonprogressors.[85] Furthermore, recent results have shown that the CXCR1-Ha haplotype of the CXCR1 chemokine receptor is more frequently found in individuals with slow disease progression and is associated with reduced expression of CD4 and CXCR4.[86] The reduced expression of CD4 and CXCR4 may result in decreased susceptibility of infection of target cells with X4-tropic strains of HIV-1.[86]

The initial studies that discovered the role of chemokine receptors as HIV-1 co-receptors originated from the observation that chemokines can potently modulate HIV-1 infectivity.[87] The β-chemokines that are 'regulated upon activation, normal T expressed and secreted' (RANTES) – macrophage inflammatory protein (MIP)-1α and MIP-1β – have been identified as major HIV-suppressive factors produced by CD8+ T cells *in vitro*. Furthermore, endogenous levels of RANTES, MIP-1α and MIP-1β expression in CD4+ T cells were much elevated in some people who remained uninfected despite multiple sexual exposures to HIV-1-infected partners.[88] The binding of one chemokine to its cognate receptor essentially mediates the downregulation of surface chemokine receptor expression. Therefore, in addition to genetic control, chemokine levels themselves may influence infectivity and disease progression. In particular, there is evidence

that very high levels of RANTES, MIP-1α and MIP-1β are detectable in persons bearing the Δ32CCR5–Δ32CCR5 homozygous genotype.[88] Similarly, unusually high levels of β-chemokines have been found in people with hemophilia who have remained uninfected with HIV-1 despite repeated exposure to contaminated blood products before HIV-1 testing became available.[89] Furthermore, levels of MIP-1β (which is the only suppressive CCR5-specific chemokine) in those who have overt AIDS can be significantly lower than those in HIV-1-infected patients who have chronic disease; moreover, higher levels of MIP-1β are associated with a lower risk of disease progression.[90] Recent studies indicate that the different levels of expression of RANTES results from the identification of different genetic variants of RANTES in its promoter region.[91,92] Certain genetic variants of RANTES have been associated with different rates of disease progression but additional studies are needed to support further these preliminary observations.[93]

Along the same line, recent studies have shown the importance of CCL3L1 which is at the same time a potent agonist of CCR5 and a potent inhibitor of R5-HIV-1 strains.[94] It has been shown that CCL3L1 high copy numbers are associated with higher levels of CCL3L1 secretion. Of interest, it was also shown that CCL3L1 low copy numbers were found in infected compared to uninfected individuals.[95]

These observations suggest that suppressive chemokines may play a role in the control of HIV-1. Production of chemokines by effector CD4+ T cells occurs at the site of virus replication, and the chemokines may protect local target cells and activated effector cells by downregulating CCR5 in an autocrine manner. The varying extents to which these mechanisms are put in motion may explain the varying levels of protection against disease progression.

Recent studies have highlighted the importance of endocellular factors and their impact on HIV-1 replication. The host factor APOBEC3G mediates strong antiviral activity and its antiviral activity is suppressed by the Vif HIV-1 protein.[96] Similar antiviral activity has been shown for the host factor TRIM5α.[97] However, contradictory results have been obtained in different *in vitro* systems or patient populations and therefore the antiviral effects of TRIM5α need further confirmation.[98]

In summary, host genetic factors do play a role in modulating the course of HIV-1 infection. Furthermore, the potential role of chemokines in affecting infectivity and disease progression may further widen our therapeutic options along with HAART.

Virologic factors

As discussed above, interaction among different host factors helps to determine a certain virologic set-point in each HIV-1-infected person after the transition from primary to chronic HIV-1 infection.[54,55] This set point represents the level of plasma viral RNA that accurately predicts disease progression (i.e. the level of plasma viremia that corresponds to a risk of progression to either AIDS or death). In the past, many predictors have been identified – clinical, biologic and virologic. The CD4+ T-cell count is historically the most important and widely used predictor. However, the load of plasma RNA is an accurate predictor, especially when used along with the CD4+ T-cell count.[54] Therefore, the higher the plasma viral RNA load, the greater the risk of rapid progression to AIDS and death. It is worth noting that the power of association between levels of plasma HIV-1 RNA and risk of progression does not significantly vary if viremia is measured after seroconversion (i.e. knowing the date and duration of HIV-1 infection) or during the established chronic asymptomatic phase (i.e. with no available information about the duration of the infection, as is often the case in clinical settings).[55] Viral load is therefore a very powerful predictor if measured during the chronic asymptomatic phase, once the virologic set-point has been reached.

However, the level of plasma viral RNA lacks accuracy and reliability as a predictor if measured during primary HIV-1 infection.[99] In this phase, rapid disease progression is predicted by:

- a retroviral syndrome lasting more than 14 days;
- the number and the intensity of clinical signs and symptoms;

- central nervous system involvement; and
- viral phenotype.

The viral phenotype is an important virologic factor that can contribute to the rate of disease progression. R5 HIV-1 strains are non-syncytium-inducing strains, whereas X4 HIV-1 strains are syncytium-inducing strains. Syncytium-inducing strains tend to emerge during the late phase of the disease and a shift in viral phenotype from non-syncytium-inducing strains to syncytium-inducing strains heralds disease progression. The viral phenotype of the non-syncytium-inducing strains is associated with prolonged AIDS-free survival and is more commonly found in long-term nonprogressors.[100]

IMMUNE CORRELATES OF PROTECTION

Functional and phenotypic patterns of HIV-1-specific CD4 T-cell responses

The pattern of the HIV-1-specific CD4 T-cell response during primary infection is typical of an effector response, i.e. IFN-γ/TNF secreting CD4 T-cell response.[101–104] The patterns of HIV-1-specific CD4 T-cell responses in the chronic phase of infection are strictly dependent on a series of factors,[105] including the lack of control of virus replication, the initiation of antiviral therapy during the acute phase and treatment-mediated virus suppression, and the spontaneous control of virus replication as it may occur in a small (1%) percentage of subjects known as long-term nonprogressors (LTNP).[106] In the absence of control of virus replication, the HIV-1-specific CD4 T-cell response during chronic infection remains unchanged compared to the acute infection phase, i.e. typical effector IFN-γ/TNF response.[104,105] Following antiviral therapy-mediated virus suppression and in LTNP, who spontaneously control virus replication with viremia levels <50 HIV-1 RNA copies per ml of plasma (the limit of detection of the standard polymerase chain reaction assay), the HIV-1-specific CD4 T-cell response is composed of single interleukin (IL)-2, IL-2/IFN-γ/TNF and IFN-γ/TNF secreting cell populations similar to the CD4 T-cell response in chronic CMV infection.[104,105,107–109]

With regard to virus-specific proliferation, HIV-1-specific proliferating CD4 T cells are generally not detected during acute infection.[102] The detection of virus-specific proliferative CD4 T-cell responses is consistently associated with the presence of virus-specific IL-2 secreting CD4 T-cell populations during chronic infection.[105] With regard to HIV-1 infection, they are found in LTNP and in a proportion (about 40%) of subjects following antiviral therapy.[110]

The phenotype of HIV-1-specific CD4 T cells during primary infection is typical of effector cells, i.e. CD45RA⁻CCR7⁻.[105] Therefore, HIV-1-specific CD4 T cells with the CD45RA⁻CCR7⁻ phenotype belong to the IFN-γ/TNF secreting cells.[104,105] The phenotype of virus-specific CD4 T cells is substantially different during the chronic phase of infection.[104,105] These changes are consistent with the presence of functionally distinct CD4 T-cell populations and of cell populations at different stages of differentiation. The phenotype of HIV-1-specific CD4 T cells remains unchanged compared to primary infection in the absence of control of virus replication, i.e. CD45RA⁻CCR7⁻, consistent with the presence of effector IFN-γ/TNF secreting cells.[104,105]

Functional and phenotypic patterns of virus-specific CD8 T-cell responses

HIV-1-specific CD8 T cells during primary infection are typical effector cells, i.e. IFN-γ/TNF secreting cells. The patterns of the HIV-1-specific CD8 T-cell response during the chronic phase of infection generally correlate with the extent of virus control. The HIV-1-specific CD8 T-cell response remains predominantly an effector response, i.e. IFN-γ/TNF secreting cells, in association with uncontrolled virus replication. Both IL-2/IFN-γ/TNF and IFN-γ/TNF secreting CD8 T cells are found in LTNP in association with controlled virus replication.[104,105] The presence of both IL-2/IFN-γ/TNF and IFN-γ/TNF

secreting HIV-1-specific CD8 T cells was found only in 30–40% of subjects following successful suppression of virus replication by antiviral therapy. Therefore, antiviral therapy-mediated suppression of virus replication is not associated with consistent detection of the IL-2 CD8 T-cell response as is the case for the HIV-1-specific CD4 T-cell response that is constantly associated with the detection of single IL-2 and IL-2/IFN-γ/TNF cells. HIV-1-specific CD8 T-cell proliferation was dependent upon the presence of the IL-2/IFN-γ/TNF secreting cells and thus was consistently observed in the LTNP and in the 30–40% of subjects successfully treated with antiviral therapy.[111]

The phenotype of HIV-1-specific CD8 T cells during primary infection is typical of effector cells, i.e. CD45RA⁻CCR7⁻. The phenotype of virus-specific CD8 T cells is substantially different during the chronic phase of infection.[111] As in the case of CD4 T cells, the changes were consistent with the presence of functionally distinct CD8 T-cell populations at different stages of differentiation. The phenotype of HIV-1-specific CD8 T cells in chronic infection with uncontrolled virus replication remains unchanged compared to primary infection, i.e. CD45RA⁻CCR7⁻.[111] The phenotype of HIV-1-specific CD8 T cells in LTNP was mostly composed of two cell populations (CD45RA⁻CCR7⁺ and CD45RA⁻CCR7⁻) that contained both IL-2/IFN-γ/TNF cells and IFN-γ/TNF cells.

Protective T-cell response

Recent studies have provided evidence for both functional and phenotypic heterogeneity of Ag-specific CD4 and CD8 T-cell responses observed in different virus infections.[112–122] A number of hypotheses have been proposed such as:

- the virus hypothesis proposing that the heterogeneity of the virus-specific immune response is strictly dependent on each virus;[123]
- the maturation hypothesis proposing that certain viruses such as HIV-1 may skew the maturation of HIV-1-specific T cells as compared to other viruses such as CMV and EBV;[102,124] and
- the senescence hypothesis proposing that the functional loss of HIV-1-specific T cells is due to the rapid senescence of T cells which is selectively induced by HIV-1.[123]

The above hypotheses were originally proposed to explain the functional impairment of CD8 T cells in HIV-1 infection but can also be applied to CD4 T cells. The different observations and hypotheses are not mutually exclusive, and indeed what they reflect is the existence of different functional/phenotypic patterns of T-cell responses that can be explained through a single mechanism. The likely mechanism is that the functional/phenotypic heterogeneity of virus-specific CD4 and CD8 T-cell responses is predominantly dependent on, and modulated by, different levels of Ag load.

In support of this mechanism, different functional patterns of CD4 and CD8 T-cell responses can be observed within the same virus infection.[104,105,107,111] The effector IFN-γ/TNF CD4 and CD8 T-cell response during primary HIV-1 infection associated with high Ag load switches to a memory response composed of single IL-2, IL-2/IFN-γ/TNF and IFN-γ/TNF CD4 T cells and of IL-2/IFN-γ/TNF and IFN-γ/TNF CD8 T cells after the transition to the chronic phase of infection associated with virus control and very low levels (not detectable) of Ag load.[102,104,105,107,108,111] The HIV-1-specific CD4 T-cell response is an effector IFN-γ/TNF response during primary infection and chronic infection with uncontrolled virus replication. It shifts to a memory response composed of single IL-2, IL-2/IFN-γ/TNF and IFN-γ/TNF CD4 T cells either in LTNP or subjects treated with antiviral therapy, i.e. conditions with controlled virus replication and low/undetectable Ag load. The interruption of antiviral therapy causes the loss of control of virus replication, high Ag load and the shift back to the effector IFN-γ/TNF CD4 T-cell response.[104]

The differences in the functional patterns of CD8 T-cell response observed between chronic HIV-1 infection with uncontrolled virus replication and high Ag load and chronic HIV-1 in LTNP associated with virus control/elimination and low/undetectable Ag load support the hypothesis that HIV-1-specific CD8 T-cell responses are also modulated by Ag load.[111,125] Overall, the functional and the phenotypic patterns of CD4 and CD8 T-cell responses reflect different levels of virus replication and Ag load and different stages of T-cell differentiation, i.e. effector cells and, within memory cells, T_{CM}, T_{EM} and T_{ET}. The functional T-cell patterns seem to follow the rule: high Ag load = effector IFN-γ/TNF T-cell response while low/undetectable Ag load = single IL-2 (only for CD4 T cells) plus IL-2/IFN-γ/TNF plus IFN-γ/TNF T-cell memory response.

The investigation of the functional patterns of virus-specific CD4 and CD8 T-cell responses against the most common human viruses has provided substantial advances in the identification of the T-cell immune responses that may be effective in the control of virus replication and in the prevention of establishment of persistent chronic infection and virus-associated disease.[105] In this regard, it has been instrumental in determining the functional characterization of virus-specific CD4 and CD8 T cells on the basis of their ability to secrete IL-2, TNF and IFN-γ following Ag-specific stimulation for several reasons. These include:[104,105,107,108,111]

- a strong correlation between the presence of virus-specific CD4 and CD8 IL-2 secreting T cells and virus control;
- the presence of CD4 and CD8 IL-2 secreting T cells being always associated with the proliferation capacity; and
- no correlation between the presence of IFN-γ/TNF secreting CD4 and CD8 T cells and also the presence of cytotoxic function in CD8 T cells and virus control.

Therefore, protective CD4 and CD8 T-cell responses are characterized by the presence of multiple cytokine secreting cells, i.e. single IL-2, IL-2/IFN-γ/TNF and IFN-γ/TNF CD4 T cells and IL-2/IFN-γ/TNF and IFN-γ/TNF CD8 T cells, and by the proliferation capacity of these cells.[104,105,111] It is important to mention that the two cytokines secreting CD8 T-cell populations are also cytotoxic.[126]

The ability of CD4 and CD8 T cells to mediate multiple functions identifies functional signatures of CD4 and CD8 T-cell responses (Fig. 88.5). We have termed these responses polyfunctional. The presence of only effector IFN-γ/TNF CD4 and CD8 T-cell responses and of cytotoxic function in CD8 T cells may correspond to an effective response during the effector phase of the response, i.e. during primary infection or virus re-activation in chronic infection, but it is invariably a non-effective immune response in persistent chronic infection with uncontrolled virus replication. The effector IFN-γ/TNF CD4 and CD8 T-cell responses have been termed monofunctional. Although there is no formal demonstration that polyfunctional CD4 and CD8 T-cell responses

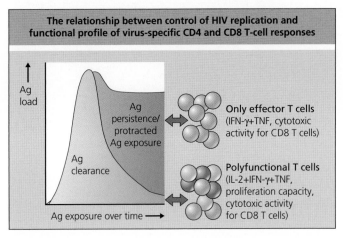

The relationship between control of HIV replication and functional profile of virus-specific CD4 and CD8 T-cell responses

Fig. 88.5 Schematic representation of the relationship between control of HIV replication and functional profile of virus-specific CD4 and CD8 T-cell responses. Only effector T cells secrete only inflammatory cytokines, lack proliferation capacity, are cytotoxic (for CD8 T cells) and are at a more advanced stage of differentiation. Polyfunctional T cells secrete IL-2 in addition to inflammatory cytokines, are endowed with proliferation capacity, are cytotoxic (for CD8 T cells) and also contain cells at an earlier stage of differentiation.

are directly responsible for control of virus replication and prevention of virus-associated disease, polyfunctional T-cell responses may certainly be used as markers of effective antiviral immunity. The advances in the delineation of antiviral protective T-cell responses may provide important insights in the evaluation of the so-called T-cell vaccines.

REFERENCES

References for this chapter can be found online at http://www.expertconsult.com

Primary HIV infection

INTRODUCTION

Although primary HIV infection (PHI) is a rarely diagnosed, self-limiting disease, it is a topic of considerable interest, since the first encounter of HIV with the immune system sheds light on many aspects of pathogenesis. As the severity of PHI predicts progression to immunodeficiency years later, it is reasonable to hope that treatment of PHI can delay or even prevent progression to AIDS. From a public health perspective, a diagnosis of PHI is important because such patients are highly infectious.[1,2] To miss a diagnosis of PHI is to miss an opportunity both for intervention and for prevention of further transmission.

Experience shows that the diagnosis is not difficult to make; education is the key.

EPIDEMIOLOGY

Primary HIV infection is often asymptomatic but sometimes it presents with dramatic manifestations requiring hospital admission. There is a spectrum between complete absence of symptoms during the time of seroconversion and severe disease; therefore, it is not surprising that opinions vary about the percentage of patients who have symptomatic PHI. A physician's previous experience with PHI and a high index of suspicion greatly increase the rate of recognition of PHI. Retrospective analysis from the US armed forces showed that 33% of patients suffered from an identifiable disease between their last seronegative and first seropositive serum sample. At the other extreme, in Australia,[3] 93% of seroconverting persons reported having been 'sick' compared with 40% of controls; 12% of seroconverting patients were hospitalized as a result of symptomatic PHI.

It is not known what factors determine the severity of PHI. Theoretically, the size of the inoculum, the virulence of the infecting HIV strain (including such factors as cellular tropism and cytopathogenicity) and the patient's immune status could be involved, but evidence as to whether these factors are important is lacking. One series of transfusion-associated cases found that symptomatic PHI was more frequent among those infected by people who had late-stage disease (and presumably high circulating viral loads). There is little evidence that the frequency or severity of PHI differs between transmission categories or between men and women. Symptomatic PHI can occur with HIV-2 infection and in children, although almost all cases have been reported in adults infected with HIV-1. There are theoretic reasons to believe that co-infection with other viruses, particularly from the herpes group, might enhance the proliferation of HIV, and patients who are simultaneously co-infected with cytomegalovirus have had particularly severe symptoms of PHI.

Symptoms typically start 2–4 weeks after infection, with extremes of 5 and more than 90 days. The median duration of symptoms is estimated between 12 and 28 days.[4] Moderate and subjective symptoms such as fatigue may persist for months, although almost all patients eventually enter an asymptomatic phase lasting years.

PATHOGENESIS AND PATHOLOGY

Studies of acute simian immunodeficiency virus (SIV) infection have elucidated aspects of HIV and AIDS. Weeks after inoculation, SIV causes massive loss of memory CD4+ cells in many tissues,[5] but particularly in the intestinal tract.[6] Increased permeability of the gut permits translocation of microbial products, resulting in chronic immune activation which is a hallmark of progressive HIV infection.[7]

Because PHI most often presents as a benign self-limiting disease, pathologic information is only available from easily biopsied tissues. The skin rash is caused by a dermal perivascular lymphohistiocytic infiltrate around vessels of the superficial dermis; the epidermis is normal. The inflammatory cells are predominantly of the CD4+ phenotype, and may represent a T-cell-mediated reaction to HIV and to the p24 antigen, which can be detected in Langerhans cells.

Lymph node biopsies reveal abundant HIV, including the envelope proteins gp120 and gp160 in dendritic reticulum cells, as well as in lymphocytes. The structure of the germinal centers is relatively normal and quite unlike the follicular hyperplasia of established HIV-1 infection, but extrafollicular B lymphocytes are reduced in number and the follicles are infiltrated by CD8+ T cells.[8,9]

Therapy has a pronounced effect on the quantity of HIV detectable in lymph nodes. There is a lag of more than 6 months between disappearance of the virus from plasma and disappearance from lymph nodes. However, even patients who have no detectable viremia for several months while being treated for PHI, and whose lymph node biopsies are apparently free from HIV, relapse after discontinuing medication. These findings emphasize the essential role of a virus reservoir for HIV provided by memory T cells.[10]

CLINICAL FEATURES

During PHI, HIV floods the blood with massive viremia,[11] spreading to the central nervous system (CNS)[12] and the lymphatic system, and invades a number of other tissues. Not surprisingly, PHI is a disease with protean clinical manifestations. Three main presentations have been described.

Cutaneous presentation

This is characterized by a maculopapular rash, 'roseola' and mucosal ulcerations (Figs 89.1–89.4). The rash affects the face, neck and trunk more than the limbs, although the palms and soles may be involved. Individual lesions are usually less than 1 cm in diameter and confluence is rare. Case reports have mentioned pustular eruptions, urticaria, erythema multiforme and, during the healing phase of PHI, alopecia and desquamation. Ulceration may occur on the genital and oral mucosa, including the esophagus, where differentiation from herpetic lesions or esophageal candidiasis is difficult.

Presentation resembling infectious mononucleosis

This is characterized by fever, pharyngitis, arthralgia, myalgia and lymphadenopathy. Although the expression 'mononucleosis-like illness' is firmly established, there are many differences from classic

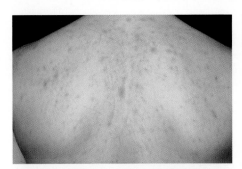

Fig. 89.1 Maculopapular rash during primary HIV infection.

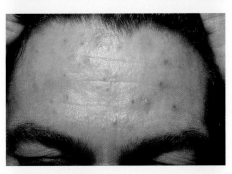

Fig. 89.2 Acneiform lesions during primary HIV infection.

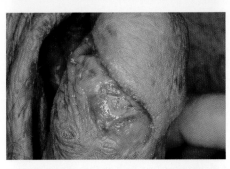

Fig. 89.3 Penile ulcer during primary HIV infection.

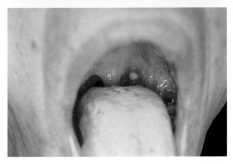

Fig. 89.4 Mucosal ulcerations during primary HIV infection.

Table 89.1 Signs and symptoms of primary HIV infection*

	Symptom/sign	%
Reported by more than 50%	Fever	77
	Lethargy/fatigue	66
	Rash	56
	Myalgia	55
	Headache	51
Reported by 20–50%	Pharyngitis	44
	Cervical adenopathy	39
	Arthralgia	31
	Oral ulcer	29
	Pain on swallowing	28
	Axillary adenopathy	24
	Weight loss	24
	Nausea	24
	Diarrhea	23
	Night sweats	22
	Cough	22
	Anorexia	22
Reported by 5–20%	Abdominal pain	19
	Oral candidiasis	17
	Vomiting	12
	Photophobia	12
	Meningitis	12
	Genital ulcer	7
	Tonsillitis	7
	Depression	7
	Dizziness	6

*These signs and symptoms are reported by at least 5% of patients.[1,2]

infectious mononucleosis, most notably the lack of prominent tonsillar involvement. In a large series (Table 89.1), only 20% of patients had a fever in combination with sore throat and enlarged cervical lymph nodes, whereas 10% did not have fever, sore throat or cervical lymphadenopathy.

Meningoencephalitis

Meningoencephalitis is characterized by photophobia and neck stiffness, headaches and disordered consciousness. The headache is typically retro-orbital and exacerbated by eye movements. Depression and changes in mood are frequent and may reflect underlying encephalitis.

Other symptoms

Table 89.1 shows the frequencies of signs and recorded symptoms in the medical charts of more than 200 patients from Switzerland and Australia. Digestive manifestations have not been well recognized in the past, but they are quite common. In exceptional cases, esophageal candidiasis (an AIDS-defining disease) may occur with a transient decline in CD4+ lymphocyte count.

Unusual manifestations associated with PHI include:

- neurologic syndromes such as radiculopathy, peripheral facial neuropathy and Guillain–Barré syndrome, and severe encephalitis with prolonged coma and seizures; and
- pulmonary involvement, which may be more frequent in intravenous drug users where PHI can be associated with bacterial pneumonia; severe pneumonitis leading to intubation and *Pneumocystis jirovecii* (formerly *P. carinii*) pneumonia[13] (with CD4+ lymphocyte counts of <100/mm³) has been described but is exceptional.

Table 89.2 Important differential diagnoses

Clinical features	Epstein–Barr virus infection	Primary HIV infection
Onset	Gradual	Abrupt
Tonsil involvement	+++	+
Pharyngeal exudate	+++	–
Rash	Rare except in patients treated with antibiotics	Frequent
Jaundice	10%	Never
Diarrhea	Rare	25%

Clinical features	Syphilis	HIV infection
Serology	Always positive	At first negative
Chancre: timing	Before generalized rash	At the same time as rash
Chancre: pain	Painless	Painful

Clinical features	Enterovirus meningitis	HIV meningitis
Population	Young adults	Young adults
Diarrhea	Rare	23%
Season	Summer–autumn	None in particular
Duration	<8 days	Often >20 days
Encephalitis	None	Frequent
Skin lesions	Rare	Frequent
Pain on swallowing	None	Frequent

Differential diagnosis

Important differential diagnoses are listed in Table 89.2; PHI must be distinguished from Epstein–Barr virus infection (infectious mononucleosis) and enterovirus meningitis, and according to the local epidemiologic context, typhoid fever, rickettsial infections and many others. The relatively few primary HIV infections easily get lost among the multitudes who present with fever, rash and pharyngitis. For instance, an estimated 6.4 million patients seeking ambulatory care present with pharyngitis each year in the USA; of these, 8500 (0.13%) have primary HIV infection.[13]

DIAGNOSIS

Seroconversion (i.e. the documented first appearance of HIV antibodies in the serum) occurs days after the beginning of the symptoms of PHI. Therefore, the usual antibody tests for HIV are not entirely reliable; they are expected to be negative during the first few days of PHI (Fig. 89.5). Assays differ in the duration of this 'seronegative period'; with the currently used sensitive tests it is usually less than 1 week after the start of symptoms of PHI.

The p24 antigen is positive when the antibody test is still negative during PHI, and the same is true of HIV viremia. Whereas both tests can be used to screen for PHI, the p24 antigen test is considerably cheaper.[14] Viremia levels reach extremely high values, often in excess of 10^6 viral genomes/ml,[15] and high titers of infectious virus have been isolated from many tissues, including seminal fluid, corroborating the epidemiologic evidence that patients who have PHI are highly infectious. Viremia decreases rapidly – at least 100-fold within days after seroconversion – but remains detectable in more than 95% of patients. Steady-state plasma viremia levels predict progression to advanced immunodeficiency and death.[16] Levels tend to remain higher in those who have symptomatic PHI.[17]

Despite the relatively short duration of PHI, a substantial percentage of newly diagnosed HIV infections are acquired from patients who are themselves recently infected.[17,18]

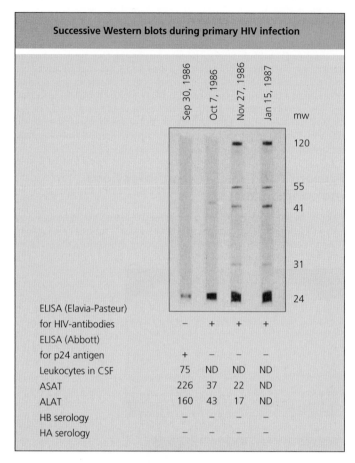

Successive Western blots during primary HIV infection

	Sep 30, 1986	Oct 7, 1986	Nov 27, 1986	Jan 15, 1987
ELISA (Elavia-Pasteur) for HIV-antibodies	–	+	+	+
ELISA (Abbott) for p24 antigen	+	–	–	–
Leukocytes in CSF	75	ND	ND	ND
ASAT	226	37	22	ND
ALAT	160	43	17	ND
HB serology	–	–	–	–
HA serology	–	–	–	–

Fig. 89.5 Successive Western blots during primary HIV infection. Note that on September 30, 1986, when the patient presented with fever, rash, meningitis and subclinical hepatitis, the screening enzyme-linked immunosorbent assay (ELISA) test for HIV antibodies was negative, while the Western blot showed only a single weak band corresponding to the p24 antigen. CSF, cerebrospinal fluid; ASAT, aspartate transaminase; ALAT, alanine transaminase; H, hepatitis (A or B); ND, not done.

Like viremia levels, lymphocyte subsets undergo rapid changes during PHI (Fig. 89.6). During the first 5–10 days, lymphopenia characteristically affects both CD4+ and CD8+ lymphocytes, with levels[13] that may be as low as those observed in AIDS. Although opportunistic infections are rare, in-vitro tests of both B and T cells show immunosuppression. Within another 2–3 weeks there is a lymphocytosis. The CD8+ lymphocyte count expands more than the CD4+ lymphocyte count, leading to a CD4+/CD8+ lymphocyte ratio of less than 1. This low ratio persists even in patients whose CD4+ lymphocyte count subsequently rises to normal.

Many other laboratory values may be abnormal during PHI, reflecting the acute inflammatory response (e.g. high erythrocyte sedimentation rate, increase in C-reactive protein) and involvement of the bone marrow (thrombocytopenia), the liver (increase in hepatic transaminases) and the CNS (pleocytosis of the cerebrospinal fluid).

MANAGEMENT

Although PHI can be severe and prolonged, it is most often a self-limiting disease. The symptoms eventually abate and the patient becomes asymptomatic. Years later, immunosuppression may appear and AIDS may develop.

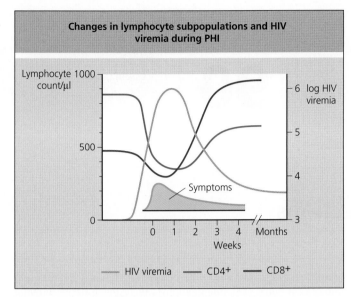

Fig. 89.6 Changes in lymphocyte subpopulations and HIV viremia during primary HIV infection.

Features of primary HIV infection that may predict the subsequent course toward AIDS

A considerable body of evidence suggests that more severe and more prolonged PHI indicates a more unfavorable course toward AIDS.[18,19] For instance, in patients who were followed after seroconversion, 58% of those who had had symptomatic PHI had developed AIDS 7 years later compared with 28% of those who had asymptomatic PHI.[20] Another study suggested that the presence of neurologic signs at the time of PHI predicted accelerated immunosuppression,[19] although there was no specific relation to the neurologic signs of AIDS, such as AIDS-related dementia or opportunistic infections of the CNS.

Does treatment of primary HIV infection improve the long-term outcome?

This is a critically important question that regrettably remains unanswered. Comparative studies between a treated group and an untreated control group face considerable practical obstacles, including the need for a large sample, extremely long follow-up and ethical issues.

Primary HIV infection is a self-limiting disease, usually of only slight or moderate severity. The balance has shifted back and forth between advocates and opponents of treatment.

Arguments in favor are:
- the association of symptomatic PHI with a worse prognosis;
- the limited heterogeneity of the viral population,[21] which should theoretically diminish the probability of emergence of resistance to antiviral drugs;
- the potential impact on infectivity and transmission;[1]
- the generalization of the HIV infection during PHI with invasion of the CNS[12] and lymphoid tissues; and
- the availability of more effective and better tolerated antiviral drugs.[22]

After pilot studies suggested that zidovudine was well tolerated and possibly effective in PHI, a prospective randomized trial in 77 patients compared placebo and zidovudine given for 6 months.[4] An effect on CD4+ lymphocytes and a statistically significant decrease in minor opportunistic infections in patients treated with zidovudine were demonstrated.

Several uncontrolled trials have been conducted in PHI with combinations of antiviral drugs:
- with highly active antiretroviral treatment, including two inhibitors of reverse transcriptase and an inhibitor of the HIV protease, viremia decreases to undetectable levels in practically all compliant patients;[23,24]
- progression to AIDS is less than in historical control groups;[25]
- the CD4+/CD8+ lymphocyte ratio normalizes; and
- lymph node biopsies of some of the patients who have persistent suppression of viremia show disappearance of virus, and proviral DNA decays faster than in patients who start treatment during chronic HIV infection.[23,26]

However, the hope of viral eradication remains unfulfilled, as discussed below.

Opponents of antiviral treatment for primary HIV infection point to the lack of studies showing clinical benefits, the high incidence of side-effects, possible increased risk of development of resistance to antiretroviral agents, expense and problems with compliance. Some 6 months or so after having started treatment during PHI, patients often have high CD4+ counts and would not otherwise qualify for antiretroviral treatment. Should they stop?

Firm recommendations await the results of properly controlled trials. After years of attempts, the SPARTAC trial in South Africa and the UK has now succeeded in recruiting several hundred patients. The study randomized participants to treatment for 3 or 12 months, or no treatment, with a planned follow-up of several years. Results are not expected before 2011 (see http://www.ctu.mrc.ac.uk/studies/spartac.asp).

REFERENCES

References for this chapter can be found online at http://www.expertconsult.com

Prevention of opportunistic infections

INTRODUCTION

One of the major clinical advances in the management of patients who have HIV infection has been the implementation in the mid-1980s of antimicrobial prophylaxis for patients with severe immune impairment. Together with the use of antiretroviral drugs, this has led to decreased morbidity from opportunistic infections (OIs) and improved survival in patients with AIDS.

Such prophylaxis requires regular measurements of CD4+ lymphocyte counts and compliance on the part of the patient, who must take many pills each day for the rest of his/her life. There are also issues of tolerance, drug interactions, emergence of resistance and cost.

Since the extensive use in Western countries of highly active antiretroviral therapy (HAART), a further marked decrease in the occurrence of AIDS-related opportunistic infections has been noted and the question of continuing or stopping prophylactic regimens has been raised in patients who have CD4+ counts increasing beyond the critical level of 200 lymphocytes/mm³.[1] Figure 90.1 summarizes the evolution of the incidence of most opportunistic infections among a cohort of 2000 patients followed at CHU Saint-Pierre hospital in Brussels.

Although prophylactic regimens against most of the opportunistic infections that occur in patients who have HIV infection exist, the decision to use prophylaxis should consider factors such as:

- the incidence and prevalence of specific infections in HIV infected individuals;
- the potential severity of disease in terms of morbidity and mortality;
- the level of immunosuppression at which each disease is likely to occur;

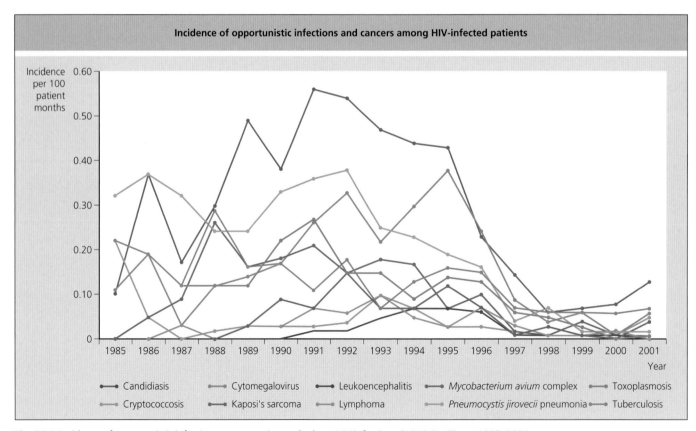

Fig. 90.1 Incidence of opportunistic infections among patients who have HIV infection. CHU Saint-Pierre, 1985–2001.

- the feasibility and efficacy of preventive measures, and their impact on quality of life and survival;
- the potential for emergence of organisms resistant to the agents used for prophylaxis;
- the risk of toxicities and drug interactions with antiretrovirals and other needed medications;
- the issue of compliance; and
- the cost-effectiveness of prophylaxis.

Prevention of infection with hepatitis B virus (HBV), hepatitis C virus (HCV), human papilloma virus (HPV) and herpes viruses through sexual contact should also be part of the long-term management of the patient. The role of newly introduced HPV vaccination in HIV patients remains unknown.

Efforts should also be made to improve early diagnosis of HIV disease, to avoid immunodeficiency or to implement prevention of opportunistic infections.

INCIDENCE AND PREVALENCE OF OPPORTUNISTIC INFECTIONS

There is a wide geographic variability in the epidemiology of opportunistic infections. The probability of developing a given disease depends on the risk for exposure to potential pathogens, the virulence of the pathogens and the level of immunosuppression of the patient.

In the USA and Northern Europe, *Pneumocystis jirovecii* pneumonia (PJP), oropharyngeal or esophageal candidiasis, cytomegalovirus disease and infections caused by *Mycobacterium avium* complex (MAC) are common. The incidence of toxoplasmosis and tuberculosis is higher in central and southern Europe and in the developing countries, depending on the prevalence of latent infection in the general population.

This geographic heterogeneity has important implications for prophylaxis. In the case of low incidence, prophylactic measures should be targeted to high-risk patients such as those who have a positive antitoxoplasma serology, a positive polymerase chain reaction for cytomegalovirus or a positive cutaneous tuberculin test for tuberculosis. In addition, for tuberculosis, epidemiologic assessment of risk should be used for some high-risk populations (intravenous drug users, migrants from an endemic area).

LEVEL OF IMMUNOSUPPRESSION

Blood CD4+ lymphocyte levels is the best marker for immune status. It has been clearly established that the number of circulating CD4+ lymphocytes is closely correlated with the risk of developing several opportunistic infections (Fig. 90.2). Once the CD4+ lymphocyte count falls below 200 cells/µl, the cumulative risk for developing an AIDS-defining opportunistic infection is 33% by year 1 and 58% by 2 years. Therefore, CD4+ lymphocyte counts remain an important parameter for monitoring patients who have HIV infection because of their predictive value for both opportunistic infections and mortality.

EFFICACY OF PROPHYLACTIC MEASURES AND IMPACT ON SURVIVAL

The survival benefit of prophylaxis for opportunistic infections has been demonstrated in a number of studies, particularly in patients who have severe immunosuppression. In the early 1980s, before the widespread use of antiretroviral therapy, it was demonstrated that trimethoprim–sulfamethoxazole (TMP–SMX) use for prevention of PJP significantly prolonged survival. A similar impact has been shown with MAC prophylaxis with clarithromycin or rifabutin.

It is clear that a prophylactic regimen that prolongs survival should be used in preference to one that does not. In this setting, the use of fluconazole for prophylaxis of systemic mycoses and oral ganciclovir for cytomegalovirus disease have failed to demonstrate a clear survival benefit and are not widely recommended.

EMERGENCE OF DRUG RESISTANCE

The development of resistance to the most commonly used agents is one of the major concerns with the use of long-term antimicrobial prophylaxis in patients who have HIV infection.

Resistance or cross-resistance has become increasingly common with prophylaxis for MAC, fungal infections and PJP. The major consequence is that, when the specific drugs are needed to treat acute infections, resistance hinders their use and alternative, less effective, or more toxic agents are the only option.[2]

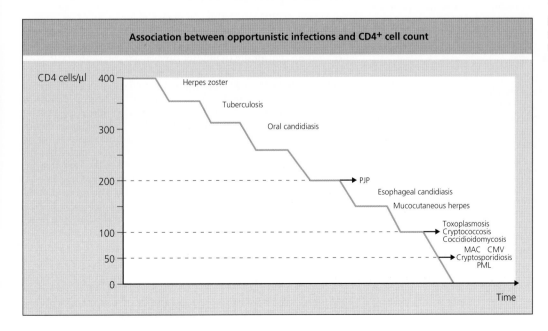

Fig. 90.2 Association between opportunistic infections and CD4+ cell count.

This issue was well illustrated with clarithromycin as prophylaxis for MAC. Despite receiving prophylaxis, 58% of the patients developing MAC had clarithromycin-resistant isolates.[3]

Prophylactic treatment of non-life-threatening infections, such as oral thrush with fluconazole, has probably contributed to the emergence and spreading of azole-resistant fungi.

Prophylactic regimens may also lead to the development of cross-resistance against more common pathogens. For example, rifabutin used for MAC prophylaxis may result in the emergence of rifampin (rifampicin)-resistant strains of *M. tuberculosis*.[4] Likewise, the widespread use of broad-spectrum antibiotics, such as clarithromycin, azithromycin or TMP–SMX, may lead to the development of resistance among organisms such as pneumococci that were not the primary targets of prophylaxis. An increasing prevalence of *Streptococcus pneumoniae* resistant to TMP–SMX, for example, could decrease the effectiveness of this agent in preventing community-acquired pneumonia in advanced HIV patients and limit therapeutic options for treating common outpatient illnesses such as respiratory, skin and soft tissue infections.[2]

DRUG TOXICITY AND DRUG INTERACTIONS

Drug toxicity can be a major factor limiting the usefulness of widely used agents. The incidence of adverse drug reactions in patients who have HIV infection varies with the type of drug and dosages used, the interactions between drugs and the stage of HIV infection.[5]

HIV-related idiosyncratic factors, organ dysfunction in late-stage disease and multiple drug therapy are the primary reasons for the increased risk of drug toxicities in HIV patients.

The issue of drug interactions has become particularly critical in the era of protease inhibitors. However, although the number of potential drug interactions is substantial, few require dosage modifications. Among these, clinicians should be vigilant when using concomitant prophylaxis and treatment of mycobacterial diseases with rifamycin, macrolides and HIV protease inhibitors.

COMPLIANCE ISSUES

The use of combination therapy for prophylaxis against multiple opportunistic pathogens significantly increases the complexity of treatment of HIV patients. In particular, it may increase the number of pills that are necessary in combination antiretroviral regimens. Such regimens may lead to patient noncompliance and inability to tolerate other therapeutic regimens, inducing antiretrovirals.

COST-EFFECTIVENESS

To be most cost-effective, prophylaxis should be directed at the most common infections in the patient population. However, an expensive prophylactic regimen may be cost-effective if it has a positive impact on quality and duration of life or if it reduces other costs. This is particularly true in severely immunocompromised HIV patients, in whom any intervention, even costly prophylaxis, that significantly reduces the incidence of hospitalization will have a favorable impact on the costs of caring. Studies have shown that prophylaxis for PJP and MAC is cost-effective, whereas prophylaxis for fungal disease and cytomegalovirus is not.[6]

DURATION OF PROPHYLAXIS AGAINST OPPORTUNISTIC INFECTIONS

Since HAART was introduced, it has become clear that prophylaxis against opportunistic infections need not necessarily be life long. As mentioned above, susceptibility to opportunistic infections can be assessed accurately by the CD4+ T-cell count. It is thus logical to stop primary or secondary prophylaxis in patients whose immunity has improved as a consequence of HAART.

Data generated until now support this approach and recommendations concerning the safety of stopping primary or secondary prophylaxis can now be made for many pathogens.

By contrast, no data are available regarding the re-initiation of prophylaxis when the CD4+ lymphocyte count decreases again to levels at which the risk for opportunistic infections exists. In particular, it is unknown whether it is better to use the threshold at which prophylaxis was stopped or the threshold below which initial prophylaxis is recommended.[7]

RECOMMENDATIONS FOR PROPHYLAXIS AGAINST OPPORTUNISTIC INFECTIONS

The US Public Health Services and the Infectious Diseases Society of America have established disease-specific recommendations for the prevention of opportunistic infections in individuals who have HIV infection, which were updated in June 2002. These recommendations include guidelines for preventing exposure to pathogens as well as on specific regimens for preventing initial episodes.[8]

Category I regimens are strongly recommended as standard of care. Category II should be strongly considered in eligible patients. Category III regimens are not routinely recommended but may be considered for use in selected patients (Table 90.1). Recommendations on prophylactic regimens to prevent recurrence of opportunistic infections have also been updated (Table 90.2).

PREVENTION OF OPPORTUNISTIC INFECTIONS IN PREGNANT WOMEN

Recommendations are the same as in other groups. Because of concerns related to administering drugs during the first trimester of pregnancy, certain health-care providers might choose to withhold prophylaxis during the first trimester of pregnancy.

DISEASE-SPECIFIC CONSIDERATIONS

Pneumocystis jirovecii

Prophylaxis of PJP has been shown to be highly cost-effective. A meta-analysis of 35 studies of PJP prophylaxis in 6583 patients showed that TMP–SMX was superior to dapsone or aerosolized pentamidine but there was no statistically significant survival advantage for TMP–SMX versus alternative agents. An advantage of TMP–SMX over alternative drugs is a significant reduction in bacterial infections. Side-effects are sufficiently severe to require discontinuation of the drug in 25–50% of TMP–SMX recipients compared to 25–40% of dapsone recipients and 2–4% of recipients of aerosolized pentamidine. There is good evidence that lower doses of TMP–SMX are better tolerated, and many advocate either the use of the lower-dose regimens using one single-strength tablet daily or one double-strength tablet thrice weekly. Patients who have adverse reactions to TMP–SMX usually tolerate dapsone.

Primary and secondary prophylaxis against PJP should be discontinued in patients treated with HAART who show an increase in CD4+ T cells to above 200/mm³ for at least 3 months. Prophylaxis should be reintroduced if the CD4+ T-cell count decreases to less than 200/mm³.[9,10]

Toxoplasma gondii

Toxoplasma seropositive patients who have a CD4+ T-cell count below 100/mm³ or who have had a previous episode of toxoplasmic encephalitis should receive prophylaxis against toxoplasmic encephalitis.

Table 90.1 Prophylaxis of first episode of opportunistic infections in adults and adolescents with HIV infection

Pathogen	Target population	First-choice regimen	Alternative regimens
Category I: recommended as standard of care			
Pneumocystis jirovecii	CD4$^+$ lymphocyte count <200/mm^3 *and/or* oropharyngeal candidiasis	TMP–SMX 1 DS q24h or 1 SS q24h	Dapsone 100 mg q24h or 50 mg q12h Dapsone 50 mg q24h *plus* pyrimethamine 50 mg weekly *plus* leucovorin 25 mg weekly Dapsone 200 mg weekly *plus* pyrimethamine 75 mg weekly *plus* leucovorin 25 mg weekly Aerosolized pentamidine 300 mg monthly by nebulizer Atovaquone 1500 mg q24h TMP–SMX 1 DS three times a week
Toxoplasma gondii	CD4$^+$ lymphocyte count <100/mm^3 *and* positive anti-*Toxoplasma* IgG	TMP–SMX 1 DS q24h	TMP–SMX 1 SS q24h Dapsone 50 mg q24h *plus* pyrimethamine 50 mg weekly *plus* leucovorin 25 mg weekly Dapsone 200 mg weekly *plus* pyrimethamine 75 mg weekly *plus* leucovorin 25 mg weekly
Mycobacterium tuberculosis	Positive PPD (5 mm) *and/or* previous positive PPD without treatment *and/or* contact with active case (regardless of PPD result)	Isoniazid 300 mg q24h *plus* pyridoxine 50 mg q24h for 9 months or isoniazid 900 mg and pyridoxine 50 mg twice weekly with directly observed therapy for 9 months	Rifampin (rifampicin) 600 mg q24h for 4 months *If isoniazid resistance*: rifampin 600 mg q24h for 12 months or rifabutin 600 mg q24h for 12 months *If multidrug resistance*: choice of drugs depends on susceptibility of isolate from source patient
Mycobacterium avium complex	CD4$^+$ lymphocyte count <50 cells/mm^3	Clarithromycin 500 mg q12h *or* azithromycin 1200 mg weekly	Rifabutin 300 mg q24h or azithromycin 1200 mg weekly *plus* rifabutin 300 mg q24h
Varicella-zoster virus (VZV)	Exposure to chickenpox or shingles *and* no history of either or negative serology	Varicella-zoster virus Ig, 5 vials im within 96h of exposure (preferably within 48h)	
Category II: generally recommended			
Streptococcus pneumoniae	CD4$^+$ lymphocyte count >200 cells/mm^3	23-valent polysaccharide vaccine 0.5 ml im (single dose); repeat in 4–5 years time	
Hepatitis B virus	All anti-HBV-negative patients	Hepatitis B vaccine 10 mg im (three doses)	
Influenza virus	All patients	Inactivated trivalent Influenza vaccine 0.5 ml im each year in autumn	Oseltamivir 75 mg q24h (influenza A or B) Amantadine 100 mg q12h Rimantadine 100 mg q12h (influenza A only)
Hepatitis A virus	All anti-HAV-negative patients at increased risk (injection drug users, men who have sex with men, hemophiliacs) or with chronic liver disease, including chronic hepatitis B or C	Hepatitis A vaccine (two doses)	
Category III: not recommended for most patients. To be considered in selected patients only			
Cytomegalovirus	CD4$^+$ lymphocyte count <50 cells/μl *and* positive cytomegalovirus antibodies	Oral ganciclovir 1 g q8h	
Bacteria	Neutropenia	G-CSF 5–10 μg/kg sc q24h for 2–4 weeks *or* GM-CSF 250 μg/m^2 iv q24h for 2–4 weeks	
Cryptococcus neoformans	CD4$^+$ lymphocyte count <50 cells/mm^3	Fluconazole 100–200 mg q24h *or* itraconazole 200 mg q24h	
Histoplasmosis	CD4$^+$ lymphocyte count <100 cells/mm^3 *and* residence in endemic area	Itraconazole 200 mg q24h	

DS, double strength; G-CSF, granulocyte colony-stimulating factor; GM-CSF, granulocyte–macrophage colony-stimulating factor; PPD, purified protein derivatives; SS, single strength; TMP–SMX, trimethoprim–sulfamethoxazole. Adapted from USPHS/IDSA guidelines.[8]

Table 90.2 Prophylaxis to prevent recurrence of opportunistic disease in adults and adolescents with HIV infection

Pathogen	Indication	First-choice regimen	Alternative regimens
Category I: Recommended as standard of care			
Pneumocystis jirovecii	Previous PJP	TMP–SMX 1 SS q24h or 1 DS q24h	Dapsone 50 mg q12h or 100 mg q24h Dapsone 50 mg q24h *plus* pyrimethamine 50 mg weekly *plus* leucovorin 25 mg weekly Dapsone 200 mg *plus* pyrimethamine 75 mg *plus* leucovorin 25 mg weekly Aerosolized pentamidine 300 mg monthly by nebulizer Atovaquone 1500 mg q24h TMP–SMX, 1 DS three times weekly
Toxoplasma gondii	Prior toxoplasmic encephalitis	Sulfadiazine 500–1000 mg q6h *plus* pyrimethamine 25–50 mg q24h *plus* leucovorin 10–25 mg po q24h (confers protection against PJP)	Clindamycin 300–450 mg q6–8h *plus* pyrimethamine 25–50 mg q24h *plus* leucovorin 10–25 mg q24h Atovaquone 750 mg q6–12h *with or without* pyrimethamine 25 mg q24h *plus* leucovorin 10 mg q24h
Mycobacterium avium complex	Documented disseminated disease	Clarithromycin 500 mg q12h *plus* ethambutol 15 mg/kg q24h (*with or without* rifabutin 300 mg q24h)	Azithromycin 500 mg q24h *plus* ethambutol 15 mg/kg q24h (*with or without* rifabutin 300 mg q24h)
Cytomegalovirus	Previous end-organ disease	Ganciclovir 5–6 mg/kg iv q24h 5–7 days/week *or* 1000 mg po q8h *or* foscarnet 90–120 mg/kg q24h *or* (for retinitis) ganciclovir sustained-release implant every 6–9 months *plus* ganciclovir 1.0–1.5 g po q8h	Cidofovir 5 mg/kg every 2 weeks (with probenecid) Fomivirsen 1 vial (330 µg) injected into the vitreous, then repeated every 2–4 weeks Valganciclovir 900 mg q24h
Cryptococcus neoformans	Documented disease	Fluconazole 200 mg q24h	Amphotericin B 0.6–1.0 mg/kg weekly Itraconazole 200 mg q24h
Histoplasma capsulatum	Documented disease	Itraconazole 200 mg q12h	Amphotericin B 1.0 mg/kg weekly
Coccidioides immitis	Documented disease	Fluconazole 400 mg q24h	Amphotericin B 1.0 mg/kg weekly Itraconazole 200 mg q12h
Salmonella spp. (non-*typhi*)	Bacteremia	Ciprofloxacin 500 mg q12h for several months	Antibiotic chemoprophylaxis with another active agent
Category II: Recommended only if subsequent episodes are frequent or severe			
Herpes simplex virus	Frequent/severe recurrences	Aciclovir 200 mg q8h *or* 400 mg q12h *or* Famciclovir 250 mg q12h	Valaciclovir 500 mg q12h
Candida (oropharyngeal, vaginal or esophageal)	Frequent/severe recurrences	Fluconazole 100–200 mg q24h	Itraconazole solution 200 mg q24h

DS, double strength; SS, single strength. Adapted from USPHS/IDSA guidelines.[8]

The double-strength tablet daily dose of TMP–SMX is recommended. Alternative regimens in patients who cannot tolerate TMP–SMX include dapsone–pyrimethamine or atovaquone (with or without pyrimethamine). Prophylactic monotherapy with dapsone, clindamycin, pyrimethamine, azithromycin or clarithromycin is not recommended.

Primary prophylaxis against toxoplasmic encephalitis should be discontinued in patients treated with HAART showing an increase in CD4+ T cells to above 200/mm³ for at least 3 months. Discontinuation of prophylaxis in patients where CD4+ counts have increased to 100–200 cells/mm³ has not been carefully evaluated. No firm recommendation can be made regarding discontinuation of secondary prophylaxis, but it appears reasonable to consider discontinuation in patients who have CD4+ T cells above 200/mm³ for at least 3 months. Prophylaxis should be re-introduced if the CD4+ T-cell count decreases to below 100–200/mm³.[10,11]

Mycobacterium tuberculosis

Latent tuberculosis infection should be treated in all patients who have HIV infection and a positive tuberculin skin test, with no evidence of active tuberculosis and no history of treatment for active or latent tuberculosis.

Regimens include:
- daily or twice weekly isoniazid (plus pyridoxine) for 9 months; and
- daily rifampin (or rifabutin) for 4 months.

Rifampin (or rifabutin) plus pyrazinamide for 2 months should not be given because severe liver injury has been associated with this combination.

In patients whose initial skin test is negative and whose CD4+ T-cell count has increased to above 200/mm³ with HAART, a repeat tuberculin skin test should be considered.[12]

Mycobacterium avium complex

Patients who have a CD4$^+$ T-cell count below 50/mm^3 should receive clarithromycin (500 mg q12h) or azithromycin (1200 mg weekly). Combination with rifabutin is not recommended. Both macrolides confer protection against respiratory bacterial infections. Rifabutin is an alternative in patients who cannot tolerate macrolides.

Primary prophylaxis should be discontinued in patients treated with HAART who show an increase in CD4$^+$ T cells to above 100/mm^3 for at least 3 months and should be re-introduced if the CD4$^+$ T-cell count decreases to less than 50–100/mm^3.[13]

Patients who have disseminated MAC should receive maintenance therapy with clarithromycin (or azithromycin) and ethambutol with or without rifabutin. It is reasonable to consider discontinuation of treatment in patients who have completed a course of at least 12 months of therapy, have no symptoms and show a CD4$^+$ T-cell count above 100/mm^3 following HAART for at least 6 months.[14]

Streptococcus pneumoniae

Patients who have a CD4$^+$ T-cell count greater than 200/mm^3 should receive a single dose of 23-valent polysaccharide pneumococcal vaccine every 4–5 years. If the CD4$^+$ T-cell count is below 200/mm^3, vaccination should be considered (with revaccination when the count increases to above 200/mm^3).[15]

Cryptococcosis

Primary prophylaxis should not be used routinely. Patients who have had cryptococcosis should receive lifelong suppressive treatment with fluconazole unless they have a sustained (≥6 months) increase in the CD4$^+$ T-cell count following HAART. Suppressive therapy should be reinitiated if the CD4$^+$ T-cell count decreases to less than 100–200/mm^3.[16]

Cytomegalovirus

Patients who have had active cytomegalovirus disease should receive maintenance therapy with any of the following regimens: parenteral or oral ganciclovir, parenteral foscarnet, combined parenteral ganciclovir and foscarnet, parenteral cidofovir or oral valganciclovir. Administration of ganciclovir via intraocular implant or repetitive intravitreous injections of fomivirsen may be used in patients who have retinitis only, and are generally combined with oral ganciclovir. Repetitive intravitreous injections of ganciclovir, foscarnet and cidofovir have been shown to be effective in uncontrolled case series.[17,18]

Discontinuation of secondary prophylaxis should be considered in patients who have received HAART and show an increase in CD4$^+$ T cells to above 100–150/mm^3 for at least 6 months. All these patients should continue to undergo regular ophthalmologic examination. Secondary prophylaxis should be restarted when the CD4$^+$ T-cell count falls to below 100–150/mm^3.[19]

Varicella-zoster virus disease

HIV adults who have no history of chickenpox or are seronegative for varicella-zoster virus (VZV) should receive VZV immunoglobulin as soon as possible but within 96 hours after exposure to a patient who has chickenpox or shingles. The efficacy of aciclovir in this setting is unknown.

REFERENCES

References for this chapter can be found online at http://www.expertconsult.com

Opportunistic infections

INTRODUCTION

The major cause of death in patients with AIDS had been the opportunistic infections (OIs) that arose as a consequence of the severe immunodeficiency characteristic of HIV infection.[1] Since the advent of the era of potent antiretroviral therapy (ART), there has been a marked decrease in the occurrence of AIDS-related opportunistic infections and a consequent increase in survival.[2] Nevertheless, there is great variability in access to ART and consequently significant AIDS-associated OIs continue. In the Western world, this is largely a consequence of delayed diagnosis, with patients presenting with an OI as the first recognition of HIV infection; in resource-poor situations, availability of ART is more of a problem. The number of circulating CD4+ lymphocytes is closely correlated with the risk of developing several opportunistic infections (see Fig. 90.2). Once the CD4+ lymphocyte count falls below 200 cells/mm³, the cumulative risk for developing an AIDS-defining OI is 33% by year 1 and 58% by 2 years. Therefore, CD4+ lymphocyte counts are the critical parameter for monitoring patients who have HIV infection because of their predictive value for both opportunistic infections and mortality. Two patterns of OI development exist – re-emergence of infections acquired early in life (often in childhood) as the CD4+ lymphocyte count falls, and newly acquired infection by organisms that become pathogenic in the setting of progressive immunodeficiency.

The probability of developing a given disease depends on the risk for exposure to potential pathogens, the virulence of the pathogens and the level of immunosuppression of the patient. There is a wide geographic variability in the epidemiology of opportunistic infections. In the USA and Northern Europe, pneumonia caused by *Pneumocystis jirovecii*, oropharyngeal or esophageal candidiasis, cytomegalovirus disease and infections caused by *Mycobacterium avium* complex (MAC) are common. The incidence of toxoplasmosis and tuberculosis is higher in Eastern and Southern Europe and in the developing countries, depending on the prevalence of latent infection in the general population.

Pneumocystis jirovecii **Pneumonia**

Pneumocystis jirovecii (previously known as *Pneumocystis carinii*, and still often referred to as PCP for *p*neumo*c*ystis *p*neumonia) is a fungal pathogen associated with opportunistic infections, especially pneumonia (PCP) in patients with altered cell-mediated immunity. Historically, the occurrence of PCP in American gay men who had no previously known immune deficiency was the first signal of the AIDS epidemic.[3] Although the implementation of prophylaxis and the advances in ART have markedly decreased its incidence, PCP remains an important OI. Its epidemiology is uncertain; although generally thought to be due to reactivation of latent infection acquired during childhood or adolescence, genetic studies of *P. jirovecii* isolates suggest that recent exposure to environmental strains may be a factor in acquisition of infection. PCP typically occurs when the CD4+ lymphocyte count is less than 200/mm³. The rate of relapse after a first episode of PCP is high (approximately 60% incidence within 1 year) when neither specific prophylaxis nor highly active antiretroviral therapy (HAART) is initiated.[4]

CLINICAL FEATURES

Pneumocystis jirovecii infection is restricted to the lung in more than 95% of cases. Disseminated infection (bone marrow, spleen, liver, retina and skin) can occur spontaneously or is associated with the use of aerosolized pentamidine. The most common clinical presentation of PCP is a progressive dyspnea with dry cough, fever (often mild) and weight loss. The mean duration of breathlessness is 3–4 weeks at presentation. On examination, fever and tachypnea are common, whereas lung auscultation may be normal or reveal only basal crepitations.

Chest radiography is an important step in the diagnosis procedure of lung diseases in AIDS. The chest radiograph is normal in less than 5% of cases. The most common pattern is a fine bilateral interstitial and then alveolar–interstitial infiltrate progressing from the perihilar to the peripheral regions (Fig. 91.1). Without therapy, or even during the first days of treatment, the alveolar–interstitial pattern worsens.

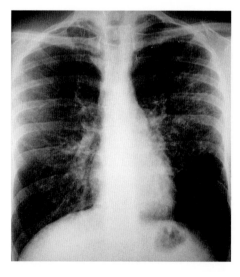

Fig. 91.1 Mild *Pneumocystis jirovecii* pneumonia. There are bilateral micronodular lesions. Courtesy of Pierre-Marie Girard.

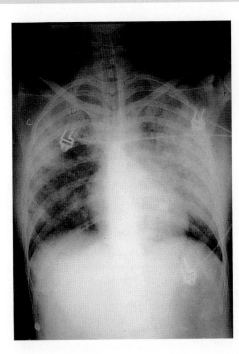

Fig. 91.2 Severe *Pneumocystis jirovecii* pneumonia. This shows an extensive alveolar interstitial infiltrate with consolidation of the left lung and upper right lobe. Courtesy of Pierre-Marie Girard.

In advanced cases, progressive consolidation with air bronchograms and complete opacification of the lungs may develop (Fig. 91.2). Numerous atypical patterns of PCP may occur. They include localized infiltrates, cavitary lesions, solitary lung nodules, spontaneous pneumothoraces and pleural effusions. Hilar or mediastinal lymphadenopathy is very rare.

Establishing a diagnosis of PCP requires the morphologic demonstration of the micro-organism. Arterial blood gases must be measured to assess the severity of the disease, but have no diagnostic value. Sputum examination is the least invasive procedure for collecting lower respiratory specimens. Because patients who have PCP generally do not have a productive cough, an induced sputum can be obtained after aerosolization of hypertonic saline, ideally under the supervision of a physiotherapist. In routine practice, the sensitivity of the test is approximately 50–60%. Fiberoptic bronchoscopy with bronchoalveolar lavage is the reference routine diagnostic procedure because its sensitivity is more than 95% and its specificity is 100%. When the diagnosis cannot be obtained from bronchoalveolar lavage fluid, transbronchial lung biopsy may help, although it is more invasive and is associated with a risk of bleeding and pneumothorax.

MANAGEMENT

The measurement of arterial gas is used routinely to define mild (Pao_2 ≥70 mmHg), moderate (Pao_2 50–70 mmHg) and severe (Pao_2 <50 mmHg) PCP. In mild PCP, outpatient management with oral therapy is often possible providing no other disease is present, there is low risk of drug malabsorption, the management strategy is well understood and the patient is aware of the potential side-effects of therapy.

Hospitalization is required for moderate and severe PCP to ensure careful monitoring of treatment, which should be administered intravenously, at least during the first days.

Trimethoprim–sulfamethoxazole (TMP–SMX) is the drug of choice for PCP whatever its severity, and no other drug or combination of drugs has demonstrated improved efficacy in control trials.[5,6] The drug is given as 15 mg/kg/day trimethoprim with 75 mg/kg/day sulfamethoxazole (in three divided doses). Side-effects include rash, fever, pruritus, digestive disturbances and cytopenia usually after 7–10 days of therapy. Approximately 10–20% of patients will need to be switched to another treatment because of TMP–SMX intolerance. It is important to determine the nature of intolerance to TMP–SMX. In practice,

contraindication to reintroduction of TMP–SMX or to the use of a combination with potential cross-intolerance to sulfonamide is based on a history of anaphylaxis or exfoliative dermatitis or other life-threatening toxicity such as severe cytolytic hepatitis. Whenever possible, the first-line therapy for PCP is always TMP–SMX. For cases of mild PCP alternates include dapsone plus trimethoprim, and clindamycin plus primaquine or atovaquone.[6] For more severe PCP, alternates include clindamycin plus primaquine or intravenous pentamidine.[6]

In addition to anti-*P. jirovecii* therapy, corticosteroids are administered as soon as possible in patients who have moderate to severe disease. The use of corticosteroids is recommended in patients whose Pao_2 is less than 65 mmHg and has been shown to improve oxygenation, reduce the risk of fibrosis, decrease the need for mechanical ventilation and reduce the case fatality rate.[7] The recommended corticosteroid regimen is:

- on days 1–5, 40 mg oral prednisone (prednisolone) q12h;
- on days 6–10, 40 mg oral prednisone/day; and
- on days 11–21, 20 mg oral prednisone/day.

In most cases, respiratory symptoms and oxygenation improve after 5–10 days. If a patient has been treated empirically (without defintive diagnosis) failure to improve after 5–7 days of treatment should trigger a re-evaluation, usually with bronchoscopy. Early mild deterioration is not infrequent during the first days of treatment. The duration of treatment is classically 21 days. When TMP–SMX is initiated intravenously, it can be switched to an oral formulation after a few days. Secondary prophylaxis is required after treatment of the attack (see Table 91.2).

PREVENTION (SEE TABLES 91.1 AND 91.2)

Prophylaxis against PCP is indicated for all HIV-infected patients with a CD4+ count less than 200 cells/μl or those with a history of oropharyngeal candidiasis or an AIDS-defining illness.

Viral Infections

Most clinically important viral infections in HIV disease are caused by DNA viruses, the majority belonging to the Herpesviridae family. The role of viral infections such as human herpes virus 8, Epstein–Barr virus and human papillomavirus in HIV-related neoplastic disorders is discussed elsewhere (see Chapter 94).

CYTOMEGALOVIRUS INFECTIONS

Serologic evidence of cytomegalovirus (CMV) infection can be detected in approximately 60% of the adult population in the USA. The prevalence of infection is strongly influenced by socioeconomic status and sexual practices; up to 95% of men who have sex with men (MSM) are seropositive for CMV. In patients who have AIDS, CMV disease usually results from reactivation of latent infection. Progressive loss of cell-mediated immunity in patients abrogates the immunologic suppression of CMV replication (see also Chapter 155). Asymptomatic excretion of CMV in urine can be detected in approximately 50% of patients who have advanced HIV disease, and over half of the patients who have CMV viremia go on to develop clinical CMV disease within 8–12 months. Cytomegalovirus end-organ disease usually occurs when the CD4+ lymphocyte count falls below 50 cells/mm³.[8]

Cytomegalovirus retinitis

Retinitis is the commonest manifestation of CMV infection in patients who have HIV infection or AIDS, accounting for 85% of CMV disease. The virus causes a relentlessly progressive, necrotizing retinitis. Cytomegalovirus retinitis is usually unilateral in the first instance,

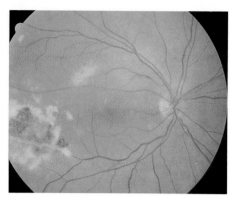

Fig. 91.3
Cytomegalovirus retinitis, with characteristic perivascular hemorrhages and exudates. Courtesy of Maurice E Murphy and Bruce Polsky.

progressing to affect the contralateral eye if untreated. Patients may be initially asymptomatic but may subsequently experience blurring of vision, floaters and painless progressive visual loss.

Diagnosis of CMV retinitis is made by systematic funduscopic examination by direct or indirect ophthalmoscopy. Characteristically, white, fluffy or granular lesions with perivascular white exudates associated with retinal hemorrhages are seen (Fig. 91.3).

Cytomegalovirus lesions may be categorized as occurring in three arbitrarily defined anatomic zones. Retinitis located in the immediate vicinity of the macula or optic disc (zone 1) is sight-threatening and should prompt immediate initiation of treatment. Lesions outside the major vascular vessels (zones 2 and 3), commonly referred to as 'peripheral retinitis', are not immediately sight-threatening but will progress if left untreated.

Gastrointestinal cytomegalovirus disease

In the upper gastrointestinal tract, CMV causes discrete esophageal ulcers, diffuse esophagitis, gastritis, gastric ulcers, duodenal ulcers and enteritis. Esophageal CMV infection usually presents with painful dysphagia; diagnosis is established by endoscopic examination showing inflammation and ulceration, with characteristic pathologic features on tissue biopsy. Cytomegalovirus enterocolitis usually presents with abdominal pain and persistent small-volume diarrhea. Endoscopic examination of the colon typically reveals plaque-like pseudomembranes, multiple erosions and ulcers.

Cytomegalovirus disease of the central nervous system

The two major CMV neurologic syndromes associated with HIV disease are CMV polyradiculopathy and CMV ventriculoencephalitis. Polyradiculopathy is seen in patients who have advanced AIDS. Approximately 50% have an associated myelitis. It is characterized by lower extremity pain, sensory deficits, weakness that can rapidly progress to flaccid paralysis, and bowel and bladder dysfunction. The most marked pathologic changes in CMV polyradiculomyelitis are found in the cauda equina and lumbosacral roots. In the appropriate clinical setting, findings on MRI of diffuse enhancement of the cauda equina and the surface of the conus strongly support the diagnosis. Cerebrospinal fluid (CSF) findings include a polymorphonuclear pleocytosis, raised protein concentration and moderately low glucose concentration. Culture of CSF may be negative but CMV antigen assays and polymerase chain reaction (PCR) for CMV DNA are more sensitive techniques (Chapter 155).

Ventriculoencephalitis usually occurs in the setting of a diagnosis of CMV disease elsewhere. Patients present with fever, lethargy and confusion. Characteristic neurologic findings include nystagmus and cranial nerve palsies. MRI with gadolinium enhancement may demonstrate periventricular enhancement. Cytomegalovirus DNA can often be detected in CSF using PCR.

Pulmonary cytomegalovirus disease

There are no particular distinguishing clinical or radiologic features to differentiate CMV pneumonitis from other causes of pneumonitis in HIV disease. Patients present with shortness of breath, dyspnea on exertion and a dry, nonproductive cough. Chest radiographs show diffuse interstitial infiltrates, and hypoxemia is usually present. Definitive diagnosis of pulmonary CMV disease in patients who have advanced HIV disease is difficult to establish because of a high incidence of asymptomatic CMV shedding – CMV can be isolated in approximately 50% of HIV-infected patients undergoing bronchoscopic examination. However, the true incidence of CMV pneumonitis is less than 10% in patients who have diagnostic bronchoscopy for evaluation of pulmonary infiltrates of unknown origin.

Management of cytomegalovirus infections[6]

Cytomegalovirus retinitis can be managed effectively with either local or systemic therapy; however, local therapy should be accompanied by some form of systemic treatment to control viremia and prevent retinitis in the contralateral eye. Oral valganciclovir, intravenous ganciclovir, intravenous ganciclovir followed by oral valganciclovir, intravenous foscarnet, intravenous cidofovir, and the ganciclovir intraocular implant combined with valganciclovir have all been shown in randomized trials to be effective treatment for CMV retinitis; balance should be maintained between ease of administration, side-effects and need for intravenous therapy. ART should be initiated promptly, and if effective in controlling HIV disease, CMV therapy can usually be discontinued after 6 months.

Intravenous ganciclovir (or oral valganciclovir in less ill patients) is the agent of choice for the treatment of CMV gastrointestinal disease.

HERPES SIMPLEX VIRUS INFECTIONS

Reactivation of herpes simplex virus (HSV) occurs frequently in patients who have advanced HIV disease, particularly in those who have low CD4+ lymphocyte counts (<100 cells/mm³). The hallmark of herpetic lesions is painful vesicular formation at a mucocutaneous site, progressing rapidly to ulceration with an erythematous base, followed by eventual healing and re-epithelialization.

As patients become more immunosuppressed, infections are characterized by prolonged viral shedding, more frequent episodes, and severe and persistent clinical disease. Recurrent genital and perirectal ulcerative lesions are the most common manifestations of HSV infection in patients who have HIV disease and are usually due to reactivation of HSV-2. Lesions may be atypical and severe in patients who have advanced disease. Prolonged new lesion formation, with continued tissue destruction, persistent viral shedding and severe local pain, is common.

HSV infections can be treated either with episodic therapy when lesions occur or with daily therapy to prevent recurrences – this decision should be individualized based on the frequency and severity of recurrences. Most infections can be treated with oral valaciclovir, famciclovir or aciclovir for 5–14 days. Severe mucocutaneous HSV lesions are best treated initially with intravenous aciclovir.

VARICELLA-ZOSTER VIRUS INFECTIONS

In the USA and Europe, most adults who have HIV disease have previously been infected with varicella-zoster virus (VZV). Owing to impaired cellular immunity, HIV-infected patients who have primary VZV are at risk of prolonged new lesion formation and are at higher risk of life-threatening visceral dissemination.

Herpes zoster may be the first indication of HIV disease and can occur at any stage of HIV infection. It usually appears as a localized or segmental painful erythematous maculopapular eruption along a single dermatome. In HIV-infected patients, zoster lesions may be bullous, hemorrhagic or necrotic. Patients infected with HIV are at risk of recurrent episodes of herpes zoster. Occasionally, widespread cutaneous and visceral dissemination may occur. Visceral dissemination to the lungs, the liver and the central nervous system (CNS) may cause life-threatening disease.

HIV-infected patients should receive prompt antiviral therapy with oral valaciclovir, or famciclovir, for 7–10 days. More severe disease (extensive skin or visceral involvement) should be treated initially with intravenous aciclovir (10 mg/kg q8h).

PROGRESSIVE MULTIFOCAL LEUKOENCEPHALOPATHY

Progressive multifocal leukoencephalopathy (PML) is an opportunistic demyelinating infection caused by JC virus, a ubiquitous DNA papovavirus for which over 70% of adults are seropositive (see also Chapter 157). PML occurs in patients who have deficient cell-mediated immunity and is estimated to affect up to 4% of patients who have AIDS. Mortality is high, and average reported survival in AIDS patients is 2–4 months. The symptoms and characteristic radiologic findings of PML are due to virus-induced lysis of oligodendrocytes, resulting in microscopic foci of myelin breakdown that coalesce to produce larger white matter lesions (Fig. 91.4). Definitive diagnosis requires tissue from brain biopsy but the identification of JC virus in the CSF by PCR has a high specificity for active disease. There is no definitive antiviral treatment for PML and optimal ART is the treatment of choice.[9] A paradoxical response to ART can be seen in some patients with PML with unexpected neurologic deterioration (see Chapter 92).

Fungal Infections

Fungi are among the most ubiquitous pathogens seen in patients who have HIV disease but are not the most common causes of mortality. Virtually all major fungal pathogens cause disease in patients who have HIV infection.

CANDIDIASIS

Candidal infection in AIDS is almost exclusively mucosal – systemic invasion is a rare and late event. Oropharyngeal candidiasis occurs in about three-quarters of all those who have HIV infection. In about

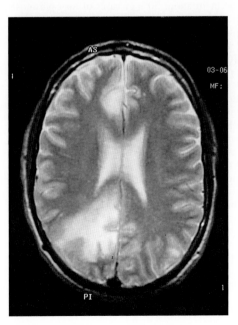

Fig. 91.4 Progressive multifocal leukoencephalopathy. MRI scan showing frontal and occipital white matter lesions. Courtesy of Maurice E Murphy and Bruce Polsky.

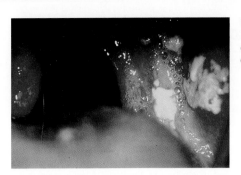

Fig. 91.5 Pseudomembranous oral candidiasis ('thrush').

one-third it tends to be recurrent and becomes progressively more severe with increasing immunodeficiency. Esophageal involvement occurs in 20–40% of all AIDS patients, predominantly in patients who have advanced disease and severe depletion of CD4+ lymphocytes. Vulvovaginal candidiasis occurs in about 30–40% of women who have HIV infection; it appears that HIV infection per se is not an important risk factor for vaginal infection, although it may influence the severity and persistence of disease.

Most candidal disease, especially initial episodes, is associated with infection by *Candida albicans*. Other species, notably *C. glabrata*, *C. dubliniensis* and *C. parapsilosis*, tend to cause infection in patients who have very advanced disease and have had extensive previous exposure to antifungal agents.

Most patients with oral candidiasis are symptomatic and complain of some oral discomfort. The classic presentation is of creamy-white plaques on an erythematous base – the pseudomembranous form of thrush (Fig. 91.5). Other manifestations include:

* an atrophic form that presents as erythema without plaques (often associated with patchy atrophic glossitis); and
* angular cheilitis, which appears as cracking, fissuring, ulceration or erythema at the corner of the mouth.

Most patients who have vaginal candidiasis present with vaginal itching, burning or pain, and usually complain of a vaginal discharge. Examination of the vaginal cavity usually reveals thrush, similar to that seen in the oropharynx.

Patients who have esophageal candidiasis develop ulcers and erosions of the esophagus and experience odynophagia or dysphagia. The combination of oral candidiasis and esophageal symptoms is both specific and sensitive in predicting esophageal involvement. Patients can be treated empirically with antifungal therapy. Endoscopy is reserved for those patients who fail to respond to evaluate for other diagnoses such as herpetic or cytomegalovirus esophagitis, idiopathic ulceration or resistant candidiasis.

The development of oral candidiasis in an HIV-positive patient should be taken as a sign of progressive immunodeficiency. Patients should have a CD4+ count measured. If they are not currently receiving ART, it should be initiated. If they are on ART, it should be reassessed and, if necessary, changed. A number of options – both local and systemic – are available for the treatment of oral candidiasis. Initially, most patients respond well clinically to any form of antifungal therapy, although mycologic responses are less common. Esophageal disease requires systemic therapy.[6] Fluconazole 200–400 mg q24h orally for 2–3 weeks is probably the therapy of choice; itraconazole 100–200 mg q12h orally is also effective.

Relapses are common if effective ART is not given and at least one-third of patients develop recurrent mucosal candidiasis. One approach to management is to treat each episode as it occurs. However, in many patients, recurrent symptomatic disease may be sufficiently severe to warrant considering chronic suppression. Fluconazole 100–200 mg q24h has proved highly successful in suppressing recurrent oropharyngeal disease and preventing esophagitis,[10] and a dose of 100 mg per week can prevent vaginal candidiasis. The major risk of this approach is the possibility of developing azole-resistant disease. However, resistant infection has become very unusual in the era of potent effective ART.

CRYPTOCOCCOSIS

Virtually all HIV-associated infection is caused by *Cryptococcus neoformans* var. *neoformans*. About 5% of patients who have advanced HIV infection in the Western world develop disseminated cryptococcosis; the disease is more prevalent in sub-Saharan Africa and southern Asia. Most cases of infection occur in patients who have very low CD4+ lymphocyte counts (<50 cells/mm³).

Cryptococcosis most commonly presents as a subacute meningitis or meningoencephalitis with fever, malaise and headache. Symptoms are usually present for 2–4 weeks before diagnosis. Classic meningeal symptoms and signs (such as neck stiffness or photophobia) occur in about one-third of patients. Some patients may present with encephalopathic symptoms such as lethargy, altered mentation, personality changes and memory loss. Analysis of the CSF usually shows mildly elevated serum protein, normal or slightly low glucose, a few lymphocytes and numerous organisms.

The CSF opening pressure is elevated in 25% of patients, and this has important prognostic and therapeutic implications.

About one-half of patients have evidence of pulmonary involvement with cough or dyspnea and abnormal chest radiographs. Most patients who have cryptococcal meningitis have positive blood cultures. Skin involvement is common and several types of skin lesion have been described; the most common form is that resembling molluscum contagiosum.

Cryptococcal antigen is almost invariably detectable in the CSF at high titer. A positive serum cryptococcal antigen titer of more than 1:8 is presumptive evidence of cryptococcal infection. The serum cryptococcal antigen can therefore be used as a screening test for the presence of cryptococcal infection in febrile patients who have HIV infection. The finding of a positive cryptococcal antigen titer in this setting is sufficient to warrant antifungal therapy.

An algorithm for the treatment of cryptococcal meningitis is shown in Figure 91.6. Untreated, cryptococcal meningitis is fatal. Amphotericin B (0.7 mg/kg intravenously) given for 2 weeks followed by fluconazole 400 mg orally for a further 8 weeks is associated with the best outcome in prospective trials, with a mortality of less than 10% and a mycologic response of approximately 70%.[7] The addition of flucytosine 100 mg/kg q24h with amphotericin B does not improve immediate outcome but may decrease the risk of relapse.[11]

Clinical deterioration may be due to cerebral edema, which may be diagnosed by a raised opening CSF pressure. Elevated opening pressures (>200 mmH$_2$O) have been linked with an increased risk of early mortality and/or blindness.[12] The opening pressure of all patients who have cryptococcal meningitis should be measured when a lumbar puncture is performed, and strong consideration should be given to reducing such pressure (by repeated lumbar puncture, a lumbar drain or a shunt) if the opening pressure is high (>200 mmH²O).[11]

All patients who have cryptococcal infection should receive optimal ART. An immune reconstitution syndrome has been described in some patients who initiate potent ART after cryptococcal infection. Cryptococcal meningitis requires long-term suppressive therapy (fluconazole 200 mg daily), unless there is improvement in immune function (undetectable plasma HIV viral RNA and a persistent rise in CD4+ lymphocyte count to at least 200 cells/mm³).

HISTOPLASMOSIS, COCCIDIOIDOMYCOSIS AND PENICILLIOSIS

Histoplasmosis is caused by the dimorphic fungus *Histoplasma capsulatum*, which is endemic in the Mississippi and Ohio river valleys of North America as well as in certain parts of Central and South America, Asia, Africa and the Caribbean. *Coccidioides immitis* is a dimorphic fungus found in the soil in the desert around the south-western USA and northern Mexico, as well as focal areas of Central and South America.

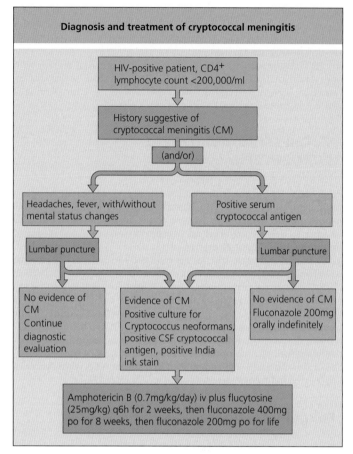

Fig. 91.6 Algorithm for the diagnosis and treatment of cryptococcal meningitis. *Continue unless CD4 T cells recover (>200 cells/mm³ for >3 months with antiretroviral therapy).

Penicilliosis is caused by the dimorphic fungus *Penicillium marneffei*, which is endemic in South East Asia (especially northern Thailand and southern China). These fungi cause disseminated infection in patients who have AIDS in endemic areas, as well as sporadic infection among HIV-positive migrants from and visitors to endemic areas.

The most common presentation is fever and weight loss. Pneumonia is usual in coccidioidomycosis and respiratory symptoms (cough, shortness of breath) occur in about 50% of cases of histoplasmosis and penicilliosis. Local or generalized lymphadenopathy, hepatosplenomegaly, colonic lesions and skin and oral ulcers also occur. Skin involvement is more common in penicilliosis. Involvement of the gastrointestinal tract (usually as ulcers) is a feature of histoplasmosis and may present with abdominal pain or gastrointestinal bleeding. Between 5% and 10% of patients with histoplasmosis have an acute septic-shock-like syndrome that includes hypotension and evidence of disseminated coagulopathy. Meningeal disease, with symptoms of lethargy, fever, headache, nausea, vomiting and/or confusion, occurs in about 10% of patients with coccidioidomycosis. Cerebrospinal fluid analysis typically reveals a lymphocytic pleocytosis with a lymphocyte count greater than 50/mm³.

Diagnosis is made by culturing the organism from clinical specimens or by demonstrating it on histopathologic examination. In histoplasmosis a peripheral blood smear may show intracellular organisms in white cells in many patients, and blood cultures, especially when collected using the lysis centrifugation system, are positive in over 90% of patients. Antigen detection in either urine or serum is an excellent method for diagnosing disseminated histoplasmosis.

For all infections, the management strategy is similar.[6] Patients should receive an initial period of treatment with amphotericin B (for 1–2 weeks) until there is clinical resolution. For histoplasmosis[13] and penicilliosis, this should be followed by itraconazole 200 mg orally q12h. For coccidioidomycosis, fluconazole, 400–800 mg q24h orally, may be an alternative for patients who have mild disease. Complete eradication is unlikely and chronic suppressive therapy with either fluconazole 200–400 mg q24h or itraconazole 200 mg q12h is needed. Successful treatment with itraconazole or fluconazole has been reported in approximately 80% patients who have *C. immitis* meningitis.

ASPERGILLOSIS

Infection with *Aspergillus* spp. is seen in patients who have advanced HIV disease. Specific risk factors that have been identified include neutropenia, use of corticosteroids and broad-spectrum antibacterial therapy and previous pneumonia, especially *Pneumocystis jirovecii* pneumonia. Typically, patients have extremely low CD4+ lymphocyte counts and a history of other AIDS-defining opportunistic infections.

Two major syndromes predominate:
- respiratory tract disease; and
- central nervous system infection.

Patients with pulmonary involvement often present with cough, shortness of breath and fever. Chest pain and hemoptysis are common. Nodular infiltrates, which may be localized or diffuse and commonly cavitate, are seen on chest radiography. Additional respiratory syndromes of pulmonary aspergilloma and localized tracheobronchial aspergillosis have been reported occasionally in patients who have AIDS. Patients who have CNS aspergillosis usually present with symptoms and signs of a mass lesion or with features of a stroke due to invasion of blood vessels. Therefore, seizures, hemiparesis and focal abnormalities are common. CT scan or MRI of the head may show single or multiple lesions, usually nonenhancing, with surrounding edema. Bony invasion is common and, because the disease may have spread from involved sinuses, the sinuses may be abnormal. Patients who have fungal sinusitis usually have the classic features of sinusitis (fever, facial pain and swelling, nasal discharge and headache). CT scan of the sinuses will usually show bony erosion, and penetration into adjacent tissues such as the brain or orbit can occur.

The prognosis of aspergillosis is poor, in part because of the fungal infection itself and in part because it tends to occur in patients who have advanced AIDS and many other complications of end-stage HIV infection. There is a poorer response to therapy in patients who have AIDS than in other immunocompromised patients. Voriconazole is the treatment of choice for invasive aspergillosis[6,14] (see Chapter 149).

Nontuberculous Mycobacterial Infections

Mycobacterium avium complex (MAC) bacteria are ubiquitous in the environment and have been isolated from a variety of sources around the world, including soil, natural water, municipal water systems, food, house dust and domestic and wild animals. These isolates are thought to be the source of most human infections but there is no evidence of MAC transmission from person to person. In untreated HIV-infected patients in the Western world, the incidence of MAC disease increases with falling CD4+ lymphocyte counts, with a cumulative probability of disseminated disease due to MAC in subjects who have CD4+ lymphocyte counts less than 50 cells/mm³ of 20–30%, and 10–20% in those who have CD4+ lymphocyte counts of 50–100 cells/mm³.

CLINICAL FEATURES

MAC infection is acquired through inhalation or ingestion of the organism, with most infections in HIV-infected patients believed to occur through colonization and invasion of the gut mucosa. Disseminated MAC disease is characterized by fever, night sweats and weight loss. The gastrointestinal tract is frequently involved and

clinical manifestations include nausea, vomiting, watery diarrhea and abdominal pain. At physical examination hepatomegaly, splenomegaly and lymphadenopathy are very common, and elevations of serum alkaline phosphatase, lactate dehydrogenase and anemia are the most frequent laboratory findings. Other nontuberculous mycobacteria, including *Mycobacterium genavense*, *M. intracellulare*, *M. haemophilum*, *M. simiae*, *M. xenopi*, *M. scrofulaceum*, *M. marinum* and *M. fortuitum*, have also been described as a cause of disseminated infection in HIV-infected patients.

Although MAC can commonly be isolated from sputum, pulmonary disease associated with MAC is rare. Patients should have a repeatedly positive culture in sputum, an infiltrate on chest radiograph, absence of other lung pathogens and preferably biopsy specimens showing acid-fast bacilli in abnormal lung tissue. However the isolation of MAC in the respiratory or gastrointestinal tract in those patients who have CD4+ lymphocyte counts less than 50 cells/mm³ represents a high risk for the development of MAC bacteremia. In this case prophylaxis or treatment should be considered.

Diagnosis of disseminated disease caused by MAC requires the isolation of the organism from a sterile site. A single blood culture has a high diagnostic yield, which is 90–95% sensitive. Once sufficient growth is achieved, the diagnosis of MAC can be made in few hours with the use of DNA probes (see Chapter 174). The diagnosis can also be made by identification of MAC from other sterile sites such as bone marrow, liver or lymph node biopsy.

The most frequent nontuberculous mycobacterium isolated from sputum in HIV-infected patients is *Mycobacterium kansasii*. Patients who have *M. kansasii* infection tend to have a low CD4+ lymphocyte count (<50 cells/mm³) and the clinical and radiologic manifestations are not different from tuberculosis. The isolation of *M. kansasii* from sputum is always considered diagnostic of pulmonary disease, since colonization is uncommon.

TREATMENT

Therapy for *Mycobacterium avium* complex

Treatment regimens should include a macrolide (clarithromycin or azithromycin) plus ethambutol.[6] The addition of rifabutin should be considered, since triple therapy has been associated with a reduction in relapses and in the emergence of resistant strains.[15] Aminoglycosides and quinolones may be useful in macrolide-resistant cases. If ART is to be used, it is important to recognize potential drug interactions between clarithromycin and both non-nucleoside reverse transcriptase inhibitors (NNRTIs) and protease inhibitors (see Practice Point 45).

In general, as with other opportunistic infections, therapy for disseminated MAC is for life. However, in situations where CD4+ T-cell counts remain greater than 100 cells/mm³ after 6–12 months of ART, patients are at low risk of recurrence of MAC and the treatment can be stopped.

Treatment of other nontuberculous mycobacterias

Mycobacterium kansasii is the second most frequent cause of pulmonary and disseminated nontuberculous mycobacterial disease. The treatment consists of a daily regimen of rifampin (rifampicin) or rifabutin, isoniazid and ethambutol for 12–18 months. *Mycobacterium genavense* and *M. haemophilum* are resistant to isoniazid, pyrazinamide and ethambutol. *Mycobacterium genavense* may be treated with a regimen similar to MAC and *M. haemophilum* with a combination of rifampin plus another active antituberculosis drug (ciprofloxacin, doxycycline, clarithromycin or amikacin). *Mycobacterium simiae* and *M. xenopi* are susceptible to isoniazid, rifampin and ethambutol and should be treated for 12 months. *Mycobacterium scrofulaceum* therapy requires surgery and isoniazid plus rifampin for 24 months with amikacin for 2–3 months. *Mycobacterium marinum* is resistant to isoniazid and pyrazinamide. Minocycline or clarithromycin or rifampin plus ethambutol for 3 months are possible therapies. *Mycobacterium fortuitum* therapy consists of amikacin plus cefoxitin plus ciprofloxacin for 1 month followed by quinolone plus clarithromycin for 3–6 months.

PREVENTION (SEE TABLE 91.1)

Prophylaxis for MAC is recommended for all AIDS patients who have CD4+ lymphocyte counts lower than 50 cells/mm³. In randomized, placebo-controlled trials, clarithromycin 500 mg/day and 1200 mg azithromycin once a week, were effective in reducing MAC bacteremia.[16,17] Before starting prophylaxis, MAC bacteremia and active tuberculosis should be ruled out. Discontinuation of MAC prophylaxis can occur in patients on ART with sustained viral suppression and a CD4+ T lymphocyte count greater than 100 cells/mm³.

Parasitic Infections

TOXOPLASMOSIS

Toxoplasmosis, caused by *Toxoplasma gondii*, an obligate intracellular protozoan, is a common OI in patients with AIDS. It has a prevalence ranging from 10% to 40% in Europe, the Caribbean area and Africa, to 5–10% in USA. This is due to the different prevalence of *T. gondii* infection in the general population of these areas. Toxoplasmosis occurs as a result of the reactivation of latent *T. gondii* infection that has persisted in the CNS or extraneural tissues after earlier acute infection. Toxoplasmosis usually occurs late in HIV disease, when the CD4+ lymphocyte count is less than 100/mm³.

The CNS is by far the most common site of toxoplasmosis and the majority of patients have encephalitis. Retinitis, pneumonitis and myocarditis are less common manifestations. Toxoplasmic encephalitis (TE) commonly manifests as single or multiple intracerebral abscesses, with focal neurologic signs and constitutional symptoms that progress over a few days or weeks. Fever and headaches are present in 40–70% of cases, neurologic dysfunction including confusion and lethargy in 40% of cases, focal CNS deficits in 50–60% of cases, and seizures in 30–40% of cases. The constellation of fever, headaches, mild neurologic deficit or any unexplained neurologic symptoms should suggest the diagnosis of TE (Fig. 91.7), and prompt CT scanning or MRI should be undertaken. MRI is more sensitive than CT scanning. Toxoplasmic abscesses are typically contrast-enhancing lesions surrounded by edema; there may be a mass effect, with displacement of the ventricles. MRI may also reveal hemorrhages, which are highly suggestive of toxoplasmic necrosis.

Most patients will have specific anti-toxoplasmal antibodies, indicating past infection (see Chapter 183). In most of cases of encephalitis, the diagnosis of toxoplasmosis is presumptive, made on clinical–radiologic criteria and confirmed by the therapeutic response. Appropriate treatment is therefore especially important, both because the response to therapy is the main criterion for diagnosis of TE, and because early initiation of therapy gives the best prognosis. Treatment consists of initial acute therapy over 3–6 weeks followed by lifelong maintenance therapy to prevent further reactivation. The combination of pyrimethamine 50–75 mg/day orally and sulfadiazine 4–6 g/day is the first-line acute therapy.[6,18] These drugs act synergistically by blocking the folic acid pathway of tachyzoites, but have no effect on the cyst forms of the parasite. Folinic acid 25 mg/day orally should be given as well to prevent bone marrow toxicity. Clinical improvement occurs within 5–10 days; the diagnosis of TE is confirmed by a decrease in both neuroradiologic and clinical abnormalities. The duration of acute therapy is 3–6 weeks. Suppressive therapy is with pyrimethamine 25 mg/day orally plus sulfadiazine 2 g/day orally lifelong or until a CD4 cell count of greater than 200/mm³ for more than 3 months is reached with ART. This combination is also effective as primary prophylaxis for *P. jirovecii* pneumonia.

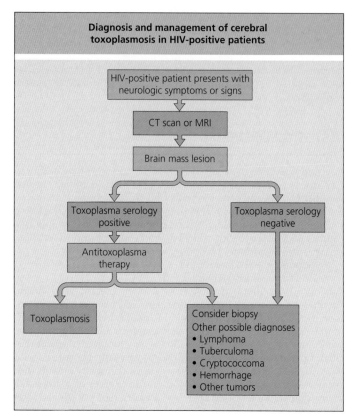

Fig. 91.7 Diagnosis and management of cerebral toxoplasmosis in HIV-positive patients. Courtesy of Christine Katlama.

CRYPTOSPORIDIOSIS

Cryptosporidiosis is a worldwide protozoan infection that is more prevalent in poorly developed countries (see also Chapter 181). It can affect normal hosts but is particularly severe in immunodeficient patients. Human cryptosporidiosis is generally caused by *Cryptosporidium parvum*, which is transmitted primarily by the fecal–oral route through person to person transmission or indirectly; outbreaks from municipal water, person-to-person transmission and animal-to-person transmission have been described. The illness is an acute enteritis. Diarrhea is the main clinical symptom, ranging in severity from mild diarrhea to cholera-like, watery diarrhea. Abdominal cramps, nausea, vomiting and anorexia usually accompany the diarrhea when it is moderate or severe. Fever is uncommon and may be due to other concurrent infections. The severity of the disease is more pronounced in patients with CD4+ lymphocyte counts less than 50/mm³. Cryptosporidiosis may rarely involve the gallbladder, the biliary tract, and the pancreatic ducts (leading to cholecystitis and pancreatitis). Diagnosis is based on the identification of the parasite in feces, in tissue specimens or in other fluids, using a modified acid-fast stain such as the Ziehl–Neelsen stain (Chapter 181).

Treatment of cryptosporidiosis is essentially symptomatic and the best option for therapy and prevention is the restoration of immune function using potent ART.

Bacterial Infections

Bacterial infections as a group, however, are the most common infectious complication of HIV disease. Patients with HIV infection are at greater risk for infections caused by common bacterial pathogens (e.g. *Streptococcus pneumoniae*, *Haemophilus influenzae*, *Salmonella* spp.) than are HIV-seronegative persons. The introduction of potent ART has been associated with a decline in the incidence of community-acquired and nosocomial bacterial pneumonia. However, the proportion of hospitalizations due to bacterial infections has increased as rates of PCP and other more opportunistic infections have declined to a greater extent. The increased rate of bacterial pneumonia in HIV-infected patients without AIDS, in comparison to HIV-negative persons, serves to emphasize that pyogenic bacterial infections may occur when immunity is relatively intact owing to the virulence of these organisms compared with other more opportunistic pathogens.

BACTERIAL PNEUMONIAS

The incidence of community-acquired bacterial pneumonia is markedly higher (three- to fivefold) among HIV-infected patients than among HIV-negative persons. Risk factors for the development of bacterial pneumonia include lower CD4+ lymphocyte counts, intravenous drug use and cigarette smoking.

In addition, risk factors for pneumococcal infection specifically include any previous history of pneumonia, low serum albumin and a lack of receipt of the pneumococcal vaccination when the patient had a CD4+ lymphocyte count greater than 200/mm³.

The clinical presentation of bacterial pneumonia in HIV-infected patients is indistinguishable from that in HIV-negative patients. The history usually reveals an acute onset of symptoms, including fever, productive cough, dyspnea and pleuritic chest pain. Physical examination commonly shows localized pulmonary findings, and laboratory evaluation may show leukocytosis and hypoxemia. Typical chest radiograph findings are of focal infiltrates, although diffuse disease may be seen. Sputum Gram stain will show multiple polymorphonuclear leukocytes, and sputum cultures are usually positive. These findings differ from the classic presentation of PCP, the most common nonbacterial cause of pneumonia in HIV-infected patients, in which the presentation is more often subacute with a nonproductive cough, a paucity of physical findings and diffuse interstitial infiltrates on chest radiograph. Nevertheless, there are frequently cases in which induced sputum examination or bronchoscopy with bronchoalveolar lavage are necessary to obtain a microbiologic diagnosis.

The pathogens most commonly responsible for bacterial pneumonia are *S. pneumoniae*, *H. influenzae* and *Haemophilus* spp. other than *H. influenzae*.[19] Other organisms that may cause disease include *M. catarrhalis*, *Klebsiella pneumoniae* and *Staphylococcus aureus*. Empiric therapy usually includes a second- or third-generation cephalosporin. If there is a lack of clinical response, other bacteria that may not respond to such treatment must be considered as possible causes (e.g. *Chlamydia pneumoniae*, *Nocardia* spp. and *Legionella* spp). In addition, in HIV-infected patients *Pseudomonas aeruginosa* frequently occurs as a community-acquired pneumonia. There are also data that suggest a shift in bacterial pathogens since the introduction of ART. A decline in *P. aeruginosa* infections has been reported, and seems to be associated with both generally higher CD4 lymphocyte counts and a reduction in the use of trimethoprim–sulfamethoxazole prophylaxis.[20]

An unusual organism responsible for bacterial pneumonia in HIV-infected patients is *Rhodococcus equi*. This bacterium is a Gram-positive rod usually associated with infections of domestic animals. In HIV-infected patients, the clinical presentation is often subacute and characterized by fever, cough, pleuritic chest pain, fatigue and weight loss. Chest radiographs often show cavitating lesions. Blood cultures may be more sensitive for diagnosis than sputum cultures – 83% sensitivity compared with 33% in one study. Treatment is usually with vancomycin (intravenously 1 g q12h), but ciprofloxacin (orally 750 mg q12h) or imipenem (intravenously 500 mg q6h) may also be used; duration of therapy is 2–4 weeks.

Bacteremia in the setting of pneumonia occurs more commonly in HIV-infected than in HIV-negative patients – increased rates of bacteremia with pneumococcal and *H. influenzae* pneumonia have been documented. Bacteremia may also occur with other pathogens responsible for pulmonary infections (e.g. *P. aeruginosa*).

SKIN INFECTIONS

Bacterial skin infections in HIV-infected patients may vary from impetigo to folliculitis to cutaneous abscesses; cutaneous abscesses are often associated with intravenous drug use as well. Recurrences may be more frequent than in the HIV-negative population, but physical findings and responsible organisms (*S. aureus* and *Streptococcus* spp.) are similar. A significant increase in subcutaneous and soft tissue abscesses associated with community-acquired methicillin-resistant *S. aureus* (MRSA) has been noted in the last few years in the USA among HIV-infected individuals.[21] Aggressive treatment with surgical drainage and appropriate antimicrobials is necessary.

Bacillary angiomatosis is a distinct skin infection specifically associated with HIV disease. (See Chapter 95.) The condition is caused either by *Bartonella henselae*, the organism also responsible for cat-scratch disease, or by *Bartonella quintana*. The clinical appearance is of very erythematous subcutaneous nodules that may occasionally resemble Kaposi's sarcoma (Fig. 91.8). Lymphadenopathy may be associated with these skin findings. Much less frequently, *B. henselae* has been identified as the cause of more deeply seated infections, including endocarditis, osteomyelitis and hepatic lesions (peliosis hepatis). Diagnosis of the skin infection may be based on the characteristic appearance, but biopsy may be carried out to rule out other causes, and it is necessary to diagnose solid-organ involvement. Histology shows vascular proliferation and mixed inflammatory cells. Warthin–Starry staining reveals the organism. Treatment is with a macrolide (erythromycin orally 250–500 mg q6h) or a tetracycline (doxycycline orally 100 mg q12h) for 1–2 months for skin disease, and longer for other sites of infection.

ENTEROCOLITIS

Among the bacterial pathogens causing diarrhea in HIV-infected patients are nontyphoidal *Salmonella* spp., *Shigella flexneri*, *Campylobacter jejunii* and *Clostridium difficile*. *Shigella* and *Campylobacter* spp. infections manifest similarly – patients note severe diarrhea (which may be bloody) associated with abdominal cramping, nausea and fever. Diagnosis is by stool culture. These infections may both be treated with oral quinolones, although resistance to quinolones is increasing (see Chapter 35).

Nontyphoidal *Salmonella* spp. infections may present either with or without diarrhea and other symptoms of colitis. In patients without gastrointestinal symptoms, the infection may manifest solely as fever without any localizing findings. The occurrence of *Salmonella* bacteremia is more common in patients with HIV infection than in HIV-seronegative groups. In addition, relapses of bacteremia are common. Unlike the recommendations for patients who are not immunosuppressed, even *Salmonella* infections limited to the gastrointestinal tract should be treated in HIV-infected patients. Treatment is usually with ciprofloxacin (500 mg q12h for 2–4 weeks), and suppressive therapy with ciprofloxacin is often used because of the risk of relapse.

Infection due to *C. difficile* may be more severe in HIV-infected patients, and these patients are more likely to have relapses and

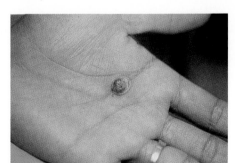

Fig. 91.8 Typical appearance of bacillary angiomatosis. Courtesy of Christine Katlama.

chronic symptoms. Antibiotic use and hospitalization are associated with the development of infection, just as they are in HIV-negative patients. *Clostridium difficile* may also occur as a community-acquired infection in HIV-infected patients. Treatment is with oral metronidazole or vancomycin.

BACTEREMIA

As discussed above, bacteremia may frequently occur as a result of *Salmonella* spp. infections and pneumonia. Bacteremia may also be associated with soft tissue infections and urinary infections. Intravenous drug use is associated with the development of *S. aureus* bacteremia and endocarditis. In addition, bacteremia may be a complication of the use of long-term intravenous catheters, which may be needed in the management of HIV-infected patients (e.g. for the intravenous treatment of CMV retinitis). The causative organisms most frequently isolated were *S. aureus* and coagulase-negative staphylococci, although infection with Gram-negative bacilli is also seen. Empiric therapy of line infections while culture results are awaited should therefore involve vancomycin and an aminoglycoside (or vancomycin and a β-lactam with broad Gram-negative coverage). As with other infections, the incidence of HIV-associated bacteremia declined in the era of potent ART, in part because of fewer hospitalizations and a reduction in the use of central venous catheters and in neutropenia.

Use of Antiretroviral Therapy During Management of Acute Opportunistic Infections

Antiretroviral therapy should be initiated as soon as possible in patients with OIs for which treatment is limited or not effective and for whom the overall improvement of immune function would be beneficial. Examples of such conditions include cryptosporidiosis,

microsporidiosis, progressive multifocal leukoencephalopathy and HIV-associated dementia.

For patients for whom definitive anti-infective therapy is available, the benefit of immediate initiation of ART in increasing CD4+ cell count and improving the patient's immunologic status must be weighed against the possibility of increased adverse effects, toxicities or drug–drug interactions. A randomized clinical trial demonstrated a clinical and survival benefit of starting ART early, within the first 2 weeks, of initiation of treatment for an acute OI.[22] The majority of OIs in this study were PCP and serious bacterial infections, and some caution must be taken extending this recommendation to OIs (such as cryptococcosis and mycobacterial infection) where the risk of immune reconstitution inflammatory syndrome (IRIS) may be higher (see Chapter 92).

The choice of regimen should follow relevant guidelines; however, in the acute setting, results of resistance testing may not be available and a boosted protease inhibitor regimen may be preferable.

Paradoxical reactions can occur in patients with active (or unrecognized) infection in whom ART can lead to an improved immune response to the underlying infective organism. This can, in turn, lead to an inflammatory response with adverse, sometimes severe, clinical consequences. These consequences of immune recovery are discussed in detail in Chapter 92.

PROPHYLAXIS OF OPPORTUNISTIC INFECTIONS

Preventive therapy for OIs was the mainstay of treatment in HIV prior to the introduction of effective ART and remains important for patients with severe immunodeficiency, even when ART-associated immune recovery can be expected. Guidelines for the primary prevention of OIs are given in Table 91.1 and recommendations for secondary prophylaxis (prevention of recurrence of OIs) are given in Table 91.2.

Table 91.1 Prophylaxis of first episode of opportunistic infections in adults and adolescents with HIV infection

Pathogen	Target population	First-choice regimen	Alternative regimens
Category I: recommended as standard of care			
Pneumocystis jirovecii	CD4+ lymphocyte count <200/mm³ and/or oropharyngeal candidiasis	TMP–SMX 1 DS q24h or 1 SS q24h	Dapsone 100 mg q24h or 50 mg q12h Dapsone 50 mg q24h plus pyrimethamine 50 mg weekly plus leucovorin 25 mg weekly Dapsone 200 mg weekly plus pyrimethamine 75 mg weekly plus leucovorin 25 mg weekly Aerosolized pentamidine 300 mg monthly by nebulizer Atovaquone 1500 mg q24h TMP–SMX 1 DS three times a week
Toxoplasma gondii	CD4+ lymphocyte count <100/mm³ and positive anti-*Toxoplasma* IgG	TMP–SMX 1 DS q24h	TMP–SMX 1 SS q24h Dapsone 50 mg q24h plus pyrimethamine 50 mg weekly plus leucovorin 25 mg weekly Dapsone 200 mg weekly plus pyrimethamine 75 mg weekly plus leucovorin 25 mg weekly Atovaquone 1500 mg q24h with or without pyrimethamine 25 mg and leucovorin 10 mg q24h

Table 91.1 Prophylaxis of first episode of opportunistic infections in adults and adolescents with HIV infection—cont'd

Pathogen	Target population	First-choice regimen	Alternative regimens
Mycobacterium tuberculosis	Positive PPD (5 mm) and/or previous positive PPD without treatment and/or contact with active case (regardless of PPD result)	Isoniazid 300 mg q24h or isoniazid 900 mg twice weekly for 9 months either plus pyridoxine 50 mg q24h *If resistance*: choice of drugs depends on susceptibility of isolate from source patient; consult with public health authorities	Rifampin (rifampicin) 300 mg q24h for 4 months Rifabutin (dose based on antiretroviral therapy) for 4 months
Mycobacterium avium complex	CD4+ lymphocyte count <50 cells/mm³ (need to rule out active mycobacterial infection before starting prophylaxis)	Clarithromycin 500 mg q12h or azithromycin 1200 mg weekly	Rifabutin 300 mg q24h
Varicella-zoster virus (VZV)	Exposure to chickenpox or shingles and no history of either infection, vaccination or negative serology	Varicella-zoster virus 1 g, 5 vials im within 96 hours of exposure (preferably within 48 h)	
Category II: generally recommended			
Streptococcus pneumoniae	CD4+ lymphocyte count >200 cells/mm³	223-valent polysaccharide vaccine 0.5 ml im (single dose); repeat in 5 years	
Hepatitis B virus	All anti-HBV-negative patients	Hepatitis B vaccine 10 mg im (three doses)	Anti-HBs should be obtained 1 month after completion of the vaccine series Nonresponders should be revaccinated with a second vaccine series
Influenza virus	All patients	Inactivated trivalent Influenza vaccine 0.5 ml im each year in autumn	
Hepatitis A virus	All anti-HAV-negative patients at increased risk (intravenous drug users, men who have sex with men, hemophiliacs) or with chronic liver disease, including chronic hepatitis B or C	Hepatitis A vaccine (two doses)	
Category III: not recommended for most patients. To be considered in selected patients only			
Cytomegalovirus (CMV)	CD4+ lymphocyte count <50 cells/ml and positive CMV viremia	Oral valganciclovir 900 mg q24h	
Cryptococcus neoformans	CD4+ lymphocyte count <50 cells/mm³	Fluconazole 100–200 mg q24h	
Histoplasmosis	CD4+ lymphocyte count <100 cells/mm³ and residence in endemic area	Itraconazole 200 mg q24h	

DS, double strength; PPD, purified protein derivatives; SS, single strength; TMP–SMX, trimethoprim–sulfamethoxazole.
Adapted from USPHS/IDSA guidelines.[6]

Certain principles underlie the decision to use prophylaxis for different pathogens:

- the incidence and prevalence of specific infections in HIV-infected individuals;
- the potential severity of disease in terms of morbidity and mortality;
- the level of immunosuppression at which each disease is likely to occur;
- the feasibility and efficacy of preventive measures, and in particular their impact on quality of life and survival;
- the potential for emergence of organisms resistant to the agents used for prophylaxis;
- the risk of toxicities and drug interactions with antiretrovirals and other drugs used by HIV-infected patients;
- the issue of compliance; and
- the cost-effectiveness of prophylaxis.

As an example, PCP is very common, causes significant mortality and can be easily prevented; as a result routine prophylaxis is recommended for all HIV-positive patients with CD4+ T-cell counts less than 200 cells/mm³. In contrast, candidiasis is also very common, but rarely causes mortality, is easily treated and prophylactic antifungals are associated with a significant risk of resistance, so prophylaxis is rarely given. Cryptococcal meningitis is associated with significant mortality and is preventable using fluconazole; however, prevention is not regarded as cost-effective in the West because it is relatively rare; in contrast primary prophylaxis is justified in areas such as sub-Saharan Africa and South Asia.

Table 91.2 Prophylaxis to prevent recurrence of opportunistic disease in adults and adolescents with HIV infection

Pathogen	Indication	First-choice regimen	Alternative regimens
Category I: Recommended as standard of care			
Pneumocystis jirovecii (PCP)	Previous PCP	TMP–SMX 1 SS q24h or 1 DS q24h	Dapsone 50 mg q12h or 100 mg q24h Dapsone 50 mg q24h plus pyrimethamine 50 mg weekly plus leucovorin 25 mg weekly Dapsone 200 mg plus pyrimethamine 75 mg plus leucovorin 25 mg weekly Aerosolized pentamidine 300 mg monthly by nebulizer Atovaquone 1500 mg q24h TMP–SMX, 1 DS three times weekly
Toxoplasma gondii	Prior toxoplasmic encephalitis	Sulfadiazine 500–1000 mg q6h plus pyrimethamine 25–50 mg q24h plus leucovorin 10–25 mg po q24h (confers protection against PCP)	Clindamycin 300–450 mg q6–8h plus pyrimethamine 25–50 mg q24h plus leucovorin 10–25 mg q24h Atovaquone 750 mg q6–12h with or without pyrimethamine 25 mg q24h plus leucovorin 10 mg q24h
Mycobacterium avium complex	Documented disseminated disease	Clarithromycin 500 mg q12h plus ethambutol 15 mg/kg q24h (with or without rifabutin 300 mg q24h)	Azithromycin 500–600 mg q24h plus ethambutol 15 mg/kg q24h (with or without rifabutin 300 mg q24h)
Cytomegalovirus	Previous end-organ disease	Valganciclovir 900 mg q24h Ganciclovir sustained-release implant every 6–9 months plus valganciclovir 900 mg q24h	Ganciclovir 5 mg/kg/q24h iv 5–7 days/week or foscarnet 90–120 mg/kg iv q24h or cidofovir 5 mg/kg iv every 2 weeks (with saline hydration probenecid)
Cryptococcus neoformans	Documented disease	Fluconazole 200 mg q24h	Itraconazole 200 mg q24h
Histoplasma capsulatum	Documented disease	Itraconazole 200 mg q12h	Amphotericin B 1.0 mg/kg weekly
Coccidioides immitis	Documented disease	Fluconazole 400 mg q24h	Itraconazole 200 mg q12h
Salmonella spp. (non-*typhi*)	Bacteremia	Ciprofloxacin 500 mg q12h for several months	Antibiotic chemoprophylaxis with another active agent
Category II: Recommended only if subsequent episodes are frequent or severe			
Herpes simplex virus	Frequent/severe recurrences	Valaciclovir 500 mg q12h or aciclovir 400 mg q12h or famciclovir 500 mg q12h	
Candida (oropharyngeal, vaginal or esophageal)	Frequent/severe recurrences	Fluconazole 100–200 mg q24h	

DS, double strength; SS, single strength.
Adapted from USPHS/IDSA guidelines.[6]

DURATION OF PROPHYLAXIS AGAINST OPPORTUNISTIC INFECTIONS

Susceptibility to opportunistic infections can be accurately assessed by the CD4+ T-cell count. It is therefore possible to stop primary or secondary prophylaxis in patients whose immunity has improved as a consequence of HAART and whose T cells have risen above the threshold of increased susceptibility. This is particulary true for patients with complete viral suppression, as ongoing improvements in immune function can be expected.

By contrast, no data are available regarding the re-initiation of prophylaxis when the CD4+ lymphocyte count decreases again to levels at which the risk for opportunistic infections exists. In particular, it is unknown whether it is better to use the threshold at which prophylaxis was stopped or the threshold below which initial prophylaxis is recommended.

REFERENCES

References for this chapter can be found online at http://www.expertconsult.com

Chapter | **92** | *Martyn A French*
Graeme Meintjes

Disorders of immune reconstitution in patients with HIV infection

INTRODUCTION

Suppression of HIV infection by combination antiretroviral therapy (ART) usually results in the reversal of HIV-induced immune defects, leading to at least partial reconstitution of the immune system and the prevention or regression of immunodeficiency disease. However, those patients who were very immunodeficient prior to commencing ART are susceptible to disorders of immune reconstitution that may cause disease.[1] These disorders most often present clinically as inflammatory and/or autoimmune immune disease and are often referred to collectively as the immune reconstitution inflammatory syndrome (IRIS).[2] This syndrome consists of more than one disorder, which may have different pathogenic mechanisms. These are:

- immune restoration disease (IRD) resulting from the restoration of pathogen-specific immune responses that cause inflammatory or cellular proliferative disease;
- immune-mediated inflammatory disease (IMID), in which immune mechanisms are implicated but the triggers are poorly understood; and
- autoimmune disease, predominantly Graves' disease.

In addition, persistent deficiency and/or dysfunction of T and B cells are other disorders of immune reconstitution that may increase the risk of illness in patients receiving ART. As increased numbers of HIV-infected individuals throughout the world receive ART, many patients will experience disorders of immune reconstitution and physicians managing patients with HIV infection should become familiar with their presentation, assessment and management.

IMMUNE RESTORATION DISEASE

History and immunopathogenesis

When zidovudine was introduced as the first antiretroviral drug in the late 1980s, it was observed that *Mycobacterium avium* complex (MAC) disease sometimes occurred during the first weeks to months of treatment. This had an atypical clinical presentation for MAC disease complicating AIDS because it was usually localized in distribution and associated with more inflammation than usually occurred in MAC disease complicating AIDS. Furthermore, it was associated with the restoration, rather than absence, of a cellular immune response to mycobacterial antigens. This type of MAC disease therefore appeared to reflect the restoration of a cellular immune response against subclinical MAC infection that resulted in immunopathology.[3] Similar observations were made when ART was introduced in the latter half of the 1990s[4,5] but the range of pathogens that could provoke an inflammatory response was much larger. Indeed, virtually any pathogen that can cause an opportunistic infection can provoke IRD when pathogen-specific immune responses are restored by ART (Table 92.1). As can be seen from Table 92.1, the nomenclature used for these disorders often reflects the clinical perspective from which they were described. Immune restoration disease can be differentiated from immunodeficiency disease based on clinical, histopathologic and immunologic characteristics (Table 92.2).

The anatomic site and clinicopathologic characteristics of the inflammation in IRD are largely determined by the provoking pathogen.[6] For example, *Mycobacterium tuberculosis* IRD mainly affects lymph nodes and lung, cryptococcal IRD usually affects the meninges and JC polyomavirus IRD (inflammatory progressive multifocal leukoencephalopathy after ART) affects the brain. Histopathology of affected tissues often reveals granulomatous inflammation when IRD is associated with an infection by mycobacteria, fungi or protozoa, and a CD8+ T-cell response when associated with infection by viruses, such as JC polyomavirus.

Mycobacterial IRD is associated with an increase in circulating T cells reacting with mycobacterial antigens, which has been demonstrated by skin testing, lymphoproliferation assays and interferon gamma (IFN-γ) release assays (IGRAs).[6,7] Restoration of mycobacteria-specific immune responses may not be associated with an increase in total circulating CD4+ T cells. For example, about 10% of patients with IRD provoked by nontuberculous mycobacteria (NTM) do not experience an increased blood CD4+ T-cell count[8] and several studies have not shown an association between *M. tuberculosis* IRD and the magnitude of the CD4+ T-cell count increase.[9] The role that restoration of pathogen-specific immune responses plays in IRD related to other pathogens is less clear. However, what evidence there is, along with the clinical features and timing of disease onset, suggest that pathogenic mechanisms are similar.[1,6]

Most cases of IRD present during the first 3 months of ART and usually during the first few weeks (early IRD). Some present later and up to 2 years after commencing ART (late IRD). The infection by the provoking pathogen may not be apparent before ART is commenced and is 'unmasked' by the immune response against it. Viable pathogens are usually isolated from the affected tissues of this 'unmasking' type of IRD but isolation from blood cultures is unusual. In other patients, IRD is provoked by an infection for which the patient is on treatment or that has recently been treated. Pathogens are usually not cultured, or are very difficult to culture, from specimens taken from the site of the IRD. It appears that there is an immune response against the antigens of nonviable pathogens. In this situation, there often appears to be a paradoxical worsening of the opportunistic infection when ART is commenced and, therefore, the term 'paradoxical IRD' is often used. It is important to recognize that this does not represent failure of treatment for the opportunistic infection, but rather an immunopathologic reaction to residual antigens of the pathogen. As there are currently no confirmatory diagnostic tests for IRD, it is necessary to use diagnostic criteria and exclude differential diagnoses that may account for the clinical deterioration before making the diagnosis of paradoxical IRD (Table 92.3).

Table 92.1 Pathogens that may provoke IRD when pathogen-specific immune responses are restored by antiretroviral therapy (ART)

Pathogen	Typical disease presentation/nomenclature
Mycobacteria	
M. avium	MAC IRD
M. tuberculosis	Mtb IRD or TB-IRIS
M. leprae	Leprosy reversal reaction after commencing ART
Bacille Calmette–Guérin	BCG lymphadenitis after ART or BCG IRIS
Other nontuberculous mycobacteria	
Fungi and yeasts	
Cryptococcus spp.	Cryptococcal IRIS or IRD (mainly meningitis)
Histoplasma spp.	
Malasezia furfur	Inflammatory seborrheic dermatitis after ART
Pityrosporon spp.	Folliculitis after ART
Pneumocystis jirovecii	'Relapse' of pneumonitis after ART
Candida	
Aspergillus	
Penicillium	
Dermatophytes	Inflammatory tinea corporis after ART
Protozoans	
Toxoplasma gondii	Exacerbation or presentation of cerebral toxoplasmosis after ART
Leishmania spp.	
Microsporidia	
Cryptosporidium parvum	
Viruses	
Cytomegalovirus (CMV)	CMV immune recovery uveitis
Varicella-zoster virus	Cutaneous zoster or CNS disease
Herpes simplex virus 1 and 2	Mucocutaneous herpes (which may be necrotizing or hemorrhagic) or CNS disease
Human herpesvirus 8	Exacerbation or presentation of Kaposi's sarcoma
Molluscum contagiosum virus	Inflammatory molluscum contagiosum
JC polyomavirus	Inflammatory progressive multifocal leukoencephalopathy
BK polyomavirus	
Hepatitis B virus	ART-associated hepatotoxicity
Hepatitis C virus	ART-associated hepatotoxicity
Parvovirus B19	Exacerbation of red cell aplasia, encephalitis
Human papillomavirus	Wart enlargement or inflammation
HIV	Exacerbation of HIV encephalitis after ART
Helminths	
Schistosoma	
Strongyloides	
Bacteria	
Bartonella	

IRD, immune restoration disease; IRIS, immune reconstitution inflammatory syndrome; MAC, Mycobacterium avium complex.

Table 92.2 Comparison of immune restoration disease and immunodeficiency disease in patients with HIV infection

Immune restoration disease	Immunodeficiency disease
Restoration of a pathogen-specific 'protective' immune response that causes immunopathology*	Failure of 'protective' immune responses to control pathogen replication
Always associated with a decline in the plasma HIV RNA level	Usually associated with a high plasma HIV RNA level†
Usually associated with an increased circulating CD4+ T cell count‡	Associated with a low circulating CD4+ T cell count
Inflammation usually greater than in immunodeficiency disease, e.g. painful tissue lesions	Tissue inflammation may be absent
Tissue lesions exhibit changes of an immune response, e.g. scarcity of pathogens, and of immunopathology, e.g. granulomatous reaction, suppuration or necrosis	Histopathology of tissue lesions demonstrates changes of an impaired immune response, e.g. abundance of pathogens, poorly formed granulomata in mycobacterial disease

*Immune restoration disease (IRD) provoked by infections with nontuberculous mycobacteria and M. tuberculosis has clearly been associated with restoration of cellular immune responses to mycobacterial antigens. The evidence for other pathogens is circumstantial or unclear.
†Persistent immune defects in patients with long-term optimal control of HIV replication may rarely be complicated by opportunistic infections.
‡The circulating CD4+ T cell count may not be increased in some patients with IRD, e.g. about 10% of patients with Mycobacterium avium complex IRD do not have an increased count.[8]

Table 92.3 Key diagnostic features of immune restoration disease

- Proven HIV infection
- Temporal relationship to antiretroviral therapy initiation
- Evidence or inference of immune recovery, for example:
  - Increase of the circulating CD4+ T cell count
  - Decrease of plasma HIV RNA level
  - Evidence of increased pathogen-specific immune response, e.g. tuberculin skin test conversion
  - Evidence of an immunopathologic 'protective' pathogenic-specific immune response in tissues affected by immune restoration disease
- Presentation characterized by prominent inflammatory features clinically or radiologically
- Exclusion of other causes for clinical deterioration, which may include:
  - Resistance of opportunistic pathogens to antimicrobial drugs
  - Another infection or malignancy
  - Adverse drug reactions
  - Poor compliance with or malabsorption of treatment for the opportunistic infection

The major risk factors for the development of paradoxical IRD are a very low CD4+ T-cell count, disseminated infection by the provoking pathogen and a short time of therapy for the opportunistic infection before ART is commenced.[4,9,10] All of these risk factors are probably markers of a high pathogen load. A low CD4+ T-cell count may also be a marker of an increased susceptibility to immune dysregulation during immune reconstitution.

The incidence of IRD amongst cohorts of patients initiating ART has been reported to be between 10% and 45% for those with a documented underlying opportunistic infection and between 10% and 25% amongst unselected patients in retrospective studies. A prospective study from South Africa reported an incidence of 10.4% in an unselected cohort of 423 patients during the first 6 months of ART.[11] In this study, *M. tuberculosis* IRD (which is commonly known as TB-IRIS) was the commonest type of IRD. This presents in many ways (Table 92.4) and is the most significant type of IRD in areas where co-infection with HIV and *M. tuberculosis* is common.[12,13]

Management

The important principles in managing IRD are to ensure that the patient is on appropriate antimicrobial therapy to suppress replication of the provoking pathogen and reduce pathogen load, continue ART unless disease is life threatening, and consider the use of anti-inflammatory therapy to control inflammation and provide symptom relief. Symptom relief might also require other medication (e.g. analgesics) or drainage of inflammatory fluid collections.

Several characteristics of IRD are relevant to making decisions about treatment: most cases are self-limiting, mortality is uncommon and corticosteroid therapy (the most frequently used anti-inflammatory therapy) has important adverse effects. In a minority of cases, IRD may present with severe and potentially life-threatening manifestations. This is especially the case when there is central nervous system (CNS) involvement. Systemic corticosteroids have been used in patients with IRD related to infection with *M. tuberculosis*, MAC and *Cryptococcus neoformans*, with several reports of a favorable response. Nonsteroidal anti-inflammatory drugs (NSAIDs) have also been used to treat IRD. However, no prospective controlled clinical trials regarding the treatment of IRD have been published so far and treatment guidelines are therefore informed by case series.

Table 92.4 Common manifestations of *M. tuberculosis* IRD (TB-IRIS)

- Worsening or recurrence of TB symptoms
- Weight loss
- Fever and/or systemic inflammatory syndrome
- Lymph node enlargement
- Cold abscess formation
- Respiratory manifestations
  - Progressive pulmonary infiltrates on chest radiography (several patterns described, including miliary infiltrates and alveolitis)
  - Pleural effusions
  - Lymph node compression of airways
- Abdominal manifestations
  - Hepatic enlargement and abscesses
  - Splenic enlargement, rupture and abscesses
  - Intestinal involvement, e.g. ileocecal perforation
  - Peritonitis
  - Ascites
  - Psoas and intra-abdominal abscesses
- Central nervous system manifestations
  - Tuberculoma enlargement
  - Meningitis
  - Myeloradiculitis
- Genitourinary tract manifestations
  - Renal involvement with acute renal failure
  - Ureteric compression
  - Epididymo-orchitis
- Other system involvement
  - Arthritis and osteitis
  - Pericardial effusion
  - Bone marrow involvement

ART is continued in most settings, but some authorities have suggested interrupting ART if IRD is life threatening or unresponsive to corticosteroids. However, interruption of ART places the patient at risk of other opportunistic infections and the development of antiretroviral resistance, and IRD may still recur when ART is re-initiated.

Corticosteroid therapy for *M. tuberculosis* IRD

Corticosteroids have been used to treat *M. tuberculosis* IRD more than any other type of IRD.[13,14] However, the risks and benefits of corticosteroid therapy are unclear and need to be carefully weighed up. Because of the immunosuppressive effect of corticosteroid therapy, its use has been associated with an excess of Kaposi's sarcoma and herpes virus reactivations in HIV-infected patients. Also, if the diagnosis of IRD is incorrect and the cause for deterioration is drug resistance, or an additional unrecognized infection, corticosteroids could compound the diagnostic error.

Given that most cases of *M. tuberculosis* IRD are self-limiting, corticosteroids are usually reserved for patients with more severe manifestations and in whom the diagnosis is certain. Such patients include those with CNS involvement, airway compression due to enlarging lymphadenopathy, refractory or debilitating lymphadenitis, or respiratory distress. The duration of corticosteroid therapy required is variable. Some patients only require a few weeks whereas a subgroup of patients with *M. tuberculosis* IRD may require prolonged courses to control symptoms. Prednisone is the most frequently used corticosteroid and has been used at doses varying from 10 to 120 mg daily.

Clinical presentation

The great majority of pathogens that cause opportunistic infections (OIs) in patients with HIV infection may also provoke IRD. Consequently, the clinical presentation of IRD can vary greatly.

Central nervous system disease

IRD involving the CNS is potentially life threatening and can result in permanent neurologic disability. Manifestations include new or recurrent meningitis and inflammation involving the brain parenchyma, spinal cord (myelitis) or nerve roots (radiculitis). A number of pathogens have been associated with IRD of the CNS and, like other forms of IRD, disease may present as an unmasking of a previously untreated OI or paradoxical deterioration or recurrent manifestations of a treated infection. The interruption of ART should be seriously considered in these patients, particularly those who have a depressed level of consciousness and those who do not respond to other measures such as corticosteroid therapy.

Meningitis

Patients with cryptococcal meningitis who have been appropriately treated with antifungal therapy may experience a recurrence of meningitis after commencing ART.[15–17] This occurs in up to 30% of patients and typically manifests with recurrent headaches and features of raised intracranial pressure. Cerebrospinal fluid (CSF) fungal culture is usually negative, but the Indian ink and cryptococcal antigen tests are usually positive, reflecting persistence of nonviable organisms. The meningitis usually occurs around 4 weeks after ART is started but cases presenting months to years after ART initiation are described. The reported mortality rate has varied from 9% to 66%. Risk factors identified are disseminated disease, higher cryptococcal antigen titer at diagnosis of cryptococcal disease and a shorter time between starting antifungal therapy and ART. Treatment should include analgesia, therapeutic lumbar punctures to reduce raised intracranial pressure and corticosteroid therapy in refractory cases. ART interruption is seldom necessary.

Similarly, patients receiving treatment for tuberculosis (TB) may present with TB meningitis (TBM) after ART initiation. In some patients this will be recurrent TBM, but others will have had TB at an extraneural site and present with new TBM as an IRD phenomenon. Treatment is with corticosteroids, for which there is evidence of efficacy in TBM.[18]

Inflammation of the brain parenchyma

Inflammation of the brain parenchyma due to IRD may manifest as focal mass lesions (granulomas, such as tuberculomas, or brain abscesses) or a diffuse process (encephalitis). Both processes may be complicated by cerebral edema. Mass lesions tend to present with focal neurologic deficits or seizures. *M. tuberculosis* IRD may present with the emergence or enlargement of cerebral tuberculomas (Fig. 92.1). This may occur in patients already on treatment for TB. Cases of cerebral toxoplasmosis, cryptococcomas and abscesses associated with infection by NTM emerging or enlarging due to IRD are also described. Treatment of these conditions involves appropriate treatment of the infection and corticosteroid therapy, particularly when there is significant cerebral edema and mass effect.

Patients with encephalitis caused by IRD may present with multiple focal deficits or a disturbance of higher cerebral functions. JC polyomavirus infection of oligodendrocytes typically results in progressive multifocal leukoencephalopathy (PML) in patients with severe HIV-induced immunodeficiency. In patients not receiving ART, this is a subacute illness with progressive neurologic deterioration. Brain imaging typically does not demonstrate significant inflammation. In patients who develop IRD related to known or previously undiagnosed JC polyomavirus infection, the clinical progression is typically accelerated and imaging demonstrates prominent inflammation. Histopathology of brain biopsies in such patients shows a perivascular mononuclear cell infiltrate consisting predominantly of CD8+ T cells.[19,20]

Rare cases of encephalitis resulting from IRD associated with infections by varicella-zoster virus (VZV), herpes simplex virus (HSV), cytomegalovirus (CMV), parvovirus B19, BK virus and HIV itself have been described. In HIV-associated encephalitis, patients have experienced rapid deterioration of HIV dementia, which has been ascribed to an inflammatory response against HIV itself in brain parenchyma. In the few cases reported to date, histopathology on brain samples obtained by biopsy or at post-mortem showed infiltration with mononuclear cells (particularly CD8+ T cells), which in some instances was demonstrated to be associated with HIV DNA.[21]

Myelitis and radiculitis

Myelitis caused by IRD has been described in association with VZV and HSV infection. The pathogen associated with the IRD may be identified by examination of CSF for DNA by polymerase chain reaction (PCR). Spinal cord intramedullary abscess due to cryptococcal IRD has also been reported.

Myeloradiculitis may rarely be a complication of meningitis in *M. tuberculosis* IRD. Inflammation in the meninges results in nerve root inflammation causing neurologic fall-out in the nerve roots affected, most frequently lumbosacral nerve roots.

Eye disease

CMV eye disease typically manifests as necrotizing retinitis without significant inflammation in patients with advanced HIV infection who are not receiving ART. After commencing ART, retinitis may result from the unmasking of subclinical CMV infection of the eye[22] or present as a paradoxical 'relapse' of retinitis in patients with treated CMV retinitis.[4,6] This is usually associated with an increased circulating CD4+ T-cell count. Frequently, uveitis characterized by prominent inflammation also occurs in association with the retinitis.

Uveitis related to CMV may also present in patients with healed retinitis and is the most common form of ocular IRD. There may be intense inflammation in the absence of active CMV infection and it appears that the uveitis results from an immune response against retained CMV antigens. This condition has therefore been referred to as immune recovery uveitis (IRU).[23] It may result in vitritis, papillitis, macular edema and epiretinal membranes, and can be sight threatening. Furthermore, retinal neovascularization may be a late complication and occur over 4 years after cessation of anti-CMV therapy.[24] The incidence of IRU is highest in patients with the largest areas of previous retinitis and may be reduced by giving therapy for CMV retinitis prior to commencing ART,[25] suggesting that the amount of residual antigen is a determinant of disease onset. Many cases are self-limiting, but orbital floor corticosteroid injections may be necessary, especially if there is declining visual acuity. The condition should be managed by an ophthalmologist.

Uveitis may also result from IRD associated with other pathogens including mycobacteria, *Histoplasma* spp. or *Leishmania major*. Anterior stromal keratitis resulting from IRD associated with VZV infection has also been described.

Lymphadenitis and soft tissue abscesses

Lymphadenitis resulting from IRD may develop in any region of the body and is often painful (Fig. 92.2). Multiple nodes that suppurate and coalesce may form inflammatory masses or cold abscesses, common sites being in the omentum and retroperitoneal space. The latter may form a psoas abscess. Cold abscesses (e.g. subcutaneous cold abscesses) may also form *de novo* in soft tissues, unrelated to lymph nodes.

In developing countries, *M. tuberculosis* is the most frequent underlying infection and lymphadenitis is the most frequent clinical manifestation of *M. tuberculosis* IRD, occurring in up to 70% of patients.[12] Patients are usually receiving treatment for TB and present with recurrent, new or worsening node enlargement after starting ART (paradoxical IRD). This is most frequently in the cervical region. Nodal masses can enlarge to greater than 10 cm in diameter. Often the lymphadenitis has prominent acute inflammatory features with tenderness and red

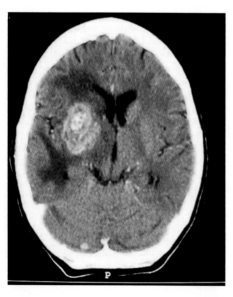

Fig. 92.1 Tuberculoma with surrounding edema in *M. tuberculosis* IRD (TB-IRIS).

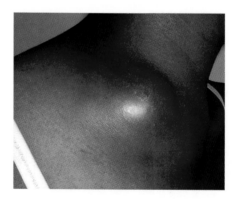

Fig. 92.2 Lymphadenitis in *M. tuberculosis* IRD (TB-IRIS).

discoloration of the overlying skin and suppuration. These features would be unusual for TB lymphadenitis in a patient not receiving ART. Large amounts of pus may be aspirated from these nodes and draining sinuses may form. The pus is typically negative for *M. tuberculosis* cultures, but may be smear-positive, reflecting the presence of non-viable mycobacteria.

Lymphadenitis is also a frequent manifestation of IRD associated with infection by NTM, such as MAC and *M. scrofulaceum*. Lymphadenitis due to MAC IRD may persist for months or even years in some patients despite treatment for the MAC infection and corticosteroid therapy.[8] IRD related to bacille Calmette-Guérin (BCG) infection following BCG vaccination of children with HIV infection has also been described.[26] This condition manifests as an inflammatory reaction at the vaccination site as well as lymphadenitis involving the regional draining lymph nodes.

Lymphadenitis and subcutaneous abscesses have also been reported in IRD associated with infection by fungi, specifically cryptococci and *Histoplasma* spp.[27] and the protozoan pathogen *Leishmania* spp.

Potential complications of IRD lymphadenitis are airway compression, venous compression resulting in deep vein thrombosis, ureteric compression and chronic draining sinuses. Compression of airways or other vital structures is usually treated with corticosteroids.

Mucocutaneous disease

A wide variety of skin conditions have been reported to present or worsen after ART is commenced.[28] Most of these conditions cause minor morbidity and usually respond to specific therapy for the associated infection. An important clinical issue is the differentiation of IRD manifestations such as acne, papular pruritic eruption of AIDS and eosinophilic folliculitis from a drug hypersensitivity reaction in the skin in order to avoid unnecessary interruption of that drug.

Both herpes simplex and herpes zoster have been reported to occur with increased frequency during early ART compared to HIV-infected patients not receiving ART. In one study, herpes zoster was found to occur five times more frequently from weeks 4 to 16 after ART initiation.[29] Herpes zoster usually manifests as typical monodermatomal lesions that respond to antiviral therapy, but disseminated cases are reported. Herpes simplex manifests with either nasolabial or anogenital ulceration, which may be necrotizing and hemorrhagic. It typically responds to appropriate systemic antiviral therapy, although refractory cases are described.

Exacerbations of Kaposi's sarcoma (KS) due to IRD occur in a minority of patients starting ART (7% in one study[30]) but may result in tumor enlargement, new lesions, inflammation and edema. Although most cases involve the skin, rapid and fatal progression of visceral KS due to IRD has been described. It is probable that the restoration of an immune response against antigens of human herpesvirus 8 (the causative agent of KS) or possibly tumor antigens provokes this IRD. Resolution without treatment may occur but severe cases may require treatment with systemic chemotherapy.

Mycobacterium leprae infection of the skin is recognized in the setting of HIV disease and has been documented to present as unmasking IRD. The reported cases have manifested with inflammatory reversal reactions involving skin lesions or neuritis.[31]

Liver disease

Hepatotoxicity or a hepatitis flare presenting as an increase in the serum transaminase levels is a well-recognized adverse effect of ART. Many studies have examined risk factors for hepatotoxicity and demonstrated that drug hypersensitivity reactions and drug-induced mitochondrial toxicity are implicated in some cases. Hepatitis C virus (HCV) and hepatitis B virus (HBV) co-infection are also important risk factors.[32] However, the pathogenesis of the liver disease is debated. The timing of hepatotoxicity after ART in patients with HIV and HCV or HBV co-infection is similar to other cases of IRD, suggesting that it might be a manifestation of IRD in the liver. Supportive evidence

is provided by reports of the exacerbation of hepatitis on liver biopsy and changes in serologic immune markers in HIV/HCV co-infected patients[33,34] and case reports of clearance of the hepatitis virus infection after the hepatitis flare for both co-infections. However, definitive studies of the immunopathogenesis have not yet been reported.

Infection of the liver by mycobacteria, fungi and protozoa may also provoke IRD after ART is commenced. The inflammation may cause right upper quadrant pain, fever and an inflammatory infiltrate in the liver that is characterized by granulomas or abscess formation. *M. tuberculosis* is the most common pathogen[35] but MAC, *Leishmania* spp., *Histoplasma* spp. and *Cryptococcus neoformans* have also been implicated.

Abdominal and renal disease

Abdominal pain is a common manifestation of intra-abdominal lymphadenitis resulting from IRD, which is usually associated with mycobacterial infection. Pain may also result from hepatitis caused by IRD (see above). It may also be a manifestation of IRD associated with infections by *Histoplasma* spp. resulting in infarction of the spleen or intestinal inflammation.[36] Peritonitis due to *M. tuberculosis* IRD may also result in abdominal pain and even mimic a 'surgical abdomen'.

Acute renal failure may result directly from granulomatous inflammation in the kidneys caused by *M. tuberculosis* IRD.

Lung disease

Paradoxical *M. tuberculosis* IRD frequently presents with a recurrence of cough and other respiratory symptoms after patients on treatment for *M. tuberculosis* infection start ART. This may be associated with new or worsening radiographic features of TB, including expanding pulmonary infiltrates, progressive cavitation, enlarging thoracic lymph nodes and enlarging pleural effusions.

In addition, patients with undiagnosed *M. tuberculosis* infection prior to ART may present with pulmonary disease soon after starting ART. This often presents in an accelerated way with prominent inflammatory features and appears to result from *M. tuberculosis* infection being unmasked by restoration of *M. tuberculosis*-specific immune responses. This presentation may mimic that of a community-acquired bacterial pneumonia and may be associated with a systemic inflammatory syndrome and respiratory failure.

MAC IRD may manifest with thoracic involvement including pulmonary infiltrates, endobronchial lesions and thoracic node enlargement. Other NTM such as *M. celatum*, *M. xenopi* and *M. kansasii* have also been associated with focal pulmonary infiltrates due to IRD.

Pneumonitis associated with *Pneumocystis jirovecii* infection has also been reported as a manifestation of IRD. Patients who have been treated for *P. jirovecii* pneumonitis (PJP) have developed a self-limiting or corticosteroid-responsive pneumonitis days to weeks after starting ART. Presentation has been with recurrent fever, dyspnea and cough, and chest radiography demonstrating alveolar infiltrates. Bronchoscopy at the time of IRD typically demonstrates an unusually vigorous inflammatory response but few or no *Pneumocystis* organisms, suggesting that this is an inflammatory response to residual *P. jirovecii* antigens.[37] Treatment is with appropriate antibiotics for PJP, usually TMP–SMX, and corticosteroid therapy.

Cryptococcal IRD has also been reported to present as necrotizing pneumonitis and thoracic lymphadenitis.[38]

Serous effusions

M. tuberculosis IRD may manifest as new or enlarging serous effusions (pleural effusions, pericardial effusions and ascites). Pleural effusions may cause respiratory distress due to compression of the underlying lung and pericardial effusions may result in cardiac tamponade, necessitating needle aspiration. Peritonitis and chylous ascites due to IRD associated with infection by NTM have also been described.

IMMUNE-MEDIATED INFLAMMATORY DISEASE IN HIV PATIENTS RESPONDING TO ANTIRETROVIRAL THERAPY

Immune-mediated inflammatory disease (IMID), in which inflammation is the result of immune responses that are apparently not precipitated by infections, may also present in HIV patients responding to ART. There are many reports of sarcoidosis presenting in this context[39] and Reiter's syndrome, lymphoid interstitial pneumonitis, Peyronie's disease, foreign body reactions and photodermatitis have also been described. Sarcoidosis may present up to 3 years after commencement of ART. Most cases present with thoracic disease but extrathoracic disease also occurs in the skin, liver, spleen, kidneys, peripheral lymph nodes, eyes, muscle and salivary glands. In some cases, the use of interleukin (IL)-2 or interferon alpha (IFN-α) therapy appears to have been a precipitating factor.[39]

The immunopathogenesis of sarcoidosis in HIV patients receiving ART is unclear but it is most likely to reflect an increased susceptibility to dysregulation of granulomatous inflammatory responses in the reconstituted immune system, which can be increased further by cytokine therapy that enhances Th1 immune responses, such as IL-2 and IFN-α.

ART-associated sarcoidosis may resolve without treatment but corticosteroid therapy is sometimes necessary. It is therefore important to differentiate sarcoidosis from IRD associated with infections that has resulted in granulomatous inflammation, such as mycobacterial IRD. Measurement of the cutaneous delayed-type hypersensitivity (DTH) response to tuberculin may be informative in this situation because it is usually absent in ART-associated sarcoidosis[39] but often present in mycobacterial IRD.[6]

AUTOIMMUNE DISEASE IN HIV PATIENTS RECEIVING ANTIRETROVIRAL THERAPY

Several types of autoimmune disease have been reported in HIV patients who have experienced immune reconstitution on ART. However, most are single case reports and it is unclear whether their occurrence during ART is merely a coincidence. In contrast, there is compelling evidence that Graves' disease is truly a disorder of immune reconstitution in HIV patients. Thus, there are over 40 cases reported in the literature, including cases in different racial groups.[40,41] It occurs predominantly in patients who had a very low CD4+ T-cell count at the time of commencing ART and who experience a substantial increase of the count on ART. Unlike IRD, ART-associated Graves' disease presents at a median time of almost 2 years after commencing ART. The immunopathogenesis therefore appears to be different from IRD and is most likely to be the result of an acquired defect of immune tolerance.

Systemic or cutaneous lupus has also been reported to present in HIV patients on ART.[42] Those cases presenting during the first 3 months of ART have had serologic evidence of lupus before treatment and it appears that the immunologic changes immediately after ART precipitate presentation with clinical disease. The other cases have presented after 9 months of ART and the lupus appears to have been acquired.

The management of autoimmune disease in HIV patients receiving ART is similar to non-HIV patients but caution has to be exercised if corticosteroid and immunosuppressant therapy are used in patients with HIV infection.

PERSISTENT DEFICIENCY AND/OR DYSFUNCTION OF T CELLS AND B CELLS

Contemporary ART is both effective and tolerable for long periods of time. It is therefore possible to suppress HIV replication for many years and realistic to aim for full reconstitution of the immune system.

The majority of HIV patients will experience a continuing increase in the circulating CD4+ T-cell count over the first 5 years of ART, which generally plateaus thereafter.[43,44] Patients who achieve a CD4+ T-cell count of >500/μl after 6 years of ART may have a life expectancy that is similar to the general population.[45] However, despite long-term control of HIV replication, some patients do not achieve a normal CD4+ T-cell count (approximately >500/μl). Data from the Swiss HIV Cohort Study indicated that 36% of patients had a CD4+ T-cell count of <500/μl after 5 years of effective ART.[46] CD4+ T-cell counts below 500/μl were associated with a low CD4+ T-cell count and older age at the time of starting ART. Patients with a CD4+ T-cell count of <350/μl on ART continue to have an increased risk of AIDS-related disease and also non-AIDS related disease.[47]

CD4+ T-cell deficiency in HIV patients receiving effective ART has several possible causes. The most common causes are a low number of circulating naive CD4+ T cells, which in part is a consequence of failure to regenerate the thymus,[48] and ongoing immune activation, which results in CD4+ T-cell apoptosis and senescence.[49] The immune activation may be a consequence of HIV replication in reservoirs, such as gut-associated lymphoid tissue.[50]

Persistent CD4+ T-cell deficiency on ART can substantially be avoided by starting ART before the onset of severe immunodeficiency. The CD4+ T-cell count that is achieved after 4–7 years of ART is related to the CD4+ T-cell count at the time of starting ART.[43–46] In one study, the median CD4+ T-cell count after 7 years of continuous ART was 870/μl in patients with a baseline count of >500/μl and 73% of patients with a baseline count of >350/μl achieved a count of ≥800/μl.[44] The findings of this study provide support for recommendations that ART should be started before the CD4+ T-cell count drops below 350/μl.

Some patients with very low CD4+ T-cell counts may achieve substantial increases in the count on ART. In the ATHENA study, the median CD4+ T-cell count after 7 years of therapy in patients with a baseline count of <50/μl was 410/μl.[44] Furthermore, 20% of patients with a baseline CD4+ T-cell count of <50/μl achieved a count of ≥800/μl after 7 years. Therefore, even patients who are severely immunodeficient when ART is commenced have the potential to achieve a normal CD4+ T-cell count. Failure to do this is more common in patients who have periods of HIV replication and who are older than 50 years of age when ART is commenced. It is therefore important to maintain long-term control of HIV replication and reasonable to consider starting ART earlier than usually would be done in patients over the age of 50.

For those patients who do not experience an increase in the CD4+ T-cell count to above 350/μl, several therapeutic strategies to increase CD4+ T-cell counts are under investigation. These are recombinant IL-2 to increase counts by enhancing cell proliferation, recombinant human growth hormone to increase thymus size and naïve T cell production, and intensification of ART to reduce immune activation and CD4+ T-cell loss. At present, none can be recommended for routine use.

In patients who had a very low CD4+ T-cell count before commencing ART and achieve a normal or near normal CD4+ T-cell count on ART, CD4+ T-cell dysfunction may persist and occasionally be associated with opportunistic infections.[51] Persistent depletion and/or dysfunction of CD4+ T cells and memory B cells in HIV patients receiving effective ART may result in impaired antibody responses to vaccines in some patients.

REFERENCES

References for this chapter can be found online at http://www.expertconsult.com

Tuberculosis in HIV

EPIDEMIOLOGY

HIV and TB risk

HIV infection is a potent risk factor for the development of active tuberculosis (TB). This may result from:

- high risk of reactivation of latent *Mycobacterium tuberculosis* infection;
- increased risk of exposure to TB;
- greater risk of infection with *M. tuberculosis* following exposure to an infectious source; and
- progression of *M. tuberculosis* infection to primary active TB.

HIV-seronegative individuals who have latent infection with *M. tuberculosis* have a lifetime risk of developing active TB of approximately 10–15%. Following HIV seroconversion, however, TB risk doubles and progressively increases with advancing immunodeficiency. The overall risk of developing active TB in HIV-infected individuals with latent *M. tuberculosis* infection is approximately 10% per year. However, the risk among patients with AIDS living in communities with high TB burden in sub-Saharan Africa may exceed 30% per year.[1]

HIV-infected patients may be at increased likelihood of exposure to TB at health-care settings,[2] for example, or through social mixing with high-risk groups such as intravenous drug users. However, it is not clear whether for a given exposure their susceptibility to *M. tuberculosis* infection is also increased. Although prospective studies of intravenous drug users in New York, USA, suggested that this was not the case, these data were confounded by the insensitivity of tuberculin skin tests (TSTs) in HIV-infected people.

HIV infection not only increases the risk of reactivation of latent *M. tuberculosis* infection, but also increases the risk of progressive primary disease following exogenous infection. Outbreaks in health-care settings in high-income countries have been characterized by attack rates of 30–40% among HIV-infected patients exposed to TB, with many developing disease within 1–2 months.

HIV and the global burden of TB

Outbreaks of HIV-associated TB – often with multidrug-resistant (MDR) disease – in New York, USA, and other cities in developed countries in the early 1990s heralded the growing recognition that TB was resurgent worldwide. In 1993, the World Health Organization (WHO) declared that TB was a global emergency, with HIV infection being identified as one of the key underlying factors that subsequently fueled a 1% annual increase in global TB incidence between 1990 and 2003.[3]

India is the country with the largest number of new TB cases each year and approximately 5% of these are estimated to be HIV co-infected. However, it is the countries of sub-Saharan Africa that have borne the brunt of the dual TB/HIV epidemics (Fig. 93.1).[4] Here the HIV epidemic is generalized within the population and high HIV prevalence rates have intersected with poor existing TB control. Worldwide it is estimated that one in three people have latent TB infection and yet the proportion in the highest burden communities in sub-Saharan Africa exceeds 60%.

Since 1990, annual TB notification rates have increased two- to threefold in many countries in sub-Saharan Africa. Although Africa contains just 10% of the world's population, it accounts for over a quarter of the global burden of TB and a majority of the world's cases of HIV-associated TB. In 2000, 31% of all adult TB cases in the African region were estimated to be attributable to HIV infection. Countries in the southern African region have been hardest hit and here HIV prevalence among new TB cases exceeds 50% (Fig. 93.2).[5] In some impoverished communities in South Africa HIV prevalence rates among antenatal women are approximately 30% and annual TB notification rates as high as 1500/100 000 population have been recorded.[6]

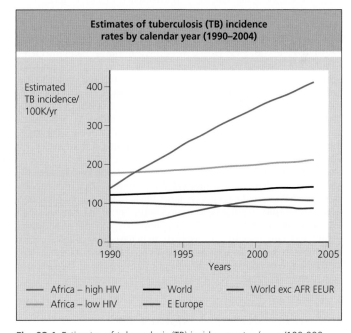

Fig. 93.1 Estimates of tuberculosis (TB) incidence rates (cases/100 000 population) by calendar year between 1990 and 2004. 'Africa – high HIV' refers to all countries in sub-Saharan Africa where HIV prevalence in adults aged 15–49 years was <4% and 'Africa – low HIV' refers to those countries where this rate was >4%. 'World exc AFR EEUR' refers to the world excluding the countries of Africa and Eastern Europe. Reproduced with permission from the World Health Organization.[5]

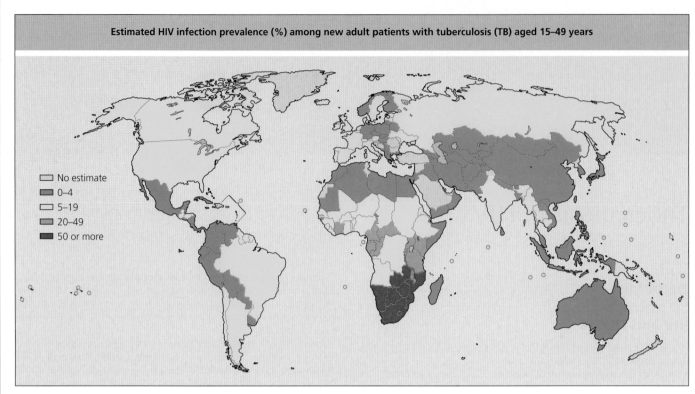

Fig. 93.2 Estimated HIV infection prevalence (%) among new adult patients with tuberculosis (TB) aged 15–49 years. Reproduced with permission from the World Health Organization.[5]

Mortality and TB transmission risk

Patients with HIV-associated TB have high mortality risk. In sub-Saharan Africa in the pre-antiretroviral therapy (ART) era, such patients had case fatality rates that were approximately fivefold higher than HIV-seronegative patients during the course of TB treatment (16–35% versus 4–9%).[7] Data from a randomized placebo-controlled trial in West Africa, however, found that mortality among patients with HIV-associated TB could be halved by trimethoprim–sulfamethoxazole (TMP–SMX) prophylaxis.[8] This suggests that many deaths result from other HIV-associated opportunistic bacterial infections and co-morbidities associated with immunodeficiency. Since TB is more difficult to recognize and diagnose in HIV-infected patients, much of the overall burden of disease may remain unascertained. In a hospital-based post-mortem study of patients in West Africa dying with AIDS, over 50% of patients were found to have previously unrecognized TB, which was often disseminated.[9]

Surprisingly, HIV-infected patients with TB are, on average, actually less infectious than those without HIV co-infection. This is due to the fact that HIV-infected patients are more likely to have either noninfectious extrapulmonary disease or noncavitating pulmonary disease with low concentrations of bacilli in the sputum (Fig. 93.3). In addition, debilitated patients with advanced HIV may have poor cough strength and therefore generate infectious aerosols less efficiently. Nevertheless, TB/HIV patients collectively are an important source of TB transmission at the community level and within health-care settings.[2]

HIV and multidrug-resistant TB

Multidrug-resistant TB (MDRTB) is caused by strains of *M. tuberculosis* that are resistant to at least isoniazid and rifampin (rifampicin) and has emerged as a global epidemic, with over 400 000 cases developing each year.[10] While this has largely resulted from deficiencies in TB case management and TB control programs, important synergies with the HIV epidemic are emerging. Institutional outbreaks of MDRTB have

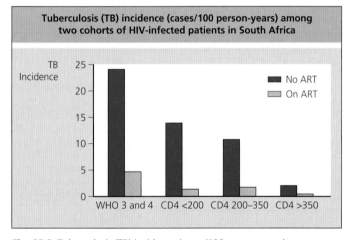

Fig. 93.3 Tuberculosis (TB) incidence (cases/100 person-years) among two cohorts of HIV-infected patients in South Africa who were or were not receiving antiretroviral treatment (ART). Patients are stratified according to baseline CD4 cell count (cells/µl) and World Health Organization clinical stage. Those receiving ART had incidence rates that were approximately 80% lower than the untreated group. Adapted from Badri *et al.*[18]

primarily affected HIV-infected patients with high attack rates and mortality. These outbreaks have been linked to poor infectious control practices in hospitals and prisons where patients with unrecognized TB and those with HIV-infection were mixed and where diagnoses of MDRTB were often delayed.

In Eastern European countries of the former Soviet Union, the epidemic of HIV-associated TB has been associated with very high rates of MDRTB and has been particularly concentrated among intravenous drug users within prisons.[10] In 2005, a large outbreak of MDRTB and extensively drug-resistant (XDR) TB cases was identified among

HIV-infected patients in rural Kwazulu, Natal Province, South Africa.[11] Again, nosocomial transmission played a key role in this outbreak (see Chapter 143 for a detailed description of therapy for MDRTB).

Although many reported TB outbreaks have been associated with the Beijing genotype of *M. tuberculosis*, drug-resistant strains do not appear to be inherently more likely to cause infection and disease in HIV-infected persons.[10] It is possible that TB drug malabsorption in HIV-infected individuals might provide a mechanism favoring the development of drug resistance. In addition, TB services in some areas of sub-Saharan Africa have been overwhelmed by the escalating case load caused by HIV, thereby undermining TB treatment completion rates and cure rates. In the South African outbreak of MDR- and XDRTB, laboratory data suggest that, in the absence of routine drug susceptibility testing, drug pressure from inappropriate treatment regimens led to sequential acquisition of resistance. Emerging data suggest an association between HIV and MDRTB at the population level, but overall most evidence suggests the association is closely related to environmental factors such as transmission in congregate settings rather than biologic factors.[10]

PATHOGENESIS

The immune response to *M. tuberculosis* is multifaceted, engaging several arms of the immune system (see also Chapters 30 and 174). CD4 T-helper cell function is central to the orchestration of cell-mediated responses to *M. tuberculosis*, culminating in the formation of epithelioid granulomas, which restrict growth of the organism. The role of CD4 cells within these processes is fundamentally undermined by HIV-1 infection.[12] In addition, the host response to *M. tuberculosis* at the site of disease provides an immunologic environment that promotes HIV replication and pathogenesis. As a result, the interaction between these diseases is bi-directional.

Impaired immune responses to *Mycobacterium tuberculosis*

Formation of immunologically competent granulomas is essential to the initial containment of *M. tuberculosis* infection and the later prevention of reactivation of latent infection. HIV-1 infection impairs a series of key elements needed to generate this immune response.[12] Antigen presentation, cytokine secretion and intracellular killing of mycobacteria by mononuclear phagocytes may be impaired. Most importantly, HIV infection also leads to numeric depletion and functional impairment of CD4 cells. In particular, HIV inhibits interleukin (IL)-2 signaling, causing impairment of T cell proliferation and activation. In addition, there is loss of secretion of type 1 cytokines such as interferon gamma (IFN-γ) and IL-12 and failure of mononuclear cell recruitment to sites of *M. tuberculosis* infection. Rates of CD4 cell loss are also greatly increased due to virus-mediated cytolysis and activation-induced apoptosis. Impaired chemotaxis, cytokine dysregulation, T-cell depletion and mononuclear cell dysfunction culminate in failure of granuloma formation and the host response to *M. tuberculosis* is thereby undermined.[12]

Impact of tuberculosis on HIV-1 pathogenesis

A substantial body of literature including *in vitro* and *ex vivo* laboratory studies and epidemiologic data collectively suggest that TB may serve as a co-factor that accelerates the rate of immunologic decline in co-infected patients.[13] While the laboratory data are clear, however, the population level impact is debated.[14] Any co-factor effect is thought to be primarily mediated by the impact of TB on HIV replication. *In vitro*, *M. tuberculosis* increases HIV production from chronically infected cell lines, enhances the infectivity of mononuclear cells for HIV and promotes HIV transmission between cells.[15]

Increases in viral load have been documented in patients upon development of TB, especially among those with relatively well preserved CD4 cell counts. Compared to the systemic circulation, HIV load is specifically increased at sites of active TB such as in the pleural space.[13] Development of TB also leads to genotypic diversification of HIV-1, both in the systemic virus pool and at the site of disease. Expression of new or more virulent HIV-1 quasi-species has the potential to permit immune escape, thereby accelerating HIV-1 disease progression.[13]

The effects of TB on HIV progression can be understood in the context of the HIV-1 life cycle, which is intimately related to the activation state of the host cell.[15] Mononuclear cell activation may upregulate expression of chemokine co-receptors such as CCR5 that enhance viral uptake into the cell and may also promote reverse transcription of HIV-1 RNA. Perhaps most importantly, the rate of transcription of proviral DNA within the host cell genome is regulated by sequences within the long terminal repeat (LTR) at the 5′ end of the HIV-1 genome. Proinflammatory cytokines such as tumor necrosis factor (TNF) lead to activation of receptors in the LTR, causing massive upregulation of HIV-1 transcription.[15,15]

Sites of TB disease and granulomas provide a favorable environment for HIV-1 replication. The host response to *M. tuberculosis* involves the recruitment and activation of large numbers of mononuclear cells and the secretion of TNF and other proinflammatory cytokines. These create a highly permissive environment for HIV, thereby maximizing the deleterious impact of HIV at the interface between *M. tuberculosis* and the host.

PREVENTION

Isoniazid preventive therapy

Many studies from around the world have shown that isoniazid preventive therapy (IPT) is an effective intervention that can substantially reduce risk of TB in HIV-infected patients.[16] A large meta-analysis that included studies with a variety of preventive regimens found an overall risk reduction of 36% in comparison with placebo.[17] The greatest reduction in TB incidence (62%) was observed among patients with a positive TST whereas the reduction among TST-negative individuals (17%) was not statistically significant. Isoniazid alone given for 6–12 months reduced TB incidence by 33% overall and by 63% in those with positive TST results. Multidrug regimens given for 2–3 months were as effective as isoniazid alone for 6–12 months. IPT has also been shown to be effective in reducing high TB recurrence rates following completion of TB treatment (secondary prophylaxis) in high TB prevalence settings where rates of exogenous re-infection are likely to be high.[16]

The durability of the benefits of IPT is unclear but is likely to be strongly dependent upon the risk of re-infection with *M. tuberculosis* following completion of therapy and may also be affected by the rate of HIV progression. The benefits are likely to be shorter lived in high TB prevalence settings; data from Zambia found a sustained benefit for approximately 2.5 years.

Overall, a strong trend towards a reduction in mortality has been observed with the use of preventive therapy (RR=0.8, 95% CI 0.63–1.02). Significant reductions in mortality have been observed in a study of HIV-infected children in South Africa and in studies of combined isoniazid and rifampin in adults.[16] Rates of hepatotoxicity are overall very low but are higher for regimens using a combination of rifampin and pyrazinamide.

Although IPT is an effective intervention, it has not been widely implemented in resource-limited settings for several reasons:
- limited health-care capacity to deliver this intervention;
- difficulties in excluding active TB prior to initiating IPT;
- associated concerns about development of isoniazid resistance; and
- limited patient adherence under program conditions.

Although patients with advanced immunodeficiency potentially have the most to gain from IPT, they also present a challenge as they are the patients in whom it is most difficult to exclude active TB prior to initiation of IPT. Ongoing research is needed to overcome these hurdles so that the benefits of this intervention can be realized. In addition, randomized controlled trials are needed to determine whether IPT used concurrently with ART reduces TB rates more than ART alone.

Antiretroviral therapy

Cohort studies in both high-income and resource-limited settings have shown reduction in TB incidence of approximately 80–90% with ART in the short term (Fig. 93.4);[18,19] further small reductions may accrue during the first few years of ART. ART is therefore the most effective available intervention for reducing TB risk in HIV-infected patients. However, during long-term therapy, TB risk does not decrease to background rates observed in HIV-negative individuals living in the same communities; in South Africa, rates remained approximately fivefold higher despite excellent long-term virologic responses.[20]

It is as yet unclear whether incident TB results from a persisting high rate of latent *M. tuberculosis* infection, high rates of nosocomial exposure or frequent exogenous re-infection in the community. However, since incident TB developing during long-term ART often occurs in the context of rising CD4 cell counts, recent exogenous exposure is perhaps a more likely infection source than reactivation disease. Ongoing risk is largely determined by a patient's absolute CD4 cell count during ART.[20] Some evidence also suggests that underlying specific defects in immune responses to *M. tuberculosis* may persist during long-term ART.[19] Such defects may be greater for those patients with the lowest pre-ART nadir CD4 cell counts, potentially highlighting the importance of earlier initiation of ART.

Infection control

The dangers of TB transmission within health facilities have long been recognized.[2] In 1928, for example, 95% of 220 student nurses in Norway acquired TB infection by their graduation as shown by TST conversion and 22% developed TB disease. Transmission risk decreased dramatically in the era of TB chemotherapy administered on an ambulatory basis rather than in hospitals. However, in the 1990s a global resurgence of TB was heralded by many reports of nosocomial outbreaks of TB (mostly MDRTB) in HIV care settings in the USA and elsewhere. In more recent years, rapid expansion of ART in resource-limited countries with high TB burden has paradoxically created unprecedented opportunities for HIV-infected patients and health-care personnel to be exposed to TB in health-care settings.[2] This was most vividly highlighted by an outbreak of XDRTB at a hospital in rural South Africa first reported in 2005.[11] By 2008, over 200 patients had died, including some hospital staff.

Infection control within health-care settings requires a tiered approach of:
- administrative controls, leading to prompt identification and separation of individuals with potentially infectious TB;
- environmental controls, such as adequate natural or mechanical ventilation or ultraviolet light germicidal irradiation; and
- respiratory protection using a face mask or respirator.[2]

How to implement infection control cost-effectively within health-care facilities in resource-limited settings is an urgent research priority.

TB control in settings with high TB/HIV prevalence

The WHO DOTS (directly observed therapy, short course) strategy is regarded as having contributed to decreases in TB notification rates in many areas of the world. However, in sub-Saharan Africa where HIV prevalence rates are high, DOTS has failed to control the TB epidemic, even in those countries such as Malawi and Tanzania which have long-standing, well-functioning, national TB control programs.

The DOTS strategy targets those with sputum smear-positive pulmonary disease who are likely to transmit TB most efficiently. DOTS, however, does not reduce the number of individuals who remain highly susceptible to TB in the community and herein lies a

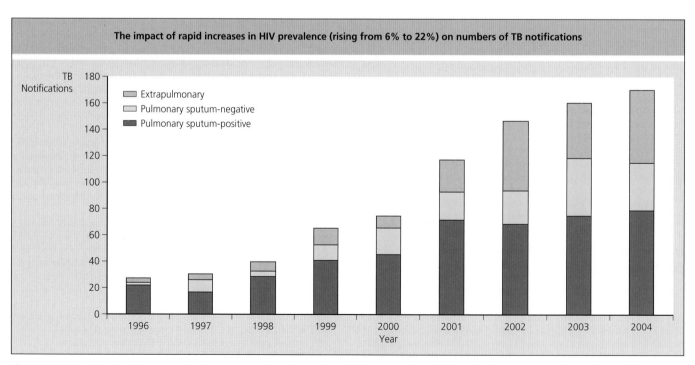

Fig. 93.4 The impact of rapid increases in HIV prevalence (rising from 6% to 22%) on numbers of TB notifications among adults in a South African community of 13 000 people between 1996 and 2004. Case numbers increased steeply as the HIV epidemic evolved, with disproportionate increases in sputum smear-negative pulmonary TB and extrapulmonary TB. Adapted from Lawn *et al.*[6]

key underlying reason for the failure of DOTS as a single intervention to stem this epidemic in sub-Saharan Africa.[21] DOTS programs must clearly be strengthened and optimized and yet this strategy must also be accompanied by other adjunctive interventions. These might include intensified TB case-finding in the community, more widespread use of HIV testing, targeted active case-finding among HIV-infected individuals, implementation of isoniazid prophylaxis and expansion of ART access. However, how these interventions can be implemented programmatically on a large scale is not clear and optimal models need to be developed.

The potential impact of scale-up of ART in sub-Saharan Africa on TB control has yet to be determined. However, since ART greatly prolongs patient survival but the long-term risk of ART remains chronically elevated (more than fivefold greater than that of HIV-seronegative people), ART is unlikely to contribute substantially to TB control.[20,22] It is therefore inevitable that combinations of interventions will be required.

CLINICAL FEATURES

M. tuberculosis causes disease across the full spectrum of HIV-associated immunodeficiency and the impact of HIV on the clinical manifestations of TB is directly related to the degree of immunodeficiency.[23] The median CD4 cell count at presentation appears to vary greatly between published series and may depend on the specific patient population and the maturity of the HIV epidemic. In a report from San Francisco in 1990, for example, the median CD4 cell count at TB presentation was 326 cells/µl, compared to <200 cells/µl in countries of southern Africa in more recent times. TB is commonly the first clinical manifestation of HIV infection, highlighting the great importance of HIV testing of all TB patients.

The spectrum of clinicopathologic manifestations of TB directly relate to blood CD4 cell counts.[23] Features of TB in individuals with well-preserved CD4 cell counts are indistinguishable from those of HIV-seronegative individuals with TB. Progressive immunodeficiency is associated with an increasing frequency of anergic TST responses, atypical presentations of pulmonary TB and sputum smear-negative disease, and an increased frequency of extrapulmonary, miliary and disseminated disease (see Fig. 93.4).

Irrespective of the site of TB, a majority of patients have systemic manifestations with fever, night sweats or weight loss. Unexplained systemic symptoms such as these in the absence of organ-specific symptoms are a not uncommon presentation of TB. In studies in Asia and sub-Saharan Africa, in which HIV-infected patient populations have been actively investigated for TB, substantial rates of subclinical TB have been documented. Although cough, for example, is strongly predictive of TB among selected TB suspects, used as a single screening symptom in active screening fails to identify approximately 20–30% of cases of pulmonary TB in HIV-infected patients.

Pulmonary disease is the major manifestation of TB in both HIV-infected and noninfected patients. Symptoms and clinical findings, however, generally have low sensitivity and specificity for diagnosis of pulmonary TB in the HIV-infected patient. Radiographic appearances of pulmonary TB with HIV co-infection reveal a lower frequency of upper lobe disease, cavitation, parenchymal opacification and fibrosis, but an increased frequency of mediastinal lymphadenopathy, small pleural effusions and miliary disease.[24] Normal radiographs may be observed in a proportion (0–30%) of patients with sputum culture-positive disease. The spectrum of appearances correlates strongly with the degree of immunodeficiency; those with high CD4 cell counts usually have a typical pattern of postprimary disease whereas those with low CD4 cell counts have a higher proportion with a primary disease pattern.

Hematogenous and lymphatic dissemination of mycobacteria in HIV-infected patients increases the risk of extrapulmonary TB. This is strongly related to the degree of immunodeficiency, with the risk particularly increasing as the CD4 cell count falls below 200 cells/µl. The relative frequency of reported extrapulmonary disease also relates to the intensity of the available diagnostic workup. Autopsy specimens from patients who died of TB and AIDS show a high frequency of

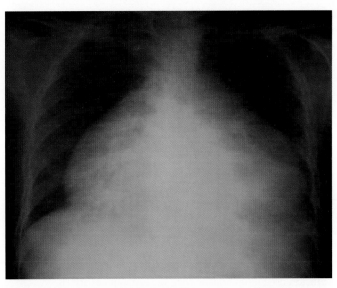

Fig. 93.5 Chest radiograph of a South African patient with HIV infection and a large tuberculous pericardial effusion. Image kindly supplied by Mpiko Ntsekhe, Division of Cardiology, Department of Medicine, Groote Schuur Hospital, University of Cape Town.

extrapulmonary and disseminated disease with multiorgan involvement. Moreover, occult disseminated TB is a frequent finding in postmortem studies of people from sub-Saharan Africa who died with AIDS or 'slim disease'.[9]

Lymphadenitis is the most common form of extrapulmonary TB; cervical nodes are most frequently involved, but disease also often occurs in inguinal, mesenteric and mediastinal nodes. Miliary radiographic shadowing has been reported in up to 38% of AIDS patients with extrapulmonary TB and typically presents with marked constitutional symptoms. HIV infection increases the risk of TB meningitis several-fold, but does not substantially alter the clinical and laboratory manifestations.

Pleural effusions were detected radiographically in one-fifth of a series of consecutive TB/HIV patients in South Africa and were more common than disseminated or miliary TB in patients with higher CD4 cell counts. Pericardial TB is strongly associated with HIV co-infection (Fig. 93.5) and is associated with a pleural effusion in up to approximately one-third of cases.

TB may involve any part of the gastrointestinal tract due to either ingestion of infected sputum or hematogenous dissemination. Whereas mediastinal adenopathy is frequently detected by thoracic radiologic imaging, mesenteric TB lymphadenitis may remain undiagnosed until initiation of ART triggers the clinical presentation as TB immune restoration disease (see also Chapter 92). Development of abscesses in the liver, spleen and other intra-abdominal organs is also a frequent finding.

DIAGNOSIS

The increased likelihood of atypical clinical presentations and subclinical TB requires a high clinical index of suspicion for TB in the HIV-infected patient. All current diagnostic tests for TB, however, have limited performance characteristics when applied to HIV-infected patients.[25] As described above, the frequency of atypical radiologic appearances of pulmonary TB increases with declining immune function.[24] Histopathologic examination of tissue specimens is similarly less likely to show granulomatous inflammation typical of TB.[26] Diagnosis is highly dependent upon obtaining multiple good quality clinical samples for laboratory analyses, which must be interpreted in the light of their known limited sensitivity.

Detection of acid-fast bacilli by light microscopy has been the cornerstone of TB diagnosis worldwide since Koch's discovery of *M. tuberculosis* in 1882. However, the average sensitivity of sputum microscopy in research settings is <60% in immunocompetent patients with pulmonary TB and is reduced to 20–50% in HIV-infected patients due to lower concentrations of bacilli in the sputum. This may be improved to a degree by use of fluorescence staining. Whereas positive sputum smears have low specificity in industrialized countries, they have good specificity in settings such as Africa where TB is far more common than nontuberculous mycobacterial disease.

Mycobacterial culture in selective media remains the most sensitive means of detecting *M. tuberculosis* bacilli in clinical specimens. This is the gold standard for diagnosis but is not available in most resource-limited regions of the world.[25] Although patients with advanced immunodeficiency may have high mycobacterial loads, bacillary numbers in sputum nevertheless tend to be low. As a result, the high sensitivity of culture diagnosis is particularly important for analysis of sputum specimens and, furthermore, culture of other specimens such as urine, blood or bone marrow may also have a useful diagnostic yield. Blood cultures have been found to be positive in up to one-third of patients with advanced immunodeficiency and extrapulmonary TB.

At present there are no serologic or antigen detection assays that offer a means of improving the diagnosis of HIV-associated TB. However, nucleic acid amplification tests (NAATs) for *M. tuberculosis* have provided a significant advance and offer the prospect of far more rapid diagnosis and rapid genotypic assessment of drug susceptibility.[25] These tests are increasingly used in high-income settings and countries with centralized laboratory services (see Chapter 174). However, their cost and complexity are currently beyond the scope of most resource-limited countries. NAATs have extremely high specificity (98–100%) and their sensitivity in sputum smear-positive specimens is also extremely high (>95%), permitting rapid diagnosis. However, their sensitivity does not yet match that of liquid culture in smear-negative specimens (60–70%), although new generations of tests are improving.

TSTs have limited utility in the investigation of the HIV-infected patient. Cutaneous anergy to purified protein derivative (PPD) has been observed in more than 50% of North American and African patients with TB and advanced immunodeficiency. In high TB prevalence settings, TSTs have some role in TB diagnosis in children but not in adults due to poor specificity for active disease. In low TB prevalence settings, use of TSTs is increasingly being superseded by the use of *in vitro* IFN-γ release assays (IGRAs). Responses assessed by the enzyme-linked immunospot (ELISpot) assay in particular appear to be preserved with HIV and advanced immunodeficiency. Positive IGRA responses support a diagnosis of either latent *M. tuberculosis* infection or active TB. However, the utility of these assays in clinical practice has yet to emerge fully.

MANAGEMENT

Patients with HIV-associated TB require optimized antituberculosis treatment and TMP–SMX prophylaxis, and should be considered for antiretroviral therapy.[27]

TB treatment

The key tenets of TB treatment in HIV-infected patients are:
- the need for a rifampin (or alternative rifamycin)-containing intensive phase administered on a daily basis to optimize smear and culture conversion rates;
- the use of rifampin throughout the continuation phase wherever possible to minimize treatment failure and risk of relapse; and
- administration of the continuation phase at least thrice weekly to reduce the risks of development of rifampin resistance and relapse.[27,28]

Early in the HIV epidemic, it was thought that patients with HIV-associated TB had similar responses to antituberculosis treatment. However, TB

recurrence rates are often higher than the rate of <5% typically observed in HIV-seronegative TB patients.[29] This may be due to either incomplete clearance of the infection and relapse or new disease resulting from high rates of exogenous re-infection. Recurrence rates may primarily be reduced by optimizing the TB treatment regimen and using ART. Additional strategies might include extending the duration of TB treatment (some guidelines suggest increasing the duration of treatment from 6 to 9 months in patients who have evidence of slow response to treatment) or the use of secondary isoniazid prophylaxis after completion of TB treatment in settings where risk of exogenous re-infection is high.[30]

Trimethoprim–sulfamethoxazole prophylaxis

TMP–SMX has been widely used in developed countries for prophylaxis of HIV-infected patients against *Pneumocystis jirovecii* pneumonia, *Toxoplasma gondii* encephalitis and bacterial sepsis. However, this was little used in resource-limited settings until a randomized placebo-controlled trial in Cote D'Ivoire in 1999 showed a 46% lower mortality rate among HIV-infected TB patients receiving TMP–SMX.[8] Further studies demonstrated that prophylaxis in TB/HIV co-infected patients increased survival by 60% and that this survival benefit continues during ART. Despite WHO recommendations, routine TMP–SMX prophylaxis has remained at a low level in sub-Saharan Africa and other resource-limited settings. Concerns over emerging resistance to this drug are not well founded since survival benefit has been demonstrated in countries even with high rates of drug resistance.[27]

Antiretroviral therapy

Benefits of ART

Development of combination ART in the mid-1990s has transformed HIV/AIDS from a fatal infectious disease into one that is potentially chronic and manageable. Early reports of combining TB treatment with ART in industrialized countries reported high rates of adverse effects and treatment switching. However, as experience has grown and the range of antiretroviral agents has expanded, good outcomes of concurrent treatment for TB and HIV are now achievable.[30]

The benefits of ART for TB/HIV patients are great. Mortality risk is substantially reduced, with a 20-fold lower adjusted hazard risk of death being reported among Thai TB patients with CD4 cell counts around 50 cells/μl at baseline. Observational data from the USA suggest that mean times to conversion of sputum smears and cultures are shortened. Since ART also decreases the incidence of TB by around 80–90%, it is very likely that ART will also greatly reduce TB recurrence rates. The full benefits of ART, however, have yet to be realized fully as a number of issues concerning concurrent administration of TB treatment with ART are still to be resolved and optimal drug regimens are lacking in resource-limited regions of the world.[30]

Pharmacokinetic interactions

Pharmacokinetic interactions between rifamycins (rifampin, rifapentine and rifabutin), non-nucleoside reverse transcriptase inhibitors (NNRTIs) and protease inhibitors (PIs) are mediated by the complex effects of these drug classes on the hepatic cytochrome P450 (CYP450) enzyme system. NNRTIs and PIs are substrates for these enzymes but also act as inducers or inhibitors.[31] In contrast, the rifamycins act only as potent inducers of this enzyme system, with rifampin having the greatest effect and rifabutin the least. They therefore cause reductions in plasma concentrations of the NNRTIs nevirapine and efavirenz by 30–40% and 20–25%, respectively.[31] In addition, with the exception of ritonavir, plasma concentrations of PIs are reduced by approximately 80% due to enhanced hepatic metabolism and increased activity of the efflux multidrug transporter P-glycoprotein.[31]

Various TB and ART regimens can be successfully combined (Table 93.1). Despite reductions in concentrations of NNRTIs, excellent

Table 93.1 Recommended regimens for the concurrent treatment of tuberculosis and HIV infection

Combined regimen for treatment of HIV andtuberculosis	PK effect of rifamycin	Tolerability/toxicity	Antiviral activity when used with rifampin (rifampicin)	Recommendation (comments)
Efavirenz-based antiretroviral therapy* with rifampin-based TB treatment	Well-characterized, modest effect	Low rates of discontinuation	Excellent	Preferred (efavirenz should not be used during the first trimester of pregnancy)
Protease inhibitor (PI)-based antiretroviral therapy* with rifabutin-based TB treatment	Little effect of rifabutin on PI concentrations, but marked increases in rifabutin concentrations	Low rates of discontinuation (if rifabutin is appropriately dose-reduced)	Favorable, though published clinical experience is not extensive	Preferred for patients unable to take efavirenz[†]
Nevirapine-based antiretroviral therapy with rifampin-based TB treatment	Moderate effect	Concern about hepatotoxicity when used with isoniazid, rifampin and pyrazinamide	Favorable	Alternative for patients who cannot take efavirenz and if rifabutin not available
Zidovudine/lamivudine/abacavir/tenofovir with rifampin-based TB treatment	50% decrease in zidovudine, possible effect on abacavir not evaluated	Anemia	No published clinical experience	Alternative for patients who cannot take efavirenz and if rifabutin not available
Zidovudine/lamivudine/tenofovir with rifampin-based TB treatment	50% decrease in zidovudine, no other effects predicted	Anemia	Favorable, but not evaluated in a randomized trial	Alternative for patients who cannot take efavirenz and if rifabutin not available
Zidovudine/lamivudine/abacavir with rifampin-based TB treatment	50% decrease in zidovudine, possible effect on abacavir not evaluated	Anemia	Early favorable experience, but this combination is less effective than efavirenz-based regimens in persons not taking rifampin	Alternative for patients who cannot take efavirenz and if rifabutin not available
Super-boosted lopinavir-based antiretroviral therapy with rifampin-based TB treatment	Little effect	Hepatitis among healthy adults, but favorable experience, among young children (<3 years)	Good among young children (<3 years)	Alternative if rifabutin not available; preferred for young children when rifabutin not available

* With two nucleoside analogues.
[†] Includes patients with non-nucleoside reverse transcriptase inhibitor-resistant HIV, those unable to tolerate efavirenz, women during the first or second trimester of pregnancy. Reproduced with permission from Centers for Disease Control and Prevention.[31]

virologic outcomes have been reported using the standard 600 mg dose of efavirenz in combination with rifampin, and this is the first-choice recommendation in international guidelines.[32] Outcomes of nevirapine therapy may be undermined if the usual 200 mg per day lead-in dose is used in patients already receiving rifampin; preinduction of hepatic enzymes may reduce drug concentrations to subtherapeutic levels. Increased doses of nevirapine, however, are associated with greater toxicity and current WHO recommendations are to use NNRTIs at standard doses when combined with rifampin.[32] A useful alternative strategy is to use rifabutin which has less impact on the metabolism of NNRTIs.[31] This agent, however, is not widely available in resource-limited settings.

Protease inhibitors do not achieve adequate plasma concentrations when combined with rifampin except when lopinavir or saquinavir is used in combination with ritonavir. However, this frequently results in hepatotoxicity and there is substantial interpatient variability in plasma concentrations, requiring therapeutic drug monitoring wherever possible.[31] A much better alternative is to use rifabutin, which is an effective alternative to rifampin that can be combined with most protease inhibitors.

Immune restoration disease

TB treatment in HIV-negative patients may be associated with a transient worsening of clinical disease (paradoxical reactions) within the first weeks of initiation of therapy. However, the frequency of these reactions is greatly increased by concurrent use of ART, and these demonstrate a strong temporal relationship with ART initiation. These immune restoration disease (IRD) events are believed to be due to the restoration of cell-mediated immunity in response to mycobacterial antigens.[33] IRD has been reported to occur in up to one-third of TB patients initiating ART in high-income settings, and most commonly presents with fever, worsening respiratory manifestations and lymphadenopathy (Fig. 93.6).[33] Initial reports from resource-poor countries to date have found lower rates.

Fig. 93.6 Chest radiographs illustrating tuberculosis (TB) immune restoration disease (IRD). This HIV-infected patient with advanced immunodeficiency had culture-confirmed drug-sensitive TB involving the right middle lobe of the lung and right hilar lymph nodes. This responded well to TB treatment with substantial resolution of the radiographic appearance over the first few weeks of treatment (a). Subsequent initiation of antiretroviral therapy resulted in a clinical and radiologic deterioration (b) and the tuberculin skin test converted from negative to strongly positive. Reproduced with permission from Lawn & French.[35]

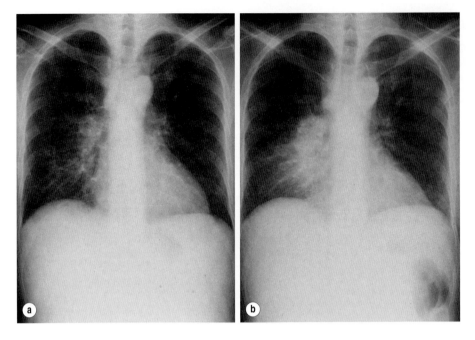

In a study from South Africa, the timing of ART initiation was the overriding determinant of risk for TB-IRD; patients starting in the first month of anti-TB treatment had a 70-fold greater adjusted risk of developing IRD compared with patients starting ART beyond 3 months of treatment. Other risk factors for IRD include low baseline CD4-cell count, disseminated/extrapulmonary TB and rapid immunologic and virologic responses to ART.[33] Although some patients with TB-IRD die, the background mortality risk of these patients is also high as they typically have very advanced immunodeficiency and disseminated TB. No data have yet shown that development of TB-IRD is associated with a substantially increased mortality risk.

Results from randomized controlled trials are needed to determine the optimal management of TB-IRD. Symptoms and signs of TB-IRD can usually be controlled by nonsteroidal anti-inflammatory drugs or by use of corticosteroids in more severe cases. Doses of corticosteroid must be adjusted for rifampin interaction and tapered according to response. ART should be continued unless severe or life-threatening IRD develops because of the ongoing risk of immunodeficiency-associated mortality.

Optimal timing of ART initiation

The optimal time to initiate ART among patients with HIV-associated TB is an important but complicated issue. Expert opinion and various national and international guidelines differ in their recommendations, and randomized controlled trials are needed to provide definitive data. Many factors favor either early or delayed initiation of ART (Table 93.2). In resource-limited settings, the mortality associated with delays in ART initiation appears to be substantially greater than in high-income countries. As a result, the need for early initiation of ART may be greater in resource-limited settings. WHO currently recommends that TB patients with CD4 cell counts <200 cells/μl should start ART between 2 and 8 weeks of TB treatment.[32] Observational data from South Africa suggest that those with CD4 cell counts <100 cells/μl or stage 4 disease should commence ART as early as possible within this time frame.

Drug-resistant tuberculosis

MDRTB requires the use of a combination of a minimum of four effective drugs and XDRTB requires the use of as many active drugs as can be achieved.[34] Mortality rates in HIV-infected and MDR- or XDRTB patients

Table 93.2 Factors favoring either early initiation of antiretroviral therapy (ART) (during intensive phase of TB therapy) or delayed initiation (during continuation phase)

Favors early initiation of ART	Favors delayed initiation of ART
• Risk of further morbidity associated with advanced immunodeficiency • Risk of mortality associated with advanced immunodeficiency • Immune recovery may enhance mycobacterial clearance with the potential to shorten sputum conversion times and reduce risk of relapse	• Avoids high pill burden during intensive phase of TB therapy, potentially improving tolerability and adherence • Easier to diagnose and manage drug toxicities and risk of toxicity may be decreased • Avoids pharmacokinetic drug interactions during intensive phase of TB therapy • Lower risk of TB immune restoration disease

are very high, even in specialized management programs. ART should improve the prognosis of such patients, although there are no data to confirm this. Due to slow clearance of mycobacterial antigen load, such patients may be at greater risk of developing TB-IRD compared to those with drug-sensitive TB. Second line anti-TB drugs are associated with considerable adverse effects that overlap with those of ART drugs. However, the absence of rifampin from the regimens does simplify the issue to some extent. In view of the high mortality risk, delays in initiation of ART should probably be minimized in those with MDRTB.

REFERENCES

📖 References for this chapter can be found online at http://www.expertconsult.com

Chapter | **94** | Emanuela Vaccher
Umberto Tirelli

Neoplastic disease

INTRODUCTION

Widespread access to highly active antiretroviral therapy (HAART) has significantly changed the spectrum of HIV-related malignancies in the industrialized countries. Among AIDS-defining cancers, Kaposi's sarcoma (KS) and non-Hodgkin's lymphoma (NHL) incidences have significantly decreased in the HAART era. The risk of invasive cervical cancer, however, has remained stable over time. The overall risk of certain non-AIDS defining cancers in HIV-infected persons is two to three times that in the general population, with no beneficial effect from HAART. Hodgkin's lymphoma is the most common non-AIDS defining cancer, with standardized incidence ratios ranging from 8 to 16, followed by cancer of the anus, lung, liver and skin.[1-5]

Malignant disease has now become a major cause of death among HIV-infected patients. Whereas KS and NHL are associated with advanced immunosuppression, Burkitt's lymphomas, Hodgkin's disease (HD) and solid tumors can occur in patients with controlled HIV infection.[6-8]

In this chapter, we will describe the epidemiology, pathology, clinical features and treatment of the two most common malignant tumors in patients with HIV infection: KS and NHL.

Cervical cancer which is related to human papillomavirus (HPV) infection (see Chapter 59) should be anticipated because of the high prevalence of HPV infection and persistence among HIV-infected women. Cervical cancer screening should be considered a must in the HAART era.

Kaposi's Sarcoma

EPIDEMIOLOGY

In industrialized countries, decline in KS incidence began in the early 1990s, but risk fell sharply in 1996 after the introduction of HAART. Among adults with AIDS, the risk for KS has currently decreased by approximately 90% compared with the pre-HAART era.[1-4] Among patients receiving HAART, there continues to be an increased risk for homosexual men and for patients with low CD4 cell counts.[8] Immune restoration induced by protease inhibitor (PI)-based and non-nucleoside reverse transcriptase inhibitor (NNRTI)-based HAART regimens appears to be equally effective in preventing KS.[9,10] However, patients with AIDS remain at significant risk compared with the general population.[1-4] The standardized incidence ratio (SIR) ranges from 3600 in the United States to 1749 in Europe.[1-4,10] The geographic distribution of KS closely reflects the prevalence of sexually acquired HIV infection worldwide. KS tends to be much higher in countries where most individuals with AIDS are homosexual than, for instance, in Italy and Spain where intravenous drug users account for the majority of cases. In contrast, in Africa, where HAART is not readily available, KS has reached epidemic proportions.

PATHOLOGY AND PATHOGENESIS

KS is a multifocal angioproliferative disease characterized histologically by neoangiogenesis and proliferating spindle-shaped cells, admixed with a variable chronic inflammatory infiltrate.[11] Spindle tumor cells express many endothelial markers and human herpesvirus 8 (HHV-8) can infect endothelial cells and induce KS-like spindle cell morphology *in vitro*. It has recently been shown that circulating endothelial precursor cells in patients with KS have evidence of HHV-8 infection. HHV-8, a member of the transforming family of gamma herpes viruses, has been found in all forms of KS and in two lymphoproliferative diseases: primary effusion lymphoma (PEL) and multicentric Castleman's disease. The virus encodes a number of genes homologous to human genes involved in cell proliferation, anti-apoptosis, angiogenesis and cytokine action. Multiple signal transduction pathways are activated by HHV-8 and both latent and lytic viral replicative cycles contribute significantly – but differently – to KS development (Table 94.1).

Extensive evidence indicates that HIV trans-activating protein Tat plays an oncogenic role in the development of KS. Tat promotes tumorigenesis of endothelial cells via stimulation of vascular endothelial growth factors, anti-apoptotic activity and HHV-8 replication.[11,12] A model of KS pathogenesis involves exposure to HHV-8, alteration in cytokine expression and response to cytokine, modulation of growth by HIV Tat and, finally, malignant transformation.

CLINICAL FEATURES

KS ranges from an indolent to an aggressive disease with significant morbidity and mortality. However, KS exhibits a less aggressive presentation in patients already receiving HAART compared with patients who are naive to HAART at KS diagnosis.[13]

Typically, the disease presents with disseminated skin lesions, often with lymph node and visceral involvement such as the gastrointestinal tract and lungs. Skin lesions arise as macular or papular eruptions, which progress to nodular plaques or lesions (Fig. 94.1); any area of the skin may be involved. Nodular KS does not usually cause necrosis of overlying skin and rarely invades underlying bone structure.

Lymphedema, particularly of the face, genitalia and lower extremities, may be out of proportion to the cutaneous disease and may be related to lymphatic obstruction and the expression of cytokines involved in the pathogenesis of KS. Lymphadenopathic KS primarily affects peripheral

Table 94.1 Major HHV-8 genes associated with tumorigenesis

Genes	Major functions
Latent genes	
LANA	Maintenance viral latency, interaction with p53 and pRB
V-Cyclin	Cell cycle progression
vFLIP	Inhibition of Fas-induced apoptosis Activation of nuclear factor kappa B (NF-κB) pathways
VIRF$_1$	Inhibition of interferon-induced gene expression Activation of myc Interaction with p53
Kaposin (K12)	Interaction with MAPK signaling pathway
Lytic genes	
VGPCR	Homologue of cellular interleukin (IL)-8 receptor Stimulation of MAPK pathway and VEGF secretion
vIL6	Homologue of cellular IL-6 Cell cycle progression Anti-apoptotic action
K4, 4.1, 6	Homologue of cellular chemokines (i.e. RANTES, MIP-1) Activation angiogenesis

K, genes unique to HHV-8; LANA, viral latency-associated nuclear antigen; MAPK, mitogen-activated protein kinase; VEGF, vascular endothelial growth factor; vFLIP, viral Fas-associated death domain-like interleukin 1β-converting enzyme; VGPCR, viral G protein-coupled receptor; VIRF, viral interferon regulatory factor.

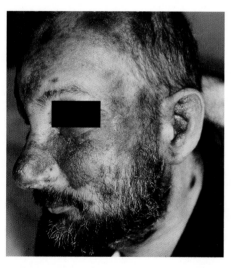

Fig. 94.1 Kaposi's sarcoma. There are large confluent hyperpigmented patch-stage lesions with lymphedema.

lymph nodes, sometimes causing massive nodal enlargement, and it may be present in the absence of mucocutaneous disease.

Oral cavity KS occurs in approximately 35% of patients and is the initial site of disease in about 15%. Intraoral lesions most commonly affect the palate and gingiva, and may interfere with nutrition and speech.

Over 50% of patients with skin disease have gastrointestinal lesions. Any segment of gastrointestinal tract may be involved, although the stomach and duodenum are most commonly affected. Gastrointestinal KS is seldom symptomatic, but may cause bowel malabsorption or obstruction, and, rarely, bleeding.

Pulmonary involvement is also quite common and may be life threatening. In approximately 20% of cases it may occur in the absence of skin lesions. The symptoms, including shortness of breath, fever, cough, hemoptysis and chest pain, and radiologic appearance of pulmonary KS are indistinguishable from those of the more common opportunistic infections. Radiographic findings vary greatly and can include nodular, interstitial and alveolar infiltrates, pleural effusion, hilar and mediastinal adenopathy, and even an isolated pulmonary nodule. The pleural effusions of KS are typically serosanguinous in nature and are associated with KS lesions on the visceral pleura.

DIAGNOSIS

Although a presumptive diagnosis of KS can often be made readily by a trained observer, a simple skin biopsy can confirm the diagnosis. It is especially important to biopsy lesions that are less typical of KS because other conditions, such as bacillary angiomatosis, may be confused with KS.

Occult blood testing is an excellent screening method for gastrointestinal tract lesions and endoscopy should be reserved for patients with positive test and/or gastrointestinal symptoms. Lesions in the gastrointestinal tract are often recognized easily on endoscopy; however, because the lesions tend to be submucosal, biopsies may not demonstrate KS.

Bronchoscopy is the procedure of choice for pulmonary KS, but gallium–thallium scanning may also be helpful in evaluating an abnormal radiograph. Kaposi's sarcoma is usually thallium avid and gallium negative, whereas infections are usually gallium avid and thallium negative.

The AIDS Clinical Trial Group (ACTG) classification groups patients according to the extent of the tumor, immune status and severity of systemic illness[14] (Table 94.2). A re-evaluation of the TIS staging system during the HAART era suggested that only the high tumor burden (T_1) and the poor systemic disease status (S_1) could identify patients with a poor prognosis.[15]

MANAGEMENT

Treatment of KS has changed substantially in the HAART era. The degree of immunocompetence, the extent of tumor burden (T) and its rate of progression, HIV comorbidity and the patient's performance status (PS) dictate the choice of treatment. However,

Table 94.2 Staging system for HIV-associated Kaposi's sarcoma

	Good risk	Poor risk
Tumor	Confined to skin and/or lymph nodes and/or minimal oral disease (confined to palate)	Tumor-associated edema or ulceration; extensive oral Kaposi's sarcoma; gastrointestinal Kaposi's sarcoma; Kaposi's sarcoma in visceral organs
Immune system	CD4+ lymphocytes ≥150/μl	CD4+ lymphocytes <150/μl
Systemic illness	No history of opportunistic infection or thrush; no systemic B symptoms; Karnofsky performance status	History of opportunistic infection or thrush; systemic B symptoms; Karnofsky performance status <70%; other HIV-related illness

optimal antiretroviral therapy is a key component of KS management. Regression of KS with HAART has already been documented in many studies and HAART has been associated with prolonged time-to-treatment failure and longer survival among KS patients who have received chemotherapy. The available evidence suggests that HAART leads to regression of limited KS. Thus, HAART may be the only anti-neoplastic therapy in the early stage of disease (T_0) and/or for slowly proliferating disease, when tumor growth is consistent with the long time interval to the development of HAART anti-KS activity (median 8–12 months).[16–19]

KS may have a recrudescence during the first 2–3 months of HAART, as an immune reconstitution inflammatory syndrome (IRIS). The potential additive effects of IRIS with steroid use in KS contraindicate its use as an anti-inflammatory therapy.

There are several mechanisms by which HAART may be active in KS, including the increase of CD4 cell count, the suppression of HIV replication and the induction of an anti-angiogenic effect, which is mediated by PIs.[12,20]

In patients with T_1 and/or rapidly proliferating disease, the first-line treatment is chemotherapy plus HAART, followed by maintenance therapy with HAART. Although several chemotherapeutic agents (i.e. bleomycin, vinblastine, vincristine, vinorelbine, doxorubicin and etoposide) were noted to be efficacious against KS in the past, current systemic cytotoxic therapy comprises liposomal anthracyclines – pegylated liposomal doxorubicin (PLD) and liposomal daunorubicin – and taxanes. Liposomal encapsulation alters drugs kinetics, resulting in a prolonged half-life. In two pre-HAART randomized studies PLD (20 mg/m^2 intravenously every 2 weeks) had activity superior to combination of ABV (doxorubicin, bleomycin, vincristine) or BV (bleomycin, vincristine), with an overall response rate ranging from 46% to 59% and a better safety profile. Liposomal daunorubicin at an intravenous dose of 60 mg/m^2 every 2 weeks in patients with pulmonary KS has resulted in clinical benefit and objective response in 59% and 32% of cases, respectively.

Myelosuppression remains the most important dose-limiting toxicity of these drugs. Peripheral neuropathy and palmar–plantar erythrodysesthesias occur infrequently and cardiotoxicity is rare. Currently, these liposomal drugs are considered the best first-line chemotherapy for the majority of advanced KS patients.[19,21,22] Preliminary evidence indicates that the combination of liposomal anthracyclines and HAART is safe and effective.

Paclitaxel, a microtubule-stabilizing drug known to inhibit Bcl-2 anti-apoptotic activity, is effective even in patients with anthracycline resistant-KS. The drug (100 mg/m^2 intravenously every 2 weeks) results in an overall response rate of 56–59%, with a median duration response of 10.4 months. The major side-effects include myalgias, arthralgias and myelosuppression. Based on these data, paclitaxel is now used after failure of first-line systemic chemotherapy. Since the metabolism of paclitaxel involves the cytochrome P450 pathway, as does PIs and NNRTIs, caution is necessary when the drug is co-administered with HAART.

The growing knowledge of KS biology provides multiple opportunities for rational targeted therapies. However, preliminary results of these clinical trials and the complexity of KS pathogenesis suggest that effective treatment strategies will require a combination of agents targeting multiple pathogenetic pathways.[22]

PROGNOSIS

Although KS sometimes has a rapid course with extensive visceral involvement in some patients, in others it is an indolent disease for many years.

In the pre-HAART era, the ACTG TIS classification predicted survival in KS patients, and CD4 count (I stage) and T stage provided the most predictive information.[14] In the HAART era, only T and S stages maintained their correlation with survival. Two different risk categories are identified: a poor risk (T_1S_1) and a good risk (T_0S_0, T_1S_0, T_0S_1), with a 3-year survival rate of 53% versus 80–88%, respectively.

Furthermore, pulmonary involvement predicts survival better than tumor extension, independent of the S stage, and identifies the poorest category.[15]

Non-Hodgkin's Lymphoma

EPIDEMIOLOGY

The incidence of NHL in HIV-infected individuals is over 100 times the incidence among the general population. NHL accounts for AIDS-defining illness in about 3% of patients in the USA and 3–6% in Europe. In the HAART era, the incidence of NHL has decreased by approximately 50%; the decline has been marked for primary central nervous system lymphoma (PCNSL) and immunoblastic lymphoma, but not for Burkitt's lymphoma (BL). The risk factors for the majority of NHLs are severe immunodeficiency, prolonged HIV infection and older age.[1–4,8]

NHL occurs among all population groups at risk for HIV infection, in all age groups and in different countries, with similar epidemiologic and clinical pathologic features.

Systemic NHL constitutes 80% of all cases; the remaining 20% are PCNSL and PEL (<5%).

PATHOLOGY AND PATHOGENESIS

According the World Health Organization, NHLs are divided into three categories:

- lymphomas occurring in immunocompetent patients, such as BL and diffuse large B-cell lymphomas (DLBCL), including centroblastic, immunoblastic and anaplastic variants;
- lymphomas occurring more specifically in HIV-infected patients, such as PEL and plasmoblastic lymphoma of the oral cavity; and
- lymphomas also occurring in other immunodeficiency states, such as polymorphic or post-transplant lymphoproliferative disorders.[23]

The pathologic heterogeneity of HIV-associated NHL reflects the heterogeneity of their associated molecular lesions. In BL, the genetic lesions involve activation of c-myc, inactivation of p53 and infection with Epstein–Barr virus (EBV) in approximately 30% of cases. Immunoblastic lymphoma, infected by EBV in 90% of cases, is characterized by frequent expression of latent membrane protein-1 (LMP-1), an EBV oncoprotein. PEL, typically growing as lymphomatous effusions, is consistently associated with HHV-8 infection. Morphologically, PEL shows features bridging immunoblastic and anaplastic large-cell lymphomas and frequently displays a certain degree of plasma cell differentiation. Recently, HHV-8 has also been detected in solid extracavitary-based lymphomas. Plasmoblastic lymphoma, a rare (~3%) distinct type of DLBCL occurring often in the oral cavity or jaw, is associated with EBV in 50–100% of cases, but usually lacks expression of LMP-1 and EBV nuclear antigen-2. Several studies have recently shown that NHLs derive from two distinct cellular pathways: lymphomas that derive from germinal center (GC) B cells are unlikely to be EBV associated, whereas those from post-GC B cells are more likely to show immunoblastic histology and to be EBV associated.[24]

CLINICAL FEATURES

One of the distinguishing features of NHL is the widespread extent of disease at initial presentation and the frequency of systemic 'B' symptoms, including fever, night sweats and weight loss of more than 10% of the normal body weight. At the time of diagnosis approximately 75% of patients have advanced disease with frequent involvement

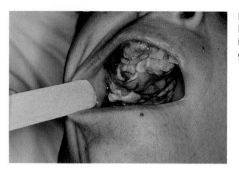

Fig. 94.2 Non-Hodgkin's lymphoma. Bulky disease in the gingiva.

of extranodal sites, the most common being the CNS, bone marrow, gastrointestinal tract and liver. Any site of the body, however, may be affected (Fig. 94.2).

Leptomeningeal disease, identified during routine lumbar puncture as part of the initial staging evaluation, remains asymptomatic in approximately 20% of patients. Gastrointestinal tract involvement, sometimes at multiple sites, develops in 10–40% of cases. Bulky disease can be observed in the anorectal region, particularly in homosexual men.

The PCNSL (i.e. intracranial parenchymal lymphoma limited to the CNS) is a manifestation of very advanced HIV disease. Usually the CD4+ lymphocyte count at diagnosis is less than 50/μl. The lymphoma develops as single or multiple lesions in the deep regions of white matter, in the basal ganglia and in the cerebellum. The clinical presentation of PCNSL is not specific and approximately 50% of patients present with lethargy, confusion and personality change, whereas many others lack lateralizing neurologic signs.

The PEL grows exclusively or mainly within pleural, pericardial or peritoneal cavities as lymphomatous effusions, usually in the absence of contiguous tumor mass. It usually remains strictly localized to the body cavity of origin and only infrequently spreads to local lymph nodes or distant sites.

In the setting of HIV disease, NHL can be difficult to diagnose because of its variable presentation. It can mask many conditions of both HIV disease itself and its associated opportunistic infections. For instance, systemic 'B' symptoms are frequently associated with both advanced HIV infection and opportunistic infections. These symptoms mandate a careful evaluation to exclude other causes, including the presence of *Mycobacterium avium-intracellulare*, cytomegalovirus or tuberculosis infection.

The PCNSL may be radiographically indistinguishable from cerebral toxoplasmosis or other CNS infections. It has been shown that detection of cerebrospinal fluid (CSF) EBV-DNA by polymerase chain reaction (PCR) in HIV-infected patients is reliably associated with PCNSL. By combining CSF EBV-DNA detection by PCR with 201Tl single photon emission computed tomography, the presence of increased uptake and positive EBV-DNA had 100% sensitivity and 100% negative predictive value. Thus in patients with hyperactive lesions and positive EBV-DNA, brain biopsy may be avoided and patients could promptly undergo definitive therapy.

DIAGNOSIS

A diagnosis of NHL should be made by histologic examination of the tissue obtained by incisional or excisional biopsy. It may be possible, however, to make an adequate diagnosis from needle aspiration cytology, and this may be required if the patient's clinical condition is critical or deteriorating rapidly.

In the absence of clinical suspicion for toxoplasmosis, EBV in the CSF in the presence of a brain lesion inaccessible to biopsy remains the gold standard for diagnosing PCNSL.

MANAGEMENT

The poor prognosis of NHL and the palliative approach to treatment are no longer the rule since the introduction of HAART. Patients with good performance status and without severe immunosuppression should be treated with curative intent in a manner comparable to immunocompetent patients, but with greater vigilance for the development of opportunistic infections. Long-term complete remission can be now observed with a possible cure of lymphoma.[25–28]

Although different chemotherapy regimens have been tested, there is still disagreement regarding the optimal chemotherapy even in the HAART era. A large European randomized trial, designed to evaluate different dose-intensive treatments according to HIV score, showed that HAART use, HIV score and age-adjusted international prognostic index (aa-IPI) were the strongest predictors for survival, but not the intensity of cyclophosphamide–doxorubicin–vincristine–prednisone (CHOP)-based chemotherapy.[26] Infusional chemotherapy is thought to overcome some drug resistance and possibly high tumor proliferative indices. Cyclophosphamide–doxorubicin–etoposide (CDE), as a 96-hour continuous infusion combined with rituximab, has yielded a complete response of 70% with an estimated 2-year overall survival of 62%.[27] A National Cancer Institute study demonstrated 74% complete remission and 2-year overall survival of 60% with infusional etoposide–prednisone–vincristine–cyclophosphamide–doxorubicin (EPOCH).[28] Preliminary results with rituximab-EPOCH show a complete remission of 65% and, compared with historical controls, improved survival from 16% to 57% after a median follow-up of 19 months. These survival outcomes reflect a dramatic improvement compared with pre-HAART trials.

Rituximab is a humanized anti-CD20 antibody that has revolutionized the treatment of HIV-negative NHL patients; however, it might increase the risk of life-threatening infections. Treatment-related infectious deaths occurred in 14% of patients treated with concurrent rituximab-CHOP followed by maintenance rituximab, but such infections were not increased in other studies (Table 94.3). Severe neutropenia is a common complication of rituximab chemotherapy, whereas hypogammaglobulinemia has rarely been reported.[27,29,30] Antiviral therapy with lamivudine has been shown to reduce viral reactivation in patients with chronic hepatitis B infection receiving chemotherapy and is recommended for patients treated with rituximab.

Preliminary studies show that high-dose therapy with autologous stem cell transplantation plus HAART is feasible and effective in patients with relapsed or refractory NHL or HD. Adequate stem cell collection is obtained in approximately 80% of cases with prompt engraftment in all cases and absence of toxic deaths. The disease-free survival and the overall survival rates are 55% and 60%, respectively, at a median of 36 months of follow-up.

Available data suggest that first-generation HAART regimens could be co-administered safely with chemotherapy, with the exception of zidovudine because of its myelosuppressive effects.[25] Additional studies are, however, warranted with the new boosted PI-based HAART, because of the high risk of pharmacokinetic interactions.

PROGNOSIS

In HIV NHLs the conventional prognostic factors influencing survival in lymphoma patients in the general population – age, disease stage, extranodal involvement, performance status, lactate dehydrogenase (LDH) levels or international prognostic index (IPI) score – have been used together with HIV-specific factors. In the pre-HAART era, the main unfavorable prognostic factors were presence of a severe immune deficit (CD4+ <100/μl), prior AIDS diagnosis and

Table 94.3 Rituximab in non-Hodgkin's lymphoma HIV: major series in the literature

Regimen	No. patients (%)	aa-IPI ≥2 (%)	Median CD4/μl	CR (%)	Febrile neutropenia (%)	Death due to progression
Rituximab + cyclophosphamide, doxorubicin and etoposide (R-CDE)	74	52	161	70	23	5
Rituximab + cyclophosphamide, doxorubicin, vincristine and prednisone (R-CHOP)	52	46	180	77	17	4
Rituximab + cyclophosphamide, doxorubicin, vincristine and prednisone + maintenance rituximab (R-CHOP-mR)	80	58	128	57	30	14
Rituximab + etoposide, prednisone, vincristine, cyclophosphamide and doxorubicin (R-EPOCH)				65		

aa-IPI, age-adjusted international prognostic index; CR, complete remission

poor general health.[26] The advent of HAART into clinical practice has changed outcome significantly: conventional survival-influencing lymphoma-related factors actually have a stronger impact on survival than factors associated with the underlying HIV infection.[25,26] Particularly in the most extensive surveys the age-adjusted IPI score (disease stage, performance status, LDH levels) is the most discriminating negative prognostic factor in patients with HIV NHLs, together with Burkitt subtype, and failure to obtain complete remission after first-line chemotherapy.[25–30]

REFERENCES

References for this chapter can be found online at http://www.expertconsult.com

Joseph Susa
Natalie Wright
Grace T Kho
Chris Bandel
Clay J Cockerell

Chapter | 95 |

Dermatologic manifestations of HIV infection

INTRODUCTION

The skin is commonly affected in patients who have HIV infection and AIDS.[1] The prevalence of cutaneous involvement approaches 100% and in many cases is the motivating force that causes the patient to seek medical care.

Dermatologic manifestations of HIV infection may provide the initial diagnostic clues, not only of the presence of the infection per se but also in some cases the stage of involvement.[2] Early-stage disease (CD4+ count 200–500 cells/mm³) can be associated with seborrheic dermatitis, oral hairy leukoplakia (OHL), Kaposi's sarcoma (KS), oropharyngeal or recurrent vulvovaginal candidiasis, herpes zoster or recurrent herpes simplex virus (HSV) infection. With a CD4+ count of 50–200 cells/mm³, bacillary angiomatosis, esophageal candidiasis, disseminated deep fungal infections, molluscum contagiosum, chronic herpetic ulcers and eosinophilic folliculitis become more prominent. With advanced HIV disease (CD4+ <50 cells/mm³), profound immunosuppression may lead to the occurrence of several coexisting infections and neoplasms. In general, skin infections and neoplastic conditions in patients who have AIDS are aggressive and difficult to treat. Early recognition of the different skin diseases will facilitate the use of an appropriate and timely therapeutic approach.

With the introduction of highly active antiretroviral therapy (HAART) in the mid 1990s, changes in the dermatologic manifestations paralleled the stabilization and improvement in CD4+ counts.[3,4] As CD4+ counts normalize with HAART therapy, many of the skin disorders affecting HIV-infected patients become similar to those seen in immunocompetent patients. Significant decreases in the incidence of KS, OHL, oral candidiasis, bacterial folliculitis, recurrent HSV and, to a lesser degree, seborrheic dermatitis, psoriasis, drug eruptions, dry skin and pruritus were noted. Conversely, conditions such as warts, scabies, photosensitivity and eosinophilic folliculitis did not abate significantly and, in some cases, increased in incidence. This increase in certain dermatologic diseases, mostly within the first 3 months following HAART initiation, is known as immune reconstitution disease (IRD) (see Chapter 92). Some entities, such as molluscum contagiosum, became less prevalent in some series and more in others, reflecting varying influences such as immune restoration, altered cytokine patterns, improved lifestyle and increased exposure. Effects of drug reactions can also be exacerbated or mitigated at this time.

This chapter describes the most common dermatologic manifestations of HIV infection, including skin changes present early in infection and in advanced disease, such as neoplastic, infectious and noninfectious conditions, hair, nail and oral changes and drug reactions.

EARLY DERMATOLOGIC MANIFESTATIONS OF HIV INFECTION: ACUTE EXANTHEM OF HIV INFECTION

The acute exanthem, which is symptomatic in about 80% of patients, begins 1–6 weeks after exposure to the virus and is associated with prodromal symptoms such as lymphadenopathy, fatigue, fever, headache, nausea, diarrhea and night sweats. The skin eruption consists of erythematous, round to oval macules and papules affecting the trunk, chest, back and upper back (Fig. 95.1). Less commonly, hives and pruritic papules and pustules can occur on the extremities. The syndrome generally lasts for 4–5 days and resolves with complete recovery.[5] The prognosis for patients who have a more severe form of acute HIV infection is poorer than for those who are asymptomatic or have mild symptoms (see Chapter 89).[5]

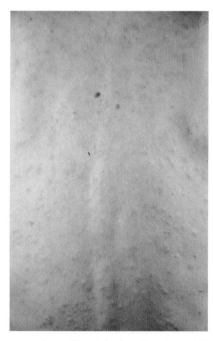

Fig. 95.1 Acute exanthem of HIV infection. There is morbilliform eruption involving the trunk and extremities. The eruption is similar to a morbilliform drug eruption and to other viral exanthemata.

NON-NEOPLASTIC INFECTIOUS DERMATOLOGIC CONDITIONS

Viral infections

Herpes simplex virus

Infections with HSV types 1 and 2 result in recurrent, severe painful grouped vesicles with an erythematous base localized mainly on the lips and genital and perianal areas. If left untreated, these lesions may enlarge and become confluent ulcerations that may persist for over 1 month, displaying slow healing and often becoming secondarily infected with bacteria. Ulcerations can occur without the patient noticing pre-existing, well-defined vesicles.[6] It is essential to establish the specific diagnosis by means of polymerase chain reaction (PCR), direct fluorescent antibody (DFA) testing, biopsies and/or viral cultures (see Chapter 155).

While the immune system is intact, the course of the disease is similar to that in noninfected individuals. Once immunosuppression sets in, the lesions can become persistent. Ulcers can expand, reach large size and even become necrotic. Nonhealing ulcers that persist for more than 1 month are one of the AIDS-defining conditions.[7] An aggressive therapeutic approach should be used with these patients, as they may be poorly responsive to standard treatment and HSV infection increases the probability of HIV transmission and shedding[8] (for therapy, see Chapter 91).

Varicella-zoster virus

The development of recrudescent varicella-zoster virus (VZV) infection in a patient at risk of HIV infection may be a sign of the presence of HIV and should alert the clinician to screen the patient.[9] It usually occurs early in the course of the disease. Varicella-zoster virus exists in a dormant state in dorsal root ganglion after the primary vesicular infection commonly known as chickenpox. With reactivation, the virus progresses downward through the nerve tracts of a solitary dermatome, leading to the characteristic zosteriform distribution of painful tense vesicles of skin (Fig. 95.2). In HIV-infected individuals, VZV infection may be recurrent and severe, with more than one dermatome involved, and may run a protracted course associated with residual postherpetic neuralgia and scarring. Disseminated herpes-zoster may occur. Atypical presentations of VZV include verrucous zoster, follicular zoster and ecthymatous or crusted zoster. Chronic lesions can be verrucous or ecthymatous and can be a presenting sign of HIV disease.[10]

Primary varicella infection can develop in previously unexposed individuals with HIV infection. The infection can be more severe, cause extracutaneous disease and be fatal.

Occurrences of VZV are common after initiation of HAART as part of IRD (Chapter 92). Diagnosis of VZV is largely clinical; however, DFA testing is a rapid and effective way to diagnose atypical presentations (see also Chapter 155; for therapy, see Chapter 91).

Cytomegalovirus

Cytomegalovirus (CMV) is the most common cause of serious opportunistic viral infection in patients who have AIDS.[11] However, cutaneous involvement is rare. In the skin, CMV has different clinical manifestations, including ulcerations, keratotic verrucous lesions, hyperpigmented plaques, morbilliform eruptions and palpable purpuric papules. Because the mucocutaneous lesions caused by CMV do not have specific features, tissue biopsy of the lesions, as well as direct viral diagnostic approaches (Chapter 155) are required to define the etiologic cause. The treatment of choice for CMV infection is intravenous ganciclovir 5 mg/kg every 12 hours. Foscarnet should be used if ganciclovir resistance is suspected (for further discussion of therapy, see Chapter 91).

Epstein–Barr virus

The majority of adults harbor latent Epstein–Barr virus (EBV) within B lymphocytes. With advanced immunodeficiency seen in HIV-infected patients, EBV replication occurs, leading to OHL, Burkitt's lymphoma or EBV-associated large cell lymphoma. Oral hairy leukoplakia manifests as single or multiple white plaques on the lateral margins of the tongue, with a verrucous surface. The presence of OHL correlates with moderate to advanced immunodeficiency.[12] Oral hairy leukoplakia responds well to systemically administered aciclovir and valaciclovir, although there is prompt recurrence after treatment.[13,14] Good response to topical application of podophyllin resin has also been reported, although recurrence is probable and podophyllin can be toxic in large doses.[15] Many clinicians elect not to treat because the lesions are asymptomatic. In some patients, OHL may regress with antiretroviral therapy alone.

Human papillomavirus

Different types of human papillomavirus (HPV) tend to cause different clinical lesions, although there is significant overlap. Infections of the skin and mucous membranes by HPV can cause widespread warts in patients who have AIDS. Types of warts observed include filiform, flat and plantar. Warts can develop in unusual locations, such as on the lips, tongue and oral mucosa (Fig. 95.3). These lesions are often treated with cryotherapy, electrocauterization or topical treatment with caustic agents such as podophyllin, imiquimod, trichloroacetic acid and 5-fluorouracil. However, the majority of these lesions are resistant to treatment and require repeated therapy.

In men, HPV affects the penis, urethra, scrotum, perianal, anal and rectal mucosa in the form of condylomata acuminata that are usually recognized as soft sessile lesions with finger-like projections. In women, the spectrum of clinical disease induced by HPV is broad, with vulvar, vaginal and cervical condylomata being observed. Cervical, vulvar and anal intraepithelial dysplasia may manifest as flat condyloma with viral cytopathic effect seen on histology but without raised warty lesions.

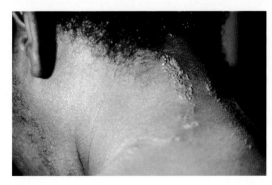

Fig. 95.2 Herpes zoster. A painful linear-zosteriform eruption of vesicles on an erythematous base is characteristic of herpes zoster. The eruption may be persistent and verrucous lesions are not uncommon.

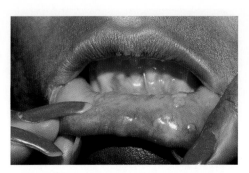

Fig. 95.3 Human papillomavirus infection. Human papillomavirus infections are common in HIV-infected patients. They may have unusual features, as demonstrated here, and may be refractory to therapy.

HIV is associated with increased incidence of high-grade dysplasia and increased risk of progression to invasive squamous cell carcinoma.[16] Human papillomavirus has been detected in more than 95% of cervical cancers and in more than 50% of anal cancers.[17] Certain subtypes of HPV (16, 18, 31, 33, 35, 39, 45 and 51) are considered to be high risk for development of anogenital intraepithelial neoplasia and associated squamous cell carcinoma. A solution of 2–5% acetic acid is helpful in delineating HPV lesions. Colposcopy or anoscopy may also reveal atypical vascular patterns in areas of intraepithelial dysplasia. As with zoster, whenever extensive warts develop in otherwise healthy patients known to be at risk of HIV infection, the patient should be screened for HIV.

Poxvirus

The most common disease caused by poxviruses is molluscum contagiosum, which develops in 10–20% of patients who have AIDS. Molluscum contagiosum is transmitted by direct skin-to-skin contact to produce cutaneous and, rarely, mucosal lesions. In adults it is most commonly transmitted by sexual contact. The lesions are characterized by dome-shaped umbilicated translucent 2–4 mm papules that develop in any part of the body but especially on the face and genital areas (Fig. 95.4). In AIDS patients these lesions are widespread, may attain immense size and can be disfiguring.[18] Most patients who have extensive molluscum contagiosum associated with HIV infection have CD4$^+$ counts well below 250 cells/mm^3. In immunosuppressed patients the diagnosis of molluscum contagiosum should be confirmed by histologic examination in any case that is questionable because it may resemble more serious infections such as cutaneous pneumocystosis, histoplasmosis and *Penicillium marneffei* infection and cryptococcosis. Toluidine or Giemsa staining can be used for cytologic examination of the white material expressed from the lesion to search for the typical large cytoplasmic inclusion bodies. Molluscum contagiosum is treated with cryotherapy, electrodessication, curettage or topical application of podophyllin, tretinoin or imiquimod cream.

Other viral infections

Several viral infections have been reported to develop with increased frequency in patients who have HIV infection. Parvovirus B19, which causes erythema infectiosum, has been reported to produce an exanthem and polyarthralgia in HIV-positive patients. Coxsackie virus and enterovirus may also lead to morbilliform or vesicular eruptions.

Bacterial infections

Folliculitis

Bacterial folliculitis is common in HIV-infected patients, appearing as widely distributed acneiform papules and pustules. Lesions may be pruritic and become excoriated. Recurrent bacterial folliculitis may serve as a clue to screen a patient for possible HIV infection. Most cases are caused by *Staphylococcus aureus*,[19] but other organisms such as *S. epidermidis* and *Pseudomonas aeruginosa* may also cause folliculitis. Nosocomial and community-acquired methicillin-resistant *S. aureus* (MRSA) should be considered when confronting folliculitis in HIV-infected individuals. Additional risk factors for MRSA exposure include intravenous drug use, men who have sex with men, recent hospitalization or incarceration.[20] Bacterial folliculitis in HIV-infected patients is often resistant to standard treatment and prolonged use of systemic antibiotics may be required.[21]

Impetigo, abscesses, cellulitis, lymphadenitis and necrotizing fasciitis

Impetigo, usually caused by *S. aureus*, is seen most commonly on the face, shoulders, axillary and inguinal areas. The infection begins with painful red macules that become vesicles and pustules and contain purulent fluid; these soon rupture and give rise to the characteristic honey-colored crust. Soft tissue and deep-seated bacterial infections such as cellulitis, abscesses and necrotizing fasciitis may also develop in HIV-infected patients and are often due to MRSA.[20] These manifest as diffuse, red, warm, tender areas in the skin, associated with severe toxemia. Streptococcal axillary lymphadenitis is a diffuse, painful swelling of lymph nodes in the axilla that is usually bilateral.

Aggressive antibiotic treatment is recommended for these processes. Excision and drainage of pus-containing abscesses has been reported as an effective treatment in community-acquired MRSA soft tissue lesions, even in the absence of antibiotic treatment.

Mycobacterial infections

Mycobacteria may produce a wide variety of skin lesions in HIV-infected individuals and infection by these organisms usually signifies severe disseminated systemic infection. Since the presenting lesions of cutaneous infections have nonspecific morphology, tissue biopsy and culture are requisite for diagnosis.

Active infection is caused primarily by *Mycobacterium avium-intracellulare* and *M. tuberculosis* and less commonly by other mycobacteria. The infection can manifest as small papules and pustules resembling folliculitis, atopic dermatitis-like eruptions, cutaneous abscesses, lymphadenitis and ulcerations.

Infections with *M. tuberculosis* may be the consequence of either primary infection at the site of broken skin that results in a local verrucous lesion, or systemic disseminated infection. Cutaneous tuberculosis is treated with the same regimen as pulmonary or extrapulmonary disease (see Chapter 93).

Bacillary angiomatosis

Bacillary angiomatosis (BA) is a pseudoneoplastic, infectious cutaneous vascular disorder[22] caused by bacteria of the genus *Bartonella*, including *Bartonella quintana* and *Bartonella henselae*.[23] There are a number of clinical manifestations of BA. The earliest and most common lesion appears as discrete pinpoint red–purple papules similar to pyogenic granulomata. These lesions may ulcerate and become crusted (Fig. 95.5). Another variant consists of subcutaneous nodules that may extend into the underlying skeletal muscle and bone. Patients who have BA may have systemic signs and symptoms, including fever, chills, night sweats and weight loss. In advanced cases, the liver and spleen may be involved. Bacillary angiomatosis occurs primarily in the context of the advanced stage of HIV infection, but may occur in patients who have other forms of immunosuppression or in a healthy host. Because the clinical presentation of this infection can easily be confused with pyogenic granuloma, biopsy should be performed. A 2- to 3-month course of erythromycin (2 g/d) or doxycycline (100 mg q12h) is effective against BA.[24,25] Recurrence is common.

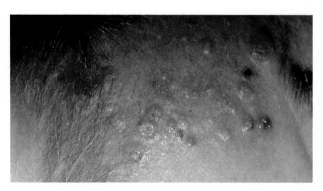

Fig. 95.4 Molluscum contagiosum. These lesions are characteristically translucent, waxy papules with central umbilication.

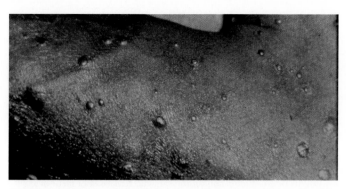

Fig. 95.5 Bacillary angiomatosis. There are elevated vascular papules of the glabrous skin. When incised, these lesions bleed profusely.

Sexually transmitted disease

The accurate diagnosis of sexually transmitted diseases (STDs) is of exceptional importance in individuals at high risk of HIV infection, because their presence increases the risk of transmitting and acquiring HIV infection.[26]

Syphilis

A high prevalence of syphilis, active as well as latent, has been found among HIV-positive patients in the USA.[26] Primary infection with *Treponema pallidum* does not show major variations, beginning with a single chancre at the site of inoculation. Chancres are 1–2 cm, painless, round to oval ulcers with raised indurated borders. Recent studies have reported multiple chancres that can be aggressive and slower to heal.[27,28] Secondary syphilis may occur in a number of forms in patients who have HIV infection, ranging from the classic papulosquamous form with involvement of palms, soles and mucous membranes to unusual forms such as verrucous plaques, extensive oral ulcerations, alopecia, keratoderma, deep cutaneous nodules and widespread gummata.

Syphilis may progress faster from secondary to tertiary disease in HIV-seropositive patients than in HIV-seronegative individuals. Those with CD4+ counts <350 cells/mm³ are at a fourfold higher risk for neurosyphilis. Early central nervous system (CNS) relapse and unresponsiveness to treatment can also be more common in HIV-infected individuals. Syphilis is a strong indicator that an individual may be infected with HIV and all patients should undergo HIV serotesting. Serologic negativity may not rule out secondary syphilis in HIV-infected individuals as true negative serologic studies can be seen with both the fluorescent treponemal antibody absorption (FTA-ABS) and VDRL tests. Skin biopsy for demonstration of spirochetes by special stains or immunohistochemical techniques may also establish the diagnosis. Current treatment involves a single dose of long-acting benzathine penicillin or ceftriaxone (1 g daily for 8–10 days).[29]

Other sexually transmitted diseases (see also Chapter 60)

Lymphogranuloma venereum (LGV) is uncommon in HIV-infected patients in the developed world, though its incidence is rising. It manifests as generalized lymphadenopathy with vulvar or penile edema with ulcerations and erosions.[30] The causative organism is one of three specific serotypes (L1, L2 and L3) of *Chlamydia trachomatis*. Diagnosis is presumptive based on clinical findings. Those thought to be infected with LGV should be started on a course of 200 mg of doxycycline daily for 21 days.[29]

Fungal infections

Candidiasis

Recurrent or persistent oral candidiasis may be the initial sign of HIV infection in many individuals and has been shown to be a predictor of progression from HIV infection to AIDS.[30] The clinical presentation is that of a whitish exudate present on the tongue or buccal mucosa that can easily be scraped away. *Candida* is also implicated in causing angular cheilitis, chronic paronychia, onychodystrophy, distal urethritis and persistent intertriginous infections. *Candida* infections are discussed in detail in Chapter 91.

Dermatophytosis

Cutaneous dermatophytosis is more common in patients with HIV than in the general population and can be extensive and severe. In any individual with extensive tinea corporis, the possibility of underlying HIV infection should be considered. Tinea corporis, often caused by *Trichophyton rubrum*, can present as a widespread dermal infection with multiple fluctuant ethematous ulcerative nodules seen mostly on the extremities.

Systemic fungal infections

Cryptococcus

The most common opportunistic fungal infection to affect the skin in HIV-seropositive patients is cryptococcosis. Umbilicated papules similar to molluscum contagiosum, nodules, pustules, ulcers and erythematous papules are all common manifestations of cutaneous cryptococcosis. If cutaneous cryptococcosis is diagnosed, a thorough investigation for extracutaneous disease should be undertaken (see Chapter 91).

Histoplasmosis

A variety of lesions are seen including nodules, plaques, vesicles, erythematous scaly plaques, necrotizing lesions simulating pyoderma gangrenosum, purpura, petechiae and pustules, with or without ulceration. Diagnosis is made through biopsy (see Chapter 91).

Coccidioidomycosis

Morbilliform eruptions, violaceous or ulcerating plaques, papules and pustules are common cutaneous lesions. If a patient has cutaneous disease, a search for other systemic manifestations should be initiated (see Chapter 91).

Other systemic fungal infections

Blastomycosis and sporotrichosis are rarely observed in HIV-seropositive patients. Mucocutaneous lesions associated with systemic fungal infections consist of pustules, ulcers, papules and nodules (Fig. 95.6). Mucocutaneous fungal infections in general may mimic other disorders such as HSV infection, cellulitis or molluscum

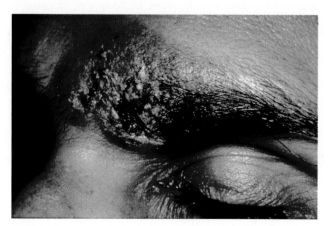

Fig. 95.6 Cutaneous histoplasmosis. These lesions are characteristically quite nondescript and may simulate other infectious disorders and verrucous neoplastic conditions.

contagiosum infection. For this reason, when the clinical diagnosis of possible fungal infection is considered, a tissue biopsy of the lesion should be performed for histologic evaluation and microbiologic cultures (see Chapter 91).[31]

Parasitic and ectoparasitic infections

HIV-seropositive individuals may present with a wide variety of parasitic and ectoparasitic infections, including scabies, demodicidosis, acanthamebiasis, leishmaniasis and toxoplasmosis. This group of infections manifests either as localized conditions or disseminated disease. The clinical presentation can be unusual and the use of cultures and skin biopsies is essential to render accurate diagnosis.[32]

Scabies

The causative agent of scabies is the mite *Sarcoptes scabei*. Scabies is one of the most frequent conditions encountered in HIV infection and is the most common ectoparasitic infection.[21] The clinical presentation can vary from discrete scattered pruritic papules and slight scale to a widespread papulosquamous eruption that resembles atopic dermatitis. A common clinical presentation is that of hyperkeratotic plaques present on the palms, soles, trunk and extremities. Patients complain of intense pruritus that is worse at night. Contacts are almost always infected. Severe scabies can lead to bacteremia and even death due to sepsis. In HIV-infected patients who have CD4+ counts <150 cells/mm³, or in patients who have advanced peripheral neuropathy and diminished sensation, scabies infection may be severe and have a much greater number of mites than normal. This presents as crusted or 'Norwegian' scabies. Microscopic examination of scrapings is used to diagnose mites or ova. Topical treatments include permethrin and benzyl benzoate. Ivermectin can be given orally.

Demodicidosis

The causative agent of demodicidosis is the mite *Demodex*. Demodicidosis has been reported only sporadically in patients who have AIDS. The clinical presentation is that of a persistent pruritic follicular eruption of the face, trunk and extremities. Demodicidosis has also been associated with the pathogenesis of rosacea-like dermatoses, perioral dermatoses and blepharitis. Diagnosis is by clinical pathologic correlation, since *Demodex* spp. are part of the normal skin microbiotica.

Leishmaniasis

Leishmaniasis has three classifications: cutaneous, mucocutaneous and visceral. The skin lesions of kala-azar with scaly lichenified depigmented plaques resemble those of lichen simplex chronicus. Nonulcerated nodules on the extensor surfaces of the limbs overlying the joints have also been described. Mucocutaneous disease begins with single or multiple lesions that heal and eventually lead to mucosal lesions. These lesions are painful and disfiguring. Leishmaniasis is more difficult to treat when associated with HIV infection. Amastigotes persist for years in macrophages and actually accelerate compromised immunity in hosts by increasing HIV viral replication.[33]

NONINFECTIOUS DERMATOSES

The noninfectious dermatoses associated with HIV infection are numerous and may occur in all stages of the disease. Although none of the disorders reported in this group has been linked directly to an infectious agent, these conditions may be in part caused by an abnormal host response to infectious agents. Noninfectious dermatoses in these patients may have atypical clinical presentations, greater severity and may fail to respond to routine treatment.[34] Because these derma-

toses often have atypical presentations in these patients, biopsies and cultures are often required for diagnosis.

Acquired xerosis and ichthyosis

HIV-infected individuals commonly complain of increased dryness of skin. Typically, xerosis is most prominent on the anterior lower legs, manifesting as diffuse dryness with focal crusting and hyperpigmented scales. In the winter it is more severe and may be associated with inflammation. Patients who have advanced AIDS may present with ichthyosis – dry, thick skin with plate-like scales. The severity of the ichthyosis correlates with the degree of wasting. Treatment includes mid-potency steroid ointments or emollients containing salicylic acid, urea or lactic acid.

Seborrheic dermatitis

This is perhaps the best known dermatosis associated with HIV infection and is seen in up to 85% of all these individuals at some point during the course of the illness.[35] The etiology of seborrheic dermatitis is poorly understood but is thought to be multifactorial. Clinically, the disease is characterized by slightly indurated, diffuse or confluent pinkish-red plaques with yellowish greasy scales and crusting in typical locations, including malar and retro-auricular areas, nasolabial folds, eyebrows and scalp (Fig. 95.7). In severe cases, which are also more common in HIV-infected patients, it extends to the chest, neck and other parts of the body. Seborrheic dermatitis in patients who have HIV infection is often resistant to treatment, which should serve as a clue that a patient might be infected. With HAART therapy, the incidence of refractory cases appears to be diminishing. For mild cases, anti-dandruff shampoo may be used. For moderate to severe disease, ketoconazole shampoo, topical steroids, coal tar, sulfur and UVB light have been reported as effective.

Psoriasis and reactive arthritis

Psoriasis develops in up to 5% of individuals with HIV infection[36] and may have a number of different manifestations. It may resemble the classic form found in immunocompetent hosts, which consists of reddish plaques with superficial gray to silver scales on the extensor surfaces and nail changes of onycholysis, pitting and subungual hyperkeratosis. Guttate psoriasis may also be seen, with or without classic psoriasis vulgaris. Severe forms, such as erythrodermic psoriasis, may be encountered. Treatment of psoriasis in these patients may be difficult, although fortunately it is one of the inflammatory conditions that responds well to therapy, especially with systemic retinoids, either isotretinoin or etretinate. Psoriasis may undergo partial remission in response to zidovudine therapy, although recurrences are common.

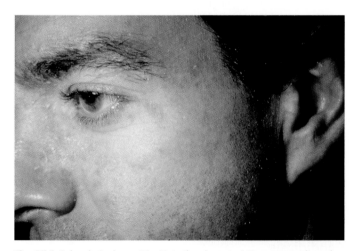

Fig. 95.7 Seborrheic dermatitis. Note the characteristic greasy scale and the erythematous plaques involving the face, especially the nasolabial folds and the eyebrows.

Other treatments that may be beneficial include systemic acitretin, topical keratolytic agents, systemic methotrexate and phototherapy.

Reactive arthritis (formerly known as Reiter's syndrome) is characterized by a triad of polyarthritis, conjunctivitis and urethritis.[37] Cutaneous manifestations include a palmoplantar pustular dermatosis that can be associated with nail dystrophy, hyperkeratosis and periungual erythema. Initially, the lesions present as erythematous macules that evolve into waxy, hyperkeratotic papules surrounded by an erythematous halo. The lesions may coalesce to form thickened plaques that are usually distributed on the palms, soles and trunk. Histologically, reactive arthritis looks identical to pustular psoriasis and relies on a clinical diagnosis. Treatments mirror those used for psoriasis in HIV-infected individuals.

Eosinophilic folliculitis

Eosinophilic folliculitis (EF), also known as eosinophilic pustular folliculitis or Ofuji's disease, is an inflammatory process of the hair follicles, the etiology of which remains undetermined. Mites, Gram-negative bacteria and fungi have all been implicated as possible etiologies. The condition is more common in men and has a peak incidence in the third decade of life. Affected patients may develop marked eosinophilia and elevated levels of IgE. Virtually all patients who have EF have CD4+ counts <200 cells/mm³; thus, it is an important cutaneous marker of advanced HIV infection.[38]

Clinically, patients develop folliculocentric pruritic urticarial papules measuring 1–4 mm in diameter on the upper trunk, face, neck and proximal extremities (Fig. 95.8). There may be coalescence of papules to form plaques. Virtually all cases are associated with lichenification secondary to chronic rubbing and scratching. In dark-skinned individuals, postinflammatory hyperpigmentation can cause considerable disfigurement.

Due to EF's clinical similarities to other pruritic papular eruptions, a biopsy should be taken of a new folliculocentric lesion to correctly diagnose EF. Therapy of EF includes exposure to ultraviolet B and natural sunlight, oral metronidazole, itraconazole, erythromycin and isotretinoin.

Papular dermatitis of AIDS

This is a nonspecific chronic papular eruption that has been reported in HIV-seropositive patients.[39] Most recently it has been termed pruritic papular eruption (PPE). The nosology of this condition has been the subject of debate and many experts consider this to represent a form of eosinophilic folliculitis. Clinically, skin-colored papules are present on

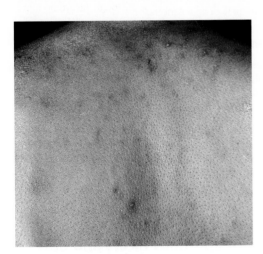

Fig. 95.8 Eosinophilic folliculitis. There are follicular papules, many of which have been excoriated, involving the upper trunk and the face. Histologically, numerous eosinophils are present within the follicular ostia.

the head, neck and upper trunk, many of which may be folliculocentric. Lesions are often excoriated, do not form confluent plaques and neglect mucous membranes. The diagnosis is made only by exclusion; thus other eruptions with similar clinical presentation should be excluded, including EF, scabies, papular mucinosis, secondary syphilis, viral exanthem and drug eruption. Treatments are anecdotal for PPE, but may include topical corticosteroids, oral antihistamines, antipruritics, UVB light and pentoxifylline given in 400 mg dosages every 8 hours for 8 weeks.[40]

Prurigo nodularis

Prurigo nodularis refers to thickened, verrucous papules and nodules and is a reaction pattern of the skin that is associated with a number of pruritic conditions. Patients who have itchy skin chronically rub and scratch, resulting in thickening with formation of typical lesions of prurigo nodularis. Although many different disorders may lead to the condition, in many patients the preceding event has long since resolved and the condition is perpetuated by the so-called itch–scratch–itch cycle.

Treatment of the disorder is based on correcting the underlying pruritus by the use of systemic and topical agents to lessen itching, such as topical corticosteroids, topical menthol- and phenol-containing lotions, topical antihistamines and systemic antipruritic agents.

Atopic dermatitis

Atopic dermatitis is seen somewhat more commonly in children who have HIV infection, having been reported in up to 20%.[41] Patients who have atopic dermatitis antedating HIV infection experience increased severity and persistence of their disease. The pathogenesis of atopic dermatitis in these patients has been associated with elevated circulating IgE antibodies to HIV and *S. aureus*. The clinical presentation is similar to that in immunocompetent hosts, with erythematous patches and plaques with fine papulovesicles associated with scaling and crusting. Treatment includes emollients, topical steroids and oral antihistamines.

Granuloma annulare

There have been a number of sporadic case reports of granuloma annulare (GA) in HIV-seropositive patients.[42] A unique feature of GA in these patients is a tendency toward widespread distribution and photoexacerbation. The clinical presentation is that of violaceous, firm papules with annular arrangement distributed on the hands, feet, arms, legs and trunk. In some patients, there may be similarity to KS. The reason for the development of GA in these patients remains unknown.

Leukocytoclastic vasculitis

Patients who have HIV disease may develop leukocytoclastic vasculitis.[43] This condition is a manifestation of immune complex-mediated disease. The clinical presentation progresses through several stages, beginning as urticarial papules or small petechiae. In most cases, characteristic palpable purpuric papules develop. Lesions are distributed on the extremities, although any body site can be affected. In HIV-infected individuals, they are more numerous and more florid than in immunocompetent hosts. The treatment of leukocytoclastic vasculitis consists primarily of identifying the underlying cause and correcting the associated abnormalities. Administration of nonsteroidal anti-inflammatory agents may be beneficial, although colchicine, dapsone or systemic corticosteroids may be required in severe cases.

NEOPLASMS

A number of different neoplastic disorders may develop in HIV-positive patients. Although lymphoreticular and vascular neoplasms are commonly observed, HIV-associated epithelial, mesenchymal and melanocytic neoplasms have also been described. The development of malignant neoplasms is of great significance because they are often sources of morbidity and mortality.[16]

Kaposi's sarcoma

Kaposi's sarcoma is a viral-associated vascular tumor that is divided into classic and epidemic forms. The classic form is an uncommon disorder that was first described in 1827 and is seen mainly in elderly men of Mediterranean origin, black equatorial Africans and patients who have lymphoma or with primary or iatrogenically induced immune deficiencies. The epidemic form of KS is associated with HIV infection.[44] Epidemic KS is associated with infection by human herpesvirus type 8 (KS-associated herpesvirus) (see Chapter 155).[45] The incidence of KS has decreased dramatically since the development of effective antiretroviral agents.

The clinical presentation may be that of single or multiple skin lesions and there may be mucosal, visceral and/or lymphatic involvement, particularly in the gastrointestinal tract and pulmonary parenchyma. Clinically, KS has three stages, including macule or patch, plaque and nodule (Fig. 95.9). Regression of KS has been seen in patients treated with effective antiretroviral combinations.

Macule or patch

These lesions are faint pink macules or patches oriented along skin cleavage lines. Initially lesions may be innocuous in appearance and are easily overlooked, being mistaken for bruises, purpura or nevi. Correct recognition of early lesions can be accomplished by performing biopsies for histopathologic examination.

Plaque

In time lesions darken and develop into raised firm indurated plaques. The color is purple to brownish because of the presence of abundant blood vessels, extravasated erythrocytes and siderophages. In some cases, lesions may ulcerate.

Nodule

Nodular lesions are dome-shaped, elevated lesions that are usually purple. On palpation they are firm and may be ulcerated. They may simulate bacillary angiomatosis and pyogenic granulomata.

Treatment

All patients should be started on effective antiretroviral therapy and skin lesions can resolve completely with HAART. For localized cutaneous disease, additional treatment of uncomplicated KS can be performed for cosmetic purposes. Local destructive measures are generally the most effective. Liquid nitrogen cryotherapy, radiation,

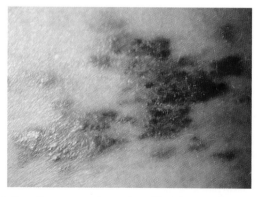

Fig. 95.9 Kaposi's sarcoma, plaque stage. There is an erythematous plaque, which is linear in shape, arranged along skin cleavage lines.

topical alitretinoin gel and intralesional injections of vinblastine sulfate 2–4 mg/ml and interferon-α-2b have all been used successfully. Pigmentary changes may occur and relapse is common.[46] For disseminated disease, antiretrovirals and chemotherapy is recommended (see also Chapter 94).[47]

Lymphomas and lymphoreticular neoplasms

A number of different lymphoreticular malignancies of both B and T cells may develop in HIV-positive patients. The majority of these are based in the lymph nodes and reticuloendothelial system, although the skin may be involved primarily or secondarily. Most are advanced at the time of diagnosis and are associated with a short median survival time (see Chapter 94).

Non-Hodgkin's lymphoma with skin manifestations in patients who have AIDS is most commonly of B-lymphocyte origin and mostly high and intermediate grade. Cutaneous T-lymphocyte lymphoma (CTCL), Hodgkin's disease, lymphomatoid granulomatosis and adult T-lymphocyte leukemia/lymphoma have also been reported. The pathogenesis of lymphoreticular neoplasms in these patients is controversial. Chromosomal abnormalities have been encountered and a possible viral etiology has also been suggested.[48] Most cases involve visceral sites and, when the skin is affected, these are usually pink–purple papules or nodules with necrosis. Deep-seated soft tissue involvement may expand superficially, forming dome-shaped nodules that often ulcerate. Hodgkin's lymphoma appears similar to non-Hodgkin's lymphoma, either as diffuse nodular lesions or as a panniculitis. CTCL may have the clinical appearance of mycosis fungoides with widespread erythematous scaly lesions distributed usually on the trunk and resembling 'eczema'. Lesions become red–brown ulcerated plaques and tumors during the more advanced stages of the disease.

The diagnosis of lymphoreticular neoplasms should be based on histopathologic examination of tissue biopsies. In many cases the use of gene rearrangement studies, flow cytometry and DNA analysis is necessary to characterize these neoplasms. Treatment consists of the usual therapy for systemic lymphoma plus antiretrovirals (see Chapter 94).

Other cancers

Several reports in the literature have described an increased incidence of intraepithelial and invasive carcinoma of the anus in patients who have AIDS-associated human papillomavirus (HPV) infection.[17] HIV is associated with increased incidence of high-grade dysplasia and increased risk of progression to invasive squamous cell carcinoma. HPV has been detected in more than 95% of cervical cancers and in more than 50% of anal cancers.

Hair and nail changes

A number of abnormalities of hair and nails may be encountered in HIV-positive patients.

Chronic inflammatory and noninflammatory alopecia has been observed. Alopecia universalis may also develop and is associated with decreased CD4+ counts.[49] Other hair changes that have been observed include premature graying, thinning and diffuse hair loss. Hypertrichosis has also been associated with HIV infection; however, the cause is unknown but is often associated with antiretroviral use.

Nail changes, including yellow discoloration, hyperpigmentation, transverse and longitudinal ridging and decreased size or loss of the lunulae, have all been reported. Longitudinal hyperpigmentation is observed in association with treatment with zidovudine.

Recurrent aphthous ulcers and other oral manifestations

Recurrent aphthous ulcers are usually idiopathic. Occurrence may represent simply as self-limited pinpoint lesions or can be progressively enlarging destructive lesions with extensive hemorrhage and necrosis. They are frequently recurrent. Pain can be quite severe and esophageal ulceration is well described. Lesions should be cultured for HSV and a biopsy may be needed to rule out malignancy (e.g. lymphoma) or infection. Smaller ulcers may be treated with a topical corticosteroid preparation. Thalidomide, 200 mg/day orally, given for 4 weeks, has been shown to be effective for larger oral and esophageal lesions.[50] It is vital that precautions are taken to avoid exposure to thalidomide during pregnancy.

Oral hairy leukoplakia and intraoral KS may be the first clue to HIV infection.

Intraoral KS may appear alone or be associated with skin or disseminated lesions. It may be flat, raised, solitary or multiple and is red–blue or purple. A biopsy may be required to distinguish it from other vascular or pigmented lesions.

Salivary gland involvement with lymphoepithelial cyst formation can lead to xerostomia and salivary gland enlargement in HIV patients. Labial salivary glands may demonstrate lymphocytic infiltrates similar to Sjögren's syndrome although the infiltrate is composed predominantly of CD8+ T cells.

Complications of antiretroviral agents

With the advent of more effective antiretroviral agents, many of the cutaneous manifestations of HIV discussed previously in this chapter occur less frequently. However, a new subset of dermatologic conditions has arisen related to the use of these drugs, namely cutaneous side-effects of antiretroviral agents. Currently there are five classes of medication used for the treatment of HIV: protease inhibitors (PIs), nucleoside analogue reverse transcriptase inhibitors (NRTIs), non-nucleoside reverse transcriptase inhibitors (NNRTIs), integrase inhibitors and entry inhibitors. Common patterns of drug eruptions include morbilliform exanthem, hyperpigmentation, urticarial eruptions, erythema muliforme minor and, rarely, Stevens–Johnson syndrome.

Morbilliform exanthems are the most common HIV-related cutaneous drug eruptions. They are characterized as a widespread, maculopapular rash that is usually found on the trunk and extremities beginning 2–10 days after drug initiation. They usually resolve on discontinuation of the offending agent. Hyperpigmentation is often related to photosensitivity and/or antiretroviral usage. Manifestations include hyperpigmentation of the palms and soles, as well as pigmented bands in the nails of the fingers and toes. Urticarial eruptions presents as wheals distributed over the face, trunk and extremities. The peak reaction is seen 1–2 days after the drug is initiated and resolves within a week after drug termination.

Erythema multiforme is an acute inflammatory reaction with characteristic patches, papules, macules and plaques that evolve into bull's eye lesions. Stevens–Johnson syndrome is a severe form of erythema multiforme. It is characterized by coalescent skin lesions and involvement of mucosal surfaces. Cutaneous manifestations include variable violaceous macules and patches originating on the face and trunk. Mucosal erosions are seen and the epidermis may peel off in large sheets.

Protease inhibitor-associated skin effects

Fixed drug eruptions have occurred as a result of therapy with saquinavir.[51] Indinavir has been associated with paronychia, alopecia, cheilitis and dry skin. Atazanavir is associated most notably with jaundice since it competitively inhibits an enzyme involved in bilirubin metabolism.[52] Fosamprenavir, darunavir, atazanavir and liponavir/ritonavir have all been associated with mild to moderate morbilliform eruptions lasting for 7–13 days.

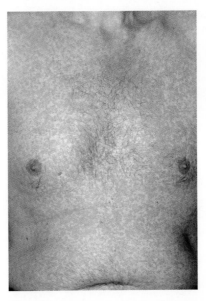

Fig. 95.10 Morbilliform drug eruption. There is a diffuse eruption of fine pink macules and papules, which have coalesced, involving the trunk and the extremities. The most common cause of these eruptions is trimethoprim–sulfamethoxazole.

Nucleoside reverse transcriptase inhibitor-associated skin effects

Morbilliform eruptions have been reported with all NRTIs but are uncommon (Fig. 95.10). Two well-known side-effects of zidovudine are nail pigmentation and hypertrichosis. Nail pigmentation may occur on several[53] or all nails of the hands and feet.[54] Emtricitabine is associated with hyperpigmentation of the palms and soles.[55]

Hypersensitivity reactions have been reported with nevirapine. These reactions are associated with fever, malaise, nausea and a mild rash that may progress to more severe cutaneous involvement, and severe fatal Stevens–Johnson reaction may occur.[56] Nevirapine hypersensitivity is more common in women and in patients with CD4+ counts >400 cells/mm³, when given as initial therapy.

Abacavir can cause a severe hypersensitivity reaction which may even be life threatening, especially if treatment is continued despite the reaction or if the patient is rechallenged with abacavir after resolution of the initial reaction.[57] Abacavir hypersensitivity has been associated with a specific human leukocyte antigen (HLA) haplotype (HLA-B*5701). Avoidance of abacavir in individuals positive for HLA-B*5701 can prevent severe hypersensitivity.

Entry and integrase inhibitor drug eruptions

Enfuvirtide is associated with drug site reactions consisting of erythema, ecchymosis, induration, nodules, cysts, pruritus, tenderness, and/or pain.[78] Rotating injection sites may reduce the severity of the reactions. Skin rash and pruritus have been rarely reported in trials of maraviroc and raltegravir.

REFERENCES

References for this chapter can be found online at http://www.expertconsult.com

HIV/AIDS-related problems in developing countries

INTRODUCTION AND EPIDEMIOLOGY

As of December 2007, an estimated 33.2 million people (30.8 million adults and 2.5 million children) were infected with HIV.[1] In 2007 alone, 2.5 million new HIV infections occurred worldwide and 2.1 million people died of AIDS. In the developing world, the majority of incident cases occur in young adults. People aged 15–24 years comprise about one-third of those living with HIV/AIDS. In 2007, illnesses associated with HIV/AIDS caused the deaths of approximately 2.1 million people, including an estimated 330 000 children younger than 15 years. More than 95% of these infections and deaths occurred in developing countries. Accompanying the morbidity and mortality borne by those infected with HIV is the dramatic alteration of the social structure attributable to the HIV epidemic. Because of the premature death of HIV-infected parents, 13 million children have been orphaned. The number of orphaned children is forecast to more than double by 2010.[2]

The contrast between the impact of HIV/AIDS in the developed world and in the developing world is striking. Figure 96.1 illustrates the discrepancy between the HIV prevalence in sub-Saharan Africa versus the rest of the world. Whereas AIDS-related mortality is declining in the USA, western Europe and Australia, it has continued to rise rapidly in sub-Saharan Africa, South East Asia and Latin America with only recent reports of optimism resulting from the scale up of antiretroviral therapy (ART).[3–6] One in 200 adults aged 15–49 years is infected with HIV in the USA and Europe, but 10–40% of pregnant women in some parts of sub-Saharan Africa are infected with HIV. Although antiretroviral therapy is given to pregnant women and their newborn infants in developed countries to prevent transmission, most pregnant women who have HIV infection in developing countries receive little or no antiretroviral therapy, creating an enormous discrepancy in perinatal transmission of HIV in these two regions of the world. In addition, recent surveys have demonstrated that nearly 75% of people with HIV infection are aware of their serostatus in the USA and Europe, whereas in a recent national serobehavioral survey in Uganda, only 21% were aware of their own status and 9% knew their partners' status, with the majority of individuals either never being tested or being unaware of their HIV status.[7]

Since the initial recognition of the AIDS epidemic, much has been done to respond to HIV infection by way of prevention and behavioral

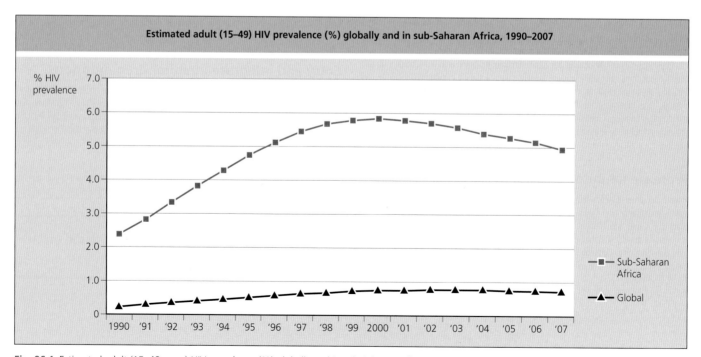

Fig. 96.1 Estimated adult (15–49 years) HIV prevalence (%) globally and in sub-Saharan Africa, 1990–2007. Data from UNAIDS Report 2007.[1]

modification. Government-supported efforts in Thailand, including HIV and AIDS surveillance systems and programs such as the '100% condom use' campaign for commercial sex, have contributed to decreased rates of HIV and sexually transmitted diseases in military recruits.[8] Similarly, in Cambodia the prevalence of HIV among pregnant women declined by almost a third between 1997 and 2000, to 2.3%. Widespread health education, increased use of condoms and voluntary HIV counseling and testing appear to have lowered the prevalence of HIV infection in some areas of sub-Saharan Africa. Recent declines in HIV prevalence among populations in Kenya, Uganda, Zimbabwe and Haiti which appear to be attributable to behavior change offer some encouraging support for the ongoing HIV prevention efforts.[9,10]

However, in the setting of this mature epidemic, declines in HIV seroprevalence have been seen in the presence of stable and high incidence.[10] Death due to HIV disease, rather than a true decrease in the incidence of HIV infection, appears to have contributed most to the reduced HIV prevalence measured in Rakai, Uganda.[11] Figure 96.2 models the lifetime risk of AIDS death for 15-year-old boys based on current HIV prevalence in adults aged 15–49 years. The upper line, based on current HIV prevalence, is compared with the lower line, which assumes that the risk for new HIV infection at each age decreases by half over the next 15 years. This indicates that, even with successful prevention campaigns, without access to treatment the proportion of young people who will die of AIDS is very high.[12]

Despite ongoing prevention efforts, the overwhelming burden of HIV disease is borne by the developing world. The factors responsible for the discrepancies between the developed and developing world in terms of the diagnosis and care of people with HIV infection and the magnitude of the HIV pandemic are multifactorial. Limited access to care, lack of diagnostic equipment and insufficient money to support either prevention or treatment programs are primarily responsible for the continuing rise in morbidity and mortality associated with HIV infection in developing countries. Underlying high prevalence rates of HIV infection and a combination of high-risk behavior and the widespread prevalence of sexually transmitted diseases act synergistically to propel the epidemic further in many areas of the developing world. Furthermore, the coexistence of other endemic diseases that are widely prevalent in developing countries, such as tuberculosis and gastrointestinal infections, complicate the care of people with HIV infection and pose additional problems for the medical personnel caring for them. Recent increases in donor resources for HIV prevention, care and treatment have dramatically changed the previously gloomy picture in developing countries. The rapid scale up of basic care and antiretroviral therapy for people infected with HIV is changing the landscape and providing optimism where previously there was little hope. This chapter reviews some of these aspects as they relate to the care of people with HIV infection living in developing countries.

CLINICAL FEATURES

The clinical manifestations of HIV infection in developing countries are diverse and reflect the wide variety of other endemic diseases within each region.[13] More than 100 pathogens, including viruses, bacteria, fungi, protozoa, helminths and arthropods, have been identified as having caused opportunistic disease in persons with HIV infection. A relatively small number of these pathogens cause a majority of the infections, yet their impact on the health of persons with HIV infection is enormous. Although the reasons for the differences between the spectrum of opportunistic infections observed in developing countries

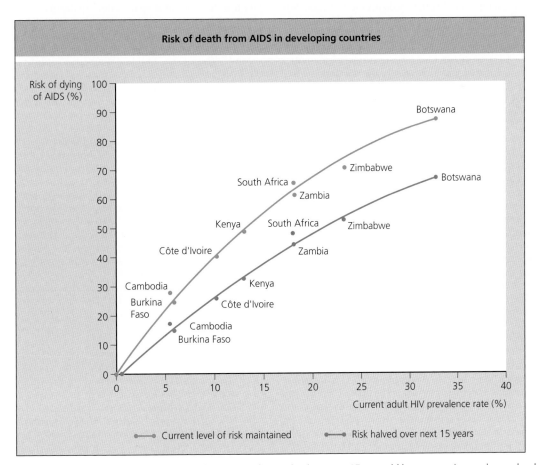

Fig. 96.2 Risk of death from AIDS in developing countries. Lifetime risk of AIDS death among 15-year-old boys, assuming unchanged or halved risk of becoming infected with HIV, in selected countries.

and in developed countries are not completely understood, they are likely to include factors such as the prevalence of pathogens in the environment, social behaviors, ecologic factors that result in exposure to these pathogens, and other undefined factors.

Determining the spectrum of opportunistic infections in a given region requires surveillance systems and diagnostic services that may not be available in many developing countries. For example, opportunistic infections that can be diagnosed with reasonable accuracy by physical examination (e.g. oral candidiasis) or by inexpensive laboratory techniques (e.g. India ink stain of cerebrospinal fluid for *Cryptococcus neoformans*) may be documented more frequently than opportunistic infections requiring more expensive diagnostic technologies (e.g. *Pneumocystis jirovecii* pneumonia, disseminated *Mycobacterium avium* complex (MAC) and cytomegalovirus disease). Because most clinical studies that document opportunistic infections are conducted in urban hospitals, those infected outside of urban centers are often not included in disease surveillance efforts. Furthermore, longitudinal cohort studies are costly to maintain in resource-poor settings. Biases in diagnosing and reporting opportunistic infections may be especially important among socially disadvantaged groups with limited access to diagnostic and health-care services. Finally, differences in clinical definitions may make comparisons between published reports difficult. For these reasons and for others, much less is known about the frequency of different opportunistic infections in the developing world than in industrialized countries.

Although it is clear that HIV infection has a definite impact on a wide variety of microbial agents in developing countries, less is known about the impact of these diseases on HIV infection. Although it has been shown that HIV disease progresses more rapidly in developing countries, recent studies report similar rates of HIV disease progression when compared with the epidemiology of HIV disease in developed countries prior to the introduction of highly active antiretroviral therapy (HAART).[14] Data quantifying the median time from seroconversion to AIDS is limited. Early studies suggested that time to AIDS was much shorter in sub-Saharan Africa and South East Asia. Obstacles included pinpointing the time of seroconversion and reconciling different definitions of AIDS. Similarly, time from seroconversion to AIDS and death has been compared with that seen in the developed world early in the HIV epidemic. In a population-based study in Uganda, the median survival from AIDS to death was 9.3 months but varied according to AIDS-defining illness.[15] Median survival associated with wasting syndrome, Kaposi's sarcoma and esophageal candidiasis was less than 3.5 months, compared with survival longer than 20 months associated with cryptosporidial diarrhea, chronic herpes simplex virus (HSV) infection and extrapulmonary tuberculosis. The median CD4+ lymphocyte count at the time of AIDS onset was 150 cells/mm³. Notably, the most common opportunistic infections in resource-poor settings, including tuberculosis and endemic bacterial infections, develop at CD4+ lymphocyte counts higher than 150 cells/mm³. A recent observational study from Uganda revealed that the median time from seroconversion to death was 9 years with a median time to CD4+ lymphocyte count of 200 was 6.3 years.[16] Evidence from Uganda also suggests that the subtype of HIV affects disease progression with subtype D progressing to AIDS more rapidly than subtype A (6.5 versus 8.0 years).[17] The recent scale up of ART access and basic HIV care including trimethoprim–sulfamethoxazole prophylaxis should ultimately have a major impact on survival in countries currently suffering high AIDS-related morbidity and death.

In addition to the clinical spectrum of disease defined by opportunistic infection, co-infection with endemic diseases and resulting immune activation may increase susceptibility to HIV infection. A person whose immune system is activated at the time of exposure to HIV may be more susceptible to infection with HIV. In this regard, the success of an aggressive sexually transmitted disease (STD) treatment program in Tanzania in decreasing the incidence of new HIV infections may be due in part to the removal of immune-activating factors. A similar community-based study conducted in Uganda and designed to evaluate the effect of STD treatment on the development of incident HIV infection found no difference.[18] The lack of a positive effect may be related to the effect of anthelmintic therapy provided to the control group. The eradication of helminths may have had an effect similar to the treatment of STDs. Furthermore, the trial did not treat for genital ulcerative disease due to HSV infection. Unfortunately, a recent clinical trial treating HSV infection among high risk women did not show any efficacy in preventing HIV acquisition. Current clinical trials are evaluating the effect of treating genital HSV infection on HIV infection and transmission as well as HIV disease progression. Chronic immune activation and infections prevalent in the developing world appear to enhance the pathogenesis of HIV.[19] Thus, both the rate of spread of the HIV epidemic as well as the clinical course in the developing world may be greatly influenced by the underlying state of heightened immune activation that exists in many people in these countries.

Tropical diseases may directly lead to an increased risk of infection with HIV. Treatment of severe anemia induced by malaria has led to HIV infection by transfusion. Female genital schistosomiasis, like other genital inflammatory conditions, may increase the efficiency of HIV transmission. Several drugs used in the treatment and prophylaxis of tropical diseases have an immunosuppressive effect and may thereby influence susceptibility to HIV. Specific interactions between HIV and infectious diseases in developing countries are listed briefly below.

Mycobacterial infections

Tuberculosis (see also Chapter 93)

Tuberculosis is the most important severe opportunistic infection observed among patients with HIV infection in developing countries because it occurs frequently, is transmissible to both people with HIV infection and uninfected persons, can be readily treated and prevented. Globally, tuberculosis is the leading cause of death among people with HIV infection, accounting for a third of deaths due to AIDS. The World Health Organization (WHO) estimates that the number of people infected with the tubercle bacillus is one-third of the world population; throughout the world a new tuberculosis infection occurs every second.[20] The greatest number of tuberculosis infections occur in people living in Asia, sub-Saharan Africa and Latin America, where about half of the adult population is infected. These are the same areas in which HIV continues to increase steadily. The WHO considers HIV as the single most important factor driving the increase in tuberculosis incidence in Africa over the past 10 years.

The increase in tuberculosis attributable to HIV has resulted in increased demand for already overburdened tuberculosis programs. During the initial stages of the HIV epidemic, when incidence rates increased dramatically, tuberculosis rates increased as well. In developing countries where young adults have high rates of infection with both HIV and tuberculosis, the risk of co-infection is correspondingly high. Worldwide, an estimated 640 000 incident cases of tuberculosis (8%) occur in the setting of HIV infection. Although the largest group of co-infected individuals lives in India, the burden of HIV infection per capita is highest in sub-Saharan Africa, with 32% of tuberculosis cases co-infected with HIV.

Infection with HIV and tuberculosis has become a particular problem in many African countries. The rates of incident tuberculosis continue to rise in Africa because of the HIV epidemic while rates are falling elsewhere because of the HIV epidemic.[21] In the central African countries of Zimbabwe and Malawi, the annual incidence of tuberculosis doubled in the 5 years 1985–90 and 20–44% of AIDS patients developed tuberculosis during the course of their infection. In contrast, only 4% of AIDS patients in the USA have tuberculosis. In a study of tuberculosis treatment in Uganda, a high prevalence (49%) of *Mycobacterium africanum* isolates was identified in patients with HIV infection who had pulmonary tuberculosis.[22] In Uganda, the prevalence of HIV infection among tuberculosis patients was 5.9 times greater than that among patients who had inactive tuberculosis. In Lusaka, Zambia, as many as 37% of hospitalized children who had tuberculosis were infected with HIV, compared with 11% of nontuberculosis controls. Cohort studies have also shown that the risk of developing active tuberculosis among persons infected with *Mycobacterium tuberculosis* is much higher in persons with HIV infection than in HIV-seronegative persons. For someone who is co-infected with HIV and tuberculosis, the annual risk of developing active tuberculosis ranges from 5% to 15%, whereas the lifetime risk among people who have tuberculosis in the absence of HIV infection is only 5–10%.

During the period 1997–2004, the estimated number of incident cases of tuberculosis increased from 8.0 million to 8.9 million, with an estimated 1.7 million deaths occurring in 2004 due to tuberculosis.[23] The progressive increase is largely due to the HIV/AIDS pandemic. In patients dying with HIV disease in Abidjan, Côte d'Ivoire, tuberculosis was present in more than half of those who had AIDS and was responsible for one-third of the deaths. The importance of tuberculosis was demonstrated in an autopsy study among patients dying of pulmonary disease in Abidjan; 40% of the HIV-positive patients died of tuberculosis, compared with only 4% of the HIV-negative patients. In Mexico, disseminated tuberculosis was found at autopsy in 25% of patients who had AIDS; this compares with 6% of patients in the USA and 5% of patients in Italy. This observation is consistent with the higher incidence of pulmonary tuberculosis in Latin America than in the USA, as well as with the higher incidence of tuberculosis in the USA among foreign-born people and people of Latin American or Asian descent.

A prospective cohort study conducted in South Africa demonstrated that the increased mortality associated with tuberculosis was observed only in patients with a CD4$^+$ lymphocyte count greater than 200 cells/mm^3 and in those without AIDS at baseline.[24] The authors proposed that the immune activation due to tuberculosis increased HIV replication and accelerated HIV disease progression.

Diagnosis, treatment and prophylaxis of HIV-associated tuberculosis are discussed in detail in Chapter 93. Meta-analyses of trials of isoniazid prophylaxis of HIV-positive populations with a positive tuberculin skin test showed a definite reduction in the development of active tuberculosis in the treated group compared with the placebo group during a period of 2–3 years.[25,26] No significant protection could be demonstrated in the groups with skin test anergy who were included in the same trials. Thus, the benefit of prophylaxis for populations that are already anergic as a result of immunosuppression is more difficult to evaluate because they indicate either no previous exposure to tuberculosis or previous infection with loss of immunologic reactivity. As with many other diseases, the cost of medication needed to carry out effective treatment of tuberculosis is lacking in many developing countries where the problem is greatest. Furthermore, patient compliance may be a limiting factor in treatment regimens of multiple drugs for periods of several months. Research priorities include the determination of the best method for detection of active tuberculosis in resource-poor settings, and optimum duration of preventive therapy.

Resistance to antituberculosis drugs has emerged as a major public health problem, particularly in settings with high HIV/tuberculosis co-infection rates. Extensively drug-resistant tuberculosis (XDR), defined by resistance to at least isoniazid and rifampicin in addition to any quinolone and at least one second-line injectable agent (capreomycin, amikacin, kanamycin). In a recent outbreak of tuberculosis among HIV-infected patients in South Africa, XDR cases comprised 24% of all multidrug-resistant isolates. These cases were virtually untreatable and 52 of 53 cases died in a median of only 16 days.[27] The strain of tuberculosis identified among these patients had the same genetic background material, suggesting that recent, possibly nosocomial transmission may have contributed to this outbreak. XDR tuberculosis has now been identified in several countries and poses a major public health threat to the fight against HIV/AIDS and tuberculosis, highlighting the need for improved diagnostic strategies, infection control measures and newer antituberculosis drugs.

In order to prevent active tuberculosis, up to 70% of the world's children are vaccinated with bacille Calmette–Guérin (BCG). Unfortunately, the efficacy of BCG in HIV-infected populations is unclear. One study found no benefit of vaccination in HIV-seropositive children; another study found a benefit of childhood vaccination in HIV-seropositive adults and protection from disease caused by *M. tuberculosis*. Recent data suggesting a beneficial effect of early BCG vaccination on mortality from all causes in children not infected with HIV indicate that measures of benefit in HIV-seropositive people need to be broader than mere prevention of tuberculosis. The WHO recommends that BCG should be given to people who have asymptomatic HIV infection in areas with a high risk of tuberculosis infection. In areas where the risk of tuberculosis is minimal, BCG is not recommended, particularly for those who are infected with HIV. Recombinant BCG vector-based vaccines are currently being evaluated in animal models for potential use in vaccination against HIV.

Mycobacterium avium complex

Although MAC is very common in advanced HIV infection in the USA and Europe, it has rarely been documented in developing countries. In one study in Uganda, none of 95 blood cultures from severely ill patients who had advanced AIDS was positive for *M. avium*; neither were any of 165 mycobacterial sputum cultures from HIV-seropositive and HIV-seronegative patients at the same hospital. In Côte d'Ivoire, none of 202 blood cultures from HIV-positive adult inpatients was positive for *M. avium*, whereas 4% grew *M. tuberculosis*. Intestinal biopsies from 98 Ugandan, Zairian and Zambian patients who had chronic HIV-related enteropathy yielded histology suggestive of *M. avium* infection in only one case. Similarly, autopsies on 78 HIV-seropositive children in Côte d'Ivoire revealed no evidence of *M. avium* infection. In Kenya and Mexico, *M. avium* has been documented in 6% of patients hospitalized with late-stage HIV disease; in Brazil it has been documented in 18% of 125 hospitalized patients. A recent study conducted in South Africa demonstrated a 10% prevalence of disseminated MAC in 10% of hospitalized patients with a CD4$^+$ lymphocyte count of less than 100 cells/mm^3.[28]

The reasons for the low frequency of disseminated disease caused by MAC in the developing world are unclear, but there are many possibilities, including less exposure to MAC, exposure to different variants of MAC, differences in host susceptibility, greater acquired immunity to mycobacteria, earlier death from infection with more virulent pathogens, and diagnostic difficulties. There may be greater acquired immunity to mycobacterial disease through BCG vaccine or previous infection with *M. tuberculosis*, but the reported BCG coverage (50%) and purified protein derivative reactivity (82%) in Uganda seem unlikely to explain the lack of any disseminated MAC.

Mycobacterium leprae

To date, there is little evidence that HIV infection has a profound effect on the frequency of *M. leprae* infection (see Chapter 103). Several studies have examined serology for HIV in newly diagnosed leprosy. In one study in Uganda of 189 new cases of leprosy matched for age, sex and district of residence, no significant difference in overall rates of HIV seropositivity was found between the patients who had leprosy (12% HIV seropositive) and the controls (18% HIV seropositive). Interestingly, HIV seropositivity was more frequent among the multibacillary cases than the paucibacillary cases. An association between HIV and leprosy was seen in studies conducted in Zambia and Nigeria. Studies in Kenya and Nigeria both support the hypothesis that HIV infection favors the multibacillary form of leprosy. A different clinical association was noted in Zambian leprosy patients who had active neuritis. The study suggested that HIV-positive patients have poorer recovery of nerve function than controls after treatment with corticosteroids.

Thus, there appears to be no striking evidence that HIV infection has an adverse effect on the course of leprosy. Multibacillary disease could possibly develop under the influence of HIV infection but, because leprosy is chronic and slow in progression, it is difficult to discern the influence of HIV on leprosy directly.

Nonmycobacterial pulmonary infections

Bacterial pneumonia

Investigations of patients with HIV who have pulmonary disease demonstrate that bacterial pneumonia caused by *Streptococcus pneumoniae* and *Haemophilus influenzae* occur as frequently in developing countries as they do in the developed world. In a study in Nairobi, Kenya, 79 episodes of invasive pneumococcal disease were seen in 587 HIV-positive women, whereas there was only one episode in 132 HIV-seronegative women.[29] Serotyping revealed that most recurrent events were related to re-infection. A wide spectrum of HIV-related pneumococcal disease was seen; 56% of cases were pneumonia, 30% were sinusitis and 11% were occult bacteremia. The mean CD4+ lymphocyte count was 302 cells/mm³ at first presentation and 171 cells/mm³ for recurrent episodes. In this study *S. pneumoniae* caused more disease at an earlier stage of HIV immunosuppression than did *M. tuberculosis*.

The importance of pneumococcal disease in the host with HIV infection cannot be underestimated. Invasive pneumococcal disease has been shown to cause significant morbidity and mortality. The use of the pneumococcal polysaccharide vaccine to prevent infection in people with HIV infection has been evaluated and generally recommended by the Centers for Disease Control and Prevention. In light of the increased prevalence of antibiotic resistance and ease of administration, this vaccine would appear to be a prudent use of resources. However, studies have shown that the polysaccharide vaccine is not beneficial in individuals with HIV infection in African populations. Conjugate pneumococcal vaccines have proven to be more immunogenic in both HIV-positive and HIV-negative children in the Gambia and South Africa and hold greater promise to reduce the incidence of invasive pneumococcal disease.

Pneumocystis jirovecii pneumonia

Several opportunistic infections that are common in developed countries are rarely identified in developing countries. For example, in Abidjan, *P. jirovecii* pneumonia accounts for only 8% of deaths from HIV-associated pulmonary disease and only 2% of all HIV-associated deaths. A recent report from Zimbabwe demonstrated that even after selecting patients who had abnormal chest radiographs that were consistent with *P. jirovecii* pneumonia, tuberculosis was still a more frequent diagnosis than *P. jirovecii* pneumonia.

Although *P. jirovecii* pneumonia appears to be infrequent in Africa and Asia, it is relatively common in Latin America and Caribbean countries, with rates similar to those documented in the USA. A retrospective case series in a clinic in London, UK, found a significantly higher rate of *P. jirovecii* pneumonia as a presenting diagnosis in non-Africans (34%) than in Africans (17%). Prevalence rates are also low in Haiti, with a case series incidence of less than 10%. Other reported rates include 7–25% in Thailand, 20–24% in Mexico and 32–45% in Brazil.

The reasons for lower rates of *P. jirovecii* pneumonia in parts of the developing world are unclear. Possible explanations include less environmental exposure to *P. jirovecii*, exposure to different strains of *P. jirovecii*, differences in host susceptibility, earlier deaths in patients in the tropics who have AIDS owing to exposure to more virulent organisms, and diagnostic difficulties. When it does occur, the clinical presentation of *P. jirovecii* pneumonia in developing countries appears to be similar to that in industrialized countries. Frequent co-infection with tuberculosis may obscure the diagnosis. The diagnosis and treatment of *P. jirovecii* pneumonia are discussed in Chapter 91.

Diarrheal disease

In addition to tuberculosis, one of the more common clinical syndromes seen in persons with HIV infection in developing countries is a diarrhea-wasting syndrome, referred to as 'slim disease'. Diarrhea lasting longer than 1 month occurs in up to 50% of patients in Africa who have AIDS, a rate that is more frequent than that observed in persons with HIV infection in industrialized countries. The diarrhea is usually intermittent and not associated with blood or mucus, and it is only rarely secretory in nature. In one-third to two-thirds of patients who have diarrhea in Uganda, Zaire and Zambia, no cause was found despite detailed examinations. In other studies, pathogens (including cryptosporidia, microsporidia, *Shigella* spp., *Salmonella* spp. and *Campylobacter* spp.) have been identified with frequencies of 7–48%.

Other diagnoses are also common among patients who have such profound wasting. In an autopsy study in Côte d'Ivoire, 44% of patients dying with HIV wasting syndrome had disseminated tuberculosis, compared with 25% without the syndrome. A chronic fever syndrome is also frequently associated with tuberculosis and non-typhoid salmonellosis. Often there is very little that can be done for patients who have this syndrome except to provide nutritional support.

Protozoan infections

Toxoplasmosis

Toxoplasma gondii is a common opportunistic infection in both developed and developing countries, and the incidence is proportional to the prevalence of latent infection in the population at risk for HIV. A higher prevalence of cerebral toxoplasmosis has been documented among Latin American patients than in the USA, which is consistent with the higher underlying prevalence of toxoplasmosis in Latin America. Although there is a suggestion that up to 50% of seropositive AIDS patients in some parts of the world may develop toxoplasmal encephalitis, its frequency in developing countries is unclear because of limited diagnostic capabilities. Autopsy series that have included examination of the brain have suggested disease prevalence rates in late-stage AIDS patients of 15% in Abidjan, 25% in Mexico City and 36% in Kampala. For more detailed information on toxoplasmosis, see Chapters 91 and 106.

Visceral leishmaniasis

The overlap of visceral leishmaniasis and AIDS is increasing because of the spread of the AIDS pandemic to rural areas and the spread of visceral leishmaniasis to suburban areas. Consequently, cases of co-infection with *Leishmania* spp. and HIV are becoming more frequent, with important clinical, diagnostic, chemotherapeutic, epidemiologic and economic implications. Co-infection with *Leishmania* spp. and HIV is now considered an 'emerging disease', especially in southern Europe, where 25–75% of adult visceral leishmaniasis cases are related to HIV infection and 1.5–9% of patients who have AIDS suffer from newly acquired or reactivated visceral leishmaniasis. The WHO reviewed 692 retrospective cases that occurred between 1985 and 1996 in southern Europe and eastern Africa.[30] Of the cases of co-infection, 90% were observed in patients with CD4+ lymphocyte counts of less than 200 cells/mm³. Bone marrow aspiration was the most frequently used technique for parasitologic diagnosis. In two-thirds of these cases, the diagnosis of HIV was made before the diagnosis of leishmaniasis.

Multiple visceral locations outside of the reticuloendothelial system are frequently involved during co-infection; these locations include the blood, skin, gastrointestinal tract, lungs and central nervous system. Because of the high frequency of leishmaniasis in the peripheral blood of these patients, transmission via blood or needles, particularly among intravenous drug users, is a major problem.

The *Leishmania* spp. frequently involved in HIV infection are those that cause visceral disease, such as *Leishmania donovani* and *L. infantum* in Asia, southern Europe and Africa, and *L. chagasi* in Latin America. Cutaneous leishmaniasis has a much wider geographic distribution than visceral disease but it is only rarely involved as a complication of HIV infection. Classic visceral leishmaniasis documented in patients with HIV infection is probably caused by reactivation of a latent infection, owing to increasing immunosuppression. In one study, the CD4+ lymphocyte count was less than 200 cells/mm³ in more than 75% of the patients with HIV infection in whom visceral leishmaniasis was diagnosed, and fewer than 5% of patients had counts of 500 cells/mm³ or greater.

The clinical presentations of visceral leishmaniasis in HIV are quite similar to that described in HIV-negative patients; clinical features include weight loss, fever, pancytopenia and hepatosplenomegaly. Diagnosis is based on a high index of suspicion in a person who has resided in or traveled to an endemic area, and treatment is similar to that employed in patients without HIV infection who have leishmaniasis (see Chapter 117). In Ethiopia, a recent clinical trial evaluated the treatment of visceral leishmaniasis in patients with and without HIV infection. Those co-infected had a greater mortality (33.3% vs 3.6%) and relapse rate (16.7% vs 1.2%). The authors expressed the concern that HIV-positive patients with relapsing visceral leishmaniasis could serve as a reservoir of resistant organisms. Treatment guidelines support the use of two drug combination therapy.

Trypanosomiasis

Trypanosoma cruzi, the cause of Chagas disease, infects millions of people in Latin America. Reports from Argentina, Brazil and Chile have described clinical and laboratory findings in about two dozen patients co-infected with HIV and *T. cruzi*.[31] These reports suggest that Chagas disease may result from reactivation of latent *T. cruzi* infection and that clinical manifestations such as meningoencephalitis may be more frequent and more severe in those infected with HIV. Activation of *T. cruzi* infection by HIV or AIDS usually presents with central nervous system manifestations, but in one review trypanosomes were demonstrated in the blood of five of six cases in whom the examination was done. In one pathologic study of 23 cases, acute myocarditis was frequently noted in those cases that were autopsied, but no information was presented as to whether clinical evidence of myocarditis was present during life.

Malaria

Initial studies examining the effect of HIV on the course of malaria found no changes in the severity, incidence or successful treatment of malaria (see Chapter 111). This may have been due to the complex immune response to malaria, which is not easily perturbed by a predominantly T-cell immunodeficiency. In one study of patients in Burkina Faso, investigators demonstrated a preservation of some components of the malaria-specific immune response in AIDS patients who were co-infected with *Plasmodium falciparum*.

Recently, a complex interplay has been found between malaria and HIV, challenging the apparent lack of a significant interaction. In Uganda, a hospital-based case-control study, a rural population-based cohort study and an urban clinic-based cohort study all showed that HIV infection was associated with increased frequency and severity of clinical episodes of malaria parasitemia.[32–34] The effect increased with declining immunosuppression as indicated by decreasing CD4+ lymphocyte counts. The interplay between malaria and HIV appears to vary with the dynamics of malaria transmission. In regions with unstable malaria transmission, HIV infection is a risk factor for severe malaria in both young children and adults.[35,36] In regions of holoendemicity, however, HIV infection appears to have only a modest effect on the risk of parasitemia and clinical malaria among semi-immune adults. Two recent studies have shown that infant mortality is higher in babies born to mothers who are co-infected with placental malaria and HIV. It was also shown that HIV infection impairs the pregnant woman's ability to control *P. falciparum* infection. Thus, there is an interaction between HIV and malaria in the placenta. In addition, malaria can contribute to the increased spread of HIV, owing to the need for more frequent transfusions to treat the anemia of malaria.

Enteric parasitic infections

Enteric parasitic infections such as isosporiasis and cryptosporidiosis may be reported in as many as 5–10% of patients who have AIDS in the tropics, compared with 0.2% of patients who have AIDS in the USA. Reports have also shown that the risk of isosporiasis among residents of the USA with AIDS is higher among those born in Latin America and Haiti than among those born in the USA. In Zambia, evaluation of persistent diarrhea in patients with AIDS revealed cryptosporidiosis (7%), microsporidiosis (16%), isosporiasis (37%) and no etiology (40%); treatment with albendazole resulted in a complete or partial response in 60% of those shown to have enteric parasitic infection.[37]

Penicillium marneffei

A common fungal pathogen in AIDS patients in South East Asia is *Penicillium marneffei*.[38] It causes the third most common opportunistic infection in HIV disease in northern Thailand, after extrapulmonary tuberculosis and cryptococcal meningitis. *P. marneffei* was first isolated in 1956 and infection was a rare event before the arrival of the AIDS pandemic in South East Asia. Since then hundreds of cases have been diagnosed, mainly in southern China, northern Thailand, Hong Kong, Vietnam, Singapore, Indonesia and Myanmar. The environmental reservoir of *P. marneffei* is unknown, but the organism has been isolated from the organs, feces and burrows of three species of bamboo rat. Exposure to soil appears to be a key factor in transmission.

Disseminated *P. marneffei* infection is characterized by fever, anemia, weight loss and papular skin lesions. Other frequent signs and symptoms include cough, generalized lymphadenopathy, hepatomegaly and diarrhea. The most common cutaneous manifestation is a generalized papular rash with a central umbilication that resembles the lesions of molluscum contagiosum. These are predominantly found on the face, scalp and upper extremities, but occur throughout the body. Chest radiographs are frequently abnormal, with diffused reticulonodular or localized alveolar infiltrates.

The mean duration of illness before presentation is 4 weeks. The incubation period of disseminated disease is unclear and the disease may be a result of reactivation of latent infection as opposed to new infection or re-infection. However, the development of clinically active disease within weeks of exposure in endemic areas, and the reports of children who have vertically transmitted HIV infection developing disease in the first months and years of life, demonstrate that primary infection can quickly lead to disseminated disease. Finally, the pronounced seasonal variation in disease incidence implies an important role for exogenous re-infection and the expression of disease with *P. marneffei* in AIDS patients in endemic areas. In addition to endemic areas, travelers from regions where *P. marneffei* is not endemic have become infected with this pathogen while traveling in South East Asia. Diagnosis and treatment are discussed in Chapter 91.

Other opportunistic infections

Other opportunistic infections, which may be similar in all areas of the world, include oral and esophageal candidiasis, cryptococcosis, cytomegalovirus infection and Kaposi's sarcoma. Herpes simplex virus infection, herpes zoster and cerebral toxoplasmosis also appear to be relatively common in most areas where diagnostic equipment is readily available. It should be noted that regional variations in frequencies of these diseases do exist within developing countries. Cryptococcosis accounted for only 2% of AIDS deaths in Abidjan but is more common in central and southern Africa.

Mycobacterial infections apart from tuberculosis, such as *Mycobacterium kansasii*, have been longstanding health problems among miners in South Africa and may now be emerging as HIV-associated infections in those miners with HIV infection.

Endemic Kaposi's sarcoma has a striking geographic distribution, being most common in central Africa. Kaposi's sarcoma associated with HIV is likely to have a similar heterogeneous disease frequency, although the incidence of Kaposi's sarcoma has increased in all countries in which HIV disease occurs. The epidemiology of the new human herpes virus, HHV-8, the viral agent causing Kaposi's sarcoma, has been the subject of intensive investigation since its discovery in 1994. Serologic studies have revealed a worldwide geographic distribution of HHV-8 with the highest seroprevalence (40–60%) in sub-Saharan Africa (see Chapter 155).

HIV TESTING

Currently, HIV testing in the developing world is done for surveillance, prevention and identification of those in need of basic care and ART. Despite improvements in the access to testing, most people still do not know their HIV status. In a recent nationwide sero-behavioral survey in Uganda, only 27% of individuals knew their HIV status. The recent efforts to scale up voluntary counseling and testing in conjunction with the expansion of antiretroviral treatment programs has greatly increased the access to HIV testing in the developing world. Unfortunately, most people still do not know their HIV status. In a recent nationwide serobehavioral survey in Uganda, only 21% of individuals knew their HIV status.[7] Rapid test formats for HIV detection of antibody have also helped improve access to HIV testing by removing the sophisticated laboratory requirements, allowing same-day provision of test results and eliminating the need for subsequent follow-up.

Despite improvements in the access to testing, the majority of people with HIV infection in the developing world do not know their HIV status. There are important reasons for knowing one's HIV status. The earlier people know they are infected, the greater the opportunity for them to access treatment, some forms of which are not expensive, and to apply pressure on communities and governments for improved access to care. The earlier people are aware of their infection, the better able they are to make informed and responsible decisions about child-bearing and avoiding transmission to spouses or partners, and to make plans for family welfare before they become ill or die. Furthermore, the one important benefit of self-knowledge of HIV status is that it helps unmask the invisible epidemic and permits a genuine community response. If people become aware of their infection early on, while they are still relatively healthy, this gives them time and energy to support one another as well as to alert the community to the epidemic.

However, these benefits to individuals, families and communities are realistically achievable only where people feel safe in finding out whether they are infected. Efforts by governments and civil society to combat rejection and discrimination directed at people who have HIV are vital (UNAIDS).

In 1998, WHO and UNAIDS issued revised guidelines for the selection and use of HIV antibody tests applicable for use in developing countries.[39] The three main objectives for HIV antibody testing are:

- screening of blood and blood products;
- unlinked and anonymous testing for the purpose of monitoring prevalence and trends of HIV infection; and
- diagnosis of HIV infection among asymptomatic people and those with clinical signs and symptoms suggestive of HIV infection.

There are three strategies recommended by the WHO. Strategy 1 applies to blood safety and surveillance in settings where HIV prevalence exceeds 10%; all serum and plasma is tested with one enzyme-linked immunosorbent assay (ELISA) or rapid assay. Serum that is reactive is considered HIV antibody positive. This strategy can be used for screening blood donors to protect the blood supply but it should not be used for notification of the blood donor unless strategy 2 or 3 is implemented.

Strategy 2 includes testing serum by one ELISA or rapid assay and, if it is reactive on the first assay, it is then retested with a second ELISA or rapid assay based on a different antigen preparation or a different test principle. Concordant results after repeat testing will indicate a positive or negative result. If the results of the two assays remain discordant, the specimen is considered indeterminate. Strategy 2 is recommended for surveillance, particularly when testing populations with a low prevalence of HIV, and for diagnosis where the prevalence of HIV among asymptomatic populations exceeds 10%. The additional test in strategy 2 compared with strategy 1 is necessary in order not to overestimate the HIV prevalence of such regions. Strategy 2 is also recommended for notification of the blood donor, particularly in developing countries, where strategy 2 is more cost-effective than strategy 3.

Strategy 3 is similar to strategy 2, except that it requires a third test if the serum is found to be reactive on the second assay. The three tests in this strategy should be based on different antigen preparations or different test principles. A specimen is considered to be antibody positive if it is reactive on all three assays. If the serum is discordant on any of the three assays, it is considered to be indeterminate. This strategy is recommended for diagnosis in settings where HIV prevalence is less than 10%.

In the selection of HIV antibody tests for use in strategies 2 and 3, the first test should have the highest sensitivity, whereas the second and third tests should have higher specificity than the first. The number of initial discordant or indeterminate results should not exceed 5%.

An HIV test kit bulk purchase program has been established by the WHO in collaboration with UNAIDS in order to provide national AIDS control programs that use tests giving the most accurate results at the lowest possible cost.

PREVENTION OF HIV INFECTION

Although the epidemic continues to spread throughout the developing world, it is also likely that increased preventive efforts could effectively limit the magnitude of the epidemic. For example, in those countries where the epidemic is still in an expansion phase but is not yet fully visible, the public health response is likely to have a decisive influence on its course. There is every reason to believe that the course of the pandemic could still be altered profoundly by the introduction of HIV prevention strategies that are within the technical reach of all countries. Several successes in slowing the HIV pandemic have provided encouragement and further stimulus for improved programs. Aggressive treatment of STDs coupled with a program of condom distribution has already been shown to be effective in decreasing HIV incidence rates in populations at high risk for HIV in sub-Saharan Africa and Asia. Needle-exchange programs have helped to stabilize and in some cases reduce HIV incidence among intravenous drug users in selected countries. HIV incidence rates can be reduced by an estimated 50% with adequately supported prevention programs. In Asia alone this could mean the prevention of several million AIDS deaths among young adults in their most productive years.

While we await the availability of a vaccine and the effect of therapeutic interventions, a primary prevention strategy must be focused on educational efforts to influence social, cultural and behavioral factors. To control the AIDS epidemic, countries will need not only to promote individual behavior change but also to address the related problems of social disruption associated with mounting unemployment, accelerated urbanization, commercial sex, rapid decline in health services and drug abuse. Fundamental social changes, such as improving the social status of women, will be required if AIDS control efforts are to succeed. In view of the rapid pace of HIV transmission in sub-Saharan Africa and Asia, implementation of these principles of AIDS prevention and care is needed urgently.

Male circumcision has emerged as a new, highly effective HIV prevention measure. Clinical trials from Uganda, Kenya and South Africa have all revealed the protective efficacy of male circumcision for HIV prevention, reducing the risk of HIV acquisition by about 60%. Access to safe male circumcision services has been endorsed by the WHO, UNAIDS and donor communities as an important component in the fight against the spread of HIV/AIDS. Several countries including Uganda, Rwanda and Kenya have incorporated male circumcision into their HIV prevention efforts and scale up of male circumcision services is currently underway.

PREVENTION OF OPPORTUNISTIC INFECTIONS

Those opportunistic infections associated with the greatest degree of morbidity and mortality, as well as available preventive and therapeutic options, include tuberculosis and bacteremia due to non-*typhi* *Salmonella* spp. and *S. pneumoniae*.[40] Tuberculosis and other endemic bacterial infections regularly occur in patients with HIV infection but without profound immunosuppression. Primary preventive therapy against tuberculosis provides an important first line of defense against the development of disease in earlier stages of HIV infection.

Recent studies have evaluated the role of trimethoprim–sulfamethoxazole (TMP–SMX) prophylaxis in reduction of infections other than *P. jirovecii* pneumonia in patients with HIV infection. A randomized trial conducted in Côte d'Ivoire showed that events leading to hospitalization or death were 43% lower in African adults with early symptomatic HIV disease treated with TMP–SMX than with placebo. The beneficial effect was due to activity of TMP–SMX against bacterial infections, malaria and isosporosis. A recent prospective cohort study conducted by the Centers for Disease Control in Uganda illustrated that TMP–SMX prophylaxis to HIV-positive individuals resulted in a 46% reduction in mortality with lower rates of malaria, diarrhea and hospital admission. Beneficial effects were also seen on the rate of CD4+ T-cell count decline and HIV viral load.[41] These findings have resulted in widespread introduction of TMP–SMX as part of basic HIV care in developing countries. Concerns cited as limitations to the use of TMP–SMX include an anticipated increase in antimicrobial resistance in pathogens such as nontyphoidal salmonellas and the pneumococcus. Of additional concern is the potential for cross-resistance between pyrimethamine and trimethoprim, as sulfadoxine–pyrimethamine is one of the most widely used treatments against *P. falciparum*.

HIV TREATMENT IN DEVELOPING COUNTRIES

On April 22, 2002, the WHO announced the first treatment guidelines for children and adults infected with HIV in the developing world.[42] This action set the stage for a tremendous increase in access to care; WHO estimated that at least 1 330 000 people needing treatment had access to antiretroviral medicines at the end of 2005. Although far below the target of 3 million, the momentum has continued, with some countries greatly expanding the numbers on treatment and hopefully able to achieve the revised WHO goal of universal access by 2010. The treatment guidelines were accompanied by the expansion of the Essential Medicines List to include antiretrovirals in addition to nevirapine and zidovudine, which were previously listed for the prevention of mother-to-child HIV transmission. The WHO public health approach to antiretroviral therapy was updated in 2006 and presents a standardization and simplification of ART. However, the complexity of providing treatment regimens to millions of people in resource-poor areas extends well beyond access to medications.

In order to ensure the safe and appropriate use of antiretrovirals, resources for evaluating patients prior to the initiation of therapy and monitoring for response to therapy, as well as for the development of potential side-effects, must also be available. The WHO recommends initiation of therapy based on clinical staging and CD4+ lymphocyte count or total lymphocyte count if CD4+ lymphocyte count is not available:

- WHO stage I includes those individuals with HIV infection who are asymptomatic or manifest persistent generalized lymphadenopathy;
- stage II includes those with weight loss (<10% body weight), minor mucocutaneous manifestations, herpes zoster and recurrent upper respiratory tract infections;
- stage III includes those with weight loss (>10% body weight), unexplained chronic diarrhea, unexplained prolonged fever, thrush, oral hairy leukoplakia, pulmonary tuberculosis, severe

Table 96.1 World Health Organization recommendations for starting HIV/AIDS therapy. Recommendations for initiating antiretroviral therapy in adults and adolescents with documented HIV infection

If CD4 testing is available	WHO stage IV disease irrespective of CD4+ lymphocyte count WHO stage I, II, III with CD4+ lymphocyte counts <200 cells/mm³
If CD4 testing unavailable	WHO stage IV disease irrespective of total lymphocyte count WHO stage II or III disease with a total lymphocyte count <1200 cells/mm³

bacterial infections and bedridden for less than 50% of the day during the past month; and

- stage IV includes those with clinical syndromes consistent with AIDS and/or bedridden for more than 50% of the day during the past month.

The guidelines, shown in Table 96.1, recommend starting ART in those who have WHO stage IV disease irrespective of CD4+ lymphocyte count and WHO stage I, II or III with CD4+ lymphocyte count below 200 cells/mm³ in areas where CD4+ lymphocyte count is available. If CD4+ lymphocyte count is unavailable, ART is recommended in those with WHO stage II or III with total lymphocyte count below 1200 cells/mm³. Assessment of HIV viral load is not considered essential for determining the need for therapy.

In addition to the assessment of immunologic function as indicated by symptoms and lymphocyte count, further testing for the safe and effective use of ART is divided into four categories as listed in Table 96.2: absolute minimum tests, basic tests, desirable tests and optional tests. Absolute minimum testing includes an HIV antibody test and hemoglobin or hematocrit level if starting a zidovudine-based regimen. Other monitoring is recommended based on the antiretroviral regimen chosen and guided by symptoms. Testing for HIV viral load is deemed to be optional.

The guidelines are based on rigorous evaluation conducted almost exclusively in developed countries. A matter for concern is whether guidelines created for the populations of developed nations are adaptable to HIV-infected populations worldwide. Specifics regarding the presence of different HIV subtypes, endemic infections such as tuberculosis, genetic determinants and environmental factors such as nutritional status may introduce factors that alter response to treatment.

Several developing countries have successfully scaled up ART including Brazil, Thailand, Senegal, Uganda and South Africa to name only a few. Numerous publications from these settings have shown that high levels of adherence and positive treatment outcomes are achievable through carefully implemented programs. With initiation of ART on a population-wide scale, continuous surveillance of drug-resistant viruses will be needed to inform treatment guidelines. Of great concern is that antiviral drug resistance due to suboptimal therapies could limit the potency of available treatments. In parallel with promulgation of the guidelines, the WHO, in collaboration with the International AIDS Society, is developing a global HIV drug resistance surveillance network.

Multiple studies conducted in developed nations have proved the tremendous benefit available to people with HIV infection by the initiation of ART. Consequently, morbidity and mortality due to HIV have declined dramatically. In developed or developing nations, ART provides the only hope of survival for those with HIV infection who are able to adhere to daily lifelong therapy. Moreover, the availability of ART can reinforce prevention activities by offering an incentive to seek HIV testing, preventing mother-to-child transmission and decreasing the risk of sexual transmission.

Table 96.2 World Health Organization guidelines for laboratory monitoring of antiretroviral (ARV) drug use

Diagnosis and monitoring laboratory tests	Pre-ART (at entry into care)	At initiation of first-line or second-line ARV regimen	Every 6 months	As required (depending on symptoms)
HIV diagnostic testing	Yes			
Hemoglobin		For AZT regimens		Yes
WBC and differential		Yes		Yes
CD4 cell count	Yes	Yes	Yes	
Pregnancy test		For efavirenz regimens		Yes
Chemistry (ALT, other liver enzymes, renal function, glucose, lipids, amylase, lipase, lactate and serum electrolytes)				Yes
Viral load measurement				Yes

ART, antiretroviral therapy.

IMPACT OF HIV AND AIDS ON HEALTH-CARE SYSTEMS

As the number of people with HIV infection in developing countries continues to increase, HIV/AIDS will continue to make increasing demands on the health-care system at all levels. The allocation of funds for prevention versus care and support varies according to region, with 66% and 32% of estimated expenditure needed for care and support in sub-Saharan Africa and Asia, respectively. AIDS prevention activities include teacher training and peer education, condom promotion and distribution, treatment of STDs, voluntary testing and counseling, transfusion screening and prevention of mother-to-child HIV transmission. Included in care and support activities are diagnostic testing, palliative care, opportunistic infection treatment, drug costs and monitoring for ART, as well as orphanage care and living assistance. Mobilization of such tremendous resources will require a considerable commitment from both domestic and donor sources.

Unfortunately, these demands come at a time of great financial vulnerability for health systems and at a stage, particularly in developing countries, when a great deal of work remains to be done to increase primary health care. Primary care is intended to be the interface of contact between communities and the national health-care system, bringing health care as close as possible to where people live and work. Diagnosis and treatment to relieve symptoms and to prevent and treat opportunistic infections can ease suffering and prolong the productive lives of people who have HIV, sometimes at a low cost. As the patient's immune system collapses, however, available treatments become increasingly more expensive. An analysis by the World Bank of alternative treatment and care options concludes that community-initiated care provided at home, although often shifting costs from the national taxpayer to the local community, also greatly reduces the cost of care and thereby offers hope of affordability in improving the quality of the last years of life of people dying with AIDS.

The epidemic will undoubtedly increase demand for medical care and reduce its supply at a given quality and price. As the number of people who have HIV infection increases, access to medical care will become more difficult and more expensive for everyone, including people not infected with HIV, and total health expenditure per capita will rise. Governments are under pressure to increase their share of health-care spending and to provide special subsidies for the treatment of HIV infection. Unfortunately, because of the scarcity of resources and the inability or unwillingness of governments to increase public health spending enough to offset these pressures, either of these policies may exacerbate the impact of the epidemic on the health-care sector.

Governments should ensure that patients who have HIV infection benefit from the same access to care as other patients who have comparable illnesses and similar ability to pay. Because of discrimination, people who have HIV are frequently denied treatment or face barriers to care that others do not encounter. Governments should also provide information about the efficacy of treatments for opportunistic illnesses, HIV infection and AIDS; subsidize the treatment of STDs and contagious opportunistic infections; subsidize the screening of the blood supply; and ensure access to health care for the poorest, regardless of HIV infection status.

REFERENCES

References for this chapter can be found online at http://www.expertconsult.com

Hepatitis B in the HIV co-infected patient

RECIPROCAL INFLUENCE BETWEEN HBV AND HIV

Extended follow-up of highly active antiretroviral therapy (HAART)-treated patients suggests that hepatitis B virus (HBV) co-infection and serum hepatitis B surface antigen (HBsAg) does not substantially affect HIV progression and HIV-related mortality.[1]

On the contrary, co-infection with HIV and treatment with HAART each modifies the natural history of HBV infection. Most of the liver damage associated with HBV infection stems from the immune system response to HBV. HIV infection can dampen this immunologic response. HAART leads to immune system reconstitution, which in HBV-infected patients can be advantageous or deleterious. These phenomena may explain some of the effects of HIV co-infection and HAART on HBV which are:[2]

- a higher risk of chronicity after acute HBV infection;
- a higher level of HBV replication and a higher rate of reactivation compared with persons without HIV co-infection;
- increased liver injury (so-called immune-reconstitution hepatitis) and liver disease progression in case of antiretroviral therapy; and
- a higher risk of liver-related death.

A lamivudine-containing HAART regimen is independently associated with a decreased risk of liver decompensation.[3] Early use of HAART containing dual-activity agents is generally positive for preventing severe immune dysfunction, controlling HBV replication, slowing liver disease progression and preventing immune-reconstitution hepatitis.

TREATMENT OF HBV IN HIV CO-INFECTED PATIENTS

Goals of therapy

The principal goals of anti-HBV treatment are to stop or decrease liver disease progression, and to prevent cirrhosis and hepatocellular carcinoma. HIV co-infected patients infrequently seroconvert to anti-HBe and anti-HBs status. Seroconversion remains an objective, but a more realistic virologic goal is prolonged suppression of HBV replication. Attaining this milestone leads to histologic improvement, significant decrease or normalization of aminotransferases and prevention of progression to cirrhosis and end-stage liver disease.

Sustained viral control requires long-term maintenance therapy. Treatment discontinuation, especially of lamivudine, has been associated with HBV reactivation, alanine aminotransferase (ALT) flares and, in rare cases, hepatic decompensation. The drawback of long-term therapy is the possibility of resistance (around 20% per year for lamivudine). Therefore, most co-infected patients require combination therapy for anti-HBV treatment.

Anti-HBV therapy recommendations

Guidelines consider two situations based on the need for anti-HIV therapy or not. The threshold of serum HBV DNA level for anti-HBV initiation is >2000 IU/ml and liver histologic evaluation may be needed in patients with serum HBV DNA >2000 IU/ml and persistently normal ALT in HIV-infected patients who do not need anti-HIV therapy (Figs PP44.1, PP44.2).[4,5]

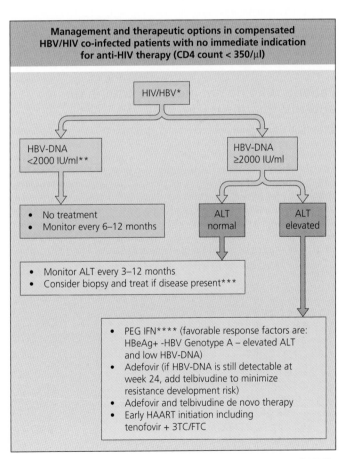

Fig. PP44.1 Management and therapeutic options in compensated HBV/HIV co-infected patients with no immediate indication for anti-HIV therapy (CD4 count >350/μl). ALT, alanine aminotransferase; 3TC, lamivudine; FTC, emtricitabine; HAART, highly active antiretroviral therapy; PEG IFN, pegylated interferon.

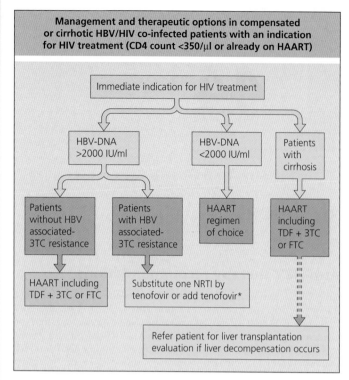

Management and therapeutic options in compensated or cirrhotic HBV/HIV co-infected patients with an indication for HIV treatment (CD4 count <350/μl or already on HAART)

Fig. PP44.2 Management and therapeutic options in compensated or cirrhotic HBV/HIV co-infected patients with an indication for HIV treatment (CD4 count <350/μl or already on HAART). 3TC, lamivudine; FTC, emtricitabine; NRTI, nucleoside reverse transcriptase inhibitor; TDF, tenofovir disoproxil fumarate.

Patients who do not meet the criteria for anti-HIV treatment (Fig. PP44.1)

These patients should not receive anti-HBV agents with dual anti-HIV activity (see Table PP44.1). Using anti-HIV therapy at this juncture raises the risk of early HIV resistance, with consequent limitations of HIV therapeutic options. In hepatitis B e antigen (HBeAg)-positive patients, pegylated interferon α-2a, adefovir dipivoxil or telbivudine should be considered. Typically, pegylated interferon is not preferred for the treatment of HBeAg-negative patients as the opportunity to achieve HBsAg seroconversion and to maintain HBV DNA suppression off therapy is low. Although not demonstrated, combination therapy of a nucleoside and a nucleotide (adefovir and telbivudine)

for such patients rather than monotherapy or pegylated interferon should be considered.

Patients who meet the criteria for anti-HIV treatment (Fig. PP44.2)

HAART, including two dual-acting drugs, constitutes the preferred option for these patients. The best choice is to combine a nucleoside and a nucleotide analogue in order to prevent long-term resistance (i.e. tenofovir plus either lamivudine or emtricitabine).

When patients change anti-HIV treatments because of intolerance or lack of efficacy, the anti-HBV component should be continued even if it is not part of the subsequent anti-HIV regimen; stopping anti-HBV therapy has been associated with reactivation of HBV infection and ALT flares.

Patients with cirrhosis

Sustained control of HBV replication in patients with cirrhosis is critical to prevent liver decompensation, hepatocellular carcinoma, and death. Preventing resistance and ensuring compliance are paramount considerations. Therefore, cirrhotic patients should receive combination anti-HBV therapy and should be monitored closely during the first 12–24 weeks of therapy, due to risk of ALT flare and immune-reconstitution hepatitis. Serum HBV DNA should be assessed every 12 weeks, especially for those with CD4 counts <200/mm³. Patients with liver decompensation should be considered for liver transplantation.

Anti-HBV therapy

Six therapeutic agents are currently approved for the treatment of chronic HBV in the USA and the European Union (Table PP44.1).

Interferon alpha

Historically, standard interferon alpha (5 MU daily or 9–10 MU three times weekly) has been the first-line therapy for HBV monoinfection. Data conflict about the value of interferon alpha in HIV-positive patients with chronic hepatitis B. The optimal dose and duration of pegylated interferon remains unknown in co-infected patients. However, pegylated interferon may be used in HBeAg patients who do not need anti-HIV therapy.

Lamivudine

This nucleoside analogue offers both anti-HIV and anti-HBV activity. It inhibits HBV replication in up to 87% of HIV/HBV co-infected patients. Rates of anti-HBe seroconversion are highly variable, ranging up to 11% of patients in some studies. HBV resistance is a major problem with lamivudine (47% of patients at 2 years and 90% at 4 years of treatment).

Table PP44.1 Responses to anti-HBV agents tested in HIV/HBV co-infected patients

	IFN	LAM	ETV	FTC	TDF	ADV*
Duration (weeks)	12–24	48	24	48	24–48	48–192
Anti-HBV activity tested in HIV patients	wt	wt	LAM-R	wt	wt, LAM-R	LAM-R
HBV DNA decline (log₁₀ copies/ml)	26%†	2.7	3.6	–	4.4	4.7–6*
HBe seroconversion (%)	9	11	–	–	4	7
ALT normalization (%)	12–20	30–50	49	–	–	35–66*
Histologic improvement	–	–	–	–	–	33–50*

IFN, standard interferon; LAM, lamivudine; ETV, entecavir; FTC, emtricitabine; TDF, tenofovir disoproxil fumarate; ADV, adefovir dipivoxil; wt, wild type; LAM-R, lamivudine HBV-resistant strain.
*Results at 48–192 weeks of ADV.
†Proportion of patients with serum HBV DNA <6 log₁₀ copies/ml.

Adefovir dipivoxil

This once-daily nucleotide analogue reverse transcriptase inhibitor is active against wild-type and lamivudine-resistant HBV. In a small series of HIV/HBV lamivudine-resistant co-infected patients,[6] adding once-daily adefovir 10 mg reduced serum HBV DNA by a median of 5.9 $\log_{10}$ copies/ml at week 144. No adefovir-associated HBV and HIV mutations surfaced during 144 weeks of follow-up. Co-infected patients generally tolerate adefovir well during short- and long-term therapy. Rare cases of renal toxicity have been reported.

HIV agents with HBV activity

Entecavir

Entecavir is a purine-derived nucleoside analogue which reduced HBV DNA by nearly 7 $\log_{10}$ copies/ml with no observed resistance over 48 weeks in HBV monoinfected, lamivudine-naive patients.

In HIV co-infected, lamivudine-resistant patients, adding entecavir reduced HBV DNA by a mean of 3.66 $\log_{10}$ copies/ml by 24 weeks of therapy. It also inhibited HIV replication with an IC_{50} lower than the plasma concentrations achieved *in vivo* at doses given for anti-HBV therapy. After 6 months of entecavir therapy, 96% of isolates from the co-infected patient contained the M184V lamivudine mutation. This variant confers high-level resistance to entecavir. Therefore, entecavir should be considered as a drug with anti-HIV activity and should be avoided in patients who do not need anti-HIV therapy.

Emtricitabine

This newer nucleoside reverse transcriptase inhibitor is a 5-fluorinated derivative of lamivudine. Emtricitabine (200 mg/day) reduces serum HBV DNA by up to 3.13 $\log_{10}$ copies/ml in HIV/HBV co-infected patients. In treatment-naive HIV/HBV co-infected patients, the incidence of mutations in the viral polymerase following 1 year of therapy with emtricitabine is around 10%. Emtricitabine is generally well tolerated.

Tenofovir disoproxil fumarate

This agent, an acyclic nucleotide reverse transcriptase inhibitor, is effective against HIV, and against wild-type and lamivudine-resistant HBV.

In HIV co-infected patients the mean $\log_{10}$ decline in HBV DNA after 48 weeks of tenofovir therapy was –4.7 with tenofovir plus lamivudine compared with –3.0 with lamivudine alone. Tenofovir anti-HBV activity was similar for patients with wild-type (–5.3 $\log_{10}$) and lamivudine-resistant HBV (–4.6 $\log_{10}$).[7]

Among HBeAg-positive patients, serum HBV DNA became undetectable in 29.6%, 7.4% lost HBeAg and 3.7% seroconverted to anti-HBe (median follow-up, 12 months).[7]

When compared to adefovir, mean $\log_{10}$ time-weighted average change from baseline to week 48 is 1 log higher with tenofovir when compared with adefovir.

No HBV resistance to tenofovir has been so far reported in HIV/HBV co-infected patients. However, almost all the HIV/HBV co-infected patients in tenofovir studies were receiving concomitant lamivudine therapy as a part of HAART. This add-on strategy may reduce the risk of HBV resistance to tenofovir.

Tenofovir use may be limited by renal toxicity (tubulopathy) that can occur even years after initiation. Creatinine and potassium levels should be monitored every 3 or 4 months.

CONCLUSIONS

The interactions of HIV, HBV and HAART complicate the disease course and management of patients co-infected with HIV and HBV. HBV co-infection does not substantially affect the course of HIV disease, but HIV co-infection does significantly alter the course of HBV disease. On the whole, early use of HAART is beneficial in co-infected patients who meet the criteria for antiretroviral therapy. Availability of agents with dual activity against HIV and HBV facilitates management of co-infected patients. It also mandates careful monitoring of treatment effects on both infections to detect and to avoid triggering resistance or relapse.

REFERENCES

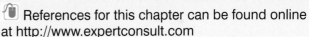 References for this chapter can be found online at http://www.expertconsult.com

HIV infection in children

Children become infected with HIV almost exclusively by the mother-to-child transmission route.[1] However, the risk of horizontal contamination, which has been little studied, has not completely disappeared in highly endemic, resource-poor countries.[2] Horizontal contamination may occur through unsafe blood transfusions or the use of nonsterile equipment for medical or traditional purposes. Child rape is also a significant risk. The progression of pediatric epidemics largely parallels that for infection in adults. However, the extremely effective prevention of mother-to-child transmission has greatly increased the gap between rich and poor countries. The World Health Organization (WHO) estimated that about two million children were infected with HIV at the end of 2007, with 420 000 new infections, leading to 330 000 deaths (Table 97.1). The proportion of pregnant women who are seropositive for human immunodeficiency virus type 1 (HIV-1) is in the range 3–8% in western and central Africa, and 15–30% in southern Africa.[3]

MOTHER-TO-CHILD TRANSMISSION

In the absence of prophylactic treatment, about 15–20% of infected mothers transmit HIV-1 to their child pre- or peripartum, with an additional risk of 10–15% associated with breast-feeding.[4] Although never strictly compared in a same cohort, the risk of mother-to-child transmission appears to be similar for the different subtypes of HIV-1 (groups A, B, C and recombinant strains), although it has been suggested that there is a higher risk associated with group D viruses.[5] HIV-2 is phylogenetically different from HIV-1 with a much lower replicative potential in humans; it also has a much lower mother-to-child transmission rate than HIV-1. Even without treatment, the transmission rate of HIV-2 is only 1–2% and mostly involves women with primary infection during pregnancy or at an advanced stage of the disease.[6]

There are several pathophysiologic mechanisms underlying transmission. In-utero contamination is possible, but occurs in only a minority of cases, despite possible HIV-1 replication in placental monocytes and CD4 cells.[4] The risk of in-utero contamination is higher in cases of chorioamnionitis and in women with very high levels of viral replication, as is observed in primary infection or in advanced stages of disease. Most infected children, however, are contaminated during labor, probably through mother-to-fetus microtransfusion.[7] The level of maternal viral replication is again a major risk factor for contamination at this point, although no lower threshold for transmission in the absence of antiretroviral prophylaxis has been established. The conditions of birth, particularly the duration of amniotic membrane rupture, can also increase the risk of transmission. Passage through the birth canal probably only makes a small contribution to the risk of infection: delivery by Caesarian section reduces the risk of transmission only if it is performed before labor begins. Premature birth is strongly associated with infection of the child, although it is unclear whether prematurity and its co-factors are a cause or consequence of infection[8] (Table 97.2). In clinical practice, viral replication detected in newborns during the first few days of life indicates in-utero replication. By contrast, peripartum infection is detected later, generally before the age of 3 months. In-utero infection is more frequently associated with a worse prognosis in children.[9,10]

ANTIRETROVIRAL PROPHYLAXIS DURING PREGNANCY

The use of antiretroviral drugs to prevent transmission has proved very effective: in optimal conditions the risk of transmission is almost zero.[1,4,11] In a recent nationwide analysis of residual transmission despite

Table 97.1 Global summary of the AIDS epidemic – December 2007

Number of people living with HIV in 2007	
Total	33.2 million (30.6–36.1 million)
Adults	30.8 million (28.2–33.6 million)
Women	15.4 million (13.9–16.6 million)
Children under 15 years	2.5 million (2.2–2.6 million)
People newly infected with HIV in 2007	
Total	2.5 million (1.8–4.1 million)
Adults	2.1 million (1.4–3.6 million)
Children under 15 years	420 000 (350 000–540 000)
AIDS deaths in 2007	
Total	2.1 million (1.9–2.4 million)
Adults	1.7 million (1.6–2.1 million)
Children under 15 years	330 000 (310 000–380 000)

The ranges around the estimates in this table define the boundaries within which the actual numbers lie, based on the best available information.

Table 97.2 Main risk factors for mother-to-child HIV-1 transmission

- Maternal viral load
- Low CD4+ cell count
- Prolonged delivery
- Chorioamnionitis
- Prematurity
- Breast-feeding

Table 97.3 Mother-to-child transmission in women receiving antiretroviral therapy

Maternal HIV-1 viral load at delivery (copies/ml)	n	% infected children
>10 000	440	6.8
1000–9999	938	1.5
400–999	440	0.7
<400	3256	0.6

From ANRS French perinatal cohort.[11]

highly active antiretroviral treatment during pregnancy and undetectable viral load at delivery, only 0.6% of children born at term were found to be infected[12] (Table 97.3). Risk factors for this residual contamination despite the full suppression of viral replication in the plasma at delivery remain to be identified. The duration of treatment and initial viral load may play a role but obstetric factors are no longer significant.[8]

The first step in prophylactic treatment is the screening of pregnant women for HIV infection at a sufficiently early stage of pregnancy. This is well managed in industrialized countries, but remains problematic in low-income countries, both for practical reasons (availability and performance of the test, collection of test results, delivery of results, the taking of appropriate therapeutic decisions in light of the results) and because such testing is not always accepted by women.[12] Potential stigmatization and the personal, familial and social consequences of testing for women are still major issues in many parts of the world.[13] Optimal prevention of transmission during pregnancy is currently based on antiretroviral therapy[14,15] (Table 97.4). Antiretroviral therapy is generally initiated at the start of the third trimester of pregnancy and continued until birth, with the aim of ensuring that maternal viral replication rates are kept below the detection threshold during the critical period for transmission to the child. If the mother is already receiving treatment or needs to be treated earlier during pregnancy, maternal treatment is continued or started without delay. During labor and until delivery, treatment is replaced by intravenous zidovudine infusion. Recent observational data have suggested that this peripartum phase of treatment may be omitted if viral replication in the mother is fully suppressed for at least a few weeks before delivery.

Alternative 'simplified' strategies have been developed for cases in which the reference treatment is not available or cannot be distributed in regions with limited access to health care.[15] These strategies – of shorter duration and inhibiting maternal viral replication less strongly – nonetheless appear to be relatively effective. Thus, the 2006 WHO recommendations for 'simplified' treatment involved zidovudine monotherapy combined with a single dose of nevirapine at birth. The transmission rate recorded with this therapy (not including the breast-feeding period) is of the order of 3–4%, versus around 20% without treatment. A single dose of nevirapine during labor alone halves the risk of transmission and remains widely used. This simple solution should, however, only be used when other options are not possible. In addition to being only moderately effective, treatment with a single dose of nevirapine favors the selection of maternal viruses resistant to this class of drug.[16] The co-administration of antiretroviral dual therapy (zidovudine–lamivudine or, more recently, tenofovir–emtricitabine) for several days after labor reduces this risk of resistance. There is no consensus on the optimal prophylactic treatment for HIV-2. An aggressive approach is certainly justified in both primary infection during pregnancy and advanced disease, both associated with a significant risk of transmission. Non-nucleoside inhibitors, such as nevirapine, have proved ineffective against HIV-2.

The dynamic nature of clinical research in this field leads to the frequent updating of these recommendations. Concerned readers are strongly encouraged to visit several dedicated sites easily accessible via the Internet.

Table 97.4 General principles for the prophylaxis of mother-to-child transmission (may vary according to national guidelines)

Prepartum

HIV-1-infected pregnant women currently receiving antiretroviral treatment

Continue the treatment if effective (plasma viral load undetectable). Avoid efavirenz if possible during the first trimester
Optimize the treatment if ineffective according to viral resistance genotype*

HIV-1-infected women who have never received antiretroviral drugs ('antiretroviral naive')

If criteria for antiretroviral (ARV) treatment initiation according to adult guidelines (clinical, immunologic, virologic) are met:
- Start without delay, as recommended for nonpregnant adults
- Select specific drug combination for pregnancy[†]
If no criteria for immediate treatment initiation, consider prophylaxis alone:
- Treatment with a combination of three drugs is preferred[‡]
- Start no later than 28 weeks

Peripartum

Zidovudine intravenous infusion during labor, until delivery[‡]
Elective Caesarian section only if uncontrolled viral replication in the plasma

Postpartum in children

Zidovudine for 4–6 weeks[‡]
Reinforced postnatal antiretroviral prophylaxis if maternal viral load uncontrolled or maternal treatment suboptimal
Bottle feeding whenever possible[§]

*If available.
[†]Main drugs selected for pregnancy (July 2008): **Nucleoside analogue**: zidovudine, lamivudine; **Protease inhibitor**: ritonavir-boosted lopinavir; **Non-nucleoside reverse transcriptase inhibitor**: nevirapine if CD4 cell count <250/mm³.
[‡]When impossible, simplified regimens are proposed (see[15]).
[§]When replacement feeding is acceptable, feasible, affordable, sustainable and safe. In other cases, consider extended ARV prophylaxis program during breast-feeding (either maternal ARV or postexposure prophylaxis in the infant).

THE RISK OF TRANSMISSION ASSOCIATED WITH BREAST-FEEDING

Eliminating the risk associated with breast-feeding is currently a major issue (see Mofenson[17] for a review). In industrialized countries, bottle feeding is advised, but the risk of nutritional infection associated with this type of feeding poses a major problem for most, but not all, children living in poor countries. According to WHO recommendations, bottle feeding should be suggested only where it can be offered at a reasonable price, for a feasible duration, with reasonable acceptance rates and with sufficient food safety and precautionary measures against infection. In all other cases, maternal breast-feeding is encouraged.

Several approaches to improving the safety of maternal breast-feeding are currently being implemented. The first involves the promotion of exclusive breast-feeding, given that mixed feeding methods increase the risk of child contamination.[18] Another approach exploits the efficacy of antiretroviral drugs, either for maternal antiretroviral treatment during breast-feeding, or for 'postexposure prophylactic' treatment of the child for the duration of breast-feeding. The preliminary findings for these two strategies are very encouraging, suggesting that it should be possible to manage the risk of transmission associated with breast-feeding effectively in the near future. The feasibility of, and tolerance of children to, this postnatal prophylactic treatment – whether given directly to the child or introduced through maternal milk – will nevertheless need to be carefully examined.

TOLERANCE OF ANTIRETROVIRAL PROPHYLAXIS IN FETUSES AND NEONATES

Fetuses and neonates generally have satisfactory tolerance to antiretroviral drugs. No evidence of teratogenesis has been found in humans.[19] Efavirenz causes neural tube defects in primates and its use in humans is contraindicated, except in cases for which no other feasible options are available. There is still some debate about the risk of prematurity associated with protease inhibitors.[20] Most recent analyses suggest that neither prematurity nor hypotrophy is linked to protease inhibitor use during pregnancy. However, current analyses are never stratified by drug and specific toxicity cannot be excluded.

The genotoxic potential of nucleoside analogues – including zidovudine, which is known to interact with both mitochondrial and nuclear DNA in humans[21,22] – merits particular attention. The main toxic effect of this molecule is reversible anemia, but the persistent inhibition of other hematopoietic lines until the age of 2 years has been observed in a number of cohorts. An impact of zidovudine on the mitochondria of treated children has been clearly demonstrated through transient biochemical abnormalities, concerning lactate concentrations, for example. A low risk of encephalopathy with persistent mitochondrial dysfunction has also been reported. A large study on cancer incidence after in-utero treatment with zidovudine alone or with lamivudine revealed no significant difference from expectations for the general population within 5 years of follow-up.[23] Tolerance to other nucleoside combinations must be evaluated. Fetal tolerance to other molecules of this class remains largely unknown, as does tolerance to new classes of drug (integrase inhibitors, fusion inhibitors).

INITIAL FOLLOW-UP OF NEWBORNS

Most children born to HIV-infected mothers are not infected by HIV, but careful management is required to optimize prevention and reduce the risk of infection further. Furthermore, the child and mother are often in a situation of social, psychological and administrative vulnerability, and may be in need of appropriate support.

All usual childcare activities can be carried out as normal. The potential benefit of an antiseptic bath with a virucidal solution has not been determined; any such act should be carried out very carefully because of the potential deleterious effects of breaks in the skin or mucous membranes in the presence of virus on these surfaces (including gastric membranes).

The continuation of prophylactic treatment must be considered, if possible, from the end of pregnancy, as the choice of treatment depends partly on the treatment already received by the mother. Treatment continued in the form of zidovudine alone is considered to be optimal in the case of maternal prophylactic treatment. Recommendations in industrialized countries suggest that this should be maintained for 4–6 weeks, but it is offered for 1 week in countries in which the full course of treatment cannot be administered. More aggressive treatment is required if the mother's treatment is considered insufficient because its duration is too short or because compliance is poor, or if there is a detectable viral load (where the test is available) before birth. There is currently no consensus recommendation concerning such intensification of treatment; it often involves triple antiretroviral therapy when such treated can be implemented, or is simplified to zidovudine for 4 weeks combined with a single dose of nevirapine when other options

are unavailable. The use of single-dose nevirapine, as for the mother, is associated with an increased risk of acquiring mutations conferring resistance to the molecule if prophylaxis fails, and this problem must be taken into account when selecting treatment.[15,16]

DIAGNOSIS IN CHILDREN AND USUAL POSTNATAL CARE

Maternal IgG antibodies cross the placenta, so the early diagnosis of infection requires a polymerase chain reaction (PCR)-based virus isolation test. PCR-based tests for DNA and those for RNA are both used and seem to give equivalent rates of diagnostic sensitivity and specificity when used for young children. These tests are ideally performed immediately after birth, but the number of infected children identified in the perinatal period is small, because most cases of contamination occur at the moment of delivery. Several weeks of viral replication are required before replication can be detected by standard methods, so screening for the virus is generally repeated at 1 and 3 months, and even at 6 months at certain centers. The sensitivity of PCR at 3 months in non-breast-fed children is close to 100%.[24] Negative serologic results at 18 months are often considered the end point in the testing process, although some centers stop follow-up after a negative PCR result at 6 months.

In cases of limited access to health care, the first PCR test is often carried out at 6 weeks, as a compromise between reducing costs and maintaining test sensitivity. In cases of breast-feeding, the risk of infection remains until weaning, and a diagnostic test (PCR before 18 months or serologic test after 18 months) must be carried out at least 4–6 after the end of breast-feeding for the valid interpretation of test results.[25] Any positive PCR result should lead to retesting without delay to confirm infection. Symptoms observed in the child may also contribute to diagnosis. Axillary adenopathy, splenomegaly and oral thrush in the first few months are highly suggestive of infection, although clearly not disease specific. A persistent cough, recurrent ENT (ear, nose and throat), skin and digestive infections, a state of malnutrition, neurologic hypertonia or hypotonia are indicative of already advanced disease. In areas in which access to PCR is restricted, a presumptive clinical diagnosis may be sufficient for the initiation of antiretroviral treatment in cases of suspected infection whilst awaiting confirmation by PCR-based diagnostic tests.

Vaccine schedules and the expanded immunization program (EIP) can be followed in each country as normal. The only vaccine posing a potential problem is bacille Calmette–Guérin (BCG), which persists in the long term, such that a subsequent vaccine disease is possible. Indeed, BCG vaccination is contraindicated for HIV-infected children in industrialized countries with a low incidence of tuberculosis. Elsewhere BCG vaccination is generally carried out in all HIV-exposed children, but recent WHO recommendations also advise against such vaccination in southern hemisphere countries in which infected children are diagnosed early.[26] Other live vaccines, such as measles–mumps–rubella (MMR) and yellow fever, do not pose the same problem of persistence and can be given normally, except to children at an advanced stage of HIV infection.

Early prevention of *Pneumocystis jirovecii* infection is offered from 1 month until 12–18 months to children exposed to HIV, while waiting for confirmation of noninfection (trimethoprim–sulfamethoxazole; 30 mg/kg sulfamethoxazole). When diagnostic procedures can easily be completed and PCR results obtained in real time, this systematic prophylaxis is offered to infected children only.

CHILDREN INFECTED WITH HIV

In the absence of antiretroviral treatment, disease progression differs between children in industrialized countries and those in countries with limited access to health care. Between 15% and 20% of infected children in Europe and North America have a risk of early and severe opportunistic infection and encephalopathy in the first 12–18 months of life.[27,28] Predictive factors for this rapid form of disease progression include the detection of in-utero viral contamination at birth, an advanced stage of illness in the mother during pregnancy and cytomegalovirus co-infection. In low-income countries, morbidity and early death rates, mostly due to infection, are much higher. In certain child cohorts from sub-Saharan Africa, the mortality rate is 50% in the first 2 years of life.[29–31] After this, disease progression tends to be slower, close to that observed in adults, although this has not been clearly demonstrated for African children.

The combination of symptoms observed in adults has also been described in children and detailed symptomatology in the WHO classification[28] (Table 97.5A). In addition to the specific risk of encephalopathy, two other complications are more frequently observed in children than in adults. The first is lymphoid interstitial pneumonia, leading to recurrent bacterial superinfections, the major clinical symptoms thus being those of the infections caused.[32] Unusual radiologic symptoms are also observed, reflecting an interstitial syndrome of variable intensity associated with mediastinal adenopathy. This can lead to the differential diagnosis of miliary tuberculosis (especially in cases of bacterial superinfection); however, the contrast between the major abnormalities observed on radiologic images and the mild symptoms can be used to exclude this diagnosis. The underlying pathophysiology remains unknown, but is often associated with bilateral parotitis, and the biologic signs include substantial CD8 hyperlymphocytosis. Co-infection may play a role and Epstein–Barr virus (EBV) has also been implicated. Bronchoalveolar lavage, when possible, reveals hyperlymphocytosis.

Another specific feature observed in children, contrasting with adults, is a higher frequency of leiomyoma or of leiomyosarcoma tumors in cases of severe immunodeficiency.[33] All organs may be affected. Here again, opportunistic EBV infection has been implicated in the pathophysiology. The proportion of children with non-progressive disease in the long term (between 10 and 15 years) has been determined in industrialized countries and found to be similar to that observed for infected adults. Predictive criteria for disease progression, in children as in adults, are CD4 levels and the viral load determined by quantitative PCR amplification of DNA. CD4 levels indicate the degree of immune deficiency and, thus, the risk of related short-term or mid-term complications.[30,34,35] The viral load indicates the rate of viral replication and probable rate of subsequent changes to the immune system. The interpretation of CD4 levels is more difficult than in adults, because of the physiologic hyperlymphocytosis observed in early life; normal adult levels are not reached until the age of 5–6 years. Counts expressed as the percentage of lymphocytes are less subject to variation and thus often preferred by pediatricians (Table 97.5B). CD4 counts are nevertheless poorly predictive during the first year of life, particularly for the prediction of early-onset severe forms of disease.

TREATMENT OF INFECTED CHILDREN

The prophylactic treatment of opportunistic or bacterial infections initially made a major contribution to reducing mortality rates in infected children. The preventive antibacterial efficacy of systematic administration of trimethoprim–sulfamethoxazole (TMP–SMX) has been demonstrated for all ages, starting as early as 1 month of age, leading to a significant decrease in mortality. It is recommended for all infected children in countries in which access to health care is limited.[36,37] Elsewhere, its prescription is more restricted: it is used either following recurrent bacterial infections despite a seemingly normal CD4 level or, more typically, following detection of CD4 lymphopenia. In countries with a high incidence of tuberculosis, the systematic prescription of isoniazid also reduces the mortality rate.[38] However, no recommendations have been established for this prophylactic treatment.

Table 97.5A WHO classification for HIV-1-infected children – clinical

Clinical stage 1

Asymptomatic
Persistent generalized lymphadenopathy

Clinical stage 2*

Unexplained persistent hepatosplenomegaly
Papular pruritic eruptions
Extensive wart virus infection
Extensive molluscum contagiosum
Recurrent oral ulcerations
Unexplained persistent parotid enlargement
Lineal gingival erythema
Herpes zoster
Recurrent or chronic upper respiratory tract infections (otitis media, otorrhea, sinusitis, tonsillitis)
Fungal nail infections

Clinical stage 3*

Unexplained moderate malnutrition not adequately responding to standard therapy
Unexplained persistent diarrhea (≥14 days)
Unexplained persistent fever (above 100°F/37.5°C, intermittent or constant, for >1 month)
Persistent oral candidiasis (after first 6 weeks of life)
Oral hairy leukoplakia
Acute necrotizing ulcerative gingivitis/periodontitis
Lymph node tuberculosis
Pulmonary tuberculosis
Severe recurrent bacterial pneumonia
Symptomatic lymphoid interstitial pneumonitis
Chronic HIV-associated lung disease including bronchiectasis
Unexplained anemia (<8.0 g/dl), neutropenia (<0.5 × 10^9/l^3) or chronic thrombocytopenia (<50 × 10^9/l^3)

Clinical stage 4*,†

Unexplained severe wasting, stunting or severe malnutrition not responding to standard therapy
Pneumocystis jirovecii pneumonia
Recurrent severe bacterial infections (e.g. empyema, pyomyositis, bone or joint infection, meningitis, but excluding pneumonia)
Chronic herpes simplex infection (orolabial or cutaneous for >1 month, or visceral at any site)
Extrapulmonary tuberculosis
Kaposi's sarcoma
Esophageal candidiasis (or *Candida* infection of trachea, bronchi or lungs)
Central nervous system toxoplasmosis (after the neonatal period)
HIV encephalopathy
Cytomegalovirus (CMV) infection, retinitis or CMV infection affecting another organ, with onset at age >1 month
Extrapulmonary cryptococcosis (including meningitis)
Disseminated endemic mycosis (extrapulmonary histoplasmosis, coccidioidomycosis)
Chronic cryptosporidiosis (with diarrhea)
Chronic isosporiasis
Disseminated non tuberculous mycobacterial infection
Cerebral or B-cell non-Hodgkin's lymphoma
Progressive multifocal leukoencephalopathy
HIV-associated cardiomyopathy or nephropathy

*Unexplained indicates that the condition is not explained by other causes.
†Some additional specific conditions may be induced in regional classifications (e.g. penicilliosis in Asia, HIV-associated rectovaginal fistula in Africa).

Table 97.5B WHO classification for HIV-1-infected children – immunologic

Classification of HIV-associated immunodeficiency	AGE-RELATED CD4 VALUES			
	≤11 months (%)	12–35 months (%)	36–59 months (%)	≥5 years (cells/mm³ and %)
Not significant	>35	>30	>25	>500
Mild	30–35	25–30	20–25	350–499
Advanced	25–29	20–24	15–19	200–349
Severe	<25	<20	<15	<200 or <15%

It is antiretroviral treatments, where available, that have changed the outlook for children infected with HIV by greatly decreasing morbidity and mortality rates.[35,39] The yearly mortality in an HIV-infected cohort of children in Europe and North America decreased from 7–10 per 100 patient-years in 1994 to less than 0.5 in 2006. Antiretroviral treatment leads to chronic, stable disease in these children, compatible with balanced and satisfactory development. The toxicity profile is globally similar to that observed in adults, but with a lower drug-induced morbidity rate, probably through lower co-morbidity (alcohol, tobacco, aging).[40,41] Compliance and adherence to the treatment regimen is critical and may require specifically tailored interventions, such as individual or group support.[42,43] The risk of AIDS has now been virtually eliminated in antiretroviral-treated children, at least in the medium term, with 10 years follow-up from the introduction of antiretroviral combination therapy. The main issues now concern the long-term prognosis for quality of life, particularly relating to the potentially deleterious effects of the virus and/or treatment on various organs, including the vascular endothelial and central nervous systems.

The general principles underlying antiretroviral treatment for children are the same as those for adults (Table 97.6; see also Chapter 100). In particular, viral replication should be decreased such that levels are stable and below the detection threshold – the only guarantee of long-term efficacy and prevention of the selection of resistance mutations. In infants over the age of 1 year, indications for treatment are based on CD4 levels. Before this age, most recommendations now suggest systematic treatment, given the difficulty of predicting early and severe forms of disease. However, it is still not possible to determine how long this early treatment should last. Recommendations concerning the choice of molecules and the threshold for starting treatment often change, and, therefore, the WHO guidelines and those of the health authorities in a number of countries should be consulted regularly. The first findings from poor countries are very encouraging, also showing marked decreases in mortality rates similar to those observed in more affluent countries. The main issue for the future, given the considerable number of children needing treatment, is the feasibility of implementing decentralized and long-term treatment programs on a wider scale in poor countries.[44,45]

Table 97.6 General principles of antiretroviral treatment for HIV-1 infected children

AGE-SPECIFIC RECOMMENDATIONS		
A: WHO classification (see Table 97.5A)		
Clinical stage	<12 months	>12 months
1	Treat all	CD4 guided*
2	Treat all	CD4 guided*
3	Treat all	Treat all
4	Treat all	Treat all

B: Age-specific CD4 threshold to initiate antiretroviral treatment for children >12 months			
CD4	12–35 months	36–59 months	>5 years
Percentage	<20%	<20%	<15%
Absolute number cells/mm³	<750	<350	<200

*See part B.
Adapted from WHO guidelines 2006, revised 2008. May vary according national guidelines.

REFERENCES

References for this chapter can be found online at http://www.expertconsult.com

Chapter | 98 |

Beverly E Sha
Constance A Benson

Special problems in women who have HIV disease

EPIDEMIOLOGY

The number and proportion of women who have HIV-1 infection in the USA have been gradually increasing. Of 39 002 persons reported to the Centers for Disease Control and Prevention (CDC) who had AIDS in 2006, 10 591 (27.2%) were women.[1] This contrasts with 1985 statistics, when 7% (534/8153) of people reported to the CDC who had AIDS were women. In 2004, HIV-1 infection was the fifth leading cause of death for white women aged 35–44 years, the leading cause of death for African-American women aged 25–34 years, and the fourth leading cause of death for Hispanic women aged 35–44 years. The racial distribution of women who were diagnosed with HIV/AIDS in 2006 was 65.2% African-American (56.2/100 000), 18% white (2.9/100 000) and 15.1% Hispanic (15.1/100 000).

Heterosexual transmission has surpassed intravenous drug use as the primary route for women acquiring HIV-1 infection in the USA. Current estimates are that 40 000 new infections occur annually in the USA, of which 30% are in women. Of newly infected women, estimates are that more than 80% acquired HIV-1 through heterosexual sex and less than 20% through intravenous drug use.

Worldwide 2007 UNAIDS estimates are that, of the 30.8 million adults living with HIV-1/AIDS, 15.4 million (50%) are women.[2] Of these, 68% live in sub-Saharan Africa. Nearly one (0.8%) in every 100 adults worldwide aged 15–49 years is HIV-1 infected. In sub-Saharan Africa, 5% of all adults in this age group are HIV-1 infected. More than 80% of all adults worldwide acquired HIV-1 infection via heterosexual intercourse.

TRANSMISSION

Factors that are important in male-to-female transmission of HIV-1 infection include:
- advanced disease in the infected source partner;
- plasma HIV-1 RNA level (and virus shedding in genital secretions);
- anal receptive intercourse;
- presence of genital ulcers;
- absence of condom use; and
- absence of zidovudine use.[3–6]

Factors associated with heterosexual female-to-male transmission of HIV-1 infection include:
- advanced disease in the infected source partner;
- plasma HIV-1 RNA level (and virus shedding in genital secretions);
- presence of genital ulcers;
- sexual intercourse during menses; and
- absence of condom use.

In developing countries, observational studies have also suggested an association of nonulcerative sexually transmitted diseases with increased rates of HIV-1 transmission. For women, *Candida* vaginitis, bacterial vaginosis and use of depot medroxyprogesterone acetate have been associated with an increased incidence of HIV-1 infection. The efficiency of male-to-female transmission of HIV-1 has been estimated to be twice that of female-to-male transmission, although some studies have found equal rates.[4,5] Suppression of herpes simplex virus (HSV)-2 infections in HIV-negative women did not decrease the risk of HIV acquisition.[8] Cellulose sulfate as a vaginal microbicide was ineffective, but women who applied 0.5% PRO 2000/5 Gel vaginally every day had a 30% lower rate of HIV acquisition (p =0.06).[8A]

CLINICAL FEATURES

Disease manifestations and progression

Overall, there are few differences in the incidence of nongynecologic opportunistic diseases between men and women who have HIV-1 infection, except for a higher incidence of esophageal candidiasis as an AIDS-defining condition and a lower incidence of Kaposi's sarcoma in women.[9] It is speculated that the higher incidence of candidiasis in women might be due to vaginal colonization with yeast or perhaps hormonal influences.

Several studies have now demonstrated that women have lower plasma HIV-1 RNA levels than do men after controlling for age, the interval from seroconversion and the CD4+ lymphocyte count.[10] Another study found that this sex difference in plasma HIV-1 RNA levels disappeared 5–6 years after seroconversion. Although women may progress to AIDS with lower viral loads, the time to progression to AIDS appears to be similar for men and women. Similarly, for HIV-1-infected men and women who have adequate access to health care and treatment, treatment response and survival appears to be equivalent.[11,12]

Gynecologic manifestations

Infection

Gynecologic disorders are common in women who have HIV-1 infection.[13] Up to 50% of HIV-1-infected women develop recurrent *Candida* vaginitis, which often precedes the development of oral or esophageal candidiasis. Several longitudinal cohorts have reported that 14–18% of women who have HIV-1 infection have or develop recurrent genital HSV infection, which can be more severe or refractory to treatment than among HIV-1 seronegative women.[12]

The relationship between HIV-1 and pelvic inflammatory disease (PID) in women is less clear. Several retrospective studies suggest that women presenting with PID have a high rate of co-infection with HIV-1 and that women who have HIV-1 infection with PID require surgical intervention more frequently because of abscess formation.[14] Prospective studies will be necessary to define this relationship and determine whether there are differences in response to therapy, microbiologic etiology and risk of recurrence or long-term sequelae.

Genital dysplasia

Cervicovaginal dysplasia is common in women who have HIV-1 infection.[13,15] Abnormal Papanicolaou smears were found in 38.3% of 1713 HIV-1-infected women and 16.2% of 482 women uninfected with HIV-1 but at risk, in the Women's Interagency HIV-1 Study cohort.[15] In multivariate analyses, risk factors for abnormal cytology included HIV-1 infection, low CD4+ lymphocyte counts, high plasma HIV-1 RNA levels and detection of human papillomavirus (HPV). In follow-up of this cohort, HPV detection, CD4+ lymphocyte count and plasma HIV-1 RNA levels predicted regression.[16] Rates of incidence, progression and regression of abnormal cytology did not differ between the HIV-1-uninfected controls and HIV-1-infected women with CD4+ lymphocyte counts >200 cells/mm³ and plasma HIV-1 RNA levels below 4000 copies/ml. In another study, 20% (80/398) of HIV-1-seropositive women compared with 4% (15/357) of HIV-1-seronegative women had cervical intraepithelial neoplasia (CIN) confirmed by colposcopy.[17] The presence of CIN was found to be independently associated with:

- HPV infection (odds ratio 9.8);
- HIV-1 infection (odds ratio 3.5);
- CD4+ lymphocyte count <200/mm³ (odds ratio 2.7); and
- age greater than 34 years (odds ratio 2.0).

The rate of CIN in women who have HIV-1 infection with <200 CD4+ lymphocytes/mm³ was 28% (27/95) compared with 19% (45/236) for those with higher CD4+ lymphocyte counts.

Conflicting data exist regarding whether CIN and invasive cervical cancer have a more aggressive course or a less favorable response to therapy among women who have HIV-1 infection. In one study prior to the availability of highly active antiretroviral therapy (HAART), 62% of 127 women who had HIV-1 infection with CIN developed recurrent CIN within 36 months of treatment compared with 18% of HIV-1-seronegative controls.[18] During the 36-month follow-up period, progression to higher grade dysplasia, including one invasive cancer, occurred in 25% of women who had HIV-1 infection compared with 2% of controls. Recently, HIV-1-infected women in New York were reported to be at higher risk than HIV-1-seronegative women for other HPV-associated malignancies, including vulvar and anal cancers. HAART that reverses immunosuppression is likely to impact favorably on the rate of HPV detection and prevalence of genital tract and anal dysplasia. Indeed, more recent studies have found a lower prevalence of CIN II and III and HPV DNA positivity among women treated with HAART.[19,20] A new quadrivalent HPV vaccine approved for HIV-uninfected females 9–26 years of age has been shown to reduce the risk of high-grade dysplasia, CIN and cervical cancer. Whether the same degree of protection will be observed among HIV-1-infected women has yet to be determined.

The 2006 Consensus Guidelines for the management of women who have cervical cytologic abnormalities are detailed in Table 98.1.[21] These guidelines now state that immunosuppressed women should be managed as per guidelines for the general population of women. These Consensus Guidelines reflect updated terminology for reporting cervical cytology results, recent availability of HPV DNA testing and further follow-up data on the natural history of atypical squamous cells of undetermined significance/low-grade squamous intraepithelial lesions.[22]

Because *Candida* vaginitis, genital HSV disease, PID and cervical dysplasia are common in women who have HIV-1 infection, these conditions, along with other common sexually transmitted diseases such as gonorrhea, chlamydial infection and syphilis, should prompt a determination of HIV-1 risk factors and appropriate HIV-1 screening as part of routine care for women.

Table 98.1 Guidelines* for cervical cancer screening of women with HIV-1 infection

Initial gynecologic examination with Papanicolaou smear	If normal, repeat in 6 months If atypical squamous cells of uncertain significance (ASCUS), three options exist for women >20 years: • repeat Pap smear at 6 and 12 months; if abnormal proceed to colposcopy • colposcopy • HPV (high-risk types) DNA testing; if positive proceed to colposcopy If atypical squamous cells cannot rule out high-grade SIL (ASC-H), proceed to colposcopy If low-grade SIL, proceed to colposcopy If high-grade SIL, immediate loop electrosurgical excision or proceed to colposcopy If atypical glandular cells (AGC), proceed to colposcopy
If initial two Papanicolaou smears are normal	Repeat annually as long as Pap smears remain normal

*Based on the 2006 Consensus Guidelines and the United States Public Health Service Guidelines.[21,22]
SIL, squamous intraepithelial lesion.

Menstrual cycle and menopause

The impact of HIV-1 infection on the menstrual cycle appears to be limited. Reports of increased rates of dysmenorrhea, oligomenorrhea, amenorrhea or menorrhagia exist, but these have been discounted by other studies.[23] A combined analysis from the Women's Interagency HIV Study (WIHS) and the Heart and Estrogen/progestin Replacement Study (HERS) with 802 HIV-infected women and 273 high-risk seronegative women found little relationship between HIV status and amenorrhea, menstural cycle length or variability.[24]

Limited data exist on the effect of HIV infection on menopause. Some studies have suggested a slightly earlier onset of menopause among HIV-infected women (46 years vs 47 years) but this may be more related to other factors known to predict earlier onset of menopause such as substance use, tobacco smoking, low relative body weight, low socioeconomic status, depression and African-American ethnicity.

PREVENTION

Contraception

Condoms are important for preventing the transmission of HIV-1 and other sexually transmitted diseases. However, alone they may not be adequate to prevent pregnancy. Reported breakage rates for male condoms are less than 2% for vaginal and anal intercourse. An evaluation of the effectiveness of the female condom at preventing pregnancy in 147 women over a 6-month period demonstrated an annual failure rate of 26%. Among 86 women who reported using the condom consistently and correctly, the annual failure rate was still 11%.[25]

Hormonal contraceptives should be considered in addition to condoms for women who have HIV-1 infection, are sexually active and wish to avoid pregnancy. In view of the wide array of potential drugs available for antiretroviral therapy and prevention and treatment

Table 98.2 Drug interactions between antiretrovirals and oral contraceptives and recommended adjustments

Agent	Effect on oral contraceptive	RECOMMENDATION		
		No dose adjustment	No data	Use alternative agent or second method
Indinavir	Norethindrone levels ↑26% Ethinylestradiol levels ↑24%	X		
Ritonavir	Ethinylestradiol levels ↓40%			X
Saquinavir			X	
Nelfinavir	Norethindrone levels ↓18% Ethinylestradiol levels ↓47%			X
Fosamprenavir	↑ in ethinylestradiol with APV ↑ in norethindrone with APV APV levels ↓20%			X
Lopinavir	Ethinylestradiol levels ↓42%			X
Atazanavir	Ethinylestradiol AUC ↑48% Norethindrone AUC ↑110%			Use lowest dose
Tipranavir	Ethinylestradiol C_{max} and AUC ↓50%			X
Darunavir	Potential for interaction from ritonavir			X
Nevirapine	Ethinylestradiol levels ↓20%			X
Delavirdine	Ethinylestradiol levels may ↑		X	
Efavirenz	Ethinylestradiol levels ↑37% No data on norethindrone levels			X
Etravirine	Ethinylestradiol AUC ↑22%	X		
Maraviroc	No significant interaction	X		
Raltegravir	No significant interaction	X		

APV, amprenavir; AUC, area under the curve.
Data from Panel on Antiretroviral Guidelines for Adult and Adolescents.[26]

of opportunistic infections, the medications of women receiving hormonal agents should be critically reviewed to avoid drug–drug interactions such as:

- those that might lead to a reduction in the efficacy of hormonal agents; and
- those that may reduce the efficacy or increase the toxicity of other drugs in the presence of hormonal agents.

In particular, protease inhibitors and non-nucleoside reverse transcriptase inhibitors (NNRTIs) can affect the levels of hormonal agents. Table 98.2 details these interactions and recommendations for their concomitant use.[26]

Pregnancy

In the USA, in 1993, the rate of HIV-1 infection among women of child-bearing age was 1.7 per 1000 and there were between 1000 and 2000 perinatally infected infants born to 6000–7000 HIV-1-infected women. UNAIDS estimates for 2007 are that, worldwide, 330 000 children under 15 years of age died in 2007, and another 2.5 million children are currently living with HIV-1/AIDS, of whom 420 000 were infected in 2007.[2]

Perinatal transmission can occur in utero and during labor and delivery, as well as postpartum, primarily through breast-feeding.[27,28] Excluding postpartum transmission through breast-feeding, data suggest that 80% of maternal–infant transmission occurs late in gestation or during labor

and delivery.[29] Several studies have found that breast-feeding increases the rate of transmission by 16% over 2 years and thus breast-feeding is not recommended when safe alternatives are available.[28] The majority of infections transmitted through breast milk occur during the first few weeks or months of life.[30] Extending prophylaxis with nevirapine ± zidovudine for the first 14 weeks of life was shown to significantly reduce postnatal HIV-1 infection in 9-month-old infants.[30A] Risk factors associated with transmission via breast-feeding include level of virus in the breast milk, mastitis, breast abscesses, maternal seroconversion during lactation, duration of feeding and mixed feeding.

A number of maternal and delivery factors appear to influence the risk of transmission and are listed in Table 98.3.[27,31] In addition, the rate of maternal–infant transmission has been reported to be increased when maternal virus exhibits rapid or high titer replication in human peripheral blood mononuclear cells, T-cell line tropism or resistance to neutralization by maternal serum. Interventions currently recommended to reduce transmission include:

- avoidance of invasive monitoring whenever possible;
- avoidance of breast-feeding;
- the use of zidovudine with or without other antiretroviral therapy during pregnancy for the mother and in the peripartum and postpartum period for the infant;
- treatment of sexually transmitted disease or vaginitis; and
- elective Caesarian section if plasma HIV-1 RNA level remains above 1000 copies/ml near term.

Table 98.3 Maternal, labor and delivery factors that increase the risk of maternal–infant transmission

Maternal factors	Labor and delivery factors
Advanced maternal HIV disease	Chorioamnionitis
Maternal p24 antigenemia	Prolonged rupture of membranes
Low maternal CD4$^+$ lymphocyte	(>4 hours)
counts	Premature delivery before
High maternal plasma HIV-1 RNA	34 weeks' gestation
levels	Use of fetal scalp electrodes
Acute maternal HIV infection	Episiotomy with severe lacerations
during pregnancy	Non-elective Caesarian section
Genital inflammation or	delivery
maternal sexually transmitted	
disease at the time of delivery	
Detectable genital tract HIV-1	
RNA near delivery	
Lack of antiretroviral therapy	
Breastfeeding	

Antiretroviral therapy to prevent perinatal transmission

The landmark AIDS Clinical Trials Group (ACTG) 076 trial demonstrated a 66% reduction in maternal–infant HIV-1 transmission with zidovudine use in the mother during pregnancy, labor and delivery, and in the baby for the first 6 weeks of life (7.6% zidovudine vs 22.6% placebo). Since that study was reported, advances have occurred in our understanding of the pathogenesis of HIV-1 disease and its treatment and management.[32] The precise mechanisms by which zidovudine diminishes maternal–infant transmission of HIV-1 remain unclear but probably include:

- decreased maternal plasma HIV-1 RNA levels;
- decreased exposure of the fetus to the virus in utero; and/or
- decreased HIV exposure of the infant at delivery or in the neonatal period.

The end result is prevention of infection from becoming established in the fetus or infant. Additional analyses have now shown that transmission of HIV-1 occurs at all levels of CD4$^+$ lymphocyte counts and even in some women who have undetectable plasma HIV-1 RNA levels, although overall the risk of transmission is greater in women who have lower CD4$^+$ lymphocyte counts and higher plasma HIV-1 RNA levels, particularly at the time of delivery.[33] Detectable virus in the female genital tract at 38 weeks gestation has also been independently associated with maternal–infant transmission of HIV-1.[34]

It is important to stress that even intervening late in pregnancy (including initiating therapy in the peripartum period) can diminish the risk of transmission.[35-37] In developing countries, a two-dose nevirapine regimen (oral nevirapine, 200 mg as a single dose given to the mother at the onset of labor and oral nevirapine 2 mg/kg given to the infant within 72 hours of birth) is widely used based on a randomized comparison that demonstrated the two-dose nevirapine regimen reduced the risk of maternal–infant transmission by 47% compared with a truncated zidovudine regimen.[38] Follow-up data from this study, however, documented the occurrence of K103N mutations in virus recovered from up to 15% of women who were randomized to nevirapine, a mutation conferring cross-class resistance to NNRTIs (with the exception of etravirine).[39] Fortunately, later data have shown that this resistance has not affected subsequent perinatal transmission rates when nevirapine is again used as the mode for prevention. The predominant circulating strain of virus generally reverts to wild-type once nevirapine is cleared. More concerning is that women randomized to receive nevirapine + tenofovir–emtricitabine for treatment of their HIV 6 or more months after receiving single-dose nevirapine for prevention of maternal–infant

HIV transmission did worse than women randomized to lopinavir–ritonavir + tenofovir–emtricitabine.[39A] After a median follow-up of 73 weeks, 26% of women receiving nevirapine developed virologic failure or death compared with 8% in the lopinavir arm. Similarly, response to nevirapine-based treatment regimens have not been compromised if initiated 6–12 months postexposure to single-dose nevirapine, although the durability of the response longer term compared with other regimens that do not contain NNRTIs remains to be established in ongoing clinical trials.[40]

All pregnant women should be offered HIV-1 testing. Repeat HIV antibody testing is now recommended in the third trimester (preferably before 36 weeks gestation) for women at high-risk of acquiring HIV infection who have negative tests earlier in their pregnancy. Women who present to labor and delivery without prior HIV testing should be offered a rapid HIV test to guide decisions. In general, current recommendations are to approach the treatment of the HIV-1-infected pregnant woman as if she were not pregnant and strive for maximal suppression of viral replication. Nevertheless, knowledge that limited data exist regarding toxicity of the 23 Food and Drug Administration (FDA)-approved antiretroviral agents to the developing fetus and the infant must also be taken into account. Tables 98.4–98.7 summarize the current information known about reverse transcriptase inhibitors, protease inhibitors, entry inhibitors and integrase inhibitors with regard to FDA approval status, placental transfer and carcinogenicity data.

To date, neither pre-term delivery nor birth defects have been clearly associated with any antiretroviral agent; however, data are limited, particularly for infants exposed to combination therapy. Only efavirenz is listed as a class D drug based on four retrospective case reports of neural tube defects (n = 3) and a case of Dandy–Walker malformation (n=1). As of 1/31/07, the prospective Antiretroviral Pregnancy Registry reported seven birth defects in 281 women with first trimester efavirenz exposure.[41] This 2.5% prevalence rate falls within the expected rate of 3.0/100 live births and no neural tube defects were reported. Currently, efavirenz should be avoided in the first trimester, because of evidence of teratogenicity in rhesus macaques at human doses.

From September 2007 through March 2008, nelfinavir was not recommended for pregnant women or women who might become pregnant due to the presence of low levels of ethyl methane sulfonate (EMS) in nelfinavir. EMS is a process-related impurity that is known to be teratogenic, mutagenic and carcinogenic in animals. The manufacturing process has been modified and nelfinavir is again safe to use in women and children. The Women's and Infants Transmission Study (WITS) found an increased rate of hypospadias only in first trimester zidovudine-exposed boys but not in the rate of hypospadias among zidovudine-exposed boys overall. A French group reported 12 cases of mitochondrial dysfunction among 2644 uninfected infants who received zidovudine or the combination of zidovudine and lamivudine in utero and/or after birth. Two of these children developed progressive neurologic dysfunction and died. This syndrome has not been detected in over 20 000 children born to HIV-1-infected women in the USA.

On the basis of this information, the US Public Health Service (USPHS) has drafted the following guidelines for the treatment of HIV-1-infected pregnant women.[42]

If the woman has had no prior antiretroviral therapy, treatment should be based on standard indications. However, at a minimum, the three-part zidovudine regimen as outlined in ACTG 076 should be administered. In a meta-analysis, antenatal antiretroviral prophylaxis primarily with zidovudine alone was shown to reduce transmission for women who have plasma HIV-1 RNA levels below 1000 copies/ml at or near delivery compared with no antenatal therapy (1% vs 9.8%, respectively).[43] Most experts feel comfortable substituting zidovudine 300 mg q12 h orally for the maternal component. Combination therapy is recommended for women who have a plasma HIV-1 RNA level over 1000 copies/ml. Consideration can be given to delaying the initiation of therapy until after 10–12 weeks gestation, which is thought to be the critical time for fetal organogenesis.

If the HIV-1-infected pregnant woman is already receiving antiretroviral therapy when pregnancy is diagnosed, then therapy is generally continued, even in the first trimester. Although not recommended

Table 98.4 Reverse transcriptase inhibitors

Agent	Studies showing transmission to fetus prevented	FDA APPROVED		FDA pregnancy category*	Placental transfer (%)
		Neonates	Children		
Zidovudine	Yes	Yes	Yes	C	80
Didanosine	No	Yes	Yes	B	50
Lamivudine	Yes	Yes	≥3 months	C	100
Stavudine	No	Yes	≥1 month	C	80 (rhesus monkeys)
Abacavir	No	No	≥3 months	C	Yes (rats)
Emtricitabine	Yes	No	≥3 months	B	40 (mice)
Tenofovir	No	No	≥18 years	B	95
Nevirapine	Yes	Yes	≥2 months	C	100
Delavirdine	No	No	No	C	?
Efavirenz	No	No	≥3 years	C	100 (rhesus monkeys)
Etravirine	Yes	No	≥18 years	B	?

*FDA pregnancy categories:
A Adequate and well-controlled studies of pregnant women fail to demonstrate a risk to the fetus during the first trimester and no evidence of risk during later trimesters.
B Animal studies fail to demonstrate a risk to the fetus but no adequate studies exist in pregnant women.
C Animal studies demonstrate risk or have not been conducted and safety in human pregnancy has not yet been determined. However, the benefit of the drug may still outweigh the risk.
D Positive evidence of human fetal risk exists based on adverse reaction data but benefits may still outweigh the risks.
Data from Panel on Antiretroviral Guidelines for Adult and Adolescents[26] and from Guidelines for the Use of Antiviral Agents in Pediatric HIV Infection.[26A]

Table 98.5 Protease inhibitors

Agent	Studies showing transmission to fetus prevented	FDA APPROVED		FDA pregnancy category*	Placental transfer
		Neonates	Children		
Nelfinavir	No	No	≥2 years	B	Minimal
Indinavir	No	No	≥18 years	C	Minimal
Ritonavir	No	No	>1 month	B	Minimal
Saquinavir	No	No	≥16 years	B	Minimal
Fosamprenavir	No	No	≥2 years	C	?
Lopinavir/ritonavir	No	≥14 days	Yes	C	20%
Atazanavir	No	No	≥6 years	C	10%
Tipranavir	No	No	≥2 years	C	?
Darunavir	No	No	≥3 years	B	?

*FDA pregnancy categories – see Table 98.4.
Data from Panel on Antiretroviral Guidelines for Adult and Adolescents[26]and from Guidelines for the Use of Antiviral Agents in Pediatric HIV Infection.[26A]

Table 98.6 Entry inhibitors (FDA approved)

Agent	Studies showing transmission to fetus prevented	Neonates	Children	FDA pregnancy category*	Placental transfer
Enfuvirtide	No	No	≥6 years	B	None
Maraviroc	No	No	≥16 years	B	?

*FDA pregnancy categories – see Table 98.4.
Data from Panel on Antiretroviral Guidelines for Adult and Adolescents[26]and from Guidelines for the Use of Antiviral Agents in Pediatric HIV Infection.[26A]

Table 98.7 Integrase inhibitors (FDA approved)

Agent	Studies showing transmission to fetus prevented	Neonates	Children	FDA pregnancy category*	Placental transfer
Raltegravir	No	No	≥16 years	C	Y (rats)

*FDA pregnancy categories – see Table 98.4.
Data from Panel on Antiretroviral Guidelines for Adult and Adolescents[26] and from Guidelines for the Use of Antiviral Agents in Pediatric HIV Infection.[26A]

(particularly for women with CD4$^+$ lymphocyte counts <200 cells/μl), if the decision is made to stop therapy during the first trimester owing to concerns about teratogenicity, all drugs should be stopped and then restarted simultaneously in order to minimize the development of resistance. Women on efavirenz should stop their antiretroviral therapy until past the first trimester and then restart a new regimen.

Zidovudine should be incorporated into the regimen whenever feasible; however, if resistance or intolerance precludes its use, zidovudine should still be administered intravenously intrapartum and to the baby as outlined above. Additionally, zidovudine and stavudine should not be co-administered. Some experts would also recommend zidovudine in combination with other antiretroviral agents for infants born to mothers who have known or suspected zidovudine resistance.

For women receiving standard antenatal antiretroviral therapy, the addition of the two-dose nevirapine regimen did not further reduce transmission rates and, as previously discussed, resulted in the development of mutations conferring resistance to NNRTIs.[44,45] Thus, for women who do not achieve adequate viral suppression near delivery, Caesarian section is recommended without the addition of the two-dose nevirapine regimen.

If an HIV-1-infected woman presents in labor and no prior antiretroviral therapy has been given, two antiretroviral treatment options are recommended:

- intrapartum intravenous zidovudine until delivery, and zidovudine to the newborn for 6 weeks; or
- the two-dose nevirapine regimen combined with intrapartum intravenous zidovudine and 6 weeks of zidovudine for the newborn.

If nevirapine is administered, consider adding lamivudine to zidovudine intrapartum or soon therafter for 7 days to limit the development of resistance to nevirapine. This is the preferred option at our institutions. Results from a recent study completed in pregnant women in South Africa indicated that this strategy reduced the frequency of nevirapine resistance compared with the two-dose nevirapine regimen without lamivudine and zidovudine.[46] Another study added a single dose of tenofovir and emtricitabine at delivery to nevirapine and found that this approach decreased resistance to nevirapine by 53% 6 weeks after delivery.[47]

Infants born to HIV-1-infected mothers who have received no antiretroviral therapy during pregnancy or intrapartum should still receive zidovudine for the first 6 weeks of life. Consideration may also be given to treating the infant with additional antiretroviral medications. The mother's therapy should be re-evaluated after delivery in both these situations.

Resistance testing is available to guide antiretroviral therapy choices. The International AIDS Society–USA Panel and EuroGuidelines Group for HIV-1 Resistance recommend that all pregnant women who have detectable viremia have resistance testing performed prior to initiating or changing antiretroviral therapy. The USPHS recommends resistance testing for HIV-1-infected pregnant women prior to initiating therapy and for those entering pregnancy with a detectable HIV-1 RNA level while on therapy. While underlying resistance can affect the ability to achieve maximal viral suppression, it is not clear that the presence of mutations increases the likelihood of transmission to the infant. Resistant virus has been transmitted to infants; however, women who have zidovudine resistance mutations have not consistently transmitted infection to their infants at higher rates and, in some cases where transmission has occurred, wild-type virus was transmitted. When less than potent antiretroviral regimens (zidovudine monotherapy or dual nucleoside analogues) are administered to pregnant HIV-1-infected women because antiretroviral therapy is not indicated for the women themselves or women choose to minimize exposure to antiretroviral therapy during pregnancy, development of resistance can occur and can potentially limit future treatment options.

A meta-analysis of 15 prospective cohort studies, conducted in an era when pregnant HIV-1-infected women received no antiretroviral therapy or zidovudine monotherapy, showed that elective Caesarian section decreased the risk of maternal–infant transmission of HIV-1 compared with other modes of delivery.[48] For women on zidovudine, transmission was 2% with elective Caesarian section and 7.3% with other modes of delivery. Because transmission rates are expected to be below 2% for women on potent antiretroviral therapy with controlled viremia, the American College of Obstetricians and Gynecologists' Committee on Obstetric Practice recommends Caesarian section before the onset of labor for women who have plasma HIV-1 RNA levels above 1000 copies/ml near term. The Caesarian section should be performed at 38 weeks gestation without amniocentesis to assess for fetal lung maturity. For a scheduled Caesarian section, intravenous zidovudine should be started 3 hours before surgery. Caesarian section has greater morbidity than vaginal delivery but current data suggest that HIV-1-infected women have similar complications to those in uninfected women except for those with advanced disease where the complication rates are higher.

Duration of ruptured membranes is also associated with an increased risk of transmission. A meta-analysis of the same 15 studies used to assess the benefit of Caesarian section showed, for the first 24 hours after membrane rupture, a 2% increase in transmission for every additional hour of membrane rupture.[49] Cleansing the birth canal with a 0.25% chlorhexidine solution every 4 hours until delivery did not reduce transmission in one study, except when membranes were ruptured more than 4 hours before delivery.[50] Whether or not nonelective Caesarian section to shorten the duration of ruptured membranes or labor will further reduce transmission rates is currently unknown.

Safety monitoring guided by the pregnant woman's specific antiretroviral therapy should be performed. Routine hematologic and hepatic enzyme monitoring is recommended for women on zidovudine. Liver function should be monitored in all women receiving antiretroviral therapy. Women receiving nucleoside reverse transcriptase inhibitors (NRTIs) should also be assessed for development of lactic acidosis and hepatic steatosis with frequent liver enzyme and electrolyte monitoring in the third trimester. Cases of fatal lactic acidosis have been reported in pregnant women receiving prolonged courses of didanosine and stavudine. When other alternatives are available, this combination should be avoided during pregnancy. Women initiating nevirapine should have frequent monitoring of transaminase levels due to the risk of hepatotoxicty that can occur within the first 18 weeks. Standard glucose tolerance testing is recommended at 24–28 weeks gestation. Some experts recommend earlier testing for women on chronic protease inhibitor therapy begun prior to pregnancy. In general, the plasma HIV-1 RNA level should be monitored 2–6 weeks after initiating or changing antiretroviral therapy, monthly until undetectable and then every 2 months until delivery. The CD4$^+$ lymphocyte count should be monitored every 3 months. A plasma HIV-1 RNA level should be obtained at 34–36 weeks gestation to guide decisions on mode of delivery. A first trimester ultrasound is recommended to guide dates. A second trimester, level II ultrasound is recommended to assess the fetus for women on combination antiretroviral therapy.

In the future, ongoing or planned studies will certainly provide more information regarding the use of the newer reverse transcriptase inhibitors, protease inhibitors, entry inhibitors, integrase inhibitors and combination regimens for the treatment of pregnant women and the prevention of transmission to the fetus/infant. In the meantime, HIV-1-infected pregnant women should be referred for participation in clinical trials whenever possible and be reported to the appropriate agencies that collect safety and teratogenicity data. In the USA, the Antiretroviral Pregnancy Registry can be reached at http://www.apregistry.com.

In general, pregnant women who have HIV-1 infection should receive prophylaxis for opportunistic infections appropriate for their stage of disease.[22] For *Pneumocystis jirovecii* pneumonia prophylaxis, some experts recommend avoiding trimethoprim–sulfamethoxazole and dapsone in the first trimester, and trimethoprim–sulfamethoxazole close to term to reduce the risk of kernicterus in the infant. Aerosolized pentamidine can be substituted during these time periods. While rifabutin and the macrolides have not been studied in pregnant women, those at high risk of disseminated *Mycobacterium avium* complex disease may benefit from the use of these medications after the first trimester. Azithromycin is favored owing to its safety profile because clarithromycin is teratogenic in animals. Pregnant women who have a positive purified protein derivative skin test for tuberculosis should also receive isoniazid prophylaxis after the first trimester. Pregnant women should also avoid eating raw or undercooked meat and avoid contact with cat feces to diminish the risk of toxoplasmosis. Good handwashing techniques should be employed for prevention of cytomegalovirus (CMV) disease, particularly in women who are health-care workers or who have children in day-care settings.[22] For CMV-seronegative women who require blood transfusions, only CMV-seronegative blood products should be used.[22]

Several studies have now demonstrated no adverse effect of pregnancy on the progression of HIV-1 disease for women who have CD4+ lymphocyte counts >200 cells/μl.[51] Unfortunately, women who have more advanced HIV-1 disease may not tolerate pregnancy as well and may have a higher rate of spontaneous abortion, prematurity, low birth weight infants and other complications of pregnancy.[52]

REFERENCES

 References for this chapter can be found online at http://www.expertconsult.com

Mark W Hull
Marianne Harris
Julio SG Montaner

Chapter | **99** |

Principles of management of HIV in the developed world

INTRODUCTION

The management of HIV infection continues to evolve as a result of a better understanding of HIV pathogenesis and with the emergence of new drugs, treatment strategies and laboratory monitoring tools. Antiretroviral therapy has advanced considerably since the first introduction of highly active antiretroviral therapy (HAART).[1,2] Regimens have become simpler, better tolerated and safer.[3] HAART-related immune reconstitution reliably prevents AIDS-related morbidity and mortality and furthermore allows discontinuation of primary and secondary prophylaxis for AIDS-related opportunistic infections in some settings.[4,5] Life expectancy of HIV-infected individuals in the modern HAART era is now measured in decades.[6,7] Improved longevity has been associated with the emergence of new challenges, including newly recognized adverse effects of long-term exposure to antiretroviral drugs. These include disorders of fat accumulation and fat wasting (lipodystrophy), dyslipidemias and glucose intolerance, hypertension, osteoporosis and increased risk of myocardial infarction.[8,9] Treatment interruptions, once considered a possible means of mitigating adverse events, have now been shown to be associated with increased morbidity and mortality.[10]

Management strategies now focus on preparing patients for initiation of antiretroviral therapy, and for long-term use of HAART with its possible concomitant metabolic effects. Patients who do not yet meet criteria for starting antiretroviral therapy must be protected from other infectious diseases by vaccination or prophylaxis when appropriate, and must be followed closely from a laboratory perspective to determine the optimal time of intervention with antiretroviral therapy.

Traditionally, the CD4+ lymphocyte (CD4 cell) count has been regarded as the key surrogate marker for prognostic staging and therapeutic monitoring of HIV-infected individuals. CD4+ lymphocyte loss is linked to the rate of HIV viral turnover, and the interaction between the quantifiable plasma HIV RNA level (i.e. the HIV viral load) and CD4+ lymphocyte production will ultimately determine CD4 cell loss.[11,12]

BASELINE EVALUATION OF THE HIV-INFECTED INDIVIDUAL

History and physical examination

The history should elicit the date of diagnosis and, if available, information regarding prior negative tests in order to estimate the length of time since infection. Symptoms related to progression of HIV infection and manifestations of opportunistic infections should be explored. For patients who had previously received antiretroviral therapy, detailed information regarding CD4 cell nadir, prior drug regimens, adherence, CD4 and viral load response and adverse effects should be documented. In addition, details regarding co-morbidities and concomitant medication should be well documented. A detailed history of drug and environmental allergies should be elicited.

Personal lifestyle, history of prior sexually transmitted diseases, safer sex, harm-reduction practices and reproductive history and expectations should be discussed in detail. Prior immunizations should be documented.

The physical examination should focus on clinical manifestations of HIV disease and those of AIDS-related opportunistic infections or malignancies. The oropharynx and dermis should be closely examined, and in patients with more advanced disease (CD4 cell count <50 cells/mm³) it may be necessary to arrange proper ophthalmologic assessment with a slit-lamp examination to rule out cytomegalovirus (CMV) retinitis. In female patients, Papanicolaou (Pap) testing should be performed to assess for cervical dysplasia.

General laboratory tests are also very important, particularly before the start of a treatment program. These should include those listed in Table 99.1. Abnormalities of the complete blood count are common, and updated serologic testing for co-infections such as hepatitis B and C and toxoplasmosis is required.

Prognostic laboratory markers

The CD4 cell count and plasma HIV viral load are the key prognostic markers for disease progression to AIDS or death among untreated HIV-infected individuals. These remain the essential components of laboratory monitoring. The initiation of antiretroviral therapy depends primarily on the CD4 cell count and to a lesser extent on the plasma HIV viral load among asymptomatic HIV-infected individuals.

CD4 cell counts are reported in absolute numbers and as the percentage (fraction) of total lymphocytes that are CD4 positive. The CD4 fraction is directly measured, while the absolute count is calculated as the product of the absolute lymphocyte count and the CD4 percentage. The CD4 cell count reflects the level of immune suppression. In adults, the CD4 cell count is normally between 400 and 1400 cells/mm³. As the CD4 cell count falls below normal, and particularly once thresholds of 200 cells/mm³ or a CD4 percentage of 15% are reached, the risk of opportunistic infection rises.[13,14]

There is substantial diurnal variation in the CD4 cell count; it is lowest in the morning and highest in the evening. As a result, clinical specimens are best collected consistently in the morning. The CD4 cell count can also be influenced by exercise, acute illness, co-morbidities or drugs such as systemic corticosteroids. In some patients, the CD4 percentage may serve as a better prognostic marker for progression to AIDS or death than the absolute count; this would include patients with splenectomy and pregnant women.[15,16] Short-term CD4 fluctuations of up to 30% have been shown to occur in HIV-infected individuals who are clinically stable.[17,18] As a result, it is important to monitor

Table 99.1 Laboratory tests for baseline evaluation of HIV-infected individuals

Test	Comment
HIV-specific tests	
Plasma HIV RNA (viral load)	
CD4+ lymphocyte count (absolute and percentage)	
General laboratory profile	
Complete blood count	Evaluates baseline abnormalities such as anemia or HIV-related thrombocytopenias
Electrolytes, creatinine, urinalysis	Baseline renal abnormalities may require further investigation and influence choice of antiretrovirals
Liver profile (alanine aminotransferase, aspartate aminotransferase, alkaline phosphatase, total bilirubin), amylase	Abnormalities may require further hepatic investigations. Elevated baseline liver profile may affect antiretroviral choice (avoidance of agents associated with higher rate of hepatotoxicity)
Fasting lipid profile, fasting blood sugar	Future risk of cardiac-related morbidity may require early interventions and influence the choice of antiretrovirals
Co-infection/opportunistic diseases assessment	
Urine, urethral or cervical screens for sexually transmitted infections as indicated by history and examination	
Serologic testing for syphilis	Rapid plasma reagin (RPR)
Serologic testing for hepatitis A, B and C	If hepatitis B serology is in keeping with chronic infection or resolved infection, consider hepatitis B DNA screen. Vaccinate nonimmune individuals
Toxoplasma and cytomegalovirus serology	
Tuberculin skin test (± sputum smears and cultures for mycobacteria, as indicated by history and physical examination)	If >5 mm and no signs of active infection, consider isoniazid prophylaxis
Chest radiography	
Cervical Papanicolaou smear	
Pregnancy test	

trends in the CD4 cell count over time rather than placing too much emphasis on a single reading. Similarly, two CD4 cell counts, separated by at least 1–4 weeks should be obtained at baseline, prior to initiating antiretroviral therapy.

Plasma viral load has been shown to be an independent predictor of disease progression and death in untreated HIV-infected individuals.[11,19,20] Plasma viral load is also a factor in deciding when to initiate antiretroviral therapy.[3,21] From a practical standpoint it is useful to consider the CD4 cell count as indicative of the level of immunologic suppression or 'damage that has already occurred' and the viral load as indicative of the level of disease activity or the 'damage that is about to occur'. Three assays are currently available to quantify plasma HIV-1 viral load. These are the HIV RNA polymerase chain reaction (PCR), the branched-chain DNA and the nucleic acid sequence-based amplification assays. Ultrasensitive assays have lower limits of detection of 50 copies/ml. The variability of the assay is approximately $0.3 \log_{10}$ copies/ml and, as a result, a $0.5 \log_{10}$ change in HIV RNA level is regarded as a significant viral load change in the context of antiretroviral therapy. Among patients on HAART, the plasma viral load is the primary laboratory marker of treatment efficacy. A treatment-induced 10-fold ($1 \log_{10}$) reduction in plasma HIV-1 RNA is associated with a decrease of approximately 50% in the relative risk of death.[1,22]

Resistance testing

A baseline genotypic resistance test should be performed in patients with recent infection (i.e. less than 3 years) to evaluate for transmission of drug-resistant virus.[23] Determination of resistance at this stage will help to guide future therapy, and resistance mutations should be taken into account even if later testing reveals wild-type virus. Baseline resistance testing is also recommended in all individuals before selection of the first HAART regimen. Baseline resistance testing has been shown to be cost-effective once prevalence of primary resistance reaches 5%.[23–25] In addition, baseline resistance testing is particularly important if the initial regimen will contain a non-nucleoside reverse transcriptase inhibitor.

FOLLOW-UP ASSESSMENT

Asymptomatic, untreated patients with CD4 cell counts >500 cells/mm³ should be monitored every 3–4 months both clinically and with CD4 cell counts and plasma viral load.[21,25] In patients with CD4 cell counts between 350 and 500 cells/mm³, similar monitoring every 2 months is warranted.[26] Once the CD4 cell count is <350 cells/mm³ (or below 15%), patients should be offered initiation of therapy. If this is deferred for any reason, monthly monitoring should be recommended. In addition, among patients with high CD4 cell counts (>500 cells/mm³), and CD4 declines in excess of 100 cells/year or plasma HIV RNA >100 000 copies/ml, more frequent (i.e. monthly) monitoring is also warranted.

Asymptomatic individuals with CD4 cell counts within the normal range are considered to have adequate immune function; opportunistic infections are therefore rare in this setting, except for tuberculosis, Kaposi's sarcoma or lymphomas. However, common infections, in particular respiratory and dermatologic conditions, are frequent in this setting. Management of nonopportunistic common infections in otherwise healthy HIV-infected individuals should follow the same protocols as in uninfected individuals. Pap testing, screening for sexually transmitted infections and tuberculin skin tests should be performed annually in at-risk patients.

Metabolic testing

Lipid abnormalities are common in HIV infection, with perturbations in triglyceride and high-density lipoprotein (HDL) values.[27] Antiretroviral therapy can lead to further abnormalities with increases in total cholesterol and triglyceride levels.[28,29] Fasting lipid profiles should be obtained at baseline, in conjunction with an assessment of overall cardiovascular risk using the Framingham risk assessment score.[30] Furthermore, lipid values should be monitored every 2–3 months after initiating antiretroviral therapy. Patients with abnormal lipid profiles should be managed according to the underlying targets set by the updated National Cholesterol Education Program guidelines. In this setting, revision of the HAART regimen in favor of a similarly active but more lipid-friendly option should be considered. Alternatively, lipid-lowering strategies recommended for HIV-infected individuals with dyslipidemia should be pursued[31–33] (see Practice Point 47).

HIV-infected patients may be at increased risk for osteopenia and osteoporosis.[34] This may again reflect underlying HIV effects, although antiretroviral drugs have also been implicated.[35,36] Patients with other risk factors for bone loss should be screened using dual-energy X-ray absorptiometry (DEXA). Some would advise that this test be repeated every few years, particularly in high-risk patients; however, routine use of DEXA scans remains controversial.[25,37]

Counseling

The need for risk reduction counseling should be assessed at all encounters. This should include assessment of higher-risk sexual activities, substance use and other factors that may influence adherence to antiretrovirals such as psychiatric disorders and depression. When issues are identified, patients should receive targeted counseling or referral to multidisciplinary care teams. Patients should have the opportunity to discuss the most recent trends in management and antiretroviral therapy.

PROPHYLACTIC MANAGEMENT

Tuberculin skin test

A tuberculin skin test should be performed at baseline and annually in patients at risk for exposure. Induration >5 mm is considered positive, and should prompt evaluation for possible active tuberculosis prior to consideration of treatment for latent tuberculosis infection (tuberculosis chemoprophylaxis). Chemoprophylaxis is also recommended for patients with recent exposure to a documented case of active tuberculosis, chest radiography supportive of previous tuberculosis or a history of untreated or inadequately treated previous tuberculosis. A 9-month course of isoniazid in conjunction with pyridoxine to reduce the risk of isoniazid toxicity is recommended.[38,39]

Vaccinations

While antigen recognition is still intact, it is essential to boost humoral immunity against common pathogens. Standard vaccines such as the tetanus–diphtheria toxoid vaccine should be updated as necessary. Influenza vaccine has been shown to be safe and immunogenic in the setting of HIV, and should be administered annually at the beginning of the winter season.[40,41] The polyvalent polysaccharide *Streptococcus pneumoniae* vaccine (Pneumovax) should be administered at least once, and repeated after 5 years.[42] Hepatitis A and B vaccines should be encouraged in susceptible patients, and in particular in at-risk individuals such

as intravenous drug users, those with multiple sexual partners, men who have sex with men and individuals co-infected with hepatitis C.[43,44]

Prophylaxis (see also Chapter 91)

As seen in Table 99.2, as HIV disease progresses, prophylaxis for opportunistic infections becomes increasingly important. Once the CD4 cell count decreases below 200 cells/mm³ the risk for *Pneumocystis jirovecii* (previously *P. carinii*) pneumonia rises, and more than 80% of individuals with untreated HIV will experience an episode of *Pneumocystis* pneumonia over their lifetime.[13] Prophylaxis is indicated if the CD4 cell count is <200 cells/mm³, the CD4 percentage is below 15% and in patients with recurrent oral thrush.[39]

Patients with other AIDS-defining illnesses should also be offered primary prophylaxis, and patients experiencing *Pneumocystis* pneumonia should be placed on secondary prophylaxis after completion of acute treatment. The preferred regimen consists of one double-strength (DS) tablet of trimethoprim–sulfamethoxazole (TMP–SMX) daily. The use of intermittent dosing (3 days each week) for the DS tablet, or the use of one single-strength tablet of TMP–SMX daily, have been shown to be less effective than a regimen of 1 DS tablet daily.[45] Alternatives include dapsone 100 mg or atovaquone 1500 mg daily or inhaled pentamidine 300 mg monthly.

Prophylaxis for toxoplasmosis is indicated for those individuals who have positive serum IgG for toxoplasmosis and CD4 cell counts <100 cells/mm³.[39] Trimethoprim–sulfamethoxazole remains the first-line regimen for primary prophylaxis. Dapsone with pyrimethamine, and folinic acid or single agent atovaquone are possible alternatives. As HIV disease progresses, prophylaxis for *Mycobacterium avium* complex (MAC) with weekly azithromycin should be initiated once CD4 cell counts

Table 99.2 Prophylaxis and treatment for opportunistic infections	
CD4+ lymphocyte cell count	Management strategy
Any	If needed, update standard diphtheria–pertussis–tetanus and inactivated polio vaccines Annual influenza vaccine 23-Valent pneumococcal polysaccharide vaccine. Responses may be better if CD4 >200 cells/mm³. Revaccination should be considered after 5 years Hepatitis A and B vaccines Tuberculin skin test and 9 months isoniazid prophylaxis if ≥5 mm induration
<500	Monitor CD4 cell count and viral load every 3–4 months
<350	Consider monitoring CD4 cell count and viral load every 1–2 months, and discuss antiretroviral initiation
<200	Initiate *Pneumocystis jirovecii* prophylaxis. Trimethoprim–sulfamethoxazole 160 mg/800 mg (1 double-strength tablet) q24 h is first-line agent
<100	Start prophylaxis for toxoplasmosis if seropositive, if not on trimethoprim–sulfamethoxazole
<50	*Mycobacterium avium* complex prophylaxis with azithromycin 1200 mg po weekly Ophthalmologic screening for cytomegalovirus retinitis (repeat at 6-monthly intervals)

drop to <50 cells/mm³ but only after active MAC has been excluded.³⁹ Routine ophthalmologic assessment for CMV retinitis is indicated at 3- to 6-month intervals while the CD4 cell count is <50 cells/mm³.

Both primary and secondary prophylaxis for these common opportunistic infections can be discontinued in patients who experience HAART-related consistent increases in their CD4 cell counts to levels >100 cells/mm³ for MAC, and >200 cells/mm³ for toxoplasmosis and *Pneumocystis jirovecii*.[4,46,47]

INITIATION OF ANTIRETROVIRAL THERAPY

The objective of antiretroviral therapy is to prevent disease progression and prolong survival while maintaining quality of life. Long-term nonprogression will be achieved by reducing plasma viral load to below 50 copies/ml on a sustained basis. The use of combinations of antiretroviral agents with no overlapping toxicity and demonstrated additive to synergistic antiviral effect is recommended to maximize the duration of the virologic response.[3,21] Since 1996, triple drug combination antiretroviral therapy has been shown to decrease morbidity and mortality dramatically in symptomatic and asymptomatic HIV-1-infected individuals.[1,2,48–52]

The Department of Health and Human Services and the International AIDS Society–USA have produced comprehensive consensus guidelines for the management of HIV, including issues around the initiation of therapy.[3,21] These are generally consistent with guidelines published by a number of national societies.[53,54] An approach to antiretroviral therapy is suggested in Figure 99.1.

WHEN TO START THERAPY

General principles

Antiretroviral therapy should be commenced in any patient with HIV-related symptoms or signs, opportunistic infections or cancers.[3,21,53] For asymptomatic patients, recommendations for the initiation of therapy are based primarily on thresholds of CD4⁺ lymphocyte counts and to a lesser extent on plasma HIV-1 RNA; these have been identified as key prognostic markers of the risk for disease progression in natural history and observational studies as well as randomized clinical trials.[11,55–57] Cohort studies have characterized rates of disease progression to AIDS or death based on CD4⁺ and plasma viral load thresholds in treated patients, and have long demonstrated that 200 cells/mm³ represents a critical threshold. CD4 cell levels below 200 cells/mm³ identify patients who are at high short-term risk of developing AIDS-defining illnesses and death, and for whom the effectiveness of antiretroviral therapy is partially compromised.[58–60] Recent data from large cohort studies and observations from clinical trials suggest that HIV-related morbidity and mortality may occur more commonly at higher CD4 strata than previously recognized, and that HAART may also reduce non-AIDS-related morbidity and mortality at CD4 cell counts above 200 cells/mm³.[61-63] Thus, current treatment guidelines consistently recommend that all individuals with CD4 cell counts <350 cells/mm³ should be encouraged to start therapy.[3,21]

Of note, among individuals with CD4 cell counts of 200 to 350/mm³, a CD4 cell count fraction ≤15% of the total lymphocyte count has been shown to be an independent predictor of short-term risk of developing an AIDS-defining illnesses or death, and decreased effectiveness of antiretroviral therapy.[64]

If a decision is reached to defer initiation of antiretroviral therapy in this setting, this decision should be re-evaluated frequently (i.e. monthly) with clinical and laboratory evaluation.

There is growing recognition of the deleterious consequences of chronic inflammatory states due to uncontrolled HIV replication. As such, although currently it is generally recommended that initiation of therapy be deferred among asymptomatic patients with CD4 cell counts >350 cells/mm³,[3,21] guidelines do recognize the need for earlier initiation of antiretroviral therapy in the presence of conditions that may be exacerbated by chronic HIV-related inflammatory states

or ongoing uncontrolled viral replication. These conditions include underlying cardiovascular disease, hepatitis B or C co-infection, and HIV-associated nephropathy. In these cases, consideration should be given to initiation of HAART regardless of CD4 cell count.[3] Other features that may lead to consideration of HAART therapy at CD4 cell counts >350 cells/mm³ include an HIV-1-RNA level that is consistently above 100 000 copies/ml or rapid CD4 cell loss (≥100 cells per year). However, the issue of when to start HAART remains a matter of some debate; ongoing cohort analyses suggests that there may be benefit to initiating therapy at CD4 cell counts in excess of 500 cells/mm³.[65] Other theoretical benefits of earlier HAART initiation include greater immunological preservation or restoration, and potential for reduced HIV transmission.[66,67] New simpler, safer and better-tolerated regimens make earlier treatment a more attractive proposition today. However, the potential benefits of earlier treatment initiation need to be weighed against the risks associated with longer duration of drug exposure, such as drug toxicities, emergence of resistance, and cost. This strategy needs to be tested in controlled clinical trials before being widely adopted in clinical practice.

The effectiveness of antiretroviral therapy is also critically dependent on maintaining a nearly perfect level of adherence to therapy. Incomplete adherence is a key determinant of the emergence of drug-resistant HIV,[68,69] increased risk for CD4⁺ cell decline, progression to AIDS, and death.[70–72] HIV drug resistance is typically associated with cross-resistance to other members of the same class,[73,74] limiting future treatment options. Thus, it is critical that patients have access to optimal adherence support before initiating antiretroviral therapy.

Special considerations

Gender

Study results are conflicting as to whether there are gender-specific differences in the natural history of HIV disease.[75,76] However, the effectiveness of antiretroviral therapy as measured by the risk of progression to AIDS or death is independent of gender.[51,58,59,77] There is general agreement among guidelines that timing of HAART initiation should be the same in men and women.

Intravenous drug users

With regard to the critical role of adherence in treatment success, physician perception of a patient's potential ability to adhere to HAART does not justify withholding HAART when medically indicated, even in patients with relatively chaotic lifestyles or active intravenous drug use.[78] Rather, adherence should be optimized in all patients starting HAART, through counseling, education and addressing relevant co-morbidities, including psychosocial issues (e.g. addictions, depression) that might pose barriers to adherence. Whenever possible, selection of compact once-daily regimens is to be encouraged, as long as it is deemed clinically appropriate. Assisted therapy programs, such as directly observed therapy or programs that link daily HAART and methadone dispensing, have proven of great value in some settings.[79,80]

Co-infection with viral hepatitis

Co-infection with hepatitis C and/or B virus is common among HIV-infected individuals. Co-infection with HIV may accelerate the progression of liver disease due to viral hepatitis[81,82] and conversely may enhance the risk of hepatotoxicity of some antiretroviral agents.[83] An additional consideration is the risk for exacerbation of hepatitis, and potentially hepatic failure, due to immune reconstitution syndrome occurring early after starting antiretroviral therapy. Nonetheless, control of HIV replication by initiating antiretroviral therapy has been shown to decrease mortality due to liver disease in the setting of hepatitis C co-infection.[84,85]

Hepatitis C treatment, while potentially curative, can be associated with substantial adverse effects and tolerability issues, particularly

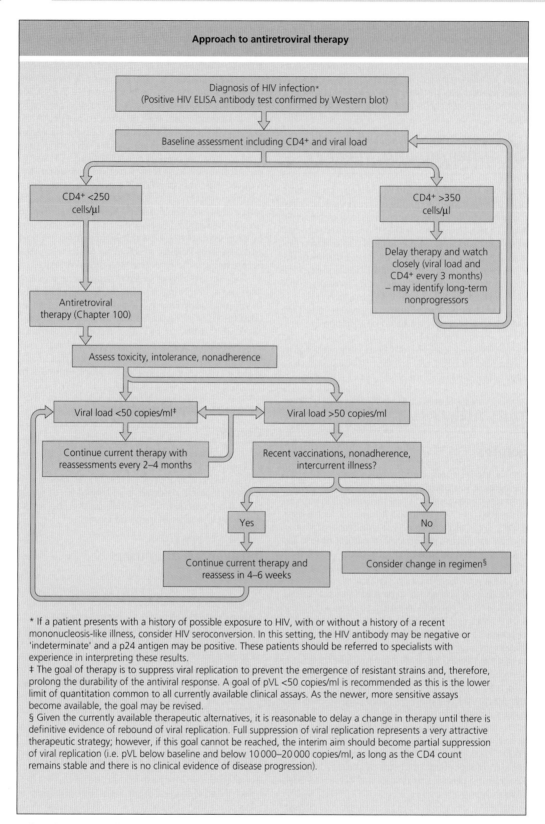

Approach to antiretroviral therapy

Diagnosis of HIV infection*
(Positive HIV ELISA antibody test confirmed by Western blot)

Baseline assessment including CD4+ and viral load

CD4+ <250 cells/μl

CD4+ >350 cells/μl

Delay therapy and watch closely (viral load and CD4+ every 3 months) – may identify long-term nonprogressors

Antiretroviral therapy (Chapter 100)

Assess toxicity, intolerance, nonadherence

Viral load <50 copies/ml‡

Viral load >50 copies/ml

Continue current therapy with reassessments every 2–4 months

Recent vaccinations, nonadherence, intercurrent illness?

Yes

No

Continue current therapy and reassess in 4–6 weeks

Consider change in regimen§

* If a patient presents with a history of possible exposure to HIV, with or without a history of a recent mononucleosis-like illness, consider HIV seroconversion. In this setting, the HIV antibody may be negative or 'indeterminate' and a p24 antigen may be positive. These patients should be referred to specialists with experience in interpreting these results.
‡ The goal of therapy is to suppress viral replication to prevent the emergence of resistant strains and, therefore, prolong the durability of the antiviral response. A goal of pVL <50 copies/ml is recommended as this is the lower limit of quantitation common to all currently available clinical assays. As the newer, more sensitive assays become available, the goal may be revised.
§ Given the currently available therapeutic alternatives, it is reasonable to delay a change in therapy until there is definitive evidence of rebound of viral replication. Full suppression of viral replication represents a very attractive therapeutic strategy; however, if this goal cannot be reached, the interim aim should become partial suppression of viral replication (i.e. pVL below baseline and below 10 000–20 000 copies/ml, as long as the CD4 count remains stable and there is no clinical evidence of disease progression).

Fig. 99.1 An approach to the initiation of antiretroviral therapy. pVL, plasma viral load.

when given in combination with HIV treatment. Thus when the CD4 cell count is >350 cells/mm³, it is preferable to initiate (and, if possible complete) therapy for hepatitis C first, prior to initiating HAART. On the other hand, a co-infected patient with a CD4 count <350 cells/mm³ should be stabilized on HAART before therapy for hepatitis C is undertaken.[83–85] Patients with CD4 cell count >350 cells/mm³

who are unable to receive hepatitis C therapy should be evaluated for early initiation of HAART according to current guidelines due to recognition of improved liver-related mortality. (See Practice Point 46.)

In the setting of co-infection with HIV and hepatitis B, it is noteworthy that some antiretroviral agents have activity against both HIV and hepatitis B virus (HBV), notably tenofovir, adefovir, lamivudine and emtricitabine. As a result, HAART regimens containing tenofovir in combination with either lamivudine or emtricitabine are expected to suppress serum hepatitis B DNA levels in a durable fashion, with associated biochemical and clinical improvements, even in patients with advanced liver disease.[21] Use of lamivudine, emtricitabine or tenofovir as the only active hepatitis B agent should be avoided due to risks of development of hepatitis B resistance.[21] Significant rebound in hepatitis B viral load and even clinical hepatitis can occur if one or both of these agents is discontinued without replacement by another anti-HBV agent.[21]

More recently, the anti-HBV drug entecavir was also found to have some (still poorly characterized) anti-HIV activity, resulting in emergence of nucleoside-associated resistance mutations among patients who were not on suppressive antiretroviral therapy for HIV.[86] For co-infected patients requiring treatment for hepatitis B but not immediately for HIV, agents without crossover anti-HIV effect (such as interferon) are preferable, to avert the emergence of drug-resistant HIV.[21] While adefovir has modest anti-HIV activity, it does not appear to select for significant drug-resistant HIV mutations at the doses used for treatment of hepatitis B[87,88] (see Practice Point 44).

CHOICE OF INITIAL ANTIRETROVIRAL REGIMEN

Current guidelines advise that regimens consist of a backbone of two nucleoside or nucleotide reverse transcriptase inhibitors (NRTIs) plus either a non-nucleoside reverse transcriptase inhibitor (NNRTI) or a ritonavir-boosted protease inhibitor (PI).[3,21] The choice of specific regimens and agents should be individualized, taking into account results of testing for primary resistance, patient preferences and life-style, co-infections (e.g. viral hepatitis), co-morbidities (e.g. diabetes, kidney disease), cardiovascular risk factors and concomitant medications. Considerations for selecting individual agents are outside the scope of this chapter. Guideline recommendations for specific preferred agents are revised regularly based on new information and the availability of new agents and fixed-dose formulations which enhance convenience and compliance. Specific antiretroviral agents are described in detail in Chapter 100.

MONITORING PATIENTS ON INITIAL ANTIRETROVIRAL THERAPY

After starting a new antiretroviral regimen, the patient should have the plasma HIV RNA level checked every 4–8 weeks until a target of <50 copies/ml is achieved, a threshold typically reached within 24 weeks. Viral load monitoring can then be decreased to approximately 3-monthly intervals, along with CD4 cell counts in stable patients. Adherence, drug intolerance, drug toxicities and clinical disease status should also be re-evaluated at each visit.

CHANGING ANTIRETROVIRAL THERAPY

When to change

Treatment failure

From a practical standpoint, treatment failure is defined in virologic terms as either the failure to achieve a viral load <50 copies/ml or the occurrence of a confirmed viral load rebound above 50 copies/ml in the absence of other obvious explanation (e.g. treatment interruption, intercurrent illness or immunizations).

It is critically important to understand and correct the determinants of treatment failure in any given individual. This must be done

before a change in therapy is implemented. If the plasma viral load rebounds despite ongoing therapy, consider imperfect adherence to the antiretroviral regimen as the most likely cause.[69] The 'forgiveness' of a regimen to breakdowns in adherence is dependent to some degree on the pharmacokinetics and barrier to resistance posed by the regimen. However, in many cases, even relatively minor degrees of nonadherence can lead to viral breakthrough and ultimately emergence of resistance.[89] If suboptimal adherence is identified, the pattern of and reasons for missed doses should be evaluated. Alternative dosing regimens can often be accommodated to better suit an individual's lifestyle. Intolerance to medications may be mitigated by altering the time of dosing, administering with food and, if possible, altering dosing interval. Other issues such as depression or substance use, which can negatively impact adherence, may need to be addressed.

Another major cause of treatment failure is reduced susceptibility of the virus to one or more antiretroviral drugs in the regimen. Patients can be initially infected with drug-resistant strains of HIV.[24] Resistant strains can also emerge when the virus is allowed to replicate in the presence of drug, as in the case of incomplete adherence, insufficiently potent regimens or suboptimal drug levels. Considerable cross-resistance exists within antiretroviral drug classes, so patients may harbor virus resistant to an agent as a result of exposure to another agent within the same drug class.[23] Resistance to multiple classes of antiretrovirals severely limits the chances of success with future regimens. Resistance testing should be performed as soon as virologic failure is established, and the results used to design an alternative fully suppressive regimen to avoid further development of resistance. Additional discussion of HIV drug resistance appears in Practice Point 48.

Treatment failure may also be due to inadequate drug levels. Most antiretroviral agents are prescribed without regard to individual patient characteristics such as weight; however, for many of these agents, notably the protease inhibitors, there is considerable interindividual variation in pharmacokinetics. This can only be assessed by therapeutic drug monitoring (TDM), i.e. directly measuring plasma drug levels. However, optimal target levels for antiretroviral drugs are not always well defined. Another common cause of inadequate antiretroviral drug levels is unrecognized drug–drug interactions, either with other antiretrovirals within the regimen or with concomitant medications taken for other indications.[90] Dose adjustments may overcome some of these interactions; however, in the case of multiple drug regimens with complicated potential interactions, TDM will be necessary to establish the direction of the interaction and make appropriate adjustments.

A change in therapy in the setting of failure of previous treatment should only be carried out after careful evaluation of prior drug exposure, prior response to therapies, prior tolerability and toxicity issues, as well as the results of resistance testing done on a real-time basis and on relevant stored samples, if available. Failure to address these issues effectively will invariably compromise the chances of success with the new regimen. Whenever possible, pharmacokinetic issues (past and present) should also be evaluated. Multiple variables must be considered when changing regimens in the context of virologic failure in a given clinical case. As such, guidelines cannot replace expert advice in this setting. It is critical, therefore, that the decision of when to change and what to change to be arrived at under the guidance of an experienced practitioner.

Toxicity

Tolerability issues are a frequent reason for modification of HAART regimens. When the causal agent responsible for a given toxicity is known, replacing that single agent is relatively simple and usually effective. The issue is more challenging if the link between the responsible agent and the emerging toxicity is not clear. At times it is difficult to differentiate specific antiretroviral drug toxicity from a co-morbid condition or toxicity due to a concomitant medication, for example in the case of hepatic transaminase elevations. In such instances, other potential causes should be evaluated and managed if possible, or ruled out prior to implementing changes in the antiretroviral regimen.

Significant toxicities may also develop due to drug–drug interactions, particularly if the exposure to one agent is substantially increased in the presence of another, for example rhabdomyolysis due to increased levels of certain statins in the presence of ritonavir-boosted protease inhibitors.[91] Management of patients in a multidisciplinary setting with access to specialized pharmacists with a thorough knowledge of potential drug interactions can alleviate these problems.

ALTERATION OF ANTIRETROVIRAL REGIMENS

The composition of a new regimen will depend on the underlying reasons for changing therapy. If a patient experiences drug toxicity, brief cessation of all medications is recommended. Decreasing dosages or discontinuing a single medication should be discouraged, as this will compromise the potency of the regimen and eventually promote the development of resistance. In general, as long as the antiviral potency of the regimen is preserved, exchanging an individual component of the regimen to deal with a toxicity problem is acceptable. The closer the agents are in terms of their potency and resistance profile, the easier and safer the change will be. Drug substitutions become more complicated when the patient presents with a history of prior drug exposure and/or failure of multiple regimens. In such cases, changes in therapy should only be performed under the guidance of an experienced physician.

When a decision is made to change therapy for confirmed virologic failure, the new regimen should be one with the highest probable effectiveness, as predicted by the patient's complete drug history and the resistance test results, as well as the highest likelihood of tolerability and adherence. New regimens should contain at least two (and if possible three) drugs deemed to be fully active.[3,21] It is important to emphasize that HIV isolated particularly early on during virologic treatment failure is often not resistant to all of the drugs in the failing regimen. In addition, latently infected lymphocytes may harbor archived viruses resistant to drugs used in the past which are not detected by routine resistance testing in the plasma.

Cross-resistance among drugs in the same class may be extensive and this often limits the number of fully active alternative regimens. With the currently approved first generation NNRTIs, the risk of cross-resistance is high after an NNRTI-containing regimen fails.[23] With protease inhibitors, intraclass cross-resistance is less predictable. Depending on the pattern of resistance, an alternative protease inhibitor can often be selected. With NRTIs, the extent of class cross-resistance varies from drug to drug and is poorly reflected by genotype or phenotype testing results. In rare circumstances, multidrug resistance to NRTIs may develop through a unique mutational pathway.[23] Maximal activity would be expected from drugs belonging to a new class to which the patient's virus has not previously been exposed and would not be expected to have any mutations conferring resistance. Cross-resistance is also known to occur within newer classes of drugs, including fusion inhibitors, CCR5 receptor antagonists and integrase inhibitors.

Monitoring patients after regimen change

As with a first regimen, the patient should have the plasma HIV RNA level checked 4–8 weeks after starting a new regimen to ensure the desired early response, and followed closely (i.e. monthly) until the viral load is below 50 copies/ml. Adherence, drug tolerance and emerging toxicities with the new regimen will also need to be monitored as well as any changes in clinical disease status. Such follow-up is best undertaken in close collaboration with an experienced physician.

TREATMENT INTERRUPTIONS

CD4 cell count-guided treatment interruptions have been considered as a means of sparing patients from the adverse effects of long-term exposure to antiretrovirals. However, a recent large controlled clinical trial has shown conclusively that structured treatment interruptions are associated with AIDS-related events and significant drops in CD4 cell counts, as well as AIDS- and non-AIDS-related mortality.[10] Currently structured treatment interruptions are not recommended except in cases of treatment-limiting intolerance or toxicity, and then under close expert medical supervision.

REFERENCES

References for this chapter can be found online at http://www.expertconsult.com

Chapter | **100** | David Asboe
Anton Pozniak

Antiviral therapy

INTRODUCTION

HIV infection is a chronic disease in which, if left untreated, high-level viral replication occurs continuously for years, even during the clinically latent phase. Without optimal antiviral therapy opportunistic infections or malignancies characteristic of AIDS typically start occurring 10–12 years after HIV infection, although may occur much sooner. Viral replication drives the progression of HIV disease and leads to worsening immunodeficiency as measured by decreasing CD4+ lymphocyte cell counts which are highly predictive of the subsequent risk of disease progression and death. Suppression of HIV replication to levels in plasma below the limit of detection is the primary objective of antiretroviral (ARV) treatment as this is associated with durable clinical, virologic and immunologic responses. Residual viral replication due to incomplete suppression in the presence of drugs is responsible for the development of viral resistance to antiretroviral drugs, thereby contributing to treatment failure and disease progression. Inability to maintain full virologic suppression is most commonly related to suboptimal adherence but may be due to viral mutations leading to decreased drug susceptibility and resistance.

Thus virologic failure is defined as either treatment being unable to reduce plasma HIV viral load to below the limit of detection or the development of virologic rebound in someone who previously was fully suppressed. With virologic failure, resistance mutations may be selected which usually decrease the susceptibility of virus to the relevant drug(s) and often will also result in decreased susceptibility to other drugs within the same class (cross-class resistance). The impact of individual mutations will depend on the mutation and the drug and class affected. For example, the mutation Y181C is selected very early in patients failing nevirapine and results in loss of susceptibility to all available members of the non-nucleoside reverse transcriptase inhibitor class.

Most individuals commencing ARV treatment will be expected to have successful, durable responses to treatment. In clinical trials after long periods of follow-up virologic undetectable rates at 3–5 years of 60–70% have been reported. However, for individuals who subsequently develop virologic failure on these initial treatments and for those who were previously treated with suboptimal therapies, the availability of new drugs with activity against resistant viruses is important in order to construct effective regimens. Also critical is the development of new drugs with better or different tolerability/toxicity profiles and with better, more patient-friendly formulations, as regimen switches are commonly related to drug intolerance or toxicity.

There are now 22 licensed drugs available for the treatment of HIV infection (Table 100.1), including six different classes acting at different sites of HIV cell entry and replication (Fig. 100.1). (See Chapter 145 for detailed discussion of antiretroviral drugs.) The availability of an increasing number of drugs and the rapidly evolving scientific information have made HIV treatment an extremely complex field. Treatment should be supervised by experts, and several national and international guidelines have been developed in order to help in the clinical management of HIV-infected adults and adolescents, pregnant women, infants and children, those with hepatitis and tuberculosis co-infections and uninfected individuals who have occupational exposure to HIV.

Table 100.1 Currently licensed antiretroviral drugs by class

NRTIs	NNRTIs	Protease inhibitors	Entry inhibitors	Integrase inhibitors
Zidovudine (ZDV)	Nevirapine	Saquinavir	Enfuvirtide	Raltegravir
Stavudine	Efavirenz (EFV)	Indinavir	Maraviroc	
Lamivudine (3TC)	Delavirdine*	Nelfinavir		
Emtricitabine (FTC)	Etravirine	Fosamprenavir		
Abacavir (ABC)		Amprenavir*		
Zalcitabine*		Lopinavir (LPV)		
Didanosine		Ritonavir (RTV)		
Tenofovir (TDF)		Atazanavir		
		Tipranavir		
		Darunavir		

Six fixed-dose combinations are approved: ZDV + 3TC; ZDV + 3TC + ABC; ABC + 3TC; FTC + TDF; LPV + RTV; TDF + FTC + EFV.
*No longer commercially available.

The replication of HIV within CD4⁺ lymphocyte and target sites of antiretroviral drugs

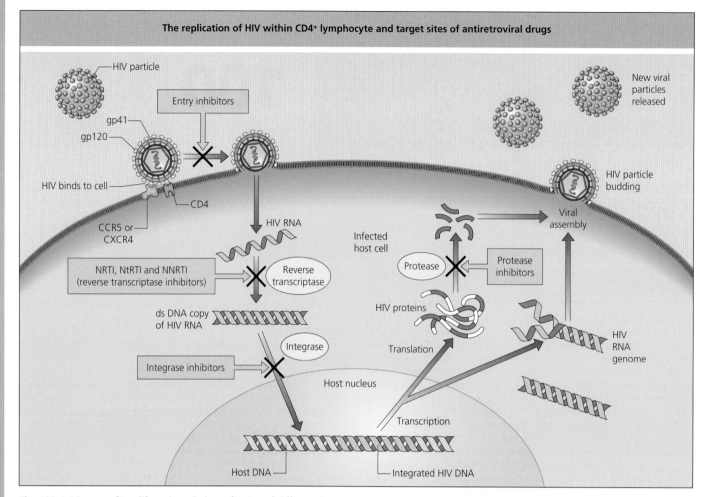

Fig. 100.1 Diagram of HIV life cycle and place of action of different drugs. With permission from Bolognia JL, Jorizzo JL, Rapini RP, *et al.*, eds. Dermatology, 2nd ed. London: Mosby; 2008.

WHEN SHOULD ANTIRETROVIRAL DRUGS BE STARTED?

Established HIV infection

Until recently, most guidelines suggested commencing treatment if individuals had symptomatic disease or if asymptomatic when the CD4 count declined to between 200 and 350 cells/mm³. In practice many started with CD4 counts of approximately 200 cells/mm³ or lower (particularly in those presenting late with advanced immunosuppression). More recently, guidelines have been recommending earlier treatment (Table 100.2). For example the European AIDS Clinical Society (EACS) recommend treating all individuals with a CD4 between 200 and 350 cells/mm³ but also to consider treatment in those with CD4 counts up to 500 cells/mm³ in presence of any of the following:

- a high viral load (greater than 100 000 copies/ml);
- a rapidly declining CD4;
- older age; or
- hepatitis C co-infection.

The trend to recommend earlier treatment has been informed by several studies which indicate that the risk of clinical disease at higher CD4 counts is greater than previously thought. This may be driving the finding that even HIV-positive individuals with high CD4 counts have raised standardized mortality ratios compared with the general population. In the SMART study of treatment interruption, individuals with CD4 counts >350 cells/mm³, including those not on treatment and those randomized to interrupt treatment, experienced more clinical disease than those who remained on treatment throughout.[2] Surprisingly, this excess of clinical disease comprised not only conditions considered to be HIV related but also such diverse conditions as cardiovascular disease, renal and hepatic disease. The US Department of Health and Human Sciences (DHHS) guidelines now specify that if HIV-related renal disease is present, early commencement of ARVs should be recommended. The International AIDS Society (IAS) USA guidelines suggest that therapy should be considered and decision individualized if an individual's CD4 count is >350 cells/mm³ and there is the presence of, or high risk for, cardiovascular disease, active hepatitis B virus (HBV) or hepatitis C virus (HCV) co-infection or HIV-associated nephropathy. There are studies planned to further examine even earlier commencement of ARVs.

Acute HIV infection

Overall there are no convincing data that treating patients during acute HIV infection has led to any substantial long-term benefits in terms of their immune system recovery. However, there are data suggesting that if patients were treated in the very early stages of acute HIV infection, they may preserve immune function, especially in the gut, and may also prevent dissemination of virus to sanctuary sites such as the brain. Treatment for acute HIV infection should be undertaken within a clinical trial or perhaps considered in an individual with moderate to severe symptoms, those who have a precipitous fall in CD4 count to <200 cells/mm³ or those with neurologic involvement (see also Chapter 89).

Table 100.2 Guidelines for when to start antiretroviral treatment

Guidelines	Symptomatic	Asymptomatic	Other
European AIDS Clinical Society[1]	CDC stage B	CD4 <200: start without delay CD4 201–350: treatment recommended CD4 350–500: may be offered	Consider at higher CD4 if: • viral load >100 000/ml • rapid CD4 decline • age >55 years
US Department of Health and Human Sciences	Symptomatic	CD4 <350 cells/mm³: treatment recommended CD4 >350 cells/mm³	Patient scenarios and comorbidities should be taken into consideration
International AIDS Society, USA	Symptomatic	CD4 <350 cells/mm³ CD4 >350 cells/mm³	Co-morbidities Patient willingness Rapid decline CD4 (>100 cells/year) Plasma viral load >100 000 copies Therapy should be considered and decision individualized

WHICH ANTIRETROVIRAL DRUGS TO START?

Individuals commencing ARV therapy for the first time will usually start with a combination of two nucleoside reverse transcriptase inhibitors (NRTIs) and either a non-nucleoside reverse transcriptase inhibitor (NNRTI) or a protease inhibitor (PI), boosted with low-dose ritonavir (Table 100.3). Before selecting a combination, it is important to take account of several pieces of clinical and laboratory information.

Baseline resistance testing

Transmission of drug-resistant virus is well documented, with up to 15% of ARV-naive individuals in some studies being found to harbor

Table 100.3 Which antiretroviral drugs to start

Guidelines	A	B
EACS, recommended	Efavirenz Nevirapine Fosamprenavir–ritonavir Lopinavir–ritonavir Saquinavir–ritonavir Atazanavir–ritonavir	Abacavir–lamivudine Tenofovir–emtricitabine
EACS, alternative	Darunavir–ritonavir	Zidovudine–lamivudine Didanosine–lamivudine or didanosine–emtricitabine
IAS-USA	Efavirenz Atazanavir–ritonavir Lopinavir–ritonavir Darunavir–ritonavir Fosamprenavir–ritonavir Saquinavir–ritonavir	Tenofovir–emtricitabine Abacavir–lamivudine
DHHS preferred	Efavirenz Atazanavir–ritonavir Darunavir–ritonavir Fosamprenavir–ritonavir Lopinavir–ritonavir	Tenofovir–emtricitabine

For EACS, IAS and DHHS guidelines, one drug (or ritonavir-boosted antiretroviral) from column A should be prescribed with a combination of drugs from column B.

HIV with at least one important drug-related mutation.[3] Studies demonstrate poorer virologic outcomes for individuals commencing combinations where transmitted resistance is present. It is widely recommended that resistance testing, where available, be performed prior to commencement of first-line therapy. With time, evidence of transmitted drug resistance may be lost due to outgrowth of wild-type virus which is more fit, resulting in 'archiving' of resistant virus. It is recommended, therefore, that resistance testing is done on the earliest available sample following the diagnosis of HIV infection.

Co-infections

It is important to establish whether an individual is co-infected with HBV or HCV before commencing ARV treatment. Tenofovir, lamivudine and emtricitabine are also active against hepatitis B. When starting ARVs, it is recommended that HBV/HIV co-infected individuals should be treated with a combination that includes two agents active against HBV.[4] The usual combination is either lamivudine or emtricitabine with tenofovir. In individuals with HCV infection an assessment of whether specific HCV treatment is required should be made. Zidovudine, didanosine and stavudine should be avoided due to increased toxicity in combination with ribavirin. There is also evidence of lower sustained virologic response rates in those on abacavir treated with interferon–ribavirin.

Co-morbidities

Comorbidities should also be considered. For example some ritonavir-boosted protease inhibitors may increase insulin resistance and therefore make control of diabetes more difficult. Protease inhibitors are also associated with increases in total cholesterol and triglycerides and in cohort studies with an increased risk of myocardial infarction. Efavirenz is associated with depression and other neuropsychiatric side-effects. In a small percentage of individuals, tenofovir leads to a decline in glomerular filtration rate (GFR). Agents other than tenofovir should be considered if individuals have severe renal impairment and caution taken in patients taking other drugs known to cause renal dysfunction.

Drug interactions

It is important in assessing co-morbid conditions to also consider co-prescribed medications. NNRTIs and PIs in particular interact with numerous other medications. Interactions may lead to lower or higher levels of ARVs, risking either treatment failure or toxicity. Furthermore, as both NNRTIs and PIs can act as inducers or inhibitors of cytochrome P450, the levels of other drugs may be affected.

Lifestyle

Finally, it must always be borne in mind that HIV infection is a long-term disease, often affecting young people. Therapy for HIV (as for other chronic diseases necessitating continuous treatment), tolerability, compliance and accessibility are important factors that must carefully be considered in the design of treatment to ensure compliance and efficacy.

Most combinations of ARVs have shown broadly similar activity and efficacy in the short to medium term. Considerations in the selection of the most appropriate regimen for the individual patient may include potency, side-effect profile, patient's predicted adherence, quality of life issues and pill burden, the potential for maintenance of future options in terms of drug class sparing and cross-resistance profile, the presence of co-morbid conditions and medications. Finally, in certain clinical circumstances and geographic areas, the potential for primary acquisition of resistant viral strains needs to be considered.

SPECIFIC ANTIRETROVIRAL DRUGS

Nucleos(t)ide reverse transcriptase inhibitors

Reverse transcriptase inhibitors act through one of two mechanisms. First, as 'chain terminators', they block the elongation of the DNA chain through blockage of further nucleosides. This mechanism is characteristic of the nucleoside and nucleotide analogues and depends on the intracellular phosphorylation of the drugs into the corresponding triphosphate. Second, they act by competition/binding of the reverse transcriptase in functionally essential sites. NNRTIs act only through this mechanism and not as 'chain terminators'. In general, nucleoside analogues have good oral bioavailability, are only minimally bound to plasma proteins, do not interfere with cytochrome P450 enzyme systems and are excreted through the kidneys. Because of these metabolic characteristics, they have relatively few interactions with other drugs as compared with PIs and NNRTIs. They are generally active against HIV-1 and HIV-2.

The most widely studied and recommended nucleoside/nucleotide backbones for initial ARV treatment are zidovudine–lamivudine, abacavir–lamivudine, or tenofovir with either lamivudine or emtricitabine.

Zidovudine and stavudine

Zidovudine is a thymidine analogue and was the first ARV agent available for use. For many years it was a recommended component of first-line combination therapy. Its relegation in guidelines to that of an alternative agent has been driven by its association with lipoatrophy. This toxicity starts to manifest after 12 months on treatment and may affect up to 50–60% of those taking zidovudine in the medium to long term. In individuals with lipoatrophy, switching away from zidovudine may result in partial reversal of the subcutaneous fat loss but this is usually slow and probably incomplete. Zidovudine remains a recommended agent for use in pregnant women to prevent mother-to-child HIV transmission.

Viruses resistant to currently recommended first-line NRTIs (tenofovir, abacavir, lamivudine and emtricitabine) will usually be susceptible to zidovudine and so it is also often useful as a second-line agent in those individuals who have virologically failed their initial treatment.

Stavudine is the other thymidine analogue in use. It is associated with a higher incidence of lipoatrophy, the onset of which is more rapid. Stavudine can also cause peripheral neuropathy, hyperlactatemia and lactic acidosis. The latter is a problem particularly in resource-poor regions as it is more commonly reported in women and the diagnosis may be delayed due to lack of available testing facilities. Stavudine has been dropped from most guidelines in developed countries and its widespread use in resource-poor countries, often for reasons of cost, is being widely questioned.

Abacavir and tenofovir

Abacavir–lamivudine or tenofovir with either lamivudine or emtricitabine have become the most commonly used NRTI backbones in developed countries. The ZODIAC study (CNA 30024) demonstrated abacavir–lamivudine (given twice daily) with efavirenz was not inferior to zidovudine–lamivudine and efavirenz.[5] Although both abacavir and lamivudine have plasma half-lives that do not appear to support once-daily dosing, intracellular concentrations of the active metabolites (both drugs need to be phosphorylated intracellularly) mean once-daily dosing is feasible. The CNA 30021 study demonstrated that abacavir and lamivudine given once daily (same daily dose) was not inferior to the standard twice-daily regimen. Again this was given in combination with efavirenz.[6]

The most important adverse effect of abacavir is a hypersensitivity reaction (HSR). This syndrome consists of multisystem presentation, usually 1–4 weeks after starting abacavir. Symptoms include fever, rash, abdominal pain, cough, shortness of breath and hypotension. When they start, symptoms are often mild but escalate in severity with each dose. The most serious problems, including shock and death, occur in those who continue treatment despite the development of hypersensitivity, or in those who stop drug and then are rechallenged with abacavir.

The prevalence of HSR in different populations varies widely, being seen most commonly in those of white race. Retrospective analyses have identified HLA-B*5701 carriage as the dominant risk factor for abacavir HSR. In the Predict study subjects starting treatment with an abacavir-containing regimen were randomized to have prospective HLA-B*5701 screening. Screening reduced the incidence of HSR to zero. The negative predictive value was 100% and the positive predictive value 50%.[7] HLA-B*5701 screening prior to using abacavir has become routine in clinical practice.

Two other important issues affect the use of abacavir in current clinical practice. The first is its association seen in cohort data with worsening cardiovascular risk. This appears to be most significant in those patients who already have a high cardiovascular risk that comprises at least five risk factors. The second is in one large clinical trial (ACTG 5202) of poorer efficacy seen in those ARV-naive patients who were randomized to receive abacavir and whose baseline viral load was over 100 000 copies/ml. More data are required to understand these issues and current guidelines suggest caution in using abacavir in these situations.

Tenofovir is an NRTI that also has activity against HBV. In the GS-934 study, tenofovir, lamivudine and efavirenz were compared over 144 weeks to zidovudine, lamivudine and efavirenz. In the primary time to loss of virologic response (TLOVR) analysis the tenofovir arm performed better. Much of the difference between the arms was related to early discontinuation in the zidovudine arm due to anemia and poorer tolerability.

Tenofovir and renal function

Numerous studies, including clinical trials, observational cohorts and expanded access data, have identified serious renal toxicity in approximately 0.5% of patients on tenofovir, a rate no different from that observed with comparator NRTIs. However, other studies have demonstrated a small but significant reduction in renal function over time when compared to other nucleosides. Tenofovir should be used cautiously in patients who have, or are at risk of developing, renal disease. This includes those who are co-prescribed other potentially nephrotoxic agents.

Lamivudine and emtricitabine

Lamivudine is a cytidine analogue and an important component of several recommended first-line combinations. It is very well tolerated and can be given either 150 mg twice daily or 300 mg once daily. It is also available as a component of the fixed-dose combinations Combivir (zidovudine, lamivudine), Trizivir (zidovudine, abacavir, lamivudine) and Kivexa (abacavir, lamivudine). Lamivudine has a low barrier to resistance. Viruses which contain the M184V mutation are, however, less 'fit' than wild-type viruses. Previous studies have demonstrated that patients with the M184V mutation who fail have plasma viral loads that do not return to pretreatment levels, remaining approximately 0.5 log below baseline. Lamivudine is also active against HBV.

Emtricitabine is a cytidine analogue similar to lamivudine. These drugs should not be used together. Emtricitabine is also active against HBV. This drug has been tested in randomized controlled trials in combination with tenofovir for the treatment of ARV-naive individuals and is available as part of a fixed-dose combination with tenofovir (Truvada) and with both tenofovir and efavirenz (Atripla).

Didanosine

Didanosine is an alternative agent for treating ARV-naive individuals and is usually given in combination with lamivudine and either an NNRTI or a protease inhibitor. Its use has been relatively limited in this context because of its tolerability and toxicity profile. While reformulation has improved tolerability, it is associated with pancreatitis, lactic acidosis and peripheral neuropathy. Recent reports have linked hepatic fibrosis and portal vein thrombosis with this drug. While these adverse effects are relative rare, their potential severity limits its use.

As it has activity against some viruses with resistance it is mostly used in second and subsequent lines of treatment. Due to pharmacokinetic interactions the dose of didanosine should be reduced if used in combination with tenofovir; however, due to concerns over efficacy and toxicity this combination should, where possible, be avoided.

Choosing either an NNRTI- or PI-based combination for first-line therapy

All currently recommended first-line therapies include a drug from the NNRTI or PI class. NNRTIs nevirapine and efavirenz have the benefit of low pill burden, potential for once-daily administration (although for nevirapine this is not a licensed schedule) and good gastrointestinal profile. However, they have a low barrier to resistance and a single mutation results in high-level resistance that impacts drugs within the same class. Both drugs but particularly nevirapine are associated with rare but potentially serious hepatic and/or cutaneous toxicity.

In contrast, ritonavir-boosted PIs are relatively forgiving in the face of suboptimal adherence, with high-level resistance usually requiring more than one mutation. Sequencing of PIs, even if resistance is present, may be possible. However PI-based combinations have a higher pill burden, sometimes have food requirements and the ritonavir used for pharmacokinetic boosting requires refrigeration. As a class they are more frequently associated with abdominal bloating and diarrhea. They are also implicated in aspects of the lipodystrophy syndrome including lipohypertrophy, insulin resistance and hyperlipidemia. Hypercholesterolemia can also occur with the NNRTI efavirenz.

One large strategic study (ACTG 5142) compared outcomes in those starting a two NRTI–efavirenz combination, a two NRTI (lopinavir–ritonavir) and an NRTI-sparing (efavirenz–lopinavir–ritonavir) combination. This study found that at 96 weeks the two NRTI–efavirenz group was associated with fewest virologic failures.[8] The NRTI-sparing arm also performed better than the PI arm but was the arm in which most resistance was seen in those who failed.

NNRTIs: Selecting nevirapine or efavirenz

The 2NN study compared nevirapine with efavirenz. Both drugs were given in combination with stavudine and lamivudine in treatment-naive individuals.[9] At 48 weeks 43.7% of the nevirapine twice-daily group and 37.8% of the efavirenz group failed. This difference of 5.9% (95% CI, 0.9–12.8) just failed to reach significance and hence the

combinations were non-inferior to one another. Two patients taking nevirapine died, one from hepatic toxicity and one from sepsis related to Stevens–Johnson syndrome.

These toxicities are well-recognized side-effects of nevirapine. To reduce the risk of these toxicities nevirapine should be started at a dose of 200 mg once daily. Patients should be reviewed at 2 weeks and the dose increased to 200 mg twice daily if there is no evidence of toxicity. The risks of these toxicities are substantially higher in those with higher CD4 counts and in women, hence it is recommended that nevirapine is not used in men with CD4 counts >400 cells/mm³ and in women with CD4 counts >250 cells/mm³.

While efavirenz may also be associated with both cutaneous and hepatic toxicity, the risk of serious problems is lower. However, efavirenz is associated with neuropsychiatric effects including dizziness, abnormal dreams, insomnia, hallucination and euphoria. These side-effects are more pronounced in the first 1–2 weeks of treatment. Occasionally patients report disabling side-effects which persist beyond this induction period, necessitating switching off efavirenz.

Congenital abnormalities have been observed in cynomolgus monkeys whose mothers were treated with efavirenz during pregnancy. While prospective studies of its use in pregnant women have failed to demonstrate an excess risk of congenital abnormalities, it remains the recommendation that an alternative agent is used in women trying to conceive or in those at higher risk of unplanned pregnancy.

Protease inhibitors

Protease inhibitors act on the binding to the catalytic site of the HIV aspartic protease. This enzyme is critical in the post-translational processing of the polyprotein products of *gag* and *gag-pol* genes into the functional core proteins and viral enzymes, respectively. Its inhibition leads to the release of immature, noninfectious viral particles.

Protease inhibitors are generally dependent on the cytochrome P450 3A4 hepatic isoenzyme for metabolism and can compete with other substrates of this enzyme. When the metabolism of other drugs that are dependent on the same enzyme is inhibited, the blood levels of these drugs can increase dramatically and toxic interactions may occur. This phenomenon has been evaluated for many of the compounds that are frequently used in patients who have HIV disease, and it has been shown that the combination of nucleoside analogues and PIs does not generally lead to untoward effects, although important pharmacokinetic interactions are possible for rifabutin, ketoconazole, rifampin (rifampicin), astemizole, terfenadine, cisapride and other drugs that are dependent on the same cytochrome enzyme.

Metabolic complications have emerged in patients treated with PIs. These include glucose metabolism abnormalities (hyperglycemia or diabetes), hyperlipidemia (mainly hypertriglyceridemia, with or without associated hypercholesterolemia), lipodystrophy or abnormal fat distribution (accumulation in the posterior neck, upper back and central abdomen). The pathogenesis of these abnormalities is still unclear and further studies are needed to define the role played by HIV infection, individual predisposing factors and treatment with specific drugs in the development of these complications.

Protease inhibitors are mostly co-prescribed with ritonavir. Ritonavir even at low dose is a potent inhibitor of cytochrome P450 3A4. This results in higher drug levels of the substrate PI over the dosing period, and is associated with a lower risk of virologic failure and a lower incidence of drug resistance in those individuals who fail treatment. The strategy to use ritonavir to boost PI levels and raise the barrier to resistance is one of the principal reasons, alongside availability of new drug classes, that 'salvage' of individuals with extensive drug resistance has been possible.

Saquinavir–ritonavir

Saquinavir has had three different formulations, the latest being that of a tablet. The recommended dose is saquinavir 1000 mg with ritonavir 100 mg twice daily. If once-daily treatment is desired in

ARV-naive patients, then saquinavir can be given at a dose of 1500–2000 mg with ritonavir 100 mg once daily. In the treatment of ARV-naive individuals, boosted saquinavir was found to be non-inferior to boosted lopinavir at 48 weeks both in combination with tenofovir and emtricitabine. There were more failures in the saquinavir arm (with drug resistance demonstrated by genotyping) than in the lopinavir arm.[10] Smaller increases in triglycerides were seen in the saquinavir arm.

Lopinavir–ritonavir

Lopinavir is a potent inhibitor of HIV-1 protease. Its bioavailability is greatly enhanced by co-administration of ritonavir and is therefore co-formulated both in a soft-gel capsule and the more recently developed, heat-stable tablet formulation. Available data indicate that the drug has good efficacy in previously untreated patients. Lopinavir is principally metabolized by the liver, and shares many of the drug interactions and contraindications common to other PIs. Two recent randomized controlled trials have shown better efficacy with atazanavir–ritonavir or darunavir–ritonavir when compared to lopinavir–ritonavir, partly driven by poorer tolerability of the lopinavir–ritonavir combination.

Fosamprenavir–ritonavir

Fosamprenavir is a prodrug of amprenavir. Metabolism of fosamprenavir increases the duration that amprenavir is available, making fosamprenavir a slow-release version of amprenavir and thus reducing the number of pills required versus standard amprenavir. A head-to-head study with lopinavir–ritonavir showed the two drugs to have comparable potency.[11] Principal side-effects include nausea, vomiting, abdominal bloating and diarrhea, along with rash, hypercholesterolemia and hypertriglyceridemia.

Atazanavir–ritonavir

Atazanavir was the first licensed once-a-day protease inhibitor to become available for use. While it can be given to ARV-naive individuals without ritonavir boosting (atazanavir 400 mg once daily) it is more commonly given with ritonavir (atazanavir 300 mg/ritonavir 100 mg once daily). Studies have demonstrated that patients failing unboosted atazanavir are more likely to develop mutations not only to protease inhibitors but also to the other components of the regimen.

The most common atazanavir-related side-effect is unconjugated hyperbilirubinemia due to atazanavir inhibiting glucuronosyltransferase. Elevated plasma bilirubin is not harmful in adults; however, individuals might find this unacceptable if they are noticeably jaundiced, particularly if scleral icterus is present. Atazanavir is less likely to cause both gastrointestinal side-effects and lipid abnormalities than other PIs. It is unknown whether fat redistribution, particularly the fat accumulation seen with other PIs, is also less likely with atazanavir. In the Castle study of ARV-naive patients, atazanavir 300 mg/ritonavir 100 mg with tenofovir and emtricitabine once daily was found to be non-inferior (in fact the data showed superiority) to lopinavir–ritonavir in combination at 96 weeks.[12]

Atazanavir has several important drug interactions:

- As it requires an acid gastric environment for optimal absorption, proton pump inhibitors such as omeprazole are contraindicated as they lead to lower plasma atazanavir levels. Care must also be taken with less potent reducers of gastric acidity such as ranitidine.
- Efavirenz induces the metabolism of atazanavir and, if co-prescribed, atazanavir should be given boosted with ritonavir and at a higher dose (atazanavir 400 mg/ritonavir 100 mg).
- Tenofovir leads to reduced atazanavir levels and, if co-prescribed, atazanavir should be given with ritonavir.

Darunavir–ritonavir

This is the most recently licensed protease inhibitor. In the Artemis study of ARV-naive patients, darunavir 800 mg/ritonavir 100 mg with tenofovir and emtricitabine once daily was found to be superior to lopinavir–ritonavir in combination at 96 weeks.[13] Ritonavir-boosted darunavir also has substantial activity against viruses with drug-resistance mutations and therefore is an important component of salvage regimens. In treatment-experienced individuals the recommended dose is darunavir 600 mg q12h/ritonavir 100 mg q12h.

MONITORING FIRST-LINE ANTIRETROVIRAL TREATMENT

Virologic and immunologic responses

The primary goal of first-line ARV treatment is to reduce the plasma viral load to undetectable levels. This has been shown to minimize the risk of selecting resistant viruses and is, as a result, associated with durability of treatment response. After initiating first-line ARV treatment it can take up to 24–32 weeks to reach undetectability on an ultrasensitive viral load assay (limit of detection 40–50 copies/ml). The viral load decline after treatment initiation occurs in three phases. The first phase representing the switching off of replication in productively infected cells is dramatic, with plasma viral loads often declining by 2–3 log in 2 weeks. Most individuals who will fully suppress have a viral load <1000 copies/ml by 8 weeks. Individuals started on ARVs should be reviewed in the first 2–4 weeks to assess for side-effects, toxicity and suboptimal adherence. If available, a viral load should be checked after 1 month on treatment.

CD4 responses to treatment are less predictable. In clinical trials, ARV-naive individuals given virologically effective treatment will have average CD4 increases of 150–200 cells in 48 weeks. However inter-subject variation is large, with some having only small increases in CD4 count (so-called discordant responders) and these patients may be older or have had prolonged HIV infection prior to treatment.

Adherence

Good adherence is critical to the success of ARV treatment. However, the minimal level of adherence necessary for success will depend on several factors, including the genetic barrier of the treatment regimen and the presence of drug resistance. Also important is the timing of nonadherence in relation to starting therapy. Poor adherence during the first few weeks when there is abundant replicating virus present is likely to be more risky than similar nonadherence when patients are fully suppressed. Self-report provides a quick, inexpensive way of assessing adherence although in some individuals probably overestimates compliance. The use of a combination of questions such as 7-day recall or a 30-day visual analogue scale has been recommended.

NEW STRATEGIES

To limit toxicity and/or cost some novel strategies using protease inhibitor monotherapy have been used both in individuals commencing treatment and in those on fully suppressive regimens. The data thus far show that this is relatively successful. However, in naive patients started on PI monotherapy a substantial proportion do not fully suppress, having viral loads between 50 and 500 cells/mm^3. It is not known what proportion of these patients will go on to evolve resistance and eventual virologic failure.

Another concern about this regimen is that it may not penetrate into sanctuary sites such as the brain, genital fluids, etc. This may leave virus replicating in these areas causing local disease, transmission or the development of resistance.

Newer drugs such as the integrase inhibitor raltegravir have been used successfully in ARV-naive patients and may have potential for first-line treatment in the future. The role of CCR5 inhibitors such as maraviroc is debatable.

WHEN TO CHANGE TREATMENT

In patients with fully suppressed virus

In these patients switching of ARVs is usually done to improve the patient's quality of life, improve adherence, and to avoid or prevent worsening of long-term toxicities. It is absolutely essential that any switches do not compromise antiviral efficacy. Drugs that have been previously used and have or may have been associated with prior antiviral failure and actual or potential resistance should be avoided.

There are some data supporting the concept that in HIV-infected persons regimens with reduced dosing frequency and low pill burdens have higher levels of adherence. Switching to a newer agent, co-formulated drugs or a formulation with a lower pill burden and dosing frequency, or one that would be less likely to cause toxicity, are strategies used to both simplify therapy and avoid toxicity. For example, changing from zidovudine or stavudine to tenofovir or abacavir may allow a regimen with a lower dosing frequency (e.g. once daily) that is co-formulated and can avoid or prevent worsening of long-term toxicities such as lipoatrophy, dyslipidemia, peripheral neuropathy, etc.[14] Switching from nevirapine to efavirenz can reduce dosing frequency and co-formulated agents will reduce the pill burden.

Switching from one PI to another, or even to the same PI at a lower dosing frequency (e.g. once a day), can reduce dosing frequency, pill count, drug–drug or drug–food interactions and dyslipidemia, or can take advantage of co-formulation. In some cases, atazanavir can be given without ritonavir if there is ritonavir intolerance or toxicity, but not if the patient is taking tenofovir because of its lowering effect on atazanavir plasma concentrations.

Switching from one class of drug to another is performed for all the above reasons. The most common substitutions for regimen simplification involve a change from a PI-based to an NNRTI-based regimen. Newer agents such as raltegravir and maraviroc might also be used in switching strategies.

Virologic failure

Virologic failure is usually defined as an inability to attain an undetectable viral load within 24–32 weeks after commencing therapy or confirmed rebound from undetectable levels. If an individual has developed resistance, the initial rebound viral load is usually low, mostly less than 1000 copies/ml. In time further mutations may ensue, resulting in higher levels of replicating virus. If the initial viral load rebound is high, this is usually due to periods of poor adherence. In this setting resistance mutations may also be identified on viral genotype. Significant falls in CD4 count and clinical disease are not usually seen with low-level virologic failure.

Resistance

It has been estimated that 10^9 to 10^{10} virions of HIV are produced per day. Mutations in the HIV genome arise spontaneously during the replication process on average once each time a viral genome is replicated. In uncontrolled HIV infection, the high HIV replication rate coupled with the mutation rate generates every possible mutation in the HIV genome each day. Thus a large pool of 'quasispecies' is created. These are genetically related but distinct HIV strains, any of which has the potential to be dominant. In most patients the dominant strain prior to any drug therapy can replicate rapidly and is termed 'wild type' based on its sequence. This wild type is usually fully susceptible to antiviral drugs. A potent ARV regimen will significantly inhibit HIV replication but an ineffective regimen or inadequate adherence by the patient will result in suboptimal inhibition of viral replication, and generation and selection of resistant mutations. It has been calculated – and borne out in clinical practice – that the selection out of any quasispecies is highly unlikely in the presence of three drugs to which the virus is susceptible. If only one or two drugs to which the virus is sensitive are used, the selection of resistant mutants will occur.

Mutations that provide a growth advantage in the presence of ARVs will allow a quasispecies to outcompete the others and become the dominant viral strain in the population, and the patient will have a 'resistant' virus.

Mutations cause resistance by structural alteration of the target molecule that prevents or reduces drug binding (in the case of PIs, NRTIs, NNRTIs and entry inhibitors), or by affecting viral enzyme function in ways that reduce the effectiveness of the drugs (in the case of NRTIs or integrase). They decrease the antiviral activity of the drugs used and cause lack of virologic response.

Most mutations also reduce the viral replication rate compared with that of wild-type virus and may take a long time to emerge as the major quasispecies. Resistance to PIs usually requires the accumulation of several mutations and this may take months or even years to occur.

Mutations associated with resistance to NNRTIs (e.g. Y181C or K103N) do not appear to affect the viral replication rate and so virus can appear as the dominant quasispecies in weeks after starting nevirapine- or efavirenz-based regimens.

Without continuous pressure on the virus to maintain the dominant strain (e.g. when the drugs are stopped), the wild-type strain will re-emerge as this is usually the most efficient at replicating. The mutated strain, however, does not disappear completely but will become a minority quasispecies, only to become dominant again if the drug that selected it is restarted.

Acquired resistance develops through the mechanism described above but primary drug resistance is through transmission of a resistant strain from one individual to another sexually, vertically or through infected blood. Rates of primary drug resistance vary with the methodology used, class of drug, risk behavior, geographic distribution and over time. Many centers are reporting declining rates or stable rates of primary drug resistance. Primary resistance occurs frequently enough in high-income countries to recommend baseline resistance testing prior to starting antiviral therapy for the first time.

Resistance by drug class

There are six licensed antiretroviral classes with 22 drugs in current use. The impact of various mutations alone and in combination is continuing to evolve as new drugs and new classes of these compounds are being developed.[15] There are now more than 200 mutations associated with antiretroviral resistance drugs.[16,17]

Nucleos(t)ide reverse transcriptase inhibitors

In the NRTI class there are 50 mutations associated with resistance to thymidine analogue- and nonthymidine analogue-containing regimens, as well as multinucleoside resistance mutations and accessory mutations.

M184V, nonthymidine analogue-associated mutations such as K65R and L74V, and the multinucleoside resistance mutation Q151M act by decreasing NRTI incorporation.

By promoting a phosphorolytic reaction, thymidine analogue mutations, the triple 69 insertions associated with multinucleoside resistance and many of the accessory mutations facilitate primer unblocking and enhanced removal of incorporated NRTI.

Thymidine analogue mutations associated with zidovudine and stavudine accumulate in two distinct but overlapping patterns:

- type I pattern mutations M41L, D67N, L210W and T215Y; and
- type II mutations D67N, K70R, T215F and K219Q/E.

The type I pattern causes higher levels of phenotypic and clinical resistance to the thymidine analogues than the type II pattern and cross-resistance to abacavir, didanosine and tenofovir.

Non-nucleoside reverse transcriptase inhibitors

Non-nucleoside reverse transcriptase inhibitors have more than 40 reverse transcriptase mutations associated with resistance, some of which, when occurring as single mutations, can confer resistance and cross-resistance to at least three drugs in this class. The primary NNRTI resistance mutations are K103N/S, V106A/M, Y181C/I/V, Y188L/C/H and G190A/S/E. Any one of these will cause high-level resistance to nevirapine and variable levels of resistance to efavirenz. The newer NNRTI etravirine usually requires multiple mutations for resistance to be significant. It appears to retain good activity against common single mutations (e.g. K103N.)

Protease inhibitors

Protease inhibitor resistance is complex and there are more than 60 mutations associated with reducing susceptibility to these drugs. These include major protease, accessory protease and protease cleavage site mutations.

More mutations are selected by PIs than by any other ARV class. There are 17 primary resistance mutations and usually a combination of several of these is required to develop high-level resistance. The effect of these PI resistance mutations on any individual PI can be difficult to predict when many mutations are present in the same virus isolate or when mutations occur in unusual patterns. Gag cleavage site mutations and accessory compensatory mutations can all impact on the susceptibility of the virus to these drugs.

Integrase inhibitors

There is already much known about resistance to the recently developed integrase inhibitors raltegravir and elvitegravir, with more than 30 integrase mutations found to be associated with these agents. Common mutations include N155H and Q148H/R/K.

Entry inhibitors

At least 15 gp41 mutations are associated with resistance to the fusion inhibitor enfuvirtide, the commonest occurring between positions 36 and 45. Resistance to the entry inhibitors targeting the CCR5 receptor (e.g. maraviroc) is unusual and more complex, resulting from mutations that promote gp120 binding of the virus to the CCR5 receptor which is bound to the drug. The majority of virologic failures with this drug, however, are the outgrowth of minority species that can use the alternative CXCR4 receptor for entry.

Measuring resistance

Most resistance tests use genomic sequencing techniques ('genotyping') that are sufficiently sensitive to pick up quasispecies which comprise at least 20% of the viral swarm as long as the viral load is >1000 copies/ml. The sequences are then analyzed to produce a mutation list and this is related to whether a particular drug is predicted to be active or not. Phenotypic techniques are also available but are expensive and time consuming, and add little extra information above genotyping. More sensitive tests looking at minority quasispecies are in development.

Rates of resistance

Currently, approximately half of treated patients undergoing testing show evidence of drug resistance and around 11% have evidence of resistance mutations affecting at least three classes of antiretroviral drug. Primary resistance is found in around 5% of patients but varies from <1% to 15% depending on geography and how long ARV therapy has been available.

Use of resistance tests

The use of resistance tests allows optimal drug combinations to be selected by the physician. Most guidelines suggest that a baseline resistance test be performed at first presentation in case there has been primary transmitted resistance.

The prevalence of drug resistance has declined among treatment-experienced patients in many developed countries as a result of improved management of HIV antiviral treatment with more and better drugs being available. One important consequence has been the improved management of treatment failure.

Resistance testing is recommended in all patients experiencing virologic failure while on treatment and changes in therapy should be guided by the results of resistance testing in these patients. Other factors in choosing therapy are also important, especially drug history as some mutations are 'lost' over time. This is especially true of the M184V mutation which cannot usually be found by routine genotyping once these drugs have been discontinued. It is inferred to be present in patients who have had virologic failure on these drugs but the resistance test was performed some time after the drug was discontinued. This phenomenon is why resistance testing should be performed at the time of virologic failure when the patient is still on the drug combination.

Viral load blips

Transient rises in viral load levels to detectable from undetectable can occur frequently. They may represent 'noise' on the viral load assay or events related to viral replication such as intercurrent systemic infection or vaccination. If low-level detectable viremia represents early virologic failure, persistently detectable viral loads are usually seen, although these may remain low level for long periods despite significant development of resistance. If this is a true 'blip', a single detectable viral load is followed by a return to the undetectable state. It is controversial as to whether blips are associated with a future risk of virologic failure but most are probably bursts of replication of wild-type virus from latently infected cells.

PRINCIPLES OF SECOND- AND THIRD-LINE TREATMENTS

Individuals with virologic failure should be changed to a regimen of antiretroviral drugs based on treatment history and resistance testing, which provides two to three fully active drugs. This may result in drugs being recycled in subsequent lines of therapy if no significant resistance is present, sequencing onto new drugs in the same class if there is nonoverlapping resistance or incorporating new classes of drug. In switching for reasons of side-effects or toxicity, care needs to be taken where a particular toxicity may be a class effect. With the number of new drugs available now most patients can have three or four lines of therapy constructed in this manner.

Other drugs available to use in second and subsequent lines of therapy

Non-nucleoside reverse transcriptase inhibitors

The problems related to this class include:
- a single mutation causing high-level cross-class resistance;
- toxicity (rash and hepatotoxicity for nevirapine) and neuropsychiatric and lipid effects (efavirenz); and
- teratogenicity (CNS malformations were seen in monkey studies on efavirenz).

New generation NNRTIs have to overcome these obstacles before being acceptable and becoming drugs of choice for highly active antiretroviral therapy (HAART) regimens. Etravirine was licensed for use in 2008.

Protease inhibitors

Tipranavir is a nonpeptide protease inhibitor which is administered with ritonavir. Tipranavir has activity against viruses that are resistant to other protease inhibitors and is recommended for patients who are resistant to other treatments. Resistance to tipranavir itself seems to require multiple mutations. However, side-effects of tipranavir can be more severe than other antiretrovirals. It needs to be co-administered with ritonavir 200 mg twice daily and this exposure is tolerated poorly by a significant proportion of patients. It is associated with higher rates of liver toxicity and gastrointestinal intolerance than other PIs. There are also significant pharmacokinetic interactions with other antiretrovirals, including agents used in salvage therapy such as etravirine.

CCR5 inhibitors

Maraviroc

Maraviroc is the first CCR5 receptor antagonist licensed for the treatment of HIV infection. Co-receptor tropism should be determined prior to using maraviroc as it is not effective against CXCR4-tropic or mixed- or dual-tropic viruses. Maraviroc is a substrate of cytochrome P450 (CYP3A) and p-glycoprotein, and has clinically significant interactions with other drugs including efavirenz and rifampin.

In the MOTIVATE 1 and 2 studies that compared maraviroc with placebo, each given in combination with an optimized background regimen to patients with advanced HIV disease and CCR5-tropic HIV-1, at 48 weeks the rates of virologic suppression to <50 copies/ml were not significant, although the mean increase in CD4 cell count was greater in the maraviroc groups.[19] Virologic failure is usually associated with the emergence of CXCR4 virus as the development of resistance mutations is rare.

Maraviroc did not reach nonsignificance when compared to efavirenz, both combined with zidovudine and lamivudine in HIV treatment-naive patients. The result was influenced by the relatively low sensitivity of the tropism assay used.

Fusion inhibitors

Enfuvirtide blocks HIV-1 entry by inhibiting fusion. It is expensive and needs to be given by subcutaneous injection twice daily. These factors have limited its widespread use. Individuals frequently develop painful injection site reactions, the impact of which can to some degree be limited by careful attention to injection technique. The effectiveness of this novel agent has been demonstrated as salvage treatment of individuals with extensive, often triple class resistance. The use of enfuvirtide is largely being replaced with newer oral agents such as raltegravir, maraviroc and etravirine.

Integrase inhibitors

Integrase inhibitors target the viral integrase enzyme, which plays an important role in the viral life cycle. The integrase inhibitors the furthest in development are raltegravir (formerly MK-0518), which has been approved by the FDA, and EMEA for use in treatment-experienced patients. It is given twice daily.

OTHER AGENTS IN ADVANCED DEVELOPMENT

The need for new drugs?

Currently licensed drugs have short- and long-term toxicities. Convenience and ease of adherence are important in constructing regimens that are easy to tolerate. Once-a-day dosing and a low pill burden are important

factors in achieving these aims. Moreover, patients who have developed virologic failure, often with multiple resistant mutations, need new drugs that are active against these drug-resistant strains. New drugs that penetrate into sanctuary sites that may act as a reservoir for HIV replication such as the CNS and genital tract are much in need. Finally, new ARV drugs known to be safe in pregnancy would be a valuable addition to the currently available treatment options for HIV infection.

DRUG–DRUG INTERACTIONS

Most drug interactions with ARVs are mediated through inhibition or induction of hepatic drug metabolism. For example, all PIs and NNRTIs are metabolized in the liver by the cytochrome P450 system, particularly by the CYP3A4 isoenzyme. Some PIs may also be inducers or inhibitors of other CYP isoenzymes and of p-glycoprotein or other transporters. There is an extensive and continuously expanding list of drugs that may have significant interactions not only with PIs or NNRTIs but also with new drug classes. Some examples include medications that are commonly prescribed for non-HIV medical conditions, such as statins, benzodiazepines, calcium channel blockers, ciclosporin and tacrolimus, anticonvulsants, rifamycins, sildenafil, ergot derivatives, azole antifungals, macrolides, oral contraceptives and methadone. St John's wort, a herbal product, can cause a decrease in PI plasma levels.

The inhibitory effect of ritonavir is used to advantage in boosting concentrations of the other PIs but may cause abnormally high levels of some drugs such as simvastatin. The NNRTIs CYP3A4-inducing effect can be an issue when giving atazanavir or lopinavir–ritonavir. Efavirenz can cause PI concentration to fall.

These drug interactions are not always predictable. As an example, tenofovir interacts with didanosine, increasing didanosine intracellular levels, but will decrease atazanavir plasma concentrations.

There are web-based and other resources to help identify drug–drug interactions between antiretrovirals and between other commonly prescribed drugs. A good source is the 2008 DHHS guidelines and interactive web sites http://www.hiv-druginteractions.org and http://www.hivpharmacology.com.

HAART AND ANTITUBERCULOUS THERAPY

There are many difficulties when it comes to managing tuberculosis (TB) and HIV co-infection. When to start antiretroviral treatment in a patient on antituberculous therapy has been an ongoing issue. Studies suggest that delaying HAART can lead to a worse prognosis with progression to AIDS and death. The fear of poor adherence, drug interactions, toxicity and development of immune reconstitution inflammatory syndrome (IRIS) might be outweighed by this risk of progression and death if the HIV remains untreated in the severely immunocompromised with CD4 counts <200 cells/mm^3. Randomized controlled trials are ongoing to try to answer this question.

Drug interactions with the essential component of TB treatment – the rifamycins – are a problem.[25,26] Rifamycins are potent inducers of drug efflux p-glycoprotein and of the cytochrome P450 enzyme system, especially 3A4 which is responsible for the metabolism of PIs, NNRTIs and the CCR5 inhibitor maraviroc. Rifampin also induces metabolism of the integrase inhibitor raltegravir.

This limits the drugs that can be used with rifampin, leaving four nucleoside regimens thus far of unproven efficacy in HIV, or using efavirenz (600–800 mg/day) or nevirapine plus nucleosides. Efavirenz is preferred because of the better interaction profile and better efficacy seen in a cohort study from South Africa. Efavirenz doses are adjusted by some physicians to 800 mg if the patient is over 60 kg and the use of drug level monitoring can be useful in this situation. Protease inhibitors boosted with ritonavir can lead to significant decreases in plasma levels and a high rate of hepatotoxicity with rifampin. If they have to be used, it is better to switch to rifabutin.

There are many overlapping toxicities of HAART and antituberculous therapy. Stavudine in particular should not be used as it leads to increased rates of peripheral neuropathy and overlaps with isoniazid in terms of this side-effect. Hepatitis and rash are other common toxicities and this is another reason why nevirapine should be used with caution.

CHRONIC HEPATITIS

Co-infection of chronic HBV or HCV with HIV increases the rate of progression to cirrhosis and liver cancer by four- to fivefold compared with hepatitis monoinfected individuals. The mortality rate of untreated HIV/HBV or HIV/HCV co-infected patients is approximately 10 times higher than that of patients with either infection alone.[26,27]

Antiretroviral therapy may reduce the rate of progression to cirrhosis and death in these patients and in those with HCV infection.

There is a chance of cure with specific therapy. Zidovudine, didanosine and abacavir interact with this therapy and should be avoided.

Tenofovir, lamivudine and emtricitabine are agents that work against HIV; however, as they also suppress hepatitis B viral replication, they should be included in regimens given to patients co-infected with HIV and HBV. The treatment of these co-infections is discussed in Practice Points 44 and 46.

PREGNANCY

In pregnant women, prevention of mother-to-child transmission (PMTCT) is paramount. Maximal continual viral suppression is needed to reduce the risk of transmission of HIV to the fetus and newborn (see Chapter 98).

The choice of an antiretroviral combination in pregnant women should be based on the safety, efficacy and pharmacokinetic data of drugs used during pregnancy. Results of a baseline resistance test are important in this situation.

Efavirenz should be avoided in a pregnant woman during the first trimester and many women switch away from this to a boosted PI prior to becoming pregnant. Boosted PIs such as lopinavir–ritonavir and saquinavir–ritonavir have been used safely and effectively in pregnancy. A more detailed discussion of this issue can be found in Chapter 98 and guidelines for the management of pregnancy and HIV can be found at US Department of Health and Human Services Public Health Service Task Force *Recommendations for Use of Antiretroviral Drugs in Pregnant HIV-Infected Women for Maternal Health* and *Interventions to Reduce Perinatal HIV Transmission in the United States* (http://aidsinfo. nih.gov/ContentFiles/PerinatalGL.pdf), the British HIV Association pregnancy guidelines (http://www.bhiva.org/cms1191540.asp) and the European AIDS Clinical Society antiviral guidelines (http://www. europeanaidsclinicalsociety.org/guidelines.asp).

REFERENCES

References for this chapter can be found online at http://www.expertconsult.com

Charles W Flexner
Paul A Pham

Drug interactions in HIV and AIDS

INTRODUCTION

The recognition and management of pharmacokinetic and pharmacodynamic drug interactions is a major factor in choosing drugs and designing dosage regimens for the HIV-infected patient. Complex multidrug regimens have become the standard of care and clinicians must be aware of the potential need for dosage alterations with combination therapy. Many of the antiretrovirals in current use can alter concentrations of concomitantly administered drugs or have their own concentrations altered by other agents. These interactions can be detrimental or beneficial to the patient.

NUCLEOSIDE REVERSE TRANSCRIPTASE INHIBITORS

The nucleoside reverse transcriptase inhibitors (NRTIs) are primarily eliminated by renal mechanisms and thus they are not generally involved in clinically significant pharmacokinetic interactions. These agents can be used with protease inhibitors, CCR5 antagonist (maraviroc), integrase inhibitor (raltegravir), fusion inhibitor (enfuvirtide) and non-nucleoside reverse transcriptase inhibitors (NNRTIs) without the need for dosage alterations. Two NRTIs – zidovudine and abacavir – are eliminated in part by hepatic glucuronidation. Inducers of glucuronyl transferase activity can modestly lower plasma concentrations of these agents, although the clinical significance of this is uncertain since the active metabolites are intracellular nucleoside triphosphates.

Nucleoside reverse transcriptase inhibitors may interact pharmacodynamically with agents that have similar side-effect profiles. Increased bone marrow toxicity may be observed when zidovudine is used with other drugs capable of bone marrow suppression, such as ganciclovir, pyrimethamine, sulfamethoxazole and chemotherapy. Many NRTI-induced toxicities have been attributed to inhibition of mitochondrial DNA (mtDNA) polymerase, which results in depletion of mtDNA and consequently depletion of components of the electron transport chain encoded by mtDNA. Common examples of mitochondrial toxicity include peripheral neuropathy and lipoatrophy. Lactic acidosis, which may be accompanied by hepatosteatosis, can be fatal. Although there is a US Food and Drug Administration (FDA) black box warning for all NRTIs, zidovudine, didanosine and stavudine have been the most commonly implicated agents. The combination of didanosine plus stavudine and/or hydroxyurea has been particularly associated with pancreatitis, peripheral neuropathy and lactic acidosis, and should be avoided.

The NRTI tenofovir increases the plasma concentrations of concomitantly administered didanosine and may increase the toxicity of didanosine if standard doses are used. A dose reduction to didanosine 250 mg/day for patients >60 kg or 200 mg daily for patients <60 kg can be considered, but the co-administration of didanosine, tenofovir and an NNRTI is generally not recommended due to the high rate of virologic failure.

NON-NUCLEOSIDE REVERSE TRANSCRIPTASE INHIBITORS

Etravirine (ETR) is a CYP3A4, 2C19, and 2C9 substrate and also undergoes glucuronidation *in vitro*. Unlike efavirenz and nevirapine, etravirine does not induce its own metabolism. ETR is a mild inducer of CYP3A4, 2B6, and glucuronidation *in vitro*, but also inhibits 2C9 and 2C19. Due to ETR induction properties, co-administration of ETR with unboosted PIs is not recommended. Although co-administration with boosted darunavir resulted in a 37% reduction in the ETR AUC, the combination has performed well in clinical trials and can be co-administered in treatment-experienced patients. Potent enzyme inducers such as rifampin, rifapentine, phenobarbital, carbamazepine, phenytoin, and St. John's wort should be avoided with ETR. In a cocktail study with warfarin, a 2C9 substrate, warfarin concentrations were significantly increased; therefore, close INR monitoring with ETR co-administration is critical.

PROTEASE INHIBITORS

Etravirine (ETR) is a CYP3A4, 2C19, and 2C9 substrate and also undergoes glucuronidation *in vitro*. Unlike efavirenz and nevirapine, etravirine does not induce its own metabolism. ETR is a mild inducer of CYP3A4, 2B6, and glucuronidation *in vitro*, but also inhibits 2C9 and 2C19. Due to ETR induction properties, co-administration of ETR with unboosted PIs is not recommended. Although co-administration with boosted darunavir resulted in a 37% reduction in the ETR AUC, the combination has performed well in clinical trials and can be co-administered in treatment-experienced patients. Potent enzyme inducers such as rifampin, rifapentine, phenobarbital, carbamazepine, phenytoin, and St. John's wort should be avoided with ETR. In a cocktail study with warfarin, a 2C9 substrate, warfarin concentrations were significantly increased; therefore, close INR monitoring with ETR co-administration is critical.

The potent inhibition of CYP3A4 by ritonavir is routinely used to optimize the AUC of all protease inhibitors except nelfinavir. For example, concomitant administration with ritonavir results in a 20-fold increase in steady-state saquinavir concentrations, allowing for a dosage and frequency reduction of saquinavir, while maintaining high blood concentrations. With ritonavir co-administration, once-daily dosing of atazanavir, fosamprenavir, saquinavir and lopinavir is possible. These combinations successfully suppress HIV replication in clinical trials in protease inhibitor-naive subjects.

In addition to enzyme inhibition, ritonavir and nelfinavir possess moderate enzyme-inducing properties and decrease concentrations of a number of co-administered agents. Ritonavir, lopinavir/ritonavir and nelfinavir increase glucuronosyl transferase activity. Ethinyl estradiol and progesterone concentrations can be decreased by concomitant administration of these protease inhibitors, necessitating alternative forms of birth control.

Similar to other protease inhibitors, tipranavir (TPV) is a substrate and inhibitor of CYP3A4; however, TPV is also a substrate and potent inducer of the p-glycoprotein drug transporter, P-gp. When co-administered with ritonavir, TPV/ritonavir produces a net inhibition of CYP3A4 which results in an increased plasma concentration of CYP3A4 substrate (i.e. atorvastatin). However, for drugs that are dual substrates of CYP3A4 and P-gp, a net induction results. For example, an AUC decrease of 45%, 49% and 70% was observed with amprenavir (APV), lopinavir/ritonavir (LPV/r), and saquinavir (SQV) co-administration, respectively.

Certain enzyme-inducing agents can profoundly decrease the concentrations of protease inhibitors. For example, rifampin has been shown to decrease the saquinavir AUC by 80% and the indinavir AUC by 65%. The resulting low blood concentrations have the potential to promote drug resistance and treatment failure, so all protease inhibitors (with the possible exception of LPV/r 400/100 mg plus RTV 300 mg q12h) should be avoided in patients receiving rifampin. Rifabutin can be considered as an alternative to rifampin, but the rifabutin dose must be decreased to 150 mg three times a week with boosted protease inhibitor co-administration. Other potent enzyme inducers, such as phenytoin, phenobarbital and carbamazepine, are likely to produce similar reductions in PI concentrations.

CCR5 ANTAGONIST

Maraviroc, the first FDA-approved CCR5 antagonist, does not inhibit or induce CYP3A4 or glucuronyl transferase activity. Unlike protease inhibitor or non-nucleoside reverse transcriptase inhibitors, maraviroc does not affect the pharmacokinetics of oral contraceptives or midazolam. As maraviroc is a substrate for CYP3A4 and P-gp, the dose of maraviroc should be halved when co-administered with CYP3A4 and/or P-gp inhibitors. When maraviroc is co-administered with HIV-protease inhibitors (with the exception of tipranavir/ritonavir) a two- to eightfold elevation of maraviroc's AUC was observed. On the other hand, efavirenz and rifampin, CYP3A4 inducers, significantly decrease maraviroc's serum concentrations. Maraviroc's dose should be adjusted based on the CYP3A4 inhibitors and/or inducers with which it is combined (Table PP45.1).

Table PP45.1 Consequences of selected CYP450-mediated drug interactions

	Agents affected	Recommendations
CYP3A4 inhibitors		
All protease inhibitors (PI)* Cimetidine Clarithromycin Delavirdine Erythromycin Itraconazole Ketoconazole Nefazodone Telithromycin	*Increased concentration of co-administered drug:* Antiarrhythmics (amiodarone, disopyramide, dofetilide, flecainide, lidocaine, mexiletine, propafenone, and quinidine); calcium channel antagonists, fentanyl, maraviroc, midazolam, simvastatin, lovastatin, triazolam, pimozide, rifabutin, terfenadine, astemizole, cisapride, ergotamine, erectile dysfunction agents	Decrease maraviroc dose to 150 mg q12h Use calcium channel antagonist with close monitoring Reduce rifabutin dose to 150 mg three times a week with boosted PI co-administration Avoid midazolam, triazolam, fentanyl, terfendadine, astemizole, cisapride, ergotamine, pimozide, simvastatin, and lovastatin co-administration
CYP3A4 inducers		
Efavirenz (EFV) Nevirapine (NVP) Anticonvulsants (i.e. phenytoin, carbamazepine, phenobarbital) Rifampin (rifampicin) Rifapentine, St John's wort	*Decreased concentration of co-administered drug:* All PIs, methadone, maraviroc	With EFV or NVP co-administration, administer all PIs with ritonavir Maraviroc dose should be increased to 600 mg twice daily Methadone dose may need to be increased with EFV or NVP co-administration Consider valproic acid or levetiracetam with CYP3A4 inducers Avoid rifampin and St John's wort with PIs and methadone co-administration
P-gp inducer		
Tipranavir/ritonavir (TPV/r)	All PIs	Avoid PI co-administration with TPV/r
UGT-glucuronosyl transferase enzyme inducers		
Lopinavir/ritonavir Ritonavir Nelfinavir Rifampin (rifampicin) Phenobarbital Phenytoin	*Decreased concentration of co-administered drug:* Oral contraceptive (ethinyl estradiol and progesterone) and raltegravir	Consider alternative barrier form of contraception or medroxyprogesterone Low-dose ritonavir (100 mg q12h) can be administered with raltegravir, but rifampin, phenobarbital and phenytoin should be avoided
Acid blockers		
H₂-blockers Proton pump inhibitors (PPIs) Antacids	*Decreased concentrations of co-administered drug:* Atazanavir, nelfinavir and delavirdine	Avoid co-administration with PPIs H₂-blockers or antacids may be administered 2 hours after atazanavir, nelfinavir and delavirdine administration

*Atazanavir, darunavir, fosamprenavir, lopinavir, ritonavir, saquinavir and tipranavir.

INTEGRASE INHIBITOR

Raltegravir, the first FDA-approved integrase inhibitor, is mainly metabolized by glucuronidation (like zidovudine) and thus should be less susceptible to drug interactions. Its metabolism is partially blocked by atazanavir, a selective inhibitor of the UGT-glucuronosyl transferase enzyme UGT1A1; this resulted in a 41% increase in the raltegravir AUC, but no dose adjustment is needed. Potent inducers of UGT-glucuronosyl transferase enzymes (i.e. rifampin, phenobarbital and phenytoin) can significantly decrease raltegravir concentrations and should be avoided.

MANAGEMENT OF DRUG INTERACTIONS

A careful review of patient medication profiles is essential to managing drug interactions in the HIV-infected patient. This should include complementary and alternative medicines, since agents such as St John's wort induce CYP3A4 and can reduce concentrations of indinavir and presumably other protease inhibitors. Clinicians need to have a general understanding of certain 'red flag' drugs that are potent inhibitors and inducers of CYP450 (i.e. rifampin, ritonavir, efavirenz, etc.). In this era of complex regimens, computerized pharmacy systems can detect many drug–drug interactions and decrease the number of inappropriate prescriptions; however, a limitation of such systems is their inability to update information beyond the FDA-approved labeling. Therefore, clinicians are encouraged to use computerized and internet-based databases that are updated more regularly. In addition, clinicians should be vigilant about the potential for drug interactions.

Patient counseling is critically important when complex antiretroviral regimens are prescribed. Patients must be instructed on how to take their medications with regard to timing and content of meals. In some cases, a written daily calendar of medications and times of administration may be useful to the patient and may improve adherence. Proper separation of dosing of certain drugs (i.e. didanosine without food and atazanavir with food) must be explained and can also be documented on a daily dosage planner.

The HIV clinician can use a variety of interventions to manage drug interactions. Selection of a drug with fewer interactions should be considered if warranted by the clinical situation. For example, azithromycin is not metabolized by CYP450 and has far fewer drug interactions compared with other macrolides. Also, drugs that can be administered once or twice daily may be useful to lessen food-related interactions or dosage separation problems. Finally, clinicians should be aware of and try to avoid drugs with overlapping toxicities. However, such combinations are sometimes unavoidable and patients who receive these agents must be closely monitored for the development of toxicity.

FURTHER READING

Further reading for this chapter can be found online at http://www.expertconsult.com

Stanislas Pol
Anaïs Vallet-Pichard
Vincent Mallet

Practice point | **46** |

How to manage the hepatitis C virus co-infected HIV patient

While hepatitis C virus (HCV) infection has no clear impact on HIV infection, HIV infection clearly has a deleterious impact on the natural history of HCV infection, especially since the introduction of highly active antiretroviral therapy (HAART). The higher hepatitis C viral load leads to higher contagiosity, increased liver-related morbidity and mortality. Since the improvement in treating HCV infection paralleled the progress in treating HIV, the question now is how to manage HIV–HCV co-infected patients.

WHY EVALUATE HIV–HEPATITIS C VIRUS CO-INFECTION?

Anti-HCV antibodies are detected in around 10–30% of HIV-infected patients; they reflect active infection as assessed by detectable hepatitis C viremia in most. The impact of HIV on HCV is characterized:

- by increasing levels of hepatitis C viremia;
- by significantly increasing the risk of mother-to-child or sexual transmission (from a mean of 6–20% and from 0% to 3%, respectively); and
- by increasing (two- to fivefold) and accelerating the risk of cirrhosis and of occurrence of cirrhosis complications; the progression of fibrosis depends on the CD4 cell count level (<200 cells/mm^3), chronic alcohol consumption and steatosis.

Thus, HCV infection is, since HAART, one of the leading causes of morbidity and mortality of HIV-1-infected patients which underlines the need for early diagnostic procedures and therapeutic strategies.

The pathobiology of the severity of liver disease in co-infected patients is multifactorial, including:

- rarely immune restoration;
- direct viral cytotoxicity in immunocompromised patients;
- nonalcoholic steatohepatitis (NASH) related mainly to the metabolic syndrome which may be induced by HAART;
- all the classic causes of liver toxicity (alcohol but also vascular diseases such as nodular regenerative hyperplasia); and
- drug-related hepatic toxicity and all antiviral drugs having potential toxicity (Fig. PP46.1).

The rate of HAART withdrawal in relation to hepatotoxicity is around 2% without significant difference regarding the type of antiretroviral treatment. Nucleoside reverse transcriptase inhibitors cause rare but severe hepatitis, which is due to a mitochondrial cytopathy with severe microsteatosis and lethal lactic acidosis. Non-nucleoside reverse transcriptase inhibitors are responsible for clinical hepatitis in 2–5% of cases, which are sometimes severe (0.1% of cases) and are associated with signs of hypersensitivity in two-thirds of cases. Drug-related hepatitis in association with protease inhibitors is observed in 2–8.5% of treated patients, with a predilection for patients co-infected with HCV or HBV. In most cases of drug-related hepatitis, liver biochemical abnormalities resolve after discontinuation of the drug.

Fig. PP46.1 Potential interactions of mechanisms of liver disease in HIV-infected patients

THERAPEUTIC IMPLICATIONS

The deleterious impact of HIV on HCV infection underlines the need for reliable anti-HCV antiviral therapies. All anti-HCV-positive, HIV-co-infected patients have to be carefully evaluated. HCV RNA detection will delineate patients with complete recovery (HCV RNA-negative) from those with active infection (HCV RNA-positive). These latter patients will undergo evaluation of the liver impact of HCV infection either by a liver biopsy or by noninvasive procedures (biochemical or morphologic by evaluation of liver stiffness).

Antiviral treatment is preceded by exclusion of nucleoside analogues which may:

- enhance ribavirin-associated anemia or interferon-induced neutropenia (azidothymidine);
- interfere with ribavirin metabolism with an enhanced risk of mitochondrial toxicity (didanosine); or
- exacerbate decompensation of liver disease (didanosine, stavudine and nevirapine). The negative influence of abacavir is questioned.

In five randomized clinical trials, 27–55% of co-infected patients who received the pegylated interferon (α2a: 180 μg or α2b: 1.5 μg/kg subcutaneously weekly) plus ribavirin (800–1200 mg/day according to the weight) combination, the recommended anti-HCV therapy, attained sustained virologic response. Absence of early virologic response (a decrease in serum HCV RNA of ≥2 $\log_{10}$ from baseline or undetectable HCV RNA at week 12) has an accurate negative predictive value (98–100% of absence of sustained virologic response, SVR); on the other hand, rapid virologic response (undetectable HCV RNA at week 4 of therapy) has a high positive predictive value of approximately 90% of SVR. Because of this accuracy, the European treatment guidelines adopted the 12-week stopping rule in co-infected patients without early virologic response.

There is no deleterious impact of the interferon–ribavirin combination on immune status with a reduction of the absolute CD4 T-cell counts during treatment (the mean decrease ranging from 130 cells/mm³ to 331 cells/mm³) but the percentage of the CD4 T-cell count either increased or remained stable: CD4 T-cell counts generally returned to baseline levels after completion of therapy.

PRAGMATIC MANAGEMENT OF HEPATITIS C VIRUS CO-INFECTED PATIENTS

Pre-existing biochemical abnormalities do not contraindicate the use of antiretroviral drugs. In some difficult situations (e.g. cirrhosis, liver transplantation), the measurement of the plasma levels of antiretroviral drugs may be valuable in order to avoid any overdoses that may lead to hepatotoxicity. In HCV–HIV co-infected patients, monthly biochemical follow-up is warranted in the first 3 months after introduction of any new antiretroviral drug and then every 3 months in order to identify potential drug-related toxicity. An increase in alanine aminotransferase levels (five times the upper normal value, but the rate of increase is more important than the absolute values) should lead to a switch of the protease inhibitor or to the introduction of a non-nucleoside reverse transcriptase inhibitor. Biochemical liver abnormalities occurring with a non-nucleoside reverse transcriptase inhibitor should lead to treatment withdrawal, especially if cutaneous signs of hypersensitivity are associated. However, the interpretation of such biochemical liver abnormalities is difficult, raising not only the question of drug-related hepatitis but also of other toxic causes such as alcohol, cocaine or metamphetamine.

An unsolved question is the respective place of anti-HCV and anti-HIV therapies. In clinical practice, most HIV patients are referred to the hepatologist while receiving HAART and the question is not relevant. In the future, physicians will have to consider the priority of each treatment according to liver histology and immune status. Given the chance of complete eradication of HCV-associated chronic hepatitis (SVR), anti-HCV therapy should be considered a priority and be treated first if the CD4 lymphocyte count is not less than 300 cells/mm³. Marked necroinflammatory activity or fibrosis (A2-A3 or F3-F4) indicates a need for anti-HCV treatment in order to avoid deleterious evolution; in contrast, low inflammatory activity or fibrosis (A0-A1 or F0-F1) does not necessarily indicate anti-HCV treatment but does indicate liver follow-up by biopsy every 3 years or noninvasive biochemical or morphologic evaluation of fibrosis each year. In intermediate situations (A2-F2), the choice to treat or not to treat should be based mainly on predictive factors, including genotype and quantitative viremia (Fig. PP46.2).

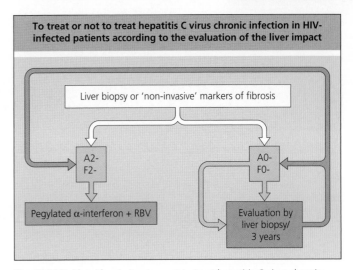

Fig. PP46.2 Algorithm to treat or not to treat hepatitis C virus chronic infection in HIV-infected patients according to the evaluation of the liver impact. RBV, ribavirin.

The newest recommendations from the 1st European Consensus Conference on the Treatment of Chronic Hepatitis B and C in HIV Co-infected Patients deal with three circumstances during the evolution of the disease:

1. during the acute phase of HCV infection (treatment outcomes are improved if treatment is initiated early);
2. during the chronic stage of hepatitis C, in which SVR rates can restrict progression to cirrhosis and hepatocellular carcinoma; and
3. finally, at the stage of cirrhosis, treatment is indicated to decrease the risk for hepatocellular carcinoma or other complications (e.g. portal hypertension and liver failure) that may necessitate liver transplantation.

In conclusion, physicians should be aware of the potential risk of:

- symptomatic liver disease in HCV–HIV co-infected patients in the era of antiretroviral therapy;
- liver deterioration paralleling immune function restoration, steatosis and immune deficiency;
- lack of clear impact of active antiretroviral therapy on HCV load; and
- potential drug-related hepatitis that may modify the natural history of HCV-related liver disease.

Liver evaluation of HCV infection should be performed regularly to identify patients with severe liver disease who require early anti-HCV therapy (see Fig. PP46.2) under close monitoring of their immune status.

FURTHER READING

🖱 Further reading for this chapter can be found online at http://www.expertconsult.com

How to manage hyperlipidemia in the HIV patient

CASE HISTORY

A 48-year-old man with HIV infection presents for routine follow-up. He was diagnosed with HIV in 2000 when he developed *Pneumocystis* pneumonia. He has maintained an undetectable HIV RNA on his current regimen of zidovudine, lamivudine and efavirenz. He has no family history of diabetes or heart disease. He smokes one pack of cigarettes per day and drinks a six pack of beer 2 nights per week. His physical examination is normal and his blood pressure is 142/80 mmHg. Fasting lipid values include triglycerides of 420 mg/dl (4.75 mmol/l), total cholesterol 260 mg/dl (6.73 mmol/l) and HDL cholesterol 28 mg/dl (0.73 mmol/l). Lipid values prior to starting treatment are not available. Does this patient have a clinically significant dyslipidemia and, if so, what are the options for management?

Dyslipidemia in HIV infection

The dyslipidemia associated with HIV infection may be a consequence of HIV infection per se, a direct effect of the antiretroviral agents used to treat HIV infection, secondary to central adiposity and insulin resistance that can occur during treatment or it may be unrelated to HIV treatment or disease. Currently marketed protease inhibitors (PIs) differ slightly in their ability to cause dyslipidemia, whereas in general non-PI-containing regimens have been found to have less of an effect on lipids. Exceptions to this include the modest triglyceride increases that have been observed with efavirenz and the increases in triglycerides associated with stavudine and zidovudine. In a recent randomized clinical trial in treatment-naive patients, increases in total cholesterol, HDL cholesterol and triglycerides were similar in patients receiving either efavirenz or lopinavir/ritonavir combined with two nucleosides. The magnitude of the effect on lipids may vary for different PI combinations. More modest increases in triglycerides have been reported with the following ritonavir-boosted protease inhibitors: atazanavir, saquinavir and fos-amprenavir. Patients with untreated advanced HIV infection have been noted to have a pattern of low HDL cholesterol and increased triglycerides.

Estimating cardiovascular risk

The long-term significance of dyslipidemia in HIV-infected individuals is not completely known; however, it has been suggested that HIV treatment-related lipid increases contribute to an increased risk for myocardial infarction associated with protease inhibitor exposure in the Data Collection on Adverse Events of Anti-HIV Drugs (DAD) study. The patterns of lipid abnormalities most commonly observed in patients with HIV infection might be expected to result in increased cardiovascular morbidity. In many cases both antiretroviral therapies

and HIV infection per se are thought to contribute. Recommendations for the management of dyslipidemia in HIV-infected individuals have been developed.

These guidelines first consider the overall risk of cardiovascular disease (CVD) and consider the following as important risk factors: current cigarette smoking, diabetes, hypertension, family history of coronary heart disease and HDL cholesterol. The first step in evaluating cardiovascular risk is to determine which risk factors are present. If so, then an estimate of the 10-year cardiovascular risk using the Framingham scoring system is suggested (see http://www.nhlbi.nih.gov/guidelines/cholesterol/index.htm). In this example, the patient has several classic risk factors for CVD: he is a smoker with untreated hypertension who also has low HDL cholesterol and elevated total cholesterol and elevated triglycerides. Using the online risk calculator available from the National Heart, Lung, and Blood Institute (NHLBI) we discover that his estimated 10-year cardiovascular risk is over 30%. This is considered a high risk, similar to that of someone with established coronary heart disease.

The reliance on LDL cholesterol complicates the use of NCEP guidelines in the management of patients with HIV infection. When the value for triglycerides exceeds 400 mg/dl (4.52 mmol/l), calculation of LDL cholesterol from the total cholesterol and HDL is not accurate. Direct measurement of LDL is not available in many settings and hence it may be reasonable to base decisions for intervention on the values of non-HDL cholesterol. The value for non-HDL cholesterol is the total cholesterol minus HDL cholesterol. In this example, the value for non-HDL cholesterol would be 232 mg/dl (6.0 mmol/l). The NCEP ATP III guidelines include goals for non-HDL cholesterol in addition to LDL cholesterol and these are included in Table PP47.1.

MANAGEMENT

Now that we have established that the patient in this example requires intervention for his dyslipidemia (and his overall cardiovascular risk), we can consider the options for management. The first steps would include discussing his diet and lifestyle. The importance of smoking cessation and treatment of his hypertension should be aggressively addressed as these factors are clearly contributing to the patient's high level of cardiovascular risk. These modifiable risk factors should be addressed prior to considering altering his currently successful antiretroviral regimen. His diet should be reviewed and he should be given information on a low-fat (with reduced saturated fat), low-cholesterol diet. It is possible that his intake of alcohol, two six packs of beer each night during the weekend, could be contributing to his hypertriglyceridemia. Given his calculated level of cardiovascular risk, additional measures to lower his non-HDL cholesterol and his elevated triglycerides are likely to be needed.

Table PP47.1 Lipid targets based on NCEP risk categories

Category	LDL-C goal	Non-HDL-C (if TG >200 mg/dl)
High risk	<100 mg/dl	<130 mg/dl
10-year risk >20% or coronary heart disease	<70 mg/dl*	<100 mg/dl*
>2 Risk factors and 10-year risk ≤20%	<130 mg/dl	<160 mg/dl
0–1 Risk factor	<160 mg/dl	<190 mg/dl

*Grundy SM, Cleeman JI, Merz CN, et al. Implications of recent clinical trials for the National Cholesterol Education Program Adult Treatment Panel III Guidelines. Circulation 2004;110:227–39. This paper includes updated targets for very high risk patients such as those who have had a recent heart attack, or those who have cardiovascular disease combined with either diabetes or severe or poorly controlled risk factors (such as continued smoking) or metabolic syndrome. Adapted from Expert Panel on Detection, Evaluation, and Treatment of High Blood Cholesterol in Adults. Executive summary of the third report of the National Cholesterol Education Program (NCEP) Expert Panel on Detection, Evaluation, and Treatment of High Blood Cholesterol in Adults (Adult Treatment Panel III). JAMA 2001;285:2486–97.

The additional measures for management of this patient's dyslipidemia include alteration in his antiretroviral regimen and the use of lipid-lowering agents. There are limited data at present to guide clinicians in this regard. The patient is currently receiving a non-nucleoside-based regimen that contains the thymidine nucleoside zidovudine; both of these drugs may be contributing to his elevated cholesterol and triglycerides. Several studies have suggested a benefit of substituting a nonthymidine nucleoside analogue such as tenofovir or abacavir as a reasonable option for patients who are well suppressed on a thymidine-based regimen with dyslipidemia. There are scant data on the impact of switching of efavirenz to either unboosted atazanavir or to nevirapine in this setting. One potential caution is the risk of a hypersensitivity reaction if nevirapine is used when CD4 cell counts are >400 cells/mm³ in men (or >200 cells/mm³ in women). If the patient is reluctant to change his therapy, and even if he does make these changes, the use of lipid-lowering agents should be considered given his high level of risk.

The HMG-CoA reductase inhibitors (statins) are generally the first-line intervention for lipid disorders in the general population, especially when the estimated coronary heart disease risk is as high as that of the patient in this example. Important drug interactions between the statin agents and the PIs have been reported and it is becoming more difficult to generalize recommendations. Simvastatin and lovastatin should not be used with protease inhibitors, pravastatin appears to be the least likely to interact with PIs with the exception of darunavir and recently, rosuvastatin was found to increase significantly when co-administered with lopinavir/ritonavir. Drug interactions are unlikely to occur with the use of the fibric acid derivatives gemfibrozil and fenofibrate. In the case above, with elevations in both triglycerides and non-HDL cholesterol and an estimated 10-year risk of 30%, therapy with a statin agent should be strongly considered. Pravastatin at a dose of 20–40 mg/day or atorvastatin at a dose of 10–20 mg/day are reasonable choices; the latter may be more beneficial for the patient's elevated level of triglycerides. In addition, consideration should be given to changing the zidovudine to either abacavir or tenofovir. If the patient does not respond to these interventions, higher doses of statin therapy can be considered. In addition, daily low-dose aspirin therapy should be considered in this middle-aged man with an elevated cardiovascular risk.

As the treatment of HIV infection has evolved into the management of a chronic disease, more emphasis is being placed on preventing long-term complications from both the disease and the therapies used to treat it. It is important for clinicians to be aware of these issues and to screen patients for lipid disorders prior to starting antiretroviral therapy and during treatment. Attention to modifiable cardiac risk factors such as smoking, diet and level of physical activity is critical and should not be overlooked. In settings where the underlying cardiovascular risk appears to be high, further interventions with lipid-lowering agents or modification of the antiretroviral regimen may be warranted.

FURTHER READING

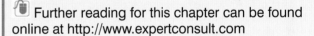 Further reading for this chapter can be found online at http://www.expertconsult.com

Multidrug-resistant HIV

FREQUENCY OF THE PROBLEM

Unfortunately, due to difficulty with adherence to antiretroviral treatment or the sequential use of partially suppressive regimens when therapy was initiated, a very significant proportion of patients with HIV infection develop multidrug-resistant HIV. In a survey of the ongoing HIV Costs and Service Utilization Study (HCSUS), approximately 63% of the patients under care had a detectable viral load at the time of the last determination, 78% of those had resistance to at least one drug and more than 50% were resistant to two. These data suggest that more than 100 000 patients in the USA alone (or half of the total number of patients in care) are infected with viruses that are resistant to antiretroviral drugs. HIV disease is similar to other infectious diseases such as tuberculosis and malaria, in which the development of resistance is a frequent clinical problem.

The problem of drug resistance in HIV is more common among subjects receiving therapy and who are in care than among patients who have never received treatment. Primary resistance to HIV therapies is rising alarmingly among new and chronically infected individuals in the developed world, and in many areas of the USA more than 15% of new HIV infection diagnoses harbor some resistance. Unfortunately, this problem will also affect the developing world when antiretroviral therapy becomes more widely available. Primary resistance is more frequently seen with nucleoside reverse transcriptase inhibitors since these are the drugs that have been used for the longest period of time, but it is increasing among non-nucleoside reverse transcriptase inhibitors and protease inhibitors. The goal is to prevent this problem by the intelligent use of antiretroviral medications and resistance testing. However, despite these efforts, the use of antiretroviral therapy will always be associated with the development of resistance, and clinicians will frequently face patients for whom no therapeutic options are readily available.

THERAPEUTIC OPTIONS FOR THE SUBJECT WITH MULTIDRUG-RESISTANT HIV

Thanks to the development of new classes of drug such as the CCR5 inhibitors (maraviroc approved in 2007), integrase inhibitors (raltegravir, 2007) the development of new agents in existing classes such as the protease inhibitors tipranavir (2005) and darunavir (2006) and the new non-nucleoside reverse transcriptase inhibitor etravirine (2008), the goal of treatment when the clinician faces a patient with multidrug-resistant virus is to resuppress HIV RNA maximally to prevent the ongoing development of viral resistance. The approach is to select at least two new active drugs in the regimen, preferably from new classes of agents. In the setting of clinical trials up to 70–80% of

the participants with extensive treatment experience may be able to reach resuppression of their HIV-RNA levels.

However it might be difficult to achieve these goals in some patients. Several considerations are important in this situation. First, virologic failure is not equivalent to immunologic and clinical failure. Deeks and colleagues have shown that the median period of time between virologic and immunologic failure is 36.4 months (3 years). The delay between virologic and immunologic failure seems to be associated with the decreased replicative fitness of viruses that harbor protease inhibitor and nucleoside-associated resistance mutations. Viruses with multiple mutations are less cytopathic *in vitro* and *in vivo* when compared to wild-type isolates. Second, discontinuing therapy in the patient with multidrug-resistant virus is associated with the overgrowth of wild-type virus after a period of approximately 12 weeks. This switch to wild type as the predominant quasispecies in the patient is associated with a significant decay in the CD4+ T-cell count, rapid progression of HIV disease and, in some cases, serious opportunistic infections. Third, there is growing evidence that the rates of clinical progression are low in patients that continue antiretroviral therapy in the presence of virologic failure, and that these subjects maintain their CD4 cell numbers, especially if the viral load is maintained below the natural set-point of the patient (the HIV RNA load before the initiation of antiretroviral therapy).

Based on the above, most experienced clinicians would maintain a partially suppressive regimen in a patient with limited therapeutic options, especially if the disease is in an advanced stage. The objective of therapy in this situation shifts from complete suppression of viral replication to partial suppression to prevent immunologic and clinical decline, and to wait until two new active therapeutic agents become available to try to achieve the goal of full viral suppression again.

Many clinicians also maintain lamivudine in these patients because the presence of the M184V mutation (usually associated with the use of lamivudine) may enhance susceptibility to zidovudine or tenofovir, drugs frequently used individually as part of combination regimens in the patient with multidrug resistance. The presence of this mutation also stabilizes the reverse transcriptase of the virus and makes it less prone to make errors, which are associated with the development of resistance. This effect may be overcome by an accumulation of nucleoside-associated mutations (also known as NAMs): M41L, E44D, D67N, K70R, V118I, L210W, T215Y/F and K219Q/E.

The development of new classes of drug has made the use of multidrug combination regimens (six or more drugs), also called 'mega-HAART regimens', very unusual and probably unnecessary.

Although some authors suggested that transient discontinuation of antiretroviral treatment might 'resensitize' the virus and make it susceptible to previously used antiretroviral agents, this phenomenon is short lived because of 'archived' resistance of the integrated HIV in the T-cell memory reservoirs. This approach was tested in several randomized trials and proved to be deleterious for the participants because of the high risk of significant clinical deterioration in the patient with advanced disease.

In the patient with multidrug-resistant HIV it is also critically important to maintain all prophylactic regimens that the subject should be taking, at the usually recommended CD4+ T-cell count thresholds. Thus, it is important to maintain *Pneumocystis jirovecii*, *Toxoplasma gondii* and *Mycobacterium avium intracellulare* prophylaxis if indicated. It is also a good idea to increase the frequency of the clinical visits to once every month or two, so that opportunistic infections can be readily identified and treated.

NEW DRUG AVAILABILITY

Before the US Food and Drug Administration (FDA) grants full approval, new drugs become available as part of compassionate use and expanded access programs. The clinician frequently is pressed and tempted to add this 'single' new drug to the regimen that the patient is taking, hoping to obtain at least a partial virologic and clinical benefit in the patient with very limited options. However, with the development of new classes of drug it has become clearly apparent that the use of at least two new agents should be tried in patients with evidence of resistance. Unless the patient is clinically deteriorating rapidly, the soundest approach might be to wait until the development of two or more new active drugs. The decision to add a single drug to a failing regimen should be based on the clinical situation of the patient and the types of drug available.

For some classes of drug (e.g. non-nucleoside reverse transcriptase inhibitors and fusion inhibitors), resistance develops very quickly if these drugs are not used as part of fully suppressive regimens. With other classes of drug (e.g. protease inhibitors or nucleoside/nucleotide analogues), resistance takes longer to develop and durable virologic and potentially clinical benefits might be obtained. So for compounds where the threshold to develop resistance is low it might be reasonable to wait until more drugs became available and a combination regimen with a good chance of response can be developed. For drugs with a higher threshold for resistance immediate use might be advisable, especially in the patient who is clinically deteriorating. For example, enfuvirtide (also known as T-20) is an injectable peptide fusion inhibitor that binds to the HR-1 domain of gp41. Its use has been associated with significant decreases in viral load when used as monotherapy and to improve the viral load response of otherwise optimized rescue regimens. HIV becomes very quickly resistant to this drug if it is not used as part of a fully suppressive antiretroviral regimen. Resistance mutations in the gp41 envelope gene have been identified primarily at positions 36–45 of the first heptad repeat (HR-1) region. On the other hand, tenofovir, a nucleotide, was evaluated as an 'intensification' (the addition of a single drug to a failing antiretroviral regimen) in Gilead study 907. The virologic benefits (approximately half a log decrease in HIV viral load) were still present after 48 weeks of treatment.

If the patient is clinically failing antiretroviral therapy, or the addition of a single drug is being considered, it is important to maximize the benefits of the background regimen that the patient is taking. Phenotypic resistance testing might have an edge over genotypic or 'virtual phenotype' testing (a genotype test with an automatic interpretation linked to a large database of geno-phenotypes) in this very complicated situation. It might identify better which drugs maintain a better residual activity *in vitro* in a patient with limited therapeutic options. It also might provide a measurement of 'replicative capacity' of the patient's virus.

THE USE OF THE REPLICATION CAPACITY ASSAY

Replicative fitness is the ability of a species or strain of virus to compete against others in a defined environment – for example, a wild-type virus is more fit than a virus with multidrug resistance in an environment where there is no drug, but the reverse is true in the presence of antiretroviral therapy. To evaluate replicative fitness, it is necessary to conduct very cumbersome assays where the two different strains to be tested compete against each other. Monogram Inc. modified their phenotypic assay and developed a 'replication capacity assay' which is provided as part of the phenotypic assay. In this assay patient-derived HIV reverse transcriptase or protease undergoes a single round of replication. The vector contains a luciferase gene that permits quantitation of replication that is then compared to the level of replication of a wild-type HIV reference strain. The result is provided as the ratio of the patient strain replication to the wild-type (reference) strain replication. Normally multidrug-resistant viruses have replication capacity values smaller than 1. Theoretically the lower the number, the less fit the virus is.

As the availability of new therapeutic agents has increased over the last years, the interest of using replication capacity as a tool for guiding therapy in the patient with multidrug resistance has decreased. A few years ago some clinicians used this assay to guide therapy in the patient with multidrug resistance, selecting combination regimens that lower the replication capacity of the predominant quasispecies of the patient. However, clinical validation of the utility of this assay is still lacking, and this approach might lead to unnecessary changes of otherwise well-tolerated regimens. Assuring the viral load is maintained as low as possible, preferably below the natural set-point of the patient, might be another approach to handle the patient who has limited therapeutic options.

FURTHER READING

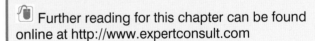 Further reading for this chapter can be found online at http://www.expertconsult.com

Section | 6 |

Jeremy Farrar & Keith PWJ McAdam

International Medicine

Geography of infectious diseases

INTRODUCTION

Infectious diseases vary by geographic region and population, and they change over time. Increasingly, humans are moving from one region to another, thereby becoming exposed to a variety of potential pathogens and also serving as part of the global dispersal process.[1] Microbes picked up at one time and in one place may manifest in disease far away in time and place. Because many microbes have the capacity of persisting in the human host for months, years or even decades, the relevant time frame for study of exposures becomes a lifetime. Furthermore, microbes also move and change and reach humans via multiple channels.

Caring for patients in today's world requires an understanding of the basic factors that underlie the geography of human diseases and events that cause shifts in the distribution and burden of specific diseases. Current technology contributes to massive population movements and rapid shifts in diseases and their distributions, but it also provides communication channels that can aid clinicians who care for patients with unfamiliar medical problems. This chapter reviews the factors that shape the global distribution of infectious diseases and the forces that are expected to shift distributions in the future. Several examples are used to illustrate the broad range of factors that affect the distribution and expression of infectious diseases.[2]

Many authors have traced the origins and spread of specific infectious diseases through human history. A century and a half ago, John Snow noted that epidemics of cholera followed major routes of commerce and appeared first at seaports when entering a new region. *Yersinia pestis*, the cause of plague, accompanied trade caravans and moved across oceans with rats on ships. Exploration of the New World by Europeans introduced a range of human pathogens that killed one-third or more of the local populations in some areas of the Americas. The plants and animals introduced as a result of this exploration have also had profound and long-lasting consequences for the ecology and economics of the new environment.[3] The speed, reach and volume of today's travel are unprecedented in human history and offer multiple potential routes to move biologic species around the globe. Pathogens of animals and plants are being transported as well, and this can affect global food security.[4] Establishment of arthopod vectors, such as mosquitoes that are competent to transmit human pathogens, in new geographic areas can expand the regions that are vulnerable to outbreaks of some vector-borne infections. This chapter focuses only on pathogens that directly affect human health and on their sources (Table 101.1). When thinking about geography of human infections, it is useful to consider both the origin of the organism and the conveyor or immediate source for the human (Fig. 101.1).

Table 101.1 Origins and conveyors of human pathogens*

Origin or carrier	Conveyor or immediate source	Examples of disease
Humans	Humans	HIV, syphilis, hepatitis B
Humans	Humans (air-borne pathogen)	Measles, tuberculosis
Soil	Soil, air-borne	Coccidioidomycosis
Soil	Food	Botulism
Animals	Water	Leptospirosis
Humans	Mosquitoes	Malaria, dengue
Humans	Soil	Hookworm, strongyloidiasis
Animals	Ticks	Lyme disease
Animals, humans	Sand flies	Leishmaniasis
Animals	Animals	Rabies
Rodents	Rodent excreta	Hantaviruses
Humans	Water, marine life	Cholera
Humans or animals (with snails as essential intermediate host)	Water	Schistosomiasis
Humans	Food, water	Typhoid fever
Animals	Water	Cryptosporidiosis, giardiasis

*Some pathogens have multiple potential sources.

This chapter addresses three key issues:
- factors influencing geographic distribution: why are some infectious diseases found only in focal geographic regions or in isolated populations?
- factors influencing the burden of disease: why does the impact from widely distributed infections vary markedly from one region or one population to another? and
- factors influencing emergence of disease: what allows or facilitates the introduction, persistence and spread of an infection in a new region and what makes a region or population resistant to the introduction of an infection?

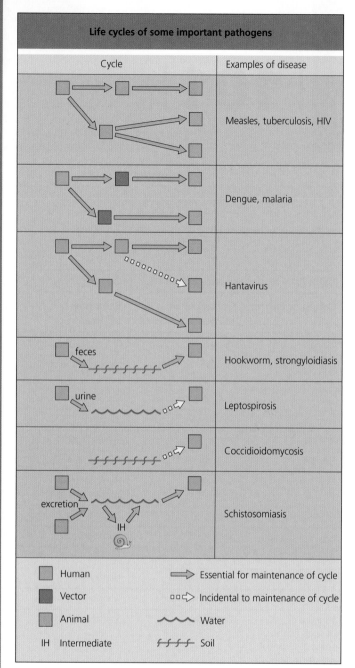

Fig. 101.1 Life cycles of some important pathogens.

Cycle	Examples of disease
	Measles, tuberculosis, HIV
	Dengue, malaria
	Hantavirus
feces	Hookworm, strongyloidiasis
urine	Leptospirosis
	Coccidioidomycosis
excretion IH	Schistosomiasis

Human — ⟹ Essential for maintenance of cycle
Vector — ⇢ Incidental to maintenance of cycle
Animal — Water
IH Intermediate — Soil

FACTORS INFLUENCING GEOGRAPHIC DISTRIBUTION

In past centuries, lack of interaction with the outside world could allow an infection to remain geographically isolated. Today, most infections that are found only in focal areas have biologic or geoclimatic constraints that prevent them from being introduced into other geographic regions. For example, the fungus *Coccidioides immitis*, which causes coccidioidomycosis, thrives in surface soil in arid and semiarid areas with alkaline soil, hot summers and short, moist winters; it is endemic in parts of south-western USA, Mexico and Central and South America. People become infected when they inhale arthroconidia from soil. An unusual wind storm in 1977 lifted soil from the endemic region and deposited it in northern California, outside the usual endemic region.[5]

In general, infection is associated with residence in or travel through the endemic region. However, because the fungus can persist in the human host for years, even decades, after initial infection (which may be mild and unrecognized), disease may be diagnosed far from the endemic regions. Although it is a 'place' disease, coccidioidomycosis has increased in the southwestern USA in recent years, in part attributable to a large influx of susceptible humans into the endemic zone and construction and other activities that disturb the soil. Outbreaks are also linked to climatic and environmental changes.[6]

Vectors

Many microbes require a specific arthropod vector for transmission or an animal reservoir host and hence inhabit circumscribed regions and may be unable to survive in other habitats. Malaria is a vector-borne infection that cannot become established in a region unless a competent vector is present. The presence of a competent vector is a necessary but not sufficient condition for human infection. The mosquito must have a source of malarial parasites (gametocytemic human or rarely other species), appropriate bioclimatic conditions and access to other humans. The ambient temperature influences the human biting rate of the mosquito, the incubation period for the parasite in the mosquito and the daily survival rate of the mosquito. Prevailing temperature and humidity must allow the mosquito to survive long enough for the malarial parasite to undergo maturation to reach an infective state for humans. Competent vectors exist in many areas without malaria transmission, because the other conditions are not met. These areas are at risk of the introduction of malaria, as illustrated by several recent examples in the USA and elsewhere.[7,8]

An estimated 77% of the world population lived in areas with malaria transmission in 1900. Today about 48% live in at-risk areas, but because of population growth and migration the total global population exposed to malaria today has increased by 2 billion since 1900.[9] Malaria was endemic in many parts of the USA into the 20th century (Fig. 101.2), with estimates of more than 600 000 cases in 1914. Even before extensive mosquito control programs were instituted, transmission declined. Demographic factors (population shifts from rural to urban areas), improved housing with screened doors and windows, and the availability of treatment were among the factors that contributed to this decrease.

The distribution of onchocerciasis in Africa is notable for its association with rivers.[10] The reason becomes clear by understanding that the vector of this filarial parasite, the black fly (genus *Simulium*), lays her eggs on vegetation and rocks of rapidly flowing rivers and usually

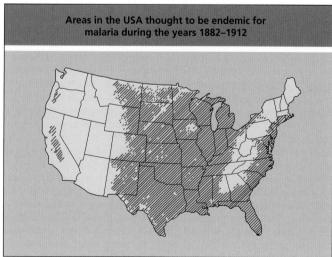

Fig. 101.2 Areas of the USA thought to be endemic for malaria during the years 1882–1912.

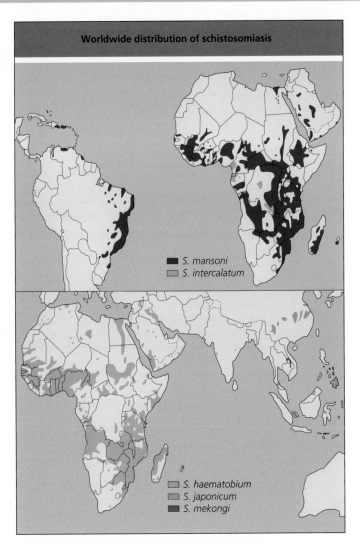

Worldwide distribution of schistosomiasis

- S. mansoni
- S. intercalatum

- S. haematobium
- S. japonicum
- S. mekongi

Fig. 101.3 Worldwide distribution of schistosomiasis.

inhabits a region within 5–10 km on either side of a river. Another name for onchocerciasis, river blindness, describes the epidemiology as well as one consequence of infection.

Some pathogens have a complex cycle of development that requires one or more intermediate hosts. Distribution may remain relatively fixed, even when infected humans travel widely, if other regions do not supply the right combination and geographic proximity of hosts (Fig. 101.3). Although persons with schistosomiasis visit many regions of the world, the parasite cannot be introduced into a new region unless an appropriate snail host is present, excreted eggs (in urine or feces) are released into water where they reach the snail hosts and humans subsequently have contact with the untreated water.[11] Local ecologic changes and climate change, however, can be associated with expansion of transmission in endemic areas or increased intensity of transmission, as has been projected as a possible consequence of warming temperatures in China.[12]

Many hantaviruses exist worldwide with distributions that are still being defined. Each hantavirus seems to have its specific rodent reservoir with which it has evolved. As with many zoonoses, humans are incidental to the survival of the virus in rodents, yet humans can develop severe and sometimes fatal disease if they enter an environment where they are exposed to the virus. Undoubtedly, other rodent-associated viruses and other pathogens (as well as pathogens associated with other animals or insects) with the capacity to infect humans will be identified as humans enter unexplored environments in the future.

Ebola and Marburg viruses are other viruses that have focal distributions but have caused dramatic human outbreaks with high mortality.

Table 101.2 Biologic attributes of organisms that influence their epidemiology

- Host range
- Duration of survival in host
- Route of exit from host
- Route of entry into human
- Inoculum need to establish infection
- Virulence
- Capacity to survive outside host
- Resistance to antimicrobials and chemicals

They also infect nonhuman primates and threaten the survival of great apes.[13] Recent studies suggest that bats may be the reservoir hosts.[14,15] Because these infections can be spread from person to person, secondary household and nosocomial spread in several instances has amplified what began as an isolated event. Lack of adequate resources in hospitals in many developing regions contributes to the spread of infections within hospitals and to persons receiving outpatient care, such as those receiving injections.

Cultural practices can lead to unusual infections in isolated areas. Residents of the highlands of Papua New Guinea developed kuru after ingestion (or percutaneous inoculation) of human tissue during the preparation of the tissues of dead relatives.

Thus, the presence of a pathogen in a region may reflect the biologic properties of the organism, its need for a certain physicochemical environment or its dependence on specific arthropods, plants or animals to provide the milieu where it can sustain its life cycle (Table 101.2). The presence of a pathogen in a region does not necessarily equate with human disease, because mechanisms must exist for the pathogen to reach a susceptible human host for human disease to occur. Sometimes it is only with exploration of new regions or changes in land use that humans place themselves in an environment where they come into contact with microbes that were previously unidentified or unrecognized as human pathogens. Preferences for specific foods, certain preparation techniques or cultural traditions may place one population at a unique risk for infection.

FACTORS INFLUENCING THE BURDEN OF DISEASE

Among the infectious diseases that impose the greatest burden of death globally, most are widely distributed: respiratory tract infections (e.g. influenza, *Streptococcus pneumoniae* and others), diarrheal infections, tuberculosis, measles, AIDS and hepatitis B.[16] Most of these infections are spread from person to person. The World Health Organization estimated that about 65% of infectious diseases deaths globally in 1995 were due to infections transmitted from person to person (Table 101.3).[16]

Table 101.3 Modes of transmission for major global infectious diseases

Mode of transmission	% of total*
Person-to-person	65
Food-borne, water-borne or soil-borne	22
Insect-borne	13
Animal-borne	0.3

*The figures are based on an estimated 17.3 million deaths due to infectious diseases in 1995, as reported by the World Health Organization.[16]

Burden from these diseases is unevenly distributed across populations and among different countries. Poor sanitation, lack of clean water, crowded living conditions and lack of vaccination contribute to the disproportionate burden from many of these infections in developing regions of the world. In industrialized countries, pockets of high risk persist. Disadvantaged populations have higher rates of tuberculosis, HIV and many other infectious and noninfectious diseases. Rates of reported cases of tuberculosis vary widely by region (Table 101.4).[17] Variation also exists within countries. Figure 101.4 shows the effect of crowded living conditions on rates of tuberculosis in England and Wales in 1992.[18] Among welfare applicants and recipients addicted to drugs or alcohol in New York City, the rate of tuberculosis was 744 per 100 000 person years or more than 70 times the overall rate for the USA.[19] The impact of an infection derives not only from the risk of exposure but also from the access to effective therapy. For example, treatment of a patient with active tuberculosis can cure the individual and eliminate a source of infection for others in the community.

Diphtheria, controlled in many parts of the world through the use of immunization, resurged in new independent states of the former Soviet Union in the 1990s, a reminder of the tenuous control over many infectious diseases. Populations in other countries also felt the impact as cases related to exposures in the Russian Federation were reported in Poland, Finland, Germany and the USA. Serologic studies in America and Europe suggest that up to 60% of adults may be susceptible to diphtheria.

Table 101.5 Factors that influence the types and abundance of microbes in a community

- Biogeoclimatic conditions
- Socioeconomic conditions
- Public health infrastructure
- Urban versus rural environment
- Density and mobility of population
- Season of the year
- Animal populations

Table 101.6 Factors that influence the probability of exposure to pathogens

- Living accommodation
- Level of sanitation
- Occupational and recreational activities
- Food preparation and preferences
- Sexual activities and other behavior
- Contact with pets, other animals, vectors
- Time spent in the area

Table 101.4 Rates of reported cases of tuberculosis worldwide by region, 1990 and 2006

Region	INCIDENCE PER 100 000 POPULATION	
	1990	2006
Africa	162	363
Americas	65	37
Eastern Mediterranean	111	105
Europe	37	49
South East Asia	200	180
Western Pacific	127	109

Data from World Health Organization.[17]

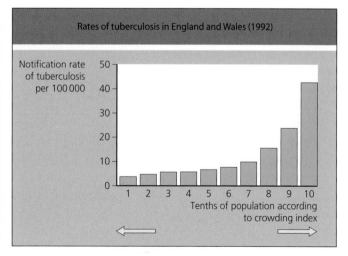

Fig. 101.4 Rates of tuberculosis in England and Wales by crowding index (1992). Adapted from Bhatti et al.[18]

Travelers to tropical and developing regions of the world can pick up geographically focal, often vector- or animal-associated infections (such as malaria and dengue),[20] but travelers most often acquire infections with a worldwide distribution that are especially common in areas lacking good sanitation.[21] Food- and water-borne infections are common and lead to travelers' diarrhea, which is caused by multiple agents (including *Escherichia coli*, *Salmonella*, *Shigella* and *Campylobacter* spp., and others), typhoid fever and hepatitis A. Respiratory tract infections may be acquired from other travelers from all over the globe during the crowding that occurs in travel (e.g. in buses, airplanes, terminals and on cruise ships) as well as from persons in the local environment. Tables 101.5 and 101.6 note factors that influence the types and abundance of microbes in a community and the probability of exposure to pathogens.

Hepatitis A virus remains a common cause of infection in developing regions of the world although it is not considered a major cause of morbidity or mortality in those regions where most persons are infected at a young age and become immune for life. The presence and severity of symptoms are related to the age at which a person becomes infected. Infection in young children is typically mild or inapparent. Persons living in areas of high transmission may be unaware of the presence of high levels of transmission, although nonimmune, older people (such as travelers) who enter the environment may develop severe, and occasionally fatal, infection. Some countries with an improving standard of living have noted a paradoxic increase in the incidence of disease from hepatitis A virus as the likelihood of exposure at a young age decreases, shifting upward the age of infection to a time when jaundice and other symptoms are more likely to occur.

Travelers may also contribute to the spread of infectious diseases and influence the global burden of these diseases.[22,23] *Neisseria meningitidis*, a global pathogen, occurs in seasonal epidemics in parts of Africa – the so-called meningitis belt (Fig. 101.5).[24] Irritation of the throat by the dry, dusty air probably contributes to invasion by colonizing bacteria. Pilgrims carried an epidemic strain of group A *N. meningitidis* from southern Asia to Mecca in 1987. Other pilgrims who became colonized with the epidemic strain introduced it into sub-Saharan Africa, where it caused a wave of epidemics in 1988 and 1989. Using molecular markers, investigators were able to trace the spread of the epidemic clone to several other countries.[25] In 1996 in Africa, major outbreaks of meningococcal meningitis occurred

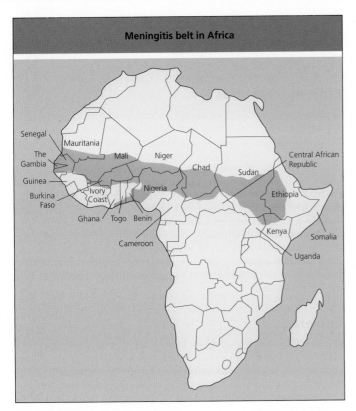

Meningitis belt in Africa

Fig. 101.5 Meningitis belt in Africa.

Table 101.7 Factors that restrict the introduction and spread of infections

- Geoclimatic factors that cannot support vector or intermediate host
- Genetics of human population, making it genetically resistant or relatively resistant
- Immunity of human population, making it not susceptible because of past infection with same or related microbe or via vaccination
- Demographic factors (e.g. size and density of population will not support sustained transmission of diseases such as measles)
- Social and behavioral factors (e.g. absence of activities such as iv drug use and unprotected sex with multiple partners)
- Food preparation habits and local traditions (e.g. certain dishes not eaten, food always well cooked)
- High-quality housing, sanitation, public health infrastructure, good surveillance
- High standard of living, good nutrition, lack of crowding, access to good medical care
- Biologic characteristics of the microbe

(>185 000 reported cases with a case fatality rate of ~10%) caused by *N. meningitidis* serogroup A, clone III-1.[26] A virulent group C, ET-15 strain of *N. meningitidis* spread in Canada and was associated with an increased case fatality rate and a higher proportion of cases in persons over the age of 5 years.[27] In these examples, the virulence of the microbe and travel and trade acted synergistically to change the epidemiology and burden of disease. In the spring of 2000 serogroup W135 *N. meningitidis* caused an outbreak of infection in pilgrims to the Hajj and subsequently spread to their contacts and others around the world. Studies using serotyping, multilocus sequence typing, multilocus DNA fingerprints and other techniques found identical W135 isolates in multiple countries. Pilgrims are required to receive a meningococcal vaccine but before this outbreak, pilgrims from many countries received a vaccine that protected against serotype A but not W135. The vaccine reduces risk of disease but does not prevent oropharyngeal carriage of *N. meningitidis*.[28]

FACTORS INFLUENCING EMERGENCE OF DISEASE

Regular, rapid movement of persons from tropical regions to major urban areas throughout the world raises concerns that unusual infections could be introduced into an environment where they could spread to large populations. In order to assess the potential for a pathogen to be introduced into a new population, information is required about the biologic properties of the organism, the region and population being considered and the mechanisms of transmission (see Table 101.1). A key factor that determines whether a pathogen can persist and spread in a new population is its basic reproductive rate, which is the number of secondary infections produced in a susceptible population by a typical infectious individual. To become established in a new host population, a pathogen must have a basic reproductive rate that exceeds one. The concept is simple but invasion and persistence are affected by a range of biologic, social

and environmental factors. Also critical in determining how easily an infection can be controlled is the proportion of transmission that occurs before onset of symptoms or during asymptomatic infection.[29]

Certain factors restrict the introduction and spread or persistence of infection in a region (Table 101.7); many of these are discussed above. Nutrition is also important in determining susceptibility to and severity of many infections. A substantial proportion of disease burden in developing countries can be attributed to childhood and maternal underweight and micronutrient deficiences.[30] Before measles vaccine was introduced, the epidemiology of measles exhibited marked periodicity in large populations, with peaks typically occurring every 2–3 years.[31] In general, a community size of about 250 000 is necessary to provide a sufficient number of susceptible people to sustain the virus. In small island communities (or other isolated populations), outbreaks typically occur only after periodic introductions from outside. Size and density of a population thus influence the epidemiology of some infections. It has been suggested that measles as it has been known in the 20th century could not have established itself much before 3000 BC because before that time human populations had not achieved sufficient size to sustain the virus. Measles could not have persisted in nomadic, hunting communities.

Examples of emerging pathogens

It is instructive to look at examples of infections that have recently undergone major shifts in distribution and to review the key factors that have influenced their geographic spread. They are a reminder of the complexity of the interactions among host, microbe and environment. A recurring theme is the movement of humans who introduce pathogens into a new region (see also Chapter 4) and human alteration of the landscape or ecology that permits contact with previously unrecognized microbes, often through interaction with animals or animal products. Many infections in humans, in the past and in recent years, have domestic or wild animals as their sources.[32]

Human immunodeficiency virus and other pathogens carried by humans

Organisms that survive primarily or entirely in the human host and are spread from person to person (e.g. by sexual or other close contact or by droplet nuclei) can be carried to any part of the world. The spread of HIV in the past three decades to all parts of the world is a reminder of the rapid and broad reach of travel networks. Although the infection has also spread via blood and shared needles, it has been the human host engaging in sex and reproduction who has been the origin for the majority of the infections worldwide. Person-to-person spread accounted for the rapid worldwide distribution of severe acute respiratory syndrome (SARS), a coronavirus infection, in the spring of 2003, after the virus emerged from an animal reservoir, most likely bats.[33]

Drugs or vaccines injected by reused inadequately sterilized needles and syringes have been and continue to be an important means of spread of blood-borne infections, such as hepatitis C, hepatitis B and HIV, in some parts of the world.[34]

Multidrug-resistant (MDR) tuberculosis has continued to increase, with World Health Organization estimates of 500 000 new cases of MDR annually (now about 5% of all new TB cases each year).[35] Extensively drug-resistant tuberculosis, which is virtually untreatable, had been reported in 45 countries by 2007. It is not only the pathogens carried by humans that are relevant. Humans also carry resistance and virulence factors that can be transferred to and exchanged with other microbes.[36]

Dengue fever

Dengue fever is a mosquito-borne viral infection that has now spread to most tropical and subtropical regions of the world and continues to increase in incidence and severity. Viremic humans regularly enter regions infested with *Aedes aegypti*, the principal vector of dengue, transporting the virus for new outbreaks. Infection can spread rapidly and outbreaks are sometimes massive, involving >30% of the population. Because four serotypes of dengue virus exist and infection with one serotype does not confer lasting immunity against other serotypes, a person can be infected more than once. The risk of developing severe dengue (e.g. dengue shock syndrome or dengue hemorrhagic fever, DSS or DHF) after repeat infection is 82–103 times greater than after primary infection.[37] In an outbreak in Cuba, 98.5% of cases of DSS or DHF were in persons with a prior dengue infection. The rate of DSS or DHF was 4.2% in persons with prior dengue infection who became infected with a new serotype.[38]

Geographic regions where multiple serotypes are circulating have continued to expand, setting the stage for more severe consequences of infection. Factors that have aided the spread of dengue include increasing (and rapid) travel to and from tropical regions; expansion of the regions infested with *Aedes aegypti*; increasing urbanization, especially in tropical areas, which has provided large, dense populations; the use of nonbiodegradable and other containers that make ideal breeding sites for the mosquito; and lack of support for vector control programs.

Most of the world population growth globally is in urban/peri-urban areas in tropical and developing regions. The expectation is that more urban areas in tropical regions will reach the critical population size, perhaps somewhere between 150 000 and 1 million people, to permit sustained transmission of dengue, and to increase the risk of the severe forms of infection, dengue hemorrhagic fever and dengue shock syndrome.

In 2001 the vector that was implicated in an outbreak of dengue in Hawaii[39] was *Aedes albopictus*, a mosquito species that has been newly introduced into many new regions in recent decades, probably primarily by shipping.[40] On phylogenic analysis the virus responsible for the Hawaii outbreak was similar to dengue, isolates from Tahiti, suggesting that viremic travelers introduced the virus from the South Pacific.

It is instructive to ask not only where dengue occurs but also where it does not. Although large dengue epidemics occurred in the USA in the 20th century, only a handful of cases have been acquired in the USA in recent years, despite the presence of epidemic disease in adjacent areas of Mexico and the presence of a competent vector (*Aedes aegypti*) in south-eastern USA (Fig. 101.6).[24] It is possible that the presence of screened dwellings and air conditioning may make

an area relatively resistant to the introduction of infection, even if a competent vector infests a region, though serologic studies have also documented that unrecognized dengue infections are occurring in Texas.[41]

Chikungunya virus

Chikungunya, a mosquito-borne alphavirus originally isolated in Tanzania in 1953, has spread from Africa, causing massive outbreaks in the Indian Ocean islands and India since 2005. Although it has typically been considered an infection of tropical regions, in the summer of 2007 an outbreak caused hundreds of cases (175 laboratory confirmed) in north-eastern Italy. The index case was a visitor from India. Of note, the vector implicated was *Aedes albopictus*, which had been first documented in Italy in 1990 and was postulated to have been introduced via used tires.[42] Mutations in the virus may have enabled it to replicate more efficiently in the mosquito vector. Chikungunya virus can be transmitted by *Aedes aegypti* and *Aedes albopictus* mosquitoes, which are now both widely distributed, so many regions of the world are vulnerable to introduction of this virus by viremic travelers.

Cholera

Cholera illustrates the complex interactions between microbe, environment and host.[43] Epidemics are seasonal in endemic regions. *Vibrio cholerae* lives in close association with marine life, binding to chitin in crustacean shells and colonizing surfaces of algae, phytoplankton, zooplankton and water plants. *V. cholerae* can persist within the aquatic environment for months or years, often in a viable but dormant state, nonculturable by usual techniques. Environmental factors, including temperature, salinity, pH and sea-water nutrients, affect the persistence, abundance and viability of the organisms, and hence have a striking influence on human epidemics.

Under conditions of population crowding, poor sanitation and lack of clean water, cholera can have a devastating impact, as was shown by the massive outbreak of El Tor cholera in Rwandan refugees in Goma, Zaire, which caused 12 000 deaths in July 1994.[44]

The organism can be carried by humans, who sometimes have few or no symptoms, and introduced into new regions. Trade probably also plays a critical role. Ballast water, picked up by boats in multiple locations and discharged at another time and place, carries a wide range of species, including many that have no direct impact on human health.[45,46] In studies of the ballast and bilge of cargo ships in the USA Gulf of Mexico, researchers were able to identify *V. cholerae* identical to the strains causing epidemic disease in Latin America.[47]

Food-borne disease

The globalization of the food market means pathogens from one region can appear in another; some are common pathogens with a worldwide distribution but others are not. An outbreak of cholera in Maryland, USA, was traced to imported, contaminated commercial frozen coconut milk.[48] Alfalfa sprouts grown from contaminated seed sent to a Dutch shipper caused outbreaks of infections with *Salmonella* spp. on two continents, in at least Arizona and Michigan in the USA and in Finland.[49] Commercial movement of fruits and vegetables redistributes resistance factors along with the microbes. Tracing the source after an infection has been diagnosed can be convoluted and often is not carried out unless disease is severe, lethal or epidemic or involves a highly visible person or population.

Travel and trade are key features in the epidemiology of the infection *Cyclospora*, a cause of gastroenteritis. Recognized for many years in

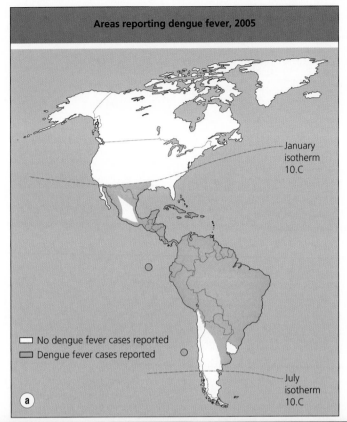

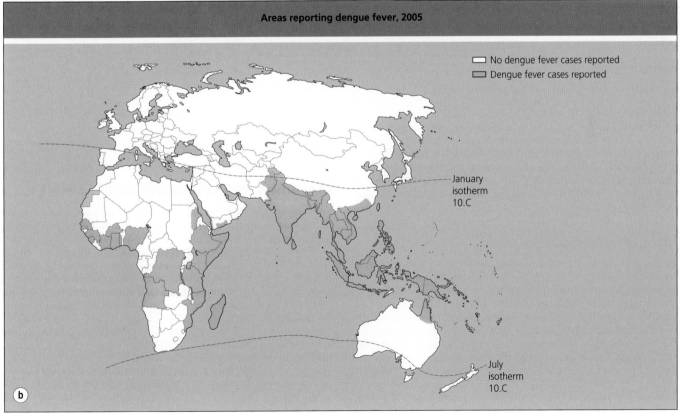

Fig. 101.6 (a, b) Areas reporting dengue fever, 2005. Many areas with a competent vector do not report dengue epidemic activity. Copyright World Health Organization 2008.

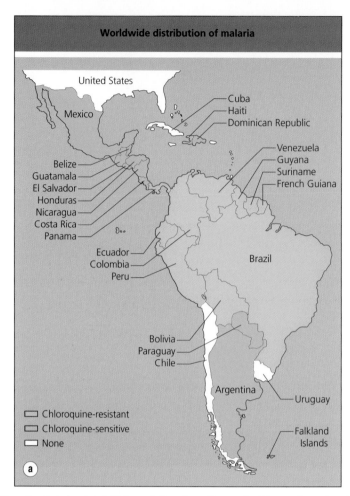

Worldwide distribution of malaria

United States

Mexico

Cuba
Haiti
Dominican Republic

Belize
Guatamala
El Salvador
Honduras
Nicaragua
Costa Rica
Panama

Venezuela
Guyana
Suriname
French Guiana

Ecuador
Colombia
Peru

Brazil

Bolivia
Paraguay
Chile

Argentina

Uruguay

Falkland
Islands

☐ Chloroquine-resistant
☐ Chloroquine-sensitive
☐ None

(a)

Fig. 101.7 (a, b) Worldwide distribution of malaria (updated CDC map). Data from Centers for Disease Control and Prevention.[24]

multiple regions of the world, cases were often associated with living in or travel to areas where sanitary facilities were poor. In the summer of 1996, a large US outbreak occurred in persons who had not traveled. Over a period of a few months, 1465 cases of cyclosporiasis were reported from 20 states. The outbreak was linked to eating raspberries imported from Guatemala.[50] During some seasons of the year up to 70% of selected fruits and vegetables sold in the USA come from developing countries.

Visceral leishmaniasis

In the past, visceral leishmaniasis in Brazil was primarily a rural disease. Recently, however, several cities have reported large outbreaks of visceral leishmaniasis.[51] Reasons for the change in epidemiology include geoclimatic and economic factors (drought, lack of farm land, famine), leading to migration of large numbers of persons, who settle in periurban areas where they live in densely crowded shanties, lacking basic sanitation. The presence of domestic animals, such as dogs, chickens and horses, in and adjacent to human dwellings provides ample sources of blood meals for the sand fly, the vector of leishmaniasis. Outbreaks have occurred in many cities in Brazil, including Teresina, São Luis and Natal. Children and young people have been most affected. Malnutrition can also contribute to the severity of the disease.

Disease–disease interactions can also alter the epidemiology of infections. Visceral leishmaniasis has become an important infection in HIV-infected people in Spain and other areas where the two infections coexist.[52] The presence of HIV leads to increased risk of progression of infection; late appearance of disease can occur

years to decades after exposure in an endemic region, leading to the appearance of cases of leishmaniasis in regions distant from endemic areas. A common consequence is missed or delayed diagnosis.

Movement of vectors and other species

Movement today involves all forms of life and the movement of nonhuman species can affect infections in humans. Importation of wild animals from Ghana into the United States led to an outbreak of monkeypox, an infection previously known to exist in Africa. Humans became infected by handling prairie dogs (sold as pets) that had been housed with the imported wild animals from Africa.[53] *Aedes albopictus* introduced into the USA via used tires shipped from Asia[54] has since become established in at least 21 contiguous states of the USA and in Hawaii. *Aedes albopictus* can transmit dengue and chikungunya viruses, as described above, and is a competent laboratory vector of La Crosse, yellow fever and other viruses. It is also hardier than many other mosquito species and therefore may spread widely and be extremely difficult to eradicate. Multiple strains of eastern equine encephalitis virus have been isolated from *Aedes albopictus* in Florida.

An example from the past illustrates the potential consequences of the introduction of a mosquito vector into a new region. In March 1930, an entomologist in Natal, Brazil, came upon *Anopheles gambiae* larvae in a small, wet, grassy field between a railway and a river.[55] He was surprised, because the usual habitat for this mosquito was Africa. Investigation revealed that the probable route of entry into South America was via boats that made mail runs between Dakar in Senegal

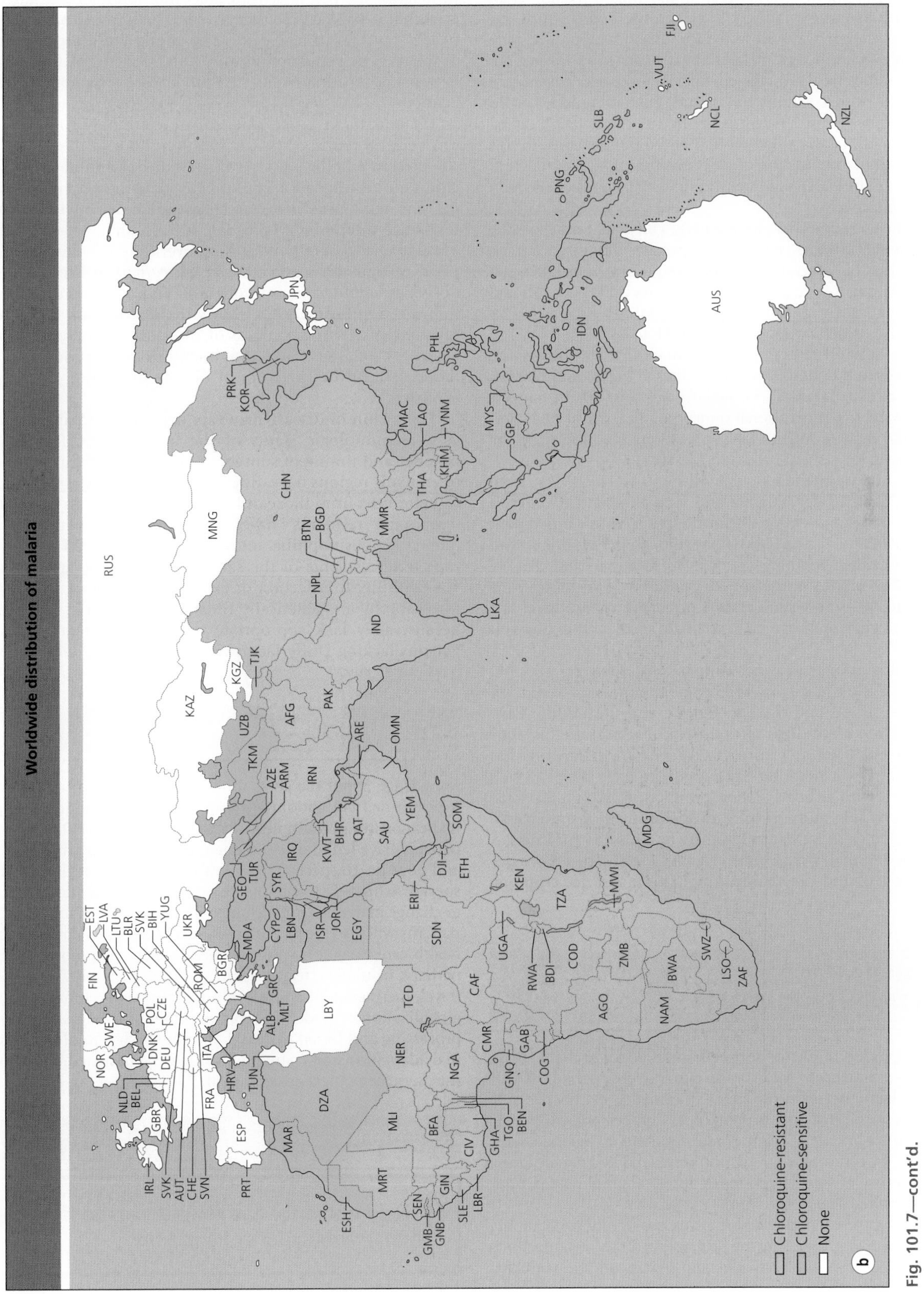

Worldwide distribution of malaria

- Chloroquine-resistant
- Chloroquine-sensitive
- None

b

Fig. 101.7—cont'd.

and Natal in Brazil, covering the 3300 km in less than 100 hours. In Dakar the boats were anchored a distance from the shore within easy flight range of *A. gambiae*. In Brazil, over the ensuing years, the mosquito spread along the coastal region and inland. Natal, as an ocean port, terminus of two railway lines and the hub of truck, car and river transportation, was well suited for dissemination of *A. gambiae* into the region. Although malaria already existed in the region, the local mosquitoes were not efficient vectors. *Anopheles gambiae*, in contrast, lived in close proximity to humans, entered houses, sought human blood and was an efficient biter. In 1938 and 1939, devastating outbreaks of malaria killed more than 20 000 persons. In this instance, the simple introduction of a new vector into a region led to severe problems. Fortunately, an intensive (and expensive) eradication campaign was effective.

Current transportation systems regularly carry all forms of life, including potential vectors, along with people and cargo. In an experiment carried out several years ago, mosquitoes, house flies and beetles in special cages were placed in wheel bays of 747 aircraft and carried on flights lasting up to 7 hours. Temperatures were as low as –62°F (–52°C) outside and ranged from 46°F to 77°F (8–25°C) in the wheel bays. Survival rates were greater than 99% for the beetles, 84% for the mosquitoes and 93% for the flies.[56] Occasional cases of so-called airport malaria – cases of malaria near airports in temperate regions – attest to the occasional transport and survival of a commuter mosquito long enough to take at least one blood meal in the new environment.

In the USA, transportation of raccoons in the late 1970s from Florida to the area between Virginia and West Virginia (in order to stock hunting clubs) unintentionally introduced a rabies virus variant into the animals of the region. From there, the rabies enzootic spread for hundreds of miles, reaching raccoons in suburban and densely populated regions of the north-east USA. Spill-over of the rabies virus variant into cats, dogs and other animal populations and direct raccoon–human interactions have had extremely costly and unpleasant consequences.[57]

Today highly pathogenic avian influenza A (H5N1) is a global concern.[58] It is entrenched in poultry populations in Asia and Africa and has caused outbreaks in Europe and the Middle East. Although the virus causes high mortality in infected humans, thus far H5N1 has not been able to establish sustained transmission from person to person. Most humans appear to have been infected via close contact with poultry or their products. Although the virus can be carried by migratory birds,[59] most introductions appear to have been related to movement of poultry and poultry products. A model designed to map risk in South East Asia found risk was associated with duck abundance, human population and rice cropping intensity.[60]

GEOGRAPHIC INFLUENCES ON DIFFERENTIAL DIAGNOSIS

Geographic exposures influence how one thinks about probable diagnoses in a given patient. In Mexico, for example, more than 50% of patients with late-onset seizures have CT evidence of the parasitic infection, neurocysticercosis.[61] In Peru, 29% of persons born outside Lima who had onset of seizures after 20 years of age had serologic evidence of cysticercosis.[62] In northern Thailand, melioidosis is a common cause of sepsis, accounting for 40% of all deaths from community-acquired sepsis.[63]

In considering the consequences of exposures in other geographic regions, relevant data in assessing the probability of various infections include the duration of visit, activities and living conditions during the stay and the time lapsed since the visit. Among British travelers to West Africa, the relative risk of malaria was 80.3 times higher for persons staying for 6–12 months than among those staying 1 week.[64] In Malawi, the risk of schistosome infection increased directly with duration of stay. Seroprevalence was 11% for those present for 1 year or less, but this increased to 48% among those present for 4 years or longer.[65] In a study of persons with cysticercosis, the average time between acquisition of infection and onset of symptoms was about 7 years.[66]

For malaria, it is necessary to know not only whether infection can be acquired in a specific location but also the specie of parasite present and the patterns of resistance to antimalarial agents. As chloroquine resistance has spread, maps now typically highlight the few remaining areas of chloroquine sensitivity. Because the resistance to antimalarial agents is a dynamic process, with levels of resistance generally increasing over time (involving *Plasmodium vivax* in some areas as well as *P. falciparum*), it is essential to base decisions about chemoprophylaxis and treatment on up-to-date information. Figure 101.7 shows the distribution of malaria and resistance patterns globally as of 2005. Recent analysis of data from a network that uses travelers as a sentinel population found marked differences in the spectrum of disease in relation to the place of exposure.[20]

Expression of disease may vary depending on age of first exposure, immunologic status of the host, genetic factors and the number and timing of subsequent exposures. Temporary residents of endemic regions have different patterns of response to a number of helminths from those of long-term residents. In cases of loiasis, temporary residents have immunologic hyperresponsiveness, high-grade eosinophilia and severe symptoms that are not seen in long-term residents of the same area.[67] Genetic factors can affect susceptibility to infection or expression of disease. Some persons, for example, are genetically resistant to infection with parvovirus because they lack appropriate receptors on their erythrocytes.[68] Persons lacking Duffy factor cannot be infected with the malarial parasite, *P. vivax*.

CONCLUSION

Knowledge about the geographic distribution of diseases is essential for informed evaluation and care of patients, who increasingly have had exposures in multiple geographic regions. Recent travel and trade patterns have led to more frequent contact with populations (human and nonhuman species) from low latitude areas, regions with greater species richness.[69] Infectious diseases are dynamic and will continue to change in distribution. Changes in virulence and shifts in resistance patterns will also require ongoing surveillance and communication to health-care providers. Multiple factors favor even more rapid change, perhaps in unexpected ways, in the future: rapidity and volume of travel, increasing urbanization (especially in developing regions), the globalization of trade, multiple technologic changes that favor mass processing and broad dispersal, and the backdrop of ongoing microbial adaptation and change, which may be hastened by alterations in the physicochemical environment.

REFERENCES

References for this chapter can be found online at http://www.expertconsult.com

Chapter | **102** | *David R Hill*

Pretravel advice and immunization

Pretravel care of international travelers is entirely preventive medicine.[1] It should be the goal of all travel medicine practitioners to maintain the health of the more than 800 million persons who cross international borders each year (World Tourism Organization, www.unwto.org). The first step in providing this care is to make a risk assessment of the traveler's journey: determining the itinerary and duration of travel, the accommodation and planned activities, and the health status of the traveler. A research expedition to the shores of Kenya's Lake Victoria will expose the traveler to more health risks than a short business trip to Nairobi. During longer trips, and especially expatriate residence, there will be a cumulative risk of disease as well as the possibility that a traveler will become lax in preventive measures such as malaria chemoprophylaxis. In order to determine destination-specific risks, the global epidemiology of infectious disease health risks can be found in several authoritative publications such as those published by the US Centers for Disease Control and Prevention (CDC)[2] and the World Health Organization (WHO)[3] and from Internet sites (see Sources of Information) (Fig. 102.1).[4]

The next step in risk assessment is to review the traveler's health. Although at least 25% of individuals travel with chronic medical conditions, these generally do not interfere with travel plans. Nevertheless, consideration of specific activities, vaccines or prophylactic medications will need to be balanced against their health.

Once a risk assessment has been made, the health professional should provide the traveler with the tools to manage this risk. These usually include vaccines, self-treatment and prophylactic medications, and preventive advice. Education about illness avoidance may be the most cost-effective measure, but it is difficult to ensure compliance.[5] Each traveler should also be informed how to access medical care during travel and on return as many travelers will need to seek medical care during and after their trip.[6,7]

With constantly changing epidemiology of disease and patterns of microbial resistance, complexity of travel itineraries, and newly released vaccines and preventive medications, most travelers should be cared for in specialized travel clinics that have trained personnel, carry all vaccines and provide accurate preventive advice.[1,8]

IMMUNIZATIONS

It is helpful to divide immunizations into three categories:
- recommended as part of routine health maintenance irrespective of international travel;
- required for entry into a country under International Health Regulations (2005) or by an individual country; and
- recommended because of risk during travel.

Immunizations are often the reason that an individual comes for pretravel care, although the risk of most vaccine-preventable illness is less than one case per 1000 journeys. Adequate records should be kept:

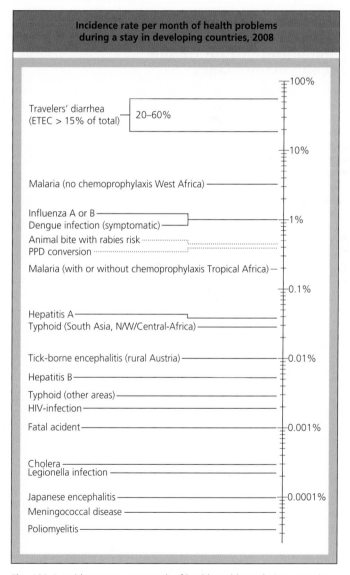

Incidence rate per month of health problems during a stay in developing countries, 2008

Fig. 102.1 Incidence rate per month of health problems during a stay in developing countries, 2008. From Steffen *et al.*[4]

the type and dose of vaccine, date of administration, manufacturer and lot number, site of administration and administrator's signature. Adverse reactions to vaccines should be reported to the appropriate national monitoring agency (e.g. in the US to the Vaccine Adverse

Event Reporting System, http://vaers.hhs.gov/, and in the UK to the Medicine and Healthcare products Regulatory Agency, www.mhra.gov.uk/index.htm). Prior to administration of any vaccine patients should undergo informed consent. The use of vaccine information sheets will help to explain to travelers the benefits and risks of each vaccine. These are often available from vaccine manufacturers and in the US can be downloaded from the CDC: www.cdc.gov/vaccines/pubs/vis/default.htm.

Most vaccines may be administered simultaneously at different sites. Patient tolerance, therefore, usually dictates how many may be given at any one time. A few rules apply. Live viral vaccines should be either given simultaneously or separated by at least 1 month. Immune serum globulin (now only rarely used for prevention of hepatitis A infection) should not be given less than 3 months before or less than 2 weeks after measles, mumps and rubella or varicella vaccines.[9] Other specific considerations are discussed later. Vaccines used in travel medicine, their administration schedule and adverse events are listed in Table 102.1. Full manufacturer's prescribing information should always be consulted before administration of a vaccine, as schedules, doses and products will often differ between countries.

Immunizations for routine health maintenance

The pretravel visit is an ideal time to update routinely recommended immunizations according to age standards. In most areas of the world this includes tetanus, diphtheria, pertussis, measles, mumps and rubella, *Haemophilus influenzae* type b, polio and pneumococcal vaccines for infants, and influenza and pneumococcal vaccines for older adults. However, standards will differ between countries: the USA includes influenza, varicella, rotavirus and hepatitis A and B vaccines for infants and quadrivalent meningococcal conjugate and human papilloma virus (HPV) vaccines for adolescents, whereas the UK provides meningococcal C conjugate vaccine and bacille Calmette–Guérin (BCG) (for high risk) for infants and has recently introduced HPV for adolescents.

Issues of inadequate coverage and waning immunity also impact the choice of vaccines. Measles is no longer endemic to the USA and nearly all cases are imported or linked to imported infections. Although important gains have been made in global control of measles, particularly in Africa, ongoing measles outbreaks in both low- and high-income regions threaten efforts to control the disease.[10,11] Waning immunity against pertussis has led to an increase in cases in older individuals and the introduction of adult formulations of pertussis vaccine combined with tetanus and diphtheria (Tdap).[12] Where available, this vaccine should be used to boost travelers in need of any one of the three antigens.

Children should receive vaccines that are age recommended; however, the schedule may be advanced if a child is traveling before they would have received a scheduled vaccine and the risk of the vaccine-preventable illness during their trip is sufficient (Table 102.2).[9] In the case of measles, a single dose may be given from 6 to 11 months for travel to high-risk destinations, with the routine schedule still administered beginning at 12–15 months.

Older adults (those ≥65 years) make up an increasing proportion (as high as 15%) of international travelers. In addition, there are many travelers with chronic medical conditions such as HIV/AIDS, diabetes or chronic pulmonary, renal, hepatic or cardiac disease. These travelers should be vaccinated with influenza and pneumococcal vaccines. The recognition that influenza is one of the most common vaccine-preventable illnesses during travel has led to the consideration of administering vaccine to healthy travelers going to areas of seasonal influenza (year round in tropical regions, December to March in the northern hemisphere and April to September in the southern hemisphere).[13] Outbreaks can occur out of season when persons from diverse regions of the world congregate in close quarters, such as on cruise ships or during mass gatherings, e.g. the Hajj. The practicalities of obtaining vaccine out of season or vaccine that is matched to influenza strains at the destination may be difficult. Seasonal influenza vaccine is not expected to provide protection against highly pathogenic avian influenza A (H5N1). The role of antivirals used as self-treatment or prophylaxis has not been thoroughly evaluated.[14]

Required immunizations

Vaccination may be required under International Health Regulations (IHR 2005)[15] or by an individual country as a condition of entry. The only vaccine that currently may be required under IHR (2005) is yellow fever (YF) vaccine. There is a risk of YF transmission in countries throughout the Amazon basin of South America, and in sub-Saharan Africa between 15° north and 10° south of the equator. YF is re-emerging and expanding into new regions, as has been seen in South America in 2008 with expansion of disease into new regions of Brazil, Argentina and Paraguay (Pan American Health Organization, www.paho.org/English/AD/DPC/CD/yf-fa.htm). Although YF disease risk maps are published by both the CDC and the WHO, determining the actual risk of a traveler's journey can be difficult.[16] In general, travelers to rural regions in areas with a risk of YF transmission (either an endemic area where there are the appropriate mosquito vectors and nonhuman primate hosts for transmission, or infected areas where there are cases of YF reported) should receive vaccine. Other countries that are not at risk of YF transmission may require vaccination of travelers arriving from YF-risk countries. Country-specific requirements can be found in the CDC[2] and WHO[17] publications, and on their respective websites (see Sources of Information). Health professionals must therefore decide if the vaccine is required for entry and/or recommended because of risk. YF vaccination must be recorded in the revised (as of June 2007) International Certificate of Vaccination or Prophylaxis (see Sources of Information).[18] In addition to vaccine, travelers should protect themselves against the daytime-biting *Aedes* spp. mosquito (Table 102.3).

In 2001 newly recognized severe adverse events following administration of YF vaccine to first-time vaccine recipients were reported. There have been two patterns, viscerotropic and neurologic. Viscerotropic reactions occur within 2 weeks following vaccination (median of 4 days) and are characterized by dissemination of vaccine virus with multiorgan failure; about 50% of cases are fatal. In these cases there are high levels of vaccine virus, prolonged viremia and an unregulated inflammatory response.[19,20] The neurologic adverse events are characterized by a meningoencephalitis that begins up to 4 weeks following vaccination (median 14 days); nearly all cases recover.[21] Acute disseminated encephalomyelitis and Guillain–Barré syndrome also occur with neurologic events. The risk factors do not appear to be related to mutation of vaccine virus, but rather to an alteration in the host response. Older age, particularly 60 years and older, and the absence of a thymus (a contraindication to vaccination) carry an increased risk for both viscerotropic and neurologic reactions.

Cholera vaccine is no longer required under IHR (2005) for international travel, and smallpox vaccine has not been required since 1982 following the global eradication of smallpox in 1977. Meningococcal vaccine is required for religious pilgrims to Saudi Arabia (see following section).

Immunizations recommended because of risk

Vaccines discussed in this section are recommended because there may be a risk of exposure during travel. There are four vaccine-preventable diseases transmitted because of poor food and water hygiene: hepatitis A, typhoid, cholera and polio.

The risk of hepatitis A during travel has declined in many countries, particularly Latin America and East and South East Asia, with transition from high to lower endemicity.[22,23] Nevertheless, vaccination can be considered for most travelers as hepatitis A vaccines are well-tolerated, highly effective, give long-term (perhaps lifelong) protection and are being incorporated into routine immunization schedules.[24]

Hepatitis A vaccines are protective even if given shortly prior to departure. Immune serum globulin that provides immediate protection, with antibodies that circulate for 2–6 months, is not usually used for protection. If available, testing for previous exposure to hepatitis A can be performed in travelers with a high likelihood of previous hepatitis A infection, i.e. those born and raised in countries with high endemicity for hepatitis A and those with a history of jaundice.

Protection against both hepatitis A and B may be achieved with the use of a combined antigen vaccine, Twinrix® (GlaxoSmithKline), in a three-dose schedule. Two doses of vaccine should be given before departure to ensure protection against hepatitis A since a lower concentration of antigen is used in this preparation compared with the single antigen hepatitis A vaccines. The course may be accelerated over 3 weeks.

Hepatitis E is enterically transmitted, particularly during periods of high rainfall. In travelers, most cases have originated from India, although mild and subclinical infection may be more common than appreciated. Pregnant women have a high mortality. Immunoglobulin and the current hepatitis vaccines do not prevent hepatitis E so food and water hygiene is the best prevention (see Chapter 154).

Typhoid and paratyphoid are imported diseases in most high-income countries. The highest risk is in travelers to South Asia (India, Pakistan and Bangladesh); however, cases also originate from Latin America and Africa.[25,26] Multidrug-resistant *Salmonella typhi* is common. There are two vaccines with similar efficacy (60–70%): an oral live-attenuated (Ty21a) vaccine and a polysaccharide (Vi antigen) injectable vaccine.[27] The Ty21a vaccine is well-tolerated, effective in children older than 4 years and provides protection for 5 years; the Vi antigen vaccine is given in a single intramuscular dose and is effective for 2–3 years. Conjugate vaccines in development should provide higher levels of protection, particularly in children under the age of 2 years. Typhoid vaccines do not reliably protect against *S. paratyphi*, which may be more commonly imported than *S. typhi*.[26]

Cholera is endemic throughout Asia and Africa and parts of the Middle East; however, it is rarely a risk for travelers. *Vibrio cholerae* 01 is endemic in all regions, whereas *V. cholerae* 0139 has circulated in Asia. More than 90% of cholera cases are reported from Africa, although some countries in Asia, such as Bangladesh which has endemic cholera, do not report cases to the WHO.[28] There is one cholera vaccine now available: an oral vaccine that combines killed *V. cholerae* with the binding (B) subunit of cholera toxin (Dukoral®, Crucell). This vaccine is well tolerated and in efficacy trials provided 60–85% protection against cholera depending upon the age of the recipient and the time interval measured.[29] Because of the very low risk of cholera in travelers, vaccine should be reserved for those who will work in refugee settings or who will travel in cholera-endemic regions and will be remote from medical care. There has been interest in the use of this vaccine to protect against the syndrome of traveler's diarrhea. While there is cross protection against *Escherichia coli* expressing the heat labile enterotoxin (LT), the protection is modest and the vaccine should not generally be used for this indication.[29]

Although global efforts at polio eradication have been successful in several WHO regions of the world (the Americas, Western Pacific and European), the disease remains endemic in India, Pakistan, Afghanistan and Nigeria, with regional spread to other countries in Africa and Asia. In addition to the endemic countries, in mid-2008 the following countries reported cases or circulation of imported poliovirus: Angola, Benin, Central African Republic, Chad, Democratic Republic of the Congo, Ethiopia, Niger and Sudan in Africa, and Burma and Nepal in Asia (World Health Organization: http://www.polioeradication.org/). Travelers to risk areas should have completed a primary series against poliomyelitis and have a booster according to their national guidelines. Saudi Arabia requires polio vaccination in travelers age 15 years and younger coming from countries reporting wild-type polio.

Other immunizations recommended because of potential exposure during travel include those against hepatitis B, Japanese B encephalitis, *Neisseria meningitidis*, rabies, tick-borne encephalitis and tuberculosis.

Many countries now administer hepatitis B vaccine as part of routine childhood immunization. Unimmunized travelers who will be exposed to blood or body fluids (e.g. health-care workers, expatriate families and children, those receiving medical or dental care and those with unprotected sexual exposure) should receive vaccine. Protection against both hepatitis A and B is available in a combination vaccine (see section on hepatitis A). The vaccination schedule for hepatitis B (Engerix® only, GlaxoSmithKline) may be accelerated to 0, 1 and 2 months with a booster at 6–12 months, and it can be further accelerated by giving doses at 0, 7 and 21 days; 65% will seroconvert at 28 days.[30]

Japanese B encephalitis is a viral encephalitis in Asia transmitted by the *Culex* spp. mosquito. The complete listing of risk areas and seasons of transmission may be found in *Health Information for International Travel*[2] or on the CDC website (wwwn.cdc.gov/travel). Prolonged residence in endemic areas or engaging in high-risk activities such as camping, bicycling or field work are indications for vaccine. Rural Asia, particularly where rice and pigs are farmed, is the highest risk area; pigs act as a reservoir for the virus and the rice fields as a breeding ground for the *Culex* mosquito vector. The most widely used vaccine, JE-VAX®, manufactured by Biken, is a mouse brain-derived vaccine whose production has been discontinued. To replace this vaccine there are two products in development: a vero cell, inactivated vaccine (Ixiaro®, Intercell) that was released in 2009, and a live-attenuated chimeric vaccine (Acambis) that uses yellow fever virus as the backbone.[31,32] JE-VAX has been associated with rare (approximately 0.1–5 episodes per 1000 doses) hypersensitivity reactions, including anaphylaxis, urticaria, angioedema and respiratory distress, that can occur at intervals ranging from minutes to as long as 1 week or more after vaccination.[33] The traveler should avoid traveling within 10 days of completing the series in case a reaction occurs during flight or on arrival in the country of destination. Patients who have a history of allergies or urticaria may be at a slightly higher risk of severe reaction, so they should be vaccinated only after careful consideration.

Meningococcal vaccine is recommended for travelers to areas highly endemic for meningococcal disease such as the meningitis belt of sub-Saharan Africa (particularly during the months from December through June). Following the global spread of meningococcal W135 disease that was traced to Hajj pilgrims in 2000, Saudi Arabia requires vaccination with a quadrivalent vaccine containing serogroups A, C, Y and W135 for religious pilgrims arriving for the Hajj or Umrah.[34] In the USA there is a conjugated quadrivalent vaccine that has been incorporated into routine immunization of adolescents. Some European countries and Canada use a conjugated group C meningococcal vaccine for protection of infants.

All travelers should be counseled about avoiding exposure to rabies virus. In most low-income regions of the world, rabies is transmitted to humans by the bite of a dog (see Chapter 160), although other mammals (e.g. bats, cats, foxes) can also transmit the virus. In North America, bat-transmitted rabies is most common. Rabies-risk countries can be determined by consulting the CDC or WHO websites or reviewing other online resources such as the Country Information Pages of the National Travel Health Network and Centre (http://www.nathnac.org/ds/map_world.aspx). Pre-exposure protection against rabies should be considered for those whose risk is increased by type of activity (e.g. running, cycling), occupation (e.g. veterinarians) and longer duration of stay. Children may be at increased risk as they are less likely to avoid contact with animals and to report a bite or lick. The intramuscular route of administration is preferred to ensure adequate development of immunity.

In order to decrease risk of transmission, all bites should be thoroughly washed with soap and water; postexposure rabies treatment should then be obtained. A traveler who has received pre-exposure vaccine will not need rabies immune globulin (RIG, either human or equine) which is difficult to obtain or unavailable in many areas of the world. If vaccine has not been received before travel, both vaccine and RIG will need to be given. Regimens may differ, but if postexposure treatment is administered properly the traveler should be protected.[35] Travelers who had an overseas rabies exposure and treatment should be evaluated upon return. They can have serology checked and postexposure treatment initiated while awaiting serologic evidence of protection (see Chapter 160).

Table 102.1 Immunizations for foreign travel*

Vaccine	Type	Route	Schedule	Indications	Precautions and contraindications†	Side-effects
Toxoids						
Tetanus–diphtheria	Adsorbed toxoid	im	Primary: 3 doses; first 2 doses, 4–8 weeks apart; 3rd dose 6–12 months later. Booster: every 10 years. A single dose may be given at age 50 years to those who have completed full pediatric schedule	All adults	GBS <6 weeks after previous dose of tetanus-containing vaccine. Severe allergic reaction to previous dose or vaccine component	Local reactions. Occasional fever, systemic symptoms. Arthus-like reactions if history of multiple boosters. Rare: systemic allergy
Tdap‡	Combination toxoids of diphtheria and tetanus with acellular pertussis	im	Primary: not used. Booster: single dose for adolescents and adults who have completed childhood DTP or DTaP course	For adolescents and adults aged 11–64 years who need boosting for any of the three antigens	Severe allergic reaction to previous dose or vaccine component. Encephalopathy within 7 days of receipt of vaccine with pertussis component. GBS <6 weeks after previous dose of tetanus-containing vaccine. History of Arthus reaction after tetanus- or diphtheria toxoid-containing vaccine administered <10 years previously	Local reactions: erythema, swelling, and pain. Occasional fever, headache, fatigue and gastrointestinal symptoms
Inactivated bacterial vaccines						
Cholera (*Vibrio cholerae*)	Killed, whole cell *V. cholerae* O1 of several serotypes and biotypes, combined with recombinant B subunit of cholera toxin	oral	Primary: 2 doses at 1 to 6 week interval. Booster: 2 years	Humanitarian or relief workers; those who will be remote from medical care in areas of cholera outbreaks. Modest protection against heat labile toxin-producing *E. coli*. No longer required under International Health Regulations. No protection against *V. cholerae* 0139	Hypersensitivity to previous dose	Mild gastrointestinal side-effects
Streptococcus pneumoniae	Polysaccharide containing 23 serotypes	sc or im	Primary: 1 dose. Booster: 1 dose recommended for high-risk patients after 5 years	≥2 years old and at increased risk of pneumococcal disease and its complications. Healthy adults 65 years or older	Severe allergic reaction to previous dose	Mild erythema and pain at injection site in about 50%. Systemic reaction in <1%. Arthus-like reaction with booster doses

	Composition	Route	Schedule	Indications	Contraindications/Precautions	Adverse reactions
Neisseria meningitis	Polysaccharide containing serotypes (A, C, Y, W135) (conjugate serotype C vaccine available in some countries)	sc	Primary: 1 dose Booster: 5 years in adults and children ≥5 years; 2–3 years in children vaccinated at 2–4 years.	Travel to areas with epidemic meningococcal disease Religious pilgrims to Saudi Arabia Asplenia or certain complement deficiency states	Severe allergic reaction to previous dose	Infrequent, mild local reactions
Neisseria meningitis	Conjugated polysaccharide containing serotypes (A, C, Y, W135)	sc	Primary: 1 dose Booster: not officially recommended	Travel to areas with epidemic meningococcal disease Religious pilgrims to Saudi Arabia Asplenia or certain complement deficiency states Children aged 11–12 years	Severe allergic reaction to previous dose	Local reactions in 10–60% Systemic reactions of fever, headache and malaise
Typhoid	Vi polysaccharide	im	Primary: 1 dose Booster: every 2 years	Risk of exposure to typhoid fever	Safety in pregnancy not known Severe allergic reaction to previous dose	Local pain and induration in 7% Headache in 16% Fever in <1%
Attenuated live bacterial vaccine						
Typhoid	Attenuated Ty21a strain of *Salmonella typhi*	oral	Primary: 1 capsule every other day for 4 doses Booster: every 5 years	Risk of exposure to typhoid fever	Safety in pregnancy not known§ Immunosuppression§ Children <6 years Acute febrile or gastrointestinal illness Antibiotics or mefloquine (separate the doses by ≥24h) Capsules must be refrigerated	Infrequent gastrointestinal upset, rash
Attenuated live virus vaccines						
Influenza (Flumist)	Attenuated live virus: trivalent	intranasal	Annual vaccination with current vaccine Age 2–8 years (no previous influenza dose), 2 doses 4–6 weeks apart Age 9–49 years one dose per season	Routinely recommended in US for persons 2–49 years Can consider for travelers at risk	Severe allergic reaction to previous dose including eggs Immunosuppression§ Persons <2 years or ≥50 years Pregnancy Children age 5–17 years taking aspirin History of GBS, asthma, chronic pulmonary, cardiac, metabolic or renal disease	Mild upper respiratory symptoms: rhinitis, nasal stuffiness, congestion

(Continued)

Table 102.1 Immunizations for foreign travel*—cont'd

Vaccine	Type	Route	Schedule	Indications	Precautions and contraindications†	Side-effects
Measles	Attenuated live virus: monovalent form or combined with rubella (MR) ± mumps (MMR)	sc	Primary: 2 doses, 1st at 12–15 months, 2nd at 4–12 years of age For adults, 2 doses separated by ≥1 month Booster: none	People born after 1956 (in US) who have not had documented measles or received 2 doses of live vaccine	Severe allergic reaction to previous dose or to gelatin or neomycin Pregnancy Immunosuppression§ (can be considered for asymptomatic HIV-infected persons) Recent (<3 months) administration of immune globulin for hepatitis A prevention	Temperature ≥39.4°C, 5–21 days after vaccination in 5–15% Transient rash in 5% Local reaction if previously immunized with killed vaccine (1963–67): 4–55%
Mumps	Attenuated live virus	sc	Primary: 2 doses (usually given as part of MMR vaccine) Booster: none	People born after 1956 (in US) who have not had documented mumps	Severe allergic reaction to previous dose or to gelatin or neomycin Pregnancy Immunosuppression§ Recent (<3 months) administration of immune globulin for hepatitis A prevention	Mild allergic reactions uncommon Rare: parotitis
Rotavirus	Attenuated live virus (2 products, RotaTeq®, Merck, and Rotarix®, GlaxoSmithKline)	oral	RotaTeq: 3 doses, 1st dose at 2 months, 2nd at 4 months and 3rd at 6 months; complete series by 32 weeks of age Rotarix: 2 doses, 1st dose at 6 weeks, 2nd at least 4 weeks later; complete series by 24 weeks of age	Must complete the series by 24–32 weeks of age depending upon vaccine product	Severe allergic reaction to previous dose Immunosuppression§ Previous history of intussusception Delay vaccination with moderate to severe gastroenteritis	Gastrointestinal upset
Rubella	Attenuated live virus	sc	Primary: 1 dose (usually given as part of MR or MMR) Booster: none	All, particularly women of child-bearing age, without documented illness or receipt of live vaccine at ≥12 months of age	Severe allergic reaction to previous dose or to gelatin or neomycin Pregnancy Immunosuppression§ Recent (<3 months) administration of immune globulin for hepatitis A prevention	Postpubertal women: up to 25% have joint pains, transient arthritis, beginning 3–25 days after vaccination, persisting 1–11 days Arthritis in <2%
Varicella	Attenuated live virus	sc	Primary: 2 doses; 1st at 12–15 months, 2nd at 4–6 years; unvaccinated older children and adults, 2 doses at 1–2 month interval	≥12 months old and no history of varicella	Severe allergic reaction to previous dose Pregnancy Immunosuppression§ Rare transmission of vaccine virus to susceptible hosts Recent (<3 months) administration of immune globulin for hepatitis A prevention	Local pain and induration in 20% Fever in 15% Localized or systemic mild varicella rash in 6%

Vaccine	Type	Route	Schedule	Indications	Contraindications/cautions	Adverse reactions
Yellow fever	Attenuated live virus	sc	Primary: 1 dose, 10 days to 10 years before travel. Booster: every 10 years	As required by individual countries or recommended because of risk	Severe allergic reaction to previous dose or to eggs; Immunosuppression (can be considered in HIV infection with specialist advice)§; Thymus disorders; Avoid in pregnant women, unless high-risk travel; Infants <9 months; Caution in persons ≥60 years old	Mild headache, myalgia, fever, 5–10 days after vaccination in 25%; Rare: immediate hypersensitivity, viscerotropic and neurologic reactions (see text)
Zoster	Attenuated live virus	sc	Primary: 1 dose ≥60 years. Booster: none		Severe allergic reaction to gelatin or neomycin immunosuppression§; Previous vaccination with varicella vaccine	Local reactions: erythema, pain, swelling; Rare varicella-like rash
Inactivated virus vaccines						
Hepatitis A	Inactivated virus; several products available (combination with hepatitis B, see below. Some countries have combination with Vi antigen typhoid vaccine)	im	Primary: 2 doses, 2nd dose after 6–24 months probably provides lifelong protection. Booster: not recommended	Travel to low-income countries; Routine childhood immunization in US; Some travelers may benefit from prevaccine hepatitis A testing (see text)	Severe allergic reaction to previous dose; Safety in pregnancy is not known	Local reaction of pain and tenderness in <20%; Occasional fever in <5%
Hepatitis B	Recombinant HBsAg; several products available (also combination with hepatitis A, see below)	im	Primary: 3 doses at 0, 1 and 6 months. Can accelerate schedule (see text). Adolescents age 11–15 years can receive 2 doses at 6-month interval. Booster: not routinely recommended	Health-care workers; Residence in areas of endemicity for HBsAg; Contact with blood, body fluids or blood-contaminated medical or dental instruments	Severe allergic reaction to previous dose	Mild local reactions in 3–30%; Occasional fever and headache
Hepatitis A and B antigens combined	Inactivated virus (A) plus recombinant HBsAg	im	Primary: 3 doses at 0, 1 and 6 months. Can accelerate schedule (see text). Booster: not currently recommended	Travelers ≥18 years at risk for both hepatitis A and B; Give at least 2 doses of vaccine before departure to protect against hepatitis A	Severe allergic reaction to previous dose; Safety in pregnancy is not known	Local reactions in ~35%; Systemic symptoms of headache and fatigue
Poliomyelitis	Inactivated virus, trivalent	sc	Primary: 3 doses, 1st two at a 4–8 week interval; 3rd 6–12 months after 2nd. Booster: 1 lifetime dose	Travel to polio-endemic countries	Severe allergic reaction to previous dose; Safety in pregnancy not known	Mild local reaction
Human papillomavirus	Inactivated virus (two products available)	im	Primary: 3 doses at 0, 2 and 6 months. Booster: none	Routine administration to females age 11–12 years. Also given to females age 13–18 years if not previously vaccinated	Severe allergic reaction to previous dose or yeast; Safety in pregnancy not known	Local reactions; Occasional systemic reactions or fever

(Continued)

Table 102.1 Immunizations for foreign travel*—cont'd

Vaccine	Type	Route	Schedule	Indications	Precautions and contraindications†	Side-effects
Influenza	Inactivated virus	im	Annual vaccination with current vaccine	Children age 6–59 months Healthy adults >50 years old Persons with chronic cardiovascular, pulmonary and metabolic conditions Health-care workers Can consider for travelers at risk	Severe allergic reaction to previous dose or eggs GBS following a previous dose of influenza vaccine	Mild local reactions in 10–60% Occasional systemic reaction of fever, malaise and myalgia
Japanese B encephalitis	Inactivated virus (tissue culture–derived virus; mouse brain purified vaccine no longer manufactured)	sc	Primary: 2 doses at days 0 and 28 Booster: not currently determined	Travelers ≥18 years to areas of risk with rural exposure or prolonged residence (see text)	Severe allergic reaction to previous dose or vaccine component Safety in pregnancy is not known	Local mild reactions Headache and myalgia common
Rabies	Inactivated virus	im or id	Pre-exposure: 3 doses at days 0, 7, and 21 or 28 Booster: not routinely recommended for travel. Other groups: depends upon risk category and is based upon serologic testing at specified intervals	Itinerary and activities that place travelers at risk of rabies	Severe allergic reaction to previous dose May be given in pregnancy if indicated id route should be completed ≥30 days before travel id route should not be used with concurrent chloroquine or mefloquine id dosing no longer available in USA	Local reactions in ~30% Mild systemic reactions: headache, nausea, aches, dizziness in ~20% Immune-complex reactions with booster doses of human diploid cell vaccine occurring 2–21 days after vaccination in 6%
Tick-borne encephalitis	Inactivated virus	im	Primary: 3 doses at 0, 1–3 months and 5–12 months (can be accelerated) Booster: 3 years	Hiking, camping in areas of risk; practice tick avoidance measures	Severe allergic reaction to previous dose or eggs Safety in pregnancy not known Hypersensitivity to previous doses	Occasional local reactions of swelling, redness or swollen regional lymph nodes Infrequent fever, headache Rare: neurologic adverse events
Passive prophylaxis						
Immune serum globulin	Fractionated Ig (primarily IgG)	im	Travel <3 months: 0.02 ml/kg Travel >3 months: 0.06 ml/kg every 4–6 months	For prevention of hepatitis A Some travelers may benefit from pretravel hepatitis A antibody testing	Not to be given less than 2 weeks after, or 3 months before, measles, mumps and rubella, or varicella vaccines	Transient local discomfort Rare: systemic reaction

*Manufacturer's full prescribing information should be consulted. Dosing and vaccines are generally for adults and based on US guidelines; pediatric doses and vaccines may vary.
†Moderate or severe acute illness with or without fever is a vaccine precaution.
‡In the UK, Td is combined with IPV for adolescent and adult boosting: TdIPV.
§Persons immunocompromised because of congenital immunodeficiency diseases, leukemia, lymphoma, generalized malignancy, and untreated HIV infection or AIDS, or persons immunosuppressed as a result of therapy with corticosteroids, alkylating agents, antimetabolites, or radiation. Persons with a history of thymectomy, thymus diseases or myasthenia gravis should not receive yellow fever vaccine.
DTP, diphtheria, tetanus, pertussis; DTaP, diphtheria, tetanus, acellular pertussis; GBS, Guillain–Barré syndrome; HBsAg, hepatitis B surface antigen; id, intradermal, im, intramuscular; IPV, inactivated polio vaccine; sc, subcutaneous.

Table 102.2 Accelerated immunization of children under 2 years of age*

Vaccine	No. of doses after which protection may be achieved	Earliest age at which dose may be given	Interval (weeks)
Diphtheria-tetanus-pertussis	3	6 weeks	≥4
Measles	1	6 months	
Polio (inactivated)	3	6 weeks	≥4
Haemophilus influenzae type b	2	6 weeks	≥4
Hepatitis A	1	6 months	
Hepatitis B	3	Newborn	≥4 for doses 1 and 2; ≥8 for doses 2 and 3

*The data shown are for children who will travel to developing areas and require protection faster than by the routine schedule. Protection conferred by these schedules may not be complete. Children vaccinated with measles at under 12 months of age should be revaccinated at 12–15 months. In polio-endemic countries, the first oral polio dose may be given in the newborn period but three additional doses should be given, the first at 6 weeks of age and then at 4-week intervals.

Tick-borne encephalitis is a viral meningoencephalitis spread by *Ixodes* spp. ticks throughout forested areas of Eastern and Central Europe, and Siberia in the spring and summer months. Unpasteurized dairy products in endemic areas may also transmit the virus.[36] There are two inactivated vaccines (Encepur®, Chiron, and TicoVac®, Baxter AG), but they have limited availability outside of continental Europe and require three doses over a year to achieve full protection, which is not practical for most travelers. Accelerated vaccine courses exist. Travelers to risk areas should exercise precautions against ticks by the use of protective clothing, repellents and insecticides. These measures will help to prevent Lyme disease, which is also transmitted by the bite of *Ixodes* ticks.

The risk of acquiring tuberculosis during travel is greatest in travelers to countries of high endemicity (e.g. incidence of >40 cases/100 000 population), those who will stay for a long period (>1–3 months) and those who will have close contact with potentially infectious persons (e.g. health-care workers, and those visiting and staying with friends and relatives). The risk of infection has ranged from about 1 case/1000 persons/month in Peace Corps volunteers to 8 cases/1000 persons/month in health-care workers.[37,38] Many children reared outside the USA have received the BCG vaccine. The UK has set guidelines for travelers: children under the age of 16 and health-care workers to high endemic regions who have not previously received BCG.[39] Travelers who are not vaccinated should be offered pre- and post-travel tuberculin (purified protein derivative) skin testing or interferon gamma testing[40] to check for conversion and, therefore, infection. The post-travel skin test should be administered 1 month or more after return.

Immunization in special groups

Two important groups of travelers require special consideration before immunization – pregnant women and immunocompromised hosts, particularly those who have HIV or AIDS. For pregnant women, inactivated vaccines can usually be given if the risk is determined to be sufficient (Table 102.4).[2,9] Measles, mumps and rubella, and the varicella vaccine should not be given, although data have not clearly demonstrated adverse outcomes when women have received rubella vaccine. Yellow fever vaccine should be avoided unless there is high-risk travel; seroconversion to YF virus during pregnancy may be lower, necessitating revaccination after delivery.[41]

HIV-infected patients are another group to consider separately (Table 102.5).[2,42] All travelers should be asked about HIV risk factors before vaccination; the safety, immunogenicity and efficacy of the vaccine being considered then need to be balanced against the risk of the disease. Vaccine immunogenicity decreases with advanced disease from HIV; a CD4 lymphocyte count of <200–400 cells/ml or <15–25% by age-specific percentages correlates with decreased immunogenicity. Although it has not been clearly studied, this may also be a cut-off point for an increased risk of adverse consequences of live viral vaccines. If assurance of immunity is needed, then postvaccination serology should be obtained.

In addition to vaccination, HIV-infected travelers should consider the health risks associated with travel to developing regions. Many enteric infections, such as *Salmonella*, *Cyclospora* and *Cryptosporidium*, and systemic infections such as leishmaniasis and tuberculosis, are more prevalent and can be prolonged and difficult to treat in HIV-infected individuals. There may also be a decreased ability to access sophisticated medical care.

Table 102.3 Mosquito avoidance*

Repellents	DEET-containing products at 20–50% give 6–12 hours protection Picaridin (20%) also effective for approximately 6 hours Lemon eucalyptus oil is effective, but requires frequent application Apply to exposed areas of skin
Protective clothing	Wear loose-fitting, long sleeves and trousers Clothing may be treated with insecticide sprays or solutions
Screens and netting	Sleeping quarters can be screened Netting should be treated with insecticides
Pyrethroid insecticide sprays and coils	May be sprayed or burned in enclosed areas

*For avoidance of *Anopheles* (malaria) and *Culex* (Japanese encephalitis) mosquitoes, precautions should be exercised from dusk to dawn. *Aedes* spp. mosquitoes (dengue and yellow fever) are active in the daytime hours.

TRAVELERS' DIARRHEA

Travelers' diarrhea (TD) is the most common illness during visits to low-income regions of the world and affects 30–60% of travelers.[43] Illness usually begins in the first week after arrival and is typically

Table 102.4 Immunization of the pregnant traveler

Vaccine		Safely given to pregnant women at risk?	Notes
Bacterial	Tetanus–diphtheria	Yes	Tdap can also be given, but preference for vaccination in second and third trimesters
	Pneumococcal polysaccharide	Yes	
	Meningococcal		
	Polysaccharide	Yes	
	Conjugate	Yes	Data on safety are not available but may be given with high-risk
	Typhoid		
	Live-attenuated	Not known	Vaccination should generally be avoided
	Vi polysaccharide	Yes	Vaccine of choice in pregnancy
	Cholera, oral killed	Not known	May be given with high-risk exposure
	BCG	No	
Viral	Hepatitis A		
	Inactivated	Yes	Data on safety not available, but may be given with risk
	Immunoglobulin	Yes	
	Hepatitis B	Yes	
	Human papillomavirus	No	
	Influenza, inactivated	Yes	
	Japanese B encephalitis	Not known	Data on safety not available, but may be given with high-risk exposure
	Measles, mumps, rubella (MMR)	No	Should wait 4 weeks after MMR before becoming pregnant
	Poliomyelitis, inactivated	Yes	
	Rabies	Yes	
	Tick-borne encephalitis	Not known	May be given with high-risk exposure
	Varicella	No	Should wait 4 weeks after varicella before becoming pregnant
	Yellow fever	Yes	Should generally be avoided, but may be given with high-risk exposure

BCG, bacille Calmette–Guérin; DTaP, diphtheria, tetanus, acellular pertussis.
Adapted from CDC and WHO guidelines: Centers for Disease Control and Prevention, 2007 #6558; World Health Organization, 2008 #7181.

mild, characterized by three or more loose to watery stools accompanied by another symptom of nausea, abdominal cramping or malaise. Fever is usually less than 101°F (38°C) and vomiting is not common. In most cases, illness is self-limiting over 3–5 days. Dysentery with tenesmus and bloody stools occurs in less than 10% of patients. Although most individuals can continue with their activities, about 25% will need to alter plans. Enterotoxigenic *Escherichia coli* (ETEC) accounts for 20–30% of the known causes, and a newly described *E. coli*, enteroaggregative *E. coli*, causes another 15–20%.[44,45] *Shigella*, *Salmonella* and *Campylobacter* spp. are the most common other bacteria (see Chapter 34). Viruses (typically rotavirus and norovirus) cause 5–20% of cases and protozoa (*Giardia*, *Cryptosporidium* and, less commonly, *Cyclospora*) cause 5% or less and are usually associated with longer duration of travel. Although the overall incidence of TD does not decline with increasing time of residence in developing areas, partial immunity will develop to ETEC diarrhea.

Prevention

A full description of the prevention and treatment of TD can be found in Chapter 34 and Practice Point 17. Taking care in the selection of food and liquids will help prevent many cases of TD; however, this is often difficult to do consistently. In addition, the risk of TD seems increasingly related to the level of sanitation at the destination.[46] Foods and liquids that are likely to be contaminated are ground-grown greens, vegetables and fruits, incompletely cooked or poorly stored meats and seafood, untreated water and ice cubes, unpasteurized milk products and food from street vendors. Travelers should restrict themselves to commercially bottled or heated beverages, recently and thoroughly cooked meats and greens, and fruits that can be peeled by the traveler. Water may be purified by bringing it to a boil or by halogenating (iodine or chlorine preparations) and then filtering it with a filter of pore size ≤1 mm.[47] The cysts of *Cryptosporidium* and *Cyclospora* (and eggs of helminths) are likely to be halogen resistant, so water potentially contaminated with these parasites should be filtered or boiled.

Several nonantimicrobial agents have been used to prevent diarrhea. Bismuth subsalicylate in tablet (2 tablets (262 mg/tablet), four times daily) or liquid form (1 oz (262 mg/15 ml), four times daily) decreases the incidence of diarrhea by about 65%. Individuals who are allergic to or taking large doses of salicylates, or who are on anticoagulant therapy should not take the drug. It can decrease the absorption of doxycycline. Ingestion of probiotics does not confer reliable protection and antimotility agents such as loperamide should not be taken preventively.

Antibiotics are effective in prophylaxis against TD, but they may be associated with adverse events, contribute to bacterial resistance and have not been studied in travelers going for more than 2–3 weeks. These factors, combined with the effectiveness of prompt self-treatment have led to the consensus that antibiotic prophylaxis should not be recommended for most travelers. For highly selected persons in whom an episode of TD would have substantial adverse consequences, it may be considered. Fluoroquinolones have an evidence

Table 102.5 Immunization in HIV infection

Vaccine		Safely given to persons with HIV infection at risk?	Notes
Bacterial	Tetanus–diphtheria	Yes	
	Pneumococcal polysaccharide and conjugate	Yes	
	Meningococcal polysaccharide and conjugate	Yes	
	Typhoid		
	Live-attenuated	No	Data on safety are not available and vaccination should be avoided
	Vi polysaccharide	Yes	
	Cholera, oral killed	Yes (see notes)	Only limited data on safety
	BCG	No	
Viral	Hepatitis B	Yes	
	Hepatitis A		
	Immunoglobulin	Yes	
	Inactivated	Yes	
	Human papillomavirus	Yes	
	Influenza, inactivated	Yes	
	Japanese B encephalitis	Yes	Data on safety are not available but may be given with risk
	Measles	Yes (see notes)	Can be given to persons who are asymptomatic and with a CD4 count ≥200 cells/mm^3
	Poliomyelitis, inactivated	Yes	
	Rabies	Yes	
	Rotavirus	Yes	
	Tick-borne encephalitis	Yes	Only limited data on safety, but may be given with risk
	Varicella (adults)	Yes (see notes)	Can be given to persons who are asymptomatic and with a CD4 count ≥200 cells/mm^3
	Yellow fever	See note	Can be given to persons who are asymptomatic and with a CD4 count ≥200 cells/mm^3

BCG, Bacille Calmette–Guérin.
Adapted from CDC and WHO guidelines: Centers for Disease Control and Prevention[2]; World Health Organization[3].

base supporting their use for most areas of the world; however, *Campylobacter* resistance limits their effectiveness in South and South East Asia. Rifaximin, a poorly absorbed rifamycin derivative, can be considered in regions where *E. coli* predominates, such as Latin America and Africa.[48]

There is no vaccine to prevent all causes of TD. The oral cholera vaccine, Dukoral, provides modest protection against LT-producing ETEC.[29] An experimental transcutaneously administered vaccine consisting of LT toxin alone has demonstrated 75% protective efficacy against moderate to severe TD.[49]

Treatment

Prompt treatment of TD should be initiated with hydration. Commercial rehydration packets combining electrolytes, sugar and buffer are easy to use and are appropriate for young children, the elderly and those with chronic medical conditions. Infants should continue breast-feeding. As diarrhea improves, the diet can be increased by adding bland foods (bread, cereals, potatoes, soups, bananas, fish and chicken) in frequent small meals.

Mild disease can be treated with bismuth subsalicylate. This reduces the number of loose stools by about 50%, but can have a delay in effectiveness of about 4 hours. The antimotility agent loperamide will rapidly decrease cramping and the number of loose stools. Loperamide should be avoided if there is blood in the stool or a fever of >101.5°F (38.5°C). Because most episodes of diarrhea are self-limiting, symptomatic therapy alone may be sufficient.

A short course of an antibiotic will improve diarrhea within 20–36 hours. Antibiotics combined with loperamide have controlled symptoms within hours.[50] The wide prevalence of sulfonamide and tetracycline resistance has made fluoroquinolones such as ciprofloxacin, norfloxacin, ofloxacin and levofloxacin the most commonly recommended antibiotics in treatment. In South and South East Asia where *Campylobacter* is a common etiology and is often resistant to fluoroquinolones, azithromycin can be used.[51] Azithromycin can also be safely given to children. Antibiotics are prescribed for up to 3 days, but single-dose therapy is often sufficient. Persons with dysentery should seek medical care if self-treatment does not result in improvement within 24 hours, or in cases of severe dehydration. Diarrhea that persists after return should be evaluated (see Chapter 36 and Practice Point 19 for a full discussion of persistent diarrhea) for causes ranging from infection with *Giardia, Cryptosporidium* or *Clostridium difficile*, to tropical sprue, to irritable bowel disease.

MALARIA PREVENTION

Malaria is one of the most important diseases to prevent as it can be fatal. The type of malaria and the risk of acquisition vary by destination and reason for travel, but worldwide there are approximately

7500 cases each year in returned travelers. Of the five recognized species of malaria in humans (*Plasmodium falciparum*, *P. vivax*, *P. ovale*, *P. malariae* and, rarely, *P. knowlesi*), *P. falciparum* is the most severe form and is also the most frequently imported species. Over 80% of *P. falciparum* cases are acquired by travelers on trips to Africa, and especially West Africa where transmission can occur in both urban and rural areas. Travelers with the highest risk for acquiring malaria are those who return to their country of birth to visit friends and relatives, termed VFR travelers; they are usually traveling to West Africa where they are most likely to acquire *P. falciparum* or to South Asia where they usually get *P. vivax*.

Malaria in travelers can almost always be prevented by following an 'ABCD' approach: 'a'wareness of the risk of malaria, mosquito 'b'ite avoidance measures, 'c'ompliance with appropriate 'c'hemoprophylaxis, and prompt 'd'iagnosis of malaria and initiation of treatment.[52]

Bite avoidance measures

Malaria is transmitted by the female *Anopheles* mosquito, which is most active during the nighttime hours from dusk to dawn. During this period travelers should wear loose-fitting cotton clothing that covers their arms and legs, apply repellents to exposed areas of skin and sleep in enclosed areas behind screens or under netting (see Table 102.3). The most effective repellents are those that contain DEET (*N,N*-diethyl-3-methylbenzamide).[53] A concentration of 20–50% will provide protection lasting from 6 to 12 hours. DEET-containing repellents are safe to use in children and pregnant women, but should be applied carefully in these hosts to avoid systemic absorption: they should not be applied to mucous membranes or irritated skin and should be washed off when coming indoors. Picaridin-based repellents are also effective. Bed nets should be treated with a residual insecticide (e.g. permethrin-containing compounds). This can also be applied to clothing and will kill insects rather than only repel them. Mosquito coils and sprays containing pyrethroids can be used in enclosed sleeping areas.

Chemoprophylaxis

Chemoprophylaxis needs to be taken on a regular basis during travel and for a period of time after return that depends on which medications are taken (Table 102.6). Most cases of malaria in returned travelers occur because the traveler fails to take any chemoprophylaxis, takes incorrect prophylaxis or does not comply with their prophylaxis. The choice of a chemoprophylactic regimen should be based on risk of exposure, types of parasite prevalent in the travel destination and health conditions of the traveler. Up-to-date sources (including authoritative websites) should be consulted before prescribing any antimalarial.[2,17]

Chloroquine as a single agent is effective only in areas where *P. falciparum* remains sensitive or is not present: Mexico, Central America west and north of the Panama Canal, the Dominican Republic and Haiti, Egypt, most areas of the Middle East and parts of China. Travelers to all other risk areas in Africa, Asia and Latin America will need to take atovaquone–proguanil (Malarone™), doxycycline or mefloquine.

Atovaquone–proguanil and doxycycline are effective in treatment and prophylaxis of all malaria species, although experience using atovaquone–proguanil with non-falciparum species is limited.[54] Both drugs are started 1–2 days before exposure to malaria and then taken daily. Doxycycline is continued for 28 days after leaving the malarious area, but atovaquone–proguanil can be discontinued after 7 days because it has a causal prophylactic effect: it kills developing hepatic stage parasites, but not the dormant, hypnozoite forms of *P. vivax* or *P. ovale*. These may emerge from the liver many months after return from the place of exposure. Atovaquone–proguanil is ideally targeted

Table 102.6 Prophylaxis of malaria*

Drug	Adult dose	Pediatric dose
Chloroquine	300 mg base (500 mg salt) po, once per week, beginning 1 week before travel, weekly whilst traveling and for 4 weeks after travel	5 mg/kg base (8.3 mg/kg salt), once per week (not to exceed adult dose)
Mefloquine	250 mg salt (1 tablet) po, once per week, beginning 1–2 weeks before travel, weekly whilst traveling and for 4 weeks after travel	≤9 kg, 5 mg salt/kg/week 10–19 kg: ¼ tablet/week 20–30 kg: ½ tablet/week 31–45 kg: ¾ tablet/week ≥46 kg: 1 tablet/week
Atovaquone/proguanil (A/P) (Malarone™)	250 mg A/100 mg P (1 adult tablet) q24h, beginning 1–2 days before travel and for 7 days after travel	62.5 mg A/25 mg P (1 pediatric tablet) 5–8 kg: ½ tablet q24h 9–10 kg: ¾ tablet q24h 11–20 kg: 1 tablet q24h 21–30 kg: 2 tablets q24h 31–40 kg: 3 tablets q24h ≥41 kg: adult dosing
Doxycycline	100 mg po q24h, beginning 1–2 days before travel and for 4 weeks after travel	≥8 years of age: 2 mg/kg po q24h, not to exceed adult dose
Proguanil	200 mg po q24h Used in combination with chloroquine for areas of low levels of chloroquine-resistant *P. falciparum* (see text)	100 mg (one tablet) 6–15 kg: ¼ tablet q24h 16–24 kg: ½ tablet q24h 25–44 kg: ¾ tablet q24h ≥45 kg: 1 tablet q24h
Primaquine (alternative for chemoprophylaxis; usually used to eradicate hypnozoites of *P. vivax* and *P. ovale*)	30 mg base (52.6 mg salt) (2 tablets) po q24h, beginning 1–2 days before travel and for 7 days after travel Must check G6PD before prescribing	0.5 mg/kg base (0.8 mg/kg salt) po q24h, beginning 1–2 days before travel and for 7 days after travel Must check G6PD before prescribing

*Full manufacturer's prescribing instructions should be consulted on dosing guidelines as they may vary between countries.
G6PD, glucose-6-phosphate dehydrogenase.

for short-term travelers to areas of risk. Doxycycline cannot be given to children under the age of 8 or to pregnant women. It should be thoroughly swallowed in the upright position to prevent esophageal irritation. Doxycycline may predispose to vaginal yeast infection and can act as a photosensitizer.

Mefloquine is highly effective in preventing malaria, including chloroquine-resistant *P. falciparum*. When it is taken in prophylactic doses, minor GI and neuropsychiatric events occur in 5–30% of users.[55] The neuropsychiatric side-effects can include sleep disturbance, vivid dreams, mood changes, anxiety, headache and dizziness. Serious adverse events such as psychosis are rare with an occurrence of about one case per 6000–20 000 users.[56] Travelers should be screened for contraindications to mefloquine before prescribing it: a known hypersensitivity to the drug, a history of seizures or psychiatric disorder, or an underlying cardiac conduction abnormality. Some travel health consultants prescribe mefloquine 2–3 weeks before departure to assess patient tolerance and allow a switch to other agents if there is a problem. Seventy per cent of adverse reactions occur during the first three doses. Loading doses of the drug are not advocated.

The combination of chloroquine plus proguanil has been recommended by practitioners in the UK for areas in which there are low levels of chloroquine-resistant *P. falciparum* malaria and only a small risk of acquisition, such as most areas of risk in India. In low risk areas, some European experts do not recommend taking any chemoprophylaxis; rather they suggest being observant to febrile episodes and carrying stand-by self treatment.[56] US and UK authorities do not advocate this approach. Health practitioners should consult the appropriate expert recommendations for their country.

Primaquine is an alternative chemoprophylactic in persons intolerant of other options and can be considered following specialist advice.[57] It is a causal prophylactic and will prevent the establishment of liver hypnozoites of *P. vivax* and *P. ovale*. The drug is taken daily beginning 1–2 days before exposure and can be discontinued 7 days after leaving the risk area. It is a requirement that glucose-6-phosphate dehydrogenase (G6PD) deficiency is ruled out in all persons for whom primaquine is prescribed.

Rural, forested areas of Thailand that border Burma and Cambodia, western Cambodia (including Siem Reap) and southern areas of Vietnam that border Cambodia, have multidrug-resistant *P. falciparum* malaria. Travelers to these areas should take atovaquone–proguanil or doxycycline for prophylaxis.

All travelers should understand that no antimalarial is 100% protective and that they can develop malaria in spite of being compliant with prophylaxis. If they develop a fever or flu-like illness overseas that could be malaria, they should seek medical care. The evaluation needs to include a blood smear performed by a competent laboratory, because the sensitivity of symptoms or physical findings alone is low. The use of self-administered rapid diagnostic kits is not generally recommended as travelers have difficulty using and interpreting these tests; they are not currently licensed for this purpose. In circumstances where travelers cannot obtain prompt medical care, self-treatment can be considered. The self-treatment drug(s) should differ from what the traveler is taking for chemoprophylaxis. Options include atovaquone–proguanil, artemether–lumefantrine (Riamet™), and quinine plus doxycycline.[56]

Travelers who have had prolonged exposure to *P. vivax* and *P. ovale* malaria can consider primaquine to eradicate dormant hepatic-stage parasites. Chloroquine-resistant *P. vivax* is unusual, but has been described from Papua New Guinea and Papua (formerly Irian Jaya) with sporadic cases from Burma, India, Guyana and Brazil.

Pregnant women should not travel to malarious areas unless absolutely necessary, because of the added risk of complications of malaria during pregnancy. Chloroquine and proguanil (with added folate) are safe. Mefloquine can be taken after the first trimester, and may be acceptable in the first trimester if there are no alternatives. Doxycycline is contraindicated and there is insufficient safety data on atovaquone–proguanil during pregnancy. Primaquine should not be given because the G6PD status of the fetus cannot be determined.

ENVIRONMENTAL RISK

Travel to the tropics is associated with increased heat and humidity; the effects that these changes can have on health should be taken into account. These range from a feeling of malaise and tiredness to increased loss of salt and water with resultant dehydration. Travelers should maintain hydration, limit exercise and sleep in a cool environment, particularly if they are elderly or have chronic medical problems. Excessive sun exposure should be avoided by wearing loose-fitting cotton clothing to cover exposed skin, wearing hats and using sunscreens with a sun protection factor of at least 15. Water insolubility may extend the life of the sunscreen. If the patient is taking doxycycline for malaria prophylaxis, it is particularly important to limit sun exposure. Skin should be kept dry and clean to avoid cellulitis and dermatophyte infection.

Travelers to altitudes above 2500–3500 meters (8200–11 500 feet) can experience acute mountain sickness (AMS) or the more severe and potentially fatal conditions of high-altitude pulmonary edema (HAPE) and high-altitude cerebral edema (HACE).[58,59] AMS is characterized by headache, nausea, vomiting, insomnia and lassitude and may affect up to 50% of persons who rapidly ascend above 4000 meters. The risk of illness can be lessened by acclimatization: spending a few days at intermediate altitudes of 1500–3000 meters and gradually ascending, sleeping at elevations no more than 300–500 meters higher each night. Acetazolamide, a carbonic anhydrase inhibitor, can be taken to assist acclimatization, particularly when persons must ascend quickly. It is given at a dose of 125–250 mg orally twice daily, starting 2 days before being at altitude and for several days at altitude.[59,60] It has also been used to treat mild symptoms of AMS. Dexamethasone can be used to treat AMS but in severe illness the safest course is always to descend. Acetazolamide is contraindicated in persons with sulfonamide allergy.

Jet lag is a common problem, particularly when more than five time zones are crossed. It is easier to travel west and lengthen the day than to travel east and shorten the day. In order to help with jet lag, several methods have been proposed: light exposure, short-acting hypnotics and melatonin.[61] When traveling east, exposure to bright light in the late morning and early afternoon may aid in the adjustment. A short- to intermediate-acting benzodiazepine or benzodiazepine receptor agonist can facilitate and maintain sleep in the new time zone, decreasing the contribution of fatigue to the effects of time zone adjustment. Melatonin, which is secreted during the night hours, has been extensively studied. A dose of 3–8 mg taken 2–3 hours before bedtime for the first few nights in the new time zone may be helpful. However, the purity and effectiveness of over-the-counter preparations have not been documented.

Deep venous thrombosis (DVT) and pulmonary embolism are recognized complications of long-haul travel. DVTs can occur in as many as 3% of persons flying for 10–15 hours and who have cardiovascular risk factors; oral contraceptive pills, pregnancy, recent surgery, certain coagulation disorders and malignancy also contribute to risk.[62,63] Some long-haul travelers will develop a pulmonary embolism.[64] In order to decrease risk, travelers should maintain their hydration and exercise their lower extremities at regular intervals. Fitted, below-the-knee support stockings will decrease the incidence of DVT and for highest risk passengers low molecular weight heparin can be considered. Aspirin is not recommended.

BEHAVIORAL RISK

Although there is much focus on infectious illness, the most important contributor to severe morbidity and mortality, particularly in young adults, is accidents and injuries, with those related to road traffic accidents and drowning most common.[65,66] Road safety can be improved by using safety belts in vehicles, avoiding excessive speed, not driving at night or after drinking alcohol, and not riding on motorcycles and mopeds. When swimming, travelers should be aware of undercurrents and never dive into unknown waters. To prevent assault and theft, travelers should not wear jewelery and clothing that draws attention, and they should travel in groups, avoiding high-risk urban areas particularly at night. The US State Department and the UK Foreign and Commonwealth Office post travel advisory and safety information (see Sources of Information). In all situations, alcohol contributes to increased risk behavior.

Sexually transmitted diseases, including HIV, gonorrhea, syphilis and chancroid, are prevalent in many destination countries in Africa, Asia and Latin America. Travelers should be counseled about safe sexual practices, and take condoms with them on their trip.[67,68] Postexposure prophylaxis against HIV may be necessary,[69] and women may need emergency contraception (information can be found on the Marie Stopes website: http://www.mariestopes.org.uk/).

OTHER DISEASES AND CONSIDERATIONS

Dengue fever, a viral disease (see Chapter 127) transmitted by *Aedes* mosquitoes, has seen a resurgence, particularly in Asia, the Caribbean and Latin America, and is a theoretical risk in the south-eastern USA. Dengue is characterized by the sudden onset of fever, headache, myalgias and arthralgias, abdominal discomfort, rash and mild liver abnormalities.[70] Severe disease (dengue hemorrhagic fever and dengue shock syndrome) is characterized by thrombocytopenia and vascular leak, and usually occurs in children following a second infection with a different dengue serotype. There is no vaccine available for prevention, so travelers need to exercise precaution against this daytime feeding mosquito. Complying with bite avoidance measures outlined in Table 102.3 will help to prevent not only dengue but a clinically similar viral infection, chikungunya virus, that in recent years has been a problem on the islands of the Indian Ocean and in countries of South and South East Asia.[71] Other less common insect-transmitted diseases such as leishmaniasis, trypanosomiasis, filariasis and rickettsial infection will also be prevented by insect bite avoidance. African trypanosomiasis has been documented in travelers to East African game parks, and African tick-bite fever caused by *Rickettsia africae* is a risk in southern Africa.[72]

Schistosoma spp. (see Chapter 112) can infect travelers who swim in fresh-water lakes and rivers, particularly in endemic areas of east and southern Africa.[73] Travelers to risk areas should avoid fresh-water swimming unless it is in a chlorinated pool. Letting water stand for 48 hours or warming it to 122°F (50°C) for 5 minutes will render it safe from the *Schistosoma* parasites. Fresh-water swimming, particularly after periods of flooding, can be a risk for acquisition of leptospirosis.

Although the viral hemorrhagic fevers, Ebola, Lassa and Marburg (see Chapter 126), garner a great deal of media attention, they are a rare risk for travelers. Current outbreaks of disease can be identified by reviewing information on ProMED or by checking the disease outbreak sites of the WHO, CDC and NaTHNaC web pages (see Sources of Information). Any returning traveler who is suspected of having a viral hemorrhagic fever should be managed according to WHO guidelines.[74]

Tattooing, injections and dental instruments should be avoided to decrease the risk of acquiring blood-borne pathogens such as hepatitis B and C and, less likely, HIV.

Travelers need to know how to access medical care during their trip. They should purchase a travel health insurance package that includes help in locating medical care, paying for the care upfront and, if necessary, providing for emergency evacuation. There are several air ambulance and insurance companies (http://travel.state.gov/travel/tips/brochures/brochures_1215.html). Embassies or consulates can assist in locating medical services, and mission hospitals can be a source of care. The International Association for Medical Assistance to Travellers (www.iamat.org) will provide a list of English-speaking physicians throughout the world. A small first-aid kit that contains analgesics, bandages, a thermometer and any frequently used over-the-counter medications is helpful as it can be difficult to find the simplest medicines overseas. All travelers should carry an extra supply of their prescription medications, and avoid putting them into checked luggage.

Post-travel illness

Travelers should report illness upon return and heath practitioners should be able to recognize common syndromes: fever, diarrhea, respiratory illness and rash.[1,7,75] Although routine post-travel follow-up for short-term travelers is usually not necessary, anyone who experienced major illness overseas or new-onset illness after return should be evaluated. A differential diagnosis can be developed by considering geography (the locations visited), activities undertaken, incubation periods of disease, frequency of occurrence, and preventive measures taken (e.g. immunizations, compliance with prophylaxis).[76] Practitioners who are not able to pursue complex investigations should refer their travelers for appropriate specialist care. A more detailed discussion of individual syndromes and diseases is provided in other chapters.

SOURCES OF INFORMATION

World Health Organization

- Home page: http://www.who.int/en
- International travel and health. Available online at: http://www.who.int/ith/en/index.html
- Disease outbreaks: www.who.int/csr/don/en/
- Weekly Epidemiologic Record: www.who.int/wer/en/
- Global Health Atlas (disease epidemiology): http://www.who.int/globalatlas/default.asp

United States

Centers for Disease Control and Prevention

- Home page: http://www.cdc.gov/
- Travel medicine home page: http://wwwn.cdc.gov/travel/default.aspx
- Health information for international travel. Available online at: http://wwwn.cdc.gov/travel/contentYellowBook.aspx
- Morbidity and Mortality Weekly Report: http://www.cdc.gov/mmwr/

US State Department

- Travel page: http://travel.state.gov/
- Medical Information for Americans Abroad (has information on travel medical insurance and air ambulance companies): http://travel.state.gov/travel/tips/brochures/brochures_1215.html

US Food and Drug Administration

- Vaccine Adverse Event Report System: http://www.fda.gov/cber/vaers/vaers.htm

Canada

- Health Canada – Travel Medicine: http://www.hc-sc.gc.ca/hl-vs/travel-voyage/index-eng.php
- Committee to Advise on Tropical Medicine and Travel: http://www.phac-aspc.gc.ca/tmp-pmv/catmat-ccmtmv/index.html
- Canada Communicable Disease Report: http://www.phac-aspc.gc.ca/publicat/ccdr-rmtc/index-eng.php
- Adverse Events Following Immunization Reporting: http://www.phac-aspc.gc.ca/im/aefi-form-eng.php

United Kingdom

- National Travel Health Network and Centre: www.nathnac.org/
- Fit for Travel (Health Protection Scotland): www.fitfortravel. scot.nhs.uk/
- Foreign and Commonwealth Office travel page: http://www. fco.gov.uk/en/travelling-and-living-overseas/
- Department of Health – Travel Advice: http://www.dh.gov.uk/ en/Healthcare/Healthadvicefortravellers/index.htm
- Health Protection Agency: http://www.hpa.org.uk/
- Vaccine Adverse Event Reporting (Medicine and Healthcare products Regulatory Agency, Yellow Card Scheme): http://www. mhra.gov.uk/Safetyinformation/Reportingsafetyproblems/ Medicines/Reportingsuspectedadversedrugreactions/index.htm

Surveillance

- European Centre for Disease Prevention and Control: http:// ecdc.europa.eu/
- European Surveillance (Eurosurveillance): www. eurosurveillance.org
- European Travel and Tropical Medicine Network: http://www. istm.org/eurotravnet/main.html
- GeoSentinel: global surveillance network of the International Society of Travel Medicine and the Centers for Disease Control and Prevention: http://www.istm.org/geosentinel/main.html
- ProMED-mail: global electronic reporting system for outbreaks of emerging infectious diseases (International Society for Infectious Diseases): http://www.promedmail.org/pls/ otn/f?p=2400:1000
- National Travel Health Network and Centre: http://www. nathnac.org/countrysearch.aspx
- TropNetEurop (European Network on Imported Infectious Disease Surveillance): http://www.tropnet.eu/
- WHO Disease outbreaks: www.who.int/csr/don/en/

International Association for Medical Assistance to Travellers

- IAMAT; advice for travelers about health risks: www.iamat.org

International Society of Travel Medicine

- Home page: www.istm.org/
- Directory of travel clinics: http://www.istm.org/clinicdir/ clinicdir.aspx
- *Journal of Travel Medicine*: http://www.istm.org/publications/ jtm.aspx

American Society of Tropical Medicine and Hygiene

- Homepage: www.astmh.org/

- Travel clinic directory: http://www.astmh.org/clinicians/ clinics.cfm
- *American Journal of Tropical Medicine and Hygiene*: http://www. ajtmh.org/

Royal Society of Tropical Medicine and Hygiene

- Home page: www.rstmh.org/
- *Transactions of the Royal Society of Tropical Medicine and Hygiene*: http://www.rstmh.org/transactions.asp

Royal College of Physicians and Surgeons of Glasgow

- Faculty of Travel Medicine: http://www.rcpsg.ac.uk/Travel%20 Medicine/Pages/mem_spweltravmed.aspx

Commercial travel medicine databases

- Gideon (Global infectious disease database): www. gideononline.com/
- Exodus Software Ltd (Ireland): www.exodus.ie
- International SOS: www.internationalsos.com/en/ emergencies.htm
- MASTA (England): http://www.masta-travel-health.com/
- Travax and Travax EnCompass (Shoreland Inc, US): www. shoreland.com/gotrav_f.html
- Travax (Health Protection Scotland): www.travax.scot.nhs.uk/
- Tropimed® (Switzerland, Germany, USA): www.tropimed. com

Travel medicine texts

- Ericsson CD, DuPont HL, Steffen R, eds. Travelers' diarrhea, 2nd ed. Hamilton, Ontario: BC Decker; 2008
- Jong E, McMullen R, eds. The travel and tropical medicine manual, 4th ed. Philadelphia: Saunders, 2008.
- Jong EC, Zuckerman JN. Travelers' vaccines. Hamilton, Ontario: BC Decker; 2004.
- Keystone JS, Kozarsky PE, Nothdurft HD, Freedman DO, Connor BA, eds. Travel medicine, 2nd ed. St Louis: Mosby; 2008.
- Schlagenhauf-Lawlor P. Travelers' malaria, 2nd ed. Hamilton, Ontario: BC Decker; 2008.

REFERENCES

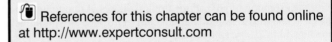 References for this chapter can be found online at http://www.expertconsult.com

Fever in a returned traveler from Kenya or the Congo

Patients returning from East or Central Africa with fever potentially have a very wide differential diagnosis, but it is important to get the probabilities in perspective. By some measure the most common treatable and potentially serious infection causing a fever in people recently returned from most of sub-Saharan Africa is malaria and this must always be excluded. Clinicians not working in Africa often underestimate how common this is: in many parts of Central, West and East Africa the average person will get a clinical attack of malaria several times a year. Case series from the Hospital for Tropical Diseases in London suggest that around one in five travelers returning from Africa with fever will have malaria.[1]

Since it is impossible to exclude malaria on the basis of clinical symptoms or signs (see Chapter 111), a blood film for malaria should always be carried out. Clinicians should not be put off the diagnosis by other potentially localizing signs or symptoms since malaria can coexist with other infections. Clinicians should also be aware that roughly half of those with proven malaria do not have a fever at the time of presentation, so a normal temperature on presentation does not exclude the diagnosis of malaria. Around 95% of all malaria from Central and East Africa will be falciparum malaria and the great majority of cases will present within a month of return though later presentations are possible.[2]

Once malaria has been excluded, however, the two key points are to take a proper travel history and a very exact record of timings of different exposures. Many of the infections that can be acquired in East and Central Africa present simply with an undifferentiated fever and a general feeling of malaise. Initial treatment decisions therefore have to be made on the basis of probabilities, and these depend on epidemiologic exposure.

The simplest timing cut-off is between those who returned within the last 21 days and those presenting more than 21 days after return. With the exception of HIV, all the tropical viruses of importance and the great majority of tropical bacterial infections such as typhoid will present within 21 days of return.

In those presenting more than 21 days after return, three parasitic diseases dominate the common tropical presentation: malaria, amebic liver abscess and Katayama syndrome due to acute schistosomiasis exposure. Tuberculosis is the other major infection to exclude, and occasionally brucellosis, although this is relatively uncommon from this part of Africa. In those presenting more than 21 days after return from the tropics, a blood film to exclude malaria, a chest X-ray looking for the raised right diaphragm suggestive of amebic liver abscess as well as for tuberculosis, and a blood culture are the essential investigations. Katayama syndrome almost always presents with an urticarial rash and eosinophilia. A history of exposure in fresh water 3–8 weeks prior to presentation is strongly suggestive. There is currently no laboratory test that can exclude Katayama syndrome, which is generally self-limiting. Further investigations in those presenting more than 21 days after return from Kenya or the Congo are best guided by localizing symptoms or signs. The great majority of those who do not have malaria will have an infection unrelated to their travel.

In those presenting within 21 days of return from East or Central Africa, malaria remains the most likely diagnosis that requires treatment. There is, however, a much longer list. Some of the more common causes are outlined in Table PP49.1. In addition to those diagnoses mentioned above, there is a range of possible tropical arboviruses (transmitted by mosquitoes). Of these, the most important clinically (in the sense that it may require treatment) is dengue. This is much less common in Africa than in South East Asia and South America but does cause cases in travelers from this part of Africa.[3] Most arboviruses are self-limiting and missing the diagnosis makes no difference to patient outcome.

Table PP49.1 Approximate incubation periods for febrile illnesses from East and Central Africa

Incubation period	Infection
Short (<10 days)	Acute gastroenteritis (bacterial, viral) Respiratory tract infection (bacterial, viral including avian influenza) Meningitis (bacterial, viral) Arboviral infections, e.g. dengue, chikungunya Rickettsial infection, e.g. tick typhus, scrub typhus Relapsing fever (*Borrelia*)
Medium (10–21 days)	Protozoal • Malaria (*Plasmodium falciparum*) • *Trypanosoma rhodesiense* • Acute Chagas disease Viral • HIV, CMV, EBV, viral hemorrhagic fevers Bacterial • Enteric fever (typhoid and paratyphoid fever) • Brucellosis • Q fever • Leptospirosis
Long (>21 days)	Protozoal • Malaria (including *Plasmodium falciparum*) • Amebic liver abscess • Visceral leishmaniasis Viral • Viral hepatitis • HIV

CMV, cytomegalovirus; EBV, Epstein–Barr virus.

Several bacterial diseases are also possible, and these generally will need treatment. Typhoid and paratyphoid occur in this part of Africa, although they are rare compared to other bacterial diseases and are a much less common cause than in, for example, patients returning from South East Asia with a fever.[4] Typhoid is often overdiagnosed in travelers in Africa, and patients having had a fever investigated locally are often told that they have typhoid based on a positive Widal test. As this is almost invariably positive because people have typhoid vaccinations prior to travel, this should not be overinterpreted. Typhoid and paratyphoid do occur in East and Central Africa but they are very rare. Non-typhi *Salmonella* infections are much more common, and in immunocompetent people tend to present with a food-poisoning picture rather than as an undifferentiated fever.

Four things are worth asking about specifically:

- travel in game parks;
- swimming in fresh water;
- whether the returned traveler was caring for sick people; and
- high-risk sexual encounters.

Fresh-water exposure increases the risk of Katayama syndrome. Exposure in game parks increases the risk of one common and unpleasant (although generally self-limiting) infection, African tick typhus. It also increases the risk of a very rare but potentially very serious infection, trypanosomiasis. Typhus is suggested by a combination of a rash (occurring in about 90% of classic African tick-typhus cases) or having seen ticks, or an eschar. The only way of excluding tick typhus is a serologic test; however, as the results may take some time to get back to most centers, if tick typhus is suspected, treatment with doxycycline is worth trying presumptively. It is one of the most common causes of febrile illness in travelers from Africa.[3] If the patient is not better within 48 hours, tick typhus is essentially excluded. Human African trypanosomiasis should be considered but is extremely unlikely.[5] The acute rhodesiense trypanosomiasis which is found in Kenya and in game parks more generally will normally be diagnosed on a blood film. Serologic tests from trypanosomiasis have a very low positive predictive value, with the great majority of positives being false-positives in travelers.

Patients who are also health-care workers returning from East and Central Africa are clearly at higher risk of a wide range of infections than the general population. Generally, these are obvious and not specifically tropical – examples are fecal–oral infections, meningococcus and tuberculosis. In rural areas the exceptionally low probability of viral hemorrhagic fever (Marburg, Ebola) should be considered in health-care workers, especially those working in rural parts of the Democratic Republic of Congo (DRC). Lassa is not thought to occur in this part of Africa. If this seems a possibility, do not take blood tests, and telephone a specialist centre for advice. However, do keep the risk in perspective – it is exceptionally unlikely.

A surprisingly large number of travelers choose to have unprotected sexual contacts in Africa, despite knowing that HIV and other sexually transmitted infections are common in most East and Central African countries.[6] HIV seroconversion and secondary syphilis should be considered, especially where there is a rash. Those who are known to be HIV positive who travel to East and Central Africa are not at particularly increased risk of exotic tropical infections, but non-typhi *Salmonella* infections (especially *S. typhimurium*), pneumococcal infections and tuberculosis are all more common than in Europe in HIV-positive individuals.

Clinical signs can be helpful in diagnosing some of the tropical infections. Where patients present with a rash or jaundice with a fever, having recently returned from East or Central Africa, this may point to particular diagnoses and some of the possibilities are outlined in Table PP49.2. Jaundice and fever should be assumed to be complicated malaria until proved otherwise. Leptospirosis and ascending cholangitis are other common causes. In most cases of viral hepatitis, fever precedes the jaundice, and thinking on the basis of jaundice that a patient has hepatitis A when they have malaria is a potentially fatal mistake.

It is important to stress that, once malaria has been excluded, the great majority of those with an acute fever returning from East and Central Africa will have a self-limiting infection, most of which are nonspecific viral illnesses which they probably would have had as much chance of catching in the UK as when in Africa itself.

Table PP49.2 Acute fever and rash, ulcer or jaundice in those returning from East or Central Africa

Rash	Infection
Maculopapular	Drug reaction, e.g. antimalarials Arboviral infection, e.g. dengue, chikungunya 'Childhood viral illness', e.g. measles, rubella, parvovirus (all more common in Africa) Infectious mononucleosis group, e.g. EBV, CMV, HIV seroconversion Rickettsial spotted fevers, e.g. African tick typhus Secondary syphilis Viral hemorrhagic fever, e.g. Ebola
Vesicular	Rickettsial spotted fever Monkeypox (very rare)
Erythroderma	Sunburn Early dengue
Purpuric	Meningococcal infection Gonococcal infection Hemorrhagic herpes zoster Dengue hemorrhagic syndrome Viral hemorrhagic fever, e.g. Lassa, Ebola, Congo–Crimean hemorrhagic fever, Rift Valley fever Rickettsial spotted fevers (severe) Severe sepsis ± disseminated intravascular coagulation
Ulcer	Eschar: rickettsiosis, anthrax Chancre: *Trypanosoma rhodesiense*, bubonic plague Skin ulcer: superinfected bacterial ulcer, anthrax, cutaneous diphtheria Genital ulcer: syphilis
Jaundice	Severe *Plasmodium falciparum* malaria Hepatitis A–E, but generally the fever precedes the jaundice Leptospirosis (Weil's disease) Septicemia including pneumococcal sepsis EBV, CMV Enteric fever (typhoid and paratyphoid) Typhus Relapsing fevers (*Borrelia* spp.) Viral hemorrhagic fever Ascending cholangitis Malaria *Mycoplasma* *Bartonella* Hemolytic–uremic syndrome (*Shigella*, *Escherichia coli*) Sickle cell crisis with infective trigger

CMV, cytomegalovirus; EBV, Epstein–Barr virus.

REFERENCES

References for this chapter can be found online at http://www.expertconsult.com

Skin rashes in a returned traveler from Ecuador

DEFINITION OF THE PROBLEM

X is a 38-year-old male who returned from a visit to Ecuador 2 weeks ago. He presents to your clinic with a 10-day history of a moderately itchy rash, worse on his right lower leg. He is otherwise fit and has not been taking medications. What are the possible diagnoses and implications for management?

HISTORY TAKING

In any patient with skin disease it is important to follow a logical history-taking format. This must include finding out about a past history of skin problems as, in many patients presenting with skin lesions after travel, the travel is incidental and they have a relevant past history (e.g. eczema or acne), possibly exacerbated by a hotter climate.

In addition, it is important to establish some key facts relevant to their recent travel which include:

- *Where has the patient been?* Try to establish the nature of the travel and determine, for instance, if they were trekking 'up country' or staying in a four-star city hotel. In addition, the type of terrain they have visited (e.g. camping by a fast-running river) may be important.
- *Has anyone else on the trip been affected?* Knowing that others have a similar problem is useful and also potentially indicative of common exposure
- *Have they been taking any medications?* This includes both recent and long-term treatments. Sun sensitivity conditioned by drugs, photodermatitis, can appear first after prolonged sun exposure.

CLINICAL EXAMINATION

Examine the patient, noting the morphology and distribution of the rash. Particularly look for evidence of rash affecting sites exposed to the sun or to insect bites

Key steps in the examination involve answering the following questions:

Is there a rash?

No evidence of rash

Pruritus may be the first sign of evidence of internal disease often not relevant to travel (e.g. chronic renal failure, liver disease). However, it may also be a sign of urticaria (symptomatic dermographism). Itching may also be the earliest sign of skin invasion by schistosomes, including nonhuman pathogens such as avian cercariae contracted while swimming, which do not cause further problems.

There is a rash but is it generalized or localized?

Localized itchy rash

Localized severe itching may be the earliest sign of acute papular onchodermatitis, the early phases of onchocerciasis. The rash is subtle with diffuse dermal edema and papule formation, often confined to one limb or body region (Fig. PP50.1); the shoulder or head may be involved in South American infections. Look for evidence of nodules (unlikely in a traveler) but a skin snip or skin biopsy from a papule is potentially diagnostic (Fig. PP50.2). A history of exposure by a river is important.

Plant- or animal-induced allergy may present with a localized itchy rash. Sometimes in the former case sun exposure may accentuate the rash which present with blisters or bullae. Jellyfish stings present with an itchy localized rash which is often arranged in linear streaks, reflecting the distribution of tentacles. The patient will have been sea bathing.

New dermatophyte infections are unusual in a patient after a short visit overseas. However, exposure to a warm climate may trigger tinea pedis or tinea cruris. Look for an inflammatory raised margin to the rash. Secondary Gram-negative infection of tinea pedis is also common in a warm humid environment. In such cases the itching may diminish and local tenderness or frank pain develops. The skin between the toe webs is eroded and raw but sometimes there is a diagnostic green

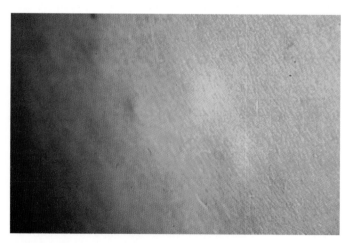

Fig. PP50.1 Acute papular onchodermatitis in a traveler.

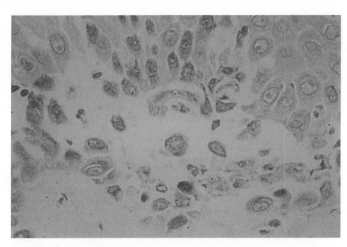

Fig. PP50.2 Skin biopsy (hematoxylin and eosin) showing edema and inflammatory infiltrate near the dermal–epidermal junction. A microfilaria can be seen.

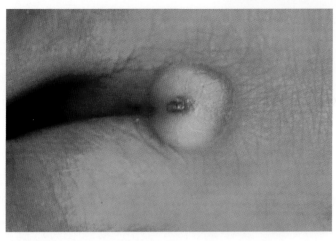

Fig. PP50.4 Local lesion of tungiasis.

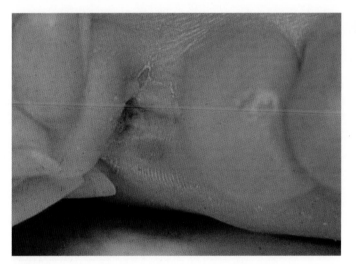

Fig. PP50.3 *Pseudomonas* infection secondary to tinea pedis.

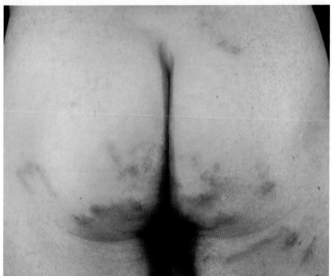

Fig. PP50.5 Cutaneous larva migrans.

tinge, indicating the presence of *Pseudomonas* (Fig. PP50.3). This is important to recognize as antifungals alone are ineffective and it is necessary to use an antiseptic such as povidone–iodine or 1% acetic acid.

If the itch is localized or confined to the foot and there is a visible nodule, ask about other sensations such as a feeling of movement; in myiasis (*Dermatobia* spp.) infection often presents in this way. Tungiasis, due to *Tunga penetrans*, may present in travelers with a localized pustular lesion, usually on the foot, with a central dark area (Fig. PP50.4). If the rash is localized to the legs or buttocks but has a sinuous morphology, cutaneous larva migrans is a possibility. The patient will usually have been sitting or lying on a beach (Fig. PP50.5).

There are other diseases that may affect a visitor to Ecuador that present with a localized skin rash which is only moderately itchy. Contrary to classic teaching, itching may be an early presenting sign, although it is seldom severe, in certain tropical conditions.

Cutaneous leishmaniasis. This sometimes starts as an itchy localized nodule which develops slowly into an indurated lesion or a localized ulcer. Patterns vary but multiple lesions may develop (Fig. PP50.6) or a lymphangitic form can present. Patients often ascribe the lesion to unresolved insect bites. Taking a biopsy or a curetting from such lesions for histology or polymerase chain reaction (PCR) can be very helpful.

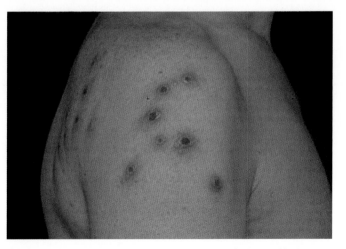

Fig. PP50.6 Cutaneous leishmaniasis presenting with clustered lesions (*Leishmania braziliensis* complex).

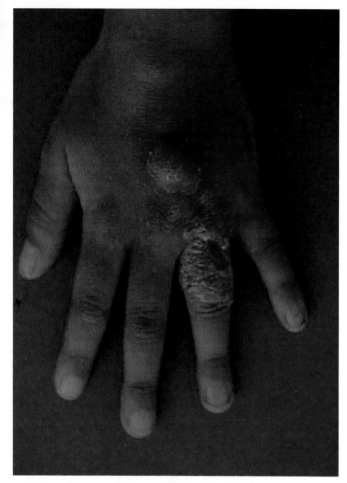

Fig. PP50.7 Lymphangitic sporotrichosis.

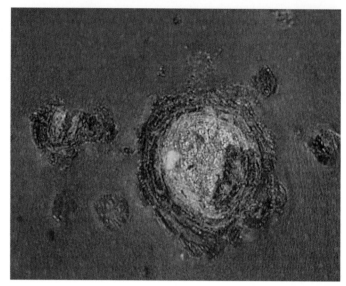

Fig. PP50.8 Streptococcal ecthyma.

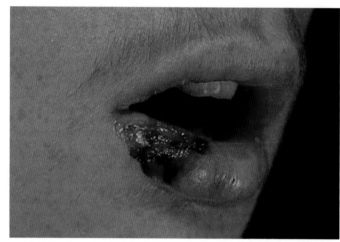

Fig. PP50.9 Early erythema multiforme triggered by human herpesvirus 1.

Sporotrichosis. This may start as a localized itchy nodule. While less common in travelers it is well recognized on those staying for a longer period and particularly those doing volunteer work in rural areas. Sporotrichosis classically presents with an ascending lymphangitic pattern of clinical lesions with nodules or ulcers along the course of a lymphatic and a primary distal lesion (Fig. PP50.7). On the face it also develops induration or ulceration and can closely resemble leishmaniasis. Sporotrichosis is often sparsely populated with yeast form fungi and culture is the best way of reaching a diagnosis.

Open wounds/sores. Open wounds or sores that itch seen in the more adventurous traveler who has been trekking may suggest a potential diagnosis of ecthyma (Fig. PP50.8). Again, these are often described as nonhealing bites but they may be covered by a dark crust which overlies a deep but regular crater. In a tropical environment streptococcal infection is the common cause.

Generalized itchy rash

It is important to note the morphology of the lesions. Possibilities in a traveler from Latin America include the following:

- Widespread insect bites. These are usually papular but may have necrotic centers. If some persist, consider cutaneous leishmaniasis (see above).
- Small target-like lesions symmetrically distributed on the face and peripheries and shallow oral ulcers might suggest

erythema multiforme. This is most commonly triggered by reactivation of human herpesvirus 1 infection following sun exposure (Fig. PP50.9). However, some endemic mycoses may trigger this response – for example, histoplasmosis in the acute phase may present with erythema multiforme. A history of cave exploring might suggest this possibility.

While ultimately diagnosis will often depend on appropriate investigations, a careful history may well provide the clue to the diagnosis.

FURTHER READING

🖱 Further reading for this chapter can be found online at http://www.expertconsult.com

Jaundice in a returned traveler from Nepal

BACKGROUND

Nepal is an increasingly popular destination for travelers attracted by its spectacular scenery and culture. There are 500 000 tourist visitors each year, and the number is rising with the ending of political conflict. Although a major earner of foreign currency, the average spend per tourist is low at around 50 USD/tourist/day, and Nepal remains extremely poor. There has been improvement in access to drinking water, but problems remain, including contamination with arsenic and human waste. Moreover, ancient traditional water sources such as the spouts in Figure PP51.1 remain popular, often prized for their taste. Outside Kathmandu the mountainous terrain is a major obstacle to communication and the development of modern sanitation and safe water supplies. Thus water-borne disease is an important cause of illness. In the south of the country where the elevation is lower the climate is more tropical and malaria is endemic. Comparative country health indicators are illustrated in Table PP51.1.

POTENTIAL CAUSES OF JAUNDICE IN NEPAL

There is a multitude of causes of jaundice. In addition to contact with pathogens perhaps not found in the traveler's normal environment (e.g. hepatitis E virus, *Salmonella enterica* serovar Typhi), holiday travel is associated with increased recreational risk-taking behavior, including sexual activity and drug taking (alcohol included).

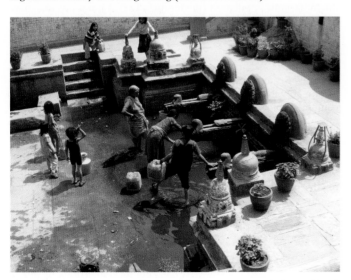

Fig. PP51.1 Collecting water from traditional water spouts in Patan, Nepal.

NON-INFECTIOUS CAUSES OF JAUNDICE

This section focuses on the differential diagnosis of infectious causes of jaundice, but of course there are many non-infectious causes. Additional non-infectious causes for the tropical traveler include drug-related hepatitis which has been described in patients using mefloquine, amodiaquine and atovaquone–proguanil for malaria chemoprophylaxis. It is also well recognized with fluoroquinolones, sometimes prescribed for self-treatment of travelers' diarrhea. Sale of pharmaceuticals is less regulated than in industrialized countries, with increased opportunity for self-medication.

INFECTIOUS CAUSES OF JAUNDICE

Potential infectious causes of jaundice are listed in Table PP51.2. This is not exhaustive! Early diagnosis and treatment are key in obtaining a good outcome from most infectious diseases. Treatable potentially fatal diseases such as malaria and enteric fever should always be considered and excluded in any patient returning from the tropics.

Table PP51.1 Comparative country indicators 2006 (UNICEF)			
	Nepal	**Vietnam**	**USA**
Gross national income per capita, US dollars	290	690	44 970
Infant mortality rate/1000 live births	46	15	6
Life expectancy at birth, years	63	74	78
Proportion of population using improved drinking water, percent	89	92	100
Proportion of population with improved sanitation, percent	27	65	100
Proportion of government expenditure allocated to health, percent	5	4	24
Total adult literacy rate, percent	49	90	–

Table PP51.2 Infectious causes of jaundice

Pathogen		Comment
Viral	Hepatitis A virus Hepatitis B virus Hepatitis C virus Hepatitis D virus Hepatitis E virus Epstein Barr virus Cytomegalovirus Human immunodeficiency virus	Requires co-infection with HBV
Bacterial	Listeria monocytogenes Neisseria spp. Pneumococcus Coxiella burnetti Rickettsia conori Treponema pallidum Chlamydia spp. Brucella spp. Leptospira spp. Salmonella enterica Mycobacterium tuberculae	As part of disseminated disease, i.e. severe sepsis Cause granulomatous hepatitis but jaundice rare. No reported Coxiella infections from Nepal In secondary syphilis. Primary disease may be asymptomatic depending upon the site of the lesion Fitz-Hugh–Curtis syndrome Typhi and Paratyphi A The commonest cause of granulomatous hepatitis worldwide
Parasitic	Entamoeba histolytica Falciparum spp. Leishmania spp. Fasciola hepatica/gigantica	If there is compression of bile ducts by abscess The presence of jaundice defines severe malaria Can cause granulomatous hepatitis, jaundice is rare Abnormal liver enzymes common in acute disease, jaundice can be a feature of established infection

Hepatitis E

Hepatitis E virus (HEV) is endemic in the developing world and is the commonest viral cause of acute hepatitis in Nepal. Probably only one-quarter of infections are symptomatic, but disease can be severe, particularly in pregnant women, with a death rate up to 25%. There have been large-scale outbreaks reported from several countries in recent years, including Nepal, but the vast majority of disease burden is accounted for by sporadic cases. The predominant route of infection is fecal–oral, but parenteral, vertical, person-to-person and zoonotic (domestic swine and rodents) routes may also be important.

In Nepal, some reports have attributed up to 90% of cases of acute infectious jaundice to HEV, but the incidence (and relative prevalence) seems to vary from year to year. The incidence is higher in the rainy season, perhaps related to fecal contamination of drinking water. Four genotypes of HEV have been described, but only one serotype, which offers the hope of development of a broadly specific vaccine.

The presentation and clinical course of hepatitis E disease, with the exception of the high mortality in pregnancy, is similar to that of hepatitis A. Large outbreaks are not such a feature of hepatitis A, and knowledge of any outbreak in the country visited by the traveler is helpful. The incubation period is in the range of 2–8 weeks. However, HEV cannot be distinguished clinically from other causes of acute hepatitis, and definitive diagnosis relies on serologic testing. Some reports have suggested the period of viremia can be prolonged; however, resolution of biochemical hepatitis seems to correlate strongly with clearance of virus from stool.

There is no specific treatment for HEV. Vaccines are in development, and a recent study in Nepal found good tolerability and efficacy from a course of three doses with a recombinant HEV vaccine.

Hepatitis A

Hepatitis A virus (HAV) is endemic in Nepal. One survey found between 3% and 8% of acute hepatitis to be due to HAV. It would be expected that the incidence of this disease would be falling in travelers thanks to the availability of effective vaccines. Spread is fecal–oral, and the incubation period is 2–6 weeks. Most infected adults (70%) become jaundiced, although children under 2 years are usually asymptomatic. Fulminant hepatic failure is rare (0.2%).

A study in 1995 found HAV to be the predominant cause of acute jaundice in foreigners in the Kathmandu valley, which contrasted with the indigenous population (predominantly HEV), but this may have changed with increased HAV vaccination.

Hepatitis B

Hepatitis B vaccination is increasingly offered to travelers. Risk factors for HBV infection are clearly defined – sex, contaminated medical equipment/blood products, intravenous drug use and vertical transmission – and a careful history may be revealing. The sex tourism industry is a growth area in South Asia. Diagnosis is through serologic testing. The incubation period is 2–6 months.

HBV accounts for between 2% and 15% of cases of acute infectious hepatitis in Nepalese patients, but the risk for local Nepalese of HBV infection is unlikely to be the same as that for visitors to the country.

Hepatitis C

Hepatitis C virus (HCV) accounts for 3–5% of acute infectious hepatitis cases in Nepal. There are few data, but most infections are due to genotypes 1 or 3. HCV is predominantly transmitted via blood, blood products and intravenous drug use. There is a very low risk of sexual transmission. In addition, virus can be transmitted through tattooing, but this risk is often not recognized by travelers. The incubation period is between 2 weeks and 6 months. Most infections with HCV lead to chronic disease (80%) and are initially asymptomatic. Less than 25% of infections are acutely jaundiced.

Early diagnosis and treatment of HCV may result in increased cure rates, and the diagnosis should be excluded in any jaundiced patients or any asymptomatic patient with a significant exposure history.

Enteric fever

Enteric fever is the commonest identifiable cause of fever in patients presenting to Patan Hospital in Lalitpur, Kathmandu. A survey of febrile patients in 2001 identified a pathogen in 37%, and 13% of all patients had culture-confirmed enteric fever. Between 1% and 2% of patients with enteric fever are jaundiced. The incubation period is 1–4 weeks.

The past 10 years have seen the increasing importance of *Salmonella enterica* serovar Paratyphi A as a cause of enteric fever, and worryingly rates of drug resistance for this organism seem to be outstripping those of *Salmonella enterica* serovar Typhi. However, later generation fluoro-quinolones, such as gatifloxacin, are effective. Marrow culture is the most sensitive diagnostic test for enteric fever. There may be only one colony-forming unit of *S. enterica* in 5 ml of blood, and diagnostic sensitivity is improved through taking a large volume of blood for culture. In Patan, about a third of patients with a clinical diagnosis of enteric fever have positive blood cultures.

Leptospirosis

Leptospirosis is widely distributed in both temperate and tropical countries and has been associated with recreational activities in travelers, including white water rafting, canoeing and triathlons. One survey of blood donors and army recruits in eastern Nepal found 12% of the population to be seropositive. Jaundice occurs in a subset of patients, although many infections are subclinical. Serologically confirmed leptospirosis accounted for 4% of all cases of fever in adults at Patan Hospital. The incubation period is between 5 and 14 days.

Headache and fever are the most frequent symptoms; other manifestations include cough, pharyngitis, myalgia, abdominal pain, hepatosplenomegaly and conjunctival suffusion. Clearly the clinical features are very similar to enteric fever, although jaundice is more common.

Diagnosis is made through paired sera; isolation of the organism is difficult but blood cultures may be positive if taken early in disease. Nucleic acid amplification techniques, including real-time polymerase chain reaction (PCR), have been developed as diagnostic tests, but are not widely available. Doxycycline or benzyl penicillin are commonly used for treatment.

Malaria

Hyperbilirubinemia is a manifestation of severe malaria. There are around 10 000 cases of malaria each year in Nepal. Most of these (90%) are *Plasmodium vivax*; *P. falciparum* accounts for the remainder. Transmission is limited to elevations of less than 1500 m, and there is seasonal variation in the transmission rate, the incidence being highest in June and August, and lowest from November to March. The Terai region has the highest transmission rates.

The risk to travelers is low; the Kathmandu valley and Himalayan districts, most frequently visited by tourists, are probably malaria free. However, travelers cannot always accurately recall their travel itinerary, exclusion of malaria is cheap and simple, and failure to diagnose malaria results in delay in treatment with potentially fatal consequences. Malaria should be excluded from all unwell travelers returning from endemic countries. If there is doubt about the infecting species, the patient should receive therapy active against *P. falciparum*, i.e. an artemisinin derivative or quinine. The SEAQUAMAT trial demonstrated the superiority of artesunate over quinine for the treatment of severe malaria.

Rickettsial disease

There is serologic evidence of possible acute infection with *Rickettsia typhi* (murine typhus) or *Orientia tsutsugamushi* (scrub typhus) in up to 27% and 23% of patients, respectively, presenting with febrile illness to hospitals in the Kathmandu area. Polymerase chain reaction for *R. typhi* is less frequently positive – 7% of febrile patients presenting to Patan Hospital. There are no data for *O. tsutsugamushi*.

In a series from Thailand, jaundice occurred in 35% of patients with scrub typhus, but this seems to be a rare feature in Nepal, where the presenting syndrome is similar to enteric fever. Treatment is with doxycycline.

Brucellosis

Granulomatous hepatitis can be a feature of brucellosis. The prevalence of brucellosis in Nepal is not known, but it has been reported. Presentation can be similar to enteric fever. The diagnosis should be considered in those with an appropriate exposure history. Risk factors for exposure are consumption of unpasteurized milk products and contact with animal carcasses or aborting animals. The incubation period is variable, and can be protracted, but is usually between 5 and 60 days.

Diagnosis is through culture of the organism – from marrow, blood or other affected tissue. Persistent negative serology excludes infection, but interpretation of low-level positive serologic results is difficult. A recent Cochrane meta-analysis found combined treatment with a tetracycline and streptomycin to be associated with better cure and lower relapse rates than treatment with rifampin (rifampicin)-based regimens.

SUMMARY

The most likely infectious cause of acute jaundice in Nepal is hepatitis E virus. While rare, potentially life-threatening infections that less commonly cause jaundice, such as malaria and enteric fever, must be excluded in all patients. Meticulous history taking with particular attention to exposures and risks is key in developing a coherent differential diagnosis and instituting timely treatment.

FURTHER READING

Further reading for this chapter can be found online at http://www.expertconsult.com

Sexually transmitted infection in a returned traveler from Durban

CASE STUDY

A 42-year-old man seeks medical assistance because of the development a single lesion on his penis. Three weeks ago he returned home from a 3-day business trip to Durban, South Africa. He noticed the lesion 3 days ago. He admits that he had unprotected sex with a South African woman whom he met in a bar. The lesion is painful, bleeds easily and its edges are undermined (Fig. PP52.1). Your clinical diagnosis is chancroid. You collect a specimen from the ulcer base and send this to the diagnostic laboratory for polymerase chain reaction (PCR) together with a blood specimen for syphilis and HIV serology. The results of the laboratory tests are shown in Table PP52.1.

BACKGROUND INFORMATION

Durban is the second largest city in South Africa and has the largest harbor on the African continent. It is situated in the province of KwaZulu-Natal. The province has the highest prevalence of HIV in South Africa and, although no recent comparative surveys have been done, it is likely to have the highest prevalence of other sexually transmitted infections (STIs) as well.

The general concept is that STIs circulate within a limited number of individuals in a population. However, the existence of such a core group in KwaZulu-Natal is challenged by the presence of nonulcerative STIs in 35% of consecutive first-time antenatal clinic attendees who perceive themselves as asymptomatic. These figures show that STIs are widespread among members of the KwaZulu-Natal population and are not restricted to individuals that seek medical care for such a disease.

Studies on the prevalence of the different organisms that cause the different syndromes in patients attending the specialized STI clinic in the centre of Durban are shown in Table PP52.2. Although these

Table PP52.1 Results of laboratory tests

PCR	*Haemophilus ducreyi*	Negative
	Treponema pallidum	Negative
	Herpes simplex virus 2	Negative
	Chlamydia trachomatis, biovar LGV	**Positive**
Serology	HIV	Negative
	Fluorescent treponemal antibody absorption (FTA-ABS)	Negative
	Rapid plasma reagin	1:1

relative prevalences change over time, all known causative agents of STIs are present in the KwaZulu-Natal population and Table PP52.2 shows the most recent available data. *Haemophilus ducreyi*, the most prevalent cause of genital ulcers a decade ago, has disappeared. Multiple infections are found in approximately 10% of patients.

Table PP52.2 Etiology of the three main STI syndromes in Durban, South Africa

	PREVALENCE (%) IN PATIENTS WITH		
	Male urethritis	**Vaginal discharge**	**Genital ulcer syndrome**
Neisseria gonorrhoeae	52	5	
Chlamydia trachomatis, biovar OG	16	5	
Mycoplasma genitalium	5		
Trichomonas vaginalis		20	
Bacterial vaginosis		52	
Chlamydia trachomatis, biovar LGV			6
Treponema pallidum			4
Haemophilus ducreyi			0
Herpes simplex virus 2			34
Calymmatobacterium granulomatis			6

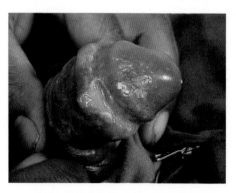

Fig. PP52.1
Lymphogranuloma venereum with chancroid-like ulcers.

Susceptibility testing of *Neisseria gonorrhoeae* isolates reveals high levels of resistance to penicillins, tetracycline and fluoroquinolones, borderline susceptibility for spectinomycin but susceptibility to cephalosporins. Therefore, the only effective treatment available for a patient with gonorrhea contracted in Durban is a third-generation cephalosporin (cefepime or ceftriaxone).

GENERAL APPROACH

Since STIs are so prevalent in KwaZulu-Natal, each traveler to Durban who is sexually active during this visit with a South African partner can become infected with one or more STI pathogens. This is not restricted to sex with a commercial sex worker. The infections result in one or more of three clinical syndromes: male urethritis (MUS), vaginal discharge (VDS) and genital ulcer syndrome (GUS). MUS and VDS are caused by the same group of microbes while GUS has a different spectrum of pathogens. Although each of these infections has their 'textbook' clinical presentation, it has been well established that the clinical presentation is a poor predictor of the etiology for all three syndromes. Apart from atypical presentations, pathogens causing MUS and VDS also cause asymptomatic infections in a significant proportion of infected individuals.

An etiologic diagnosis is dependent on the laboratory diagnosis. Since microscopy and culture has low sensitivity or is not available, nucleic acid amplification tests need to be performed. This technology is only available in specialized laboratories except for *Chlamydia trachomatis*. In patients with GUS who have acquired their infection in Durban, asymptomatic MUS or VDS should also be considered.

PRINCIPLES OF MANAGEMENT OF SEXUALLY TRANSMITTED INFECTIONS

There are two approaches to management of STIs: a syndromic approach and an etiologic approach. Which one to apply is determined by the prevalence of STIs in the patient population and the availability of advanced laboratory tests.

The syndromic approach is practiced in the public health sector in South Africa since the prevalence is high and the availability of diagnostic laboratory capacity is limited. The government advocates this approach for use in the private sector also. In this approach, patients are diagnosed at syndrome level and treated for all causes of that particular syndrome in the part of the world where the acquisition of infection took place. The organisms to be covered for the different syndromes for disease acquired in Durban are summarized in Table PP52.2. Syndromic management protocols need regular revision based on local surveillance data.

Table PP52.3 Differential diagnosis for nonhealing genital ulcers

Sexually transmitted infection	Other causes
Noncompliance to treatment Inadequate duration of treatment Resistant STI microbes Herpes simplex virus in an immunocompromised patient Secondary bacterial infection	Malignancy Tuberculosis Hydradenitis in the groin Pyodermas Behçet's disease

For patients developing symptomatic STIs in countries like the UK where the prevalence of these infections is much lower and laboratory capacity higher, the etiologic approach is more appropriate.

MANAGEMENT OF THE PATIENT PRESENTED IN THE CASE STUDY

The results of the laboratory tests indicate that this patient has lymphogranuloma venereum (LGV). The PCR applied includes a restriction step that allows differentiation between the different biovars of *C. trachomatis*. A rapid plasma reagin (RPR) test of 1:1 with a negative fluorescent treponemal antibody absorption (FTA-ABS) test is not in keeping with syphilis as positivity in the FTA-ABS precedes a positive RPR, the RPR titer is very low and the *Treponema pallidum* PCR on ulcer secretions was negative. Repeat syphilis serology on the follow-up visit at 3 weeks should be considered.

The classic clinical presentation of LGV is a small, self-healing ulcer followed by lymphadenopathy. However, in Durban LGV presents with chancroid-like ulcers. Management of patients with LGV is 3 weeks of doxycycline or erythromycin. Patients should be seen weekly for follow-up till the ulcer has healed. If no healing tendency is observed at 2 weeks from the start of treatment, an alternative diagnosis should be entertained (Table PP52.3). The approach to possible asymptomatic infection of the urethra in this patient is to collect a urethral specimen for diagnosis.

FURTHER READING

Further reading for this chapter can be found online at http://www.expertconsult.com

Eosinophilia in a returned traveler from West Africa

INTRODUCTION

Eosinophils are bone marrow-derived leukocytes that have differentiated into first myeloid and then granulocyte (basophil/eosinophil) lineages. They are present in body tissues, especially those of the gut and lungs, at concentrations much higher than the peripheral circulation. They are produced and activated through stimulation from interleukin (IL)-4, IL-5 and IL-13 which are secreted by type 2 T-helper lymphocytes (Th2). These cells have differentiated from T-helper lymphocytes under direction from IL-4. In contrast, cytotoxic Th1 responses are driven by interferon gamma which also cross-inhibits Th2 responses.

Eosinophils seem to have evolved to defend against the tissue stages of parasitic invasion where the organism is too large to be phagocytosed. IgE is synthesized by activated plasma cells which initially become attached to the membranes of mast cells and basophils. Once the parasite has been opsonized by IgE the mast cell degranulates, releasing inflammatory mediators. One of the main cells drawn to the site of this mediatory release is the eosinophil. The parasite is also opsonized by IgG and complement which, together with IgE, activate the eosinophil, causing release of lytic proteins and superoxides. One by-product of this response is the development, in certain individuals, of hypersensitivity to non-pathologic antigens, leading to allergy, atopy and high circulating levels of IgE, mast cells and eosinophils.

Eosinophilia is generally defined as the presence of greater than 450–600 eosinophils/mm³ of peripheral blood. Although this absolute number is probably of most value, a white blood cell count in which greater than 7% are eosinophils is also significant.

DEFINITION OF THE PROBLEM

A 26-year-old aid worker returned from Ghana where he had spent 9 months working on a rural development project. Prior to departure there were no outstanding health problems and he had taken appropriate malaria prophylaxis for the duration of his trip. During his time there he had stayed in fairly basic accommodation, eaten locally produced food, walked barefoot on numerous occasions and had swum in freshwater rivers and lakes.

Two weeks after return he started to develop headaches, evident in the morning but resolving during the day. He had episodes of sweating and fever as well as sore muscles and joints. After a further 2 days he woke with an urticarial rash over his torso, which came and went as the day progressed. The next morning he woke with mild swelling of his lips and tongue. At this point he decided to consult his general practitioner who sent him to hospital for investigation. A malaria slide was negative but a full blood count revealed an eosinophil count of 900 eosinophils/mm³ with a 14% fraction.

CAUSES

Without any history of travel, a raised eosinophil count would probably hint towards an atopic condition such as hay fever, asthma or eczema. However, in a traveler returning from a developing country it should suggest helminth infection to the investigating physician. Nevertheless, it is important not to miss other causes, some of which may be as a consequence of the travel and some incidental to it. It is also important to bear in mind that the absence of a raised count in no way excludes a helminth infection. A full list of causes of a raised eosinophil count is provided in Table PP53.1, with the pathophysiology, epidemiology and treatment of the infectious causes being detailed more extensively in the main text.

HIV and human T-cell lymphotrophic virus 1 (HTLV-1) may be accompanied by a raised eosinophil count in certain situations. Resolving scarlet fever is said to be associated with eosinophilia, as are brucellosis and lepromatous leprosy. Unicellular protozoan parasites almost never cause eosinophilia, the occasional exceptions being *Isospora belli* and *Dientamoeba fragilis*. Aspergillosis, in the form of allergic bronchopulmonary aspergillosis, and primary or disseminated coccidioidomycosis can be associated with an elevated eosinophil count, as can scabies and myiasis infestations.

In terms of non-infectious causes, it is always important to consider drug reactions, especially as travelers have often been taking unfamiliar medications. Common culprits are sulfa-based drugs, which include Septrin and Fansidar, but quinine, β-lactams and tetracyclines have also been implicated. Adrenal insufficiency, as well as numerous inflammatory, neoplastic and hypersensitivity conditions, should be considered; however, in the majority of cases, in those returning from the tropics, the cause will be helminthic.

INVESTIGATION AND MANAGEMENT

Any patient found to have eosinophilia needs to be questioned carefully and examined thoroughly. Whilst the history should be comprehensive, there are certain useful questions that should be considered which may direct the physician to a particular diagnosis. These are outlined in Table PP53.2 with the indicated diagnosis. In a similar way the examination needs to be complete, covering all systems but certain findings may indicate a specific condition. These are outlined in Table PP53.3.

Table PP53.1 Causes of a raised eosinophil count

Non-infectious causes

Drug reactions	Sulfa-based drugs • Fansidar (pyrimethamine–sulfadoxine) • Septrin (trimethoprim–sulfamethoxazole) β-Lactams Quinine and quinidine Non-steroidal anti-inflammatory drugs Tetracyclines Aspirin Beta-blockers
Atopic/allergic conditions	Urticaria Pemphigoid Asthma/hayfever Eczema Loeffler's syndome Chronic eosinophilic pneumonia Tropical pulmonary eosinophilia Idiopathic hypereosinophilic syndrome
Neoplasms	Lymphoma – especially Hodgkin's Chronic myeloid leukaemia Acute myeloid leukaemia Eosinophilic leukaemia Some solid-organ malignancies
Connective tissue diseases	Rheumatoid arthritis Churg–Strauss syndrome Midline granuloma Sarcoid Polyarteritis nodosa Dermatomyositis Wegener's granulomatosis
Endocrine	Addison's disease

Non-helminth infectious causes

Fungal	Aspergillosis – allergic bronchopulmonary aspergillosis Coccidioidomycosis – primary or disseminated
Ectoparasites	Scabies Myiasis
Bacterial and viral	Scarlet fever – resolving Brucellosis Leprosy – lepromatous HIV Human T-cell lymphotropic virus 1
Protozoa	*Isospora belli* *Dientamoeba fragilis*

Helminth causes

Nematodes (roundworms)	Intestinal	*Ascaris lumbricoides* Hookworms • *Ancylostoma duodenale* • *Necator americanus* *Strongyloides stercoralis* *Oesophagostomum bifurcum* Visceral larva migrans • *Toxocara canis* • *Toxocara cati* Cutaneous larva migrans • *Ancylostoma braziliense*

Table PP53.1 Causes of a raised eosinophil count—cont'd

	Tissue	*Wuchereria bancrofti* *Brugia malayi* *Mansonella perstans* *Loa loa* *Onchocera volvulus* *Trichinella spiralis* *Gnathostoma* spp.
Trematodes (flukes)		*Schistosoma mansoni, haematobium, japonicum, mekongi* • Chronic infections • Acute infections – Katayama fever Avian and mammalian schistosomiasis – swimmers' itch (schistosome dermatitis) *Clonorchis sinensis* *Opisthorchis viverrini* *Fasciola hepatica* *Paragonimus westermani*
Cestodes (tapeworms)		*Taenia saginata* *Taenia solium* *Diphyllobothrium latum* *Hymenolepis nana* *Echinococcus granulosus*

Table PP53.2 History to be considered

Geography traveled	Equatorial West Africa Sub-Saharan Africa, Arabian peninsula and some areas of elevated Central America	*Loa loa* Onchocerciasis
	Southwestern United States, northern Mexico South East Asia	Coccidioidomycosis *Gnathostoma* spp. and *Clonorchis*
Activities	Swimming in fresh water Walking barefoot Sheep-rearing	Schistosomiasis Cutaneous larva migrans, hookworm, *Strongyloides* *Echinococcus granulosus*
Food	Pork Boar, bear, horse, walrus, wart hog Beef Crab Fish, seafood or animals fed on fish Watercress Horse chestnuts	Trichinosis, *Taenia solium* Trichinosis *Taenia saginata* *Paragonimus* Fish tapeworm, *Gnathostoma* *Fasciola* *Fasciolopsis*

Investigations

Various approaches to investigation have been proposed but it is probably best to start with a basic laboratory workup. Other tests can then be added if there are specific findings on history and examination, or if something is discovered on the initial tests (Fig. PP53.1).

It is obviously better to identify a specific cause and treat it with targeted anthelmintics as this leads to more effective treatment and less unnecessary toxicity. However, if no diagnosis is forthcoming

Table PP53.3 Examination findings and possible pathology

Hydroceles, unilateral lower limb swelling	Lymphatic filariasis
Myositis, periorbital edema, splinter hemorrhages	*Trichinella*
Nodules	Onchocerciasis, *Loa loa*
Rash, pruritus	Onchocerciasis, *Loa loa*, cutaneous larva migrans, allergy (particularly to foods), vasculitis
Subcutaneous swellings	*Loa loa* or *Gnathostoma*
Larva currens	*Strongyloides*
Pulmonary findings – wheeze/cough/shortness of breath	*Ascaris*, *Strongyloides*, *Paragonimus*, tropical pulmonary eosinophilia, filariasis, asthma, aspergillosis
Hepatomegaly/tender right upper quadrant	Visceral larva migrans, schistosomiasis, liver flukes
Neurologic signs	Cysticercosis, trichinosis, schistosomiasis, strongyloidiasis

after extensive investigation or if resources are limited, then two options are available depending on the clinical status of the patient:

- first, the tests are repeated after an interval of 3 months; and
- second, presumptive treatment with albendazole and/or praziquantel can be given, targeted towards the perceived likely pathogens.

Complications

Normally eosinophilia does not lead to complications. However, if the levels have been severely raised or raised for a prolonged period of time, such as with the idiopathic hypereosinophilic syndrome, then organ damage can occur. The heart is the organ most commonly affected, resulting in endomyocardial fibrosis, pericarditis and valvular pathology. Other organs can also be involved, leading to neuropathy, skin lesions, encephalopathy, respiratory problems, enteritis, hepatitis and cholangitis.

FURTHER READING

Further reading for this chapter can be found online at http://www.expertconsult.com

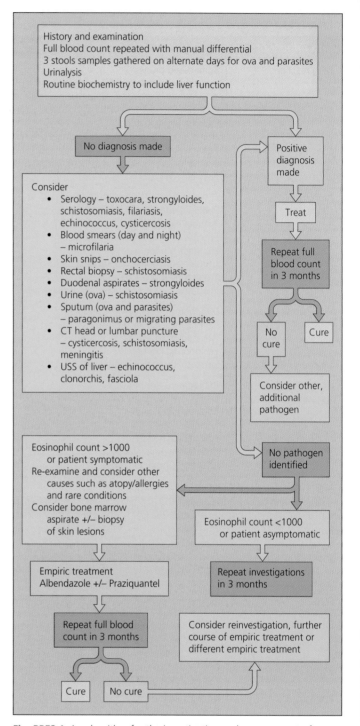

Fig. PP53.1 An algorithm for the investigation and management of eosinophilia.

Practice point | 54 |

Tom Doherty

Lymphadenopathy, splenomegaly and anemia in a returned traveler from Sudan

CASE HISTORY

A 32-year-old Caucasian man who had worked for an international aid agency in rural parts of Sudan for the last 3 years presented to hospital. He had grown up in the UK but had spent considerable periods of his working life overseas, mostly in East Africa. He complained of a fever with night sweats for the previous 6 weeks and, despite maintaining his appetite, had lost 8 kg in weight. He had no significant past medical history and, apart from doxycycline as prophylaxis against malaria, he was taking no regular medication. He smoked 10 cigarettes a day, drank alcohol in moderation and had no concerns regarding the possibility of having acquired HIV infection. He had no cough or other respiratory complaints and had not experienced any gastrointestinal symptoms.

On examination, he looked pale and unwell. He had an axillary temperature of 101.3°F (38.5°C) but his pulse rate and blood pressure were normal. He had generalized, nontender lymphadenopathy with palpable nodes in his neck, both axillae and groin, none of which was more than 1 cm in diameter. There were no peripheral stigmata to suggest HIV/AIDS. His throat looked normal, his chest was clear and examination of his cardiovascular system was unremarkable. He had marked splenomegaly with a spleen that was palpable 8 cm below the left costal margin, but no hepatomegaly. He was oriented in time, place and person and had no neurologic deficit.

Preliminary investigations revealed a pancytopenia, with a hemoglobin of 11 g/dl, total white cell count of 2.4×10^9/l and a platelet count of 131×10^9/l. A malaria parasite screen was negative on both thick and thin films. Both his erythrocyte sedimentation rate and his C-reactive protein were elevated above 100. His renal function was normal and, apart from a slight elevation in his alanine transaminase concentration, his liver function tests were unremarkable. However, his albumin concentration was low at 28 g/l. His international normalized ratio (INR) was 0.97. Chest X-ray was reported as normal.

DISCUSSION

In the context of any patient with suspected imported infection, it is often helpful to answer the four questions which comprise the maxim attributed to Professor Eldryd Parry: 'Why does this person, from this place, develop these symptoms at this time?' With regard to this case, the 'person' was a Caucasian professional who would be expected to have little or no immunity to malaria; in addition,

he did not appear to be at particularly high risk of HIV infection. The 'place' was rural Sudan, an area where many of the classic tropical diseases such as malaria, tuberculosis, leishmaniasis, brucellosis, relapsing fever and schistosomiasis would all be highly prevalent. The 'symptoms' were a febrile illness, characterized by generalized systemic upset with night sweats and weight loss, with anemia and splenomegaly as prominent signs. The duration of the symptoms, 6 weeks, would imply that this was a significant illness rather than a simple viral infection, for example. Taken together, the history, physical findings and laboratory investigations would strongly suggest a diagnosis of visceral leishmaniasis in an HIV-negative individual.

Other diagnoses would need to be considered. Apart from visceral leishmaniasis, the three other recognized causes of splenomegaly of this magnitude would be hyperreactive malarious splenomegaly (previously known as tropical splenomegaly syndrome), chronic myeloid leukemia and myelofibrosis. Hyperreactive malarious splenomegaly is thought to be more common in women than men, would be uncommon among a Caucasian population and might have been prevented by the antimalarial prophylaxis that this man was taking. Chronic myeloid leukemia would be unusual in a man of 32 and, like myelofibrosis, would not be expected to present with such florid systemic symptoms, nor with pancytopenia. In this particular case, the diagnosis was confirmed both serologically and by performing a splenic aspirate. The serologic tests comprise a direct agglutination test (DAT) looking for IgG against *Leishmania donovani* and a commercial K39 strip test (DiaSys Europe Ltd, Wokingham, Berkshire, UK) which detects 39 consecutive amino acids from the kinetoplast of *L. donovani*; taken together, these two serologic tests are virtually 100% sensitive and specific in an HIV-negative individual. The splenic aspirate using a 21-gauge needle and 0.5 ml of normal saline which is then stained with Giemsa permits a quantification method of the number of amastigotes found in the spleen.

An HIV test would be necessary as, if this were positive, this would have implications for his treatment. Chronic schistosomiasis secondary to *Schistosoma mansoni* would also need to be excluded and brucellosis is another possibility. A lymphoproliferative disorder should also be included in the differential diagnosis of anyone presenting with systemic symptoms, lymphadenopathy and splenomegaly.

A list of conditions that are associated with lymphadenopathy is given in Table PP54.1. Table PP54.2 lists those conditions associated with splenomegaly with some reference to the degree of splenic enlargement, and Table PP54.3 outlines a schedule for investigations for splenomegaly and/or anemia in a patient recently returned from abroad.

Table PP54.1 Causes of lymphadenopathy

	Causes	Notes
Common	Local sepsis	Cause is usually obvious
	Tonsillitis	Particularly streptococcal
	Epstein–Barr virus	Palatal petechiae, splenomegaly, atypical lymphocytes
	Nonspecific viral infection	
Less common but important	HIV seroconversion illness	Transient lymphadenopathy
	HIV (established disease)	Permanent lymphadenopathy
	Kaposi's sarcoma	
	Tuberculosis	
	Trypanosomiasis	Localized lymphadenopathy in early infection with chancre; generalized lymphadenopathy in late infection
	Toxoplasmosis	
	Secondary syphilis	
	Dengue fever	Lymphadenopathy occurs in 50% of cases; usually mild
	Chancroid	Usually inguinal lymphadenopathy
	Lymphoproliferative disorder	
	Neoplasia	Usually metastatic lymphadenopathy
	Sarcoidosis	Particularly hilar lymphadenopathy
	Leishmaniasis	Cutaneous and visceral
	Typhus	Usually painful eschar
Uncommon	*Wuchereria bancrofti*	
	Brugia malayi	
	Parvovirus	
	Q fever	
	Lymphogranuloma venereum	
	Castleman's disease	
	Rheumatoid arthritis	
	Systemic lupus erythematosus	
	Leptospirosis	
	Still's disease	
	Pityriasis rosea	
	Cat-scratch fever	

Table PP54.1 Causes of lymphadenopathy—cont'd

	Causes	Notes
Rare	Lepromatous leprosy	
	Erythema nodosum leprosum	
	Bartonellosis	Often tender
	Tularemia	
	Anthrax	
	Diphtheria	
	Plague	Extremely tender 'buboes'
	Kikuchi's disease	
	Ehrlichiosis	
	Behçet's syndrome	
	Wegener's granulomatosis	
	Midline granuloma	
	Whipple's disease	
	Weber–Christian disease	
	Podoconiosis	
Infections usually not associated with lymphadenopathy	Brucellosis	
	Loiasis	
	Onchocerciasis	Secondary infection of scratched skin may result in lymphadenopathy
	Malaria	
	Hepatitis	
	Typhoid	Lymphadenopathy has been reported in chronic salmonellosis
	Tuberculoid leprosy	May occur in acute disease
	Schistosomiasis	
	Flaviviruses	
	South American trypanosomiasis (chronic form)	
	Intestinal helminths	
	Strongyloides spp.	
	Hydatid disease	
	Cholera	
	Tetanus	
	Melioidosis	
	Cysticercosis	
	Amebiasis	
	Fascioliasis	

Table PP54.2 Causes of splenomegaly*

Mild splenomegaly	Malaria
	Epstein–Barr virus
	Hepatitis
	Typhoid and other salmonelloses
	Tuberculosis
	Dengue fever
	Katayama fever
	Toxoplasmosis
	Cytomegalovirus
	HIV
	Leptospirosis
	Brucellosis
	Sepsis
	Trypanosomiasis
	Histoplasmosis
	Rheumatoid arthritis/Still's disease
	Systemic lupus erythematosus
	Hemoglobinopathies
	Sarcoidosis
	Lepromatous leprosy and erythema nodosum leprosum
	Amyloidosis
Moderate splenomegaly	Lymphoproliferative disorder
	Subacute bacterial endocarditis
	Splenic abscess
	Portal hypertension due to chronic schistosomiasis
Marked splenomegaly	Visceral leishmaniasis
	Hyperreactive malarious splenomegaly
	Myelofibrosis
	Chronic myeloid leukemia
	Glycogen storage diseases

*Each section reflects the importance and/or frequency of the various conditions. The italic type shows the conditions that are more likely to occur in travelers.

FURTHER READING

Further reading for this chapter can be found online at http://www.expertconsult.com

Table PP54.3 Suggested investigations for splenomegaly and/or anemia in a patient recently returned from abroad

Initial investigations	Thick and thin blood films for malaria (repeated several times) Blood cultures (repeated several times) Full blood count (red cell indices, white cell count, evidence of hypersplenism) Blood film examination (atypical lymphocytes; red cell morphology; evidence of hemolysis)
If anemia predominates	Serum iron Transferrin, total iron binding capacity Red cell folate Vitamin B12 Fecal occult blood (repeated several times) Hemoglobin electrophoresis Also consider: bone marrow aspirate endoscopy
Serologic investigations	Epstein–Barr virus Toxoplasmosis Cytomegalovirus Malaria immunofluorescent antibody test Schistosomal ELISA Brucella Leishmania HIV Histoplasmosis Acute and convalescent sera for dengue fever and other flaviviruses Beware false-positive autoimmune disease serology
Imaging	Abdominal ultrasound and CT Chest radiography Indium-labeled white blood cell scan
Tissue diagnosis	Liver biopsy Splenic aspiration

ELISA, enzyme-linked immunosorbent assay.

History of an animal bite in a returned traveler from Burma

DEFINITION OF THE PROBLEM

A 26-year-old female presents to acute medical services 14 days after returning from a year long back-packing trip; for the past 7 weeks she has been in rural Burma. She reports being bitten by a stray but friendly dog on her ankle about 3 weeks ago. There is a visible bite wound and she complains of some pain around the bite area. She otherwise feels well. She is unsure of her pretravel immunization history.

HISTORY TAKING

When approaching this clinical scenario, the most crucial aspect of initial assessment is a detailed history of events. In this case we know the animal involved was a dog and therefore the most important aspect immediately becomes assessment of the risk of rabies. Successful management involves minimizing the patient's risk of developing symptomatic rabies. It is relatively common for an individual not to be clear about what has bitten them and then a much wider range of possibilities needs to be considered including snake, spider and scorpion bites as well as mammal bites. Terrestrial animals in the majority of South East Asia, Africa and South America are classed as high risk for rabies (see http://www.who-rabies-bulletin.org for up-to-date information by country). Bats can also carry classic and rabies-related lyssaviruses depending on species and location.

Rabies accounts for between 40 000 and 70 000 deaths per year and dog bites are responsible for 99% of these deaths.[1] Once symptomatic, apart from one or two documented exceptions, rabies is fatal; however, prompt postexposure prophylaxis is effective. The incubation period from bite to symptomatic diseases is usually between 3 and 12 weeks but has been documented up to 19 years.[2]

INITIAL ASSESSMENT (SEE ALSO FIG. PP55.1)

The location of the bite is important as the rabies virus reaches the brain by traveling centripetally along the peripheral nerves. This means bites on the neck or face have a shorter incubation time than those on hands or feet. Rabies cannot be transmitted through intact skin; however, infection has been documented after mucous membrane exposure as well as superficial scratches and licking episodes.[2]

The behavior of the biting animal is also important (Fig. PP55.2); did it appear sick, was it obviously limping or was it being uncharacteristically friendly? Did it appear to be coughing or have something stuck in its throat (hydrophobia)? In rabies-endemic countries, dogs are often reluctant to approach humans because of mistreatment; if a dog approaches humans it may be a sign that it is unwell.

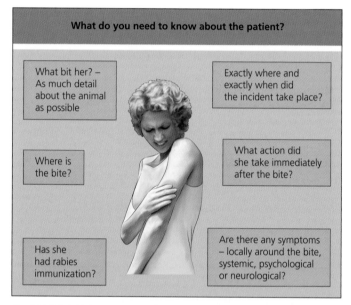

What do you need to know about the patient?

What bit her? – As much detail about the animal as possible

Exactly where and exactly when did the incident take place?

Where is the bite?

What action did she take immediately after the bite?

Has she had rabies immunization?

Are there any symptoms – locally around the bite, systemic, psychological or neurological?

Fig. PP55.1 Initial assessment of a patient bitten by an animal.

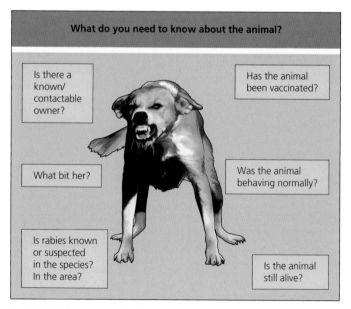

What do you need to know about the animal?

Is there a known/contactable owner?

Has the animal been vaccinated?

What bit her?

Was the animal behaving normally?

Is rabies known or suspected in the species? In the area?

Is the animal still alive?

Fig. PP55.2 Description of the biting animal.

If the owner of the animal is known, is it possible to contact them and establish if it has been vaccinated? If it is still alive, is it being kept under observation? If a dog or cat remains healthy for 15 days after the incident it is unlikely that it was infected with rabies at the time of the bite.[1]

MANAGEMENT OF ANY BITE WOUND

Initial management

- Wash thoroughly, ideally for ~15 minutes.
- Clean with chlorhexidine.
- Do not suture.
- Assess tetanus need.
- Assess need for antibiotics.
- Assess need for rabies postexposure prophylaxis.

Rabies-specific management

Postexposure prophylaxis consists of vaccination and administration of human rabies immunoglobulin (HRIG) (Table PP55.1). As the patient described above has never been vaccinated, HRIG should be administered immediately based on her weight at a dose of 20 IU/kg.[3] As much as possible of the dose should be infiltrated around the site of the wound, the remainder given as an intramuscular injection. HRIG is not necessary if the patient has completed a full vaccination course or received a booster within the previous 5 years, however high the risk or if more than 7 days have elapsed since the first dose of postexposure vaccination.

Postexposure vaccination should be commenced as soon as possible. This consists of five doses of 1 ml of vaccine intramuscularly (not gluteal); however, only two doses are necessary if the patient has been previously vaccinated. Postexposure prophylaxis should be administered if indicated irrespective of the time delay to presentation as incubation periods can be prolonged.[4] The two products licensed in the UK are human diploid cell vaccine (HDCV) and purified chick embryo cell vaccine (PCEC) although other efficacious vaccines (e.g. Vero cell vaccines) are available.[3]

DIAGNOSIS

Virologic diagnosis of rabies during life can be difficult; in most cases it is the characteristic clinical picture and history which make the diagnosis (Table PP55.2). Saliva, cerebrospinal fluid (CSF) and skin biopsies taken from the nuchal area of the neck containing hair follicles and peripheral nerves and corneal impression smears can all be tested using various methods. Fluorescent antibody testing to detect viral antigen is most commonly used; however, sensitivity is limited. Antibody tests are available but can be difficult to interpret in the immunized patient. Reverse transcriptase polymerase chain reaction (RT-PCR) can be done on saliva, CSF and skin biopsies and is available in some countries via national reference laboratories.

TREATMENT

Symptomatic furious rabies can be very distressing with a combination of painful muscle spasms, hydrophobia and feelings of terror. There is no known curative treatment so symptom control with heavy sedation and analgesia is the mainstay of treatment. There have been recent reports of survival of a very limited number of patients by implementation of what has become known as the Wisconsin protocol.[5] The utility of this approach remains unproven.

OTHER CONSIDERATIONS

Macaque monkeys found in Burma and much of South East Asia, India and Japan commonly carry B virus. This is predominantly asymptomatic in monkeys but can rarely cause human disease through bites, scratches and mucous membrane splashes. Incubation is between

Table PP55.2 Clinical presentation of rabies

Furious	Paralytic
Confusion, agitation, aggression	Ascending paralysis
Autonomic stimulation – sweating, excess saliva, terror	Fasciculation
Phases of arousal and lucid intervals	Loss of reflexes
Spasms, hydrophobia, aerophobia	Sphincter dysfunction
Cranial nerve lesions	Sweating, fever
Paralysis	Bulbar paralysis
Coma	Respiratory paralysis

Table PP55.1 Postexposure prophylaxis

IMMUNIZATION STATUS		Full pretravel immunization*	No or inadequate/unclear pretravel immunization
Location	**Type of exposure**		
Any	Contact, licks to skin but no scratch or bite	No treatment	No treatment
High- or low-risk country	Licks, scratches or abrasions, minor bites, i.e. covered areas of arms, trunk or legs.	Commence postexposure vaccine only: two doses days 0 and 3	Commence postexposure vaccine: five doses days 0, 3, 7, 14 and 28 (plus rabies immunoglobulin if high-risk country†)
High- or low-risk country	Licks of mucosa or any major bite, or any exposure where animal known to have rabies	Commence postexposure vaccine only: two doses days 0 and 3	Commence postexposure vaccine: five doses days 0, 3, 7, 14 and 28 and rabies immunoglobulin

*Full pretravel immunization = three doses on days 0, 7 and 28.
†Use of rabies immunoglobulin may sometimes be restricted to high-risk cases when shortages occur.
Adapted from Health Protection Agency guidelines.[3]

2 days and 5 weeks and end-stage disease consists of diffuse encephalomyelitis with an untreated mortality rate of 80%.[5] Prevention is predominantly by prompt and through cleaning and irrigation of the wound. Postexposure prophylaxis with valaciclovir is recommended for high-risk exposures; however, it is unproven in humans. Treatment with intravenous aciclovir or ganciclovir if central nervous system signs are present improves survival.[6]

Controversy still exists about whether to give prophylactic antibiotics to bite patients. It is generally agreed that high-risk bites such as facial or hand injuries, extensive or crush injuries and those with deep penetration warrant antibiotic prophylaxis. The drug of choice is co-amoxiclav in view of its effectiveness against the bacterial flora of animal mouths commonly implicated in these infections, such as *Pasteurella multocida* and anaerobes, as well as streptococci and staphylococci.

REFERENCES

References for this chapter can be found online at http://www.expertconsult.com

Leprosy

EPIDEMIOLOGY

Leprosy is a chronic infection of the skin and nerves with *Mycobacterium leprae*, which, although rarely fatal, is a significant cause of disability. Over the past 15 years there have been dramatic changes in the prevalence of leprosy since the introduction of multidrug therapy (MDT).[1,2] As a result of the shorter duration of therapy and more intensive control programs, the number of registered leprosy patients receiving chemotherapy has fallen from 10–12 million to 225 000 in 2006.[3] The annual case detection rate of new cases remained high for many years, but this has recently fallen from 763 000 in 2001 to 259 000 in 2006. This rapid fall may reflect reduced active case finding activities following the integration of leprosy control into general health services, as well as a true decline in the incidence of leprosy worldwide. In addition, there is a pool of 2–3 million patients with permanent nerve impairment as a consequence of leprosy.

Leprosy is widely distributed in tropical and warm temperate countries and >1 billion people live in regions where there is active transmission of *M. leprae*. There has been a reduction in the number of endemic countries (prevalence rate >1/10 000) from 122 in 1985 to 4 in 2006,[3] mainly Brazil, Democratic Republic of Congo (DRC), Mozambique and Nepal. Currently 85% of registered cases occur in only six countries:

- India (accounting for 54% of all registered cases); and
- Brazil, Indonesia, DRC, Bangladesh and Nepal in order.[3]

Because of the long incubation period of leprosy an individual from an endemic country may develop leprosy years after migration elsewhere. Delay in diagnosis is usually longer in nonendemic than endemic regions, and therefore leprosy should be considered as a diagnostic possibility in any person who is from an endemic country and has chronic lesions of the skin or impaired function of peripheral nerves.

Subclinical infection with *M. leprae* is far more common than overt disease.[4] Analysis of *M. leprae*-specific immune responses[5,6] has demonstrated that *M. leprae* infection is common after exposure, but the majority of individuals control the infection. Currently there is no specific test to distinguish latent leprosy infection from latent tuberculosis infection, but *M. leprae*-specific T-cell assays are being developed.[7]

The major mechanism of transmission of *M. leprae* is thought to occur through nasal secretions, particularly from lepromatous patients.[4] Organisms probably enter through the mucosa of respiratory tracts and, if not controlled, disseminate to the skin and peripheral nerves. Other possible modes of transmission include breast milk from mothers with untreated lepromatous disease and uncommon cases of cutaneous inoculation. Although infection with *M. leprae* has been documented in wild armadillos in the USA and some primates, zoonotic transmission does not contribute to human disease.[6]

Proximity to leprosy patients is important in transmission, and the relative risk for disease for household contacts is 8- to 10-fold greater for lepromatous cases and 2- to 4-fold greater for tuberculoid cases.[4] Nevertheless, the majority of leprosy cases are sporadic.

Genetic factors influence both the development of leprosy and the pattern of disease. Genome-wide linkage analysis in multicase families has defined susceptibility alleles in the genes for lymphotoxin-α and the ubiquitin and proteosome related enzymes, PARK2 and PACRG.[8] Susceptibility loci have also been identified on chromosome 10p13, close to the gene for the mannose receptor C type 1,[9] and the HLA region with linkage to both the HLA Class II and tumour necrosis factor genes,[10] in Indian and Brazilian patients respectively. The HLA locus also affects the pattern of disease: HLA-DR2 and -DR3 are associated with tuberculoid disease and HLA-DQ1 with lepromatous leprosy. Racial and geographic factors also influence the type of leprosy, with lepromatous leprosy being less common in Africans than Indians, and most common in Chinese and Caucasians.

The incidence of leprosy peaks in two age groups (10–15 and 30–60 years of age) and there is a male predominance in most regions of about 2:1.[4] The incubation period varies widely from months to over 30 years, but is usually prolonged, averaging 4 years for tuberculoid and 10 years for lepromatous leprosy. In contrast to tuberculosis there is no definite evidence for increased HIV prevalence in leprosy patients or a change in the clinical spectrum of leprosy among co-infected patients, although some studies suggest there is an increase in leprosy reactions in HIV-infected patients.[11] Leprosy can occur as an immune reconstitution syndrome in co-infected patients after starting highly active antiretroviral therapy.

PATHOGENESIS AND PATHOLOGY

Although *M. leprae* was the second bacterium to be associated with a human disease, it still cannot be cultivated *in vitro*. The organism is capable of limited multiplication in mouse footpad, with a doubling time of 11–13 days, and this has permitted drug sensitivity studies.[6,12] *M. leprae* is an acid-fast Gram-positive bacillus and is an obligate intracellular parasite with tropism for macrophages and Schwann cells. The bacilli show preference for growth in cooler regions of the body. The unique characteristic of *M. leprae* is its predilection to infect Schwann cells. The receptor complex on the Schwann cell is the G-domain of the laminin α2 chain in the basal lamina of Schwann cells and the laminin receptor, α-dystroglycan.[13] A number of ligands on the surface of *M. leprae* bind to this complex including the specific trisaccharide of PGL-I and a 21 kDa surface protein.

Genetic and structural analyses have confirmed that *M. leprae* is a member of the family Mycobacteriacae. A major advance has been the sequencing of the genome of an Indian isolate of *M. leprae*.[14] The genome contains 1605 genes encoding proteins and 50 genes for stable RNA molecules. Remarkably, half the functional genes in the *M. tuberculosis* genome are absent, being replaced by many inactivated or pseudogenes. This gene decay has removed entire metabolic pathways and regulatory genes, particularly those involved in catabolism. This may render the leprosy bacillus dependent on host metabolic products and may explain its long generation time and inability to grow in culture.[14] Comparison of single nucleotide polymorphisms in the *M. leprae* genome between multiple isolates from different continents suggests that leprosy infection of humans originated in East Africa or the Near East and then spread through successive human migrations.[15] Individual isolates of *M. leprae* can be distinguished by the variable number of tandem repeat sequences within their genome, but the extent of variability within individual patients for isolates collected from different sites or at different times limits the use of these repeat tandem sequences as tools for molecular epidemiologic studies.[16]

The availability of the *M. leprae* and other mycobacterial genomes has major implications for the development of new antimycobacterial drugs and *M. leprae*-specific diagnostic reagents.[6,7] The complex cell wall contains important targets of the immune response, including a species-specific phenolic glycolipid-I (PGL-I) and immunomodulatory lipoarabinomannan. The cell wall biosynthetic pathways are relatively intact in *M. leprae*, despite the loss of other genes, indicating that these represent the essential genes for the formation of a minimal mycobacterial cell wall.[17] *M. leprae* is relatively inert, and the host immune response is responsible for most of the tissue damage.

The manifestations of leprosy form a wide clinical spectrum determined by immunopathologic responses to the organism (Fig. 103.1).[18] Patients who have the polar forms of tuberculoid (TT) and lepromatous leprosy (LL) are immunologically stable, but those who have the intermediate types of borderline-tuberculoid (BT), mid-borderline and borderline-lepromatous (BL) leprosy are immunologically unstable and subject to either a gradual decline towards the lepromatous pole or upgrading reversal reactions (RRs; see Fig. 103.1). In TT

a vigorous cellular response to *M. leprae* limits the disease to a few well-defined skin patches or nerve trunks.[5] The lesions are infiltrated by interferon gamma secreting CD4+ T lymphocytes, which form well-demarcated granulomas containing epithelioid and multinucleate giant cells around dermal nerves. Few, if any, bacilli are demonstrable. Cellular immunity may be confirmed by *in-vitro* lymphocyte responses to *M. leprae* antigens or skin test reactivity. Intradermal injection of heat-killed *M. leprae* causes a transient swelling at 48 hours in a sensitized subject (Fernandez reaction), followed by the development of a granulomatous nodule at 3–4 weeks (Mitsuda reaction).[5] The latter confirms an individual's capacity to mount a T-lymphocyte response to *M. leprae*. Antibody responses to *M. leprae* are absent or low titer.

The hallmark of LL is the absence of *M. leprae*-specific cellular immunity, and this results in uncontrolled proliferation of the bacilli with extensive infiltration of the skin and nerves and numerous lesions.[5] Histologically, the dermis contains foamy macrophages filled with multiple bacilli and a scattering of CD4+ and CD8+ lymphocytes, but no organized granulomas.[18] There are high titers of antibodies to *M. leprae*-specific PGL and protein antigens. In borderline cases a progressive reduction in cellular responses is associated with a greater bacillary load, more frequent skin and nerve lesions, and increasing antibody levels.

The dynamic nature of the immune response to *M. leprae* is responsible for spontaneous fluctuations in the clinical pattern, termed leprosy reactions[5]:

- a type 1 reaction is usually an 'upgrading' RR caused by increased cellular reactivity to mycobacterial products, results in edema and acute inflammation of skin lesions and nerves, is most common in borderline patients and is a major cause of nerve damage[19]; and
- a type 2 reaction or erythema nodosum leprosum (ENL) is a systemic inflammatory response associated with the deposition of extravascular immune complexes leading to neutrophil infiltration and activation of complement in multiple organs.[20] This is accompanied by high circulating levels of tumor necrosis factor with systemic toxicity.

PREVENTION

The chief means of preventing leprosy is the interruption of transmission by treating those with infectious leprosy early. Multidrug therapy was introduced because of the increasing spread of primary and secondary dapsone resistance worldwide.[1] Its advantages are its proven efficacy[2] and improved compliance, which is related to the limited duration of therapy and its monthly observed component (see Management, below). Furthermore, early treatment before the onset of nerve damage reduces the long-term disability associated with leprosy.[21] The effectiveness of MDT prompted a World Health Organization co-ordinated campaign to implement MDT in all endemic countries, with the aim of reducing the prevalence rate of leprosy to less than 1/10 000.[3] This has been successful, with only four countries left to attain this goal. Importantly, the case detection rate has been slower to fall, probably because of the prolonged incubation period of clinical leprosy, indicating that leprosy control must be sustained through case detection and treatment of leprosy within integrated health programs.

The response to immunization with *M. leprae* bacille Calmette–Guérin (BCG) has been variable, but in a major trial in Malawi, BCG induced 50% protective efficacy against clinical leprosy, both tuberculoid and lepromatous forms.[22] Re-immunization enhanced the protective effect by a further 50%. Recent meta-analysis has confirmed the significant protective effect of BCG against leprosy in both clinical trials and case-control studies.[23] Extensive BCG immunization of children in endemic countries has probably made a significant contribution to the decline of leprosy. The addition of heat-killed *M. leprae* to BCG did not increase the observed protective efficacy of BCG in two trials.[22] Other experimental vaccines are being tested against leprosy infection at present.

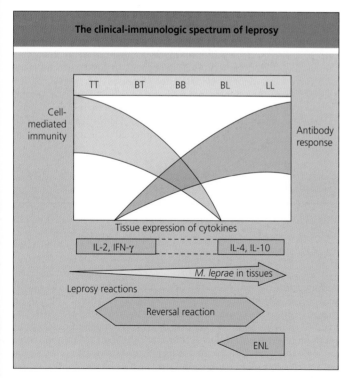

The clinical-immunologic spectrum of leprosy

Fig. 103.1 The clinical–immunologic spectrum of leprosy. This reflects the underlying host immunity as measured by the T-cell and antibody responses to *M. leprae*. Spontaneous fluctuations in the immune response are responsible for reversal reactions and erythema nodosum leprosum (ENL). TT, tuberculoid leprosy; BT, borderline tuberculoid; BB, mid-borderline leprosy; BL, borderline lepromatous leprosy; LL, lepromatous leprosy; IFN, interferon; IL, interleukin.

Chemoprophylaxis may also be useful in the control of leprosy, particularly in low endemic regions. A large, randomized control trial in Bangladesh showed that a single dose of rifampicin given to the close contacts of newly diagnosed leprosy patients resulted in a significant reduction of 57% (95% CI 33–72) in the incidence of leprosy in the contacts at 4 years.[24] Leprosy is commonly associated with poverty and overcrowding, and improved socioeconomic conditions have also contributed to the decline of leprosy in Europe and some Asian countries.

CLINICAL FEATURES

Types of leprosy

Indeterminate leprosy

This is the earliest form and occurs as a single, slightly hypopigmented ill-defined macule in children, who are often contacts of leprosy patients.[25] The majority of these lesions are self-limiting and resolve without therapy. A minority (<25%) develop into defined lesions within the clinical spectrum.

Tuberculoid leprosy

These lesions occur as one to three large asymmetric macules or plaques with sharply defined borders and hypopigmented anesthetic centers (Fig. 103.2).[25,26] Although leprosy lesions are usually hypopigmented, in light skins the macules may appear erythematous or dyschromic. Involvement of sweat glands and hair follicles results in dryness and loss of hair. Enlarged cutaneous nerves may be palpable at the edge of the lesion, but nerve trunk involvement is minimal.

Borderline tuberculoid leprosy

This is the commonest form of leprosy. The skin lesions resemble those in TT leprosy, but are more frequent and variable in appearance and their borders are less well demarcated (Fig. 103.3). The outline may be irregular with adjacent 'satellite' lesions suggesting local spread. Occasionally, large patches of BT leprosy may involve a whole limb. Asymmetric enlargement of several peripheral nerves is usual and patients may present with muscle weakness or trauma secondary to sensory impairment. Progressive nerve damage is common.

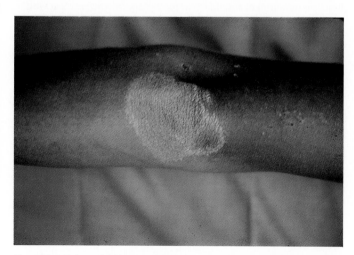

Fig. 103.2 Tuberculoid leprosy. Single hypopigmented anesthetic plaque with raised border and dry surface.

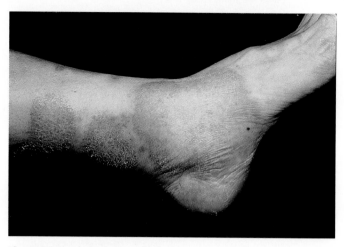

Fig. 103.3 Borderline tuberculoid leprosy. Three large well-defined erythematous patches with reduced sensation, spreading borders and satellite lesions.

Mid-borderline leprosy

This is the most immunologically unstable form with the propensity to shift rapidly towards BT leprosy during a reversal reaction or to downgrade towards BL leprosy. The skin lesions are numerous and vary in size, shape and distribution. They may be hypopigmented or erythematous. The characteristic 'target' lesion has a broad, erythematous border with a vague outer edge and 'punched-out' pale center with sensory impairment (Fig. 103.4).

Borderline lepromatous leprosy

In borderline lepromatous leprosy there are numerous small erythematous macules, which initially may be limited in distribution, but become progressively more symmetric.[25] Papules, nodules and succulent plaques may develop and, in contrast to tuberculoid leprosy, the lesions have normal sensation. The intervening skin is normal. Widespread nerve involvement is typical, especially if the patient has downgraded from BT leprosy.

Lepromatous leprosy

This is a systemic disease with a generalized bacteremia leading to widespread involvement of the skin and other organs.[25,26] The first manifestation may be a diffuse infiltration of the dermis causing a smooth shiny appearance of the skin. More typically, there are numerous symmetrically distributed macules, papules or nodules, and sensation may be retained in lepromatous lesions (Figs 103.5, 103.6). Progressive thickening of the skin results in coarsening of the facial features and nodular thickening of the ear lobes. With time the eyebrows and eyelashes become thinned.

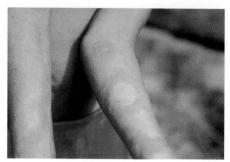

Fig. 103.4 Mid-borderline leprosy. Characteristic target lesion with raised erythematous annular border and 'punched-out' central area with impaired sensation.

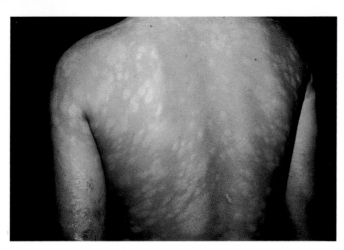

Fig. 103.5 Lepromatous leprosy. Multiple, small, slightly erythematous macules with intact sensation and symmetric distribution. The skin smears of both the lesions and intervening skin are positive for acid-fast bacilli.

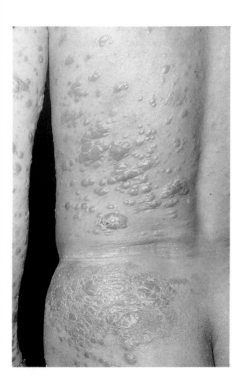

Fig. 103.6 Nodular lepromatous leprosy. Diffuse infiltration of the skin by multiple nodules of varying size, each teeming with bacilli.

Bacillary infiltration is responsible for gradual tissue damage in the involved organs. The nasal mucosa is infiltrated at an early stage, resulting in discharge and obstruction. Erosion of the cartilage and nasomaxillary bones results in perforation of the nasal septum, collapse of the nose and saddle-nose deformity. Laryngeal involvement produces hoarseness and stridor. Direct bacillary involvement of the eye causes keratitis and iritis.

Infiltration of the dermal nerves results in a peripheral sensory loss similar to that of a 'glove and stocking' neuropathy,[25] which leaves the skin susceptible to ulceration and secondary infection. Reactional episodes cause edema of the feet, shins and hands. Dactylitis develops in the hands and feet, and, together with trauma and osteomyelitis, results in phalangeal erosion.

Both testicular infiltration and orchitis contribute to testicular atrophy and secondary gynecomastia. Glomerulonephritis may occur and is usually associated with ENL. Secondary amyloidosis is a consequence of recurrent ENL reactions.

Peripheral nerve involvement

The nerves of predilection occur at superficial sites where the nerve trunks are cooler, more readily traumatized and often anatomically constricted.[25] These include the:
- ulnar nerve at the medial epicondyle of the humerus;
- median nerve at the wrist;
- Lateral popliteal nerve at the neck of the fibula;
- posterior tibial nerve behind and inferior to the medial malleolus; and
- radial nerve in the humeral groove posterior to the deltoid insertion.

Easily palpated superficial cutaneous nerves include the:
- superficial radial nerve at the wrist;
- greater auricular nerves;
- supraorbital nerve; and
- sural nerves.

These nerves should be examined for enlargement and associated weakness and sensory loss. The resulting muscle imbalance results in the characteristic deformities of clawhand, footdrop, clawtoes and wristdrop. Autonomic nerve dysfunction contributes to impaired sweating and dry skin, which is subject to cracking, infection and poor healing. The combination of insensitive feet and clawtoes leads to recurrent plantar ulceration, a major cause of disability.

In pure neural (PN) leprosy the nerve trunks are affected without any skin lesions. On biopsy the neural lesions tend to be 'lepromatous' in appearance and PN leprosy involving more than one nerve should be treated as multibacillary (MB).

Before and during therapy the function of the commonly involved nerves should be assessed at regular intervals by voluntary muscle and sensory testing (preferably with nylon monofilaments) to determine whether there is ongoing nerve function impairment. This may presage the onset of a reversal reaction before nerve pain or typical skin lesions develop. Nerve conduction studies commonly detect subclinical neuropathy in BT–BL leprosy patients and these tests may become abnormal weeks before the development of clinical neuropathy.[27] Nerve function impairment may develop or worsen despite effective chemotherapy, and early recognition and therapy prevent permanent nerve damage.[19,21] Patients with pre-existing nerve damage at diagnosis and MB patients are at greatest risk for new nerve function impairment and should be carefully monitored.[28]

Leprosy reactions

Reversal reactions

These develop in about one-third of patients who have BT–BL leprosy, usually within the first year of treatment, but monitoring for new nerve function impairment should occur for 2 years.[27,29] They present with:
- increased inflammation in established BT–BL skin lesions or new swollen lesions in BL and subpolar LL patients (Fig. 103.7);
- acute neuritis with pain or tenderness in the involved nerve and loss of function; and
- recent (<6 months) or progressive nerve function impairment in the absence of painful nerves.

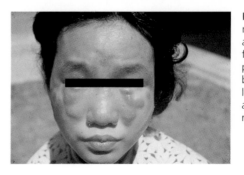

Fig. 103.7 Reversal reaction. Erythema and edema in the facial lesions of a patient who has borderline-tuberculoid leprosy undergoing an upgrading reversal reaction.

Silent neuritis responds to therapy for the RR.[30] Patients at particular risk for developing RR are those who have MB leprosy involving more than two body areas, established nerve function impairment at diagnosis, facial patches or *M. leprae*-specific IgM anti-PGL antibodies.

Erythema nodosum leprosum

This once affected 30–50% of BL and LL patients, but the frequency and severity of ENL have reduced since the regular use of clofazimine in MDT.[2] ENL may develop at any stage of therapy, but usually within the first year and is often recurrent.[31] An episode begins with fever and malaise and the rapid emergence of painful erythematous nodules, typically over the extensor surfaces of the limbs.[5,25] In severe cases widespread nodules may form pustules and ulcerate (Fig. 103.8). Painful neuritis is the most common complication. Erythema nodosum leprosum has features of widespread immune complex deposition and these may include small vessel vasculitis, iridocyclitis, polyarthritis, orchitis, lymphadenitis and glomerulonephritis.

Recurrent or uncontrolled ENL reactions can result in the development of secondary amyloidosis (amyloid A protein) within 3 months.

Eye involvement

Involvement of branches of the facial and trigeminal nerves results in lagophthalmos and corneal anesthesia, respectively, and if combined there is a considerable risk of ulceration and infection of the exposed insensitive cornea.[32]

In 25–30% of patients who have LL, infiltration of the anterior segment of the eye causes a superficial punctate keratitis and iridocyclitis, which may be painless and only recognized by slit-lamp examination. Iridocyclitis is exacerbated during episodes of ENL, but can occur independently of overt reactions. The iritis may be complicated by glaucoma or cataract, both of which contribute to leprosy-associated blindness (see Chapter 17).

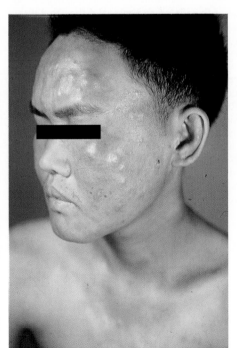

Fig. 103.8 Erythema nodosum leprosum. Tender papules associated with fever, arthralgia and acute neuritis in a patient who has lepromatous leprosy.

DIAGNOSIS

A diagnosis of leprosy is usually straightforward if it is suspected as a cause of any skin or peripheral nerve lesion in a person from an endemic country. The cardinal signs of leprosy[5,33] are:

- skin patch with sensory loss;
- nerve enlargement; and
- acid-fast bacilli (AFB) in the skin.

The presence of one or more of these features establishes the diagnosis, which should be confirmed with a full-thickness skin biopsy. Approximately 70% of all leprosy patients can be diagnosed by the single sign of a skin patch with sensory loss, but 30% of patients, including many MB patients, may not present with this sign, indicating the importance of nerve enlargement as an additional sign and the importance of clinical suspicion for the diagnosis.[33]

Acid-fast bacilli are best demonstrated in slit-skin smears, which should be taken from the edges of at least two lesions and both ear lobes. If these are not available a skin biopsy should be stained for AFB with a modified Wade–Fite stain. The extent of the bacillary load can be quantitated as a bacterial index[12] on a logarithmic scale of 1+ to 6+. The percentage of solid staining AFB in smears, the morphologic index,[12] is an indirect measure of the viability of leprosy bacilli. In PN leprosy a biopsy from a sensory nerve such as the superficial radial nerve may be diagnostic. Polymerase chain reaction (PCR) can be used to identify *M. leprae* DNA and, together with PCR-based detection of rifampin (rifampicin)-resistant strains, it is a valuable tool for epidemiologic studies.[6,34]

Lepromin testing and serology may be used for accurate classification of patients in research studies. Antibodies to PGL and other *M. leprae*-specific protein antigens are present in MB patients and their titer falls with effective therapy.[5] In patients who have BL and LL, evidence of chronic inflammation includes anemia, hypergammaglobulinemia, elevated serum amyloid A protein and positive antinuclear and anticardiolipin autoantibodies.

Other skin diseases can be differentiated from tuberculoid leprosy by the absence of anesthesia in the lesions and the presence of nerve involvement elsewhere.[25,26] Lepromatous skin lesions are not anesthetic and biopsy may be necessary to distinguish these from those due to other systemic infections, such as leishmaniasis and secondary syphilis and other nodular or infiltrative skin conditions. Other causes of nerve enlargement, such as primary amyloidosis and familial polyneuropathy, are excluded by biopsy and family history.

MANAGEMENT

Successful management of leprosy requires prolonged drug treatment and careful monitoring for complications, and it is essential to enlist the patient as an ally in this process. The patient should be educated about:

- the importance of compliance;
- the first symptoms of a reaction; and
- the elements of self-care needed to prevent secondary tissue damage if there is sensory nerve impairment.

The most important step in disability prevention is the early initiation of bactericidal drug therapy.

Antileprosy drugs

Dapsone

This is an important antileprosy drug because of its bactericidal effect at full dosage, low cost and low toxicity.[2] When used alone, stepwise dapsone resistance emerges as a major problem, owing to mutations in *folP1*, encoding dihydropteroate synthase,[6,35] but this is prevented by combination therapy. Mild hemolytic anemia is common, but is only severe in the presence of glucose-6-phosphate dehydrogenase deficiency, which should be excluded where possible. Occasionally dapsone allergy, and rarely agranulocytosis, may develop after 2–6 weeks of therapy.

Rifampin

Rifampin (rifampicin) is a key component of MDT because it is the most effective bactericidal drug against *M. leprae* when given either daily or monthly.[2,12] Toxicity is low with monthly dosage, although thrombocytopenia, hepatitis and a flu-like syndrome occasionally occur. It must be used with at least one other effective drug to prevent rifampin resistance owing to mutations in RNA polymerase.[34] Tuberculosis should always be excluded before monthly rifampin is started (see Chapters 30 and 143). Rifapentine is a long acting rifamycin-derivative, which is more bactericidal than rifampin in mice, and is currently being tested in humans.

Clofazimine

This is a fat-soluble dye that is deposited within the skin, fat stores and macrophages. It has similar bactericidal activity to that of dapsone[2,12] and also a significant anti-inflammatory effect. It is relatively nontoxic and its only disadvantage is the associated development of a reddish skin pigmentation, which resolves after the drug has been discontinued. When used in high doses for prolonged periods clofazimine is deposited in the small intestinal wall and can cause diarrhea and pain.

Other drugs

Three additional drugs have proved effective against *M. leprae* in human and mouse studies:[5,6]
- the fluoroquinolones, ofloxacin and moxifloxacin, have moderate bactericidal activity and infrequent side-effects involving the gastrointestinal tract and central nervous system;
- minocycline, the only fat-soluble tetracycline, has moderate anti-*M. leprae* activity. It has proved effective as an alternative drug in patients with LL and has low toxicity in adults when used as long-term therapy for acne, and so is a useful alternative drug for leprosy; and
- clarithromycin has modest bactericidal activity.

Multidrug therapy

The principle underlying MDT is the use of three drugs when the bacterial load is high in MB leprosy to treat and prevent the emergence of dapsone-resistant strains. Two drugs are sufficient for paucibacillary disease. Since its introduction in 1982,[1] MDT has proved highly effective and over 10 million patients have been treated with few treatment failures and remarkably low relapse rates of about 0.1/100 patient years.[3,36]

Multibacillary multidrug therapy

This is recommended for adult patients with BB, BL, LL, smear-positive BT and PN leprosy. In leprosy control programs in endemic countries, a simplified form of classification is employed, based on the number of patches so that MB leprosy >5 patches and paucibacillary (PB) ≤5 patches. Multibacillary MDT comprises:
- rifampin, 600 mg once a month, supervised administration;
- dapsone, 100 mg/day, self-administered; and
- clofazimine, 300 mg once a month, supervised administration; 50 mg/day, self-administered.

Originally MB-MDT was continued for at least 2 years and then until the skin smears became negative.[1] In subsequent field trials a fixed duration of MB-MDT for 2 years was as effective[2] and was utilized in control programs with very low rates of relapse.[36] Patients who have MB leprosy and a skin smear bacterial index of 4+ or over may require

a longer duration of therapy.[2] In 1998, WHO recommended MB-MDT of 12 months duration for use in control programs,[36] and 12-month MB-MDT is currently used in leprosy control programs in endemic countries.

Some authorities in developed countries prefer to use more frequent doses of rifampin and continue to treat until the smears are negative, which can take many years. One approach is to double the dose of rifampin to 600 mg daily for two consecutive days each month, while others use daily rifampin 450–600 mg for 2 years with dapsone and clofazimine. There is no evidence, however, that daily rifampin is more effective than when given once monthly.

If clofazimine is unacceptable because of pigmentation or if dapsone hypersensitivity occurs, minocycline (100 mg daily) or ofloxacin (400 mg daily) may be substituted.[36] Patients who have rifampin intolerance require two new drugs, minocycline and ofloxacin, along with clofazimine (50 mg/day) for 6 months and then either drug with clofazimine for another 18 months.

Paucibacillary multidrug therapy

This is recommended for indeterminate, TT and smear-negative BT leprosy[2] and in the control programs for patients with 5 patches. PB-MDT comprises of:
- rifampin, 600 mg once a month, supervised administration; and
- dapsone, 100 mg/day, self-administered.

This is continued for 6 months. If the skin smear is positive at any site, the patient is given MB-MDT. If a RR develops after completion of chemotherapy, MDT should be recommenced while on prednisone.

In some countries patients with solitary leprosy skin lesions are common. A large field study in India established that a single dose of the combination of rifampin (600 mg), ofloxacin (400 mg) and minocycline (100 mg) (ROM) was almost as effective as PB-MDT in the treatment of patients with single smear-negative skin lesions and no nerve involvement, although the follow-up period was only for 18 months.[37] This regimen should be reserved only for carefully selected patients in endemic countries with a high proportion of single lesion cases.

Treatment for reactions

Patients who have RRs, including silent nerve function impairment, require high-dose corticosteroids for a prolonged duration to permit nerve function recovery.[19] Prednisone is started at 40 mg/day and increased to 60 mg/day if there is no response, and then to 120 mg/day if necessary. Once there is evidence of improvement on serial voluntary muscle and sensory testing, the dose is reduced over 6 weeks to 20 mg/day and this is continued for some months before gradual removal. There are few clinical trials on the therapy for RRs, but one randomized study demonstrated that outcome is improved if corticosteroids are continued for at least 5 months.[38] Longer durations are often required for RRs complicating MB leprosy. It is important to maintain treatment with antimycobacterial drugs to reduce the bacillary load. Adequate analgesia is essential along with physical support during the period of active neuritis. This therapy can be successfully administered without admission if other infections and medical problems are excluded. The overall recovery rate for nerve function is 60–70%,[39] but may be up to 88% in patients with no nerve damage at diagnosis who develop acute neuropathy during MDT.[21] Recovery is less in those with pre-existing nerve function impairment or with chronic or recurrent reactions.

Mild ENL may respond to aspirin or nonsteroidal anti-inflammatory drugs, increased clofazimine dosage and rest. Moderate or severe episodes and those with neuritis require prednisone, usually starting at 40–60 mg/day. The response is rapid, but as ENL is liable to become corticosteroid dependent, the prednisone should be withdrawn over 2–3 months. Clofazimine at a higher daily dose of 300 mg suppresses ENL after 4–6 weeks, and can be used to prevent further episodes.

If the ENL is poorly controlled or recurs, it usually responds to thalidomide, 400 mg/day for 2–3 weeks, and then 100–200 mg/day as maintenance.[40] Thalidomide inhibits the release of tumor necrosis factor from macrophages and modulates T-cell function, and is of proven and prompt efficacy for ENL in clinical trials. Its use, however, is severely limited by its teratogenicity, and thalidomide should be restricted to male and postmenopausal patients under strict supervision. Thalidomide may cause a peripheral neuropathy, but this neurotoxic effect has not been evaluated in leprosy patients.

Eye involvement is common and iritis requires local treatment with corticosteroid and atropine drops.[32]

Other therapies

Prevention of disability is an important component of care.[41] Regular monitoring of nerve function will reveal early reversible RRs. Patients with irreversible nerve function impairment must learn to care for insensitive hands and feet and be provided with appropriate footwear. Plantar ulceration requires prolonged rest for healing. Physiotherapy and reconstructive surgery for clawhands and clawfeet, footdrop and lagophthalmos may prevent further tissue damage and restore appearance, and facial deformity can be corrected by plastic surgery.[41] Community-based rehabilitation is proving effective in assisting patients with persistent nerve impairment to return to full participation in their own communities.[42]

Websites

- http://www.who.int/lep/: Provides access to WHO documents on the current epidemiology, clinical features and treatment of leprosy with detailed information on MDT and leprosy control.
- http://www.ilep.org.uk/fileadmin/uploads/Documents/techforum.pdf: International Leprosy Association Technical Forum: critical evaluation of clinical diagnostic criteria and therapy for leprosy.
- http://www.leprosy-review.org.uk/: Website of *Leprosy Review* – a journal contributing to the better understanding of leprosy and its control.

REFERENCES

References for this chapter can be found online at http://www.expertconsult.com

André Z Meheus
Jai P Narain
Kingsley B Asiedu

Chapter | **104**

Endemic treponematoses

The endemic treponematoses include yaws (also known as buba, framboesia, parangi and pian), endemic syphilis (also known as bejel, dichuchwa and sklerjevo) and pinta (also known as azul, carate and mal de pinto), all of which are chronic bacterial infections. The causative organisms (*Treponema pallidum* subsp. *pertenue*, *T. pallidum* subsp. *endemicum* and *T. carateum*, respectively) are morphologically and serologically indistinguishable from *T. pallidum* subsp. *pallidum*, which is the causative organism of venereal syphilis.[1]

In the 1990s, small genetic differences (single base pair changes) were identified between the organisms of the venereal and nonvenereal treponematoses but these genetic variations did not allow differentiation of one *T. pallidum* subsp. from another.[2] Recent molecular genetic studies indicate that *T. pallidum* subsp. *pallidum*, subsp. *pertenue*, subsp. *endemicum* and a simian *T. pallidum* (Fribourg–Blanc) strain can be differentiated through subspecies-specific genetic signatures in multiple genes.[3,4]

A phylogenetic analysis indicates that *T. pallidum* subsp. *pertenue* arose first in history causing yaws in our anthropoid ancestors in the tropical belt of the Old World; it spread as yaws to the New World and as endemic syphilis to North Africa, Eastern Europe and the Middle East (through divergence of subsp. *pertenue* to subsp. *endemicum*). It finally evolved in the Americas as the modern subsp. *pallidum* strain (or a progenitor) which was introduced into the Old World as a result of the European exploration of the Americas, and disseminated as venereal syphilis all over the world.[4]

Nevertheless, in clinical practice the treponematoses (venereal and nonvenereal) continue to be diagnosed based on their distinctive clinical and epidemiologic characteristics.[1]

EPIDEMIOLOGY

Historic perspective

The endemic treponematoses, because of the disfigurement and disability they cause, were a major public health problem in the pre-antibiotic era. In 1948, the World Health Organization (WHO) and the United Nations International Children's Emergency Fund (UNICEF) sponsored a global control program. This involved 46 countries and brought these diseases under control with the help of long-acting penicillin. Unfortunately, the diseases were not eradicated and the lack of continuing vigilance allowed persistence of endemic foci in some countries, resulting in localized resurgence of these diseases since the 1980s. In 2007, WHO launched a renewed attempt to eliminate yaws.[5]

Geographic distribution

The endemic treponematoses are now largely confined to communities in remote rural areas living in poor, overcrowded and unhygienic conditions. Yaws occurs mainly in the warm, humid areas of Africa, South East Asia and the Pacific, the Caribbean and Central and South America. In the South East Asia region, India successfully eliminated yaws in 2006, and yaws now remains present only in two countries, Indonesia and Timor-Leste.[6,7] Endemic syphilis occurs mainly in the arid areas of sub-Saharan Africa and among the nomadic people of the Arabian peninsula. Pinta occurs mainly in Central and South America (among Indian tribes in the Amazon region and adjacent areas). Cases of imported yaws and endemic syphilis are sometimes encountered in the countries of the northern hemisphere, where clinicians may need to include them in the differential diagnosis.

INCIDENCE AND PREVALENCE

Accurate incidence and prevalence data are unavailable. The last estimate by WHO in 1995 yields a global prevalence of 2.5 million cases, including 460 000 infectious cases. The situation today remains unknown.

Age and sex

Yaws and endemic syphilis usually occur in children aged 2–14 years. For pinta the range is 10–30 years. Yaws affects boys more than girls; for the other diseases there is probably no sex difference.

Mode of transmission

Yaws and pinta are transmitted by direct skin-to-skin contact with infectious lesions, transmission being facilitated by a breach in the skin of the recipient. The role of nonbiting flies in the transmission is uncertain. In the case of endemic syphilis, because the initial lesions are often in or around the mouth, the infection spreads by direct contact (e.g. older children kissing their younger siblings) and by indirect contact through infected communal eating or drinking utensils.

PATHOLOGY

Yaws and endemic syphilis affect skin and bones, whereas pinta is confined to the skin.

The basic pathology in endemic treponematoses is the same as in venereal syphilis. However, the vascular changes in the endemic treponematoses are less marked. Skin biopsies from yaws patients show numerous plasma cells but few T and B cells; the treponemes are found mostly in the epidermis, whereas in venereal syphilis they are demonstrated mainly in the dermis and dermal–epidermal junction.[8] Because these differences are relative, they cannot be used to differentiate yaws from venereal syphilis.

In pinta, there is loss of melanin in basal cells, the presence of many melanophages in the dermis and the absence of inflammatory cells and treponemes in the achromic lesions.[9]

Endemic treponematoses are not believed to be associated with congenital transmission or with involvement of the cardiovascular and nervous systems.

PREVENTION

Essential in prevention of the endemic treponematoses is not only to identify and treat clinical cases but also to recognize that the presence of clinical cases in a community necessitates an immediate search for further clinical and latent cases, which also must be treated.

The supportive measures for control include:

- strengthening and improving accessibility of the primary health-care facilities;
- training of clinicians to detect and treat patients and to examine and treat household and other obvious contacts;
- health education of the population;
- improvement in the standard of living and in personal and environmental hygiene; and
- provision of soap and water and clothing to children.

CLINICAL FEATURES

The incubation period is 9–90 days (mean 21 days).

Yaws

Early stage

The initial or primary lesion ('mother yaw') appears at the site of infection on an exposed part of the body. It may be a localized maculopapular eruption or a papule, which may develop into a large papilloma 2–5 cm in diameter. It is painless but itchy and may ulcerate as a result of scratching. It may heal in 3–6 months with or without scarring. Secondary lesions, which are the result of lymphatic and hematogenous spread of organisms, appear a few weeks to 2 years after the primary lesion. They may consist of multiple excrescences, often resembling the initial papilloma. The papillomas may ulcerate and the exudate may dry to form a yellow crust which, when removed, gives the lesion an appearance of a raspberry (hence the name 'framboesia'). The lesions may be irregular, crescentic or discoid in shape and on moist areas may mimic condylomata lata of venereal syphilis. They are rather florid and become more numerous in the rainy season (Fig. 104.1). They may last up to 6 months and heal with or without scarring. Infectious relapses may occur for 5 years and, rarely, for 10 years.

Other manifestations include:

- regional lymphadenopathy;
- palmar and plantar lesions, which may be painful, resulting in a crab-like gait; and
- osteoperiostitis of the proximal phalanges of the fingers (dactylitis) or of long bones, causing nocturnal bone pains.

The patient may at any time enter latency, with only serologic evidence of the infection.

Late stage

About 10% of patients develop late lesions after 5 years or more of untreated infection. The late stage is characterized by gummatous lesions of skin, bones and overlying tissues. The manifestations, some of which also occur in early stage but are now more destructive, include:

- hyperkeratosis of palms and soles with deep fissuring;
- juxta-articular subcutaneous nodules;

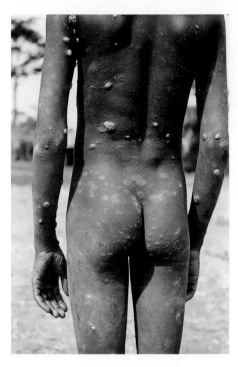

Fig. 104.1 Mixed early yaws lesions: papillomata, ulceropapillomatous lesions and squamous macules. Courtesy of WHO, Geneva.

- more extensive osteoperiostitis of long bones (e.g. sabre tibiae);
- hyperostosis of the nasal processes of the maxillae ('goundou'); and
- ulceration of the palate and nasopharynx (rhinopharyngitis mutilans; Fig. 104.2) with secondary infection resulting in foul-smelling discharge ('gangosa').

Endemic syphilis

The primary lesion is seldom seen. The early manifestations include mucous patches (i.e. shallow painless ulcers on the lips and in the

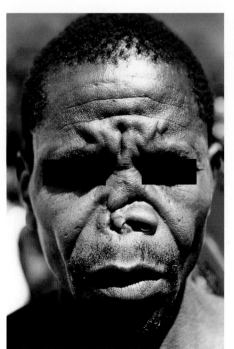

Fig. 104.2 Gangosa in late stage of yaws (rhinopharyngitis mutilans; occurs also in endemic syphilis). Courtesy of WHO, Geneva.

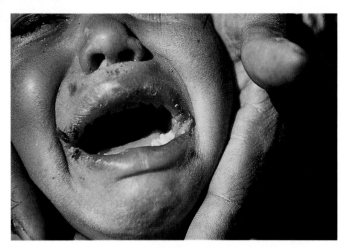

Fig. 104.3 Angular stomatitis (also called split papules) of endemic syphilis; these lesions are also found in early yaws. Courtesy of Dr GM Antal.

oropharynx) and other mucocutaneous and bone lesions resembling those of venereal syphilis and yaws. Papillomata favor warm and moist areas and occur as split papules or angular stomatitis at the labial commissures (Fig. 104.3). Later, the patient may enter the latent phase, which may be prolonged; after this some patients develop late lesions, which are similar to those seen in yaws.[11,12]

Pinta

Pinta is confined to the skin and is the mildest of all treponematoses. The primary lesion, appearing at the site of entry of *T. carateum* on an exposed part of the body, is an itchy, red, scaly papule, sometimes associated with satellite lesions and regional lymphadenopathy. The secondary stage develops several months later, in other areas, with the appearance of pintids, which are similar to the initial lesions. These are also itchy. In due course, they undergo a variety of color changes from red to copper-colored, gray and bluish-black. The lesions remain infectious for many years.

The late lesions are characterized by varying degrees of hypochromia, discoloration, atrophy and achromia. Sometimes these features are seen in the same area.

Attenuated endemic treponematoses

In areas of reduced transmission, the clinical expression of endemic treponematoses can be much milder (a few or even a single papilloma) or many of the infected subjects can be asymptomatic.[1,10] In the Gambia, 9.3% of pregnant women were seropositive for a treponemal infection; children of seropositive mothers showed no signs of congenital syphilis and there was no increase in perinatal, neonatal or child deaths. No clinical signs of endemic treponematoses were found, indicating the asymptomatic nature of the infection.[11,12]

In a number of countries of West and Central Africa, high prevalence rates for syphilis have recently been found in pregnant women based on rapid treponemal tests; clinical cases of endemic treponematoses (yaws or bejel) are not reported or not known to exist in those areas. A serosurvey in children 2–15 years of age could help to indicate that this seroreaction is probably due to past (asymptomatic) endemic treponematoses or might be venereal (latent) syphilis.

HIV infection and endemic treponematoses

As yet, no information is available on any interaction between HIV infection and endemic treponematoses.

DIFFERENTIAL DIAGNOSIS

In endemic areas, an accurate clinical diagnosis can be made in the presence of classic lesions. This will, however, necessitate appropriate training of clinicians, especially in view of the rather milder forms being encountered. The difficulties arise when there are no clinical lesions (i.e. latent cases), when venereal syphilis is also locally prevalent and when the patient is an immigrant from an endemic area presenting at a clinic in a nonendemic country. Differentiation from venereal syphilis is important because of social stigma implications. A careful and detailed history (including that of mother, father and siblings when appropriate) and thorough physical examination are always essential.

Apart from venereal syphilis, the conditions to be considered for differential diagnosis include:

- skin sepsis, scabies, fungal infection, lichen planus, plantar warts, psoriasis and tungiasis in a patient who has early skin lesions;
- tropical ulcer, cutaneous leishmaniasis, mycotic lesions and leprosy in a patient who has gummatous ulceration; and
- tuberculosis and sickle cell disease in a patient who has dactylitis.

Pinta may need to be differentiated from pityriasis versicolor, tinea corporis, vitiligo, leprosy and chloasma.

DIAGNOSIS

There is no test that can differentiate the treponematoses (including venereal syphilis) from one another. The diagnosis of treponemal infection is confirmed by the demonstration of treponemes (but beware of nonpathogenic commensals) in a wet preparation of the material from early lesions by darkfield microscopy or in the biopsy material stained by the silver impregnation technique.

Serologic tests – rapid plasma reagin (RPR) or VDRL nontreponemal tests, *T. pallidum* hemagglutination assay (TPHA) or fluorescent treponemal antibody absorption (FTA-ABS) treponemal (i.e. specific) tests – should be carried out in all cases, but their interpretation requires expertise. The treponemal tests are particularly useful to confirm a reactive nontreponemal test (exclusion of false-positives). A reactive treponemal test may indicate a current infection or a past infection ('serologic scar'). Simple and rapid treponemal tests became recently available in the form of immunochromatographic strips; as they can use whole blood and do not require refrigeration they are extremely useful in the field.[13] Radiologic evidence of osteoperiostitis may assist in the diagnosis.

If the differentiation from venereal syphilis is difficult, the patient should be managed as for venereal syphilis.

MANAGEMENT

Penicillin remains the drug of choice. Long-acting benzathine penicillin G, given intramuscularly in a single session, is preferred. The dose is 600 000 units for children under the age of 6 years, 1.2 million units for those aged 6–15 years and 2.4 million units for those over 15 years. The dose may be divided, half to be given into each buttock. While it is recognized that treponematoses have remained exquisitely sensitive to penicillin, there is a report of penicillin treatment failures of yaws in Papua New Guinea.[14] A few penicillin treatment failures have also been observed in Ecuador.[15]

The distinction between relapse, re-infection or true resistance is difficult to make but these clinical failures are worrisome and should be further researched. Oral penicillin V (50 mg/kg in four divided doses) for 10 days was used in rural Guyana and 16 out of 17 children with yaws were cured.[16] However, such a regimen with multiple doses has a potential compliance problem and is not suitable as epidemiologic treatment (e.g. in elimination campaigns).

There is little information on the use of drugs other than penicillin to treat these conditions in case of penicillin allergy, but regimens recommended for treatment of venereal syphilis should be efficacious. Azithromycin in a single dose of 2 g orally was shown to be highly efficacious in adults but emergence of azithromycin-resistant *T. pallidum* should be monitored.[17] Oral erythromycin or tetracycline 500 mg every 6 hours for 15 days or oral doxycycline 100 mg every 12 hours for 15 days is also likely to be effective; children between 8 and 15 years of age should receive half that dose. Tetracyclines (including doxycycline) are not recommended for pregnant and breast-feeding women and for children under the age of 8 years. For children younger than 8 years, azithromycin and erythromycin should be given in doses adjusted for their body weight.

Contacts

Arrangements should be made to examine and, if appropriate and after proper explanation, to treat the household contacts and other close contacts.

Prognosis and follow-up

The lesions become noninfectious within 24 hours after the injection of penicillin. Whereas treatment in early stages should result in cure in almost 100% of patients, it will not reverse any destructive change in late stages. Rapid plasma reagin (or VDRL) titers should decline within 6–12 months, becoming negative in about 2 years. However, in a small proportion of cases, especially if treated in late stages, the RPR (or VDRL) may remain positive, albeit in low titer (below 1:8). The specific tests (i.e. TPHA, FTA-ABS, rapid treponemal tests) will remain positive throughout life.

REFERENCES

References for this chapter can be found online at http://www.expertconsult.com

African trypanosomiasis

EPIDEMIOLOGY

African trypanosomiasis (sleeping sickness) causes considerable mortality and morbidity across much of the African continent. Approximately 18 000 cases are reported annually to the World Health Organization (WHO) and the estimated burden of disease is 50 000–70 000 cases annually.[1] The number of new cases has fallen over the past 10 years due to intensive control activities.

African trypanosomiasis occurs in two distinct clinical forms: an acute form, caused by *Trypanosoma brucei rhodesiense*, transmitted in endemic situations by savanna *Glossina morsitans* group flies and in epidemic situations by a 'riverine' species, *Glossina fuscipes*; and a more chronic form caused by *Trypanosoma brucei gambiense*, transmitted by the riverine species *Glossina palpalis*, *G. tachinoides* and *G. fuscipes* (Fig. 105.1).[2] *T. b. rhodesiense* occurs in east and central Africa between Ethiopia and Botswana. It is a zoonosis with several game animal reservoirs; cattle are important reservoirs in epidemics. *T. b. gambiense* occurs from Uganda west to Senegal and south through Zaire to Angola; humans are the prime reservoir of infection (Fig. 105.2, Table 105.1). Over 95% of reported African trypanosomiasis cases are caused by *T. b gambiense*.

PATHOGENESIS

Trypanosomes are blood and tissue parasites of vertebrates and are transmitted by blood-sucking insects. A developmental cycle occurs in the gut and sometimes in the salivary glands of the insect vectors,

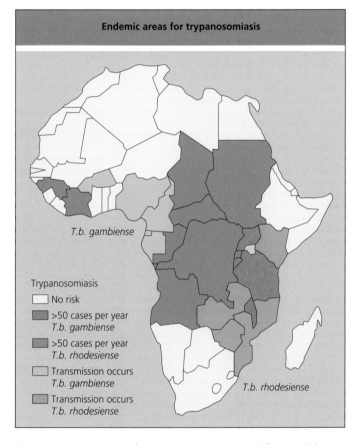

Endemic areas for trypanosomiasis

T.b. gambiense

T.b. rhodesiense

Trypanosomiasis

☐ No risk

■ >50 cases per year *T.b. gambiense*

■ >50 cases per year *T.b. rhodesiense*

☐ Transmission occurs *T.b. gambiense*

☐ Transmission occurs *T.b. rhodesiense*

Fig. 105.2 Endemic areas for trypanosomiasis. Adapted from World Health Organization.[1]

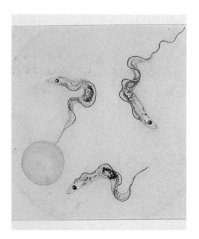

Fig. 105.1 The causative organisms of sleeping sickness in humans. Reproduction of Dutton's original drawing of *Trypanosoma brucei gambiense* from the blood of a man. The organisms possess nucleus kinetoplast and flagella, and their relative size can be assessed from the red blood cell diameter of 7 μm.

producing infective metacyclic trypanosomes; mammals acquire the infection by the bite of the tsetse fly vector. Trypanosomes are microscopic, varying in length from 15 μm to 35 μm, and are highly active when observed under the microscope.

Metacyclic trypanosomes inoculated during tsetse feeding multiply locally in extracellular spaces and induce the typical 'chancre' (Fig. 105.3), with a marked local tissue response characterized by vasculitis, perivascular mononuclear cell infiltration, edema and local tissue damage. Trypanosomes enter the lymphatics and multiply within lymph nodes, leading to parasitemia 5–12 days after infection. Antigenic variation of the surface glycoproteins causes successive waves of parasitemia as the parasite evades the host immune response.[3]

Table 105.1 Epidemiology and distribution of the human trypanosomiases

	Trypanosoma brucei gambiense	*Trypanosoma brucei rhodesiense*
Distribution	Uganda to Senegal and Angola	Ethiopia south to Botswana and east of Rift Valley
Vector	*Glossina palpalis, tachinoides, fuscipes*; feed on any available host	*Glossina morsitans, pallidipes, swynnertoni, (fuscipes* in epidemics); host is game or cattle
Acquisition	Sites of high human–vector contact: river crossings, sacred groves, streams; end of dry season in Guinea savannas; peridomestic transmission in derived humid savanna; plantations of coffee and cocoa	Human penetration into savanna woodland; associated occupations (e.g. hunting, fishing, gathering of firewood and honey)
Epidemic characteristics	Lack of control (surveillance, diagnosis, treatment and vector control) as a result of expansion of human reservoir	Changes of habitat; intense human–fly–cattle contact for *G. fuscipes* transmission; encroachment on human habitation for *G. morsitans* transmission
Animal reservoirs	Pigs; to a lesser extent other domestic animals, rarely game animals	Game animals in endemic situation (bushbuck and hartebeest); cattle in epidemic situation

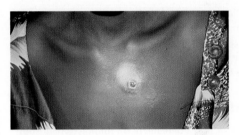

Fig. 105.3 Typical chancre of a patient infected with *Trypanosoma brucei rhodesiense*. The chancre develops at the site of the infecting fly bite.

Parasites enter the central nervous system (CNS) via the choroid plexus or by transcytosis across endothelial cells to cause a lymphocytic meningoencephalitis, which particularly affects the brain stem, although cortical areas and the cerebellum are also involved.[4] Perivascular infiltration with lymphocytes, plasma cells, macrophages and characteristic morular cells occurs; microglia and astrocytes proliferate and there is neuronal destruction and demyelination. Similar lesions also occur in the heart, serous membranes and endocrine organs.

Polyclonal activation of B lymphocytes leads to elevation of IgM concentrations. Heterophile antibodies, rheumatoid factor, immune complexes and autoantibody production may occur. Some neuropsychiatric manifestations may be biochemically induced; elevated prostaglandin D_2 concentrations have been found in advanced *T. b. gambiense* infection, which may be responsible for the circadian sleep disorders.[4,5]

PREVENTION

There are two major components of sleeping sickness control: detection and treatment of cases, and vector control. In *T. b. rhodesiense* areas, patients who present with symptoms of early parasitemia (passive surveillance) can be treated at local rural centers. In epidemics, rapid deployment of active surveillance using blood film screening and the establishment of local treatment centers is important (Fig. 105.4). In *T. b. gambiense* areas, limited clinical symptoms in the early stages require active surveillance. Individuals can be screened using gland aspiration or rapid antigen tests (e.g. the card agglutination test for trypanosomes, CATT). Although prophylactic measures such as 6-monthly intramuscular injections of pentamidine have been suggested for populations most at risk, concerns about development of drug resistance and the masking of second-stage infections means that this is no longer advocated.[6]

Vector control using insecticide-impregnated traps and targets has been demonstrated to be effective in epidemics of *T. b. gambiense* in the Congo[7] and in epidemics of *T. b. rhodesiense* transmitted

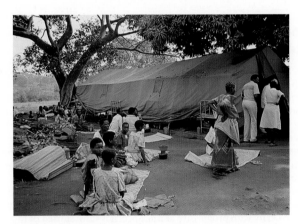

Fig. 105.4 Emergency treatment center Uganda. This center was established to provide facilities for the care and treatment of patients with sleeping sickness during the epidemic in Busoga.

by *G. fuscipes* in Uganda.[8] Sterile insect release methods may also be useful in reducing vector populations.[9] Residual insecticide application to *Glossina* resting sites, insecticide spraying and the clearing of riverine habitats have been used in the past but resource and environmental considerations mean that these can no longer be considered. In *T. b. rhodesiense* epidemics, treatment of the cattle reservoir with trypanocides may prevent human sleeping sickness.[10]

CLINICAL FEATURES

A local skin lesion, the chancre, may develop at the site of inoculation (see Fig. 105.2). This is a raised, tender, edematous papule that rapidly increases in size with surrounding local edema, erythema and local lymphadenopathy. Chancres resolve after 2–3 weeks; they are common in *T. b. rhodesiense* infections, but rare in *T. b. gambiense* infections. Trypanosomes subsequently invade lymphatics and blood, leading to the hemolymphatic stage (stage I) and may invade the central nervous system and cerebrospinal fluid (CSF), leading to meningoencephalitis (stage II). *Trypanosoma b. gambiense* causes a mild but protracted illness over months or years, which is followed by the late development of meningoencephalitis. In contrast, *T. b. rhodesiense* causes a severe, acute, febrile disease, with rapid progression to meningoencephalitis and death within months.[6,11]

Hemolymphatic trypanosomiasis (stage I)

The characteristic clinical features of hemolymphatic trypanosomiasis comprise:

- episodes of fever, often accompanied by chills and rigors, malaise and prostration;
- headache;
- joint pains; and
- loss of weight.

In *T. b. gambiense* infections the disease slowly increases in severity as it progresses. Lymphadenopathy occurs in *T. b. gambiense* infections and enlargement of the posterior cervical glands is characteristic (Winterbottom's sign). Lymph nodes are moderately enlarged, firm and discrete. Splenomegaly occurs in around one-third of cases, and may be associated with hepatomegaly. A fleeting erythematous rash ('circinate erythema') on the trunk or upper extremities is evident in light skinned people. There are focal areas of edema, facial puffiness, dependent edema and serous effusions including ascites, pleural effusions and pericardial effusions. Myocarditis occurs especially in *T. b. rhodesiense* infections.[11]

Meningoencephalitic trypanosomiasis (stage II)

In *T. b. rhodesiense* infections, cerebral involvement occurs within weeks of the onset of infection, whereas in *T. b. gambiense* infections meningoencephalitis may be delayed several years after initial infection. Headache becomes more severe and protracted. Personality changes may occur early, especially in *T. b. gambiense* infections, with apathy, lack of attention, loss of appetite, antisocial behavior and paranoid or delusional states. Abnormalities of sleep are characteristic and result from disturbance of normal circadian rhythms; daytime inappropriate somnolence is often associated with nocturnal insomnia.

Neurologic features include tremors, muscle fasciculation, increased muscle tone and rigidity, choreic and athetotic movements. The gait is affected early with progressive ataxia. Speech is slow, slurred or incoherent. Convulsions and hemiplegia can occur. Pyramidal tract and cranial nerve lesions are less common. Kerandel's sign refers to deep hyperesthesia, often with a delayed response to painful stimuli. Intractable pruritus is a feature of *T. b. gambiense*, especially in the later stages. Ocular manifestations can include iritis, chorioretinitis and papilledema.

The course of the disease is a relentless deterioration to a stuporose state, with cachexia, wasting and progressive malnutrition (Fig. 105.5). Patients become increasingly difficult to rouse and pass into deepening coma and death. This is relatively rapid in *T. b. rhodesiense* but may be protracted over months or years in *T. b. gambiense*. Intercurrent infections, especially bronchopneumonia, are common in the late stages of the disease. In *T. b. gambiense*, amenorrhea and impotence are common.[11,12]

Sleeping sickness in special groups

Although sleeping sickness is less common in children than adults, the clinical course of infection in children may be more severe and, with *T. b. rhodesiense* infection, progression to meningoencephalitis may be even more rapid than in adults.[13] Congenital infection has been described in *T. b. gambiense*.

Trypanosomiasis caused by *T. b. rhodesiense* or *T. b. gambiense* may occur in tourists and visitors to endemic areas. Severe early infections with high peripheral parasitemia are most common, characterized by a severe systemic illness with fever, anemia, biochemical abnormalities and circulating immune complexes. Thrombocytopenia is common and coagulopathy and disseminated intravascular coagulation may occur. Most travelers do not develop CNS involvement; however, delayed diagnosis may be a problem outside endemic areas, especially if no chancre is present.[14]

DIAGNOSIS

Routine laboratory tests demonstrate normal white cell counts, raised erythrocyte sedimentation rate, anemia, thrombocytopenia, low serum albumin and elevated serum IgM.

Parasitologic diagnosis[15]

Diagnosis of sleeping sickness is dependent on finding trypanosomes in the chancre, blood, lymph gland juice or CSF – either in unfixed or unstained preparations, when moving parasites are observed, or in stained preparations. Blood films are usually positive in *T. b. rhodesiense* infection but parasitologic diagnosis may be difficult in chronic *T. b. gambiense* disease; repeated examination and concentration techniques such as microhematocrit centrifugation or the quantitative buffy coat (QBC) improve diagnostic sensitivity. *Trypanosoma b. gambiense* may also be diagnosed by finding parasites in aspirates from enlarged cervical lymph glands.

Diagnosis of second stage (CNS) disease requires examination of CSF. Before lumbar puncture, a single dose of suramin eliminates trypanosomes from the blood, avoiding the risk of contamination of CSF with trypanosoma.[6] Parasites may be found in the centrifuged deposit, which should be examined within 15 minutes of the lumbar puncture. A raised CSF cell count (>5/mm³) or raised CSF protein also indicates CNS infection.

Immunologic diagnosis

A number of serologic tests have been developed; CATT is particularly useful for rapid preliminary screening of large populations for *T. b. gambiense* infection, but positive results must be confirmed parasitologically.[16] An antigen detection test (CIATT) can detect *T. b. rhodesiense* in serum and CSF. This may be useful for following the response to therapy.[17]

Differential diagnosis

In endemic areas, *T. b. rhodesiense* is most common in occupational groups such as hunters, game wardens and fishermen, although all members of the community may be affected. Transmission of *T. b. gambiense* occurs where there is contact between humans and water, and both sexes and all age groups are affected. Outside endemic areas, trypanosomiasis caused by *T. b. rhodesiense* should be considered in travelers from eastern and southern Africa (especially those who have visited game parks) who present with an acute severe febrile illness. *Trypanosoma b. gambiense* infections may present months or years after exposure, with a febrile illness or neuropsychiatric features.

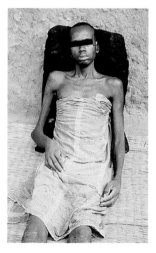

Fig. 105.5 Comatose terminal stage patient with sleeping sickness. Note the degree of cachexia.

Chancres may be confused with insect bites, skin infections, an eschar or cutaneous anthrax. Early hemolymphatic disease mimics a wide range of febrile illnesses, especially malaria, relapsing fever, typhoid, brucellosis and arboviral infections. Occasionally, myocarditis may dominate the clinical picture. The differential diagnosis of meningoencephalitis includes a wide range of inflammatory cerebral infections; in particular, cryptococcal or tuberculous meningitis complicating HIV infection needs to be excluded. The neuropsychiatric presentations of trypanosomiasis may be confused with a variety of psychiatric syndromes, especially when personality change or psychotic behavior predominates. Late-stage disease may also mimic focal neurologic disorders, parkinsonism and space-occupying cerebral lesions.

MANAGEMENT

Treatment of sleeping sickness depends upon the stage of disease; a lumbar puncture is therefore crucial to determine whether there is evidence of CNS involvement. At least one dose of suramin or pentamidine should be given to clear blood parasites before a lumbar puncture is performed to prevent inoculation of parasites into the CSF at the time of lumbar puncture. There have been few recent advances in the chemotherapy of trypanosomiasis and the number of available drugs is limited (Table 105.2).[18]

Most treatment regimens are relatively toxic and it is therefore important to diagnose and treat nutritional deficiencies or intercurrent infections; routine anthelmintic and antimalarial treatment is often given. Hemolymphatic trypanosomiasis is treated with suramin or pentamidine; the latter is only effective in *T. b. gambiense* infection. Meningoencephalitis requires treatment with drugs that cross the blood–brain barrier in trypanocidal concentrations. The mainstays of therapy are arsenical drugs, particularly melarsoprol, used since the beginning of the 20th century. Eflornithine and nifurtimox are also used for the treatment of late-stage *T. b. gambiense* infections. In most individuals, drugs rapidly clear parasitemia or CNS parasites, but relapses occur and 2-year cure rates are the best estimate of drug efficacy. Treatment responses vary according to the drug, severity of illness and geographic location.

Hemolymphatic trypanosomiasis

Suramin is given intravenously as a 10% solution. Fever, nausea, vomiting and urticaria are common but the most severe side-effect is an idiosyncratic anaphylactic reaction, which is infrequent (1 in 2000–4000) but may be more common in the presence of onchocerciasis. Proteinuria and renal failure may also occur. Intramuscular or intravenous pentamidine are alternatives to suramin in *T. b. gambiense* infection and are usually well tolerated. Side-effects include a histamine-like reaction with hypotension and circulatory collapse, hypoglycemia and, after prolonged administration, hyperglycemia and diabetes; adrenaline (epinephrine) and glucose should be available when pentamidine is administered.

Meningoencephalitic trypanosomiasis

Melarsoprol is a trivalent arsenical compound that crosses the blood–brain barrier. A number of treatment schedules have been used, most lasting for 4–5 weeks. However, shorter 10-day treatment regimens have recently been shown to be effective in *T. b. gambiense* infection.[19,20] Thrombophlebitis and cellulitis following extravascular leakage are common (Fig. 105.6). The most important side-effect is reactive arsenic encephalopathy, which occurs in 2–10% of patients, usually after the third or fourth dose. Presentation is usually as an acute deterioration in conscious level, often heralded by convulsions. There is an associated case fatality rate of 10–50%. Prophylactic prednisone (prednisolone) reduces the incidence of reactive arsenic encephalopathy in *T. b. gambiense* (but not *T. b. rhodesiense*) infection.[21] Other toxicity is also common – a peripheral neuropathy occurs in up to 10% of patients and skin reactions, hepatic and renal toxicity are also seen; hemolysis may occur in glucose-6-phosphate dehydrogenase deficiency. Treatment with melarsoprol normally leads to a striking improvement in the mental and physical condition of patients with sleeping sickness. However, recent data suggest that rates of relapse following melarsoprol therapy are increasing.[18]

Eflornithine (difluoromethyl-ornithine, DFMO) is an ornithine decarboxylase inhibitor that is effective in the treatment of stage I and stage II *T. b. gambiense* infection but is poorly effective against *T. b. rhodesiense*. Most current regimens use intravenous administration,

Table 105.2 Drugs currently used for the treatment of sleeping sickness

Drug	Species	Indication	Route	Typical dosage regimen	Side-effects
Suramin	*Trypanosoma brucei rhodesiense* (*Trypanosoma brucei gambiense*)	Stage I	Slow iv infusion	Day 1: 5 mg/kg test dose Days 3, 10, 17, 24, 31: 20 mg/kg Alternative: 5 mg/kg day 1 10 mg/kg day 3 20 mg/kg days 5, 11, 17, 23, 30	Anaphylaxis Cutaneous reactions
Pentamidine	*T. b. gambiense*	Stage I	im/iv	7–10 doses of 4 mg/kg q24h (or alternate days)	Local reactions (im) Hypotension Hypoglycemia
Melarsoprol	*T. b. rhodesiense*	Stage II	iv infusion	Three series of four daily doses of 1.2–3.6 mg/kg, each separated by 7–10 days	Arsenical encephalopathy
	T. b. gambiense			As for rhodesiense or short course 2.2 mg/kg q24h for 10 days	Peripheral neuropathy Dermatitis
Eflornithine	*T. b. gambiense*	Stage II	iv infusion (po)	400 mg/kg q24h in four divided doses for 7–14 days	Diarrhea Pancytopenia Convulsions
Nifurtimox	*T. b. gambiense*	Stage II	po	15–20 mg/kg q24h in three divided doses for 14 days	Anemia Neurologic side-effects

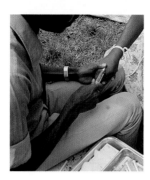

Fig. 105.6 Treatment of a patient with an intravenous injection of melarsoprol. It is vital to adhere to the schedules of treatment and to have a scrupulous technique of injection in order to avoid destruction of local tissue as a result of leakages of the melarsoprol suspended in propylene glycol.

although oral preparations are being evaluated. The drug is less toxic than melarsoprol. Standard courses last 14 days; 7-day courses have been advocated but appear to be less effective in new cases of sleeping sickness.[22] Eflornithine may be safer and more effective than melarsoprol in some settings, although it is not as effective in those who are HIV positive.[23,24] It may also be useful for the treatment of late-stage *T. b. gambiense* infection when the organism has become resistant to melarsoprol.

Nifurtimox is a drug that has occasionally been used in the treatment of arsenic-refractory *T. b. gambiense*. On its own, it has high relapse rates, but a low-dose melarsoprol regimen combined with nifurtimox was superior to standard dose regimens.[25] Combination with nifurtimox allows a reduction in the dose and duration of eflornithine therapy with no loss of efficacy and lower adverse event rates.[26]

Post-treatment follow-up

Following treatment, patients should be reviewed every 3 months for 6 months and then 6-monthly for 2 years to identify episodes of relapse, which may occur after both early- and late-stage disease. In late-stage infection, the CSF abnormalities improve slowly after treatment and values usually return to normal within 1–2 years. CSF examination should be repeated before discharge and routinely at follow-up to detect parasites or a rising cell count. Relapse in *T. b. gambiense* following treatment with suramin or pentamidine is often treated with melarsoprol; eflornithine can also be used. Relapse in *T. b. rhodesiense* is usually treated with a second course of melarsoprol; nifurtimox may be effective if further relapse occurs but data are limited. Combination therapy has also been used in the treatment of relapse but there are inadequate data to determine its role at present.

REFERENCES

References for this chapter can be found online at http://www.expertconsult.com

Other parasitic infections of the central nervous system

This chapter reviews parasitic infections of the central nervous system (CNS), with brief reference to trypanosomiasis and cerebral malaria (see Chapters 105, 111 and 118).

EPIDEMIOLOGY

Numerous species of protozoa and helminths parasitize man, especially in tropical and developing countries where environmental conditions promote mass transmission. Many sources of infection exist (Table 106.1). Table 106.2 lists parasites that can invade the CNS as adults, larvae or ova, depending upon the species, and gives their principal geographic distribution. It excludes parasitic Diptera, whose maggots occasionally invade the brain from the eye, nose or ear, and ticks that cause tick bite paralysis.

Many parasitic diseases that may affect the CNS are zoonoses. Examples, identifying the mammalian hosts, include:

- toxoplasmosis (cats and rodents);
- South American trypanosomiasis (domestic and wild animals);
- Rhodesian trypanosomiasis (antelopes, cattle);
- angiostrongyliasis (rodents);
- gnathostomiasis (fish-eating mammals);
- trichinosis (pigs and rats);
- toxocariasis (dogs and cats);
- schistosomiasis japonica (domestic animals and rodents); and
- echinococcosis (dogs and herbivores).

Gambian trypanosomiasis, schistosomiasis mansoni and schistosomiasis haematobium are essentially anthroponotic. In taeniasis solium (*Taenia solium*) humans are the definitive host but the larval cysticerci are found in pigs.

Relatively few parasites commonly involve the CNS. In some (e.g. *Plasmodium falciparum*, *Trypanosoma* spp., *Toxoplasma gondii*, *Angiostrongylus cantonensis* and *Taenia solium* (cysticercosis)), it is part of the life cycle. In others, it is accidental (e.g. eosinophilic meningo-encephalitis caused by the raccoon ascarid *Bayliscaris procyonis*).

Because CNS involvement is often underdiagnosed and silent, it is difficult to estimate prevalence and incidence rates. However, autopsy studies of patients with cysticercosis in Peru, Mexico, India and Zimbabwe have shown CNS infection rates of 0.5–3%, usually without clinical sequelae; in Mexico, 80% were asymptomatic.[2] Schistosomiasis japonica affects 70 million people and 2–5% of cases develop CNS complications.[3] Clinical evidence of CNS involvement is uncommon in infections with *S. mansoni* and *S. haematobium*, but autopsy studies in Zimbabwe, Nigeria, Egypt and Brazil have revealed ova in the brain in 3–28% and in the spinal cord in 0.3–2% of cases.[4] Worldwide, cerebral malaria is the most commonly diagnosed manifestation of CNS parasitism; in African children with severe falciparum malaria, 30–70% have this complication.[5]

PATHOGENESIS AND PATHOLOGY

Parasites invade the CNS as adults, larvae or ova, through the systemic circulation or retrogradely via the vertebral venous system (Fig. 106.1). Clinical sequelae depend upon the nature and number of parasites and the immune response. Immune evasion is exhibited by many parasites (e.g. *Toxoplasma gondii*, *Trypanosoma* spp.), with minimal tissue reaction.

In falciparum malaria, maturation of the trophozoite to the schizont requires sequestration of the parasitized erythrocyte by cytoadherence in capillaries, including those of the CNS. This is usually without clinical sequelae in immune subjects, but in cerebral malaria massive sequestration obstructs capillaries, the most plausible explanation for coma.[5] In acute African trypanosomiasis, trypomastigotes rapidly invade the brain. They may become dormant but later, in stage II of the disease, especially in Gambian trypanosomiasis, they cause nonsuppurative encephalomyelitis (see Chapter 105).

Migrating larvae of the nematodes *Angiostrongylus cantonensis*, *Gnathostoma spinigerum*, *Toxocara canis* and *Toxocara cati*, *Trichinella spiralis*, occasionally *Loa loa*, *Mansonella perstans*, *Ascaris lumbricoides* and *Dirofilaria immitis* (the dog heartworm) produce transient focal cerebral lesions or eosinophilic meningoencephalitis.[6,7] *Bayliscaris procyonis* and the saprophytic soil nematode *Micronema deletrix* have also been incriminated. *Angiostrongylus cantonensis*, and others that cannot complete their life cycle in humans, die after a few weeks.

Certain trematode ova and larvae can involve the CNS. In early schistosomiasis, anomalous migration of worms to the CNS is followed by a cell-mediated response to ova deposition to form a periovular granuloma.[8] When the subsequent humoral response to adult worms and egg antigens is excessive, Katayama fever occurs, especially in *Schistosoma japonicum* infection, with fever, eosinophilia and self-limiting encephalopathy or myelopathy. In chronic schistosomiasis retrograde passage of ova and occasionally worms through Batson's vertebral venous plexus may result in myelopathy or cerebral lesions. This also occurs in *S. haematobium* infection with obstructive uropathy. When hepatosplenic schistosomiasis develops, ova pass through portopulmonary anastomoses to the lungs and reach the systemic circulation through arteriovenous shunts or by pulmonary veins (see Fig. 106.1). Schistosomal cor pulmonale also promotes cerebral embolization of ova. Ova in the CNS may incite little histologic reaction, but the development of a granuloma, focal vasculitis, localized infarction or rarely subarachnoid or cerebral hemorrhage can result.[4] In paragonimiasis, flukes migrate from lung to brain through the soft tissues of the neck.

In cysticercosis, the larval oncospheres reach cerebral and meningeal capillaries and mature to cysticerci in the gray matter and meninges. The spinal cord is largely spared. Cysticerci survive silently for 2–10 years. Intense inflammation follows their death and antibodies appear in the cerebrospinal fluid (CSF). Healing, with fibrosis

Table 106.1 Sources of parasite infection and resulting disease

Source of Infection		Disease
Food	Salads	Amebiasis, angiostrongyliasis, ascariasis, cysticercosis
	Raw aquatic plants	Fascioliasis
	Uncooked vegetables	Angiostrongyliasis, echinococcosis, cysticercosis
	Uncooked pork	Trichinosis, taeniasis solium, sparganosis
	Uncooked beef	Toxoplasmosis
	Uncooked freshwater fish	Gnathostomiasis, diphyllobothriasis, heterophyiasis, meganonimiasis
	Uncooked freshwater crayfish or crabs	Paragonimiasis, angiostrongyliasis
	Uncooked snakes, frogs*	Sparganosis
	Uncooked land molluscs (e.g. *Achatina fulica* snails)	Angiostrongyliasis
Fresh water	Skin contact	Schistosomiasis
	Nasal contact	*Naegleria fowleri* meningoencephalitis
	Consumption	Sparganosis, dracontiasis, amebiasis
Other environmental sources	Geophagy	Toxoplasmosis, toxocariasis, ascariasis, hydatidosis
	Soil	Strongyloidiasis
	Airborne	*Acanthamoeba castellani* meningoencephalitis, ascariasis
Arthropods	Mosquito (*Anopheles* spp.)	Falciparum malaria
	Mosquito (*Culex* spp.)	Bancroftian filariasis, dirofilariasis
	Midge (*Culicoides* spp.)	Mansonellosis
	Tsetse fly (*Glossina* spp.)	Rhodesian and Gambian trypanosomiasis
	Blackfly (*Simulium* spp.)	Onchocerciasis
	Chrysops flies	Loiasis
	Reduviid bugs (e.g. *Triatoma* spp.)	American trypanosomiasis (Chagas' disease)
Other sources	Blood transfusion/contaminated syringes and needles	Falciparum malaria, American trypanosomiasis, toxoplasmosis
	Cardiac, renal transplant	Toxoplasmosis
	Lung, liver, kidney	Microsporidiosis
	Transplacental	American trypanosomiasis (Chagas' disease), toxoplasmosis
	Autoinfection†	Cysticercosis, strongyloidiasis

*In South East Asia, frogs applied as a poultice may transmit sparganosis.
†Patient with taeniasis solium inadvertently consumes eggs he or she has passed in feces.

and calcification, follows. If the oncosphere enters the subarachnoid space or ventricles, then chronic meningitis with hydrocephalus may result.[2] Rarely, parasites produce large cystic lesions (e.g. in paragonimiasis, hydatidosis and coenurosis). In dracontiasis an extradural abscess containing an adult worm may compress the spinal cord, and in diphyllobothriasis an adult tapeworm competes with the host for vitamin B12 and can produce myelopathy (see Chapter 113).

Immunodeficiency and central nervous system parasitism

Immunodeficient patients are susceptible to the same parasites as the immunocompetent. Falciparum malaria is not more common in patients with HIV/AIDS but the parasite count may be increased and vertical transmission of the virus from mother to baby enhanced. In toxoplasmosis, following acute infection, cysts containing the resting phase bradyzoites remain dormant in muscle, heart, brain or choroid for decades. (The risk of a nonimmune subject developing toxoplasmosis following organ transplant from a seropositive donor is 50% for cardiac and 20% for renal transplant.) In immunosuppressed states (e.g. AIDS, leukemia and lymphomas, inherited immunodeficiency syndromes, systemic lupus erythematosus, immunosuppressive drug therapy, radiotherapy, etc.), reactivation of bradyzoites produces multiplying tachyzoites, with cerebral abscess formation. Reactivation

results from impaired interferon gamma (IFN-γ) dependent cell-mediated and humoral immunity.[9] In AIDS, this occurs when the CD4 lymphocyte count falls below 350 cells/mm³. Other parasite infections have followed transplantation, including microsporidiosis (lung, liver, kidney) and malaria (kidney and bone marrow).[10] *Trypanosoma cruzi* spares the brain in the immunocompetent, except children, but in immunodeficiency (in AIDS, CD4 cell count <200/mm³), often after symptom-free decades, reactivation produces cardiomyopathy and/or acute, multifocal, necrotizing meningoencephalitis or a cerebral granuloma.[11] Although *Leishmania* spp. have been incriminated in various neurologic manifestations including peripheral neuropathy, optic nerve involvement, and even meningitis, reported from India, Egypt and the Sudan,[10] in most cases supportive evidence is not strong since other unidentified, opportunistic infections might have been responsible. Other opportunistic parasites that invade the CNS include free-living amoebae (e.g. *Acanthamoeba culbertsoni* and *Balamuthia mandrillaris*), which produce chronic granulomatous meningoencephalitis,[12] and the intestinal microsporidium *Encephalitozoon cuniculi*, which disseminates to produce encephalopathy.[13] *Strongyloides stercoralis* larvae normally hatch in the small intestine, penetrate the mucosa, migrate through the lungs and return to the jejunum as adults. In immunodeficiency, especially in human T-cell lymphoma virus 1 (HTLV-1) infection, *Strongyloides* hyperinfection may develop with massive tissue invasion, encephalitis and complicating *Escherichia coli* meningitis.

Table 106.2 Parasites that cause generalized or focal or space-occupying lesions and their principal geographic distribution

Parasite		CNS disease	Geographic distribution
Protozoa	Acanthamoeba castellani*	Meningoencephalitis	Worldwide
	Balamuthia mandrillaris	Meningoencephalitis	Worldwide
	Encephalitozoon cuniculi	Encephalitis	Worldwide
	Entamoeba histolytica*	Meningoencephalitis	Tropics, subtropics
	Naegleria fowleri*	Meningoencephalitis	Worldwide
	Plasmodium falciparum	Cerebral malaria	Tropics, subtropics
	Toxoplasma gondii	Encephalitis, SOL brain	Worldwide
	Trypanosoma brucei gambiense	Encephalitis	West Africa eastward to Rift Valley
	Trypanosoma brucei rhodesiense	Encephalitis	Central and East Africa
	Trypanosoma cruzi	Meningoencephalitis	Central and South America
Helminths Nematodes	Angiostrongylus cantonensis	Meningoencephalitis	South East Asia, Oceania
	Ascaris lumbricoides*	SOL brain	Worldwide
	Bayliscaris procyonis*	Meningoencephalitis	North America
	Mansonella perstans*	Meningoencephalitis	Tropical Africa
	Dirofilaria immitis*	Meningitis	Worldwide
	Dracunculus medinensis*	SOL spinal cord	Tropical Africa, Asia and Brazil
	Loa loa*	Meningoencephalitis	Central and West Africa
	Gnathostoma spinigerum	Meningoencephalitis	Far East
	Micronema deletrix*	Meningoencephalitis	North America
	Onchocerca volvulus*	SOL brain	West Africa, South America, Yemen
	Strongyloides stercoralis*	Meningoencephalitis	Tropics, subtropics
	Trichinella spiralis	Meningoencephalitis	Worldwide
	Toxocara canis, Toxocara cati	SOL brain	Worldwide
	Wuchereria bancrofti*	SOL brain	Tropics, subtropics
Trematodes	Fasciola hepatica*	SOL brain	Worldwide, sheep-farming countries
	Heterophyes heterophyes*	SOL brain and cord	Far East, Middle East
	Metagonimus yokogawi*	SOL brain and cord	Far East, Europe
	Paragonimus westermani	SOL brain and cord	Far East, tropical Africa, South America
	Schistosoma japonicum	SOL brain and cord	Far East, Philippines, Indonesia (Sulawesi)
	Schistosoma mansoni	SOL brain and cord	Africa, Middle East, South America
	Schistosoma haematobium	SOL brain and cord	Africa, Middle East
	Schistosoma intercalatum	Myelopathy	Sâo Tomé e Príncipe
Cestodes	Diphyllobothrium latum*	Myelopathy	Russia, Canada and subarctic Europe
	Echinococcus granulosus (hydatidosis)	SOL brain and cord	Worldwide
	Echinococcus multilocularis*	SOL brain and cord	Northern Europe, Canada, Japan
	Spirometra spp. (sparganosis)*	SOL brain and cord	South East Asia, North America
	Taenia multiceps (coenurosis)*	SOL brain and cord	Worldwide
	Taenia solium (cysticercosis)	SOL brain and cord	Worldwide, South America

Parasites of the order Diptera, whose maggots may invade the CNS, and ticks that cause tick bite paralysis are excluded. Note that related species of some parasites listed produce similar symptomology (e.g. *Angiostrongylus mackerrasae* in Queensland, Australia, *Angiostrongylus malayensis* in Malayasia and Indonesia, and numerous *Paragonimus* spp. in different parts of the world).
*CNS disease is infrequent or rare. SOL, space-occupying lesion.

PREVENTION

Important personal precautions (see also Chapter 102) for the control and prevention of parasite infestations are outlined in Table 106.3.

CLINICAL FEATURES

Most parasitic CNS infections lack specific diagnostic features. Diagnosis depends on suspecting a parasitic etiology and obtaining a history of residence in an endemic area (at any time from recent to remote, depending upon the parasite suspected), when exposure to infection may have occurred. The latter often requires a searching inquiry because patients are usually ignorant of the ways in which infection is contracted. Clinicians unfamiliar with this complex field must refer to a differential diagnosis checklist, remembering that multiple parasite infections are common in the tropics.

Major neurologic syndromes

Cerebral malaria

Fever, coma, absence of meningitis or focal neurologic signs (in the early stages) and presence of falciparum trophozoites in the blood suggest cerebral malaria. Alternative causes in a person who coincidentally has falciparum parasitemia include encephalitides, various systemic and toxic infections, and heat stroke.[5]

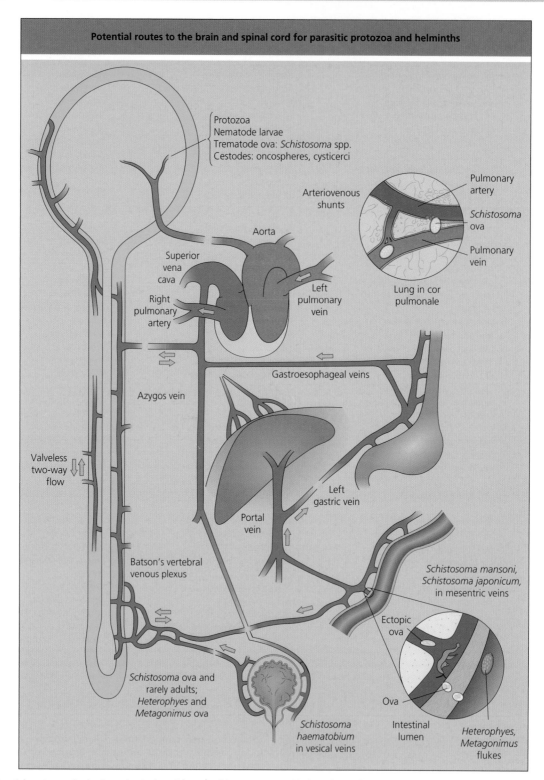

Potential routes to the brain and spinal cord for parasitic protozoa and helminths

Protozoa
Nematode larvae
Trematode ova: *Schistosoma* spp.
Cestodes: oncospheres, cysticerci

Arteriovenous shunts

Pulmonary artery

Schistosoma ova

Pulmonary vein

Lung in cor pulmonale

Aorta

Superior vena cava

Left pulmonary vein

Right pulmonary artery

Gastroesophageal veins

Azygos vein

Left gastric vein

Valveless two-way flow

Portal vein

Batson's vertebral venous plexus

Schistosoma mansoni, Schistosoma japonicum, in mesentric veins

Ectopic ova

Ova

Schistosoma ova and rarely adults; *Heterophyes* and *Metagonimus* ova

Intestinal lumen

Heterophyes, Metagonimus flukes

Schistosoma haematobium in vesical veins

Fig. 106.1 Potential routes to the brain and spinal cord for parasitic protozoa and helminths. Collateral circulation (e.g. in hepatosplenic schistosomiasis with portal hypertension) allows ova to embolize via portopulmonary anastomoses to the lung and thence to the systemic circulation. Batson's vertebral venous plexus allows retrograde access to the spinal cord and brain by parasites and/or ova.

Trypanosomiasis

In stage II of African trypanosomiasis (sleeping sickness), chronic encephalomyelitis develops. This presents with change of personality, apathy, extrapyramidal signs including tremor, chorea, expressionless facies and reversal of sleep rhythm (see Chapter 105). Acute American trypanosomiasis causes meningoencephalitis in children.

Meningitis or meningoencephalitis

A specific helminthic cause is suggested by periorbital edema and generalized myositis (trichinosis) or subcutaneous migratory swellings followed by CNS complications (gnathostomiasis).[6] In angiostrongyliasis – history of consumption of uncooked *Achatina* or (in Thailand) *Pila* snails, or paratenic hosts of the nematode (e.g. freshwater prawns)

<table>
<tr><td colspan="2">**Table 106.3** Important personal precautions for the control and prevention of parasite infestations</td></tr>
<tr><td colspan="2">

- Avoidance of drinking water or eating salads or uncooked food (vegetables, meat, freshwater fish, crustaceans or terrestrial molluscs) in regions where contamination by various protozoa and helminths is probable
- Efforts to discourage children from geophagy (risk of toxoplasmosis and toxocariasis from cat and dog excreta, respectively)
- Regular anthelmintic treatment of pet dogs and cats
- Prevention of skin exposure to fresh water in regions endemic for schistosomiasis
- Prevention of arthropod bites (protective clothing, use of insect repellent creams and mosquito nets)
- Effective prophylaxis for falciparum malaria
- Screening patients who have been exposed to strongyloidiasis prior to immunosuppressive therapy
- Trimethoprim–sulfamethoxazole prophylaxis for toxoplasmosis in AIDS when the CD4 count falls below 350 cells/mm³.

</td></tr>
</table>

– signs may fluctuate markedly; the patient may have headache, confusion, severe generalized dysesthesia, neck stiffness and various focal neurologic signs but later the same day the patient may be almost symptom free. Fever is often absent.[1,7] Other migrating larval nematodes can produce similar variable features.

Focal or space-occupying lesions

Parasitic space-occupying lesions in the CNS are usually without diagnostic features (see Table 106.2). However, cysts in the third ventricle (e.g. cysticercus, hydatid or coenurus cysts) cause intermittent internal hydrocephalus with periodic headache and loss of consciousness.

Toxoplasmosis

Immunodeficient patients developing reactivation toxoplasmosis, with abscess formation usually in the basal ganglia, present with low-grade fever, headache, seizures, raised intracranial pressure and hemiparesis. Diffuse encephalitis is less frequent.

Cysticercosis

Acute infection presents with headache, diffuse hyperesthesia and myalgia. The first manifestation may be seizures, developing months or years after exposure to infection. Careful examination of the whole skin surface may reveal firm, painless, pea-sized, subcutaneous nodules in 50% or more of patients.[2] Differentiation from other causes of seizures is required.

Schistosomiasis

In *S. japonica* infection, and less frequently in *S. mansoni* and *S. haematobium* infections, ova in the CNS may cause seizures or present as a space-occupying lesion. There may be no other evidence of schistosomiasis.

Myelopathy

Myelopathy is uncommon in parasitic infection, except in schistosomiasis.[14] Asymptomatic deposition of ova in the spinal cord is frequent in *S. haematobium* infection but *S. mansoni* is the usual cause of myelopathy; it is uncommon in *S. japonicum* infection. *S. intercalatum* was incriminated in two cases from São Tomé e Príncipe. The usual presentation is acute, flaccid, areflexic paraparesis caused by a granuloma in the conus medullaris but spasticity is present in higher lesions. Acute massive necrosis of the lower cord, presumably immunologically mediated, has been described in Brazil. The differential diagnosis includes tuberculosis, neoplasia and HTLV-1 infection. In diphyllobothriasis, megaloblastic anemia is present in association with posterior column degeneration.

Table 106.4 Ophthalmic involvement by parasites

Disease	Parasite
Iritis	*Toxoplasma gondii, Trypanosoma gambiense* and *rhodesiense, Leishmania donovani, Onchocerca volvulus, Wuchereria bancrofti, Dirofilaria immitis, Toxocara* spp., *Gnathostoma spinigerum* and cysticerci
Choroidoretinitis	*T. gondii* (bilateral, congenital; unilateral, acquired), *O. volvulus, Angiostrongylus cantonensis, Toxocara* spp., *Loa loa, Schistosoma mansoni*, cysticerci and *Armillifer armillatus* (pentastomid larvae)
Optic neuritis	*T. gondii , Trypanosoma gambiense* and *rhodesiense, O. volvulus, A. cantonensis* and *Paragonimus westermani*
Orbital myositis	*Trypanosoma cruzi*
Orbital or retro-orbital mass or lesion	*Leishmania* spp., *Trichinella spiralis, G. spinigerum, S. mansoni, Fasciola hepatica, P. westermani, Echinococcus granularis* cyst, cysticerci and *Taenia brauni* coenurus (in tropical Africa)

Ophthalmic involvement by parasites

Reports of direct or immunologic involvement of the eye by parasites are extensive; specific diseases are outlined in Table 106.4. In addition, the maggots of various Diptera can invade the eye (e.g. *Oestrus ovis*), ear or nose (e.g. *Cochliomyia hominivorax*), rarely extending to the brain.

Tick bite paralysis

In Australia, Africa, America and south east Europe, various hard (ixodid) and soft (argasid) ticks possess salivary neurotoxins. Between 1 and 6 days after it starts feeding, symmetric, ascending, flaccid paralysis appears, reaching the facial and bulbar muscles. Pain, fever and sensory abnormalities are absent. Death may result from respiratory failure. Recovery follows early removal of the tick.

DIAGNOSIS

Cerebral malaria

The demonstration of ring forms of *Plasmodium falciparum* in the blood and exclusion of other causes of coma (including normal CSF) are the basic diagnostic criteria.

African trypanosomiasis: sleeping sickness

Trypanosomes may be present in blood films. The enzyme-linked immunosorbent assay (ELISA) IgM is positive in 90%. Suramin is given prior to lumbar puncture (LP) to destroy blood trypomastigotes that might otherwise enter the CSF. The CSF contains lymphocytic pleocytosis, raised protein and normal glucose levels and occasionally motile trypomastigotes. Polymerase chain reaction (PCR) may detect *Trypanosoma* DNA in CSF. CT and MRI scans show brain edema (see also Chapter 105).

Meningitis or meningoencephalitis

Examination of the CSF is essential. This is often deferred if papilledema or CT scan evidence of raised intracranial pressure is present, but if an early diagnosis is critical (e.g. to exclude tuberculous meningitis) cisternal or LP to aspirate a small sample of CSF is justified. In protozoal infections, lymphocytosis, normal glucose and mildly raised protein levels are typical. Similar findings are present in helminthic meningoencephalitis, but eosinophilia is usually present. Nonparasitic causes of eosinophilic meningitis include Hodgkin's disease, polyarteritis nodosa and occasionally bacterial or viral meningitis. Micro-organisms observed include amebae in primary amebic meningoencephalitis, trypomastigotes in African trypanosomiasis and in *T. cruzi* infections in children (and immunodeficient adults), and occasionally larval worms in angiostrongyliasis and in disseminated strongyloidiasis.

Other investigations may point to the diagnosis. Stool may contain larvae in strongyloidiasis and sputum ova or larval worms in many helminthic infections (see Chapters 108 and 184). In filarial diseases, microfilariae may appear in the peripheral blood at night (Bancroftian filariasis), at noon (loiasis) or at any time (mansonellosis) or in a skin snip (onchocerciasis). In trichinosis, biopsy of a tender muscle may reveal larvae.

Focal or space-occupying lesions

Basic parasitologic investigations may explain focal or space-occupying lesions. The stool may contain ova in *S. mansoni* and *S. japonicum* infections, paragonimiasis, fascioliasis, heterophyiasis, metagonimiasis and diphyllobothriasis. The terminal drops of urine may contain ova of *S. haematobium*. Multiple rectal snips may reveal schistosome ova of all species. In paragonimiasis, and occasionally schistosomiasis, the sputum contains ova.

The CSF in toxoplasmosis and cysticercosis reveals a lymphocytic pleocytosis and raised protein and occasionally reduced glucose levels. In schistosomiasis, a modest lymphocytosis is typical and protein and glucose levels are usually normal, whereas in paragonimiasis, eosinophilia is accompanied by raised protein levels. Eosinophilia is present in only 25% of cases of cerebral hydatidosis.

Immunodiagnostic tests for *protozoa* and helminths (see Chapters 183 and 184)

When organisms cannot be detected, antibody or antigen detection tests in serum and/or CSF confirm exposure or support diagnosis.[14] Immunodiagnosis is especially useful in the following:

* toxoplasmosis (ELISA, PCR for antigens);
* trypanosomiasis;
* neurocysticercosis (ELISA is 90% specific in blood and almost 100% in CSF; immunoblot may be negative if few cysticerci are present);
* echinococcosis (indirect hemagglutination test positive in 60% of sera); and
* schistosomal myelopathy (ELISA in the CSF is positive in >75% of cases).

To confirm active infection with *T. cruzi*, xenodiagnosis is performed utilizing laboratory-raised vector reduviid bugs to feed on the patient (see Chapter 118).

Ultrasonography of the liver or CT or MRI scans of the abdomen detect amebic and hydatid hepatic cysts (the latter calcify), *Fasciola hepatica* flukes in bile ducts or periportal fibrosis (pathognomonic of hepatosplenic schistosomiasis). Chest radiography and CT scans may reveal pulmonary paragonimiasis, hydatid cyst (non-calcifying) or schistosomal cor pulmonale. In schistosomal myelopathy, myelography typically reveals an intramedullary lesion of the conus with a complete block between T12 and L1. CT or MRI may identify a granuloma; occasionally diffuse cord edema is observed, as in the Katayama syndrome.

CT and MRI scans assist diagnosis of cerebral parasitic space-occupying lesions. Toxoplasmosis presents as one or more low-density lesions, usually ring enhancing (Fig. 106.2). In early cysticercosis, small nonenhancing hypodense lesions are present. Later, a hyperdense center (the scolex) develops (Fig. 106.3), with ring enhancement when it dies (Fig. 106.4). Finally, calcification supervenes.[2] Plain radiographs may show multiple calcified cysticerci in muscle. In hydatid cysts,

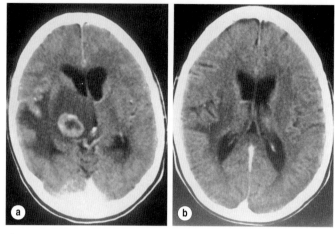

Fig. 106.2 *Toxoplasma* abscess. (a) This CT brain scan shows a *Toxoplasma* abscess in the left internal capsule, compressing the lateral ventricles. Contrast demonstrates a typical ring-enhancing effect. (b) Same patient after 17 days of treatment with pyrimethamine and sulfonamide showing resolving abscess.

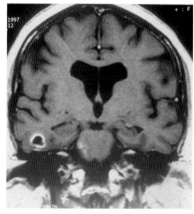

Fig. 106.3 Coronal MRI of brain showing living cysticercus, with the scolex appearing as a hyperintense center ('pea in the pod' appearance). There is no visible inflammatory reaction.

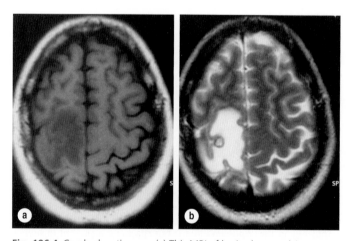

Fig. 106.4 Cerebral cysticercus. (a) This MRI of brain shows a dying cysticercus surrounded by intense inflammation. (b) Postcontrast MRI T2-weighted image demonstrating the isointense wall of the cyst and surrounding hyperintense edema.

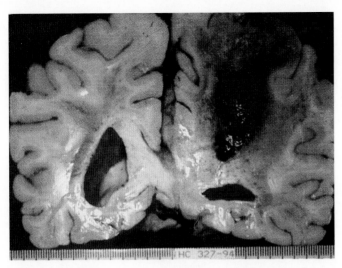

Fig. 106.5 Extensive necro-hemorrhagic lesions of the right cerebral hemisphere in an AIDS patient with reactivated acute Chagas' disease. Courtesy of Professor L Chimelli.

CT scan is the most definitive investigation; dead cysts calcify. The CT/MRI scan in paragonimiasis reveals cystic calcified lesions containing flukes, in schistosomiasis a contrast-enhancing granuloma, and in sparganosis a granuloma containing a worm. Other investigations (e.g. gallium-67 scans and positron emission tomography) are useful but nonspecific for identifying inflammatory foci.

Finally, whenever the diagnosis is in doubt, brain or spinal cord biopsy under CT guidance is required.

Immunodeficient patients

Meningitis in immunodeficiency (e.g. AIDS) is more likely to be caused by cryptococcosis or tuberculosis than parasites. In meningoencephalitis in South or Central American patients, Chagas' disease should be considered. Rarer causes include chronic granulomatous meningoencephalitis (caused by *Acanthamoeba culbertsoni* or *Balamuthia mandrillaris*) diagnosed by brain biopsy. Encephalopathy in disseminated microsporidiosis is diagnosed by identifying *Encephalitozoon cuniculi* cysts in the urine, and neuroimaging may show multiple ring-enhancing lesions in gray and white matter.

Cerebral space-occupying lesions are most likely to be caused by toxoplasmosis (10% of cases in North America, up to 50% in Africa) or tuberculoma. In North America, 2% are due to primary CNS lymphomas; the specific investigation is thallium-201 single photon emission CT. In South America, a 'chagoma' caused by *T. cruzi* should be considered (Fig. 106.5). Many other opportunistic infections can produce space-occupying lesions (e.g. nocardiosis, cryptococcoma, aspergilloma and syphilitic gumma). Myelopathy is most likely to be caused by tuberculosis but many other causes, including toxoplasmosis and HTLV-1 infection, must be considered.

MANAGEMENT

Specific treatment of parasite infections listed in Table 106.1 is discussed in the relevant chapters. Here, the management of the major CNS parasitic disease syndromes is summarized.

Cerebral malaria

Any comatose patient who has suspected or diagnosed falciparum malaria should be treated at once with intravenous quinine (or in North America, quinidine), while monitoring blood glucose, pending further evaluation (see Chapter 111). Corticosteroid drugs are withheld as they worsen the prognosis.

African trypanosomiasis: sleeping sickness

Suramin is given to clear trypanosomes from the blood. After 1 week, melarsoprol is administered. Eflornithine is effective in Gambian trypanosomiasis only (see Chapters 105 and 150).

Meningitis and meningoencephalitis

When a parasitic cause (excluding cerebral malaria) is diagnosed, corticosteroid treatment (prednisolone 1–2 mg/kg/day) should be considered if there is raised intracranial pressure or if the patient is seriously ill. If specific treatment is lacking (e.g. in angiostrongyliasis, trichinosis, gnathostomiasis and toxocariasis), it may be the only option other than repeated LP to reduce pressure. Diethylcarbamazine and thiabendazole have been tried in toxocariasis and albendazole in gnathostomiasis (together with corticosteroids) with some evidence of benefit.

Focal or space-occupying lesions

In cystericercosis, when living cysticerci are present, praziquantel (without corticosteroids, which reduce its efficacy) 10–20 mg/kg q8h for 21 days, sometimes increased to 25 mg/kg q8h for up to 30 days,[2] is advocated. Albendazole (with preceding corticosteroid therapy) 15 mg/kg/day for 1 week has replaced praziquantel in some centers. Seizures are controlled by anticonvulsants. Despite the apparent benefit of these drugs, if untreated, the majority of cysts disappear without sequelae within 1 year. Surgery should be avoided unless the cysticercus is blocking the third ventricle.

In schistosomiasis, praziquantel 40 mg/kg is routinely given as a single dose; 60 mg daily for 3 days may eradicate worms more completely. Suspected schistosomal myelopathy should be treated conservatively with praziquantel. When this develops acutely in the Katayama syndrome, with edema of the spinal cord (Fig. 106.6), adjunctive, high-dose corticosteroid treatment is essential. Schistosomal myelopathy may improve even after several months of paraplegia. Surgery is required if there is deterioration despite treatment. If schistosomal myelopathy is encountered unexpectedly at operation, only a biopsy should be obtained.[4] It is difficult to know when schistosomiasis has been cured; antibody titers decline slowly and antigen detection may be negative although some worms persist (see Chapter 112).

Cerebral paragonimiasis is treated conservatively with praziquantel or bithionol. Hydatid cysts are completely excised, first administering praziquantel or albendazole. Surgical resection is required for a sparganum and for a coenurus (with adjunctive praziquantel).

Treatment of central nervous system parasitism in immunodeficiency

Standard treatment applies for most parasitic infections. The immune status should be improved if possible (e.g. administer highly active antiretroviral treatment in AIDS). If brain biopsy is not possible, empiric treatment for suspected toxoplasmosis in an IgG-seropositive patient (IgM remains negative) is pyrimethamine and sulfadiazine or high-dose trimethoprim–sulfamethoxazole. A convincing response within 7–10 days supports the diagnosis. Lifelong trimethoprim–sulfamethoxazole prophylaxis follows recovery. When *Toxoplasma* IgG is negative, an intracerebral space-occupying lesion is treated as either a tuberculoma or a primary CNS lymphoma. In South America, early treatment of Chagas'

Fig. 106.6 MRI of the spinal cord of a 9-year-old Omani boy with acute schistosomiasis mansoni, who presented with transverse myelitis (vertical scale in cm). Extensive cord edema from the first thoracic vertebral level to the conus medullaris is present (arrows). He improved and was ambulant after 2 weeks treatment with prednisone and praziquantel but had persistent incontinence of urine.

meningoencephalitis (which may coexist with toxoplasmosis) with benznidazole is imperative. No effective treatment for chronic granulomatous meningitis exists (see Chapters 118 and 182). Cerebral microsporidiosis (*Encephalitozoon cuniculi*) is almost invariably fatal, but has responded temporarily to albendazole 400 mg q12h (Chapters 150 and 181). Hyperinfection with strongyloidiasis responds to ivermectin, and broad-spectrum antibiotics for the usual coexistent *E. coli* meningitis.

REFERENCES

References for this chapter can be found online at http://www.expertconsult.com

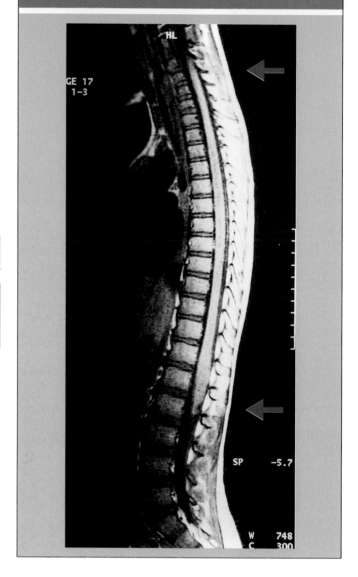

MRI of the spinal cord of a 9-year-old boy with acute schistosomiasis mansoni

Eye infections in the tropics

This chapter discusses the contribution of infection to the major blinding diseases of the tropics and the ocular features associated with common tropical infections. In tropical practice, visual prognosis in both major blinding infections and simple trauma is often worsened by late presentation, secondary infection and inappropriate use of traditional eye medicines.

Major Blinding Infections of the Tropics

Cataract, vitamin A deficiency, trachoma and onchocerciasis are classically considered to be causes of blindness in developing countries. An increasing number of countries, including recently Pakistan, Nigeria and Ethiopia,[1–3] have now undertaken community-based surveys to identify the causes of blindness, showing that cataract, universally, is by far the greatest cause of blindness. Trachoma and onchocerciasis are considered to account for 3.6% and 0.8%, respectively, of the global burden of blindness.[4] In these two diseases, and in two other important tropical infectious diseases, leprosy and measles, infection and the host response to it play prominent and contrasting roles in the pathogenesis of blindness and other ocular complications. These are discussed below.

TRACHOMA

Trachoma is a chronic follicular keratoconjunctivitis caused by infection with *Chlamydia trachomatis*, almost exclusively of serotypes A, B, Ba and C (the 'genital' *C. trachomatis* serotypes D–K may cause disease that is indistinguishable from trachoma, but this is rare). Host tissue tropism in *C. trachomatis* is strongly related to the capacity to synthesize tryptophan, with all ocular strains having inactivating mutations in the *trpBA* tryptophan synthetase genes.[5] Trachoma is characterized by scarring sequelae in the conjunctiva after repeated infections.

Epidemiology

Trachoma is one of the most common infectious diseases: the WHO estimates (2008) that there are 84 million people infected worldwide and that 8 million people are irreversibly visually impaired due to trachoma. Several million more individuals are projected to become visually impaired due to trachoma in the next 20 years as a result of demographic trends.[6] The global picture of trachoma has changed considerably in recent decades but information from a number of countries remains scanty. India and China in particular have some evidence of a trachoma problem, and because of their very large populations, could be very influential in the estimates if accurate data on their trachoma burden were forthcoming. It is a disease of poverty, associated with poor personal and environmental hygiene, and it was common in much of Europe and North America during the 19th century. The map (Fig. 107.1) represents the best available information on the current distribution of active trachoma. Trachoma is found principally in sub-Saharan Africa, with additional foci in Asia, in South America and among aboriginal Australians.

In trachoma-endemic communities, the main reservoir of infection is the eyes of affected children: active trachoma is unusual among adults, and there is evidence that most transmission of trachoma occurs within the family[7,8] as a result of close contact between young children and their mothers and other caregivers. Transmission is favored by poor environmental and personal hygiene, lack of water for washing, inadequate sleeping space, inadequate disposal of rubbish or sewage, and the proximity of domestic animals. It is considered to take place via fingers, fomites and flies: the relative importance of these means of transmission probably varies from one community to another.

Pathogenesis

There is evidence that the pathologic features of trachoma are not the result of direct tissue damage but are immunologically mediated. A single infection with *C. trachomatis* usually leads to a self-limiting follicular conjunctivitis, and repeated episodes may be necessary for the development of intense inflammation and scarring sequelae. The most characteristic histologic finding in active trachoma is the presence of follicles, which resemble germinal centers in the superior tarsal conjunctiva. Subsequently subconjunctival scarring occurs and contraction of scars causes distortion of the tarsal plate, entropion and trichiasis.

Evidence from animal models suggests that cellular immune mechanisms are of primary importance in limiting and clearing chlamydial infection. Why some individuals clear infection without sequelae, while others develop scars is not known. There is some evidence that scarred subjects have a reduced capacity for clearance of chlamydial infection, which occurs by way of specific T helper-1 lymphocyte and interferon gamma responses.[9] Genetic variants at the interleukin (IL)-10 locus which potentiate IL-10 transcription increase the risk of scarring.[10,11] A series of other observations implicate tumor necrosis factor (TNF), which has proinflammatory and antichlamydial activity, and matrix metalloprotease 9 (MMP-9; a mediator in the extracellular matrix breakdown pathway linking inflammation and tissue remodeling) in the process by which repeated episodes of intense disease and infection lead to scarring.[12–16] Antibodies to a chlamydial heat shock protein, Hsp 60, are also associated with scarring sequelae of infection in both the eyelid and the genital tract, but it is uncertain whether these reflect a causal role for this antigen or an epiphenomenon.

Prevention

The goal of prevention is to reduce transmission to such a level that exposure to reinfection does not occur often enough to cause blinding trachoma. Measures focused on improving personal and community

Fig. 107.1 Current distribution of active trachoma (WHO).

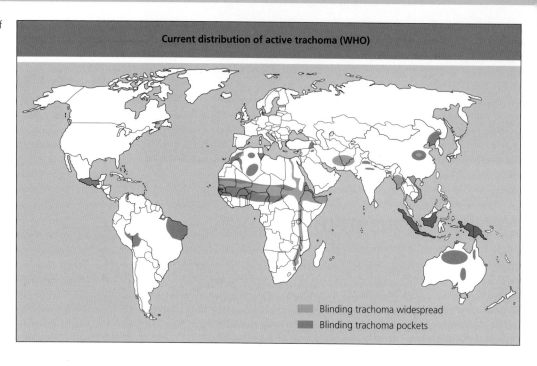

Current distribution of active trachoma (WHO)

Blinding trachoma widespread
Blinding trachoma pockets

hygiene such as the provision of adequate water supplies, fly control and latrines are likely to reduce the incidence of trachoma. A study of community education targeted at face washing showed that, with intense effort, reductions in trachoma prevalence are possible but not well sustained.[17] Treatment of active cases with antibiotics may be effective temporarily but even high coverage mass treatment may fail due to re-exposure to untreated individuals.[18] The WHO-endorsed strategy is known by the acronym SAFE: Surgery, Antibiotic treatment, Facial cleanliness and Environmental improvement. There is no vaccine at present.

Clinical features

In endemic communities *C. trachomatis* infection is usually acquired early in childhood and the progressive scarring and distortion of the eyelid may lead to corneal scarring and blindness, usually in late middle age. In severely affected communities signs of trachoma can be found in over 90% of children aged between 1 and 2 years and blindness rates may approach 25% in those over 60 years. In most endemic areas, there is no sex difference in prevalence or incidence until after adolescence, but both active trachoma and its scarring sequelae are commoner in women, probably reflecting their closer contact with children.

Subjects who have trachoma typically have few symptoms until the final stages when inturned eyelashes (trichiasis) develop. Secondary bacterial infection may play a role in this progression, and in the mucopurulent conjunctivitis, nasal discharge and chronic otitis media seen in some patients.

The most prominent sign of active trachoma is the presence of lymphoid follicles, which are usually found on the superior tarsal conjunctiva. These can be easily visualized by everting the upper eyelid, although they may occasionally be found at the corneoscleral junction (limbal follicles). The presence of five or more of these pale off-white spots with a diameter <0.5 mm is needed in the central area of the superior tarsal conjunctiva to meet the accepted definition of trachomatous inflammation of follicular grade (TF) (Fig. 107.2). Active trachoma is also associated with capillary congestion of the conjunctiva, visible either as small red dots (papillae) or as obscuration of the normally visible tarsal blood vessels by inflammatory thickening. If these blood vessels are obscured over more than half of the central area over the tarsal plate, trachomatous inflammation of intense grade

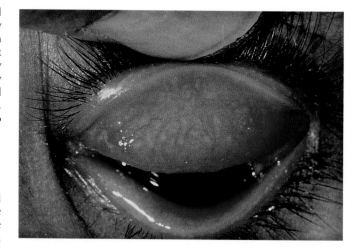

Fig. 107.2 Everted eyelid showing follicular trachoma (TF). Courtesy of the WHO Program for the Prevention of Blindness.

(TI) is said to be present (Fig. 107.3). Neovascularization of the cornea or 'pannus' is associated with active *C. trachomatis* infection and in trachoma typically involves the superior corneal margin.

Conjunctival scars – which, if clearly visible, would be graded trachomatous scarring (TS) – are initially small and stellate, but eventually become broad and confluent (Fig. 107.4). The scars contract, causing distortion of the tarsal plate and loss of its normal protective functions, resulting in inturning of the lashes (trichiasis, which is graded TT if any lash is deviated towards the eyeball), which rub on the cornea (Fig. 107.5). This can lead to corneal opacity and ultimately to blindness from abrasion of the cornea. Limbal follicles resolve to leave small depressions at the limbus known as 'Herbert's pits' (see Fig. 107.4).

Trachoma may be confused with other conditions producing a follicular conjunctivitis (Table 107.1). With the exception of viral conjunctivitis, which is acute and self-limiting, the other conditions in Table 107.1 are never endemic in a community. However, limbal follicles or Herbert's pits (see Fig. 107.4) are the only clinical sign unique to trachoma[19] and these do not occur even in a majority of cases.

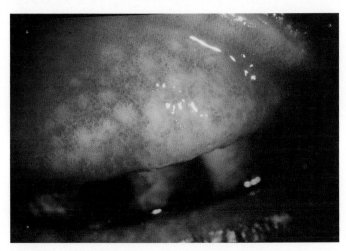

Fig. 107.3 Everted eyelid showing intense inflammatory trachoma. Follicles are also present.

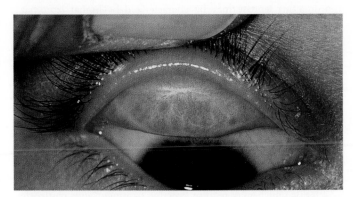

Fig. 107.4 Everted eyelid showing trachomatous scarring (TS). There are also Herbert's pits visible at the corneoscleral junction. Courtesy of the WHO Program for the Prevention of Blindness.

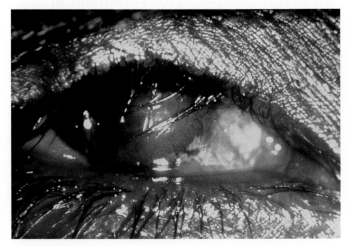

Fig. 107.5 Trachomatous trichiasis (TT) and secondary corneal opacity. Courtesy of the WHO Program for the Prevention of Blindness.

Diagnosis

Trachoma is usually diagnosed on clinical grounds. The simplified grading scheme including TF, TI, TS and TT has been developed by the World Health Organization for public health purposes.[20] Several laboratory tests can be used to confirm a diagnosis of trachoma, but these are rarely available in endemic areas. Chlamydial infection is

Table 107.1 Causes of follicular conjunctivitis

Cause	Comments
Folliculosis	Follicles are few and occur in the inferior fornix without inflammation or hyperemia; a common finding
Viral infections	Acute, self-limiting with signs of resolution in 2 weeks
Trachoma	
'Inclusion conjunctivitis' and other ocular chlamydial infections	Also caused by ocular chlamydial infection, often with genital serotypes; frequently unilateral

'Toxic' follicular conjunctivitis:
    Molluscum contagiosum
 	
    Drug induced
 	
    Eye cosmetics
	
	Caused by spillage of contents of molluscum lesions on eyelids
	Follows use of eye medications for months or years
	Granules of cosmetics seen in follicles

Bacterial infections: *Moraxella* spp. and others	Angular blepharitis with *Moraxella lacunata*; seen in adolescent girls who share eye make-up
Axenfeld's chronic follicular conjunctivitis	Reported in institutionalized children and native Americans, probably a mild form of trachoma[13]
Chronic follicular conjunctivitis of Thygeson	Outbreak in a Californian high school that contained trachoma cases; features compatible with mild active trachoma[13]
Parinaud's oculoglandular syndrome	Associated with pathogens invading through the conjunctivae; associated with systemic malaise and gross pre-auricular lymphadenopathy; some cases associated with exposure to cats and may be due to feline strains of *Chlamydia psittaci*; many other causes (e.g. syphilis, lymphogranuloma vereneum, tuberculosis, tularemia, cat-scratch disease)
Vernal catarrh	Occurs in atopic subjects; characteristic appearance with giant 'cobblestone' papillae

characterized by blue intracytoplasmic inclusions in Giemsa-stained epithelial cell scrapings. The organism can be cultured in cell monolayers, visualized in smears using direct fluorescent antibody methods or detected by enzyme immunoassay. Nucleic acid amplification tests (NAATs) targeting DNA sequences in either the common plasmid pCT1 of *C. trachomatis* or, more recently, ribosomal RNA sequences[21] are the most sensitive methods for demonstrating ocular chlamydial infection.

Management

Individual sporadic cases may be treated with 1% tetracycline eye ointment topically q12h for 6 weeks. A single oral dose of azithromycin (20 mg/kg) is just as effective.[22] Mass treatment with azithromycin is recommended by WHO for all inhabitants of any district, neighborhood or community in which the prevalence of TF exceeds 10% in children aged 1–9 years. As of 2008, over 77 million doses of azithromycin, donated by the manufacturer, have been distributed through the International Trachoma Initiative for this purpose.

Trichiasis can be treated by epilation, but this normally provides only temporary relief and lid surgery is usually needed to prevent blindness. Tarsal rotation[23] is the operation of choice.

ONCHOCERCIASIS

Pathogenesis

In the eye, as in the rest of the body, pathology is due to an inflammatory reaction to dead microfilariae of *Onchocerca volvulus*. As these can be found in the cornea, the anterior chamber, the iris, the lens, the retina and the choroids, onchocercal lesions may involve all these sites. In the conjunctiva and iris, an immunohistochemical study has found that chronic ocular onchocerciasis is associated with predominant infiltration by CD8+ lymphocytes and is associated with major histocompatibility complex class II expression in the resident cell population, suggesting activation.[24] Regulatory T cells may have a role in suppressing the immune response.[25]

Clinical features

Eye involvement in onchocerciasis is usually bilateral and affects men more commonly than women.

Punctate or 'snowflake' keratitis occurs as inflammatory cells accumulate around dead microfilariae and it may respond to topical corticosteroids. Sclerosing keratitis, in which neovascularization and scarring develop nasally and temporally in the cornea and then extend inwards from the inferior limbal margin to involve the whole surface in a total corneal scar, has been a common cause of blindness, particularly in savannah regions. Microfilarial movement may be visible in the anterior chamber with a slit-lamp, often closely associated with the posterior corneal surface. Inflammatory reactions may produce iritis, and cataract may also contribute to reduced vision. In the posterior segment of the eye, choroidoretinal atrophy, with clumping and breaking up of the retinal pigment epithelium, and associated optic atrophy may follow. These changes contribute further to visual loss and have no specific treatment.

MEASLES

Pathogenesis

Measles virus infection and its consequences are a major risk to sight in tropical practice. In Africa they cause about 50% of childhood blindness, usually from corneal scarring.[26] Although measles virus infects the corneal epithelium and the conjunctiva, its devastating effects on the cornea are the results of secondary processes which include infection, acute vitamin A deficiency, exposure and the effects of traditional eye medicines. Measles virus-associated immunosuppression appears to be responsible for reactivation of herpes simplex virus, which has been found in corneal ulcers after measles,[27] and gut involvement appears to precipitate acute vitamin A deficiency in those with marginal reserves.

Clinical features

The direct effects of measles on the eye are a punctuate keratitis and sometimes conjunctival lesions that are analogous to Koplik's spots, which normally resolve without sequelae. Corneal ulceration and keratomalacia with liquefaction of the cornea and the whole eye may supervene in acute vitamin A deficiency. Secondary ulceration due to herpes simplex may be typically dendritic or modified by other factors as discussed below. If subjects are too sick or too dehydrated to close their eyes, corneal dryness and exposure ulceration may result, and in tropical practice, traditional medicines are frequently applied and may

contribute to secondary infection and a worse prognosis. Subjects who have ocular complications of measles should be treated with vitamin A, topical antibiotics and measures to avoid corneal exposure.

LEPROSY

Pathogenesis

In leprosy three main mechanisms operate in the eye to cause pathology. Overwhelming bacterial infection in lepromatous leprosy may lead to atrophy of the involved tissues. The eye may be involved in type 1 reactions (reversal reactions), in which motor and sensory nerve loss is prominent, and in type 2 reactions, in which inflammation within the eye is prominent. As elsewhere in the body, it is the reactions that cause most damage, manifesting as visual loss and blindness in the case of the eye.

Clinical features (see also Chapter 103)

Lepromatous leprosy may be characterized by limbal lepromata, painless yellow or pink nodules at the corneoscleral junction. Chalky deposits may be associated with corneal invasion by *Mycobacterium leprae*. The iris may become thin and atrophic, and pathognomonic 'iris pearls' (which are calcified foci of dead leprosy bacilli) appear as white nodules on the surface of the iris.[28] Type 1 reactions involving the fifth cranial nerve can result in corneal anesthesia, and lagophthalmos (inability to close the eyes) may occur if the seventh cranial nerve is involved. Together, they produce a cornea that is both anesthetic and exposed, and therefore requires protection. Eye health education, blinking exercises, protective spectacles and surgical procedures such as tarsorrhaphy may all be needed.[28] Type 2 erythema nodosum leprosum (ENL) reactions may also cause acute or chronic iritis, which requires treatment with topical corticosteroids, or scleritis which may require systemic treatment with corticosteroids and clofazimine.

Clinical Aspects of Eye Involvement in Common Tropical Infections

BACTERIAL INFECTIONS

Tuberculosis

Primary tuberculosis may affect the conjunctiva with nodular lesions and associated chronic conjunctivitis that is not responsive to standard topical treatment. In miliary disease, tubercles may be found in the conjunctiva, the iris or the choroid. Phlyctenular conjunctivitis and granulomatous uveitis may be associated with tuberculosis but are not specific for it. Optic neuritis may complicate tuberculous basal meningitis.

Sexually transmitted diseases

Ocular gonococcal infection, usually as a result of autoinoculation from the genital tract, causes an acute purulent conjunctivitis that may progress rapidly to corneal ulceration and perforation in the absence of appropriate treatment.

Gonococcal ophthalmia neonatorum, acquired by an infant passing through an infected birth canal, is similarly threatening to sight and usually presents in the first week of life as a bilateral purulent conjunctivitis.[29]

Ocular autoinoculation from genital *C. trachomatis* infection causes a clinical picture identical to trachoma, except that it is commonly unilateral. Among infants born to infected mothers, 30% develop chlamydial ophthalmia neonatorum, which is usually a self-limiting bilateral mucopurulent conjunctivitis presenting within 2 weeks of delivery. In a small proportion of cases, pneumonia and permanent lung sequelae follow. Thus chlamydial and gonococcal ophthalmia neonatorum require both systemic and topical therapy.

Iritis, retinal vasculitis, optical neuritis and disseminated chorioretinitis may be features of secondary acquired syphilis.

Other bacterial infections

Petechiae may be seen at the conjunctiva in meningococcal meningitis: conjunctivitis, anterior uveitis and even panophthalmitis may complicate meningococcaemia. Diphtheria may present with a membranous conjunctivitis, lid edema and the local effects of exotoxin. Cholera with rapid dehydration has been associated with the acute development of cataracts. Rose spots in typhoid fever may involve the conjunctiva. The clinical picture known as Parinaud's syndrome (follicular or granulomatous conjunctivitis and preauricular lymphadenopathy, often with systemic malaise) is associated with pathogen invasion via the conjunctiva and may be seen with a number of infections, including tuberculosis, syphilis, tularemia, cat-scratch disease and lymphogranuloma venereum. Brucellosis has been associated with chronic granulomatous uveitis. Dilatation of the conjunctival vessels and subconjunctival hemorrhages may be presenting features of leptospirosis or typhus.

PARASITIC INFECTIONS

Retinal hemorrhages and retinal whitening are components of a specific malarial retinopathy[30] and may be the earliest sign of cerebral involvement. Unilateral edema of the eyelid (Romana's sign) may be seen in American trypanosomiasis if the inoculation site is in the region of the eye. Chorioretinitis is the most common ocular manifestation of toxoplasmosis. An ocular larva migrans syndrome (larvae migrating within the eye) may be seen with *Toxocara* and *Gnathostoma* spp., and *Loa loa* typically migrates under the conjunctiva. Egg granulomas may occur in the conjunctiva or choroids in schistosomiasis. Cysticerci of *Taenia solium* may occur within the eye, often subretinally.

VIRAL INFECTIONS

Herpes simplex virus, which has a worldwide distribution, can have devastating effects on the eye. In many tropical environments this is the commonest cause of corneal ulceration, often occurring as a complication of measles or causes of high fever such as malaria. A narrow, branching dendritic ulcer that is best seen with fluorescein staining is typical (Fig. 107.6); however, in tropical practice the time to presentation and inappropriate use of traditional eye medicine often modify this, leading to larger ameboid ulcers. If available, idoxuridine or aciclovir drops should be given very frequently until epithelial healing takes place.

Infection with HIV may itself cause a retinopathy with cotton wool spots, indicating damage to the retina. Cytomegalovirus retinopathy

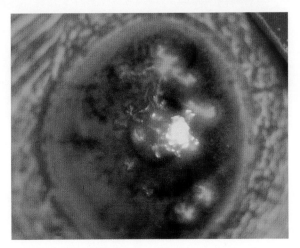

Fig. 107.6 Typical dendritic ulcer caused by herpes simplex virus, visualized with fluorescein staining.

does not seem to be common in tropical practice, but syphilis, tuberculosis and herpes simplex virus and their associated ocular manifestations are commoner among HIV patients. Kaposi's sarcoma may involve the eyelid or conjunctiva.

MICROBIAL KERATITIS

Although contact lens use is the most important predisposing factor for microbial keratitis in developed country settings, in tropical practice microbial keratitis is usually the result of corneal trauma, and may have been mismanaged in the traditional sector before presentation. Patients present with a history of preceding trauma, together with photophobia, pain, loss of vision and purulent discharge in the affected eye, with cells and pus in the anterior chamber (hypopyon). The corneal defect may contain bacteria (*Staphylococcus aureus*, *Streptococcus*, *Proteus* or *Pseudomonas* spp. are commonly reported) or fungi.[22] Fungal keratitis, often with *Aspergillus* and *Fusarium* spp., has been reported associated with trauma involving plant or organic matter. If available, microscopy or culture of a corneal scrape, or local knowledge,[31] may help to diagnose the cause. Medical treatment with frequent application of topical antibiotic solutions and/or antifungals may prevent corneal scarring or perforation.

REFERENCES

References for this chapter can be found online at http://www.expertconsult.com

Managing an outbreak of meningococcal disease in an African village

For over 100 years, major epidemics of meningococcal disease have occurred every few years in countries of the African Sahel and sub-Sahel, the African 'meningitis belt' (Fig. PP56.1). Epidemics, which may be very large, start during the hot, dry season and subside with the coming of the rains. Epidemics often have a focal start, beginning in a cluster of villages, before spreading rapidly to involve a district, region or country. This review addresses the management of a local outbreak involving a cluster of villages within a country of the African meningitis belt.

In countries of the African meningitis belt, since the clinical features of meningitis are well recognized by the community, the first indication of an imminent outbreak may be a community-based report of cases of meningitis within a group of villages. In several countries of the meningitis belt, a more formal, facility-based reporting system has been established through which cases of meningitis are reported to a national center on a weekly basis. Thus, the first indication that a district medical officer receives of a possible outbreak may come either directly from the community or from an increase in the number of cases of meningitis reported from an individual health center during the preceding week. Deciding when to raise the alarm is a difficult decision but some simple guidelines have been devised by the World Health Organization to help. Based on past experience, these set out the attack rates which, in different epidemiologic circumstances, are likely to predict an epidemic (Fig. PP56.2).

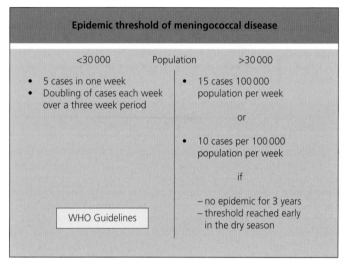

Fig. PP56.2 Numbers of cases of meningitis predicting an outbreak of meningococcal disease in a country in the African meningitis belt.

Table PP56.1 Steps to be followed on the report of a suspected outbreak of meningococcal disease

- Confirm that the cases being reported have meningitis
If this is the case:
- Determine the cause of the meningitis
If this is a meningococcus:
- Notify local, national and international authorities using established reporting procedures
- Establish or activate an epidemic management team
- Establish additional treatment facilities and obtain the necessary supplies of drugs
- Make urgent arrangements for vaccination of the affected communities if the outbreak is caused by serogroup A, C or W135 meningococcus

Once it has been established that an outbreak is likely, the district health team must undertake a number of actions (Table PP56.1). Urgency is essential as outbreaks can progress with frightening speed.

Step 1

Step 1 involves establishing that the cases being reported are cases of meningitis and, if so, determining their cause. This requires lumbar puncture in a selected number of patients at the health facility where cases are being seen and examination of their cerebrospinal fluid

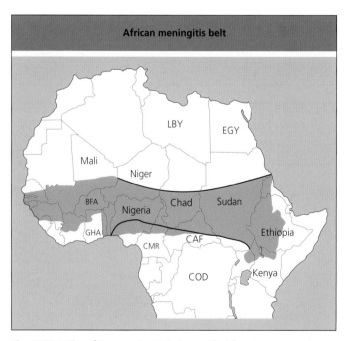

Fig. PP56.1 The African meningitis belt, modified from Lapeysssonnie.

(CSF). Detection of turbid CSF confirms the diagnosis of meningitis, and rapid diagnostic tests can be used for determination of the cause if conventional microbiologic support is not available. It cannot be assumed that clusters of cases are caused by the meningococcus as, within the meningitis belt, pneumococci (especially those of serotype 1) can cause similar outbreaks. Rapid diagnostic tests that are currently commercially available are based on latex technology and are relatively expensive; work is in progress to develop simpler dipstick assays.

Collection of CSF into transport medium allows bacteria to survive transport to a central laboratory where they can be cultured and further characterized using serologic and molecular biologic methods. Determination of the capsular serogroup of the meningococcus responsible for the outbreak is essential in order to guide vaccination policy (see below). Isolates may be sent to an international reference laboratory for more detailed molecular typing. Collection of laboratory samples should be accompanied by acquisition of simple epidemiologic data on the cases such as their age, sex, residence and recent travel history.

Step 2

If an outbreak of meningococcal disease is confirmed, regional, national and international authorities should be informed using established reporting procedures.

Step 3

Confirmation of an outbreak that has passed the epidemic threshold should initiate epidemic control procedures. In many epidemic-prone regions, a standing committee will be in place which needs only to be activated. In other areas, an emergency committee may need to be established. This committee must be broad based and include representatives of all groups likely to be affected by an epidemic (Table PP56.2).

Step 4

An epidemic of meningococcal disease can rapidly gain momentum and overwhelm the ability of dispensaries or a small district hospital to cope with the large number of sick patients that it generates. Thus, emergency treatment facilities may be needed, utilizing school buildings, tents or other convenient places. For many years, the standard treatment for cases of epidemic meningococcal disease has been oily chloramphenicol given as a single injection but this is being superseded by a single injection of ceftriaxone, which is easier to give and which is becoming cheaper. It may be necessary to recruit relatively untrained staff (e.g. teachers) to help with simple patient care such as ensuring that patients are well hydrated.

Step 5 – Chemoprophylaxis

Because outbreaks often cover an area with rapidly expanding and ill-defined boundaries, chemoprophylaxis is not usually recommended for outbreak management unless this occurs in a defined institution,

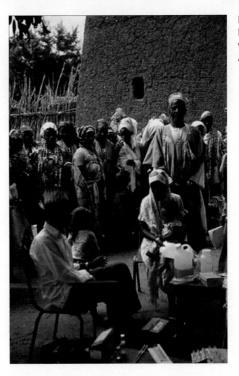

Fig. PP56.3
Meningococcal vaccination in an African village.

such as a residential school or military barracks, when chemoprophylaxis with rifampin (rifampicin) might be used.

Step 6 – Vaccination

Bivalent (serogroup A + C), trivalent (serogroup A, C, W135) and quadrivalent (serogroup A, C, W135, Y) meningococcal polysaccharide vaccines are available but the last is too expensive for epidemic control and is used primarily for vaccination of pilgrims. Both the bivalent and trivalent vaccines have been used in epidemic control and shown to be partially effective. Thus, if initial investigation shows that the outbreak is caused by a serogroup A, C or W135 meningococcus, vaccination of the affected communities should be undertaken as soon as possible (Fig PP56.3).

Vaccination is usually given to those aged 1–29 years old, the main group at risk. Defining the extent of the population to be vaccinated can be difficult. Speed is essential if vaccination is to have its maximum impact. Obtaining the vaccine and syringes needed for epidemic control rapidly has been facilitated by the creation of the International Coordinating Group (ICG), a group of donors and implementing agencies.

When implemented rapidly, vaccination with polysaccharide vaccines can halt an epidemic and save many lives; however, there is no evidence that the widespread use of polysaccharide vaccines in the meningitis belt over many years has reduced the frequency of epidemics. A more effective preventive strategy is needed. The dramatic success of a serogroup C meningococcal polysaccharide/protein conjugate vaccine in eliminating serogroup C meningococcal disease in the UK and elsewhere in Europe has raised expectations that the serogroup A vaccine, currently being developed by the Meningitis Vaccine Project, will be equally successful when deployed in mass vaccination campaigns in countries of the African meningitis belt. Immunization campaigns using this vaccine will commence in 2010.

FURTHER READING

Table PP56.2 Potential members of an epidemic management team

- District medical officer
- Officer in charge of the local hospital or dispensaries
- Senior nursing officer
- Pharmacist
- Officer responsible for the local expanded program on immunization
- Representative of the civil administration
- Representative of the traditional leaders
- Representative of the local educational authority
- Religious leaders
- Representative of the World Health Organization
- Representative of any local nongovernmental organizations involved in health-care delivery
- Representative of the local media – newspaper, radio

Further reading for this chapter can be found online at http://www.expertconsult.com

Parasitic infections of the gastrointestinal tract

INTRODUCTION

This chapter examines the parasitic causes of gastrointestinal infection in the nonimmunocompromised host. The organisms involved are a very heterogeneous group of protozoa and helminths. They vary in size from microsporidia, which are barely visible using light microscopy, to long multicellular organisms such as *Taenia saginata*, which can reach 25 m in length (Fig. 108.1). The clinical approach is emphasized here because the parasites themselves are discussed elsewhere (see Chapters 180, 181 and 184), and diagnosis in amebic infections is covered in Chapter 110. Parasitic gastrointestinal infections in HIV infection are discussed in Chapter 91. The parasites discussed in this chapter are listed in Table 108.1. Bacterial causes of chronic diarrhea and tropical sprue are discussed in Chapter 36.

EPIDEMIOLOGY

In affluent settings, parasitic infections appear to be uncommon causes of gastrointestinal illness. Certain populations are particularly likely to be affected:
- returned travelers;
- day-care workers and patients;
- migrant workers; and
- men who have sex with men.

The most common causes of parasitic gastrointestinal infection are *Giardia intestinalis* and *Cryptosporidium* spp.

In resource-poor settings the impact of parasitic infections is of much greater significance in relation to morbidity, mortality and economic impact. Their epidemiology is varied and their control presents a complex sociopolitical problem. The most important infections are *Entamoeba histolytica*, *G. intestinalis*, hookworms, *Ascaris* spp. and tapeworms.

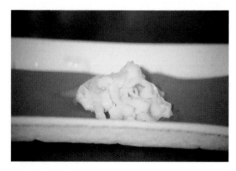

Fig. 108.1 Adult beef tapeworm (*Taenia saginata*) passed in a patient's feces.

Geographic distribution of parasites

The distribution of a parasite depends upon:
- human behavior;
- the physical environment; and
- the biologic environment.

Human behavior

Behavioral factors are often dominant but the distribution of vectors, intermediate hosts and reservoir hosts is also to some extent under human control. Some parasites are worldwide in their distribution, such as *E. histolytica* and *G. intestinalis*, whereas others are very localized.

Table 108.1 Gastrointestinal parasites

Intestinal protozoa	Amebae	*Entamoeba histolytica*; *Entamoeba dispar*
		Commensals *Entamoeba coli*
		Entamoeba hartmanni
		Endolimax nana
		Iodamoeba butschlii
	Bigyra	*Blastocystis hominis*
	Flagellates	*Giardia intestinalis*
		Dientamoeba fragilis
	Ciliate	*Balantidium coli*
	Coccidia	*Cryptosporidium parvum/C. hominis*
		Cyclospora cayetanensis
		Isospora belli
	Microsporidia	*Enterocytozoon bieneusi*
		Encephalitozoon intestinalis (formerly *Septata intestinalis*)
Intestinal helminths	Nematodes (round worms)	*Ascaris lumbricoides*
		Enterobius vermicularis
		Hookworms: *Ancylostoma duodenale*
		Necator americanus
		Trichuris trichiura
		Strongyloides stercoralis
	Trematodes (flukes)	*Fasciolopsis buski*
		Heterophyes heterophyes
	Cestodes (tapeworms)	*Taenia solium*
		Taenia saginata
		Hymenolepis nana
		Diphyllobothrium latum

Physical environment

The physical environment also affects the distribution of parasites. Temperature and humidity affect the viability of parasites in the external environment; viability is lost in cold or over-hot temperatures and most parasites require moist, aerobic conditions. Examples of parasites for which these factors are critical include:

- the cysts of protozoa with direct life cycles, such as *E. histolytica*, *G. intestinalis, Balantidium coli* and the various gut commensal species (*Entamoeba coli, Entamoeba hartmanni, Endolimax nana, Iodamoeba butschlii*);
- the oocysts of *Isospora belli*;
- the eggs and larvae of soil-transmitted nematodes (*Ascaris* spp., hookworm[1] and *Strongyloides stercoralis* (see Fig. 108.3));
- the eggs of trematodes (*Fasciolopsis buski* and *Heterophyes heterophyes*) and cestodes before their entry into the aquatic environment; and
- the eggs of cestodes before their ingestion by the intermediate hosts (*Taenia solium* and *Taenia saginata*).

Temperature and humidity also affect sporulation of oocysts, the rates of embryonation of nematode, cestode and trematode eggs, and the development times for hookworm and *Strongyloides* larvae. Parasites that have a soil stage are affected by the particular physical properties of the soil, including its particle size and water-holding capacity, and by factors such as rainfall. Susceptibility to anaerobic conditions is important for some parasites when 'night soil' (human feces) is used raw or after composting as a fertilizer.

The aquatic environment is important in the life cycle of many parasites. In the trematodes, the cercariae of *Heterophyes* spp. must survive long enough to infect the fish or shrimp and the metacercariae of *F. buski* must survive long enough to infect the human or pig hosts. *Strongyloides* larvae live in the capillary water films in soil and on low vegetation.

Biologic environment

The biologic environment also affects the epidemiology of these gastrointestinal parasites. The distribution in nature of appropriate vectors, intermediate hosts and reservoir hosts can obviously affect the distribution of parasites. Examples of animal reservoirs are *F. buski* in dogs, pigs or rabbits; *B. coli* in pigs; *C. parvum* in domestic animals, particularly cattle; and *H. heterophyes* in fish-eating mammals. Secondary hosts include snails for *F. buski* and freshwater fish for *H. heterophyes*. An important biologic factor is the presence of dung beetles that take the parasitic ova or larvae underground to a more favorable physical environment.

Human factors

Population density and urbanization

The agricultural revolution in developing countries has produced large resident human populations with the potential for direct person-to-person spread of infection and greater environmental contamination by feces. In addition, animal husbandry has created other cycles for parasite transmission, for example *Cryptosporidium* spp. in calves. Rapid urbanization, especially in the tropics, is often associated with increased poverty, poorer housing and unsanitary conditions. The result is that people may be living in a more fecally polluted environment than in rural areas, encouraging such diseases as amebiasis and giardiasis. Epidemics, such as outbreaks of cryptosporidiosis, may occur when public water supplies become fecally contaminated. *Cyclospora cayetanensis* is transmitted via contaminated produce and contaminated drinking water.[2] The soil-transmitted nematodes *Ascaris lumbricoides* and *Trichuris trichiura*[3] are often more common in towns and cities. Overcrowding favors direct transmission of *Hymenolepis nana* and *Enterobius vermicularis*, especially in children when levels of hygiene and sanitation are poor.[4]

Population movements

Population changes associated with mining, political unrest or industrialization may cause people to move into at-risk areas; travelers may also visit such areas.

Dams and irrigation

Development programs in the tropics frequently involve irrigation projects, where contaminated water supplies reach greater numbers of people and larger water-borne outbreaks may occur. Irrigation and poor drainage facilitate the breeding of flies that may have a role in spreading fecal material.

Agriculture

Cattle raising may be complicated by bovine cysticercosis (*T. saginata*), which renders carcasses unsaleable, and calves may be a source of human infection. Pigs can allow *T. solium*, the pork tapeworm, to be spread and *F. buski*, the intestinal fluke, to prosper. *Balantidium coli* is also acquired from close contact with pigs. Fish farms in which water plants such as water calthrop are grown transmit *F. buski*, especially if human or pig feces are used as fertilizer. Foods implicated in outbreaks of cyclosporiasis in the USA include fresh raspberries, mesclun lettuce and Thai basil.[5] In endemic areas cases of cyclosporiasis have also been associated with drinking contaminated water or to recreational water contaminated with human sewage. To date there is no known association with animal husbandry or animal feces.[6] The use of untreated human night soil enables soil-transmitted helminths to enter the human food chain.

Domestic environment

Sanitation, water supplies and domestic customs in hygiene and food preparation are all very important. Children are at risk of parasitic infections because of poor hand washing after defecation, finger sucking and playing with soil. Local dietary behavior is critical for parasite transmission. Ingestion of certain fish, crustacea, mollusks and aquatic vegetation can lead to fluke infection. Tapeworms are contracted by ingestion of undercooked pork or beef (*Taenia* spp.) or certain freshwater fish (*Diphyllobothrium* spp.). People who have occupations involving sewage, water or soil contact are at increased risk of parasitic infection.

Host susceptibility

Host susceptibility is affected by many factors such as nutritional status, intercurrent disease, pregnancy, immunosuppressive drugs and malignancy. Previously mild or clinically inapparent infections can produce dangerous disease when host immunity falls, such as occurs in strongyloidiasis, in which the parasite is capable of multiplying by autoinfection within its host, and fatal amebiasis that may occur if corticosteroids are administered in error.

Some protective immunity is usually acquired by the host but its effectiveness is variable. The absence of symptomatic giardiasis in adults in places where the infection is common is good evidence for acquired immunity. Re-infection and superinfection, possibly by different gastrointestinal parasite strains, is certainly common in areas of endemic infection. Immunodeficiency associated with HIV infection is of paramount importance in some of the more recently recognized gastrointestinal parasitic diseases such as cryptosporidiosis and microsporidiosis (see Chapter 91).

PATHOGENESIS AND PATHOLOGY

Gastrointestinal parasites cause disease in a variety of ways. Most are present in the lumen of the gut or attached to the mucosa of the gut wall and are not capable of invasion. The coccidian parasites such

Table 108.2 Anatomic location of gastrointestinal parasites		
Lumen only	Small bowel (normally)	*Ascaris lumbricoides*
	Large bowel	*Entamoeba histolytica/dispar*
		Balantidium coli
		Enterobius vermicularis
Mucosal attachment	Small bowel	*Giardia intestinalis*
		Tapeworm
		Hookworm
		Fasciolopsis buski
		Heterophyes heterophyes
	Large bowel	*Trichuris trichiura*
Epithelial cell invasion	Small bowel	*Isospora belli*
		Cyclospora cayetanensis
		Cryptosporidium parvum/ C. hominis
		Microsporidia
Mucosal invasion	Small bowel	*Strongyloides stercoralis*
	Large bowel	*Entamoeba histolytica*
		Balantidium coli

as cryptosporidia can invade the epithelial cells of the small bowel. Others, such as *E. histolytica*, *S. stercoralis* and occasionally *B. coli*, do invade the mucosa (Table 108.2).

Gastrointestinal protozoa

Amebiasis

Amebic ulcers mostly develop in the cecum, appendix or adjacent ascending colon, although the sigmoidorectal region can be involved.[7] Amebic ulcers are formed on the mucosa. They are usually flask shaped with a small, raised opening and a larger area of mucosal destruction below. The mucosa between abscesses is normal but lesions can be confluent. Pathogenic amebae are able to resist complement-mediated lysis and they possess other virulence factors such as attachment lectins, cysteine proteases and other enzymes[8] which, it is believed, assist the trophozoites with apoptosis of mammalian intestinal cells. Amebae have tissue-lysing enzymes on their surfaces that can be released from lysosomes or after amebic rupture. Recent studies *in vitro* and in mice have suggested that alterations in intestinal permeability may be mediated by pore-forming proteins called amebapores as well as alterations in tight junction proteins; this has yet to be confirmed in humans.[9]

In a study in Bangladeshi children, acquired immunity to amebiasis was associated with the appearance of an intestinal IgA response to the parasite Gal/GalNAc lectin, the virulence factor required for attachment of *E. histolytica* trophozoites to human cells. An intestinal IgA response to this lectin was associated with a 70% reduction in infections in children over the 2-year study period. On the other hand, those children who developed anti-amebic IgG antibodies in the serum were more susceptible to amebiasis. Interestingly, serum anti-lectin IgG antibodies cluster in families, supporting the presence of an inherited component to susceptibility to amebic disease.[10] Based on work with *Entamoeba invadens*, a parasite of reptiles, Eichinger has suggested that interactions of amebae with intestinal mucin glycoproteins promote encystment of the parasite and thus prevent invasion.[11] This is in keeping with the finding that *E. histolytica* cyst passers are asymptomatic.[12]

Giardiasis

The histopathology of the upper small bowel varies from normal to subtotal villous atrophy in giardiasis. *Giardia* spp. seem unable to penetrate the mucosal wall in humans but are able to attach to the mucosa of the small bowel. In symptomatic cases there is increased mucus secretion and dehydration.[13] *Giardia intestinalis* may undergo antigenic variation, thereby evading the human immune response.[14] Giardiasis is more common in the immunodeficiency syndromes, particularly in common variable hypogammaglobulinemia, although there is no particular increase in incidence among the HIV-infected population.

Balantidium coli

The trophozoite of *Balantidium coli* causes mucosal inflammation and ulceration, invading the distal ileal and colonic mucosa. Ulceration may be superficial or involve the full thickness of the bowel, leading to perforation.[15] Invasion may be enhanced by hyaluronidase produced by the parasite. Other products liberated by the parasite as well as host factors, such as the recruitment of mucosal inflammatory cells, may also be important.[16]

Cryptosporidiosis

Cryptosporidial infection in humans is most commonly due to *Cryptosporidium parvum* and *Cryptosporidium hominis* (formerly *Cryptosporidium parvum* genotype 1,[17] but *C. felis*, *C. muris*, *C. canis* and *C. meleagridis* have been identified in immunocompromised individuals.[17] *C. hominis* has been linked to more severe symptoms in sporadic outbreaks, in HIV-positive individuals and in a study of Brazilian children. In a study of more than 500 Peruvian children, *C. hominis* was the predominant cryptosporidial species and subtype Ib was associated with more symptoms of nausea, vomiting and general malaise in association with diarrhea than other subtypes (Ia, Id and Ie).[18] Different subtypes of *C. hominis* have varying effects in those patients with HIV-associated cryptosporidiosis (see Chapter 91).

Cryptosporidium infects the intracellular, extracytoplasmic area of host epithelial cells of the small bowel. The intracellular stage of *C. parvum* resides within a parasitophorous vacuole in the microvillus region of the host cell. Oocysts undergo sporogony while in the host cells. Approximately 20% of the oocysts do not form the usual environmentally resistant oocysts but are released as sporozoites that are capable of penetrating the microvillus regions of other cells within the intestine. This explains the ability of *C. parvum* to cause severe diarrhea in some patients, particularly in the immunocompromised.[19] Small bowel histology shows villous atrophy and crypt hyperplasia, usually with a mixed inflammatory cell infiltrate in the lamina propria. There is impaired absorption and enhanced intestinal secretion. There appears to be *Cryptosporidium*-associated apoptotic epithelial cell death.

The precise molecular mechanism for cryptosporidial diarrhoea is not yet elucidated. There appears to be enterotoxin-like activity and it appears that attachment of *Cryptosporidium* to epithelial cells induces survival signals in those cells so that the organism is able to multiply, while at the same time causing alterations such as apoptosis in adjacent uninfected cells which impair absorption and secretion by those cells and result in clinical disease; however, no enterotoxin has yet been isolated.[20]

Cyclosporiasis

The mechanism of diarrhea production has not been clearly established for *Cyclospora cayetanensis*. The organism is found within enterocytes. There is reduction in villus height with associated mucosal inflammation and increased numbers of intraepithelial lymphocytes, which suggests a direct effect on the intestinal mucosa.[21]

Isosporiasis

Mild to subtotal villous atrophy and crypt hyperplasia occurs in *I. belli* infection. Histologically, there may be infiltration of the lamina propria with large numbers of eosinophils, plasma cells, lymphocytes and polymorphs. Dilated lymphatics may be seen.[22]

Microsporidiosis

Intestinal microsporidia infect enterocytes in the small bowel and undergo sporogony, which leads to enterocyte degeneration, vacuolation and loss of the brush border. These cells are sloughed off and the spores are capable of infecting further enterocytes.[23,24]

Gastrointestinal helminths

Nematode infections

Ascariasis (roundworm infection)

The embryonated eggs of *A. lumbricoides* are ingested and hatch in the stomach and duodenum, from where the larvae penetrate the intestinal wall (Fig. 108.2). They are carried to the lungs in the circulation and usually cause no symptoms unless there are a large number of larvae, in which case pneumonitis can ensue. The larvae then break out of the lung tissue and may cause some bronchial epithelial damage. Intense tissue reaction with infiltration of eosinophils, macrophages and epithelioid cells occurs.[25] Jejunal histology shows shortened villi, a decrease in the villus:crypt ratio and cellular infiltration of the lamina propria.[25]

Hookworm infection

Hookworm disease is caused by *Ancylostoma duodenale* and *Necator americanus*. Vesiculation and pustules can occur on the skin at the site of entry of the filariform larvae. Asthma and bronchitis occur during migration through the lungs, with small hemorrhages into the alveoli and infiltration of eosinophils and leukocytes. Adult hookworms attach firmly to the small bowel mucosa; *A. duodenale* does this by means of well-developed mouth parts and *N. americanus* by means of cutting plates. There tends to be chronic blood loss at the site where the worm attaches.

Trichuriasis (whip worm)

The egg of the nematode *T. trichiura* hatches in the small intestine and the larva penetrates the villi causing no pathologic reaction. It re-emerges after 1 week and migrates to the cecum and colorectum. When few worms are present there is little damage, but with heavy infections there is hemorrhage, mucopurulent stools and symptoms of dysentery, sometimes with rectal prolapse (the *Trichuris* dysentery syndrome).[26]

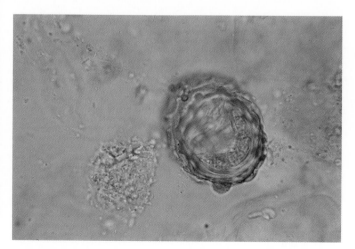

Fig. 108.2 *Ascaris lumbricoides* ovum in feces. The ovum measures 50–70 × 40–50 μm and is elliptical. The rough albuminous coat gives it a mammillated appearance.

Strongyloidiasis

The life cycle of *S. stercoralis* is complex (Fig. 108.3). Human infection is acquired when filariform larvae in the soil penetrate the skin. This can cause petechial hemorrhages, congestion and edema at the site of entry. The larvae migrate into cutaneous blood vessels and are carried to the lungs, where they break out of the pulmonary capillaries and sequentially enter the alveoli, trachea, pharynx and then the mucosa of the duodenum and upper jejunum. There can be pathologic findings similar to those of bronchopneumonia with lobar consolidation. The females mature in the intestine, invade the tissues of the bowel wall and lay their eggs, which hatch and release first-stage (rhabditiform) larvae in the feces (Fig. 108.4). In certain situations, the rhabditiform larvae mature in the intestine to the filariform stage, and these parasites bore into the wall of the duodenum and jejunum and initiate another cycle of infection, which eventually results in there being more adult worms in the small bowel. Filariform larvae that penetrate the bowel wall can spread throughout the lymphatic system to the mesenteric lymph glands and can enter the general circulation and hence the liver, lungs, kidneys and gallbladder. They can cause granulomas in the gastrointestinal tract and mesenteric glands. There are abscesses in the lungs and there may be granuloma in the liver. Migrating larvae may cause the patient to die from sepsis arising from the normal intestinal bacterial flora.

Trematode infections (flukes)

Fasciolopsis buski *infection*

The giant intestinal fluke *F. buski* is contracted by humans and pigs through eating metacercariae attached to water plants. The parasite excysts and attaches to the mucosa of the jejunal and duodenal wall causing mechanical injury and inflammation, which can lead to ulcers, bleeding or abscesses. There may be a mild anemia and low levels of serum vitamin B12, owing to the parasite's competition for the vitamin or impairing its absorption.

Heterophyes heterophyes *infection*

Heterophyes heterophyes is a trematode that infects humans and is found mainly in Asia. The pathology depends on the degree of infection acquired through ingestion of pickled or raw fish. The metacercariae excyst and attach to the walls of the small intestine. The adults may cause only a mild inflammatory reaction. Eggs may enter the circulation because the adults are attached deeply into the intestinal wall. Ectopic eggs can provoke granuloma formation, especially if they lodge in the heart or brain.[27]

Cestode infections (tapeworms)

Taenia solium *and* Taenia saginata

The pork tapeworm (*T. solium*) and the beef tapeworm (*T. saginata*)[28] are acquired by the human host by ingestion of poorly cooked meat that contains the encysted larvae (cysticerci). The larva is digested in the stomach and the head of the tapeworm evaginates in the upper small intestine, attaches via the scolex to the intestinal mucosa and feeds by absorbing nutrients from the bowel. The scolex of *T. solium* has four suckers and a rostellum that contains a double row of hooks; *T. saginata* has the suckers only. Very little pathology is caused by these well-adapted adult worms, which may reach 7 m and 25 m in length, respectively. The pathologically significant stage for humans is the cysticercus of *T. solium*. The eggs passed in feces are ingested and hatch when they are exposed to gastric juice. The oncospheres that are released penetrate the intestinal wall and are carried via the bloodstream and can potentially form a cysticercus in any organ. The cysticercus is an ovoid, milky-white bladder with the parasite head invaginated inside. The pathology is described in detail in Chapter 113.

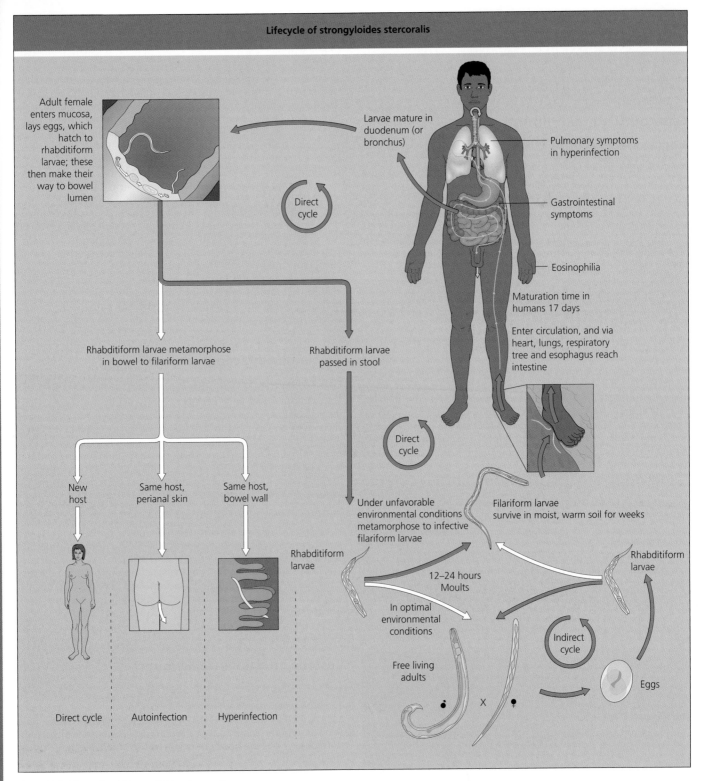

Fig. 108.3 Life cycle of *Strongyloides stercoralis*.

Dwarf tapeworm (Hymenolepis nana)

Once the ova of the dwarf tapeworm *H. nana* are ingested they encyst in the small intestinal villus mucosa. The adult worm reaches a length of 3–4 cm and begins egg production. Heavy infections of more than 100 worms can cause some symptoms, and the competition for nutrients has been linked with growth retardation in children, although this may be more the result of unsanitary conditions, poverty and malnutrition.

Fish tapeworm (Diphyllobothrium latum)

The fish tapeworm *D. latum* has a life cycle involving a first intermediate host of tiny aquatic invertebrates, a second intermediate host of predominantly freshwater fish and a definitive host that includes humans, other terrestrial mammals and less commonly marine mammals (believed to become infected by eating anadromus fish). The tapeworm attaches to the small intestinal mucosa by means of two longitudinal slit-like suckers (bothria). Infections are commonly

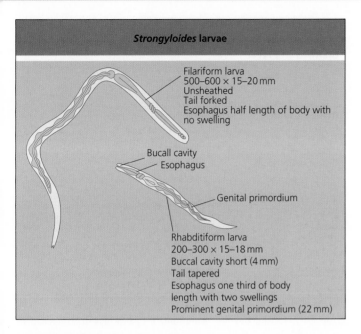

Strongyloides larvae

Filariform larva
500–600 × 15–20 mm
Unsheathed
Tail forked
Esophagus half length of body with no swelling

Bucall cavity
Esophagus

Genital primordium

Rhabditiform larva
200–300 × 15–18 mm
Buccal cavity short (4 mm)
Tail tapered
Esophagus one third of body length with two swellings
Prominent genital primordium (22 mm)

Fig. 108.4 *Strongyloides* larvae.

multiple and may reach more than 100 individual worms, each measuring up to 10 m in length. The pathology is minimal from the local effects. Tapeworm anemia has been described exclusively in Finland and has now all but died out as a result of control measures. The anemia is caused by vitamin B12 deficiency, with worms competing for the limited dietary vitamin B12, and it is strongly associated with gastritis and achlorhydria; there is probably a genetic predisposition to this condition.

PREVENTION

The prevention and control of parasitic gastrointestinal disease can be achieved through improvement of living standards, personal hygiene and better sanitary conditions.[29] In immunocompromised patients, different recommendations need to be considered (see Chapter 90).

Public health hygiene measures

Disposal of human sewage and waste water is fundamental to the control of parasitic gastrointestinal infections. Fecal material contaminates agricultural food crops or water supplies if it is passed promiscuously in the fields or close to habitation or if it is deliberately used unprocessed on fields as fertilizer ('night soil'). Any of the gastrointestinal parasites can be transferred in this way. Following rain, fecal material is washed into rivers and pools. *Giardia* cysts are found in surface water in many parts of the world.

The provision of latrines can reduce these sources of environmental contamination but, unfortunately, unless they are well constructed and maintained, latrines can themselves become important foci of infection. The prevalence of *Ascaris* infection is often higher among urban latrine users than among rural nonusers. The eggs of *A. lumbricoides* and also those of *T. trichiura* are very often resistant and can remain viable in the latrine environment for long periods. In addition, the moist soil around a latrine favors the survival of hookworm larvae[30] and the free-living cycle of *S. stercoralis*.

Domestic waste water (and the excreta that it accompanies) when used for irrigation puts crops and workers at risk. Sewage may enter lakes, rivers and ponds and the water then be used for drinking or irrigation. *Cryptosporidium* oocysts are particularly difficult to eliminate from water and require an efficient filtration system. Boiling water is the most reliable method of killing oocysts.

Composting is another reliable way of killing the infective forms of parasites. This takes 3–4 months. Cysts, eggs and larvae are quite rapidly killed at temperatures of 131°F (55°C) and die within a few days at 113°F (45°C). The compost heap needs turning and good maintenance or the periphery may become an intense transmission focus. Chemical treatment of excreta has been used, for example 12–24 hours in ammonium sulfate, but proper control is important to maintain efficacy and avoid toxicity to fish and plant life. Solid waste from sewage treatment plants is used as agricultural fertilizer and can contain viable parasites if inadequately processed. Sewage treatment removes or destroys parasites by sedimentation and the creation of completely anaerobic conditions. The eggs of *Taenia* spp. and *A. lumbricoides* are notoriously resistant and sometimes survive in the solid wastes taken from sedimentation tanks or ponds.

Personal hygiene measures

Most gastrointestinal diseases could be prevented if it were easy to modify human behavior. In practice this is often very difficult, but health education can be very effective and it can take many forms. Schools can be targeted or the local press used for a health awareness campaign. The fecal–oral route of transmission is very important, especially for intestinal protozoa. For example, infected food handlers are disseminators of *G. intestinalis* and *E. histolytica* cysts. There is high prevalence of infection in institutions for children or the mentally subnormal, where personal hygiene is poor. Those intestinal helminths whose life cycles can lead to fully embryonated eggs being released or formed very soon after entry into the environment (*H. nana* and *E. vermicularis*) are also spread in this way. Microsporidia are probably spread by the fecal–oral or urinary–oral route. Simple hand washing before preparing and eating food prevents transmission of these infections. The soil-to-skin route of infection can be inhibited by wearing shoes.[31] Infective forms of hookworm and *Strongyloides* larvae will be stopped from entering the skin. Persons dealing with composted human feces must use boots and gloves.

Good food hygiene is essential. Prevention of most of the parasites transferred by the fecal–oral route can be achieved by washing all salad vegetables and fruit before consumption. Kitchen utensils and hands should be washed frequently. Avoidance of wild-grown watercress and other water plants prevents *F. buski* infections. Proper cooking of meat and fish removes the risk of flesh-derived parasites such as *H. heterophyes* and tapeworms. Problems arise when cultural preferences dictate consuming these products raw, undercooked, salted, dried or pickled. The inspection of meat can detect the presence of cysticerci in the carcasses and allow infected meat to be condemned. Stopping the consumption of fish that is raw, pickled or salted is often impossible if it is part of a deep cultural tradition. Deep freezing of meat and fish at temperatures colder than –4°F (–20°C) for 24–48 hours kills all these parasites.

Prevention by chemotherapy

The treatment of these gastrointestinal parasites with appropriate chemotherapy is helpful in the prevention of further cases. This is particularly so in developed parts of the world. In areas where parasitic disease is endemic, generally only symptomatic patients are treated. Patients that are asymptomatic, those in whom the diagnosis is incidental and those who do not have heavy infections are usually not treated, as re-infection is probably inevitable. Mass chemotherapy has been used in amebiasis, soil-transmitted nematodes (*A. lumbricoides*,[32] hookworm, *T. trichiura*) and tapeworms (*T. saginata*, *T. solium*, *D. latum*).[33] Success depends upon several factors:

- the chemotherapeutic agent used should have a broad spectrum of activity and be given annually as a single oral dose;
- the drugs should be cheap to purchase and administer; and
- the drugs should have few side-effects.

In the past, mass chemotherapy was used in an attempt to eradicate amebiasis but, because treatment required a prolonged course of luminal amebicides, compliance was poor and reinfection in endemic areas was high. *Fasciolopis buski* infection in Indonesia has been treated by community-based praziquantel treatment but rapid re-infection followed. Selective or targeted chemotherapy may be of more use. *Enterobius vermicularis* infection in one child requires treatment not only of that child but also all family contacts together with education in personal hygiene. In 2003 a national program of soil-transmitted hookworm control (*A. lumbricoides* and *T. trichiura*) was implemented in Uganda, which has shown a sharp reduction in intensity of infection following annual mass drug administration of albendazole to children and high-risk adults. By 2006–2007 approximately 43 million treatments had been administered/[34] Ivermectin (in two separated doses) has been used successfully as mass treatment in north-east Brazil to control both intestinal helminths (including strongyloidosis) and ectoparasites including scabies.[35] A more recent study in Ecuador of school-age children demonstrated that treatment annually and biannually with ivermectin over a period of up to 17 years may have had a significant impact on *T. trichiura* infection.[36]

Vaccines

As yet no vaccines have been used in humans for the control of gastrointestinal parasitic diseases.[37]

Role of prophylaxis

There is no evidence for prophylactic use of chemotherapy being helpful in prevention of these gastrointestinal parasitic diseases.

Advice for travelers on preventive measures is discussed in Chapter 102.

CLINICAL FEATURES

The symptoms produced by gastrointestinal parasites are diverse. The most common presentation is of poorly localized abdominal pain; less commonly there is nonspecific diarrhea (Table 108.3). The severity varies from asymptomatic carriage to life-threatening gastrointestinal disease, as occurs in amebiasis and cryptosporidiosis. It is important to emphasize that the identification of an infection by stool microscopy does not necessarily imply that it is the cause of a patient's symptoms. This is particularly so in the case of light helminth infections, which are often completely symptomless. Other pathologies should be excluded before attributing the patient's symptoms to the gut parasite. Some of these infections present with extraintestinal manifestations, such as iron-deficiency anemia, wasting or (in the case of hookworm infection) growth retardation.

Gastrointestinal disease caused by protozoa

Amebiasis (*Entamoeba histolytica*)

It is now recognized that there are two species of amebae that were formerly termed pathogenic and nonpathogenic *E. histolytica*.[38] Methods used to separate these include biochemical, immunologic and genetic data. These are now called *Entamoeba histolytica* and *Entamoeba dispar*. Only *E. histolytica*

Table 108.3 Gastrointestinal parasites associated with diarrhea

Diarrhea and fever	*Entamoeba histolytica* *Cryptosporidium parvum/C. hominis* *Isospora belli* *Cyclospora cayetanensis* (occasionally)
Diarrhea with blood in stool	*Entamoeba histolytica* *Trichuris trichiura* *Strongyloides stercoralis* (rarely)
Chronic diarrhea	*Entamoeba histolytica* *Giardia intestinalis* *Cryptosporidium parvum* *Isospora belli* *Cyclospora cayetanensis* Microsporidia *Trichuris trichiura* Hookworm (*Necator americanus* and *Ancylostoma duodenale*) *Strongyloides stercoralis*

is capable of causing disease. Asymptomatic cyst carriers may excrete cysts for a variable length of time, usually only a few weeks. Confirmation that the parasite previously described as *Entamoeba histolytica* is in reality two species, *Entamoeba dispar* which is nonpathogenic and *Entamoeba histolytica* which is a pathogen, meant that the natural history of amebiasis needed reassessment.[12] Haque *et al.* studied 300 preschool children in Dhaka, Bangladesh.[10] Over a 2-year period, new *Entamoeba histolytica* infections were found in half the children. Of those who were asymptomatic cyst passers, one in 10 subsequently developed diarrhea within 2 months of the start of infection; 10% of the children had diarrhea in association with *E. histolytica* and 4% were found to have amebic colitis.

Amebic intestinal disease

The incubation period of invasive amebiasis varies from a few days to 1–4 months. There is a good correlation with the presence of *E. histolytica* trophozoites containing ingested red blood cells. Patients may be asymptomatic or present with colicky abdominal pain, frequent bowel movements and tenesmus. Amebic dysentery is characterized by blood-stained stools with mucus occurring up to 10 times a day. The duration of the dysentery can be very variable and may last for only a few days or for several months with concomitant weight loss and debility. The symptoms may be confused with inflammatory bowel disease. In acute cases the clinical picture may mimic appendicitis, cholecystitis, intestinal obstruction or diverticulitis.

Amebic extraintestinal disease

Amebic dysentery progresses to invasive amebic disease in between 2% and 8% of patients. Symptoms can be gradual in onset, with right upper quadrant pain and fever. Weakness, weight loss, dry cough and sweating are less common. Tender hepatomegaly is often seen with liver function tests that are normal or only slightly abnormal. Jaundice is very unusual. The site most commonly involved is the upper right lobe of the liver, and abscesses are mostly solitary. A raised right diaphragm may be found on chest radiograph. The abscess is visualized by ultrasound, CT or MRI. Hematogenous spread to the brain (see Chapter 106), lung, pericardium and other sites is possible.

Giardiasis (*Giardia intestinalis*)

The clinical spectrum of giardiasis ranges from asymptomatic infection, through acute gastrointestinal infection to severe chronic diarrhea[39] with intestinal malabsorption.[40] The average incubation period is 9 days and the acute infection is self-limiting.[41] Common symptoms include nausea, diarrhea, flatulence and upper abdominal cramps with distention and nausea. Weight loss is common and there can be signs of malabsorption (steatorrhea, disaccharidase deficiency and vitamin B12 deficiency).

Blastocystis infection (*Blastocystis hominis*)

There is controversy surrounding *B. hominis*; it is unclear whether it causes gastrointestinal disease or not. When large numbers are found in stool in the absence of other parasites, bacteria or viruses it may be the cause of diarrhea, cramps, nausea, fever, vomiting and abdominal pain. Data from Canada indicate that, although it is commonly seen in stools, it is not pathogenic.[42] This finding is further supported by a large Australian study which found no correlation between clinical symptoms and the presence of *B. hominis* in immunocompetent adults.[43] It is possible that a small subset of *B. hominis* organisms have virulence factors that are missing in most.[44]

Dientamoeba fragilis infection

Like *Blastocystis*, the pathogenicity of *Dientamoeba fragilis* is uncertain. It has been associated with a wide range of symptoms. In children, symptoms may include intermittent diarrhea, abdominal pain, nausea, anorexia, malaise, fatigue, poor weight gain and unexplained eosinophilia.[45]

Cryptosporidiosis (*Cryptosporidium parvum* and *C. hominis*)

The incubation period of *Cryptosporidium* infection averages 3–6 days. Symptoms include a flu-like illness, diarrhea, malaise, abdominal pain, anorexia, nausea, flatulence, malabsorption, vomiting, mild fever and weight loss. In the 1993 Milwaukee water-borne outbreak of cryptosporidiosis, which affected around 403 000 people, the mean duration of illness was 12 days and the median maximum number of stools per day was 12.[20] Oocyst excretion generally occurs for 3–30 days (average 12 days) and occurs at the same time as the symptoms. Generally the symptoms are self-limiting, and prolonged disease is uncommon.[46] In immunocompromised patients the situation is different and there can be intractable, profuse, life-threatening diarrhea.[47,48]

Cyclosporiasis (*Cyclospora cayetanensis*)

There is epidemiologic evidence that *Cyclospora cayetanensis* is the cause of persistent diarrhea in immunocompetent patients as well as in immunocompromised patients. Initially, the clinical findings do not distinguish cyclosporal diarrhea from other causes of diarrhea. Other common symptoms are abdominal pain, nausea, vomiting and anorexia.[49] *Cyclospora* infection can last for 1–8 weeks.[21]

Isosporiasis (*Isospora belli*)

The predominant clinical symptom is diarrhea, which may be intermittent and last for months or even years. Stools are watery, soft, foamy and offensive, which may suggest malabsorption. There is associated weight loss, abdominal pain and fever.[50,51] In HIV-infected patients, chronic infection occurs.

Microsporidiosis

Microsporidia may cause acute self-limiting diarrhea in immunocompetent persons,[23] in patients who have immunodeficiency other than AIDS and in the elderly.[24] In HIV infection, chronic diarrhea and wasting are common.[52] *Enterocytozoon bieneusi* is one of the most important intestinal pathogens in severely immunodeficient HIV-infected patients; it is present in 7–50% of those who have otherwise unexplained chronic diarrhea. In one large Australian study there has been a reported decline in incidence of microsporidiosis from 11% in 1995 to 0% in 2004.[53] There are also increasing reports of intestinal microsporidial infections in immunocompetent people.[54] *Encephalitozoon intestinalis* (formerly *Septata intestinalis*) is a less commonly recognized cause of chronic diarrhea. *Encephalitozoon cuniculi* intestinal infection has been reported. These are covered in Chapter 181.

Balantidiasis (*Balantidium coli*)

Balantidium coli, the largest and least common of the human protozoan pathogens, is capable of causing an infection resembling amebic colitis. It is particularly prevalent among people living in close association with pigs in South America, Iran, Papua New Guinea and the Philippines. Up to 80% of persons carrying the organism are asymptomatic carriers.[16] Acute diarrhea with blood and mucus begins abruptly and is associated with nausea, abdominal discomfort and marked weight loss. There can be inflammatory changes and ulceration in the proctosigmoid region. Peritonitis and colonic perforation can progress rapidly to death. A chronic infection occurs with intermittent diarrhea and infrequent bloody stools.

Helminthic gastrointestinal disease

The World Bank regards intestinal helminth infections as the main cause of disease burden in children from 5 to 14 years old in developing countries.

Ascariasis (*Ascaris lumbricoides*)

Most cases of ascariasis are asymptomic; symptomatic infections are more common in children than adults. When large numbers of larvae migrate to the lungs in a short time period, *Ascaris* pneumonitis can result. This is the clinical picture of Löffler's syndrome, which is characterized by dyspnea, dry cough, wheezing or coarse rales, fever up to 104°F (40°C), transient eosinophilia and a chest radiograph that is suggestive of viral pneumonia and that resolves within a couple of weeks. In addition, eosinophils, Charcot–Leyden crystals and larvae may rarely be found in the sputum. Symptoms of asthma and urticaria may continue during the intestinal phase of ascariasis. The adult worms occasionally migrate from the small bowel and cause biliary or hepatic ascariasis. Rarely, adult worms migrate into the biliary tree with secondary sepsis and abscess formation. Pancreatitis may result from migrating ascarids that obstruct the pancreatic duct. In people who have large numbers of adult worms intestinal obstruction can occur owing to the sheer bulk of worm bodies. Adult worms migrate more in the presence of a stimulus such as a fever of over 102°F (38.9°C) or the use of a general anesthetic, and they may block the bile duct or pancreatic duct or enter the liver or peritoneal cavity. In children, nutritional deficiencies such as reduced appetite, kwashiorkor (protein-energy malnutrition), vitamin A deficiency and growth deficit are related to the burden of the adult worms.[55]

Enterobiasis (*Enterobius vermicularis*)

Infection with *Enterobius vermicularis* (threadworm or pinworm) causes few or no symptoms in the vast majority of people. The predominant symptom is nocturnal pruritus ani, caused by migration of the female worms from the anus to the perianal skin in the process of laying their eggs. Scratching may be intense and secondary infection may ensue. Pruritus vulvae caused by pinworms entering the vulva is occasionally seen. In children, insomnia, loss of appetite, loss of weight, emotional instability, enuresis and irritability may also be found.[55]

Hookworm infection (*Ancylostoma duodenale, Necator americanus*)

Hookworm causes ground itch, a moderate-to-severe pruritus of the skin, usually of the feet, as the hookworm larvae penetrate. Secondary infection can occur if the vesicular lesions are excoriated by scratching. A pneumonitis, caused by alveolar migration of larvae, is less common, less severe and causes less sensitization than that seen with *Ascaris* or *Strongyloides* infection. Symptoms of the intestinal phase are fatigue, nausea, vomiting, abdominal pain, diarrhea with occult bleeding, and weakness. Heavy worm burdens may have serious sequelae in young children.[56] This is particularly problematic with *A. duodenale* infection. Eosinophilia is usually present. According to the degree of worm burden, chronic infection leads to an iron deficiency anemia[30] and hypoproteinemia with pallor, edema of the face and feet, listlessness, koilonychia, cardiomegaly, heart failure and rarely mental retardation. Iron deficiency in children is associated with impaired academic performance at school and in adults with weakness and fatigue, leading to reduced productivity.

Trichuriasis (*Trichuris trichiura*)

Light infections with this common, ubiquitous infection rarely cause symptoms. In heavy infections (more than 10000 eggs per gram of feces), epigastric pain, vomiting, distention, flatulence, anorexia and weight loss may occur. Rarely the *Trichuris* dysentery syndrome may occur, with blood and mucus in the stools and, in heavy infections, prolapse of the rectum. Reduced childhood growth rates, reduced food intake, iron deficiency and gastrointestinal protein loss are seen in heavy infections. The diagnosis is made when numerous worms are seen on the rectal mucosa or eggs are found in the stool. A 'honeycomb' effect of the small intestine has appearances similar to Crohn's disease. There may be deformity of the proximal colon and also the ileum or appendix.

Strongyloidiasis (*Strongyloides stercoralis*)

Strongyloides stercoralis largely causes asymptomatic infection of the small intestine, which can last for 30 years or longer.[57] The prepatent period from infection through the skin to the appearance of rhabditiform larvae in the stools is 1 month or more. Symptoms only develop with high intestinal worm loads, which can be the result of several factors. In people debilitated by concurrent disease or malnutrition, there may be massive invasion of the tissues by *S. stercoralis*. Treatment with immunosuppressive drugs in a patient harboring *S. stercoralis* can also lead to the same effect.[58] Infection with human T-cell leukemia virus 1 is important in predisposing to massive infection by *S. stercoralis*. Interestingly, infection with HIV is not a common cause of the *Strongyloides* hyperinfection syndrome; this may be due to the decreased likelihood of intestinal larval migration in the presence of CD4 lymphopenia seen in HIV infection.[59] Symptoms include watery mucous diarrhea, with the severity depending on the intensity of the infection. Sometimes diarrhea alternates with constipation. Malabsorption of fat and vitamin B12 with a chronic diarrhea and protein-losing enteropathy has also been described and is rapidly reversed by treatment.

There are two types of skin rash. The first is larva currens, which occurs on the trunk or near the anus, and is a linear eruption in which the larvae migrate under the skin causing an itchy, nonindurated wheal with a red flare that moves rapidly and disappears in a few hours. This contrasts to the indurated and persistent track of nonhuman hookworm larvae (cutaneous larva migrans). The second type of rash is urticaria.

Features of the strongyloidiasis hyperinfection syndrome (see Fig. 108.3) include severe diarrhea, malabsorption, edema, hepatomegaly and paralytic ileus. Gram-negative sepsis is a recognized complication. In very severe cases encephalopathy and even secondary pyogenic meningitis have been described.

Fasciolopsis buski infection

Fasciolopsis buski is confined to Asian countries, particularly Thailand. Symptoms are more frequent in children than adults owing to their greater exposure to water plants while at play. Like many other intestinal parasites, the majority of infected people have very minor symptoms or none at all. In heavier infections, clinical features can include diarrhea, abdominal pain, vomiting, flatulence, poor appetite, fever and eosinophilia. In very severe cases there may be ascites, edema of the face, abdomen and legs, anemia, anorexia, weakness and even intestinal obstruction. Intestinal ulceration may cause malabsorption and lead to malnutrition and wasting.[27]

Heterophyes heterophyes infection

Heterophyes heterophyes causes few symptoms unless the infection is heavy, which is dependent on the quantities of pickled or uncooked fish eaten in endemic areas (mostly the Middle and Far East). The adult worms produce abdominal pain, diarrhea with mucus and ulceration of the intestinal wall.

Beef and pork tapeworm infection (*Taenia saginata* and *Taenia solium*)

The clinical features of *T. saginata*, the beef tapeworm, and *T. solium*, the pork tapeworm, are similar. The adult worms in the gastrointestinal phase of both organisms usually cause no symptoms, but carriers can sometimes feel a proglottid emerging from the anus; the motile proglottid may be upsettingly obvious in the feces. Other associated symptoms, such as abdominal pain and distention, nausea and anorexia have been attributed to the tapeworm. There is occasionally a mild eosinophilia but there is no anemia, even in long-term infection. Cysticercosis complicates infection with *T. solium* only. Ingestion of *T. solium* eggs leads to the dissemination of oncospheres in the bloodstream; these can become lodged anywhere in the subcutaneous and intramuscular tissues,[60] where they become cysticerci; symptoms depend on the particular body site involved. The clinical findings of neurocysticercosis are discussed in detail in Chapter 113.

Dwarf tapeworm infection (*Hymenolepis nana*)

As with other tapeworms, there are usually few symptoms in *H. nana* infection. Symptoms that may occur include abdominal pain, anorexia, irritability and headache. Eosinophilia is common. Symptoms are more common in heavy infections and may cause growth retardation in children.

Fish tapeworm infection (*Diphyllobothrium latum*)

There are few if any symptoms from infection with *D. latum*. Symptoms including diarrhea, headache and nonspecific malaise all appear to be somewhat more common than in uninfected people. Tapeworm-associated anemia is probably related to vitamin B12 deficiency caused by competition for the vitamin between the tapeworm and a genetically predisposed host; however, this is now exceedingly rare.

DIAGNOSIS (TABLE 108.4)

Microscopic examination of the stool is fundamental to the diagnosis of all the gastrointestinal infections. A minimum of three stool specimens, examined by trained personnel using a concentration and a permanent stain technique, should be used.

An ELISA for *Strongyloides* is useful in screening patients who have suggestive symptoms or eosinophilia. In microscopically proven

Table 108.4 Methods of diagnosis of gastrointestinal parasites

Intestinal protozoa	
Entamoeba histolytica and nonpathogenic amebae (*E. dispar*, *E. hartmanni*, *Entamoeba coli*, *Iodamoeba butschlii* and *Endolimax nana*) Methods to differentiate *Entamoeba histolytica* and *E. dispar*	Fecal microscopy for cysts Also possible to scrape or aspirate material from mucosal surfaces at sigmoidoscopy for microscopic examination Microscopy of fresh feces (within 20 min) which must contain blood and mucus to detect trophozoites containing ingested red cells enables *E. histolytica* to be distinguished from *E. dispar* ELISA of fecal samples (to detect galactose adhesin) PCR (often only available in reference centers) Culture and zymodeme pattern analysis (reference standard test)[61] Serologic tests are valuable in cases of suspected amebic abscess (and ameboma); the indirect fluorescent antibody test is positive in over 95% of cases after 14 days but should be confirmed by the cellulose acetate precipitin test
Giardia intestinalis	Fecal microscopy for cysts (and occasionally trophozoites); if negative, a string test, duodenal aspirate or biopsy may be positive ELISA to detect *Giardia* antigens in fecal specimens (sensitivity and specificity of 87–100%) Indirect immunofluorescence test on fecal specimens using a cyst-specific monoclonal antibody[62] Direct fluorescent antibody test (MERIFLUOR DFA) against cell wall antigens to *Giardia* in fecal specimens demonstrated increased sensitivity and specificity of over 95%[63] Immunochromatographic assays are also available for qualitative detection in fecal specimens[63] Serology tests are also available
Blastocystis hominis *Dientamoeba fragilis* *Balantidium coli* *Cryptosporidium parvum/C. hominis*	Fecal microscopy with Romanowsky stain Fecal microscopy with Romanowsky stain Fecal microscopy Fecal microscopy or intestinal biopsy. Staining of oocysts (~5 µm) with auramine, modified ZN or immunofluorescence using monoclonal antibodies[64] Immunochromatographic assays are also available for qualitative detection in stool specimens[63] PCR is still principally reference laboratory technique
Cyclospora cayetanensis	Fecal microscopy or intestinal biopsy. Cysts are visible using auramine, modified ZN (~8 µm) and are bright blue autofluorescent under UV light (330–380 nm)
Isospora belli	Fecal microscopy or intestinal biopsy. Stain with modified ZN or auramine under UV light
Enterocytozoon bieneusi and *Encephalitozoon intestinalis* (formerly *Septata intestinalis*)	Fecal microscopy with a modified trichrome stain or a fluorescent chromotrope stain Electron microscopy or PCR is needed for species identification
Nematodes (roundworms)	
Ascaris lumbricoides *Ancylostoma duodenale* *Necator americanus* (hookworms) *Trichuris trichiura* *Enterobius vermicularis* *Strongyloides stercoralis*	Depends on identification of ova, larvae or worms in feces on light microscopy Samples should be mixed well before examination and a concentration method is usually used Parasites are identified by appearance and size Visualized by Sellotape slide or perianal swab Fecal microscopy for larvae and fecal culture can also be performed A string test can also be undertaken as can serologic tests
Trematodes (flukes)	
Fasciolopsis buski	Fecal microscopy looking for ova and identification of worms Serology is also available in some centers
Heterophyes heterophyes	Fecal microscopy for ova and identification of worms
Cestodes (tapeworms)	
Taenia solium	Fecal microscopy for ova and proglottids to differentiate between the pork and beef tapeworm Serology available for cysticercosis but not for intestinal tapeworm infection
Taenia saginata	Fecal microscopy for ova and segments
Hymenolepis nana	Fecal microscopy for ova
Diphyllobothrium latum	Fecal microscopy for ova and segments

ZN, Ziehl–Neelsen stain.

disease, the sensitivity of *Strongyloides* serology has been shown to be best in immigrants with chronic infection when compared to travellers to endemic countries.[65] Cross-reactions occur occasionally with ascariasis and filarial infection. The filarial ELISA cross-reacts in some cases of strongyloidiasis. Serum antigiardial antibody detection is not clinically useful in highly endemic areas because people may be seropositive from past infection. The giardial immunofluorescent antibody test gives good titers if the disease has caused mucosal damage, and it is helpful in the investigation of parasite-associated malabsorption.

MANAGEMENT

Gastrointestinal protozoa

The management of gastrointestinal protozoa is summarized in Table 108.5. Treatment regimens are discussed in detail in Chapter 150.

Entamoeba histolytica (see Chapter 110)

Treatment of *E. histolytica* infection is divided into two types. Luminal amebicides, such as diloxanide furoate, act on organisms in the intestinal lumen and are not effective against organisms in tissue. Tissue amebicides, such as metronidazole and tinidazole, are effective in treating invasive amebiasis but less effective in the treatment of organisms in the bowel lumen. There is some controversy about treating asymptomatic patients. Ideally, any amebic cysts should be tested to identify whether they are *E. histolytica* (in which case the infection should be treated to avoid the risk of developing invasive disease and to prevent secondary spread) or *E. dispar* (which does not require any treatment). However, until ELISA or PCR tests become widely deployed it will continue to be usual to treat asymptomatic patients in nonendemic areas with diloxanide furoate (see Table 108.5). When asymptomatic cyst carriage persists after treatment for amebic dysentery or liver abscess, further treatment with a luminal amebicide is mandatory, otherwise relapse is frequent. The treatment of asymptomatic cyst carriers in endemic areas is of questionable value because of the high rate of re-infection. A second-choice intraluminal amebicide is paromomycin.[66] New broad-spectrum antiparasitic agents are being introduced as infection with multiple parasites is a common occurrence in the tropics. Nitazoxanide, a compound structurally similar to nitrobenzamide, is reported to act on a wide range of intestinal parasites, including some cestodes, nematodes and protozoa. In a study in Mexican children, Davila-Gutierrez reported a higher eradication rate for treatment of *E. histolytica*/*dispar* with nitazoxanide 100 mg twice daily for 3 days than with quinfamide 100 mg as a single dose.[67] Further work is needed to determine whether or not nitazoxanide will become a first-line treatment for amebic cyst passage.

Proven amebic dysentery should always be treated. Drugs of choice are metronidazole or tinidazole followed by diloxanide furoate (see Table 108.5). Amebic liver abscess is treated with metronidazole, 400–500 mg orally q8h, followed by diloxanide furoate as above. Tinidazole is an alternative; chloroquine (150 mg base q6h for 2 days, then 150 mg base q12h for 19 days) can also be used.

Giardia intestinalis (see Chapter 180)

Treatment is often unnecessary because most healthy, immunocompetent patients have a self-limiting disease and recover by their own natural host defense mechanisms. Treatment of symptomatic patients reduces the duration and severity of symptoms. The treatment of asymptomatic cyst carriers is controversial in endemic areas. Generally, in a nonendemic area, asymptomatic *Giardia* cyst carriers are treated. The 5-nitroimidazole derivatives metronidazole or tinidazole are the treatment of choice and can be used in short courses.[41] Albendazole, 400 mg daily for 5 days, has been shown to have useful antigiardial activity. Mepacrine, an acridine dye, has a similar efficacy but is generally less well tolerated with an incidence of 1.5% of acute psychosis. Furazolidone, a nitrofuran, has lower efficacy but is well tolerated. Newer thiazolide antiparasitic agents such as nitazoxanide, which is licensed by the Food and Drug Administration (FDA) for the treatment of *G. intestinalis* in children, appear well tolerated with good oral bioavailability.[68] *In-vitro* and *in-vivo* resistance of *G. intestinalis* has been demonstrated, although rarely, to conventional therapy, particularly to the 5-nitroimidazoles such as metronidazole and tinidazole.[69–71]

Table 108.5 Treatment of gastrointestinal protozoal infection*

Condition	Drug	Dosage
Amebiasis		
Asymptomatic carrier of intestinal cysts		
1st choice	Diloxanide furoate	500 mg q8h for 10 days
2nd choice	Paromomycin (aminosidine)	500 mg q8h for 10 days
Intestinal infection (amebic dysentery or ameboma)	Metronidazole or	750–800 mg q8h for 5 days
	Tinidazole followed by	2 g daily for 2–3 days
	Diloxanide furoate or	500 mg q8h for 10 days
	Paromomycin	500 mg q8h for 10 days
Amebic liver abscess	Metronidazole or	400–500 mg q8h for 5–10 days
	Tinidazole followed by	2 g daily for 3–5 days
	Diloxanide furoate	500 mg q8h for 10 days
Giardiasis		
1st choice	Tinidazole or	2 g single dose
	Metronidazole	400–500 mg q8h for 3 days
2nd choice	Nitazoxanide	500 mg q12h for 3 days
3rd choice	Albendazole	400 mg q24h for 5 days
4th choice	Mepacrine	100 mg q8h for 5–7 days
Balantidium coli **infection**		
1st choice	Tetracycline	500 mg q6h for 10 days
Alternatives	Ampicillin, metronidazole or paromomycin	
Cyclospora cayetanensis **infection**		
1st choice	Trimethoprim–sulfamethoxazole (co-trimoxazole)	960 mg q12h for 7 days
Alternatives	Ciprofloxacin	500 mg q12h for 7 days
Isospora belli **infection**		
1st choice	Trimethoprim–sulfamethoxazole (co-trimoxazole)	960 mg [160 mg (TMP)/800 mg (SMX)] q12h for 7–10 days (q6h in immunosuppressed patients)
2nd choice (if intolerant to sulfonamides)	Furazolidone	100 mg q6h for 10 days

*All treatments are adult dosage and given orally unless stated otherwise.

Blastocystis hominis

If *B. hominis* is present in the stool, the physician must not stop looking for another cause of diarrhea. Whether any treatment is required is controversial. Metronidazole seems to be the most appropriate drug.

Dientamoeba fragilis

In adults infected with *D. fragilis*, improvement can be seen with tetracycline; in children, metronidazole is appropriate.

Balantidium coli

Tetracycline is effective against *B. coli*. Doxycycline 100 mg daily for 10–14 days is an alternative. Other drugs to which *B. coli* is sensitive are ampicillin, metronidazole and paromomycin. Surgery may be required for fulminant disease with perforation or abscess formation.

Cryptosporidium spp. (see Chapter 91)

Cryptosporidium spp. infection is self-limiting in those who have normal immunity. It presents a severe problem when it occurs in patients who have AIDS.[47] Where available, treatment is with HAART (highly active antiretroviral therapy) with or without antiparasitic agents. No currently available drug reliably eradicates cryptosporidial infection, but suppression of infection is possible. Agents currently in use are paromomycin, azithromycin[72] and nitazoxanide.[73] In one randomized control trial of immunocompetent adults and children with *C. parvum* infection, the parasitologic and clinical cure rate with nitazoxanide (500 mg q12h for adults, 100–200 mg q12h for children) was significantly greater than placebo.[74]

Cyclospora cayetanensis

Many cases of *C. cayetanensis* infection are self-limiting. When treatment is felt to be necessary trimethoprim–sulfamethoxazole (co-trimoxazole) has been found to be effective, eradicating the oocysts from 94% of 16 patients in 7 days compared with 12% of 17 patients who received placebo.[75] Relapse is common in the immunocompromised but responds to a second course of treatment. Given the propensity of sulfonamide-containing drugs to cause side-effects in HIV-infected individuals, an alternative agent to co-trimoxazole is required. Verdier *et al.* compared the activity of trimethoprim–sulfamethoxazole (TMP–SMX) 160/800 mg orally twice daily for 1 week with ciprofloxacin 500 mg twice daily for 1 week in HIV-positive patients infected with *Cyclospora cayetanensis*.[76] Nine received TMP–SMX and 11 received ciprofloxacin. Diarrhea ceased in all patients receiving TMP–SMX and in 10 of 11 patients receiving ciprofloxacin. At 7 days all those who received TMP–SMX had negative stool examinations, four of 11 treated with ciprofloxacin had persisting oocysts, one of whom still had diarrhea. All four responded to open treatment with TMP–SMX. Patients who had shown a complete response at 7 days were given maintenance therapy with TMP–SMX 160/800 mg three times weekly or ciprofloxacin 500 mg three times weekly for 10 weeks. No recurrences were observed in the TMP–SMX group but one of seven patients who received ciprofloxacin experienced a recurrence after 4 weeks. Whilst ciprofloxacin is not as effective as TMP–SMX against *Cyclospora*, it provides an acceptable alternative for individuals who cannot tolerate a sulfonamide.

Isospora belli

Treatment of *I. belli* infection may be necessary in the immunocompromised, and oral trimethoprim–sulfamethoxazole eliminates the parasite in most cases; relapse is common but retreatment is usually effective. Prophylactic trimethoprim–sulfamethoxazole may then be necessary. Pyrimethamine–sulfonamide combinations have also proven to be effective.[77] If the patient is intolerant to sulfonamides, furazolidone 100 mg four times daily for 10 days is an alternative. The macrolide antibiotic roxithromycin (2.5 mg/kg q12h) was reported to be successful in a single patient with AIDS and *I. belli* infection who had not responded to co-trimoxazole or pyrimethamine therapy. The 5-nitrothiazole derivative nitazoxanide is also reported to be effective in isosporiasis in a dose of 7.5 mg/kg (500 mg for adults; 200mg for children less than 12 years of age) twice daily for 3 days. Biliary isosporiasis may require intravenous co-trimoxazole as both oral co-trimoxazole and oral nitazoxanide have been reported to fail in the presence of malabsorption and cholangitis due to *I. belli*.[78,79]

Microsporidia

The treatment of microsporidiosis in the immunocompetent patient is not required. Evidence and experience in treating these infections comes from HIV-infected patients where albendazole has been shown to be useful with some species of microsporidia, notably *Encephalitozoon intestinalis*.[80] Fumagillin has shown activity against *Enterocytozoon* bieneusi,[81] as has nitazoxanide, although the evidence has been limited to case reports.[82]

Gastrointestinal helminths

The management of gastrointestinal helminths is summarized in Table 108.6 (see Chapter 150).

Table 108.6 Treatment of gastrointestinal helminthic infection*

Condition	Drug	Dosage
Nematodes		
Round worms		
Ascaris lumbricoides	Albendazole	400 mg, single dose
	Mebendazole	100 mg q12h for 3 days
	Levamisole	150 mg, single dose
	Piperazine hydrate	4.5 g, single dose
Enterobius vermicularis	Mebendazole	100 mg, single dose
	Piperazine phosphate	4 g, single dose
	Pyrantel pamoate	10 mg/kg, single dose
Hookworms		
Ancylostoma duodenale	Mebendazole	100 mg q12h for 3 days
Necator americanus	Albendazole	200 mg q24h for 3 days
	Levamisole	150 mg, single dose (less effective against *N. americanus*)
	Pyrantel pamoate	10 mg/kg, single dose
Trichuris trichiura	Mebendazole	100 mg q12h for 3 days or 600 mg, single dose
	Albendazole	400 mg, single dose
Strongyloides stercoralis	Ivermectin	200 µg/kg, daily for 2 days
	Albendazole	400 mg q12–24h for 3 days
	Thiabendazole	25 mg/kg (max 1.5 g) q12h for 3 days
Trematodes (flukes)		
Fasciolopsis buski	Praziquantel	15 mg/kg, single dose
Heterophyes heterophyes	Praziquantel	10–20 mg/kg, single dose
Cestodes (tapeworms)		
Taenia solium	Praziquantel	10 mg/kg, single dose
	Niclosamide	2 g, single dose
Taenia saginata	Praziquantel	10 mg/kg, single dose
	Niclosamide	2 g, single dose
Hymenolepis nana	Praziquantel	20 mg/kg, single dose
	Niclosamide	2 g on day 1 then 1 g/q24h for 6 days
Diphyllobothrium latum	Praziquantel	10 mg/kg, single dose
	Niclosamide	2 g, single dose

*All treatments are adult dosage and given orally unless stated otherwise.

Ascaris lumbricoides

Treatment is effective only against the adult worm. It is usual to treat any established infection. The drugs used are albendazole, mebendazole, levamisole or piperazine in a single adult dose of 4 g of piperazine phosphate or 4.5 g of piperazine hydrate, or pyrantel pamoate. *Ascaris* pneumonitis responds dramatically to prednisolone therapy and anthelmintics should be given 2 weeks after lung involvement. Surgery is sometimes required for bowel perforation or obstruction.

Enterobius vermicularis

Enterobius vermicularis infection is treated with mebendazole (100 mg, single dose, which is repeated if necessary after 2–3 weeks), piperazine phosphate (4 g, single adult dose repeated after 14 days) or pyrantel pamoate (10 mg/kg, single dose). The whole family should be treated simultaneously, fresh bed linen and night clothes should be provided and the nails kept short and scrubbed. Repeat treatment may be required because recurrence is common.

Hookworm

Hookworm infection is treated by eliminating the adult worms and treating anemia if present; these treatments can be carried out concurrently. In endemic countries where re-infection is inevitable, light infections are treated only in children, not in adults. Mebendazole and albendazole are effective against both *A. duodenale* and *N. americanus*. In a single-dose comparison of albendazole and mebendazole, albendazole gave better cure and egg reduction rates.[83] Levamisole is less effective against *N. americanus*, and pyrantel pamoate is preferred. In a study from Ivory Coast, Utzinger *et al.* reported a reduction in the prevalence and intensity of hookworm infections in schoolchildren receiving praziquantel for *Schistosoma mansoni* infection. If their results are replicated they will have a significant impact upon helminth control programs.[84]

Trichuris trichiura

In symptomatic patients and in asymptomatic carriers who have high numbers of eggs, trichuriasis is treated with mebendazole or albendazole. In undernourished children who have moderate infection intensities in Jamaica, albendazole treatment also resulted in improvement in some tests of cognitive ability and in school attendance and school performance, even after controlling for socioeconomic status.[85]

Strongyloides stercoralis

Strongyloides stercoralis infection should be treated in both symptomatic and asymptomatic people because of its ability to cause hyperinfection if immunosuppression occurs. Ivermectin is the drug of choice. This regimen has proven very effective in a prospective randomized trial comparing the efficacy of ivermectin and thiabendazole in Cambodian refugees who had symptomatic chronic strongyloidiasis[86] and in a prospective randomized trial comparing a 7-day course of oral albendazole with a single dose of ivermectin in 42 Thai adults with chronic *Strongyloides*.[87] Ivermectin also looks very promising in HIV-positive patients infected with *S. stercoralis*. Albendazole is also effective. Thiabendazole, orally twice daily for 3 days, is effective but often poorly tolerated. Subcutaneous ivermectin (unlicensed in humans) has proven effective in a case of life-threatening *Strongyloides* hyperinfestation.[88,89] Although there are no currently known minimally effective concentrations of ivermectin for *Strongyloides* treatment in humans, repeated doses subcutaneously[90] and orally[91] appear to have a cumulatively increasing antiparasitic effect.

Fasciolopsis buski

Fasciolopsis buski infection is treated with praziquantel which is highly effective. Niclosamide has also been used.

Heterophyes heterophyes

Heterophyes heterophyes infection is treated with a single dose of praziquantel. Niclosamide is an alternative.

Taenia solium and Taenia saginata

Patients who have *T. solium* infection should be evaluated for the presence of cerebral cysticercosis before commencing therapy against the intestinal tapeworm. Praziquantel is effective therapy for the adult worm. Niclosamide has also been widely used.

Hymenolepis nana

Hymenolepis nana infection can be treated with a single oral dose of praziquantel. Niclosamide is also successful.

Diphyllobothrium latum

Diphyllobothrium latum infections are treated with praziquantel. Niclosamide was extensively used in the past.

REFERENCES

References for this chapter can be found online at http://www.expertconsult.com

Chapter | 109 |

Christiane Dolecek
We wish to acknowledge the contribution of John Richens, the author of the previous chapter.

Typhoid fever and other enteric fevers

EPIDEMIOLOGY

Typhoid fever and paratyphoid fever are Gram-negative septicemias caused by *Salmonella enterica* serovar Typhi (*S. typhi*) and *Salmonella enterica* serovar Paratyphi (*S. paratyphi*) A, B and C. Typhoid and paratyphoid fever are summarized as enteric fevers. Whilst *S. typhi* and *S. paratyphi* A and B infections are restricted to humans, *S. paratyphi* C can affect a variety of animals.

Typhoid fever is endemic in Africa, Asia, Central and South America and is found in parts of the Middle East, southern and eastern Europe.[1] Infections seen in Europe, Australia and North America are usually acquired abroad, mostly from the Indian subcontinent, South East Asia and South America (Fig. 109.1).

Estimates from the World Health Organization (WHO) suggest that the worldwide incidence of typhoid fever is approximately 21 million cases annually with 210 000 deaths and paratyphoid fever causes an additional 5 million diseases.[2] It is likely that the proportion of disease caused by *S. paratyphi* A has been underestimated; recent data show that enteric fevers were caused in 64% in China, in 24% in India and in 33% in Nepal by *S. paratyphi* A.[3,4]

In population surveillance studies from Asia the typhoid incidence (per 100 000 persons per year) among 5–15 year olds in Vietnam and China was low (24 and 29, respectively) and high in Indonesia, Pakistan and India (180, 413 and 493, respectively).[5] In endemic areas typhoid fever has been considered to be a disease of schoolchildren and young adults; however, recent data emphasize that it is a common cause of morbidity in children between 1 and 5 years. Transmission of typhoid fever occurs via the fecal–oral route by ingesting contaminated water or food or through direct person-to-person contact. Risk factors for acquiring enteric fever are contaminated water (Fig. 109.2), eating food prepared outside the home, shellfish from polluted water, vegetables fertilized with human waste and having a relative with a recent history of typhoid fever living in the same house. Chronic typhoid carriers involved in food handling are an important reservoir of infection.

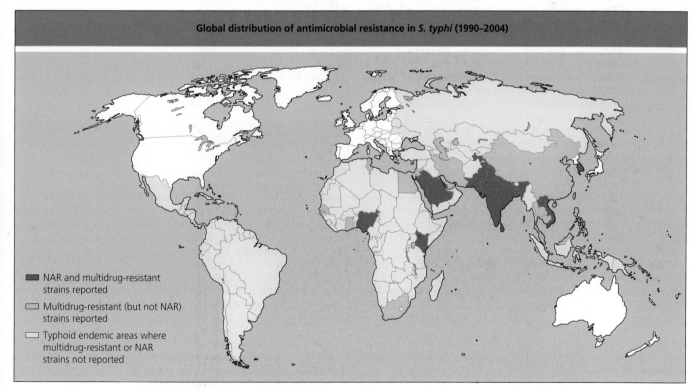

Global distribution of antimicrobial resistance in *S. typhi* (1990–2004)

- ■ NAR and multidrug-resistant strains reported
- □ Multidrug-resistant (but not NAR) strains reported
- □ Typhoid endemic areas where multidrug-resistant or NAR strains not reported

Fig. 109.1 Global distribution of antimicrobial resistance in *Salmonella typhi* (1990–2004). Reproduced with permission from Bhan *et al.*[9]

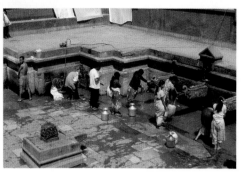

Fig. 109.2
Community water spouts in Kathmandu, Nepal. Villagers, mostly women and children, are seen collecting their daily water provision from the community's stone spouts. This water is usually not boiled.

PATHOGENESIS AND PATHOLOGY

The species *Salmonella enterica* (see Chapter 169) is divided into six subspecies (*enterica, salamae, arizonae, diarizonae, houtenae* and *indica*) and contains more than 2400 serotypes.[6] Most of the Salmonellae that cause disease in humans (including *S. typhi, S. paratyphi* and *S. typhimurium*) are in the subspecies *enterica*.

S. typhi and *S. paratyphi* are flagellated, non-spore-bearing, facultative anaerobic Gram-negative bacilli, identified by a characteristic biochemical pattern and confirmed by serologic identification of their somatic lipopolysaccharide (O) and flagellar protein (H) antigens. *S. typhi* and *S. paratyphi* C sometimes possess a polysaccharide capsular Vi (virulence) antigen that coats the O antigen and potentially protects it from antibody attack.

The genome of *S. typhi* is 4.8 million base pairs in length and encodes approximately 4000 genes.[7] There are several large insertions, believed to originate from bacteriophages or plasmids, termed the *Salmonella* pathogenicity islands which encode genes that are important for survival in the host. *Salmonella* has two type III secretion systems (TTSS) encoded by *Salmonella* pathogenicity islands SPI-1 and SPI-2. The invasion of epithelial cells is mediated by the SPI-1 TTSS which injects virulence proteins into the host cell, leading to macropinocytosis of the bacteria and cytoskeletal rearrangement of the host cell to allow translocation. SPI-2 TTSS secretes effectors required for survival and replication in *Salmonella*-containing vesicles inside phagocytes and epithelial cells.[8]

S. typhi also has more than 200 pseudogenes. The inactivation of these genes may explain the host restriction of *S. typhi*.

Volunteer studies have shown that the infective dose of *S. typhi* is 10^3 to 10^9 bacteria. Gastric acidity destroys the organisms but gastric hypoacidity (following gastrectomy, intake of histamine-2 receptor antagonists or proton pump inhibitors) allows a greater number of organisms to enter the small intestine. In a study from India, *Helicobacter pylori* infection has been associated with an increased risk of typhoid fever.[9]

After ingestion in water or food, *S. typhi* bacteria reach the small intestine where they adhere to the mucosal epithelial cells. They penetrate the mucosal epithelium via the M (membranous) cells (specialized cells overlying the Peyer's patches), enterocytes or via a paracellular route. They are taken up by macrophages and multiply in the mononuclear phagocytic cells of the small intestine, are drained into mesenteric lymph nodes and reach the general circulation (causing an asymptomatic primary bacteremia) by lymph drainage from the thoracic duct. During the incubation period, which varies between 7 and 14 days, the bacteria reside and multiply within the organs of the reticuloendothelial system (spleen, liver, bone marrow and lymph nodes, especially the Peyer's patches of the terminal ileum). Bacteria are then shed into the bloodstream, marking the onset of fever and symptomatic disease. During the symptomatic stage, *S. typhi* can be cultured from blood, although this is made difficult by the low bacterial load that characterizes this infection (less than one colony-forming unit per ml of blood).

If left untreated, the *S. typhi* bacteremia persists for several weeks. In this phase the organism disseminates widely to the organs of the reticuloendothelial system. *S. typhi* infection produces hyperplasia of the Peyer's patches in the first week, which can resolve or progress to necrosis. Ulcers can lead to perforation and hemorrhage, usually in the third week, although these may occur earlier or later during the disease.[1]

The majority of patients mount local and systemic humoral and cellular immune responses but these do not confer complete protection against relapse or re-infection. The mortality of untreated typhoid used to be about 10–20%.

PREVENTION

Typhoid and paratyphoid fever can be prevented by the provision of safe water, good food hygiene and safe sewage disposal. As chronic carriers pose a special risk to the community, programs to detect and treat chronic carriers are needed.[10]

Vaccines are another tool to prevent enteric fever. There are two licensed vaccines for typhoid fever, the parenteral Vi polysaccharide and the oral Ty21 vaccines.

The live oral Ty21 vaccine is available in enteric-coated capsules or liquid formulation. It is administered in three doses (four doses in the USA and Canada) 2 days apart and is licensed for adults and children above 6 years. Field studies with the oral Ty21 vaccine in the 1980s showed a protective efficacy of 96% after 3 years in Egypt, 77% in Chile after 3 years when using the liquid formulation and 53% in Indonesia after 2.5 years.[1] Herd protection was demonstrated during the field trials in Chile. Ty21a cannot be used in immunocompromised patients and pregnant women, and antibiotics should be avoided 7 days before and after immunization. Booster doses are recommended every 5 years.

The injectable capsular polysaccharide Vi vaccine is given in a single dose (25 µg) and is immunogenic and licensed above 2 years of age. A single intramuscular injection conferred a protective efficacy of 55% after 3 years in South Africa and 72% after 17 months in Nepal.[10] Booster doses are recommended every 3 years.

The Vi conjugate vaccine is immunogenic in children under 2 years and had a protective efficacy of 91.5% after 27 months in field trials in Vietnam,[10] but is not yet commercially available.

None of the currently licensed typhoid vaccines protects against *S. paratyphi* A, an emerging infection in Asia, and there is no licensed paratyphoid vaccine available. A polyvalent panenteric vaccine is urgently needed.

CLINICAL FEATURES

Enteric fever presents with fever, headache, anorexia and abdominal discomfort with either diarrhea or constipation. This can be accompanied by nausea, vomiting and a dry cough. Profuse diarrhea has been described in typhoid patients with HIV infection.[1] Abdominal tenderness, hepatomegaly (40–70% of patients) and splenomegaly are common. It is rare for patients with typhoid fever not to have any abdominal symptoms, but even in the absence of these symptoms typhoid fever cannot be excluded.

Less than 5% of patients show rose spots, small blanching erythematous maculopapular lesions of about 2–4 mm diameter on the trunk (Fig. 109.3). Hemoglobin levels, white cell counts and platelet counts are normal or reduced. Liver enzymes (aspartate aminotransferase, alanine aminotransferase) are often elevated two to three times the upper limit of normal and bilirubin is normal or slightly raised. Abdominal sonography may demonstrate enlargement of liver and spleen and prominent mesenteric lymph nodes.

Although it has been frequently cited in the literature that *S. paratyphi* causes a milder disease, recent prospective clinical trials have

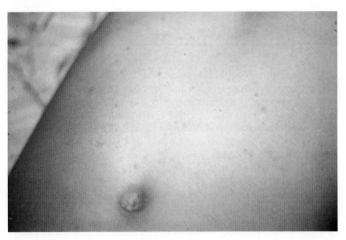

Fig. 109.3 Typhoid rose spots. These are small, blanching maculopapular lesions, ~1–4mm in size, usually seen on the trunk. They may also take on a more purpuric, nonblanching character. Courtesy of CM Parry, Liverpool, UK.

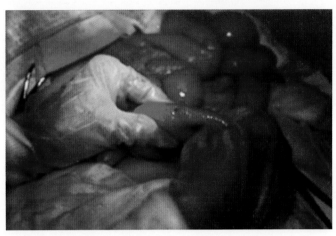

Fig. 109.4 Gastrointestinal perforation, usually of the terminal ileum, is one of the most serious complications of typhoid fever. The picture shows the surgical inspection of a perforating necrotic ulcer. Courtesy of John Wain, Cambridge, UK.

reported that enteric fever caused by *S. typhi* and *S. paratyphi* A are clinically indistinguishable.[4,11] *S. paratyphi* A has also been described as a cause of severe enteric fever in Indonesia.[12]

Complications and severe typhoid fever

Complications of typhoid fever are more likely to occur in patients who have been sick for longer periods without receiving treatment and in patients with nonsusceptible *S. typhi* isolates who do not receive appropriate treatment (Table 109.1), and may develop in up to 10% of hospitalized patients.[10]

Septic shock and acute respiratory distress syndrome are serious complications when treatment is delayed.

Table 109.1 Important complications of typhoid fever
Abdominal complications
Gastrointestinal bleeding
Intestinal perforation and shock
Hepatitis with/without jaundice
Cholecystitis
Genitourinary complications
Retention of urine
Glomerulonephritis
Cardiovascular complications
Asymptomatic ECG changes
Myocarditis
Sudden death
Respiratory complications
Pneumonia
Bronchitis
Hematologic complications
Anemia
Disseminated intravascular coagulation (DIC)
Focal infections
Abscesses of brain, liver, spleen etc.
Neuropsychiatric complications
Encephalopathy – reduced consciousness levels
Meningitis
Seizures

Gastrointestinal bleeding (occurs in about 10% of patients), intestinal perforation and typhoid encephalopathy are the most common complications. Gastrointestinal bleeding results from a necrotic Peyer's patch eroding the wall of an enteric blood vessel. Often the bleeding resolves without intervention, but in about 2% of cases the bleeding requires blood transfusion. Gastrointestinal perforation, usually at the terminal ileum (Fig. 109.4), is the most serious complication; it occurs in about 1–3% of hospitalized cases.[1] It manifests as acute abdomen or as worsening of abdominal pain accompanied by shock. Perforation is associated with a high mortality and needs urgent surgical intervention.

A reduced level of consciousness or encephalopathy, often accompanied by shock, is a serious complication, associated with a mortality of up to 50%.[12] Typhoid encephalopathy encompasses a wide range of symptoms ranging from agitation to delirium and coma. These symptoms might be possibly caused by liver failure, hematogenic dissemination to the brain or other unknown mechanisms.

The incidence of this presentation varies between different countries, ranging from 10% to 40% of hospitalized cases in Indonesia and Papua New Guinea but less than 2% in Pakistan and Vietnam. This variation is unexplained.[1] In patients with encephalopathy, cerebrospinal fluid should be obtained and meningitis (including tuberculous meningitis) and encephalitis excluded.

The prognosis of typhoid fever during pregnancy has been improved through antimicrobial treatment. Typhoid fever acquired through intrauterine infection can lead to neonatal typhoid fever, a severe sepsis with a mortality of up to 10% or to asymptomatic persistent secretion.[1]

Relapse

The recurrence of symptoms within 1 month after treatment has been completed and symptoms have resolved is considered a relapse. Relapse rates vary considerably (between 0% and 10%) and are related to the efficacy of the antibiotic treatment.[1,13,14]

Chronic carriage

Between 1% and 5% of patients with a history of enteric fever become chronic carriers, harboring *S. typhi* or *S. paratyphi* in their gallbladder and shedding bacteria intermittently in their stools after the illness.[10] These carriers are an important reservoir of infection and are usually asymptomatic. Up to 25% of chronic carriers do not have a history of typhoid infection. The rate of carriers is higher among females and patients with cholelithiasis. An association between urinary carriage of *S. typhi* and *S. paratyphi* A and schistosomiasis has been described, caused by obstructive lesions of the urinary tract.

Case fatality

A recent WHO report has estimated the case fatality rate in typhoid fever at 1%.[2] There seems to be considerable geographic variation; in Vietnam and Pakistan the case fatality rate among hospitalized patients is less than 2%, but in patients with severe typhoid fever in Papua New Guinea and Indonesia it can be as high as 30%.[1] The most important contributor to a poor outcome is probably a delay in instituting effective antibiotic treatment.

Differential diagnosis

Typhoid fever presents with unspecific symptoms and this makes the diagnosis difficult. Other endemic illnesses, most importantly malaria, have to be ruled out. Typhoid can occasionally present as a gastroenteritis with vomiting and diarrhea at its initial presentation. Differential diagnosis includes leptospirosis, typhus (rickettsial disease), tuberculosis, brucellosis, other bacterial sepsis, encephalitis, amebic liver abscesses, visceral leishmaniasis, viral diseases (dengue fever, infectious mononucleosis, hepatitis, influenza) and lympho-proliferative disease.

ANTIMICROBIAL DRUG RESISTANCE

In 1948 the introduction of chloramphenicol revolutionized the management of typhoid fever.[15] Chloramphenicol was effective for more than 20 years, but then in the 1970s outbreaks of chloramphenicol-resistant typhoid fever occurred in Mexico, India and Vietnam. In the late 1980s there were outbreaks of typhoid fever that were resistant against all 'first-line' antimicrobials (multidrug resistance is defined as resistance to chloramphenicol, ampicillin and trimethoprim–sulfamethoxazole).[1] These multidrug-resistant (MDR) *S. typhi* isolates have been responsible for numerous outbreaks in countries in the Indian subcontinent, South East Asia and Africa.[9] All MDR strains so far examined have been harboring plasmids of the incHI1 incompatibility group.

The fluoroquinolone class of drugs has become the treatment of choice for typhoid fever. The fluoroquinolones show excellent tissue penetration, accumulation in monocytes and macrophages and high drug levels in the gallbladder. However, there have been reports from Vietnam, India and Tajikistan of the emergence of *S. typhi* isolates that respond less well to the fluoroquinolones.[1,9] In 1997, an epidemic in Tajikistan caused by resistant strains caused illness in more than 10 000 people and 108 deaths. Technically these isolates are still within the breakpoints set for fluoroquinolone susceptibility by the Clinical Laboratory Standard Institute (CLSI),[16] but they are resistant to nalidixic acid (the prototype quinolone) and show higher minimum inhibitory concentrations (MICs) to the fluoroquinolones. Patients infected with these isolates show a poor clinical response when treated with ciprofloxacin or ofloxacin.

Nalidixic acid resistance is usually caused by single point mutations in the bacterial target enzyme *gyrA*, either at codon 83 or 87.[17] High-level ciprofloxacin-resistant *S. typhi* with double mutations at position 83 and 87 from the Indian subcontinent has been described.

Recently there have been reports of *S. typhi* isolates with reduced susceptibility to the fluoroquinolones that test nalidixic acid sensitive,[9] suggesting another mechanism of resistance. There have been sporadic reports of ceftriaxone-resistant *S. typhi* fever, but these isolates remain rare.[18] A decreasing trend of chloramphenicol-resistant *S. typhi* has been reported in recent years from the Indian subcontinent.[9]

MDR as well as nalidixic acid-resistant *S. paratyphi* A is an emerging problem in the Indian subcontinent.[3,4]

DIAGNOSIS

The diagnosis of enteric fever requires the isolation of *S. typhi* or *S. paratyphi* from blood, bone marrow or an anatomic lesion. Blood culture is the gold standard in the diagnosis of enteric fever. As a low bacterial load is a characteristic feature of typhoid fever, obtaining a large volume of blood – ideally 10–15 ml for schoolchildren and adults and 2–4 ml for preschool children – is recommended. The sensitivity of blood culture is estimated to be 50–60%; bone marrow culture is more sensitive (up to 80%), because of the higher concentration of bacteria in the bone marrow.[10]

Serology

The Widal tube agglutination test, described more than 100 years ago, is based on the presence of agglutinating antibodies to the O and H antigens of *Salmonella*. It is usually performed in settings where culture facilities are not available. In the original format, paired sera (acute and reconvalescent) were required and a fourfold increase of antibodies (to O and H antigens) supported the diagnosis of typhoid fever. However, the test is usually performed on acute serum and lacks sensitivity and specificity. This is because not everybody mounts a detectable antibody response to *S. typhi*, healthy populations in endemic areas and people who received typhoid vaccine show a high level of antibodies and there is cross-reactivity to other *Salmonella* serotypes. Rapid tests (Tubex, Typhidot and Typhidot M) have been developed with varying sensitivity and specificity.[19]

MANAGEMENT

Enteric fevers are systemic infections and antimicrobial treatment should be initiated early. It is important to provide supportive measures, such as oral and intravenous fluids, appropriate nutrition and antipyretics. More than 90% of patients are managed at home with oral antibiotics, and reliable and close medical follow-up for complications or failure to respond to therapy. Patients with persistent vomiting, severe diarrhea and abdominal distention need admission to hospital.[10]

The management of patients with enteric fever should include blood and stool cultures after completion of treatment to check for convalescent stool carriage, as well as follow-up to identify chronic fecal carriage.

The choice of treatment depends on the antimicrobial susceptibility of the isolates, but is also influenced by cost and availability, which are important factors, especially in endemic regions.

Table 109.2 shows the recommendations of the World Health Organization for the treatment of typhoid fever, updated with evidence from recent randomized controlled trials.[13,14,20]

The fluoroquinolones are the most effective treatment for typhoid fever. In patients infected with nalidixic acid-susceptible isolates, fever usually resolves within 4 days, cure is achieved in 96% of patients and rates for fecal carriage and relapse are below 2%.[1]

The fluoroquinolones are also recommended for the treatment of children with typhoid fever. Concerns that the fluoroquinolones might cause cartilage damage in children have led to their cautious use in many countries. However, extensive experience with the fluoroquinolones in children with cystic fibrosis, typhoid fever and bacillary dysentery has provided a body of evidence suggesting that these antibiotics are safe in children.[1,10]

For infections with nalidixic acid (quinolone)-resistant *S. typhi* and *S. paratyphi*, azithromycin, newer generation fluoroquinolones (gatifloxacin) and third-generation cephalosporins (ceftriaxone) are effective.

Two trials[13,20] and one recent trial from Nepal (Basnyat B, unpublished results; this trial included monitoring for dysglycemia) show that the 8-methoxy-fluoroquinolone gatifloxacin is safe and efficacious in patients with enteric fever (91% and 96% overall treatment success, respectively). A retrospective study from Canada reported a high risk

Table 109.2 Treatment of uncomplicated typhoid fever*

Susceptibility	OPTIMAL THERAPY			ALTERNATIVE EFFECTIVE DRUGS		
	Antibiotic	Daily dose (mg/kg)	Days	Antibiotic	Daily dose (mg/kg)	Days
Fully sensitive	Fluoroquinolone, e.g. ofloxacin or ciprofloxacin[†]	15	5–7[‡]	Chloramphenicol Amoxicillin Trimethoprim– sulfamethoxazole	50–75 75–100 8/40	14–21 14 14
Multidrug resistance	Fluoroquinolone	15	5–7	Azithromycin Ceftriaxone	10–20 75	7 10–14
Quinolone (nalidixic acid) resistance[§]	Azithromycin or newer fluoroquinolone, e.g. gatifloxacin[#]	10–20

10 | 7

7 | Ceftriaxone | 75 | 10–14 |

*Based on the World Health Organization (WHO)[10] recommendations for the treatment of typhoid fever, updated with evidence from recent randomized controlled trials in typhoid fever.[13,14,20] Cefixime, an oral third-generation cephalosporin that was included in the WHO recommendations of 2003, has been removed due to recent evidence.[20]
[†]The available fluoroquinolones (ofloxacin, ciprofloxacin, fleroxacin, pefloxacin) are all highly active and equivalent in efficacy, with the exception of norfloxacin, which has inadequate oral bioavailablity and should not be used in typhoid fever.[10]
[‡]Three-day courses have also been shown to be effective, but should be reserved for epidemic containment.[10]
[§]Prolonged courses of high-dose fluoroquinolones (e.g. ofloxacin 20 mg/kg q24h) have been recommended[10] and are standard treatment in many contries for nalidixic acid-resistant *S. typhi* and *S. paratyphi* A; however, a recent trial using ofloxacin at 20 mg/kg q24h for 7 days has shown treatment success in only 64% of patients and high rates of convalescent fecal (19%) carriage (at day 8).[14]
[¶]Azithromycin used at 20 mg/kg q24h for 7 days achieved better cure rates (93% and 91%, respectively)[13,22] than azithromycin 10 mg/kg q24h in multidrug-resistant and nalidixic acid-resistant typhoid fever.
[#]Two published trials[13,20] and one recent trial from Nepal (Basnyat B, unpublished results; this trial included monitoring for dysglycemia) show that the newer 8-methoxy-fluoroquinolone gatifloxacin is safe and efficacious in patients with typhoid fever (91% and 96% overall treatment success, respectively). A retrospective study from Canada reported that gatifloxacin used in elderly patients (mean age 77 years) with type 2 diabetes has a high risk of inducing dysglycemia;[21] this was not seen in the typhoid treatment trials in young and otherwise healthy patients.

of gatifloxacin-induced dysglycemia in elderly patients (mean age 77 years) with type 2 diabetes.[21] These side-effects were not seen in the young and otherwise healthy patients in these trials.

Prolonged courses of fluoroquinolones (e.g. ofloxacin 20 mg/kg/day) have been recommended[10] and are standard treatment in many countries for nalidixic acid-resistant *S. typhi* and *S. paratyphi* A. However, a recent trial using ofloxacin at 20 mg/kg/day for 7 days has shown treatment failure in 36% of patients and high rates (19%) of immediate post-treatment fecal carriage (at day 8).[14]

Cefixime (oral third-generation cephalosporin) should not be used. A recent trial observed high treatment failure rates of 38% and the trial was stopped early by the trial's Independent Data Safety and Monitoring Board.[20]

Ceftriaxone should be used for 10–14 days. Ceftriaxone therapy for 7 days was associated with a relapse rate of 14%.[9]

There are few data on the treatment of typhoid fever in pregnancy. Ampicillin for fully susceptible isolates and ceftriaxone are considered safe for this indication.[10]

Management of severe typhoid fever

Both inpatients and outpatients should be closely monitored for the development of complications. The parenteral fluoroquinolones are probably the first choice for the treatment of severe typhoid fever[10] and should be given for a minimum of 10 days, but there are no randomized trials to date. For patients infected with nalidixic acid-resistant isolates, ceftriaxone is effective.[10]

A trial conducted in the 1980s showed a dramatic beneficial effect of high-dose dexamethasone treatment (3 mg/kg for the first dose given over 30 minutes and 1 mg/kg every 6 hours for 48 hours) in severe typhoid fever patients with encephalopathy and shock, given in addition to chloramphenicol. Dexamethasone treatment reduced the mortality from 56% to 10% when compared to placebo.[12] Hydrocortisone at a lower dose was not effective.

Intestinal perforation is a surgical emergency. Early intervention is crucial, and mortality rates increase as the delay between perforation and surgery lengthens, varying between 10% and 32%.[10] Metronidazole should be added to the antibiotic regimen.

Patients with intestinal hemorrhage need intensive care, monitoring and blood transfusion. Intervention is not needed unless there is significant blood loss, but cross-matched blood should be ready and the surgical team alerted.

In patients presenting with a relapse, which is defined as the re-occurrence of acute illness after the patient has been treated successfully, cultures should be obtained and patients should be treated according to the susceptibility pattern of the infecting isolate.

Typhoid carriers

Chronic carriers play an important role in the transmission of typhoid and paratyphoid fever. As *S. typhi* and *S. paratyphi* are only shed intermittently in the feces, a series of stool cultures should be obtained to detect typhoid carriers. In order to eradicate carriage, long antimicrobial treatment courses of 6 weeks should be given according to the susceptibility of the isolates. In susceptible isolates, clearance was achieved in up to 80% with the administration of 750 mg ciprofloxacin or 400 mg norfloxacin twice daily for 28 days.[10] If cholelithiasis is present the patient may require cholecystectomy as well as antibiotic therapy.

REFERENCES

References for this chapter can be found online at http://www.expertconsult.com

Chapter | **110** |

David C Warhurst

In memory of Peter Sargeaunt and Mehreen Zaki, who died in 2008.

Amebic infections

INTRODUCTION

Amebiasis ranks as the fourth most common protozoan cause of death, behind malaria, African trypanosomiasis and leishmaniasis.[1] The motile trophozoites (amebae) live in the lumen of the large intestine, where multiplication by binary fission takes place. Trophozoites of *Entamoeba histolytica* can invade the colonic mucosa producing ulceration and dysentery (Fig. 110.1). Through blood-borne spread they can give rise to extraintestinal lesions, usually abscesses in the liver (see Fig. 110.5). The course of dysentery is usually self-limiting, but amebic liver abscess is potentially fatal unless diagnosed promptly and treated appropriately. During their life in the large intestine, the trophozoites of *Entamoeba* spp. develop into cysts, a dormant stage, resistant to environmental stress, which is passed out in the feces and serves to infect other humans after ingestion in contaminated water or food.

This organism was first observed by Lösch[2] in 1875, who reported from St Petersburg on a fatal dysentery in a patient with persistent diarrhea, fever, general weakness and tenesmus. However, not until the last decade of the 20th century was it generally accepted that amebae termed *E. histolytica* living in the human colon and producing 4-nucleate cysts between 10 and 20μm in diameter comprised three distinct species, *E. histolytica*, *E. dispar* and *E. moshkovskii*, of which only *E. histolytica* was capable of causing dysentery and other pathologic manifestations. *E. dispar* had been proposed as a nonpathogen, separate from but morphologically identical to *E. histolytica*, by Brumpt in 1925:[3] the separation of potentially pathogenic *E. histolytica* from morphologically similar amebae was supported by Sargeaunt and colleagues[4] in 1978 on the basis of isoenzyme patterns, then on nucleic acid sequence by Diamond & Clark[5] in 1993. The World Health Organization (WHO)[6] redefined amebiasis in 1997 as infection with *E. histolytica*, with or without clinical manifestations, and noted the importance of distinguishing it from the morphologically identical but nonpathogenic *E. dispar*.

It has since become clear that *E. moshkovskii* represents a third morphologically similar nonpathogenic species, isolated from humans, but able to grow in culture at ambient temperatures (10–25°C) as well as 37°C, unlike *E. histolytica* or *E. dispar*.[7] Although initially it was thought that human infections with *E. moshkovskii* might be rare and restricted to temperate zones, it now appears that the organism may infect humans over a much wider geographical range.[8,9] Worldwide *E. histolytica* prevalence data gathered from stool examinations for cysts during the last century are therefore misleading. However, mortality data from confirmed cases of invasive disease are likely to be reliable. Similarly, prevalence data based on serology remain valuable indicators of distribution because natural infections with noninvasive species of *Entamoeba* do not elicit an antibody response.[10]

Clinically it is clearly desirable, when symptoms such as bloody diarrhea or colitis are seen and amebae are present, that:

- we should be able to confirm the presence of the pathogen, *E. histolytica*, ideally by reliable specific tests; and
- in the absence of a confirmed *E. histolytica* infection, the true cause of the symptoms (e.g. shigellosis) should be found and treated, incidentally avoiding unnecessary chemotherapy for amebiasis.

Because the three species have only recently been differentiated, it is an epidemiologic priority to understand their worldwide distribution and fully evaluate their individual significance.[11]

DIAGNOSIS

Amebic colitis

Although diarrhea alone may be the presenting feature, amebic colitis, like shigellosis, classically presents with bloody diarrhea or dysentery; this should be differentiated from carcinoma, necrotizing colitis, cytomegalovirus (CMV) colitis (in AIDS), antibiotic-associated colitis and inflammatory bowel disease (misdiagnosis and corticosteroid treatment can be fatal here). Laboratory tests are essential for definitive diagnosis. Detection of specific antibody (IgG) in serologic tests can be extremely valuable for confirming invasive amebic disease of the colon or extraintestinal amebiasis.

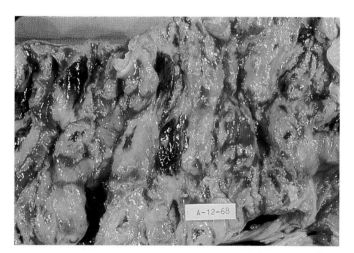

Fig. 110.1 Pathology specimen from a fatal case of human amebic colitis. Deep ulcerations into the submucosa have produced abundant hemorrhages. Courtesy of Dr Jesús Aguirre García, Hospital General de México, Secretaria de Salud.

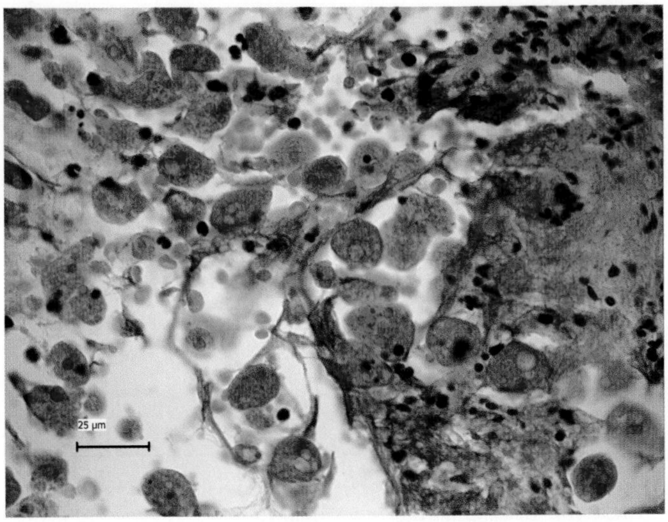

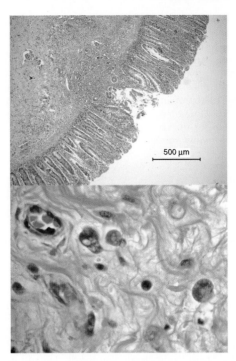

Fig. 110.2 Section through bleeding colonic ulcer showing *E. histolytica* trophozoites with ingested red blood cells in human colonic submucosa and undermined mucosa. Leukocytes from the cellular reaction are visible, and they show typically strongly stained nuclei and sparse cytoplasm. The technique is Ehrlich's alum hematoxylin with eosin, which stains erythrocytes well but does not clearly show the amebic nuclei. Courtesy of John Williams, LSHTM.

In classic fecal microscopy, nonpathogenic *Entamoeba* spp. such as *E. coli*, *E. hartmanni*, *E. polecki*-like amebae (including *E. chattoni*)[12] and also *Iodamoeba butschlii* and *Endolimax nana* can be distinguished from *E. histolytica*, *E. dispar* and *E. moshkovskii* by the size of cysts, nuclear number and/or nature of inclusions. Cysts of the last three species are all quadrinucleate and average 12 µm in diameter (10–20 µm). Morphology of the trophozoite is usable, since to find amebae which have ingested erythrocytes in fresh samples of mucoid or bloody mucoid stools, or in a rectal scrape/rectosigmoidoscopy sample from suspected amebic colitis (Fig. 110.2) is diagnostically highly predictive of *E. histolytica* infection.[13] However, the laboratory worker must be sufficiently skilled not to mistake erythrophagocytosis in human leukocytes with densely staining polymorphic or monocytic nuclei for the same process in the generally larger, vacuolated and motile amebic trophozoites, each with a poorly staining nucleus which is difficult to detect. When recognizable amebic trophozoites without ingested red blood cells are seen well away from bleeding areas, in advance of the main inflammatory response, it can also be strongly suggestive of invasive disease (Figs 110.3, 110.4). The nonmicroscopic molecular biologic technique of nested polymerase chain reaction (PCR) and the simpler, but still expensive, technique of specific *E. histolytica* antigen detection, which can both be carried out on stool samples, are recommended[14] in preference to microscopy. Buss *et al.*[15] found that the TechLab *E. histolytica* II antigen-detection test based on Eh-adherence lectin detected *E. histolytica* infections more accurately than another similarly based test. Antigen detection test kits are unfortunately not as sensitive as PCR.

Amebic liver abscess diagnostics

Amebic liver abscess is usually accompanied by right hypochondrial pain and tender liver. The diaphragm is often seen to be raised on chest X-ray. A neutrophil leucocytosis (>10 000) and a raised alkaline phosphatase may be detected (see Table 110.2). There is usually a space-occupying lesion in the liver on ultrasound and CT scan. If an aspirate is done, amebic trophozoites may be detected microscopically, by antigen detection or by PCR, in the atypical 'pus' (mainly necrotic liver parenchyma with few neutrophils or macrophages). Serology for antiamebic antibody, which is elevated in more than 90% of cases, is very helpful.[16]

Fig. 110.3 Small mucosal ulcer, with early submucosal spread. Deep in the submucosa, all we see suggestive of a cellular response is in lymphatic vessels, near the blue arrow which shows the position of the advancing front of invading amebae. In the detail of this area (below) no leakage of blood or obvious damage to tissues has taken place, and the amebae have ingested no red blood cells. The technique is Ehrlich's alum hematoxylin with eosin, which stains erythrocytes well but does not clearly show the amebic nuclei. Courtesy of John Williams, LSHTM.

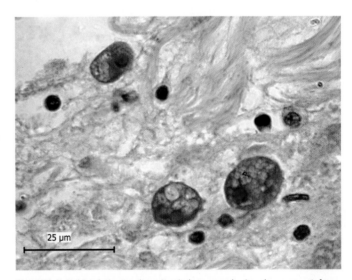

Fig. 110.4 *E. histolytica* trophozoites in human colonic submucosa. A few leukocytes from the cellular reaction, with heavily stained nuclei and sparse cytoplasm, are visible. Weigert's iron hematoxylin and eosin highlights the dark staining of a chromatin ring just inside the nuclear membrane in each ameba. The abundant cytoplasm contains vacuoles with host-cell material in the process of digestion. Courtesy of John Williams, LSHTM.

Differential diagnosis

Pyogenic abscess and neoplasm of the liver are commonly the alternative diagnoses. Pyogenic abscess is more common in older patients with a previous history of hepatobiliary or abdominal disease. The presenting features may be jaundice, pruritus and septic shock, with no hepatomegaly or elevated diaphragm in the chest X-ray, while amebic serology is negative. Needle aspiration allows microscopy and culture in such circumstances.

Where the patient is febrile and wasted and has vague abdominal discomfort, liver neoplasm is suspected. On CT scanning, the distinct image may be indicative, and blood samples may test positive for alpha-fetoprotein, carcinoembryonic antigen or other tumor markers.[16] Stool microscopy, antigen testing or PCR should be carried out, to search for the concomitant asymptomatic intestinal ameba infection commonly found in amebic liver abscess cases.

EPIDEMIOLOGY

Entamoeba histolytica (*sensu lato*) is one of the 10 most common intestinal infections in the world. Recent WHO[1] estimates give 48 million clinical cases per year, resulting in at least 70 000 deaths (mortality in clinical disease = 0.15%). Using recent advances in molecular genetics, the potentially pathogenic *E. histolytica* can be distinguished from the nonpathogenic similar species. This allows scrutiny of important and previously obscure pathogen–host interactions, and a number of studies from around the world are now available to provide a better understanding of the epidemiology of the disease (see website for further information).

Although invasive amebiasis is much less common in industrialized countries than in the developing world, it is still important to identify an *E. histolytica* infection there, as misdiagnosis can lead to death. Missed intestinal amebiasis, mistaken for chronic ulcerative colitis, may be treated disastrously with corticosteroids. Infection rates in immigrant groups can be significant, and outbreaks can occur in institutions such as schools or psychiatric hospitals where hygiene is compromised. A major increase in intestinal amebic infections reported in male homosexual populations in USA, Canada and England has mainly been asymptomatic, caused by the nonpathogenic *E. dispar*. In 136 suspected or confirmed HIV-positive inpatients in Tanzania, *E. histolytica*, *E. moshkovskii* and *E. dispar* were all detected without evidence of invasive amebic disease.[9] In Japan and Taiwan, however, invasive amebiasis due to *E. histolytica* is certainly found in groups of sexually active male homosexuals, though there is no evidence that symptoms are more serious in HIV.

PATHOGENESIS

Stanley,[17] Ackers & Mirelman[18] and Guo *et al.*[19] have recently reviewed amebiasis in general, and in particular the expanding scenario of pathogenesis and invasion.

The first stage in pathogenesis is the attachment of the trophozoite to the human target cell, erythrocyte, enterocyte or leukocyte which is made by a surface-located Eh-adherence lectin and is necessary for all subsequent changes. The adherence of the binding domain to target cells can be inhibited experimentally by D-galactose or N-acetyl D-galactosamine, and naturally by colonic mucin. This lectin, often termed 'Gal/GalNAc lectin' or 'Eh-adherence lectin' is also used by the amebae for binding bacteria prior to phagocytosis. The heavy subunit of the Eh-adherence lectin has a carbohydrate recognition domain (CRD) of 104 residues which is only 89% conserved in the homologous sequence expressed by nonpathogenic *E. dispar*.[20,21]

It is probable that Eh-adherence lectin responds to attachment by stimulating cytoskeletal changes in the ameba, associated with phagocytosis of the target cell and also the transfer of cysteine proteinases (EhCP-) and amebapores (EhAP-) from granules in the amebic cytoplasm to the membrane or external medium.

Subsequently, amebae produce a range of neutral cysteine proteinases[18] which are expressed on the cell membrane or are secreted to the exterior. They have the ability to break down matrix collagen, allowing the spread of amebae in the submucosa. Attracted (and activated) by interleukin 8 (IL-8) or other cytokines, neutrophils (and to a lesser extent macrophages) invade the mucosa and ease the entry of the amebae to the submucosa and deeper layers of the colonic wall.

The transcriptional framework of virulence[22]

Recent studies have shed considerable light on the molecular basis of virulence in amebiasis (see website for additional information), and now that the draft genome sequence of *E. histolytica* has been obtained[23] and is undergoing secondary editing, comparison with nonvirulent *E. histolytica* clones, *E. dispar* and *E. moshkovskii* is progressing. New regulatory genes,[24] retrotransposons and new attachment proteins are being discovered.

TRANSMISSION AND PREVENTION

Although the organism can infect other animals, there is effectively no reservoir of *E. histolytica* other than humans. All age groups are susceptible to infection with *E. histolytica*; persons with asymptomatic intestinal infection are most likely to be excreting cysts. Young children in particular are likely to infect their carers (mainly mothers and female relatives) and healthy infected adults (male or female) capable of work may be involved under relatively insanitary conditions in preparing food sold on the streets or in small retail outlets. In endemic areas poor education, poverty, overcrowding, inadequate washing facilities and shortage of uncontaminated water supplies for washing and drinking, together with poor sanitation, favor fecal–oral transmission.

When the fully developed and infective cysts are passed in the stools, they can be killed by desiccation. Cysts in fecal material die within 10 minutes on the surface of the hands, but can survive under (long) fingernails for 45 minutes. Conditions of high relative humidity will prolong these survival times. Although the cysts are killed by freezing, they may survive for more than 100 hours at 25°C in moist conditions or in water. Survival in water at low temperatures above freezing can be for at least 3 months, but above 50°C it is a matter of minutes. Pasteurization or brief boiling is sufficient to eliminate the possibility of transmission from milk or water. Residual concentrations of chlorine sufficient to eliminate bacterial contamination from drinking water supplies will not kill the cysts: 3 mg/l is needed for 30 minutes. Cysts may be removed from water by slow filtration through biologic sand filters or rapid sand filtration after flocculation.

Feachem *et al.*[25] classify *Entamoeba* spp. on the basis that the cysts are infective when passed, and they are resistant to stomach acid. Thus the direct fecal–oral route is probably more important than for geohelminths (where development to the infective stage generally needs to take place outside the body) and compared to bacteria the inoculum size can be small (<<100). Since the cysts are susceptible to desiccation their persistence in the environment is limited. When, eventually, uncontaminated water supplies for drinking and hand washing become available, and health education increases personal hygiene, the importance of the direct fecal–oral route would be expected to diminish together with the prevalence of infection. Risk factors for infection in endemic areas have been reported to be crowding, illiteracy, lack of safe drinking water and inadequate disposal of human waste. It appears that focusing on availability of suitable water supplies for drinking and hand washing, as well as health education, should be the priority, together with early diagnosis and treatment.[26]

Apart from the desirability of preventive treatment of asymptomatic persons in an endemic area,[27] there will be reservations over its practicality in view of the high re-infection rate. Recommendations for treatment of asymptomatic carriers in nonendemic areas do not usually include a tissue amebicide, which avoids major ethical objections on the grounds of side-effects. Two alternatives are available:[29] paromomycin 25–35 mg/kg q8h for 7–10 days, or diloxanide furoate (if available) 500 mg q8h for 10 days.

Some success has been achieved in the laboratory, using recombinant preparations of the Eh-adherence lectin to immunize experimental animals. However, the method will need much more development before it is ready for preventive trials in humans.

CLINICAL FEATURES

Amebic invasion more commonly remains localized in the colon but can metastasize via the portal vein to the liver and more rarely, by extension from a liver abscess into pleura, lungs and/or pericardium. The amebae invade the colonic mucosa through small punctures in the mucosal surface and spread laterally into the submucosa, producing typical flask-shaped ulcers (see Fig. 110.3). Extension may occur rarely from the colon to large abdominal vessels and other viscera including the urogenital system, or extremely rarely to the brain by hematogenous spread. Extension to the skin can take place through rupture of an untreated liver abscess or from a perforated colonic segment. Primary infection of the skin can also be acquired by direct contact with an infected subject during vaginal or anal intercourse.[16]

Intestinal amebiasis (Table 110.1)

The spectrum of invasive disease ranges in severity from mild diarrhea to life-threatening fulminating necrotic colitis (see Fig. 110.1) and perforation of the colon, which are the main causes of death in invasive intestinal amebiasis. Other complications include direct extension to the skin and dissemination, mainly to the liver (Figs 110.5, 110.6). Severe intestinal amebiasis is twice as frequent in adults as in children,[16,28] where it may be associated with undernourishment.

Usually an acute rectocolitis characterizes invasive intestinal disease. Most patients present with a nontoxic dysenteric syndrome (a 'walking dysentery') and general symptoms are not as prominent as in *Shigella* dysentery. The onset of acute rectocolitis is gradual and 85% of patients develop intense abdominal pain (Table 110.1).[16,28]

Initially there are loose watery stools, but these rapidly become blood-stained and contain mucus. Tenesmus associated with rectosigmoidal involvement occurs in 50% of patients. Watery diarrhea or loose stools without blood may be present for a few days, particularly if the distal colon is involved. Ameboma is an abnormal response,

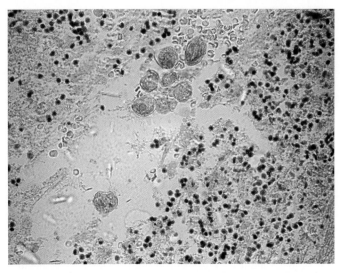

Fig. 110.6 Liver abscess section stained with Ehrlich's hematoxylin and eosin. Many dark-stained nuclei of necrotic liver cells are seen around the liquid content of the abscess. A group of amebic trophozoites is seen adjacent to an area of bleeding.

Table 110.1 Clinical features of acute amebic colitis	
Clinical feature	**Percentage of cases**
Symptoms for 0–1 week	48
2–4 weeks	37
>4 weeks	15
Diarrhea	100
Dysentery	99
Abdominal pain	85
Lower back pain	66
Fever	38
Abdominal tenderness	83
From Adams & McLeod.[30]	

probably to prolonged infection and manifesting as a marked granuloma, mimicking colon carcinoma, except in its rapid response to metronidazole. Usually there is a marked serologic antiamebic titer. With some symptoms resembling the toxic colon of nonspecific ulcerative colitis, invasive amebic colitis is an emergency which may progress to life-threatening fulminant colitis with perforation and development of amebic peritonitis, the most serious condition associated with invasive amebiasis of the intestine. This is apparently influenced by nutritional factors, age and susceptibility, and, probably, strain differences in virulence. Ulceration and necrosis can affect all layers of the colon wall; perforations can be multiple and can give rise to purulent peritonitis. In a series of 62 patients with fulminant amebic colitis seen by Guarner[31] from 1963 to 1970, 57.5% showed a single perforation, 28% multiple perforations and none were found in 14.5%.

When the luminal surface of the mucosa has been damaged, the amebae may undermine the mucosa to give more ulceration, producing abundant microhemorrhages. Normal mucosa can still be seen macroscopically between the sites of invasion. Ulcers are initially superficial, with hyperemic borders and a necrotic base (see Fig. 110.3). Progression of the lesions may result in a loss of mucosa and submucosa covering the muscle layers and lead to rupture of the serosa.

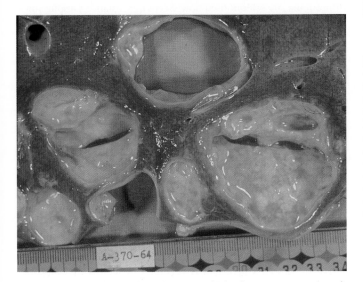

Fig. 110.5 Human amebic liver abscess. Multiple abscesses, one cavitated, can be observed occupying virtually all lobes of the liver parenchyma, which is replaced by a semisolid material. Courtesy of Dr Jesús Aguirre García, Hospital General de México, Secretaría de Salud.

Amebic liver abscess

Liver abscess is the most common extraintestinal form of invasive amebiasis, which may occur in all age groups, but is 10 times more frequent in adults, with three to five times as many cases seen in men.[16] Lesions are usually single and localized to the right lobe of the liver in the posterior, external and superior portions.[28]

Amebae probably spread from the intestine to the liver through the portal circulation. Although liver abscess develops after intestinal infection, patients rarely have associated amebic rectocolitis, but the large intestine is colonized with *E. histolytica* in more than 70% of cases.

In most patients, mainly those under 30 years of age and children,[16] the clinical presentation and course of the disease are typical (Table 110.2). The onset is abrupt, with pain in the upper abdomen and high fever. The pain is intense and constant, radiating to the scapular region and right shoulder; it increases with coughing, deep breathing or when the patient rests on the right side. When the abscess is located in the left lobe, the pain tends to be felt in the epigastrium and may radiate to the left shoulder. Fever is present in most cases; it varies between 100°F (38°C) and 104°F (40°C), frequently in spikes, but is sometimes constant over several days, with rigors and profuse sweating. There is anorexia and rapid weight loss and approximately one-third of patients have a nonproductive cough. Nausea and vomiting may occur and in some cases there may be diarrhea or dysentery. Physical examination reveals a pale wasted patient who has an enlarged tender liver. Digital pressure in the right lower intercostal spaces produces intense pain and there is often marked tenderness on percussion over the right lower ribs in the posterior region. Movement of the right side of the chest and diaphragm is greatly restricted, as is the intensity of respiratory sounds. Older patients may present with a chronic and milder nonspecific febrile illness, hepatomegaly, anemia and abnormal liver function tests.[16]

Table 110.2 Clinical features of amebic liver abscess

Clinical feature		Percentage of cases
Symptoms for	<2 weeks	37–66
	2–4 weeks	20–40
	4–12 weeks	16–42
	>12 weeks	5–11
Fever		71–98
Abdominal pain		62–98
Diarrhea/dysentery		14–66
Cough		10–32
Weight loss		33–53
Tender liver		80–95
Hepatomegaly		43–93
Epigastric tenderness		22
Rales, rhonchi		8–47
Jaundice		10–25
White cell count >10 000/mm³ (10 × 10⁹/1)		63–94
Elevated transaminases		26–50
Elevated alkaline phosphatase		38–84
Elevated bilirubin		10–25
Increased erythrocyte sedimentation rate		81
Based on Martínez-Palomo & Ruíz-Palacios G.[28]		

Complications

Amebic liver abscesses commonly produce thoracic complications, particularly pleurisy with a nonpurulent pleural effusion, rupture into the bronchial tree and, less commonly, rupture into the pleural cavity or amebic pericarditis. Rupture into the abdomen occurs in approximately 8% of patients who have amebic liver abscess; only rarely do abscesses rupture into the gallbladder, stomach, duodenum, colon or inferior vena cava. Occasionally, an abscess may erode through the abdominal wall and reach the skin. Secondary infection of amebic liver abscesses is an uncommon complication, which can be suspected when the patient presents with a severe toxic state and there is lack of response to antiamebic chemotherapy.[28] Although acute appendicitis is a common cause for emergency surgery, amebic appendicitis, even in Mexico City where amebic colitis is endemic, is a rare ocurrence (see website for further information).

MANAGEMENT

Because they are efficiently absorbed from the small intestine and reach high concentrations in the tissues, metronidazole and related 5-nitroimidazole compounds are the drugs of choice for treatment of invasive amebiasis. They are termed 'tissue amebicides'. Concentrations in the large intestinal content do not reach amebicidal levels, and only those trophozoites invading the mucosa and deeper tissues are affected. Since they do not prevent the production of infective cysts in the lumen, the tissue amebicides are often reported to be 'inactive against the cysts'. Actually, none of the available amebicides is active against the cysts themselves. The 5-nitroimidazoles have few negative features: adverse interactions are seen with alcohol (also warfarin and phenytoin) and they are known to be mutagenic against bacteria in the Ames test. Although cancer has been reported in mouse testing, no carcinogenic effects have been reported in humans. Although their effect on fetal development is unknown, it is recommended that, because of their ability to cross the placental barrier and rapidly enter the fetal circulation, they should be avoided in the first trimester and prescribed under strict supervision during the second and third trimesters. Similarly, because of secretion in breast milk, breast-feeding should be suspended if 5-nitroimidazoles are prescribed.

The tissue amebicides emetine hydrochloride and dehydroemetine (cardiovascular and gastrointestinal adverse effects), combined with chloroquine, are seldom used now except in resistance. Despite some isolated reports of failure in the treatment of amebic liver abscess with metronidazole, and even though *in-vitro* studies confirm that some established and long-cultivated isolates of the organism are indeed metronidazole resistant,[32] clinical metronidazole resistance is vanishingly rare.

Use of luminal amebicides after treatment with tissue amebicides for elimination of intestinal infection with *E. histolytica*

Since 5-nitroimidazole tissue amebicides are ineffective against the trophozoites in the colonic lumen, complete treatment for both intestinal and extraintestinal infection should be followed by a course of a luminal amebicide. Two alternatives are available[29] (see above): diloxanide furoate (if available) in adults, 500 mg orally q8h for 10 days, or paromomycin 25–35 mg/kg orally q8h for 7–10 days. Both these agents are poorly absorbed from the intestine and so reach optimal amebicidal concentrations within the intestinal lumen, without troublesome side-effects. Paromomycin is the usual choice, as the availability of diloxanide is patchy. These have also been recommended for the treatment of asymptomatic infections in food handlers and when infection control measures are being applied within families and close associates of infected persons. The use of these agents in asymptomatic persons is controversial in endemic areas, considering the high risk of re-infection. However, the approach, when operationally possible, appears to be ethical in view of the safety of these drugs.

Fulminant amebic colitis

Guarner[31] reports on a series of 47 patients with known or suspected perforation who had surgical treatment. Of 20 who received conservative surgery (i.e. without removal of part of the colon), 16 (80%) died (7 had colostomy, 6 ileostomy, 1 exteriorization of the affected segments, 5 suture of a single perforation and 1 surgical drainage). Where the treatment included resection (i.e. removal of a damaged part or whole of the colon), mortality was 56%. He stresses the importance of making an adequate evaluation of the magnitude of the colonic lesions, as well as the possibility of liver lesions: 'Surgery should be immediate and radical.' When the right colon is involved, right colectomy is indicated; when both sides are involved, total colectomy is indicated. In a total colectomy, ileostomy and suprapubic exteriorization of the rectal segment ought to be performed. Primary anastomosis is not advised; it is better to exteriorize. The patients should always be nursed in intensive care to allow maintenance of vascular tone and osmotic pressure, and to avoid respiratory problems. Antibacterial and antiamebic therapy should be instituted at an early preoperative stage, using a broad-spectrum antibiotic and 500 mg metronidazole intravenously q8h with intravenous fluid replacement. Guarner supports the use of high-dose corticosteroids if the patient enters a state of shock.[31]

Further advice on amebic peritonitis supporting the above surgical approach is given by Cook[33] who refers to case reviews by Shukla et al.[34] Gastric suction is recommended. Overall mortality may be over 50%, but resection of the necrotic area with exteriorization of both cut ends of the bowel allowed survival in six of nine cases.

Ameboma

This amebic granuloma often localizes in the ascending colon. Guarner[31] recommends the physician should make a precise clinical diagnosis and take a cautious attitude to surgical intervention in ameboma. He reports a series of 71 cases, 42 treated medically and 29 surgically. In the surgical group, 16 had exploratory laparotomy, 8 required hemicolectomy, and in 5 drainage of a concurrent amebic liver abscess was carried out. All of those medically treated were cured by chemotherapy, whereas there was 17% mortality in the surgical group. (Among these may, of course, have been the worst cases.)

Amebic liver abscess

Amebic liver abscess should be treated with chemotherapy; surgery is rarely indicated. It is not recommended to remove the 'pus' from an amebic liver abscess (as is often seen in pyogenic abscesses). Only 2% of amebic liver abscesses are reported to be contaminated with bacteria, and surgical intervention itself can be responsible. A marked reduction in amebic liver abscess mortality followed introduction of metronidazole and reduction in surgical intervention.[31] Aspiration of the abscess might be necessary in some cases where the abscess is more than 10 cm

in diameter and also when in the left liver lobe. Percutaneous drainage is usually sufficient and safer than the open surgical approach, which may be needed if the abscess is ruptured.[35] Surgery should be reserved for patients with a ruptured abscess, with bacterial superinfection or with abscesses that cannot be reached safely by the percutaneous route.

Since those who develop amebic liver abscess are usually carrying an asymptomatic intestinal infection of E. histolytica, the importance of elimination of intestinal carriage using luminal amebicides in addition to tissue amebicides has been emphasized, to prevent recurrence of the abscess, which occasionally does happen, and to protect the close associates of the patient from infection.

A prompt diagnosis and adequate chemotherapy will control most cases of liver abscess produced by E. histolytica. In general, a full clinical recovery and disappearance of the liver lesions (as confirmed by CT scanning) can be expected for uncomplicated cases. In 85% of cases liver imaging reveals resolution of amebic abscesses within 6 months of treatment; the remaining 15% of cases still show imaging defects 3 years after treatment.[28]

Percutaneous drainage

Indications for percutaneous drainage[31] of an amebic liver abscess are:

- imminent rupture of a large abscess;
- as a complementary therapy to shorten the course of the disease when the response to chemotherapy has been slow; and
- when pyogenic or mixed infection is suspected (e.g. persisting fever on treatment).

Drainage should be carried out under ultrasound or CT guidance. Catheters should *not* be left in for drainage and should be rapidly removed to avoid contaminating the track and skin.

Surgical drainage

Indications for surgical drainage[31] include:

- imminent rupture of an inaccessible liver abscess, especially of the left lobe;
- a risk of peritoneal leakage of necrotic fluid after aspiration;
- rupture of a liver abscess.

When surgical drainage is indicated in abscess of the left lobe, with the patient lying supine, a 5–10 cm incision on the midline will isolate the drainage point.

The study of Guarner[31] should be consulted in case of pleuropulmonary complications or amebic pericarditis. Similarly, for advice on extremely rare cases of hematogenously spread cerebral amebiasis, see also Guarner.[31]

REFERENCES

 References for this chapter can be found online at http://www.expertconsult.com

Diarrhea in a returned traveler from Mexico

DEFINITION OF THE PROBLEM

A 21-year-old woman returned from Mexico with diarrhea which had started 10 weeks previously while she was attending a summer course in Cuernavaca. The initial episode started abruptly with 5–10 bowel movements (BM) per day, accompanied by intestinal cramps, fever of 39°C and mild headache. The feces were watery at first, and then turned mushy. No blood was observed. She consulted a local physician who prescribed ciprofloxacin 500 mg twice daily for 3 days, which she took faithfully. The diarrhea improved, but remained at 3–5 BMs per day with mild cramps until she returned to the USA 2 weeks later, and then persisted for an additional 8 weeks, at which time she consulted another physician.

Her history revealed that she had been in good health without any bowel disorders. While in Mexico she ate at local restaurants for most lunches and dinners but carefully avoided fresh fruits and vegetables and drank only bottled water. Her only medication was a birth-control pill. Physical examination by her physician was unremarkable except for some mild periumbilical tenderness. Rectal examination and later colonoscopy were normal. Her laboratory values, including complete blood count and differential, liver function tests and hepatitis screens, were all negative. Stool examination on three occasions for bacterial pathogens (including *Clostridium difficile*) and for parasites were all negative.

She was treated with azithromycin, followed by metronidazole, without any change in her symptoms. She did gain some relief with loperamide. She was seen by a gastroenterologist at 3 months and then 6 months later. Many gastrointestinal studies, including small bowel radiographs and CT scan of the abdomen as well as repeats of the earlier studies were all negative. She continues to have 3–5 BMs per day without blood, mild abdominal pain, occasional constipation, but mostly mushy stools. Her weight has remained stable at 60 kg.

EPIDEMIOLOGY

Persistent diarrhea is a common occurrence in travelers returning from a journey to a high-risk area, such as Mexico, where up to 40–50% of visitors from North American are stricken with acute travelers' diarrhea.[1] When strict Rome criteria[2] are applied to make a diagnosis of what is now recognized as irritable bowel syndrome (IBS), a recent meta-analysis of eight studies found an incidence of 9.8% in persons with a history of acute infectious gastroenteritis compared to 1.2% in controls.[3] In two prospective studies specifically done in returning travelers,[4] the incidence of IBS was 10%[5] and 14%.[6] The diarrhea symptoms tend to predominate in the returning traveler with only occasional intervals of constipation (alternating cycles of diarrhea/constipation are more frequent in noninfectious IBS). Care in eating and drinking should be followed by travelers to high-risk areas, as practiced by our patient, since it may prevent serious illness; however, such virtue is not rewarded by avoidance of diarrhea, as has been shown in several studies.[1] She had a particularly severe and prolonged course of travelers' diarrhea in Mexico and this is known to increase the risk of IBS.[4]

IBS should be a diagnosis of exclusion in a returning traveler since it is based on clinical criteria without the support of any specific laboratory or imaging tests and many other causes must be considered (Table PP57.1). An alternative diagnosis in the returning traveler with diarrhea is a persistent intestinal pathogen, either bacterial or parasitic. (Viral pathogens do not tend to persist, except cytomegalovirus, which is rare in a normal host; fungal pathogens are also unlikely in a previously healthy person.) Among the bacteria, *Campylobacter*, *Salmonella* and *Shigella* can cause symptoms and continuing pathology for weeks and months until they are treated with an appropriate antibiotic. *Giardia* is arguably the most common cause of persistent diarrhea in a traveler.[7]

INVESTIGATIONS AND MANAGEMENT

Our patient underwent several stool examinations in expert laboratories and was also treated expectantly with metronidazole. *Entamoeba histolytica* is frequently diagnosed clinically but rarely present by

---

Table PP57.1 Causes of persistent diarrhea in a returning traveler

- Bacterial infection, which may be untreated or associated with an antibiotic-resistant strain, most commonly *Campylobacter*, *Shigella* or *Salmonella*
- Parasitic infection, especially *Giardia lamblia*, followed by *Cryptosporidium parvum*, *Cyclospora cayetanensis* or *Entamoeba histolytica*
- Acquired disaccharidase deficiency, especially lactase deficiency
- Postinfectious irritable bowel syndrome
- Inflammatory bowel disease, new onset of Crohn's disease or ulcerative colitis
- *Clostridium difficile* diarrhea or colitis
- Medication-associated diarrhea (e.g. magnesium, sorbitol, various antibiotics)
- Tropical sprue (also known as tropical malabsorption)
- Bowel carcinoma

laboratory testing – amebiasis has been called by Elsdon Dew, 'the refuge of the diagnostically destitute'. *Cryptosporidium* and *Cyclospora* were also excluded by stool examination. Acquired lactase deficiency is surprisingly common in returning travelers and it can be a permanent condition. It can be suspected in the first instance by relief upon avoidance of dairy products, and proven by a hydrogen breath test. Many patients with Crohn's disease or ulcerative colitis date the onset of their symptoms to an episode of acute gastroenteritis and these conditions must be ruled out by endoscopy and imaging studies.

Diarrhea and colitis caused by *C. difficile* have been reported in returning travelers who have been treated with antibiotics such as a fluoroquinolone. In one report, the symptoms persisted in five of six patients for 25–62 days before gaining relief.[8] Other drugs, herbs and micronutrients (e.g. magnesium) have been implicated in persistent diarrhea. Tropical sprue (also known as tropical malabsorption) has been diagnosed in returning travelers, usually those on long journeys or expatriates. Weight loss is a common finding and the condition is associated with laboratory studies showing malabsorption of fat, carbohydrates and/or vitamin B12. A final consideration is an occult bowel cancer.

In our patient the other diagnoses were excluded and the clinical picture fitted the persistent diarrhea form of IBS. Continued symptoms for more than 6 months and even for years has been reported in other forms of postinfectious IBS,[9] including IBS following *Salmonella* gastroenteritis.[10] While some relief is gained with loperamide and similar drugs, the long-term prognosis for persistence of grinding diarrhea remains grim.

REFERENCES

References for this chapter can be found online at http://www.expertconsult.com

Amebic cysts in the stool

INTRODUCTION

Amebiasis is considered by the World Health Organization as one of the top three causes of mortality from parasitic disease with estimates of 40 000–100 000 deaths per year. Approximately 10% of the world's population is thought to be infected and although occasional cases in animals have been recorded, humans are thought to be the definitive host. The causative agent is the protozoan parasite *Entamoeba histolytica* and it presents as either amebic colitis or amebic abscess. It is most commonly spread via fecal–oral means through the contamination of food and water sources with infectious cysts from human feces. Less developed regions with poor sanitation and hygiene have a high prevalence of amebic illness. Person-to-person spread within families and amongst other household contacts is also well documented. Transmission between men who have sex with men (MSM) is increasingly recognized, but is still a minor route of infection worldwide. This condition should also not be forgotten in the returning traveler who has visited an endemic area.

Other amebae present in the stool that are considered nonpathogenic include *Entamoeba dispar, Entamoeba coli, Entamoeba hartmanni, Iodamoeba butschlii* and *Endolimax nana*. It is now commonly recognized that the majority of people with detectable *Entamoeba* are colonized with *E. dispar* which is nonpathogenic and nondisease causing, even in the most immunocompromised patients with AIDS.[1] These organisms in the stool are, however, a marker that the patient has come into contact with water or food contaminated with human feces.

PATHOGENESIS

Entamoeba histolytica exists in two stages within the human host, the ameboid trophozoite and the infectious cyst. The conditions that cause the transition from one form to the other are poorly understood. Once the cysts are ingested by the host they are protected from gastric acid degradation by the cyst wall. They then pass through the small intestine and excyst in the colon into the trophozoite stage where they multiply by binary fission. Trophozoites are motile, engulfing bacteria and food particles, and can potentially invade the host gut mucosal wall using a combination of proteolytic, phagocytic and cytolytic properties, disrupting tight junctions causing changes in permeability, and ultimately resulting in host cell apoptosis.[2] The trophozoites can exit via the stool and although they can be seen occasionally, they do not survive outside the body. More typically they encyst within the colon and are excreted in large numbers in host feces.

CLINICAL FEATURES

Many *E. histolytica* infections are asymptomatic or self-limiting. The incubation period is thought to be a minimum of 7–10 days after cyst ingestion, although it can extend longer than that. The acute intestinal form of infection results in a diarrheal illness (often but not always with blood and mucus) and an acute proctocolitis, with inflamed, edematous mucosa and numerous discrete flask-shaped ulcers which develop as the disease progresses. These are often separated by normal tissue and the findings are not grossly dissimilar to the appearance of inflammatory bowel disease. Typically there is also associated abdominal tenderness and colicky pain. If the infection is prolonged and severe, peritonitis, intussusception and hemorrhage may occur. Fever and an associated leukocytosis are more commonly seen in a more fulminant course of the infection, which, although rare, is sometimes associated with severe malnutrition and in those who are immunocompromised or on steroid treatment. It manifests as areas of confluent ulceration and colonic necrosis and has a significant associated mortality. Chronic intestinal sequelae include colonic stricture and post-amebic colitis.

Amebic infection can also become invasive either through direct invasion through the gut wall or via hematogenous spread. Breaches in the gut mucosal surface and spread through the portal circulation can result in the formation of a liver abscess. They commonly present with fever, right upper quadrant pain, rarely with jaundice and if left untreated can discharge through the skin, rupture into the peritoneum or extend through the diaphragm. Approximately 20% of cases have a history of dysentery and 10% have a history of diarrhea at presentation. Abscesses have also been identified in both the lung and brain, although these are much rarer.

DIAGNOSIS OF CYST TYPE

The diagnosis of amebic dysentery and amebic liver abscess is discussed in Chapter 110. This practice point deals only with the detection of amebic cysts (Fig. PP58.1). Light microscopy of fecal specimens remains the traditional mainstay of amebic cyst diagnosis, but has the limitation of being unable to differentiate between *E. histolytica* and the nonpathogenic *E. dispar*, the cysts of which are morphologically identical. The importance of identifying pathogenic species is clear as there is both a requirement to minimize unnecessary treatment and a need to delineate the epidemiology. The cysts of nonpathogenic amebae other than *E. dispar* can be distinguished by their size and morphology.

E. histolytica/E. dispar cysts are typically round, approximately 10–15 µm in diameter and have four nuclei, each with a central karyosome, when mature (Fig. PP58.2). A trichrome stain is required to

A key to the identification of amebic and flagellate cysts

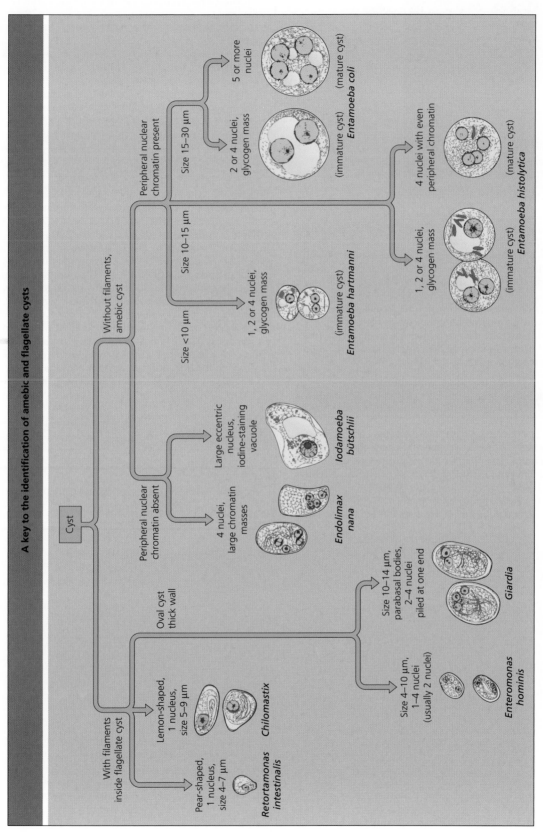

Fig. PP58.1 A key to the identification of amebic and flagellate cysts. (Courtesy of WHO – http://whqlibdoc.who.int/publications/9241544104_(part 2).pdf.)

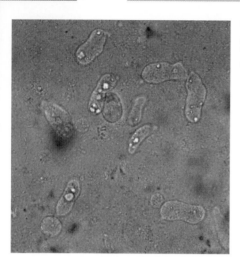

Fig. PP58.2
Entamoeba histolytica trophozoites in culture.

Essential points

- *Entamoeba histolytica* is the most significant amebic cyst in the stool
- Microscopy does not differentiate between *E. histolytica* and *E. dispar*
- ELISA stool antigen detection tests or PCR are needed to separate *E. histolytica* from *E. dispar*
- *E. dispar* cysts do not need treatment
- Metronidazole or tinidazole (used to treat amebic dysentery and abscess) do not kill luminal forms of *E. histolytica* reliably
- The agent of choice for *E. histolytica* cyst passage is diloxanide furoate. Alternatives are paromomycin or nitazoxanide

demonstrate detailed nuclear morphology which shows fine peripheral chromatin and a central karyosome.

Many diagnostic laboratories now use a commercially available enzyme-linked immunosorbent assay (ELISA) stool antigen detection method (to detect galactose adhesin) to differentiate *E. histolytica* from *E. dispar*.

More recently, polymerase chain reaction (PCR) assays have reportedly shown improved sensitivity and specificity over other methods of cyst detection,[3] although the data are somewhat conflicting between different centers.[4] Currently many of these molecular assays are only performed in reference laboratories.

MANAGEMENT

The presence of *E. histolytica* cysts in the stool does not necessarily indicate the presence of amebic dysentery, for which the presence of trophozoites is required (see Chapter 110). Furthermore, the absence of intestinal cysts does not exclude a diagnosis of amebic dysentery or amebic liver abscess. *Entamoeba histolytica* is detected in the stools of patients with amebic liver abscess less than 50% of the time using light microscopy, although in studies this rises to 75% if the stool is cultured.[5]

Asymptomatic cyst passers of *E. histolytica* can be treated with diloxanide furoate 500 mg q8h for 10 days for adults and 20 mg/kg for children in three divided doses. An alternative is paromomycin 25–30 mg/kg/day in three divided doses for 7 days. A new agent available for luminal use is nitazoxanide 500 mg q12h for 3 days.[6] The decision whether or not to treat asymptomatic carriage with *E. histolytica*/*E. dispar* partly depends on whether or not the person lives in an endemic area and is likely to become re-infected fairly quickly. Consideration also needs to be given to the cost which may outweigh any benefit to the individual, given that many cases of *E. histolytica*/*E. dispar* infection are in fact *E. dispar* which would lead to unnecessary drug administration. However, elimination of cyst passage is clearly indicated following treatment for amebic dysentery or amebic liver abscess where failure to eradicate the intestinal phase of the infection can lead to relapse.

Treatment of amebic dysentery and amebic abscess are discussed in Chapter 110.

REFERENCES

References for this chapter can be found online at http://www.expertconsult.com

Malaria

INTRODUCTION

Malaria is a parasitic disease caused by the coccidian protozoa of the genus *Plasmodium*, and transmitted by *Anopheles* spp. Human malaria can be caused by *Plasmodium falciparum*, *P. ovale*, *P. vivax* and *P. malariae* (Fig. 111.1), but clusters of malaria caused by *P. knowlesi* jumping species from long-tailed macaque monkeys to men have been described in South East Asia.[1] The life cycle of the parasite is summarized in Figure 111.2. Although it is increasingly recognized that *P. vivax* is able to cause severe disease in humans, including severe anemia, pulmonary edema, hemoglobinuria and rarely coma,[2] the vast majority of severe disease is caused by *P. falciparum*, resulting in 1–2 million deaths per annum. The majority (>90%) of these casualties are children in sub-Saharan Africa, where transmission intensity is high. The total burden of malaria disease, however, is similar in Asia, where transmission is low, but the population size much larger.

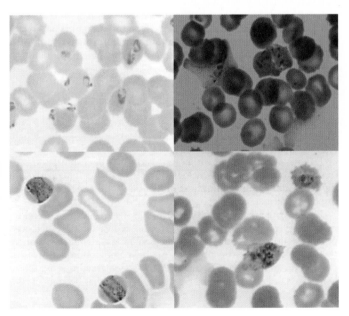

Fig. 111.1 Asexual stages of (clockwise, starting left upper corner) *Plasmodium falciparum*, *P. vivax*, *P. ovale* and *P. malariae*. Courtesy of Dr Kesinee Chotivanich.

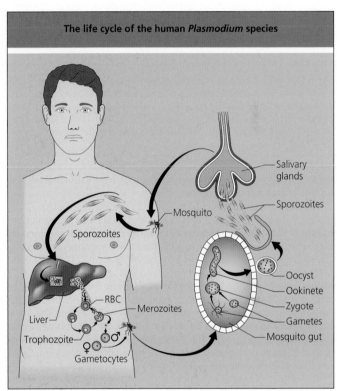

The life cycle of the human *Plasmodium* species

Fig. 111.2 The life cycle of the human *Plasmodium* species. Adapted from White NJ. Antimalarial drug resistance. J Clin Invest 2004;113:1084–92.

EPIDEMIOLOGY

Geographic distribution

Malaria control efforts during the last century eliminated malaria from North America, Europe and Russia, but it has remained a major problem throughout the tropics. At the end of the 20th century, with increasing problems of antimalarial drug and insecticide resistance, childhood mortality caused by malaria was on the increase. However, at the beginning of this millennium a surge in efforts towards malaria control, including the wide distribution of impregnated bed nets and

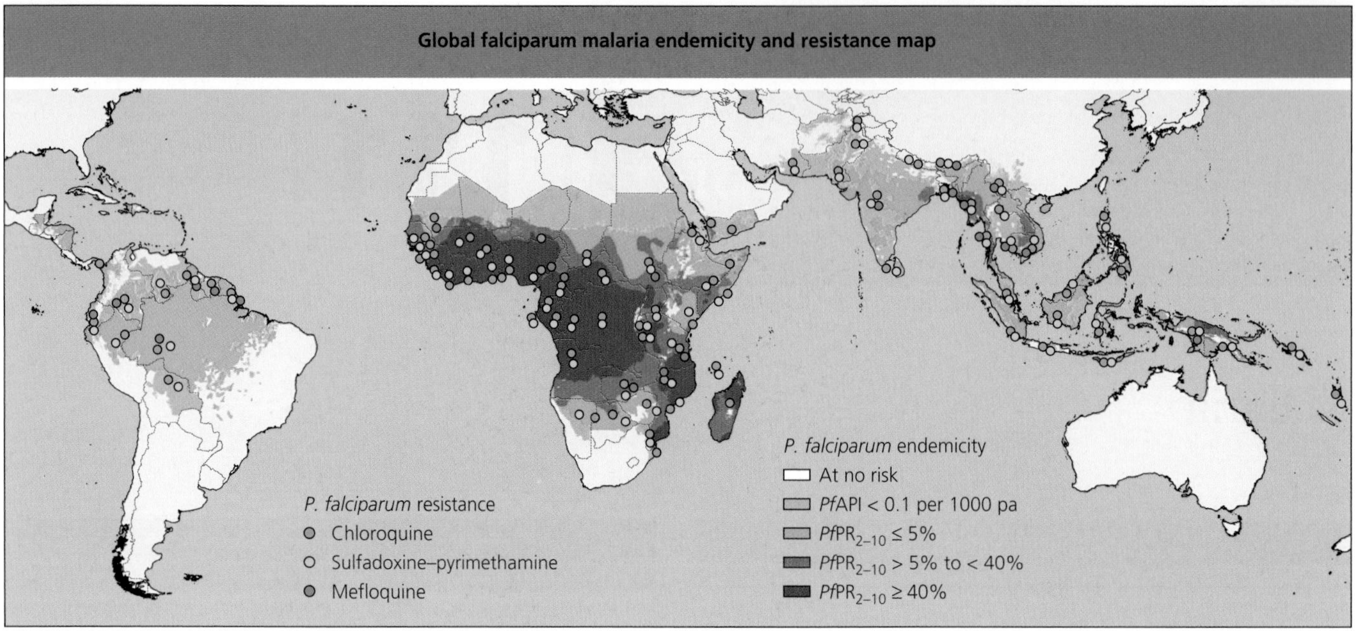

Fig. 111.3 Global falciparum malaria endemicity and resistance map. Endemicity data were compiled using both prevalence data and climatologic information. The spatial distribution of *P. falciparum* malaria prevalence rates, age standardized to 2–10 years (*Pf*PR$_{2-10}$) are categorized as low risk *Pf*PR$_{2-10}$ ≤5%, light red; intermediate risk *Pf*PR$_{2-10}$ >5% to <40%, medium red; and high risk *Pf*PR$_{2-10}$ ≥40%, dark red. The rest of the land area was defined as unstable risk (medium gray areas, where *Pf*API <0.1 per 1000 pa) or no risk (light gray). From Hay *et al*.[4] Data on resistance are from the WHO.[5] Mefloquine resistance data outside South East Asia are currently under review.

the deployment of effective treatment with artemisinin-based combination therapy, has started to reduce malaria-attributable mortality in several African and Asian countries.[3]

Measuring the malaria burden of disease is difficult. Modern epidemiologic methods estimate malaria incidence and its distribution from a combination of case-incidence data and parasite prevalence, medical intelligence and the use of plausible biologic constraints for malaria transmission by the *Anopheles* vector based on temperature data and information on vegetation and population[4] (Fig. 111.3). In 2007, 2.37 billion people lived in areas at risk for *P. falciparum* transmission. In large parts of sub-Saharan Africa transmission is moderate to high, with *P. falciparum* malaria prevalence rates above 50%, and the number of infectious mosquito bites (expressed as the entomologic inoculation rate or EIR) ranging between 10 and 1000 per year. Outside Africa, *P. falciparum* malaria prevalence is largely hypoendemic, with less than 10% parasite rates, corresponding to an EIR of <1 per year.

In Asia *P. vivax* malaria is responsible for approximately 50% of the total malaria prevalence, and is also common in Central and South America, North Africa and the Middle East. Mixed infection with *P. falciparum* is common in South East Asia. *P. vivax* is rare in West Africa, where the majority of people lack the erythrocyte surface Duffy-antigen/chemokine receptor (Duffy blood group negative), which is required for red cell invasion. The prevalence of malaria caused by *P. ovale* (mainly West Africa and Asia) and *P. malariae* is always much lower than the other species. Mixed infection with *P. falciparum* occurs frequently.

With modern air travel, individuals with malaria can be rapidly transported within hours to any part of the world, and malaria is a common imported infection occurring in travelers (import malaria). Occasionally airplanes carry infected mosquitoes, which can give unexpected infections in the neighborhood of airports in nonendemic countries (airport malaria). Malaria can also be transmitted by blood and blood products (transfusion malaria).

Epidemiologic factors

Malaria epidemiology depends upon a complex interplay between the vector (female *Anopheles* mosquitoes), the host (humans) and the malaria parasite. Malaria transmission does not occur at temperatures below 61°F (16°C) or above 91°F (33°C) ambient temperature, and at altitudes above 2000 m of sea level, because sporogony (the development of the sporozoite in the mosquito) cannot take place. Longevity of the vector, which is climate dependent, has to be at least a week, since after the sexual forms of the parasite (gametocytes) are engulfed during a blood meal, sporogony takes 6–12 days (shorter at higher temperatures). Of the over 400 species of *Anopheles*, only 80 of these can transmit malaria, and approximately 45 are considered important vectors. Each vector has its own behavior and blood-feeding patterns, although most bites occur in the evening, at night or in the early morning. For example *Anopheles gambiae*, an important malaria vector in Africa, feeds mainly on humans (anthropophilic), bites mainly after 23:00 hours and mostly indoors (endophagic) where it also tends to rest (endophilic).

Seasonal rainfall dramatically increases the breeding of mosquitoes. Depending on the *Anopheles* species, larvae spend most of their time at the surface of fresh water and salt water marshes (mal-aria means 'bad air'), mangrove swamps, grassy ditches, rice fields, puddles or other water collections, like discarded car tires. In the human host a subpopulation of gametocytes appears after a series of asexual cycles in *P. falciparum*, but earlier in *P. vivax*, another important factor in malaria transmission. Gametocyte density is higher in patients with high parasitemia, in nonimmune individuals (children) and with the use of an antimalarial drug in the presence of drug resistance.

Certain genetic hemoglobinopathies protect against the development of severe falciparum malaria. This has led to a state of 'balanced polymorphism' in populations living in malaria endemic areas, where the disadvantage of the presence of the hemoglobinopathy, especially in the homozygotes, is balanced by the malaria protective effect, which is mainly evident in the heterozygotes. This has been most convincingly shown for sickle cell disease, thalassemia and Melanesian ovalocytosis.

Where malaria prospers, human societies prosper the least, and there is a striking correlation between malaria and poverty. The effects of malaria are felt on diverse areas including fertility, population growth, savings and investments, worker productivity, medical costs, absenteeism, subtle developmental retardation in children and premature mortality.

PATHOGENESIS AND PATHOLOGY

The parasite

The sporozoite form of the parasite is injected into the host when the female *Anopheles* mosquito is probing for a blood meal. After inoculation the parasite hides and replicates in the liver for 5–7 days in *P. falciparum*, after which between 10^5 and 10^6 merozoites are released into the bloodstream. In malaria caused by *P. vivax* and *P. ovale*, but not *P. falciparum*, some parasites stay behind in the liver; these hypnozoites can cause a relapse of the disease long after treatment of the blood stage infection. The merozoites quickly invade circulating erythrocytes, where the erythrocytic cycle of the parasite begins. The parasite matures from a small ring form to the pigment-containing trophozoite, and develops into the mature schizont after division of the nucleus. In *P. falciparum* after 48 hours the erythrocyte ruptures and 6–36 merozoites are released, which will invade passing erythrocytes (Fig. 111.4). In *P. vivax* and *P. ovale* infections this cycle also takes 48 hours, whereas it takes 72 hours in *P. malariae*. There is then a massive expansion of the infection in the human host, with a multiplication factor of around 8 to 10, but sometimes up to 20, per new generation, as observed in early studies with *P. falciparum* as a treatment for syphilis. About 12–13 days after inoculation the parasite number has increased from about 10 parasites to between 10^8 and 10^{10} parasites, and the patient starts to have fever. In the nonimmune patient the disease can quickly progress into severe disease if the infection is not treated, with an increase in the total number of parasites in the body up to 10^{12} to 10^{13}.[6]

Cytoadherence

Plasmodium falciparum is the human *Plasmodium* species responsible for the vast majority of severe disease and is also the only species that induces cytoadherence to vascular endothelium of erythrocytes containing the mature forms of the parasite. As the parasite matures, parasite proteins are transported and inserted into the erythrocyte membrane. The high molecular transmembrane protein *P. falciparum* erythrocyte membrane protein 1 or *Pf*EMP1 is the most important ligand for cytoadherence.[7] Cytoadhesion begins at approximately 12 hours of parasite development, 50% of the maximum effect is obtained at 14–16 hours, and adherence is highly effective in the second half of the parasite life cycle.[8] As a result, late stages of the parasite are only sparsely detected in a peripheral blood slide, and when they do appear in significant numbers (>20% of the total parasites) this is a poor prognostic sign representing a large sequestered parasite load.[9]

*Pf*EMP1 is encoded by the highly variable *VAR* gene family, comprising around 60 genes. The high switch rate between these genes gives rise to a new variant *Pf*EMP1 in 2% of the parasites every new cycle, and this clonal antigenic variation helps the parasite escaping the immune system.[10] *Pf*EMP1 is expressed on the surface of 'knobs', which can be identified by electron microscopy as protrusions from the erythrocyte membrane acting as points of attachment to the vascular endothelium (Fig. 111.5). Other surface proteins that might play a role in cytoadherence are sequestrin, rifin and surfin. On the vascular endothelium numerous receptors that can bind *Pf*EMP1 have been

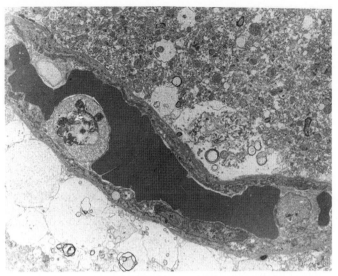

Fig. 111.5 Microcirculatory obstruction in falciparum shown in a post-mortem needle specimen from a fatal case of adult severe malaria. The capillary lumen is reduced by the rigid sequestered erythrocyte containing the mature parasite. Rigid uninfected cells will be hampered in squeezing through the narrowed lumen that remains. Adhesive forces between infected and uninfected red blood cells (rosetting) and between adjacent infected red blood cells (autoagglutination) could further reduce microcirculatory flow. Courtesy of Dr Emsri Pongponrat. Reproduced with permission from Dondorp AM, Pongponrat E, White NJ. Reduced microcirculatory flow in severe falciparum malaria: pathophysiology and electron-microscopic pathology. Acta Trop 2004;89(3):309–17.

identified, with different distributions in various organs and different contributions to rolling, tethering and finally stable binding of the parasitized erythrocyte. Of these, only CD36, which is constitutionally expressed on most vascular beds but remarkably absent in brain vessels, and chondroitin sulfate A (CSA), the main receptor in the placenta, are able to support firm adhesion under flow conditions.[11] The intercellular adhesion molecule 1 (ICAM-1) is the most important receptor on brain endothelium, and its expression is upregulated by the proinflammatory cytokine tumor necrosis factor (TNF).

Recently it has been suggested that platelets, which express CD36, might serve as a sticky bridge between infected erythrocytes and the endothelium, which could be particularly important in the brain microvasculature lacking CD36.[12] (11). Sequestration of parasitized erythrocytes in capillaries and post-capillary venules causes heterogenic blockage of the microcirculation, which can be demonstrated in living patients by video microscopy[13] and is the cause of retinal bleaching on ophthalmoscopy.[14] Sequestration is not distributed equally throughout the body and is greatest in the brain; however, it is also prominent in the heart, eyes, liver, kidneys, intestines and adipose tissue.[15] Autopsy studies have found that patients dying from cerebral malaria have more prominent sequestration in the brain microvasculature compared to severe but noncomatose fatal cases.[16,17] Autopsy studies

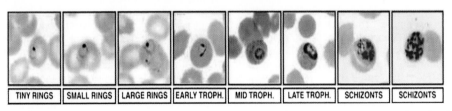

| TINY RINGS | SMALL RINGS | LARGE RINGS | EARLY TROPH. | MID TROPH. | LATE TROPH. | SCHIZONTS | SCHIZONTS |

Fig. 111.4 Developmental stages of *Plasmodium falciparum* during the 48-hour asexual life cycle. Mature stages, trophozoites (troph.) and schizonts efficiently adhere to the endothelial lining in the microcirculation, so that these stages are rarely seen in the peripheral blood. If present in the peripheral blood, this denotes a large parasite biomass, associated with severe disease. Courtesy of Dr Kamolrat Silamut.

in children dying from cerebral malaria in Malawi describe, in addition to erythrocyte sequestration, intravascular accumulation of platelets, as well as mononuclear leukocytes and fibrin deposition.[18]

Red cell deformability, rosetting and autoagglutination

Sequestration of parasitized erythrocytes will compromise the microcirculation in vital organs. In addition, the deformability of both parasitized and uninfected erythrocytes is markedly reduced in severe malaria.[19] Acting synergistically with the reduction in lumen caused by sequestration, rigid erythrocytes presumably further reduce blood flow in the microcirculation of vital organs, causing dysoxia with lactic acidosis, organ dysfunction and death. Lactic acidosis is a strong and reproducible predictor for death in falciparum malaria, both in children and adults.[20] In addition, formation of erythrocyte clumps through rosetting and autoagglutination could further compromise flow. Rosette formation is the in-vitro phenomenon in which uninfected red blood cells adhere to erythrocytes containing the mature forms of the parasite. However, whereas all erythrocytes containing the mature parasite cytoadhere, not all rosette. Rosette-forming strains are associated with severe disease,[21] although other studies have not found this association[22] and their pathophysiologic role is not clearly established.

Autoagglutination is the aggregation of parasitized red blood cells, which is mediated via platelet CD36. Presence of this phenotype has been associated with disease severity in both Kenya and Thailand.[23] In general, hemodynamic shock is not a contributor to microcirculatory failure until very late in the disease (<10%). Cerebral blood flow in larger vessels is not decreased in cerebral malaria.[24] Axonal accumulation of β-amyloid precursor protein as a measure of impaired axonal transport observed in autopsy studies may represent a final common pathway leading to, in essence, reversible neurologic dysfunction in cerebral malaria. Whether focal dysoxia is the cause of this axonal dysfunction has not been established.

Permeability and intracranial pressure

There is a mild generalized increase in systemic vascular permeability in severe malaria, but the blood brain barrier (BBB) in adults with cerebral malaria is functionally grossly intact.[25] Studies in African children with cerebral malaria do show a subtle increase in BBB permeability with a disruption of endothelial intercellular tight junctions. Imaging studies reveal that most adults with cerebral malaria have no cerebral edema. In African children cerebral edema is a more frequent, although not a consistent finding. Similarly, opening pressures on lumbar puncture are usually normal in adult patients, but are elevated in over 80% of children with cerebral malaria.[26]

There is only one published controlled trial evaluating the use of mannitol in pediatric cerebral malaria, which did not show a beneficial effect.[27] Additionally, raised intracranial pressure in children is more likely a feature developing in the later stages of cerebral malaria, rather than a primary cause for coma.

Immunologic factors and cytokines

Despite the enormous intravascular antigenic load in malaria, with the formation and deposition of immune complexes and variable complement depletion, there is little evidence of a specific immunopathologic process in severe malaria. As in other severe infections, blood concentrations of proinflammatory cytokines like TNF, interleukin (IL)-1, interferon gamma (IFN-γ), IL-6 and IL-18 are raised, as well as anti-inflammatory Th2 cytokines (IL-4, IL-10), but there is an imbalance in patients with a fatal course of the disease.[28]

A potent stimulator inducing proinflammatory cytokine production by leukocytes is the glycosylphosphatidylinositol (GPI) anchor of *P. falciparum*. GPI stimulates the production of TNF and possibly also the lymphokine 'lymphotoxin'. Both cytokines can upregulate the expression of ICAM-1 and vascular cell adhesion molecule 1 (VCAM-1) on endothelium cells, and could thus promote sequestration of parasitized erythrocytes in the brain, contributing to coma. High plasma concentrations of TNF in patients with falciparum malaria correlate with disease severity, including coma, hypoglycemia, hyperparasitemia and death. However, a trial using monoclonal antibodies against TNF did not show a beneficial effect on either mortality or coma duration, but was associated with a significant increase in neurologic sequelae.[29] Moreover, concentrations of TNF are also high in paroxysms of uncomplicated vivax malaria.

Further downstream in the cytokine cascade, nitric oxide (NO) production is increased via inducible NO synthase (iNOS), and iNOS expression is increased in the brain in fatal cerebral malaria. NO has been proposed as a cause for coma through interference with neurotransmission, but more recent studies have shown reduced levels of NO and its precursor, L-arginine, in severe malaria, related to endothelial dysfunction in these patients.[30] With our present knowledge proinflammatory cytokines seem to be related to overall disease severity, and are clearly involved in the pathogenesis of fever and possibly other complications like dyserythropoiesis, adult respiratory distress syndrome (ARDS), renal failure and hypoglycemia, but not in the pathogenesis of coma per se. Other researchers in the field contest this view.[31]

PREVENTION AND MALARIA CONTROL

Malaria prevention and control have three principal components:
- reduction of contact between vector and human host;
- prevention of disease through prophylactic use of antimalarial drugs; and
- adequate treatment (described below) of malaria episodes to minimize the risk for transmission.

Currently no vaccines to protect against malaria are licensed but promising candidates are in development (see below).

Minimizing contact between vector and human host

The affluent traveler has a range of effective options to prevent mosquito bites, which include screened windows, air conditioning, protective clothing and insect repellents (e.g. DEET). Few of these are permanently available to the majority of residents in malaria endemic regions who depend on indoor residual insecticide spraying (IRS) and bed nets impregnated with insecticides (ITNs) to prevent mosquito bites. IRS is highly effective as long as vectors remain susceptible and insecticides are funded and delivered, neither of which has been the case in sub-Saharan Africa. Sophisticated IRS programs rotate insecticides which usually include pyrethroids and dichlorodiphenyltrichloroethane (DDT) to minimize the emergence of resistance. IRS can be highly effective[32] but has not been sustainable and has therefore mixed popularity among malaria control experts. Despite these concerns the current wave to support for malaria control programs has led to a renaissance of IRS programs in sub-Saharan Africa.

A second approach to prevent mosquito bites is the use of insecticide-impregnated bed nets. A series of randomized trials have clearly demonstrated the high effectiveness of ITNs, and wide scale introduction has importantly contributed to a decrease in malaria transmission in many African countries. Bed nets requiring regular dipping in insecticide solutions are now being replaced by 'long-lasting insecticidal nets', which remain effective for extended periods (years). Delivery of these nets through social marketing has been advocated, but increasingly experts think that free distribution of nets is needed to show impact.[33] Efficacy of bed nets will depend on the timing of biting of the predominant Anopheles vector, since ITNs can only protect as long as the individual is covered by the bed net.

Prevention of disease through prophylactic use of antimalarial drugs

Travelers visiting malaria endemic countries are recommended to take prophylactic antimalarial drugs. The choice of drug will depend on pharmacokinetic/dynamic properties, safety profiles and the prevailing drug resistance patterns in the area. Since these patterns change over time, the recommendations in Table 111.1 can only serve as a guideline. For people living in malaria endemic countries, targeted prophylactic use of antimalarial drugs, rather than widespread drug administration, has recently gained popularity as a measure for malaria control in the form of intermittent presumptive treatment (IPT). IPT targets two populations at high risk for malaria attacks: infants (IPTi) and pregnant women (IPTp). The experience of IPT is mostly based on use of sulfadoxine–pyrimethamine (S/P) in sub-Saharan Africa, which is increasingly losing its efficacy on the continent.[34] As widespread use of S/P is likely to accelerate the emergence of S/P resistance, the balance between benefit and risk of adverse effects becomes more important. Trials using drugs other than S/P are currently in progress.[35]

Vaccine development

Despite the accepted need and great promises of a vaccine that can protect against malaria there is still no malaria vaccine licensed. *Plasmodium falciparum* is genetically complex and antigenic surface proteins are highly variable. Yet protective immunity can be obtained with age in populations residing in malaria endemic areas. Immunoglobulin purified from the blood of immune adults from endemic regions can passively transfer protection against *P. falciparum*,[36] but cell-mediated immunity is thought to also play an important role.

The current most promising vaccine candidate is known as RTS,S, a recombinant protein pre-erythrocytic stage vaccine, based on *P. falciparum* circumsporozoite antigen. RTS,S, combined with the ASO1E adjuvant, has an adjusted vaccine efficacy of 53% (95% CI 28–69) against developing clinical malaria in children aged 5–17 months during a mean duration of 8 months follow-up. In addition, early phase trials with vectored vaccines aiming at liver stage parasites are currently underway.[37] Vaccinations with irradiated sporozoites have been shown to be highly protective. Producing irradiated sporozoites in sufficient quantities, which have to be isolated from infected mosquitoes, is a daunting challenge. However, the persistence of the developers and the increased availability of funds for malaria vaccines have resulted in plans for clinical trials with this candidate vaccine in the near future.[38]

A malaria vaccine cannot replace other malaria control efforts since no malaria vaccine candidate will be 100% protective or provide lifelong protection. No malaria vaccine on its own can reduce transmission sufficiently to eliminate malaria. However, the addition of a vaccine to other tools for malaria control has the potential to drive malaria transmission to very low levels, even in high transmission areas.

CLINICAL FEATURES

The clinical manifestations of malaria are critically dependent on the immune status of the host. In areas of stable high transmission (sub-Saharan Africa) severe falciparum malaria occurs predominantly between 6 months and 3 years of age; mild symptoms are seen in older children, and a state of partial immunity (or 'premunition') means that adults are usually asymptomatic. With transmission intensity decreasing (moderate transmission) the period with symptomatic disease shifts to a slightly older age. In low transmission areas, severe and symptomatic disease occurs at all ages, and will affect especially young adults. Pregnant women are at increased risk of developing symptomatic and severe malaria in all transmission settings.

Uncomplicated malaria

In most cases, the incubation period for falciparum and vivax malaria is around 2 weeks, but this can vary widely. The majority (>90%) of *P. falciparum* infections in travelers occur within 8 weeks of leaving an epidemic area. Some *P. vivax* strains (var. *hibernans*) in a few areas of China and North and South Korea have extremely long incubation times (up to 9–12 months).

The clinical features of all four human malarias start nonspecifically and resemble influenza. Headache, muscular ache, vague abdominal discomfort, lethargy and dysphoria often precede the fever. Rising temperatures initially cause shivering, mild chills, worsening headaches, malaise and loss of appetite. If the infection is untreated, the fever in *P. vivax* and *P. ovale* regularizes to a 2-day cycle (tertian malaria; fever on the third day if the starting day is counted as number one) and *P. malaria* fever spikes occur every 3 days (quartan malaria; fever on the fourth day). The fever pattern in *P. falciparum* is generally much more variable, since the infection tends to be less synchronized. Classic 'paroxysms' are therefore more common in tertian and quartan malaria, and consist of an abrupt steeply rising temperature to >102°F (39°C), with intense headache and highly uncomfortable 'cold chills' with peripheral vasoconstriction, and dramatic rigors with shaking limbs and teeth chatter. This is followed by a 'hot stage' during which the patient may have a temperature well over 104°F (40°C), with peripheral vasodilatation, often with restlessness and vomiting. During defervescence, the patient has profuse transpiration and feels exhausted. As the infection continues,

Table 111.1 Currently available drugs with antimalarial activity	
Arylaminoalcohols	
4-aminoquinolines	Chloroquine
	Amodiaquine
	Amopyraquine
	Pyronaridine
	Piperaquine
	Quinine
	Quinidine
	Mefloquine
	Halofantrine*
	Lumefantrine (Benflumetol)
8-aminoquinolines	Primaquine
	Tafenoquine (Etaquine)
Dihydrofolate reductase inhibitors	Pyrimethamine
	Proguanil
	Chlorproguanil
	Pyrimethamine–sulfadoxine
	Chlorproguanil–dapsone
Artemisinin and derivatives	Artemisinin
	Artemether
	Artesunate
	Artemether
	Dihydroartemisinin
Hydroxynaphthaquinones	Atovaquone
	Atovaquone–proguanil
Antibiotics with antimalarial activity	Sulfonamides
	Tetracycline–doxycycline†
	Chloramphenicol
	Fluoroquinolones (weak)
	Rifamycins (weak)
	Macrolides
	Clindamycin
	Lincomycin

Drugs in italics are either still investigational or are not widely available.
*Halofantrine is not recommended as first-line treatment for uncomplicated malaria because of cardiotoxicity.
†Doxycycline should not be used in children under 8 years of age.

the spleen and liver enlarge and anemia develops. Mild abdominal discomfort is common in malaria. In routine clinical practice in malarious areas malaria is rarely the cause of lymphadenopathy, pharyngitis or a rash.

Severe malaria

The vast majority of severe malaria is caused by falciparum malaria in nonimmune individuals, although severe vivax malaria is relatively common in areas with chloroquine resistance.[2] Severe malaria is a multisystem disease. In a minority of patients cerebral malaria is an isolated presentation and generally combined with other severity signs. In areas of high transmission in sub-Saharan Africa severe malaria is mainly a pediatric disease. Important symptoms in children are severe anemia, hypoglycemia and coma with convulsions. Main prognostic indicators are coma, respiratory distress (which includes a Kussmaul pattern breathing related to metabolic acidosis) and to a lesser extent severe anemia.[39]

In low transmission areas such as South East Asia, young adults are the most affected group. Cerebral malaria, metabolic acidosis, renal failure, severe jaundice and ARDS are the most prominent complications in this group. Coma and acidosis have the strongest prognostic significance, whereas patients developing ARDS or renal failure have a high risk of dying. Definitions of the clinical manifestations of severe falciparum malaria are summarized in Table 111.2.

Cerebral malaria

The clinical picture is that of a diffuse encephalopathy with unrousable coma; focal signs are relatively uncommon. In young children coma can develop rapidly, with a mean onset after only 2 days of fever. One or more generalized seizures, which cannot be distinguished clinically from febrile convulsions, often precede the coma. In adults the onset in usually more gradual, with high fever (mean duration of 5 days) and increasing drowsiness, but sometimes agitation. Convulsions are present in about 15% of the cases, whereas more than 50% of pediatric cases have convulsions. Convulsions are most frequently generalized, but in small children approximately 25% have subtle or subclinical convulsions, with seizure activity on electroencephalography, but only minor convulsive movements of limbs or facial muscles. These patients often have deviated eyes, excessive salivation and irregular breathing patterns. Signs of meningism are absent, although passive resistance to neck flexion is not uncommon. The eyes often show a divergent gaze. Bruxism with grinding of the teeth and a positive pout reflex are common in cases with deep coma. Various forms of abnormal posturing can be present, with either a decorticate pattern with flexor rigidity of the arms and extension of the legs or a decerebrate pattern with abnormal extensor responses in arms and legs with or without opisthotonos.[40]

In areas of high transmission a high background prevalence of peripheral parasitemia can hamper the diagnosis of 'cerebral malaria'. A positive blood slide in a febrile comatose child in this setting does

Table 111.2 Manifestations and complications of severe falciparum malaria, including current opinions about pathophysiology and treatment

Manifestations and complications	Pathophysiology	Treatment
Coma (Glasgow Coma Score <11; Blantyre Coma Score <3) and convulsions	Sequestration of parasitized red blood cells in the cerebral microcirculation and other factors	Hypoglycemia and other causes of meningo/encephalitis should be excluded Good general intensive nursing care, including close observation of breathing, eye care Give nasogastric tube, Foley catheter If feasible: intubation to protect airway Frequent monitoring of blood glucose Treat convulsions (e.g. diazepam); prophylactic anticonvulsive treatment is not recommended
Anemia (Hct <20%, in presence of parasitemia >100 000/μl)	Loss of parasitized red blood cells, increased splenic clearance of uninfected red blood cells (decreased red cell deformability, immunologic factors?), dyserythropoiesis	General recommendation: transfusion if in distress, or Hct <20% (adults), or Hb <5 g/dl in children
Hyperparasitemia (>10% infected red blood cells)	Host immunologic factors and parasite virulence factors (multiplication rate, red cell selectivity)	Start parenteral antimalarial drugs promptly in effective doses (artemisinins; if quinine: give loading dose) Exchange transfusion (?)
Hypoglycemia (blood glucose <40 mg/dl)	Increased use, decreased production (?) Quinine-related hyperinsulinism	Glucose 10%, 4 mg/kg bodyweight
Acute renal failure (plasma creatinine >3 mg/dl)	Acute tubular necrosis Prerenal component (dehydration)	Record input/output (Foley catheter) Check biochemistry (BUN, electrolytes), start or transfer for renal replacement therapy (hemofiltration or hemodialysis preferred over peritoneal dialysis)
Severe jaundice (bilirubin >3.0 mg/dl, with parasitemia >100 000/μl)	Mainly in adults; multifactorial	No specific treatment Monitor blood glucose
Fluid/electrolyte imbalances, metabolic acidosis (venous plasma bicarbonate <15 mmol/l or lactate >4 mmol/l)	Dehydration, SIADH (?) Only minor increase in capillary permeability, compromised microcirculation by sequestration and other factors causing anaerobic glycolysis	Careful fluid resuscitation Bicarbonate administration only if pH ≤7.15 Dialysis as treatment for severe acidosis has been advocated

Table 111.2 Manifestations and complications of severe falciparum malaria, including current opinions about pathophysiology and treatment—cont'd

Manifestations and complications	Pathophysiology	Treatment
Respiratory distress and pulmonary edema	Acidosis-related deep breathing Pulmonary edema (ARDS) mainly in adults and pregnant women Etiology unknown; cytokine mediated (?)	See also acidosis ARDS: do not overfill, positive pressure mechanical ventilation with PEEP etc. Do not allow 'permissive hypercapnia' (brain swelling) Distinguish from pneumonia
Black water fever	Related to severe malaria, quinine use and G6PD deficiency	Transfusion if needed Bicarbonate administration (?)
Circulatory shock (systolic BP <90 mmHg [80 mmHg in children] with cold extremities)	Rare in malaria (nitric oxide binding by free hemoglobin?) Consider concurrent septicemia	Fluids, inotropic drugs (do not use adrenaline [epinephrine] because of lactic acidosis), antibiotics
Abnormal bleeding	Diffuse intravascular coagulation: consider concomitant sepsis Isolated thrombocytopenia (very common) not enough explanation	No specific treatment Packed red cell transfusion if indicated

Aspects of pathophysiologic mechanisms or treatment that are still controversial are marked with a '?'.
ARDS, adult respiratory distress syndrome; G6PD, glucose-6-phosphate dehydrogenase; Hct, hematocrit; PEEP, positive end-expiratory pressure; SIADH, syndrome of inappropriate antidiuretic hormone secretion.
Adapted from White et al.[52]

not always adequately exclude other possible diagnoses, and bacteremia can be present in up to 20% of these patients.[41] The presence of retinal hemorrhages on ophthalmoscopy can sometimes be useful here because of its specificity for malaria, although a majority of patients will lack this finding[18] (Fig. 111.6).

In surviving patients the median time to full recovery of consciousness is approximately 24 hours in children, compared to 48 hours in adults. Neurologic sequelae are rare in adults recovering from cerebral malaria (<1%) (Fig. 111.7), but more frequent in children, with approximately 12% still having symptoms at the time of discharge, including hemiplegia, cortical blindness, aphasia and cerebellar ataxia.[42] These symptoms will completely resolve over a period from 1 to 6 months in over half of the children, but a quarter will be left with

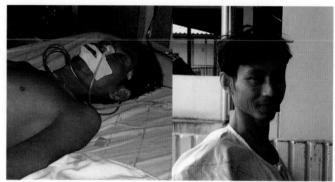

Fig. 111.7 Adult severe malaria has a high case fatality rate of around 20% in developing countries. However, surviving patients, even those presenting with a deep coma (left), usually recover without sequelae (right). Neurologic sequelae are more common in pediatric cases.

major residual neurologic deficits. More subtle cognitive impairments as a late consequence of cerebral malaria are common in children, especially in those cases presenting with a combination of coma, hypoglycemia and seizures.[43]

Acidosis

Metabolic acidosis is a major cause of death in severe malaria.[20] Acidosis results from accumulation of lactic acid and other unidentified organic acids as a result of tissue ischemia, compounded by reduced hepatic clearance. Renal impairment can further aggravate the metabolic acidosis. Lactic acidosis is often associated with hypoglycemia.

Anemia

Anemia is mainly a complication in young children and its pathogenesis is multifactorial. Red cells will be destroyed at the moment of schizont rupture, but the rapid decline in hematocrit is more importantly determined by an accelerated destruction of nonparasitized red

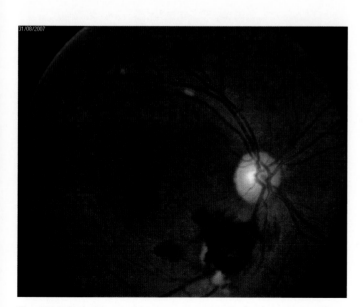

Fig. 111.6 Retinal hemorrhages are a common finding in patients with severe and cerebral malaria (around 15%). Because of its specificity, it can sometimes be a useful tool to distinguish malaria from other causes of febrile illnesses with coma. Courtesy of Dr Abdullah Abu Sayeed.

cells. Moreover, reticulocyte counts are low in the acute phase of the disease because of bone marrow dyserythropoiesis. Increased clearance of uninfected erythrocytes is associated with their increased rigidity and possibly with neomembrane antigens resulting from aborted merozoite invasion, which makes them more prone to removal in the sinusoids of the spleen.[44]

Anemia in African children is only partly explained by malaria. In addition, bacteremia, hookworm, HIV infection and deficiency of vitamin A and vitamin B12 are all associated with severe anemia.[45]

Hypoglycemia

Hypoglycemia is most prominent in small children and pregnant women with severe malaria. Demand is increased because of increased anaerobic glycolysis (also causing lactic acidosis), increased metabolic demands of the febrile illness, and the malaria parasites which use glucose as their major fuel. Supply is reduced as a result of reduced oral intake, vomiting, and failure of hepatic gluconeogenesis, although this has been contested. Hepatic glycogen is exhausted rapidly. The net result is hypoglycemia in 20–30% of children with severe malaria. In patients treated with quinine, this is compounded by quinine-stimulated pancreatic β-cell insulin secretion.[46] Untreated hypoglycemia can cause neurologic damage and is associated with residual neurologic deficit in survivors.

Renal impairment

Acute renal failure is a feared complication of adult severe malaria and most frequently results from acute tubular necrosis. Usually the patient is oliguric for a median of 4 days, but nonoliguric renal failure may also occur. Renal microvascular obstruction and cellular injury consequent upon sequestration in the kidney and the filtration of free hemoglobin, myoglobin and other cellular material are contributing factors.[47] Elevated plasma TNF has also been associated with renal impairment. Significant glomerulonephritis is very rare, except in chronic *P. malariae* malaria which can cause an immune complex glomerulonephritis with a nephrotic syndrome.

Respiratory distress

Respiratory distress manifesting as deep breathing or tachypnea is associated with poor outcome in children with severe malaria.[39] There may be intercostal recession, use of the accessory muscles of respiration and flaring of the alae nasi.

Respiratory distress is often present as respiratory compensation for a profound metabolic acidosis, but can also be caused by the presence of severe anemia or a concomitant lung infection. Pulmonary edema is rare in children. Respiratory depression can be caused by an overuse of anticonvulsants, particularly phenobarbital in combination with benzodiazepines. Identification of these different causes of respiratory distress is important as each requires a different treatment modality.

In adults with severe falciparum malaria, but occasionally in severe vivax infections, ARDS with increased pulmonary capillary permeability can develop, which has a high mortality (Fig. 111.8). Pregnant women are especially prone to this complication. Overhydration aggravates the condition, but is not the cause; the pulmonary capillary wedge pressure is usually normal.

Blackwater fever

A minority of patients (6% in adult severe malaria) develop massive intravascular hemolysis and the passage of 'Coca-Cola'-colored urine (Fig. 111.9). The pathogenesis of Blackwater fever could be related to a build-up of oxidative stress in the erythrocyte membrane. Risk factors are glucose-6-phosphate dehydrogenase (G6PD) deficiency and the use of oxidative drugs such as primaquine.[48] Blackwater fever may contribute to the development of acute renal failure, although in the majority of cases renal function remains normal.

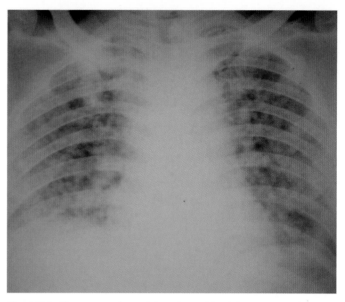

Fig. 111.8 Chest X-ray of an adult patient with adult respiratory distress syndrome (ARDS), a feared complication of severe falciparum malaria in adults.

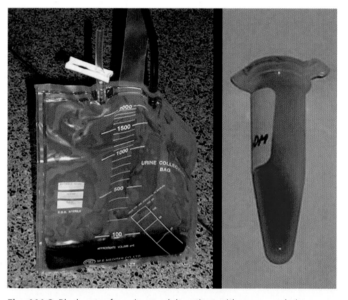

Fig. 111.9 Blackwater fever in an adult patient with severe malaria. Massive intravascular hemolysis of both infected and uninfected erythrocytes causes 'Coca-Cola'-like discoloring of the urine.

Shock

Shock or 'algid malaria' is relatively rare in severe malaria (<10%). In most cases the blood pressure of patients with malaria is at the lower end of the normal range, probably due to vasodilatation. Marked hypotension in a few cases may be the result of dehydration, but is more commonly due to concomitant sepsis, and possible sources (e.g. respiratory and urinary tract infections) should be investigated.

Bleeding

Bleeding due to the commonly occurring thrombocytopenia in malaria is rare. Bleeding is more likely to occur in the setting of disseminated intravascular coagulation, which should prompt the clinician to consider concomitant sepsis as a cause. More often there is only subtle activation of the coagulation cascade with a reduction in anti-thrombin III concentration, an increase in thrombin–antithrombin III complexes and a reduction in factor XII and prekallikrein activities, which do not appear to be clinically significant.[49]

Differential diagnosis

Malaria is a great mimic and must enter the differential diagnosis of a number of clinical presentations.

- In the acute presentation, fever due to malaria needs to be differentiated from typhoid, viral illnesses such as dengue fever and influenza, leptospirosis, brucellosis and respiratory and urinary tract infections. Less common causes of tropical fevers include leishmaniasis, trypanosomiasis, rickettsial infections and relapsing fevers.
- In the case of cerebral malaria, it is of utmost importance to exclude the presence of hypoglycemia as a contributing factor. The principal differential diagnosis in tropical areas is of a bacterial or viral meningoencephalitis. If the patient presents with any sign of meningeal involvement a lumbar puncture should be performed. Especially in small children this implies that in most cases a lumbar puncture will be necessary. Some African centers treating pediatric cerebral malaria postpone lumbar puncture fearing herniation related to raised intracranial pressure which is present in a majority of their cases. These centers start empiric antibiotic coverage in all children until results of lumbar puncture become available. Other differential diagnoses include enteric fevers, trypanosomiasis, brain abscess and other causes of coma.
- The anemia of malaria can be confused with other common causes of hemolytic anemia in the tropics such as that due to the hemoglobinopathies (e.g. sickle cell disease, thalassemia), G6PD deficiency and the South East Asian form of ovalocytosis. The anemia of malaria must be differentiated from that of iron, folate or vitamin B12 deficiency. Hookworm and HIV infection are also associated with severe anemia.
- The renal failure of malaria must be distinguished from renal impairment due to sickle cell disease, leptospirosis, use of traditional herbal medicines and chronic renal disease resulting from glomerulonephritis and hypertension.
- The jaundice and hepatomegaly of malaria must be distinguished from that of viral hepatitis (A, B and E, cytomegalovirus and Epstein–Barr virus infections), leptospirosis, yellow fever, biliary disease and drug-induced disease, including alcohol.

DIAGNOSIS

Because of the high prevalence of the disease in the tropics and the danger of developing severe disease, a traveler with fever who has been in a malarious area within the previous 2 months must be considered to have malaria unless proved otherwise. Similarly, in patients living in endemic countries who present with a fever the suspicion of malaria should be high. On the other hand there tends to be overdiagnosing of malaria in high transmission malarious countries, partly because of the lack of diagnostic facilities. A clinical diagnosis of both uncomplicated and severe malaria is not reliable because of the nonspecific presentation of the disease.

As such, the diagnosis malaria should be confirmed by either a rapid diagnostic test or microscopy of stained thin and thick blood films, at a magnification of 1000. The intraerythrocytic parasites must be identified and counted. In severe malaria, the developmental stage of the parasites and the percentage of neutrophils containing malarial pigment have prognostic significance. A negative blood smear makes the diagnosis very unlikely, unless the patient has received antimalarial treatment before presentation. If there is still uncertainty the slide should be repeated every 12 hours for 48 hours. Microscopy with fluorescent staining of the buffy coat (quantitative buffy coat analysis or QBC) has a higher sensitivity to detect low parasitemias, but this is seldom needed. Dipstick detection of the *P. falciparum* antigens *Pf*HRP2 and *p*LDH (Paracheck, Binax NOW, ParaSight-F, ICT Malaria Pf, OptiMAL) has a diagnostic sensitivity similar to that of microscopy, but does not require an experienced microscopist. Parasitemia and parasite stages cannot be assessed in this way. *Pf*HRP2 remains circulating weeks after cure, which can lead to false-positive results in high transmission settings in patients with a recent malaria attack.

MANAGEMENT

Uncomplicated malaria

Malaria caused by *Plasmodium falciparum*

Today, resistance of *P. falciparum* against chloroquine has reached most parts of the tropics and resistance against the usual next alternative, sulfadoxine–pyrimethamine, is rapidly spreading. To ensure efficacy and to limit the chances of de-novo appearance and spread of antimalarial drug resistance, falciparum malaria should be treated with combinations of two or more blood schizontocidal drugs with independent modes of action. Artemisinin combination therapy (ACT) has become the standard recommendation for treatment of uncomplicated malaria, endorsed by the WHO.[5] The potent antimalarial capacity of the artemisinins quickly reduces the total body parasite number, which will not only relieve symptoms rapidly, but will also reduce the chance of emergence of clones resistant against the partner drug. The partner drug mutually protects the artemisinin component against resistance development.[50]

To ensure treatment courses that do not exceed 3 days, the partner drug to the artemisinin derivative should have a longer half-life in order to kill the remaining parasites (about 10^3 to 10^5 of the initial 10^8 to 10^{13}). Possible partner drugs in ACT regimens include amodiaquine, atovaquone–proguanil, clindamycin, doxycycline, lumefantrine, mefloquine, piperaquine, pyronaridine, chlorproguanil–dapsone, proguanil–dapsone, sulfadoxine–pyrimethamine, and tetracyclines. Of these partner drugs, lumefantrine, mefloquine and piperaquine have proven efficacy even in areas of multidrug-resistant *P. falciparum*, although piperaquine is presently only licensed in Asia. The combination of an artemisinin derivative with amodiaquine or sulfadoxine–pyrimethamine has been shown to be effective only in areas where amodiaquine and sulfadoxine–pyrimethamine monotherapy failure rates do not exceed 20%. Chloroquine cannot be recommended because of widespread high-level resistance. Of these combinations, artemether–lumefantrine, dihydroartemisinin–piperaquine, artesunate–mefloquine and artesunate–amodiaquine are now available as fixed combinations. Artesunate–pyronaridine will be registered in the near future. Wide deployment of fixed combinations will preclude the use of artemisinin monotherapy, which is an important strategy to reduce the spread of drug resistance. In 2008 the first well-documented cases of reduced *in-vivo* sensitivity of *P. falciparum* for artesunate were reported.

The following ACTs are currently recommended for treatment of uncomplicated falciparum malaria:[5]

- artemether + lumefantrine
- artesunate + amodiaquine
- artesunate + mefloquine
- artesunate + sulfadoxine–pyrimethamine.

An effective combination therapy not containing an artemisinin derivative is atovaquone–proguanil (Malarone), which can be used in the treatment of imported uncomplicated falciparum malaria in returning travelers in nonendemic countries.

Tables 111.1 and Tables 111.3–111.6 summarize the different drug combinations and dosing schemes for the treatment of uncomplicated falciparum malaria. Table 111.7 summarizes treatment of uncomplicated falciparum malaria in returning nonimmune adult travelers and Table 111.8 in pregnant women. If the patient is vomiting and not

Table 111.3 Dosing schedule for artemether–lumefantrine (fixed combination)

Body weight in kg (age in years)	NO. OF TABLETS RECOMMENDED AT APPROXIMATE TIMING OF DOSING*					
	0h	8h	24h	36h	48h	60h
5–14 (<3)	1	1	1	1	1	1
15–24 (3–9)	2	2	2	2	2	2
25–34 (9–14)	3	3	3	3	3	3
>34 (>14)	4	4	4	4	4	4

*The regimen can be expressed more simply for ease of use at the program level as follows: the second dose on the first day should be given any time between 8h and 12h after the first dose. Dosage on the second and third days is twice a day (morning and evening). The drug should be taken with food or milk.
Adapted from White et al.[52]

Table 111.4 Dosing schedule for artesunate plus amodiaquine

Age	DOSE IN NO. OF TABLETS ARTESUNATE (AS)/AMODIAQUINE (AQ) FIXED COMBINATION			
		Day 1	Day 2	Day 3
5–11 months	AS: 25mg with AQ: 67.5mg	1	1	1
1–6 years	AS: 25mg with AQ: 67.5mg	2	2	2
7–13 years	AS: 100mg with AQ: 270mg	1	1	1
>13 years	AS: 100mg with AQ: 270mg	2	2	2

Table 111.5 Dosing schedule for artesunate plus mefloquine*

Age	DOSE IN MG (NO. OF TABLETS)					
	ARTESUNATE			MEFLOQUINE (BASE)		
	Day 1	Day 2	Day 3	Day 1	Day 2	Day 3
5–11 months	25 (½)	25	25	–	125 (½)	–
1–6 years	50 (1)	50	50	–	250 (1)	–
7–13 years	100 (2)	100	100	–	500 (2)	250 (1)
>13 years	200 (4)	200	200	–	1000 (4)	500 (2)

*A fixed combination is now also available.
Adapted from White et al.[52]

Table 111.6 Dosing schedule for artesunate plus sulfadoxine-pyrimethamine

Age	DOSE IN MG (NO. OF TABLETS)					
	ARTESUNATE			SULFADOXINE–PYRIMETHAMINE		
	Day 1	Day 2	Day 3	Day 1	Day 2	Day 3
5–11 months	25 (½)	25	25	250/12.5 (½)	–	–
1–6 years	50 (1)	50	50	500/25 (1)	–	–
7–13 years	100 (2)	100	100	1000/50 (2)	–	–
>13 years	200 (4)	200	200	1500/75 (3)	–	–

Adapted from White et al.[52]

Table 111.7 Recommendations on the treatment of falciparum malaria in nonimmune adult travelers

For travelers returning to nonendemic countries	• Atovaquone–proguanil (1 g/400 mg q24h for 3 days) • Artemether–lumefantrine (1.5 mg/12 mg/kg q12h for 3 days) • Quinine (10 mg/kg q8h) plus doxycycline* (3.5 mg/kg q24h) or clindamycin (10 mg/kg q12h) • All drugs to be given for 7 days
For severe malaria	• The antimalarial treatment of severe malaria in travelers is the same as the general recommendation for severe malaria • Travelers with severe malaria should be managed in an intensive care unit • Hemofiltration or hemodialysis should be started early in acute renal failure • Positive pressure ventilation should be started early if there is any breathing pattern abnormality, intractable seizure or acute respiratory distress syndrome

*Doxycycline should not be used in children under 8 years of age.

Table 111.8 Treatment of uncomplicated falciparum malaria in pregnancy

First trimester	Quinine (10 mg/kg q8h), preferably plus clindamycin (5 mg/kg q8h) for 7 days An artemisinin-based combination therapy (ACT) should be used if it is considered that the benefits of treating outweigh the risks of not treating when the only drug option available is an ACT
Second and third trimesters	ACT known to be effective in the country/region or artesunate (2 mg/kg q24h) plus clindamycin for 7 days, or quinine plus clindamycin for 7 days
Severe malaria	As in non-pregnant individuals (see Table 111.7) Increased risk of hypoglycemia in quinine-treated patients
Vivax malaria Chloroquine sensitive	Chloroquine 25 mg base/kg divided over 3 days Primaquine is contraindicated during pregnancy Chloroquine prophylaxis (300 mg base once per week) should be continued until delivery
Chloroquine resistance	No clear guidelines Quinine, artesunate and amodiaquine can be used

tolerating oral treatment, parenteral treatment with artesunate, artemether or quinine is warranted. Hyperparasitemia above 4% is, for some authors, also an indication for parenteral treatment, even in the absence of any other severity sign. Others recommend an oral ACT under close supervision.[5] Hyperparasitemia above 10% should be treated with parenteral antimalarials.

Malaria caused by *P. vivax*, *P. ovale* and *P. malariae*

P. vivax and *P. ovale* form hypnozoites, parasite stages in the liver that can result in multiple relapses of infection, weeks to months after the primary infection. Radical cure of the infection targets both the blood stage and the liver stage, preventing relapse as well as recrudescence. In general, *P. vivax, ovale* and *malariae* are sensitive to chloroquine, which remains the treatment of choice; however, radical cure can only be achieved by the addition of primaquine. Important chloroquine-resistant vivax malaria has been reported, especially from Papua New Guinea and parts of Indonesia. In these settings, dihydroartemisinin–piperaquine and artemether–lumefantrine are an effective treatment for vivax malaria.[51]

The following are currently recommended for treatment of uncomplicated vivax malaria (Table 111.9):

- chloroquine + primaquine
- amodiaquine + primaquine (for chloroquine-resistant), *or*
- artemisinin-based combination therapy (dihydroartemisinin + piperaquine or artemether + lumefantrine; not recommended is artesunate + sulfadoxine–pyrimethamine).

The recommended treatment for malaria caused by *P. ovale* is the same as that given to achieve radical cure in vivax malaria, i.e. with chloroquine and primaquine. *P. malariae* should be treated with the standard regimen of chloroquine as for vivax malaria, but does not require radical cure with primaquine.

Severe malaria

Antimalarial treatment

Prompt start of parenteral antimalarial treatment in full doses is essential in this life-threatening condition. Available recommended parenteral drugs include artesunate, artemether and quinine. Chloroquine and sulfadoxine–pyrimethamine are no longer recommended for the treatment of severe malaria because of widespread resistance. Treatment of the acute phase of severe vivax malaria is the same as for severe falciparum malaria. If the patient is recovering and able to take oral medication, parenteral treatment can be changed to oral treatment. A full course of an ACT can be chosen as follow-on oral treatment.

Quinine

Parenteral quinine or artesunate are the drugs of choice for treating severe malaria in African children, and the results of a large trial comparing these two treatments can be expected in 2010. Because of its cardiotoxicity, intravenous infusion should be carried out over 4 hours. Where intravenous infusion is not practical, quinine can be given by deep intramuscular injection in the upper thigh. Quinine is a relatively toxic drug with a narrow therapeutic ratio.

Table 111.9 Treatment of uncomplicated vivax and ovale malaria

- Chloroquine 25 mg base/kg divided over 3 days, combined with primaquine 0.25 mg base/kg, taken with food once daily for 14 days is the treatment of choice for chloroquine-sensitive infections. In Oceania and South East Asia the dose of primaquine should be 0.5 mg/kg
- Amodiaquine (30 mg base/kg divided over 3 days as 10 mg/kg single daily doses) combined with primaquine should be given for chloroquine-resistant vivax malaria
- In moderate glucose-6-phosphate dehydrogenase (G6PD) deficiency, primaquine 0.75 mg base/kg should be given once a week for 6 weeks. In severe G6PD deficiency, primaquine should not be given
- Where artemisinin combination therapy has been adopted as the first-line treatment for *Plasmodium falciparum* malaria, it may also be used for *P. vivax* malaria in combination with primaquine for radical cure. Artesunate plus sulfadoxine–pyrimethamine (S/P) is the exception, since S/P is generally not effective against *P. vivax*

Table 111.10 Antimalarial treatment of severe malaria

Artesunate*	2.4 mg/kg iv or im stat, at 12 and 24 h, then daily (artesunic acid (60 mg) is dissolved in 0.6 ml 5% sodium bicarbonate and injected iv as a bolus, or diluted to 5 ml with 5% dextrose for im injection; 1 ampoule = 60 mg)
Artemether	3.2 mg/kg im stat, followed by 1.6 mg/kg daily; **not** for iv administration (1 ampoule = 80 mg)
Quinine	20 mg/kg dihydrochloride salt by iv infusion over 4 h, followed by 10 mg/kg infused over 2–8 h q8h
Quinidine	10 mg base/kg infused at constant rate over 1–2 h, followed by 0.02 mg/kg/min as constant infusion, with electrocardiographic monitoring

*Parenteral artesunate is the drug of choice for the treatment of severe malaria in low transmission areas or outside malaria endemic areas. For children in high transmission areas there is as yet insufficient evidence to recommend any of the above antimalarial medicines over another.

Quinine-induced hyperinsulinemic hypoglycemia is a particular problem in patients with severe malaria, especially during pregnancy, and is impossible to diagnose clinically in the already unconscious patient. Frequent monitoring of blood glucose concentrations is therefore essential.[46] It is also important that parasitocidal drug levels are obtained as quickly as possible, so in patients who have not been given a dose of quinine <12 hours before admission an initial loading dose of 20 mk/kg should be administered.[52] In severe malaria the dose should be reduced by one-third after 48 hours if there is no clinical improvement or if there is renal failure. Dosing schemes are summarized in Table 111.10.

Artesunate and artemether

The artemisinin derivatives are rapidly parasitocidal, and crucially unlike quinine they kill young circulating parasites before they sequester in the deep microvasculature. In adult patients with severe malaria, treatment with intravenous artesunate is importantly superior over quinine in preventing death[53] and is the drug of choice for the treatment of severe malaria in low transmission areas and in pregnancy in the second and third trimesters.[5] For pediatric severe malaria the results of a large African trial comparing artesunate with quinine are awaited. A good manufacturing practice (GMP) formulation of artesunate has recently become available for compassionate use in the USA.

Intramuscular (fat-soluble) artemether, unlike intramuscular (water-soluble) artesunate, is erratically absorbed in patients with severe disease, and might explain why trials in both adults and children have shown similar mortality in patients treated with intramuscular artemether compared to quinine.[54] There are insufficient trials with the other parenteral fat-soluble artemisinin derivative artemotil (artemether) to allow firm recommendations. Dosing schemes of artesunate and artemether are summarized in Table 111.10.

Convulsions

Seizures in cerebral malaria should be treated with rectal diazepam, intravenous lorazepam, paraldehyde or other standard anticonvulsants, after high flow oxygen and appropriate airway management have been initiated. Prophylactic phenobarbital was shown to reduce seizure incidence in adult cerebral malaria, but a study in children using a single intramuscular dose of 20 mg/kg increased mortality, possibly through respiratory depression caused by an interaction with diazepam.[55] Prophylactic anticonvulsive therapy is therefore currently not recommended.

Anemia

Benefits of blood transfusion should outweigh the risks (especially HIV and other pathogens). There is no clear evidence supporting specific hemoglobin cut-off levels, and a number of figures are quoted in reviews and guidelines. In adults the threshold for blood transfusion is commonly set at a hematocrit below 20%, in African children at a hemoglobin level below 4 mg/dl (absolute threshold) or 5 mg/dl if there is coexisting respiratory distress, impaired conscious or hyperparasitemia.

Acute renal failure

Renal replacement therapy can save lives in those cases with acute renal failure, a common complication in adult patients, with an untreated mortality of over 70%. Hemofiltration, when available, is superior to peritoneal dialysis in terms of mortality and cost-effectiveness.[56]

Hemodynamic shock

Shock in severe malaria ('algid malaria') should be treated initially with oxygen and fluids (with monitoring of central venous pressure if available). A septic screen including blood cultures should be performed, and appropriate broad-spectrum antibiotics commenced to cover the possibility of bacterial sepsis. Massive hemorrhage from the gastrointestinal tract or rarely a ruptured spleen should be excluded. Dopamine, dobutamine and noradrenaline (norepinephrine) can be used as inotropic medication, but adrenaline (epinephrine) should be avoided as it induces serious lactic acidosis.[57]

Bacterial superinfection

Bacterial superinfection is common in malaria and must be suspected, particularly if the fever remains high despite antimalarial treatment or if there is evidence of septicemia or focal sepsis (e.g. pneumonia or urinary tract infection).

Supportive treatment

Severe malaria is a multiorgan disease and adequate supportive treatment is crucial for survival. Good nursing care is essential, with particular attention to fluid balance, management of the unconscious patient, and detection of potentially lethal complications such as hypoglycemia. Mechanical ventilation in the unconscious patient helps to protect the airway. The role of aggressive fluid resuscitation in the management of severe malaria, particularly in children, is unclear. The debate centers around whether children with severe malaria are intravascular hypovolemic and to what extent this contributes to impairment of the microcirculation. Many 'resource poor' countries are at a stage where basic intensive care support in regional hospitals is becoming feasible, a development which has great potential to further reduce mortality.

Other adjunctive treatments

Many adjunctive treatments have been tried in often underpowered clinical trials, but none has been shown convincingly to improve survival in severe malaria. Exchange blood transfusion is a popular adjunctive therapy, particularly in well-resourced settings. There are a number of rationales for its use in severe malaria, including removal of parasitized erythrocytes, removal of cytokines and other soluble toxins and mediators, and improving the rheology of the blood unparasitized erythrocytes by replacing unparasitized erythrocytes with reduced deformability. However, a meta-analysis of small studies and case series showed no clear benefit.

REFERENCES

📖 References for this chapter can be found online at http://www.expertconsult.com

Schistosomiasis

INTRODUCTION

Schistosomiasis or bilharzia, caused by infection with trematode *Schistosoma* spp., is one of the most debilitating helminthic diseases among rural populations, particularly in sub-Saharan Africa. Schistosomiasis can cause a wide range of symptoms and consequences depending on the species, the worm burden and the length of time infected. There are three major species which affect humans, of which two are predominant in Africa (*Schistosoma haematobium* and *Schistosoma mansoni*) and one is only found in the Far East, e.g. China and the Philippines (*Schistosoma japonicum*). Another two less widespread species – *Schistosoma mekongi* in South East Asia and *Schistosoma intercalatum* in Africa – are considered to be less of a public health problem.

EPIDEMIOLOGY

Schistosomiasis is prevalent in 76 countries and territories in tropical and subtropical regions (Fig. 112.1), with an estimated 207 million people infected and 779 million people at risk.[1] Approximately 85% of infections are found in sub-Saharan Africa.[2] The geographic distribution of *S. haematobium* and *S. mansoni* within endemic areas is dependent on the presence of suitable aquatic intermediate host snails (*Bulinus* and *Biomphalaria* spp., respectively). Human water contamination activities, such as urination and defecation, lead to infection in these snails while exposure during activities such as swimming, fishing or irrigation lead to cercariae from snails infecting humans and completing the cycle. In the case of *S. japonicum*, a reservoir of infection exists in domestic and wild animals and the snail intermediate hosts are amphibious *Oncomelania* species.

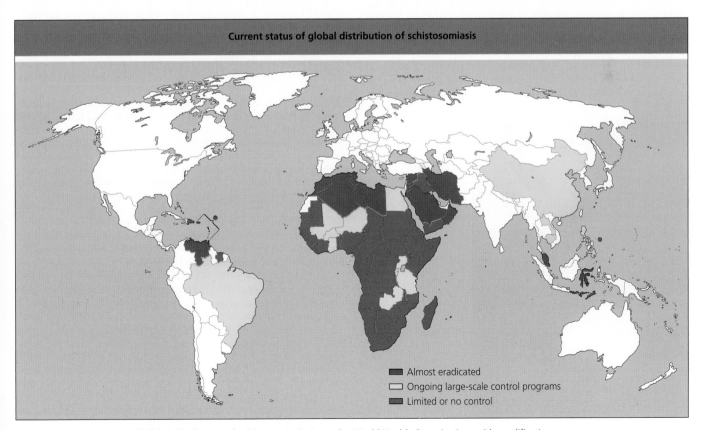

Current status of global distribution of schistosomiasis

■ Almost eradicated
□ Ongoing large-scale control programs
■ Limited or no control

Fig. 112.1 Current status of global distribution of schistosomiasis. From the World Health Organization, with modification.

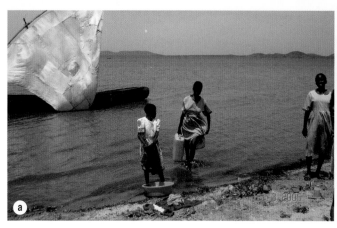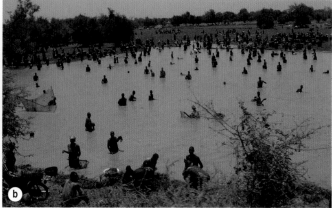

Fig. 112.2 Water contact activities. (a) Girls collecting water and washing in Lake Victoria in Uganda. (b) Mass fishing activities in Burkina Faso.

Transmission levels are determined by cultural, social and behavioral activities (Fig. 112.2). Recent infections in new areas have resulted from new irrigation projects[3] and may probably be accelerated by climate change.[4] Detailed information on geographic distribution in each endemic country/area has been obtained through rapid epidemiologic mapping[5] or using geographical information system (GIS) technology.[6] *S. mekongi* is present only in the Mekong River basin in South East Asia, though latest research suggests that the distribution may be a little wider, with intermediate host *Neotricula aperta* snails. Finally, *S. intercalatum* is present in limited areas in Central and West Africa with *Bulinus* spp. as snail host.

In endemic areas, children may acquire infection in infancy,[7] much earlier than previously believed, probably through being bathed in the infested water by their mothers (Fig. 112.3). Prevalence of infection usually increases with age, peaks in age 10–20 years and then decreases in adults. Intensity of infection, which is measured as the number of eggs excreted (a surrogate estimate of worm load) in urine (*S. haematobium*) or feces (*S. mansoni*, *S. japonicum*, *S. mekongi* and *S. intercalatum*), follows a similar pattern to prevalence: increasing with age through childhood and then decreasing in adults. Schistosomiasis does, however, result in exceptional consequences when epidemiologic conditions are extreme – for example, car washers in Kenya present a unique situation of repeated heavy infections,[8] despite frequent treatment.

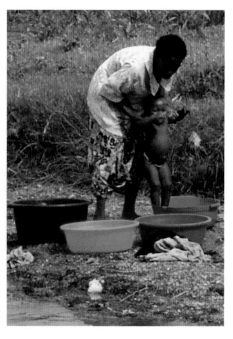

Fig. 112.3 Water contact – baby bathing. A baby is being washed by the mother near Lake Victoria in Uganda. Courtesy of Dr J Russell Stothard.

There are two schools of thought about this 'normal' age-specific pattern of prevalence and intensity whereby peak infection in children and decline in adults may be explained by either acquired immunity due to existing infections, or a reduction in water contact patterns in older age groups. Those who favor the second argument of water contact as a major factor point to the gender-related patterns in prevalence and intensity of infection which vary in different areas according to behavioral, professional, cultural and religious factors.

Another epidemiologic feature of schistosome infections is that the frequency distribution of the number of worms in individuals in endemic areas is aggregated or overdispersed.[9] This means that in most populations the majority of infected individuals harbor a relatively low worm burden and only a minority (5–15%) are heavily infected (as measured by eggs in stool or urine). Consequently, this minority group of individuals is most likely to show severe morbidity. What determines the predisposition to heavy or light infection is not known, but may be attributed to age, innate and acquired immunity and/or genetic background of individuals.[10]

PATHOGENESIS AND PATHOLOGY

Disease manifestations caused by schistosome infections are multiple, depending on the parasite species, but can be divided into acute and chronic phases.

Acute schistosomiasis is seen most commonly soon after exposure to an infested water body by previously unexposed individuals, and is more common in *S. japonicum* and *S. mansoni*. The typical acute symptoms are observed after the percutaneous penetration of cercariae which can cause cercarial dermatitis, a local hypersensitivity reaction to the penetrating parasites at the site of entry. Subsequently, Katayama fever, a systemic hypersensitivity reaction, can then occur during the next month as larvae migrate through the lungs. The exact pathogenesis is still unknown, but is probably a serum sickness-like illness caused by circulating immune complexes and proinflammatory cytokines in response to the migrating schistosomula and the egg antigens.[11] Classically, egg laying begins approximately 6 weeks after infection, and the onset of oviposition can cause severe bloody diarrhea.

In chronic schistosomiasis, caused by continued infection with mating worm pairs, pathologic lesions are mainly localized in specific sites within infected individuals. While the adult worms are living in the blood vessels and are feeding on blood, it is the eggs and the subsequent host granulomatous reactions to the eggs trapped in tissues which cause the damage. Mature worms reside in the venous tributaries of the vesical (*S. haematobium*) or mesenteric (*S. mansoni*, *S. japonicum*, *S. mekongi* and *S. intercalatum*) plexuses and continue oviposition for life. Through the secretion of proteolytic enzymes, and perhaps aided by urinary tract or intestinal movement, the eggs rupture capillary vessels and then pass

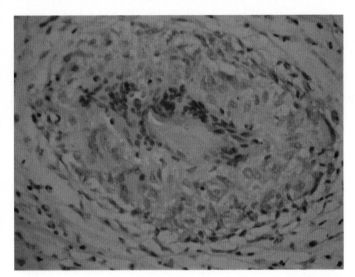

Fig. 112.4 Multiple granulomata surrounding eggs. Courtesy of Dr Robert Goldin.

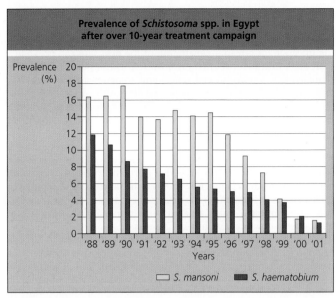

Fig. 112.5 Decreasing prevalence of *Schistosoma* spp. in Egypt (1988–2001) in the course of an ongoing treatment campaign. Redrawn from Fenwick *et al.*[14] Copyright Elsevier 2003.

through the tissues to the lumen of these viscera where they are carried to the outside via urine or stools. This process causes bleeding, which in the short term causes overt blood in the urine and blood in the stool (less easily visible) and in the longer term contributes to anemia. A significant proportion of parasite eggs, however, are either retained in local tissues (bladder or gut walls) or carried via venous blood to distant organs such as the liver and lung, and are trapped there due to their relatively large size (60–170 μm). As long as the worms are alive, the numbers of trapped eggs continue to accumulate in the tissues. At these sites, miracidia in the trapped eggs secrete soluble antigens which diffuse out of the egg shell, triggering a marked inflammatory and granulomatous response from the host immune system. As a result, the individual eggs (or cluster of eggs in the case of *S. japonicum*) are enclosed by the aggregated immune cells, including eosinophils, forming granulomas (Fig. 112.4).

The granulomatous response is a form of delayed-type hypersensitivity reaction and is dependent predominantly on CD4+ T cell-mediated mechanisms.[12] Granulomas are tumor-like inflammatory nodules which can cause intrahepatic portal vein obstruction, leading to portal hypertension, or obstruct urine flow through the ureters, leading to hydroureters and hydronephrosis. The miracidia within the eggs, however, survive for only 6–8 weeks and then die, thus eliminating the continuous antigenic stimulation. The granulomas may then disperse and fibrous tissues form. The tissue damage caused by scattered eggs does not cause a significant problem, but when numerous eggs are trapped the damage becomes significant. Therefore, the severity of morbidity is closely related to the intensity of infection and the passage of time.

PREVENTION

Prevention of infection by improved water supplies and sanitation is fundamental to the elimination of schistosomiasis, as was achieved several decades ago in Japan and more recently in Puerto Rico.[13] In the meantime, current control programs in less developed countries target prevention of morbidity using chemotherapy, with elimination some way in the future. After 20 years of regular chemotherapy, Egypt has significantly reduced the prevalence of infection and reduced the public health importance of schistosomiasis (Fig. 112.5).[14]

Without human contact with fresh water there would be no infection. For nonindigenous travelers into endemic areas, avoidance of all freshwater sources is most prudent, because a single exposure to many cercariae can have severe consequences. However, for indigenous residents in endemic areas the risks are more complex and multifaceted, often reflecting the degree of education, socioeconomic status and cultural

and recreational practices. In many areas in sub-Saharan Africa, the snail-infested water bodies may be the only water sources in their daily life, and for fishermen, farmers and domestic washing, contact is unavoidable. How can people with regular water contact escape infection? Strategies considered for prevention may include mollusciciding to kill intermediate host snails, chemotherapy of infected individuals to reduce transmission sources, health education to improve hygiene, provision of latrines and sewage disposal, installation of a clean water supply, and economic and social development in general. Each of these strategies has its limitations and should be used in conjunction with others in an integrated manner according to local conditions. In recent years, despite investments to develop antischistosome vaccines, and promise in laboratory studies using a mouse model, a successful vaccine and a practical vaccination strategy are still some way away.

To reduce morbidity, a preventive chemotherapy strategy has been recommended by the World Health Organization[15] to reduce the intensity of infection in the population by targeted mass chemotherapy. This strategy to prevent morbidity should be based first on targeting school-aged children and populations at high risk. Since children can acquire infection at a very young age and severe morbidity usually takes years to develop, repeated annual treatment during school-aged years should prevent the devastating consequences of organ damage at a later stage of life. Since 2002, the Schistosomiasis Control Initiative (SCI) based at Imperial College London, has implemented a sustainable integrated chemotherapy strategy using praziquantel against schistosomiasis and adding in albendazole to control the concurrent intestinal helminth infections,[16] and approximately 40 million treatments were dispensed in six countries by mid 2008. Since 2006, control of schistosomiasis by chemotherapy has been 'absorbed' into a rapid-impact package covering seven major neglected tropical diseases including schistosomiasis, and this is now being implemented in several sub-Saharan African countries.[17]

CLINICAL FEATURES

The clinical manifestations of schistosomiasis are related not only to the parasite species but also to the intensity of infection and genetic make-up of the infected individuals. Disease manifestations have multiple stages and also interact with other co-infections such as HIV and malaria, and nutritional conditions.

The first clinical manifestations occur as individuals are acquiring infection, as cercarial penetration of the host skin can provoke a temporary urticarial rash that can manifest within hours of exposure (contacting cercariae-infested water) and sometimes persist for days as maculopapular lesions. Such cercarial dermatitis, also called 'swimmers' itch', usually occurs in those who have not previously been exposed, e.g. tourists and migrants. The lesions are usually self-limited and often go unrecognized in endemic areas.

Interestingly, in temperate climate zones (e.g. in the lakes in North America) a similar 'swimmers' itch' is seen and is due to penetration of skin by schistosomal cercariae that normally infect birds or other small animals and cannot fully develop in humans. The severity of the lesions is dependent on the degree of exposure. After heavy exposure to the infested water, a delayed-onset dermatitis as urticaria or angioedema may occur within 1–12 weeks.

A few weeks to months after a primary schistosome infection, systemic manifestations of acute schistosomiasis, Katayama fever, can develop. Early infections are mostly asymptomatic, but in some cases of heavy naive infections the disease starts suddenly with nonspecific symptoms, such as fever, fatigue, myalgia, malaise, nonproductive cough, eosinophilia and patchy pulmonary infiltrates on chest radiography. Abdominal symptoms may develop later when egg deposition begins. Most patients recover spontaneously after 2–10 weeks, but some may develop persistent and more serious disease with weight loss, dyspnea, diarrhea, diffuse abdominal pain, bloody diarrhea, hepatosplenomegaly and widespread rash.

Chronic schistosomiasis and its liver and bladder sequelae may develop within months but usually it takes years after infection depending on the accumulated intensity of infection or the length of exposure to infection. Symptoms, signs and pathologic lesions are species specific.

Urinary schistosomiasis

Urinary schistosomiasis is caused by infection with *S. haematobium*. Most infected individuals show some symptoms, the most common of which is blood in the urine – haematuria (Fig. 112.6a). Other early signs include frequency of urination, dysuria and proteinuria. Haematuria in school-aged children in sub-Saharan Africa, although usually present, is not considered important, because it is often unrecognized as a disease symptom. In girls, it may be confused with menstruation; in boys, it may be considered as a sign of puberty in local perception. The prevalence of these symptoms varies according to the degree of endemicity in each local setting but rates of almost 100% in infected children are not unusual.

Ultrasound examination of the urinary tract in longstanding infections usually indicates thickening of the urinary bladder wall (Fig.

112.6b) and granulomas, and sometimes hydronephrosis and evidence of bladder and ureteric calcification can be seen. Kidney function is usually well preserved, but may be complicated by frequent urinary tract bacterial infection and bladder or ureteric stone formation. There is strong epidemiologic association with squamous bladder cancer, which occurs characteristically in older age groups, especially historically in Egypt, where there is now evidence that with the recent decline of *S. haematobium*, the cancer has decreased.[18]

Intestinal/hepatic schistosomiasis

Intestinal/hepatic schistosomiasis is caused by infection with *S. mansoni*, *S. japonicum*, *S. mekongi* or *S. intercalatum*, with most of the reports of the former two species. There is no definitive symptom such as blood in the urine, and so in many cases with light infections, symptoms and signs are nonspecific and unrecognized. In a relatively small proportion of individuals with heavier infections and/or with a long history of exposure, chronic or intermittent abdominal pain and discomfort, loss of appetite and diarrhea with or without blood may be common.

The serious long-term consequences of infection are liver disease which manifests as early inflammatory and late fibrotic stages. The early stage is typified as hepatomegaly due to the granulomatous response – sharp-edged enlargement of the left liver lobe and perhaps splenomegaly. At this stage liver function can be normal. Ultrasound examination may reveal mild forms of diffuse fibrosis. With the progression of the disease, massive deposition of the diffuse collagen deposits in the periportal spaces leads to pathognomonic periportal or Symmer's pipe-stem fibrosis (which is classic *S. mansoni* pathology). This in turn leads to portal hypertension, splenomegaly, collateral venous circulation and esophageal varices. The liver is not necessarily enlarged and may even be shrunk, and liver function tests remain largely unaffected, in contrast to other causes of liver disease. Ultrasonography will reveal typical fibrotic streaks and portal vein dilatation. The late stage of liver disease may be associated with extensive splenomegaly, ascites and repeated episodes of hematemesis which is often fatal (Fig. 112.7).

Unusual consequences of schistosomiasis

Schistosomiasis may also appear in other forms, e.g. pulmonary, genital or neurologic. These are caused by the deposition of schistosome eggs or worms in these organs/systems and subsequent host granulomatous responses. A common and yet only recently recognized complication is female genital schistosomiasis, which is caused by *S. haematobium* infections in women, with up to 75% of those infected having schistosome eggs in the uterine cervix, vagina or vulva. It usually manifests as mucosal grainy sandy patches, mucosal bleeding and inflammation, and later as ulcerative lesions in these genital areas.

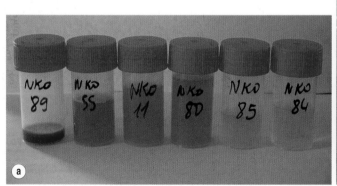

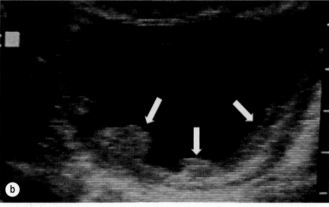

Fig. 112.6 Urinary schistosomiasis. (a) Blood in urine samples collected during a school survey in Burkina Faso. (b) Ultrasound image of the bladder wall from a child infected with *S. haematobium*.

Investigations have shown that genital schistosomiasis can significantly increase the chances of HIV infection.[19]

Another serious possible complication is neurologic schistosomiasis, which can be present in infections with all three main species.[20] Cerebral complications associated with *S. japonicum* can occur during all phases of infection from acute to chronic. These include delirium, loss of consciousness, seizures, dysphasia, visual field impairment, focal motor deficits and ataxia. Spinal complications such as myelopathy are primarily caused by *S. mansoni* but can complicate later stages of *S. haematobium* infection and occur during the acute phase of egg production (see Chapter 106). Severe myelopathy can provoke a complete flaccid paraplegia with areflexia, sphincter dysfunction and sensory disturbances.

DIAGNOSIS

Travelers from nonendemic areas reporting with nonspecific malaise after visiting Africa need to be questioned about water contact. Apart from blood in the urine, infection with different schistosome species manifests only a variety of nonspecific clinical features, and therefore a personal history of possible contact with infested water in endemic areas in tropical or subtropical regions is an important indicator for a suspicion of schistosomiasis.

Parasitologic examination of urine (for distinctive eggs of *S. haematobium*) or stool (for *S. mansoni*, *S. japonicum*, *S. mekongi* and *S. intercalatum* eggs) by microscopy is still the gold standard for the diagnosis of schistosomiasis (see also Chapter 184). However, it must be noted that in some cases with advanced stage of infection the eggs may not be present in urine or stools. In addition, microscopic examination of stool has a relatively low sensitivity and repeated samples or multiple tests may be required to detect eggs in those with low intensity of infection. For *S. haematobium*, urine should preferably be collected around noon, when egg passage is maximal, and generally 10 ml should be concentrated through filtration onto a nitrocellulose filter for examination under a microscope and eggs counted. The intensity of infection can be expressed as number of eggs per 10 ml urine. A less sensitive but useful method for *S. haematobium* is detecting hematuria with a reagent strip which reacts to blood. This practice, however, is more useful for survey work in highly endemic areas than for returning occasional travelers in the developed world because of the multiple etiologies of hematuria.

For intestinal schistosomes, eggs in the feces is the definitive diagnosis; unfortunately, failure to find these eggs does not necessarily mean that the individual is negative. The most commonly used stool examination method is the Kato–Katz thick smear, which examines 41.7 mg feces in each smear, so when the number of eggs are counted, the egg load can be quantified. The intensity of infection is then expressed as number of eggs per gram of feces, and this is assumed to be proportional to the number of worms.

Serologic tests using schistosome antigens to detect antibodies are sensitive but cannot distinguish current from past infection as antibodies can remain in circulation for a long period, even after chemotherapeutic cure, and can also cross-react with other helminth infections. Antigen detection techniques which use labeled monoclonal antibodies to detect circulating anodic antigens or circulating cathodic antigens in serum or urine have been developed. The methods are quantitative and can be used to estimate the worm burden, but they have low sensitivity for light infections.

Clinical diagnosis by ultrasonography of the liver or urinary tract pathology is a valuable tool. Standard protocols (Niamey protocols)[21] for ultrasound examination have been developed to classify schistosome hepatic fibrosis and urinary tract lesions. It is very useful for evaluating the treatment effect and the reversal of schistosome pathology, but requires specific expertise. In hospital settings, cystoscopy and endoscopy may be used to visualize tissue lesions. Tissue samples may be obtained from rectal mucosa, bladder and liver biopsies, and examined for schistosome eggs.

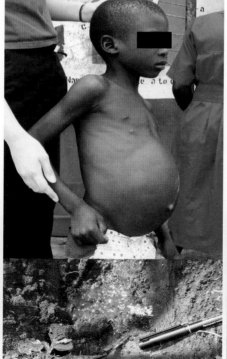

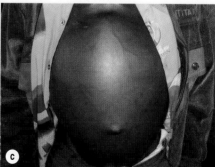

Fig. 112.7 Intestinal/hepatic schistosomiasis. (a) Ultrasound image of the liver of a child infected with *S. mansoni*. (b) Advanced case of *S. mansoni* infection of a child with blood in the stool and ascites. (c) Advanced case of *S. mansoni* infection of an adult.

MANAGEMENT

Treatment of schistosomiasis is relatively inexpensive and safe using the drug praziquantel, which is active against all adult schistosome species at a single oral dose of 40 mg/kg given after food. Praziquantel rarely causes significant side-effects; however, in those with heavy worm burdens, abdominal pain, nausea and vomiting may occur. Recently the World Health Organization has declared that praziquantel is safe for pregnant women and young children (≤4 years of age or ≤94 cm in height). The drug is not effective against eggs and immature worms. After a single treatment, 70–100% of individuals cease to excrete eggs in urine or feces; in those not cured, the intensity of infection (egg counts) should be reduced by over 90%. Artemisinin (or one of its derivatives) has been reported as effective against immature schistosome worms, but not against adult worms. This is a drug currently in use against malaria and so a minor effect on prevalence in endemic areas may be observed.

For acute early cases, treatment should be given to suppress the hypersensitivity reaction, and a combination of praziquantel and artemisinin might be given to kill adult and immature worms. Praziquantel therapy in early chronic infections will result in reversal of pathologies such as hepatomegaly, bladder wall thickening or hydroureters. However, in late stage infections with severe pathologic conditions, such as portal hypertension or extensive hydronephrosis, general medical care will be required. In extreme cases, corrective surgical procedures for portal hypertension or urinary tract anatomic alterations may be necessary.

REFERENCES

References for this chapter can be found online at http://www.expertconsult.com

Cestode and trematode infections

INTRODUCTION

Cestodes (tapeworms) and trematodes (flukes) are ubiquitous flat-worms that are able to infect both vertebrates and invertebrates. The life cycles of both types of helminth are complex and are character-ized by morphologically distinct developmental stages of the para-site being harbored by different host species. Most of these worms are restricted in the range of host species that they can infect, particularly in the definitive host of the adult reproductive worms. From among the large number of parasitic flatworms, humans are the preferred host of just a few, although more are capable of causing incidental (paratenic) human infection.

Despite this variety, the life cycles of the flatworms that infect humans have several features in common:

- all trematodes undergo asexual reproduction in aquatic snails, the intermediate host, and sexual reproduction in a definitive mammalian host;
- the geographic distribution of infections with the various host flukes corresponds to the range of their intermediate snail; and
- when eggs passed in the waste products (usually feces) from a definitive host infected with an adult fluke come into contact with fresh water, they hatch to release larvae that then infect snails.

Flukes are categorized according to their habitat in the human host: blood flukes (*Schistosoma* species), intestinal flukes (*Fasciolopsis*), liver flukes (*Clonorchis*, *Opisthorchis* and *Fasciola*) and lung flukes (*Paragonimus*). In the case of schistosomiasis, larvae (known as cercar-iae) released by snails penetrate skin or mucous membranes that come into contact with infected water. Other human trematode parasites cause infection through consumption of food – usually a form of fish or seafood – contaminated with encysted intermediate stages (meta-cercariae). They are mainly found throughout the tropics and sub-tropics, although a few species are also found in temperate climates.

Adult cestodes are tapeworms that are parasitic in the intestinal tracts of various vertebrate hosts. Intermediate hosts are infected by ingesting eggs, which develop into a cystic larval form in host tissues. The life cycle is completed when these infected tissues are eaten by a suitable definitive host. Tapeworms are flat, segmented worms, com-posed of a head (scolex) and a series of symmetric segments, known as proglottids. The scolex may be equipped with hooks, suckers or elongated grooves to facilitate attachment to the host's intestine. Each segment possesses a complete set of both male and female reproduc-tive organs; sperm are typically transferred between adjacent segments, giving rise to gravid proglottids that contain thousands of embryo-nated eggs. Gravid segments detach from the parent worm and either exit intact via the feces, or disintegrate before leaving the host, releas-ing embryonated eggs. Cestodes lack a functional digestive tract; the tegument, or body covering, serves as a metabolically active layer through which nutrients are absorbed. Although adult tapeworms do not cause much pathology, the encysted larval forms of cestode para-sites (termed cysticerci) often have serious adverse consequences for the intermediate human host, especially neurocysticercosis caused by the larval stages of the pork tapeworm, *Taenia solium*.

Schistosomiasis is discussed in Chapter 112 and echinococcosis in Chapter 114.

TAPEWORM INFECTIONS

Taeniasis

For both the beef tapeworm, *Taenia saginata* (Fig. 113.1), and the pork tapeworm, *T. solium*, humans are the only definitive hosts. Infection is acquired by eating raw or undercooked beef or pork, respectively, that contain living cysticerci. The clinical consequences of taeniasis are usually mild and are limited to minor abdominal symptoms, such as epigastric fullness, nausea and vomiting with *T. saginata*, and abdomi-nal pain, distention and diarrhea with *T. solium*. *T. saginata* proglottids tend to migrate spontaneously from the anus, causing considerable alarm in the host. *Taenia* spp. do not appear to have any significant nutritional effect on their host. The principal complication of infec-tion with *T. solium* is that eggs may be passed in the feces and subse-quently be ingested and cause cysticercosis (see below) either in the same host or in others living in close proximity.

DIPHYLLOBOTHRIASIS

Diphyllobothrium latum is the longest parasite that infects humans: adult worms can achieve a length of more than 33 feet (10 m) in the small intestine. Maintenance of the life cycle of *D. latum* requires that feces of infected hosts be discarded into fresh water that contains the appro-priate crustacean and fish intermediate hosts and that the infected fish be eaten raw by definitive hosts. Although *D. latum* was previously

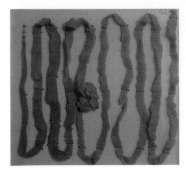

Fig. 113.1 *Taenia saginata.* A mature worm may be up to 33 feet (10 m) long. Courtesy of Guy Baily.

a common infection in Scandinavia, the incidence there has been reduced markedly because of improved sanitation, so that most cases now occur in Russia, Brazil and Japan.[1] Humans are the most important definitive host for this tapeworm, although bears, dogs and other carnivores may serve as reservoir hosts. Adult worms cause minimal clinical disease, although they may compete with the host for absorption of vitamin B12 from the intestinal lumen. Megaloblastic anemia due to depletion of vitamin B12 has been reported in the past as a consequence of infection with *D. latum*, but this is now rarely seen. Various other *Diphyllobothrium* spp. that usually occur in wild animals may infect humans incidentally, principally in the sub-Arctic and the northern Pacific areas. Clinical consequences of these infections appear to be relatively minor.

Hymenolepis

Infection with the dwarf tapeworm (so-called because of its small size) *Hymenolepis nana* occurs worldwide, mostly in children living in conditions with poor sanitation. Rodents are the main reservoir. Infection is acquired either by ingestion of embryonated eggs (from rodents or humans) or an infected insect containing cysticercoid metacestodes. Ingested eggs hatch in the small intestine, releasing larvae that penetrate the lamina propria of the small bowel epithelium where they differentiate into cysticercoids that re-enter the intestinal lumen and attach to the surface of the villous tissue. These develop into new tapeworms approximately 4 cm in length. If an intact cysticercus is ingested, it attaches directly to the small intestinal wall and matures into an adult worm. Although most infections are asymptomatic, heavy infections may result in diarrhea.

Zoonotic tapeworms

Several tapeworms that are not primarily adapted to humans may nevertheless cause incidental human infection after accidental exposure. *Hymenolepis diminuta* is a tapeworm of rodents that uses their fleas as an intermediate host. Similarly, *Dipylidium caninum* passes between dogs and their fleas. Both are occasional sources of human infection worldwide, principally in children, through the accidental ingestion of fleas. There are no known serious clinical consequences with either tapeworm infection.

Diagnosis and management of tapeworm infections

Diagnosis of tapeworm infection is made by microscopic identification of characteristic eggs in the feces, although the species cannot be determined based on morphology since members of the genera *Taenia* and *Diphyllobothrium* produce identically shaped eggs (Fig. 113.2). Speciation can be made by examination of entire proglottids which may sometimes be found in the feces. Treatment with a single dose of praziquantel at 10 mg/kg is effective for all human tapeworms except *H. nana*, for which at least 25 mg/kg should be administered.

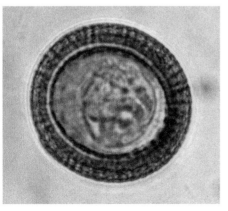

Fig. 113.2 *Taenia* egg. Speciation cannot be done based on morphology. Eggs measure between 30 and 40 μm in diameter.

CYSTICERCOSIS

Epidemiology and prevention

Cysticercosis is caused by ingestion of eggs of the pork tapeworm *T. solium*. Although food and water contaminated with human feces were previously thought to be the primary source of tapeworm eggs, recent evidence indicates that the most common source is an asymptomatic tapeworm carrier in the household.[2] Infected pigs serve to perpetuate the infection: pigs have access to contaminated human feces by their coexistence with humans in the domestic setting and the lack of adequate sanitation and sewage facilities. Cysticercosis remains endemic in most low-income countries, especially in Latin America and Asia (particularly China and South East Asia). The World Health Assembly in 2003 recommended several measures to control *T. solium* infection with the aim of reducing the incidence of neurocysticercosis, including mass or selected treatment with praziquantel to reduce the prevalence of adult worm infection in endemic areas, improved pig husbandry, enforced meat inspection and control, and treatment of infected animals.[3]

Pathogenesis

After ingestion, *T. solium* ova hatch upon exposure to gastric and duodenal contents, releasing oncospheres (embryos) that invade the intestinal wall, enter the vasculature and migrate to host tissues where they develop into larval cysts. In most tissues, cysts are eliminated by the host's immune system, except for sites such as the central nervous system and the eye, which are immunologically privileged, and both striated and cardiac muscle where development to the cysticercus stage is rapid. Cysts are normally approximately 1 cm in diameter and consist of a scolex (head) of the tapeworm larva that is surrounded by a vesicle formed by extension of the parasite's tegument, all of which is enclosed by a host-derived capsule.

Cysts can be found in any part of the central nervous system, although the majority are located in the brain parenchyma, where they initially form viable vesicles which may remain alive for years. However, the host's immune system eventually prevails and the cysticercus dies, a process called involution. First, the vesicular fluid becomes turbid and a thick collagen capsule forms around the dying cyst together with diffuse edema (colloidal stage). The scolex then shows signs of degenerating into coarse granules (granular stage), corresponding to resolution of the surrounding edema and eventual formation of a calcified nodule that represents a dead cysticercus. Significant clinical consequences of cysticercosis are related to this neurologic involvement (Fig. 113.3).

Clinical features

Most of the morbidity and mortality due to this infection is caused by neurocysticercosis, with seizures and sequelae of raised intracranial pressure being the most common clinical manifestations. Symptomatic

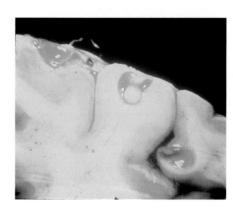

Fig. 113.3 Cysticerci in the brain. Courtesy of Guy Baily.

neurocysticercosis results from a combination of factors, including the number, stage and location of the cysts, together with the severity of the host's immune response against the parasites. As many as 70% of individuals with neurocysticercosis will present with seizures.[4] Other manifestations include those of intracranial hypertension (focal signs, dementia and seizures), caused primarily by hydrocephalus but also rarely by cysticercotic encephalitis. Hydrocephalus occurs most commonly with cysts that are located in the ventricles or subarachnoid space. If untreated, hydrocephalus may lead to permanent loss of cerebral function with dementia and cortical blindness. Various focal neurologic findings may also occur and usually follow a subacute or chronic course, although acute signs may arise due to a stroke.

Ophthalmic cysticercosis is not uncommon and typically manifests as intraocular cysts floating freely in the vitreous or the subretinal space, where they give rise to visual field defects or scotomata (Fig. 113.4). Development of uveitis or retinitis may result in permanent loss of vision.

Extraneural cysticercosis is usually asymptomatic and consists initially of nontender subcutaneous nodules or discrete swellings of particular muscles in which cysticerci have embedded. Several months after initially being noticed, the nodules may swell and become tender as the cysts begin to involute and die. Ultimately, the cysts will calcify; subcutaneous and intramuscular calcifications may persist for years after cysticercal death.

Diagnosis

Diagnosis of neurocysticercosis is usually made on the basis of imaging studies – CT or MRI – and confirmatory serology. Although MRI has better accuracy in making a diagnosis – especially for cysts in the ventricles or basal cisterns – CT is more commonly used in most endemic areas. On CT, viable cysts appear as hypodense lesions whereas degenerating cysts appear as contrast-enhancing lesions with a surrounding ring of edema (Fig. 113.5). The scolex may sometimes be visualized in the interior of viable cysts, but usually not in degenerating ones. The most commonly used serologic test is the enzyme-linked immunoelectrotransfer blot, which has a specificity of 100% and reported overall sensitivity of 98%, although the sensitivity is considerably less for individuals with a solitary lesion.[5]

Occasionally, evidence of extracranial cysticercosis may aid in the diagnosis, particularly direct visualization of ophthalmic cysticerci, palpation of subcutaneous cysticerci or evidence of cigar-shaped intramuscular calcifications seen on plain radiography (Fig. 113.6). A set of diagnostic criteria has been formulated to aid in the diagnosis of neurocysticercosis, which permits classification as either definitive or probable disease.[6]

Management

Treatment of neurocysticercosis consists of a combination of antiparasitic and symptomatic modalities and should involve specialists in infectious diseases, neurology, neuroimaging and neurosurgery.

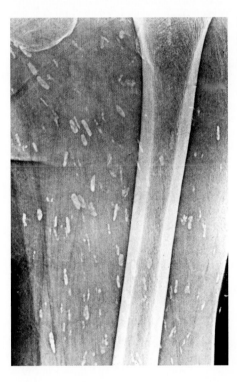

Fig. 113.5 CT image of neurocysticercosis. Viable cysts appear as radiolucent defects (arrowhead). The central protoscolex may be visualized as a radiodense spot (small arrow). Cysts that show ring enhancement are probably degenerating. Calcified cysts (large arrow) are dead and will not benefit from specific therapy. Courtesy of Guy Baily.

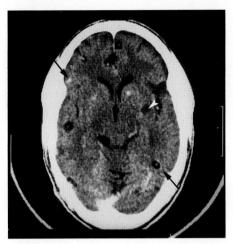

Fig. 113.6 Plain radiograph of lower leg with numerous calcified cysticerci of *Taenia solium*.

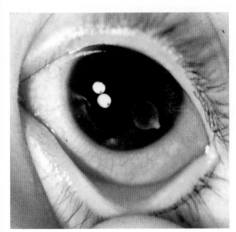

Fig. 113.4 Cysticercus of *Taenia solium* floating in the anterior chamber of the eye.

Antiparasitic measures include cysticidal medications (albendazole or praziquantel) and surgical resection of cysts, whereas symptomatic interventions can include antiepileptics, analgesics and placement of ventricular shunts.[7]

There has been considerable controversy over the use of cysticidal medications, mostly because treatment-associated parasite death can lead to an acute inflammatory reaction in the surrounding brain tissue which can result in seizures, raised intracranial pressure and even death. However, studies have now shown that treatment of viable intraparenchymal cysts results in reduced numbers of seizures and faster resolution of cysts.[8] Although in most cases single enhancing lesions resolve spontaneously,[9] many experts maintain the value of cysticidal treatment. Albendazole (15 mg/kg daily for 7 days) is preferred over praziquantel (100 mg/kg daily in three doses for 15 days) because of its higher cysticidal effect and the fact that serum concentrations of praziquantel are decreased with concomitant use of corticosteroids. Simultaneous administration of corticosteroids reduces the headache, vomiting and other complications that may result from the inflammation induced by dying parasites; their use is indicated in treatment of multiple intraparenchymal cysts.

Cysticercotic encephalitis should not be treated with cysticidal drugs because this may result in increased intracranial pressure. Treatment for this condition is with high-dose steroids and diuretics. Cysticidal treatment is also not indicated for individuals with calcified lesions alone since these represent degenerated parasites.

Treatment of extraparenchymal cysts is considerably more complex. Subarachnoid and Sylvian fissure cysts should be treated with cysticidal drugs and high-dose steroids, although placement of a ventricular shunt should be performed first in cases with hydrocephalus. Ventricular cysts should be excised surgically or by neuroendoscopy; adjunct antiparasitic treatment is controversial.

OTHER LARVAL CESTODE INFECTIONS

Coenurosis

Humans are occasionally accidentally infected with the metacestode (juvenile stage) of *Taenia multiceps*, *T. brauni*, *T. serialis* or other *Taenia* spp., the adult form of which normally infects dogs. Intermediate hosts include cattle and sheep or goats. The metacestode, known as a coenurus, often invades the central nervous system where it forms a large cyst, often more than 2 cm in diameter, with multiple invaginated protoscolices.

Human cases are rare and largely occur in Africa, although infections have been reported worldwide. Diagnostic criteria include epidemiologic, clinical, radiologic and, most often, biopsy findings; serology is not available. Treatment usually involves surgical excision if the cyst is accessible; specific anthelmintic therapy is unavailable.

Sparganosis

Infection by the migratory plerocercoid larvae of the cestodes *Spirometra mansonoides* and other *Spirometra* spp. is termed sparganosis. Although the definitive hosts remain unknown, intermediate hosts include reptiles, amphibians, birds and some mammals. Humans become infected from ingestion of the raw or undercooked flesh of an intermediate host such as inadequately cooked frog or snake meat, or from using the skin or flesh of such animals as a poultice for wounds or sore eyes, as is customary practice in parts of eastern Asia.

Clinically, a localized subcutaneous inflammatory swelling forms from entry of the larva into host tissue, which can slowly migrate and contains a single worm-like sparganum (Fig. 113.7). If the worm enters via a dressing placed over the eye, migration into the brain may occur along the optic nerve, with occasional devastating results. Treatment consists of surgical excision.

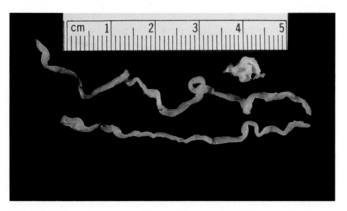

Fig. 113.7 Sparganum worm dissected from an inguinal mass. Courtesy of Guy Baily.

Trematode Infections

LIVER FLUKE INFECTIONS

Epidemiology

Clonorchis sinensis, *Opisthorchis viverrini* and *Opisthorchis felineus* are three closely related species which, for clinical purposes, can be considered as one. *C. sinensis* (Fig. 113.8) is the most common of the three, with over 25 million people infected in Japan, Korea, China, Cambodia, Laos and Vietnam. *O. viverrini* is found in northern Thailand and Laos, whereas *O. felineus* occurs throughout the Philippines, Japan, Vietnam, India and eastern Europe. All three species are acquired by ingesting raw or undercooked fresh water fish or crab harboring metacercariae, with dogs and cats serving as the most common reservoir hosts. Adult worms living in definite hosts produce eggs that are excreted in feces. Eggs that reach fresh water are eaten by the intermediate aquatic snail host, stimulating the miracidia to hatch and develop; motile cercariae subsequently released from the snails encyst under the scales of appropriate fresh water fish or crustaceae, completing the life cycle.

Pathogenesis and pathology

Ingested larvae excyst in the small intestine and transform into immature flukes that then migrate into the biliary tract, where they develop into hermaphroditic adult flukes that begin producing eggs after about 4 weeks. Adult worms may survive for decades within small bile ducts in the liver, where they feed on epithelium. Pathologic consequences arise from the mechanical injury and eosinophilic inflammatory reaction caused by adult worms present in the bile ducts. Over time, heavy infections lead to desquamation of the biliary epithelium, leading to hyperplasia, and eventual fibrosis or metaplastic changes that can lead to cholangiocarcinoma. This is especially true for heavy *O. viverrini* infections that may be associated with a 15-fold increase in the risk of developing cholangiocarcinoma.[10]

Clinical features

Most liver fluke infections are light and asymptomatic. Heavier infections may be associated with nonspecific epigastric or right upper quadrant pain, nausea, anorexia and diarrhea.[11] Heavy infections are also associated with recurrent ascending cholangitis and pancreatitis due to secondary bacterial infection and stone formation in chronically infected, fibrosed bile ducts.

Diagnosis and management

Eggs of liver flukes can be detected by microscopic examination of a concentrated sample of feces; differentiation between the eggs of the various species is often difficult. Eosinophilia and elevated levels of serum IgE are often present in heavy infections. On ultrasound, aggregates of flukes may be visualized as echogenic foci within bile ducts. Treatment with praziquantel 75 mg/kg/day in three doses for 2 days is highly effective, as is albendazole for 7 days.

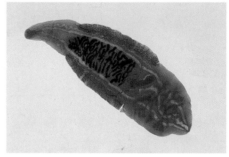

Fig. 113.8 An adult liver fluke (*Clonorchis sinensis*). The worm is typically about 2 cm in length. Courtesy of Guy Baily.

FASCIOLIASIS

Humans are occasionally infected with the sheep liver fluke, *Fasciola hepatica* (Fig. 113.9), or the closely related cattle fluke, *F. gigantica*. Both are acquired by eating contaminated leafy wild plants (especially watercress) that grow in standing bodies of fresh water. *F. hepatica* is found worldwide, whereas *F. gigantica* is endemic in Africa and Asia. After excysting in the small intestine, metacercariae penetrate the intestinal wall and migrate to the surface of the liver which they penetrate to enter the parenchymal tissue. Migration of the immature worms to the liver can be associated with fever, eosinophilia and painful hepatomegaly that usually subsides within a month.[12] Ingested metacercariae occasionally migrate to tissues other than the liver such as the brain or kidney, where they may present as a small mass lesion.

Microscopic identification of eggs in the feces is the definitive method of diagnosis, although the sensitivity can be low because eggs are produced only intermittently. Ultrasonography or CT scan may reveal hepatic or biliary abnormalities due to fascioliasis. If no eggs are found in the stool, diagnosis can be made using serology (an ELISA), even in the acute stage of infection, although there is some cross-reactivity with antigens of other trematodes.[13] *Fasciola* is the only human flatworm that is not effectively treated with praziquantel. Bithionol is the recommended treatment, although side-effects are frequent and it is not readily available. Nitazoxanide and the veterinary drug triclabendazole have also been successfully used to treat fascioliasis.

LUNG FLUKE INFECTIONS

Epidemiology

The lung fluke, *Paragonimus westermani*, is found throughout eastern Asia and infects a wide variety of mammalian reservoir hosts. Numerous fresh water crustaceans such as crabs and crayfish serve as intermediate hosts and infection occurs when these are eaten raw or lightly cooked. Several other members of the *Paragonimus* genus routinely cause human infection, mostly in areas of eastern Asia, central and western Africa, and Latin America.

Pathogenesis and pathology

Ingested metacercariae excyst in the small intestine and penetrate into the abdominal cavity where they develop into immature flukes before crossing the diaphragm to enter the lungs and mature into reproductive

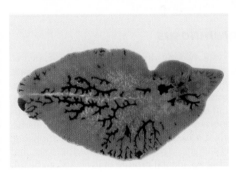

Fig. 113.9 A typical adult of *Fasciola hepatica*, measuring 30 × 14 μm.

adults within 2–3 months. *P. westermani* usually lives as pairs of worms within a host-derived fibrous capsule at the periphery of the lungs. Pathology results from the local effects of established adult worms and the surrounding inflammatory reaction characterized by eosinophilic infiltration. Occasionally, worms develop in ectopic sites such as the brain, muscle, liver or skin. Other species of *Paragonimus* can cause significant tissue damage as the larvae migrate through the viscera.

Clinical features

Adult *P. westermani* worms may cause progressive disease characterized by chronic cough that is productive of blood-tinged sputum. Complications include recurrent bacterial pneumonia and lung abscess formation. Larval migration due to non-*P. westermani* species, especially in Asia, may give rise to migratory subcutaneous nodules and more seriously to an eosinophilic meningitis.[14]

Diagnosis and management

Diagnosis is by microscopic identification of eggs in the sputum or feces (due to swallowed sputum). Serologic tests are also available but do not differentiate between current and past infection. Chest radiography may reveal cavitary disease that must be distinguished from lung abscess due to other causes, especially tuberculosis. Eosinophilia is common. Praziquantel at a dose of 75 mg/kg in three divided doses for 2 days is the drug of choice and is effective against extrapulmonary disease.

INTESTINAL FLUKE INFECTIONS

Over 50 species of intestinal flukes have been reported in humans, but most cases are due to *Fasciolopsis buski*, *Echinostoma* and *Heterophyes* species. All are found throughout eastern Asia, whereas *Heterophyes* is also found in the Middle East and North Africa. All are zoonoses and infect humans only incidentally; for *F. buski*, the reservoir hosts include pigs and dogs. Humans acquire infection by consuming contaminated aquatic plants (especially bamboo shoots and water chestnuts for *F. buski*) or fish (*Echinostoma* and *Heterophyes*). Infections are usually asymptomatic, although heavy *Fasciolopsis* infections, often with more than 500 worms, can result in diarrhea alternating with constipation, abdominal pain, nausea and vomiting.[15] Intestinal obstruction or malabsorption may develop in the most severe cases.

Diagnosis is based on identification of characteristic operculated eggs on microscopic examination of feces. The treatment of choice for all intestinal flukes is praziquantel 75 mg/kg in three divided doses given in one day.

REFERENCES

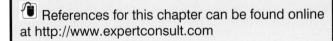

References for this chapter can be found online at http://www.expertconsult.com

Hydatid disease

Echinococcus spp. are cestode parasites commonly known as small tapeworms of carnivorous animals. Their medical importance lies in the infection of humans by the larval stage of the parasites, predominantly including two species:

- *Echinococcus granulosus*, which is the causative agent of cystic hydatid disease (or cystic echinococcosis, CE);[1] and
- *Echinococcus multilocularis*, which causes alveolar echinococcosis (AE).[2]

A few other species or genotypes, namely *E. equinus*, *E. ortleppi*, *E. vogel* (*vogeli*), *E. oligarthrus* and *E. shiquicus*, are only very rarely or not found in humans at all, and will thus not be covered in the present chapter.

EPIDEMIOLOGY

Echinococcus granulosus

Echinococcus granulosus parasitizes as a small tapeworm the small intestine of dogs and occasionally other carnivores. The shedding of gravid proglottids or eggs in the feces occurs within 4–6 weeks after infection of the definitive host (Fig. 114.1). Ingestion of eggs by intermediate host animals or humans results in the release of oncospheres into the gastrointestinal tract, which then migrate to primary target organs such as liver and lungs, and less frequently to other organs (Fig. 114.2). Usually, the fully mature metacestode (i.e. hydatid cyst) develops within several months or years.

Infections with *E. granulosus* occur worldwide, predominantly in countries of South and Central America, the European and African part of the Mediterranean area, the Middle East and some sub-Saharan countries, Russia and China. The annual incidence rates of diagnosed human cases/100 000 inhabitants vary widely, for example 13 in Greece, 143 in some provinces of Argentina, 197 in the Hinjang province of China and 220 in the Turkana district of Kenya. Most cases observed in Central Europe and the USA are associated with immigrants from highly endemic areas. Various strains of *E. granulosus* have been described, and differ especially in their infectivity for intermediate hosts such as humans. The most important strains for human infection include sheep (G1) and cattle (G5) as intermediate hosts.

Echinococcus multilocularis

The natural life cycle of *E. multilocularis* involves predominantly red and arctic foxes as definitive hosts (Fig. 114.3), but domestic dogs can also become infected and represent an important infection source for humans in highly endemic areas.[3] In the definitive host, egg production starts as early as 28 days after infection. After egg ingestion by a rodent or a human, larval maturation will occur practically exclusively within the liver tissue (see Fig. 114.2); subsequent metastases may affect adjacent or distant tissues, such as lungs or brain. Proliferation occurs by exogenous budding of metacestode tissue with a progressive tumor-like growth; central necrotic cavities may develop and cause differential diagnostic problems.

The geographic distribution of *E. multilocularis* is restricted to the northern hemisphere. In North America, the cestode is mainly present in the subarctic regions of Alaska and Canada, but an apparent expansion of distribution within the North–Central American continent was documented. In Europe, relatively frequent reports of AE in humans occur in central and eastern France, Switzerland, Austria and Germany. Within the past 10 years, the endemic area of Europe now includes many more countries such as Belgium, The Netherlands and Italy, and most former Eastern bloc countries as far up as Estonia. The Asian areas where *E. multilocularis* occurs include the whole zone of tundra, from the White Sea eastward to the Bering Strait, covering large parts of Russia, China and northern Japan.

Worldwide there are scant data on the overall prevalence of human AE. Some well-documented studies demonstrate a generally low prevalence among affected human populations. The annual mean incidence of new cases in different areas including Switzerland, France, Germany and Japan has therefore been reported to vary between 0.1 and 1.2/100 000 inhabitants.[1,2] The incidence of human cases correlates with the prevalence in foxes and the fox population density. Recently, a study documented that a fourfold increase of the fox population in Switzerland resulted in a statistically significant increase of the annual incidence of AE cases.[4]

PATHOGENESIS AND PATHOLOGY

Echinococcus granulosus

Cystic echinococcosis (cystic hydatid disease) is clinically related to the presence of one or more well-delineated spherical primary cysts, most frequently formed in the liver, but other organs such as the lungs, kidney, spleen, brain, heart and bone may also be affected (see Fig. 114.2). Tissue damage and organ dysfunction result mainly from this gradual process of space-occupying displacement of vital host tissue, vessels or parts of organs. Consequently, clinical manifestations are primarily determined by the site, size and number of the cysts, and are therefore highly variable. Accidental rupture of the cysts can be followed by a massive release of cyst fluid and hematogenous or other dissemination of protoscolices. This can result in anaphylactic reactions and multiple secondary cystic echinococcosis (as protoscolices can develop into secondary cysts within the same intermediate host).

The histology of a typical hydatid cyst exhibits the germinal layer as the primary site of parasite development (see Fig. 114.1). It is surrounded by a parasite-derived thick laminated layer, which is rich in aminocarbohydrates, as shown by periodic acid–Schiff (PAS) positivity. The germinal layer forms protoscolices and brood capsules within the

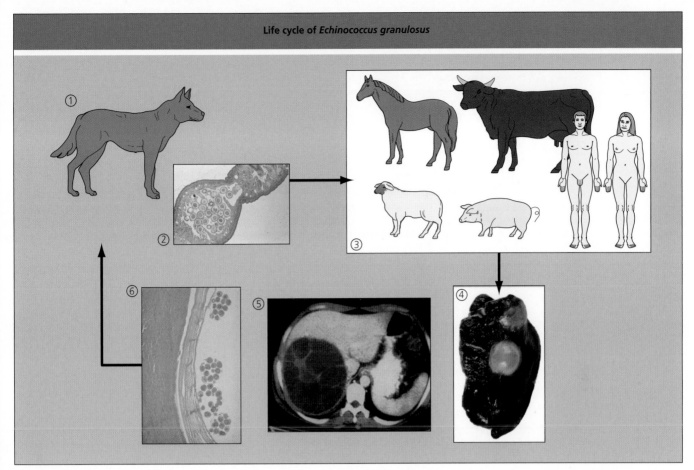

Life cycle of *Echinococcus granulosus*

Fig. 114.1 Life cycle of *Echinococcus granulosus*. Adult tapeworms parasitize the small intestine of definitive hosts, mainly dogs (1). Parasite proglottids and eggs are shed with the feces (2), such eggs being infectious for intermediate hosts including humans (3). Hydatid cyst formation occurs predominantly in the liver (4), but also in lungs and other organs. Imaging techniques such as CT (5) demonstrate well-delineated, fluid-filled, usually unilocular bladder-like lesions. Internal daughter cysts may be visible in larger cysts as septated segments within the primary cyst. Histologically, the cyst by itself consists of a very thin inner germinal and nucleated layer with a predominantly syncytial structure (6). The germinal layer is externally protected by an acellular laminated layer of variable thickness. The endogenous formation of brood capsules and protoscolices is a prerequisite for completion of the life cycle (6), which occurs when definitive hosts ingest protoscolex-containing hydatid cysts.

cyst lumen. Granulae, calcareous corpuscles and occasionally free daughter cysts are often observed. The parasite evokes an immune response, which is involved in the formation of a host-derived adventitious capsule. This often calcifies uniquely in the periphery of the cyst, one of the typical features found in imaging procedures. In the liver there may be cholestasis. Commonly, there is pressure atrophy of the surrounding parenchyma. Immunologically, the coexistence of elevated quantities of interferon (IFN)-γ, interleukin (IL)-4, IL-5, IL-6 and IL-10 observed in most of hydatid patients supports Th1, Th17 and Th2 cell activation in CE. In particular, Th1 cell activation seemed to be more related to protective immunity, whereas Th2 cell activation was related to susceptibility to disease.[5]

Echinococcus multilocularis

In infected humans the *E. multilocularis* metacestode (larva) develops primarily in the liver (see Fig. 114.2). Occasionally, secondary lesions form metastases in the lungs, brain and other organs. The typical lesion appears macroscopically as a dispersed mass of fibrous tissue with a conglomerate of scattered vesiculated cavities with diameters ranging from a few millimeters to centimeters in size. In advanced chronic cases, a central necrotic cavity containing a viscous fluid may form, and rarely there is a bacterial superinfection. The lesion often contains focal zones of calcification, typically within the metacestode tissue and not in the periphery as in CE.

Histologically, the hepatic lesion is characterized by a conglomerate of small vesicles and cysts demarcated by a thin PAS-positive laminated layer with or without an inner germinative layer (see Fig. 114.3). Parasite proliferation is usually accompanied by a granulomatous host reaction, including vigorous synthesis of fibrous and germinative tissue in the periphery of the metacestode, as well as necrotic changes centrally. In contrast to lesions in susceptible rodent hosts, lesions from infected human patients rarely show protoscolex formation within vesicles and cysts.

Genetic and immunologic host factors are responsible for the resistance shown by some patients in whom there is an early 'dying out' or 'abortion' of the metacestode.[6] Therefore, not everyone infected with *E. multilocularis* is susceptible to unlimited metacestode proliferation, developing symptoms on average within 5–15 years after infection.[2,3] The host mechanisms modulating the course of infection are most likely of an immunologic nature, including primarily suppressor T-cell interactions. Thus, the periparasitic granuloma, mainly composed of macrophages, myofibroblasts and T cells, contains a large number of CD4+ T cells in patients with abortive or died-out lesions, whereas in patients with active metacestodes the number of CD8+ T cells is increased. An immunosuppressive process is assumed to downregulate the lymphoid macrophage system. Conversely, the status of cured AE is generally reflected by a high *in-vitro* lymphoproliferative response. The cytokine mRNA levels following *E. multilocularis* antigen stimulation of lymphocytes show an enhanced production of

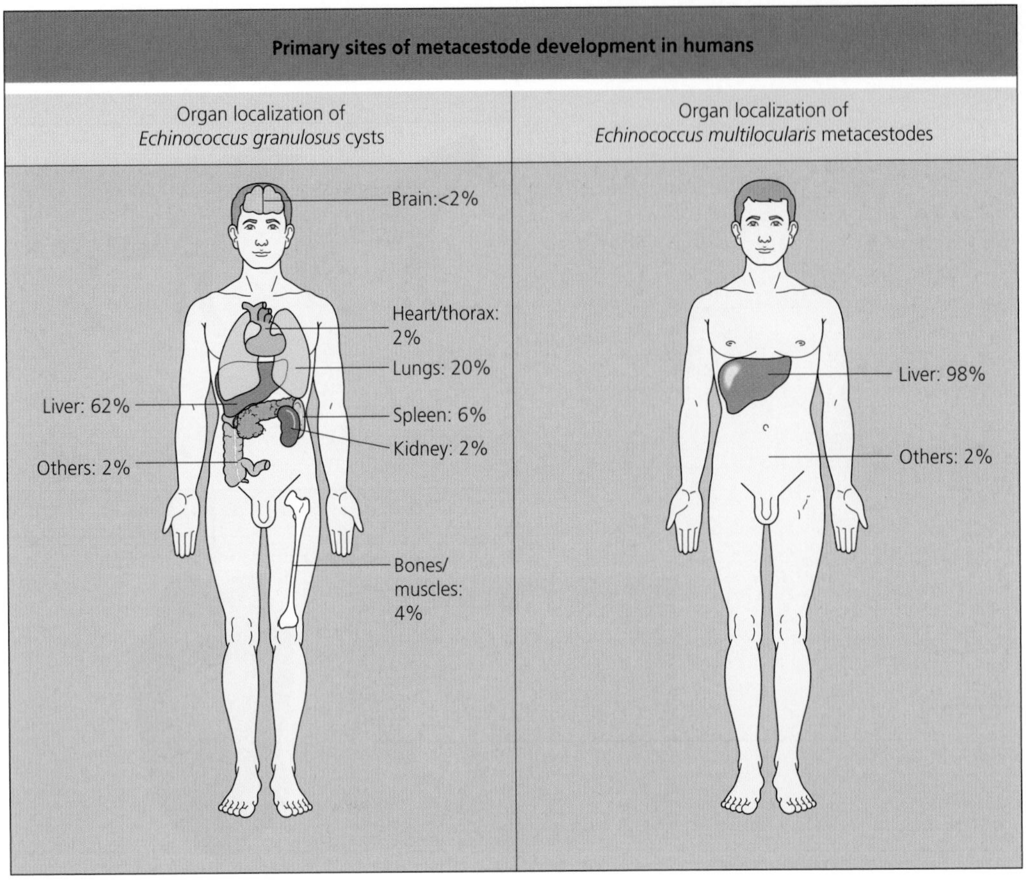

Fig. 114.2 Primary sites of metacestode development in humans. Organ distribution of the primary sites of metacestode development for *Echinococcus granulosus* (cystic echinococcosis) and *Echinococcus multilocularis* (alveolar echinococcosis) in human disease.

Th2-cell cytokine transcripts of IL-3, IL-4 and IL-10, including significant IL-5 mRNA expression in patients and not in healthy control donors.[7] A lack or deficiency of T helper (Th) cell activity such as in advanced AIDS is associated with a rapid and unlimited growth and dissemination of the parasite in AE,[8] and recovery of the T cell status in AIDS is prognostically favorable.[9]

PREVENTION

Prevention of both CE and AE focuses primarily on veterinary interventions to control the extent and intensity of infection in definitive host populations, which may be approached indirectly by controlling the prevalence in animal intermediate hosts. This includes regular pharmacologic treatment and taking sanitary precautions for handling domestic dogs to prevent infection and egg excretion, respectively.[10] Regular praziquantel treatment of wild-life definitive hosts may contribute to lowering of the prevalence in affected areas.[11] Finally, a vaccine to protect ruminant intermediate hosts from *E. granulosus* infection is available.[12]

CLINICAL FEATURES

The initial phase of primary infection is always asymptomatic. The infection may then remain asymptomatic for years or even decades depending upon the size and site of the developing cyst or metacestode mass. After a highly variable incubation period, the infection may become symptomatic due to a range of different events.

Cystic echinococcosis

The growing cyst can exert pressure on or induce dysformation of adjacent tissues, thus inducing dysfunction of the affected organ or vascular compromise. In the case of hepatic CE, signs and symptoms may include hepatomegaly with or without a palpable mass in the right upper quadrant, right epigastric pain, nausea, vomiting and occasionally cholestatic jaundice. In inoperable cases, hepatic compromise may lead to biliary cirrhosis and the Budd–Chiari syndrome.

Infestation of the lungs may present with chronic cough, hemoptysis, bilioptysis, pneumothorax, pleuritis, lung abscess and parasitic lung embolism.

Rare but often catastrophic infestations can affect the heart or the brain. In the heart this can present as a tumor, pericardial effusion including tamponade, complete heart block and sudden death. In the spine and brain presentation is as a tumor with neurologic symptoms. Hydatid disease should be considered as a cause of stroke in young patients.

A cyst may rupture and spill its content into the adjacent site. Rupture into the biliary tree will mimic biliary colic or result in cholestatic jaundice and cholangitis or pancreatitis. This is the presenting symptom in 5–25% of patients. Rupture in the liver but also in the lungs and other organs may result in acute anaphylactic shock reactions, which usually represent the initial and life-threatening manifestation. Each spilled protoscolex can develop into a secondary cyst. This is the most frequent reason for relapses that occur after surgical interventions.

A cyst can become superinfected; in hepatic CE this occurs in about 9% of patients and is an indication for rapid surgical intervention.[13]

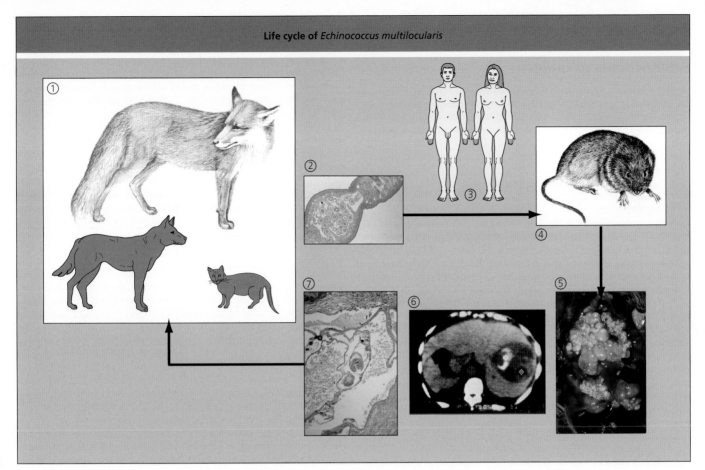

Life cycle of *Echinococcus multilocularis*

Fig. 114.3 Life cycle of *Echinococcus multilocularis*. This involves predominantly foxes as definitive hosts (1) and occasionally other carnivores such as domestic dogs or house cats. Egg production by the tapeworm starts as early as 28 days after infection (2). Eggs must be ingested by a suitable intermediate host, including humans (3) and various rodent species (4). As a result, the parasite metacestode primarily becomes established in the liver. Macroscopically, the typical lesion is characterized by a dispersed mass of fibrous tissue with a multitude of interconnected vesicles ranging from a few millimeters to centimeters in size (5). The lesion often contains focal necrotic zones with scattered calcifications, as demonstrated by CT (6). Histologically, the hepatic lesion consists of a conglomerate of small vesicles and cysts demarcated by a thin laminated layer with or without an inner germinal layer and, predominantly in the rodent intermediate host, protoscolex formation (7). Oral ingestion of protoscolex-containing metacestodes by definitive hosts completes the life cycle.

The majority of patients with CE have single organ involvement with solitary cysts. Simultaneous involvement of two or more organs is observed in 10–15% of patients, depending on the geographic origin of the patient and the strain of the parasite. In hepatic CE, the right lobe is more frequently affected than the left. Cyst size usually varies between 1 and 15 cm in diameter. Cyst growth ranges between a size increase of a few millimeters (1/3 of the patients) to approximately 10 mm (most of the patients); 1/10 of the patients exhibit a rapid increase with an annual average of 30 mm. In Europe, the average age of patients at diagnosis is 36 years. Approximately 10% of the CE cases occur in children, and the rate of lung involvement is significantly increased among this group. Pulmonary cysts occasionally become superinfected and this is best detected by CT scanning. The ratio of males to females may vary depending on the geographic area but is statistically not significant overall.

Hepatic alveolar echinococcosis

In patients with hepatic AE, the size of the liver lesion will range between a few millimeters up to 50 cm or more when patients present. A classification of the different types and stages of AE has recently

been released.[14] Typical calcifications occur in 70% of cases and central or peripheral necrotic cavities are also found in approximately 70% of cases. Clinical signs at diagnosis include hepatomegaly–cholestasis–jaundice, secondary biliary cirrhosis, liver abscess, portal hypertension and Budd–Chiari syndrome. The disease starts frequently with nonspecific symptoms such as epigastric pain or cholestatic jaundice. In complicated cases, evidence of secondary biliary cirrhosis and/or cholangitis will be found. Evidence of cholestasis is frequently present, while transaminases are only rarely and moderately elevated, in particular when there is central necrosis. One of the most feared complications is infection of a necrotic cavity and/or obstructed bile ducts, which are associated with very high mortality due to development of septic shock. Distant metastases can occur late in the disease; these have been described in brain, spine, lung and bone. Metastatic disease occurs in approximately 10–20% of patients.

The growth rate of the metacestode tissue is usually slow in immunocompetent patients. Analysis by CT scans indicated an average volume increase of 15 ml/year for progressive forms of AE. In Europe, the average age of AE patients at diagnosis is 55 years.[2] Young children rarely develop AE, unless the cellular immune system is compromised.[8] The ratio of males to females varies geographically, but any variation is not statistically significant.

DIAGNOSIS

Echinococcus granulosus

In many cases, imaging procedures together with serology will yield the diagnosis. Sonography is the primary diagnostic procedure of choice for hepatic cases, although false-positives occur in up to 10% of cases due to the presence of nonechinococcal serous cysts, abscesses or tumors. An international classification of ultrasound images in CE has been released.[15] The main diagnostic features of hydatid disease include:

- separation of the membrane from the wall;
- daughter cysts; and
- ruptured cysts.

Computed tomography is the best investigation for detecting extra-hepatic disease and volumetric follow-up assessment; MRI assists in the diagnosis by identifying changes in the intra- and extrahepatic venous systems. Ultrasonography is also helpful in following up treated patients as successfully treated cysts become hyperechogenic. Calcification of variable degree occurs in about 10% of the cysts.

Aspiration cytology appears to be particularly helpful in the detection of pulmonary, renal and other nonhepatic lesions for which imaging techniques and serology do not provide appropriate diagnostic support. The viability of aspirated protoscolices can be determined by microscopic demonstration of flame cell activity and trypan blue dye exclusion. Anti-Ag5 monoclonal antibody has been used for the detection of the respective antigen in diagnostic fine-needle aspiration biopsies (FNABs) from patients with suspected CE.[16] Immunodiagnostic tests to detect serum antibodies are used to support the clinical diagnosis of CE.[17] The indirect hemagglutination tests and the enzyme-linked immunosorbent assay using E. granulosus hydatid fluid antigen are diagnostically relatively sensitive for hepatic cases (85–98%). For pulmonary cysts and for cases in children the diagnostic sensitivity is markedly lower (50–60%); multiple organ involvement yields a very high sensitivity (90–100%). These tests are usually used for primary serologic screening. Specificity is low for other cestode infections. To increase specificity, primary seropositive sera are retested using a confirmation test such as immunoblotting for 8 kDa/12 kDa subunits of E. granulosus antigen B.[17]

Serologic studies to follow-up patients with CE postoperatively have shown that only a few antigens correlate with the activity status of a treated cyst, including antigen B[18] and antigen P29.[19]

Besides skin tests and basophil degranulation tests, diagnostic cellular immunodiagnosis has focused on in-vitro lymphoproliferative responses to E. granulosus antigens. The diagnostic sensitivity of cell-mediated immunodiagnosis is 75%, including the finding of sero-negative patients with a positive proliferation test.[17]

Echinococcus multilocularis

Among the imaging procedures, ultrasonography, CT and MRI are of greatest diagnostic value, none of those being uniquely superior.[20] Irregularly dispersed clusters of calcifications on plain abdominal radiographs may give the first clue as to the etiology of the disease; the percentage of calcifications within the lesions increases from 30% to nearly 100% as the disease progresses. Hyperechogenic and hypoecho-genic zones characterize the lesions. The cystic appearance may reflect central necrotic cavities. Similar findings can be found on CT and the lesions are typically not enhanced with contrast medium. The lesions are heterogeneous hypodense masses with irregular contours and lacking well-delineated walls. Hilar involvement can lead to liver atrophy, which is easily visualized by CT. Ultrasonography is the preferred imaging procedure for mass screening programs. Magnetic resonance imaging adds to diagnosis, in particular in cases with appropriate organ localization such as brain and bone, and to visualize pathologically altered microstructures in certain affected organs. Thus, MRI can give a precise analysis of the different components of the parasitic lesions

such as necrosis and fibrosis.[20] However, in contrast to CT, microcalcifications are not visualized by MRI.

Assessing the parasite viability in vitro following therapeutic interventions may be of tremendous advantage when compared with the invasive analysis of resected or biopsied samples. Such alternatives may be offered by magnetic resonance spectrometry or positron emission tomography (PET). The latter technique has recently been used for assessing the efficacy of chemotherapy in AE.[21] PET positivity actually demonstrates periparasitic inflammatory processes due to remaining activity of the metacestode tissue.

Immunodiagnosis represents a valuable secondary diagnostic tool complementary to imaging procedures and is useful for confirming the nature of the etiologic agent.[17] Serologic tests are more reliable in the diagnosis of AE than CE. The use of purified E. multilocularis antigens such as the Em2 antigen and recombinant antigens from the family of EMR proteins (EmII/3-10, EM10, EM4 and Em18, all four of them harboring an identical immunodominant oligopeptide sequence) exhibits diagnostic sensitivities ranging between 91% and 100%, with overall specificities of 98–100%.[17] These antigens allow discrimination between the alveolar and the cystic forms of disease with a reliability of 95%. Seroepidemiologic studies reveal asymptomatic preclinical cases of human AE as well as cases in which the metacestode has died at an apparently early stage of infection (see above).[3] Serologic tests are of value for assessing the efficacy of treatment and chemotherapy only when linked to appropriate imaging investigations. Prognostically, disappearance of anti-II/3-10 or anti-Em18 antibody levels coupled to PET negativity indicates inactivation of AE.[22] Cellular immune tests show that the in-vitro lymphoproliferative response to E. multilocularis antigen stimulation is high in cured patients who have had radical surgery and in patients with dead lesions, and is significantly lower in patients who have had partial or no surgical resection.

Histopathologic and immunohistochemical procedures to analyze surgically resected samples or biopsies obtained by FNAB include the use of species-specific MAbs such as MAbG11 or polymerase chain reaction.[16]

MANAGEMENT

The management of CE and AE follows the strategy recommended in the manual on echinococcosis published in 2001 by the Office International des Epizooties and the World Health Organization.[10]

Echinococcus granulosus

Surgery remains the mainstay in the treatment of hepatic hydatid disease. Cystectomy and pericystectomy offer a good chance for cure and should be undertaken wherever possible. Occasionally, formal hepatic resection will be required. Radical surgery – either pericystectomy or resection – is possible in 50–85% of cases. In the absence of complications this can be achieved with little mortality and an acceptable morbidity. Laparoscopic pericystectomy has been demonstrated to be as safe and effective as open laparotomy in selected cases with hepatic and/or splenic involvement.[23]

If surgical removal of the cyst is contraindicated, treatment of CE has several alternatives such as PAIR (Puncture, Aspiration, Injection of a helminthicide and Re-aspiration), chemotherapy or 'wait and observe' approach.

Indications for hepatic surgery include:

- large liver cysts with putatively multiple daughter cysts;
- single liver cysts, situated superficially, which may rupture spontaneously or as a result of trauma;
- bacterially superinfected cysts;
- cysts communicating with the biliary tree and/or exerting pressure on adjacent vital organs;
- brain, heart and kidney cysts, and spinal and bone cysts.

Relative contraindications are inoperable cases as defined for surgical procedures in general, patients with cysts difficult to access and abortive cysts that are either partly or totally calcified.

A direct communication between the hydatid cyst and the biliary tree may contraindicate the use of protoscolicidal solutions, which can cause chemical cholangitis leading to sclerosing cholangitis. Formalin should not be used for this reason. Protoscolicides with a relatively low risk of toxicity are 70–95% ethanol or 15–20% hypertonic saline solution; effective killing of protoscolices is only achieved after a long-term contact with the agent. Thus, double percutaneous aspiration and injection of alcohol into the cyst without re-aspiration of the ethanol, which remains *in situ*, may prove more efficacious than PAIR (see below).[24]

Preoperative chemotherapy with albendazole for up to 3 months (with a minimum of 4 days) is indicated for reducing the risk of secondary echinococcosis after operation.[25] Therapy may additionally include praziquantel that exhibits a good antiprotoscolicidal activity. Diagnostic puncture of hydatid cysts increases the risk of cyst rupture and dissemination of protoscolices and is therefore not recommended.

PAIR has become well justified in selected cases (Table 114.1).[26]

Treatment with benzimidazoles (preferably albendazole) is highly recommended for 4 days prior to intervention. After successful instillation of protoscolicides and re-aspiration, benzimidazoles should be given for 3 months.

Treatment of nonresected cysts with benzimidazoles (albendazole or mebendazole) results in cyst disappearance in 30% of cases; in 30–50% of patients there is cyst degeneration or a significant reduction in cyst size and in 20–40% of patients the cysts show no morphologic change.[10] Indications for chemotherapy include inoperable patients as listed above.

The formerly conventional dosage of albendazole (10–15 mg/kg/day in several 1-monthly courses with 14-day intervals) included three courses at minimum, and more than six courses were usually not necessary. This strategy is more commonly replaced by continuous treatment, which demonstrated equal or improved efficacy without increased adverse effects when compared with cyclic treatment.[27] For mebendazole, the usual dosage is 40–50 mg/kg/day for at least 3–6 months. Praziquantel has been proposed as an additional antiprotoscolicidal drug to be given once a week in a dose of 40 mg/kg along with benzimidazoles. It is also recommended before and after surgery/PAIR when there is a risk of cyst rupture and release of protoscolices.

Echinococcus multilocularis

The following strategies are commonly accepted for treatment of AE:

- the first choice of treatment is radical surgical resection of the entire parasitic lesion from the liver and other affected organs in all operable cases, with excision of the parasitic lesion following the rules of radical tumor surgery;
- concomitant chemotherapy is mandatory for all cases after radical surgery or after nonsurgical interventional procedures;[27] and
- long-term chemotherapy for inoperable or only partially resectable cases and all patients after liver transplantation.[10]

Presurgical chemotherapy is not indicated for AE. The daily dosage for albendazole and mebendazole treatment is the same as for CE. For albendazole, continuous treatment is well tolerated for a duration up to 6 years, and is replaced by the former discontinuous scheme (see above) only in cases with side-effects related to medication. For mebendazole, plasma drug levels should be over 74 ng/ml (250 nmol/l). Generally, the duration of treatment is at least 2 years after radical surgery or continuously for many years for inoperable cases or if resection is incomplete. In experimental trials, alternative compounds have been used to treat AE. Experimental studies included amphotericin B[28] and nitazoxanide.[29]

As an ultimate goal, liver transplantation has been proposed for a selected group of patients who have inoperable AE and chronic liver failure. However, the indications are limited and focus on cases with extensive lesions restricted to the liver and secondary liver disease leading to chronic liver failure;[30] relapse is frequent and caused by extrahepatic metacestodes, which rapidly proliferate under immunosuppressed conditions.

REFERENCES

🖰 References for this chapter can be found online at http://www.expertconsult.com

---

Table 114.1 Indications and relative contraindications for PAIR

Indications

- Patients refusing surgery
- Infected cysts not communicating with the biliary vessel system
- Inoperable patients (see contraindications for surgery, above)
- Pregnant patients
- Anechoic lesion ≥5 cm in diameter
- Cysts with a regular double laminated layer
- Cysts with more than five septal divisions
- Multiple cysts (≥5 cm in diameter) in different liver segments
- Relapse after surgery
- Failure to respond to chemotherapy

Relative contraindications

- Inaccessible or risky location of the cyst in the liver
- Multiple septal divisions
- Cysts with echogenic lesions
- Inactive cysts or calcified lesions
- Communicating cysts; cysts located in the lung and bones; and some others
- Presence of exophytic cysts or dilated bile ducts on preoperative imaging

Filariasis

INTRODUCTION

Lymphatic filariasis (LF), onchocerciasis and loiasis are the three most important filarial infections of humans (Table 115.1) and for two of these (lymphatic filariasis and onchocerciasis) there are now major public health initiatives to control or eliminate them completely.[1–3] All of these infections are caused by parasites transmitted by biting arthropods (mosquitoes or flies). Each goes through a complex life cycle that includes a slow maturation (often 3–12 months) from the infective larval stage carried by the insects, to the adult worm that resides either in the lymph nodes and adjacent lymphatics or in the subcutaneous tissue. The offspring of the adults, the microfilariae, are 200–350 μm in length and either circulate in the blood (lymphatic filariasis and loiasis) or migrate through the skin (onchocerciasis), awaiting ingestion by the insect vectors in which they develop infectivity for humans to continue this complex life cycle.

EPIDEMIOLOGY

Lymphatic filariasis

There are 120 million people in at least 80 countries of the world who are infected with lymphatic filarial parasites, and it is estimated that 1.2 billion people (20% of the world's population) are at risk of acquiring infection.[1] Of these infections, 90% are caused by *Wuchereria bancrofti*, whose only host is humans, and most of the remainder are caused by *Brugia malayi*. The major vectors for *W. bancrofti* are culicine mosquitoes in most urban and semiurban areas, anopheline mosquitoes in the more rural areas of Africa and elsewhere, and *Aedes* spp. in many of the endemic Pacific islands. For the *Brugia* parasites, *Mansonia* spp. serve as the major vector, but in some areas anopheline mosquitoes are responsible for transmitting the infection. *Brugia* parasites are confined to areas of eastern and southern Asia, especially India, Malaysia, Indonesia and the Philippines.

Onchocerciasis

There are almost 18 million people in 37 endemic countries who are infected with *Onchocerca volvulus*; 99% of these people live in sub-Saharan Africa.[2] Humans are the exclusive host for *O. volvulus*; there is no nonhuman reservoir of infection. Blackflies of several *Simulium* species are the vectors of infection, and because the larvae of these flies require fast-flowing water for their development, transmission is limited to those areas within the flight range of the flies that breed in such rivers. Thus, the distribution of onchocerciasis ('river blindness') is very much determined by river systems and tributaries in Africa, Yemen and the Americas, where the infection is endemic.

Loiasis

Loa loa infects approximately 12 million people in the rainforest belt of western and central Africa and equatorial Sudan, where the *Chrysops* vector flies can easily find breeding spots.[3] Although *L. loa*

Table 115.1 Principal filarial diseases

Disease	Number of people infected worldwide	Parasite	Vector	Principal clinical manifestation	Distribution	Location of micro-filariae within the body	Periodicity
Lymphatic filariasis	120 million	*Wuchereria bancrofti*	Mosquitoes	Lymphedema, elephantiasis, genital pathology (hydrocele)	Tropics worldwide	Blood	Nocturnal (95%), 'subperiodic' (5%)
		Brugia malayi	Mosquitoes	Lymphedema, elephantiasis	Asia, India, Philippines	Blood	Nocturnal (75%), 'subperiodic' (25%)
Onchocerciasis	18 million	*Onchocerca volvulus*	Blackflies	Dermatitis, blindness	Africa (99%), Americas, Yemen	Skin	Minimal
Loiasis	12 million	*Loa loa*	Deer flies	Angioedema, 'eyeworm'	Africa	Blood	Diurnal

can be found in a number of nonhuman African primates, there is little or no cross-infection between the cycles of *L. loa* in humans and in nonhuman primates.

PATHOGENESIS AND PATHOLOGY

Pathology associated with the filariases results from a complex interplay of the pathogenic potential of the parasite (and its endosymbionts), the immune response of the host and external ('complicating') bacterial and fungal infections.[1–6]

Lymphatic filariasis

Although genital abnormalities (especially hydrocele) and lymphedema or elephantiasis are the most recognizable clinical entities associated with lymphatic filarial infections (Fig. 115.1), earlier changes can be detected when lymphoscintigraphy or ultrasound techniques are used,[4] including lymphatic dilatation with abnormal lymphatic function. Such subclinical changes can be seen even in young children[7] and can occur with or without a localized inflammatory response. Secondary host inflammation, including responses to bacterial and fungal superinfections of tissues with compromised lymphatic function, causes most of the progression and physical destruction associated with elephantiasis. Endotoxins released when the *Wolbachia* endosymbionts of the parasite are killed during natural or drug-induced parasite death may also play a role in inducing this local inflammation.

The pathology in lymphatic filariasis that is immune mediated most commonly derives from the lymphatic dysfunction consequences of the responses to dead or dying worms in the lymphatics; however, for the syndrome of tropical pulmonary eosinophilia, the pathogenesis is distinctly different,[8] the inflammation resulting from immunologic (allergic) hyperresponsiveness to the microfilaria-stage parasites.

Onchocerciasis

Most of the significant pathology in onchocerciasis affects the skin (Fig. 115.2) or the eyes.[2] There are both noninflammatory and inflammatory routes to tissue damage.[5] In 'steady-state' chronic *O. volvulus* infections, between 10 000 and 500 000 microfilariae are produced each day. These microfilariae migrate through the skin, inducing little inflammatory response; however, the elaboration of collagenases, elastases and other enzymatic molecules leads to hyperpigmentation, atrophy and thinning of the skin (see Fig. 115.2). Superimposed inflammatory reactions to dying microfilariae result in episodic papular

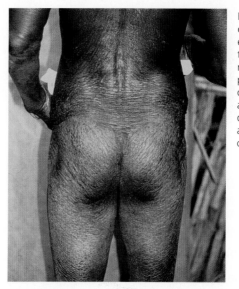

Fig. 115.2 Onchocerciasis. Evidence of excoriation caused by the patient's trying to relieve the maddening pruritus caused by onchocerciasis. Note also the marked dermal atrophy associated with chronic infection.

dermatitis. In the eyes, these inflammatory responses result either in a characteristic punctate keratitis and, ultimately, anterior segment blindness or in uveitis and retinal lesions that can lead to posterior segment blindness. Again, the endosymbiont bacterium (*Wolbachia* spp.) within *O. volvulus* adult worms and microfilariae might also play a role in the pathogenesis of onchocerciasis skin and eye disease.[9]

Loiasis

'Calabar' swellings, the angioedematous lesions characteristic of loiasis, have been less well studied. Presumably, these are immune-mediated inflammatory responses to migrating subcutaneous adult worms (Fig. 115.3). Not common in untreated patients, but increasingly problematic in populations receiving ivermectin for co-endemic onchocerciasis, is a central nervous system (CNS) depression syndrome leading to coma or even death.[3] Its pathogenesis is suspected to involve inflammatory responses to dying microfilariae in cerebral vessels, but the details remain uncertain.

PREVENTION

Filarial infections can be acquired only from vector-borne infective larvae. Therefore, prevention of infection can be achieved either by decreasing contact between humans and vectors, generally through vector control efforts, or by decreasing the amount of infection the vector can acquire to pass on to uninfected individuals, through treating the human host.

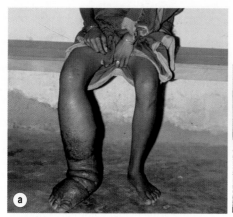

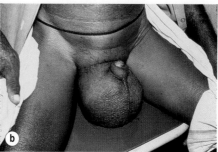

Fig. 115.1 Elephantiasis. (a) Already advanced elephantiasis in a 14-year-old Indian girl who has bancroftian filariasis. Although such clinical expression of filarial disease is more commonly seen in adults, infection in endemic areas is usually established in early childhood. (b) Scrotal elephantiasis in an adult man who has bancroftian filariasis.

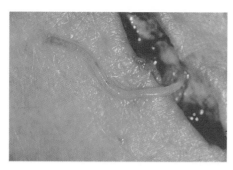

Fig. 115.3 *Loa loa* adult worm. The worm has been teased from the subcutaneous tissue after incision was made through a small pruritic papule (0.5 cm in diameter) in an expatriate patient who had loiasis. Such papules can occur spontaneously or after treatment with DEC.

Lymphatic filariasis

Population-based prevention

Efforts to decrease filariasis in populations through mosquito-vector control have usually proved ineffective owing to high cost and the long lifespan of the parasite (4–8 years). With the advent of extremely effective single-dose, once-yearly, two-drug regimens (albendazole 400 mg plus either ivermectin 200–400 µg/kg or diethylcarbamazine (DEC) 6 mg/kg), the alternative approach of treating whole populations (and thereby decreasing microfilariae available to the vectors) has become the norm.[10] Indeed, it is this strategy that forms the basis of the new Global Program to Eliminate Lymphatic Filariasis undertaken by the World Health Organization (WHO) and a Global Alliance of public and private sector partners.[1,10]

Individual-based prevention

Contact with infected mosquitoes can be decreased through the use of personal insect repellents, bed nets or insecticide-impregnated materials. Alternatively, suggestive evidence from animal models and some limited experience in human populations indicate that a prophylactic regimen of DEC (6 mg/kg/day for 2 days each month) could provide effective protection against infection.

Onchocerciasis

Population-based prevention

Despite its considerable expense, a highly successful program to prevent onchocerciasis based on large-scale insecticiding to control the vector blackflies was undertaken in 11 West African countries by the WHO, the United Nations Development Program and the World Bank. In its 27 years of existence this 'Onchocerciasis Control Program' was extraordinarily successful in 'reclaiming' both land and lives of people otherwise severely compromised by onchocercal disease.[2] However, this expensive and difficult approach to population-based prevention of onchocerciasis has been superseded by a new strategy that both treats and prevents infection through the use of once-yearly ivermectin in affected populations of all countries where onchocerciasis is endemic.[2]

Individual-based prevention

Decreased contact with infected blackflies through protective clothing and repellents is helpful in preventing infection. Although no prophylactic treatment regimen has yet been defined, studies employing monthly doses of ivermectin in cattle exposed to the related parasite *O. ochengi* show a dramatic prophylactic effect of ivermectin,[11] but studies have not yet been undertaken to see whether similar prophylactic efficacy can be shown for ivermectin in humans as well.

Loiasis

Population-based prevention

No specific prevention efforts in populations have been undertaken.

Individual-based prevention

There are good data that repeated use of DEC (300 mg weekly or 6 mg/kg/day for 2 days each month in adults) is effective prophylaxis against acquisition of *L. loa* infection.[12]

CLINICAL FEATURES

Lymphatic filariasis

Chronic manifestations

Hydrocele, even though found only with *W. bancrofti* (and not *Brugia*) infections, is the most common clinical manifestation of lymphatic filariasis. It is seen principally after puberty and there is a progressive increase in prevalence with age.[13] In some endemic communities, as many as 40–60% of all adult males have hydrocele. It often develops in the absence of overt inflammatory reactions and, indeed, many patients who have hydrocele also have microfilariae circulating in the blood. The localization of adult worms in the lymphatics of the spermatic cord leads to a thickening of the cord so that the cord is palpable on physical examination of most patients. Hydroceles can become massive but still occur in the absence of any lymphedema or elephantiasis in the penis and scrotum (see Fig. 115.1).[14]

Although lymphedema can also develop in the absence of overt inflammatory reactions and in the early stages be associated with microfilaremia, the development of elephantiasis (either of the limbs or the genitals) is most frequently associated with a history of recurrent inflammatory episodes. Patients who have chronic lymphedema or elephantiasis are rarely microfilaremic. Very important in the progression of these lesions is the fact that the redundant skin folds, cracks and fissures of the skin provide havens for bacteria and fungi to thrive and intermittently penetrate the epidermis, leading to either local or systemic infections.

Chyluria, another of the chronic filarial syndromes, is caused by the intermittent flow of intestinal lymph (chyle) through ruptured lymphatics into the renal pelvis and subsequently into the urine. The mechanisms underlying this have not been well defined and the clinical course is known to be intermittent. Nutritional compromise can, however, be severe in patients who have chronic chyluria; special diets (low-fat and high-protein, supplemented with fluids) can often be helpful.[1]

Acute manifestations

There are four distinct acute manifestations of lymphatic filariasis, each with a different set of causative mechanisms and pathogenic implications.

The first and most important is acute inflammation of the limbs or scrotum (sometimes with systemic symptoms) that is related to bacterial or fungal superinfection of tissues with already compromised lymphatic function.[14]

Often confused with this picture in the past, a second type of acute syndrome is characterized by initiation of inflammation in the lymph nodes (commonly the inguinal or axillary node) with 'retrograde' extension down the lymphatic tract and an accompanying 'cold' edema. Here the inflammation appears to be immune mediated around dying parasites in the nodes; it is much less frequent than the episodes of inflammation initiated by dermal infection.[14]

A third acute filarial syndrome is tropical pulmonary eosinophilia (Weingarton's syndrome), a distinctly different syndrome caused by an immunologic hyperresponsiveness to filarial infection.[8] It is characterized by:

- extremely high levels of peripheral blood eosinophilia;
- asthma-like symptoms;
- restrictive (and often obstructive) lung disease;
- very high levels of specific antifilarial antibodies; and
- an excellent therapeutic response to appropriate antifilarial treatment with DEC.

While occurring with a frequency of less than 1% of all cases of clinical filariasis, it is nevertheless a severe condition that can lead to chronic interstitial fibrosis and pulmonary failure.

The fourth (and least commonly recognized) form of acute inflammatory reaction is that seen early after infection, particularly in expatriates who are exposed to and acquire filarial infection for the first time. Lymphangitis occurs around developing larval and early adult stages in these patients, associated with acute eosinophilic inflammation.[8]

Asymptomatic presentations

Of all the patients who have lymphatic filariasis, at least half appear clinically asymptomatic. Some of these have microfilariae circulating in their blood, while others have infections identifiable only by filarial antigen in the circulation. Essentially all have hidden damage to their lymphatic or renal systems.[7,15] A precise understanding of the natural history of these 'asymptomatic' infections is still not available, despite their obvious importance in the development of clinical disease.

A variety of other syndromes coexisting with filariasis are found in filarial-endemic regions; because they sometimes show evidence of therapeutic response to DEC they have been regarded as possible manifestations of lymphatic filariasis. These include arthritis (typically monoarticular), endomyocardial fibrosis, tenosynovitis, thrombophlebitis, lateral popliteal nerve palsy and others. Although future studies may strengthen an etiologic relationship with filariasis, such presentations cannot now be confidently attributed to lymphatic filarial infection.

Onchocerciasis

Chronic presentations

Most damage from onchocerciasis occurs in the skin and eye. Subcutaneous nodules (generally 1–6 cm in diameter) can be palpated superficially, but most skin involvement is a waxing and waning of maculopapular rashes, essentially always accompanied by itching (see Fig. 115.2),[2] likely because of allergic responses to dying microfilariae. During the long course of infection, the skin becomes extensively damaged, losing much of its elasticity and even pigmentation. Indeed, when the skin over the inguinal nodes (which are often enlarged by their continued stimulation from dying microfilariae) becomes so atrophic that it cannot support the underlying lymph nodes, the clinical presentation of 'hanging groin' occurs.

In the eye, acute changes are those associated with dying microfilariae and the local inflammatory reactions that they induce.[2] In the cornea, 'fluffy opacities' (inflammatory cells associated with the dying microfilariae) can lead to punctate keratitis, and in prolonged and heavy infection inflammation in the cornea results in sclerosing keratitis; inflammatory responses localized elsewhere in the eye lead to iridocyclitis, choroidoretinitis or optic atrophy. Longer-term complications of these inflammatory eye processes also include glaucoma and cataract.

Loiasis

The two most characteristic clinical features of loiasis are the passage of an adult filarial worm across the eye ('eye worm'), often in an otherwise asymptomatic person, and Calabar swellings.[3] The latter are localized areas of erythema and angioedema that may be 5–10 cm or more in size. Often they occur in the extremities and may last for several days before regressing spontaneously. If the inflammatory reaction extends to nearby joints or peripheral nerves, corresponding symptoms may develop. Routine radiographs of people in endemic areas may reveal calcified dead worms lying between the metacarpals.

Expatriate syndrome

'Expatriate syndrome' is a term to describe the clinical and immunologic hyperresponsiveness found in expatriate visitors to regions endemic for loiasis and other filariases. These people manifest prominent signs and symptoms of inflammatory reactions (including allergic reactions) to the mature or maturing parasites. In loiasis, these manifestations have included primarily Calabar swellings, hives, rashes and occasionally asthma.[12] In bancroftian filariasis (when military personnel or other migrants to endemic areas have acquired these infections), the manifestations have usually been lymphangitis, lymphadenitis and genital pain (from inflammation of the associated lymphatics), with hives, rashes and other 'allergic-like' manifestations, including blood eosinophilia.[8]

DIAGNOSIS

Except for *W. bancrofti* infections, diagnosis of filarial infections depends principally on the direct demonstration of the parasite (almost always microfilariae) in blood or skin specimens using relatively cumbersome techniques and having to take into account the periodicity (nocturnal or diurnal) of microfilariae (see Table 115.1). Most alternative methods based on detection of antibodies by immunodiagnostic tests have not proved to be satisfactory because of their failure to distinguish between active and past infections and their problems with specificity. There is good evidence, however, that recombinant antigens will greatly improve the value of such antibody-based immunodiagnostics in the future.

Lymphatic filariasis

Antigen detection

Circulating filarial antigen detection, with its very high specificity and sensitivity, should now be regarded as the 'gold standard' for diagnosing *W. bancrofti* infections.[16] Two commercial forms of this assay are available: one is based on the methodology of an enzyme-linked immunosorbent assay and yields semiquantitative results; the other is based on a simple card (immunochromatographic) test and yields only qualitative (positive or negative) answers. No such test is currently available for brugian filariasis.

Microfilaria detection

Before the development of the circulating filarial antigen assay, detection of microfilariae in blood was the standard approach to diagnosing lymphatic filarial infection, and it is the one still required today for both brugian filariasis and those situations where the antigen detection test is not available for bancroftian filariasis. Such assessments must take into account the possible nocturnal periodicity of the parasites when choosing the optimal time for drawing blood; namely, between 10.00 pm and 2.00 am for most brugian filariasis and bancroftian infections.[8] The simplest technique for examining blood or other fluids (e.g. hydrocele fluid or articular effusions) is to spread 20 μl evenly over a clean slide that is dried and then stained with Giemsa or a similar stain. A wet smear may also be made by diluting 20–40 μl of anticoagulated blood with water or 2% saponin, which will lyse the red blood cells but allow the microfilariae to remain motile and thus more readily identifiable. The larger the blood volumes examined, the greater will be the likelihood of detecting low levels of parasitemia. Other concentration techniques are also available.[8]

Clinical diagnosis

Many lymphatic filariasis patients are amicrofilaremic and therefore the diagnosis of these infections must be made 'clinically'. For amicrofilaremic syndromes other than tropical eosinophilia syndrome, serologic findings based on detecting IgG$_4$ antibodies have proved helpful, because this subclass of IgG has greater diagnostic specificity and is stimulated by the presence of active infection. Such antibody analyses also are particularly helpful in diagnosing the 'expatriate syndrome', in which background (i.e. pre-exposure) levels of IgG and especially of IgG_4 antibodies to filarial antigens are very low, so that elevated levels have significant diagnostic implications in association with the clinical presentation.[16]

Eosinophilia is a frequent concomitant of all filarial syndromes but is diagnostically helpful only when the eosinophil levels are extremely high (as in tropical eosinophilia or the expatriate syndrome).

Onchocerciasis

Parasitologic techniques are most commonly used to diagnose onchocerciasis.[2] Microfilariae can be visualized directly in the anterior chamber fluid of the eye by slit-lamp examination of patients who have been 'prepared' by remaining for 2 minutes in a head-down position to allow microfilariae to drift forward into the anterior chamber. Skin microfilariae can be visualized after a skin snip has removed the most superficial layers of skin with either a corneoscleral punch or a small needle and disposable razor blade to obtain approximately 1 mg of a bloodless piece of skin. This sample is then placed in saline or water for examination for the emergence of microfilariae after 30 minutes to 24 hours. Alternative tests include a polymerase chain reaction on skin-snip specimens or a patch test, in which DEC is incorporated into a cream that is placed on the skin, covered by gauze and the area later observed for development of papular dermatitis resulting from the death of the microfilarial parasites. Also, subcutaneous or deep nodules (generally 1–6 cm in size) can be detected by palpation or ultrasound, and the adult worms they contain can be identified histologically in specimens that have been removed surgically.

Loiasis

Diagnosis of loiasis remains dependent on direct parasitologic identification (most frequently microfilariae in the blood) or indirect serologic approaches in association with a compatible clinical presentation and exposure history.[3,17] *Loa loa* microfilarial periodicity in the blood means that blood sampling must be done near midday (usually between 12.00 pm and 2.00 pm). Treatment with DEC of some amicrofilaremic patients who have suspected loiasis can induce an inflammatory nodule which, on biopsy, frequently discloses an adult worm surrounded by acute inflammatory cells. Eosinophilia and antifilarial antibodies are important diagnostic tools in expatriates with extensive exposure to infection.[18] Radiographic assessment is of little diagnostic value in these patients, but because hypereosinophilia resulting from loiasis has been associated with endomyocardial disease, echocardiography is of value in establishing whether cardiac damage has occurred.

MANAGEMENT

Lymphatic filariasis

Treatment of the infection

Remarkable advances in treating lymphatic filarial infection have recently been achieved,[19] but most of these have focused not on individual patients but on the community reduction of microfilaremia through once-yearly treatment, as described above. As few clinical trials have focused on optimizing treatment for the individual patient, there are still insufficient data to permit formal recommendation for a change from the older treatment regimens (DEC 6 mg/kg/day for 12 days in bancroftian filariasis and for 6 days in brugian filariasis); importantly, however, essentially the entire effectiveness of such a 'course' of DEC results from the first dose.[20] Ivermectin, although very effective in decreasing levels of microfilaremia, appears not to kill adult worms and thus it cannot be expected to cure infection

completely. Albendazole, on the other hand, appears to kill the adult worms after prolonged courses (2–3 weeks) and to inhibit production of microfilariae after single doses (400 mg).[19]

Therefore, for treating infection in individual patients, in spite of the older textbook advice to use 6- or 12-day courses of DEC, more recent expert opinion[20] recommends use of either of the two single-dose, two-drug regimens currently employed in the Global Program to Eliminate Lymphatic Filariasis. These are DEC (6 mg/kg) plus albendazole (400 mg), and ivermectin (200–400 µg/kg) plus albendazole (400 mg). Because the use of DEC in patients who have either onchocerciasis or loiasis can be unsafe (see below), it is important that individual patients who have bancroftian filariasis and who live in areas endemic for these other infections be examined for co-infection with these parasites before being treated with DEC. While there may, in addition, be a role for multi-week doxycycline treatment of individual patients to cure infections,[21] additional studies are required before such a recommendation can be advanced.

Both diethylcarbamazine and ivermectin, given at the doses necessary to treat microfilaremic patients, cause minimal or no drug-induced side-effects. However, their rapid killing of microfilariae releases enough antigen to overwhelm the modulating effects of the host's immune system and to induce a variety of side reactions.[22] These occur in proportion to the pre-treatment microfilarial levels and include headaches, fever, myalgia, lymphadenopathy and occasionally rash, itching and other symptoms. Although the most severely affected patients can also experience postural hypotension, generally these reactions are well managed through the use of antipyretics, antihistamines or, in the most severe instances, corticosteroids. In the tropical eosinophilia syndrome, as there are no microfilariae in the blood, there is no exacerbation of symptoms, but rather a steady improvement over the 2–4 weeks during which DEC is administered.

Treating the disease

Although it is important to cure the infection, management of the consequences of that infection (particularly the lymphedema, elephantiasis and genital pathology) is what is often of greatest concern to the patient. For early disease manifestations, it has been shown repeatedly that treatment of communities with either intermittent (monthly, 6-monthly or yearly) drug administration or the steady use of DEC-fortified table or cooking salt leads to clinical improvement, with decreases in hydrocele size and prevalence and in regression of early lymphedema.[14]

In more chronic states, patients with hydroceles or related urogenital pathology must be subjected to surgical procedures in order to obtain relief.[14]

The most dramatic change in managing patients with lymphatic filariasis has come from the recent recognition that bacterial and fungal superinfections of tissues with compromised lymphatic function play a prominent and progressively exacerbating role in disease development, so that careful attention to these infections can dramatically improve the outcome.[8,14] Rigorous hygiene in the affected limbs removes much of the excess stress on the lymphatic system and allows it (although still functionally compromised) to handle much more of the extracellular fluid effectively. Management regimens should include the following:

- twice-daily washing of the affected parts with soap and water;
- raising the affected limb at night;
- regular exercising of the affected limb to promote lymph flow;
- keeping the nails clean;
- wearing shoes; and
- using antiseptic or antibiotic creams to treat small wounds or abrasions.

The addition of elastic bandages and other adjunctive measures can further improve results.

These same intensive local hygiene efforts and antibiotic ointments can also decrease the frequency of recurrent infection episodes in patients who have elephantiasis of the penis or scrotum. Unfortunately, however, specific guidelines for management have not yet been developed for successfully reversing such anatomic distortions caused by the infection.

Noninvasive management of chyluria relies on nutritional support, especially replacement of fat-rich diets with high-protein, high-fluid diets supplemented where possible with medium-chain triglycerides.[8] Surgery, the sclerosing effects of lymphangiography or, often, time alone can also lead to the cessation of the leakage of lymph into the renal pelvis, collecting system and urine.

Onchocerciasis

Complete cure of *O. volvulus* infections, though not yet the goal of public health programs or most physicians, is now very feasible for individual patients, since long-term treatment with doxycycline (100 mg/day for 6 weeks) kills the adult parasite by depleting it of its essential endosymbiont (*Wolbachia*) bacterium.[21]

However, for most patients, because the pathology is generally associated with the microfilarial stage of the parasite, treating to kill the microfilariae rids the patients of existing symptoms and protects them from development of further eye lesions. The safest, most effective microfilaricide is ivermectin at the recommended dosage of 150–200 μg/kg; in various settings it has been repeated at 12-, 6- or even 3-month intervals. For individual patients, the frequency of treatment can best be determined by the rate at which symptoms (primarily itching and rash) recur. For individual patients, optimal management requires a thorough eye examination before initial treatment to ensure that no microfilariae are present, since it is the inflammatory complications of treatment with microfilaricides that must be avoided, especially in the eye. If there are microfilariae in the eye, the most conservative approach to treatment would include administration of prednisone 1 day before the dose of ivermectin is given and for 2 days after it. Short courses of corticosteroids have little negative effect on the microfilaricidal activity of ivermectin, and they are clearly effective in diminishing the side reactions caused by killing the microfilariae.

The side reactions that follow treatment of onchocerciasis with ivermectin (or, earlier, with DEC) have been termed the Mazzotti reaction. They result from the rapid killing of microfilariae and consist primarily of headache, fever, pruritus, adenopathy, rash and, occasionally, postural hypotension.[23] Although pronounced after DEC, they are much milder after ivermectin and are self-limiting (beginning within hours of treatment and persisting as long as 4–5 days); they can be managed satisfactorily with antipyretics, analgesics, antihistamines and, if necessary, systemic corticosteroids.

Because adult worms, which are generally not killed by either ivermectin or DEC, continue to shed microfilariae for up to 12–15 years, symptoms may recur and require additional 'microfilaricidal' treatment over an extended period of time.

Loiasis

The approach to treatment of loiasis depends on the clinical presentation. In patients who do not have microfilaremia, DEC 6–8 mg/kg/day for 3 weeks is the optimal treatment and results in cure of approximately half of the patients. Repeated courses of the drug are indicated when patients become symptomatic again and each repeated treatment results in additional patient cures.[24]

For microfilaremic patients, the approach to treatment is more difficult because the side reactions induced by the dying microfilariae can include CNS complications and even death. Such severe reactions rarely, if ever, occur in patients who have blood microfilaria counts of less than 2000/ml of blood (drawn at the time of day for peak parasitemia). However, even in a very controlled hospital setting, when highly microfilaremic loiasis patients were treated with DEC (initially at very low dosages – 0.25 mg/kg – and then increased progressively), there were still some patients in whom there was development of a post-treatment encephalopathy and death. This was not prevented even when corticosteroids were co-administered.[25]

When ivermectin is used instead of DEC, the clearance of microfilaremia from the blood is very much slower and not so complete. While it is much safer than DEC, both in terms of the systemic side reactions that it elicits (similar to those of the Mazzotti reaction) and in terms of avoiding the catastrophic neurologic complications in patients with extremely high levels of microfilaremia (especially 15 000–100 000 mf/ml), ivermectin has still led to instances of CNS deterioration, coma and death. With optimal clinical care, the transient CNS compromise of such ivermectin-treated patients can be managed successfully and catastrophic results minimized.[3] However, the treatment of loa-endemic populations with ivermectin (usually as part of national programs linked to the African Program for Onchocerciasis Control[2] or the Global Program to Eliminate Lymphatic Filariasis[1]) often must be rendered in remote areas without access to optimal medical management. Therefore, this potential complication of treatment provides a major challenge that must be overcome before these massive public health initiatives can be successfully implemented in the loa-endemic regions of Africa.

If patients experience an adult *L. loa* crossing the eye below the conjunctiva, such worms can be removed through simple surgical incision of the conjunctiva, but because usually there are multiple parasites within the patient, a single procedure may not be curative.[26]

REFERENCES

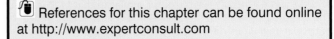 References for this chapter can be found online at http://www.expertconsult.com

Infections in sickle cell disease

DEFINITION

Sickle cell disease is a 'generic' term that includes a group of geno-types characterized by pathology associated with the presence of sickle hemoglobin (HbS). This abnormal hemoglobin results from a single amino acid substitution of valine for glutamic acid at position 6 in the β-chain. Inheritance of this abnormal gene from one parent and a normal gene for HbA from the other results in the harmless carrier state, the sickle cell trait. Sickle cell trait (AS genotype) is excluded from the definition of sickle cell disease because it causes no clinical problems in the great majority of subjects unless they are exposed to hypoxic environments such as high altitude or respiratory depression. The principal genotypes of sickle cell disease include:

- homozygous sickle cell (SS) disease, in which the abnormal HbS gene is inherited from both parents;
- sickle cell-hemoglobin C (SC) disease, in which the gene for HbS is inherited from one parent and the gene for HbC from the other. HbC is the second most common abnormal hemoglobin among people of West African origin; and
- inheritance of the sickle cell gene with one of the genes for β-thalassemia.

The β-thalassemia genes reduce the synthesis of β-chains, the degree of reduction determining the presence and amount of HbA. In sickle cell β⁰-thalassemia there is total suppression of β-chain synthesis, no HbA and a generally severe course similar to that of SS disease. The spectrum of sickle cell β⁺-thalassemia results from a variety of molecular mutations differing in different populations and result-ing in variable amounts of β-chain synthesis and hence HbA. Most common among peoples of African origin are mutations resulting in 20–30% of HbA and a very mild clinical course. In India, a more severe mutation results in only 3–5% HbA and in Greece, the com-monest mutation results in 10–15% HbA. In both these phenotypes, there does not appear to be enough HbA to significantly reduce sick-ling and sickle cell β⁺-thalassemia in both regions has a relatively severe clinical course, often similar to SS disease.

DISTRIBUTION AND PREVALENCE

In equatorial Africa, the prevalence of the sickle cell trait commonly reaches 20–30% (Fig. 116.1). Contrary to the common belief that the sickle cell gene is confined to peoples of African ancestry, the gene is widespread in populations around the Mediterranean (Sicily, north-ern Greece, southern Turkey, the Levant and northern Africa), Saudi Arabia (especially eastern Saudi Arabia and the Arabian Gulf) and central India. HbC is a marker of west African ancestry, reaching a

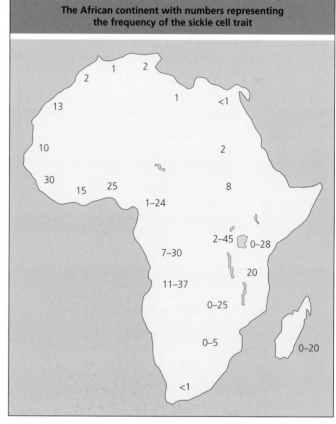

The African continent with numbers representing the frequency of the sickle cell trait

Fig. 116.1 The African continent with numbers representing the frequency of the sickle cell trait. Note the low levels in northern and southern Africa and high but variable levels in equatorial Africa.

prevalence of 20% in parts of Ghana and Burkina Faso, falling to 3–5% in Nigeria, and not occurring in central or east Africa, Saudi Arabia, Greece or central India.

In Nigeria, where approximately 25% have the sickle cell trait, it is estimated that SS disease occurs once in every 50 births, or 100 000 births annually. The prevalence of SS disease at later ages is deter-mined by the mortality of this genotype, which in Africa is often very high with infrequent survival to adult life. In Jamaica, the relative fre-quencies of the four major genotypes at birth (Table 116.1) are also influenced at later ages by their relative mortality which is greater in SS disease and Sβ⁰-thalassemia. The prevalence of these four major genotypes among African-Americans and among the UK population

Table 116.1 Relative frequency of principal genotypes of sickle cell disease in Jamaica*

Genotype	Frequency at birth
Homozygous sickle cell (SS) disease	1 in 300
Sickle cell-hemoglobin C (SC) disease	1 in 500
Sickle cell β$^+$-thalassemia	1 in 3000
Sickle cell β^0-thalassemia	1 in 7000

*In these data, sickle cell β$^+$-thalassemia refers to the common Jamaican form with 20–25% HbA.

of Afro-Caribbean origin are similar to those in Jamaica (because of similar gene frequencies) although the increasing population of direct African origin has markedly increased trait and disease frequencies in the UK. In all populations, the prevalence of sickle cell disease at birth is determined by the gene frequency but at later ages is influenced by the relative survival of affected patients and by the relative severity which determines presentation in hospital-based populations.

PATHOGENESIS AND PATHOLOGY

On deoxygenation, HbS molecules form rigid linear structures (polymers), which increase the intracellular viscosity and deform red cells into an abnormal 'sickled' shape. This can be reversed on oxygenation but after several sickle–unsickle cycles, these cells may become permanently deformed. These less deformable red cells have difficulty negotiating the capillary beds where normal red cells with an average diameter of 7 μm have to bend and fold to traverse a capillary measuring 3 μm. As a result, these abnormal red cells become prematurely destroyed (hemolysis) and may also block blood flow (vaso-occlusion).

Accelerated hemolysis results in anemia, jaundice, an increased prevalence of pigment gallstones and marked bone marrow expansion with high metabolic demands. The consequences of vaso-occlusion are determined by the site of the occlusion, but may include strokes, retinal ischemia, acute chest syndrome, a variety of splenic pathologies and chronic leg ulcers. Some manifestations, such as bone marrow necrosis, are influenced by both the hemolytic and vaso-occlusive components which give rise to dactylitis, the painful crisis, avascular necrosis of the femoral head and of the sternum and ribs which may precede the acute chest syndrome. In these conditions, the pathology is initially confined to areas of active bone marrow and is presumed to be precipitated by the high metabolic demands outstripping the supply. The mechanism is still controversial but may result from vaso-occlusion or, more likely, by shunting of blood away from the active marrow.

The pathologies of particular relevance to infections in sickle cell disease are the accelerated bone marrow activity, the prevalence of leg ulcers, acute chest syndrome and – most important of all – the early loss of splenic function. These processes are most marked in SS disease, sickle cell β^0-thalassemia and severe forms of sickle cell β$^+$-thalassemia, and less in SC disease and mild forms of sickle cell β$^+$-thalassemia.

The spleen in sickle cell disease

The spleen acts like a filter in the circulation, removing damaged red cells and bacteria from the bloodstream. It achieves this function by requiring red cells to squeeze between endothelial cells (Fig. 116.2) as the blood traverses from the cordal tissue to the splenic sinuses before returning to the circulation.[1] In addition to the filtering mechanism,

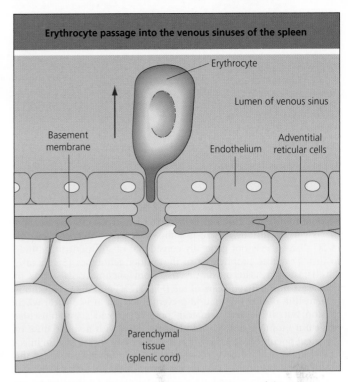

Erythrocyte passage into the venous sinuses of the spleen

Fig. 116.2 Erythrocyte passage into the venous sinuses of the spleen. A red cell passing between endothelial cells (arrow shows direction of movement) from the cordal tissue to the vascular sinus. Sickle cells do not have this deformability, so they accumulate in the spleen. Modified from Weiss.[1]

the spleen also represents a large mass of reticuloendothelial tissue in intimate contact with the circulation and is important in the production of specific antibodies. These are especially important if the liver is to participate actively in the removal of blood-borne antigens. Splenectomy removes these protective mechanisms and in patients without sickle cell disease has been calculated to increase the risk of sepsis 50- to 60-fold.

In sickle cell disease, the abnormal red cells damage splenic function early in life. Even when clinically enlarged, splenic uptake of ^{99m}technetium sulfur colloid is abnormal;[2] elevated pitted red cell counts, which suggest abnormal splenic function, may occur as early as 6 months of age and are seen in 20% of SS children by 1 year of age and in 40% by 2 years of age.[3] This loss of splenic function appears to be directly related to the susceptibility to infection[4] and may be reversed by transfusion in young children (Fig. 116.3).[5] It is also delayed in SS patients with high levels of fetal hemoglobin (HbF), which inhibit sickling and allow persistence of splenic function in SS patients in eastern Saudi Arabia.[6]

CLINICAL FEATURES

Bacterial infection

Streptococcus pneumoniae

The susceptibility to invasive pneumococcal infection in SS disease is well recognized and was first reported in 1928. The relative risk has been calculated to be at least 20 times that in the general population, and age-specific incidence rates are highest before the age of 2 years and fall sharply after 5 years.[7] Infection is closely linked to the appearance of clinical splenomegaly before 6 months of age.[8]

Prophylactic penicillin markedly reduces this risk, whether given orally[9] or by depot monthly intramuscular injection,[10] and has now

Fig. 116.3 [99m]Technetium sulfur colloid scans (posterior view) in a 2-year-old child with SS disease and splenomegaly. (a) The scan shows hepatic uptake but no splenic uptake. (b) A repeat scan 6 days after a blood transfusion shows restoration of splenic uptake of colloid. From Pearson *et al.*[5]

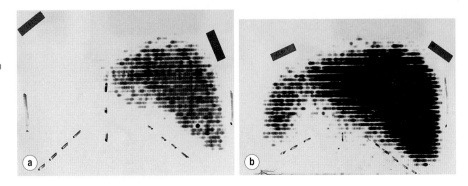

become routine for children with severe genotypes (SS disease, Sβ⁰-thalassemia). Although there is some evidence of an increased risk in SC disease, it is not generally considered of sufficient magnitude to justify routine prophylaxis in the milder genotypes (SC disease, Sβ⁺-thalassemia). The maximum risk from pneumococcal sepsis in Jamaica is in the first 3 years of life (Fig. 116.4) and depot injections of penicillin during that period prevent infection. It is unclear when to stop but the current Jamaican protocol provides intramuscular penicillin monthly from 4 months to 4 years with a single dose of 23-valent pneumococcal vaccine at the time of the last penicillin injection. Intramuscular injections are preferred in Jamaica to avoid the problems of compliance which may compromise the twice daily oral penicillin generally favored in the USA. Twice daily erythromycin may be given in children who are allergic to penicillin. The nonconjugated capsular polysaccharide pneumococcal vaccine does not confer adequate protection in young children, but its immunogenicity improves with the age of the patient, and preliminary data suggest that protective levels against many of the serotypes are achieved by the vaccine given at 4 years of age.

Two recent factors may cause these policies to be reassessed: the increasing prevalence of penicillin-resistant pneumococci, which may account for 20–50% of isolations in children with SS disease in the USA; and the development of a conjugate pneumococcal vaccine, which may be effective given at 2, 4 and 6 months. The availability of this vaccine has been associated with a significant decline in invasive disease[11] but potential disadvantages are the high cost and the less comprehensive coverage (7- or 9-valent) compared with the standard 23-valent nonconjugate vaccine.

This susceptibility to the pneumococcus has not been shown in all sickle cell populations and studies on the bacteriology of sepsis in SS disease in Nigeria[12–15] and Uganda[16] revealed a paucity of *Streptococcus pneumoniae*, the most common agents being *Klebsiella*, staphylococci, *Salmonella* and *Escherichia coli*. Possible interpretations of this infrequency of pneumococci include the early use of over-the-counter penicillin, the rapid demise of septicemic patients before they reach hospital, the environmental dominance of Gram-negative organisms or the intriguing postulate that malaria-induced splenomegaly may allow persistence of splenic function.[14] Regardless of the potential

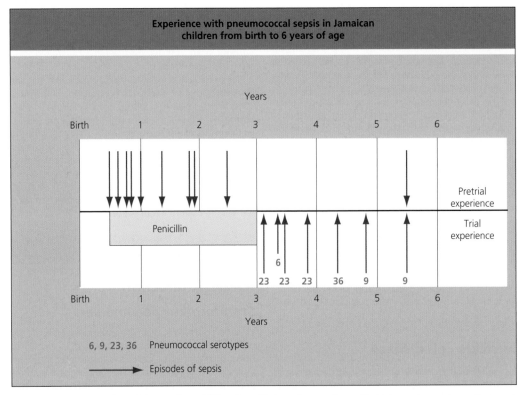

Fig. 116.4 Experience with pneumococcal sepsis in Jamaican children from birth to 6 years of age. Pretrial experience shows that sepsis episodes commenced at 6 months and 9 or 10 episodes occurred before 3 years. During penicillin prophylaxis from 6 months to 3 years, no episodes occurred but seven episodes occurred after cessation of penicillin. The numbers by the arrows refer to pneumococcal serotypes.

mechanism, there seems to be enough doubt to justify a trial of pneumococcal prophylaxis in SS disease in equatorial Africa if governments are to be persuaded to spend limited resources on pneumococcal prophylaxis in sickle cell disease.

Haemophilus influenzae type b

It seems likely that children with SS disease are also more prone to *Haemophilus influenzae* type b (Hib) infection, which has been increasing in importance with the advent of effective pneumococcal prophylaxis.[17] Extensive data from the US Cooperative Study of Sickle Cell Disease showed an incidence rate of 0.45 per 100 patient-years under 6 years of age, not significantly different from the incidence in the normal black population;[6] however, a susceptibility of 20–60 times that in the normal population has been proposed from other studies.[18] Although the risks of Hib infection in SS disease are unclear, prophylaxis appears justified and may be effected by conjugated Hib vaccines given between 2 and 6 months of age.[19]

Salmonella

Susceptibility to *Salmonella* osteomyelitis in SS disease has long been documented but an association with *Salmonella* sepsis in the absence of clinical bone involvement is less familiar. In a Jamaican study, half of the *Salmonella* isolations from blood occurred without obvious bone involvement and were associated with a 22% mortality because the potential significance of *Salmonella* spp. in a septic patient often went unrecognized.[20] On the other hand, none of the patients with *Salmonella* isolations associated with bone involvement died because the increased awareness of the association led to the early use of specific therapy against *Salmonella* spp.

Salmonella osteomyelitis is believed to be a secondary infection of avascular bone marrow and its distribution reflects that of the underlying bone marrow necrosis. The complication may become superimposed upon dactylitis in young children and should be suspected if the swelling is marked or there is high fever, in which case a surgical opinion should be sought regarding drainage; infection may be followed by a premature epiphysial fusion and a permanent shortening of affected small bones (Fig. 116.5). At later ages, osteomyelitis may follow bone marrow necrosis in the shafts of the long bones, ribs or sternum, pelvis and vertebrae. Infection of the avascular femoral head may be particularly difficult to diagnose, but this can lead to very rapid dissolution and extensive bone damage. Diagnosis depends on positive blood culture, and the diagnostic yield may be increased by invasive procedures such as bone marrow aspirate or trephine biopsies. The differential diagnosis of sterile avascular necrosis and osteomyelitis is a difficult clinical challenge and even bone scanning techniques have generally been unhelpful, the diagnosis resting on clinical judgment. Treatment is by specific antibiotics against *Salmonella* spp., such as chloramphenicol, ampicillin, trimethoprim–sulfamethoxazole (co-trimoxazole) or third-generation cephalosporins. Surgical drainage and the removal of sequestra may be necessary for complete healing and, even after apparent recovery, patients are prone to recurrence, sometimes years later, suggesting that the organisms remain dormant or loculated.

The source of *Salmonella* organisms in SS disease remains unknown, but common speculations include microinfarction of the gut wall in patients carrying *Salmonella*, or gallbladder colonization associated with gallstones and an abnormal gallbladder wall. However, a recent study showed no association with gallstones or with indices of vaso-occlusion, and *Salmonella* isolation from stools is only occasionally reported in patients with *Salmonella* osteomyelitis. The high prevalence of *Salmonella enteritidis*, which accounted for one-third of all isolations in the Jamaican series, suggests a dietary source and the possibility that *Salmonella* spp. may be carried by white cells raises the intriguing possibility that the organism could be introduced to the site of initially sterile avascular necrosis by the inflammatory process. More work is needed on the method of acquisition of *Salmonella* spp. in SS disease.

Escherichia coli

The extent of the increased risk of *Escherichia coli* infections in SS disease is unknown, but a significant excess of the SS genotype has been noted among black children admitted to hospital with serious infection and diagnosed as having *E. coli* sepsis.[21] *Escherichia coli* sepsis has also been associated with osteomyelitis and stroke. Urinary tract infections appear more common in SS disease and are a likely origin of *E. coli* sepsis.

Splenectomy and infection

Splenectomy, which may avoid morbidity and potential deaths in acute or chronic red cell sequestration, may be deferred because of concerns over loss of the splenic contribution to immune competence. However, the immune functions of the spleen in such patients are already compromised and no increase in severe infections or deaths occurred in 130 splenectomized SS patients when compared with 130 age and sex-matched SS controls followed over the same period.[22] If splenectomy is indicated in SS disease, either prophylactically in acute splenic sequestration or therapeutically in chronic hypersplenism, splenectomy should not be deferred for fear of losing any persisting splenic immune function. This practice has been satisfactory in nonmalarial areas but insufficient data on which to base recommendations are available in malarial environments, and both the role of splenectomy and of malarial prophylaxis should be studied separately in these areas.

Malaria

There is a special relationship between malaria and the HbS gene initially noted because malaria endemicity tended to coincide with high frequencies of the sickle cell trait in Africa. This has been the basis of many studies which have reached general agreement that during a critical period in early childhood (between the loss of passively acquired maternal immunity and the development of active immunity), the presence of the sickle cell trait confers some protection. The mechanism remains controversial and may be multifactorial, but increased sickling of parasitized red cells has been demonstrated and may serve to identify the host cell to the spleen and bring about its more effective removal. The maintenance of high frequencies of the sickle cell gene in areas of falciparum malaria led to the hypothesis of balanced polymorphism, proposing that a survival advantage in the sickle cell trait was balanced by the disadvantage and presumed loss of two genes in the early deaths occurring in SS disease. This protection is usually considered confined to the sickle cell trait but there is recent evidence that some resistance to infection may also occur in

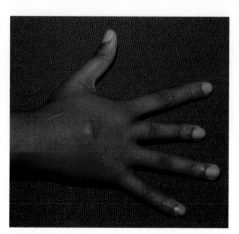

Fig. 116.5
Shortened third finger following infection complicating dactylitis. The scar represents surgical drainage of an apparent abscess.

SS disease. Once established in SS disease, malaria is believed to be a major cause of morbidity and mortality, exacerbating the already rapid hemolysis. It is unclear whether such patients die of malaria or succumb to symptoms of sickle cell disease precipitated by malaria.

Viral infection

Patients with SS disease are not believed to be intrinsically more prone to viral infections. Antibody responses to viral vaccines appear normal and infection rates by human parvovirus are similar in SS disease and AA controls.[23] More frequent transfusion-acquired viral infections such as hepatitis C virus and HIV may simply reflect the greater exposure to blood transfusion.

Human parvovirus infection appears to be the cause of aplastic crisis in SS disease, but this reflects a difference in response rather than an increased susceptibility. Human parvovirus infection colonizes and destroys red cell precursors in the bone marrow, but as the virus becomes neutralized by specific antibody, bone marrow function returns usually after 7–10 days. In SS disease, the red cell survival may be as short as 7–10 days and, unless oxygen delivery is maintained by transfusion, the aplastic crisis may result in death. Human parvovirus displays the general characteristics of a viral infection – most affected patients are under 15 years of age, in Jamaica epidemics occur at 3- to 4-year intervals and infectivity reaches 70–80% among nonimmune siblings. Close monitoring of at-risk siblings of affected cases is therefore recommended. A human parvovirus vaccine has been developed but it is still awaiting clinical trial. Human parvovirus infection in SS disease may be followed by cerebrovascular or renal complications in some cases.

Infection with atypical organisms

Mycoplasma pneumoniae and *Chlamydia pneumoniae* have been associated with the acute chest syndrome in patients with SS disease, especially in the autumn. The clinical course of these infections may be severe but it is unknown whether patients are more prone to develop these infections. The increased rate of hospital admission among SS patients also exposes them to an increased chance of hospital-acquired infections.

Other mechanisms of infection

Gallstones

The rapid hemolysis and consequent high excretion of bilirubin increases gallstones which occurred in 50% of SS patients in the Jamaican Cohort Study by the age of 25 years.[24] Jamaican experience suggests that most are asymptomatic, but complications include acute or chronic cholecystitis. The organism involved is usually *E. coli*, although anaerobes may also occur.

Leg ulceration

Chronic leg ulceration, a feature of SS disease, affects approximately 70% of Jamaican SS patients; they occur most commonly for the first time between 15 and 20 years of age and run a healing–relapsing course. The ulcer surface is commonly colonized by *Staphylococcus aureus*, *Pseudomonas aeruginosa* and β-hemolytic streptococci, but these ulcers are rarely associated with evidence of systemic infection. A possible association between ulcer-borne β-hemolytic streptococci and glomerular disease with proteinuria has been suggested, similar to the association between skin carriage of this organism and acute glomerulonephritis described from Trinidad; however, since both leg ulceration and proteinuria increase with age, correction for age in analyses did not confirm this relationship. Leg ulcers occasionally act as a portal of entry for tetanus.

The lack of evidence for systemic infection in leg ulceration suggests a limited role for antibiotic therapy, although infection with *P. aeruginosa* may occasionally be associated with ulcer deterioration and poor healing.

Acute chest syndrome

The acute chest syndrome is a pneumonia-like pathology with elements of infection, infarction, pulmonary sequestration and fat embolism. It is a major cause of morbidity and the commonest single cause of mortality at all ages after 2 years. The contribution of primary infection is controversial, and, although early studies reported pathogens in approximately half the cases in children aged under 3 years, recent studies have found evidence of bacterial infection in only 4–14% of episodes. Furthermore, the poor response to antibiotics and the striking improvement in many cases following transfusion has favored a vascular pathology rather than an infective one. Infections with the atypical agents *Mycoplasma pneumoniae* and *Chlamydia pneumoniae* have been mentioned above.

CONCLUSION

Patients with sickle cell disease are susceptible to some but not all infections. However, any infective illness coinciding with sickle cell disease may precipitate sickle-related complications, such as painful crisis, by inducing fever and possibly dehydration from vomiting and diarrhea.

REFERENCES

 References for this chapter can be found online at http://www.expertconsult.com

Leishmaniasis

EPIDEMIOLOGY

Leishmania can cause cutaneous (CL), mucocutaneous (MCL) and visceral (VL, kala-azar) disease. The distribution of leishmaniases is shown in Figure 117.1; ~1.5 million cases of CL and 500 000 cases of VL occur annually.[1] Phlebotomine sandflies transmit leishmaniasis from a range of infected animals (= zoonotic) or from human to human (= anthroponotic). Transmission varies according to climate, habitat, season and occupation. All forms of leishmaniasis are increasing in many areas. In Brazil, the increase in VL and CL is due to deforestation, which brings humans into close contact with animal reservoirs and forest vectors of *Leishmania braziliensis* and other species. In North Africa and the Middle East, irrigation projects resulted in increased numbers of gerbils and construction of townships in these areas has led to increases in endemic CL caused by *Leishmania major*. Breakdown of the infrastructure in Afghanistan caused outbreaks of urban CL due to *Leishmania tropica*.

Visceral leishmaniasis

This is caused by *Leishmania donovani*, *Leishmania infantum* and *Leishmania chagasi* (see Fig. 117.1); the latter two species are indistinguishable. A reduction of dichlorodiphenyltrichloroethane (DDT) spraying against malaria vectors in India and Bangladesh heralded the start of the present epidemic of *L. donovani* VL, which affects hundreds of thousands annually. Population movement, famine, civil war and ecologic change caused epidemics of VL (*L. donovani*) in Sudan and Somalia.[2,3] In Europe prior to effective antiretrovirals, 20–70% of cases of VL (due to *L. infantum*) were co-infected with HIV, and 1.5–9% of AIDS patients had VL.[4] Co-infections of HIV and *Leishmania* are increasing in Africa (especially Ethiopia), India and South America.

Subclinical or self-healing infection occurs more frequently than clinical VL, particularly where *L. infantum* or *L. chagasi* is involved.[5] In epidemics involving *L. donovani*, most infections are symptomatic, and the mortality rate is high.[6]

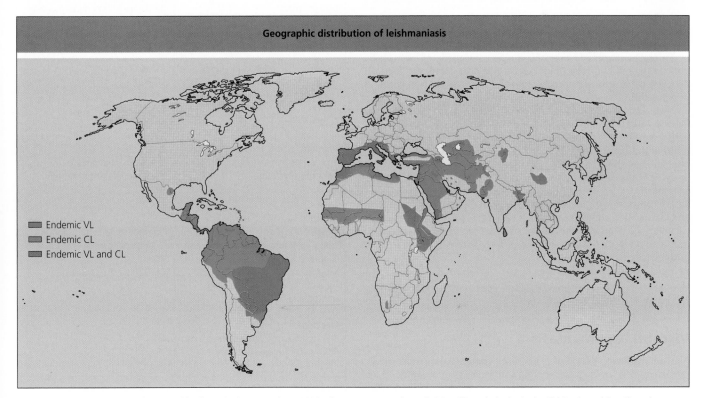

Geographic distribution of leishmaniasis

■ Endemic VL
■ Endemic CL
■ Endemic VL and CL

Fig. 117.1 Geographic distribution of leishmaniasis. More than 90% of VL cases occur in India/Nepal/Bangladesh, Sudan/Ethiopia and Brazil, and more than 90% of CL cases occur in Brazil/Peru, Algeria, Saudi Arabia and Syria/Iraq/Iran/Afghanistan. Courtesy of Pablo Martín-Rabadán and Emilio Bouza.

Cutaneous leishmaniasis

In the Old World, *L. tropica* causes anthroponotic CL in villages, towns and cities; *L. major* causes zoonotic CL in those living or working near gerbil burrows. Smaller numbers of CL cases are caused by *L. infantum* in Europe and *L. aethiopica* in Ethiopia and parts of Kenya. In the New World, CL is mainly caused by members of the *Leishmania mexicana* complex (*L. mexicana mexicana*, *L. m. amazonensis*, *L. m. venezuelensis*) and the *Leishmania braziliensis* complex (*L. braziliensis braziliensis*, *L. b. panamensis*, *L. b. guyanensis*, *L. b. peruviana*).[7]

PATHOGENESIS AND PATHOLOGY

Infected macrophages produce nitric oxide as an innate mechanism for killing *Leishmania* amastigotes; this is inhibited by the parasite, which multiplies in the parasitophorous vacuole. Eventually, infected macrophages rupture and amastigotes are taken up by new phagocytes. Macrophages and dendritic cells present *Leishmania* antigens to T cells and this results in either:

- an effective cellular immune response – a T-helper (Th)1 pattern; or
- an ineffective humoral response – a Th2 pattern.

In the Th1 response, T cells activate macrophages by releasing the cytokines interferon (IFN)-γ and interleukin (IL)-2. In the Th2 response, T cells release cytokines IL-4, IL-5, IL-10 and transforming growth factor (TGF)-β, which inhibit macrophages from killing amastigotes (see Chapter 2). Each *Leishmania* spp. produces a typical pattern of disease, and host cellular immunity (genetic factors, nutrition and co-morbidities all contribute) at the time of infection will determine whether:

- a clinical or subclinical infection results;
- the disease is visceral, cutaneous or mucocutaneous;
- lesions are few or diffuse; and
- response to treatment is complete or partial.[8]

PREVENTION

Individual protection against nocturnal sandfly bites is provided by insecticide-impregnated bed nets. Long sleeves and trousers, and permethrin-impregnated clothing may also help.[9]

Animal reservoirs of *Leishmania* can be controlled, for example by bulldozing gerbil burrows or killing infected dogs. Domestic dogs can be given deltamethrin-impregnated collars or 65% spot-on solution of permethrin.[10] Active case finding and treatment of patients with VL and post-kala-azar dermal leishmaniasis (PKDL) caused by *L. donovani* and CL caused by *L. tropica* reduce human-to-human transmission. Early case finding is possible using serologic tests, for example the direct agglutination test (DAT) and rapid test strips using a recombinant antigen, rK39.[11] Sandflies are susceptible to residual insecticides; spraying homes or fogging streets reduces the density of peridomestic sandflies.

Two doses of a vaccine, combining killed *Leishmania* promastigotes and live bacille Calmette–Guérin (BCG) were >70% protective against CL in Ecuador;[12] in Iran one dose of a similar vaccine was ineffective.[13] In Sudan a similar vaccine did not prove effective against VL,[14] but boosted cure rates in PKDL.[15]

CLINICAL FEATURES

Visceral leishmaniasis

After an incubation period of 2–8 months (range 10 days to >2 years), the patient develops pyrexia, wasting and hepatosplenomegaly, which may become massive (Fig. 117.2). Males outnumber females in Africa and India, partly because outdoor activities expose males to sandfly

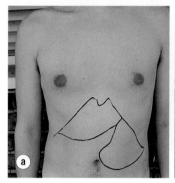
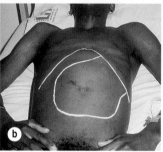

Fig. 117.2 Visceral leishmaniasis. (a) Hepatosplenomegaly and pallor in a 29-year-old Italian man. (b) Splenomegaly and pallor in a 23-year-old Angolan. Both complained of weight loss, fatigue and fever of several weeks' duration.

bites, but mainly because females are denied access to diagnosis and treatment. When treatment is provided free, or active case-finding done, the ratio of male:female cases approaches 1:1.[16] In Europe or Brazil, VL affects mainly infants (hence the name *L. infantum*) or adults co-infected with HIV.

Visceral leishmaniasis in India, Kenya and Somalia often has an ill-defined onset, and months elapse before the patient presents with fever, discomfort from an enlarged spleen, abdominal swelling, weight loss, epistaxis, cough or diarrhea. Conversely, patients in Sudan or those affected during an epidemic characteristically experience high fever, progressing over a few weeks to prostration, weakness, dyspnea and acute anemia.

The physical signs (Table 117.1) depend upon the duration of the disease, the nutritional state of the patient and the presence of

Table 117.1 Features of visceral leishmaniasis (*Leishmania donovani*)*

Clinical feature	Proportion affected (%)
Age <9 years	22 (*L. infantum* and *L. chagasi* more commonly affect children and infants)
Age <15 years	44
Fever	83–100
Wasting	70–100
Uncomfortable spleen	81–88
Cough	72–83
Epistaxis	44–55
Diarrhea	25–55
Vomiting	2–37
Splenomegaly	93 (adults), 98 (children)
Lymphadenopathy	55–86 (uncommon outside Africa)
Jaundice	2–7
Edema	2–7

Laboratory findings	Proportion (%)
Globulin >30 g/l	98
Anemia	61–92
Albumin <30 g/l	88
Leukopenia	84
Thrombocytopenia	73
Elevated bilirubin	17
Elevated alkaline phosphatase	40
Positive *Leishmania* serology	95
Parasitologically proven	96

*The duration of symptoms is 2–4 months but is shorter in children

complications. Late cases are thin, wasted and cannot walk unaided. Hair changes and pedal edema accompany hypoalbuminemia, but ascites is rare. Nonspecific hyperpigmentation of the face, hands, feet and abdomen occurs ('kala-azar' means 'black sickness'). The spleen is enlarged in >90% of cases. Though massive spleens are often photographed, reaching the left or right iliac fossa, the average spleen in VL only reaches 5–10 cm below the left costal margin. It is smooth, firm and nontender unless there has been a recent infarct. The liver is moderately enlarged in one-third of cases. Lymphadenopathy is common only in African patients, in whom unimpressive, peanut-sized lymph nodes are often palpable in the groins. Jaundice, mucosal and retinal hemorrhage, and episcleritis are occasional features. Neurologic complications, such as confusion, tremor and ataxia, convulsions, foot-drop and nerve deafness, are occasionally seen. After weeks to months of illness, most VL patients die, often as a result of uncontrolled bleeding (nasal, intestinal, intracranial), secondary bacterial pneumonia, anemic heart failure, tuberculosis or dysentery, or other infections (e.g. cancrum oris).

Leishmaniasis in patients who are immunosuppressed or have HIV infection

Visceral leishmaniasis is an AIDS-defining opportunistic infection. Currently, HIV/VL is commonest in north-eastern Africa (especially Ethiopia), India and Brazil.[4] In southern Europe numbers of co-infected cases fell dramatically after the adoption of highly active antiretroviral treatment (HAART). VL in HIV co-infected patients in Europe characteristically occurs at very low CD4 counts, and affects injecting drug users disproportionately because shared syringes spread the infection. The clinical features of HIV/VL in Europe are often atypical: the symptoms vague, the laboratory abnormalities nonspecific, and hepatosplenomegaly absent or unimpressive. *Leishmania* amastigotes may be found unexpectedly in circulating neutrophils or bone marrow aspirates of febrile HIV-positive patients, or in rectal, gastric or skin biopsies. *Leishmania* serology is negative in one-third of such patients. During treatment, patients may experience drug toxicity (especially pancreatitis on antimonials) and even if apparently responding well they are prone to relapse. With HAART, many HIV-infected patients with *L. infantum* achieve long-term cure; the danger of relapse recedes once their CD4 count is >200 cells/mm[3] for >3 months. A minority of HIV/VL patients never achieve a good CD4 response, despite effective HIV suppression, and relapse repeatedly. Eventually such patients become nonresponsive to all antileishmanial drugs.

L. donovani in Africa and India is more virulent than *L. infantum* in Europe, and the clinical picture of HIV/VL is indistinguishable from VL in HIV-negative patients. Those with HIV co-infection have high mortality during and after treatment, and higher rates of relapse and PKDL.[16,17] In Ethiopia, even good CD4 responses may not protect against repeated relapses.[18] Cutaneous leishmaniasis has been reported in patients who have HIV infection in Africa and South America. The lesions often resemble those of diffuse cutaneous leishmaniasis (DCL, see below).

VL may occasionally occur in patients immunosuppressed by drugs or who have undergone organ transplantation or thymectomy. There is usually no prior history of leishmaniasis, and travel to endemic areas may have been years previously.

Post-kala-azar dermal leishmaniasis

After successful treatment for VL due to *L. donovani* (but not *L. chagasi*/*L. infantum*), patients may develop a prolonged inflammatory reaction in skin and/or mucosae called post-kala-azar dermal leishmaniasis (PKDL).

In Sudan, PKDL occurs toward the end of apparently successful treatment or weeks to months later. Mild PKDL affects ~55% of VL patients, including those with subclinical VL.[19] In India, PKDL is less common, and occurs months to years after VL. Occasionally, PKDL is acute and severe, resulting in desquamation of skin and mucosae. More

commonly, it is characterized by the development of hypopigmented patches, nodules and plaques. Parasites are infrequent or absent from the biopsies. Patients with PKDL are infectious to sandflies and may be the reservoir of *L. donovani* between outbreaks.

Cutaneous leishmaniasis

In CL (Fig. 117.3) amastigotes multiply in dermal macrophages near the site of inoculation, typically on the arms, legs, face or ears. The lesions may be:

- nodular or ulcerative; and
- single or with multiple satellite nodules or lymphangitic spread.

The most typical lesion of CL is a nodule or chronic ulcer with a diameter of 2–5 cm and indurated margins. The ulcer may be covered by a fibrinous crust or exudate. It is painful if large or secondarily infected.

The histologic picture is of an intense lymphoid and monocytic infiltrate with granulomas. A 'tissue-paper' scar remains after healing. The median spontaneous healing rate differs for each species and is typically:

- <5 months for *L. major*;
- <8 months for *L mexicana*; and
- ~1 year for *L. tropica* and *L. braziliensis*.

There are two chronic forms of CL. Diffuse cutaneous leishmaniasis is rare but disfiguring. Widespread plaques containing huge numbers of amastigotes persist for decades. People with DCL are anergic to leishmanin, but do not have visceral dissemination or systemic symptoms. DCL is caused mainly by *L. aethiopica* in Africa and *L. amazonensis* in South and Central America. Leishmaniasis recidivans is a chronic, nonhealing or relapsing cutaneous infection, seen mainly with *L. tropica* infection in the Middle East. These patients are hypersensitive to leishmanin and organisms are rarely identified (see Fig. 117.3).

Mucocutaneous leishmaniasis

Mucocutaneous leishmaniasis (MCL; Fig. 117.4) occurs in ~3–10% of cases of CL due to *L. b. braziliensis*, especially in Peru and Bolivia. MCL usually occurs months to years after CL has healed, but simultaneous CL and MCL can occur, as can MCL without previous CL. Usually the tip of the nose, nasal cartilage or upper lip are

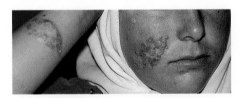

Fig. 117.3 Cutaneous leishmaniasis. *Leishmania tropica* recidivans leishmaniasis lesions on the face and forearm of a Syrian girl. These had been present for 4 years with slow healing in the center and multiple recurrences despite courses of intralesional meglumine antimonate.

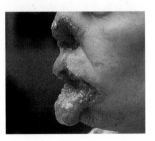

Fig. 117.4 Mucocutaneous leishmaniasis. A young man from Peru who had a 2-year history of slow enlargement of the lips and ulceration of the nostrils. Courtesy of Professor Luis Valda Rodriguez.

involved first with a painless induration or ulceration. The condition may remain static or may extend over months to years into the nasopharynx, palate, uvula, larynx and upper airways. The nose may be destroyed.

Biopsies show a chronic inflammatory and granulomatous infiltrate with very few amastigotes. Cultures of biopsies are usually positive for *L. braziliensis* but this may require repeated attempts. Less severe oral (e.g. tongue), nasal or laryngeal involvement occasionally occurs with other species (e.g. *L. infantum*) and this often indicates an underlying immune defect.

DIAGNOSIS

Parasitologic diagnosis

Clinical leishmaniasis is supported by serologic or skin tests but is ideally confirmed by finding or culturing the parasite. *Leishmania* spp. may be isolated from material taken from reticuloendothelial tissue or from biopsies of skin or mucosal lesions. Some of the sample is smeared onto glass slides stained with Giemsa and examined for amastigotes (Fig. 117.5). The rest of the sample is inoculated into suitable media and cultured at 78.8–82.4°F (26–28°C); a positive culture produces motile promastigotes within 2 weeks.

In VL, positive yields from smears of aspirates are of the following order: spleen, >95%; bone marrow or liver, 70–85%; lymph node (Africa), 58–65%; and buffy coat of blood (HIV/VL), ~70%.[11] Cultures yield about another 10% in good hands. The technique of splenic aspirate is shown in Figure 117.6.

In CL, DCL, PKDL and MCL, slit skin smears are taken from the raised edge of the CL ulcer or center of the CL nodule (Fig. 117.7; see Chapter 103). Amastigotes are most abundant in fresh CL lesions and are very numerous in DCL. Conversely, they are infrequent in old CL lesions, in MCL and in PKDL.

Immunologic diagnosis

In VL, 95% of cases have high titers of anti-*Leishmania* antibodies by the direct agglutination test (DAT), immunofluorescent antibody test (IFAT) or enzyme-linked immunosorbent assay. A major advance is the dipstick test using the rK39 antigen, which gives sensitivity and specificity for VL of >90% in India.[11] In Europe, ~30% of HIV/VL

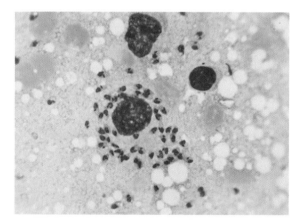

Fig. 117.5 Amastigotes (Leishman–Donovan bodies) in bone marrow aspirate from a patient who had *Leishmania infantum* visceral leishmaniasis and AIDS. The nucleus and kinetoplast stain deeply with Giemsa and give the organism its characteristic appearance. *Histoplasma* spp. are the main source of mistaken identification in bone marrow smears, but lack these structures. Amastigotes measure 2–3 mm in length and are found within macrophages in tissue sections, but usually lie free in smears because infected macrophages burst as they are smeared.

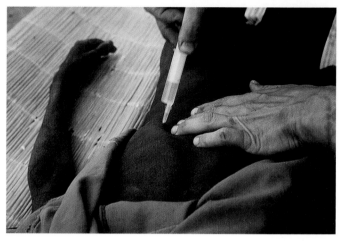

Fig. 117.6 Splenic aspiration. The picture shows a splenic aspirate being performed under field conditions on a child suffering from *Leishmania donovani* kala-azar in south Sudan. The procedure is simple, painless and safe if the prothrombin time is normal and the platelet count is above 40 × 10⁹/l. Palpate the spleen and mark its outline. Using a 30 mm long 21-gauge needle attached to a 5 ml syringe, penetrate the skin over the spleen. Withdraw the plunger 1 ml and plunge the needle into the spleen upwards at an angle of 45°and withdraw immediately, maintaining suction. The tiny amount of material obtained is sufficient for culture and smear. Courtesy of Drs Robert Wilkinson and Jill Seaman.

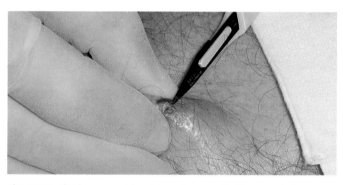

Fig. 117.7 Slit skin smear. The picture shows a slit skin smear being taken from the edge of a chronic *Leishmania infantum* ulcer obtained in Malta. Smears are taken from the raised edge of the ulcer or center of the nodule, where amastigotes are most abundant. The skin is cleaned and then firmly pinched throughout the procedure to squeeze away blood. A 5 mm long and 3 mm deep incision is made and then the scalpel is turned through 90° and the blade is used to scrape the edge of the slit. A line of tissue scrapings is gently streaked on to a slide and the process is repeated until two or three lines of scrapings are present on at least two slides. Further scrapings and fluid oozing from the pinched slit are put into culture medium.

patients have negative serology for *Leishmania*; in Africa, *Leishmania* serology is positive in most HIV/VL patients.[18] In VL, the leishmanin skin test is invariably negative, indicating antigen-specific anergy. In CL, *Leishmania* serology may be weakly positive and the leishmanin skin test is usually positive. In MCL and PKDL, both serology and the leishmanin skin test are usually positive. In DCL, there is anergy and both serology and the leishmanin skin test are negative.

MANAGEMENT

Ideally, VL, like other life-threatening infections, should be treated with combination chemotherapy to improve cure rates, reduce duration and toxicity of treatment, reduce relapses and (in areas of zoonotic transmission) delay the development of drug-resistant *L. donovani*. However, despite agreement among all experts on this principle, combination treatment has only been adopted in a few situations.[16]

Antileishmanial drugs

Pentavalent antimonials

Pentavalent antimonials (Sb^v) have been used since the 1940s. Sodium stibogluconate contains Sb^v 100 mg/ml; meglumine antimonate contains 85 mg/ml. In the systemic treatment of VL, CL and MCL, a single daily dose of 20 mg Sb^v/kg is used for 28 days. Intravenous injections are less painful than intramuscular injections. Courses of up to 3 months are used for PKDL. Primary resistance to Sb^v is seen in ~1% of cases in Africa and up to 60% in parts of India. Relapse rates should be <5%, but secondary Sb^v resistance is likely to develop in patients who relapse unless they are retreated very thoroughly.

Toxicity

Sb^v is reduced by parasite reductases to SbIII, and human reductases might perform a similar function. This may account for the unpredictable toxicity of Sb^v, as well as explaining why toxicity is rare in 'well' patients treated for PKDL, but common in 'ill' patients with VL, particularly those with HIV/VL. Sb^v-induced hyperamylasemia is common, and pancreatitis may be symptomatic and even fatal, especially in those co-infected with HIV.[20] Elevated liver enzymes, arthralgia and myalgia, thrombocytopenia, leukopenia, anorexia and thrombophlebitis all occur. Patients may experience symptoms indistinguishable from VL itself: lethargy, headache, nausea, vomiting. Electrocardiograph (ST-segment and T-wave) changes occur commonly; prolongation of the corrected QT interval to >0.5 s is an indication to temporarily discontinue therapy.[21] Acute renal failure, thrombocytopenia, arthritis, tremors and exfoliative dermatitis occur occasionally. If toxicity occurs, treatment should be changed to another agent. If only Sb^v is available, treatment should be stopped for 1–2 days; if toxicity recurs, the daily dose should be reduced.

Before starting treatment, ideally a full blood count, biochemistry profile and electrocardiograph should be obtained. Patients should be hospitalized during systemic Sb^v therapy where possible, and biochemical and hematologic parameters monitored twice weekly. This is usually impossible in endemic countries, where Sb^v is administered by a nurse to outpatients without the facilities for monitoring toxicity. Sudden deaths, thought to be due to arrhythmias, occur occasionally in VL patients. It is unclear what proportion of deaths in VL is due to Sb^v. However, in a randomized controlled study involving 580 VL patients, many of whom were HIV positive, the mortality was 10% among patients treated with Sb^v versus 2% among miltefosine recipients.[22]

Intralesional administration

When used intralesionally, ~1 ml of undiluted Sb^v is infiltrated into the base and edges of a CL lesion. The injections are repeated every 2–3 days for up to 2–3 weeks. There are no systemic side-effects, but the injections are painful.

Amphotericin B

Amphotericin B deoxycholate is a very powerful antileishmanial and a first-line drug in India, with good efficacy in Uganda, Nepal and elsewhere. Amphotericin B is remarkably nontoxic in the regimen of 15 doses of 1 mg/kg on alternate days.[23] The main limitation is the need for hospitalization and slow intravenous infusions. Where possible, renal function and electrolytes should be monitored weekly. Amphotericin B is the drug of choice for advanced MCL, for which Sb^v treatment is often ineffective, and total doses of 30 mg/kg are

used. Amphotericin B has not been systematically assessed for CL or PKDL.

Lipid-associated amphotericin B

These particulate preparations of amphotericin B are taken up by macrophages and therefore target amphotericin B to the site of infection, achieving very high levels in liver and spleen. They have lower renal and infusion toxicity than amphotericin B but are more expensive. Liposomal amphotericin B (AmBisome®) has been extensively used, and is licensed for VL in many countries. It is rapidly effective and nontoxic for VL in Europe,[24] Sudan[25] and India.[26] The licensed regimen is a total dose of 20–30 mg/kg, given as at least five daily doses of 3–4 mg/kg over a period of 10–21 days. Liposomal amphotericin B can be dosed flexibly, since the drug has very low toxicity and a prolonged tissue half-life in spleen and liver (and, presumably, bone marrow).[27]

Very short courses of liposomal amphotericin B (two doses of 10 mg/kg) have been used in Europe.[27] While total doses as low as 5 mg/kg as a single dose have a high cure rate in India,[26] liposomal amphotericin B is not as effective in Sudan.[25,28] A few complicated cases of CL have been successfully treated with long courses of liposomal amphotericin B.

Amphotericin B cholesterol dispersion (Amphocil®) and amphotericin B lipid complex (Abelcet®) have also been used successfully in VL.

Combination therapy

Liposomal amphotericin B would be ideally suited as part of a combination therapy. Regimens currently under consideration are a single dose of AmBisome 5 mg/kg plus a short course of either intramuscular paromomycin sulfate or oral miltefosine.

Miltefosine

Miltefosine is an oral drug with good efficacy against VL;[29] it is licensed in several countries. The common side-effects are mild to moderate vomiting and diarrhea and modest elevation of liver enzymes. More rare are anorexia, nausea, abdominal pain and increase of urea and creatinine. Miltefosine should be avoided in pregnancy, and women of child-bearing potential must use effective contraception during and for 2 months after treatment.

The duration of miltefosine treatment is 28 days. The daily dose for adults and children >25 kg is 100 mg/day; for children 2–12 years (8–25 kg) it is 2.5 mg/kg/day (max 50 mg/day). Miltefosine should be taken in divided doses with meals.

Miltefosine (same regimen as above) is highly effective against *L. braziliensis* CL and MCL in South America[30,31] and against *L. major* CL in Iran.[32]

Paromomycin (aminosidine)

Paromomycin sulfate (previously called aminosidine sulfate) is an aminoglycoside antibiotic used since the 1950s, which is a highly effective and cheap antileishmanial for VL, though it has little efficacy in CL or MCL. It is licensed in India in the dose of paromomycin sulfate 15 mg/kg/day for 21 days.[33] This dose is equivalent to paromomycin (base) 11 mg/kg/day.

Paromomycin is well-tolerated. In clinical trials, no cases of renal impairment occurred, and subclinical ototoxicity (which was reversible) occurred in only 2%, with 6% developing mild, reversible elevation of liver enzymes.[33]

Combination treatment

A combination of Sb^v and paromomycin has been used extensively in Sudan with good effect.[16,34] The regimen is sodium stibogluconate 20 mg/kg/day plus paromomycin sulfate 15 mg/kg/day, both given intramuscularly daily for 17 days.

Pentamidine

Pentamidine is not routinely used for VL, although short courses – seven doses of 2 mg/kg on alternate days, or four doses of 3 mg/kg on alternate days – are effective for New World CL.[35]

Second-line oral agents

Ketoconazole is effective for CL caused by *L. major* and *L. mexicana*, but is less effective against *L. tropica*, *L. aethiopica* and *L. braziliensis*. Fluconazole[36] and itraconazole have similar efficacy and are better tolerated. Imidazoles cannot reliably cure VL or PKDL.

Topical treatment

Topical paromomycin in the treatment of CL has been evaluated in many studies. At best, it shows a modest benefit over placebo and is usually less effective than Sb^v.[37]

Monitoring response to treatment

Visceral leishmaniasis

Intercurrent infections such as malaria, tuberculosis and dysentery must be treated, and good hydration and nutritional supplements provided. Severely ill patients should receive empiric broad-spectrum antibiotics (e.g. ceftriaxone) to cover sepsis.

With effective antileishmanial treatment, the patient will be afebrile within 1 week and clinical and laboratory abnormalities will improve within 2 weeks. Liposomal amphotericin B acts faster than Sb^v.

After successful treatment, amastigotes will be absent from aspirates and cultures will be negative; a test-of-cure aspirate is not needed unless the patient has previously relapsed or has not shown a full clinical recovery. The patient should be reviewed during 6–12 months after treatment. Slight splenomegaly may persist for several months. A relapse rate of less than 5% is expected for immunocompetent patients but more than 80% for patients who also have HIV infection; most relapses occur within 6 months. Body weight, spleen size, full blood count, serum albumin concentration and erythrocyte sedimentation rate are all sensitive markers of recurrent VL.

Maintenance with intravenous pentamidine every 2–4 weeks or liposomal amphotericin B weekly may be useful to prevent or delay relapse for patients who have HIV infection, but efficacy is unproven. HIV co-infected patients should be started on HAART, irrespective of the CD4 count, since relapsing VL carries a high morbidity and mortality.

When treating a relapse of VL, a drug combination is advised, and parasite clearance should be confirmed by a test-of-cure aspirate.

Cutaneous leishmaniasis

Treatment is necessary if the lesions are large, multiple, disfiguring or overlie a joint. Intralesional Sb^v is cheap and usually effective but CL due to *L. braziliensis* should be treated systemically to reduce the risk of subsequent MCL. Most relapses of CL will occur within 12 months.

Mucocutaneous leishmaniasis

Untreated MCL will slowly progress to produce extensive mutilating lesions. Early lesions respond better to treatment[37] but the response is slow and relapses are common. Corticosteroids should be added if the larynx or airways are involved, to prevent edema complicating the start of treatment. Relapse may occur up to several years after treatment, so prolonged clinical follow-up is necessary.

REFERENCES

References for this chapter can be found online at http://www.expertconsult.com

Iveth J González
Michael A Miles
Mark D Perkins

Chapter | 118 |

Chagas disease (American trypanosomiasis)

DEFINITION

Chagas disease, first described by the Brazilian scientist Carlos Chagas in 1909,[1] is a vector-borne anthropozoonosis caused by the protozoan parasite *Trypanosoma cruzi*. Infection with *T. cruzi*, which is life-long, is characterized by three clinical phases:

1. acute phase which may be present with edema at the cutaneous or conjunctival portal of entry of the parasite;
2. indeterminate or latent phase which is asymptomatic and of a median duration of 10 years; and
3. chronic phase with the appearance of cardiac (chagasic cardiopathy) and digestive (megaesophagus and megacolon) pathology.

EPIDEMIOLOGY

Although control of Chagas disease has dramatically improved in the past two decades, this parasitic disease is widely disseminated in Latin America and is considered as a public health problem in many of its countries.[2] By the end of the 1980s it was estimated that 16–18 million people were infected, that 90–100 million more were at risk of infection, and that 450 000 new cases occurred each year. However, after the launch of the Southern Cone Initiative by six endemic countries in 1991 (Argentina, Bolivia, Brazil, Chile, Paraguay and Uruguay) and similar initiatives in Central America and the Andean Pact countries in 1997, Chagas disease cases have been declining.[3] Currently it is thought that less than 9 million people are infected, and Brazil, Uruguay and Chile have been declared free of transmission due to domestic *Triatoma infestans* (Fig. 118.1). Nevertheless, around 40 million people remain at risk of infection, transmission is still present and national programs for the control of this disease are not present in countries such as Mexico, Peru, Colombia and Costa Rica.[2] In the USA it is estimated that around 100 000 persons are infected.[4] Although most of them are migrants who acquired the diseases during their childhood, vectors and animals infected with *T. cruzi* can be found in many parts of the country and at least six documented cases of autochthonous transmission have been reported.[5]

ETIOLOGIC AGENT

The causative agent of Chagas disease is the protozoan parasite *Trypanosoma cruzi*. Similar to other parasites of the order Kinetoplastida, *T. cruzi* is characterized by the presence of the kinetoplast, a DNA-containing organelle located within the mitochondrion at the posterior end of the parasite close to the flagellar base.

Biochemical and genetic studies have demonstrated that *T. cruzi* is actually a group of genetically diverse parasite populations. Isoenzyme and other analyses have led to classification of *T. cruzi* parasites in two major lineages, *T. cruzi* I and *T. cruzi* II, with the latter containing five subgroups (a–e).[6] In the Southern Core region, *T. cruzi* IIb, IId and IIe are the predominant agents although sporadic cases of *T. cruzi* I occur.[7] However, *T. cruzi* I is the predominant cause of Chagas disease in the Amazon region and in countries north of the Amazon region, where megasyndromes seem to be less commonly associated with chronic disease.[8]

Chagas disease is primarily a zoonosis in which wild and domestic animals serve as reservoirs. All mammals, but not birds or reptiles, are considered to be susceptible to *T. cruzi* infection. Mammals typically involved in sylvatic transmission include opossums, armadillos, raccoons, monkeys, wood rats and others. Domestic dogs, guinea pigs, cats, rats and mice may in some situations be important reservoirs. Chickens, although not infected, are a significant factor because they can sustain large infestations with the reduviid vectors.[9]

The life cycle of the parasite is complex. It circulates in the blood of infected mammals in an elongated trypomastigote form, about 20 μm long, and characterized by the presence of a flagellum that goes over an undulating membrane from the kinetoplast to the anterior end of the parasite (Fig. 118.2). Triatomine insects may ingest the parasite during a blood meal and in the midgut of the insect trypomastigotes transform into epimastigotes and multiply by binary fission. Epimastigotes then migrate and attach to the walls of the rectal sac where they produce nondividing metacyclic trypomastigotes that are eliminated with the insect feces. Infective metacyclic trypomastigotes gain entry into the mammalian host by penetrating mucous membranes or abraded skin. Trypomastigotes can then enter nonphagocytic or phagocytic cells, in which they transform into round amastigotes, without flagellum and of 0.5–4 μm in diameter, and divide by binary fission to produce a pseudocyst. Before rupture of the pseudocyst, amastigotes transform into trypomastigotes, which upon release re-enter cells or circulate in the blood, thus completing the life cycle (Fig. 118.3).

TRANSMISSION

The transmitting vectors of *T. cruzi* parasites are blood-sucking triatomine bugs of the order Hemiptera, family Reduviidae, subfamily Triatominae, and primarily genera *Rhodnius*, *Triatoma* and *Panstrongylus*. Around half of the 130 known triatomine species have been found to be naturally infected, although due to their physiologic similarities all of them are considered as potential vectors of Chagas disease.[10] The most common species are *Triatoma infestans* (Argentina, Bolivia, Brazil, Chile, Paraguay, Peru and Uruguay), *Rhodnius prolixus* and *Triatoma dimidiata* (northern South America and Central America), *Panstrongylus megistus* (central and eastern Brazil) and *Triatoma brasiliensis* (northeastern Brazil) (Fig. 118.4).

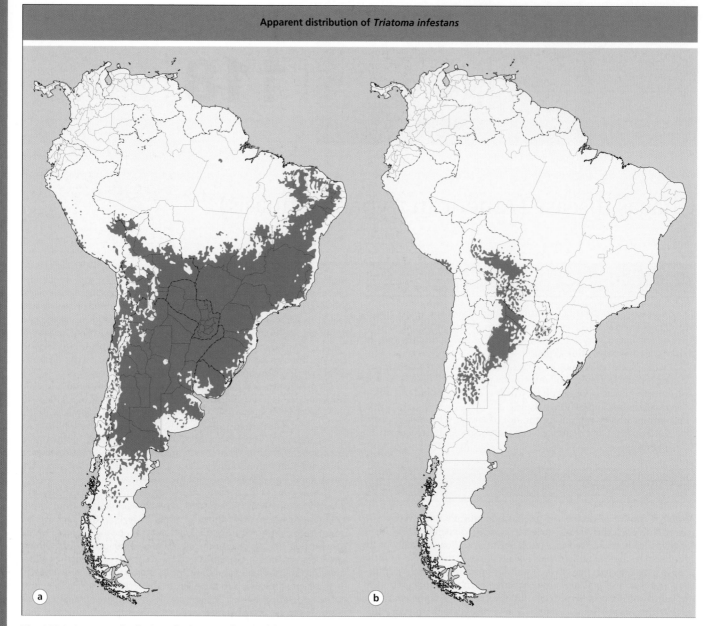

Fig. 118.1 Apparent distribution of *Triatoma infestans*. (a) Maximum predicted distribution in the absence of control interventions. (b) An estimate of current distribution based on report from the Intergovernment Commission for the Southern Cone Initiative. Reproduced with permission from Schofield *et al.*[2] Copyright Elsevier 2006.

Eggs from these insects reach complete development in around 134 days and adult forms can live for around 1 year. Adult triatomines are 1.5–3 cm long, with an elongated head, chitinous thorax and double wings. The natural habitats of triatomines are trees, burrows and rocks, where they feed on mammals, birds and reptiles. However, the presence of triatomines inside houses or huts constructed with vegetal materials favors the domestic transmission (Fig. 118.5).

Infection of triatomines with *T. cruzi* parasites occurs during a blood meal from a mammalian reservoir. Generally the vector is infective 20 days after ingesting parasites and continues to be infective for the rest of its life. Transmission of parasites occurs when infected triatomine insects defecate during a blood meal, depositing parasites close to the conjunctiva, mucosal tissues or the bite wound in the skin. Secondary routes of transmission to humans include blood transfusion, organ transplant and transplacental transmission. *Trypanosoma cruzi* can also be transmitted when mammalian hosts ingest infected insects or insect feces. This mechanism may be important in maintaining the sylvatic cycle[11,12] and occasionally causes significant outbreaks in humans.

PATHOGENESIS AND CLINICAL SYMPTOMS

Acute phase

The initial acute phase of *T. cruzi* infection may be asymptomatic and is not commonly reported, being diagnosed mainly in children younger than 10 years old. The incubation period between exposure to infection and the appearance of symptoms may be as short as 2 weeks. Metacyclic trypomastigotes that enter the organism are phagocytosed and multiply in local macrophages, inducing a localized inflammatory response causing unilateral conjunctivitis and periophthalmic edema (Romaña's sign) if parasites enter the conjunctiva (Fig. 118.6) or a cutaneous lesion (chagoma) if the portal of entry is the skin. Occasionally multiple chagomas may be seen in infants. Regional lymphadenopathy often accompanies acute infection, and systemic migration of parasites and invasion of other organs may result in fever, hepatosplenomegaly, generalized

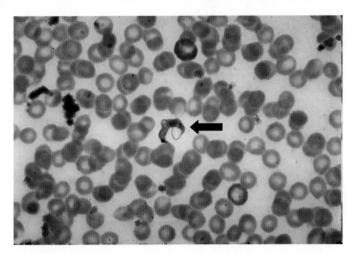

Fig. 118.2 *Trypanosoma cruzi* trypomastigote. Micrograph of *T. cruzi* (arrow) in a blood smear using Giemsa staining technique. Source: US Centers for Disease Control and Prevention (CDC), Atlanta, GA, USA. Public Health Image Library ID#3013.

lymphadenopathy, facial or generalized edema, rash, vomiting, diarrhea and anorexia. Acute infection in the heart may cause an acute myocarditis, with cellular infiltrate and patchy areas of necrosis and infected cells. There may be early ECG abnormalities, including sinus tachycardia, increased PR interval, T-wave changes and low QRS voltage. Acute phase infections are fatal in around 10% of cases in children. Once *T. cruzi* infection has been acquired, in the absence of treatment it is usually retained for life.[13]

Indeterminate or latent phase

In those surviving acute phase infection, intracellular multiplication and parasitemia in the blood subside, although trypomastigotes may still be detectable by sensitive methods. The majority of individuals who recover from the acute phase lead entirely normal lives without any further sequelae. However, after a symptom-free indeterminate phase of unpredictable duration which may last many years, ECG abnormalities typical of chronic Chagas disease arise in up to 30% of patients. There is no way to predict which individuals will progress to develop chronic Chagas.

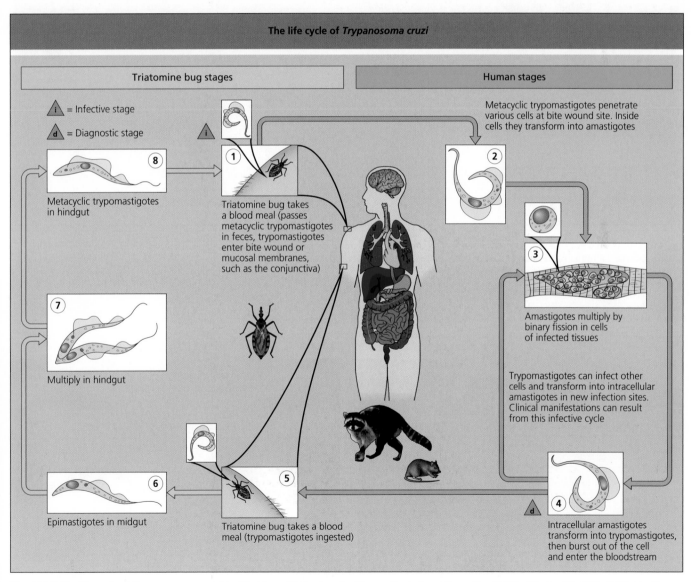

Fig. 118.3 The life cycle of *Trypanosoma cruzi*. Modified from US Centers for Disease Control and Prevention (CDC), Atlanta, GA, USA. Public Health Image Library ID#3384.

Geographical distribution of Chagas vectors

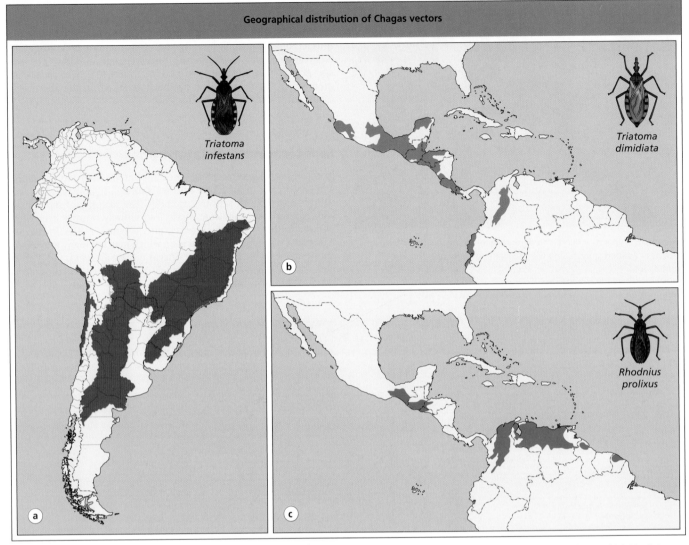

Fig. 118.4 Distribution of Chagas vectors. Maps indicating the historical distribution of (a) *Triatoma infestans*, (b) *Triatoma dimidiata* and (c) *Rhodnius prolixus*. Source: Pan American Health Organization/World Health Organization. 1989. Unpublished document WHO/VBC/89.967. Geneva, Switzerland.

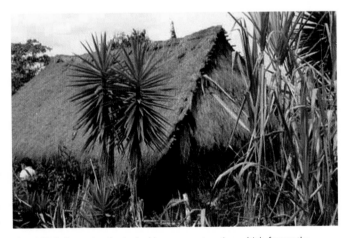

Fig. 118.5 Example of a typical house construction which favors the domestic transmission of *Trypanosoma cruzi* parasites.

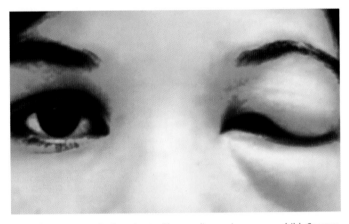

Fig. 118.6 Romaña's sign. Acute Chagas disease in a young child. Source: Special Programme for Research and Training in Tropical Diseases (TDR). World Health Organization Image ID#9305157.

Chronic phase

The pathogenesis of chronic Chagas disease is still somewhat enigmatic. Pathogenesis has been described as involving an inflammatory response, focal neurologic damage and, sometimes, autoimmunity.[14] *Trypanosoma cruzi* invades and replicates in macrophages, fibroblasts, Schwann cells, and smooth and striated myocytes, and parasite DNA can be found in heart muscle and smooth muscle of the alimentary tract in the chronic phase. It is known that antigens released from ruptured pseudocysts may spread from the immediate site of infection and be adsorbed to uninfected cells. This may lead to an extension of focal damage and the release of normally sequestered host antigens, which could precipitate autoimmunity. Candidate cross-reactive epitopes between *T. cruzi* and mammalian tissues have also been described, such as B13 and cruzipain in *T. cruzi* and host antigens in cardiac cells.[15] It is not clear whether autoantibodies are markers of pathology or have a causal role.

Focal lesions in the conducting system of the heart are associated, both clinically and experimentally, with corresponding ECG abnormalities. The pathogenesis of this 'neurogenic' form of chronic Chagas disease is thought to depend upon irreversible neuron loss in the acute phase, exacerbated by further loss with age, such that a threshold is reached beyond which organ function is perturbed. Gross pathology of the heart consists of megacardia and focal thinning of the myocardium, especially at the apex of the left ventricle, which may lead to apical aneurysm formation, which is considered to be pathognomonic of chronic chagasic cardiomyopathy (Fig. 118.7). Cardiac signs include dysrhythmias, palpitations, chest pain, edema, dizziness, syncope and dyspnea. The most typical ECG changes are right bundle branch block and left anterior hemiblock, but there may also be atrioventricular (AV) conduction abnormalities, including complete AV block. Many different types of dysrhythmia may occur, including sinus bradycardia, sinoatrial block, ventricular tachycardia, primary T-wave changes and abnormal Q waves.[16]

Associated chronic phase gastrointestinal symptoms result from denervation of hollow viscera and consequent dysfunction. Chagasic megaesophagus (Fig. 118.8) is more common than chagasic megacolon (Fig. 118.9) and either or both may be associated with chagasic cardiomyopathy.[17] Signs of megaesophagus include loss of peristalsis, regurgitation and dysphagia. Constipation and abdominal pain are typical symptoms of megacolon. Advanced megacolon may be associated with obstruction, perforation and sepsis.

The differential diagnosis of Chagas disease includes distinction from all other types of heart disease and ECG abnormalities, but changes such as right bundle branch block and left anterior hemiblock associated with a history of exposure to *T. cruzi* infection are indicative. Megacolon due to Hirschsprung's disease is usually recognizable, in part because of its rarity in adults.

Congenital infection

Perinatal transmission of *T. cruzi* parasites may occur in 2–10% of women of child-bearing age with indeterminate or chronic Chagas disease.[18] Characteristic signs of congenital infection are: hepatosplenomegaly, jaundice, anemia, interstitial pneumonia, myocarditis and neurologic signs. The ECG in congenital cases is usually normal but there may be low-voltage complexes, decreased T-wave height and increased AV conduction time.

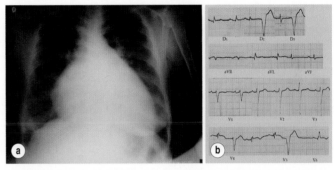

Fig. 118.7 Patient with advanced Chagas cardiomyopathy. (a) Radiography showing enlargement of heart. (b) ECG showing ventricular extrasystoles, atrioventricular block, ischemia and myocardial fibrosis in chronic Chagas' heart disease. Reproduced with permission from Coura.[31]

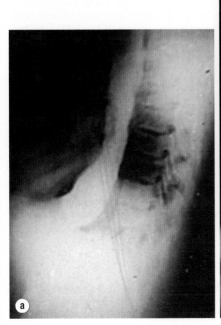
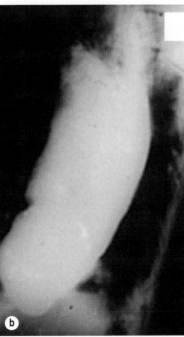

Fig. 118.8 Chagasic megaesophagus. Barium contrasted radiographs showing (a) megaesophagus grade III and (b) megaesophagus grade IV in a patient with chronic Chagas disease. Modified with permission from Coura.[31]

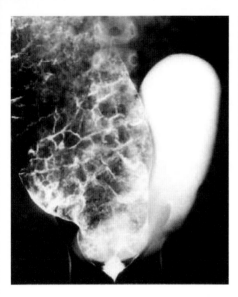

Fig. 118.9 Chagasic megacolon. Barium contrast radiography from the large intestine presenting a very large rectum–sigmoid segment filled with fecal mass. Reproduced with permission from Da-Costa-Pinto et al.[32]

Post-transfusion

Transfusion can be considered the second most common form of transmission for *T. cruzi*. The risk of parasite transmission by one unit of blood fluctuates between 12% and 20%.[18] The appearance of symptoms such as general lymphadenopathy and splenomegaly are common and occur several months after the blood transfusion. This is possibly due to the fact that trypomastigotes in contaminated transfused blood may less efficiently invade the heart or other organs.

Immunodeficient patients

An immunocompromised state may lead to reactivation of infection, producing symptoms typical of the acute phase. Meningoencephalitis is infrequent in immunocompetent adults but more common in infants and in immunocompromised adults. Chagas disease in HIV-infected patients is associated with advanced disease with CD4 counts <200 cells/mm³. The central nervous system (CNS) and the heart are the most commonly affected sites and may account for 75% and up to 44% of chagasic disease in HIV patients, respectively.[19] CNS manifestations can include acute fatal meningoencephalitis, tumoral lesions or a granulomatous encephalitis called 'brain chagoma'. Cardiac manifestations are heart failure and arrhythmias.

Reactivation of Chagas disease is always associated with high parasitemias in contrast to the low parasitemias found in chronic immunocompetent patients. Treatment of *T. cruzi* infection in HIV-positive individuals should be started early in the reactivation process, although meningoencephalitis carries a very poor prognosis.[20]

DIAGNOSIS

The World Health Organization (WHO) recommends that individual diagnosis must be based on two conventional tests based on different principles and different antigens.[21] This is due to the suboptimal sensitivity and/or specificity reported for the existing tests. The diagnosis of acute, congenital and reactivated forms of Chagas disease is based on direct detection of parasites, while the diagnosis of chronic infection is generally based on serologic testing.[13]

Parasitologic diagnosis

Direct microscopy

Circulating trypomastigotes may be detectable by direct microscopy of unstained wet-blood preparations in around 90% of acute cases and virtually never in chronic cases. Several methods can be attempted to improve the sensitivity of parasitologic diagnosis. These include microscopic examination of Giemsa-stained thick blood films, buffy coat layer after centrifugation of hematocrit capillaries (with care to avoid exposure to infection), centrifugation sediment from recently separated serum (Strout's method) and centrifugation sediment after lysis of red blood cells with 0.87% ammonium chloride. All these methods may fail, even in the acute phase of infection, if the parasitemia is low. Microscopic examination of biopsies from lymph nodes is an alternative in cases of undetectable parasitemia.

Xenodiagnosis

A more sensitive method of parasitologic diagnosis is the process known as xenodiagnosis, in which triatomine insects from laboratory colonies maintained on birds are fed on the suspect patient. The sensitivity of this method is close to 90% during the acute phase and between 20% and 50% during the chronic phase of the disease. The insects are dissected about 20–25 days after feeding and the hind gut contents are examined for the presence of *T. cruzi* epimastigotes. Care must be taken to avoid infection during this procedure and insects should be dissected in a microbiologic safety cabinet. It is also necessary to ensure that insects in the colony are not infected with the monoxenous flagellate *Blastocrithidia triatomae*, which may be found in *T. infestans*.

In the chronic phase of Chagas disease, xenodiagnosis is still the parasitologic method of choice throughout most of Latin America. In areas where *R. prolixus* is a vector of *T. cruzi*, xenodiagnosis may yield the nonpathogenic human trypanosome *Trypanosoma rangeli*. Frequently, *T. rangeli* infections in *Rhodnius* spp. can be identified by the presence of long, slender (up to 80 mm) epimastigotes invading the insect salivary glands (*T. rangeli* is transmitted by inoculation, not by contamination).

Culture

Culture of venous blood on to a blood agar base medium may be used as an alternative to xenodiagnosis but demands better laboratory facilities, is difficult to perform under field conditions and seldom achieves the sensitivity of xenodiagnosis.

Serologic tests

Specific antibodies to *T. cruzi* are usually detectable within a few days of infection and usually persist for life unless the infection is eliminated by chemotherapy. Rarely, serologic reversion may occur without treatment. There is an initial IgM response and a sustained IgG response, which is detectable by a variety of assays. Commonly used tests include the immunofluorescent antibody test (IFAT), enzyme-linked immunosorbent assay (ELISA) and the indirect hemagglutination test (IHAT). Most of these tests use lysates of epimastigotes as target antigens but several are based on recombinant proteins. Their sensitivity ranges from 96.5% to 100% and their specificity from 87% to 98.9%. Cross-reactions may occur, especially with visceral and cutaneous leishmaniasis, which may coexist in the same geographic area with Chagas disease.[22] Infants born of seropositive mothers may be seropositive until up to 9 months of age due to transplacental transfer of IgG. Seropositivity in such infants using an IgM-specific conjugate suggests congenital infection. Short-term visitors to endemic areas are extremely unlikely to acquire Chagas disease and, if infection is suspected through exposure to triatomine bites or blood transfusion, serologic status may be used to exclude more likely causes of heart disease.[23]

Molecular methods

Detection of *T. cruzi* DNA by polymerase chain reaction (PCR) may be an adjunct to parasitologic diagnosis. Different assays targeting DNA sequences such as the 195 base pair satellite repeat or the kDNA minicircle conserved region have been evaluated.[24] Although PCR-based assays have better sensitivity rates than xenodiagnosis, PCR methods have not been standardized and no kits are available commercially. For these reasons and because of the technical complexity of the testing, PCR is limited primarily to research settings and clinical utilization is minimal.[25]

Although several methods are available, current diagnostic approaches are insufficient to respond to the global Chagas disease challenge. There is an urgent need to develop and market new diagnostic tests that may be used in the remote areas where the disease is endemic and which perform well enough to direct clinical care.[26]

TREATMENT

Currently there are only two drugs available to treat Chagas disease: benznidazole and nifurtimox.[27] It has been estimated that both drugs produce parasitologic cure in 60–85% of acute cases. The use of either of these two drugs is recommended during the acute phase of infection and for chronic cases in patients under 15 years of age. Chemotherapy for chronic Chagas disease in adults is more controversial as the pathogenesis might be largely attributable to acute phase damage. Adult chronic cases are thus not always treated because the contribution of continued low-level infection to pathogenesis is uncertain, side-effects may cause interruption of treatment, treatment often fails to eliminate the organism and cure is difficult to prove (negative parasitology is not sufficiently sensitive to prove absence of infection and reversion of serology may take decades). Immunocompromised patients must be treated, and double or even higher dose rates, if tolerated, may be recommended to treat meningoencephalitis. Similarly, congenital cases also demand treatment. New therapeutic alternatives for *T. cruzi* elimination are being evaluated and work in this area has recently been extensively reviewed.[28]

Benznidazole

This orally delivered nitroimidazole should be used at doses from 5 to 10 mg/kg/day in two divided doses for 60 days. Children tolerate higher doses than adults. Common adverse events are rashes, fever, nausea, anorexia, weight loss, headache and insomnia. After 4 weeks of treatment dermatologic adverse events and peripheral neuropathy could occur and this should lead to treatment discontinuation. Laboratory testing for blood cell count should be performed before the start of treatment and every week during treatment to detect possible bone marrow suppression. This drug is contraindicated during pregnancy, in cases of hepatic or renal failure, and in cases of hematopathology or neuropathology.

Nifurtimox

Similar to benznidazole, nifurtimox is better tolerated by children. Recommended doses differ with age and are 15–20 mg/kg for children, 12.5–15 mg/kg for adolescents below 16 years old and 8–10 mg/kg for adults. Nifurtimox should be used at 25 mg/kg for the treatment of meningoencephalitis and at 10–20 mg/kg for congenital cases. The drug should be administered in three divided doses for 90 days in acute cases and 120 days in chronic cases. In adults it is recommended to start the treatment with low doses and increase by 2 mg/kg per week until reaching the maximal dose. Adverse events produced by nifurtimox are anorexia, weight loss, nausea, vomiting and abdominal discomfort. In some patients, symptoms of central nervous system toxicity could be present. These could be irritability, insomnia, disorientation, tremors, polyneuropathy, dizziness, vertigo and mood changes. Reversible psychiatric symptoms could also be present in elderly patients. This drug is not recommended during pregnancy.

Supportive treatment

Chemotherapy is often required for the treatment of adverse events such as fever, vomiting, diarrhea and convulsions. Management of acute meningoencephalitis may require anticonvulsants, sedatives and intravenous mannitol. Management of chronic chagasic heart disease may be a balancing act between patient management, drug administration and use of a pacemaker.[16] Sodium intake is restricted if there is acute-phase heart failure and diuretics and digitalis may be indicated.

Vasodilatation (angiotensin-converting enzyme inhibitors) and maintenance of normal serum potassium may be required initially; digitalis is advisable only as a last resort because it may aggravate dysrhythmias. Bradycardia that does not respond to atropine, atrial fibrillation with a slow ventricular response or complete AV block may necessitate a pacemaker. Surgical resection of dysrhythmic endocardial regions and of ventricular aneurysms has been suggested. Heart transplantation for end-stage chagasic cardiomyopathy has been shown to be a valuable treatment option.

Megaesophagus may improve with dietary control or respond to dilatation of the cardiac sphincter using probes, air or hydrostatic pressure. The surgical procedure for alleviating advanced megaesophagus involves selective removal of a portion of muscle at the junction between the esophagus and stomach. Severe megaesophagus may demand replacement of the distal esophagus with another part of the alimentary tract such as the jejunum.[17] The recommended surgical treatments for megacolon are the anterior rectosigmoidectomy and the modified Duhamel–Haddad operation.[29]

Table 118.1 Screening of blood donors for *Trypanosoma cruzi* in Latin America

	Coverage (%)	Seropositive (%)
Southern Cone countries		
Argentina	100	4.50
Bolivia	86	9.90
Brazil	100	0.61
Chile	75*	0.47
Paraguay	99	2.80
Uruguay	100	0.47
Andean Pact countries		
Colombia	99	0.98
Ecuador	100	0.15
Peru	99	0.26
Venezuela	100	0.67
Central America		
Belize	100	0.40
Costa Rica	100	0.34
El Salvador	100	2.46
Guatemala	100	0.79
Honduras	100	1.40
Nicaragua	100	0.49
Panama	98	0.90

* 98% in endemic regions.
From Schofield *et al.*[2] Copyright Elsevier 2006.

PREVENTION

There is no vaccine for Chagas disease. Crude or fractionated antigens can protect experimental animals against a fatal challenge infection. However, prospects for vaccine development are remote because of the alleged autoimmune pathogenesis of Chagas disease and the impracticality of vaccine trials.[30] Current preventive measures are focused on four main strategies:[3]

- the elimination of domestic vectors;
- the screening of blood donors;
- maternal screening and treatment of infected newborns; and
- active case detection and treatment among school-age children.

Chagas disease is maintained by poverty and poor housing (see Fig. 118.5), which prevent families and communities from controlling domestic triatomine populations. Prevention of new cases of vector-borne *T. cruzi* infection relies on insecticide spraying, health education and improved housing. Pyrethroids, which have low toxicity and high residual activity, are the insecticides of choice for killing triatomines.

Blood for transfusion and organ donors should be screened by one of the available serologic methods. In Latin America, ELISA is the principal method for the current extensive screening of blood donors for *T. cruzi* (Table 118.1). Chemical methods to sterilize donated blood were previously recommended; however, universal blood donor screening for *T. cruzi* infection is now the preferred strategy for the prevention of transfusion- and transplant-related Chagas disease.[23] In 2006, the US Food and Drug Administration (FDA) approved an ELISA from Ortho-Clinical Diagnostics for blood screening prior to transfusion.

REFERENCES

References for this chapter can be found online at http://www.expertconsult.com

Chapter | **119** | *Sharon J Peacock*

Melioidosis

Melioidosis is a serious bacterial infection caused by the Gram-negative bacillus *Burkholderia pseudomallei*. This organism has been designated a select agent by the US Centers for Disease Control and Prevention.

EPIDEMIOLOGY

The global distribution of melioidosis is shown in Figure 119.1. Most cases are diagnosed in South East Asia and Northern Australia, but the disease is underrecognized in many parts of the world (reviewed in[1]). Imported infection is seen mainly in immigrants or soldiers serving in endemic areas, but occasionally occurs in tourists.[1]

Melioidosis occurs as a result of inoculation, inhalation or ingestion of *B. pseudomallei* present in the environment. In Asia, melioidosis is most commonly seen in agricultural workers who probably acquire disease following contamination of existing wounds or new penetrating injuries. Evidence for infection via the respiratory route includes the development of melioidosis in US helicopter crews and servicemen during the war with Vietnam, and the shift towards more pneumonic melioidosis observed in Northern Australia during periods of extreme weather including heavy rainfall and winds.[2] Ingestion was implicated as the route of infection during an outbreak associated with contaminated drinking water,[3] although this appears to be rare. Near-drowning led to a cluster of melioidosis cases in survivors of the 2004 tsunami.[4] Mother-to-child and person-to-person transmission are very rare, while patient-to-patient transmission in the hospital setting has not been reported in the published literature. Rare laboratory-acquired infections have been described (reviewed in[5]).

Melioidosis is seasonal in the tropics where most cases present during the rainy season.[1] Males are more often affected than females, and infection can occur at any age with a peak incidence in people aged 40–60 years. Risk factors include diabetes mellitus, chronic lung or kidney disease, thalassemia, alcohol excess, malignancy and immunosuppressive treatment (including corticosteroids) (reviewed in[1]). An associated predisposition is present in around three-quarters of adults presenting with melioidosis.

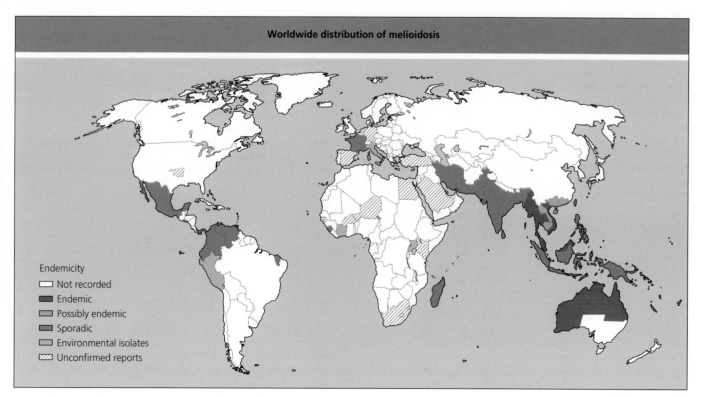

Worldwide distribution of melioidosis

Endemicity
- ☐ Not recorded
- ■ Endemic
- ▨ Possibly endemic
- ▨ Sporadic
- ☐ Environmental isolates
- ▨ Unconfirmed reports

Fig. 119.1 Worldwide distribution of melioidosis. Reproduced with permission from Cheng & Currie.[1]

PATHOGENESIS AND PATHOLOGY

Study of the pathogenesis of melioidosis is in its infancy compared with many other infectious diseases. Key questions are:

- How does *B. pseudomallei* interact with the host immune response, and how does this relate to specific conditions that predispose to melioidosis?
- What is the basis for bacterial latency and persistence *in vivo*?

Putative virulence factors include quorum sensing, a type III secretion system (TTSS3) that shares homology to the *inv/spa/prg* TTSS of *Salmonella enterica* serovar Typhimurium and the *ipa/mxi/spa* TTSS of *Shigella flexneri*, capsular polysaccharide, lipopolysaccharide and flagella (reviewed in[6]).

Burkholderia pseudomallei is a facultative intracellular pathogen that can invade nonphagocytic cells and persist in phagocytes. Following uptake, the organism can escape endosomes and propel itself within and between cells by polar nucleation of actin and induce cell fusion. TTSS3 is central to this process (reviewed in[6]), and BimA is required for actin-based bacterial motility.[7] Reversible colony morphology switching associated with complex alterations in protein expression has been described, and this may be associated with adaptive changes that facilitate bacterial survival *in vivo*.[8] The cytokines interferon gamma (IFN-γ), tumor necrosis factor (TNF) and interleukins (IL)-12 and IL-18 play an important role in early resistance against experimental *B. pseudomallei* infection. These cytokines are expressed during human melioidosis, and may contribute to pathogenesis since high plasma levels of several cytokines are correlated with mortality.

The macroscopic pathology of melioidosis is primarily one of abscess formation. These may be single or multiple, and present in one or more organs. The histopathologic appearance of infected human tissue forms a spectrum from acute to chronic granulomatous inflammation. Samples taken at post-mortem were reported to show focal or diffuse acute necrotizing inflammation with varying numbers of neutrophils, macrophages, lymphocytes and 'giant cells' of unknown cell type.[9] Intracellular bacteria have been observed within macrophages and giant cells.[9]

PREVENTION

Burkholderia pseudomallei is ubiquitous in the environment in areas where disease is endemic and avoidance of the organism is virtually impossible. Protective gear (waterproof shoes or boots and protective gloves) are recommended for agricultural workers in affected geographical regions, but are rarely used because they cause discomfort when worn for prolonged periods in tropical climates. People with risk factors for melioidosis should be advised to stay indoors during periods of heavy wind and rain due to the potential for aerosolization of *B. pseudomallei*. These recommendations are based on known routes of transmission but their efficacy has not been evaluated to date. No *B. pseudomallei* vaccine is available for human use.

CLINICAL FEATURES

The period between an exposure event that results in melioidosis and clinical features of infection is highly variable and often difficult to define. A history of a specific inoculation event is often absent. In one study, 25% of cases reported a specific event from which an incubation period of 1–21 days (mean 9 days) was derived.[10] The incubation period following a high inoculum event such as near-drowning may be short, with a period of less than 24 hours from event to bacteremia in some cases. By contrast, exposure may be followed by a prolonged period of latency, the maximum recorded being 62 years.[11]

Time from onset of clinical manifestations to presentation to a medical facility is also highly variable. In northeast Thailand, around a third of patients have symptoms for less than 7 days, one half report being unwell for 7–28 days, and the remainder have symptoms for more than 28 days.[12] In Northern Australia, 13% of patients presenting for the first time had symptoms for more than 2 months.[10]

Manifestations of disease are extremely broad and range from an acute fulminant bacteremia to a chronic localized infection. Melioidosis is a great mimicker, and it is often impossible on clinical grounds to differentiate between this and other acute and chronic bacterial infections, including tuberculosis. The majority of adult patients develop an acute septicemia associated with bacterial dissemination that most commonly manifests as pneumonia and/or hepatosplenic abscesses. Multiple organ involvement, and the development of additional organ involvement following presentation, are common.

Bacteremia is detected in around half of patients with melioidosis. Septic shock is common in this group and is frequently complicated by the development of organ dysfunction. The lung is involved in approximately half of all cases, manifesting as pneumonia and/or lung abscess(es) (Fig. 119.2). Large or peripheral lung abscesses may rupture into the pleural space to cause thoracic empyema. Solitary or multiple abscesses are detected in the liver and/or spleen in around one-quarter of cases in Thailand when abdominal imaging is performed as routine. More than half of patients with hepatosplenic abscess(es) lack abdominal signs and symptoms. Renal abscesses are often associated with calculi and urinary tract infection. Infection involving the urinary tract is present in at least one-quarter of Thai patients based on a urine culture positive for *B. pseudomallei*, although only a quarter of positive cases have urinary symptoms such as urinary frequency, dysuria, haematuria, or flank or back pain.[13] Genitourinary infection is common in Australia, with prostatic abscesses occurring in 18% of male patients.[14]

A neurologic syndrome of meningoencephalitis with varying involvement of the brain stem, cerebellum and spinal cord has been reported in 5% of melioidosis cases in Darwin, Australia.[15] Prominent features on presentation were unilateral limb weakness, predominant cerebellar signs, mixed cerebellar and brain stem features with peripheral weakness, or flaccid paraparesis.[15] Peripheral motor weakness may mimic Guillain–Barré syndrome and unilateral limb weakness may mimic a stroke. Focal suppurative infections involving the central nervous system with or without meningitis have been reported. CNS infections occur in around 1.5% of melioidosis patients in Thailand,[16] but the syndrome of meningoencephalitis has not been defined in this setting.

Figure 119.3 shows serial CT brain scans with contrast performed on a patient with neurologic melioidosis. The patient initially presented with fever and a hemiparesis. Blood, throat swab and urine cultures were negative for *B. pseudomallei*. A CT scan was performed (a), and the patient was treated for a urinary tract infection and a cerebrovascular accident. The patient re-presented 2 months later with worsening headache, confusion and hemiparesis. Repeat CT scan (b) showed a ring-enhancing lesion with surrounding edema in the right frontoparietal lobe, pus from which grew *B. pseudomallei*. The patient went on to make a full recovery after prolonged parenteral antimicrobial treatment.

Osteoarticular involvement is diagnosed in around one-sixth of patients in Thailand, but only 4% of those affected in Australia.[14] The knee is the most common site for septic arthritis, and more than one joint is involved in a quarter of affected cases. Osteomyelitis is often secondary to infection of another organ, although localized osteomyelitis does occur.

Melioidosis in Thai children presents as acute suppurative parotitis in around one-third of cases, but this is uncommon in Thai adults and very rare in Australia. Parotitis is bilateral in 10% of cases and may be complicated by rupture into the auditory canal, facial nerve palsy and necrotizing fasciitis.[17]

Skin and soft tissue infections are found in a quarter of melioidosis patients in Thailand and one-sixth in Australia. This includes superficial pustules, subcutaneous abscesses and pyomyositis. Such foci may represent the source of systemic infection, or may result from hematogenous or local spread (Fig. 119.4). Soft tissue infection may run an aggressive course similar to that seen for necrotizing

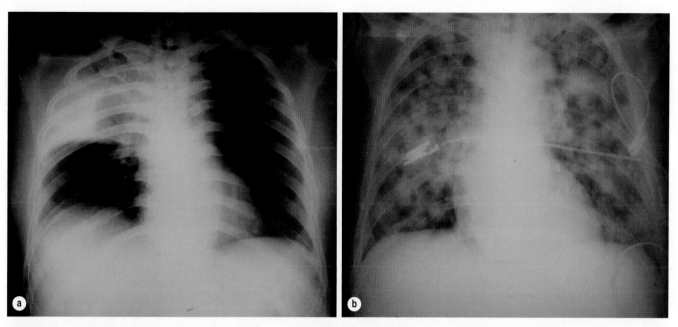

Fig. 119.2 Chest radiographs of two patients with melioidosis. (a) Right upper lobe consolidation in a patient with bacteremia, pneumonia, pyelonephritis and subcutaneous abscesses. (b) Widespread bilateral shadowing in a patient with bacteremia, pneumonia and multiple abscesses in liver and spleen. Courtesy of Dr Gavin Koh.

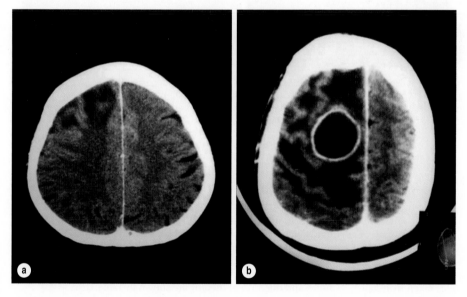

Fig. 119.3 CT brain scans. (a) Hypodensity in the right frontal lobe. (b) Ring-enhancing lesion with surrounding edema in the right frontoparietal lobe. Reproduced with permission from Limmathurotsakul *et al.*[16]

fasciitis caused by other organisms. Infections involving many other sites have been described, including lymphadenitis, mycotic aneurysm, mediastinal infection, pyopericarditis, orbital cellulitis, corneal ulcers, acute otitis media, sinusitis, and abscess formation in the breast, scrotum and deep tissues of the neck.

DIAGNOSIS

Given the myriad of possible presentations, a high index of suspicion is essential for clinicians working in areas that are endemic for melioidosis. This infection should also be considered when investigating the

cause of fever in returning travelers or army personnel who could have been exposed to a contaminated environment. Microbiologic culture and identification of *B. pseudomallei* represents the diagnostic gold standard (Fig. 119.5).

A direct immunofluorescent microscopy assay has been described that provides a rapid presumptive diagnosis of melioidosis,[18] but the antibody used is not commercially available and the assay is restricted to a small number of laboratories in Thailand. Unlike the investigation of many other bacterial infections, culture should be performed on all available specimens including blood, urine, throat swab, respiratory secretions, pus and swabs from surface wounds. Growth of even a single *B. pseudomallei* colony from any sample is

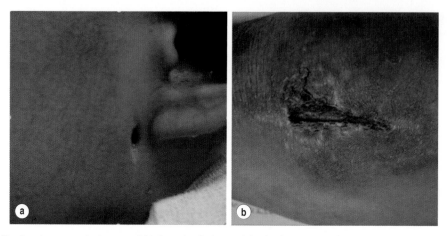

Fig. 119.4 (a) Abscess affecting the pre-auricular area. (b) Infected soft tissue of the heel. Courtesy of Drs Rapeephan Rattanawongnara and Ekamol Tantisattamo.

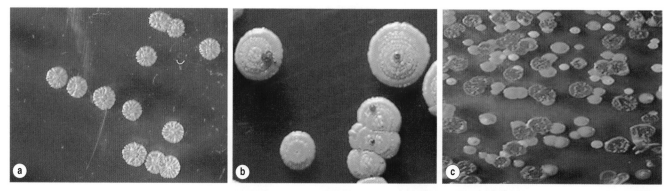

Fig. 119.5 Colony variation is commonly seen during culture of clinical isolates on Ashdown's agar. (a) Typical colony appearance of *B. pseudomallei* after incubation at 37°C in air for 3 days. (b) Colony variation within a single colony in which the parental colony (pink) has given rise to a second morphotype (red). (c) Variable colony morphology from a single sample; genotyping confirmed the presence of a single clonal type. Reproduced with permission from Wiersinga *et al.*[6] Original pictures courtesy of Mrs Vanaporn Wuthiekanun and Dr Narisara Chantratita.

diagnostic for melioidosis in patients presenting to hospital with a febrile illness, since the organism is not a member of the normal human flora. Because the organism can become disseminated in the host, the site of culture positivity may not necessarily reflect the major site of clinical infection. For example, a throat swab may be positive for *B. pseudomallei* in a patient who presents with a liver or splenic abscess. It is important to alert the laboratory to the suspicion of melioidosis because the organism can easily be overlooked as a contaminant (especially in cultures of samples taken from colonized sites) and because cultures should be handled in biosafety containment level 3 facilities. Preliminary culture results should be available within 48 hours, although identification may be delayed when microbiologists are not familiar with the organism. Speed to blood culture positivity has prognostic significance, and the bacterial count of *B. pseudomallei* in blood and urine are positively associated with outcome (reviewed in[12]).

Polymerase chain reaction (PCR) has been evaluated for the diagnosis of melioidosis but is not in routine use. Serologic assays such as the indirect hemagglutination (IHA) test have no role in the diagnosis of melioidosis where infection is endemic since anti-*B. pseudomallei* antibodies are common in the general population.[19] A single IHA titer of >1:40 or a rising titer in an individual who has not previously resided in areas where melioidosis is endemic may be diagnostically useful but requires careful interpretation based on a detailed travel and medical history.

MANAGEMENT

Appropriate parenteral antimicrobial agents should be commenced immediately on suspicion of the diagnosis of melioidosis. Ideally, culture should be performed prior to their administration but treatment should not be delayed if culture cannot be performed rapidly, as in the case of aspiration of pus under imaging or operative procedure. Choice and duration of therapy are shown in Table 119.1.

A retrospective study of the effect of granulocyte colony-stimulating factor (G-CSF) in patients with septic shock due to melioidosis at the Royal Darwin Hospital, Northern Australia demonstrated a dramatic decrease in mortality from 95% to 10% concurrent with its introduction.[20] However, a randomized placebo-controlled trial of G-CSF for severe melioidosis in northeast Thailand failed to show an effect on mortality.[21] No other adjunctive therapies have been shown to improve outcome from melioidosis. Patients with severe melioidosis associated with septic shock, respiratory failure associated with severe infection or acute respiratory distress syndrome, acute renal failure and other manifestations of a severe septic illness require intensive care management where this is available. The availability of intensive care facilities is an important contributor to the marked difference in outcome for high-income versus low- or lower-middle-income countries. Predictors of mortality from melioidosis include APACHE II and a scoring system based on a smaller number of readily available parameters.[22]

Table 119.1 Antimicrobial treatment of melioidosis

Drug	Dose	Duration
Initial parenteral treatment		
Ceftazidime Meropenem	50 mg/kg/dose (up to 2 g) q6–8h*, *or* 25 mg/kg/dose (up to 1 g) q8h*	Minimum 10–14 days, or longer (4–8 weeks) for deep-seated infection
Oral eradicative treatment		
Trimethoprim–sulfamethoxazole	Weight-based regimen for adults (q12h): • 2 × 160–800 mg (960 mg) tablets if >60 kg • 3 × 80–400 mg (480 mg) tablets if 40–60 kg • 1 × 160–800 mg (960 mg) *or* 2 × 80–400 mg (480 mg) tablets if <40 kg *with or without*	At least 3–6 months
Doxycycline	2.5 mg/kg/dose up to 100 mg po q12h†	

Notes:
1. Amoxicillin–clavulanate is an alternative treatment for pregnant women and children younger than 8 years and as an alternative to first-line therapy in other patient groups. Amoxicillin–clavulanate dosing for melioidosis is reviewed in[23]. For intravenous-phase treatment, the recommended dose is 20/5 mg/kg q4h. Parenteral amoxicillin–clavulanate is associated with higher rates of treatment failure, so avoid if first-line drugs can be given. For oral eradicative treatment, use amoxicillin–clavulanate at a dose of 20/5 mg/kg q8h. For adult patients <60 kg a dose of 1000/250 mg q8h is suggested. For patients >60 kg, the recommended maximum dose is 1500/375 mg q8h. Oral amoxicillin–clavulanate is associated with higher rates of relapse.
2. Adjust drug dosages as necessary in patients with renal failure, a common complication of melioidosis.
*Consider addition of trimethoprim–sulfamethoxazole 8/40 mg/kg (up to 320/1600 mg) q12h for treatment of patients with neurologic, prostatic, bone or joint melioidosis.
†Doxycycline is not used as part of oral treatment of melioidosis in Australia but is routinely used in Thailand. The equivalence of trimethoprim–sulfamethoxazole versus trimethoprim–sulfamethoxazole plus doxycycline is the subject of a randomized clinical trial in Thailand.

Hematologic and biochemical blood tests should be performed to detect the onset of acute renal failure, abnormal liver function tests and anemia, all of which are well recognized during severe melioidosis. Arterial blood gases should be taken in patients with lung involvement and/or any evidence of respiratory impairment. Admission C-reactive protein may be normal or only mildly elevated, including patients with severe sepsis, fatal cases and in relapsed melioidosis.

A chest radiograph should be taken in all patients with suspected melioidosis. Common radiographic patterns include localized patchy alveolar infiltrate, focal, multifocal or lobar consolidation, diffuse interstitial shadowing considered consistent with blood-borne spread of infection, pleural effusion, and upper-lobe involvement which may include cavitation. The radiographic pattern may mimic tuberculosis. The development of empyema and/or lung abscess(es) is well recognized, and repeat chest radiographs are indicated for patients with respiratory involvement.

Abdominal ultrasound or CT scan should be performed on all patients with melioidosis to exclude the presence of abscesses in liver and spleen. The finding of a 'Swiss cheese' appearance on ultrasound or a 'honeycomb' appearance on CT scan are characteristic for melioidosis. Clinical evidence of prostatic involvement requires appropriate imaging. Transrectal ultrasound findings include solitary and multiple abscesses. Early brain CT scan may be normal in patients with neurologic melioidosis, but MRI often shows dramatic changes.[15,16] The need for other imaging will depend on clinical features and organ involvement.

Parenteral antibiotics are required for a minimum of 10–14 days or until clear clinical improvement is observed (whichever is the longer). This is followed by oral antibiotics to complete 12–20 weeks of therapy (or more if clinically indicated), as described in Table 119.1. Melioidosis is characterized by difficulty in eradicating the causative organisms. Fever clearance is often slow (median fever clearance time of 9 days), and without evidence of clinical deterioration is not normally sufficient to indicate the need for a change in therapy. Sputum and draining abscess cultures may remain positive for several weeks in a patient who is otherwise responding to treatment. A patient who has clinical deterioration or persistently positive blood cultures should be viewed as failing treatment, at which stage the need for imaging, drainage of collections and change in antimicrobial therapy should be considered.

Death from melioidosis occurs in around 50% of cases in Thailand and 19% in Australia.[12,14] The majority of deaths are due to uncontrolled sepsis and/or organ dysfunction, including respiratory and renal failure. The single most important complication for patients who survive the first episode is recurrent melioidosis, which may occur despite prolonged appropriate oral antimicrobial treatment. This occurs in around 13% of patients followed for 10 years, half of which occurs within 12 months of the primary episode.[24,25] Recurrence represents either relapse following failure to eradicate bacteria responsible for the primary infection, or re-infection with a new strain. Three-quarters of recurrent cases are due to relapse and one-quarter to re-infection.[26] Time to recurrence is significantly shorter for episodes due to relapse compared with those due to re-infection.[24] Choice and duration of oral antimicrobial therapy are the most important determinants of relapse, followed by the presence of a positive blood culture and multifocal distribution.[24]

REFERENCES

References for this chapter can be found online at http://www.expertconsult.com

Plague

Plague is an acute, life-threatening zoonosis caused by the bacterium *Yersinia pestis*.[1-3] The disease is best known for three devastating pandemics, including the Black Death of the Middle Ages. The last of these pandemics, which began in southwest China in the late 1800s, was largely over by the end of World War II but human cases of plague continue to occur in many regions. Plague is primarily a disease of rodents, and humans typically acquire infection as a result of being bitten by rodent fleas, less commonly by handling infected animals, and rarely by inhaling infectious respiratory particles. Historically, urban, rat-borne plague outbreaks have been responsible for most human plague cases and widespread epidemics. Over the past half century, however, most human plague outbreaks have occurred in remote, rural populations.[3,4] The three principal clinical forms of plague are bubonic plague, septicemic plague and pneumonic plague. The most common of these is bubonic plague, an acute illness characterized by fever and enlarged tender lymph nodes (buboes) that usually appear in the groin, axillary or cervical regions proximal to the site of inoculation. Bacteremia and sepsis occur when lymphatic defenses have been breached (septicemic plague) and plague pneumonia can arise from inhaling infectious respiratory droplets or secondarily as a result of blood-borne invasion of the lungs. Occasionally, pneumonic plague spreads from person to person, most often in crowded, substandard living conditions.[5]

Plague is often fatal when not diagnosed and treated appropriately early in the course of infection.[1,3] The aminoglycosides, tetracyclines and chloramphenicol are the antibiotics most commonly used to treat human plague.[1,6,7] Prevention and control of plague during outbreaks relies on prompt identification and treatment of human cases, isolation of pneumonic cases and identification of their contacts, and use of flea control measures.[5] Pneumonic plague patients should be isolated under respiratory droplet precautions until no longer infectious.[1,7] Persons who have been in close contact (<2 m) with pneumonic plague patients should be placed on antimicrobial prophylaxis. Others who have more distant contact should be monitored for fever. Human plague risks can be reduced further by environmental sanitation measures intended to reduce rodent populations.[5] Plague is considered to be an important potential weapon of bioterrorism.[2,7]

EPIDEMIOLOGY

Agent

Yersinia pestis is a Gram-negative, microaerophilic coccobacillus belonging to the Enterobacteriaceae. Molecular studies, including genomic sequencing of a few *Y. pestis* strains, indicate that this bacterium has recently evolved from the enteric pathogen, *Y. pseudotuberculosis*.[8] *Y. pestis* is nonmotile, nonsporulating, does not ferment lactose and exhibits bipolar staining with Wayson, Wright or Giemsa stain. Growth occurs in a variety of media at a wide range of temperatures (4–40°C; optimal 28–30°C) and pH values (5.0–9.6; optimal 7.2–7.6).[9]

The plague bacterium produces many factors that enable it to survive in and cause disease within its mammalian hosts (virulence factors) and be transmitted by flea vectors (transmission factors) (Table 120.1).[2,9] Some factors are expressed selectively at temperatures and environments encountered in fleas or mammals. For example, hemin storage locus (*hms*) products are expressed in the low temperature environment of the flea and produce a biofilm that enables plague bacteria to form blockages in the flea's gut. These blockages hamper the flea's ability to ingest blood and cause it to starve. Starving fleas repeatedly attempt to feed and often regurgitate in an effort to clear the blockage from their guts, a behavior that can flush *Y. pestis*-containing material from the blockage into the bite wound and result in infection of the host. At typical mammalian body temperatures biofilm production ceases, causing dissolution of blockages and occasionally clearance of *Y. pestis* infection from fleas. Murine toxin (*ymt*), which is highly toxic in mice and rats but has little effect on other mammals, also is required for survival of *Y. pestis* within flea midguts.

In mammals, plasminogen activator (*pla*) degrades blood clots and helps plague bacteria escape from the site of initial inoculation. YopM, which is resistant to *pla* activity, competes for thrombin and inhibits its activation of platelets, further promoting dissemination of *Y. pestis* within the host. Early in infection, *Y. pestis* behaves as a facultative intracellular pathogen, invading and multiplying within host phagocytes. Survival of plague bacteria within the host is made possible by a type III secretion system composed of various Yops that can interfere with the production of proinflammatory cytokines, impair the cytoskeletal dynamics of phagocytes and cause immune cell death by apoptosis. At mammalian host temperatures *Y. pestis* produces a capsular antigen (*caf1*) that renders it resistant to further phagocytosis and, along with the effects of various Yops, allows it to multiply extracellularly. Various iron uptake systems, including one that utilizes the siderophore yersiniabactin, enable the plague bacterium to compete with its hosts for this essential nutrient.

Three biovars (biotypes) of *Y. pestis* have been recognized according to the ability of the bacteria to ferment glycerol and reduce nitrate, distinctions that have also been supported by various molecular analyses.[8,9] These biotypes (Antiqua, Medievalis and Orientalis) originally were thought to have been correlated respectively with the three principal plague pandemics – Justinian's Plague, the Black Death, and the Modern (Third) Pandemic. More recent analyses have complicated this picture, calling into question these biovar–pandemic associations and establishing the presence of a previously unrecognized Microtus biovar and atypical isolates that have been termed pestoides group.[8]

Although plague is global in its distribution, the majority of its spread occurred during the Third Pandemic. As a consequence, strains

Table 120.1 Proposed virulence and transmission factors for *Yersinia pestis*

Genomic element	Virulence or transmission factor	Proposed role in virulence or transmission
9.5 kb plasmid (pesticin plasmid; a 19 kb dimer of this plasmid also exists)	Pesticin sensitivity (*pst*)	Loss of sensitivity to pesticin (a bacteriocin) is associated with reduced siderophore binding capability (affects iron uptake)
	Plasminogen activator (*pla*)	Fibrinolytic activity (important for dissemination)
70–75 kb plasmid (low calcium response plasmid)	*Yersinia* outer proteins (Yops – genes found in the Yop virulon, a type III secretion system; includes *IcrV* or V antigen)	Proposed functions vary among Yops and include: translocation of other Yops (effectors) across cell membranes; disturbance of phagocyte cytoskeleton dynamics (interferes with phagocytosis); blocking production of proinflammatory cytokines and interfering with ability of B and T cells to be activated by means of antigen receptors (immunosuppression); or binding thrombin (interferes with thrombin–platelet aggregation)
100–110 kb plasmid	Murine toxin (*ymt*)	Required for survival in fleas; also has β-adrenergic antagonist activity in rats and mice but not guinea pigs, rabbits, dogs or nonhuman primates
	F1 'capsular' antigen (*caf1*)	Resistance to phagocytosis by monocytes
Chromosomal	Pigmentation (*pgm* locus, includes genes of *hms* locus, high pathogenicity island and *ybt* operon)	Pigment-positive strains bind hemin and appear pigmented on culture media containing Congo Red; *pgm* locus contains genes of the high pathogenicity island (HPI), which is found in other Yersiniae and certain related enteric bacteria; the HPI contains the *ybt* (yersiniabactin) operon, which encodes genes of a siderophore-based iron uptake system; the *pgm* locus also contains the *hms* locus, which produces biofilm and must be functional for 'blocking' to occur in the flea vector (blocking increases efficiency of *Y. pestis* transmission by fleas)
	Endotoxin (lipopolysaccharide)	Lipopolysaccharide release associated with major pathogenic effects of plague sepsis, systemic inflammatory response syndrome and associated adult respiratory distress syndrome, cytokine activation, complement cascade, disseminated intravascular coagulation, bleeding, unresponsive shock and organ failure
	Serum resistance (lipopolysaccharide in part)	Resistance to complement-mediated lysis; proposed to be related in part to lipopolysaccharide structure
	pH 6 antigen (*psa*)	Entry into naive macrophages; assists in delivery of Yops into phagocytic cells

from the Americas demonstrate very little genetic diversity in comparison to those of central and eastern Asia which display rich biochemical, genetic and host diversities.[10,11]

Life cycle

Yersinia pestis is maintained in cycles involving transmission between rodents and their fleas and through long-term survival of infectious fleas in burrows or other off-host environments. (Fig. 120.1).[12] Other proposed means of maintenance include survival of *Y. pestis* in soils or in chronically infected rodents,[13] but evidence that either of these is important under natural conditions is limited. Humans and other incidental hosts of *Y. pestis* are not directly involved in maintaining its natural cycle.

Although most foci are maintained by transmission between wild rodents and their fleas, commensal rats (*Rattus rattus*, *R. norvegicus*, etc.) and their fleas (especially Oriental rat fleas, *Xenopsylla cheopis*) remain the principal sources of large epidemics. In a few areas, such as Madagascar, commensal rats also act as the primary rodent hosts of *Y. pestis*.[5] The most critical role played by susceptible rodents in the natural plague cycle is to serve as sources of infection for feeding fleas.[12] Although virtually any rodent can be infected with *Y. pestis*, not all succumb to plague, and the susceptibility of rodent populations and species can vary greatly. Only those fleas that feed on dying rodents with very high (>10^6 *Y. pestis*/ml blood) bacteremias are likely to become infected. Besides enabling infection of fleas by *Y. pestis*, fatal bacteremias in rodents force infected fleas to abandon their dead hosts and seek new ones, thus promoting spread of the disease among wild animals and humans.

Geographic distribution

Plague foci are widely distributed throughout the world, and human cases are typically reported from 10 or so countries each year.[14] Selected countries reporting significant human or animal plague outbreaks during the interval from 1988 to 2007 are shown in Figure 120.2.

Populations affected

Plague mostly affects impoverished populations of developing countries living in rural villages that are heavily infested with rodents

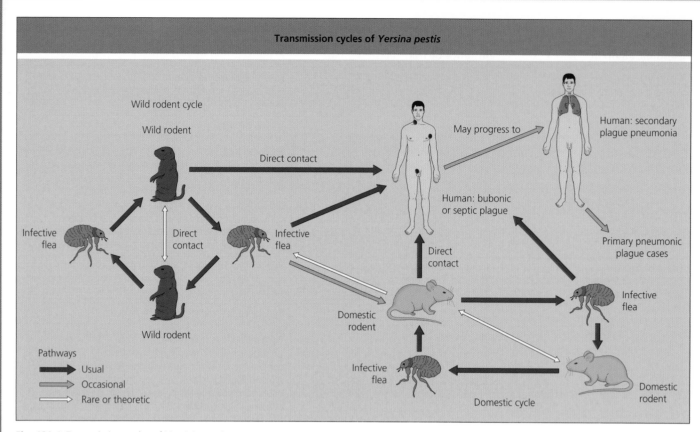

Fig. 120.1 Transmission cycles of *Yersinia pestis*.

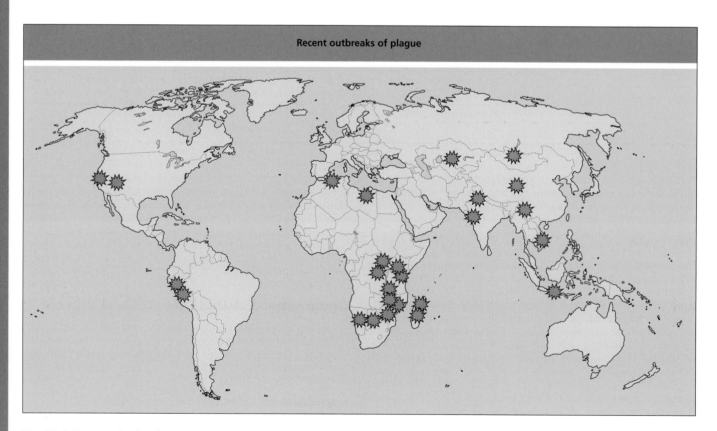

Fig. 120.2 Recent outbreaks of plague. Compiled from sources of the WHO, the Centers for Disease Control and Prevention, and the individual countries.

(particularly commensal rats) and their fleas. Urban rat-borne plague is now unusual, but still occasionally occurs in developing countries.[1,4] In the USA, most persons are exposed to infection around rural residential properties that are often poorly maintained and provide shelter and food for rodents.[4] Cases also occasionally occur among campers, hikers, hunters, pet owners, veterinary staff or others exposed to plague in natural settings or through handling infected animals.[5,15]

In the absence of control measures, plague can spread from rural areas to major cities and ports, either through unintended transport of rats or other animals, or by passage of infection between adjoining rodent populations.[4,5] Occasionally, persons who travel during the incubation phase later develop plague pneumonia and transmit the disease to others encountered along their way. Plague risks for persons visiting endemic areas for business or tourism are extremely low because these persons typically stay in relatively modern hotels and spend little time in the rural villages most likely to be affected by the disease.

Disease incidence

Virtually all plague cases reported to the World Health Organization (WHO) in recent decades have come from Asia, Africa and the Americas. While the last great pandemic originated in Asia, over the last 20 years there has been a striking shift in distribution of cases from that continent to Africa.[3,4,14] Based on the latest WHO statistics, 25 countries reported a total of 38 359 cases (mean of 2557 cases per year) and 2845 deaths (7.4% fatality rate) from 1989 to 2003 (Table 120.2).[14] During this 15-year period, nine countries in sub-Saharan Africa and nearby Madagascar reported 81% of the world's cases, with the remaining cases occurring in Asia (14.2%) and the Americas (4.3%). Madagascar alone reported over 34% of all cases and Tanzania accounted for 14%. In 2003, five African countries (Algeria, Democratic Republic of the Congo, Madagascar, Mozambique and Uganda) reported 98.7% of global plague cases and 98.8% of plague deaths.[14] At present, plague in Asia and the Americas occurs only sporadically, although large

Table 120.2 Reported cases of plague in humans by country, 1989–2003			
Region	**Country**	**Number of cases**	**Number of deaths**
Africa	Algeria	11	1
	Botswana	173	12
	Democratic Republic of Congo	4935	616
	Kenya	44	8
	Madagascar	13148	1132
	Malawi	907	16
	Mozambique	2387	28
	Namibia	2012	80
	Tanzania	5249	335
	Uganda	821	130
	Zambia	1169	29
	Zimbabwe	417	34
	Total	**31 273**	**2421**
Americas	Bolivia	37	6
	Brazil	105	0
	Ecuador	14	14
	Peru	1380	60
	USA	101	10
	Total	**1637**	**90**
Asia	China	519	52
	India	892	58
	Indonesia	6	0
	Kazakhstan	24	7
	Laos	10	0
	Mongolia	115	36
	Myanmar	761	6
	Vietnam	3122	175
	Total	**5449**	**334**
World totals		**38 359**	**2845**

outbreaks remain a possibility, as demonstrated by an epidemic of more than 1200 cases that occurred in Peru from 1992 to 1995.

Although large outbreaks have not been reported in the USA since the early 1900s when the disease was first introduced, plague still represents an emerging disease in this country,[4] with more than 420 cases of human plague reported since 1950. The most recent outbreak occurred in 2006 when 17 cases were reported from seven states, equaling the highest number of reported cases in any year since 1984.[16] Although plague remains enzootic and occasionally causes epizootics in rural areas within the 17 western-most states, about 90% of all human cases reported in the past three decades have occurred in four states (New Mexico, Colorado, Arizona and California).[4,16]

Sources of infection and risks for humans

Flea bites are the most common source of human *Y. pestis* infection.[1] Plague also can be acquired through handling infected animals, which is an important source of exposure among persons who hunt and skin marmots (*Marmota* spp.) in central Asia and among similar groups in the USA who handle carcasses of prairie dogs, ground squirrels, rabbits and wild carnivores.[1,5] Pet owners and veterinary staff may become infected with *Y. pestis* while caring for infected domestic cats.[15] Outbreaks of plague have occurred in Saudi Arabia, Libya, Jordan and Kazakhstan as a result of persons handling or consuming infected camel or goat meat.[2,5]

Human risks of exposure to infectious fleas or animals are typically greatest during epizootics when *Y. pestis* spreads rapidly through rodent populations, causing high mortality among these animals and abandonment of dead hosts by fleas. Even in the presence of efficient flea vectors, epizootics probably occur only when rodent host densities exceed certain threshold levels, presumably because of the increased likelihood of host-to-host contact and transfer of infectious fleas between hosts. Among the most important factors affecting rodent populations and the occurrence of plague are those related to climate,[17] particularly precipitation and temperature, both of which can influence plague transmission through their impacts on rodent food availability, rodent host population dynamics, vector flea abundance, blockage of flea guts by biofilm and survival of infectious fleas.

Primary pneumonic plague occurs when persons inhale infectious respiratory secretions.[1,7] This usually arises during the course of an outbreak of bubonic plague in which persons develop secondary pulmonary infection and then spread plague to others through infectious respiratory droplets, starting a chain of airborne transmission. Persons living in the same home as a pneumonic plague patient or attending the sick are especially at risk. Unfortunately, plague can be spread intentionally as an aerosol, cause severe outbreaks (most likely pneumonic plague outbreaks) with many fatalities, create panic and require special preparations to ensure effective responses to bioterrorism attacks (see also Chapter 71). For these reasons *Y. pestis* is classified as a category A agent (highest bioterrorism risk), along with the agents of anthrax, smallpox, tularemia and viral hemorrhagic fevers.[2,7] *Yersinia pestis* strains could also be genetically modified so they would be resistant to the antibiotics commonly used to treat plague.

Under natural conditions, primary pneumonic plague comprises only a small fraction of the total number of cases in any plague-endemic region. In the USA primary pneumonic plague cases represent only about 2% of total cases, nearly all of which were associated with handling cats that had plague pneumonia and cough.[15] Human-to-human spread of plague through respiratory contact has not been documented in the USA since 1924,[7] but the likelihood of pneumonic plague outbreaks remains high in many developing countries.

Seasonality

Flea-borne cases of human plague in the northern hemisphere are most likely to occur between late spring and the end of summer when epizootic transmission peaks.[1] In tropical and semitropical plague foci, transmission may vary between a wet, relatively cool season and another season of hotter, drier weather, with the numbers of cases being lower during the latter period.[17] Occasional winter cases of human plague occur in temperate regions among hunters, trappers, pet owners or veterinary staff handling infected animals.

PATHOGENESIS AND PATHOLOGY

Yersinia pestis is among the most pathogenic bacteria known, using numerous chromosomal and plasmid-encoded gene products to cause severe disease and promote its establishment and spread within the host (see Table 120.1).[2,9]

Yersinia pestis organisms inoculated through the skin or mucous membranes travel to and multiply within regional lymph nodes.[1] In the early stages of infection, nodes are found to be edematous and congested with minimal inflammatory infiltrates and vascular injury. Fully developed buboes are surrounded by serous fluid, contain large numbers of plague bacteria and exhibit considerable vascular damage, hemorrhagic necrosis and neutrophil infiltrates. In later stages, abscess formation and spontaneous rupture of lymph nodes may infrequently occur.

Plague sepsis in the absence of signs of localized infection, particularly a bubo, is termed primary septicemic plague and can result from direct entry of *Y. pestis* through broken skin, mucous membranes or the bite of an infectious flea.[1] Septicemic plague can also occur secondarily to bubonic or pneumonic plague when lymphatic or pulmonary defenses are breached and *Y. pestis* enters the bloodstream and multiplies en masse. Bacteremia commonly occurs in all forms of plague, while septicemia occurs less commonly and can be immediately life threatening.

Yersinia pestis can cause serious disease in almost any organ. Fatal cases commonly experience diffuse interstitial myocarditis with cardiac dilatation, multifocal necrosis of the liver, diffuse hemorrhagic splenic necrosis and fibrin thrombi in renal glomeruli.[1] Disseminated intravascular coagulation (DIC) can occur, resulting in thrombosis within the microvasculature, necrosis and bleeding, and widespread cutaneous, mucosal and serosal petechiae and ecchymoses, as well as occasional gangrene of acral parts, such as the fingers and toes (see Fig. 120.4).

Primary plague pneumonia, which usually results from inhalation of infective respiratory particles,[1] often begins as a lobular process and then extends by confluence, becoming lobar and then multilobar. Typically, plague organisms are numerous in the alveoli and pulmonary secretions. Secondary plague pneumonia arising from hematogenous spread of *Y. pestis* typically begins as a diffuse interstitial process, with plague bacilli appearing most numerous in interstitial spaces. Pathologic findings in untreated cases of plague pneumonia usually include edema, diffuse pulmonary congestion, hemorrhagic necrosis and scant infiltration by neutrophils.[1]

PREVENTION AND CONTROL

Rapid identification and treatment of cases is of utmost importance to limit fatalities and prevent human-to-human spread of plague.[1,5] In endemic regions, human and animal-based plague surveillance should be done to identify areas at risk. Epidemiologic investigations of human cases and threatening epizootics must also be conducted to effectively target control actions. Rapid implementation of flea control measures to reduce risk of infectious flea bites is also critical. Other environmental measures include reducing sources of food and shelter for rodents, and occasionally selective use of rodenticides. Flea control should always be undertaken before the killing of rodents to reduce the chances that infected fleas will leave dying hosts and feed on humans.[5]

Health providers also need appropriate education and consultation so that they can help others protect themselves. Personal protective measures and preventive actions should be encouraged, including avoidance of sick or dead animals, use of insect repellents (*N,N*-diethyl-M-toluamide, DEET), flea control for pets, use of rubber gloves by hunters, and provision of prompt veterinary care for cats that might be ill with plague. A plague vaccine is no longer available commercially, although clinical trials of recombinant vaccines containing F1 (*caf1*) and V antigens of *Y. pestis* are currently underway.[2]

CLINICAL FEATURES

Bubonic plague

The incubation period of bubonic plague is usually 2–6 days but occasionally longer. Typically, patients experience acute onset of fever, chills, myalgias, arthralgias, headache and lethargy.[1] Tenderness and pain often occur within 24 hours in a regional lymph node(s) proximal to the initial site of inoculation. The femoral and inguinal groups of nodes are most commonly affected, axillary and cervical nodes less so, depending on the site of inoculation and geographic location of the cases. Cervical lymph node involvement is more commonly observed in countries where individuals sleep on hut floors, presumably because this behavior results in a greater risk of being bitten in the neck region by infectious floor-dwelling fleas. Enlarging buboes become progressively swollen, painful and tender, sometimes exquisitely so. Typically, the patient avoids movement, stretching and pressure near the bubo and guards against palpation. Tissues surrounding the bubo often becomes edematous and the overlying skin may be reddened (Fig. 120.3). Although relatively uncommon, inspection of the skin around the bubo or distal to it may reveal a flea bite marked by a small scab, papule, pustule or ulcer. Larger furuncular lesions, sometimes with tularemia-like eschars, also can occur rarely. Plague buboes differ from lymphadenitis of most other causes by their rapid onset, extreme tenderness, surrounding edema, accompanying signs of toxemia and absence of cellulitis or readily apparent ascending lymphangitis.

When treated soon after illness onset with an appropriate antimicrobial agent, bubonic plague patients usually experience defervescence and improvement of other systemic manifestations over a 2- to 3-day period.[1] Buboes frequently remain enlarged and tender for a week or more after initiation of treatment and rarely become fluctuant. Without antimicrobial treatment, bubonic plague patients typically exhibit an increasingly toxic state of fever, tachycardia, lethargy followed by prostration, agitation, confusion and, in more severe cases, convulsions and delirium. Differential diagnostic options include staphylococcal or streptococcal adenitis, tularemia, cat-scratch disease, mycobacterial infection, acute filarial lymphadenitis, chancroid and strangulated inguinal hernia.

Septic plague

Septicemic plague typically presents as a rapidly progressive, overwhelming endotoxemia that is usually fatal unless treated promptly.[1] Primary sepsis occurs in the absence of regional lymphadenitis, and a diagnosis of plague is likely to go unsuspected until results

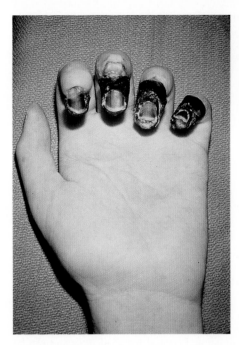

Fig. 120.4 Septic plague patient who demonstrated disseminated intravascular coagulation, bleeding into the skin and acral gangrene as a late manifestation.

are available from blood cultures. Patients with primary septicemic plague often present with gastrointestinal symptoms, including nausea, vomiting, diarrhea and abdominal pain, further complicating diagnosis. Petechiae, ecchymoses, bleeding from wounds or orifices, and ischemia of acral parts are manifestations of DIC (Fig. 120.4). Preterminal signs can include refractory hypotension, renal shutdown, obtundation and other signs of shock. Acute respiratory distress syndrome associated with septicemic plague may be confused with other conditions, including hantavirus pulmonary syndrome.

Differential diagnostic possibilities include septicemia caused by other bacterial infections, such as the agents of meningococcemia, bacterial endocarditis, tularemia or other Gram-negative bacterial infections.

Pneumonic plague

Pneumonic plague is the most rapidly developing and life-threatening form of plague.[1,7] The incubation period for primary pneumonic plague is usually 2–5 days (range 1–6 days). Illness onset is most often sudden, with chills, fever, body pains, headache, weakness, dizziness and chest discomfort. Cough, sputum production, increasing chest pain, tachypnea and dyspnea typically predominate on the second day of illness; hemoptysis, increasing respiratory distress, cardiopulmonary insufficiency and circulatory collapse can also occur. The sputum of primary plague pneumonia patients is typically watery or mucoid, frothy and blood tinged, and can be bloody. Initially, chest signs may indicate localized pulmonary involvement and a rapidly developing segmental consolidation can appear before bronchopneumonia occurs elsewhere in both lungs (Fig. 120.5). Liquefaction necrosis and cavitation can develop at sites of consolidation and result in residual scarring.

Secondary pneumonic plague resulting from metastatic spread typically manifests as a diffuse interstitial pneumonitis with sputum production that is scant and more likely to appear tenacious and inspissated than the sputum of primary pneumonic plague patients.

Differential diagnostic possibilities include other bacterial conditions such as tularemia, mycoplasma pneumonia or other community-acquired bacterial pneumonias, Legionnaires' disease, Q fever and staphylococcal or streptococcal pneumonia. Viral pneumonias requiring differentiation include influenzal pneumonitis, hantaviral pulmonary syndrome and those caused by respiratory syncitial virus or cytomegalovirus infection.

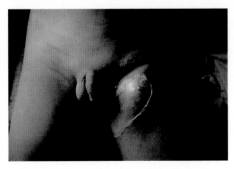

Fig. 120.3 Left inguinal and femoral buboes, demonstrating surrounding edema and overlying desquamation.

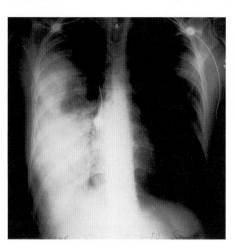

Fig. 120.5 Chest radiograph of a patient who has primary plague pneumonia, showing extensive infiltrates in the right middle and lower lung fields.

Other manifestations

Plague meningitis is unusual (3% of USA cases from 1950–1994) and typically arises as a complication among the treated survivors of bubonic plague.[1] Plague occasionally presents as pharyngitis accompanied by fever, sore throat and cervical lymphadenitis, and can be confused with other more common infectious causes of pharyngitis. Primary plague pharyngitis can result from respiratory exposures or ingestion of infected undercooked meat and is usually associated with marked cervical glandular enlargement. Oculoglandular plague can arise from inoculation of Y. pestis through the conjunctiva.

DIAGNOSIS

Except in outbreak situations, making a timely diagnosis of plague requires a high index of clinical suspicion, careful case history and physical examination. Treatment delays or misdiagnoses increase the likelihood of fatalities,[6] and infected travelers who seek medical care after returning from endemic areas are especially at risk. Laboratory tests for plague are highly reliable when conducted by experienced persons, but such expertise is usually limited to reference laboratories.

When plague is suspected, clinical specimens should be obtained promptly for microbiologic assays, chest radiographs taken and specific antimicrobial therapy initiated. Blood and other specimens, including bubo aspirates, sputum, tracheal washes, swabs of skin lesions or pharyngeal mucosa and cerebrospinal fluid, should be collected when appropriate and inoculated onto suitable media (e.g. brain–heart infusion broth, sheep blood agar, chocolate agar or MacConkey agar).[18] Bubo aspirates typically yield only small amounts of fluid and 1–2 ml of saline may need to be injected first to obtain adequate material. Smears of each specimen should be stained with Gram, Wayson or Giemsa stain. An acute-phase serum specimen should be collected for Y. pestis antibody testing, followed 3–4 weeks later by a convalescent-phase specimen. For fatal cases, samples from buboes, liver, spleen, lungs and bone marrow should be collected at autopsy for culture, fluorescent antibody or immunohistochemical staining, and histologic studies. Yersinia pestis-infected tissues can be transported in Cary Blair or similar holding medium. Presumptive identification of Y. pestis can be made by direct immunofluorescence assay, polymerase chain reaction or antigen capture enzyme-linked immunosorbent assay. A rapid immunogold dipstick assay that detects Y. pestis antigens in patient samples also appears promising,[19] providing staff are adequately trained in its application and use appropriate controls. In addition to providing rapid results, the dipstick-type assays can be used in remote village clinics, which typically lack refrigeration, extensive laboratory equipment and access to adequate microbiologic laboratories.

Laboratory confirmation of plague can be provided by isolation of Y. pestis from body fluids or tissues.[18] Plague bacteria are readily distinguished from other Gram-negative bacteria by polychromatic and immunofluorescence staining properties, growth characteristics, biochemical profiles and lysis by Y. pestis-specific bacteriophage. Laboratory mice are susceptible to Y. pestis and are used to make isolations from contaminated materials and for virulence testing. Alternatively, confirmation can be provided by demonstration of a fourfold change in serum antibodies to Y. pestis.[18] A titer of 128 or greater in a single serum sample from a patient who has a compatible illness and who has not received plague vaccine can provide presumptive evidence of infection. Less than 5% of patients fail to seroconvert and some will develop detectable antibodies within 5 days of illness onset, although most seroconvert 1–2 weeks later and a few require more than 3 weeks to seroconvert. Early antibiotic therapy may delay seroconversion by several weeks. Positive serologic titers decrease gradually over time but can be present for months to years. Passive hemagglutination assay (PHA) is used most frequently for serodiagnosis; however, enzyme-linked immunosorbent assays that detect IgM and IgG antibodies to Y. pestis are also useful as they can identify antibodies characteristic of early infection and differentiate these from antibodies resulting from previous vaccination.

White blood cell counts for plague patients typically range from 10 000 to 25 000/mm^3 and contain predominantly early stage polymorphonuclear leukocytes.[1] In some instances leukemoid reactions occur with white cell counts in excess of 50 000/mm^3.

MANAGEMENT

Untreated, plague is fatal in over 50% of patients who have bubonic plague and in nearly all patients who have septicemic or pneumonic plague. Mortality rates in the USA were reportedly 14%, 22% and 57% for cases of bubonic, septicemic and pneumonic plague, respectively.[7] Fatalities are almost always due to delays in seeking treatment or misdiagnosis, emphasizing the need for rapid diagnosis and appropriate antimicrobial therapy (Table 120.3).[1,6]

Streptomycin has long been considered the drug of choice for treating plague, but another aminoglycoside (gentamicin) is increasingly being used because of its availability and ease of administration.[1,6] Tetracyclines or chloramphenicol are also effective, and chloramphenicol is indicated for conditions that require high tissue penetration, such as plague meningitis, pleuritis, endophthalmitis or myocarditis. Although doxycycline is typically the tetracycline of choice for treating plague, clinical trials of its efficacy have not been reported. However, a recent review of 75 human plague cases in New Mexico, USA indicated that gentamicin or tetracyclines were as efficacious as streptomycin in treating human plague.[6] Trimethoprim–sulfamethoxazole (co-trimoxazole) has been used successfully to treat bubonic plague, but it is considered a secondary choice. Although fluoroquinolones have yet to be evaluated for treating human plague, animal experiments suggest these agents would be effective and ciprofloxacin has been recommended as an antimicrobial for treating human cases during bioterrorism attacks.[7] Penicillins, macrolides and cephalosporins have a suboptimal effect and should not be used to treat plague. In general, antimicrobial treatment should be continued for either 7–10 days or for at least 3 days after the patient has become afebrile. Improvement is usually evident 2–3 days from the start of treatment, although fever may persist for several more days.

Complications of delayed treatment include DIC, adult respiratory distress syndrome and other consequences of bacterial sepsis; such patients require intensive monitoring and close physiologic support. Buboes may require surgical drainage and abscessed nodes can be a cause of recurrent fever in patients. Viable Y. pestis have been isolated from buboes 1–2 weeks after clinical recovery. Although isolated reports exist of Y. pestis strains resistant to streptomycin or tetracycline, the few antibiotic-resistant Y. pestis strains isolated from humans have not been associated with treatment failure and typically have exhibited only partial resistance to a single agent. However,

Table 120.3 Treatment guidelines for plague

Drug		Dosage	Route of administration
Streptomycin	Adults Children	1 g q12h 15 mg/kg q12h*	im im
Gentamicin	Adults Children Infants/neonates	1–1.5 mg/kg q8h[†] 2.0–2.5 mg/kg q8h 2.5 mg/kg q8h	im or iv im or iv im or iv
Tetracycline	Adults Children >8 years old	0.5 g q6h 6.25–12.5 mg/kg q6h	po po
Doxycycline	Adults Children >8 years old and >45 kg Children >8 years old and >45 kg	100 mg q12h 100 mg q12h 2.2 mg/kg q12h	po or iv po or iv po or iv
Chloramphenicol	Adults Children >1 year old	12.5 mg/kg q6h[‡] 12.5 mg/kg q6h[‡]	po or iv po or iv

*Not to exceed 2 g/day.
[†]Daily dose should be reduced to 3 mg/kg as soon as clinically indicated.
[‡]Up to 100 mg/kg per day initially. Dosage should be adjusted to maintain plasma concentrations at 5–20 mg/ml. Hematologic values should be monitored closely.

a multidrug-resistant strain of *Y. pestis* isolated from a plague patient in Madagascar appeared to be highly resistant to the antibiotics typically recommended for treatment (tetracycline, streptomycin and chloramphenicol).[20] Resistance was plasmid-mediated and could be transferred to other strains of *Y. pestis* and to *Escherichia coli*. Surveillance for multidrug-resistant *Y. pestis* in Madagascar and elsewhere has not provided evidence for the spread of similar strains. Postexposure treatment for 7 days with a tetracycline, chloramphenicol or trimethoprim–sulfamethoxazole is recommended for persons who have had close contact with pneumonic plague patients in the previous 7 days.[7]

In addition to fever watch, antimicrobial prophylaxis is sometimes recommended for persons who have handled an infected animal or for household members of bubonic plague patients because of likely flea exposures.[1,6] Antimicrobial prophylaxis also might be recommended following a bioterrorism attack.[7] Isolation and respiratory droplet precautions are recommended for patients with pneumonic plague, including the use of masks for persons caring for these patients while they are infectious. The use of masks may interrupt person-to-person transmission during pneumonic plague outbreaks. Pneumonic plague patients are considered to be noncontagious following 48 hours of antibiotic treatment.

REFERENCES

References for this chapter can be found online at http://www.expertconsult.com

C Ben Beard
David T Dennis

Chapter | **121** |

Tularemia

Tularemia is an uncommon, potentially severe bacterial zoonosis caused by *Francisella tularensis*. The natural cycle of the causative organism involves maintenance of infection in a wide diversity of animal hosts and in certain hard ticks. Transmission of *F. tularensis* to humans, which are incidental hosts, occurs by several modes, including bites by infective ticks and other arthropods, direct inoculation of *F. tularensis* through skin or mucous membranes from handling infectious materials, ingestion of contaminated water or food, or by inhalation of contaminated aerosols or dusts. The agent of tularemia is widely distributed in temperate and subarctic regions of North America and Eurasia. Human infection results in various clinical presentations of varying severity depending on the route of inoculation, the dose and virulence of the infecting strain, and the host defenses. The most common clinical form, ulceroglandular tularemia, presents as an illness with fever, an ulcer at the site of inoculation and regional lymphadenitis. Several other forms occur involving various organ systems. Tularemia is considered to be an important potential weapon of bioterrorism.

EPIDEMIOLOGY

Agent

Francisella tularensis is a small, facultatively intracellular, Gram-negative coccobacillus. The organism has a lipidated envelope and is able to survive under favorable conditions for several weeks in water, moist soil and decaying animal carcasses. Within the species *F. tularensis*, there are three recognized subspecies: *F. t. tularensis* (type A), *F. t. holarctica* (type B) and *F. t. mediasiatica*. Type A isolates are known almost entirely from North America, with the single exception of a collection of isolates made in the Danube region in Slovakia.[1] Type B isolates are found throughout the northern hemisphere, both in Eurasia and widely across North America. Subspecies *mediasiatica* is limited in its distribution to central Asia.[2]

Traditionally, type A isolates have been considered more virulent than type B isolates based on observations derived primarily from animal models. Recent studies, however, have revealed genetic differences in isolates evaluated from around the USA, indicating that type A strains from western USA are less virulent than type B strains in terms of clinical outcomes in humans.[3]

In addition to the three *F. tularensis* subspecies, there are two other closely related species in the genus, *Francisella novicida* and *Francisella philomiragia*. Disease caused by these agents is rare and generally less severe. *Francisella novicida* has been seen as a cause of illness in immunocompromised patients, and *F. philomiragia* has been seen in immunocompromised patients and near-drowning vicitims.[4]

Francisella tularensis is considered to be a potential agent of bioterrorism because it can be weaponized as an aerosol, could result in large numbers of casualties, and because it requires special actions for medical and public health preparedness.[5] (See also Chapter 71.)

Life cycle

Francisella tularensis is widespread in nature and has been recovered from more than 100 species of wild mammals, at least nine species of domestic animals (including cats, dogs and cattle), numerous species of birds, some amphibians and fish, and more than 50 species of arthropods.[6] The principal natural cycles of the agent involve maintenance of infection in wild mammalian hosts, such as lagomorphs (wild hares and rabbits), terrestrial rodents (especially voles and meadow mice) and aquatic rodents (water rats, muskrats, beaver). Certain species of hard ticks are able to maintain infection from one developmental stage to another. Transmission among animals is accomplished by the bites of blood-feeding arthropods or by direct exposure to contaminated materials in the environment (Fig. 121.1).[6] Predation and cannibalism may also contribute to the natural cycle.

Humans become infected:
- when they intrude into the arthropod-borne cycle and are bitten by ticks, which are true biologic vectors, or by blood-feeding flies or mosquitoes via mechanical transmission;
- by handling or ingesting infectious animal tissues or fluids;
- by ingestion of contaminated water or food; or
- by inhalation of infective aerosols or dusts.

Occasional cases occur following infective bites or scratches by cats[7] or other carnivores or predators with contaminated mouths or claws. Although the agent is highly infectious, requiring only 10–50 organisms to regularly cause experimental infections of humans, person-to-person transmission has not been documented.

Geographic distribution

Tularemia is endemic throughout much of the Nearctic and Palaearctic regions between latitudes 30°N and 71°N. This includes all of North America from the Arctic Circle to northern Mexico, much of Eurasia and some states of northern Africa along the Mediterranean coast.[6] In North America, the highest incidence of tularemia in humans occurs in south-central, south-eastern, Great Plains and Rocky Mountain regions of the USA (Fig. 121.2),[8] but cases have been reported throughout the continental USA, across Canada and in Mexico as far south as Guadalajara. In Eurasia, the disease occurs most frequently in Scandinavia and in states of the former Soviet Union. Tularemia also occurs sporadically throughout most of Europe, in some areas of the Near East and Middle East, in Central Asia and in Mongolia. It has not been documented in Central or South America, Australia or Africa outside the Mediterranean littoral.

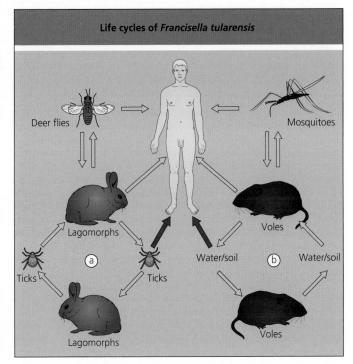

Fig. 121.1 Life cycles of *Francisella tularensis*. The two major life cycles in nature are shown. In cycle (a), which is dominant in North America, *F. tularensis* is maintained predominantly among lagomorphs and hard ticks. In cycle (b), which is dominant in Eurasia, *F. tularensis* is principally maintained among cricetine rodents, especially field voles and mice, water voles and other aquatic rodents. Humans are incidental hosts that are infected by tick vectors and by the bites of flies or mosquitoes that have contaminated mouthparts, by direct contact with infected animal carcasses or other contaminated materials, by ingestion of contaminated matter or by inhalation of infectious aerosols or dusts.

Populations affected

Tularemia is a rural disease. It affects persons of all ages and both sexes. Groups at highest risk include:[9–11]

- hunters and trappers, wildlife specialists, animal skinners and dressers, butchers and others who handle potentially infective animal carcasses;
- rural residents, especially farmers, who are exposed to water, soils and dusts contaminated by infected wild animals, such as meadow voles, lagomorphs and aquatic mammals; and
- persons exposed in enzootic areas to bites by certain hard ticks, tabanid flies or mosquitoes.

Disease incidence

Global incidence figures are not available. In Eurasia, recent outbreaks involving hundreds of cases each have been reported from Sweden,[12] Kosovo[13] and Spain,[14] and outbreaks involving thousands of persons have been reported in the past from the former Soviet Union. Tularemia incidence is relatively stable in the USA, where the disease has been in steady decline since 1945 (Fig 121.3).[8] In the period 2000–2005, a total of 778 cases were reported from 42 states, averaging 130 cases (range 90–154) per year. Four states accounted for 52% of all reported cases: Missouri (158 cases), Arkansas (117 cases), Oklahoma (76 cases) and Massachusetts (57 cases). The highest incidence among 5-year age groups was in 5–9 year olds and 75–79 year olds. Males accounted for 69% of reported cases during this period. Reported disease onset peaked in summer months, with 66% of cases occurring from May through August, although cases were reported from all months of the year (CDC, unpublished data).

Sources of human infection

Eurasia

Cricetine rodents (especially meadow voles, lemmings, water voles and muskrats), water and soil contaminated by these animals, hares (*Lepus* spp.) and bites by contaminated mosquitoes (especially *Aedes cinereus*) are the principal sources of human tularemia in Eurasia.[6] Mosquito-borne infection occurs in forested and marshy Scandinavian and Baltic regions. Sporadic cases also result in Eurasia from bites by infected ticks and by blood-feeding flies. Outbreaks of tularemia among farmers have been described in Europe following respiratory exposure to dusts from contaminated stored and fresh mown hay,[15,16] and among workers in agricultural processing plants exposed to contaminated water sprays. Ingestion of water and food contaminated by

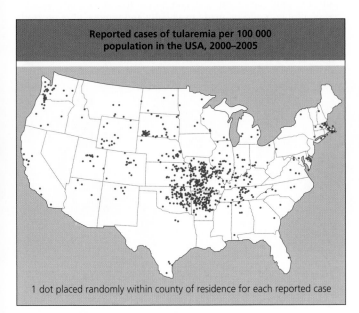

Fig. 121.2 Reported cases of tularemia per 100 000 population in the USA, 2000–2005.

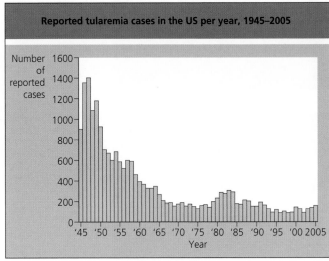

Fig. 121.3 Reported tularemia cases in the USA per year, 1945–2005.

infected rodents or hares has also resulted in outbreaks in the region, such as recently reported from Kosovo and Turkey.[13,17] In Japan, the disease has historically been associated with the trapping, handling and eating of wild hares.

North America

The principal animal sources of infection in North America are the cottontail rabbit (Fig. 121.4) (*Sylvilagus* spp.), wild hares and rodents (muskrats, beaver, voles, ground squirrels).[6,9] The agent is vectored by certain species of hard ticks, especially the dog tick, *Dermacentor variabilis* (Fig. 121.5), the lone star tick, *Amblyomma americanum*, and the Rocky Mountain wood tick, *Dermacentor andersoni*.[6] Biting tabanid flies, especially deer flies (*Chrysops* spp.) (Fig. 121.6), mechanically transmit the infection. The epidemiology of tularemia in North America has changed significantly since the 1930s and 1940s, when the disease most commonly called 'rabbit fever' had a much higher incidence and when cases were more likely to occur in the winter and be linked to the hunting, dressing and butchering of wild rabbits and hares than to arthropod bites[18,19] (CDC, unpublished data).

Seasonality

Mosquito-borne transmission in Eurasia peaks in the summer months. In North America, a peak of tularemia cases in the spring and summer months is associated mostly with bites by ticks and blood-feeding flies, and a second peak in the late autumn and winter is associated with handling infected animals, especially among hunters and trappers.[3,18]

PATHOGENESIS AND PATHOLOGY

The principal pathologic changes in localized disease occur at the cutaneous site of inoculation and in the regional lymph nodes draining the site; when the disease is disseminated, the lungs, spleen, lymph nodes, liver and skin are most often involved.[20–22] The primary skin lesion begins as a papule several days following inoculation. The papule rapidly progresses to a vesicle that erodes and develops into an ulcer, which is typically 2–3 cm in diameter with an irregular, slightly raised and erythematous border. The base is necrotic, and frequently covered with a thick dark scab that can mimic the eschar of cutaneous anthrax (Fig. 121.7). Affected lymph nodes show hemorrhagic necrosis and may suppurate. Secondary skin lesions have also been described in tularemia, including papular and papulovesicular lesions, erythema nodosum and erythema multiforme.

Francisella tularensis is an obligate intracellular organism within the vertebrate host, and the response to infection has a prominent component of cell-mediated immunopathology.[23–25] Histologically, early disease is characterized by focal suppurative necrosis. The central area of necrosis is at first composed primarily of polymorphonuclear leukocytes and macrophages, which may be replaced by epithelioid cells in more advanced lesions. A wall of fibroblasts may surround the acute inflammatory reaction. Later, smaller lesions may be indistinguishable from miliary tubercles. A frequent finding on pathologic examination of affected lungs is small (3–12 mm), yellowish, necrotic subpleural nodules. Patchy interstitial infiltrates are common in pneumonic tularemia; bronchopneumonia is found in about 30% of cases, and lobar pneumonia with consolidation of an entire lobe in about 15% of pneumonic cases. Lung abscesses occasionally occur. Hilar lymph nodes may be inflamed and enlarged.

Prevention

Persons exposed in endemic areas to ticks, biting flies or mosquitoes should, when feasible, wear protective clothing and apply repellents containing DEET (N,N-diethyl-M-toluamide) to skin and clothing as directed by the manufacturer. Permethrin-based products can be applied to clothing to kill ticks and biting flies on contact. Frequent examinations should be made to identify and remove ticks on clothing and skin. Persons should always avoid direct contact with sick or dead animals, and hunters, trappers, dressers and butchers should wear impervious gloves when skinning and handling wild animal carcasses.

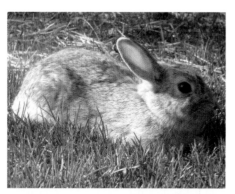

Fig. 121.4 Desert cottontail (*Syvilagus audubonii*). Important reservoir of tularemia in western USA.

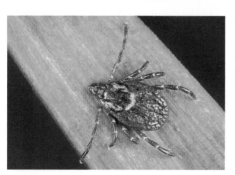

Fig. 121.5 The dog tick (*Dermacentor variabilis*). Important vector of tularemia in eastern and central USA.

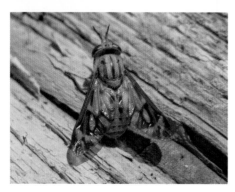

Fig. 121.6 The deer fly (*Chrysops discalis*). Primary vector of tularemia in western USA.

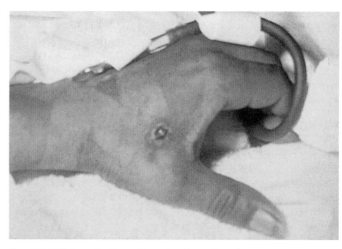

Fig. 121.7 Tularemic ulcer with eschar formation after percutaneous inoculation of *Francisella tularensis*.

The use of fine particle masks while engaged in landscaping activities has been suggested as a possible means of reducing infective inhalation exposures, such as those which can result when using power tools that generate environmental dusts. An outbreak of pneumonic tularemia occurred in Massachusetts, USA, among landscapers who were infected through this exposure route.[26]

Live attenuated vaccines have been used to protect laboratory personnel who routinely work with *F. tularensis*. Vaccines have also been used in an attempt to reduce the incidence of disease among rural residents of highly endemic areas of the former Soviet Union. The attenuated live vaccine strain (LVS) was developed by the US Department of Defense from an attenuated tularemia type B strain from the former Soviet Union and evaluated in the USA under a Food and Drug Administration investigational new drug protocol. Currently, no tularemia vaccine is licensed for general use, however, and this is an important area of active research.[25] Persons exposed to a laboratory accident possibly resulting in aerosolization or inoculation of *F. tularensis* should be considered for prophylactic antibiotic administration or placed on fever watch and closely monitored for early signs of illness.

CLINICAL FEATURES

The primary forms of tularemia include:[20–22]
- ulceroglandular tularemia (45–85% of cases);
- glandular tularemia (10–25% of cases);
- oculoglandular tularemia (<5% of cases);
- typhoidal (septic) tularemia (<5% of cases);
- oropharyngeal tularemia (<5% of cases); and
- pneumonic (inhalation) tularemia (<5% of cases).

The incubation period is usually 2–5 days (range 1–14 days). Onset is sudden; typically, the patient has fever of 100–104°F (38–40°C) and a constellation of nonspecific manifestations including chills, headache, generalized body aches (often prominent in the lumbosacral region), nausea, weakness, cough and chest pain.[20–22] Without treatment, nonspecific symptoms usually persist for several weeks. Sweats, chills, progressive weakness and weight loss characterize the continuing illness. Any of the principal forms of tularemia may be complicated by bacteremic spread that may lead to secondary sepsis, tularemic pneumonia, meningitis or other metastatic infection.

Before antibiotics became available, the overall mortality rate from infections with type A strains was in the range of 5–10%; however, a considerably higher fatality rate was reported for typhoidal and pneumonic forms of disease. A recent study was performed on 316 culture isolates that were obtained from human tularemia cases reported to the CDC from 1964 to 2004.[3] For the 235 patients for whom outcome was known, the overall case fatality rate was 9%. A molecular subtyping method that distinguished eastern and western clades of type A strains revealed that the case fatality rate for isolates that fit into the type-A-east subtype was 14%, while the case fatality rate observed in the type-A-west subtype was 0%. Type B isolates had an intermediate case fatality rate of 7%. This study suggests that significant variability exists among type A subtypes, and that the traditional view that type A is more virulent than type B is not always true.

Ulceroglandular tularemia

A local papule appears at the site of inoculation at the time of, or shortly after, the onset of fever and other generalized symptoms. This becomes vesiculated and pustular, and then ulcerates within a few days of its first appearance. Typically, the ulcer is tender, has an indolent character and may be covered by a scab (see Fig. 121.7). By the time of ulceration, painful lymphadenitis occurs in one or more adjacent nodes in the afferent pathway. In persons infected by handling contaminated materials, the epitrochlear nodes (8%) and the axillary nodes (65%) are the most commonly affected. In persons infected by arthropod bites, the femoral–inguinal nodes (64%), the axillary nodes (24%) and the cervical nodes (6%) are commonly involved.[22] In some cases, an abscessed node may suppurate, create a sinus tract and discharge purulent material to the outside.

Oculoglandular tularemia

Oculoglandular tularemia (Parinaud's syndrome) follows contamination of the conjunctival sac. Ulceration may occur on the conjunctiva, which becomes severely inflamed, with marked edema and vasculitis. Characteristically, there is painful swelling of nodes draining the periorbital tissues, such as the preauricular, submandibular and cervical chain nodes.

Glandular tularemia

Glandular tularemia differs from the ulceroglandular type only in not having the local cutaneous ulceration. It is more likely to follow arthropod-borne inoculation than direct percutaneous inoculation of the hands and fingers of persons handling infected animal tissues.

Typhoidal tularemia

Typhoidal tularemia presents as an acute illness without localizing signs.[22] The diagnosis is most often made by the identification of *F. tularensis* in blood cultures. Abdominal pain, diarrhea and vomiting may be prominent in early illness. Sepsis may occur and the systemic inflammatory response syndrome may ensue, rarely accompanied by complications such as disseminated intravascular coagulation and bleeding, acute respiratory distress syndrome, shock and organ failure. Typhoidal tularemia may result from inapparent inhalation exposures, that then progresses to pneumonia in more than 50% of cases; infection of the kidneys and the meninges may also occur. In some cases, the upper gastrointestinal tract may be the principal target organ in typhoidal tularemia.

Oropharyngeal tularemia

Oropharyngeal tularemia is acquired by ingesting inadequately cooked game, or contaminated water or food. The patient may develop a painful exudative pharyngitis or tonsillitis, or a stomatitis, sometimes with ulceration, and tender cervical lymphadenopathy. Suppuration, fistula formation and drainage of cervical nodes may occur.[13]

Pneumonic tularemia

Pneumonic tularemia is a common secondary complication of other forms of tularemia. Infrequently, primary pneumonia arises from inhalation of an infective aerosol or dust. In addition to fever, chills, fatigue and other generalized symptoms of infection, pneumonic manifestations include cough (usually with minimal sputum production), chest discomfort, sometimes with pleuritic pain, dyspnea, tachypnea and occasionally mild hemoptysis.

Francisella tularensis was weaponized for aerosol delivery by biowarfare programs during and after the Second World War, and it is assumed that this would be the most likely mode of delivery in a potential terrorism attack. The expected result would be an outbreak of pneumonic tularemia and nonspecific febrile illness (typhoidal tularemia) beginning 3–5 days after exposure; this might at first be difficult to distinguish from the many usual causes of community-acquired infection. It is possible that an aerosol exposure could also result in cases of oropharyngeal and oculoglandular disease. Since naturally acquired tularemia is most frequently a rural disease, bioterrorism might be suspected should a cluster of cases occur in an urban population. The recognition, and medical and public health management of tularemia as a weapon of bioterrorism has recently been outlined.[5]

DIAGNOSIS

The presumptive diagnosis of tularemia is made by clinical examination combined with information on potentially infective exposures. Differential diagnostic possibilities are many, as follows:

- in persons who have glandular or ulceroglandular disease they include plague, cutaneous anthrax, sporotrichosis, cat-scratch fever, lymphogranuloma venereum, streptococcal or staphylococcal lymphadenitis, toxoplasmosis, mycobacterial infection, chancre and chancroid;
- in persons who have oropharyngeal tularemia, other bacterial and viral causes of stomatitis, pharyngitis and cervical adenitis must be considered, such as streptococcal infection, infectious mononucleosis, mycobacterial infection, adenoviral infection and diphtheria;
- in persons who have pneumonia, they include mycoplasmal pneumonia, chlamydial pneumonia, Legionnaires' disease, staphylococcal or streptococcal pneumonitis, *Haemophilus influenzae* pneumonia, plague, histoplasmosis and tuberculosis; and
- in persons who have typhoidal tularemia, they include bacterial endocarditis, disseminated mycobacterial or fungal infection, typhoid fever, brucellosis, listeriosis, leptospirosis, Q fever, plague and other causes of sepsis.

The clinical diagnosis of tularemia is confirmed by culture recovery of *F. tularensis*. Alternatively, acute and convalescent serum specimens that differ in titer by fourfold, with at least one serum positive, are also considered confirmatory. *Francisella tularensis* may be present in human lesion exudates, respiratory secretions, blood, and lymph node aspirates as well as animal tissues and fluids.

Francisella tularensis can be isolated from nutrient-enriched clinical specimens on sheep blood agar (SBA), but a cysteine-enriched medium is strongly recommended for subculture as the organism will usually fail to thrive with continued passage on SBA. *Francisella tularensis* grows well on several types of cysteine-supplemented agar, including chocolate agar (CA), cysteine heart agar with 9% chocolatized blood (CHAB), buffered charcoal yeast extract (BYCE), Thayer–Martin agar and IsoVitaleX supplemented agars. For blood culture, the BACTEC system or an equivalent system is recommended. The agglutination reaction for combined IgM and IgG immunoglobulins is the routine serologic procedure used in most laboratories. Reference laboratories use microagglutination methods that are more sensitive than tube agglutination procedures. Antibody titers usually do not rise before 10 days or more of illness onset.

Direct fluorescent antibody staining, using a FITC-labeled antibody against *F. tularensis* cells, is a rapid assay for identification of *F. tularensis*. A variety of polymerase chain reaction (PCR) methods have also been described for molecular detection of *F. tularensis* and can be invaluable diagnostic tools when organisms are noncultivable. Once an isolate has been confirmed as *F. tularensis*, supplemental tests including biotyping (biochemical or molecular) and molecular subtyping can be used for additional characterization. These tests can be extremely useful for determining the source of infection, understanding transmission cycles or identifying species or subspecies.[27]

Personnel handling diagnostic cultures of *F. tularensis* are at considerable risk for infection, due to the low infectious dose for *F. tularensis*. Tularemia has been one of the most commonly reported laboratory-associated bacterial infections.[28] For diagnostic laboratories, biosafety level 2 practices, containment equipment, and facilities are recommended for activities involving clinical materials of human or animal origin suspected or known to contain *F. tularensis*. Biosafety level 3 practices, containment equipment and facilities are recommended, respectively, for all manipulations of suspect cultures, animal necropsies and for experimental animal studies.[29]

MANAGEMENT

Patients are best managed under hospital care until a full diagnostic evaluation and satisfactory treatment response has occurred. Streptomycin, which is bactericidal, has been the traditional drug of choice based on experience and efficacy.[5,30] It is given intramuscularly to adults in a dosage of 1 g and to children at 15 mg/kg (not to exceed 2 g/day), twice daily for 10 days. Gentamicin, an acceptable alternative, is given parenterally in an adult dosage of 5 mg/kg and to children at 2.5 mg/kg, per day for 10 days. A tetracycline (most commonly doxycycline) or chloramphenicol may be used in place of an aminoglycoside, especially in less severely ill patients, but use of these bacteriostatic agents occasionally results in primary treatment failures, and dosage schedules of at least 14 days are recommended to prevent relapses.

Oral or parenterally administered ciprofloxacin has been used to treat adults and children with good success in standard doses for 10 days.[31] Patients begun on parenterally administered antimicrobials can switch to oral administration when clinically indicated.

Francisella tularensis organisms routinely produce β-lactamase and are resistant to β-lactam antibiotics and azithromycin, but they are generally highly susceptible to aminoglycosides, tetracyclines, chloramphenicol and quinolones.[32,33] Penicillins and cephalosporins are not effective and should not be used.

Typically, fever and general symptoms of acute infection begin to regress within 24–48 hours of initiation of appropriate antibiotic administration. Factors associated with a poor outcome include delays in seeking medical care, or delays in diagnosis and treatment, and underlying medical disorders, such as diabetes or alcoholism.[34] Standard (universal) precautions only are required for purposes of hospital infection control.[5] Postexposure prophylactic antibiotic treatment of close contacts is not recommended because human-to-human transmission is not known to occur.

REFERENCES

References for this chapter can be found online at http://www.expertconsult.com

Nicholas PJ Day
Paul Newton
Philippe Parola
Didier Raoult

Chapter | 122 |

Scrub typhus and other tropical rickettsioses

INTRODUCTION

Tropical rickettsioses are a diverse group of zoonotic infectious diseases caused by obligate intracellular bacteria grouped in the family Rickettsiaceae of α-proteobacteria. These organisms are nonflagellate, small coccobacilli occurring within the host cytoplasm or nucleus and are not bounded by a vacuole. They are usually transmitted to humans by arthropods, in which they may be maintained by transovarial transmission. The members of the family Rickettsiaceae responsible for human disease in the tropics are:

- *Orientia tsutsugamushi*, the causative organism of scrub typhus (tsutsugamushi disease in Japan);
- the typhus group (TG) of the genus *Rickettsia*, containing *R. prowazeckii*, the agent of classic epidemic or louse-borne typhus, and *R. typhi*, which causes murine or flea-borne typhus; and
- the spotted fever group (SFG) *Rickettsia*, containing a large and ever increasing number of species. These are mostly transmitted from rodents and other animals by ticks, except for *R. akari* (mites) and *R. felis* (fleas).

Q-fever has in the past been considered a rickettsiosis and will be covered in this chapter, though its causative agent *Coxiella burnetii* has been transferred to the α-proteobacteria order Legionellales.

The agents of rickettsioses are associated with arthropods including ticks, mites, fleas and lice, which may act as vectors, reservoirs and/or amplifiers of the organisms. Most of these vectors favor specific optimal environmental conditions, biotopes and hosts. These factors determine the geographic distribution of the vector and consequently the risk area for the rickettsioses. This is particularly true when vectors are also reservoirs of pathogens, as seen in the case of ticks for most spotted fever group rickettsioses.[1] Thus, although some rickettsioses are distributed worldwide (Q-fever, murine typhus), a specific area is usually associated with specific diseases, and most rickettsioses are therefore geographic diseases. Table 122.1 summarizes the rickettsioses occurring in tropical areas of Africa, Asia, America and Australia.

There are no vaccines currently available against any tropical rickettsioses. Prevention is mainly based on avoiding the arthropod bite. The best method to avoid tick, flea and chigger bites is to use topical DEET (N,N-diethyl-m-toluamide) repellent applied to exposed skin and treat clothing with permethrin, which kills arthropods on contact. Bites may also be limited by wearing long trousers that are tucked into boots. People staying in infested areas should be advised to check their bodies routinely for the presence of arthropods. Any tick found attached should be removed immediately using blunt, rounded forceps.

Scrub Typhus

INTRODUCTION

Scrub typhus, caused by *Orientia tsutsugamushi*, is an important and widespread cause of febrile illness in rural areas of Asia and northern Australia (Fig. 122.1). It is contracted via the bite of the larval stage of several species of trombiculid mite of the genus *Leptotrombidium* ('chiggers'), which live in a wide range of vegetation types from scrub and primary forest to gardens and beaches. Infected mites are characteristically found in discrete foci called mite islands, where the risk of contracting scrub typhus is high. The bacteria are maintained transovarially in the mite population, and often infect the rodents on which the larval stage of the mite normally feeds. Humans are accidental hosts (Fig. 122.2). Scrub typhus presents as a systemic vasculitis-like infection, though the target cell along with much about the pathogenesis remains unknown.

CLINICAL FEATURES

Symptoms usually occur between 6 and 10 days after the mite bite. The presenting features are typically fever, generalized or regional lymphadenopathy, a macular or maculopapular rash (Fig. 122.3), severe headache and myalgia. Muscle tenderness is minimal or absent. Nausea and vomiting, diarrhea, constipation, conjunctival suffusion and reversable sensorineural deafness can also occur. A painless papule occurs at the bite site that later ulcerates, forming a black crust or 'eschar' (Fig. 122.4) in a variable proportion of patients – this variability probably reflects, at least in part, the extent of the physical examination. However, the eschar and rash may be absent or unnoticed.

Complications include jaundice, meningoencephalitis, myocarditis, interstitial pneumonia leading on to adult respiratory distress syndrome (ARDS), and renal failure. Animal experiments suggest that disease severity may vary widely with the strain of bacteria. In the pre-antibiotic era mortality rates as high as 35% were reported, and the disease still carries a significant risk of death in rural areas where effective treatment is unavailable or delayed.

DIAGNOSIS

The gold standard diagnostic tests for scrub typhus are the indirect immunoperoxidase and the immunofluorescent assay (IFA), based on cell-culture-derived *O. tsutsugamushi* antigens, applied to paired

Table 122.1 Tropical rickettsioses throughout the world

Location by continent	Vectors	Disease	Agent	Specific areas	Risk of exposure
Africa/Middle East	**Ticks**				
	Rhipicephalus sanguineus	Mediterranean spotted fever	Rickettsia conorii	Mediterranean area (Algeria, Tunisia, Morocco, Libya, Egypt, Israel, Turkey), Kenya, Somalia, Central African Republic, Zimbabwe and South Africa	Urban (2/3) and rural (1/3)
	Amblyomma spp.	African tick-bite fever	R. africae	Sub-Saharan Africa	Rural area. Safari
	Hyalomma marginatum	Unnamed	R. aeschlimmanii	Morocco, Zimbabwe, South Africa	
	Dermacentor marginatus*	Tick-borne lymphadenopathy	R. slovaca	Morocco*	
	Dermacentor marginatus*	Unnamed	R. raoultii	Morocco*	
	Rhipicephalus sanguineus*	Unnamed	R. massiliae	Morocco*,	
	R. muhusamae*		R. sibirica mongolotimonae	Mali*, Central African Republic*	
	H. truncatum*	Unnamed		South Africa, Algeria, Niger*	
	Ixodes ricinus*	Unnamed	'R. monacensis'	Morocco*, Tunisia*	
	Fleas				
	Xenopsylla cheopis (rat flea)	Murine typhus	R. typhi	Ubiquitous. High prevalence in coastal areas	Contact with rats and rat fleas
	Pulex irritans (human flea)*	Flea-borne spotted fever	R. felis	Tunisia, Algeria	
	Lice				
	Pediculus humanus corporis	Epidemic typhus	R. prowazekii	Ethiopia, Burundi, Rwanda, Uganda, Algeria	Civil war, refugee camps, lack of hygiene in cold or mountainous areas
Americas	**Ticks**				
	Amblyomma cajennense	Rocky Mountain spotted fever	R. rickettsii	Central America (Mexico, Panama, Costa Rica), South America (Brazil, Colombia)	Rural areas
	Amblyomma triste	Unnamed	R. parkeri	Brazil	
	Amblyomma spp.	African tick-bite fever	R. africae	West Indies	Rural areas
	Amlyomma triste*	Unnamed	R. parkeri	Brazil	
	Fleas				
	Xenopsylla cheopis (rat flea)	Murine typhus	R. typhi	Ubiquitous	Contact with rats and rat fleas
	Ctenocephalides felis (cat flea)*	Flea-borne spotted fever	R. felis	Mexico, Brazil, Peru	
	Lice				
	Pediculus humanus corporis	Epidemic typhus	R. prowazekii	Peru and Andes	Lack of hygiene in mountainous area
Asia	**Ticks**				
	Rhipicephalus sanguineus	Indian tick typhus	R. conorii indica	India. Suspected in Thailand, Korea, Laos and Sri Lanka	
	Ixodes granulatus	Flinders Island spotted fever	R. honei	Thailand	

Arthropod	Disease	Pathogen	Distribution	Risk factors
Ixodes ovatus *Dermacentor taiwanensis* *Haemaphysalis longicornis* *Haemaphysalis flava*	Oriental or Japanese spotted fever	*R. japonica*	Japan†	Agricultural activities, bamboo cutting
Ixodes ovatus, *I. persulcatus,* *I. monospinus**	Unnamed	*R. helvetica*	Japan.† Suspected in Thailand, Laos	
*Hyalomma asiaticum**	Lymphangitis-associated rickettsiosis	*R. sibirica mongolotimonae*	China (Inner Mongolia)*†	
Dermacentor nuttalli, *D. marginatus,* *Haemaphysalis concinna*	North-Asian tick typhus	*R. sibirica sibirica*	Northern China, former USSR (Asian republics, Siberia), Armenia, Pakistan	
Dermacentor silvarum	Far-Eastern tick-borne rickettsiosis	*R. heilongjiangii*	North-eastern China	
Unknown	Unnamed	'*R. kellyi*'	India	
Fleas *Xenopsylla cheopis* (rat flea)	Murine typhus	*R. typhi*	Ubiquitous	
Ctenocephalides felis (cat flea)*	Flea-borne spotted fever	*R. felis*	Thailand, Laos	
Trombiculid acarins *Leptotrombidium* spp.	Scrub typhus	*Orientia tsutsugamushi*	Asia–Pacific region from Korea to Papua New Guinea and Queensland, Australia, and from Japan to India and Afghanistan	Rural activities, Agricultural activities, Soldiers in the field
Lice *Pediculus humanus corporis*	Epidemic typhus	*R. prowazekii*	China, India (Kashmir)	Civil war, refugee camps, lack of hygiene in cold or mountainous areas
House mouse mite *Liponyssoides sanguineus*	Rickettsialpox	*R. akari*	Korea‡	
Australia				
Ticks Unknown	Flinders Island spotted fever	*R. honei*	Flinders Island, north-eastern Australia	
Ixodes holocyclus	Queensland tick typhus	*R. australis*	North-eastern Australia	
Fleas *Xenopsylla cheopis* (rat flea)	Murine typhus	*R. typhi*	Ubiquitous	Contact with rats and rat fleas
Trombiculid acarins *Leptotrombidium* spp.	Scrub typhus	*Orientia tsutsugamushi*	Northern Territory and Western Australia, Queensland, Australia	Rural activities, Agricultural activities, Soldiers in the field

*Suspected by detection of the pathogen in the relevant arthropod.
†Although not included in tropical areas, Japan and China are included as relevant to tropical travel medicine.
‡Isolated from voles (*Microtus fortis pelliceus*).
Note: Q-fever caused by *C. burnetii* is distributed worldwide (except in New Zealand).

Distribution map of scrub typhus

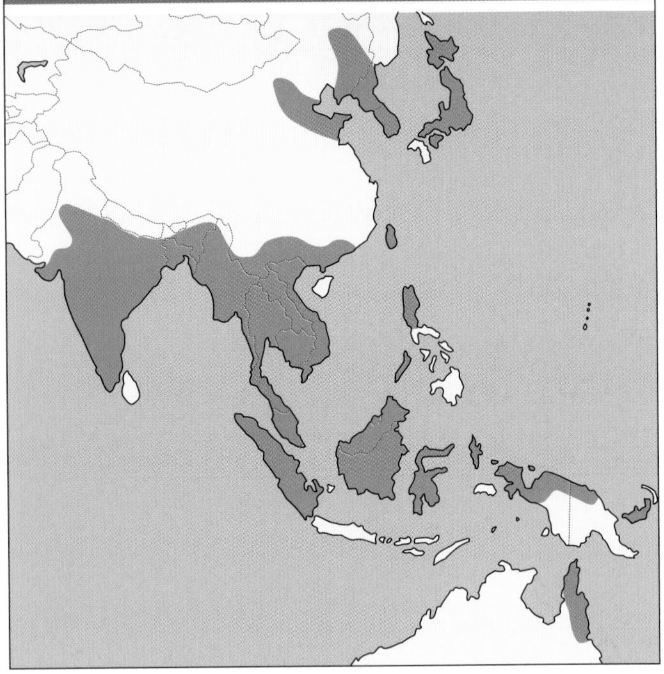

Fig. 122.1 Distribution map of scrub typhus. Scrub typhus or tsutsugamushi disease (from a Japanese word meaning 'noxious bug') is caused by infection with *Orientia tsutsugamushi* and is transmitted by larval trombiculid mites of the genus *Leptotrombidium*. The disease occurs in the Indian subcontinent, South East Asia, the Far East and islands of the south-west Pacific including the Republic of Palau. From Peters W, Pavsol G. Atlas of tropical medicine and parasitology, 6th ed. St Louis: Mosby; 2006. Copyright Elsevier 2006.

admission and convalescent samples. These tests are not standardized across laboratories and are usually unavailable in poor tropical areas. They are, however, superior to the old Weil–Felix test (based on detection of antibodies cross-reactive to antigens of the OX-K strain of the unrelated bacteria *Proteus mirabilis*). Polymerase chain reaction (PCR) methods for detection of the 47 kDa and 56 kDa protein genes of *O. tsutsugamushi* have been developed but are not standardized or in widespread use. Although *O. tsutsugamushi* can be cultured from blood, this takes several weeks and requires special tissue culture techniques and a biosafety level 3 facility. Anti-*O. tsutsugamushi* IgM- and IgG-based rapid diagnostic tests have been developed but have not been adequately assessed in the field.

TREATMENT

Scrub typhus is very responsive to treatment with appropriate antibiotics, which should be given empirically if the diagnosis is suspected. Unless contraindicated, doxycycline is the standard treatment (usual adult oral dose is 100 mg q12h for 7 days, following a 200 mg loading dose). Tetracycline 500 mg q6h for 7 days may also be used. Trials of shorter courses are underway. Azithromycin (500–1000 mg on the first day followed by 250–500 mg daily for 2 days) is an effective alternative[2] and has been shown to be effective in a single dose.[3] Azithromycin is particularly useful if doxyclines are contraindicated, such as in pregnancy. Chloramphenicol is another alternative to the tetracyclines (500 mg q6h in adults or 50–75 mg/kg/day in children for 7 days). Roxithromycin, telithromycin and rifampin have also been used successfully.

Epidemic Typhus

INTRODUCTION

Epidemic typhus, caused by *R. prowazeckii*, is one of the most dangerous of the arthropod-borne diseases and remains a major public health threat. It is transmitted by the human body louse (*Pediculus humanus corporis*), which lives in human clothing and thrives in conditions such as poverty and war where hygiene levels are poor. The bacteria are not transmitted vertically in lice and humans are the major reservoir (sporadic cases have been reported through contact with the flying squirrel *Glaucomys volans* in the USA). *R. prowazekii* is transmitted to people by infected louse feces (in which *R. prowazekii* survives for weeks), through aerosols (thought to be the main route of infection for health-care workers attending patients) or by skin autoinoculation, following scratching. Recently epidemics of epidemic typhus have occurred in Ethiopia, Burundi, Russia and Peru.[4] Sporadic cases have been recently reported in North Africa and France. Epidemic typhus must therefore still be considered a potential major health risk in tropical countries, particularly in environments such as refugee camps in cooler mountainous areas.

CLINICAL FEATURES

The incubation period is about 10–14 days. Patients develop malaise and vague symptoms before the abrupt onset of signs including fever (100%), headache (100%) and myalgia (70–100%). Other common signs include nausea or vomiting, coughing and epistaxis. Meningoencephalitis is a common complication in severe cases, with meningism, tinnitus, deafness and altered consciousness, ranging from mild confusion through agitated delirium and coma. Diarrhea, pulmonary involvement, myocarditis, splenomegaly and conjunctivitis may also occur. Most patients (20–80%) develop a skin rash that classically begins on the trunk and spreads to the limbs. It may be macular, maculopapular or petechial and may be difficult to detect on darker skin tones. The overall mortality rate is around 20%, rising to 60% in the malnourished and aged, though with appropriate antibiotic treatment mortality may be as low as 4%. Recrudescence of epidemic typhus unrelated to louse infestation or Brill–Zinsser disease can appear many years after the acute disease and has milder symptoms.[4]

DIAGNOSIS

Epidemic typhus can be diagnosed serologically by IFA, though Western blot combined with cross-adsorption tests is required for differentiation from murine typhus in positives. The Weil–Felix test (based on cross-reactivity with the *Proteus vulgaris* OX-19 antigen) is even less specific and should not be used. *R. prowazeckii* can be cultured in L929 cells using blood or skin biopsy samples. Recently, a quantitative real-time PCR assay targeting the *glt*A gene specific for *R. prowazeckii* has been developed.

TREATMENT AND PREVENTION

In suspected cases antibiotics should be given prior to confirmation of the diagnosis. The following antibiotic regimens are considered effective:

- doxycycline 100 mg daily (4 mg/kg daily for children), in two divided doses if possible, for 3 days;
- tetracycline 300–500 mg q6h (children 50 mg/kg q6h) orally or intravenously; and

Epidemiologic cycle of scrub typhus

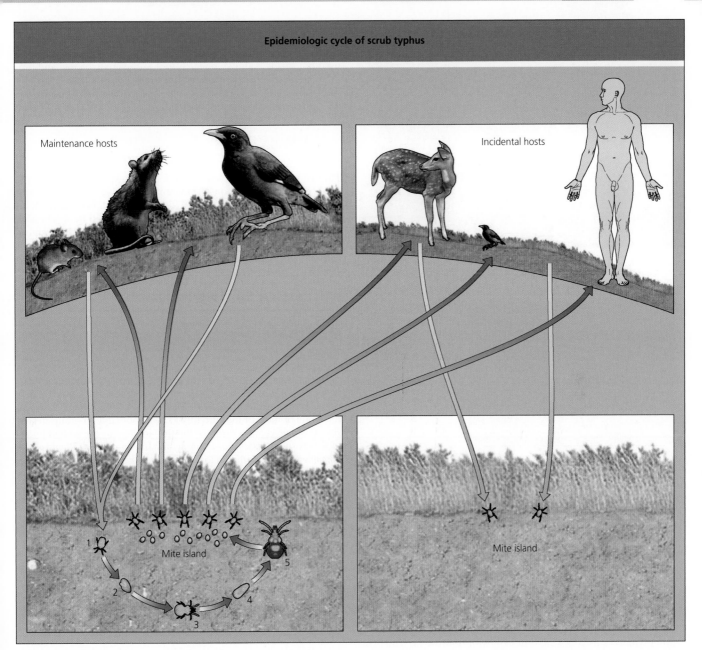

Fig. 122.2 Epidemiologic cycle of scrub typhus. *Orientia tsutsugamushi* is present in trombiculid-infested rodents. Not far from Kuala Lumpur, for example, *Leptotrombidium deliensis* is found in the forest and *Leptotrombidium akamushi* in the grass ('lalang'). The mites occur in colonies known as 'mite islands' that are associated with the nests of the rodents on which they normally feed. They pass through a cycle that includes a parasitic, blood-feeding, hexapod larva (1), a nymphochrysalis (2), followed by eight-legged, nonparasitic nymphal (3) and adult stages (5) between which is interposed an imagochrysalis (4). The cycle of infection is maintained in the focus, since engorged larvae are returned to the rodent nest, where they drop off and complete the rest of their cycle, with the adults finally laying eggs there. Vertical transmission of the Rickettsiae occurs so that the true reservoir of infection is the mite. Other mammals, humans and occasionally birds may be bitten by the larvae, which cause severe irritation. Thus, scrub typhus, although a zoonosis, can occur in small outbreaks if groups of people (e.g. soldiers in the jungle) rest in the vicinity of a mite island. IH, incidental hosts; MH, maintenance hosts; MI, mite island. adapted from Audy JR Red mites and typhus. London: Athlone Press; 1968.

- chloramphenicol 500–750 mg q6h (children 75 mg/kg q6h) orally or intravenously for 7 days.

In outbreak situations a single 200 mg dose of doxycycline is usually effective. Louse eradication (e.g. in refugee camps) is the most important preventive measure and is essential in the control of outbreaks. Since body lice live only in clothing, the simplest method of delousing is to remove and then destroy or wash and boil all clothing. Dusting of all clothing with 10% DDT, 1% malathion or 1% permethrin is also a rapid and effective method of killing body lice and reduces the risk of re-infestation.

Murine Typhus

INTRODUCTION

Murine typhus, also known as endemic typhus, is a flea-borne rickettsiosis caused by *R. typhi*. The rat flea *Xenopsylla cheopis* is the principal vector; rodents, mainly *Rattus norvegicus* and *R. rattus*, act as reservoirs. In suburban areas of the USA the cat flea, *Ctenocephalides felis*, has been

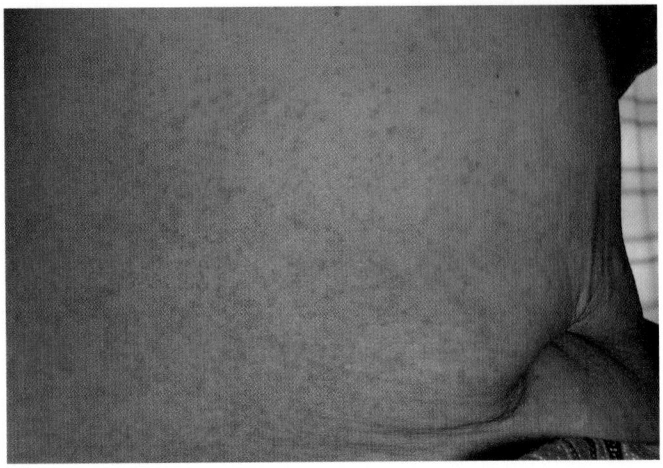

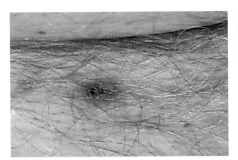

Fig. 122.3 Macular rash in a patient with scrub typhus.

Fig. 122.4 Eschar at the bite site, a hallmark of rickettsial diseases.

identified as the principal vector.[5] People become infected when flea feces containing *R. typhi* contaminate disrupted skin or are inhaled into the respiratory tract. Exposure to rat fleas is linked to exposure to rats, and high endemicity tends to occur in areas with large rat populations. Murine typhus has a worldwide distribution, occurring in urban as well as rural settings, though it probably has a higher incidence in warmer countries.

CLINICAL FEATURES

Murine typhus is usually a mild disease with nonspecific signs. The incubation period is 7–14 days and at presentation the classic triad of fever, headache and skin rash is observed in less than 15% of cases. Rash is present in less than 50% of patients and is often transient or difficult to observe. Nausea, vomiting, abdominal pain, diarrhea, jaundice, confusion, seizures and renal failure have also been reported. Peripheral lymphadenopathy is significantly less frequent in murine typhus than in scrub typhus, and eschars do not occur, useful distinguishing clinical features in areas of Asia where the two diseases coexist.[6] Mortality is low, around 1% with antibiotic treatment, and even without treatment the disease is usually a self-limiting illness lasting 7–14 days.

DIAGNOSIS

The IFA on paired admission and convalescent samples is the definitive diagnostic test, though false-positives can occur due to cross-reactivity with antigens from other bacteria. Cross-absorption of sera and Western blotting can be used to differentiate infections when cross-reactions occur. Other serologic tests exist but in general these have lower sensitivity than the IFA. PCR-based molecular methods have been devised for detecting TG organisms, though none is specific to murine typhus. Culture in vero or L929 cell lines may also be used but this is mainly a research tool as sensitivity is low and biosafety level 3 laboratory facilities are needed. Anti-*R. typhi* IgM- and IgG-based rapid diagnostic tests have been developed but have not been adequately assessed in the field.

TREATMENT

The drug of choice is doxycycline in both nonpregnant adults (100 mg q12h orally or intravenously) and children (4 mg/kg q12h up to a maximum of 100 mg per dose). The usual recommended duration of treatment is 7 days, but shorter courses may well be as effective. Chloramphenicol can be used as an alternative and may be useful in pregnancy. Whether azithromycin may be an efficacious alternative is currently unknown.

Rickettsial Spotted Fevers

INTRODUCTION

The spotted fevers are caused by a large and expanding number of rickettsial species, all of which are transmitted by ticks except for rickettsialpox caused by *R. akari*, which is mite borne, and the flea-borne infection due to *R. felis*. Ticks are not only vectors but also reservoirs of most of the currently known spotted fever group rickettsiae. Ecologic characteristics of the tick are keys to the epidemiology of tick-borne diseases. For example, the brown dog tick *Rhipicephalus sanguineus*, which is the vector of *R. conorii*, lives in dog environments (kennels and human houses) and has a low affinity for people. Cases of Mediterranean spotted fever are sporadic in endemic areas and most cases are encountered in urban areas. In contrast, *Amblyomma hebraeum*, which are heavily infected vectors of *R. africae* in southern Africa, emerge from their habitats and actively attack animals, particularly ruminants. Since they also feed readily on people that enter their biotopes, cases of African tick-bite fever often occur as grouped cases among subjects entering the bush (e.g. during a safari) and individuals can suffer several tick bites simultaneously.

CLINICAL FEATURES

The clinical symptoms of spotted fever group rickettsioses begin 6–10 days after the arthropod bite and typically include fever, headache, muscle pain, rash, local lymphadenopathy and a characteristic inoculation eschar ('tache noire') at the bite site. Despite the spotted fever appelation many patients with these infections confusingly have no rash – 'unspotted spotted fever'.

The main clinical signs vary depending on the rickettsial species involved and therefore may allow the clinician to distinguish between diseases. For example, African tick-bite fever is characterized by the occurrence of multiple inoculation eschars and grouped cases, as numerous highly infected *Amblyomma* may attack and bite many people in several places at the same time.[7] In contrast, in Mediterranean spotted fever due to *R. conorii*, a single eschar is usual because of the low likelihood of the tick biting people and a low rate of infection of the ticks. Details of each pathogen and clinical pictures are presented elsewhere (see Chapter 176).

Spotted fever group rickettsioses range from mild to severe and fatal diseases. For example, to date no mortalities or severe complications have been reported in patients with African tick-bite fever, whereas the mortality rate from Mediterranean spotted fever may be as high as 2.5%.

DIAGNOSIS

Investigations using a panoply of new molecular, immunologic and serologic tools have led to the recent dramatic expansion in the number of spotted fever rickettsial species now known to cause human disease. IFA is the most commonly used technique, though convalescent samples are usually needed. In specialist centers a panel of antigens is used for testing for a range of possible SFG pathogens. Cross-reactivity within the SFG, between the SFG and the TG, and with other unrelated pathogens is a problem, so cross adsorption assays and PCR-based techniques are often required to identify to the species level. Direct immunodiagnosis on blood and skin biopsies can be of value, as can culture of the pathogen. A real-time PCR has been developed based on 47 kDa, *glt*A and *omp*B gene targets which will distinguish scrub typhus, TG and SFG on admission blood samples.

TREATMENT

The treatment of choice for spotted fever rickettsioses is 200 mg doxycycline/day for 1–7 days depending on the severity of the disease. In children and pregnant women, macrolides including josamycin (50 mg/kg/day in children or 3 g/day in adults), roxithromycin, clarithromycin and azithromycin have all been used successfully for the treatment of Mediterranean spotted fever, as has chloramphenicol.

Q-Fever

INTRODUCTION

Q-fever is a zoonotic infection caused by *Coxiella burnetii*, usually acquired occupationally by the ingestion or inhalation of virulent organisms from infected mammals, mostly goats, sheep and cats, and their products. *Coxiella burnetii* has been found to infect more than 40 species of ticks throughout the world, but the role of ticks in human infections is not confirmed.

CLINICAL FEATURES

Acute Q-fever is usually mild, with asymptomatic seroconversion occurring in 50–60% of infected individuals.[8] A self-limited febrile syndrome occurs most frequently in symptomatic patients, but in more serious cases hepatitis, pneumonitis and prolonged fever may develop (see Chapter 176). Chronic Q-fever represents the development of the acute disease in predisposed hosts. It may present as endocarditis in patients with underlying heart valve lesions or, more rarely, as vascular aneurysms, graft infections, chronic bone infections or pseudotumors of the lung.

DIAGNOSIS

The diagnosis of Q-fever relies mainly on serology. *Coxiella burnetii* exhibits phase variation, and in acute Q-fever antibodies to phase II antigens predominate and their titer is higher than the phase I antibody titer. In chronic forms of the disease, however, elevated anti-phase I antibodies are uniformly detected. A phase I IgG titer of 800 or greater is one of the major modified Duke criteria for endocarditis. Q-fever can also be diagnosed by PCR, though this test is not widely available.

TREATMENT

The treatment of choice for acute Q-fever is doxycycline 100 mg 12 hourly for 14 days, though fluoroquinolones may also be used. The treatment of chronic disease is complex, involving long courses (≥18 months) of doxycycline + hydroxychloroquine, plus surgery if indicated.

REFERENCES

References for this chapter can be found online at http://www.expertconsult.com

Brucellosis

EPIDEMIOLOGY

Brucellosis, also known as undulant fever or Malta fever, is a zoonosis caused by bacteria of the genus *Brucella*. The disease exists worldwide, with the highest prevalence in the Mediterranean countries, Asia, Africa and Central and South America. Around 500 000 new cases are reported annually worldwide, of which only 100–200 are in the USA,[1] but brucellosis is clearly underreported.

Brucellosis is transmitted to humans by direct contact with infected animals, by ingestion of unpasteurized milk or milk products, through cuts and abrasions or by inhalation of aerosols. It is common though infrequently diagnosed in pastoral rural populations in Africa and the Middle East. In many European countries and in the USA it is mainly an occupational disease occurring in abattoir workers, butchers and farmers. Veterinary surgeons may become infected by accidental inoculation of live attenuated *Brucella* vaccine. Person–person transmission is extremely rare.

Four *Brucella* spp. can cause infection in humans:

- *Brucella melitensis*, which is found in goats, sheep and camels, is the most widespread and is the most virulent;
- *Brucella abortus*, which is found in cattle and camels, is less virulent;
- *Brucella suis*, which is found in pigs, is also less virulent; and
- *Brucella canis*, which is found in dogs, is the least common.

Other animals, including wildlife, may provide a reservoir for brucellae.[2]

PATHOGENESIS

Brucellae are facultative intracellular bacteria that are able to survive and multiply within mononuclear phagocytes. The mechanism is poorly understood but seems to include the suppression of degranulation of myeloperoxidase-containing granules, suppression of phagosome–lysosome fusion and production of protective enzymes.

The host reaction to brucellae is the formation of granulomas. *Brucella melitensis* and *B. suis* cause the most severe disease with caseating granulomas. Granulomas eventually heal with fibrosis and calcification.

Humoral antibodies seem to play some role in protection against re-infection. Control of the infection, however, depends on cell-mediated immunity.[2]

PREVENTION

The prevention of human brucellosis is dependent on the elimination of brucellosis in domestic animals. The use of veterinary vaccines for *B. abortus* and *B. melitensis* together with pasteurization of milk has resulted in a dramatic decrease in the incidence of human brucellosis. There is no effective vaccine available for *B. suis*. People at high risk of infection, such as veterinary surgeons and abattoir workers, should wear protective clothing. Laboratory-acquired brucellosis can be prevented by adherence to biosafety level 3 precautions. No effective vaccine is available for human use. Travelers to high endemic areas should be advised not to drink unpasteurized milk.

CLINICAL FEATURES

Brucellosis is a systemic infection that can involve any organ or organ system. The incubation period is normally between 2 and 4 weeks, but it may be months. The onset of clinical disease can be acute or insidious. Subclinical infection has been observed. Brucellosis is characterized by numerous somatic complaints in contrast to the few abnormal physical findings. Hepatosplenomegaly is present in 20–60%, depending on the species of *Brucella*, and mild lymphadenopathy is present in 10–20%. The nonspecific symptoms (e.g. fever, sweats, anorexia, fatigue, myalgia, malaise, headache and depression) are common and may mimic diseases such as tuberculosis, toxoplasmosis, mononucleosis, hepatitis, systemic lupus erythematosus, typhoid and many others.

When symptoms related to a single organ or organ system are dominant, it is often referred to as localized disease. The most common complications are listed in Table 123.1. The term 'chronic brucellosis' should be reserved for patients who have complaints of ill health for more than 12 months.[2] This includes patients who have relapsing illness or persisting focal infection and patients complaining of weakness, fatigue and depression, but with no objective signs of infection and no elevation of IgG antibody titer. This last group is believed to suffer from a psychoneurosis or a syndrome akin to chronic fatigue syndrome (see Chapter 70).

Table 123.1 Common complications of brucellosis

Organ system	Patients (%)
Cardiovascular	1–2
Endocarditis	0–2
Cutaneous	5–10
Gastrointestinal	50–70
Genitourinary	1–5
Orchitis	1–4
Neurologic	2–4
Osteoarticular	20–40
Sacroiliitis	10–15
Spondylitis	8–10
Pulmonary	15–25

Complications

Osteoarticular complications

Osteoarticular complications affect 20–40% of patients. Sacroiliitis is the most common reported complication, especially when *B. melitensis* predominates.[3] The characteristic radiographic findings are blurring of articular margins and widening of the sacroiliac space (Fig. 123.1). The clinical presentation is systemic symptoms and pain.

Spondylitis is most often seen in the lumbosacral region in elderly men, probably reflecting pre-existing anomalies in the spine, and it may be complicated by paraspinal abscesses (Fig. 123.2). The main symptoms are fever and vertebral pain. The typical radiographic findings are epiphysitis of vertebrae and narrowing of the intervertebral disc (Fig. 123.3). Bone scans and CT scans may detect infection earlier than radiography.[4]

Differential diagnosis includes tuberculosis, fungal and pyogenic osteomyelitis, multiple myeloma and metastatic carcinoma.

Arthritis especially involves the hips, knees and ankles.

Gastrointestinal complications

Up to 70% of patients have intestinal complaints such as anorexia, nausea, vomiting, abdominal pain, diarrhea or constipation. The liver is probably always involved, but liver function tests are usually only mildly abnormal. Cirrhosis does not seem to follow *Brucella* infection.

Pulmonary complications

Respiratory symptoms are reported in 15–25% of patients. They range from flu-like symptoms to bronchitis, interstitial pneumonitis, lung abscesses, hilar lymphadenopathy and lung effusions.

Genitourinary complications

Complications from the genitourinary tract are rare. Acute orchitis or epididymo-orchitis with signs of systemic infection do occur and interstitial nephritis, glomerulonephritis and pyelonephritis resembling tuberculosis have been described. Brucellosis during pregnancy is rare but it can result in abortion like any other systemic infection.

Neurologic complications

Depression is a common complaint, but invasion of the central nervous system occurs in only 2–4% of cases. It usually presents as acute or chronic meningitis. Encephalitis, polyradiculopathy, psychosis and meningovascular complications have also been described.[5] Analysis of cerebrospinal fluid reveals elevated protein, lymphocytic pleocytosis, low to normal glucose and most often intraspinally produced specific antibodies. Brucellae are isolated from cerebrospinal fluid in less than 30% of patients.

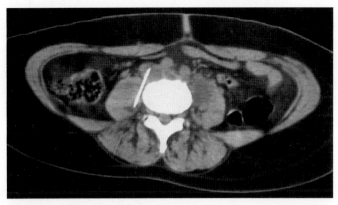

Fig. 123.2 CT scan of fine needle aspiration of paraspinal abscess (arrow) in a patient with brucellosis.

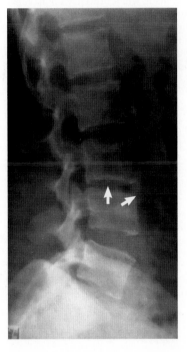

Fig. 123.3 Radiograph of the lumbar spine in a patient who has discitis and spondylitis of L3–4 caused by brucellosis. Note the reduced disc space and the destruction of the upper articular margins of L4 (arrows).

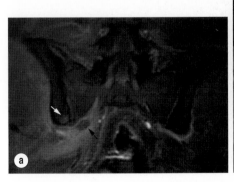
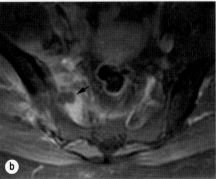

Fig. 123.1 MRI showing sacroiliitis: (a) coronal; (b) axial. T1 fat saturated images obtained after intravenous gadolinium contrast. There is osseous enhancement at the inferior part of the joint (white arrow) and huge soft tissue enhancement surrounding a non-enhancing abscess (black arrow).

Cardiovascular complications

Endocarditis, although rare, is the main cause of death related to brucellosis.[6] The aortic valve is involved more often than the mitral valve. Other complications include mycotic aneurysms, myocarditis and pericarditis.

Cutaneous involvement

Cutaneous manifestations of brucellosis consist mainly of transient nonspecific lesions including erythema nodosum, petechiae, vasculitis, papules and rashes.

DIAGNOSIS

Because the symptoms of brucellosis are nonspecific, it is crucial that the attending physician anticipate the probability of the disease. A certain diagnosis of brucellosis is made when brucellae are isolated from blood, bone marrow or other body fluids or tissues. Most laboratories employ rapid isolation methods for blood cultures. However, these cultures need to be maintained for up to 30–40 days to isolate *Brucella* spp. successfully. Bone marrow cultures are more sensitive than blood cultures in acute brucellosis and tend to remain positive later in the course of the infection, even during antimicrobial treatment.

The serum agglutination test is still the best standardized and most widely used serologic test.[7] It measures both IgG and IgM antibodies; antibodies to *Vibrio cholerae*, *Francisella tularensis* and *Yersinia enterocolitica* can give false-positive reactions. False-negative reactions due to blocking antibodies are seen and dilutions of 1:640 should be made. A titer of 1:160 is normally considered positive, as is a fourfold or greater rise in titer. Most patients who have acute infection develop IgM and IgG antibodies. The IgG antibodies persist as long as the infection is active and they increase with relapse and decrease with cure. The enzyme-linked immunosorbent assay (ELISA) appears to be more sensitive than and as specific as the serum agglutination test. It is rapid, easy to perform and can be automated.[7] Polymerase chain reaction (PCR) has also been shown to be very sensitive and specific, and appears to be a very useful test for initial diagnosis, post-treatment follow-up and early detection of relapses.[8,9]

MANAGEMENT

As single drug treatment results in a high relapse rate (5–40%), combination therapy is usually recommended. Duration of treatment is normally 6 weeks, but longer in complicated cases.[10]

Uncomplicated brucellosis is treated with oral doxycycline 100 mg q12h plus oral rifampin (rifampicin) 600–900 mg q24h, or oral doxycycline plus an intramuscular or intravenous aminoglycoside (e.g. streptomycin 1 g q24h or gentamicin 240 mg q24h) for 2–3 weeks. Children less than 8 years of age and pregnant women should not be treated with doxycycline. Instead, oral trimethoprim–sulfamethoxazole can be used (20 mg/kg sulfamethoxazole and 4 mg/kg trimethoprim q12h in children for 6 weeks, 800 mg sulfamethoxazole and 160 mg trimethoprim q12h in adults for 6 weeks) plus intramuscular gentamicin (5 mg/kg q24h in children and 240 mg q24h in adults for 1 week). Gentamicin can be replaced by oral rifampin (10–20 mg/kg q24h in children and 600 mg q24h in adults for 6 weeks).

Complications

Complications of brucellosis such as meningitis and endocarditis require prolonged courses of therapy, directed by the response.[2] In severe cases, a combination of three agents is often recommended (e.g. doxycycline or trimethoprim–sulfamethoxazole, plus an aminoglycoside and rifampin). Endocarditis often requires additional surgical intervention.[6]

Many other antimicrobial agents have shown *in-vitro* activity against *Brucella* spp., including fluoroquinolones, third-generation cephalosporins and azithromycin. However, these drugs should only be used in controlled trials or kept as second-line medication until further studies confirm their efficacy.

With chemotherapy the overall mortality rate is less than 2%.

REFERENCES

References for this chapter can be found online at http://www.expertconsult.com

Leptospirosis

INTRODUCTION

Leptospirosis, caused by pathogenic species of the bacterial genus *Leptospira*, is the most geographically widespread zoonotic disease, affecting humans in both rural and urban settings in temperate and tropical climes.[1] The disease is maintained in nature by chronic renal infection of mammals, leading to environmental contamination with infective organisms. Human infection follows exposure to infected animals, either directly or indirectly through contaminated soil and water. The majority of patients experience a mild febrile illness, while a minority develop a severe illness known as Weil's disease which is characterized by bleeding, jaundice and renal failure leading in the most severe cases to death from pulmonary hemorrhage or renal failure.

MICROBIOLOGY

Leptospires are highly motile, obligate aerobic spirochetal bacteria, about $0.25 \times 6–25\,\mu m$ in size (Fig 124.1).[2] Leptospires survive for days or weeks in warm, damp, slightly alkaline conditions, especially in still or slowly moving fresh water in the temperate summer and in damp soil and water in the tropics, particularly in the rainy season. Until recently the Leptospiraceae were classified mainly on the basis of gross

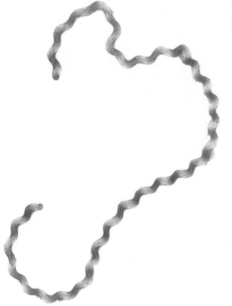

Fig. 124.1 Electron micrograph of a leptospire.

agglutination between strains, with over 200 pathogenic and 60 non-pathogenic saprophytic serovars. More recently the genus *Leptospira* has been split into species on the basis of DNA–DNA hybridization. Eighteen species are now recognized, 12 pathogenic or probably pathogenic and six saprophytic. The two classification systems are currently used side by side, somewhat uncomfortably as a number of serovars have been found in multiple *Leptospira* spp.; further (hopefully simplifying) developments are likely in the future.

EPIDEMIOLOGY

In temperate climates, leptospirosis is acquired mainly through recreational or occupational exposure, or through living in slums, but in tropical regions exposure through vocational activities such as rice farming is more widespread.[2] The burden of disease is greatly underestimated in the tropical developing world. Leptospirosis is an important cause of febrile illness in tourists returning from the tropics, particularly those involved in adventure tourism. The reported incidence of leptospirosis in developed countries is declining and the disease is no longer reportable in the USA.

The serovar classification remains useful for epidemiologic purposes, as many geographically widespread serovar–reservoir associations exist. The most ubiquitous are *icterohaemorrhagiae* with rats *Rattus* species, *hardjo* with cattle and *pomona* with pigs. Other serovars are more restricted in their distribution, such as *lai*, which causes most cases of human infection in China and the Korean peninsula. The new, more discriminative technique of multilocus sequence typing confirmed that a large outbreak of human leptospirosis in northeast Thailand lasting several years was caused by a single ecologically successful clone (sequence type 34) of *L. interrogans* serovar *autumnalis*, which was associated with bandicoot rats.[3]

PATHOGENESIS AND PATHOLOGY

Leptospires gain access to the circulation through penetration of abraded skin or intact mucous membranes, disseminate and ultimately penetrate various tissues. This action results in a systemic illness with a wide spectrum of clinical features. A systemic vasculitis with endothelial injury is the basic microscopic finding, with damaged endothelial cells usually showing varying degrees of swelling, denudation and necrosis. Leptospires have been documented in large- and medium-sized blood vessels and capillaries in various organs. The major affected organs are:

- the kidneys, with a diffuse tubulointerstitial inflammation and tubular necrosis;
- the lungs, usually congested, with focal or massive intra-alveolar hemorrhage; and
- the liver, which shows cholestasis associated with mild degenerative changes in hepatocytes.

Other systems may also be affected, with myocarditis, meningoencephalitis and uveitis all occurring in severe disease. Whether a direct toxic effect of the leptospires or the resulting immune response causes the vascular injury is unclear. *Leptospira* outer membrane proteins (OMPs) and lipopolysaccharides may elicit inflammation through a Toll-like receptor 2-dependent pathway.[4] Thrombocytopenia and activation of the coagulation cascade are also commonly seen.[5] During recovery leptospires continue to be excreted in the urine for some days.

PREVENTION

Prevention measures are based upon an awareness of the epidemiology of disease occurring in a region.

Rodent control should be attempted where appropriate and feasible. Occupational protective clothing is effective in groups at risk. In some high-risk groups (e.g. soldiers on jungle maneuvers), oral chemoprophylaxis with doxycycline 200 mg weekly is effective,[6] but there have been few attempts to use this approach on a large scale, such as after massive flooding.

Vaccines are available for use in the livestock industry, and in some countries for human use, but these have been largely unsuccessful.[7] However the identification of new surface-exposed proteins and putative virulence determinants through the availability of whole genome sequences have provided new candidates for vaccine development.[8]

CLINICAL FEATURES

Humans become ill 7–12 days after exposure to leptospires. The disease course is classically described as being biphasic, with an acute bacteremic phase and a second 'immune' phase, though clinically the two phases merge, particularly in severe disease. The acute phase is characterized by a sudden onset of fever, chills, retro-orbital headache, anorexia, abdominal pain, nausea and vomiting, and conjunctival suffusion (Fig. 124.2). Myalgia with muscle tenderness in the calves, abdomen and paraspinal region is characteristic, and when affecting the neck and nuchal region may mimic meningitis. In mild disease defervescence of fever occurs after 3–9 days.

The second or 'immune' phase starts either immediately or 2–3 days later, and is characterized by leptospiruria and the appearance of IgM antibodies. Symptoms recur and signs of meningitis may develop in up to 50% of cases. Optic neuritis, peripheral neuropathy and prolonged uveitis can also occur. In severe cases, fever may persist and be associated with renal insufficiency or failure, varying levels of jaundice, and myocarditis. Coagulopathy may occur, leading to bleeding manifestations ranging from a petechial rash and conjunctival hemorrhage through to gastrointestinal bleeding and pulmonary hemorrhage. Death, occurring in 10–15% of these severe cases, is usually due to pulmonary hemorrhage, renal failure or cardiac failure and arrhythmias secondary to myocarditis. Chest radiographs may reveal

numerous abnormalities including pulmonary infiltrates, pleural effusions or a diffuse pneumonitis.

Clinical laboratory investigations reveal red and white cells in the urine with proteinuria. An elevated white cell count, thrombocytopenia and a high creatinine phosphokinase are commonly observed. The bilirubin may be very elevated but the transaminases rarely exceed two to three times the upper limit of normal.

The differential diagnosis of leptospirosis includes dengue fever, malaria, rickettsioses, influenza and other acute febrile illnesses depending on the geographic location.

DIAGNOSIS

Because of the broad spectrum of symptoms and the wide differential diagnosis, a high index of clinical suspicion is required if appropriate diagnostic tests are to be made. Though leptospires can be isolated from blood and cerebrospinal fluid samples during the first 7–10 days of illness, and from urine during the second and third weeks, isolation of the organism requires special media and takes several weeks of incubation and thus does not contribute to individual patient care. A large number of methods for detection of leptospiral DNA by polymerase chain reaction have recently been described, and though more sensitive than culture, these have not yet been standardized and optimized for routine use.

A strong IgM antibody response, which appears about 5–7 days after onset of symptoms, can be detected using several commercial assays based on ELISA, latex agglutination and immunochromatographic rapid test technologies. Unfortunately, these have relatively poor sensitivity on admission samples. The microscopic agglutination test applied to paired acute and convalescent samples remains the gold standard, but this is a complex assay that detects antibodies against live antigen suspensions and is performed only in reference laboratories. This test yields information about the presumptive infecting serovar and thus has some epidemiologic value. In endemic areas, single elevated titers must be interpreted with caution because antibodies persist for years after acute infection.

Direct microscopic examination of clinical samples is of little value, but immunohistochemical staining of autopsy specimens is a valuable diagnostic tool.

MANAGEMENT

Patients with mild or anicteric disease usually get better without treatment. Doxycycline 100 mg/day has been shown to shorten the duration of the illness, and is as effective as cefotaxime or penicillin G while at the same time treating rickettsioses which may present in a clinically similar fashion.[9] Until the efficacy of antibiotic treatment in late-stage severe disease is resolved, patients should be treated with intravenous penicillin G (benzylpenicillin), cefotaxime or ceftazidime.[10] Hospitalization is recommended for severe cases. Excellent supportive care with particular attention to fluid and electrolyte balance and pulmonary and cardiac function is critical. Renal failure should be treated by hemodialysis or hemodiafiltration if available, though peritoneal dialysis can be used in resource-poor settings.

REFERENCES

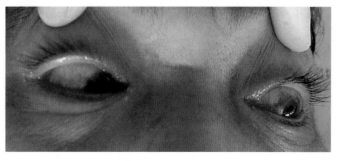

References for this chapter can be found online at http://www.expertconsult.com

Fig. 124.2 Conjunctival suffusion and jaundice.

Relapsing fevers

INTRODUCTION

Repeated abrupt episodes of fever, separated by afebrile periods, give relapsing fever its name. There are two forms:

- tick-borne relapsing fever, caused by various *Borrelia* spp.; and
- louse-borne relapsing fever, caused by *Borrelia recurrentis*.

Both diseases are transmitted by arthropod ectoparasites and, rarely, by needlestick, blood transfusion or transplacentally, but they differ in their epidemiology, clinical features and management. Sometimes, they cause fever in returned travelers.

EPIDEMIOLOGY

Tick-borne relapsing fever

Tick-borne relapsing fever is endemic in most temperate and tropical countries except in Australasia and the Pacific region. In the West African savanna region, *B. crocidurae* is the most prevalent bacterial infection, creating a medical problem second only to malaria.[1] It has increased during the recent drought. In parts of East Africa, it is an important cause of abortion and perinatal mortality.[2]

Borrelia-tick complexes

Different species of *Borrelia* spirochetes and soft ticks of the genus *Ornithodoros* (Argasidae) are associated with different parts of the world (Table 125.1).

Tick vectors are predominantly soft ticks (Argasidae) of the genus *Ornithodoros*, found in dry savanna areas and scrub, particularly near rodent burrows, caves, piles of timber and dead trees, or in cracks and crevices in walls, roof spaces and beneath the floors of log cabins, anywhere inhabited by small rodents. Unlike louse-borne relapsing fever, tick-borne relapsing fevers are zoonoses with the possible exception of *B. duttonii* infection that was thought to be transmitted only between humans. However, new evidence suggests that in central Tanzania this species may infect domestic chickens and pigs.[3] Vertebrate reservoir species are rodents such as rats, gerbils, mice, squirrels and chipmunks and also dogs and birds. Ticks ingest spirochetes while sucking blood from infected animals or humans. They attack at night, remaining attached for less than 30 minutes before retreating back to their hiding places. Infection is either by a bite, through infected saliva, or by contaminating mucosal membranes with infected coxal fluid. Borreliae are not excreted in tick feces.

Ticks remain infected for life and while starved of blood for as long as 7 years. Spirochetes can be transmitted venereally from male to female ticks and by females (but perhaps not those of the *O. moubata* complex) transovarially to their progeny.

Table 125.1 Geographic distribution of *Borrelia* and *Ornithodoros* spp.

Borrelia spp.	*Ornithodoros* spp.	Geographic distribution
New World tick-borne relapsing fever borreliae		
B. hermsii	*O. hermsi*	Canada, Central and Western United States, Mexico
B. turicatae	*O. turicata*	Southwestern United States, Mexico
B. parkeri	*O. parkeri*	Western United States, Baja California
B. mazzotti	*O. talaje*	Mexico, Central America
B. venezuelensis	*O. (venezuelensis) rudis*	Colombia, Venezuela, Argentina, Bolivia, Paraguay
Old World tick-borne relapsing fever borreliae		
B. duttonii	*O. moubata*	Sub-Saharan Africa
B. crocidurae	*O. (erraticus) sonrai*	West, North, East Africa, Middle East
B. persica	*O. tholozani*	Middle East, Central Asia from Uzbekistan to western China
B. hispanica	*O. erraticus*	Iberian peninsula, Greece, Cyprus, North Africa
B. latyschewi	*O. tartakowskyi*	Eastern Europe, Iran, Iraq, Afghanistan
B. caucasia	*O. asperus*	Iraq, Eastern Europe

Louse-borne relapsing fever

The incidence of this classic epidemic disease of armies, refugees and immigrants has fallen in the last decade, but louse-borne relapsing fever remains endemic and seasonally epidemic in the highlands of Ethiopia and adjacent areas of Sudan and Somalia, hilly areas of Yemen and perhaps some parts of the Peruvian and Bolivian Andes.[4] Serologic evidence of *B. recurrentis* infection was also found in homeless people in Marseille.[5] The human body louse, *Pediculus humanus corporis*, is an obligate blood-sucking human ectoparasite that ingests borreliae while feeding. Transmission is by scratching, which crushes lice so that their celomic fluid is inoculated through broken skin or intact mucous membranes such as the conjunctiva, or inoculates infected louse feces. Unlike ticks, lice cannot infect their progeny. Humans are the only reservoirs of this infection.

Louse-borne relapsing fever thrives in the highlands of Ethiopia during the rainy season when impoverished people, encouraged to wear clothes by the cold wet climate, are crowded together and infested with lice, but lack the facilities for controlling the infestation. More than 20 000 lice were recovered from the clothes of one infected person.

PATHOGENESIS

Relapsing fever spirochetes in the blood are lysed by specific bactericidal IgM antibodies, independent of complement and T cells. However, some spirochetes persist extracellularly in various organs: spleen, liver, kidneys, eye and especially in the brain and cerebrospinal fluid. Relapse of spirochetemia and symptoms is explained by antigenic variation, which has been investigated mainly in *B. hermsii*.[6] Transposition of silent gene sequences from an archive stored in extrachromosomal plasmids and their recombination and expression on a linear plasmid results in the synthesis of a new major outer membrane lipoprotein. The spirochete possesses virulence and protective factors. *Borrelia hermsii* surface protein CRASP-1 binds factor H (FH), FHR-1 and plasminogen. FH protects against opsonophagocytosis by inhibiting C3b. Plasminogen is bound and activated to plasmin, stimulating fibrinolysis that promotes spread. Erythrocyte rosetting shields spirochetes physically from host antibody.[7] Antigenic variation generates isogenic serotypes with properties such as enhanced invasiveness for cerebral vascular endothelium.

PREVENTION

Tick-borne relapsing fever

Tick infestation of dwellings can be reduced by improved house construction (e.g. rodent-proofing of cabins on the North Rim of the Grand Canyon), control of their peridomestic rodent hosts and use of residual insecticides (pyrethroids, benzene hexachloride, lambda-cyhalothrin, malathion or dichlorodiphenyltrichloroethane – DDT). Travelers should avoid sleeping in places where ticks and rodents are abundant, such as poorly maintained log cabins, and should apply repellents to their skin (*N,N*-diethyl-M-toluamide – DEET). Postexposure prophylaxis with doxycycline (200 mg followed by 100 mg on the next 4 days) has proved effective against *B. persica* in Israel.[8]

Louse-borne relapsing fever

Infested clothing should be de-loused using heat (>60°C), chlorine bleach or insecticide (10% DDT, 1% malathion, 2% temephos, 1% propoxur or 0.5% permethrin) and patients should be bathed with soap and 1% cresol (Lysol). Lice are abundant in hair, which should be washed or shaved off. Breaking transmission from lice to the susceptible population is essential for the control of an epidemic.

CLINICAL FEATURES

Tick-borne relapsing fever

Ticks bite painlessly and detach after only a short feed and infection produces no eschar, so exposure usually passes unnoticed. After an incubation period of 3–18 days, the illness starts with sudden fever, chills, headache, muscle and joint pains, extreme fatigue, prostration and drenching sweats.[4] Epistaxis, abdominal pain, diarrhea, cough and erythematous or petechial rashes may follow. Depending on the *Borrelia* spp. involved, up to 40% of patients may develop neurologic disturbances reminiscent of those in Lyme disease: paresthesiae, visual symptoms, lymphocytic meningitis, cranial nerve palsies (especially VII), encephalitis, myelitis, sciatica and radiculitis. Several cases of adult respiratory distress syndrome (ARDS) have been described in the United States.

The density of spirochetemia governs clinical severity. Symptoms abate after a few days, only to recur about 7–15 days later. As many as eight relapses may follow, becoming sequentially less severe. Abortion and perinatal mortality is common. In one study in Tabora, Tanzania, parturition was precipitated in 58% of infected pregnant women. Perinatal mortality was 436/1000 births; its risk related to low birth weight and gestational age, and the total loss of pregnancies including abortions was 475/1000. Spirochetemia was higher in pregnant than nonpregnant women.[2]

Louse-borne relapsing fever[4,9]

After an incubation period of 4–17 (average 7) days, the first symptoms are fever, chills, headache, muscle and body aches, fatigue, dizziness, anorexia and nightmares. At least 50% of patients develop bleeding: epistaxis, subconjunctival hemorrhage (Fig. 125.1) or petechial hemorrhages, especially on the trunk (Fig. 125.2). An enlarged and tender liver, often with an enlarged spleen, is palpable in as many as 50% of cases in some outbreaks, and about half of these are jaundiced. The respiratory system is affected in about 15% of cases. Cough may indicate pneumonia or acute pulmonary edema. Transient myocardial damage may lead to acute left ventricular failure with pulmonary edema. Neurologic signs are less common than in tick-borne relapsing fever. Confusion or coma suggests circulatory failure, cerebral hemorrhage (Fig. 125.3) or hepatic failure. Fetal loss is very common in pregnant women.

Spontaneous crisis and Jarisch–Herxheimer reaction

The clinical course of relapsing fever, especially louse-borne, usually ends either with a 'spontaneous crisis' on about day 5 of the untreated illness or by a Jarisch–Herxheimer reaction (J-HR).[9] About 1–3 hours

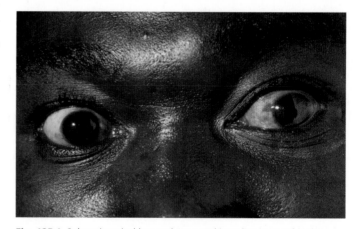

Fig. 125.1 Subconjunctival hemorrhages and jaundice in an Ethiopian patient with louse-borne relapsing fever. Copyright D.A. Warrell.

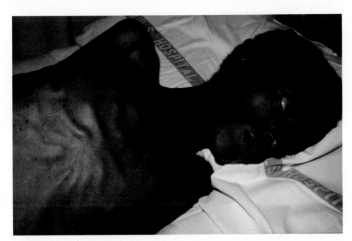

Fig. 125.2 Petechial hemorrhages in an Ethiopian patient suffering from louse-borne relapsing fever complicated by typhoid. Copyright D.A. Warrell.

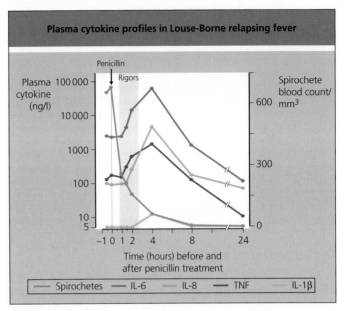

Plasma cytokine profiles in Louse-Borne relapsing fever

Fig. 125.4 Plasma cytokine profile in a patient with louse-borne relapsing fever during the Jarisch–Herxheimer reaction to penicillin treatment. Copyright D.A. Warrell.

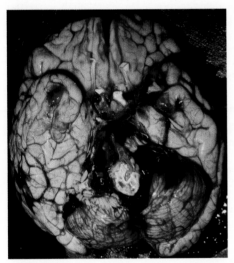

Fig. 125.3 Fatal cerebral hemorrhage in louse-borne relapsing fever. Copyright D.A. Warrell.

LABORATORY FINDINGS

In blood films, spirochetes are best demonstrated with Giemsa or Wright's stain, counterstained with 1% crystal violet (Fig. 125.5). Thick films have a 20-fold higher sensitivity than thin films. In louse-borne relapsing fever, spirochete density in peripheral blood may exceed 500 000/mm³. There is a peripheral neutrophil leukocytosis but, during the Jarisch–Herxheimer reaction or spontaneous crisis, leukocytes almost disappear transiently from the peripheral blood. Thrombocytopenia is common and there is a coagulopathy attributable partly to hepatic dysfunction and partly to disseminated intravascular coagulation with increased fibrinolytic activity. Biochemical evidence of hepatocellular damage is found in most patients.[4] A few patients show transient, mild renal impairment. A mild neutrophil–lymphocyte pleocytosis has been described.

after antibiotic treatment, the patient becomes restless. Violent rigors herald rapid increases in temperature, respiratory rate, pulse rate and blood pressure. There may be associated vomiting, diarrhea, coughing, musculoskeletal pains and delirium. Some patients die of hyperpyrexia at the height of the fever. During the ensuing flush phase of this endotoxin-like reaction, there is profuse sweating, intense vasodilatation and a fall in mean arterial pressure, and a slow decline in temperature over the next 6–12 hours. Fatalities during this phase are due to hypovolemic shock or acute pulmonary edema resulting from myocarditis, sometimes precipitated by the patient's getting out of bed and standing up. The incidence of Jarisch–Herxheimer reactions varies from 30% to almost 100% in different published reports of patients who were carefully observed.

A borrelial pyrogen, an outer membrane variable major lipoprotein[10] released by the action of antimicrobial agents, stimulates an explosive release of cytokines from macrophages through nuclear factor kappa B (NF-κB),[11] principally tumor necrosis factor (TNF), interleukin (IL)-6, IL-8 and IL-1β, just before the start of the clinical manifestations of the Jarisch–Herxheimer reaction (Fig. 125.4).[12] The reaction is unaffected by corticosteroids, but is delayed by the opiate agonist–antagonist meptazinol and can be prevented by a polyclonal antibody against TNF if this is given just before antibiotic treatment.[13]

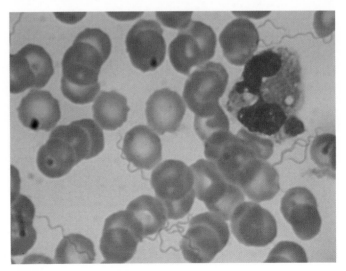

Fig. 125.5 Spirochetes of *Borrelia recurrentis* in a thin blood film. Copyright D.A. Warrell.

DIAGNOSIS

In patients with acute fevers after travel to tropical countries, it is essential to examine thick and thin blood films for malarial parasites. This may reveal relapsing fever spirochetes. Misidentification of microgametes of *Plasmodium vivax* has led to the diagnosis of 'pseudo-borreliosis'.[14] In tick-borne relapsing fever, spirochetes may be difficult or impossible to find, even at the height of a relapse and, increasingly, polymerase chain reaction (PCR) and serology are being used. However, Lyme disease borreliae may produce cross-reacting antibodies, due to expression of conserved antigenic epitopes. ELISA, using the GlpQ gene product, can distinguish relapsing fever from Lyme disease.[15] In louse-borne relapsing fever, the higher and more persistent spirochetemia is more easily detected.

In vitro culture of borreliae, including *B. recurrentis*, *B. duttonii* and *B. crocidurae*, is now possible, using Barbour–Stoenner–Kelly medium.[16]

Differential diagnosis

In a febrile patient with jaundice, petechial rash, spontaneous systemic bleeding and hepatosplenomegaly, the following differential diagnoses should be considered, depending on the geographic location: falciparum malaria, yellow fever and other viral hemorrhagic fevers (such as Rift Valley fever in the Horn of Africa), viral hepatitis, rickettsial infections (especially louse-borne typhus which has the same epidemiologic predispositions as louse-borne relapsing fever) and leptospirosis. Secondary infections, known to complicate louse-borne relapsing fever, include bacillary dysentery, salmonellosis, typhoid (see Fig. 125.2), typhus, malaria and tuberculosis.

In the differential diagnosis of travelers at risk, two less common causes of episodic recurrent fever are trench fever (caused by *Bartonella quintana*) if there was possible contact with lice, or rat-bite fever (caused by *Spirillum minus*).

PROGNOSIS

Reported case fatalities during *B. recurrentis* epidemics have exceeded 40% but this can be reduced to less than 5% with antimicrobial treatment, provided that appropriate ancillary treatment is given during the life-threatening Jarisch–Herxheimer reaction. Tick-borne relapsing fever is less dangerous. Deaths during relapses are most unusual but have been reported in tick-borne relapsing fever.

MANAGEMENT

The principles of treatment are:
- to eliminate spirochetemia and prevent relapses, using antibiotics;
- to monitor the patient very carefully through the Jarisch–Herxheimer reaction; and
- to restore and maintain circulating volume during the 24 hours after starting antibiotic treatment.

Antibiotic agents

The choice of agents is based on clinical experience.[17]

Tick-borne relapsing fever

Doxycycline 100 mg per day for 10 days is recommended for adults. For pregnant women and young children, erythromycin can be used.

Louse-borne relapsing fever

A single 500 mg oral dose of tetracycline or erythromycin stearate is effective. In severely ill patients who are likely to vomit, effective parenteral treatment consists of either a single intravenous dose of tetracycline hydrochloride (250 mg)[18] or, for pregnant women and children, a single intravenous dose of erythromycin lactobionate (300 mg for adults, 10 mg/kg for children). In mixed epidemics of louse-borne relapsing fever and louse-borne typhus, a single oral dose of doxycycline 100 mg has proved effective.[19] Penicillins and chloramphenicol are also effective.[17,18] Some experienced clinicians prefer to use a low dose of penicillin (adult dose, 100 000–400 000 units by intramuscular injection) in severe cases and pregnant women because they believe that the incidence and severity of the Jarisch–Herxheimer reaction will be less although the risk of relapse is greater.[4,20]

Supportive treatment

Postural hypotension and cardiac arrhythmias are prevented by nursing the patient flat in bed for 24 hours after antibiotic treatment. Hyperpyrexia and hypovolemia must be prevented. Acute heart failure with pulmonary edema responds to intravenous furosemide and digoxin. Bleeding and clotting problems are treated with vitamin K, platelets and clotting factor concentrates. Complicating infections, notably typhoid, salmonellosis, bacillary dysentery, tuberculosis, malaria and typhus in some endemic situations, must be treated appropriately.

REFERENCES

References for this chapter can be found online at http://www.expertconsult.com

Lisa E Hensley
Victoria Wahl-Jensen
Joseph B McCormick
Kathleen H Rubins

Chapter | **126** |

Viral hemorrhagic fevers

INTRODUCTION

Viral hemorrhagic fever (VHF) describes a syndrome which can be caused by multiple unrelated viruses. The clinical disease is often characterized by an acute onset, high fever and, in some cases, a high mortality rate. Although not fully defined for all VHFs, the bleeding manifestations are thought to be the result of capillary leakage. Death is usually attributable to multiorgan system failure and hypovolemic shock, with or without acute respiratory distress syndrome (ARDS).

VIROLOGY AND NATURAL HISTORY

To date, all known VHFs are caused by a range of single-stranded enveloped RNA viruses including arenaviruses, bunyaviruses, filoviruses, paramyxoviruses, flaviviruses and henipahviruses (Fig. 126.1; Table 126.1). Almost all of the VHFs can be described as zoonoses; these agents rely on an animal or insect reservoir for their maintenance and transmission. Therefore initial infections with these viruses are usually geographically restricted to areas where the reservoir and/or vector resides. However, the possibility of subsequent person-to-person transmission and importation outside the endemic or epidemic area(s) does exist.

VHF occurs primarily in rural or developing countries where there is substantial contact with rodents, ticks or mosquitoes and poor facilities for medical care. Only dengue, and occasionally yellow fever, are seen in populous areas. Distribution of individual VHF is often limited by reservoir/vector presence. However, as a result of the increasing mobility of populations, infected patients can and do appear almost anywhere in the world. This was highlighted recently with an imported case of Marburg hemorrhagic fever from Uganda to the Netherlands in 2008. Large epidemics of VHF can kill thousands of people, such as yellow fever outbreaks, or several hundred people, as has been the case with recent Marburg and Ebola outbreaks. However, there are often sporadic cases that go undiagnosed or fail to capture the attention of the local medical community; thus the incidence as well as the distribution of VHFs is likely underreported. Details pertaining to each family of VHF viruses are presented below.

Arenaviruses are rodent-borne pathogens that have potential to cause hemorrhagic fever (HF) infections in humans.[1,2] The viruses are classified into two categories: Old World and New World, based on geographic location. Geographic distribution of these viruses appears to be dependent on the presence of the rodent host. In West Africa, Lassa virus is the sole Old World arenavirus reported to be responsible for human infection. However, recent reports suggest that there may be additional or divergent arenaviruses circulating and potentially responsible for clinical disease.[3] Of the New World arenaviruses, Junin virus, Machupo virus, Guanarito virus and Sabia virus are the etiologic agents of Argentine HF, Bolivian HF, Venezuelan HF and Brazilian HF, respectively.

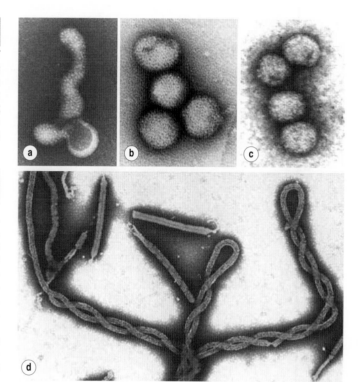

Fig. 126.1 Transmission electron micrographs of negatively stained hemorrhagic fever viral particles. (a) Junin virus. Arenavirus particles range in morphology from highly pleomorphic as shown in this field to mainly spherical. Virion sizes range from 50 to 300 nm with a mean of 100–130 nm. (b) Rift Valley fever virus. Bunyaviral particles are roughly spherical and range in diameter from 90 to 120 nm. (c) Yellow fever virus. Flaviviral particles are essentially isometric and consistent in size, ranging from 40 to 50 nm in diameter. (d) Ebola virus. Filoviral particles are mostly filamentous and vary in length up to 14 000 nm with a uniform diameter of 80 nm. Mean unit length is about 1000 nm. Other forms of filoviral particles included U shaped, '6' shaped or circular configurations; branching of filamentous particles can also occur. From Jahrling PB, Marty AM, Geisbert TW. Viral hemorrhagic fevers. In: Dembek ZF, ed. Medical aspects of biological warfare. In: Lenhart MK, Lounsbury DE, Martin JW, eds. Textbooks of military medicine. Washington, DC: Department of the Army, Office of The Surgeon General, Borden Institute; 2007:Ch. 13.

In the Bunyaviridae family,[4] Crimean–Congo hemorrhagic fever virus (CCHF),[5] hantaviruses[6] – particularly Andes virus (ANDV), Hantaan virus (HTNV), and Sin Nombre virus (SNV) – and Rift Valley fever virus[6,7] cause VHF in humans. CCHF is spread by ticks and occurs widely across Africa, south-eastern Europe, the Middle East and Asia.

Table 126.1 Epidemiologic characteristics of the most important viral hemorrhagic fevers

	ARENAVIRUSES*		FILOVIRUSES		BUNYAVIRUSES			FLAVIVIRUSES	HENIPAVIRUSES	
	Lassa virus	Junin, Machupo, Guanarito, Sabia	Ebola	Marburg	Hantavirus	Crimean–Congo	Rift Valley fever	Yellow fever	Nipah	Hendra
Geography	West Africa	South America, North America	Central and West Africa	East and Central Africa	Worldwide	Europe, Asia, Africa	Africa	South America, Africa	Malaysia, Singapore	Australia
Primary source of infection	Rodent (*Mastomys natalensis*)	Rodent (*Calomys, Zygodontomys sp.*)	Unknown; possibly bats		Rodents; species depends on location	Tick-borne (>27 species)	Mosquito	Mosquito-borne (*Aedes* and *Hemogogus* spp.)	Unknown; possibly bats	
Transmission	Nosocomial Rodent to human/person to person	Rodent to human	Nosocomial; possibly reservoir to human; person to person; also infected great apes and possibly monkeys can transmit to humans		Rodent to human; human to human for Andes virus	Nosocomial tick to human; possibly animal to human; possibly person to person	Mosquito to human; possibly animal to human via blood	Mosquito to human (human reservoir in outbreaks)	Contact with infected pigs, bats, or materials contaminated with secretions from infected bats	Contact with infected horses
Risk factors	Close contact *Mastomys* rural West Africa; close contact infected persons	Contact rodents in circumscribed agricultural areas South America, possibly North America	Close contact with infected blood or secretions from infected persons; environmental risk unknown (possibly caves for Marburg)		Contact with rodent or rodent urine in dust; laboratory	Tick bites; contact with infected livestock; contact with blood or secretions from infected persons	Mosquito bites rural Africa	Mosquito bites rural West Africa and South American rainforests	Close contact infected blood or secretions from infected animals or persons	
Treatment	Responds to ribavirin when treated early	Junin responds to immune plasma given early; all may respond to ribavirin	No currently approved treatment; does not respond to ribavirin; several therapeutics under efficacy testing in animal models		Ribavirin may be beneficial early; trial and current use in China; open-label trial in USA for acute pulmonary disease was inconclusive	Sensitive to ribavirin; several published reports of successful case treatment	Sensitive to ribavirin; limited data in monkeys; no human data	No therapy; does not respond to ribavirin	No currently approved treatment	
Vaccine	DNA and recombinant Vesicular Stomatis Virus (rVSV) vaccines under evaluation in animal models. Development of human vaccine possible	Attenuated vaccine to Junin virus has greatly reduced cases in Argentina; no vaccine available for others	rVSV and adenovirus vaccine platforms have demonstrated efficacy in nonhuman primates	rVSV adenovirus vaccine, VEE replicon and virus-like particle vaccine platforms have demonstrated efficacy in nonhuman primates	M gene DNA vaccine expressing glycoproteins 1 and 2 protects small animals from challenge and elicits neutralizing antibody in Rhesus monkeys; also formalin-inactivated vaccine but no trial data	Killed vaccine available in Eastern Europe and China, but no published trials	Attenuated vaccine for animals, none for humans	Live attenuated vaccine since 1940s; one of the most effective vaccines ever	No currently approved vaccine	

*Arenaviruses have been isolated from wood rats in the south-western USA – their capacity to cause human infection is uncertain.

Hantaviruses are found throughout the world and infection of the natural rodent host results in a chronic carrier state without pronounced pathology or signs of disease. Diseases caused by hantaviruses generally manifest as either hemorrhagic fever with renal syndrome (HFRS) or hantavirus pulmonary syndrome (HPS). Although reported worldwide, HFRS is widely distributed in eastern Asia, with particularly high prevalences observed in China, Russia and Korea. HPS has been reported in the USA as well as areas of South and Central America. Rift Valley fever (RVF) virus is mosquito borne and causes an acute illness in livestock and wild animals. RVF is described as being both endemic and epidemic in areas of Africa and the Middle East.

The filoviruses (Ebola and Marburg viruses) are responsible for some of the most lethal VHFs.[8] The Ebola viruses are comprised of four distinct species with mortality rates up to 90% while Marburg virus is a single species with different isolates having varying mortality rates (20–90%). Natural outbreaks of filoviruses in humans have been reported in the Democratic Republic of the Congo, Republic of the Congo, Sudan, Uganda, Angola and Gabon.[9] Filoviruses have been implicated in large scale die-offs of great ape populations. There is growing evidence that bats are the likely reservoir and infection of nonhuman primates represents inadvertent transmission to these animals.

The Flaviviridae which cause HF include yellow fever virus (see Chapter 164) and dengue virus (see Chapter 127), both of which are spread by mosquitoes.[10] Yellow fever is endemic in sub-Saharan Africa and tropical regions of South America with fatality rates of 5–7%. Dengue fever (DF) and dengue hemorrhagic fever (DHF) are caused by one of four closely related, but antigenically distinct, virus serotypes. Infection with one of these serotypes provides immunity to only that serotype for life, so individuals living in a dengue-endemic area can have more than one dengue infection during their lifetime. The average case fatality rate associated with DHF is 1%. Other flaviviruses can cause hemorrhagic fever, including Kyasanur Forest disease virus, Omsk hemorrhagic fever virus and Alkhurma virus, but these are confined to very local areas and are not discussed in detail here.

In the Paramyxoviridae, the genus Henipavirus composed of Nipah virus and the closely related Hendra virus (formerly called equine morbillivirus) have recently been identified as producing VHF in humans.[11] Nipah virus was first identified in an outbreak of respiratory disease and encephalitis in pigs and humans in Malaysia and Singapore. Hendra virus was isolated during an outbreak of respiratory illness and neurologic disease among horses and a small number of people in Australia. Transmission to humans is typically due to exposure to bodily fluids and excretions from infected horses for Hendra virus and to close contact with infected pigs, bats or materials contaminated with saliva or waste from infected bats for Nipah virus. Bat species, particularly flying foxes, have been implicated as potential reservoirs in the transmission of Nipah virus. Current distribution of Nipah virus includes India, Bangladesh and Singapore.

DIAGNOSIS AND CLINICAL FEATURES

The most critical element for the clinical diagnosis in nonendemic areas is a thorough case history spanning the incubation period (3 days to 4 weeks before the onset of fever). The case history must include:

- an extensive review of recent travel, particularly to endemic areas;
- contact with severely ill febrile individuals;
- contact with potential vectors (e.g. ticks or mosquitoes);
- contact with animals or animal products (e.g. animal blood or carcasses, rodent droppings, etc.);
- any entry into environments where a reservoir may be or may have been present (e.g. caves housing large bat populations or houses with large rodent infestations); and
- participation in activities that may have placed the patient in close contact with infected or diseased individuals such as traditional funeral practices or preparations.

A medical care provider or other worker who might have had contact with blood from a primary case should also alert the physician to possible VHF (see also PP60).

The essential clinical features (Fig. 126.2) are highlighted in Table 126.2. Often clinical presentations are nonspecific and include a history of sudden or rapid onset of fever, severe body pains and headache that is often described as prominent or excruciating. Other features may include confusion, severe pharyngitis, nausea and vomiting, petechiae, oozing from the gums and bradycardia (Figs 126.3, 126.4). Proteinuria is common. Peripheral white blood cell counts are often low very early in disease, but may dramatically increase later, and therefore the presence of neutrophilia may falsely indicate a bacterial disease and be misleading. Thrombocytopenia is common and platelet function is often impaired, even in the presence of low-normal platelet counts. Partial thromboplastin times may be prolonged, but prothrombin times may be relatively unaffected depending on the agent, the severity or stage of the disease (early or late).

As the disease progresses, hypovolemic shock, pulmonary edema and frank bleeding may ensue. Aspartate aminotransferase (AST) is usually raised and virtually all VHFs distinguish themselves from viral hepatitis by the disproportionately high AST levels compared with alanine aminotransferase (ALT). Ratios of AST to ALT may be as high as 11:1; the level of AST also typically reflects prognosis. Patients are rarely jaundiced (except in yellow fever) and the bilirubin is usually normal.

The viruses are pantropic. These agents typically have a period of uncontrolled viral replication with high titers of infectious virus in the blood and tissues (Fig. 126.5). Encephalopathy and neurologic sequelae such as ataxia and deafness can occur, particularly in the early convalescent phase. This phenomenon is most prominent in patients who

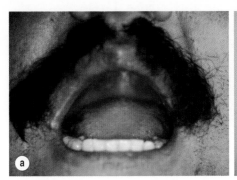
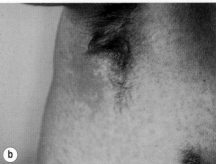
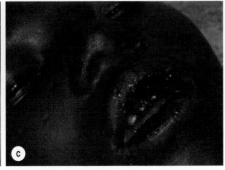

Fig. 126.2 Clinical manifestations of viral hemorrhagic fever. (a) Soft and hard palate erythema in Lassa fever. (b) Maculopapular skin rash in Lassa fever. (c) Mild oral and nasal mucosal bleeding in Lassa fever. From Schlossberg D, ed. Clinical infectious disease. New York: Cambridge University Press; 2008:1319–32.

Table 126.2 Key clinical features of viral hemorrhagic fevers

	ARENAVIRUS		FILOVIRUS		BUNYAVIRUS			FLAVIVIRUS		HENIPAVIRUSES	
	Lassa virus	South American	Ebola*	Marburg	Old World hantavirus	New World hantavirus	Crimean–Congo	Rift Valley fever	Yellow fever	Nipah virus	Hendra virus
Untreated case fatality (%)	2–20	16	25–90	20–90	1–15	45–50	10–50	1–2	20–50	40%	66%†
Cardiovascular system											
Thrombocytopenia	+	+++	+++	+++	++	+	+++	++	++		
Oozing	++	++	+++	+++	++	–	+++	++	+++		
Petechiae	–	+++	+	+	+++		+				
Ecchymoses			++	++		–	++				
Circulatory shock	+++	+++	+++	+++	+++	+++	+++	+++	+++		
Tissue edema	++		+	+	+	+					
Major hemorrhage	+	+	++	++	+	–	++	+	++		
Central nervous system											
Encephalopathy	+++	+	+	+	–	–	+			+++	+++
Ataxia	+	++			+						
Deafness	++										
Blindness			+								
Mood alteration	+	+	+	+			++			+++	+++
Intracranial bleeding					+						
Other major systems											
Renal	–	–	+/–	+/–	+++	+			+		
Pulmonary (ARDS)	+++	+	+	+	+	+++			+		
Hepatic	+	+	+	+	+	+	+	+	+++		

ARDS, adult respiratory distress syndrome.
+ Denotes present to differing degrees indicated by number of marks; – denotes absence; no mark indicates no reliable data.
*Reston is not a human pathogen.
†There have only been three reported cases of Hendra virus.

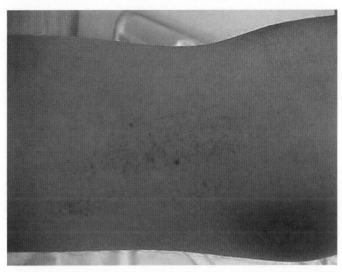

Fig. 126.3 Petechial rash in a patient with Crimean–Congo hemorrhagic fever. From Peters W, Pasvol G. Atlas of tropical medicine and parasitology, 6th ed. Philadelphia: Mosby; 2006. Copyright Elsevier 2006.

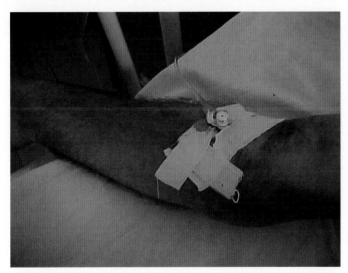

Fig. 126.4 Ecchymoses in a patient with Crimean–Congo hemorrhagic fever. From Peters W, Pasvol G. Atlas of tropical medicine and parasitology, 6th ed. Philadelphia: Mosby; 2006. Copyright Elsevier 2006.

recover from Lassa fever infections. The etiology of the central nervous system sequelae remains unclear and will likely have to be determined on an agent-by-agent basis.

Care must be taken in collecting, handling and transporting specimens, and consultation with the laboratory is essential. At a minimum, standard precautions should be implemented at all times and all potentially infectious specimens must be clearly labeled as hazardous. Blood samples should be drawn into a vacuum tube system. Specimens for transport should be transferred to a leakproof plastic container and double wrapped in leakproof containers in which they can be transported to a suitable reference laboratory (see Chapter 164).

Laboratory diagnosis utilizes several methods, including:

- presence of virus-specific IgM or IgG in the serum;
- presence of viral RNA, usually in serum or white cells, demonstrated by a reverse transcriptase polymerase chain reaction (RT-PCR) or genomic chip-based method;
- presence of viral antigen through enzyme-linked immunosorbent assay (ELISA) for specific viral antigens in serum or blood;
- isolating the virus from blood, serum, oral swab or other clinical sample;

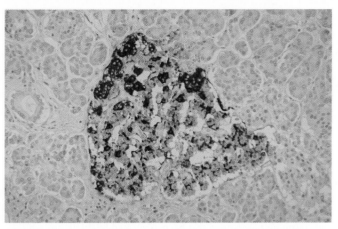

Fig. 126.5 Immunohistochemical staining for hemorrhagic fever viral antigens. Pancreas from a fatal human case of Marburg hemorrhagic fever (Ravn strain). Note that Marburg virus-positive staining (red) is limited to the pancreatic islet with multifocal distribution within the islet (streptavidin-alkaline phosphatase method, section counterstained with hematoxylin). From Jahrling PB, Marty AM, Geisbert TW. Viral hemorrhagic fevers. In: Dembek ZF, ed. Medical aspects of biological warfare. In: Lenhart MK, Lounsbury DE, Martin JW, eds. Textbooks of military medicine. Washington, DC: Department of the Army, Office of The Surgeon General, Borden Institute; 2007:Ch. 13.

- visualization using electron microscopy; and
- demonstrating a fourfold rise in antibody titer.

Sera may be inactivated for use in serologic assays by gamma irradiation; if this is unavailable, heating at 140°F (60°C) for 30 minutes is usually sufficient. Immunofluorescence assays and ELISAs may detect both virus antibody and antigen. More recently, molecular techniques such as PCR or direct sequencing performed on serum or tissues to detect viral RNA have been found to be rapid, reliable and safe. However, while these techniques or these assays are widely available in the developed world, they are not always available in the VHF endemic areas, and a combination of both traditional antigen/antibody detection methods as well as newer molecular techniques can be used. Lastly, available facilities or infrastructure may also dictate which detection methods are utilized. Recent advances in the development of field portable equipment will likely continue to increase capabilities for rapid detection and diagnosis even in remote areas.[12]

MANAGEMENT

For many of the VHFs it is likely that aggressive and appropriate clinical management can reduce reported mortality and morbidity rates. Patient travel and additional trauma should be avoided. Any surgery should be carried out using the most stringent of precautions to protect medical staff and the risk of uncontrolled bleeding in severe cases must be considered. Gentle sedation and pain relief should be implemented. Standard precautions for management of patients with bleeding diatheses should be used. Management of dehydration and bleeding such as the use of intravenous fluids, blood replacement, platelet transfusions, factor replacements or the use of anticoagulants should be evaluated on a disease-by-disease basis and use of these interventions should be closely monitored as fluid balance will likely prove to be the main challenge of acute disease management. Although patients often present with a high hematocrit due to dehydration, pulmonary edema is a real risk for many VHFs and patients should be infused with caution. Full intensive care support, where available, may include mechanical ventilation, extracorporeal membrane oxygenation, monitoring of central venous pressure and dialysis as well as equipment and medications for management of seizures and arrhythmias. Use of vasopressors as well as low-dose steroids have been suggested but to date there are no clinical data to evaluate their efficacy in these diseases.

The development of disseminated intravascular coagulation (DIC) remains a controversial observation for many of the VHFs and it may be that DIC is observed for only certain VHFs or in the most severe presentations. However, when present, effective clinical management may improve survival. For filoviruses the development of a consumptive coagulopathy, with fibrin deposition and significantly elevated levels of D-dimers and the procoagulant protein tissue factor have been documented. Recently, significant improvement in survival was observed in nonhuman primate models of filoviruses using strategies that target the activation of the coagulation pathway.[13,14]

The availability of effective antivirals is limited. Some utility has been reported for the use of ribavirin for the treatment of Lassa fever, Argentine hemorrhagic fever and CCHF (see Table 126.1). Therapy with immune plasma has also been advocated for VHFs, but efficacy has not been fully demonstrated. Recent data indicate that postexposure vaccination in filoviruses models could also reduce or prevent morbidity and mortality. Regardless of the therapeutic intervention, early implementation will likely increase efficacy. Appropriate treatment should be started as soon as possible when cases or potential cases are identified.

Pregnant patients often present with absent fetal movements and abortion is a common complication. For Lassa fever aggressive obstetric intervention to remove the deceased fetus has been shown to increase the survival of the mother. Transportation of VHF patients in rural or remote settings is contraindicated. In severe cases the cardiovascular system is often unstable and any trauma is likely to induce bleeding. Furthermore, transportation without adequate precautions has the potential to expand the epidemic area and expose a greater number of people to secondary infection. Patients may be managed quite successfully in standard hospital isolation rooms with rigorous barrier nursing techniques.

PREVENTION

Education, surveillance and early identification and management of infected patients is critical to disease control and prevention of spread. Community outreach and education should include not only the medical staff for the proper handling of patients and materials from infected patients but also the community as a whole on how these viruses are transmitted and what steps may be take to prevent infection and spread. The key to the prevention of nosocomial transmission in both endemic and epidemic areas has consistently been good hospital and laboratory practice, with strict isolation of febrile patients and rigorous use of gloves and disinfection.[15] Disinfection can be accomplished by washing/soaking with fresh solutions of 0.5% phenol in detergent, 0.5% hypochlorite solution, formaldehyde, glutaraldehyde or paracetic acid.

The 1995 interim update on the 1988 US Centers for Disease Control and Prevention guidelines for the management of patients with VHF recommend patient isolation in a single room, preferably but not necessarily with a negative air pressure gradient from the hallway through an anteroom to the patient room.[16] Past recommendations for strict isolation of patients in a plastic isolator have been abandoned in favor of straightforward strict barrier nursing. This practice presents no excess risk to hospital personnel and allows substantially better care of the patient.

REFERENCES

References for this chapter can be found online at http://www.expertconsult.com

Dengue

INTRODUCTION

Dengue is a vector-borne viral infection and a globally important public health problem.[1,2] The dengue viruses (serotypes 1, 2, 3 and 4) are enveloped, single-stranded RNA viruses of the Flaviviridae family. Transmission from human to human is predominantly by the mosquito *Aedes aegypti*, which bites in the daytime, is adapted to human habitats and has a preference for human blood meals. More than 1 billion people are at risk of dengue infection in over 100 countries (Fig. 127.1).

Any of the four serotypes of dengue virus can result in dengue, which is a systemic febrile illness lasting 3–7 days and characterized by viremia, fever, rash, headache, muscle and joint ache. Occasionally, dengue manifests as dengue hemorrhagic fever (DHF), a potentially life-threatening illness associated with capillary leakage, hemorrhagic manifestations and, in severe cases, hypovolemic shock.

TRANSMISSION

Human-to-human transmission of dengue viruses occurs through the bites of infected female *Aedes aegypti* mosquitoes and less commonly *Aedes albopictus*. The virus circulates in the blood of infected humans for 2–7 days. Mosquitoes become infected after feeding on the blood of a viremic individual. Once infected, a mosquito is capable of transmitting the virus to susceptible individuals for the rest of its life during probing and blood feeding. Transovarial transmission of dengue virus to the next mosquito generation has been observed under laboratory conditions, but the relevance of this to disease epidemiology is yet to be determined. A sylvatic (jungle) cycle of transmission occurs amongst primates in some parts of the world, but in the vast majority of endemic regions transmission is from human-to-human via the mosquito vector.

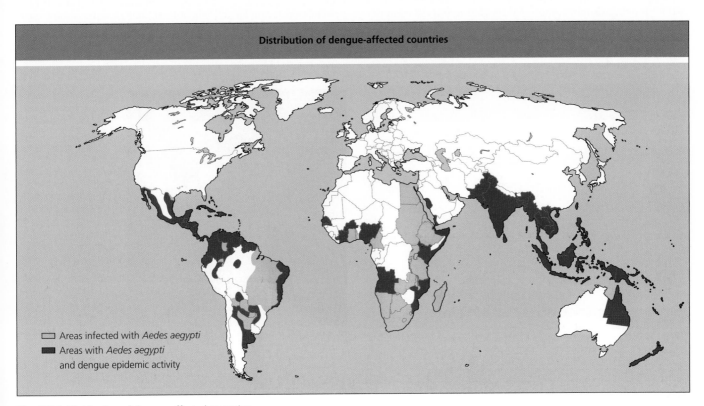

Distribution of dengue-affected countries

☐ Areas infected with *Aedes aegypti*

■ Areas with *Aedes aegypti* and dengue epidemic activity

Fig. 127.1 Distribution of dengue-affected countries.

PATHOGENESIS

Dengue hemorrhagic fever is strongly associated with secondary, so-called heterotypic infections (two sequential infections caused by different serotypes). DHF is rare given the total number of secondary infections.[3–6] In secondary infections, disease severity is linked to high initial viral loads[7,8] and robust humoral and cellular anamnestic immune responses driven by antigenic cross-reactivity between dengue viruses (DENVs).[9–13] DHF also occurs during primary DENV infection of infants born to DENV-immune mothers.[14–17] Halstead has proposed that infants born to DENV-immune mothers and previously infected children or adults have in common a single immune risk factor – DENV-reactive IgG antibodies.[18] The capacity of subneutralizing concentrations of DENV-reactive IgG antibodies to enhance DENV infections in Fc receptor-bearing cells,[18,19] a phenomenon called antibody-dependent enhancement (ADE), provides a unifying basis to explain severe dengue in secondary infections and in infants with primary infections. ADE could result in higher viral burdens *in vivo* and a host inflammatory response that might account for the capillary leakage syndrome.

Pathogenesis has also been linked to the antigenic characteristics or virulence of certain viral lineages. For example, dengue serotype 2 viruses from South East Asia may be more likely to elicit DHF. Host genetic factors may also be relevant and predispose some individuals to DHF, although definitive data in this area remain scant. There are animal models of dengue virus infection, but no model reliably replicates the clinical syndrome of DHF in such a way that it could serve to fully define its pathogenesis. The current understanding of DHF pathogenesis is summarized in Figure 127.2.

PREVENTION

Several tetravalent live-attenuated dengue vaccines are in clinical development, though none is yet close to licensure.[20] Specific antiviral therapies are also in development and these could conceivably be used for prophylaxis in the future. For travelers to tropical countries, the only practical method of prevention is to avoid mosquito bites by wearing protective clothing and using appropriate repellents.

Reduction of mosquito populations currently remains the best method of preventing dengue transmission. Vector control consists of scrupulous destruction and control of breeding sites. All unwanted containers should be discarded, buried or filled with sand. Larvivorous small fish or a crustacean called Mesocyclops can provide control of mosquito larvae. Adult mosquitoes can be destroyed by pyrethrin knock-down sprays or organophosphate sprays delivered in microdroplets. Nevertheless, the relentless increase in the geographic footprint of dengue, and the total number of affected people, indicates most vector control strategies in endemic areas are inadequate, not sustainable and/or poorly targeted.

CLINICAL FEATURES

Dengue fever

The differential diagnosis of classic dengue fever includes other arboviral infections as well as measles, rubella, enterovirus infections, adenovirus infections and influenza. Other differential diagnoses that should be considered depending on local disease prevalence include typhoid, malaria, leptospirosis, hepatitis A, rickettsial diseases and bacterial sepsis.

Most dengue infections are clinically silent or result in only mild, undifferentiated febrile illness, particularly in children. Classic dengue fever is typically seen in adolescents and adults and characterized by a sudden onset of fever with severe headache, retro-orbital pain, gastrointestinal disturbances and generalized pains in the muscles and bones ('breakbone fever'). A maculopapular rash may appear around the time of defervescence, usually 3–7 days after fever onset (Fig. 127.3). Fever is accompanied by leukopenia and moderate thrombocytopenia. Manifestations of vascular permeability are usually not present.

Dengue hemorrhagic fever/dengue shock syndrome

Dengue hemorrhagic fever is an acute vascular permeability syndrome accompanied by abnormal hemostasis. The early clinical presentation is similar to dengue fever, and includes abrupt onset of fever, malaise, vomiting, headache and anorexia. Capillary leakage begins during the febrile phase but typically manifests around

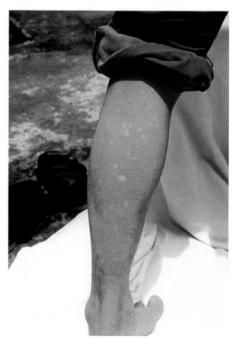

Fig. 127.3 Diffuse macular recovery rash in an adult patient with dengue. The rash may appear between 3 and 6 days after fever onset. Note the 'islands' of normal skin surrounded by erythematous skin.

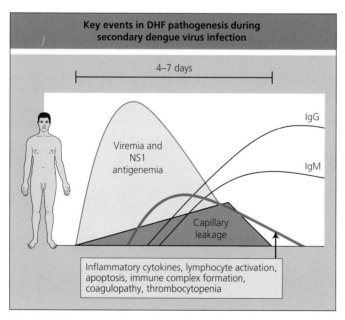

Key events in DHF pathogenesis during secondary dengue virus infection

4–7 days

IgG

IgM

Viremia and NS1 antigenemia

Capillary leakage

Inflammatory cytokines, lymphocyte activation, apoptosis, immune complex formation, coagulopathy, thrombocytopenia

Fig. 127.2 Key events in dengue hemorrhagic fever pathogenesis during secondary dengue virus infection.

the time of defervescence, the 'critical period'. Capillary leakage can be indicated by hypoproteinemia, elevated hematocrit, pleural effusions, ascites, gallbladder wall thickening and perivesicular edema. Scattered spontaneous petechiae and easy bruising at venepuncture sites are relatively common findings. Frank bleeding from mucosal sites (e.g. gastrointestinal, nose, gums, vagina) can occur in severe cases. Modest hepatic involvement is typical and the liver can be palpable and tender and accompanied by abnormal liver transaminase levels. Common laboratory abnormalities include thrombocytopenia and leukopenia with a relative lymphocytosis. Convalescence is fairly rapid and uneventful after the 1- to 2-day critical period around the time of defervescence.

Dengue shock syndrome (DSS), the most common life-threatening complication of acute dengue, occurs when excessive capillary leakage precipitates circulatory dysfunction or collapse. Circulatory dysfunction is seen as a narrowing of pulse pressure (≤20 mmHg) or hypotension for age accompanied by one or more of the following: cold clammy extremities, delayed capillary refill time, flushed face, circumoral cyanosis, diaphoresis, restlessness, irritability and midepigastric pain. Respirations and pulse are rapid. The pathophysiologic presentation of DSS (thrombocytopenia and relatively slow development of hypovolemia) is distinct from other infectious causes of cardiovascular shock.

MANAGEMENT

World Health Organization guidelines for dengue management have been published[21] and are currently being revised. There are no specific treatments for dengue. The mainstay of treatment remains good supportive care, with a particular focus on careful fluid management. Oral rehydration is usually sufficient for patients with little or no evidence of capillary permeability. Acetaminophen (paracetamol) can be used to reduce fever; however, aspirin and nonsteroidal anti-inflammatory drugs are contraindicated.

Patients with a rapidly rising hematocrit, profound thrombocytopenia, persistent vomiting, severe abdominal pain, ecchymoses or mucosal bleeding require very careful and frequent monitoring of vital signs and hematocrit (Fig. 127.4). A rapidly rising hematocrit should prompt conservative parenteral fluid therapy. Rapid but careful restoration of circulating plasma volume is the mainstay of therapy for patients with established DSS. Fluid volumes for resuscitation

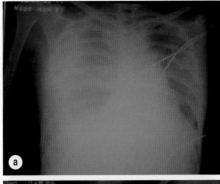
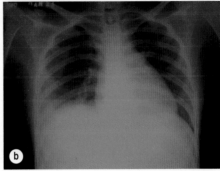

Fig. 127.5 (a) Antero-posterior chest X-ray showing a large pleural effusion on the right side in an adult patient with dengue shock syndrome. (b) The same patient at hospital discharge. Such severe radiologic findings occur in dengue patients with capillary leakage and who have received an excessive volume of intravenous fluid.

should be kept to a minimum but sufficient to maintain cardiovascular stability and adequate urine output during the phase of active leakage. As soon as re-absorption begins, intravenous fluids should be stopped. Fluid overload with respiratory compromise is a recognized complication and a contributor to mortality (Fig. 127.5). Isotonic crystalloid solutions should be the first choice for resuscitation, with colloid solutions reserved for patients presenting with severe DSS and those with repeated or prolonged cardiovascular compromise (Fig. 127.6).

In the event of significant bleeding, transfusion is indicated but with due care to the risks of fluid overload. There is no evidence from randomized controlled trials to support the use of platelet concentrates, even for profound thrombocytopenia. Similarly, there is no evidence that corticosteroids improve clinical outcome in children with established shock.

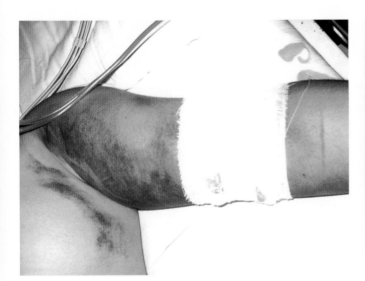

Fig. 127.4 Hematoma in a patient with severe dengue. The combination of increased vascular fragility, platelet dysfunction/thrombocytopenia and coagulation disorders is believed to explain hemorrhagic manifestations in dengue. Frank hemorrhage, as pictured here, is relatively uncommon given the overall disease burden.

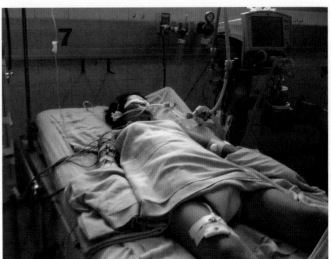

Fig. 127.6 A patient with dengue shock syndrome. As shown in this image, patients with severe dengue require fluids (or blood products in cases with severe bleeding) to maintain hemodynamic stability. Respiratory support can be required in cases with severe pleural effusion and respiratory compromise.

LABORATORY DIAGNOSIS

Laboratory confirmation of dengue is helpful to clinical management and for epidemiologic surveillance. In many settings, a presumptive diagnosis of dengue is made by detection of high levels of DENV-reactive IgM in a single acute plasma/serum sample. The interpretation of dengue serology requires an understanding that antibody responses elicited by flaviviruses can be cross-reactive. Therefore adequate controls should be included in serologic assays in settings where other flaviviruses co-circulate with dengue viruses (e.g. Japanese encephalitis virus). A definitive diagnosis of dengue can be made by reverse transcriptase polymerase chain reaction (RT-PCR), virus isolation or detection of the dengue viral antigen NS1 in plasma.

REFERENCES

References for this chapter can be found online at http://www.expertconsult.com

Anthrax

INTRODUCTION

Anthrax is primarily a disease of herbivores which can be transmitted to humans. It was one of the first zoonoses described. Currently, anthrax has assumed greater importance as a result of the potential use of *Bacillus anthracis* spores as an agent of bioterrorism and biological warfare.

EPIDEMIOLOGY

Anthrax occurs worldwide. This infection is still endemic or hyperendemic in both animals and humans in some parts of the Middle East, in West Africa, Central Asia, South America and Haiti. Soil is the reservoir for the infectious agent. Figure 128.1 shows the cycle of infection in nature. Infection in humans is correlated with the incidence of disease in domestic animals. In economically advanced countries, where animal anthrax has been controlled, it occurs only occasionally among humans. Human anthrax is most common in enzootic areas in developing countries, among people who work with livestock, eat undercooked meat from infected animals, or work in establishments where wool, goatskins and pelts are stored or processed.[1,2]

The main route of transmission is contact with or inhalation of *B. anthracis* spores. Human cases may occur in an agricultural or an industrial environment. Agricultural cases have occurred in individuals who came into contact with sick or dead animals in rural areas. In certain impoverished communities, livestock owners are forced to slaughter animals at the first sign of infection in order to salvage the meat, hair and hides because of economic problems. Farmers,

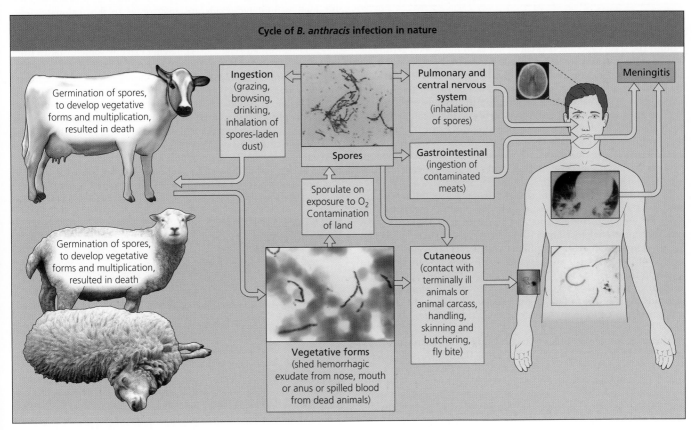

Fig. 128.1 Cycle of *Bacillus anthracis* infection in nature.

butchers, knackers, shepherds and veterinarians are therefore the most frequently infected.[1-4] Anthrax is also reported in women spinning wool with hand spindles and in carpet weavers.[5] Another route of infection is by ingestion of raw or undercooked meat from an infected carcass.[6-8] Travelers should be aware that, in certain societies, some traditional meals are made of raw meat and are consumed without any cooking or preservation methods.

There is also an infection risk after contact with a commercial product prepared from inadequately treated wool or leather. Products made from contaminated hair (e.g. shaving brushes, wool coats), skins (e.g. drums, drumheads made of animal skin) and bone meal (e.g. fertilizer) may continue to be sources of infection for many years.[1,2]

Insect vectors, such as horseflies, have been reported to transmit *B. anthracis* from an infected animal to a second animal. They could also theoretically infect humans by mechanical transfer but this has not been well documented.[1,2]

Industrial anthrax occurs as a result of the inhalation of spore-laden dust or other aerosols, or contact with spores. In the industrial environment, spores in dust clouds created from the handling of dry hides, skins, sheep wool, goat hair, bone meal and the like are inhaled or spread through contact with the skin of workers. Most cases in industrialized countries are associated with exposure to animal products, particularly goat hair imported from countries in which anthrax is endemic.[1,2,9]

The disease is generally accepted as noncontagious; records of person-to-person spread exist but are very rare. All cases were cutaneous anthrax; there are no reports of inhalation or ingestion anthrax. Occasionally, laboratory-acquired infections have occurred.[1,2,10]

In 2001 there was an outbreak of anthrax in the USA that apparently resulted from the deliberate distribution of spores in the postal system, resulting in a number of cases of both cutaneous and inhalational anthrax.[11]

PATHOGENESIS

Bacillus anthracis, the causative agent of anthrax, is a Gram-positive, aerobic or facultatively anaerobic, endospore-forming, rod-shaped bacterium. The spores lodging in a cut or abrasion in the skin germinate there and the emergent vegetative bacilli spread to the regional lymph nodes. Ingestion anthrax results if spores lodge similarly in lesions in the gastrointestinal tract or achieve access to Peyer's patches. Inhaled spores may, on occasion, lead to infection of nasal-associated lymphoid tissues; those reaching the lungs do not germinate in the alveoli but remain dormant until carried by macrophages to the tracheobronchial lymph nodes. The spores germinate inside the macrophages and the emergent vegetative forms are released from the macrophages, multiply in the lymphatic system and enter the bloodstream, causing toxemia and sepsis.[2,12]

Bacillus anthracis has two principal virulence factors: the toxin complex and the polypeptide capsule. Both are plasmid mediated. The genes for the toxin components and virulence gene regulators AtxA and PagR are located on a large (182 kb) plasmid designated pX01 and the genes for capsule synthesis and their regulators AcpA and AcpB are located on a smaller (95 kb) plasmid, pX02. Loss of either plasmid results in considerable reduction in virulence. Possibly also contributing to virulence are other proteins encoded on the chromosome or plasmids, such as cell surface S-layer extractable antigen 1 (EA1) and surface array protein (Sap), anthrolysin O, siderophores and metal cation transport proteins.[2,13]

The toxin complex consists of three synergistically acting proteins: protective antigen (PA, 83 kDa), lethal factor (LF, 90 kDa) and edema factor (EF, 89 kDa). LF in combination with PA (lethal toxin, LeTx) and EF in combination with PA (edema toxin, EdTx) are secreted during multiplication of the vegetative cells and are accepted as responsible for the characteristic signs and symptoms of anthrax. EdTx is a calmodulin-dependent adenylate cyclase that increases intracellular levels of cyclic AMP (cAMP) on entry into most types of cell, leading to impaired maintenance of water homeostasis and characteristic edema. EdTx also inhibits macrophage activity by altering their cytokine production, decreases the circulating lymphocyte population and diminishes neutrophil function. LF is a zinc-dependent metalloprotease that cleaves the amino termini from mitogen-activated protein kinase kinases (MAPKKs), thereby disrupting signaling pathways with range of resulting pathologic effects. LeTx kills or disrupts production and function of macrophages, dendritic cells, neutrophils, and some epithelial and endothelial cells, downregulates cytokine production (preventing induction of chemokines integral to responses to viral or bacterial infection), inhibits B-cell proliferation and reduces B-cell production of immunoglobulin. Inflammatory mediators released in response to LeTX may also contribute to the sudden death characteristic of systemic anthrax and its lethal effect on microvascular endothelial cells is presumed to be responsible for the also characteristic terminal hemorrhages.[2,12-14]

CLINICAL FEATURES

The disease occurs primarily in three forms: cutaneous, gastrointestinal and respiratory. Sepsis and meningitis can rarely develop after the lymphohematogenous spread of *B. anthracis* from a primary lesion (cutaneous, gastrointestinal or pulmonary).

Cutaneous anthrax

Cutaneous anthrax accounts for 95% of human cases. The spore is introduced into the skin via a cut, abrasion or insect bite. The incubation period ranges from 1 to 19 days, usually 2-7 days. The lesion begins as a pruritic papule. The papule enlarges and a ring of vesicles develops around the papule at day 2-4 of the disease. Vesicular fluid may be a hemorrhagic exudate (Fig. 128.2). This area is surrounded by a small ring of erythema and marked edema develops. Unless there is secondary infection, there is no pus and the lesion is not painful, although painful lymphadenitis may occur in the regional lymph nodes. Eventually, the vesicle or vesicular ring ruptures, discharging a clear fluid, and a central depressed black necrotic lesion known as an eschar is formed (Fig. 128.3). Edema extends some distance from the lesion. The eschar begins to resolve about 10 days after the appearance of the initial papule. Resolution is slow (2-6 weeks), regardless of treatment (Fig. 128.4).[2,12]

The lesion is usually 1-3 cm diameter and remains round and regular. Rarely, a lesion may be larger and irregularly shaped. Systemic symptoms, including low-grade fever, malaise and headache, may be present. The cutaneous reaction may be severe in some patients and is characterized by significant local and spreading edema associated with blebs, bullae, induration, chills and fever (see Fig. 128.3b). Clinical symptoms may be more severe if the lesion is located in the face, neck

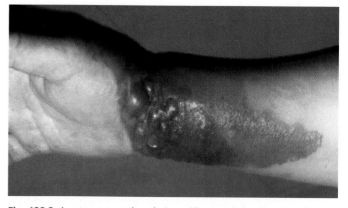

Fig. 128.2 A cutaneous anthrax lesion with extensive erythema and hemorrhagic bullae on the wrist.

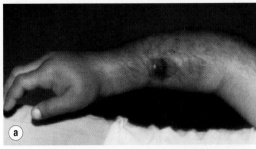

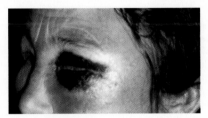

Fig. 128.3 Cutaneous anthrax. (a) A well-developed lesion on the right forearm (third day of disease). (b) The extension of the skin lesion in the same patient on the sixth day. Extensive edema, induration and bullous changes have occurred over the last 3 days despite antibiotic therapy. Antibiotic therapy does not prevent inflammatory reactions.

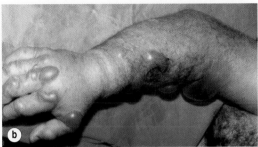

Fig. 128.4 A dried black anthrax eschar on the eyelids on the 15th day of therapy (third week of the disease). The lesion healed leaving a deep scar. Courtesy of Professor O Ural, Konya, Turkey.

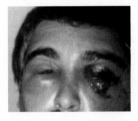

Fig. 128.5 An anthrax lesion of the eyelids surrounded by erythema and massive edema extending from the left eye to the right and down to and beyond the neck. Such extensive edema is characteristic of anthrax. This lesion healed with therapy and left a deep scar.

or chest. In these more severe forms, clinical findings are high fever, toxemia, regional painful adenomegaly and extensive edema; shock and death may ensue (Fig. 128.5).[2-4,12,15]

More than 90% of lesions occur in exposed areas such as the face, neck, arms or hand (Table 128.1). The site of infection often reflects the occupation of the patient. Workers who carry hides or carcasses on their shoulders are prone to infection on the back of the neck. Handlers of contaminated animal products tend to be infected on the arms, wrists and hands. The patients generally have a single cutaneous lesion but sometimes they have two or more. Atypical localization can also be seen.[2-4,12,15]

Gastrointestinal anthrax

Ingestion of *B. anthracis* in contaminated food or drink can cause gastrointestinal anthrax. The incubation period is commonly 3–7 days. There are two clinical forms of gastrointestinal anthrax: intestinal and oropharyngeal.[2,6-8,12]

Table 128.1 Distribution of lesions in 107 cases with cutaneous anthrax

Site of lesion	No. of cases	%
Hands and fingers	79	73.8
Wrists and arms	10	9.3
Eyelids and face	11	10.3
Neck	2	1.9
Feet and legs	5	4.7
Total	107	100
Data from Doganay.[15]		

The symptoms of intestinal anthrax are initially nonspecific and include nausea, vomiting, anorexia and fever. With progression of the illness, abdominal pain, hematemesis, bloody diarrhea and massive ascites occur, and signs suggestive of acute abdomen appear. Toxemia and shock then develop, followed by death. The lesions occur most commonly on the wall of the terminal ileum or cecum. The stomach, duodenum, upper ileum and large bowel are occasionally affected.[2,7,8,12]

Oropharyngeal anthrax is less common than the gastrointestinal form. The lesion is generally localized in the oral cavity, especially on the buccal mucosa or tongue, or the tonsils, and the posterior wall of the pharynx. In some cases, the lesion may be present in two or more places in the gastrointestinal system, oropharynx and intestine. The oral lesion is generally 2–3 cm in diameter and covered with a gray pseudomembrane surrounded by extensive edema. When infection is localized on the tonsils, the affected tonsil is also intensely edematous and covered with pseudomembrane. The main clinical features are sore throat, dysphagia, fever and painful regional lymphadenopathy in the neck. The illness progresses rapidly and edema develops around the lymph node and may extend to the upper anterior chest wall. Bacteremia may develop. The infection leads to toxemia and acute respiratory distress syndrome. Shock and coma ensue. In some cases, toxemia leads to sudden death. Despite intensive medical therapy, the mortality is about 50%.[2,6,7,12]

Inhalation anthrax

This natural form of anthrax was previously almost always caused by industrial exposure to spores; however, the most serious outbreaks of anthrax in 1979 in Sverdlovsk and in October 2001 in America are new and notable exceptions.[2,11,16]

Inhalation anthrax shows a biphasic clinic pattern with a mild initial phase followed by an acute and severe second phase. After an incubation period of 1–6 days (up to 43 days in the event at Sverdlovsk), the illness begins with mild fever, fatigue, malaise, myalgia, nonproductive cough and some chest or abdominal pain. The disease progresses to the second phase within 2–3 days. The second phase is characterized by high fever, toxemia, dyspnea and cyanosis. Hypothermia and shock develop, resulting in death. In up to half of patients, meningitis develops as a complication.[2,9,12]

Anthrax meningitis

The meningeal form of anthrax is very rare. The world's literature contains approximately 100 cases of anthrax meningitis, with a mortality rate of over 90%.[2,14] Meningitis may be a complication of the three forms of primary anthrax. The most common portal of entry is skin (52%) and then the lungs (22.9%). Anthrax meningitis also occurs in cases of gastrointestinal anthrax. The organisms can spread to the central nervous system by hematogenous or lymphatic routes. The primary focus of infection cannot be determined in about

10% of cases and it is called primary anthrax meningitis. Blood cultures are positive for *B. anthracis* in 70% of patients who have meningitis.[2,12,17,18]

The clinical presentation includes sudden onset of fever, fatigue, myalgia, headache, nausea, vomiting, agitation, seizures, delirium and meningeal symptoms. The initial signs are followed by rapid neurologic deterioration and death. The cerebrospinal fluid is often bloody and contains many Gram-positive bacilli.[2,12,17,18]

Anthrax sepsis

Sepsis may occur by spreading of *B. anthracis* via the lymphohematogenous route from a primary lesion. Sepsis is rarely seen in patients who have cutaneous anthrax; it is more commonly seen in patients who have inhalation and gastrointestinal anthrax. Clinical features include fever, respiratory distress and changing mental status. Severe toxemia and shock may lead to death in a short time.[2]

COMPLICATIONS

Some 10–20% of untreated cases of cutaneous anthrax might be expected to result in death. With treatment, the mortality rate is less than 1%. Toxemic shock due to massive edema, airway obstruction by compression on the trachea from edematous swelling around the neck, temporal artery inflammation, deep tissue necrosis and secondary infection, deep scar tissue and eyelid deformity are all recorded as complications in cases of cutaneous anthrax.[2–4,15]

Serious complications such as sepsis and meningitis can be seen in inhalation anthrax and gastrointestinal anthrax. These complications are less frequently seen in cutaneous anthrax. The mortality rate in industrial-related inhalation anthrax is over 80%, despite treatment. Gastrointestinal anthrax is also a potentially fatal disease. Mortality is greater than 50%. If an early diagnosis is made and appropriate treatment given, the disease can be cured.[2,6–8,17]

DIFFERENTIAL DIAGNOSIS

A history of exposure to contaminated animal materials, occupational exposure and living in an endemic area are all important clues for the suspicion of anthrax. The ulcerative eschar of cutaneous anthrax must be differentiated from other papular and ulcerative lesions that present with regional lymphadenopathy. If regional lymphadenopathy together with a purulent lesion is present, a cutaneous anthrax lesion may be superinfected with pyogenic bacteria such as staphylococci. The differential diagnosis should include ecthyma gangrenosum, rat-bite fever, ulceroglandular tularemia, plague, glanders, orf, rickettsialpox, erysipelas, staphylococcal skin and lymph node infection, syphilitic chancre and cutaneous tuberculosis. A severe cutaneous anthrax lesion involving the face, neck and anterior chest wall must be differentiated from orbital cellulitis, dacryocystitis and deep tissue infection of the neck. Necrotizing soft tissue infections – particularly group A streptococcal infections and gas gangrene – and severe cellulitis due to staphylococci should also be considered in the differential diagnosis of severe forms of cutaneous anthrax. Gas and abscess formation are not observed in patients who have cutaneous anthrax.[2–4,12]

Intestinal anthrax mimics food poisoning (in the early stages), acute abdomen of other causes and hemorrhagic gastroenteritis, particularly necrotizing enteritis due to *Clostridium perfringens*. In the differential diagnosis of oropharyngeal anthrax, streptococcal pharyngitis, Vincent's angina, Ludwig's angina, parapharyngeal abscess and deep tissue infection of the neck should be considered.[2,6,7]

The differential diagnosis of anthrax meningitis should include acute meningitis of other bacterial etiology and subarachnoid hemorrhage.[2,12,18] Sepsis due to other bacteria should be considered in the differential diagnosis of anthrax sepsis.[2,12]

The initial symptoms are nonspecific and clinical presentation of inhalation anthrax is similar to those of atypical pneumonia from other causes and cardiovascular collapse with noninfectious causes.[2,12]

INVESTIGATIONS

The investigation of a potential exposure to the infectious agent is very important for suspicion of anthrax. However, the source of infection cannot be determined in some cases. In cutaneous lesions, swabs are appropriate for collecting vesicular exudates for microscopy and bacterial culture. In a well-formed eschar, in which vesicular exudate is absent, the edge of the eschar can be lifted up with forceps and fluid obtained by a capillary tube. A smear is made from the material and is stained with polychrome methylene blue and examined microscopically for the presence of the pink-staining encapsulated bacilli (McFadyean reaction). The samples are also inoculated on blood agar.[2]

For the isolation of *B. anthracis* in patients who have suspected gastrointestinal anthrax, swabs from oropharyngeal lesions and samples of vomit, feces, blood and ascites should be obtained. Specimens likely to be contaminated with commensal flora should be cultured on polymyxin-lysozyme-EDTA-thallous acetate (PLET) agar as a selective medium for *B. anthracis*.[2]

Radiographic examination of the chest usually reveals widening of the mediastinum in inhalation anthrax. Parenchymal infiltration and pleural effusion can also be seen. Direct examination of a smear of pleural fluid or blood, stained with polychrome methylene blue or Gram stain, may show encapsulated bacilli. *Bacillus anthracis* can be isolated from the cultures of these specimens.[2,9,12]

Blood or cerebrospinal fluid smear stained with polychrome methylene blue should be examined for the encapsulated bacilli, and blood and/or cerebrospinal fluid cultures should be taken for isolation of *B. anthracis* in cases of sepsis or meningitis. Blood culture is also positive in many cases with systemic anthrax.[2,12,17]

Serologic tests are also useful for diagnosis of anthrax. New diagnostic techniques include immunohistochemical testing of clinical specimens by using *B. anthracis* capsule and cell wall antibody and, most recently, by *B. anthracis*-specific polymerase chain reaction. These new rapid methods may become useful in early diagnosis and in culture-negative patients.[2,12]

MANAGEMENT

In-vitro human clinical isolates of *B. anthracis* are sensitive to many antibiotics: penicillins, aminoglycosides, macrolides, quinolones, carbapenems, tetracyclines, vancomycin, clindamycin, rifampin (rifampicin), cefazolin and linezolid.[2,19] Penicillin G is still the drug of choice in the therapy of naturally occurring anthrax. In mild uncomplicated cutaneous anthrax, intramuscular procaine penicillin (800 000 to 1 million units q12–24h) or amoxicillin (500 mg orally q6–8h) is suggested for 3–5 days. *B. anthracis* cannot be isolated from cutaneous lesions 24–48 hours after antibiotic administration. Early treatment will limit the size of the lesion but will not alter the evolutionary stages (Table 128.2).[2,12]

In patients showing signs of systemic involvement, such as inhalation anthrax or gastrointestinal anthrax, meningoencephalitis, sepsis and cutaneous anthrax with extensive edema, antibiotics should be given intravenously. Penicillin G is the first choice, given at a dose of 4 million units q4–6h (total daily dose should be 20–24 million units) until the patient's symptoms resolve and fever returns to normal. At this point, the intravenous antibiotic can be switched to

Table 128.2 Suggested antibiotic therapy for anthrax in adults

Category	Antibiotic	Duration of therapy
Naturally occurring anthrax	First choice* • Penicillin G procain 0.6–1.2 mU im q12–24h • Penicillin G, sodium or potassium 4 mU iv q4–6h • Amoxicillin 500 mg po q6–8h Alternative* • Doxycycline 100 mg po q12h • Ciprofloxacin 500–750 mg po q12h, 200–400 mg iv q12h	Uncomplicated cutaneous anthrax: 3–5 days Systemic anthrax[†]: 10–14 days
Biological weapon or bioterrorism-related anthrax	Ciprofloxacin 500–750 mg po q12h, 200–400 mg iv q12h Doxycycline 100 mg iv/po q12h	60 days

*Antibiotic therapy should be given orally in mild cutaneous anthrax. In cases of severe cutaneous anthrax or systemic anthrax, initial antibiotic therapy should be given intravenously; when fever has subsided to normal, antibiotic therapy may be switch to oral.
[†]In systemic anthrax, initial antibiotic choice should be combined with one or two of the following antibiotics: penicillin, ampicillin, ciprofloxacin, imipenem, meropenem, vancomycin, rifampin (rifampicin), clindamycin, streptomycin or other aminoglycoside.
Adapted from[2,12,20].

intramuscular penicillin G or to an oral antibiotic. In the treatment of systemic anthrax, penicillin should be combined with one or two other antibiotics to which *B. anthracis* is susceptible. Penicillin G may be combined with clindamycin, clarithromycin or ciprofloxacin in treating inhalation anthrax or with an aminoglycoside (streptomycin is suggested) in gastrointestinal anthrax.[2,12]

Anthrax meningoencephalitis is a life-threatening infection. Currently, a combination of penicillin G and rifampin is the first choice of treatment. Other possible regimens would be penicillin G in combination with vancomycin, or vancomycin and rifampin.[2,12,18]

In the event of allergy to penicillin, doxycycline or ciprofloxacin is accepted as best alternative. Tetracyclines and erythromycin are also effective alternatives in mild cutaneous anthrax in developing countries. In uncomplicated cutaneous anthrax, doxycycline or ciprofloxacin is given orally. In systemic anthrax, doxycycline or ciprofloxacin should be given intravenously and may be combined with another suitable antibiotic, as with penicillin.[2,12,18–20]

Duration of treatment in uncomplicated cutaneous anthrax is suggested as 3–5 days (may be 3–7 days). Therapy in cases of systemic anthrax should be continued for 10–14 days.[2]

Supportive treatment for shock, intubation, tracheotomy or ventilatory support in respiratory problems and steroid administration or other anti-brain edema therapies for anthrax meningoencephalitis are life saving in some cases. It is noted that surgical resection of intestinal lesions with medical treatment has shown a beneficial effect.[2,8,12]

PREVENTION

The prevention of anthrax in human is based on:
• control of the infection in animals;
• prevention of contact with infected animals and contaminated animal products;
• environmental and personal hygiene;
• medical care of cutaneous anthrax; and
• disinfection of fur and wool.

Occupational groups at risk may be vaccinated. An acellular vaccine is available in the USA and the UK, and is used mostly in occupational and military settings. This vaccine is not recommended for normal travelers unless there is likely to be occupational exposure. A live spore vaccine has been produced and used in China and Russia. Accelerated development is underway to produce safer and more effective vaccines.[1,2]

REFERENCES

References for this chapter can be found online at http://www.expertconsult.com

What are the treatment options for a pregnant patient with malaria?

DEFINITION OF THE PROBLEM

Malaria is the most important parasitic infection in humans and in pregnancy is detrimental to the mother and fetus. In pregnancy the adverse effects of malaria infection result from:

- systemic infection, comparable to the effects of any severe febrile illness in pregnancy, i.e. maternal/fetal mortality, abortion, stillbirth and premature delivery; and
- parasitization, i.e. birth weight reduction, maternal/fetal anemia, interaction with HIV and susceptibility of the infant to malaria.

The hallmark of malaria in pregnancy is parasites sequestered in the placenta. Sequestered parasites evade host defense mechanisms including splenic processing and filtration. Sequestration is not known to occur in the benign malarias due to *Plasmodium vivax*, *Plasmodium ovale* and *Plasmodium malariae*. *Plasmodium falciparum* causes greater morbidity (principally low birth weight and anemia) and mortality than non-*falciparum* infections. The clinical manifestations in pregnancy depend on premunition, i.e. the degree of natural immunity to malaria (Table PP59.1).

Premunition appears slowly following continuous and numerous re-infections by malaria parasites to prevent it waning. Premunition acquired in childhood is impaired during the first pregnancy but recovers during subsequent gestations. *Plasmodium falciparum* is unique in its ability to sequester in large numbers in the placenta and placental parasites have been shown to bind preferentially to chondroitin sulfate A. During the course of pregnancy or over successive pregnancies women develop variant specific immunity to chondroitin sulfate A binding infected red blood cells (IRBC). Thus, in areas of high transmission (conferring high premunition), severe anemia is common and is associated with mortality, predominantly affecting primigravidae; on the other hand, in areas of low transmission or in epidemics, pregnant women of any gravida are at risk of severe and cerebral malaria and death.

Ideally malaria infection during pregnancy should be prevented. Failing this (an increasing problem due to drug resistance) prompt diagnosis and effective treatment will prevent fatal outcomes and help reduce morbidity in both mother and baby. Clinicians who assess and manage pregnant women with malaria in nonendemic countries will be unfamiliar with the condition. Delay and misdiagnosis, with subsequent failure to provide prompt effective treatment, are the main recurring themes in death from malaria.

CLINICAL CASES

Case 1 – severe malaria

A 37-year-old West African woman presented for the first time in pregnancy to a London maternity department at 29 weeks gestation in her first pregnancy, with a 5-day history of fever. She had recently returned to her home in London (resident 2 years) after a 1-month visit to West Africa to take care of her mother (no prophylaxis). On admission her temperature was 103.1°F (39.5°C), pulse rate 130 beats/min (bpm) and blood pressure 108/56 mmHg. She was conscious and responsive. Her urine contained protein on ward testing and was sent for culture (subsequently negative). Her uterus was soft and fetal size was appropriate for 29 weeks. There was a fetal tachycardia (180 bpm) with a suspicious cardiac rhythm: a flat trace with reduced short-term variability (<5 bpm). Her initial investigation results were as follows: hemoglobin (Hb) 8.2 g/dl, white blood cell count 18.3 × 10⁹/l and platelets 50 × 10⁹/l. Apart from her thrombocytopenia, her coagulation screen was normal. Two hours after admission her malaria film was reported to be positive with 10% *Plasmodium falciparum* IRBC including schizonts and malaria pigment. Her blood sugar was 2.6 mmol/l.

The patient was transferred to the intensive care unit and commenced on an infusion of 10% dextrose after a bolus of 50 ml of 50% dextrose. She received a loading dose of intravenous quinine 20 mg/kg over 4 hours and clindamycin 5 mg/kg. In view of the hyperparasitemia, she was transferred to a tertiary referral unit for consideration of exchange transfusion. During the transfer she became unconscious and her blood sugar was 1.4 mmol/l. She regained consciousness with 0.5 g/kg glucose. She had repeated episodes of hypoglycemia over the next few days. She required two units of blood for severe symptomatic anemia. After an initial rise in parasitemia (6-hourly blood smear) in the first 24 hours her parasitemia was down to 1% by the third day of treatment. On the fourth day she developed acute respiratory distress syndrome and despite ventilation died the next day. Fetal heart beat was not detectable before she died.

Case 2 – uncomplicated malaria

A 26-year-old Burmese woman in her third pregnancy presented at 24 weeks gestation for antenatal booking. She had arrived in the UK 1 week previously, as part of the resettlement of Karen refugees from the Thai–Burmese border. She reported having had fever in the last 24 hours with headache, muscle and joint pain for 2 days. Much to the chagrin of the physician on duty she requested a malaria smear. This was agreed to and was positive for *P. falciparum*, 1.2% IRBC, and *P. vivax*, 0.2% IRBC. Routine booking investigations were carried out. All results were unremarkable apart from the hemoglobin (9.5 g/dl with iron-deficient indices). The patient was diagnosed as having uncomplicated malaria and was treated with coartemether 4 tablets with 200 ml of milk. She vomited all the tablets 15 minutes after treatment initiation and said it was because of the milk. The physician ordered metoclopramide and repeated the dose with soya milk and without further vomiting. The patient was admitted to the ward, spiked a fever that evening of 104°F (40.0°C), treated with paracetamol and oral fluids. There were no further febrile episodes, the remaining doses of coartemether were well tolerated and

Table PP59.1 Main consequences of malaria in pregnancy in different transmission situations

	Nonimmune*	Low premunition	High premunition
Susceptibility	++++	+++	++
Risk of illness	++++	+++	+
Severe anemia	?	+++	+++
Severe/cerebral malaria	++++	+++	-
Maternal/fetal mortality	++++	+++	+
Birth weight reduction	?	++	++
Fetal wastage	++++	++++	+
Gravida at risk	All	All	Primigravidae
Placental parasitemia	?	+	+++

*Includes women never exposed to malaria and women who come from endemic areas but who have lived for a prolonged period outside a malaria-endemic area.
+, Level of severity.
?, No data available. (There are actually no collective data on the effects of malaria in nonimmune women, but the severity of the infections caused by *Plasmodium falciparum* in this group would probably mask the effect on maternal anemia and birth weight.)

the patient was blood smear negative on the second day of treatment. Ultrasound assessment revealed an appropriately grown fetus with normal amniotic fluid volume. There was bilateral notching of the uterine artery Doppler waveforms with raised resistance indices, suggesting a degree of placental dysfunction. The umbilical artery and fetal arterial Doppler studies were normal. By the next antenatal visit the uterine artery Doppler waveforms had normalized.

Six weeks later the woman complained again of headache, muscle and joint pain, no fever and again requested a malaria smear. *P. vivax* trophozoites 0.5% IRBC, schizonts and gametocytes were all reported. The physician on duty diagnosed *P. vivax* and treated the woman with chloroquine 10, 10 and 5 mg/kg once daily on days 0, 1 and 2, respectively. At 32 weeks gestation the fundal height was 27 cm. By 37 weeks gestation fundal height measurement and serial scans for growth demonstrated intrauterine growth retardation (IUGR), despite normal Dopplers. The woman had spontaneous onset of labor at 37.2 weeks gestation and a normal vaginal delivery of a term 2.3 kg normal infant. At 18 hours postpartum the midwife on the labor ward recorded the temperature of the patient as 100.4°F (38°C). As everyone was aware of the woman's history of malaria a blood smear was ordered for the mother and baby (normal vital signs) and both were positive for *P. falciparum*. Attempts to salvage the placenta to do a malaria smear were made too late and were not done. The mother and the baby were successfully treated with 3 days of atovaquone–proguanil (Malarone).

DIAGNOSIS

Failure to consider malaria as a possible diagnosis can result in death. The diagnosis of malaria in pregnancy, as in nonpregnant patients, relies on microscopic (the current gold standard) examination of thick and thin blood films for parasites, or the use of rapid diagnostic tests that detect specific parasite antigen (see Chapter 111). Microscopic diagnosis allows species identification and estimation of parasitemia, so that appropriate antimalarials can be prescribed. Always consider malaria in the febrile patient and never forget to ask for a history of travel. Thrombocytopenia, metabolic acidosis and elevated lactate levels are also highly suggestive of severe malaria. The investigation of a patient with suspected falciparum malaria in pregnancy should be treated with great urgency. Blood and urine should be cultured to exclude other infections. In the comatose patient, lumbar puncture

should be considered to exclude meningitis and encephalitis, providing there is no evidence of raised intracranial pressure.

In a woman from an endemic country with severe anemia and suspected asymptomatic disease, presumptive treatment should be given even if a blood smear is negative.

MANAGEMENT

Prompt treatment is vital in pregnancy as the disease is more severe and mortality is 2–10 times higher than in nonpregnant patients. The disease in pregnancy is associated with higher parasitemia and is dangerous for both mother and fetus. The aim of treatment of uncomplicated malaria is to cure the patient and in severe malaria to save the mother's life. Severity of malaria is determined by the symptoms and microscopic findings (Table PP59.2).

Management of malaria in pregnancy depends on the infecting species, severity of the disease, the stage of pregnancy (first trimester or other), prophylaxis or intermittent preventive therapy, and drug availability. The fast expansion of resistant isolates has compromised many of the standard antimalarials, including chloroquine, sulfadoxine–pyrimethamine and quinine monotherapy.[2] Patients may deteriorate under treatment, at which point management should be upgraded to account for severity. Drugs for treatment are summarized in Table PP59.3. Specific points related to treatment of malaria in pregnant women have been summarized in Table PP59.4.

CONCLUSION

There is a paucity of data on antimalarials used for treatment and prevention in pregnancy. Most of what we know about chloroquine in pregnancy comes from research on autoimmune disease in pregnancy and for quinine from its historical use. Sulfadoxine–pyrimethamine has been widely advocated as a preventive antimalarial in pregnancy without clear evidence of the efficacy or pharmacokinetic properties in pregnant women. There have only been 10 randomized controlled trials (RCTs) specifically involving treatment for pregnant women with acute uncomplicated falciparum malaria involving a total of 1914 patients. Much larger numbers of women must be treated and followed prospectively until the data on efficacy, outcome and drug safety

Table PP59.2 Classification of severity of malaria in pregnancy

Grade of malaria	Microscopic findings	Symptoms	Case fatality rate
Uncomplicated	Positive blood smear with parasite count <4% IRBC or parasitemia of 150 000/µl	First symptoms are usually nonspecific and similar to a minor systemic viral illness Headache, lassitude, fatigue, abdominal discomfort, dizziness and muscle and joint aches, followed by fever, chills, sweating, anorexia, vomiting and worsening malaise are the typical features of uncomplicated malaria No signs of severity* or organ dysfunction	Low: ~0.1% for *P. falciparum* infections Non-*falciparum* species are rarely fatal
Uncomplicated hyperparasitemia	*P. falciparum* asexual parasitemia with ≥4% IRBC 2% should be used in the nonimmunes from nonendemic countries	As for uncomplicated	As for uncomplicated if treated adequately
Severe (rare reports with *P. vivax* monoinfection)	*P. falciparum* asexual parasitemia (or positive rapid diagnostic test)	No other obvious cause of symptoms and with signs of severity* and/or organ dysfunction	High: 15–20% in nonpregnant patients compared with 50% in pregnancy Untreated severe malaria is always fatal

IRBC, infected red blood cells.
*Signs of severity: *Clinical manifestations*: prostration, impaired consciousness, respiratory distress (acidotic breathing), multiple convulsions, circulatory collapse, pulmonary edema (radiologic), abnormal bleeding, jaundice, hemoglobinuria; *Laboratory tests*: severe anemia, hypoglycemia, acidosis, renal impairment, hyperlactatemia, hyperparasitemia.
Adapted from WHO.[1]

Table PP59.3 Drugs for treatment of malaria in pregnancy

Species and trimester	Severity	Treatment
P. vivax, *P. ovale* and *P. malariae*, regardless of trimester	Not usually severe If severe, see *P. falciparum* (severe)	Chloroquine phosphate (1 tablet contains 250 mg salt equivalent to 155.3 mg base) Dose: 10 mg/kg base q24h on days 1 and 2, followed by 5 mg/kg base on day 3 For chloroquine-resistant *P. vivax*, amodiaquine, quinine or artemisinin derivatives can be used
First trimester: *P. falciparum* or mixed species, i.e. *P. falciparum* and non-*falciparum* (usually *P. vivax*) co-infection	Uncomplicated	1st episode: quinine 10 mg/kg q8h for 7 days, preferably with clindamycin* 5 mg/kg q8h for 7 days Subsequent episodes: repeat treatment with quinine and clindamycin* as above ACT that is locally effective or artesunate 2 mg/kg q24h for 7 days with clindamycin* as above
Second and third trimesters	Uncomplicated	1st episode: ACT that is locally effective such as artemether–lumefantrine§ or artesunate plus clindamycin* as above Malarone (atovaquone–proguanil)† alone can be used for treatment in pregnancy but it is highly recommended to use it with artesunate to maximize fever and parasite clearance times and ensure cure Subsequent episodes: artesunate plus clindamycin* as above Artesunate–atovaquone–proguanil and dihydroartemisinin–piperaquine§ can be used for *P. falciparum* recurrence in the same pregnancy
Regardless of trimester	Uncomplicated hyperparasitemia	Artesunate: 4 mg/kg po loading dose then 2 mg/kg q24h for 7 days with clindamycin* as above, *or* Quinine iv (see below)
Regardless of trimester	Severe	Artesunate‡: 2.4 mg/kg iv at 0, 12 and 24h, then q24h until the patient can tolerate oral artesunate 2 mg/kg q24h for a total of 7 days, and clindamycin* 5 mg/kg q8h for 7 days, *or* Quinine: 20 mg/kg iv loading dose given over 4h, then 10 mg/kg 8h after the loading dose was started, followed by 10 mg/kg q8h for 7 days Once the patient has recovered sufficiently to tolerate oral medication both quinine 10 mg/kg and clindamycin 5 mg/kg q8h should be continued for/until 7 days

ACT, artemisin-based combination therapy.
*When clindamycin is not available, give artesunate monotherapy.
†Malarone use in pregnancy.[2]
‡Intravenous artesunate is the best treatment[3] but unfortunately is not available routinely in the UK. Some hospitals may have their own supply.
§Prescribe artemether–lumefantrine and dihydroartemisinin–piperaquine with fat.[4]
Dosages for pregnant women are likely to be revised when all the pharmacokinetic antimalarial pregnancy data become available.[4]
Adapted from WHO.[1]

Table PP59.4 Problems pertinent to treatment of malaria in pregnant women

Adjunctive treatment	Relationship to pregnancy	Details of treatment
Antiemetics	There are no trials specifically in pregnancy but pregnant women have a higher tendency to vomit than nonpregnant women	If vomiting occurs within 30 mins, the full dose should be repeated. If vomiting occurs from >30 to 60 mins, repeat half the dose. An antiemetic (metoclopramide) can be given im or iv; wait 20 mins before repeating the dose Antiemetics are widely used for treatment in malaria although there have been no studies of their efficacy. There is no evidence to indicate harm. If a patient vomits twice they will need parenteral treatment. Oral medication can be recommended when oral fluids are well tolerated. Although these patients may show no signs of severity, the treatment regimen should be switched to that used for severe cases
Antipyretics	Fever is a cardinal feature of malaria. In pregnant women it has been associated with premature labor	Paracetamol 1 g q4–6h (maximum 4 g q24h) is safe and effective
Intravenous infusions	Due to greater circulating volume in pregnancy and increased losses, hydration is essential Quinine is still widely used in pregnancy but can be a particularly offensive drug to take due to cinchonism (tinnitus, hearing loss, nausea, uneasiness, restlessness and blurring of vision)	Febrile pregnant women with nausea and vomiting may be dehydrated and oral fluids need to be encouraged and adequate urine output confirmed. Intravenous fluids may be required, particularly on quinine
Glucose	Pregnancy can predispose to hypoglycemia and the nausea associated with malaria prevents some women from taking an adequate oral intake, thus promoting hypoglycemia Hypoglycemia in pregnancy may be profound and recurrent, particularly on quinine	Hypoglycemia may manifest as fetal brady- or tachycardia. In the most severely ill patients it is associated with lactic acidosis and high mortality In patients who have been given quinine, abnormal behavior, sweating and sudden loss of consciousness are the usual manifestations
Tocolytic therapy	Pre-term labor appears to be associated with the fever from malaria	Usual pre-term labor protocols apply Monitor uterine contractions
Fetal distress	Exclude maternal hypoglycemia, particularly if the patient is being treated with quinine and hyperthermia is the cause	Normal labor protocols should be implemented but fetal heart rate must be monitored. This may reveal fetal tachycardia, bradycardia or late decelerations in relation to uterine contractions, indicating fetal distress
Antibiotics	Secondary bacterial infection, principally Gram-negative septicemia, has been reported in pregnancy	The patient is collapsed with a systolic blood pressure <80 mmHg in the supine position Blood cultures should be taken if the patient shows signs of shock or fever returns after apparent fever clearance Hypovolaemia should be corrected and broad-spectrum antibiotics started immediately (e.g. ceftriaxone). Once the results of blood culture and sensitivity testing are available, give the appropriate antibiotic
Assisted ventilation	Pulmonary edema is a grave complication of severe malaria, with a high mortality in pregnancy (over 50%)	May be present on admission or develop suddenly and unexpectedly, or develop immediately after childbirth The first indication of impending pulmonary edema is an increase in the respiratory rate which precedes the development of other chest signs Hypoxia may cause convulsions and deterioration in the level of consciousness and the patient may die within a few hours Ensure the pulmonary edema has not resulted from iatrogenic fluid overload
Blood transfusion	Severe anemia is associated with perinatal mortality, maternal morbidity and an increased risk of postpartum hemorrhage	Women who go into labor when severely anemic or fluid overloaded may develop acute pulmonary edema after separation of the placenta Transfuse pregnant women slowly, preferably with packed red blood cells, and furosemide 20 mg iv; alternatively exchange transfusion may be given

in pregnancy (including developmental assessment of the infant) are robust, and clear guidelines can be issued.

For first trimester antimalarials, there is not a single RCT published. Given the impact of malaria in pregnancy and the huge number of women affected, this is a scandal. The collective data on epidemiology, prevention and treatment of malaria in pregnancy clearly demonstrate how dangerous malaria in pregnancy is to both the mother and the baby. Malaria in pregnancy is a medical emergency. It can be prevented and treated with reasonable confidence using Tables PP59.3 and PP59.4.

REFERENCES

References for this chapter can be found online at http://www.expertconsult.com

Management of a patient from Gabon with fever, malaise, sore throat and a negative malaria smear

Systemic illness accompanied by high fever should always prompt a search for malaria in any patient from a malaria-endemic region such as Gabon in equatorial West Africa. Once malaria has been confidently excluded, a more detailed differential diagnosis should be considered. Routine respiratory viruses, infectious mononucleosis or streptococcal pharyngitis would be the most common illnesses to account for an acute febrile illness with sore throat and malaise. Other infections such as typhoid, meningococcal meningitis, leptospirosis, dengue or plague are possible in this setting. The presence of severe prostration, myalgia, unrelenting headache followed by pharyngitis and any evidence of hemorrhagic complications should bring to mind the possibility of a hemorrhagic viral infection in this patient. Sporadic or epidemic occurrences of viral hemorrhagic fever (VHF) from arenaviruses, flaviviruses, bunyaviruses, filoviruses and hantaviruses are increasingly recognized by clinicians in specific geographic regions worldwide. Global markets for international trade in combination with improved access to remote areas by expanded transportation systems now make it feasible that these highly contagious viral illnesses could disseminate widely. Even in nonendemic regions physicians need to be cognizant of the risk of hemorrhagic viral fevers in international travelers or immigrants from tropical regions. Animal handlers in primate research laboratories throughout the world are also at risk. It is essential that health-care facilities develop a strategy to manage VHF even if the chances of seeing such patients seem remote.

It is important that physicians be aware of the potential risk of viral hemorrhagic fevers for several reasons:

- to ensure appropriate diagnosis and management of index cases;
- to provide advice, counseling and possible prophylaxis to close contacts;
- to minimize the risk of nosocomial transmission among health-care workers (HCWs) caring for such patients; and
- to alert public health authorities as soon as possible in the event of an outbreak of VHF.

Strict adherence to basic infection control techniques and some advance planning will minimize the risk to HCWs and allow rapid, compassionate and safe care of affected patients.

MICROBIOLOGY AND PATHOGENESIS

Hemorrhagic viruses in which person-to-person transmission has occurred in health-care settings include Lassa fever, Ebola virus and Marburg virus, new world arenaviruses and the tick-transmitted virus of Crimean–Congo hemorrhagic fever. These hemorrhagic fever viruses are particularly important to recognize because nosocomial transmission to HCWs is a real possibility. The animal reservoir and mode of transmission to humans is reasonably well understood for Lassa fever and other arenaviruses (contact with the excreta from rodents such as the *Mastomys* rat), Crimean–Congo hemorrhagic fever (tick transmitted from wild and domestic mammalian reservoirs) and Marburg virus (contact with African green monkeys). Recently the animal reservoir for Ebola virus has been determined to be bat species in endemic regions in Africa and possibly chimpanzees (although they may be as much a victim of Ebola virus as humans, rather than a reservoir). In a patient from Gabon, Ebola would be the most likely VHF in this region of the world although yellow fever, Marburg virus, Lassa fever or even Rift Valley fever could be possible.

These viral syndromes share many overlapping clinical features in humans. After an incubation period of between 3 and 21 days, patients develop the abrupt onset of fever, headache, myalgia, sore throat, respiratory symptoms, abdominal pain, nausea, vomiting, diarrhea and conjunctivitis with associated pharyngitis and cervical lymphadenitis. A macular skin eruption may occur in infections with Ebola and Marburg viruses. Various degrees of mucosal and cutaneous hemorrhage occur associated with thrombocytopenia and disseminated intravascular coagulation. The geographic location or travel history of the patient is most useful in the initial clinical distinction between these different types of VHF before virologic confirmation.

These viruses share rapid growth potential and the ability to invade a variety of cell types, resulting in high-grade viremia. The patient's blood and body fluids become contagious to others who come into direct contact with them. Transmission may also occur through handling of bodies during burial rituals, as demonstrated in recent Ebola outbreaks in Central Africa. Although many other nontransmissible febrile illnesses present in a similar fashion, strict infection control measures need to be instituted to guard against potential transmission of hemorrhagic fever viruses until the diagnosis is established. Health-care workers caring for patients with VHF are at risk owing to high viral concentrations present in body fluids and secretions.

DIAGNOSIS AND MANAGEMENT

Recent improvements in the serologic diagnosis of VHF now make it possible to make a specific diagnosis in the early phases of acute illness in the majority of patients. An antigen-capture enzyme-linked immunosorbent assay has been developed for Ebola virus and may allow rapid diagnosis in acutely ill patients. Specific IgM and IgG capture enzyme-linked immunosorbent assay antibody studies are available for serologic diagnosis in convalescent samples. Virus isolation from the blood and body secretions of acutely ill patients is the definitive diagnostic method. This is an extreme biohazard and should only be attempted in laboratories with biosafety level IV facilities. Reverse transcription and polymerase chain reaction for specific viral RNA is also a useful diagnostic method in patients who have VHF. Many of these methodologies are unavailable in regions of the world where these diseases are endemic. For this reason, the recent development of an immunochemical staining method for skin biopsy samples is particularly valuable. This method allows for fixation of tissues at the site of diagnosis and eliminates the biohazard of transportation of infected human tissues.

Routine diagnostic methods to evaluate other common febrile illnesses should not be delayed because of suspected VHF. In particular, care must be taken to exclude falciparum malaria which may be fatal if unrecognized and left untreated. In practice, most cases of suspected VHF turn out to have malaria. Universal precautions when handling blood and body secretions should suffice to protect HCWs from hemorrhagic viruses.

INFECTION CONTROL METHODS

These viruses are transmitted through direct contact with the patient or the patient's secretions. There is a remote risk of air-borne transmission of some strains of Ebola virus based on studies with nonhuman primates, but this has not been observed as a significant hazard in actual human outbreaks of Ebola virus infections. The primary infection control strategy is strict contact isolation, universal blood and body substance precautions, use of disposable sterile medical devices and needles, and enhanced preventive measures in the handling of blood and body fluids. Body substances are contagious during the acute febrile illness, but there is no evidence of transmission during the incubation phase of the illness. The guidelines listed in Table PP60.1 should be instituted in patients who have suspected VHF.

TREATMENT OPTIONS AND POSTEXPOSURE PROPHYLAXIS

The arenaviruses, including Lassa fever, are susceptible to ribavirin and this antiviral agent has proven to be efficacious in patients and in HCWs occupationally exposed to blood or body fluids (e.g. by percutaneous needlestick accident). Regrettably, ribavirin has been studied extensively in the laboratory and in previous outbreaks of Ebola virus and has proven ineffective in patients. New antiviral agents are desperately needed to treat Ebola and are a current area of intense research interest (Table PP60.2).

Passive immunotherapy from plasma or antibody preparations from surviving patients with high-titer antibody or experimental animals has variable and generally disappointing activity as a salvage therapy in severely ill patients with Ebola infection, but might be a consideration in a HCW following accidental exposure to the virus. Inhibitors of the tissue factor:factor VII coagulation pathway appear to be of some therapeutic benefit in experimental trials in primate studies, and some immune-based strategies against major viral glycoprotein antigens found on the surface of Ebola viruses appear promising as a preventive and even as a possible treatment option against Ebola virus.

REPORTING

All patients who have suspected viral hemorrhagic fever should be reported to public health authorities as soon as possible. This allows for a co-ordinated response to an epidemic situation and ensures that diagnostic and therapeutic efforts will be handled appropriately. Expert international assistance is necessary should a viral hemorrhagic fever occur in an international traveler.

Table PP60.1 Infection control methods for suspected viral hemorrhagic fever

Isolation method	Comments
Isolation room	Use a negative pressure room if available. Use strict contact isolation, universal blood and body substance precautions and enhanced prevention measures in the handling of blood and body fluids
Personnel and visitors	Restrict traffic flow into the patient's room. A daily record should be kept of all those who enter and leave the patient's room. Only essential personnel should be exposed to the patient and the patient's body fluids
Personal protection	Fluid-impervious gowns, gloves, face shields or surgical masks with eye protection (goggles); if the patient has cough, vomiting or extensive hemorrhage, respirators with filters (high-efficiency particulate air respirators) and shoe coverings should be worn.
Clinical samples	Clinical samples should be placed in plastic sealed bags and transported in a leak-proof container without contaminating the external surfaces. Samples should be handled in a biologic safety cabinet (biosafety level III). Serum should be pretreated with a polyethylene glycol phenolic for 1 h before handling. Automated analyzers should be disinfected with 1:100 dilution of bleach after use. Fixation of blood smears and tissue samples will inactivate the virus and can be handled in a routine manner
Decontamination of the environment and of linen	Disinfect contaminated environmental surfaces using a registered hospital disinfectant or 1:100 dilution of bleach. Soiled linens can either be decontaminated by autoclaving or incineration. Hot cycle laundering with bleach may be acceptable
Human excrement and blood and body fluids	Human excreta, blood and body fluids should be decontaminated by 1:100 dilution of bleach for 5 min before disposal
Surgical procedures and autopsy	If a surgical procedure is essential, extreme caution should be exercised to avoid blood contamination. Double gloves, full-face shields with high-efficiency particulate air filtration, water-impervious gowns and shoe covers should be worn. Avoid generation of an aerosol. Deceased persons should not be embalmed. The body should be placed in leak-proof, sealed material and cremated or buried in a sealed casket

Table PP60.2 Treatment options and postexposure prophylaxis for Ebola virus

Agent	Level of evidence	Comment
Ribavirin	No activity in animal models or uncontrolled clinical trials	Not effective against Ebola virus
S-adenosyl-L-homocysteine inhibitor	Experimental studies only	Some activity in mouse models
Interferon-α 2b	Experimental studies only	Delays illness and viremia but no survival benefit in experimental animals
Immune plasma or hyperimmune antibody preparations targeting viral glycoproteins	Variable experimental data, case reports	Variable, generally disappointing results; might decrease viremia
Small inhibitory RNAs against Ebola virus polymerase	Experimental studies only	Early promising results in guinea pig studies
Tissue factor inhibitors	Primate laboratory animals, no clinical studies	33% survival rates in primate models
Attenuated recombinant vesicular stomatitis virus (VSV) vectors expressing Ebola virus glycoproteins	Primate laboratory animals, no clinical studies	Protection when administered up to 24 h after Ebola virus challenge

FURTHER READING

Further reading for this chapter can be found online at http://www.expertconsult.com

Follow-up of the returned traveler who has swum in Lake Malawi

INTRODUCTION

Lake Malawi is a huge freshwater resource 630 km long and 50 km wide in Central Africa, providing essential food and income for a large proportion of Malawians and people of the other nations that border its shores. Over the past two decades it has become a major attraction for both 'local' tourists and for backpackers and overlanders from outside Africa, with the associated development of hotels and facilities for water sports such as scuba diving and windsurfing. These are especially found in the south around Cape Maclear and Monkey Bay, where the shores are relatively shallow and the snail vectors for *Schistosoma haematobium* have become established. Further north and centrally, the ecology of the lake differs, with deep water close to the land. Bilharzia was recognized by early European visitors to Malawi and was noted in 50% of lakeshore inhabitants in the early 1900s. It has become more widely established since then, particularly with the development of irrigation schemes. The predominant species is *S. haematobium*, but small pockets of *S. mansoni* also exist.

Schistosomiasis has become a common diagnosis in expatriates and short-term tourists in Malawi and similar risks are also recognized for travelers to Zimbabwe, the Dogon area of Mali and other freshwater lakes in Africa. A large case-control study showed that 33% of foreigners in Malawi had serologic evidence of exposure to infection, the highest risk being associated with repeated exposure to the lake, especially around Cape Maclear.[1] Our own experience of screening groups of returned travelers is that 75% of those who spend a week scuba diving at Cape Maclear will have clinical or asymptomatic laboratory evidence of infection. People are at risk from showers and swimming pools that are fed directly with unchlorinated lake water as well as from paddling and swimming. Brief exposure is sufficient; we recently screened students from the same school who had spent 48 hours only at two locations around the lake. Of those camping near Cape Maclear, 90% (19/21) had been infected, compared with none of 17 students camping on Likoma Island, another popular tourist spot.

GENERAL APPROACH TO THE TRAVELER WHO HAS SWUM IN LAKE MALAWI

The general approach to the traveler who has swum in Lake Malawi is the same as that for any other traveler, including the need to exclude malaria in febrile patients (Chapter 111). A detailed travel and exposure history must be taken, including details of travel dates; business and leisure activities undertaken; consumption of unsafe food, water and drinks; history of insect bites or animal exposures; specific infection exposures; use of health care facilities while overseas; illness in fellow travelers and sexual activities. The precise timing, frequency, type and locations of any freshwater contact should be recorded. Previous travel and possible schistosomal risk activity should be checked, along with pre-existing illnesses including atopy and urologic or gastrointestinal problems. Enquiries should routinely review adherence to antimalarial chemoprophylaxis and mosquito avoidance measures, and the use of measures that might reduce schistosomal load such as vigorous rubbing of the skin immediately after immersion, or pre- or postexposure use of antischistosomal soaps, *N,N*-diethyl-M-toluamide (DEET) or permethrin on the skin.

Only a minority of people will remember experiencing 'swimmer's itch', lasting from a few to 48 hours after swimming, caused by penetration of the skin by cercariae. This does not reliably predict later symptoms, which first appear in a substantial minority of patients 3–8 weeks after exposure, as the 'Katayama syndrome', which is related to an immunologic reaction to final migration of schistosomules around the body and the onset of oviposition by the maturing flukes (see Chapter 112). Typical symptoms include fever, headache, malaise, wheezing, dry cough and dyspnea. Transient urticarial rashes are common (Fig. PP61.1), and lymphadenopathy and hepatosplenomegaly may be found on examination.[2] Usually this is a diagnosis of exclusion, and the supportive laboratory finding of eosinophilia exceeding $440–500 \times 10^6/l$ (depending on local definitions) is not always present. We have seen cases misdiagnosed as glandular fever due to coincident lymphocytosis, false-positive slide tests for infectious mononucleosis and mild disturbance of liver function tests. Transient shadows may be seen on chest radiographs.

Whether or not patients have experienced earlier symptoms, continued oviposition from 3 to 6 months after exposure may then cause symptoms related to the organs involved. *Schistosoma haematobium* principally affects bladder, prostate and seminal vesicles, and typical complaints are of terminal hematuria, perineal discomfort and, in males, alteration in the consistency (thin or lumpy) or color (yellow or frank blood) of semen. Women occasionally notice a wart-like genital granuloma. *Schistosoma mansoni* primarily affects the large bowel, leading to blood in feces and alteration in bowel habit, but the anatomic location of both species has considerable overlap. Symptoms are more common with *S. haematobium* infections and may be associated with nonspecific fatigue.[3]

The long-term outcome of untreated, relatively light infections of visitors is unknown, but is likely to be benign and not to lead to the complications caused by chronic and repeated infections of inhabitants of endemic areas, such as bladder cancer and portal or pulmonary hypertension (see Chapter 112). However, a small minority of travelers develop central nervous system complications such as epilepsy or spinal cord damage due to ectopic deposition of ova, and the general expert consensus is that all exposed travelers should be screened and treated.

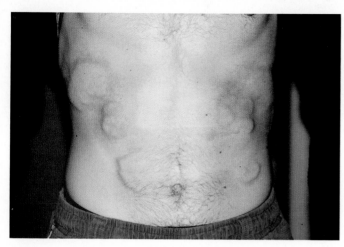

Fig. PP61.1 Giant urticaria associated with Katayama syndrome after swimming in Lake Malawi. Courtesy of Dr ME Jones, Edinburgh.

SCREENING

The minimum investigations, whether or not symptoms are present, should include an absolute eosinophil count, testing of urine for blood, and microscopy for ova in feces and on a filter of a whole urine sample collected over a period of 4 hours straddling the middle of the day (4-hour mid-day urine specimen).[3,4] If such a sample cannot be obtained, a 'terminal urine' sample should be obtained for microscopy, i.e. the last few drops of urine at the end of micturition are most likely to contain ova. 'Routine' urine microscopy is insufficiently sensitive, as egg output can vary during the day such that greater yield is found around noon. Semen microscopy may become positive earlier than urine or feces, and males can be asked to provide a sample for microscopy, particularly if being screened in the first few months after water exposure. If the index of clinical suspicion remains high and other tests are negative, a squash preparation of a fresh rectal biopsy can be examined for ova. Viability of ova, hence current infection, can be inferred from the observation of active flame cells within the miracidium developing in the ovum. Eosinophilia is only found in about 50% of patients in the chronic phase of infection.

The rather crude serologic tests available from European reference centers include an enzyme-linked immunosorbent assay (ELISA) using circumoval protein as antigen to detect circulating antischistosomal antibodies. These become positive from about the time of oviposition, but seroconversion may take up to 6 months and late follow-up screening is essential for those who are asymptomatic and who have negative tests before this time. The serologic tests available from the US Centers for Disease Control and Prevention use an ELISA based on microsomal fractions of adult *S. mansoni*, which become positive soon after exposure to infection, but a species-specific immunoblot may also be required to detect *S. haematobium* or other species. Once positive, serology remains so for years and titers may even increase during the first year after treatment. Follow-up serologic tests after treatment are not, therefore, useful as a test of cure or even for distinguishing re-infection after subsequent re-exposure of the patient to infected water. The disappearance of any symptoms or other positive tests, including eosinophilia, is more reliable for follow-up after treatment.

TREATMENT

Treatment is relatively easy and harmless, using oral praziquantel in a dose of 40 mg/kg, sometimes split into two doses 6 hours apart to reduce any associated nausea, which is usually short lived. Many scuba divers and other visitors treat themselves with locally purchased praziquantel immediately after diving, but this is useless as postexposure prophylaxis. There has been interest in the use of dimeticone or DEET-based preparations for pre- and postexposure prevention of cercarial penetration of skin, but this has not gained wide acceptance. Prophylaxis and chemosuppression with artemisinin compounds have shown more promise in field trials against *S. japonicum* and these deserve further study in African settings.

As praziquantel has limited efficacy during the incubation and invasive phases of *S. haematobium* infection,[5] patients treated at the stage of Katayama syndrome symptomatology need to be re-treated 3 months later. Patients with moderate-to-severe Katayama syndrome may also benefit from a short course of prednisone (e.g. 40 mg daily for several days), preferably started a few hours before anthelmintic treatment. However, this anecdotal recommendation merits a prospective randomized trial to establish both short- and long-term benefit in reducing chronic fatigue, which is quite common after Katayama symptomatology. Corticosteroids reduce the efficacy of praziquantel, so increased dosing of praziquantel is therefore recommended by some.

Patients who present later with symptoms such as hematuria or positive laboratory tests should also be treated and should be followed up 6 months later to establish disappearance of any previous positive findings. Asymptomatic travelers with negative screening tests 6 months or more after lake exposure do not require treatment or further follow-up. It is debatable whether every patient who presents with hematuria and ova in the urine should have further investigations such as ultrasonography or cystoscopy to exclude coincident tumors or other problems. We have a low threshold for urologic referral, which is essential if local symptoms do not resolve after antischistosomal drugs.

SUMMARY

Overall, the risk of acquiring schistosomiasis from swimming in the south of Lake Malawi is so high that screening of returned expatriates, travelers and immigrants is essential and is unlikely to yield false-positive results. Many expatriates regard the risk as so common that they bypass the screening process and treat themselves and their families as a routine every 6 months. We suggest that this approach is inappropriate for the occasional traveler who has swum in Lake Malawi (or similar freshwater bodies), who should be fully assessed before possible treatment with an anthelmintic that is only available on a named-patient basis outside the tropics.

REFERENCES

References for this chapter can be found online at http://www.expertconsult.com

Section | 7 |

Roger G Finch & Scott M Hammer

Anti-Infective Therapy

Principles of anti-infective therapy

The discovery, development and widespread use of antimicrobial drugs are counted among the major achievements of modern medicine. Not only has the outcome from life-threatening infections, such as bacterial meningitis, pneumococcal pneumonia and postpartum sepsis, been dramatically improved, but much minor morbidity arising from community-acquired infections has been controlled with benefit to the individual, society and the economic well-being of nation states. Furthermore, the infectious complications of many surgical procedures have been reduced while organ transplantation and cancer chemotherapy have become much safer procedures.

However, the very success of antimicrobial agents has led to their worldwide acceptance by health-care professionals and the public alike, with the result that much prescribing is excessive, inappropriate and unnecessary.[1] Indeed, in many countries, antimicrobial drugs can be purchased by the public without prescription, leading to so-called 'over-the-counter' selling, which is largely unregulated and poorly defined in terms of impact on patient safety and public health, as well as the inevitable pressure it places on the development of antibiotic resistance (see also Chapter 131).

Unique among therapeutic agents, antimicrobial drugs are directed not at any host-derived disease or pathophysiologic process but at an invading micro-organism. In turn, many pathogens have developed the ability to evade inhibition as a consequence of genetic modification. Resistance to antimicrobial drugs now threatens the ability to effectively treat a number of infectious diseases.[2-4] The gradual erosion of efficacy has meant that recommendations for treating specific infections need to be regularly reviewed and revised as resistance rates increase. For these reasons there is a continuous need to develop new agents, which is a costly and time-consuming process and subject to the vagaries of industrial economic priorities. In the case of antibacterial drugs there is significant concern over the current shortfall in new agents to treat an increasing number of multidrug-resistant pathogens.[5,6]

ANTI-INFECTIVE DRUGS

Anti-infective drugs are generally classified according to their major microbial targets rather than by target disease or infection. Pharmacopoeias and formularies categorize these as antibacterial, antiviral, antifungal and antiparasitic (antiprotozoal or anthelmintic) agents. Within these categories some specific indications can be found such as drugs used in the treatment of HIV/AIDS.

Among anti-infective drugs the largest proportion is for the treatment of bacterial infections. For example, in the UK more than 100 antibacterial agents are available. However, many of these are derivatives of a limited number of classes of agents. As a result, antibacterial activity is dependent upon approximately a dozen distinct targets.

This in part explains the ease with which resistance can emerge, disseminate and, in turn, often affect several agents within a single class of drug.

The burden of human infectious disease varies internationally. In tropical and subtropical countries parasitic disease is more common. However, the range of drugs available to treat these infections is limited and includes many agents that have been in clinical use for decades. The World Health Organization regularly publishes a list of 'essential' drugs.[7] The majority of such drugs are off-patent and generically available and therefore of low cost. However, this emphasis on generic well-established agents also reflects the low priority given to developing agents for diseases in resource-poor countries relative to the major markets of the world. However, more recently as a consequence of greater awareness through international travel and population migration, and the attention being paid to the HIV pandemic in the developing world, greater investment is being targeted at new drugs for diseases such as malaria and tuberculosis.

In contrast to the relative dearth of new agents to treat parasitic disease, drugs available to treat viral infections (Table 129.1), and in particular HIV/AIDS (Table 129.2), have increased remarkably in the past quarter century. There are now more than 20 agents available for managing HIV/AIDS, although none is curative. Agents effective against herpesviruses, notably herpes simplex, varicella-zoster and cytomegalovirus, have had a major impact on both primary and recurrent infections with these viruses and have been of particular benefit in controlling these infections as they occur in the context of HIV disease, transplantation and malignant disease.

GENERAL PRINCIPLES OF PRESCRIBING

The widespread availability and use of antibacterial agents to treat and prevent infectious disease needs to be balanced against the ever-present threat of drug resistance either among target pathogens or in micro-organisms making up the host normal flora. This can have impact beyond the individual patient since dissemination of either a resistant organism or a resistance mechanism can have serious consequences within hospitals and nursing homes or as a result of spread within the community at large.[6]

As a consequence a set of principles has emerged with the objective of not only ensuring safe and effective prescribing but also sustaining the efficacy of anti-infective drugs by reducing the risk of resistance emerging.[8] These principles govern such issues as when to prescribe and which agent(s) to select, as well as issues of dose, frequency and duration of therapy. The requirement for therapeutic drug monitoring applies to selected agents to ensure effective or nontoxic concentrations, or both. In addition, it is important to identify prior

Table 129.1 Antiviral drugs: non-HIV

Agent	Mechanism of action	Antiviral activity	Mechanism of resistance	Toxicity/side-effects
Aciclovir	Inhibits DNA polymerase, chain terminator. Requires viral thymidine kinase and cellular enzymes	HSV-1, HSV-2, VZV, CMV (much less activity), EBV (in vitro)	Mutations in thymidine kinase (more common) and mutations in DNA polymerase	Intravenous: phlebitis, crystalline nephropathy. Confusion, delirium, lethargy, tremors, nausea, vomiting, lightheadedness, diaphoresis, rash
Adefovir	Nucleotide analogue	HBV	Mutational resistance	Renal impairment at >30 mg q24h
Amantadine	Inhibits transmembrane protein M2, reduced uncoating of viral genome	Influenza A	Point mutation in gene encoding transmembrane domain M2 protein	Nervousness, anxiety, lightheadedness, confusion, insomnia
Cidofovir	Acyclic nucleoside phosphonate (does not require a virus-specific thymidine kinase)	HSV-1, HSV-2, VZV, EBV, CMV	Mutations in DNA polymerase	Severe nephrotoxicity, neutropenia, ocular hypotony, metabolic acidosis. Carcinogenic, teratogenic
Entecavir	Nucleoside reverse transcriptase inhibitor	HBV	Mutational resistance	Hepatotoxicity, headache, hyperglycemia, raised lipase
Famciclovir	Prodrug to penciclovir	See penciclovir	See penciclovir	Headache, nausea, diarrhea, vomiting, pruritus, LFT abnormalities
Fomivirsen (intravitreal)	Antisense oligonucleotide	CMV	In-vivo resistance not seen	Iritis, vitreitis, increased ocular pressures, visual changes
Foscarnet	Noncompetitive inhibitor of viral DNA polymerase (does not require thymidine kinase)	HSV-1, HSV-2, VZV, CMV, EBV, influenza A, influenza B, HBV, HIV	In CMV, single mutation in conserved region of DNA polymerase	Renal impairment, electrolyte disturbances, seizures, anemia, neutropenia, fever, nausea, vomiting, diarrhea, headache
Ganciclovir	Inhibitor of DNA polymerase, also competitive inhibitor of deoxyguanosine triphosphate (monophosphorylation by infection-induced kinases in HSV and VZV, and viral-encoded phosphotransferase in CMV-infected cells)	HSV-1, HSV-2, VZV, CMV, EBV, HHV-6	One or more point mutations in UL97, mutations in CMV DNA polymerase	Bone marrow suppression, fever, rash, increased LFTs, nausea, vomiting, eosinophilia, seizures, confusion, encephalopathy
Interferon-α (including pegylated interferon)	Induces changes in infected/exposed cells to promote resistance to infecting virus. Produces proteins that inhibit RNA synthesis, cleaves cellular and viral DNA, inhibits messenger RNA, alters cell membranes, inhibits release of replicated virions	Papillomavirus, HCV (pegylated), HBV, HDV, HIV		Fever, headache, chills, arthralgias, myalgias, fatigue, dizziness, neutropenia, thrombocytopenia, somnolence, depression, cognitive changes, suicidal ideation, increased LFTs, altered thyroid function, nausea, vomiting, diarrhea
Lamivudine	Competitively inhibits viral reverse transcriptase, terminates proviral DNA chain extension	HBV, HIV	Mutations at YMDD locus (conserved domain reverse transcriptase)	Low-dose equivalent to placebo. High dose: headache, fatigue, insomnia, myalgias, arthralgias, diarrhea, rash, lactic acidosis, hepatomegaly

	Mechanism	Spectrum	Resistance	Side effects
Oseltamivir	Neuraminidase inhibitor	Influenza A, influenza B	Mutations in viral neuraminidase and viral hemagglutinin	Nausea, vomiting
Penciclovir (topical)	Incorporated into DNA molecule	HSV-1, HSV-2, VZV, EBV (less so), CMV (less so), HBV (in vitro)	Mutations in thymidine kinase and mutations in DNA polymerase	Topical same as placebo
Ribavirin	Guanosine analogue, three possible mechanisms: competitive inhibition of host enzymes, inhibition of viral RNA polymerase complex, inhibition of messenger RNA formation	RSV, HCV (clinically); but also influenza A, influenza B, mumps, measles, parainfluenza, herpesviruses, togavirus, bunyavirus, adenovirus, Coxsackie virus, hemorrhagic fever virus, HAV, HBC, Lassa fever virus, Hantavirus	Anemia, hyperbilirubinemia, elevated uric acid, nausea, headache, lethargy. Teratogenic, mutagenic, embryotoxic, gonadotoxic	
Rimantadine	Inhibits transmembrane protein M2, reduced uncoating of viral genome	Influenza A	Point mutation in gene encoding transmembrane domain M2 protein	Nervousness, anxiety, lightheadedness, confusion, insomnia (much less so than amantadine)
Trifluridine (topical)	Pyrimidine nucleoside	HSV-1, HSV-2, CMV, vaccinia, some adenoviruses		
Valaciclovir	Valine ester of aciclovir	See aciclovir	See aciclovir	Headache, nausea, abdominal pain
Valganciclovir	Metabolized to ganciclovir	See ganciclovir	See ganciclovir	Bone marrow suppression, fever, nausea, headache, vomiting, insomnia, abdominal pain, peripheral neuropathy, paresthesias, potential carcinogen
Zanamivir (aerosolized/intranasal)	Neuraminidase inhibitor	Influenza A, influenza B	Mutations in viral neuraminidase and viral hemagglutinin	Nasal, throat discomfort, bronchospasm in asthmatics

CMV, cytomegalovirus; EBV, Epstein–Barr virus; HAV, hepatitis A virus; HBV, hepatitis B virus; HCV, hepatitis C virus; HDV, hepatitis D virus; HHV, human herpesvirus; HSV, herpes simplex virus; LFT, liver function test; RSV, respiratory syncytial virus; VZV, varicella-zoster virus.

Table 129.2 Antiviral drugs: HIV

Agent	Mechanism of action	Toxicity/side-effects
Abacavir	Nucleoside reverse transcriptase inhibitor	Hypersensitivity syndrome, rash, fever, nausea, vomiting, diarrhea, abdominal pain, elevated LFTs
Atazanavir	Protease inhibitor	Increased unconjugated bilirubin, gastrointestinal symptoms
DAPD	Nucleoside reverse transcriptase inhibitor	Nausea, vomiting, diarrhea, abdominal pain, hepatitis
Darunavir	Protease inhibitor	Hepatotoxicity, rash, nausea, diarrhea, erythema multiforme, lipodystrophy
Delavirdine	Non-nucleoside reverse transcriptase inhibitor	Rash, headache, Stevens–Johnson syndrome, nausea, depression
Didanosine	Nucleoside reverse transcriptase inhibitor	Nausea, vomiting, diarrhea, abdominal pain, peripheral neuropathy, pancreatitis
Efavirenz	Non-nucleoside reverse transcriptase inhibitor	Dizziness, difficulty concentrating, nausea, vomiting, diarrhea, rash, flu-like symptoms
Emtricitabine	Nucleoside reverse transcriptase inhibitor	Nausea, diarrhea, headache
Enfurvirtide	Fusion inhibitor	Injection site inflammation
Etravirine	Non-nucleoside reverse transcriptase inhibitor	Rash, hypersensitivity reaction, nausea
Fosamprenavir	Protease inhibitor	Rash, hyperlipidemia, diarrhea, lipodystrophy, headache
Indinavir	Protease inhibitor	Nephrolithiasis, nausea, dysgeusia, benign hyperbilirubinemia
Interleukin-2	Peripheral expansion of existing CD4+ lymphocytes	Nausea, vomiting, diarrhea, fever, asthenia, pruritus
Lamivudine	Nucleoside reverse transcriptase inhibitor	No significant toxicity, peripheral neuropathy, pancreatitis
Lopinavir	Protease inhibitor	Nausea, asthenia, diarrhea
Maraviroc	Co-receptor blocker	Hepatotoxicity, fever, rash, abdominal pain
Nelfinavir	Protease inhibitor	Diarrhea
Nevirapine	Non-nucleoside reverse transcriptase inhibitor	Dizziness, rash, difficulty concentrating, nausea, vomiting, diarrhea, flu-like symptoms
Raltegravir	Integrase inhibitor	Rash, hyperlipidemia, injection site pain
Ritonavir	Protease inhibitor	Dysgeusia, nausea, vomiting, diarrhea, circumoral paresthesias, increased triglycerides, LFTs, CPK and uric acid
Saquinavir	Protease inhibitor	Nausea, vomiting, diarrhea, headache
Stavudine	Nucleoside reverse transcriptase inhibitor	Peripheral neuropathy
Tenofovir	Nucleoside reverse transcriptase inhibitor	Nausea, vomiting, diarrhea, headache, elevated LFTs and CPK
Tipranovir	Protease inhibitor	Nausea, vomiting, diarrhea
Zidovudine	Nucleoside reverse transcriptase inhibitor	Anemia, neutropenia, nausea, vomiting, myositis, neuropathy

CPK, creatine phosphokinase; LFTs, liver function tests.

experience of adverse drug reactions in an individual as well as the potential future risks of toxicity from hypersensitivity or other effects. Here the importance of drug interactions is stressed. One additional issue specific to antibacterial drugs is the ability of some to select for superinfecting organisms such as *Clostridium difficile* or *Candida* spp. These pathogens also have the ability to disseminate within the hospital to cause epidemic disease.

Rationale for therapeutic prescribing

Antimicrobial prescribing should be based on clear evidence of infection established by either laboratory investigation or sound clinical criteria. In general, laboratory confirmation of infection, although desirable, is only possible in a minority of treated infections and is largely confined to hospitalized patients where access to laboratory investigation is readily available.

The majority of prescribing is based on a clinical assessment of infection where symptoms and signs point to the likely source and nature of the disease. The need to distinguish infectious from noninfectious causes of systemic inflammation is of fundamental clinical importance and has led to clear criteria which support the identification of the 'sepsis syndrome'. These have particular application in managing severe sepsis.[9] Table 129.3 summarizes the differences between the systemic inflammatory response, sepsis, severe sepsis and septic shock (see also Chapter 44).

Once a definitive or presumptive clinical diagnosis has been made, such as pneumonia or urosepsis, a putative microbiologic diagnosis can be inferred based on knowledge, preferably locally derived, of the usual microbiologic causes of a particular infection. There are only a few clinical diagnoses that can confidently predict the exact microbiologic cause of an infection; examples include erysipelas (*Streptococcus pyogenes*), cutaneous anthrax (*Bacillus anthracis*) and herpesvirus infections such as herpes simplex and varicella-zoster.

Table 129.3 Definitions of systemic inflammatory response, sepsis, severe sepsis and septic shock

Systemic inflammatory response

- Temperature >38°C or <35°C
- Heart rate >90 beats/min
- Respiratory rate >20 breaths/min or $Paco_2$ <32 mmHg
- WBC >12 000 cells/mm³ or <4000 cells/mm³ or >10% immature (band) forms

Sepsis

Clinical features of SIRS plus culture-proven infection
or
Infection identified by visual inspection

Severe sepsis

Sepsis plus one or more signs of organ hypoperfusion or dysfunction:
- Areas of mottled skin
- Capillary refilling requires 3 seconds or longer
- Urine output <0.5 ml/kg for at least 1h, or renal replacement therapy
- Lactate >2 mmol/l
- Abrupt change in mental status
- Abnormal electroencephalographic findings
- Platelet count <100 000 platelets/ml
- Disseminated intravascular coagulation
- Acute lung injury or acute respiratory distress syndrome
- Cardiac dysfunction, as defined by echocardiography or direct measurement of the cardiac index

Septic shock

Severe sepsis plus one or more of the following:
- Systemic mean blood pressure is <60 mmHg (or <80 mmHg if the patient has baseline hypertension) despite adequate fluid resuscitation
- Maintaining the systemic mean blood pressure >60 mmHg (or >80 mmHg if the patient has baseline hypertension) requires dopamine >5 μg/kg per min, noradrenaline (norepinephrine) <0.25 μg/kg per min or adrenaline (epinephrine) <0.25 μg/kg per min despite adequate fluid resuscitation

The results of microbiologic sampling may confirm the nature of an infection and support the continued use of initial empiric treatment or indicate alternative therapy. However, most prescribing is empiric, particularly in community practice, which accounts for about 80–90% of antimicrobial prescribing. Many such infections are managed satisfactorily in the absence of microbiologic investigation.

Prophylactic prescribing

In contrast to therapeutic prescribing for an established infection, antimicrobial agents are prescribed for a variety of medical and surgical indications in order to prevent infection arising as a complication of that condition or surgery. Such prophylactic use must recognize that the risk:benefit ratio must be justified since prophylactic prescribing means that a large number of patients, of whom only a proportion will be at risk of infection, will be exposed to antimicrobial agents. The selected regimen must therefore have been demonstrated to be safe as well as effective in the particular indication.

Surgical prophylaxis

Many surgical procedures such as large bowel surgery and cholecystectomy were formerly associated with high rates of infectious complications. However, short-course (single-dose) perioperative prophylaxis given at the time of induction of anesthesia substantially reduces

this risk.[10] The antimicrobial spectrum of the drug(s) selected must be appropriate for the micro-organisms most commonly responsible for complicating infections.[11] In the case of large bowel surgery an extended spectrum cephalosporin combined with metronidazole, both administered as a single dose, are effective. Amoxicillin–clavulanate, ampicillin–sulbactam, cefoxitin and cefotetan provide alternative choices.

Joint arthroplasty and cardiac valve implant surgery present a particular risk. Micro-organisms introduced at the time of surgery can have serious consequences. Coagulase-negative staphylococci and *Staphylococcus aureus* (including methicillin-resistant *Staph. aureus*, MRSA) are particularly frequent pathogens. Perioperative prophylaxis using an antistaphylococcal penicillin such as flucloxacillin or oxacillin is widely used; however, where there are concerns over the possibility of drug-resistant strains, vancomycin is preferred.[12]

Medical prophylaxis

Medical prophylaxis refers to the use of antimicrobial prophylaxis in a variety of nonsurgical conditions and procedures known to be at risk of serious infectious complications. Anatomic or functional asplenia predisposes to severe sepsis, particularly in childhood where *Strep. pneumoniae*, *Haemophilus influenzae* or *Neisseria meningitidis* is seen. Prophylaxis using long-term daily administration of low-dose oral penicillin (erythromycin in the penicillin allergic) is commonly recommended during childhood (see Chapter 82).[13,14]

Infective endocarditis complicates bloodstream infection in selected, very-high-risk patients with pre-existing valvulopathy; this risk justifies perioperative antibiotic prophylaxis for certain procedures in the oral cavity, although the efficacy of this approach has not been validated and remains controversial (see Chapter 47 for detailed discussion).[15–17] The choice of antibiotic is determined by the nature of the operative procedure and recent history of antibiotic use, as well as the potential for drug intolerance in the recipient.

Malaria is a risk to those traveling to the tropics and subtropics. The use of antimalarial agents for the period immediately prior to departure, during residence in a malaria risk country and for 4 weeks after return, is an effective and well established practice in preventing this potentially life-threatening disease.[18] The choice of regimen is determined by the itinerary of the traveler, the risk of exposure to chloroquine-sensitive or chloroquine-resistant infection, resistance to other antimalarial agents and the potential for adverse drug reactions. These regimens are discussed in Chapters 111 and 150.

A further example of medical prophylaxis is the use of postexposure prophylaxis in those exposed to HIV infection as a result of a needlestick injury. This primarily affects health-care workers who have sustained a percutaneous hollow needle injury from a known or presumptive HIV-infected source. Prompt administration of combined antiretroviral drugs (e.g. zidovudine, lamivudine and lopinavir/ritonavir) for a period of 4 weeks is currently recommended after a careful assessment of the risks (see Chapter 86).[19] Such a regimen is effective but may give rise to significant toxicity in some individuals.

Choice of agent or agents

Fundamental to the treatment of infectious diseases is the selection of an antimicrobial regimen with established efficacy against the target infection based on clinical trials and supported by widespread clinical use. The antimicrobial spectrum of activity should be based on susceptibility data from epidemiologic studies and ideally confirmed by laboratory testing of antimicrobial samples. The most frequently used methods are disc diffusion tests – such as the Kirby–Bauer method in North America or the British Society for Antimicrobial Chemotherapy (BSAC) method in Europe – and the determination of the minimum inhibitory concentration (MIC) of the antibiotic. Disc susceptibility testing involves the agar inoculation of an approximated number of bacteria as a 'lawn', with the overlaying of antibiotic-impregnated discs. After overnight incubation, zones of inhibition appear around the discs

Fig. 129.1 (a) A disc diffusion sensitivity plate showing a fully sensitive coliform tested against a typical range of first-line antibiotics. Courtesy of Dr M Cubbon, Brighton, UK. (b) An E-test showing a methicillin-sensitive *S. aureus*. The MIC of oxacillin for this strain is 0.25 mg/l, and is obtained by noting the point at which the zone of inhibition intersects with the test strip. Courtesy of Dr M Cubbon, Brighton, UK.

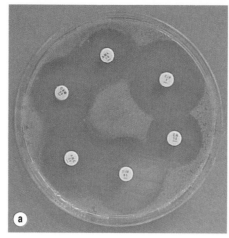
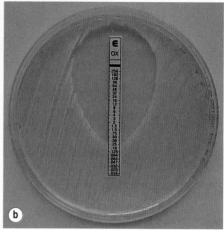

impregnated with antibiotics to which the organism is susceptible (Fig. 129.1a). MIC testing used to be done by agar or broth dilution, but now most laboratories use an ingenious antibiotic-impregnated strip, the E-test (Fig. 129.1b) or other automated techniques. In the USA, the National Committee for Clinical and Laboratory Standards Institute (CLSI) and the European Committee on Antimicrobial Susceptibility Testing (EUCAST) set 'breakpoints' for the MIC based on the integration of MICs with achievable antibiotic levels in serum and tissues, clinical pharmacology and data from *in-vitro* and animal models. Typically these results are presented to the clinician as a report of 'sensitive', 'intermediate' or 'resistant'.

For example, amoxicillin is widely used to treat mild to moderate community respiratory infections such as otitis media which is caused by *Strep. pneumoniae*, *Strep. pyogenes* or *H. influenzae* infection to which amoxicillin is active against the majority of isolates. In contrast, acute lower urinary tract infection (cystitis) is usually caused by enteric pathogens and requires agents such as trimethoprim or nitrofurantoin for its management. However, resistance to amoxicillin by *H. influenzae* and to trimethoprim among *Escherichia coli* is threatening the efficacy of these agents.

Broad-spectrum versus narrow-spectrum antimicrobial agents

The terms 'broad spectrum' and 'narrow spectrum' are widely used to distinguish between agents that target a limited range of pathogens in contrast to broad-spectrum agents to which many pathogens are susceptible. Historically, the terms have been applied to developments in the penicillin class of drugs. Penicillin G (benzylpenicillin) targeted a limited number of pathogens – for example, *Strep. pneumoniae*, hemolytic streptococci and *Neisseria* spp. (meningococci and gonococci). With the development of the aminopenicillins (e.g. amoxicillin), the spectrum increased to also include *H. influenzae* and *E. coli* and were thus considered as broad-spectrum agents; however, as stated above, with time many of these pathogens have become resistant as a result of β-lactamase production.

Among currently available agents the carbapenems (e.g. meropenem) and the ureidopenicillins (e.g. piperacillin) are truly broad-spectrum agents with activity against many Gram-positive and Gram-negative pathogens and, in the case of meropenem, many anaerobic bacteria as well. At the present time vancomycin, other glycopeptides and linezolid are considered narrow-spectrum agents. This contrasts with many other classes and individual drugs. Figure 129.2 provides a summary of the common susceptibility patterns for many commonly prescribed antibacterial drugs.[20]

The antimicrobial spectrum of an antibiotic has important practical implications. Narrow-spectrum agents have a more limited range of indications and in general require greater diagnostic precision to ensure they are used appropriately. They also require greater emphasis on documenting the microbiologic nature of an infection. In contrast, broad-spectrum agents usually capture a greater range of micro-organisms and indications. They are also widely used as initial empiric therapy of respiratory tract and intra-abdominal infections. Microbiologic sampling, although desirable, is not essential for their successful clinical use.

One of the consequences of broad-spectrum agents is their impact on the normal flora, particularly that of the gastrointestinal tract. As a consequence, microbial overgrowth by resistant organisms such as *Candida* spp. and *C. difficile* may occur and give rise to superinfection or *C. difficile*-associated diarrhea, respectively.[21]

Bactericidal versus bacteristatic activity

Antibacterial drugs act by either killing or inhibiting the growth of micro-organisms. These bactericidal or bacteristatic effects are determined by the mode of action of a drug against a particular target organism. Table 129.4 identifies the usual mode of action of commonly prescribed agents.

Cell-wall active agents, such as the penicillins, cephalosporins and glycopeptides, are largely bactericidal as are many (but not all) agents that interfere with protein synthesis. Examples of the latter include the tetracyclines. Metabolic inhibitors of folic acid synthesis, namely the sulfonamides and trimethoprim, are also bacteristatic. Cidality can be affected by drug concentration and *in-vitro* conditions of testing, and may also vary by target pathogen. Nonetheless, it is a useful distinguishing feature with clinical implications in selected circumstances.

In general, bactericidal and bacteristatic agents are equally effective in the management of many mild to moderate infections. However, bacteristatic agents are dependent upon an effective host immune response, notably the ability to phagocytose drug-exposed bacteria. There are a number of clinical conditions in which host immunity is either deficient or suppressed and where bacteristatic agents should be avoided in favor of bactericidal agents. Such immunocompromised patients may be either immunodeficient or immunosuppressed.

Immunodeficiency captures a variety of congenital and acquired defects of immunity, of which many are associated with an increased frequency and severity of infection. While immunosuppression can also arise from impaired host defenses as a result of underlying disease, it is more often a complication of cytotoxic chemotherapy, immunosuppressant treatment or radiotherapy. Patients undergoing organ or bone marrow transplantation or cancer therapy are particularly at risk of infection when profoundly neutropenic.[22] The period of immunosuppression is usually limited as the target disease responds to treatment.

For the above reasons bactericidal agents are preferred when managing infection in immunocompromised patients, especially those with neutropenia. Other circumstances where bactericidal agents are recommended are in the management of infective endocarditis.[23–25] The

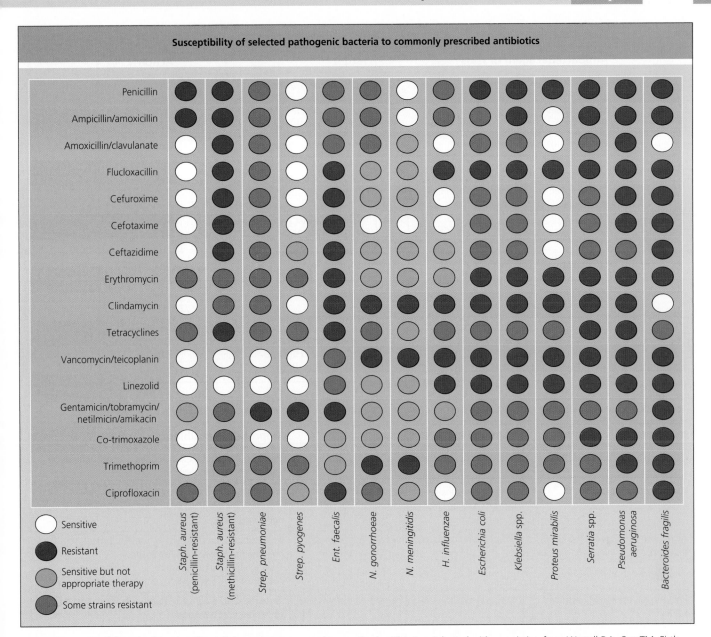

Fig. 129.2 Susceptibility of selected pathogenic bacteria to commonly prescribed antibiotics. Adapted with permission from Warrell DA, Cox TM, Firth JD, eds. *Oxford Textbook of Medicine*, 5th ed. Oxford: Oxford University Press; 2010.

infected vegetations are impermeable to phagocytic cells and require high plasma concentrations of bactericidal drug(s) to sterilize them.

Dose selections and frequency of administration

In an ideal world the correct dose and frequency of administration of an antimicrobial should be accurately defined and confirmed by clinical trials that focus on efficacy and safety in the management of most common infections. However, in the treatment of infection there are many biologic variables that are either host or pathogen derived. Furthermore, the pathophysiologic response to infection adds additional variables. Despite these caveats the selection of anti-microbial chemotherapy is supported by a matrix of information that includes *in-vitro* evaluation of antimicrobial activity, animal models of infections, pharmacokinetic studies of the drug in health and disease, and clinical trial data developed to support the approved indications. Table 129.5 identifies some common bacterial infections affecting adults and the agents used in their treatment.

Pharmacokinetics

The pharmacokinetic profile of a drug is a reflection of its absorption, distribution, metabolism and excretion. The bioavailability of a drug indicates the degree of absorption from the gastrointestinal tract. Parenterally administered agents, such as the aminoglycosides, which are not absorbed from the gut achieve 100% bioavailability. The bioavailability of orally administered antibiotics ranges from 20% for sulfasalazine to up to 100% for ciprofloxacin, nitrofurantoin and cefaclor, for example. To be effective at the site of infection, antibiotics must be well distributed in the tissues. In general, lipophilic agents (e.g. chloramphenicol) and uncharged or nonpolar drugs (e.g. fluoro-quinolones) are able to cross biologic membranes and achieve effective concentrations in tissues. The apparent volume of distribution of an antibiotic (V_d) is calculated by dose/plasma concentration and may reflect the ability of the drug to enter inflammatory cells and tissues.

Drugs once absorbed are generally distributed in the blood and tissues bound to plasma proteins, most notably albumin. The degree of protein binding varies from drug to drug. The unbound or 'free' drug is the biologically active moiety which is in equilibrium with the

Table 129.4 Examples of microbicidal and microbistatic antibacterial agents

Antibacterial agent or class	Target	Action
β-Lactams	*Peptidoglycan synthesis*	
Glycopeptides	Transpeptidases	Cidal
Daptomycin	D-alanyl-D-alanine ligase	Cidal
	Dephosphorylation of lipids	Cidal
Isoniazid, ethionamide, ethambutol	*Mycolic acid synthesis*	Cidal
Aminoglycosides, tetracyclines, oxazolidinones	*Protein synthesis*	
	Ribosomal 30S subunit	Static
Chloramphenicol, macrolides, lincosamides, streptogramins, oxazolidinones	Ribosomal 50S subunit	Static
Mupirocin	tRNA synthetase	Cidal
Fusidic acid	Elongation factor G	Cidal
Metronidazole, nitrofurantoin	*Nucleic acid synthesis*	
	DNA disruption	Cidal
Quinolones	DNA gyrase A and topoisomerase IV	Cidal
Novobiocin	DNA gyrase B	Cidal
Rifampin (rifampicin)	RNA	Cidal
Flucytosine	RNA and DNA synthesis	Cidal
Trimethoprim, *para*-aminosalicylic acid	*Folic acid metabolism*	
	Dihydrofolate reductase	Static
Sulfonamides, diaminodiphenyl sulfone	Dihydropterate synthase	Static

Table 129.5 Common clinical sites for bacterial infections in adults, frequently encountered organisms and appropriate antibiotics*

Infection site	Common bacterial etiology	Appropriate antibiotics[†]
Oropharynx, tonsil	*Streptococcus pyogenes*	Penicillin V × 10 days, macrolides, second-generation cephalosporin, clindamycin
Acute bacterial sinusitis	*Strep. pneumoniae, Haemophilus influenzae, Moraxella catarrhalis*, group A streptococcus	Amoxicillin, ampicillin–clavulanate, cefpodoxime, cefuroxime axetil, oral first- or second-generation cephalosporin
Acute exacerbation of chronic bronchitis	*Strep. pneumoniae, H. influenzae, M. catarrhalis*	Mild: amoxicillin, doxycycline, trimethoprim–sulfamethoxazole, oral cephalosporin Severe: ampicillin–clavulanate, azithromycin, oral cephalosporin, levofloxacin, gatifloxacin, moxifloxacin
Pneumonia, community-acquired, smoker	*Strep. pneumoniae, H. influenzae, M. catarrhalis*	Outpatient: azithromycin, fluoroquinolone, second-generation cephalosporin
Pneumonia, community-acquired, non-smoker	*M. pneumoniae, Chlamydia pneumoniae, Strep. pneumoniae*	As above
Pneumonia, community-acquired	As above	Inpatient: third-generation cephalosporin, plus erythromycin or azithromycin, fluoroquinolone
Urinary tract infection, uncomplicated cystitis	Enterobacteriaceae	Trimethoprim–sulfamethoxazole, trimethoprim, nitrofurantoin, fluoroquinolone
Pyelonephritis	Enterobacteriaceae, *Enterococcus* spp.	Fluoroquinolone, ampicillin plus gentamicin, third-generation cephalosporin, ticarcillin–clavulanate, ampicillin–sulbactam, piperacillin–tazobactam
Urethritis, gonococcal	*Neisseria gonorrhoeae*	Ceftriaxone, cefixime, ciprofloxacin, ofloxacin
Urethritis, nongonococcal	*Chlamydia* spp., *Mycoplasma hominis*, *Ureaplasma* spp.	Doxycycline, azithromycin
Pelvic inflammatory disease	*N. gonorrhoeae, Chlamydia* spp., *Bacteroides* spp., Enterobacteriaceae, *Streptococcus* spp.	Ofloxacin or levofloxacin plus metronidazole, ceftriaxone plus doxycycline, cefotetan or cefoxitin plus doxycycline, ampicillin–sulbactam plus doxycycline
Prostatitis, <35 years old	*N. gonorrhoeae, Chlamydia* spp.	Ofloxacin, ceftriaxone plus doxycycline
Prostatitis, >35 years old	Enterobacteriaceae	Fluoroquinolone, trimethoprim–sulfamethoxazole, aminoglycoside

Table 129.5 Common clinical sites for bacterial infections in adults, frequently encountered organisms and appropriate antibiotics*—cont'd

Infection site	Common bacterial etiology	Appropriate antibiotics[†]
Gastroenteritis	*Shigella* spp., *Salmonella* spp., *Campylobacter* spp., *Escherichia coli* O157 H7	Fluoroquinolone
Cholecystitis	Enterobacteriaceae, enterococci, anaerobes	Ampicillin–sulbactam, piperacillin–tazobactam, imipenem, meropenem
Diverticulitis	Enterobacteriaceae, anaerobes, enterococci	Ampicillin–sulbactam, piperacillin–tazobactam, imipenem, meropenem, metronidazole plus fluoroquinolone
Spontaneous bacterial peritonitis	Enterobacteriaceae, *Strep. pneumoniae*	Cefotaxime, ceftriaxone, ticarcillin–clavulanate, piperacillin–tazobactam, ampicillin–sulbactam
Cellulitis	Group A streptococcus, *Staphylococcus aureus*	Nafcillin, oxacillin, flucloxacillin first-generation cephalosporin, erythromycin, ampicillin–clavulanate
Septic arthritis, monoarticular, sexually active	*N. gonorrhoeae*	Ceftriaxone, cefotaxime, ceftizoxime
Septic arthritis, monoarticular, not sexually active	*Staph. aureus*, *Streptococcus* spp., Gram-negative *L. bacillus*	Nafcillin, oxacillin or flucloxacillin or clindamycin or vancomycin plus third-generation cephalosporin or ciprofloxacin
Septic arthritis, prosthetic	*Staph. epidermidis*, *Staph. aureus*, Enterobacteriaceae, *Pseudomonas* spp.	Vancomycin ± rifampin (rifampicin) plus ciprofloxacin or aztreonam, or ceftazidime or cefepime or aminoglycoside
Osteomyelitis	*Staph. aureus*	Nafcillin, oxacillin, first-generation cephalosporin, vancomycin
Meningitis	*Strep. pneumoniae*, *N. meningitidis*	Ceftriaxone ± vancomycin
Endocarditis, native valve	Viridans streptococcus, other streptococcal species, enterococci, staphylococci	Penicillin or ampicillin, plus nafcillin–oxacillin, plus gentamicin; vancomycin plus gentamicin
Endocarditis, prosthetic valve	*Staph. epidermidis*, *Staph. aureus*	Vancomycin plus gentamicin ± rifampin (rifampicin)

*This table is not intended to be all-inclusive. Specific infections are considered in detail in other chapters. Note that some agents have restricted geographic availability.
[†]This is a general overview; the choice of antibiotics must consider the resistance pattern in any given geographic area (e.g. penicillin and macrolide resistance in *Strep. pneumoniae*; ampicillin and trimethoprim–sulfamethoxazole resistance among *E. coli*), as well as adjustments based on the identified etiologic agent and susceptibility testing.

bound fraction. In general, the degree of protein binding has a limited impact on the outcome of most infections. However, highly bound agents (>95%) may have difficulty crossing some biologic membranes which may have clinical importance when treating infections of the joints, abscesses and the meninges.

Drugs may be excreted unchanged but in general undergo metabolism, especially in the liver for subsequent excretion in the bile. Typical metabolites are the result of glucuronidation, conjugation and acetylation. Drugs metabolized by the cytochrome P450 system may interact with other drugs which share this route. Most metabolites are microbiologically inactive. One exception is the desacetyl metabolite of cefotaxime, which contributes in part to the antimicrobial activity of the parent drug.

In those with impaired liver function, drugs excreted through the liver should be used with caution or avoided. Dose adjustment may be appropriate following careful assessment of liver function tests. The Child–Pugh assessment is often used as an indicator of the severity of liver impairment in clinical trials of new agents in order to guide dosing.[26,27]

Drug excretion is also largely the result of renal excretion. The latter may be either a metabolically active or passive process, and involve the glomeruli or renal tubules or both. Impairment of renal function often leads to a prolonged drug half-life for renally excreted drugs. Dose modification may be required to avoid drug accumulation and drug toxicity.

A clear understanding of the elimination half-life and excretion of antibiotics also influences dosage selection. Drugs with a short half-life are rapidly eliminated and need more frequent administration to produce satisfactory antibiotic concentrations at the site of infection. Drugs with a longer half-life are often more convenient, especially those where single daily dosing is effective.

Pharmacokinetic and pharmacodynamic parameters

The pharmacokinetic (PK) variables that are most useful in antibiotic chemotherapy include bioavailability (F), maximal serum concentration (C_{max}), time to reach C_{max} (t_{max}), elimination half-life ($t_{1/2}$) and area under the drug concentration curve following a dose (AUC).

Recently the pharmacodynamic (PD) characteristics of antimicrobials have become important in determining dosage schedules. In addition, they can be used as predictors of safety and the risks of selecting drug-resistant organisms. Antibiotic pharmacodynamics can be described as the interrelation between pharmacokinetics (drug concentrations) and the antimicrobial effects that result from these concentrations in, for instance, serum, tissues and body fluids. The most useful pharmacokinetic and pharmacodynamic variables are summarized in Table 129.6. These include the ratio of the area under the 24-hour concentration–time curve to the MIC (AUC_{24}/MIC) the ratio of C_{max} to MIC

Table 129.6 Pharmacokinetic and pharmacodynamic parameters that affect antibiotic therapy

Parameters		Details
Pharmacokinetic	F	Bioavailability, fraction of the administered dose absorbed intact; intravenous drugs have 100% bioavailability; oral drugs vary with absorption and are usually less bioavailable than intravenous forms
	C_{max}	Maximal serum concentration after single or multiple doses
	t_{max}	Time after drug administration to reach C_{max}
	$t_{\frac{1}{2} elim}$	Elimination half-life; time to reduce peak serum concentration by 50%
	AUC	Area under the concentration–time curve (relates to total drug exposure following a dose)
Pharmacodynamic	C_{max}/MIC, peak/MIC	Ratio of the maximum serum concentration to the MIC (predicts activity of concentration-dependent bactericidal antibiotics)
	AUC/MIC	Ratio of the area under the concentration–time curve to the MIC (also predicts activity of concentration-dependent bactericidal antibiotics)
	t >MIC, t_{eff}	Time above the MIC; the duration of time during a dosing interval that serum concentration remains above the MIC (predicts activity of time-dependent bactericidal antibiotics)

(peak/MIC) and the time during a given dosing interval that the serum concentration remains above the MIC (time above MIC, t >MIC).[8]

Data based on PK:PD parameters and timed plasma samples from volunteers and patients may be employed in mathematical models using approaches such as Monte Carlo simulations. This has greatly contributed to defining effective and safe dosage schedules for many recent antibacterial[28] and antiviral agents,[29] and most recently to define optimum schedules for antifungal drugs.[30]

Using this basic pharmacokinetic data and *in-vitro* susceptibility profiles of micro-organisms, the relationship between PK and PD variables can be characterized graphically.[31] Figure 129.3 illustrates these key parameters in relation to the MIC of a target pathogen. The relationship of C_{max} and AUC to MIC as well as t (time) above MIC can distinguish drugs which exhibit concentration-dependent killing from those characterized by time-dependent killing.[28] Examples of the former include the fluoroquinolones and aminoglycosides and, in the case of the latter, the penicillins and cephalosporins.

Such PK:PD data have supported single daily dosage regimens for the aminoglycosides[32] and dosage revisions for ciprofloxacin and more recently levofloxacin.[33] PK:PD data are also important in determining the dose and frequency of administration of new drugs and as an indicator of the emergence of resistance in marginally susceptible pathogens.

Postantibiotic effects

Bacterial growth may be inhibited following exposure to an antibiotic even after the drug concentration has fallen below the MIC. This is known as the postantibiotic effect (PAE) and is determined *in vitro* by observing bacterial growth after drug removal.[34] Animal models have been described which measure PAE *in vivo*. Postantibiotic effects can vary by drugs and micro-organism. For example, prolonged PAEs have been reported after aminoglycoside or fluoroquinolone exposure of Gram-negative *L. bacilli*, whereas most β-lactam antibiotics exhibit shorter PAEs. The prolonged PAE for gentamicin against Gram-negative bacilli has provided additional support for current once-daily dosage schedules.

Mutant preventing concentrations

Target pathogens with MICs at or below clinically achievable concentrations of drug may develop resistance. This was recognized in relation to *Pseudomonas aeruginosa* and *Strep. pneumoniae* exposed to borderline plasma concentrations of ciprofloxacin. Dosage schedules are now better designed and selected to minimize this risk by defining the mutant preventing concentration (MPC) of a drug against selected target pathogens.[35]

Drug safety

No drug is free from side-effects. Adverse reactions range from drug hypersensitivity to dose-related side-effects and unpredictable or idiosyncratic phenomena. They may be trivial and readily reversible, have more serious consequences or be life-threatening and occasionally fatal. They should be constantly under consideration by the prescriber and reported to the regulatory authorities, particularly in relation to new agents and in the case of unusual or serious side-effects. They should also be prominently and readily identified within the patient's medical record.

With regard to antibiotics, the penicillins and cephalosporins share the β-lactam ring structure and in turn have many adverse effects in common. These include hypersensitivity rashes and other reactions and toxicity to hematopoietic cells. However, there are differences between these two classes. Hypersensitivity reactions occur less commonly to the cephalosporins. This applies to anaphylaxis which is the

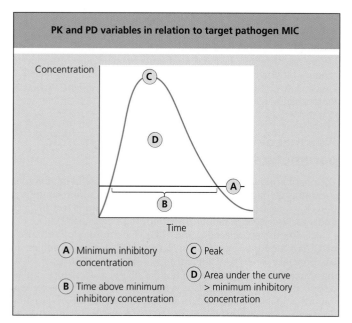

PK and PD variables in relation to target pathogen MIC

Concentration

Time

(A) Minimum inhibitory concentration

(C) Peak

(B) Time above minimum inhibitory concentration

(D) Area under the curve > minimum inhibitory concentration

Fig. 129.3 The relationship between the pharmacokinetic profile of an antibiotic and the minimum inhibitory concentration (MIC) against a hypothetical target organism. Reproduced with permission from Finch.[8]

most severe and feared hypersensitivity reaction. Any severe hypersensitivity reaction to a β-lactam is a bar to its future use and of the β-lactam agents in general. However, milder forms of hypersensitivity, such as skin eruption to a penicillin, do not necessarily preclude the use of a cephalosporin.

Many adverse drug events can be minimized in persons with known excretory organ malfunction by adjusting the dose. The aminoglycosides, such as gentamicin, have been extensively studied and dosage schedules developed which are adjusted for age, weight, gender and renal function.

Prescribing of antimicrobial drugs, as in other areas of medicine, must be based on a careful assessment of the patient, the nature and severity of the disease being treated and any identifiable predispositions to drug toxicity. Such a risk assessment may lead to the decision to use a drug with a higher adverse reactions profile in the severely ill patient which contrasts to the management of mild, often self-limiting community infections where safety has a higher priority. In relation to prophylactic use, only agents with the highest safety profiles are appropriate, since in only a proportion of recipients will clear benefit ensue.

Therapeutic drug monitoring

Therapeutic drug monitoring (TDM) aims to ensure safe and effective prescribing for drugs with a narrow therapeutic index. The latter reflects the limited margin between the therapeutic and toxic concentrations of a particular drug. In contrast, drugs such as penicillins have a wide therapeutic index and even when given in high concentration are generally safe.

In practice much TDM is directed at ensuring therapeutic nontoxic concentrations of the aminoglycosides. Other examples include TDM for antifungals such as itraconazole and most recently voriconazole[36] in the treatment of severe fungal infections as well as, in some circumstances, antiretroviral agents such as the protease inhibitors and nonnucleoside reverse transcriptase inhibitors.[37]

Combined drug regimens

In general and whenever possible it is preferable to manage an infection with a single drug. Provided the drug is effective this reduces the cost of treatment and limits the risk of adverse reactions. However, this demands that the agent selected is not only appropriate to the nature of the infection but also that there is either microbiologic documentation or strong clinical evidence as to the likely microbiologic cause and that it will be susceptible to the agent selected.

There are an increasing number of diseases and circumstances where a combination of drugs is appropriate or necessary to control the infection. Examples include tuberculosis,[38] HIV/AIDS infection[39] and, more recently, malaria.[40] However, in practice, drugs are frequently combined where there is uncertainty about the microbiologic nature of a diagnosis or where the spectrum of a single agent is inadequate, particularly in situations such as intra-abdominal sepsis. Here infection is often polymicrobial with both aerobic and anaerobic pathogens present. Combining an extended-spectrum cephalosporin, such as cefuroxime or cefotaxime, with metronidazole provides an appropriate 'broad-spectrum' regimen. Another example is in the treatment of severe community-acquired pneumonia when both atypical and conventional pathogens need to be 'covered'.[41,42]

Another important reason for combined drug regimens is to prevent resistant organisms emerging on therapy. This was first demonstrated in the treatment of tuberculosis where minority populations of organisms can become resistant to isoniazid or rifampin (rifampicin). These occur at low frequency, being of the order of 1 in 10^8 to rifampin and 1 in 10^9 to isoniazid. Single-drug therapy would eliminate the susceptible organisms and initially be accompanied by clinical improvement. However, the minority resistant populations subsequently multiply and eventually cause relapse of disease which is much harder to treat. For these reasons the standard regimen for treating pulmonary tuberculosis includes isoniazid and rifampin combined with a third

(pyrazinamide) and fourth (ethambutol) agent for the first 2 months, by which time the results of susceptibility testing are generally available. It is then usually safe to continue with a two-drug regimen of isoniazid and rifampin for the remaining 4 months of treatment (see Chapter 143).[38]

Similar principles are increasingly being applied to the treatment of severe malaria, particularly in regions of the world where chloroquine-resistant malaria is widespread. Examples include combinations of artemisinin with tetracycline or mefloquine.[40] It is surprising that it has taken so long to move from single-agent treatment of malaria to combined regimens in an era when very few antimalarial drugs are being developed and drug-resistant disease has become so widespread.

Other circumstances where combined regimens have become the norm are in the management of HIV/AIDS[39] and chronic hepatitis C.[43] In both diseases clinical trials have shown greater efficacy with combined regimens. In the case of HIV/AIDS, viral load is more rapidly controlled and sustained with faster immune reconstitution and resultant clinical well-being. By selecting two or more agents from different classes of antiretrovirals, drug resistance is delayed in addition to providing a more efficacious regimen.

In the case of hepatitis C, pegylated interferon combined with ribavirin is not only more effective than single-drug therapy in terms of disease control but also in the case of genotype 2 and 3 infection offers a prompt and sustained viral response with high cure rates.[44]

Another rationale for combined drug regimens is to achieve synergistic inhibition of a target pathogen. The combining of a penicillin (for susceptible strains) with an aminoglycoside to treat enterococcal endocarditis is now standard therapy since *in vitro* and *in vivo* the combination is more effective than a penicillin alone.

Other synergistic combinations include β-lactam/aminoglycoside regimens to treat serious *P. aeruginosa* infections of the bloodstream and lower respiratory tract infections, especially in the immunocompromised patient.[45] Likewise, amphotericin B and flucytosine are synergistic in the treatment of cryptococcal meningitis.[46]

Economic considerations

Antibiotics account for approximately 20% of all prescribed drugs. Primary care is responsible for around 90% of this prescribing, the remainder being used in the treatment of hospitalized patients. However, community prescribing relies largely on oral and, to a lesser degree, topical agents. In contrast, in hospital, parenteral administration is the dominant route. Parenteral agents are more expensive, more costly to prepare, require infusion systems and account for much staff time in their preparation and administration. With the improved oral bioavailability of agents such as the fluoroquinolones, there is an economic advantage to place less reliance on parenteral regimens, unless this is clinically unavoidable. Switching from intravenous to oral treatment is increasingly used in managing a variety of infections and can result in significant cost savings without impairing outcomes.[47]

Another factor affecting the cost of treatment is the increasing use of generic agents which account for more than three-quarters of prescribing in primary care. Generics are generally substantially cheaper than patented preparations and many hospitals permit generic substitution of a proprietary drug by pharmacists dispensing these drugs.

In addition to the cost of treatment, many health-care systems are looking critically at the total cost of managing specific infectious diseases. For example, this has led to a careful assessment of which patients justify hospital management according to diagnosis, disease severity and age. Furthermore, the choice, route and duration of treatment are also undergoing critical review. No longer can the unit cost of a medicine be seen as the sole determinant that dictates choice of therapy.

Increasingly health-care systems require an economic assessment of the performance and use of new agents at the time of licensing. In the UK the National Institute for Health and Clinical Excellence assesses the benefit of a particular drug in managing a disease in the context of health-care gain using indices such as number required to treat to achieve observed benefit. Such a macroeconomic approach has advantages and disadvantages. Approval in the context of socialized medicine means that specific treatments can be adopted. However, the purchaser is rarely the individual who remains dependent upon competing demands on health-care budgets to gain access to new medicines. Furthermore, products which are approved by the regulatory authority may not necessarily be approved for widespread use despite passing the hurdle of documented efficacy, safety and pharmaceutical quality. In other countries the availability of a new drug post-approval may be linked to an agreement on reimbursement charges from government. In general, these systems have been created to control the ever-spiraling costs of medicines and health care. However, they are also proving a disincentive to industry to develop new drugs such as antibacterials which are generally used in short courses, unlike drugs used to manage chronic disease.

Failure of antimicrobial therapy

Despite adhering to the above prescribing principles in the selection and use of antimicrobial agents, some infections still fail to respond to treatment. It is therefore important to review the response to therapy. This applies particularly to the seriously ill hospitalized patient where clinical response and laboratory monitoring, such as declining neutrophil count and other inflammatory markers provide supportive evidence of improvement. In primary care the patient should be advised about the anticipated course of their illness and to seek further medical assessment should any complications develop or the symptoms fail to respond.

Failure to respond to antimicrobial treatment may have several explanations. These include the accuracy of the primary diagnosis, the choice of initial therapy, the selection of dose and route of administration, the duration of treatment and, in the case of trauma or implant surgery, an assessment of the possible presence of deep-seated infection. Surgical drainage of pus with abscess formation is often overlooked and needs emphasis.

Failure to make a correct diagnosis may be the result of an inaccurate clinical assessment and, in turn, presumptive microbiologic assessment to guide initial empiric therapy – for example, the incorrect diagnosis of superficial cellulitis instead of more deep-seated necrotizing fasciitis. Here the selection of oxacillin or flucloxacillin alone will be ineffective, particularly against MRSA or anaerobic pathogens.[48] A careful review and further investigations, where indicated, are important in reassessing the unresponsive patient.

The dose and route of medication are also of importance. For example, pneumococcal pneumonia can be effectively managed in the community with oral agents for patients with mild to moderate infection. However, in those with bacteremic infection, parenteral therapy is preferred, especially when complications such as meningitis arise and where the choice of drug, route and dose of therapy differ.

Another example is selection of an incorrect formulation of a drug. Vancomycin is the preferred agent for managing severe C. difficile-associated diarrhea (CDAD) but needs to be prescribed orally and not intravenously as in the case of systemic staphylococcal infection. Furthermore, the oral dose of vancomycin for CDAD differs from that used to treat bloodstream staphylococcal disease.

Most mild to moderate infections respond to 5–10 days of antibiotic therapy. However, selected infections require more protracted therapy to avoid treatment failure and relapse. Severe Legionella pneumophila pneumonia may require up to 3 weeks of treatment,[42] as does meningitis caused by Listeria monocytogenes. This emphasizes the value of establishing a microbiologic diagnosis, particularly when treating severe infection.

The place of bactericidal regimens in selected patients has been emphasized, particularly in those with known defects in immune function, notably the profoundly neutropenic patient. Likewise infections at body sites relatively protected from the host immune response require bactericidal regimens for optimum control. Examples include infective endocarditis and bacterial meningitis.

Infection as a complication of the presence of foreign materials, notably vascular and articular prosthetic devices, is increasing. Infection is often caused by skin micro-organisms, notably coagulase-negative staphylococci. These are not only of variable sensitivity to many commonly used agents but also adhere to the foreign material as biofilms in which they are protected against host defenses and are less responsive to treatment. Prolonged therapy or surgical revision, sometimes with removal of the infected device, may be necessary to eliminate the infection.

Formularies, guidelines and medicines management

The complexity and ever-changing nature of disease management has given rise to a variety of prescribing support systems and initiatives which are grouped under the title of antibiotic stewardship.[49] These are now recognized as essential in health care where advances in medicine, together with education and training, often go hand in hand with patient care. Furthermore, the fiscal burden of the cost of medicines and their administration has added to the need for formularies and prescribing support systems. In the case of antimicrobial therapy the situation is further compounded by the occurrence and threat of drug-resistant pathogens to the individual patient and the wider community.

The variety of prescribing support systems varies from country to country and even within different hospitals and administrative units of health-care delivery. They include formularies, treatment guidelines, online prescribing systems, care pathways, care bundles and audit, all of which influence antimicrobial prescribing.[49]

Formularies

Formularies, in their original form, were simply a listing of drugs stocked by the pharmacy. Formularies would include agents to cover topical, oral and parenteral use. A decision to include an agent in a formulary is currently, but not universally, based on recommendations by an institutional Drug and Therapeutics Committee or its equivalent. Such decisions are influenced by medical need, cost and increasingly clear evidence of efficacy and safety for the proposed indication.[50] Many institutions distinguish between drugs that may be freely prescribed being appropriate for many common indications from those for specialist use such as antibiotics used in regimens for managing infections in neutropenic patients. In addition, some agents have restricted uses and can only be prescribed following discussion and approval by a microbiologist or infectious disease specialist.

Increasingly, national considerations are being applied to the approval and availability of treatments. These economic analyses influence prescribing, reimbursement costs and, in some countries, whether or not a drug is made nationally available or not. In the UK, the National Institute for Health and Clinical Excellence increasingly assesses medicines in the context of disease management and makes judgments on the availability of new products, notably those which carry a high cost.

Treatment guidelines

Treatment guidelines are increasingly linked to formularies.[51] Local guidelines make recommendations with regard to the preferred and alternative agents relevant to specific diseases and conditions. At institutional level such decisions require evidence based on a review of the published literature in addition to the manufacturer's dossier. Such evidence includes controlled clinical studies, meta-analyses and, whenever possible, nationally or internationally published evidence-based guidelines.

Treatment guidelines have a number of advantages. They reflect current best therapy whenever possible and identify issues relevant to cost containment such as when generics or generic substitution is appropriate. Standardization of management also supports purchasing arrangements and in particular provides an important resource for education and training of prescribing practitioners. In addition, audits of compliance by prescriber, unit and institution are possible and increasingly provide a means for measuring patient outcome according to treatment. The latter is challenging to achieve but important in order to continuously update treatment recommendations.

Implementation of guidelines has been shown to improve management, reduce inappropriate prescribing, lower costs and reduce bacterial resistance for selective indications, such as ventilator-associated pneumonia.[52] However, compliance with guidelines is often poor.[53]

Electronic prescribing support is becoming more widely available and permits an accurate recording of prescribing practice by patient and prescriber.[54] More sophisticated systems influence choice through prompts to approved drugs for given diagnoses. Others have taken this one stage further and include microbiologic data to further refine prescribing selection, or have targeted specific classes of antibiotic to improve usage and reduce adverse effects.[55]

The appointment of clinical pharmacists to support good prescribing practice is a more recent phenomenon.[56] Their knowledge of medicines and skills can improve prescribing standards, minimize prescribing errors and encourage audits. Their appointment also permits cost saving exercises such as automatic stop orders and intravenous to oral switching algorithms. Invariably they also influence decisions by Drug and Therapeutics Committees. Antimicrobial pharmacists have emerged in the UK as a further refinement of this role with particular emphasis on hospital prescribing practice. The adoption of antimicrobial management teams is increasing worldwide but does require institutional support and the correct professional expertise.[57]

SUMMARY

In conclusion, safe and effective prescribing is a professional and lifelong commitment by all prescribing professionals. The ever-changing nature of therapeutics inevitably requires a major commitment to continuous education and professional development.

The principles of good prescribing practice as described above are particularly important in relation to antimicrobial agents where the dynamics of infectious disease with regularly emerging novel pathogens, new expressions of virulence and new resistance mechanisms add further complexity to prescribing.

REFERENCES

References for this chapter can be found online at http://www.expertconsult.com

Françoise Van Bambeke
Youri Glupczynski
Marie-Paule Mingeot-
Leclercq
Paul M Tulkens

Chapter | **130** |

Mechanisms of action

ANTIBIOTICS THAT ACT ON THE CELL WALL

The basis of the bacterial cell wall is peptidoglycan, containing alternating residues of *N*-acetyl-glucosamine and muramic acid in β-1→4 linkage. The carboxyl groups of muramyl residues are substituted by short peptides (usually pentapeptides) terminated by a D-Asp-D-Ala-D-Ala sequence. Cell-wall active antibiotics act by inhibiting the activity of enzymes involved in the synthesis of the precursors or in the reticulation of peptidoglycan.

β-Lactams

The β-lactam nucleus is the basic building block of an exceptionally large class of antibiotics that all share a common mode of action but have quite distinct properties in terms of spectrum, pharmacokinetics and, to some extent, activity against resistant strains.

Chemical structure

All antibiotics in this class contain a cyclic amide called β-lactam. With the exception of the monobactams, this cycle is fused with a five- or six-membered cycle. According to the nature of the four-membered latter and/or of the heteroatom included, the following classes have been described (Fig. 130.1):

- penams – β-lactams with a five-membered ring containing a sulfur atom (penicillins);
- clavams – β-lactamase inhibitors that contain a five-membered ring with an oxygen as the heteroatom (e.g. clavulanic acid; sulfur analogues have also been reported);
- carbapenems – five-membered rings without heteroatom and with a double bond (e.g. thienamycin, imipenem);
- cephems – six-membered unsaturated rings with a sulfur atom (cephalosporins);
- oxacephems – the oxygen analogues of cephems (latamoxef);
- monobactams – cyclic amides in a four-membered ring (azetidine) with a methylcarboxylate function in the case of nocardicins and a sulfonate in the case of the other monobactams (e.g. aztreonam).

Other β-lactams include thiacephems, dethiacephems, dethiacephams, heterocephems and cephams, as well as diverse bicyclic systems.

Mode of action

β-Lactams act primarily as inhibitors of transpeptidases (specialized acyl serine transferases), thereby impairing the synthesis of the cell wall (Fig. 130.2).[1] β-Lactams mimic the D-Ala-D-Ala sequence in that the distance between the carboxylate or the sulfonate (monobactams) and the cyclic amide is similar, and act as a false substrate for D-alanyl-D-alanyl transpeptidases. The carbonyl of the beta-lactam ring reacts with a serine residue of the transpeptidases (also called penicillin-binding proteins, PBPs) to give an inactive acyl enzyme ('suicide inhibition' by formation of a covalent bond; Fig. 130.3).[2] Transpeptidases, located in the periplasmic space, are directly accessible in Gram-positive bacteria but protected by the outer membrane in Gram-negative bacteria, which β-lactams must cross (mainly via porin channels).

The impairment of cell wall formation by β-lactams explains the inhibition of the growth of bacteria, but the bactericidal effect results from indirect mechanisms (mostly the activation of autolytic enzymes). β-Lactams are usually active against rapidly dividing bacteria only.

Resistance

Resistance to β-lactams occurs by three main different mechanisms.

- First, access to the PBPs in Gram-negative bacteria might be abolished by alteration of porin channels, which affects highly water-soluble β-lactams.
- Second, resistance can be conferred through modification of PBPs, in particular PBP2 which is essential for the 'shaping' of bacteria. The most typical example is found in methicillin-resistant *Staphylococcus aureus* (MRSA) that produces an altered protein (called PBP2' or PBP2a) with a very low affinity for β-lactams. This makes the bacteria resistant to all conventional β-lactams. Recent research has shown that PBP2a is insensitive to β-lactams because the protein is in 'closed' conformation, preventing access of the drug to the reactive serine. This is circumvented if bacteria are exposed to acidic pH, which causes an opening of the enzymatic cavity.[3] This can also occur if β-lactams have a bulky hydrophobic substituent attached to the molecule in the vicinity of the carboxylate (see Fig. 130.4 for cephalosporins). These molecules typically show a loss of activity towards MRSA of only one to eight dilutions (corresponding to the energy needed to open the PBP2a) compared to fully susceptible *S. aureus* (in contrast with often more than 256-fold for conventional β-lactams). Two anti-MRSA β-lactam antibiotics (ceftobiprole and ceftaroline)[4] have been clinically developed. Penicillin-binding proteins in staphylococci or in other organisms (e.g. streptococci) can also show decreased affinity; in such cases resistance is more specific to some β-lactams but can also be only partial (decreased susceptibility).
- The third and for many years the most frequent mechanism of resistance is the production of hydrolyzing enzymes called β-lactamases.[5] The corresponding genes may be carried either on chromosomes (where their expression may be constitutive or inducible) or on plasmids, and their products are secreted out of the cell wall in Gram-positive bacteria and in the periplasmic space in Gram-negative bacteria. β-Lactamases are serine proteases that have a high affinity for β-lactams and cleave the amide bond. Although most β-lactamases open the β-lactam ring in the same way

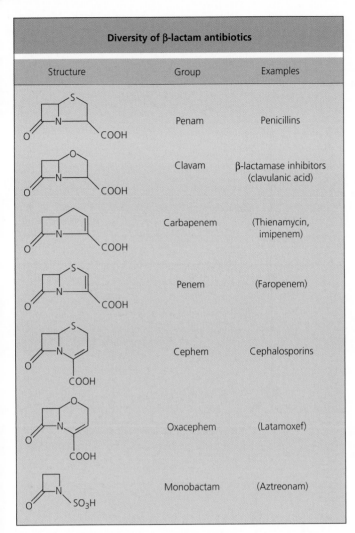

Diversity of β-lactam antibiotics		
Structure	Group	Examples
	Penam	Penicillins
	Clavam	β-lactamase inhibitors (clavulanic acid)
	Carbapenem	(Thienamycin, imipenem)
	Penem	(Faropenem)
	Cephem	Cephalosporins
	Oxacephem	(Latamoxef)
	Monobactam	(Aztreonam)

Fig. 130.1 Diversity of β-lactam antibiotics: main ring structures names and representative antibiotics. The figure highlights the fact that all drugs share a common four-piece β-lactam ring and a carboxylate (or sulfonate) function at an appropriate, similar distance. (Clavams are weak antibiotics but efficient β-lactamase inhibitors.)

as transpeptidases, the hydrolysis rate is far quicker than in PBPs (see Fig. 130.3), resulting in the regeneration of the enzyme and the production of an irreversibly inactivated antibiotic. While PBPs turn slowly (one β-lactam per hour), the β-lactamases can turn on good substrates over 1000 times per second. X-ray data and genetic studies of β-lactamases and PBPs show a high level of structural homology, suggesting that both derive from a common ancestor.

A number of β-lactams have been made to resist to β-lactamases by appropriate steric hindrance or change in conformation (Fig. 130.5), giving rise to the large number of successive generations of so-called β-lactamase-resistant penicillins and cephalosporins. β-Lactamases, however, have an extraordinary plasticity and inevitably develop activity against all new derivatives at a rapid pace (Table 130.1).

Thanks to their specific structure, clavams are poor antibiotics but bind tightly to β-lactamases and inactivate them. Given in combination with β-lactams, they provide protection unless the bacteria overproduce β-lactamases. Some β-lactamases can also hydrolyze the clavams.

Pharmacodynamics

β-Lactams are relatively slow-acting antibiotics that must be present at a concentration above the minimum inhibitory concentration (MIC) for as long as possible. Conversely, concentration above four

to five times the MIC provides little gain in activity, so that frequent dosing is more appropriate than infrequent administration of large doses. Administration of β-lactams by continuous infusion is gaining increasing popularity,[6] but care must be taken regarding the stability of the drugs when exposed to room temperature for prolonged periods of time (carbapenems are unstable and cannot be used by continuous infusion; a 'prolonged' infusion time of 3–4 hours has been proposed for doripenem as part of the drug labeling). In general, β-lactams show only a moderate postantibiotic effect.

Future developments

Efforts continue to develop β-lactams active against MRSA in order to obtain compounds with increased intrinsic activity (applying the approach used with cephalosporins to penems). In parallel, efforts are being made to develop more effective β-lactamase inhibitors (especially for Gram-negative bacteria). Faropenem, an oral penem, was halted in its development in spite of excellent activity against pneumococci, largely because of fear of triggering resistance to the whole class of penems if used indiscriminately in the community.

Hybrid molecules combining a β-lactam part and an active antibiotic part from a different class (e.g. glycopeptides, fluoroquinolones) have also been described, with some potentially promising compounds (because of markedly improved activity) in development.

Glycopeptides and lipoglycopeptides

Chemical structure

Currently available glycopeptide antibiotics (vancomycin, teicoplanin) contain two sugars and an aglycone moiety made of a relatively highly conserved heptapeptide core, bearing two chloride substituents. The aglycone fraction is responsible for the pharmacologic activity of the molecule, whereas the sugars are thought to modulate its hydrophilicity and its propensity to form dimers (see below). As a result of their large size, glycopeptides are not only unable to cross the outer membrane of Gram-negative bacteria, explaining why they are inactive against these organisms, but are also unable to penetrate inside bacteria, limiting them to an extracellular target. Lipoglycopeptides are semisynthetic derivatives characterized by the addition of a hydrophobic moiety, which confers additional properties to the drugs.

Mode of action

Glycopeptides inhibit the late stages of cell wall peptidoglycan synthesis (see Fig. 130.2) by binding to D-Ala-D-Ala termini of the pentapeptide-ending precursors localized at the outer surface of the cytoplasmic membrane. At the molecular level, glycopeptides form a high affinity complex with D-Ala-D-Ala by establishing hydrogen binding via their aglycone moiety.[7] The strength of this binding is greatly enhanced either by the dimerization of the glycopeptide molecules mediated by their sugars and the chloride atom on the aglycone (vancomycin) or by their anchoring in the membrane by a fatty acyl chain substituent.[8] The subsequent steric hindrance around the pentapeptide termini blocks the reticulation of peptidoglycan by inhibiting the activity of transglycosylases (responsible for the fixation of a new disaccharide–pentapeptide subunit on the nascent peptidoglycan) and of transpeptidases (catalyzing the formation of interpeptide bridges).

Lipoglycopeptides (telavancin, oritavancin) add membrane-destabilization effects and stronger inhibition of the transglycosidase activities to the basic mode of action of the older molecules (resulting in the leakage of ions and other small molecules, causing rapid bacterial death). This is due to their membrane-anchoring properties (favored by the abundance of acidic phospholipids in bacterial membranes) and to dimerization of molecules[9] (Fig. 130.6) and, for oritavancin and enterococci, the possibility to bind an additional site in the petidoglycan.[9a] Dalbavancin (currently under development) also has a lipophilic side chain but does not appear to destabilize bacterial membranes, and results in exceptionally low MICs and a very prolonged half-life.

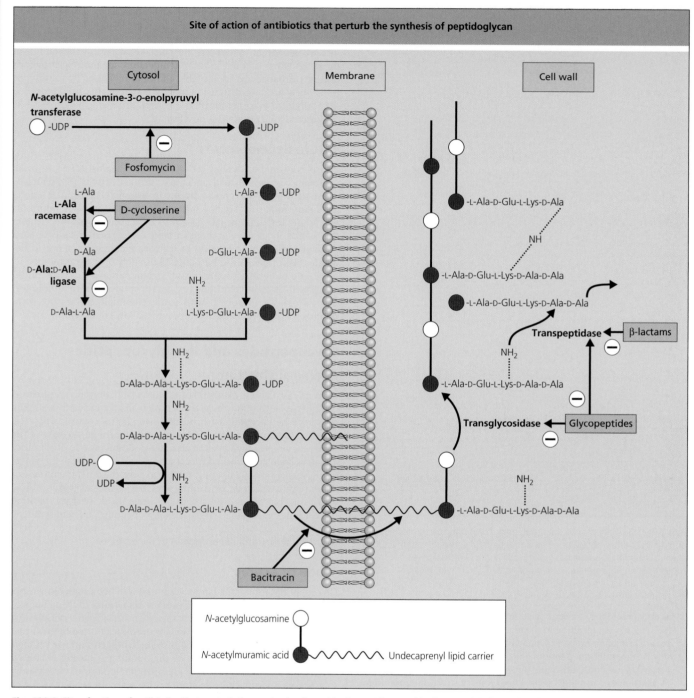

Fig. 130.2 Site of action of antibiotics that perturb the synthesis of peptidoglycan. The peptidoglycan unit is formed in the cytosol of bacteria by binding to uridine diphosphate (UDP) N-acetylmuramic acid of a short peptide (the nature of which differs between bacteria). This precursor is then attached to a lipid carrier and added to N-acetylglucosamine before crossing the bacterial membrane. At the cell surface peptidoglycan units are reticulated by the action of transglycosylases (catalyzing the polymerization between sugars) and of transpeptidases (catalyzing the polymerization between peptidic chains). The antibiotics act as follows: fosfomycin is an analogue of phosphoenolpyruvate, the substrate of the N-acetylglucosamine-3-O-enolpyruvyl transferase synthesizing N-acetylmuramic acid from N-acetylglucosamine and phosphoenolpyruvate; cycloserine is an analogue of D-Ala and blocks the action of D-Ala racemase and D-Ala: D-Ala ligase; bacitracin inhibits the transmembrane transport of the precursor; vancomycin binds to D-Ala-D-Ala termini and thus inhibits the action of transglycosylases and transpeptidases; and β-lactams are analogs of D-Ala-D-Ala and suicide substrates for transpeptidases.

Resistance

Resistance to glycopeptides results from substituting a D-lactic acid or a D-serine in place of terminal D-Ala of the pentapeptide. While this does not prevent the action of the transpeptidase, it ruins the binding of the glycopeptides because of the loss of one crucial hydrogen bond.[7] This mode of resistance is most prevalent in enterococci, but rarely in *S. aureus*. In the latter, resistance is more commonly acquired as a result of

thickening of the cell wall associated with an increased abundance of free D-Ala-D-Ala termini. As a result, the MICs of the organisms increase modestly by about two- to eightfold, producing the so-called vancomycin- or glycopeptide-intermediate phenotype (VISA and GISA), eventually reaching a value of 4 mg/l or more at which clinically achievable serum concentrations of vancomycin can no longer inhibit bacterial growth (current CLSI and EUCAST breakpoints set a limit of 2 mg/l for susceptible strains). A further difficulty is the fact that the expression of

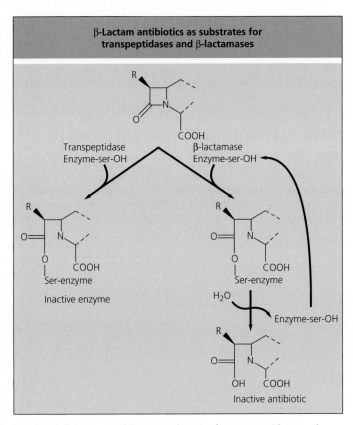

Fig. 130.3 β-Lactam antibiotics as substrates for transpeptidases and β-lactamases. The left part of the illustration shows how a β-lactam covalently binds to the transpeptidases. Hydrolysis of this acylated enzyme is very slow (one β-lactam per hour), making the enzyme inactive. The right part of the illustration shows that the same reaction occurs in the case of a β-lactamase. Hydrolysis of the acylated enzyme is, however, very rapid (1000 β-lactams per second), making the antibiotic inactive and regenerating the enzyme for a new cycle of hydrolysis.

this resistance is variable and may only affect a small proportion of a given inoculum, giving rise to a heteroresistance phenotype that makes detection by automated systems fairly unreliable.[10]

Lipoglycopeptides (telavancin, oritavancin) are partially immune to both resistance mechanisms thanks to their dual mode of action. It remains uncertain, however, whether keeping only the membrane-destabilizing effects (typically expressed only at higher drug concentrations than are needed to bind to D-Ala-D-Ala) will be sufficient to maintain clinically useful activity. Dalbavancin has variable activity against VISA strains and no useful activity against vancomycin-resistant organisms.

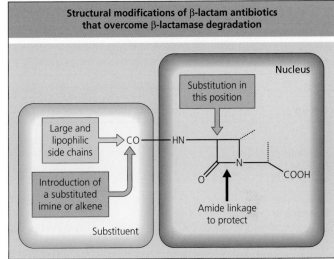

Fig. 130.5 Structural modifications of β-lactam antibiotics that overcome β-lactamase degradation. A first strategy, applied in penicillins, cephalosporins, oxacephems and monobactams consists of the introduction of a large side chain on the nucleus, possibly containing a substituted imine or alkene. A second strategy, applied in oxacephems and cefoxitin as well as in temocillin, consists of the introduction of a methoxy group on the β-lactam ring.

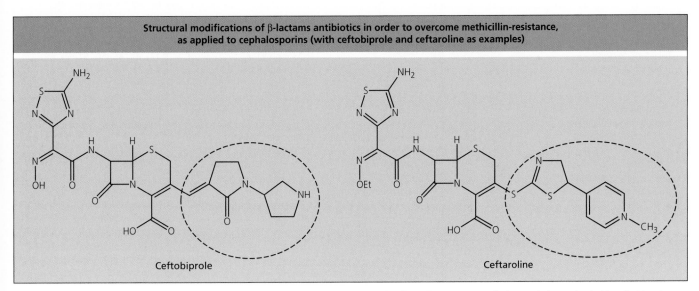

Fig. 130.4 Structural modifications of β-lactam antibiotics in order to overcome methicillin resistance, as applied to cephalosporins (with ceftobiprole and ceftaroline as examples). The bulky hydrophobic moieties (dotted-lined ellipse) added to the molecules forces a conformational change in PBP2a resulting in the opening of the active site and allowing acylation (inactivation) by the antibiotic. Although activity is largely restored towards methicillin-resistant organisms, MICs remain still typically one to four dilutions higher than for susceptible ones. The increase in lipophilicity also makes it necessary to administer the molecules as prodrugs – medocaril for ceftobiprole and fosamyl for ceftaroline (not shown).

Pharmacodynamics

Conventional glycopeptide antibiotics exhibit slow bactericidal activity, which is concentration independent. Because of their half-life (about 8 hours for vancomycin and much longer for teicoplanin), conventional glycopeptides display a 24-hour area under the serum concentration–time curve/MIC (AUC_{24h}/MIC) rather than a time above MIC phamacokinetic/pharmacodynamic pattern of activity.[11] This means that their mode of administration – whether discontinuous (q12h for vancomycin) or continuous – is similar. There is an increasing tendency to use vancomycin by continuous infusion (favored by its excellent aqueous stability) and to rely on trough rather than peak levels for optimum therapy. This contrasts with lipoglycopeptides, for which C_{max}/MIC ratios are probably more important. Lipoglycopeptides accumulate in macrophages and act on phagocytosed S. aureus.

Glycopeptides exhibit a synergistic effect with aminoglycosides, probably by facilitating the penetration of the latter drugs in bacteria.

Future developments

Talavancin has approved in 2009 for clinical use in the US, while oritavancin is still under development due to safety issues. Future developments should be geared towards clinical demonstration of superiority of these highly bactericidal molecules in comparison with vancomycin for 'difficult' indications.

Other agents acting on the cell membrane and cell wall synthesis

Daptomycin is a cyclic peptide flanked by an oxodecyl side chain conferring a strong amphiphilic character to the molecule (molecules in this group are often referred to as lipopeptides or peptolides; this erroneously suggests high lipophilicity, which is not true for daptomycin since the octanol–water partition is actually quite negative).

Table 130.1 Functional classification of β-lactamases

Group	Molecular class	Preferred substrates	Active β-lactams	Typical examples
Group 1: serine cephalosporinases not inhibited by clavulanic acid	C	Cephalosporins I, II, and III (>> cephalosporins IV, monobactams, penicillins)	Carbapenems Temocillin (cephalosporins III and IV; variable upon level of expression)	AmpC from Gram-negatives; variable upon the species
Group 2: serine β-lactamases				
2a: penicillinases inhibited by clavulanic acid	A	Penicillins (penicillin, ampicillin >> carbenicillin >> oxacillins)	Amoxicillin + clavulanic acid Cephalosporins Carbapenems	Penicillinases from Gram-positives
2b: broad-spectrum β-lactamases inhibited by clavulanic acid	A	Penicillins (penicillin, ampicillin >> carbenicillin >> oxacillins) Cephalosporins I and II	Cephalosporins III and IV Monobactams* Carbapenems Amoxicillin + clavulanic acid	TEM-1, TEM-2, SHV-1 from Enterobacteriaceae, Haemophilus spp., Neisseria gonorrhoeae
2be: extended spectrum β-lactamases inhibited by clavulanic acid (ESBL)	A	Penicillins Cephalosporins I II III (IV) Monobactams	Carbapenems Temocillin	TEM-3 to -29, 42, 43, 46–49, 52–58, 60, 61, 63, 65, 66, 72, 92 from Enterobacteriaceae SHV-2 to -9, 11–14, 18–22, 24 from Klebsiella spp. CTX-M-1 to CTX-M-54 (five phylogenetic groups) in Enterobacteriaceae K1-OXY from Klebsiella oxytoca
2br: broad spectrum β-lactamases with reduced binding to clavulanic acid	A	Penicillins	Most cephalosporins Monobactams* Carbapenems	TEM-30 to -41 (= IRT-1 to IRT-12), 44, 45, 50, 51, 59, 68, 73, 74, 76–79, 81–84 from Escherichia coli SHV-10 from Klebsiella spp.
2c: carbenicillin-hydrolyzing β-lactamases inhibited by clavulanic acid	A	Penicillins Carbenicillin (Cephalosporins I and II)	Piperacillin + tazobactam Cephalosporins III and IV Monobactams* Carbapenems	PSE-1, PSE-3, PSE-4 from Pseudomonas aeruginosa
2d: cloxacillin-hydrolyzing β-lactamases generally inhibited by clavulanic acid	D	Penicillins Cloxacillin Cephalosporins I and II	Carbapenems Cephalosporin III Monobactams* Piperacillin + tazobactam	OXA-1 to OXA-4 in Enterobacteriaceae OXA-2, OXA-10 (PSE-2) in Pseudomonas aeruginosa (penicillins, cefpirome, cefepime >> cephalosporins III) OXA-11 to -19, 28, 32, 45 are ESBLs in P. aeruginosa (R to Ceph 3, Ceph 4 and aztreonam) OXA-23, -24, -58 are carbapenemases in Acinetobacter baumannii

Table 130.1 Functional classification of β-lactamases—cont'd

Group	Molecular class	Preferred substrates	Active β-lactams	Typical examples
2e: cephalosporinases inhibited by clavulanic acid	A	Cephalosporins I and II	Cephalosporins III and IV Monobactams* Penems	FPM-1 from *Proteus vulgaris* Cep-A from *Bacteroides fragilis*[†] SME-1 to -3 from *Serratia* spp. IMI-1/2 and NMC-A from *Enterobacter cloacae* KPC-1 to -4 from *Klebsiella* spp. other Enterobacteriaceae and *Pseudomonas* GES-1 to -11 in Enterobacteriaceae, *P. aeruginosa* and *A. baumannii*
2f: carbapenem-hydrolyzing-nonmetallo β-lactamases	B	Most β-lactams, including carbapenems (low or high resistance level depending on enzyme, species and genetic environment)	Carbapenems Monobactams and β-lactam inhibitors (variable activity depending on type of enzyme, bacterial host and genetic environment)	
Group 3: metallo-β-lactamases inhibited by EDTA	B	Most β-lactams, including carbapenems	Monobactams*[‡]	L-1, XM-A from *Stenotrophomonas maltophilia* CcrA from *B. fragilis* A2h, CphA from *Aeromonas hydrophila* IMP-1 to -23, VIM-1 to -18 in *Pseudomonas*, other Gram-negative nonfermenters and Enterobacteriaceae SPM-1, GIM-1, SIM-1, DIN-1 in *P. aeruginosa* and *A. baumannii*
Group 4: penicillinases not inhibited by clavulanic acid		Penicillins, including carbenicillin and oxacillins	Monobactams*[‡] and generally carbapenems	SAR-2 from *B. cepacia*

*Monobactams are not active on Gram-positive bacteria.
[†]Penems are the only molecules active in this case.
[‡]Remain active for most of the rare published studies.
EDTA, ethylenediaminetetraacetic acid.
Compiled from [62, 63, 64, 65]. The number of enzymes as well as their spectrum of activity is continually evolving.

Daptomycin is used against vancomycin-resistant enterococci for staphylococcal infections. It has a novel mode of action, in that the molecule binds to Ca^{2+} to form an oligomeric assembly with the lipid tails pointing inwards. The loose micelles serve to deliver daptomycin to the bacterial membrane in a 'detergent-like' form, causing leakage of cytosolic contents and a rapid bactericidal effect (Fig. 130.7).[12] Daptomycin is only active against Gram-positive bacteria since it cannot cross the outer membrane of Gram-negative organisms. Daptomycin shows preferential interaction with the phospholipid, phosphatidylglycerol, which is abundant in prokaryotic cell membranes and largely absent from eukaryotic cell membranes, except in lung surfactant where it forms aggregates, thereby explaining the failure of daptomycin in treating pulmonary infections.

Resistance to daptomycin has already been described, resulting from mutations in genes that encode enzymes involved in the synthesis of phosphatidylglycerol. *Staphylococcus aureus* with a VISA phenotype (see glycopeptides section) are less susceptible to daptomycin due to impaired access through the thickened cell wall.[9]

Daptomycin activity is concentration dependent, whereas its toxicity (mainly for skeletal muscle) is more related to the frequency of exposure. As a result, daptomycin should be administered once daily. The original dose during development was 4 mg/kg. Whether this will be sufficient for difficult-to-treat staphylococcal infections and can be increased without eliciting unacceptable toxic reactions is presently investigated.

D-Cycloserine is a broad-spectrum antibiotic which has structural similarities to D-Ala (see Fig. 130.2; Fig. 130.8) and inhibits the conversion of L-Ala into D-Ala (catalyzed by a racemase) and the dimerization of D-Ala (catalyzed by the D-Ala:D-Ala ligase).[13]

Fosfomycin, which bears structural similarities to phospho-*enol*-pyruvate, inhibits very early stage synthesis of peptidoglycan by impairing the formation of uridine diphosphate (UDP)-*N*-acetyl-glucosamine-*enol*-pyruvate, a precursor of UDP-*N*-acetylmuramic acid (see Figs 130.2, 130.8).[14]

Bacitracin is a polypeptide of complex structure. It acts as an inhibitor of peptidoglycan synthesis at the level of translocation of the precursor across the bacterial membrane (see Fig. 130.2).[15]

ANTIBIOTICS THAT ACT ON PROTEIN SYNTHESIS

Bacterial ribosomes comprise:
- a 30S subunit that binds mRNA and initiates protein synthesis; and
- a 50S subunit that binds aminoacyl tRNA, catalyzes peptide bond formation and controls the elongation process.

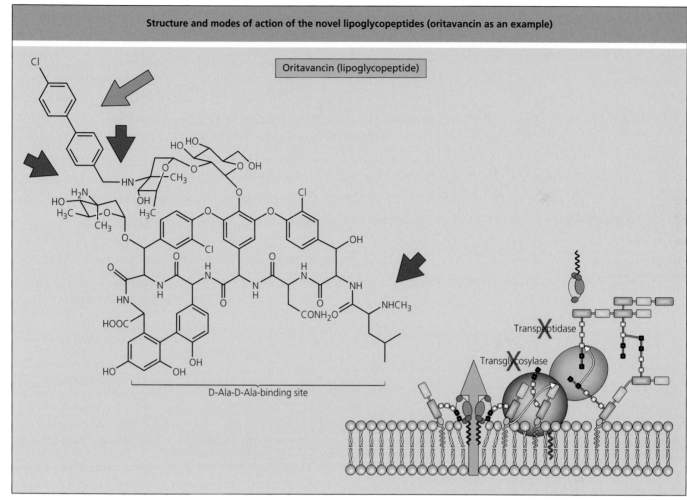

Fig. 130.6 Structure and proposed modes of action of the novel lipoglycopeptides (oritavancin as an example). Inset: the drugs are characterized by the presence of a bulky hydrophobic moiety (chorodiphenyl in this example; dark green arrow) and either additional amino groups (red arrows) or other polar groups (phosphonate for telavancin; not shown), resulting in a global amphiphilic character for the whole molecule. Note that the D-Ala-D-Ala binding site of the molecule remains unchanged. Main figure: the molecule interacts with the D-Ala-D-Ala termini of the pentapeptide (closed squares) as vancomycin, inhibiting both the transpeptidase and the transglycosidase activities, but also inserts itself into the membrane through its lipophilic side chain (this is favored, in the case of oritavancin, by its strong capacity to dimerize). As a result, lipoglycopeptides induce membrane leakage and thereby display a marked, concentration-dependent bactericidal effect. This second mode of action is exerted even if bacteria display a D-Ala-D-Lac or D-Ala-D-Ser in place of the D-Ala-D-Ala moiety, in as in vancomycin-resistant organisms. Specificity towards bacterial membranes probably stems from the fact that membrane-anchoring is enhanced by the presence of phospatidylglycerol, an acidic phospholipid abundant in bacterial but not in eukaryotic cell membranes. Adapted from Van Bambeke et al.[9]

The main sites identified in the 50S unit are the donor peptidyl site (P-site), where the growing peptide chain is fixed, and the acceptor aminoacyl site (A-site), where peptide bond formation occurs.

Aminoglycosides

Chemical structure

Streptomycin, discovered in 1944, has a limited spectrum of activity. Other aminoglycosides with a broader spectrum (kanamycins or gentamicins) have subsequently been obtained from natural sources. In the 1970s, the development of netilmicin and amikacin demonstrated the possibility of obtaining compounds active against strains resistant to earlier aminoglycosides.

Aminoglycosides comprise several aminohexoses joined by glycosidic linkages to a dibasic cyclitol.[16] The latter is streptidine in streptomycin and its derivatives, fortamine in the fortimicin series and 2-deoxystreptamine in most clinically used aminoglycosides.

This 2-deoxystreptamine moiety links to cyclic sugars either at positions 4 and 5 (neomycin and paromomycin) or 4 and 6 (kanamycin, tobramycin, amikacin and dibekacin for the kanamycin family; gentamicin C_1, C_{1a}, C_2, sisomicin, netilmicin and isepamicin for the gentamicin family; Fig. 130.9). All compounds are positively charged at physiologic pH.

Bacterial targeting

Aminoglycosides selectively inhibit bacterial protein synthesis by binding to the 30S ribosomal subunit. However, molecules displaying a hydroxyl function in C6' in place of an amino function (G-418, also known as geneticin) can also affect protein synthesis of eukaryotes.

Mode of action

Although the highly polar nature of aminoglycosides prevents diffusion through membranes, they do cross the outer membrane of

Structure and modes of action of the lipopeptide daptomycin

Daptomycin (lipopeptide)

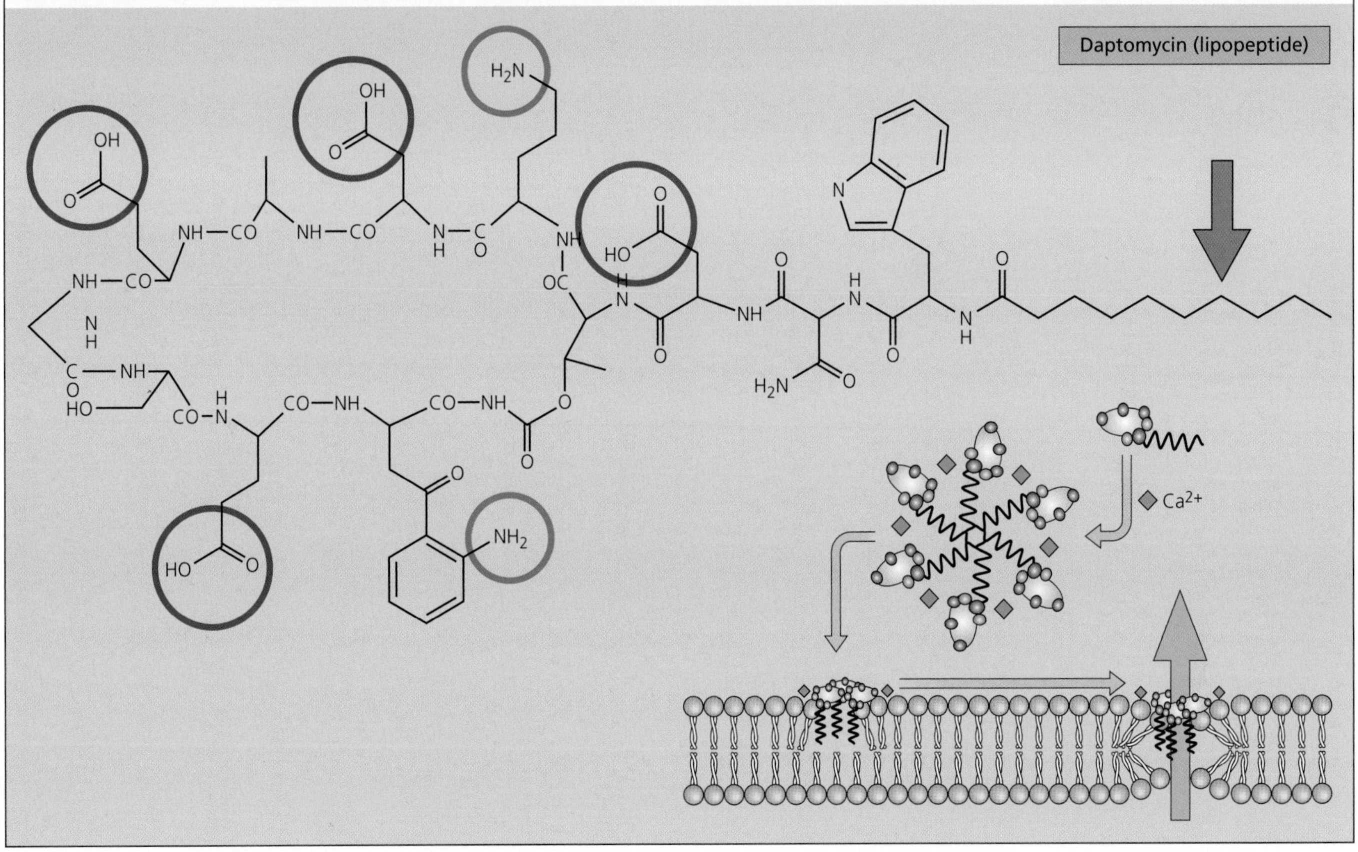

Fig. 130.7 Structure and mode of action of the lipopeptide daptomycin. The drug is a cyclic, polar depsipeptide (the ionizable residues are circled) flanked with a lipophilic oxodecyl side chain (purple arrow) conferring to the molecule a marked amphiphilic character. In the presence of Ca^{2+}, daptomycin forms loose micelles that serve as a delivery system to the bacterial membrane where the drug lipophilic side chain can then interact with the fatty acid chains of the phospholipids causing permeabilization and rapid bacterial death. As for lipoglycopeptides, specificity towards bacterial membranes stems from the fact that daptomycin–membrane interactions are favored by the presence of phosphatidylglycerol, an acidic phospholipid abundant in bacterial but not in eukaryotic cell membranes (it is, however, present in lung surfactant, causing daptomycin inactivation in this environment and explaining clinical failures in pulmonary infections). Modified from Van Bambeke *et al.*[9]

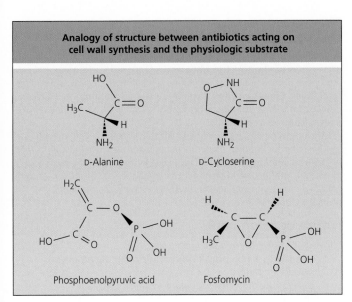

Analogy of structure between antibiotics acting on cell wall synthesis and the physiologic substrate

D-Alanine

D-Cycloserine

Phosphoenolpyruvic acid

Fosfomycin

Fig. 130.8 Analogy of structure between cycloserine and fosfomycin and the corresponding physiologic substrates involved in peptidoglycan synthesis.

Gram-negative bacteria through a non-energy-dependent process involving drug-induced disruption of Mg^{2+} bridges between adjacent lipopolysaccharide molecules. Their transport across the cytoplasmic (inner) membrane of both Gram-positive and Gram-negative bacteria is dependent upon electron transport and is therefore termed energy-dependent phase I (EDP-I). Being related to the capacity of the bacteria to maintain a transmembrane electrical potential, this transport is impaired in anaerobic environments, at low external pH or in high osmolar culture media, which explains the corresponding reductions of antibacterial activity.

Once in the bacterial cytosol, aminoglycosides bind largely to the aminoacyl site of the 30S subunit of ribosomes and, to a lesser extent, to specific sites of the 50S subunit, again through an energy-dependent process (energy-dependent phase II, EDP-II), disturbing the elongation of the nascent peptide. Their mechanism of action is complex, involving inhibition of the transfer of peptidyl tRNA from the A-site to the P-site and impairment of the proofreading process that controls translational accuracy.[17] The aberrant proteins may be inserted into the cell membrane, leading to altered permeability and further increasing aminoglycoside transport, which contributes to and explains the highly bactericidal, concentration-dependent activity of aminoglycosides. (Binding of aminoglycosides to RNA has also been related to antiviral effects and impairment of eukaryotic protein synthesis, which, however, are not observed under conditions of clinical usage of presently developed aminoglycosides.)

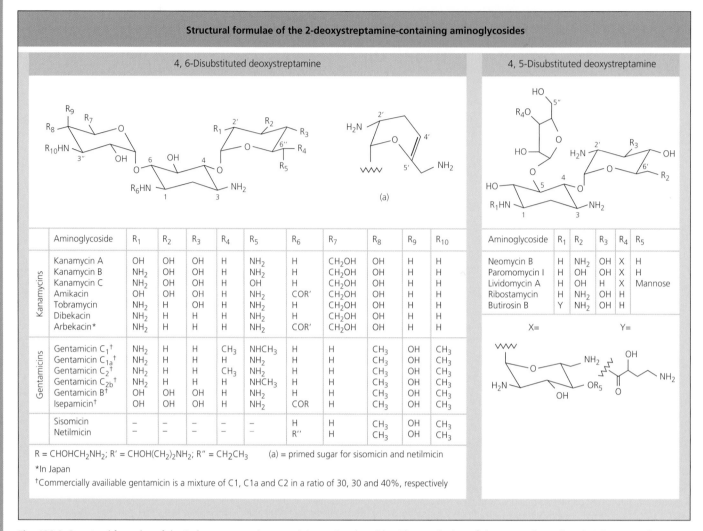

Structural formulae of the 2-deoxystreptamine-containing aminoglycosides

4, 6-Disubstituted deoxystreptamine

	Aminoglycoside	R₁	R₂	R₃	R₄	R₅	R₆	R₇	R₈	R₉	R₁₀
Kanamycins	Kanamycin A	OH	OH	OH	H	NH₂	H	CH₂OH	OH	H	H
	Kanamycin B	NH₂	OH	OH	H	NH₂	H	CH₂OH	OH	H	H
	Kanamycin C	NH₂	OH	OH	H	OH	H	CH₂OH	OH	H	H
	Amikacin	OH	OH	OH	H	NH₂	COR'	CH₂OH	OH	H	H
	Tobramycin	NH₂	H	OH	H	NH₂	H	CH₂OH	OH	H	H
	Dibekacin	NH₂	H	H	H	NH₂	H	CH₂OH	OH	H	H
	Arbekacin*	NH₂	H	H	H	NH₂	COR'	CH₂OH	OH	H	H
Gentamicins	Gentamicin C₁†	NH₂	H	H	CH₃	NHCH₃	H	H	CH₃	OH	CH₃
	Gentamicin C₁ₐ†	NH₂	H	H	H	NH₂	H	H	CH₃	OH	CH₃
	Gentamicin C₂†	NH₂	H	H	CH₃	NH₂	H	H	CH₃	OH	CH₃
	Gentamicin C₂ᵦ†	NH₂	H	H	H	NHCH₃	H	H	CH₃	OH	CH₃
	Gentamicin B†	OH	OH	OH	H	NH₂	H	H	CH₃	OH	CH₃
	Isepamicin†	OH	OH	OH	H	NH₂	COR	H	CH₃	OH	CH₃
	Sisomicin	–	–	–	–	–	H	H	CH₃	OH	CH₃
	Netilmicin	–	–	–	–	–	R''	H	CH₃	OH	CH₃

4, 5-Disubstituted deoxystreptamine

Aminoglycoside	R₁	R₂	R₃	R₄	R₅
Neomycin B	H	NH₂	OH	X	H
Paromomycin I	H	OH	OH	X	H
Lividomycin A	H	OH	H	X	Mannose
Ribostamycin	H	NH₂	OH	H	
Butirosin B	Y	NH₂	OH	H	

(a)

X= Y=

R = CHOHCH₂NH₂; R' = CHOH(CH₂)₂NH₂; R'' = CH₂CH₃   (a) = primed sugar for sisomicin and netilmicin

*In Japan

†Commercially availiable gentamicin is a mixture of C1, C1a and C2 in a ratio of 30, 30 and 40%, respectively

Fig. 130.9 Structural formulae of the 2-deoxystreptamine-containing aminoglycosides. The numbering of the atoms shown is as in Mingeot-Leclercq et al.[16] with the primed numbers (') being ascribed to the sugar attached to C4 of the 2-deoxystreptamine (as this C is of the R configuration) and the doubly primed numbers ('') being ascribed to the sugar attached to either the C6 (S configuration) for the 4,6-disubstituted 2-deoxystreptamine or the C5 (R configuration) for the 4,5-disubstituted 2-deoxystreptamine. (i) Eventually no molecule is shown in bold; (ii) the choice of one or another molecule is highly variable from one country to another (for non truly scientific reasons).

Resistance

Resistance occurs mainly from the production of aminoglycoside-modifying enzymes (Fig. 130.10). The semisynthetic derivatives (e.g. netilmicin, amikacin, isepamicin) were specifically designed to protect against the principal enzymes. However, multienzyme-producing bacteria have become increasingly common, causing multidrug resistance.[16] These enzymes may have physiologic functions against natural substrates and only target aminoglycosides opportunistically. However, point mutations and selection have quickly increased specificity and efficacy.[18]

A second mechanism of resistance causes membrane impermeabilization, the underlying mechanism of which is mainly active drug efflux, with at least five distinct systems described in bacteria of medical interest such as *Escherichia coli* and *Pseudomonas aeruginosa*.[19] Because efflux proteins seem to capture their substrate from the inner, hydrophobic core of membranes and since aminoglycosides are polar, it is believed that it is actually a combination of aminoglycosides and phospholipids that serves as a substrate for efflux.

A third mechanism involves post-transcriptional methylation of 16S rRNA occurring in Enterobacteriaceae and nonfermenters. This affects all currently used 2-deoxystreptamine-containing aminoglycosides, with at least six distinct genes reported worldwide.[20]

Pharmacodynamics

Aminoglycosides demonstrate rapid, concentration-dependent killing as well as an important postantibiotic effect, probably due to a largely irreversible binding to the ribosomes. Once-a-day regimens provide the optimal mode of administration, producing high peak serum concentrations. Simultaneously, toxicity (renal and auditory) is delayed as uptake of the drug into the target tissues is saturable. As a result, a once-daily schedule is preferred.

Aminoglycosides are synergistic with antibiotics acting on cell wall synthesis by facilitating bacterial penetration of the aminoglycoside. In contrast, their activity is antagonized by bacteriostatic agents such as chloramphenicol and tetracyclines, probably by inhibition of their energy-dependent uptake and interference with the movement of the ribosome along mRNA.

Future developments

Efforts have been directed at:
- increasing the binding affinity while retaining binding selectivity; and
- developing derivatives resistant to aminoglycoside-inactivating enzymes, with one novel molecule (ACHN-490 [6' (hydroxylethyl)-1-(haba)-sisomicin]) currently in clinical development.

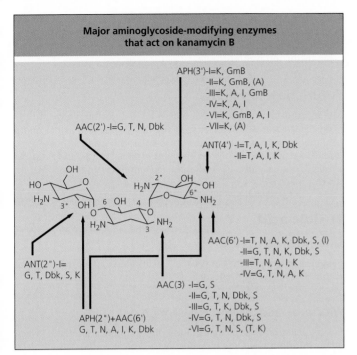

Major aminoglycoside-modifying enzymes that act on kanamycin B

Fig. 130.10 Major aminoglycoside-modifying enzymes that act on kanamycin C. This aminoglycoside is susceptible to the largest number of enzymes. The *N*-acetyltransferases (AACs) affect amino functions and the *o*-nucleotidyltransferases affect hydroxyl functions. Each group of enzymes inactivates specific sites, but each of these sites can be acted upon by distinct isoenzymes (Roman numerals) with different substrate specificities (phenotypic classification). At least one enzyme is bifunctional and affects both positions 2″ (*o*-phosphorylation) and 6′ (*N*-acetylation). The main aminoglycosides used clinically on which these enzymes act are amikacin (A), dibekacin (DbK), commercial gentamicin (G), gentamicin B (Gmb), kanamycin A (K), isepamicin (I), netilmicin (N), sisomicin (S) and tobramycin (T). The drug abbreviations that appear in parentheses are those for which resistance was detectable *in vitro* although clinical resistance was not conferred. Data from Shaw *et al.*[18]

Another approach has been to reduce aminoglycoside toxicity based on the underlying cellular and molecular mechanisms uncovered over the last 20 years.[21]

Tetracyclines and alkylaminocyclines

Chemical structure

The early tetracyclines were derived from *Streptomyces* spp. (tetracycline, oxytetracycline), in contrast to more recent semisynthetic compounds (doxycycline, minocycline). All are characterized by four hydrophobic fused rings, which are diversely substituted, but principally by oxygenated hydrophilic groups. Alkylaminocyclines possess an additional substituent with a bulky hydrophobic moiety and an ionizable amino function (Fig. 130.11). Tigecycline is often referred to as a glycylcycline based on the presence of a glycyl moiety as a spacer between the main part of the molecule and the ter-butyl-amino group. Because other derivatives with similar properties have different spacers but a similar hydrophobic amino group, a better name for the class is alkylaminocyclines.

Bacterial targeting

Tetracyclines penetrate the outer membrane of Gram-negative organisms through porins. Intracellular accumulation inside the bacteria depends on the pH gradient between the cytosol and the external medium, which may occur by diffusion or a transmembrane proton-

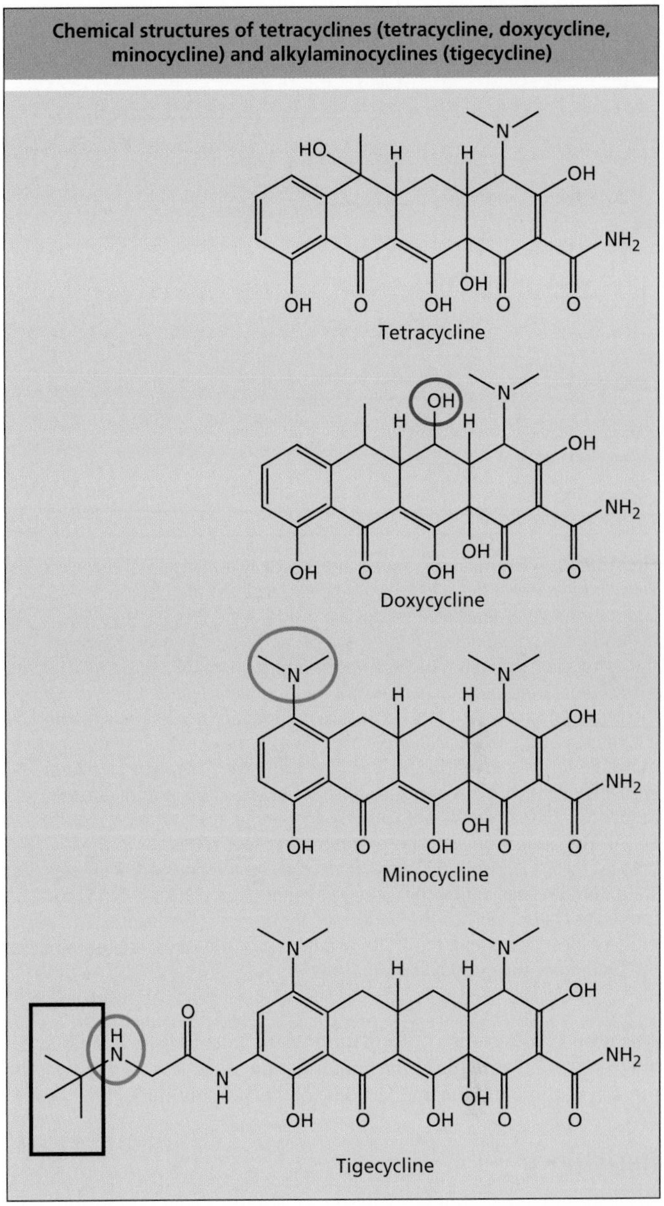

Chemical structures of tetracyclines (tetracycline, doxycycline, minocycline) and alkylaminocyclines (tigecycline)

Fig. 130.11 Chemical structures of tetracyclines (tetracycline, doxycycline, minocycline) and alkylaminocyclines (tigecycline). The figure highlights the displacement of a hydroxyl group between tetracycline and doxycycline, and the additional ionizable aminofunction in minocycline which confer a more prolonged half-life and improved activity (minocycline). Tigecycline is the first of a new group of derivatives with a bulky hydrophobic moiety (square; *ter*-butyl in the case of tigecycline) and an additional amino group (circled) that make the molecule less susceptible to efflux by tetracycline–specific transporters as well as to ribosomal protection, the two main mechanisms of bacterial resistance towards all other tetracyclines.

driven carrier. The main argument in favoring the latter is that it could explain the selective action of tetracyclines (Fig. 130.12).

Mode of action

Tetracyclines interfere with the initiation step of protein synthesis (Fig. 130.12). More precisely, they inhibit the binding of aminoacyl tRNA to the A-site of the ribosome.[22] The 7S protein and the 16S RNA show the greatest affinity for tetracyclines and are therefore the main targets. This binding inhibits the fixation of a new aminoacyl tRNA on the ribosome. In addition, tetracyclines bind, or at least protrude, in the P-site by

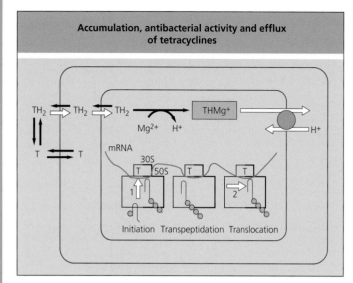

Accumulation, antibacterial activity and efflux of tetracyclines

Fig. 130.12 Accumulation, antibacterial activity and efflux of tetracyclines. Tetracyclines freely diffuse through the extracellular membrane of Gram-negative organisms. Penetration inside bacteria is an energy-dependent process, depending on the pH and Mg^{2+} gradient between the extracellular medium of Gram-positive organisms or the periplasmic medium of Gram-negative organisms and the intracellular medium. Only the protonated form is highly diffusible, so that accumulation is favored by a lowering of the extracellular pH. Once inside the cytosol, the tetracycline molecule forms a nondiffusible complex with Mg^{2+}. This type of complex with a bivalent cation is also the substrate of the efflux pumps present in the membrane of resistant bacteria and acting as H^+ antiports (purple circle). The antibacterial action of the tetracyclines (T) is due to their binding to the 30S subunit of the ribosomes. In the pretranslocational state, tetracyclines inhibit the binding of aminoacyl tRNA (arrow 1) to the A-site (yellow part of the ribosome). In the post-translocational state, tetracyclines protrude in the P-site (white part of the ribosome) and inhibit the binding of the peptidyl-tRNA (arrow 2).

alteration in ribosome conformation in the post-translocational state, and may modify the ribosome conformation at the level of the head of the 30S subunit and the interface side of the 50S subunit.

Resistance

Resistance to tetracyclines is widespread. Some 29 genes on mobile elements have been identified in the so-called 'tetracycline' (tet) family and three in the 'oxytetracycline resistance' gene family (otr).[22] Among the tet and otr genes, two main mechanisms have been described, namely efflux (which is an important and widespread mechanism of bacterial resistance, and was actually discovered with tetracyclines) and ribosomal protection. Resistance by enzymatic inactivation has been described but remains uncommon. Low levels of resistance can also result from mutations or a decrease in porin content of the outer membrane, with consequent decreased tetracycline uptake in Gram-negative bacteria.

As tigecycline increases the number of bonds to the target 16S RNA, the drug is unaffected by the ribosome protection mechanism.[23] Together with the vicinal hydrophobic moiety, it makes the molecule less susceptible to efflux, and is therefore active against many Gram-negative organisms with the exception of *P. aeruginosa* and Proteae because of a resistance nodulation cell division (RND)-type efflux pump (MexXY-OprM) constitutively expressed by these bacteria.[24]

Pharmacodynamics

Tetracyclines are essentially bacteriostatic and need to be administered at intervals determined by the drug half-life in order to maintain their serum level above the MIC of the infecting organism for as long as possible. Because of their prolonged half-life, however, $AUC_{24h}/$

MIC emerges as the main parameter driving the activity of tetracyclines (including tigecycline) *in vivo*. In contrast to conventional tetracyclines, tigecycline has no useful oral bioavailability and must be given by the intravenous route.

Future developments

Mutants resistant to tigecycline (mostly related to efflux) have already been reported in *Acinetobacter* spp. The development of efflux pump inhibitors would also be useful not only in this context but also to extend the activity of tigecycline and similar compounds against *P. aeruginosa*. Orally bioavailable alkylaminocyclines are also in development.

Fusidic acid

Chemical structure

Fusidic acid is a steroid-like structure, belonging to the fusidane class. It is used in its sodium salt form.

Mode of action and resistance

Fusidic acid prevents the dissociation of the complex formed between guanosine diphosphate, elongation factor 2 and the ribosome, thereby inhibiting the translocation step of the peptidyl tRNA from the P-site to the A-site of the ribosome.[25] Because of a lack of cross-resistance with other antistaphylococcal agents, fusidic acid is enjoying a revival in several countries in the treatment of multiresistant *S. aureus*, but always in combination because of the high rate of emergence of resistance when used as monotherapy (mainly based on data from drug usage as a topical application; this could be much less if the drug is given orally).[26] The latter seems to result from the acquisition of the *fusB* gene (located on a transposon-like element of which homologues exist in many clinically important and environmental Gram-positive bacterial species), which protects ribosomal protein synthesis inhibition from fusidic acid in a dose-dependent fashion.[27]

Pharmacodynamics

Fusidic acid is bacteriostatic but may be bactericidal at high concentrations. Although fusidic acid has been used in many countries for years, it has never been approved in the US so far. In view of the mounting epidemic of community-acquired MRSA, a clinical development of fusidic acid in the US is presently under way.

Mupirocin

Chemical structure

Mupirocin contains a short fatty acid side chain (9-hydroxynonanoic acid) linked to monic acid by an ester linkage. Mupirocin is also called pseudomonic acid because its major metabolite is derived from submerged fermentation by *Pseudomonas fluorescens*. Pseudomonic acid A is responsible for most of the antibacterial activity; three other minor metabolites of similar chemical structure and antimicrobial spectrum have been called pseudomonic acids B, C and D.

Mode of action and resistance

Mupirocin inhibits bacterial RNA and protein synthesis by binding to bacterial isoleucyl tRNA synthetase, which catalyzes the formation of isoleucyl tRNA from isoleucine and tRNA. This prevents incorporation of isoleucine into protein chains, leading to arrest of protein synthesis. Resistance to mupirocin develops through the production of a modified target enzyme.[28]

Because of its unique mechanism of action, there is no cross-resistance between mupirocin and other antimicrobial agents.[29]

Pharmacodynamics

Mupirocin is bacteriostatic at low concentration but becomes bactericidal at concentrations achieved locally by topical administration. The *in vitro* antibacterial activity is greatest at acidic pH, which is advantageous in the treatment of cutaneous infections because of the low pH of the skin.

Future developments

The peculiar mode of action of mupirocin has triggered genomic-based research to identify similar targets at the level of the other amino acids, which could lead to new compounds.

Retapamulin

Retapamulin is a semisynthetic derivative of pleuromutilin, a naturally occurring tricyclic antibiotic, diterpene, discovered in the early 1950s, and out of which only veterinary antibiotics had been developed until now. Retapamulin inhibits bacterial protein synthesis by binding to domain V of 23S rRNA, thereby blocking peptide formation directly by interfering with substrate binding. Resistance occurs through mutations in the genes encoding 23S rRNA, but is not crossed with other antibiotics as the binding site is unique compared with those of other antibiotics acting on ribosomes.[30] This makes retapamulin appealing for the treatment of a variety of susceptible Gram-positive pathogens. Retapamulin has been developed as a topical antibiotic for the management of impetigo and uncomplicated secondarily infected traumatic skin lesions.

Macrolides
Chemical structure

The main active macrolides are 14-, 15- or 16-membered lactone rings, substituted by two sugars, one of which bears an aminated function. In 15-membered macrolides (azithromycin), an additional aminated function is inserted in the lactone ring, conferring to this subclass of molecule the name of 'azalides'. Ketolides are 14-membered macrolides in which the cladinose is replaced by a keto function and which possess in their macrocycle a carbamate linked to an alkyl-aryl extension, represented by telithromycin as the only registered antibiotic (Fig. 130.13).[31]

Erythromycin, the first clinically developed macrolide, is a natural product. Most of the more recent molecules are semisynthetic derivatives designed to be stable in acidic milieu, and are therefore characterized by an improved oral bioavailability. Both 16-membered macrolides and ketolides are intrinsically acid stable.

Bacterial targeting

Macrolides specifically bind to the 50S subunit of the ribosomes (more precisely, to the 23S rRNA), which does not exist in eukaryotic cells.

Mode of action

Macrolides reversibly bind to the peptidyl transferase center, located at the 50S surface, causing multiple alterations of the 50S subunit functions. While macrolides only bind to domain V of the 23S rRNA, ketolides also bind to domain II of 23S rRNA as a result of their carbamate extension, and thus are double anchored to their target (Fig. 130.14).[32] Macrolides are classically thought to block the peptide bond formation or the peptidyl tRNA translocation from the A-site to the P-site. However, additional consequences of their binding to ribosomes have been reported. It has been proposed that they could also favor the premature dissociation of peptidyl tRNA from the ribosome during the elongation process, leading to the synthesis of incomplete peptides.[33] It has also been suggested that erythromycin prevents the assembly of the 50S subunit, a property not generalizable to other macrolides.

Resistance

Clinically meaningful resistance occurs primarily by modification of the bacterial target and therefore affects all macrolides; it can also occur by efflux.[34] Target modification also affects lincosamides and streptogramins because of the common binding site for these three classes of antibiotic and also explains why macrolides, streptogramins, lincosamides and chloramphenicol have antagonist pharmacologic activity. Resistance to macrolides may be inducible or constitutive; however, if inducible it will not affect streptogramins and lincosamides since these are not inducers.[34] Ketolides (due to their lack of cladinose) and 16-membered macrolides are not inducers and therefore show activity on a subset of resistant strains. Moreover, the double ribosomal anchoring of ketolides confers a higher affinity not only for wild-type ribosomes, but also for ribosomes of strains resistant by methylation of domain V, with consequent improved activity against resistant strains.[31]

Although efflux mechanisms are being reported, 16-membered macrolides are again spared this effect. The frequency of strains susceptible to 16-membered macrolides and resistant to 14- and 15-membered macrolides remains low, however.

Pharmacodynamics

Macrolides are essentially bacteriostatic antibiotics, except at high concentrations. Their concentration at the infected site therefore needs to be durably maintained above the MIC of the pathogen. Because of their prolonged half-life, clarithromycin, azithromycin and telithromycin have been shown to primarily reflect the AUC_{24h}/MIC parameter *in vivo*.[31]

Future developments

Efforts to develop new ketolides continue, with the aim of selecting compounds with improved intrinsic activity (especially against multiresistant pneumococci and community-acquired MRSA) and a better safety profile, as telithromycin has been severely restricted in its indications because of liver toxicity.[31]

Lincosamides
Chemical structure

Lincomycin and its 7-chloro-7-deoxy derivative, clindamycin, comprise a propylhygrinic acid linked to an aminosugar.

Mode of action

Lincosamides bind to the 50S ribosomal subunit and have a mode of action similar to that of macrolides.

Resistance

The main mechanism of resistance to lincosamides is similar to that of macrolides and streptogramins and consists of an alteration of the 50S subunit. Rare cases of enzymatic inactivation (adenylation reaction) of the antibiotic have also been described for clindamycin. Resistance dissociation is, however, observed for those strains for which macrolide resistance is inducible, as clindamycin is not an inducer.[35] Likewise, efflux-mediated resistance to macrolides does not affect lincosamides, also leading to resistance dissociation.[34]

Pharmacodynamics

Lincosamides are bacteriostatic and are antagonists of macrolides and streptogramins, which bind at the same site on the ribosomes.

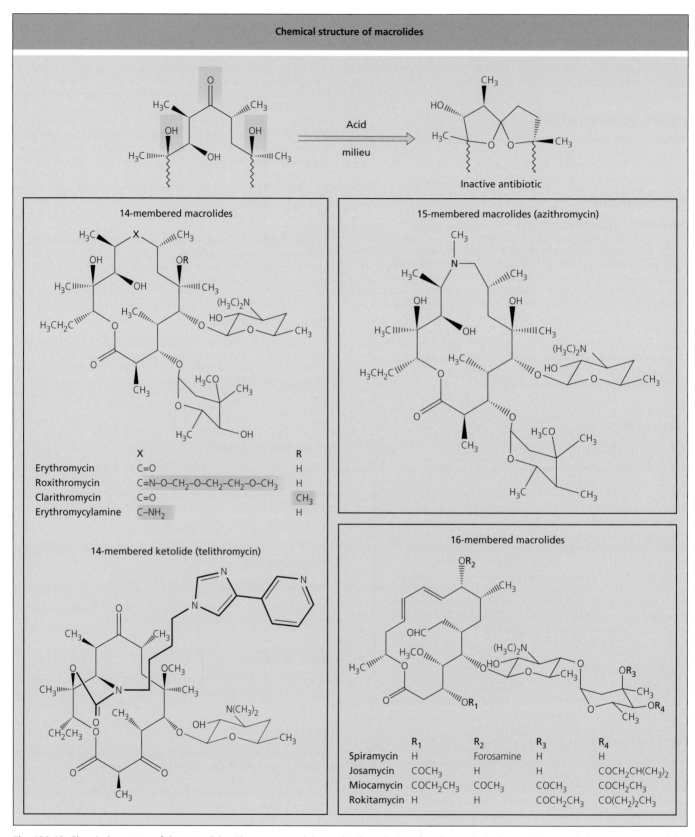

Fig. 130.13 Chemical structure of the macrolides. The upper panel shows the degradation of erythromycin in the gastric milieu (substituents responsible for the instability of the miolecule are shown in purple). 16-Membered macrolides and ketolides are intrinsically stable. The structural modifications conferring stability in acidic milieu to 14- and 15-membered macrolides are highlighted in pink in the middle panel.

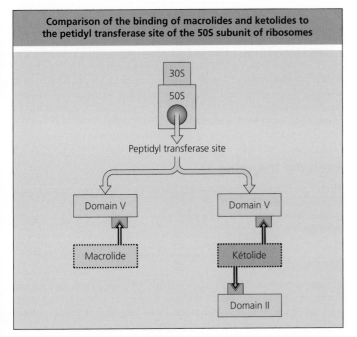

Comparison of the binding of macrolides and ketolides to the petidyl transferase site of the 50S subunit of ribosomes

Fig. 130.14 Comparison of the binding of macrolides and ketolides to the peptidyl transferase site of the 50S subunit of ribosomes. Macrolides are characterized by a single anchoring point and ketolides by a double anchoring point, which increases the affinity of ketolides for wild type and methylated ribosomes.

Streptogramins

Chemical structure

Streptogramins are antibiotics that comprise a pair of synergistic constituents, namely a depsipeptide (group I) and a lactonic macrocycle (group II). Quinupristin–dalfopristin is the only combination used in the clinic so far.[36]

Mode of action

Streptogramins bind to the 50S subunit of the bacterial ribosome. They interfere with protein synthesis by a double mechanism, involving inhibition of the incorporation of aminoacyl tRNA in the ribosome and the translation of mRNA. The synergistic effects of the two components could be due to a modification of the conformation of the ribosome caused by binding of the group I component, which exposes a site of fixation for the group II component.[33]

Resistance

Resistance is by mutation of the ribosomal target and results in cross-resistance with macrolides and lincosamides. Because of the presence of two components, however, synergistins remain active against many macrolide and lincosaminide-resistant isolates. Resistance to streptogramins alone is rare and occurs by enzymatic inactivation (hydrolase and acetylase).

Pharmacodynamics

Streptogramin constituents are highly synergistic and exhibit dose-dependent bactericidal activity in combination. In addition, they also increase the antibiotic activity of aminoglycosides and rifamycins. Streptogramins also exhibit a prolonged postantibiotic effect with delayed regrowth when the antibiotic concentration falls under its MIC. This may result from persistent binding of the drug to its target.

Future developments

Quinupristin/dalfopristin currently has limited use only. There is, however, a potential interest in novel streptogramins for the treatment of infections caused by bacteria resistant to other antibiotics, mainly multi-resistant *S. aureus* and vancomycin-resistant enterococci. At least one compound for oral administration (NX-103) is under development.

Chloramphenicol and thiamphenicol

Chemical structure

These antibiotics are constructed on a dichloroacetamide bearing a diversely substituted phenyl group.

Bacterial targeting

Chloramphenicol acts principally by binding to the 50S subunit of the bacterial ribosomes. However, it can also interact with mitochondrial ribosomes of eukaryotic cells, which results in its toxicity.

Mode of action

Chloramphenicol enters the bacteria by an energy-dependent process. Its antibiotic activity is due to competitive inhibition for the binding of aminoacyl tRNA to the peptidyltransferase domain of the 50S subunit. This induces conformational change in the ribosome, which slows or even inhibits the incorporation of the aminoacyl tRNA and in turn the transpeptidation reaction.[37]

Resistance

Resistance to chloramphenicol is mainly due to the production of a specific inactivating acetyltransferase.[38] The encoding gene is often located on plasmids that also confer resistance to other antibiotic classes. Another mechanism of resistance results in reduced drug entry into the bacterium.

Pharmacodynamics

Chloramphenicol is bacteriostatic. It competes in binding to the ribosomes with macrolides and lincosamides, making its combination with these drugs useless.

Oxazolidinones

Chemical structure

Like fluoroquinolones, oxazolidinones are synthetic molecules. The first derivatives were described in the 1970s, although linezolid, the first clinically available molecule, only became available in the 1990s (Fig. 130.15). The 5-(S)-configuration of the oxazolidinone ring is essential for activity, which is further improved by its substitution by an *N*-fluorinated aryl group and a C5 acylaminomethyl group.[39]

Mode of action

Oxazolidinones inhibit protein synthesis at an earlier step than other antibiotics acting on the ribosome. Their binding site is located in the vicinity of the peptidyl transferase with the A-site of the bacterial ribosome where they seem to interfere with the placement of the aminoacyl tRNA.[40] This interaction prevents the formation of the initiation ternary complex which associates tRNA^{met}, mRNA and the 50S subunit of the ribosome, and therefore the binding to the ribosome as well as the synthesis of peptide bonds, and the translocation of tRNA^{met} into the P-site. They can compete for binding to the 50S subunit with other antibiotics (e.g. lincosamides, chloramphenicol) without being antagonistic.

Linezolid, the only available oxazolidinone, is mainly active against Gram-positive cocci, with minimal activity against most Gram-negative bacteria as a result of drug efflux in these organisms.[41]

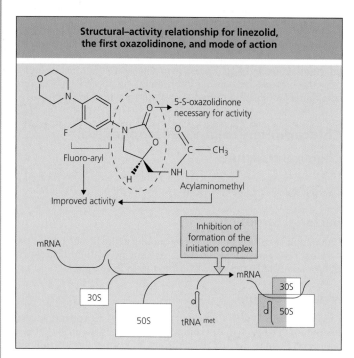

Fig. 130.15 Structure–activity relationship for linezolid, the first oxazolidinone, and mode of action. The drug prevents the formation of the ternary complex between mRNA, ribosome subunits and tRNA^{met} necessary for protein synthesis.

Oxazolidinones also interact with mitochondrial ribosomes to inhibit protein synthesis, which is probably the basis for the undesirable myelosuppressive effects of linezolid.[42]

Resistance

Because of the unique mode of action of oxazolidinones, there is no cross-resistance with other antibiotics acting on protein synthesis. Resistance develops following point mutations of the 23S rRNA[43] or deletions in the gene encoding riboprotein L4.[44]

Pharmacodynamics

Oxazolidinones are bacteriostatic against enterococci and staphylococci with a short postantibiotic effect. For streptococci, linezolid is bactericidal for the majority of strains. Because of its prolonged half-life, linezolid activity is primarily dependent on the AUC_{24h}/MIC parameter *in vivo*.[11]

Future developments

New oxazolidinones being developed have a broadened spectrum, increasing intrinsic activity and, potentially, reduced side-effects, and no new compounds (torezolid and radezolid) are currently in clinical development.

DRUGS THAT AFFECT NUCLEIC ACIDS (DNA/RNA)

Fluoroquinolones

Chemical structure

Fluoroquinolones are totally synthetic products originally derived from nalidixic acid. All current compounds have a dual ring structure, with a nitrogen at position 1, a free carboxylate at position 3 and a carbonyl at position 4. A fluor substituent at position 6 usually greatly enhances activity, whereas the substituents at positions 7, 8 and N1 modulate the spectrum, the pharmacokinetics and the side-effects of the drugs (Fig. 130.16).[45] In this respect, more recent molecules (moxifloxacin, gemifloxacin, gatifloxacin) have been designed to better cover Gram-positive organisms, while retaining activity against Gram-negative organisms and, in the case of moxifloxacin, against anaerobes. They all present a small hydrophobic substituent at N1 and a diaminated small-sized ring substituent at position 7.

Bacterial targeting

Fluoroquinolones cross the outer membrane of Gram-negative bacteria via porins. Their affinity for their bacterial target is 1000 times greater than for the corresponding eukaryotic enzyme, which ensures their specificity.

Mode of action

Fluoroquinolones inhibit the activity of topoisomerases. These enzymes are responsible for the supercoiling of DNA (DNA gyrase) and the relaxation of supercoiled DNA (topoisomerase IV). Both enzymes have a similar mode of action, implying:
- the binding of DNA to the enzyme;
- the cleavage of the DNA;
- the passage of the DNA segment through the DNA gate; and
- the resealing of the DNA break and release from the enzyme.

Gyrase and topoisomerase IV are tetramers composed of two types of subunit, namely two GyrA or ParC catalyzing the DNA cutting and resealing, and two GyrB or ParE responsible for the transduction and binding of ATP. The main target of fluoroquinolones is DNA gyrase in Gram-negative bacteria and topoisomerase IV in Gram-positive bacteria.[46]

Fluoroquinolones form a ternary complex with DNA and the enzyme (Fig. 130.17).[47] This binding site for fluoroquinolones is formed during the gate-opening step of the double-stranded DNA. Co-operatively, four fluoroquinolone molecules are fixed to single-stranded DNA. Their stacking is favored by the presence of the co-planar aromatic rings in their structure and by the tail-to-tail interactions between the substituents at N1. Interaction with DNA occurs by hydrogen bonds or via Mg^{2+} bridges established with the carbonyl and carboxylate groups. Interaction with the enzyme is mediated by fluoride at position 6 and the substituents at position 7. The binding of the fluoroquinolones stabilizes the cleavable complex (formed by the cut DNA and the enzyme) and leads to the dissociation of the enzyme subunits. The latter action is, however, observed only for potent molecules or at higher concentrations.

Fluoroquinolones are highly bactericidal, which is not explained by the above mechanisms alone and requires RNA and protein synthesis to be observed, suggesting the formation of abnormal proteins as a consequence of DNA cleavage. Quinolones also induce an SOS (DNA repair) response, which involves three proteins (RecA, LexA and RecBCD). Induced RecA cleaves the repressor of the SOS regulon (LexA), stimulating repair of damage caused by fluoroquinolones to DNA. Induced RecBCD binds to the chromosome at the double-strand break created by the ternary complex of topoisomerase–DNA–quinolone, leading to mutagenesis as well as increased cell survival in the presence of quinolones. This system therefore protects against the antibacterial activity of fluoroquinolones and could be a basis for emergence of resistance.[48]

Resistance

Resistance was long considered to be only chromosomally mediated from mutation of the topoisomerases (reducing drug-binding ability), porin impermeabilization (for Gram-negative bacteria) or

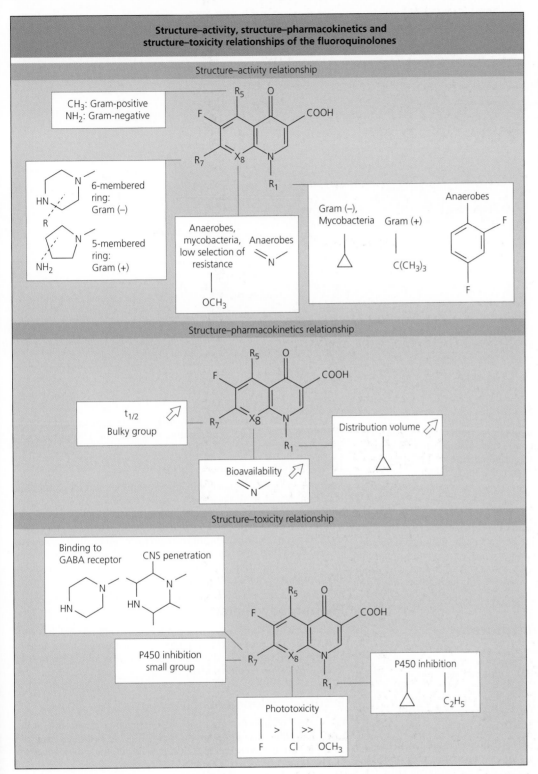

Fig. 130.16 Structure–activity, structure–pharmacokinetics and structure–toxicity relationships of the fluoroquinolones. These considerations form the basis of the rational development of the new molecules of this class, which have a very extended spectrum (including Gram-positive bacteria and anaerobes), a long half-life and minimal phototoxicity and metabolic interactions.

efflux.[45] A methoxy substituent at position 8 (see Fig. 130.16) lowers the ratio of the MIC in gyrase mutant strains to the corresponding MIC in the wild type, thereby reducing the risk of selecting resistant mutants during therapy. Plasmid-mediated resistance, however, is now increasingly observed,[49] related to the production of:

- Qnr proteins capable of protecting DNA gyrase from quinolones (which have homologues in water-dwelling bacteria where they probably serve as chaperones); and
- AAC(6′)-Ib-cr, a variant aminoglycoside acetyltransferase capable of acetylating ciprofloxacin.

Pharmacodynamics

The activity of fluoroquinolones is largely both concentration dependent (which drives the bactericidal effect) and proportional to the amount of drug administered (which drives the global efficacy *in vivo*), making these drugs C_{max}/MIC and AUC_{24h}/MIC dependent for their activity. For older fluoroquinolones that have a short half-life (e.g. ciprofloxacin), this imposes the use of repeated doses per day (combining all doses in a single administration would favor bactericidal effects but would risk toxic reactions). For newer fluoroquinolones with more prolonged

Fig. 130.17 Ternary complex formed between DNA, DNA–gyrase or –topoisomerase IV and stacked fluoroquinolones. Subunits A form covalent bonds via Tyr122 with the 5′ end of the DNA chain. The binding site for fluoroquinolones is located in the bubble formed during the local opening of the DNA molecule. The right panel shows the parts of the antibiotic molecules interacting with DNA, with the enzyme, or favoring the stacking of the fluoroquinolone molecules. Adapted from Shen et al.[47]

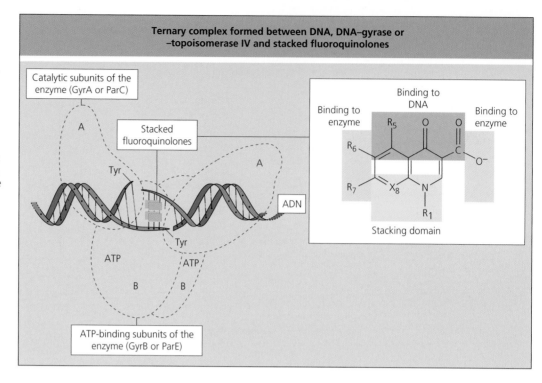

Ternary complex formed between DNA, DNA–gyrase or –topoisomerase IV and stacked fluoroquinolones

half-lives (levofloxacin, moxifloxacin, gemifloxacin), once-daily administration is possible, with the aim of obtaining both C_{max}/MIC (>8) and AUC_{24h}/MIC (from 30 to 125 or more) ratios, offering optimal efficacy and minimizing selection of resistant subpopulations.[45,50] The European breakpoints (usually ≤2 mg/l) have taken this into account.

Future developments

New molecules with extended spectra, still greater intrinsic activity and resistance to efflux transporters are being sought, although a major difficulty is to avoid increases in toxicity. Molecules with enhanced activity at acid pH (for urinary tract, intracellular or stomach infections) or much lower MICs than registered fluroquinolones are currently being developed.

Nitroimidazoles and nitrofurans

Chemical structure

The nitroheterocyclic drugs include nitrofuran and nitroimidazole compounds (Fig. 130.18).

Mode and spectrum of action

The activity of the nitroheterocyclic drugs requires activation of the nitro group attached to the imidazole or furan ring, which must undergo single- or two-electron enzymatic reduction in the bacteria.[51] Although the nitro radicals generated by reduction of the parent drugs are similar for the nitroimidazoles and the nitrofurans, these drugs differ by their reduction potential, and therefore their spectrum of activity. Thus nitroimidazoles must be fully reduced to generate the highly reactive species (hydroxylamines) that cause damage, whereas singly reduced nitrofurans may directly inhibit the activity of enzymes involved in the degradation of glucose and pyruvate and covalently bind to proteins and DNA by an alkylation reaction. Nitroimidazoles will, therefore, express activity only towards truly anaerobic and microaerophilic bacteria, and to other parasitic organisms such as *Trichomonas vaginalis*, capable of generating a sufficiently low redox potential thanks to the

presence of an H_2-generating organelle (hydrogenosome), whereas nitrofuranes are equally active against anaerobic and aerobic bacteria.

Resistance

Resistance to nitroimidazoles in true anaerobic bacteria is rare, but has been described in *Bacteroides fragilis* (combination of decreased antibiotic uptake, reduced nitroreductase and pyruvate:ferredoxin oxidoreductase activity and increased lactate dehydrogenase activity).[52] It has become significant in *Helicobacter pylori* (null mutations in *rdxA* encoding an oxygen-insensitive nitroreductase that normally prevents reoxidization of metronidazole in the microaerophilic environment of this bacterium).[53]

Pharmacodynamics

Nitroimidazoles show concentration-dependent killing, which is consistent with the current clinical pattern of dispensing a large dose in a single administration (although more frequent administration of lower dose is also recommended).

Future developments

The variety of substitutions that can be attached to the ring structures may allow new drug development. This has not been explored so far for antibacterial therapy, although finding new derivatives for amebiasis and giardiasis is being actively pursued.

Ansamycins

Chemical structure

These macrocyclic antibiotics are lipophilic and therefore easily diffuse through membranes. They comprise two aromatic rings (containing a quinone), connected by a long chain (or 'ansa' – hence the name given to this class of antibiotics), which confers a rigid character to the whole molecule. The first clinically developed and major antibiotic in this class is rifampin (rifampicin). Successful successors have been rifapentin, rifamixin and rifabutin.

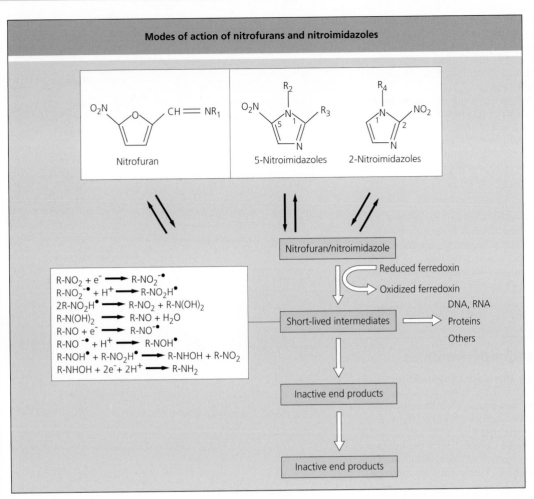

Fig. 130.18 Structures and modes of action of nitrofurans and nitroimidazoles. The molecules must be reduced to form highly reactive products that interact with intracellular targets.

Mode of action

Ansamycins inhibit the initiation of the transcription of DNA in mRNA and therefore subsequent protein synthesis. The RNA polymerase is made up of five subunits ($\alpha_2\beta\beta'\sigma$):

- α subunits establish contact with transcription factors;
- β′ subunit is a basic polypeptide that binds DNA;
- β subunit is an acidic polypeptide and is part of the active site; and
- σ initiates transcription and then leaves the polymerase nucleus.

The core polymerase ($\alpha_2\beta\beta'$) therefore retains the capacity to synthesize RNA but is defective in its ability to bind and initiate DNA transcription.

Inhibition by rifamycins follows binding of the antibiotic to the β subunit of the RNA polymerase or, to a lesser extent, of the DNA–RNA complex. This binding is mediated by hydrophobic interactions between the aliphatic ansa chain and the β subunit. The precise site of binding has been identified only partly, by studying mutants in RNA polymerase that have acquired resistance to rifampin. All the mutations affecting drug binding belong to three clusters of amino acids in the central domain of the β subunit. Specificity of action depends on the fact that ansamycins alter mammalian cell metabolism only at concentrations 10 000 times those necessary to cause bacterial cell death (Fig. 130.19).

Pharmacodynamics

Rifamycins are bactericidal. This effect could be due to either the high stability of the complex formed between rifampin and the enzyme or the formation of superoxide ions of the quinone ring of the antibiotic molecule. Because their action is to hinder bacterial multiplication,

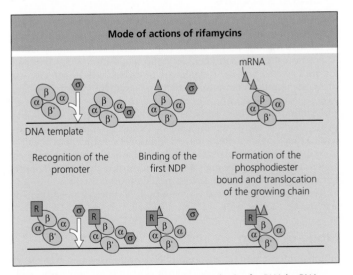

Fig. 130.19 Mode of action of rifamycins. Synthesis of mRNA by RNA polymerase is shown in the upper panel and inhibition by rifamycins (R in the green squares) is shown in the lower panel. The RNA polymerase core is made up of four subunits, of which the β′ subunit binds to the DNA template and the β subunit binds the ribonucleotide diphosphate (NDP; triangle). The σ factor only participates to the initiation step by allowing for the recognition by the enzyme core of promoter sequences on the DNA template. Rifamycins bind to the β subunit. They do not interfere with the binding of the nucleotide diphosphate, but rather inhibit the transcription initiation either by impairing the formation of the first phosphodiester bond or the translocation reaction of the newly synthesized dinucleotide.

they are, at least *in vitro*, antagonists to antibiotics requiring active bacterial growth to exert their activity (β-lactams) or to other antibiotics acting on protein synthesis (macrolides and aminoglycosides). This antagonism is, however, not observed *in vivo* because of the different distribution of these antibiotics (intracellular for rifamycins vs extracellular for β-lactams and aminoglycosides).

Rifamycins show a long postantibiotic effect because of the irreversible character of their binding. The excellent penetration of rifamycins in eukaryotic cells has often been a major argument for supporting their use against intracellular organisms, including mycobacteria (exposure to critical concentrations of rifampin may be sufficient to kill intermittently metabolizing mycobacterial populations).[54]

Future developments

Benzoxazinorifamycins constitute a new group of semisynthetic molecules with development oriented towards *Chlamydia* infections and other intracellular organisms.[55] Of note, diarylquinolines, inhibitors of mycobacterial ATP synthase,[56] have now emerged as novel tuberculostatic agents acting even on dormant organisms, with TMC207 (R207910) having reached a clinical stage.

ANTIMETABOLITES

Sulfonamides and diaminopyrimidines

Prontosil (sulfamidochrysoidine) – a synthetic compound with antibacterial activity found by Domagk in 1932 – was a prodrug which led to the development of the sulfonamides. With diaminopyrimidines, they inhibit the folate pathway in bacteria. For many years, diaminopyrimidines were used in combination with sulfonamides except for specific indications (parasitic diseases) or for the treatment of uncomplicated cystitis. A recent revival of diaminopyrimidines has been the discovery and development of iclaprim (not yet approved).

Chemical structure

Sulfonamides are derived from *p*-aminobenzenesulfonamide which is a structural analogue of *p*-aminobenzoic acid, a factor required by bacteria for folic acid synthesis (Fig. 130.20). A free amino group at position 4 and a sulfonamide group at position 1 are required for antibacterial activity. Heterocyclic or aromatic rings substituting the sulfonamide enhance this activity by modifying absorption and gastrointestinal tolerance.

Diaminopyrimidines such as trimethoprim (Fig. 130.20) and pyrimethamine are pyrimidines substituted at position 5 by an aromatic group. Pyrimethamine has an additional substituent at position 6. Iclaprim (Fig. 130.20) is the result of pharmacochemical research aimed at selecting compounds not only more active than trimethoprim but also expanding activity against trimethoprim-resistant strains. It is a racemic mixture of two enantiomers, both of which show equipotent activity.

Mode of action

Sulfonamides inhibit tetrahydrofolic acid synthesis, acting at the level of dihydropteroate synthetase as analogues of *p*-aminobenzoic acid, and as alternative substrates to become incorporated into a product with pteridine.[57,58]

Diaminopyrimidines are specific competitive inhibitors of bacterial dihydrofolate reductase.[57,58] Selectivity of action is achieved as trimethoprim in establishing more binding interactions with the bacterial than with the corresponding eukaryotic enzymes. In addition, the NADPH co-factor may stabilize the enzyme–trimethoprim complex in bacteria. Iclaprim shows additional increased binding and the ability to inhibit the trimethoprim-resistant enzyme, based on the lipophilic interactions of the cyclopropyl ring with two hydrophobic amino acids (Leu54 and Ile50) of the target enzyme.[59]

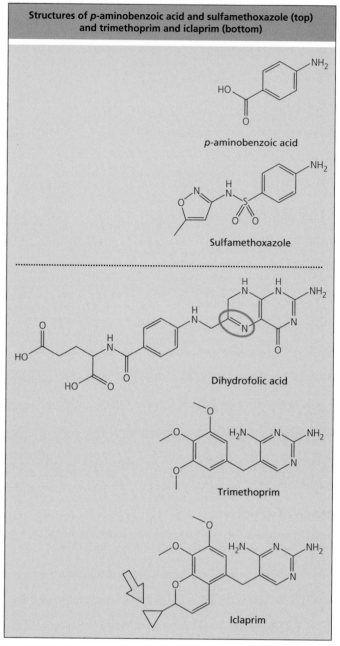

Structures of *p*-aminobenzoic acid and sulfamethoxazole (top) and trimethoprim and iclaprim (bottom)

p-aminobenzoic acid

Sulfamethoxazole

Dihydrofolic acid

Trimethoprim

Iclaprim

Fig. 130.20 Structures of *p*-aminobenzoic acid and sulfamethoxazole, and trimethoprim and iclaprim. The figure highlights the similarity between *p*-aminobenzoic acid (a sulfonamide) and dihydrofolic acid and trimethoprim, which are the basis for the activity of these drugs (in dihydrofolic acid, the red circle outlines the positions that are reduced for conversion into tetrahydrofolic acid); this part of the figure also shows the differences between trimethoprim and iclaprim, for which the bulky cyclopropyl moiety (block arrow) strengthens the interactions with the target enzyme and helps to overcome resistance to trimethoprim.

Resistance

For sulfonamides, resistance mainly occurs from hyperproduction of *p*-aminobenzoic acid or a reduced affinity of dihydrofolate reductase for the antibiotic, causing resistance to the whole class. For diaminopyrimidines, resistance mostly occurs via enzyme mutations which prevent binding, but this can be reversed by suitable modification such as that made with iclaprim.[59]

Pharmacodynamics

Sulfonamides are bacteriostatic; however, in combination with diaminopyrimidines they are bactericidal. The pharmacodynamics of iclaprim are poorly defined, mainly because of low blood levels and interference by thymidine on its activity.

ANTIBIOTICS ACTING ON THE MEMBRANE

Cyclic polypeptides (polymyxins/colistins)

Chemical structure

These are a collection of cyclic, branched polypeptides (molecular masses about 1000 Da) containing both cationic and hydrophobic amino acids. Some of these are of the D configuration or are non-DNA coded, which confers resistance to mammalian peptide-degrading enzymes. Polymyxins are obtained from *Bacillus polymyxa* and colistins from *Aerobacillus colistinus*. Only polymyxin B and colistin (identical to polymyxin E) are used in clinical practice. Commercial colistin contains at least two components (E1 and E2, also called colistin A and colistin B) differing by the length of the fatty acid chain.

Mode of action

Because of their amphipathic character, polymyxins and colistins act as detergents and alter the permeability of the cytoplasmic membrane.[60] They therefore act at all stages of bacterial development. However, they cannot diffuse easily through the thick peptidoglycan layer of Gram-positive bacteria. In contrast, they bind easily to the outer membrane of Gram-negative bacteria (interacting with the lipopolysaccharide (LPS) and triggering a 'self-promoted uptake' process) from where they reach the cytoplasmic membrane through polar as well as nonpolar channels. These properties explain their strong and fast bactericidal activity through disruption of the inner membrane and their essentially Gram-negative spectrum.

Resistance

Acquired resistance to polymyxins and colistins is chromosomal and results from decreased permeability of the outer membrane secondary to changes in its biochemical composition. Bacteria with decreased sensitivity are characterized by a decreased phospholipid/lipid ratio and a higher content of divalent cations (Ca^{2+}, Mg^{2+}). Protein H1 from *P. aeruginosa* (OprH) prevents binding of polymyxins and colistins to lipopolysaccharide, and its overproduction correlates with reduced sensitivity. However, this change is not sufficient per se and must be combined with other modifications of the membrane; two genes downstream to OprH (PhoP and PhoQ) co-regulate OprH and polymyxin B resistance. Resistance to polymyxins and colistins was previously uncommon but is now increasingly described in strains exhibiting multiple resistance to β-lactams and aminoglycosides. A puzzling observation is that the regrowth is easily observed *in vitro*, suggesting the occurrence of a so-called 'adaptive resistance', the mechanism of which is still uncertain.

Pharmacodynamics

Colistin A and polymyxin B show concentration-dependent activity but little or no postantibiotic effect, justifying the administration of repeated daily doses.[61] The pharmacodynamic parameters governing the activity of colistin are still undefined as both C_{max}/MIC and time above MIC are critical not only for efficacy but also to prevent regrowth.

Nonantibiotic pharmacologic and toxicologic properties related to chemical structure

As membrane-disrupting and lipid-binding agents, polymyxins and colistins display a number of non-antibiotic effects. Some of them are potentially useful, such as inactivation of endotoxins and synergy with serum bactericidal activities. Others, however, are highly detrimental to the host and include activation of the alternate complement pathway, mastocyte degranulation with histamine release, decreased production of cytokines (but increased tumor necrosis factor release), increased membrane conductance in epithelia, and apoptosis.

Future developments

Because of the widespread emergence of resistance to other antimicrobials, colistin B has become more frequently used in chronic, difficult-to-treat infections (e.g. pulmonary infections in cystic fibrosis patients). Polymyxin B has also been investigated as an anti-endotoxin agent.[54] New, potentially less-toxic derivatives of these molecules and other membrane-destabilizing peptides have also been isolated or synthesized recently with some of them being under clinical development.[53]

REFERENCES

References for this chapter can be found online at http://www.expertconsult.com

Mechanisms of antibacterial resistance

INTRODUCTION

Although treatment of infections is often initiated empirically, the laboratory determination of bacterial susceptibility to an antimicrobial agent is essential because of widespread resistance to all classes of antimicrobial agents. Standardized methods for determining susceptibility and resistance have been formulated.[1] Bacterial isolates considered resistant to an antibiotic by these methods usually cannot be treated by this antibiotic, although the successful clinical outcome for isolates deemed susceptible likewise cannot be guaranteed.

There is a strong correlation between the presence of some determinants of bacterial resistance and the outcome of antimicrobial therapy. The presence of a β-lactamase in *Neisseria gonorrhoeae* strongly correlates with penicillin treatment failure. The presence of the *mecA* gene in *Staphylococcus aureus* is highly predictive of treatment failure with oxacillin, and in fact oxacillin-resistant *Staph. aureus* (usually called methicillin-resistant *Staph. aureus*, MRSA) is by definition also considered resistant to all β-lactam antibiotics.

However, the presence of a resistance gene is not equivalent to treatment failure. The gene should also be expressed in sufficient amounts to lead to phenotypic resistance. Expression may differ depending on culture conditions or site of infection. For example, β-lactamase production is common among Enterobacteriaceae but resistance to penicillins depends on the mode and degree of expression.

Antibiotic resistance can be divided into eight basic groups depending on the mechanism involved:

- the presence of an enzyme that inactivates the antibiotic;
- the presence of an alternative enzyme to that inhibited by the antibiotic;
- target mutation, which reduces binding of the antibiotic to the target;
- target modification, which reduces binding of the antibiotic to the target;
- reduced uptake of the antibiotic,
- active efflux of the antibiotic,
- removal by binding of the antibiotic, and
- protection of the target enzyme by binding another protein.

The genetic determinants for resistance against antimicrobial agents can be located on the bacterial chromosome or on plasmids. The analysis of resistance genes and their distribution through the use of modern DNA techniques has provided new insights into the mechanisms of resistance and the spread of resistance genes in hospitals and the community.

RESISTANCE TO β-LACTAM ANTIBIOTICS

Penicillin is the oldest β-lactam antibiotic; subsequent developments have included a whole array of β-lactam-based antibiotics, such as the first-generation through to the fourth-generation cephalosporins, monobactams and carbapenems. Almost immediately after the introduction of penicillin, resistance was observed in staphylococci. The β-lactam antibiotics interfere with cell wall synthesis by binding enzymes called penicillin-binding proteins (PBPs). Resistance to β-lactams is mainly caused by either the presence of β-lactamases, which destroy the lactam ring, or the presence of altered PBPs, which are not inhibited by these antibiotics. In Gram-positive bacteria the β-lactamase is excreted into the extracellular environment, and in Gram-negative bacteria it is excreted into the periplastic space. Whether the β-lactam antibiotic is effective against the bacterium depends on a number of factors (Fig. 131.1), including:[2]

- the concentration of the antibiotic in the environment;
- the rate of entry through the outer membrane (in the case of Gram-negative bacteria);
- the amount of β-lactamase;
- the hydrolysis rate for the antibiotic by the β-lactamase; and
- the affinity of the PBPs for the antibiotic.

The number of β-lactamases has risen steadily since the introduction of penicillin. The β-lactamases have been classified according to their

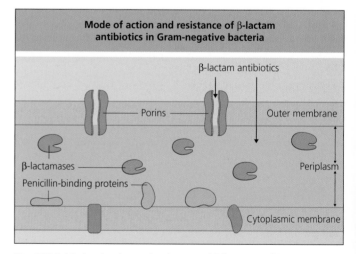

Fig. 131.1 Mode of action and resistance of β-lactam antibiotics in Gram-negative bacteria.

functional aspects.[3] This system is based on hydrolysis rates for a number of substrates and the level of inhibition by clavulanic acid, but simple point mutations may alter the classification. They have also been classified according to the nucleotide sequences that encode β-lactamases.[4] Classes A, C and D have a serine at their active site, whereas class B has a zinc atom at the active site. Class A enzymes are encoded mostly on plasmids, whereas class C enzymes are generally chromosomally encoded, although the genes for these β-lactamases are also found increasingly on plasmids. Class A enzymes are generally constitutively expressed. Class C enzyme genes are present in almost all Gram-negative bacilli, except *Salmonella* spp., but their presence does not necessarily lead to resistance. Class C enzymes are usually inducible and a total of four genes are required for expression of β-lactamase activity. *Escherichia coli* possesses the *ampC*, *ampD* and *ampG* genes, but lacks the *ampR* gene. Why *E. coli* possesses three of these genes and lacks the fourth is unclear. Class D is a limited group of enzymes able to hydrolyze oxacillin; they are related to class C enzymes. Class B is of increasing importance because many act as carbapenemases. The β-lactamases range between 30 and 40 kDa in size.

The commonest β-lactamases in Enterobacteriaceae are TEM-1, TEM-2 and SHV-1 (TEM are the first three letters of the name of the patient from whom the isolate was obtained; SHV stands for sulfhydryl variable). These are simple penicillinases and their activity can be inhibited by compounds such as clavulanic acid and tazobactam, thereby rendering penicillin derivatives active again. However, TEM and SHV enzymes can easily obtain a broader spectrum through mutations, which may lead to resistance against third-generation cephalosporins. Inactivation of aztreonam, ceftazidime, cefotaxime or ceftriaxone is considered an indicator for the presence of such an extended-spectrum β-lactamase (ESBL). However, these antibiotics can also be inactivated by the overproduction of ampC.

Resistance to third-generation cephalosporins was first described in 1983 and was mediated by a plasmid encoding for a TEM-related β-lactamase. The majority of ESBLs are found in *Klebsiella pneumoniae*, but also increasingly in other Enterobacteriaceae. Extended-spectrum β-lactamases are encoded by plasmids and are highly transmissible. More than 160 TEM-type and 100 SHV-type β-lactamases have been described; nearly half are ESBLs, but at least 10 members of the TEM family are no longer inhibited by clavulanic acid (inhibitor-resistant TEM). In addition, 60 CTX-M-type, and 10 OXA-type ESBLs are known. Besides these commonly occurring ESBL families, other ESBLs have been described.[5]

Some plasmid-encoded cephalosporinases, which are also called cephamycinases, are derived from plasmid-encoded ampC β-lactamases, but are produced constitutively. The prevalence of plasmid-encoded ampC β-lactamases among Enterobacteriaceae is increasing. Further spread of these genes through the hospital or the community may further endanger the use of cephalosporins.

Another group comprises the carbapenemases. These enzymes inactivate the highly active carbapenems such as imipenem and new carbapenems such as ertapenem and doripenem. In the past these enzymes were only encoded chromosomally, but increasingly the genes encoding these β-lactamases are also found on plasmids. This will lead to an increase in resistance against carbapenems. However, resistance is still rare with the exception of *Pseudomonas aeruginosa* and *Acinetobacter* spp. Many carbapenemases belong to Class B. However, an OXA carbapenemase, which is a Class A enzyme, has been reported. In addition, three *K. pneumoniae* carbapenemases (KPC) are known. These enzymes have also been reported in other Enterobacteriaceae, including *Salmonella*, and have caused several outbreaks in the eastern USA.

Altered PBPs are also a major reason for resistance against β-lactam antibiotics. An altered PBP is involved in methicillin resistance in staphylococci. Both MRSA and methicillin-resistant *Staphylococcus epidermidis* (MRSE) are important causes of nosocomial infections. These infections are difficult to treat because both MRSA and MRSE are generally multiresistant and susceptible to only a limited number of antibiotics.

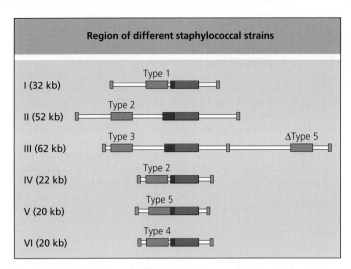

Fig. 131.2 *MecA* region of different staphylococcal strains. Red: *mecA*, methicillin-resistance gene; purple: regulatory genes *mecI/R*; gray: *ccr* genes with indication of type; green: direct repeats; white: variable sequences.

This PBP2a is encoded by the *mecA* gene. Regulation of methicillin resistance is complex. Expression can be heterogeneous and only a few cells express the phenotype, although all cells are genotypically identical and possess the *mecA* gene. Through mutation the resistance phenotype may become homogeneous, which is the case in the majority of isolates. Expression is also influenced by the plasmid-encoded β-lactamase regulatory (blaR) systems blaR1 and blaI inducer-repressor system, which interacts with the mec-associated mecR1 and mecI system.[6] The *mec* determinant appears to originate in coagulase-negative staphylococci, which have a much higher prevalence of the gene, and horizontal transfer appears to take place on a regular basis.

The *mecA* gene is located on a staphylococcal chromosome cassette (SCC*mec*). Six basic types of SCC*mec* have been described based on the type of *ccr* genes and the presence or absence of the complete *mecI* and *mecR* genes (mec complex A and B, respectively) (Fig. 131.2). Within these basic types considerable variation has been observed. This is in part due to the insertion of resistance plasmids and/or transposons into some SCC*mec*. The *ccr* genes are site-specific recombinases which recognize the direct repeats and are involved in the mobilization of SCC elements and thereby their transfer between different staphylococci. SCC*mec* is always integrated in the *orfX* gene of staphylococci.[7] Besides the presence of *mecA*, some methicillin-resistant strains are overproducers of β-lactamases.[8,9]

Resistance to penicillin in *Streptococcus pneumoniae* is also due to the presence of altered PBPs, and this mechanism can be responsible for chromosomally mediated penicillin resistance in *N. gonorrhoeae*. In *Enterococcus faecium* mutations in PBP5 are responsible for resistance to ampicillin. Ampicillin resistance is frequently found in hospital-associated strains. Vancomycin-resistant clinical isolates are often also ampicillin resistant.

A reduction in porins in Gram-negative bacteria such as Enterobacteriaceae, and in particular in *P. aeruginosa* and *Acinetobacter* spp., contributes to β-lactam resistance, but by itself is insufficient to account for resistance.

RESISTANCE TO AMINOGLYCOSIDES

The first clinically effective aminoglycoside, streptomycin, was found in *Streptomyces griseus* in 1944. Numerous aminoglycosides have since been isolated from species belonging to the genera *Streptomyces*, *Micromonospora*, *Bacillus* and *Pseudomonas*. Synthetic derivatives, such as amikacin, were also produced. Clinically, the most important aminoglycoside antibiotics are gentamicin, tobramycin, amikacin and streptomycin. They have a broad antimicrobial spectrum and are effective against both Gram-positive and Gram-negative organisms; however, they are ineffective against anaerobes. Aminoglycosides bind to ribosomes and thus interfere with protein synthesis.

Resistance to aminoglycoside antibiotics is widespread and of clinical importance. It is observed in both Gram-negative and Gram-positive bacteria. Aminoglycosides enter the bacterial cell in several phases. In the first phase the aminoglycosides bind to anionic sites on the cell and, after binding, diffuse through outer membrane proteins. In *P. aeruginosa* the entry is enhanced; the lipopolysaccharides of *P. aeruginosa* are rich in phosphate groups to which the aminoglycosides bind. This binding displaces magnesium ions, thus allowing entry of the aminoglycoside. The second and third phases are energy dependent and transport the aminoglycoside molecules across the cytoplasmic membrane. The lack of activity of aminoglycosides against anaerobes is explained by the fact that their transport across the cytoplasmic membrane depends on aerobic respiration.

Inactivation of aminoglycosides is the major mechanism of resistance against these antibiotics; others include ribosomal modification and reduced permeability. The enzymes responsible for aminoglycoside inactivation belong to three classes, depending on the type of modification that causes inactivation: phosphotransferases (APH), acetyltransferases (AAC) and nucleotidyltransferases (ANT). Each class is subdivided on the basis of the site of modification on the substrate and substrate specificity (Table 131.1). Often these enzymes are able to modify several structurally related aminoglycosides. The enzymes have to inactivate their targets before they reach the ribosomes and they appear to be either located inside the cell or associated with the cytoplasmic membrane.[10]

Studies concerning the evolution of resistance using nucleotide sequencing clearly show that, at least within enzyme classes, the genes are related. For example, immunologic and hybridization tests have shown that the APH(3′) enzymes from streptococci and staphylococci are closely related, as are those enzymes on the Gram-negative transposons (Tn), Tn5 and Tn903. However, there is far less homology between enzymes from Gram-negative bacteria compared to enzymes from Gram-positive bacteria. Nevertheless, the genes from Gram-negative bacteria appear to be more closely related to a gene of *Streptomyces fradiae*. It is likely that gene transfer has taken place between these species. Aminoglycoside resistance genes are believed to originate from genes involved in the production of aminoglycosides in aminoglycoside-producing species.[11]

Table 131.1 Characteristics of a selected set of aminoglycoside-modifying enzymes. Only the clinically relevant antibiotics are listed

Enzyme subclass	Number of different genes described that encode enzymes capable of the same aminoglycoside modification	Modification	Distribution
AAC(1)	1		
AAC(3)-I	2	Gentamicin	Gram-negative bacteria
AAC(3)-II	3	Gentamicin, tobramycin	Gram-negative bacteria
AAC(3)-III	3	Gentamicin, tobramycin	Gram-negative bacteria
AAC(3)-IV	1	Gentamicin, tobramycin	Gram-negative bacteria
AAC(3)-VI	1	Gentamicin	Gram-negative bacteria
AAC(3)-VII	1		Fungi
AAC(3)-VIII	1		Fungi
AAC(3)-IX	1		Fungi
AAC(3)-X	1		Fungi
AAC(6′)-I	9	Amikacin	Gram-negative and Gram-positive bacteria
AAC(6′)-II	2	Gentamicin, tobramycin	Gram-negative bacteria
AAC(6′)-III	1		Gram-negative bacteria
AAC(6′)-APH(2″)	1	Amikacin, gentamicin, tobramycin	Gram-positive bacteria
AAC(2′)I	1	Gentamicin, tobramycin	Gram-negative bacteria
ANT(2″)-I	3	Gentamicin, tobramycin	Gram-negative bacteria
ANT(3″)-I	1	Streptomycin	Gram-negative bacteria
ANT(4′)-I	1	Amikacin, tobramycin	Gram-positive bacteria
ANT(4″)-I	1	Amikacin, tobramycin	Gram-negative bacteria
ANT(6)-I	1	Streptomycin	Gram-positive bacteria
ANT(9)-I	1		Gram-positive bacteria
APH(3′)-I	3		Gram-negative bacteria
APH(3′)-II	1		Gram-negative bacteria
APH(3′)-III	1	Amikacin	Gram-positive bacteria
APH(3′)-IV	1		Gram-positive bacteria
APH(3′)-V	3		Fungi
APH(3′)-VI	2	Amikacin	Gram-negative bacteria
APH(3′)-VII	1		Gram-negative bacteria
APH(3″)-I	2	Streptomycin	Fungi
APH(6)-I	4	Streptomycin	Fungi
APH(4)-I	2		Gram-negative bacteria, fungi

AAC, acetyltransferase; ANT, nucleotidyltransferase; APH, phosphotransferase.

Besides the transfer of genes between bacteria and aminoglycoside-producing species, transfer between Gram-positive and Gram-negative species has been documented.[12] It should be noted, however, that transfer of a functional resistance gene from one species to another does not assure the expression of resistance.

Aminoglycoside resistance in staphylococci is well documented[13] and up to six genes have been identified. Often more than one resistance gene is present. One of the most remarkable aminoglycoside enzymes is the bifunctional AAC(6′)-APH(2″) enzyme, which is found on Tn4001 of Staph. aureus and in Enterococcus faecalis isolates. Nucleotide sequencing data suggest that the enzyme arose through the fusion of two genes, each encoding one of the partners. The epidemiology of Tn4001 is well studied and illustrates that substitutions, insertions and deletions play an important role in the adaptation of these elements to new hosts.

Hybridization studies in Australia showed that Tn4001 could be present on the bacterial chromosome as well as on a number of structurally related plasmids, and this was linked to the rapid spread of gentamicin- and tobramycin-resistant Staph. aureus in Australia. The same transposon was also observed in the USA but with shorter inverted repeats and insertion sequences flanking the resistance gene.

Initially, only resistance against the naturally occurring aminoglycosides was observed and only APH(3′)-II and APH(3′)-III were capable of modifying amikacin in vitro, but the introduction of this antibiotic quickly changed this. In the San Juan Veterans Administration Medical Center, the prevalence of amikacin resistance increased from 0.2% to 3.6% among aerobic Gram-negative bacilli in 4 years through the use of amikacin as a first-line antibiotic. Analysis of plasmids obtained from amikacin-resistant Serratia marcescens and K. pneumoniae showed that these were almost identical. This suggested that the plasmid disseminated through the hospital and that this dissemination occurred quickly.[14]

Besides antibiotic modification, alteration of the binding site for aminoglycosides can play a role in Gram-negative bacteria. 16S rRNA methylation as protection against aminoglycosides has been reported, but is not widespread. Resistance to streptomycin is often caused by mutation of the S12 protein in the small ribosomal subunit (30S subunit).

RESISTANCE TO MACROLIDES, LINCOSAMIDES AND STREPTOGRAMINS

Macrolide, lincosamide and streptogramin (MLS) antibiotics are chemically distinct inhibitors of bacterial protein synthesis. Macrolides are composed of a minimum of two amino sugars or neutral sugars attached to a lactone ring of variable size. Macrolides can be subdivided according to the chemical structure of their lactone ring into 14-membered, 15-membered or 16-membered lactone ring macrolides. These classes differ in their pharmacokinetic properties and in their responses to bacterial resistance mechanisms. Lincosamides are alkyl derivatives of proline and are devoid of a lactone ring. Streptogramin antibiotics are mixtures of naturally occurring cyclic peptide compounds. They are composed of two factors, A and B (e.g. pristinamycin II and I, virginiamycin M and S), with synergistic inhibitory and bactericidal activities[15,16] (see Chapter 135).

Intrinsic resistance to macrolide, lincosamide and streptogramin B (MLS_B) antibiotics in Gram-negative bacilli is due to low permeability of the outer membrane to these hydrophobic compounds.

Three different mechanisms of acquired MLS resistance have been described in Gram-positive bacteria. First, target modification alters a site in 23S rRNA that is common to the binding of MLS_B antibiotics. Modification of the ribosomal target confers cross-resistance to MLS_B antibiotics (MLS_B-resistant phenotype) and remains the most frequent mechanism of resistance, although enzymatic modification of the antibiotics and active efflux appear to be increasing.[15,17,18]

Target modifications

Macrolide, lincosamide and streptogramin antibiotics bind to 50S ribosomal subunits and inhibit elongation of peptide chains. Resistance to MLS_B antibiotics is mostly due to acquisition of erythromycin resistance methylase (erm) genes that encode enzymes that N^6-dimethylate an adenine residue of 23S rRNA. The precise site of methylation has been located in a highly conserved region of the rRNA. Nucleotide alterations in 23S rRNA, both mutational and post-transcriptional, cluster in the peptidyltransferase region in 23S rRNA domain V, providing a physical basis and a common location for MLS_B antibiotic sites of action. Methylation of rRNA probably leads to a conformational change in the ribosome that results in decreased affinity and leads to co-resistance to all MLS_B antibiotics. This suggests that the binding sites for these drugs overlap or at least functionally interact. Streptogramin A-type antibiotics are unaffected, and synergy between the two components of streptogramin against MLS-resistant strains is maintained.

A sequence comparison of erm genes from various bacterial species and results of hybridization experiments under stringent conditions led to the recognition of at least nine classes of resistance determinants (Table 131.2). Because a number of these genes cross-hybridize, clinical isolates can be assigned to one of four hybridization classes: ermA, ermC, ermAC, and ermF. This gene distribution is relatively species specific. The amino acid sequences of the methylases encoded by these determinants are related, indicating that the erm genes are derived from a common ancestor, possibly belonging to an antibiotic producer.

Table 131.2 Distribution of erm genes in clinically important bacterial species

Hybridization class	Gene	Host
ermA	ermA	Staphylococcus aureus Coagulase-negative staphylococci Enterococcus faecium Streptococcus pyogenes
	ermTR	Streptococci (including S. pneumoniae and S. pyogenes)
ermAM	ermP ermZ	Clostridium perfringens Clostridium difficile Enterococcus faecalis
	ermBC	Escherichia coli Lactobacillus reuteri
	ermAM	Streptococcus sanguis Streptococcus pneumoniae Streptococcus agalactiae Streptococcus pyogenes Streptococci (including S. pneumoniae and S. pyogenes) Enterococci
ermC	ermB	Staphylococcus aureus Bacillus subtilis Lactobacillus spp. Enterococcus faecium
	ermC	Staphylococcus aureus Coagulase-negative staphylococci
	ermM	Staphylococcus epidermidis
ermF	ermF	Bacteroides fragilis Bacteroides ovatus

Data from Leclercq & Courvalin.[15]

Expression of MLS$_B$ resistance can be constitutive or inducible. The character of resistance is not related to the class of *erm* determinant but, rather, depends on the sequence of the regulatory region upstream from the structural gene for the methylase. Regulation by these regions occurs by a translational attenuation mechanism in which mRNA secondary structure influences the level of translation. In laboratory mutants and clinical isolates, single nucleotide changes, deletions or duplications in the regulatory region convert inducibly resistant strains to constitutively resistant ones that are cross-resistant to MLS$_B$ antibiotics.

Expression of MLS resistance in staphylococci may be constitutive or inducible. When expression is constitutive, the strains are resistant to all MLS$_B$ antibiotics. Streptogramin A-type antibiotics escape resistance, and synergy with streptogramin B-type antibiotics is retained. When expression is inducible, the strains are resistant to 14- and 15-membered macrolides only. The 16-membered macrolides, the commercially available lincosamides and the streptogramin antibiotics remain active. This dissociated resistance is due to differences in the inducing abilities of MLS antibiotics; only 14- and 15-membered macrolides are effective inducers of methylase synthesis in staphylococci.

Resistance to MLS antibiotics in streptococci can also be expressed constitutively or inducibly. However, unlike the situation with staphylococci, various macrolides or lincosamides may act as inducers to various degrees. Thus, in streptococci, whether inducible or constitutive, ribosomal methylation leads to cross-resistance among macrolides, lincosamides and streptogramin B antibiotics.

In addition, alterations in ribosomal protein L4 account for resistance in pneumococcal strains selected *in vitro* by macrolide passage. The presence of alterations in the L4 ribosomal protein is consistent with the interpretation that this protein is in contact with or near the peptidyltransferase region in domain V of 23S rRNA. Thus, this alteration may act indirectly to alter 23S rRNA conformation.[19] In some cases, these modifications also reduce the *in vitro* activities of ketolides, derivatives of macrolides, which were designed in order to act against macrolide-resistant micro-organisms.

Mutations in domain V of the 23S rRNA genes resulting in resistance to erythromycin have been reported for *Campylobacter* spp. For *Helicobacter pylori* three point mutations in the same domain have been associated with clarithromycin resistance: A2142G, A2143G, and A2142C. In addition, a T2183C mutation has been described, but its influence on the susceptibility to clarithromycin is unknown.

Antibiotic inactivation

Unlike target modification, which causes resistance to structurally distinct antibiotics, enzymatic inactivation confers resistance only to structurally related drugs.[15,17–20]

Enzymes (ErmA and ErmB) that hydrolyze the lactone ring of the macrocyclic nucleus and phosphotransferases (type I (*mphA*) and type II) that inactivate macrolides by introducing a phosphate on the 2′-hydroxyl group of the amino sugar have been reported in members of the family Enterobacteriaceae and in *Staph. aureus*. The gene *linA* mediates resistance to lincosamides. The product of *linA* has been partially purified and demonstrated to act as a lincosamide O-nucleotidyltransferase. Lactonases that are capable of cleaving the macrocyclic lactone ring structure of type B streptogramins have been identified in staphylococci (*vgb* and *vgbB* genes). Two staphylococcal-related determinants, *vat*, *vatB*, *vatC*, and *satA* encoding an acetyltransferase that inactivates type A streptogramins, have been characterized. In addition, the *vga* and *vgaB* genes encode resistance to type A streptogramins. The *vat* and *vgb* genes are adjacent to each other on plasmid pIP630. This vat–vgb region is flanked by inverted copies of the insertion sequence IS*257*, suggesting a role for this element in dissemination of these determinants. In enterococci the *vatD* gene has been described. A *vatE* gene has also been reported. Both *vatD* and *vatE* confer resistance to streptogramin A compounds.

Active efflux

The presence of multicomponent macrolide efflux pumps in staphylococci (*msrA*, *msrB*) and *N. gonorrhoeae* (*mtr*), as well as an efflux system in streptococci (*mefA*, *mefE*), has also been documented.[21–24] *msr* genes confer resistance only to 14- and 15-membered ring macrolides. Recent epidemiologic surveys have shown that some erythromycin-resistant strains of pneumococci and group A streptococci have been shown to have the M phenotype, namely resistance to macrolides but susceptibility to lincosamide and streptogramin B antibiotics. These strains contain the *mefA* or *mefE* gene coding for an efflux pump for 14- and 15-membered macrolides. The presence of a plasmid-mediated gene, *vga*, encoding for a putative ATP-binding protein, has been associated with an active efflux of streptogramin A group compounds. An overview on macrolide resistance genes was published in 2001.[19]

RESISTANCE TO FLUOROQUINOLONES

Fluoroquinolone antibiotics exert their antibacterial effects by inhibition of certain bacterial topoisomerase enzymes, namely DNA gyrase (bacterial topoisomerase II) and topoisomerase IV.[13,24–27] These essential bacterial enzymes alter the topology of double-stranded (ds) DNA within the cell. In most bacteria, the chromosome exists as a single circle of dsDNA, which is maintained in a highly negatively supercoiled state. This energetically activated form is required for critical cellular processes such as replication and transcription.

Deoxyribonucleic acid gyrase and topoisomerase IV are heterotetrameric proteins composed of two subunits, designated A and B. The genes encoding the A and B subunits are referred to as *gyrA* and *gyrB* (DNA gyrase) or *parC* and *parE* (DNA topoisomerase IV; *grlA* and *grlB* in *Staph. aureus*).

Deoxyribonucleic acid gyrase is the only enzyme that can affect supercoiling of DNA. Inhibition of this activity by fluoroquinolones is associated with rapid killing of the bacterial cell. Topoisomerase IV also modifies the topology of dsDNA, but whereas DNA gyrase seems to be important for maintenance of supercoiling, topoisomerase IV is predominantly responsible for separation of daughter DNA strands during cell division.

In Gram-negative organisms, DNA gyrase is the primary target for quinolones, whereas topoisomerase IV appears to be the primary target in *Staph. aureus* and *Strep. pneumoniae*. In Gram-positive species, mutations in genes encoding topoisomerase IV appear to precede mutations in DNA gyrase. Nevertheless, in *Strep. pneumoniae* it has been shown that different quinolones can have different primary targets in the same bacterial species (i.e. quinolone structure determines the mode of antibacterial action). Thus, the primary target seems to be dependent on the bacterial species as well as on the quinolone structure.

Target modification

Alterations of the target enzymes appear to be the most dominant factors in expression of resistance to quinolones.[13,24–28] Many Gram-negative fluoroquinolone-resistant organisms contain a *gyrA* mutation, resulting in inhibition of supercoiling of DNA and elevated minimum inhibitory concentrations (MICs; Table 131.3). The first molecular characterization of a quinolone resistance mutation in *gyrA* was reported in 1988 from *E. coli*. The mutations found were situated in a relatively hydrophilic region of the polypeptide and close to a tyrosine residue at amino acid 122 at the active site, which has been shown to be the site covalently bound to the DNA. The small region from codon 67 to 106 was designated the quinolone resistance-determining region (QRDR). In almost all instances, amino acid substitutions within the QRDR involve the replacement of a hydroxyl group with a bulky hydrophobic residue. This suggests that mutations in *gyrA* induce changes in the binding site conformation or charge (or both) that may be important for interactions between quinolones and DNA gyrase.

Although quinolones are thought to interact primarily with the A subunit of DNA gyrase, there are mutations in the B subunit that also confer quinolone resistance in some species, such as *E. coli*. However, the frequency of *gyrB* mutations has been shown to be relatively low compared with the frequency of *gyrA* mutations in clinical isolates of *E. coli* and other Gram-negative organisms. No *gyrB* mutations have been reported as resulting in cross-resistance between quinolones and

Table 131.3 Alterations in DNA gyrase subunit A conferring quinolone resistance

Organism	Amino acid substitution
Acinetobacter baumanni	Gly 81 → Val Ser 83 → Leu
Aeromonas salmonicida	Ser 83 → Ile Ala 67 → Gly
Coxiella burnetti	Glu 87 → Gly
Campylobacter jejunii	Ala 70 → Thr Thr 86 → Ile
Campylobacter lari	Ser 83 → Arg Thr 86 → Ile Glu 87 → Lys, Gly Thr 86 → Ile Asp 90 → Ala, Asn Pro 104 → Ser
Enterobacter cloacae	Ser 83 → Leu
Escherichia coli	Ala 51 → Val Ala 67 → Ser Gly 81 → Cys, Asp Asp 82 → Gly Ser 83 → Leu, Trp, Ala, Val Ala 84 → Pro Asp 87 → Asn, Val, Thr, Gly, His Gln 106 → Arg, His Ala 196 → Glu
Enterococcus faecalis	Ser 83 → Ile Gln 106 → His, Arg
Enterococcus faecium	Glu 87 → Lys
Helicobacter pylori	Asp 86 → Asn Asn 87 → Lys, Ile, Tyr Ala 88 → Val Asp 91 → Gly, Asn, Tyr Ala 97 → Val
Mycobacterium avium	Ala 90 → Val
Mycobacterium smegmatis	Ala 90 → Val Asp 94 → Gly
Mycobacterium tuberculosis	Gly 88 → Ala, Cys Ala 90 → Val Ser 91 → Pro Asp 94 → Asn, His, Gly, Tyr, Ala, Val Ser 95 → Thr
*Neisseria gonorrhoeae**	Ser 83 → Phe Asp 87 → Asn
Pseudomonas aeruginosa	Thr 83 → Ile Asp 87 → Tyr, Asn, Gly, His

Table 131.3 Alterations in DNA gyrase subunit A conferring quinolone resistance—cont'd

Organism	Amino acid substitution
Shigella dysenteriae	Ser 83 → Leu Asp 87 → Asn, Gly
Salmonella	Ala 67 → Pro Asp 72 → Gly Val 73 → Ile Gly 81 → Asp, Cys, His, Ser Ser 83 → Ala, Asp, Phe, Tyr Asp 87 → Gly, Tyr, Asn Leu 98 → Val Ala 119 → Glu, Ser, Val Glu 139 → Ala
Staphylococcus aureus	Ser 84 → Leu, Ala, Phe Ser 85 → Pro Glu 88 → Lys, Gly
Staphylococcus epidermidis	Ser 84 → Phe

*The substitutions for *Neisseria gonorrhoeae* are based on *Escherichia coli* sequence.
Adapted from Everett & Piddock.[25]

the B subunit inhibitors coumermycin and novobiocin. This is consistent with evidence which suggests that the GyrB protein comprises two distinct domains: an *N*-terminal domain containing the sites for hydrolysis of adenosine triphosphate and binding of coumermycin, and a *C*-terminal domain containing the QRDR of GyrB.

Topoisomerase IV is a secondary target for fluoroquinolone action in *E. coli* in the absence of a sensitive DNA gyrase. Mutations in *parC* result in further decreased susceptibility. These mutations in *parC* have been shown to occur at Ser80 and Glu84, which are analogous to codons Ser83 and Asp87 of *E. coli* gyrA, and to be common in fluoroquinolone-resistant clinical isolates of *E. coli*. A mutation has also been reported in the *parE* gene that results in decreased fluoroquinolone susceptibility. However, as in the case with *gyrB*, such mutations appear to be rare in clinical isolates.

In *Staph. aureus*, topoisomerase IV is the primary target of fluoroquinolones. Strains with mutations in *gyrA* and *gyrB* without *grlA* mutations resulting in high-level fluoroquinolone resistance can be isolated by single-step selection with fluoroquinolones in *E. coli* but not in *Staph. aureus*. Previously, 116 clonally unrelated *Staph. aureus* isolates originating from nine different countries were screened for mutations in the *gyr* and *grl* gene loci.[28] In correlating the characterized mutations to the resulting MIC of ciprofloxacin, it is clear that all studied isolates without the *grlA* mutation at position Ser80 were susceptible to ciprofloxacin. All ciprofloxacin-resistant isolates had the *grlA* mutation Ser80 in combination with either a Ser84 mutation or a Glu88 mutation within the *gyrA* gene. In two isolates a Ser80 to Phe mutation was combined with no mutations in the *gyrA* gene, resulting in a MIC value for ciprofloxacin of 2 µg/ml, which, although elevated from a wild-type level, is still below the breakpoint for resistance. These data support the finding that in *Staph. aureus*, *grlA* mutations precede *gyrA* mutations in developing resistance to ciprofloxacin.

Combinations of single point mutations within the *gyrA* gene from various species have been shown to be associated with higher MIC values for ciprofloxacin than single point mutations. Similarly, two combinations of single point mutations within *grlA*, of a Glu84 to Val mutation or an Ala48 to Thr mutation in combination with a Ser80 to Phe mutation, were associated with relatively higher ciprofloxacin MIC values (64–256 µg/ml) than only a single Ser80 to Phe mutation

(8–64 µg/ml). Sequence data show that some *grlA* and *gyrA* mutations are conserved in both MRSA and methicillin-sensitive *Staph. aureus* from unrelated clones of *Staph. aureus* isolated from different countries.

Topoisomerase IV mutations have now been characterized in several other organisms. In *Strep. pneumoniae* topoisomerase IV also appears to be the primary target for fluoroquinolone action. Ciprofloxacin-resistant mutants of *Strep. pneumoniae* were generated by stepwise selection at increasing drug concentrations. First-step mutants exhibiting low-level resistance had no detectable changes in their topoisomerase QRDR, suggesting altered permeation or another novel resistance mechanism. Second-step mutants exhibited an alteration in ParC at Ser79 to Tyr or Ser79 to Phe or at Ala84 to Thr. Third- and fourth-step mutants displaying high-level ciprofloxacin resistance were found to have, in addition to ParC alteration, a change in GyrA at residues equivalent to *E. coli* GyrA resistance hotspots Ser83 and Asp87 or in GyrB at Asp435 to Asn, equivalent to *E. coli* Asp426. ParC mutations preceded those in GyrA, suggesting that topoisomerase IV is the primary topoisomerase target and gyrase the secondary target for ciprofloxacin in *Strep. pneumoniae*. Additionally, it has been shown that in *Strep. pneumoniae* different quinolones can have different primary targets. The targeting of DNA gyrase by sparfloxacin in *Strep. pneumoniae* but of topoisomerase IV by ciprofloxacin indicates that target preference can be altered by change in quinolone structure.

Decreased uptake

Deoxyribose nucleic acid gyrase and topoisomerase IV are both located in the cytoplasm of the bacterial cell. In order to reach their targets, fluoroquinolone antibiotics must traverse the cell envelope. In Gram-positive bacteria this consists of the cell wall and a single membrane, whereas in Gram-negative bacteria the fluoroquinolone must first cross the outer membrane. Changes in the outer membrane of Gram-negative bacteria have been associated with decreased uptake and increased resistance to fluoroquinolones.[24–27] Some of these changes may be due to the effect of quinolones or *gyrA* mutations, or both, on differential expression of outer membrane proteins, because it has been shown that *gyrA*-mediated changes in supercoiling of DNA can affect the expression of porin genes.

Active efflux

Increased efflux as a mechanism of fluoroquinolone resistance has been reported in fluoroquinolone-resistant *Staph. aureus*. The *norA* gene encodes the multidrug efflux pump NorA.[29] The NorA protein has a hydropathic amino acid profile consistent with a location in the cytoplasmic membrane and it exhibits a low level of fluoroquinolone efflux, with a preference for hydrophilic fluoroquinolones. Efflux is an active process and can be inhibited by protonophores. NorA-mediated fluoroquinolone resistance is due to overexpression of the wild-type gene *norA*. In *P. aeruginosa*, resistance to fluoroquinolones as well as to a number of other antimicrobial agents has often been associated with decreased accumulation and increased expression of outer membrane proteins, often with concomitant increase in cytoplasmic membrane proteins. Resistance is due to overexpression of one or more efflux systems (i.e. OprK) capable of removing fluoroquinolones and other antibiotic compounds. *E. coli* has also been shown to possess efflux systems, notably EmrAB and AcrAB.[25]

Protection of gyrase and topoisomerase IV

Plasmid-encoded quinolone resistance was discovered in the late 1990s. The responsible gene, *qnrA1*, encodes a pentapeptide repeat protein that binds to gyrase and protects it from the action of quinolones. Remarkably, another member of the pentapeptide-repeat family, encoding a microcin, kills bacteria by inhibiting gyrase, which is also the mode of action for quinolones. Organisms that produce this microcin make another pentapeptide repeat protein that protects gyrase from the microcin and also some quinolones. The *qnr* gene product leads to a 10- to 100-fold increase in the MIC for quinolones. Because MIC values for quinolones are often extremely low, the expression of the *qnr* gene may be insufficient to reach the breakpoint for resistance or even intermediate resistance. Nevertheless, it has been speculated that this may offer the bacterium a larger time window to develop mutations in gyrase or topoisomerase and thereby higher levels of resistance.

A number of variants of *qnrA1* have been reported, as well as more distant relatives called *qnrB* and *qnrS*. Variants of the latter types are also known. Isolates harboring *qnr* genes have been reported worldwide and the mechanism seems of growing importance. At least one large national outbreak with an *Enterobacter* strain has been reported.[30]

MAR operon

Escherichia coli and a number of other organisms possess mechanisms that provide intrinsic protection against a wide range of chemically unrelated toxic substances, including quinolone antibiotics. Multiple antibiotic resistance (MAR) in *E. coli* has been shown to be the result of mutations in the *mar* locus of the *E. coli* chromosome. A homologue of the *mar* locus exists in other members of the Enterobacteriaceae as well as in other bacteria. In *E. coli*, the *mar* locus consists of two divergently expressed operons, *marC* and *marRAB*, both of which are required for full expression of the MAR phenotype. Expression of the MAR phenotype, whether by induction or mutation, protects the cells from fluoroquinolone killing at up to four times the MIC. This may be more clinically important than the relatively modest increases in MIC associated with MAR because cells that escape death would have the potential to mutate to higher levels of fluoroquinolone resistance.[24,25,31]

RESISTANCE TO TETRACYCLINES

Tetracyclines probably penetrate bacterial cells by passive diffusion. Tetracycline acts by reducing the affinity of the A and P sites of the 30S ribosomal subunit for aminoacyl transfer RNA, resulting in the inhibition of protein synthesis.[13,24,32–35]

A growing number of bacterial species are acquiring resistance to the bacteriostatic activity of tetracycline. To date, at least 38 tetracycline-resistance (Tet) determinants and three oxytetracycline-resistance (Otr) determinants, first found in oxytetracycline-producing *Streptomyces* spp., have been described and characterized, with new Tet determinants being identified regularly. Most are associated with plasmids, whereas others are on the chromosome. Resistance to tetracyclines is primarily due to acquisition of Tet determinants rather than to mutation of existing chromosomal genes.[36]

The two most widespread mechanisms of bacterial resistance are:
- energy-dependent efflux pumps; and
- an elongation-factor G-like protein that confers ribosomal protection.

Both mechanisms are widespread among Gram-negative and Gram-positive bacteria (Table 131.4). Oxidative destruction of tetracycline has been found in a few species. Nevertheless, the enzymatic inactivation of the antibiotic is not thought to be important in nature.

The classification of Tet determinants according to their mechanism of resistance is shown in Table 131.5. Resistance to tetracycline may result in cross-resistance to the second-generation tetracyclines doxycycline and minocycline. Resistance to tigecycline, the newest generation of tetracyclines (i.e. glycylcycline), has been reported.

Reduced intracellular concentration of tetracycline

Because the ribosome is the target, antibiotic activity of tetracycline depends on the presence of the drug in the cytoplasm. A reduced

Table 131.4 Distribution of tetracycline-resistance determinants

Genus	Tet determinant
Acinetobacter	Tet A, B, M, 39
Actinobacillus	TetB, H, L
Actinomyces	TetL, W
Aerococcus	TetM, O
Aeromonas	TetA, B, C, D, E, 34
Afipia	TetM
Alteromonas	TetD
Arcanobacterium	TetW
Bacillus	TetK, L, W
Bacteroides	TetM, Q, X, 36
Brevundimonsa	TetB
Butyrivibrio	TetW
Campylobacter	TetO
Chlamydia	TetC
Citrobacter	TetA, B, C, D
Clostridium	TetK, L, M, P, W, 32, 36
Corynebacterium	TetM, 33
Edwardsiella	TetA, D
Eikenella	TetM
Enterobacter	TetB, C, D, M
Enterococcus	TetK, L, M, O
Erypsipelothrix	TetM
Escherichia	TetA, B, C, D, E, G, M
Eubacterium	TetK, M
Fusobacterium	TetM
Gardnerella	TetM
Gernella	TetM
Haemophilus	TetA, B, M
Kingella	TetM
Klebsiella	TetA, D, M
Lactobacillus	TetK, M, O, S, W, 36
Lactococcus	TetM, S
Listeria	TetK, L, M, S
Megasphaera	TetO, W
Microbacterium	TetM
Mitsuokella	TetM, W
Mobiluncus	TetO
Moraxella	TetB, H
Morganella	TetL
Mycobacterium	TetK, L, OtrA, B
Mycoplasma	TetMa
Neisseria	TetB, M, O, Q, W
Nocardia	TetK, L
Pasteurella	TetB, D, H
Peptostreptococcus	TetK, L, M, O
Photobacterium	TetB, M
Plesiomonas	TetA, B, D
Porphyromonas	TetM, W
Prevotella	TetM, Q, W
Proteus	TetA, B, C
Providencia	TetG
Pseudomonas	TetA, B, C, M, 34
Ralstonia	TetM
Roseburia	TetW
Salmonella	TetA, B, C, D, E, L
Selenomonas	TetM, W
Serratia	TetA, B, C, 34
Shigella	TetA, B, C, D

Table 131.4 Distribution of tetracycline-resistance determinants—cont'd

Genus	Tet determinant
Staphylococcus	TetK, L, M, O, U, W, 38
Stenotrophomonas	Tet35
Streptococcus	TetK, L, M, O, W
Streptomyces	TetK, L, M, W, OtrA, B, C
Ureaplasma	TetMa
Veillonella	TetA, L, M, S, W
Vibrio	TetA, B, C, D, E, G, M, 34, 35
Yersinia	TetB

Data from Roberts.[32]

Table 131.5 The mechanism of resistance for different tetracycline determinants

Efflux	*tet*(A), *tet*(B), *tet*(C), *tet*(D), *tet*(E), *tet*(G), *tet*(H), *tet*(J), *tet*(K), *tet*(L), *tet*(V), *tet*(Y), *tet*(Z), *tet*(30), *tet*(31), *tet*(33), *tet*(35), *tet*(38), *tet*(39), *tetA*(P), *otr*(B), *otr*(C), *tcr3*
Ribosomal protection	*tet*(M), *tet*(O), *tet*(Q), *tet*(S), *tet*(T), *tet*(W), *tet*(32), *tet*(36), *tetB*(P), *otr*(A)
Enzymatic	*tet*(X), *tet*(34), *tet*(37)
Unknown	*tet*(U)

Data from Roberts.[36]

tetracycline concentration in the cytoplasm can be achieved by two mechanisms:[13,24,32–35]

- the permeability of the cell envelope may be lowered; or
- tetracycline may be pumped out of the cytoplasm in an energy-dependent fashion.

Bacteria differ in their cell wall composition, causing differences in permeability and hence insensitivity to antibiotics. The peptidoglycan layer surrounding most Gram-positive bacteria does not reduce cytoplasmic accumulation of low molecular weight antibiotics such as tetracycline. In contrast, the outer membrane of Gram-negative bacteria is an effective permeability barrier for hydrophobic compounds. The effects of permeability barriers are usually supported by additional resistance mechanisms to achieve high-level resistance. Energy-dependent efflux of tetracycline causes high-level resistance in bacteria by itself.

Two different types of efflux pump are involved in tetracycline resistance: multidrug-resistance pumps and tetracycline-specific transporters. A multidrug-resistance pump belonging to the Acr family is responsible for the reduced tetracycline accumulation in *P. aeruginosa*. Furthermore, *E. coli* has a chromosomal multidrug-resistance efflux system that is associated with the *mar* locus. Multidrug efflux pumps transport their substrate straight out of the cell into the surrounding medium. In contrast to the broad substrate range of multidrug transporters, many of the efflux pumps identified in Gram-positive and Gram-negative bacteria specifically transport tetracycline. The efflux proteins exchange a proton for a tetracycline–cation complex and are antiporter systems. Efflux determinants from Gram-negative bacteria (TetA–E, TetG–H) share a common genetic organization, which is different from the one in Gram-positive bacteria. Both Gram-negative and Gram-positive bacteria contain a structural and a repressor gene that are expressed in opposite directions from overlapping operator regions. The Gram-positive *tetK* and *tetL* genes encoding tetracycline efflux proteins are regulated by mRNA attenuation in a similar way to that described for Gram-positive *erm* genes encoding rRNA methylase and *cat* genes encoding chloramphenicol acetyltransferases. Tetracycline-specific exporters pump their substrate into the periplasm and not across the outer membrane, as found for the multidrug efflux pumps.

Protection of the ribosome

Protection of the ribosome from the action of tetracycline as a mechanism of tetracycline resistance was discovered in streptococci. Tetracycline resistance can result from production of a protein that interacts with the ribosome such that protein synthesis is unaffected by the presence of the antibiotic. To date, six classes of Tet determinants that confer tetracycline resistance on the level of protein synthesis have been identified. Most of the work on the mechanism of ribosomal protection has been done on TetM. The ribosomal protection proteins encoded by the other classes have an amino acid sequence similarity of at least 40% to TetM. Therefore, the mechanism of action may be similar for all ribosomal protection proteins. TetM ribosomal protection protein resembles elongation factors (EFs) in three properties:

- it has amino acid sequence similarity to EF-G (which translocates the peptidyl transfer RNA during protein synthesis) and EF-Tu;
- it has a ribosome-dependent guanosine triphosphatase activity; and
- it seems to confer resistance by reversible binding to the ribosome.

However, to date, the biochemical basis of tetracycline resistance mediated by TetM remains unclear. One possibility is that TetM stabilizes the ribosome–tRNA interaction in the presence of tetracycline.[13,24,32–34,36]

RESISTANCE TO CHLORAMPHENICOL

Chloramphenicol is a bacteriostatic antibiotic that binds to the 50S ribosomal subunit and inhibits the peptidyltransferase step in protein synthesis. Resistance to chloramphenicol is mostly due to inactivation of the antibiotic by a chloramphenicol acetyltransferase (CAT) enzyme that acetylates the antibiotic. Chloramphenicol resistance most commonly results from the acquisition of plasmids that encode CAT; however, in certain Gram-negative bacteria, decreased outer membrane permeability can confer resistance to chloramphenicol and structurally unrelated compounds.[13,24]

Enzyme inactivation

Chloramphenicol contains two hydroxyl groups that are acetylated in a reaction catalyzed by CAT. Monoacetylated and diacetylated derivatives are unable to bind to the 50S ribosomal subunit to inhibit prokaryotic peptidyltransferase. Expression of the *cat* genes in *Staph.*

aureus, *Strep. pneumoniae* and *Enterococcus faecalis* is typically inducible, and expression appears to be regulated by translational attenuation in a similar manner to the *erm* genes conferring resistance to macrolides. The *cat* gene is preceded by a nine amino acid leader peptide, and the leader mRNA can form a stable stem-loop structure, which masks the ribosome binding site of the *cat* gene. Chloramphenicol appears to cause the ribosome to stall on the leader sequence, opening the stem-loop structure, thereby exposing the *cat* ribosome binding site and allowing *cat* expression. In Gram-negative bacteria, resistance to chloramphenicol is usually mediated by plasmid-mediated or transposon-mediated genes that are generally expressed constitutively.

Decreased permeability

In Gram-negative bacteria, resistance may also be due to chromosomal mutations that result in decreased outer membrane permeability. In *P. aeruginosa*, nonenzymatic chloramphenicol resistance is associated with the presence of the *clmA* gene. The ClmA protein appears to effect reduced expression of the outer membrane porins OmpA and OmpC and decreased chloramphenicol uptake. In *E. coli*, resistance to chloramphenicol and structurally unrelated antibiotics is part of the MAR phenotype.[37]

RESISTANCE TO GLYCOPEPTIDES

The glycopeptide antibiotics vancomycin and teicoplanin inhibit cell wall synthesis in Gram-positive bacteria by interacting with the terminal D-alanyl-D-alanine (D-Ala-D-Ala) group of the pentapeptide side chains of peptidoglycan precursors. This interaction prevents the transglycosylation and transpeptidation reactions required for polymerization of peptidoglycan. Almost all bacteria synthesize peptidoglycan terminating in D-Ala-D-Ala, but the exclusion limits of the porin proteins of Gram-negative outer membranes prevent transport of the glycopeptides, and so only Gram-positive species are susceptible to clinically achievable concentrations of this class of antibiotics.

Glycopeptide resistance in enterococci

The vancomycin-resistant enterococci (VRE) can be divided into six different phenotypic groups: A, B, C, D, E and H (Table 131.6).[13,24,38–43]

The origin of the *van* genes in enterococci is not known. The *vanA* gene has 52% amino acid sequence identity to the D-Ala-D-Ala ligase of *Salmonella* spp. and can complement a temperature-sensitive ligase mutant of *E. coli*. The D-Ala-D-Ala ligase is responsible for the production of the D-Ala-D-Ala dipeptide, which in Gram-positive bacteria is the target for glycopeptide antibiotics. The *vanB* and *vanC* genes are also both highly comparable in sequence to D-Ala ligases.

Table 131.6 Resistance to enterococcal glycopeptides

Resistance	ACQUIRED					Intrinsic
Phenotype	VanA	VanB	VanD	VanG	VanE	VanC
MIC (mg/l) Vancomycin Teicoplanin	64–1000 16–512	4–1000 0.5–1	64–128 4–64	8–16 0.5	16 0.5	2–32 0.5–1
Expression	Inducible	Constitutive	Constitutive	Inducible	Constitutive	Inducible
Location	Plasmid Chromosome		Chromosome	Chromosome	Chromosome	Chromosome
Modified target	D-Ala–D-Lac	D-Ala–D-Lac	D-Ala–D-Lac	D-Ala–D-Ser	D-Ala–D-Ser	D-Ala–D-Ser

Adapted from Shlaes & Rice[38] and Courvalin.[44]

VanA resistance phenotype

The *vanA* gene is carried within a transposon together with several other genes, many but not all of which are required for the expression of resistance to vancomycin. The VanA product is a D-Ala-D-lactate (D-Lac) ligase. The *vanH* gene apparently encodes an enzyme that catalyzes the conversion of pyruvate to D-lactic acid. The VanA ligase uses this as a substrate to form the depsipeptide D-Ala-D-Lac, which is then incorporated into an alternative, vancomycin-resistant peptidoglycan precursor (Fig. 131.3). The VanX protein appears to cleave the D-Ala-D-Ala dipeptide, decreasing the amount of substrate that is available for the formation of the normal pentapeptide. The VanX protein does not hydrolyze the D-Ala-D-lactate pentapeptide or pentadepsipeptide.

Most vancomycin-resistant strains of enterococci also produce a carboxypeptidase. The structural gene for this carboxypeptidase in VanA-harboring strains is *vanY*. The carboxypeptidase may reduce the levels of the normal precursor so that the alternative precursor predominates. The *vanY* gene, however, is not required for resistance to cyclic glycopeptides. The inducible nature of glycopeptide resistance in most VanA enterococci suggests that expression is regulated at the genetic level. The genes *vanR* and *vanS* are involved in the regulation of VanA resistance, and the analysis of the amino acid sequences of the gene products has indicated similarity with two-component signal transducing regulatory systems that sense and respond to environmental stimuli. VanR appears to act as a transcriptional activator and seems to be stimulated by VanS. The phosphorylated VanR peptide acts on a promoter that lies between *vanS* and *vanH* and from which the *vanH*, *vanA* and *vanX* genes are co-transcribed. The environmental stimulus that triggers the initial phosphorylation of VanS has not been identified, but it is probably related to the presence of vancomycin and its interaction with the D-Ala-D-Ala target site, which inhibits transglycosylation.

In addition to the high-level glycopeptide resistance mediated by the *vanH*, *vanA*, *vanX* and *vanY* genes, a second mechanism of resistance exists. The *vanZ* gene mediates resistance to teicoplanin while vancomycin MICs are unaffected. The mechanism by which the VanZ peptide confers this low-level teicoplanin resistance has yet to be established.

Other Van resistance phenotypes

The drug resistance of VanB-harboring strains appears to be similar to that of VanA-harboring strains, except that the VanB-harboring strains originally described remained susceptible to teicoplanin. However, it has become clear that glycopeptide-resistant enterococci containing the *vanB* gene are phenotypically diverse, exhibiting a wide range of vancomycin MICs, including high-level resistance. In addition, the emergence of mutants that express *vanB* constitutively has been described. Resistance mediated by *vanB* may also be transferable, with the gene located either on the chromosome or on plasmids.

The *vanC* resistance determinants are present on the chromosome in *Enterococcus casseliflavus* and *Enterococcus gallinarum* and are intrinsic characteristics of these species. VanC-harboring enterococci have low-level resistance to vancomycin and remain susceptible to teicoplanin. The pentapeptide that results from the action of the VanC ligase terminates in D-Ala-D-Ser. This substitution probably reduces vancomycin binding, albeit not to the same degree as the depsipeptide found in VanA and VanB enterococci. Insertional inactivation of *vanC* caused reversion to vancomycin susceptibility, suggesting the existence of a second chromosomal ligase that synthesizes vancomycin-susceptible precursors.

VanC-harboring strains with high-level resistance to glycopeptides as a result of the acquisition of the *vanA* gene cluster have also been isolated. The biochemical basis for the VanC phenotype displayed by

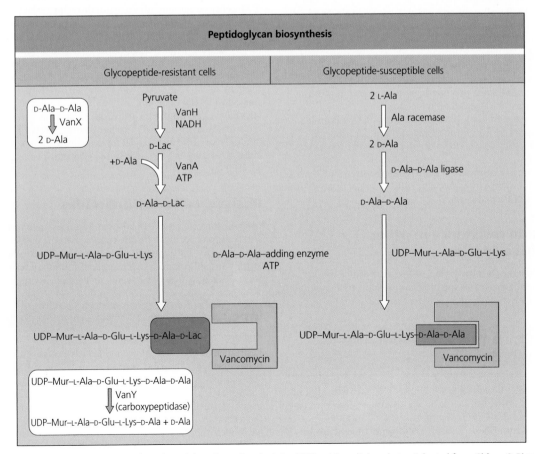

Fig. 131.3 Peptidoglycan biosynthesis. ATP, adenosine triphosphate; Lac, lactate; UDP, uridine diphosphate. Adapted from Shlaes & Rice.[38]

most isolates of *Enterococcus casseliflavus* and *Enterococcus flavescens* remains to be clarified in detail. Two genes, designated *vanC-2* and *vanC-3*, have been identified in these species. There is extensive similarity between the *vanC-2* or *vanC-3* gene and the *vanC* gene, now designated *vanC-1*, from *Enterococcus gallinarum*, although they do not cross-hybridize.

A third mechanism of vancomycin resistance is VanD. Resistance levels for vancomycin and teicoplanin are 64–128 and 4–64 µg/ml, respectively. The genes are located chromosomally and are constitutively expressed. Conjugative transfer has not been demonstrated. VanE and VanG are two mechanisms that yield low-level vancomycin resistance and teicoplanin is unaffected. Both mechanisms are inducible and located on the chromosome. The VanG cluster can be transferred by conjugation.[44]

Glycopeptide resistance in staphylococci

Resistance to glycopeptides among staphylococci is phenotypically diverse.[43] *Staph. aureus* strains of intermediate resistance to glycopeptides have been obtained *in vitro* and *in vivo* by the selection of resistant mutants. Vancomycin-intermediate *Staph. aureus* (VISA) or glycopeptide-intermediate *Staph. aureus* (GISA) isolates show a thicker cell wall which presumably binds the vancomycin before it reaches its target.[45] Furthermore, most GISA isolates show reduced cross linking when compared with isogenic revertants. Interestingly, only some of them (Michigan, New Jersey, Düsseldorf) showed a reduction in D-glutamic acid amidation.[43] The genetic mechanism for this cell-wall thickening has not been resolved. Comparison of a *Staph. aureus* isolate before vancomycin treatment and its vancomycin intermediate descendent after treatment by whole genome sequencing showed 37 differences between the isolates. However, the relevance of these changes has not been demonstrated.[46]

It is likely that the following mechanisms are associated with the appearance of the GISA strain:[43]

- accelerated cell wall synthesis, which leads to a thickened cell wall capable of affinity trapping large amounts of vancomycin and shielding the membrane-associated lipid II target molecules;
- in addition, impaired cross linking, most probably caused by the accelerated cell wall synthesis, will be reduced due to the fact that nonamidated precursors are poor substrates for the staphylococcal transpeptidation reaction; and
- since lower nonamidation and lower cross linking both lead to even higher consumption of vancomycin per unit cell wall weight, they also contribute positively to the resistance phenotype.

High-level vancomycin resistance has also been reported and is caused by acquisition of the VanA transposon by MRSA, almost certainly from vancomycin-resistant enterococci.[45]

Glycopeptide resistance in other Gram-positive species

Glycopeptide resistance is intrinsic in some Gram-positive species such as *Lactobacillus* spp., *Leuconostoc* spp., *Pediococcus* spp. and *Erysipelothrix rhusiopathiae*; the mechanism has yet to be clarified.

RESISTANCE TO TRIMETHOPRIM AND SULFONAMIDES

Trimethoprim and sulfonamides are synthetic agents that affect the biosynthesis of tetrahydrofolic acid, an essential derivative used in amino acid and nucleotide synthesis.[13,24,47–49] Sulfonamides are analogues of *para*-aminobenzoic acid. They competitively inhibit the enzyme dihydropteroate synthase (DHPS), which catalyzes the condensation of dihydropteridine with *p*-aminobenzoic acid synthesis.

Trimethoprim is an analogue of dihydrofolic acid. It competitively inhibits the enzyme dihydrofolate reductase (DHFR). Dihydrofolate reductase catalyzes the reduction of dihydrofolic acid to tetrahydrofolic acid, the final step in tetrahydrofolic acid synthesis. Trimethoprim–sulfamethoxazole (co-trimoxazole) is a combination of trimethoprim with a sulfonamide.

Intrinsic resistance to trimethoprim and sulfonamides

Outer membrane impermeability results in trimethoprim and sulfonamide resistance in *P. aeruginosa*. Intrinsic resistance to trimethoprim in a number of species is due to host DHFR enzymes with low affinity for the drug. Folate auxotrophs such as *Enterococcus* spp. and *Lactobacillus* spp. that are able to use exogenous preformed folates exhibit reduced susceptibilities to sulfonamides and trimethoprim.

Resistance to trimethoprim

Both high- and low-level resistance has been reported in several species. In some cases, chromosomally encoded trimethoprim resistance may be due to:

- overproduction of the host DHFR;
- mutations in the DHFR structural gene *folA*; or
- mutations that inactivate thymidylate synthetase, an enzyme that converts deoxyuridylate to thymidylate.

The thymidylate mutants require exogenous thymine or thymidine for DNA synthesis and are thus resistant to folate pathway antagonists.

High-level resistance to trimethoprim in enterobacteria is almost always caused by the acquisition of DNA that specifies a trimethoprim-resistant DHFR with an altered active site. At least 11 modified DHFRs have been characterized in Gram-negative organisms. In staphylococci, trimethoprim resistance is encoded by the *dfrA* gene, which encodes a trimethoprim-resistant type S1 DHFR. The transposon-encoded *dfrA* gene appears to be responsible for both high- and low-level trimethoprim resistance in *Staph. aureus* and coagulase-negative staphylococci. The differences in resistance level correlate with differences in transcription caused by deletions adjacent to a copy of IS*257* in Tn*4003*, which affects the promoter used by *dfrA*. The *Staph. epidermidis* trimethoprim-sensitive chromosomal DHFR gene *dfrC* differs from *dfrA* by only four base pairs, strongly suggesting that *dfrA* originated from the *Staph. epidermidis* chromosomal gene. Site-directed mutagenesis of *dfrA* and kinetic analyses of the purified DHFRs indicate that a single alteration (Phe98 to Tyr) is responsible for trimethoprim resistance of type S1 DHFR.

Resistance to sulfonamides

Chromosomally encoded sulfonamide resistance has been described and resistance seems to be due to increased production of *para*-aminobenzoic acid. Furthermore, alterations of DHPS could lead to low affinity for sulfonamides. Acquired sulfonamide resistance can result from the acquisition of plasmids that encode a drug-resistant DHPS.

RESISTANCE TO OTHER ANTIBIOTICS

Resistance to linezolid, a recently licensed oxazolidinone, has already been reported. Linezolid is used to treat infections with enterococci and staphylococci, and in both genera resistance has been reported. In enterococci, a G2505A or G2576T mutation in the 23S rRNA gene has been described. The latter mutation has also been reported for staphylococci and streptococci. In addition, G2447T and C2534T mutation have been reported for the latter species.[50–52] Plasmid-mediated linezolid resistance has also been described. The plasmid encodes a Cfr methyltransferase which modifies 23S rRNA.

Fusidic acid inhibits elongation factor G (EF-G), a protein of the ribosome, and thereby protein synthesis. Many resistant isolates have mutations in the *fusA* gene, which encodes EF-G. Reduced uptake and efflux have been reported, but details are largely unknown.

Mupirocin inhibits isoleucyl RNA synthetase to inhibit protein synthesis. Low-level resistance is caused by mutations in the gene of this enzyme on the chromosome. Acquisition of a novel isoleucyl tRNA synthetase encoded by *mupA* leads to high-level resistance.

Metronidazole resistance in *H. pylori* is the result of the disruption of the *rdxA* gene that encodes NADPH nitroreductase. This enzyme converts metronidazole in a metabolite that is toxic for the bacterial cell. Only a small percentage of isolates lack mutations in the *rdxA* gene; it is speculated that mutations affecting its expression are involved.[53]

RESISTANCE IN *MYCOBACTERIUM TUBERCULOSIS*

Mycobacterial resistance to first-line antimicrobial agents is a major concern. The slow growth rate of *M. tuberculosis* and the serious consequences of inappropriate therapy make the study of the mechanisms of antibiotic resistance of particular importance.

The main antibiotics for the treatment of mycobacterial infections are isoniazid and rifampin (rifampicin). Resistance was reported soon after the introduction of isoniazid in 1952. Isoniazid acts by inhibiting an oxygen-sensitive pathway in the mycolic acid biosynthesis of the cell wall. The mechanism of resistance appears to be multifactorial, and genetic modifications in a number of genes may have an effect. Some of these effects have only been observed in *in-vitro* generated mutants. The genes involved include the *katG* gene-encoded catalase-peroxidase, the isoniazid target-encoding *inhA* gene and the upstream region of the neighboring *mabA* gene, upstream of the *aphC* gene and the *kas* gene.[54] Mutations in *katG* are the most important for clinical resistance. The product of the *katG* gene is essential to convert isoniazid to its active form.

The molecular basis of rifampin resistance is understood better. Rifampin interferes with RNA synthesis. At least eight amino acid substitutions in the *rpoB* subunit of RNA polymerase have been described as conferring resistance.[55]

Resistance to aminoglycosides has been reported for *M. tuberculosis* and is caused by an rRNA gene mutation. Resistance to pyrazinamide is most commonly caused by mutations in the *pncA* gene or its upstream region. The *pncA* product is required to convert pyrazinamide into its active form. Tolerance to isoniazid and ethambutol can probably be caused by an efflux mechanism, but details are lacking.

MULTIPLE RESISTANCE

Bacteria are often resistant to more than one antimicrobial agent. Multiple resistance is conferred by three mechanisms:
- reduced permeability;
- active efflux; and
- multiple resistance genes.

Reduced permeability is generally caused by alteration in the cell wall of the bacterium, especially the reduced expression of porins. The best known is the reduction of the outer membrane protein (omp) ompF, from *E. coli*. In general, it can be said that reduction in porin numbers leads to a decreased uptake of antibiotics. The resulting lower concentration of antibiotics can be frequently dealt with by a resistance mechanism that, without a reduced number of porin proteins, only results in a slight increase in MIC.

Efflux of antibiotics is a common resistance mechanism. Often an efflux pump is only able to pump out a single antibiotic and its close structural homologues (e.g. pumps dedicated to tetracycline efflux). However, more general-purpose efflux systems are also known. These

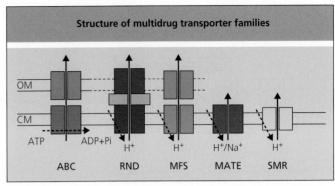

Fig. 131.4 Schematic structure of multidrug transporter families. Different subunits are indicated by different colors. Efflux is indicated by arrow. Energy source for efflux is indicated by broken arrow. The cellular membrane (CM) is present in all cells, but Gram-positive bacteria lack an outer membrane (OM). Some multidrug transporter families are present in both Gram-positive and Gram-negative bacteria as indicated by dotted lines for the OM. (See text for details.)

pumps can handle a wide variety of different compounds including many antibiotics. The efflux systems belong to a number of families:
- ATP-binding cassette (ABC) superfamily of transporters;
- major facilitator (MSF) superfamily;
- resistance-nodulation-division (RND) superfamily;
- small multidrug resistance (SMR) family;
- drug metabolite transporter (MDT) superfamily; and
- multidrug and toxic compound extrusion (MATE) family.

ABC and MSF transporters are not only broadly distributed among prokaryotes, but also among eukaryotes. The transporters can be composed of either a single polypeptide or multiple polypeptides depending on the family (Fig. 131.4). Gram-negative bacteria as well as mycobacteria have an inner and outer membrane and the compounds must be transported across both. The ABC transporters are dependent on ATP for their activity, whereas the proton-motive force is used by other transporters. Mutations are usually required for constitutive expression of these pumps and, in turn, high-level resistance. However, mutations may also affect the substrate specificity facilitating the efflux of novel substrates. The AcrAB of the MAR system in *E. coli* and the MexAB pumps of *P. aeruginosa* belong to the RND superfamily. Multidrug resistance among *P. aeruginosa* is caused in large part by the latter system, but a significant contribution is made by acquired resistance genes. Resistance to disinfectants is usually also mediated by efflux pumps.[56]

The MAR system in *E. coli* is one of the best studied systems and reduced uptake and active efflux are combined in a single regulatory system. The MAR system was discovered by Levy and coworkers, who observed that resistant mutants were obtained at a frequency of 10^{-7} when *E. coli* was plated on agar media containing either tetracycline or chloramphenicol. Usually, mutants obtained with one antibiotic were also resistant to the other, but cross-resistance to β-lactams, puromycin, rifampin and nalidixic acid was also observed. A three-gene operon containing *marRAB* is essential for drug resistance by this mechanism (Fig. 131.5). Sequencing studies revealed that resistant mutants had mutations either in the putative operator–promoter region of the operon or in the *marR* gene. The MarR product acts as a negative regulator for the *mar* operon. The MarA product is required for resistance. The MarA product is supposed to act on at least two different promoter regions. The first is involved in the expression of OmpF protein. Expression of OmpF is regulated by the *micF* gene. Transcription of this gene leads to the production of an antisense RNA for the *ompF* mRNA. Stimulation of *micF* RNA production by the MarA product causes reduced translation of the OmpF mRNA owing to its blockage by the *micF* antisense RNA and thereby reduced permeability through OmpF.

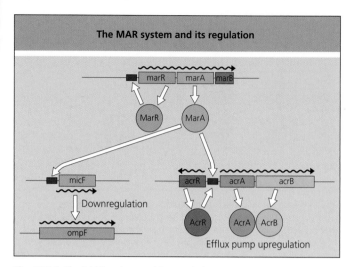

Fig. 131.5 The MAR system and its regulation.

The MarA product also interacts with the *acr* operon. This operon encodes two subunits of an efflux pump. Inactivation of this efflux system results in hypersensitivity to a wide variety of antimicrobial agents. The expression of the *acr* operon appears to be regulated by AcrR, the product of the third gene of this operon. MarA apparently interacts with the binding of AcrR to its operator, resulting in increased expression of the two subunits of the efflux pump. However, the expression of the pump is also increased by a variety of environmental stimuli, such as ethanol and high concentrations of salt, but these stimuli apparently do not operate through either MarA or AcrR. Despite the detailed molecular knowledge about this mechanism of multiple resistance, its clinical impact is not clear.[57]

Multiple resistance caused by the presence of a number of different resistance genes can originate from the sequential acquisition of mutations or resistance genes, but often these genes are transferred as part of complete units. These units are located either on transposons or multiresistance plasmids that have acquired these genes over time. Transposons, easily mobilizable genetic elements that range in size from a few to more than 150 kilobases, are an important source for the spread of antibiotic resistance. Numerous different transposons have been described and many of them carry one or more antibiotic-resistance determinants. Resistance to any class of antimicrobial agent may be encoded on a transposon. Transposons may integrate either in plasmids or the bacterial chromosome and may be present in multiple copies, thereby enhancing their effectiveness in the expression of resistance.

A number of transposons have been well studied. These include Tn*5*, Tn*7*, Tn*10* and Tn*21* from Gram-negative bacteria and Tn*554*, Tn*916* and Tn*4001* from Gram-positive bacteria.[58] Transposition may be very efficient and the spread of Tn*4001* described above is an example. Tn*916* and its derivatives, found in enterococci, lactococci and staphylococci, was one of the first conjugative transposons discovered. It encodes resistance against tetracycline and chloramphenicol. Tn*916* is a member of a large family of related conjugative transposons, but other families have also been described. Conjugative transposons are not limited to Gram-positive bacteria; they are also present in Gram-negative bacteria. Tn*916* has also been found in *N. gonorrhoeae* for example. Conjugative transposons have a somewhat different mechanism of transfer from the more common transposons such as Tn*5* and Tn*10*, but they are well equipped for dissemination between species, although transfer is regulated. For some conjugative transposons, this transfer may be upregulated (by up to 10 000 times) by antibiotics, which enhances the dissemination of antibiotic-resistance determinants. In addition, these conjugative transposons may mobilize co-resident plasmids, which also may carry antibiotic-resistance determinants, resulting in the transfer of multiple antibiotic resistance.[59]

Integrons are a special group of genetic elements. There are two groups of integrons: resistance integrons and superintegrons. Superintegrons are found in many Gram-negative species and are located on the chromosome. These integrons contain tens to hundreds of gene cassettes, which encode for a large variety of different functions. Resistance integrons contain up to 10 gene cassettes. Nearly all known gene cassettes in these integrons encode for resistance to antibiotics or disinfectants. The most common resistance integrons belong to class 1, but two other classes are known as well. The class 1 integrons are characterized by two conserved sequences (CSs). The 5'-CS contains the *int* gene, which encodes a protein homologous to other members of the integrase family. The 3'-CS consists of the *qacEΔ1* and *sulI* genes and an open reading frame, *orf5*.[60] The *qacEΔ1* and *sulI* genes define resistance against quaternary ammonium compounds and sulfonamide, respectively (Fig. 131.6).

Integration of gene cassettes by the integrase takes places between the conserved segments, preferentially at a position at the end of the 3'-CS called the *attI* site. Cassettes can also be excised by the integrase and can exist as free circular DNA molecules. This process can also lead to rearrangement of the order of cassettes in an integron. Each gene cassette has an imperfect inverted repeat element. This so-called 59-base pair element, which may vary in length between 57 and 141 base pairs, is unique for each gene cassette.[61] At least 100 gene cassettes have been described, including genes defining resistance against β-lactam antibiotics, aminoglycosides, trimethoprim, chloramphenicol and antiseptics and disinfectants (Table 131.7).[60] Generally the

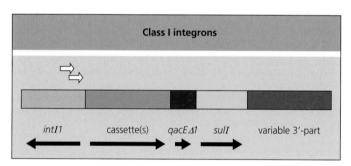

Fig. 131.6 Class 1 integrons. Open arrows indicate the promotors P1 and P2 and point in the direction of transcription from each promotor site; black arrows indicate the direction of open reading frames (orf) (see text for details).

Table 131.7 Resistance and mechanism of resistance for gene cassettes

Resistance	Enzyme
β-Lactams	Class A β-lactamases Class B β-lactamase Class D β-lactamases
Aminoglycosides	Aminoglycoside adenylyltransferases Aminoglycoside acetyltransferases
Chloramphenicol	Chloramphenicol acetyltransferases Chloramphenicol exporter
Trimethoprim	Class A dihydrofolate reductases Class 8 dihydrofolate reductases
Rifampin (rifampicin)	ADP ribosylation
Streptothricin	Streptothricin acetyltransferase
Antiseptics and disinfectants	Quaternary compound exporter
Unknown function	Not applicable

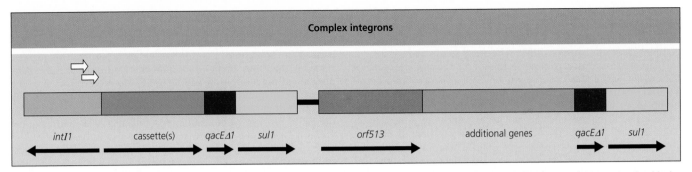

Fig. 131.7 Complex integrons. Open arrows indicate the promotors P1 and P2 and point in the direction of transcription from each promotor site; black arrows indicate the direction of open reading frames (orf) (see text for details).

cassettes do not have promoters, but transcription occurs from one of two promoter sequences present in the 5'-CS. Integrons are widespread in Enterobacteriaceae but are also found in pseudomonads. Isolates may carry more than one integron.[60]

Class 1 integrons can also form complex integrons. In complex integrons an integron is normally followed by *orf513*, a number of

additional genes and a second copy of the 3'-CS (Fig. 131.7). The additional genes are not gene cassettes, but have their own promoters and often encode resistance to antibiotics including third-generation cephalosporins. The first complex integron was described in 2000.[62] Subsequently, numerous complex integrons have been found worldwide. Their prevalence seems to be increasing, probably through

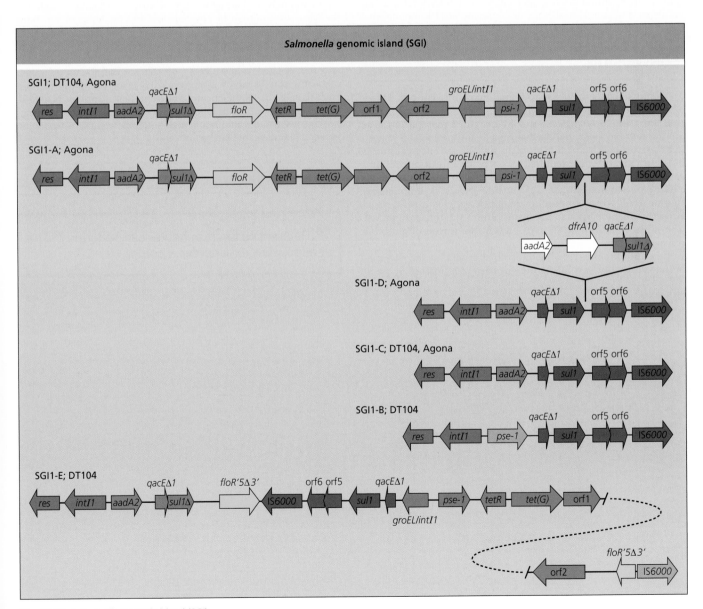

Fig. 131.8 *Salmonella* genomic island (SGI).

selection by cephalosporin use. Complex integrons appear to be frequently linked to an atypical class of insertion elements. These elements are mobile and may also help to explain the mobility of complex integrons between different bacterial strains and species.

Class 1 integrons can also be found on the chromosome of *Salmonella*, where they are present on *Salmonella* genomic island 1 (SGI1). SGI1 is formed by a variable stretch of DNA, which may be up to 43 kb in length. It is located on the *Salmonella* chromosome between the *thdf* and the *yidY* genes, which are present in all *Salmonella enterica* serovars. SGI1 can contain a variety of different resistance genes. All resistance genes are grouped in one region called the multidrug resistance (MDR) region. Seen from the *thdf* gene, the MDR region is located in the distal part of SGI1. In *Salmonella enterica* serovar Typhimurium DT104 SGI1 is frequently present. The MDR region consists of two integrons and a number of intervening genes, including resistance genes. It can be considered as an archetype for SGI1 and is designated SGI1 without further additions. Variations on this theme are found in other serovars. Only one integron may be present and variation in gene cassettes is observed (Fig. 131.8).[63] More than a dozen different SGI1 variants have been described. The MDR region of SGI1 seems to be an important hotspot for the collection of resistance genes. Although resistance to mostly older antibiotics is encoded, some of these antibiotics (e.g. ampicillin and tetracycline) are commonly used in animal husbandry and humans. SGI1 is mobile when helper functions are provided by plasmids.

CONCLUSION

Antibiotic resistance is ubiquitous and increasing. The best-known examples are MRSA, vancomycin-resistant enterococci, penicillin-resistant *Strep. pneumoniae* and ESBL-carrying Enterobacteriaceae. Studies into the molecular mechanisms of antimicrobial resistance help us to understand the problem and to monitor outbreaks, but other measures are required to quell the spread of resistance genes. Local, national and international antimicrobial surveillance studies are required to gain insight into trends in antimicrobial resistance on which empiric treatment of patients can be based. However, only the prudent use of antibiotics and infection prevention measures will limit or even prevent the spread of antibiotic resistance.

It is not only the use of antimicrobial agents for the treatment of humans that plays a role in the spread of resistance; their use for the treatment of animals also plays a role. The practice in animal husbandry of using antibiotics in subtherapeutic concentrations as growth enhancers is a particular cause for concern, although now banned in the European Union and other countries. This practice started in the 1950s. In the 1960s it became controversial and experts questioned the wisdom of adding antibiotics to feed owing to the emergence of multidrug-resistant Enterobacteriaceae. (In fact, the first multidrug-resistant Enterobacteriaceae had been observed in the 1950s.) In 1966 a multidrug-resistant *Salmonella* strain ingested via food caused an outbreak that resulted in six deaths. Many studies were issued, but on a political level little action was taken and the controversy continues today. An example is avoparcin, which gives rise to cross-resistance to vancomycin. Evidence was recently provided that transfer of vancomycin-resistant enterococci from animals to humans may be possible.[64] Although transfer of resistant strains from animals to humans has been demonstrated, it is often contended that strains of bacteria living in animals are not able to survive in humans because they are not well adapted. However, animal strains of at least some multiresistant strains are able to survive for weeks in humans. They may not cause disease directly, but they provide a reservoir of resistance determinants, which can spread easily between strains and species.[65]

Interestingly, in Europe the use of avoparcin has been high and the use of vancomycin in hospitals low, but the levels of vancomycin-resistant enterococci causing infections in patients are low. In the USA, although avoparcin is not used in feed, the amount of vancomycin used in hospitals is high and vancomycin-resistant enterococci are often isolated from patients. This suggests that the use of antibiotics in hospitals may pose a greater threat for the spread of resistance than use of subtherapeutic concentrations of antibiotics in feed. Inappropriate use of antibiotics in both veterinary and medical practice thus contributes to the spread of antibiotic resistance, leading to potentially untreatable infections.

REFERENCES

References for this chapter can be found online at http://www.expertconsult.com

E Yoko Furuya
Christine J Kubin

Chapter | **132** |

Antibiotic prophylaxis

INTRODUCTION

Surgical site infections (SSIs) are a major source of morbidity and mortality and represent the second most common cause of health-care-associated infections (HAI) after urinary tract infections.[1] Depending on the type of surgery, 2–20% of patients develop SSIs, with risk being highest for cardiac and intra-abdominal surgeries.[2] SSI is the most common postoperative complication, and there are published data to show that postoperative complications can have a significant impact on the patient and on hospital resources, with reported increases in length of stay, hospital costs and mortality. Length of stay can increase by 4–11 days compared to patients without complications after surgery.[3,4] Recent studies from the US National Surgical Quality Improvement Program (NSQIP) have shown that postoperative complications can increase hospital costs by US$1398 (for infectious complications) and mortality may increase by 69%.[3,5]

Moreover, an increasing proportion of SSIs are now being caused by multidrug-resistant organisms such as methicillin-resistant *Staphylococcus aureus* (MRSA) and fungi such as *Candida albicans*.[6] Consequently, the selection of appropriate antimicrobial prophylaxis is becoming an increasingly complex issue. In this chapter we highlight the general principles of antibiotic prophylaxis and summarize the recommendations for major types of surgery and other invasive procedures.

PATHOGENESIS

Surgical site infections develop due to microbial contamination of the surgical wound, most commonly from patients' endogenous flora or from an exogenous source, such as personnel in the operating room or the environment. The role of wound contamination during the postoperative period, from direct inoculation or from hematogenous seeding, is less clear but is thought to be involved in late infections of prosthetic devices.

The risk of SSI is due to a combination of factors as follows:[7]

$$\frac{\text{Dose of bacterial contamination} \times \text{virulence}}{\text{Resistance of the host patient}} = \frac{\text{Risk of surgical}}{\text{site infection}}$$

Preoperative antisepsis and antimicrobial prophylaxis are performed to decrease the bacterial load in the wound; however, it is not possible to completely sterilize it, as up to 20% of skin flora resides beneath the surface in sebaceous glands and hair follicles. Regarding the bacterial 'dose', studies demonstrate that a concentration of $>10^5$ organisms per gram of tissue is the critical threshold above which risk of SSI increases significantly.[8] As shown in the above equation, however, this dose could be lower if the virulence of the organism is high, host immunity is low or prosthetic material (including suture material) is in place.

Since the microbiology of SSIs is usually a function of the patient's skin flora, the causative organisms are most often staphylococci: *S. aureus* and coagulase-negative staphylococci. However, some patients can also be colonized with a variety of other organisms including Gram-negative bacilli and *Candida* species which can then lead to infection of the wound. Finally, in intra-abdominal surgeries, gastrointestinal flora such as enteric bacteria and anaerobes can contaminate the wound and cause infection.

SSI RISK CLASSIFICATION SYSTEMS AND SSI RISK FACTORS (TABLE 132.1)

Since 1964, surgical wounds have been categorized by the traditional wound classification system, which stratifies wounds into four categories based on the expected bacterial dose that would contaminate the wound: clean, clean–contaminated, contaminated and dirty–infected. Data show that these wound categories have different associated infection rates, ranging from 5% for clean surgeries and up to 22% for the contaminated category, if antimicrobial prophylaxis is not administered (down to 0.8% and 10% respectively if antibiotics are administered).[10]

However, surveillance systems that track SSI rates have moved away from stratifying wounds based on this classification, as it fails to account for patient- and procedure-related factors. The system that is most widely used at present is the National Nosocomial Infection Surveillance (NNIS) risk index; this index was itself based on an index developed during the Study on the Efficacy of Nosocomial Infection Control (SENIC) project which was the first study to demonstrate efficacy of SSI surveillance.[11] The NNIS risk index counts the number of risk factors present among the following:

- an American Society of Anesthesiologists (ASA) preoperative assessment score of 3, 4 or 5;
- an operation classified as either contaminated or dirty–infected; and
- an operation with duration of >T hours, where T depends on the type of operative procedure.

After a recent assessment by the Centers for Disease Control and Prevention (CDC) in patients across the US,[12] the latest addition to this score has been the subtraction of a point if the procedure was performed laparoscopically (as more and more procedures are). This index has been shown to be useful in performing risk adjustment when benchmarking SSI rates. The NNIS risk index is used by the CDC's National Healthcare Safety Network (NHSN) for surveillance in the US, as well as by national surveillance systems in most countries in Europe and elsewhere around the world. Finally, in addition to the risk factors present in the NNIS risk index, there are additional host factors that may place a patient at higher risk for developing SSIs, in particular diabetes mellitus and malnutrition.[13]

Table 132.1 Surgical site infection risk classification systems

Wound classification system[9]	
I. Clean	An uninfected operative wound in which no inflammation is encountered and the respiratory, alimentary, genital or uninfected urinary tract is not entered. In addition, clean wounds are primarily closed and, if necessary, drained with closed drainage. Operative incisional wounds that follow nonpenetrating (blunt) trauma should be included in this category if they meet the criteria
II. Clean–contaminated	An operative wound in which the respiratory, alimentary, genital or urinary tract is entered under controlled conditions and without unusual contamination. Specifically, operations involving the biliary tract, appendix, vagina and oropharynx are included in this category, provided no evidence of infection or major break in technique is encountered
III. Contaminated	Open, fresh, accidental wounds. In addition, operations with major breaks in sterile technique (e.g. open cardiac massage) or gross spillage from the gastrointestinal tract, and incisions in which acute nonpurulent inflammation is encountered are included in this category
IV. Dirty–infected	Old traumatic wounds with retained devitalized tissue and those that involve existing clinical infection or perforated viscera. This definition suggests that the organisms causing postoperative infection were present in the operative field before the operation
SENIC (Study on the Efficacy of Nosocomial Infection Control) index[11]	
1 point	Operative time >2h
1 point	Abdominal procedure
1 point	Contaminated or dirty procedure
1 point	≥Three discharge diagnoses
NNIS (National Nosocomial Infection Surveillance) risk index[12]	
1 point	ASA score of 3, 4 or 5
1 point	Contaminated or dirty procedure
1 point	Length of procedure >T hours (75th percentile duration of specific procedure)
Minus 1 point	Use of laparoscope

ASA, American Society of Anesthesiologists.

SURVEILLANCE FOR SSI

Given the potential consequences of SSIs and other HAIs, substantial resources have been put toward surveillance and prevention programs in the US and other countries in order to monitor and reduce infection rates. In the US, the CDC developed the National Nosocomial Infection Surveillance (NNIS) system as early as the 1970s as a voluntary reporting system. This system has since been renamed the National Healthcare Safety Network (NHSN) and enables confidential data exchange and analysis within its information technology architecture. In the 1990s, a number of European countries established national or regional HAI surveillance systems, largely modeled on the NNIS system. More recently, an initiative known as Hospitals in Europe Link for Infection Control through Surveillance (HELICS) was created in order to establish a surveillance system supported by the European Union.[14]

There is some suggestion that surveillance can help improve practice by promoting awareness of HAI rates and potential problems. According to data from the NNIS system, SSI rates in most patient groups have declined since the 1990s as surveillance has progressed.[15]

One key component of good SSI surveillance is having a case definition that is applied accurately and consistently. Comparing data across different institutions, regions or countries is complicated by potentially variable application of case definitions, along with fundamental differences in health-care systems. Postdischarge surveillance has represented one of the more problematic aspects of SSI surveillance, as it is difficult to achieve consistent case identification methods among postoperative patients who have been discharged and found to have an SSI at an outpatient visit.

INDICATIONS FOR ANTIBIOTIC PROPHYLAXIS

In most instances, antibiotic prophylaxis is administered to prevent an SSI by decreasing the microbial burden at the surgical site. While there is fairly good agreement between consensus statements regarding which surgery types require prophylaxis, the increase in less invasive procedures, including laparoscopic procedures and procedures performed by interventional radiology, has led to some controversy regarding the necessity of prophylaxis. We will address these less invasive procedures in detail. Finally, in some instances, antibiotic prophylaxis is administered not to prevent an SSI, but rather to prevent endocarditis from procedure-induced transient bacteremia in patients with underlying cardiac disease.

GENERAL PRINCIPLES OF ANTIBIOTIC PROPHYLAXIS

Choice

The choice of antibiotic should ideally be one which is 'safe, inexpensive, and bactericidal with an *in vitro* spectrum that covers the most probable intraoperative contaminants for the operation' as noted by the CDC's SSI guidelines.[7] Thus the antibiotic choice will vary depending on the type of procedure. Cephalosporins appear to be effective in a wide variety of surgery types, and they fit the criteria listed above. Additional reasons for their attractiveness are their relatively long duration of action and comparatively low cost. First-generation cephalosporins, such as cefazolin, are frequently used for clean procedures (and some clean–contaminated procedures) due to their adequate coverage of Gram-positive organisms, as well as some Gram-negative organisms. For surgeries involving the distal intestinal tract, second-generation cephalosporins, such as cefoxitin, are frequently used for their additional anti-anaerobic spectrum of activity.

Dose

It is crucial to achieve and maintain levels of the antibiotic in the serum and at the surgical site that exceed the minimum inhibitory concentration (MIC) for likely pathogens, from the time of incision until the incision is closed. Therefore, both the dose and timing of administration of the antibiotic are important. The dose may need to be individualized based on a given patient's weight; this is particularly important in the setting of rising rates of obesity worldwide. Based on pharmacokinetic principles, lean body weight and volume of distribution are related, suggesting that larger doses are necessary for larger patients. For example, it is currently recommended to increase the cefazolin dose from 1 g to 2 g for patients weighing >80 kg to increase the likelihood of serum and adipose tissue concentration above the MIC of likely organisms.[16] Moreover, cefazolin concentrations in patients undergoing gastric bypass surgery after a 2 g preoperative dose were found to be insufficient and decreased as patient body mass index increased.[17] Redosing of the antibiotic is key if the procedure extends beyond 4 hours and/or major blood loss occurs. The goal is to redose every 1–2 half-lives of the drug being used; assuming normal renal function, this is approximately every 4 hours for most cephalosporins.

Timing

In order to allow the antibiotic adequate time to distribute to the site of action and to maintain adequate levels throughout the procedure, guidelines recommend that most intravenous antibiotics should begin infusing within 1 hour of surgical incision time. The exceptions to this recommendation are vancomycin and fluoroquinolones, which should begin infusing within 2 hours prior to surgical incision to minimize the potential for adverse reactions associated with rapid infusion and to ensure adequate tissue levels. However, a more precise or optimal time within this 1-hour window remains somewhat controversial. Guidelines, including the US National Surgical Infection Prevention Project, recommend administering antibiotics 'as near to the incision time as possible to achieve low SSI rates'.[18,19]

Earlier studies determined that antibiotics given 1–2 hours preoperatively were more effective at preventing SSIs than were antibiotics given 2–24 hours preoperatively or postoperatively (in fact, antibiotics given after surgery resulted in SSI rates no different than if no antibiotics were given at all).[20,21] It is unclear, however, whether data support administering antibiotics within 5–10 minutes of incision time. As mentioned above, antibiotics must have time to achieve adequate levels in serum and local tissues; whether 5 minutes is sufficient is uncertain and this optimal time may vary among different antibiotics.

In a recent study, Garey et al. found that, with regard to vancomycin prophylaxis for cardiac surgery, administration within 16–60 minutes before incision was associated with the lowest SSI rate, and administration within 0–15 minutes prior was associated with a relative risk of 7.8 by comparison.[22] Weber et al. retrospectively reviewed 3836 consecutive surgical procedures, including gastrointestinal, vascular and trauma surgeries, and found that SSI risk was lowest when cefuroxime was administered 59–30 minutes prior to incision (adjusted odds ratio=1.95 when cefuroxime was administered less than 30 minutes prior).[23] Hence, administration of prophylactic antibiotics 'as near to the incision time as possible' may not be optimal; instead, administration 30 minutes to an hour prior may be more ideal. Further studies are needed to clarify this issue.

Duration

Antibiotic prophylaxis continued for more than 24–48 hours after surgery does not further decrease SSI rates, but rather increases the emergence of antibiotic-resistant bacteria.[7,18,24,25] In fact, it is unclear whether any antibiotic is necessary beyond the time of wound closure. Nonetheless, it is variable from surgery to surgery as to whether guidelines recommend single dose or continuation for 24 hours postoperatively based on the methods in published literature. The exception is cardiac surgery, where most guidelines recommend prophylaxis for 48 hours, although it is very possible that 24 hours would be just as effective in preventing SSIs.[26,27]

β-Lactam allergy

Because β-lactams, such as cephalosporins, are often the drugs of choice for surgical prophylaxis, it is important to elucidate the type of reaction that is being labeled as a 'penicillin' or 'β-lactam' allergy. Unless there has been a true, major allergic reaction (e.g. urticaria, angioedema, anaphylaxis, toxic epidermal necrolysis, Stevens–Johnson syndrome), the patient may be able to safely tolerate a cephalosporin. It is now recognized that the cited cross-reactivity to cephalosporins in penicillin-allergic patients of 10% is an overestimate and primarily based on data from the 1960s and 1970s.[28]

The incidence of true adverse reactions to cephalosporins is low in patients with reported penicillin allergies and this cross-allergenicity is now thought to be related to side chain similarity to penicillin or amoxicillin.[28] This similarity is diminished in second- and third-generation cephalosporins. Moreover, the lack of allergic reactions after receiving cefazolin preoperatively in patients who report a non-severe penicillin allergy has been documented.[29] Usual alternatives to β-lactams in patients with severe allergies are vancomycin and clindamycin. If Gram-negative pathogens are also of concern, however, an additional agent such as an aminoglycoside (e.g. gentamicin) may need to be added.

Methicillin-resistant *Staphylococcus aureus*

In recent years, given the increase in methicillin-resistant *Staphylococcus aureus* (MRSA) in both the hospital and the community, the issue of MRSA coverage for surgical prophylaxis has arisen, particularly in the cardiac surgery population. It is well known that hospitalized patients colonized with *S. aureus* (methicillin-susceptible or -resistant) are at higher risk of developing subsequent *S. aureus* infections than are noncolonized patients, usually with their colonizing strains.[30] This has been demonstrated for SSIs as well.[31] Well-described risk factors for MRSA carriage include recent hospitalization or surgery, dialysis, the presence of chronic open wounds and antibiotic use.[32]

In general, however, glycopeptides such as vancomycin are not recommended as first-line prophylaxis. For patients known to be colonized with MRSA, consideration should be given towards using vancomycin for prophylaxis as opposed to a β-lactam such as cefazolin. Guidelines and the literature, however, remain unclear regarding when vancomycin should be used as a preferred first-line agent for prophylaxis. In 1999, the CDC's SSI prevention guidelines stated that 'a threshold has not been scientifically defined that can support the decision to use vancomycin' for surgical antibiotic prophylaxis.[7]

In the intervening decade, no new studies have been published to delineate this threshold. However, there have been several studies directly comparing the efficacy of vancomycin versus a β-lactam in preventing SSI. Finkelstein et al. conducted a study in an Israeli hospital with a 'high' prevalence of MRSA infections (rate was not specified) in which patients were randomly assigned to receive vancomycin or cefazolin prior to cardiac surgery.[33] They found that overall SSI rates were similar in the two groups and that infections due to methicillin-susceptible staphylococci were more common in the vancomycin group (there was a nonsignificant trend towards more infections caused by methicillin-resistant organisms in the cefazolin group). A meta-analysis by Bolon *et al.* included this study as well as six other randomized trials (total 5761 procedures) and similarly found that neither antibiotic class (glycopeptides or β-lactams) was superior in preventing cardiac SSIs.[34] In fact, in subgroup analysis β-lactams appeared to be superior to glycopeptides in preventing chest SSIs. This may be due to the fact that, while glycopeptides are more broad-spectrum for Gram-positive coverage than β-lactams, they appear to have poorer tissue penetration and slower bacterial killing.[35]

More recently, Garey *et al.* reported that when their hospital switched from cefuroxime to vancomycin, their monthly coronary artery bypass graft (CABG) SSI incidence decreased significantly (as compared to their valve replacement SSI rates).[36] However, this was not a prospective, randomized study. Hence, while further research is needed on this topic, currently cephalosporins (usually cefazolin) remain the first-line agents for prophylaxis in cardiac surgery.

Non-systemic agents

Topical *Staphylococcus aureus* decolonization

Because *S. aureus* is one of the most significant pathogens causing SSIs, much attention has been paid to strategies for the prevention of *S. aureus* infections, both methicillin-susceptible and methicillin-resistant. These strategies have mainly focused on topical *S. aureus* decolonization using chlorhexidine gluconate or mupirocin.

Chlorhexidine gluconate

Chlorhexidine gluconate is an antiseptic agent that has been shown to decrease microbial flora on the skin and prevent infection risk in various settings, including as a skin preparatory agent for surgical procedures and for insertion of vascular access devices, as a surgical hand scrub, and for oral hygiene. Numerous studies have been published regarding its use in preoperative bathing, the hypothesis being that by decreasing overall microbial skin colonization there is less opportunity for the surgical wound to become contaminated by the patient's endogenous flora. A recent Cochrane Collaboration review evaluated data from six randomized controlled trials with a total of >10 000 participants; pooled data did not show any significant decrease in SSI rates with antiseptic bathing or showering.[23] Although the studies included in this review varied in their methodologic quality, the two largest trials (with >6000 subjects) were deemed to be of high quality.

Nevertheless, many institutions continue to practice this intervention for their patients preoperatively, particularly in light of numerous recent studies indicating chlorhexidine bathing's efficacy in other settings (e.g. prevention of catheter-associated bloodstream infections and of transmission of vancomycin-resistant enterococci in the intensive care unit[37,38]). Currently there is interest in the use of chlorhexidine-impregnated wipes as an alternative to bathing or showering with chlorhexidine soap. Although the wipes only contain 2% chlorhexidine, they have been shown to achieve higher chlorhexidine concentrations on the skin than the 4% chlorhexidine soap,[39] and may represent an attractive alternative for patients who are unable to shower or bathe thoroughly. Preoperative chlorhexidine bathing may be considered if other measures have been instituted and SSI rates remain high.

Finally, Segers *et al.* studied the effects of preoperative decontamination of the nasopharynx and oropharynx using 0.12% chlorhexidine gluconate.[40] Patients received an oropharyngeal rinse and nasal ointment containing either chlorhexidine or placebo prior to cardiac surgery and continuing until the nasogastric tube was removed (usually the day after surgery). The intervention decreased the overall nosocomial infection rate, but did not significantly decrease the SSI rate. More data are needed to make conclusive recommendations regarding nasopharyngeal and oropharyngeal decontamination with chlorhexidine.

Mupirocin

Mupirocin is a topical antibiotic that can be administered intranasally in an attempt to eradicate a significant reservoir for *S. aureus* (patients who develop *S. aureus* infections are often colonized in their nares at the time of infection). As the incidence of infections due to MRSA has increased, there has been growing interest in the use of mupirocin preoperatively for the purposes of preventing postoperative *S. aureus* and MRSA infections. One of the largest studies looking at this issue was published by Perl and colleagues in 2002, in which >4000 preoperative patients were enrolled in a randomized, placebo-controlled trial.[41] They found that intranasal mupirocin did not significantly reduce the rate of *S. aureus* SSIs overall, but that there was a significant reduction in *S. aureus* SSIs specifically for *S. aureus* carriers. Since then, many other smaller studies have been published on this theme, and recently two systematic reviews were performed on some of these studies. In one review by Trautmann *et al.*, the authors concluded that mupirocin prophylaxis did not reduce the overall *S. aureus* SSI rate in patients undergoing orthopedic, gastrointestinal and cardiothoracic surgery, although the MRSA SSI rate was reduced.[42] However, this review did not look at the effect of mupirocin on *S. aureus* carriers specifically and excluded non-English language papers. By contrast, the review by van Rijen *et al.* focused solely on patients who were *S. aureus* carriers and found that mupirocin significantly reduced the overall rate of postoperative *S. aureus* infections.[43] Interestingly, however, there was no significant decrease in SSIs due to *S. aureus*. The main limitation of this analysis was the fact that its outcome was mostly determined by the results of the study by Perl *et al.*,[41] as they had by far the largest study group. The use of prophylactic intranasal mupirocin has been widely adopted for preoperative patients and is recommended by the Society of Thoracic Surgeons' practice guidelines for all patients undergoing cardiac surgery 'in the absence of a documented negative test for staphylococcal colonization'.[27]

RECOMMENDATIONS FOR SPECIFIC PROCEDURES (TABLES 132.2, 132.3)

One of the most important principles in the selection of an antimicrobial for prophylaxis is to effectively provide coverage for the most common pathogens associated with wound infections following the specific surgical procedure. Basic principles of pharmacokinetics and pharmacodynamics dictate that the agent chosen should have effective tissue penetration, a relatively long half-life, minimal toxicity and minimal side-effects. Published literature supports the use of many different regimens for the prophylaxis of any one surgical procedure (see Tables 132.2 and 132.3). Other factors such as cost and antimicrobial resistance, however, tilt the pendulum towards more narrow-spectrum, older antimicrobial agents.

Cardiothoracic surgery

Antimicrobial prophylaxis for cardiac procedures is addressed in all standard guidelines as well as specifically in a statement from the Society of Thoracic Surgeons.[27,44] Antimicrobial prophylaxis should be administered for all cardiac procedures with median sternotomy. The incidence of deep sternal wound infections is reported to be between 0.25% and 4%,[44] and the consequences of these infections can be devastating. Two recent reviews of deep sternal wound infections, one during 1990–2003 and the other during 2001–2005, reported in-hospital mortality rates of 6.9% and 9.2%, respectively.[45,46]

Prophylaxis should target staphylococcal species, namely *S. aureus* and coagulase-negative staphylococci. As mentioned above, the increasing prevalence of MRSA complicates antimicrobial choices and some guidelines have recommended the use of vancomycin in institutions with a 'high rate' of infection due to MRSA, but the threshold for a 'high rate' has not been established (see section on MRSA above).

Table 132.2 Antibiotic prophylaxis recommendations for selected surgical procedures (superscripts denote source of recommendations; see footnote below)

Type of surgery	Recommended drugs	Alternative drugs	Duration
Cardiothoracic	Cefazolin*[†‡] or cefuroxime[†‡] or cefamandole* or vancomycin (if high risk for MRSA) [†‡]	*β-Lactam allergy:* Vancomycin[†‡] ± gentamicin* or clindamycin[†]	Single-dose[‡], ≤48h[†], ≤72h*
Gastrointestinal			
Gastroduodenal	Cefazolin* (high risk only[‡])	*β-Lactam allergy:* Clindamycin + gentamicin[†] or ciprofloxacin[‡] or levofloxacin[‡] or aztreonam[‡]	Single dose*[‡]
Biliary			
Open procedures	Cefazolin*	*β-Lactam allergy:* Clindamycin + gentamicin or ciprofloxacin or levofloxacin or aztreonam	Single dose*
Laparoscopic procedures	Cefazolin (high risk only)[‡]	*β-Lactam allergy:* Clindamycin + gentamicin[‡] or ciprofloxacin[‡] or levofloxacin[‡] or aztreonam[‡]	Single dose[‡]
Appendectomy for uncomplicated appendicitis	Cefoxitin*[‡] or cefotetan* or cefmetazole* or cefazolin + metronidazole[‡] or ampicillin–sulbactam[‡]	*β-Lactam allergy:* Clindamycin + gentamicin[‡] or ciprofloxacin[‡] or levofloxacin[‡] or aztreonam[‡] or gentamicin + metronidazole*	Single dose*[‡]
Colorectal	*Oral:* Neomycin + erythromycin base*[†‡] or neomycin + metronidazole[†‡] *Parenteral:* Cefotetan*[†] or cefoxitin*[†‡] or cefmetazole* or cefazolin + metronidazole[†‡] or ampicillin–sulbactam[†‡]	*β-Lactam allergy:* Clindamycin + gentamicin[†‡] or fluoroquinolone[†‡] or aztreonam[†‡] or metronidazole + gentamicin[†] or fluoroquinolone[†]	*Parenteral:* Single dose (≤24 h)*[†‡]
Head and neck			
Clean with prosthesis placement	Cefazolin*	Clindamycin	Single dose*
Incisions through oral or pharyngeal mucosa	Cefazolin*[‡] or clindamycin*	Cefazolin + metronidazole* or clindamycin + gentamicin*[‡]	Single dose*[‡]
Neurosurgery			
Elective craniotomy or cerebrospinal fluid shunting	Cefazolin*[‡] or vancomycin (if high risk for MRSA or β-lactam allergy)*[‡]	Oxacillin* or nafcillin*	Single dose*[‡]
Obstetrics/gynecology			
Caesarian delivery	Cefazolin*[‡]	*β-Lactam allergy:* Clindamycin + gentamicin[†] or ciprofloxacin[†] or levofloxacin[†] or aztreonam[†]	Single dose*[‡]
Hysterectomy	Cefotetan*[†] or cefazolin*[†‡§] or cefoxitin*[†§] or ampicillin–sulbactam[†‡] or metronidazole[§] or tinidazole[§]	*β-Lactam allergy:* Clindamycin + gentamicin or fluoroquinolone or aztreonam or metronidazole + gentamicin or fluoroquinolone or clindamycin monotherapy	Single dose (≤24 h)*[†‡§]
Ophthalmic	Topical gentamicin*[‡] or tobramycin*[‡] or ciprofloxacin[‡] or gatifloxacin* or levofloxacin* or moxifloxacin[‡] or ofloxacin[‡] or neomycin–gramicidin–polymyxin B*[‡] or cefazolin by subconjunctival injection[‡]	Addition of tobramycin by subconjunctival injection*	Prior to procedure*, 2–24 h[‡]
Orthopedic			
Hip fracture repair	Cefazolin*	Vancomycin*	24 h*
Implantation of internal fixation devices	Cefazolin*	Vancomycin*	24 h*
Total joint replacement	Cefazolin*[†‡] or cefuroxime[†‡] or vancomycin (if high risk for MRSA)*[†‡]	*β-Lactam allergy:* Vancomycin*[†‡] or clindamycin[†]	Single dose (≤24 h)*[†‡]

(Continued)

Table 132.2 Antibiotic prophylaxis recommendations for selected surgical procedures—cont'd

Type of surgery	Recommended drugs	Alternative drugs	Duration
Urologic (high risk patients only)	*Oral:* Trimethoprim–sulfamethoxazole* or ciprofloxacin‡ *Parenteral:* Cefazolin* or ciprofloxacin‡	*Oral or parenteral:* Levofloxacin	Single dose*‡
Vascular	Cefazolin*†‡ or cefuroxime†‡ or vancomycin (if high risk for MRSA)†‡	Vancomycin ± gentamicin* *β-Lactam allergy:* Vancomycin†‡ or clindamycin†	Single dose (≤24 h)*†‡
Transplantation			
Heart	Cefazolin*	Cefuroxime* or cefamandole* or vancomycin ± gentamicin*	48–72 h*
Lung and heart–lung	Cefazolin*	Cefuroxime* or cefamandole* or vancomycin*	48–72 h*
Liver	Cefotaxime + ampicillin*	*Beta-lactam allergy:* clindamycin + gentamicin or ciprofloxacin or levofloxacin or aztreonam	48 h*
Pancreas and pancreas–kidney	Cefazolin*	*β-Lactam allergy:* Clindamycin + gentamicin or ciprofloxacin or levofloxacin or aztreonam	Single dose*
Kidney	Cefazolin*	*β-Lactam allergy:* Clindamycin + gentamicin or ciprofloxacin or levofloxacin or aztreonam	Single dose*

MRSA, methicillin-resistant *Staphylococcus aureus*.
*As recommended by the American Society of Health-System Pharmacists (ASHP) Therapeutic Guidelines on Antimicrobial Prophylaxis in Surgery.
†As recommended by the National Surgical Infection Prevention Project[18,19]
‡As recommended by The Medical Letter.
§As recommended by the American College of Obstetrics and Gynecology[49]

Table 132.3 Recommended initial dose, half-life and time to redosing intraoperatively[18,19]

Antimicrobial	Usual half-life with normal renal function (hrs)	Infusion time (min)	Usual intravenous dose (weight-based dosing)	Redosing interval (hrs)
Ampicillin	1–1.8	10–30	1–2 g (50 mg/kg/dose)	4
Ampicillin–sulbactam	1–1.8	10–30	1.5–3 g (50 mg/kg/dose ampicillin component)	4
Aztreonam	1.5–2	3–5 (slow iv push) 15–60 (intermittent infusion)	1–2 g (30 mg/kg/dose)	3–5
Cefamandole	0.5–2.1	3–5 (slow iv push) 15–60 (intermittent infusion)	1 g (20–40 mg/kg/dose)	3–4
Cefazolin	1.2–2.5	3–5 (slow iv push) 15–60 (intermittent infusion)	1–2 grams (20–30 mg/kg/dose)	2–5
Cefotaxime	1.5–6	3–5 (slow iv push) 15–60 (intermittent infusion)	1–2 g (50 mg/kg/dose)	4
Cefuroxime	1–2	3–5 (slow iv push) 15–60 (intermittent infusion)	1.5 g (50 mg/kg/dose)	3–4
Clindamycin	2–5.1	10–60 (do not exceed 30 mg/min)	600–900 mg (3–6 mg/kg/dose)	3–6
Ciprofloxacin	3.5–5	60	400 mg (10–15 mg/kg/dose)	4–10
Gentamicin	2–3	30–60	1.5 mg/kg/dose*	3–6
Levofloxacin	6–8	60	500 mg (10 mg/kg/dose)	12–18
Metronidazole	6–14	30–60	500 mg–1 g (15 mg/kg/dose)	6–8
Nafcillin	0.5–1.9	30–60	1–2 g (12–50 mg/kg/dose)	2–4
Oxacillin	0.5–1.8	10–30	1–2 g (12–50 mg/kg/dose)	2–4
Vancomycin	4–6	60 (≥60 min if >1 g)	1 g (10–15 mg/kg/dose)	6–12

Recommendations from the US Surgical Infection Prevention and Surgical Care Improvement Projects prefer cefazolin or cefuroxime, but suggest the use of vancomycin in patients at high risk for MRSA. Similarly, the Society of Thoracic Surgeons recommends consideration for the use of vancomycin combined with a β-lactam for patients with either presumed or known staphylococcal colonization, institutions with a 'high incidence' of MRSA, patients susceptible to colonization (hospitalized >3 days, transfer from another inpatient facility, already receiving antibiotics) or a procedure involving insertion of a prosthetic valve or vascular graft. This recommendation, however, is less well established.

Duration of prophylactic antibiotics beyond 48 hours does not decrease the potential for SSIs but rather increase the potential for antimicrobial resistance, and should be avoided. Continuation of antimicrobial prophylaxis until chest tubes or other indwelling catheters are removed is not warranted.[44]

Gastrointestinal surgery

Prophylaxis is recommended for most gastrointestinal procedures. The biliary tract is considered a sterile site, and the stomach contains few bacteria due to the highly acidic environment. However, the density of bacteria progressively increases from the small bowel to the colon, as does the proportion of anaerobic to aerobic bacteria. Prophylaxis is recommended for all procedures that enter the small bowel and colon. The intrinsic risk of infection associated with entry into other areas of the gastrointestinal tract is considered low and does not support routine antibiotic prophylaxis except in high-risk patients (see Less invasive procedures, discussed later in this chapter). In gastroduodenal surgeries, patients at a higher risk of infection include those with achlorhydria, decreased gastric motility, gastric outlet obstruction, morbid obesity, gastric bleeding or cancer.[47] For biliary procedures, high-risk patients may include the elderly, those with recent symptoms of inflammation, common duct stones, jaundice or those with a history of previous biliary surgery. Colorectal procedures have a high risk of infection and warrant routine antibiotic prophylaxis in all patients.

In gastroduodenal procedures, first- and second-generation cephalosporins have demonstrated effectiveness and are the most widely used, but the number of studies is limited compared to other types of surgery. In these cases, SSIs caused by *Bacteroides* species are rare. The need to cover anaerobic bacteria increases in distal areas of the gastrointestinal tract, and antibiotics for prophylaxis of colonic procedures should be directed at both Gram-negative aerobes and anaerobic bacteria.

Head/neck surgery

Antimicrobial prophylaxis is recommended for all head and neck procedures that involve entry into the oropharynx (clean–contaminated procedures). Antimicrobial prophylaxis is not warranted for patients undergoing clean procedures of the head and neck.[48] Antimicrobial choice should target the normal flora of the mouth and oropharynx, especially streptococci and oropharyngeal anaerobes, as postoperative wound infections are frequently polymicrobial.

Neurosurgery

Clean neurosurgical procedures are associated with a relatively low risk of SSI, usually less than 5%. Nonetheless, antimicrobial prophylaxis is recommended for clean procedures, which include craniotomies, laminectomies and ventricular fluid-shunt placements. Surgical site infections in this population are primarily associated with Gram-positive bacteria, especially *S. aureus* and coagulase-negative staphylococci.

Obstetric/gynecologic surgery

Antimicrobial prophylaxis is recommended for hysterectomies (vaginal, abdominal) and Caesarian deliveries. For most SSIs following gynecologic procedures, the bacterial source is the skin or the vagina. Aerobic Gram-positive cocci (e.g. staphylococci) predominate from the skin, but the potential for exposure to Gram-negative aerobes and anaerobic bacteria can be expected when the vagina is opened or incisions are made near the perineum or groin.[7,49] Postoperative infections associated with hysterectomies are often polymicrobial. Cephalosporins have been the most widely studied in these procedures and studies comparing different cephalosporins have not shown differences in rates of infection. Cefazolin, cefotetan, cefoxitin and ampicillin–sulbactam have been recommended.

For Caesarian sections, a first-generation cephalosporin is the drug of choice. Unlike in other surgical procedures, current guidelines recommend that the timing of antimicrobial administration for Caesarian deliveries should be delayed until after cord clamping to avoid effects on the child's normal bacterial flora. This delay in administration is supported by a few studies including a large, randomized trial in 642 women that demonstrated no differences in infectious morbidity between women administered antimicrobials preoperatively compared to after cord clamping.[50] However, based on newer studies that have shown otherwise,[51,52] a recent joint publication by the American College of Obstetricians and Gynecologists and the American Academy of Pediatrics stated that administering antibiotics pre-incision appears to be more effective in preventing SSIs than post-cord clamping.[53]

Orthopedic surgery

Clean orthopedic procedures not involving implantation of foreign materials do not require routine antimicrobial prophylaxis as the risk of an SSI is low. Any possible benefit is not considered significant enough to outweigh antimicrobial cost and potential for toxicity and antibiotic resistance. There are additional orthopedic procedures, however, where the use of antimicrobial prophylaxis significantly decreases the incidence of SSIs. These procedures include the insertion of a prosthetic joint, ankle fusion, revision of a prosthetic joint, reduction of hip fractures, reduction of high-energy closed fractures and reduction of open fractures. Such procedures are associated with a risk of infection of 5–15%, which is reduced to less than 3% by the use of prophylactic antimicrobials.[54]

Skin organisms account for most SSIs in orthopedic surgery, with *S. epidermidis* and *S. aureus* accounting for >70% of infections following total joint replacements. First-generation cephalosporins are the most widely studied antimicrobials for prophylaxis in this population. While second-generation cephalosporins offer no clear advantage, either cefazolin or cefuroxime is recommended as the preferred antimicrobial for prophylaxis in patients undergoing hip or knee arthroplasty without a β-lactam allergy. Similar to cardiac procedures, vancomycin is an alternative to consider in institutions with a 'high rate' of MRSA.

The duration of antimicrobial prophylaxis following orthopedic procedures has been debated. There is no evidence that extension of antimicrobial prophylaxis duration beyond 24 hours or until drains or catheters are removed is beneficial in reducing infections.[55]

Urologic surgery

The most common infectious complication following urologic surgery is bacteriuria. More importantly, however, antimicrobial prophylaxis prevents bacteremia and SSIs with the secondary goal of preventing bacteriuria. Most urologic procedures do not require prophylaxis in patients with sterile urine. The notable exceptions are in patients undergoing transurethral prostatectomy, transrectal prostatic biopsies and insertion of urologic prostheses.[56–58]

A wide range of antimicrobials has been studied as prophylaxis in urologic procedures. Current recommendations include the use of trimethoprim–sulfamethoxazole, cefazolin or a fluoroquinolone as the preferred antimicrobials in high-risk patients only (i.e. positive or unavailable urine culture, preoperative urinary catheter, transrectal prostatic biopsy or insertion of prosthetic material) and in patients undergoing a transurethral prostatic biopsy. *Escherichia coli* is the most common organism complicating these procedures, but other Gram-negative bacilli and enterococci also cause infection. The choice of agent for urologic procedures must be dictated by patient-specific and local susceptibility data, given that significant increases in trimethoprim–sulfamethoxazole and fluoroquinolone resistance in *E. coli* have been noted.

Vascular surgery

Antimicrobial prophylaxis is indicated for abdominal and lower extremity vascular procedures including aneurysm repair, thrombo-endarterectomy and vein bypass. Infection involving vascular graft material can be particularly devastating. It appears that patients undergoing vascular-access surgery for hemodialysis also have a decreased rate of infection following the administration of antimicrobial prophylaxis compared to placebo.[59] The most common organisms associated with infections following vascular procedures include *S. aureus*, *S. epidermidis* and enteric Gram-negative bacilli. Cefazolin and cefuroxime remain the drugs of choice, with the option to use vancomycin in institutions with a 'high rate' of infections caused by MRSA.

LESS INVASIVE PROCEDURES

The purpose in administering antibiotic prophylaxis for most of the procedures listed above is to prevent the development of an infection at the surgical site. One additional purpose for antibiotic prophylaxis is to prevent bacteremias that could lead to endocarditis. Guidelines on endocarditis prevention in dental and other procedures have recently been revised and are described here in detail.

Furthermore, as technology advances, the ability to perform procedures in a minimally invasive way is progressively increasing. Many procedures that previously could only be performed openly in an operating room setting can now be performed laparoscopically or by a nonsurgical interventionalist. These procedures are associated with their own, usually lower, risk of infection. Because most of these procedures involve newer technology, there is a smaller body of literature associated with their infection risk and antibiotic prophylaxis. Here we discuss what is available for selected procedure types.

Prevention of infective endocarditis in dental and other procedures

Previous guidelines from the American Heart Association (AHA) published in 1997 were somewhat complex and recommended antibiotic prophylaxis for the prevention of infective endocarditis (IE) in numerous settings.[60] In recent years, however, it has been acknowledged that IE is much more likely to result from randomly occurring bacteremias (such as from brushing teeth) than from dental, gastrointestinal or genitourinary tract procedures, and that ongoing maintenance of good oral hygiene is likely to have a greater beneficial effect than antibiotic prophylaxis pre-procedure. Moreover, as prophylaxis is likely to prevent very few cases of IE, the risks associated with prophylaxis probably outweigh the benefits.

In 2006 the British Society for Antimicrobial Chemotherapy issued guidelines recommending prophylaxis only for patients with a history of previous IE or who have had cardiac valve replacement or surgically constructed pulmonary shunts or conduits.[61] Similarly, in 2007 the AHA released revised and simplified guidelines which have greatly narrowed the settings in which antibiotic prophylaxis is recommended for IE prevention[62] (see Tables 132.4 and 132.5 for specific recommendations). Prophylaxis is indicated for all dental

---

Table 132.4 Cardiac conditions for which prophylaxis is reasonable with dental procedures[62]

- Prosthetic cardiac valve or prosthetic material used for valve repair
- Previous infective endocarditis
- Congenital heart disease (CHD). Only patients with the following conditions are candidates for prophylaxis:
  - Unrepaired cyanotic CHD, including palliative shunts and conduits
  - Completely repaired congenital heart defect with prosthetic material or device, whether placed by surgery or by catheter intervention, during the first 6 months after the procedure. After 6 months, prophylaxis is *not* recommended because endothelialization of prosthetic material occurs within this time
  - Repaired CHD with residual defects at the site or adjacent to the site of a prosthetic patch or prosthetic device (which inhibit endothelialization)
- Cardiac transplantation recipients who develop cardiac valvulopathy

---

Table 132.5 Prophylactic regimens for dental, oral, respiratory tract or esophageal procedures

Situation	Agent	DOSING REGIMEN: SINGLE DOSE 30–60 MIN BEFORE PROCEDURE	
		Adults	Children
Oral prophylaxis			
Standard	Amoxicillin	2 g	50 mg/kg (max 2 g)
Penicillin allergy	Clindamycin *or*	600 mg	20 mg/kg (max 600 mg)
	Cephalexin*† *or*	2 g	50 mg/kg (max 2 g)
	Azithromycin *or* clarithromycin	500 mg	15 mg/kg (max 500 mg)
Parenteral prophylaxis			
Standard	Ampicillin	2 g iv or im	50 mg/kg (max 2 g) iv or im
Penicillin allergy	Clindamycin *or*	600 mg iv	20 mg/kg (max 600 mg) iv
	Cefazolin†	1 g iv or im	50 mg/kg (max 1 g) iv or im
	Ceftriaxone†	1 g iv or im	50 mg/kg (max 1 g) iv or im

*Or other first- or second- generation oral cephalosporin in appropriate equivalent dosage.
†Cephalosporins should not be used in individuals with immediate-type hypersensitivity reaction (urticaria, angioedema or anaphylaxis) to penicillins.
Adapted from Wilson *et al.*[62]

procedures that involve manipulation of gingival tissue or the periapical region of teeth or perforation of the oral mucosa (including standard dental cleanings) in patients at risk. Viridans group streptococci are the most common cause of endocarditis following these procedures. Prophylaxis is not recommended, however, for routine anesthetic injections through noninfected tissue, taking dental radiographs, placement of removable prosthodontic or orthodontic appliances, placement of orthodontic brackets, bleeding from trauma to the lips or oral mucosa, orthodontic appliance adjustment or shedding of deciduous teeth.[62]

Pacemaker/cardioverter-defibrillator implantation

Along with a worldwide aging population, the incidence of cardiac device implantation is increasing, along with an increasing risk of infection. The estimated rate of infection after implantation of permanent endocardial leads is 1–2%, although published rates vary.[63] While there are few large-scale randomized controlled trials evaluating the efficacy of antibiotic prophylaxis in this setting, there is a meta-analysis pooling data from >2000 patients in seven trials which suggested a protective effect of antibiotic prophylaxis in patients undergoing permanent pacemaker implantation.[64] Antibiotics used in the trials were either a penicillin with activity against *S. aureus* or a first-generation cephalosporin, but duration of therapy varied considerably, ranging from 6 hours to 8 days. In most studies the antibiotic was administered within the 2 hours preceding the incision.

More recently, a large prospective survey (the PEOPLE study) in patients with implantation of pacemakers and cardioverter-defibrillators reported that antibiotic prophylaxis appeared to have a protective effect (adjusted odds ratio 0.4) against the development of a cardiac device-related infection.[63] Nonetheless, there was variability in type and duration of antibiotic prophylaxis (antibiotics were administered according to local guidelines). Hence, while it remains unclear as to the optimal duration and choice of antibiotics, there does appear to be a body of literature suggesting that antibiotic prophylaxis is beneficial in preventing cardiac device-related infections. A single dose of a β-lactam antibiotic such as cefazolin is probably appropriate to cover skin flora.

Gastrointestinal endoscopy

Antibiotic prophylaxis has been used in the setting of gastrointestinal endoscopy for two purposes:
- to prevent endocarditis from bacteremia; and
- to prevent gastrointestinal or intra-abdominal infections from local seeding.

It is no longer recommended for the prevention of IE (see Prevention of infective endocarditis in dental and other procedures, above). Here we will discuss settings in which prophylaxis has been used to prevent local infections.

Endoscopic retrograde cholangiopancreatography

Cholangitis and pancreatitis can occur as a result of endoscopic retrograde cholangiopancreatography (ERCP), particularly when biliary drainage is incomplete.[65] Antibiotic prophylaxis is a common practice for some of these patients, but practices and guidelines vary widely as to which specific subsets of patients should receive antibiotics. Most randomized controlled trials investigating this issue are relatively small, and since infection rates are low it is probable that they were not adequately powered to detect a difference in infection rates. A meta-analysis by Harris *et al.* summarized the results of five randomized controlled trials and found no significant difference in infection rates between the group that received prophylaxis and the group that did not.[66] A recent retrospective review followed outcomes over an 11-year period during which the use of prophylaxis was sequentially scaled back. Initially all patients with biliary or pancreatic obstruction, those likely to need therapeutic intervention and those with immunosuppression received prophylaxis. By the end of the study period, the only patients who received prophylaxis were those in whom drainage was suspected to be incomplete, or were considered immunosuppressed. The authors found no significant difference in infection outcomes during this time.[67] Finally, a review by Subhani *et al.* examined the evidence for antibiotic prophylaxis in ERCP and stated that prophylaxis for all patients was not beneficial. However, they suggested that if prophylaxis were given to patients with incomplete drainage, that 80% of cholangitis episodes would be prevented.[68]

The American Society for Gastrointestinal Endoscopy (ASGE),[69] the British Society of Gastroenterology Endoscopy Committee[70] and the European Society of Gastrointestinal Endoscopy[71] all recommend antibiotic prophylaxis when ERCP is performed for pancreatic pseudocyst drainage or biliary obstruction (ASGE narrows the latter criterion to those in whom incomplete drainage is anticipated, as is recommended by Subhani *et al.*[68]). The antibiotic chosen should cover biliary organisms, including enterococci and enteric Gram-negative bacteria. Fluoroquinolones or β-lactam/β-lactamase inhibitor combinations, such as ampicillin–sulbactam, are sometimes used.

Endoscopic ultrasound-fine needle aspiration

With regard to endoscopic ultrasound-fine needle aspiration (EUS-FNA) procedures, antibiotic prophylaxis is often administered when FNA of cystic lesions along the GI tract is performed so as to prevent cyst infection; however, these infections are rare and there are no randomized studies evaluating the efficacy of antibiotic prophylaxis in these patients, despite the fact that expert opinion frequently recommends it.

Percutaneous endoscopic gastrostomy

Antibiotic prophylaxis is recommended for percutaneous endoscopic gastrostomy (PEG) tube placements, typically with single-dose cefazolin. A recent Cochrane Review did find a significant decrease in peristomal infections with antibiotic prophylaxis.[72]

Interventional radiology

There are no randomized controlled trials in the interventional radiology (IR) arena proving the efficacy of antibiotic prophylaxis. Nonetheless, it has become a standard of care in many institutions to administer antibiotics in this setting. In a recent review by Ryan *et al.*,[73] it is acknowledged that the benefit of antibiotic prophylaxis for central venous access is unproven, and antibiotics are not recommended for routine vascular access procedures such as angiography, angioplasty, stent placement and peripheral access (the authors leave open the option of single-dose cefazolin for tunneled central venous access although there are no specific data to support this recommendation). Nonetheless, Ryan *et al.* do recommend antibiotic prophylaxis for other IR procedures such as embolization procedures (uterine fibroid, hepatic chemoembolization, splenic, renal) and tube placements (cholecystostomy, gastrostomy, nephrostomy). Again, however, few studies exist in the IR realm to support these recommendations. When prophylaxis is given, a single-dose antibiotic covering the local organisms is sufficient (frequently used options include cefazolin for skin flora and ampicillin–sulbactam or ceftriaxone for gastrointestinal or genitourinary organisms).

Laparoscopic cholecystectomy

Most randomized controlled trials looking at the utility of antibiotic prophylaxis for laparoscopic cholecystectomy have included only a small number of patients. However, a meta-analysis combining results from five studies with a total of 899 patients found no significant difference in wound infection rates between those that received antibiotic prophylaxis and those that did not.[74] Hence, most experts do not recommend routine prophylaxis for laparoscopic cholecystectomy.

REFERENCES

References for this chapter can be found online at http://www.expertconsult.com

Non-inpatient parenteral antimicrobial therapy

INTRODUCTION

Most antibiotics given at home are administered orally. However, over the past 20 years, intravenous antimicrobial therapy delivered either at home or in the non-inpatient setting has developed as an important component of health-care delivery. This type of service has been termed outpatient parenteral antimicrobial therapy (OPAT), but the more general term of non-inpatient parenteral antimicrobial therapy (NIPAT) will be used in this chapter.

Over a quarter of a million patients are treated in the USA annually in this manner.[1] Indeed, it is estimated that in the 1990s up to 1 in 1000 North Americans each year received outpatient parenteral therapy. The use of home intravenous antimicrobial therapy was first reported in 1974 for children who had cystic fibrosis-associated pneumonia and subsequently for patients who had osteomyelitis.[2,3] In addition to the USA, NIPAT is now a common treatment modality in many regions, including Europe[4] and Australia.[5] These programs are useful both for patients who have infections requiring prolonged intravenous antibiotic therapy (e.g. osteomyelitis, septic arthritis or endocarditis) and for patients who have common acute infections such as skin and soft tissue infections (SSTIs) or pyelonephritis, in whom in-hospital admission may be avoided entirely. Increasingly, patients with device or prosthesis infections, wound infections and line-related bacteremia are amenable to non-inpatient therapy.

In two large recent US studies of the experience of infectious disease consultants and geriatricians with NIPAT, the four commonest infections treated, in descending order, were bone and joint infections, endocarditis, SSTIs and bacteremia. Prosthetic or orthopedic device infections, line infections and intra-abdominal infections are also important emerging disorders treated in the outpatient setting.[6,7] The potential advantages and disadvantages of NIPAT are summarized in Table 133.1. A crucial component for successful and safe treatment is that patients are clinically stable and have appropriate home circumstances and support.

This chapter focuses on the core aspects of delivering parenteral antimicrobials in the non-inpatient setting and summarizes current guidance on good practice. Key areas include patient evaluation and selection, including typical models of care, the technology that is needed to deliver this, different indications for non-inpatient therapy and attributes of key antimicrobials for such therapy, monitoring treatment and measuring outcomes. However, related topics such as duration of therapy, when to switch from intravenous to oral therapy, and the pharmacologic details of the infusions are not addressed here although are available in published guidelines.

Table 133.1 Potential advantages and disadvantages of outpatient parenteral antimicrobial therapy

Potential advantages	Potential disadvantages
Patient at home with family	Increased patient/family stress
Continue work, school	Nonadherence with therapy
Decreased nosocomial infections	Misuse of intravenous access
Fewer cannula-associated infections	Decreased supervision
Improved utilization of hospital beds	Feeling of abandonment
Patient sense of empowerment	Inappropriate antibiotic selection
Reduced health care costs (possible)	Nonadherence to bed rest, leg elevation
	Potential for unnecessarily prolonged duration of OPAT because of less medical incentive to stop treatment

Adapted from Howden & Grayson.[8]

EVIDENCE BASE AND CLINICAL PRACTICE GUIDELINES

Although there have been very few randomized trials of non-inpatient therapy, those that have been done have primarily compared inpatient treatment to home therapy; these and many published case series in diverse settings have generally reported good treatment outcomes.[8–10] A recent primary care randomized controlled trial of intravenous antibiotic treatment of cellulitis confirmed that intravenous antibiotic therapy can be safely and effectively delivered at home and is preferred by patients. Up to one-third of the patients in this study were deemed unsuitable because of co-morbidities or lack of home support.[11] While the primary driver for non-inpatient treatment has been cost containment, increasingly there is widespread acceptance by patients, caregivers, clinicians and payers that it is a safe, successful and cost-effective option with enhanced quality of life compared to inpatient hospital treatment. The other benefits include a reduced risk of health-care-acquired infections.

While experience over nearly 25 years has demonstrated the benefits of non-inpatient parenteral therapy for a variety of infections, high-grade evidence-based guidelines are lacking. However, there are a number of guidelines or good practice statements to assist physicians and other health-care professionals with various aspects of the administration of NIPAT. These are outlined in Table 133.2 [4,8,10,12,13]

Table 133.2 Guidelines for the administration of NIPAT

Guideline	Country of origin	Year	Reference	Comment
Practice guidelines for outpatient parenteral antimicrobial therapy	USA	2004	Tice et al.[10]	The most complete updated guideline on all aspects of NIPAT but primarily aimed at the US health-care system
Hospital-in-the home treatment of infectious diseases	Australia	2002	Howden & Grayson[8]	Good practice statement written by two Australian experts; provides good practical advice. Emphasis on home therapy and infusion options
Outpatient and home parenteral antibiotic therapy (OHPAT) in the UK: a consensus statement by a working party	UK expert panel	1998	Nathwani & Conlon[12]	Good practice statement with UK focus, written by multidisciplinary team of authors. Broad applicability
Advisory group on home-based and outpatient care (AdHOC): an international consensus statement on non-inpatient parenteral therapy.	International (non-US)	2000	Nathwani et al.[4]	Useful perspective on models of care and how to overcome clinical, logistic, fiscal and political barriers to setting up non-inpatient services globally
Managing skin and soft tissue infections: expert panel recommendations on key decision points	USA and UK	2003	Eron et al.[13]	Skin and soft tissue infection focus on management with particular emphasis on severity classification to determine site of care

NIPAT, non-inpatient parenteral antimicrobial therapy.

and provide a resource for good practice in a variety of clinical settings; they can also be adapted for different geographic regions and health-care systems. A good resource for updated guidance, presentation and outcomes research, as well as access to the OPAT handbook, is http://www.opat.com. The updated US guidelines[10] provide an excellent summary of reports that support the effectiveness of non-inpatient parenteral therapy for a variety of conditions. Many more such studies or reports can be added to this literature, particularly with newer antibiotics such as ertapenem, daptomycin and caspofungin.

MODELS FOR NON-INPATIENT INTRAVENOUS ANTIMICROBIAL THERAPY AND PATIENT SAFETY

The delivery of high-quality, safe home therapy is best achieved by a NIPAT team consisting of physicians, nurses and pharmacists who use clearly delineated treatment protocols.[6,10,12] Physicians should be experienced in the treatment of infection and have a good understanding of antimicrobial dynamics and pharmacokinetics to allow appropriate decisions regarding the selection and duration of therapy, as well as drug monitoring. For more complex, life-threatening infections such as endocarditis it is important to select patients carefully to minimize the risk of harm. Strict criteria[14] for defining the most appropriate patients are therefore evolving, thereby giving greater reassurance about safety to infection specialists, cardiologists, patients and their caregivers.

Since nursing staff usually administer therapy, they have regular contact with the patient and caregivers and are often the initial contact when problems arise. NIPAT pharmacists assist in the choice and mode of therapy, drug supply and the stability of the drug in the ambulatory setting.

This multidisciplinary team approach is essential to ensure safe and effective functioning of an NIPAT program. Key generic considerations that govern this include the following.

- Is parenteral therapy needed and, if so, is this decision based on medical need and appropriateness and not driven by bureaucratic or economic factors?
- Are appropriate resources available for delivering the service?

- Is the type of ambulatory setting safe, adequate and supported?
- Are the patient and caregivers willing to participate safely, effectively and reliably?
- Is there an effective communication system between all members of the team and the patient?
- Is there an understanding by the patient and caregivers of the risks and benefits of the treatment?
- Is there a clear, unequivocal, 24-hours-a-day mechanism of support for dealing with patient or caregiver queries and emergencies?
- Is there a care pathway where all key decisions around treatment and monitoring are documented confidentially and are easily accessible?
- Is there a quality assurance system[15] in place with specific program outcomes to evaluate the effectiveness and safety of the program?

Many NIPAT units have an infusion center (generally located within a hospital or clinic) where patients can be medically reviewed and receive directly observed therapy. NIPAT can be administered by a nurse visiting the patient at home, the patient receiving treatment in an infusion center or patients (or their relatives) self-administering therapy. Self-administration requires a well-motivated patient and caregiver who are capable of being educated regarding safe drug administration. It can be particularly useful for patients requiring prolonged or multi-dose therapy, or for those who require repeated courses of intravenous therapy (e.g. patients who have cystic fibrosis). In some countries (e.g. Italy) general practitioners often deliver therapy in the patient's home, particularly for lower respiratory tract infections.[16] The use of the intramuscular route is not uncommon in this country.

TECHNOLOGY USED IN NON-INPATIENT PARENTERAL ANTIMICROBIAL THERAPY

Recent advances in medical technology have allowed development of new venous access devices and drug delivery systems that have improved the safety of NIPAT.

Venous access devices

The optimal choice of vascular access is generally based on a number of factors, including the proposed treatment duration, the medication to be infused and the type of delivery system to be used.

Peripherally inserted central catheters

Peripherally inserted central catheters (PICCs) are a convenient form of intravenous access for NIPAT. They are made of flexible silicone, are introduced into the antecubital vein and advanced into the superior vena cava, and are easily held in position with an adhesive dressing. Advantages of PICCs include the fact that they can be inserted and removed in the outpatient setting, are very durable, can be kept patent with an infrequent saline flush and have a relatively low infection rate.[17] Because of their central positioning, they are suitable for administration of concentrated antibiotic solutions such as used in continuous-infusion dosing.

Peripheral intravenous cannulae

Peripheral intravenous cannulae are generally used for short-duration therapy, but to minimize the risk of phlebitis they should be changed every 2–3 days. Thus, nursing staff need to be skilled in cannula insertion and care.

Long-term central venous catheters

These catheters (e.g. Hickman's, Port-A-Cath) are occasionally used in patients who have few other options for intravenous access, or who require them for administration of parenteral nutrition or cancer chemotherapy. In-hospital admission and anesthesia are generally required for insertion; however, they have a low infection rate and provide effective access for patients who require prolonged or repeated intravenous therapy.

Drug delivery systems

Like the choice of intravenous access, the optimal NIPAT drug delivery system is influenced by the agent to be delivered and the proposed treatment duration.[8,18]

Direct push

Intravenous injection over 5–10 minutes is useful for antibiotics such as cephalosporins, penicillins and teicoplanin. Spring-loaded devices are available that can deliver an intravenous push using small (e.g. 10–20 ml) syringes.

Gravity

Drug administration by gravity is usually used for agents that require dilution in larger volume solutions (e.g. 100–1000 ml) before infusion, or where infusions require administration over an extended period of time (e.g. vancomycin, amphotericin B, ertapenem, daptomycin).

Controlled-rate infusion devices

A number of compact, battery-operated, computerized infusion pumps are available that can be programmed to deliver the antibiotic by either continuous infusion or intermittent bolus. They can be readily carried in a small bag around the waist or neck, and allow the patient to continue with normal activities while receiving therapy. These pumps are generally expensive to purchase but are reusable and most models will alarm if the intravenous line becomes blocked or develops in-line air bubbles. Nonprogrammable continuous-infusion devices are also available that are either spring loaded or elastomeric – in these the tension in either the spring or the elastomeric 'bladder' propels the infusion. Although these pumps are cheaper, they are generally not reusable and will not alarm if the infusion is interrupted. Both devices are ideal for the continuous infusion of antimicrobials that are stable in solution over a 24-hour period and that have optimal activity when stable high serum concentrations are maintained (e.g. antistaphylococcal penicillins).[19–22]

INTRAVENOUS ANTIBIOTIC REGIMENS

Ideally, the principles used for appropriate antibiotic prescribing should be similar to those applied to patients managed in hospital. Appropriate antimicrobial agent(s) include those with the narrowest antibacterial spectrum appropriate for the responsible pathogen, most practical dosing regimen and lowest purchase and delivery costs. Patient-specific factors are also important, such as avoiding aminoglycosides in patients who have significant renal impairment or β-lactams in penicillin hypersensitive patients. However, in the non-inpatient setting it is important to consider a number of pragmatic considerations which may determine the ultimate antimicrobial choice. Although most antibiotics, like the semisynthetic penicillins, can be administered three or four times a day or through continuous infusions by using controlled-infusion devices, long-acting agents such as ceftriaxone or the glycopeptides make once daily or less frequent (e.g. teicoplanin) dosing possible, and are often favored as they are convenient and reduce overall resource use such as the need for high technology infusion devices. Such agents are also preferred as they do not require an infusion but rather can be given easily by a bolus (direct push).

Other important considerations include using agents that have a proven track record of safety, stability and effectiveness in the ambulatory setting. While many currently used antimicrobials in the ambulatory setting often have an antimicrobial spectrum that is broader than necessary for many indications, there is presently no evidence that such agents (e.g. cephalosporins) are promoting antimicrobial resistance, increasing *Clostridium difficile* diarrhea or are less effective than their narrow-spectrum counterparts.[16,23] In many countries where the non-inpatient infrastructure is less well developed or resources are scarce, drugs that do not require technologic support, infusion pumps or close therapeutic monitoring, and can be given simply, are deemed attractive. Indeed, the cost-effectiveness of NIPAT is an important consideration for drug choice in many health-care facilities.[24]

A core group of antimicrobials have been used in the NIPAT setting, with more antibiotics being added to the core list with broadening worldwide experience and the emerging clinical application of new agents. These are summarized in Table 133.3. The antibiotic groups below summarize key features of some of the agents in used in NIPAT.

β-Lactams

The clinical efficacy of β-lactams against many pathogens is related to the proportion of the dosing interval during which the serum drug concentrations are maintained above the minimum inhibitory concentration (MIC) of the infecting pathogen(s).[19] Thus, β-lactams with a short half-life (e.g. penicillin, ampicillin, antistaphylococcal penicillins) should either be dosed frequently (e.g. q4–6h), which is generally impractical for NIPAT, or administered by continuous infusion. There is increasing experience with the successful use of continuous-infusion antistaphylococcal penicillins (e.g. oxacillin, flucloxacillin) and some cephalosporins (e.g. ceftazidime) for the treatment of a range of conditions, including osteomyelitis, endocarditis and pneumonia.[19,20,21,25] Limiting factors with continuous-infusion administration include the availability and cost of accurate drug delivery devices and the instability in solution of some agents (e.g. ampicillin) after compounding.

Cephalosporins such as ceftriaxone, which allow for once-daily dosing, can be extremely useful for NIPAT.[23] Similarly, recent studies in which oral probenecid used to prolong the half-life of

Table 133.3 Parenteral antibiotics commonly used in the non-inpatient setting

Antibiotic	$t_{1/2}$ (h)	Stability (90% at 20°C)	Usual dosing	Monitor	Phlebitis risk* and main side-effects	Main clinical indications	Comment
Aminoglycosides	2–3	30 days	q24h	Renal levels	1; Nephrotoxicity, vestibular toxicity	Cystic fibrosis, pyelonephritis; endocarditis (q8–12h)	Once daily; increasingly used except for endocarditis
Amphotericin B (deoxycholate)	24–360	5 days	Three times weekly	Renal, electrolytes	3; Nausea, chills, nephrotoxicity	Invasive fungal infections	Still commonly used but superseded by lipid-based amphotericin or caspofungin
Caspofungin	>48	1 day	q24h (higher first loading dose)	Renal, electrolytes	1; Mainly GI, sometimes electrolyte imbalance	Invasive fungal infections, Candida spp. endocarditis	Limited experience in NIPAT
Cefazolin	1–2	1 day	q8–12h q24h with probenecid	WBC	1; Similar to ceftriaxone	SSTIs, osteomyelitis, pyelonephritis	Narrower spectrum than ceftriaxone Longer half-life/less frequent dosing when added to probenecid
Ceftriaxone	5–11	3 days	q24h	WBC	1; Mainly GI Monitor for Clostridium difficile diarrhea	SSTIs, osteomyelitis, Lyme disease, pyelonephritis, meningitis, pneumonia, endocarditis	Extensive experience of safety and effectiveness in non-inpatient setting
Ertapenem	4	6 hours	q24h	WBC	2; Mainly GI Monitor for C. difficile diarrhea	SSTIs, intra-abdominal infections, diabetic foot ulcer infections, some complicated UTIs	Expanding experience for a variety of infections in the non-inpatient setting
Ganciclovir	3	5 days	q24h (maintenance therapy)	WBC	1; Mainly GI Marrow toxicity (e.g. neutropenia)	CMV invasive infections, e.g. retinitis	Less used due to the availability of oral valganciclovir
Teicoplanin	40	48 hours	q24h iv, or higher dose two to three times a week parenterally	Renal, WBC	1; Fevers, anemia and rash	SSTIs, osteomyelitis, bacteremia, endocarditis	Extensive experience in bacteremia, endocarditis, non-inpatient setting outside USA
Vancomycin	6	7 days	q12–24h	Renal, WBC	2; Nephrotoxicity, rash	SSTIs, bacteremia, osteomyelitis, endocarditis	Extensive experience in treating Gram-positive infections in the non-inpatient setting
Cidofovir	40	24 hours	Once weekly (induction); once every 2 weeks (maintenance)	Renal, WBC	1; Nephrotoxicity, neutropenia, fever	CMV retinitis	Limited experience but alternative to ganciclovir in the non-inpatient setting, infrequent dosing
Daptomycin	38–48	2 hours	q24h	Renal, WBC, weekly CPK levels	2; GI, myopathy	SSTIs, right-sided endocarditis, bacteremia	Emerging agent, limited experience in non-inpatient setting Off label use in bone and joint infections
Dalbavancin (not yet licensed for clinical use)	6–10 days	Not known	Two doses, 1 week apart	WBC	1; GI, fever, endocarditis	SSTIs, catheter-related bacteremia	New agent, very limited experience of use in non-inpatient setting High potential for use, e.g. in emergency departments

Phlebitis risk: 1 = mild; 2 = moderate; 3 = severe.
CMV, cytomegalovirus; CPK, creatinine phosphokinase; GI, gastrointestinal; NIPAT, non-inpatient parenteral antimicrobial therapy; SSTIs, skin and soft tissue infections; UTIs, urinary tract infections WBC, white blood cell count.

the first-generation cephalosporin cefazolin have established that this combination given once daily is effective in the treatment of conditions such as cellulitis.[24]

More recently, ertapenem, a long-acting carbapenem that can be given once daily by infusion, has been used to treat skin and soft tissue infections, intra-abdominal and pelvic infections and diabetic foot ulcer infections caused by polymicrobial infections or extended-spectrum β-lactamase (ESBL)-producing coliforms.[26,27]

Aminoglycosides

A number of clinical studies suggest that administration of aminoglycosides (e.g. 4–5 mg/kg/day or fixed 7 mg/kg/day gentamicin) as a once-daily dose rather than as two or three divided doses is associated with similar efficacy and probably reduced toxicity as compared with multidosing regimens when treating Gram-negative infections.[28,29] Once-daily gentamicin is preferred when treating infections such as pyelonephritis, cholangitis and moderate–severe Gram-negative pneumonia. However, they remain unpopular with elderly patients,[7] and data regarding their efficacy – including settings such as pregnancy, neonates, burns patients, cystic fibrosis and some cases of endocarditis – are limited or lacking.

Glycopeptides

Glycopeptides (e.g. vancomycin, teicoplanin) are effective against many Gram-positive pathogens. Vancomycin generally needs to be administered twice daily over at least 1–2 hours, while teicoplanin, after initial loading, may be given rapidly once daily or in some cases less frequently.

Vancomycin can often be given once daily in elderly patients whose renal function has declined with age. Although glycopeptides have been used in NIPAT, because of their infrequent dosing requirements they are usually only an appropriate choice when used to treat resistant bacteria such as methicillin-resistant *Staphylococcus aureus* (MRSA), or in patients who are allergic to β-lactams. The efficacy of teicoplanin in some situations has been questioned although the published experience of this agent in the non-inpatient setting is highly effective.[30]

The emergence of resistant pathogens such as vancomycin-resistant enterococci reinforces the view that glycopeptides should only be used when clearly indicated although in our experience this resistance is primarily seen in critical care facilities in hospitalized patients rather than the ambulatory setting and the exact role of glycopeptide use is as yet unclear.[31]

Dalbavancin, an investigational, long-acting glycopeptide analogue that can be administered in two single doses a week apart for SSTIs, appears to exhibit many ideal properties for a NIPAT agent.[32,33] However, its cost-effectiveness, potential for promoting resistance due to long-acting, subinhibitory tissue concentrations and the possibility of protracted adverse reactions due to the very long half-life remain concerns. Other long-acting, investigational glycopeptides such as oritavancin and telavancin may be potential candidates for use in the ambulatory setting.

More recently daptomycin, a new once-daily cyclic lipopeptide, has been used to treat complicated SSTIs.[34] and bacteremia due to endocarditis. It requires monitoring with weekly creatine phosphokinase to predict rare myopathy. Its potential for use as an alternative to the glycopeptides in the ambulatory setting for SSTIs, right-sided endocarditis[35] and other infections (e.g. bone and joint infections) is likely to expand.

Antiviral agents

Ganciclovir is effective for both acute treatment and long-term suppression of serious cytomegalovirus disease and is administered once or twice daily. Such regimens are suitable for NIPAT, although the availability of oral ganciclovir and the highly bioavailable valganciclovir have reduced the need for long-term intravenous suppressive therapy and may avoid the need for intravenous induction therapy in some patients.[36] Other intravenous antiviral agents (e.g. foscarnet and cidofovir) may occasionally be used in NIPAT.

Antifungal therapy

While parenteral amphotericin B deoxycholate has been the main agent used to treat serious fungal infections in the non-inpatient setting,[37] concerns about nephrotoxicity remain. Once daily caspofungin is increasingly used in the treatment of serious invasive candidal infections such as fungemia and endocarditis.[38]

INDICATIONS FOR HOME INTRAVENOUS ANTIMICROBIAL THERAPY

A wide variety of infections can be safely and conveniently treated with NIPAT, should such treatment be appropriate. Commonly used antibiotics and their likely indications are outlined in Table 133.3 although many of these patients may be treated effectively with oral antibiotics with high bioavailability where indicated. Infections that are relatively common and generally require only brief NIPAT include skin and soft tissue infections, pyelonephritis, pneumonia, bacterial meningitis, infective exacerbations associated with chronic lung disease and, increasingly, line-related bacteremia and late-stage Lyme disease. Such patients do not generally need long-term venous access and ideally can be treated with agents that require only infrequent dosing (e.g. once or twice daily). Serious diseases that are often suitable for NIPAT include endocarditis, osteomyelitis, septic arthritis, prosthetic device infections, deep-seated diabetic foot infections, deep abscesses (e.g. brain, psoas, liver – generally after initial drainage), invasive fungal and cytomegalovirus disease in transplant recipients and HIV-infected patients. Since these conditions usually need prolonged intravenous antibiotic therapy, long-term venous access (e.g. PICC) is often required and innovative treatment regimens (e.g. continuous-infusion agents or twice or thrice weekly agents) may be appropriate, depending on the responsible pathogen(s). Although these conditions are not common, they are often large consumers of in-hospital bed days; hence, NIPAT may substantially improve in-hospital bed utilization by treating this relatively small number of patients.

Patient selection

Appropriate patient selection is a crucial component in ensuring a safe and successful NIPAT program. Both patient-specific and disease-specific factors are important in the decision to accept a patient for NIPAT. In particular, special care should be taken when assessing elderly or isolated patients for NIPAT, who often do not cope well with medical illness, and patients who have serious diseases such as endocarditis, where potentially catastrophic complications can occur.

Patient-specific factors

Factors that may be potential contraindications to NIPAT include:
- patients who live alone or in isolated areas, or who do not have a telephone or other means of rapid communication;
- active substance abuse;
- aggressive patients, relatives or pets (these generally argue against patient suitability for NIPAT care, since the safety of members of the NIPAT team is crucial); and
- the presence of a language barrier between patient and staff that cannot be overcome with the assistance of interpreters or family members (this suggests that safety at home cannot be assured and that in-hospital therapy may therefore be more appropriate).

Disease-specific factors

A clearly defined diagnosis is important before embarking on NIPAT. Patients who have common, less serious conditions such as cellulitis can often be transferred directly from the emergency department or general practitioner to the NIPAT program, avoiding in-hospital admission. Patients who have more serious conditions such as endocarditis, osteomyelitis and meningitis generally require a period of inpatient assessment, treatment and stabilization before transfer to a NIPAT program to complete their treatment course.

Disease-specific indications

Specific common and emerging infections that can be treated with NIPAT are discussed in more detail below.

Skin and soft tissue infections

Bacterial skin and soft tissue infections collectively refer to a variety of microbial invasions of the skin layers (epidermis, dermis and subcutaneous tissues), inducing a host response. Infections may present either as cutaneous abscesses with a collection of pus surrounded by an area of erythema and swelling or as diffuse, spreading infections as in cellulitis or erysipelas. Bacterial skin and soft tissue infections occur frequently and range in severity from superficial infections of mild to moderate severity to deeper, occasionally necrotizing, infections. Although SSTIs represent a common indication for antibiotic therapy, an etiologic diagnosis is often difficult and most patients are treated empirically. As the description implies, complicated SSTIs are usually more severe, progress rapidly, involve deeper tissues and possess a greater risk of limb loss than uncomplicated SSTIs. Complicated cellulitis, complex abscesses, post-traumatic or surgical site infections, and infected diabetic and ischemic ulcers are commonly encountered examples. Hospitalization along with surgical debridement or drainage, parenteral antibiotic therapy, and management of co-morbid conditions such as peripheral vascular disease or diabetes mellitus is usually necessary.

Many SSTIs may be amenable to NIPAT and the key decision issues in these cases are around the need for hospitalization and supportive therapy and the most appropriate antibiotic therapy. The Eron classification for SSTIs based on severity assessment and the presence of stable co-morbidities provides a useful practical guide to determining the most appropriate site of care and antibiotic choice.[39]

Numerous US studies have demonstrated the efficacy of once-daily ceftriaxone 1–2 g for cellulitis, although the appropriateness of this relatively broad-spectrum agent for this indication has been questioned.[10] The first-generation cephalosporin, cefazolin, when given in a dose of 2 g twice daily,[40] or 2 g once daily together with oral probenecid 1 g once daily, is effective.[41] Both regimens have comparable clinical efficacy to that of once-daily ceftriaxone and represent practical, appropriate NIPAT options. Subsequent switching to oral agents such as dicloxacillin (500 mg q6h), cephalexin (500 mg q6h) or clindamycin (300 mg q6h) after initial improvement usually results in cure.

Pyelonephritis and complicated urinary tract infections

Gentamicin (4–7 mg/kg intravenously q24h), ceftriaxone (1 g intravenously q24h) or ciprofloxacin (500–750 mg orally q12h) are appropriate empiric single agents for pyelonephritis, since the usual pathogens are often Gram-negative bacilli. Ampicillin or penicillin may also be given empirically to treat possible enterococcal infections, although this is an uncommon pathogen in young patients. Antibiotic selection should be reviewed once the results of urine and blood cultures are available.

Studies have demonstrated that oral fluoroquinolones are highly effective in treating pyelonephritis, and they may be considered as an alternative to parenteral therapy for patients in whom adherence is assured.[42] Although ciprofloxacin would not usually be the first-line choice for in-hospital care of pyelonephritis, the fact that its use may avoid the need for intravenous access offers a significant practical advantage.

Recently, outbreaks of multiresistant ESBL-producing *Escherichia coli* infections, or sometimes *Klebsiella* spp., have caused urinary tract infections in the community.[43] Many of these patients have been effectively treated with parenteral once daily ertapenem as resistance to aminoglycosides and quinolones has increased.

Community-acquired pneumonia

Ceftriaxone 1–2 g once daily is widely used for the home intravenous treatment of pneumonia. However, in many regions ceftriaxone would not be the drug of first choice for in-hospital care of community-acquired pneumonia and the drug's broad spectrum of activity may be unnecessary. Furthermore, the availability of highly effective oral therapy, the need for oxygen support and close monitoring in patients who are deemed of need for parenteral drugs makes this a less attractive therapeutic indication for NIPAT.

Endocarditis

Increasingly, a large and significant number of patients with endocarditis are treated in the non-inpatient setting and account for a higher proportion of treatment days.[44] Indeed, the ambulatory intravenous therapy option is now included in some key guidelines for the treatment of endocarditis.[45] Although endocarditis can be successfully treated with NIPAT it can pose problems because of the risk of life-threatening complications and for this reason strict selection criteria for patients who have endocarditis have been proposed.[14,45] They suggest that most patients who have endocarditis should generally be managed in hospital for the initial 2 weeks. One exception may be patients with uncomplicated viridans streptococcal endocarditis who rapidly become afebrile and clear their bacteremia; such patients may be suitable for transfer home after 1 week. Patients who have complicated endocarditis (heart failure, conduction abnormality, perivalvular abscess), aortic valve disease, prosthetic valve endocarditis, acute endocarditis or infection caused by virulent organisms such as *Staphylococcus aureus* should generally be managed primarily as inpatients.

Ceftriaxone (2 g/day) has been most commonly used for the home treatment of uncomplicated viridans streptococcal endocarditis; it appears to be effective when given either alone for 4 weeks or together with an aminoglycoside for 2 weeks.[14,44,45] Monitoring of renal and auditory function is particularly important if aminoglycosides are being used for prolonged periods. There are also infrequent case reports of treatment with intermittent-dose (and occasionally continuous-infusion) penicillin via a computerized pump for viridans streptococcal endocarditis in the NIPAT setting.

There are also a number of reports of successful NIPAT for staphylococcal endocarditis. Treatment options include the use of antistaphylococcal penicillins given by computerized pump as a continuous infusion or by intermittent bolus.[20,21,25] Vancomycin may be used in β-lactam-allergic patients but appears to be less effective than β-lactams for susceptible staphylococcal strains.[46]

Daptomycin is another potential option for methicillin-resistant or methicillin-susceptible *S. aureus* bacteremia secondary to right-sided endocarditis.[35] There are very limited NIPAT data for endocarditis caused by other organisms such as enterococci, HACEK organisms and fungi. Outpatient parenteral antimicrobial therapy for endocarditis generally requires central venous access (e.g. PICC) and close weekly clinical and drug monitoring.

Osteomyelitis

Most forms of osteomyelitis require 4–6 weeks of parenteral antimicrobial therapy, although the treatment choice, duration and need for surgery may differ depending on the responsible pathogen(s), host factors and the bone involved. *Staphylococcus aureus* is the most common cause of osteomyelitis, but other pathogens such as coagulase-negative staphylococci, *Pseudomonas* spp. and Enterobacteriaceae may be involved when osteomyelitis is nosocomial in origin or associated with foreign bodies or intravenous drug abuse.[47] Thus, various treatment options may need to be considered.[48] Long-term intravenous access is generally required unless oral fluoroquinolones are considered appropriate.[47–49]

Prosthetic device infections

Prosthetic orthopedic infections and other device-related (e.g. endovascular) infections, primarily due to *S. aureus* or coagulase-negative staphylococci, continue to increase and often require prolonged antibiotic therapy. They represent a significant clinical and health-care resource challenge.[50] Oral options are often limited; oral linezolid is less desirable because of potential hematologic, metabolic and neurologic side-effects with protracted therapy. Therefore, glycopeptides or lipopeptides are attractive options, usually in combination with oral rifampin (rifampicin). These infections represent a major future opportunity for NIPAT.

MONITORING PATIENTS RECEIVING NON-INPATIENT PARENTERAL ANTIMICROBIAL THERAPY

Patients require careful monitoring while receiving both NIPAT and oral therapy. Although the home environment has many advantages for the patient, the careful regular monitoring that generally occurs in hospital is not present at home. In general, patients should be reviewed by the NIPAT physician at least once a week, usually in the outpatient department or office. Specific factors to assess on review include:

- patient's reaction to NIPAT;
- response to therapy;
- drug side-effects; and
- other complications (e.g. venous cannula infection).

Routine hematology and biochemistry, as well as serum drug levels, are also often monitored weekly.

Since in some situations more frequent reviews, or even emergency assessments, may be necessary, all good NIPAT programs should have a system to manage these.

SUMMARY

Given recent trends worldwide, an increasing proportion of medical care that previously would have been administered in hospital is likely to be delivered at home or in other ambulatory care settings. Patient selection should be based primarily on medical suitability rather than economic considerations. However, ensuring appropriate antibiotic selection and providing safe delivery systems and continuity of care by a multidisciplinary team are key challenges. The importance of evaluating key patient and program outcomes cannot be overemphasized if NIPAT programs are to remain a safe, effective and high quality standard of care.

REFERENCES

References for this chapter can be found online at http://www.expertconsult.com

Gary J Noel
Jason S Kendler
Barry J Hartman
Mark Macielag
Karen Bush

Chapter | **134** |

β-Lactam antibiotics

INTRODUCTION

Although Alexander Fleming observed that a *Penicillium* mold inhibited the growth of bacteria in culture in 1928, it was not until 1941 that Florey, Chain and Abraham used penicillin for the first time to treat patients with staphylococcal and streptococcal infections.[1] More than 60 years later, the β-lactam antibiotics remain the mainstay of treatment for a variety of bacterial infections (Table 134.1) and now include:

- penicillins;
- cephalosporins;
- monobactams;
- carbapenems; and
- β-lactamase inhibitor combinations.

Table 134.1 Clinical use of β-lactam antibiotics by site of infection

Infection site	β-Lactam used
Skin/soft tissue infections	Cephalosporins, penicillins, carbapenem (ertapenem)

Head and neck infections
  Dental infections
  Pharyngitis
  Sinusitis
  Meningitis
	
	Penicillins
	Cephalosporins, penicillins
	Penicillins, cephalosporins
	Cephalosporins (third- and fourth-generation agents), carbapenem (meropenem)

Lower respiratory tract infections	Penicillins, cephalosporins, carbapenems (especially for hospital-acquired infections)
Urinary tract infections	Penicillins, cephalosporins, monobactam, carbapenems (especially for infections due to multidrug-resistant Gram-negative bacilli)
Intra-abdominal infections	Cephalosporins (in combination with agent anaerobic activity), carbapenems, ureidopenicillin with β-lactamase inhibitor
Bone and joint infections	Penicillins, cephalosporins

PENICILLINS

The natural penicillins such as penicillin G are used primarily for the treatment of selected Gram-positive as well as selected Gram-negative infections. The penicillinase-resistant penicillins, including nafcillin and oxacillin, had been used for the treatment of infections due to staphylococci prior to the emergence of widespread resistance among staphylococci due to the acquisition of low-affinity penicillin-binding proteins. These agents are active against other Gram-positive organisms and continue to remain agents of choice in treating methicillin-susceptible staphylococci. The aminopenicillins such as ampicillin and amoxicillin have a similar spectrum of activity as the natural penicillins, but have additional activity against Gram-negative organisms including many Enterobacteriaceae. When used together with β-lactamase inhibitors, they have good activity against Gram-positive, Gram-negative and anaerobic organisms that produce β-lactamases, enzymes which can hydrolyze these agents. The carboxypenicillins (ticarcillin) and ureidopenicillins (piperacillin) have activity against aminopenicillin-resistant Gram-negative bacilli, especially *Pseudomonas aeruginosa*, and can also be used in conjunction with β-lactamase inhibitors for extended activity against β-lactamase-producing organisms.

Cephalosporins

Cephalosporins are frequently designated as belonging to a generation, first through fourth, to suggest a general spectrum of activity of the agents. In this categorization, first-generation cephalosporins had activity against Gram-positive cocci, but had limited activity against Gram-negative pathogens. The second-generation cephalosporins had improved Gram-negative activity compared with that of the first-generation cephalosporins. Selected second-generation cephalosporins (i.e. cefoxitin and cefotetan) also had activity against anaerobes. Third-generation cephalosporins had further improved Gram-negative activity, but their activity against Gram-positive bacteria was variable (e.g. cefotaxime, ceftazidime and ceftriaxone). Cefepime (primarily USA) and cefpirome (Europe) are known as fourth-generation cephalosporins with demonstrated efficacy against most clinically important Gram-positive and Gram-negative bacteria.

Another useful categorization of cephalosporins is based on chemical structure[2,3] and could become more widely accepted with the emergence of new agents having a unique microbiologic spectrum, such as ceftobiprole and ceftaroline with anti-methicillin-resistant *Staphylococcus aureus* (MRSA) activity. As cephalosporin resistance increases due to extended spectrum β-lactamases and carbapenemases, the antimicrobial spectrum of agents categorized within these generations will need to be redefined, especially for Gram-negative bacteria.

Monobactams

Monobactams, with aztreonam as the only commercially available agent, are effective only against aerobic Gram-negative organisms and have no activity against Gram-positive organisms or anaerobes.

Carbapenems

The carbapenems (imipenem, meropenem, ertapenem and doripenem) have the broadest bacterial coverage of the β-lactam antibiotics. These agents have been used to treat patients with infections caused by Gram-positive, Gram-negative and anaerobic bacteria.

Mechanism of action

β-Lactam antibiotics inhibit bacterial cell wall synthesis, a bactericidal mechanism of action. These agents bind tightly to proteins known as penicillin-binding proteins (PBPs) on the inner surface of the bacterial cell membrane, thereby interrupting the terminal transpeptidation process in bacterial cell wall biosynthesis. Ultimately, loss of viability and, in some bacteria, lysis, occurs as the result of the activation of autolytic enzymes.

Bacterial resistance

Four major mechanisms lead to bacterial resistance to β-lactam antibiotics:

- failure of the antibiotic to penetrate the bacterial cell membrane;
- efflux of the antibiotic from the periplasmic space by specific pumping mechanisms;

- alterations in PBPs that reduce the binding affinities of the β-lactams (intrinsic resistance);[4] and
- bacterial production of β-lactamases, which hydrolyze the β-lactam ring and render the antibiotics microbiologically inactive. This is the most important and most common cause of resistance, especially in Gram-negative bacteria.[5]

Strategies to combat resistance, including the use of β-lactamase inhibitors, are discussed later in this chapter.

PHARMACOKINETICS AND DISTRIBUTION

Absorption

The β-lactams have variable absorption from the gastrointestinal tract. Some agents, such as the antipseudomonal penicillins and methicillin, are acid-labile and cannot be taken orally. The absorption characteristics and pharmacokinetics of the β-lactams are shown in Table 134.2. Of note, amoxicillin is almost totally absorbed when administered orally whereas ampicillin is only partially absorbed. The presence of food in the stomach can delay absorption and can lower the peak serum concentration for some β-lactams, such as ampicillin, cefaclor, cephalexin and ceftibuten, but can increase the absorption of cefuroxime and cefpodoxime.

Distribution

Following absorption, β-lactams are variably and reversibly bound to serum proteins, mostly albumin. Protein-bound drug does not exert antimicrobial activity. Excretion of the β-lactams is primarily renal (glomerular filtration and tubular secretion) and, in general, the serum half-life of these drugs is short, often 1 hour or less.

Table 134.2 Pharmacokinetics of selected β-lactam antibiotics

Generic name	Oral absorption (%)	Effect of food on absorption	Protein binding (%)	Serum half-life (h)	Biliary excretion (% of dose)
Penicillins					
Amoxicillin–clavulanate	75/–	Minimal/increases	20/30	1.3/1.0	2–3/<1
Ampicillin–sulbactam	40/–	Decreases/–	28/38	1.1/1.0	3/0.24
Azlocillin	NA		30	0.8–1.5	5.3
Bacampicillin	87–95	None	28	1.1	0.1
Carbenicillin (Indanyl)	30–40		50–60	1.0	Minimal
Cloxacillin	50	Decreases	90–98	0.5	2–10
Dicloxacillin	35–76	Decreases	95–97	0.7	Some penetration into bile
Methicillin	NA		17–45	0.5–1.0	2–3
Mezlocillin	NA		16–42	1.1	2.5
Nafcillin	10–20	Decreases	90	0.5	8
Oxacillin	30	Decreases	94	0.5	2–10
Penicillin G	15	Decreases	65	0.5	5
Penicillin V	60	Lowers and delays peak	80	0.5	
Piperacillin–tazobactam	NA		26–33/31–32	1.0/0.7–0.9	20
Ticarcillin–clavulanate	NA		45/30	1.2/1.0	4/<1

Table 134.2 Pharmacokinetics of selected β-lactam antibiotics—cont'd

Generic name	Oral absorption (%)	Effect of food on absorption	Protein binding (%)	Serum half-life (h)	Biliary excretion (% of dose)
Cephalosporins					
Cefaclor	52–95	Lowers and delays peak	22–25	0.6–0.9	Some penetration into bile
Cefadroxil	90	None	20	1.5	High conc. in bile
Cefazolin	NA		73–87	1.4–2.0	0.03
Cefditoren (pivoxil)	14–16	Increased with fatty meal	88	1.6	Some penetration into bile
Cefdinir	16–25	Reduced after a fatty meal	60–70	1.7	
Cefepime	NA		20	2.0	Some penetration into bile
Cefixime	40–50		65	3–4	5
Cefoperazone	NA		82–93	1.9	20–30
Cefotaxime	NA		30–51	1.0–1.5	0.1
Cefotetan	NA		78–91	3–4.6	13
Cefoxitin	NA		65–79	0.7–1.1	High conc. in bile
Cefpodoxime (proxetil)	46–50	Increases	18–40	2.1–2.8	Some penetration into bile
Cefprozil	95	None	35–45	1.3–1.8	
Ceftazidime	NA		10–20	1.5–1.8	0.21
Ceftibuten	>90	Lowers peak	65–77	2–2.4	
Ceftizoxime	NA		30	1.3–1.9	0.2–7.8
Ceftobiprole (medocaril)	NA		16	3.0	<1%
Ceftriaxone	NA		85–95	5–11	10–65
Cefuroxime (axetil)	52	Increases	33–50	1.5	0.13
Cephalexin	90	Lowers and delays peak	5–15	0.7–1.1	0.29
Cephalothin	NA		65–80	0.5–1.0	High conc. in bile
Loracarbef	~90	Decreases	25	1.2	
Monobactam					
Aztreonam	NA		56	1.7–2.9	<1
Carbapenems					
Doripenem	NA		5–15	1.0	<1%
Ertapenem	NA		85–95	4	Some penetration into bile
Imipenem–cilastatin	NA		15–25	1.0	<0.3
Meropenem	NA		2	1.0–1.5	Some penetration into bile

Pharmacokinetic data as per references 6–32.
NA, not applicable because agent is administered by parenteral route only.
Absence of information is due to lack of published data.

Procaine penicillin G and benzathine penicillin G are intramuscular preparations that are absorbed slowly, allowing for longer dosing intervals. Nafcillin, the ureidopenicillins (20–30%), cefoperazone (20%), ceftriaxone (10–65%) and cefotetan (13%) have significant excretion in bile.[13]

Imipenem, a carbapenem, is inactivated by dehydropeptidase I, an enzyme present on the renal brush border and other tissues. Cilastatin, a dehydropeptidase inhibitor and nephroprotectant, is administered along with imipenem to prevent subtherapeutic levels of the antibiotic. Cilastatin is not microbiologically active nor does it alter the pharmacokinetics of other drugs.[33]

The β-lactam antibiotics achieve therapeutic concentrations in most tissues including lung, kidney, bone, muscle and liver, and in secretions such as synovial fluid, pleural fluid, pericardial fluid,

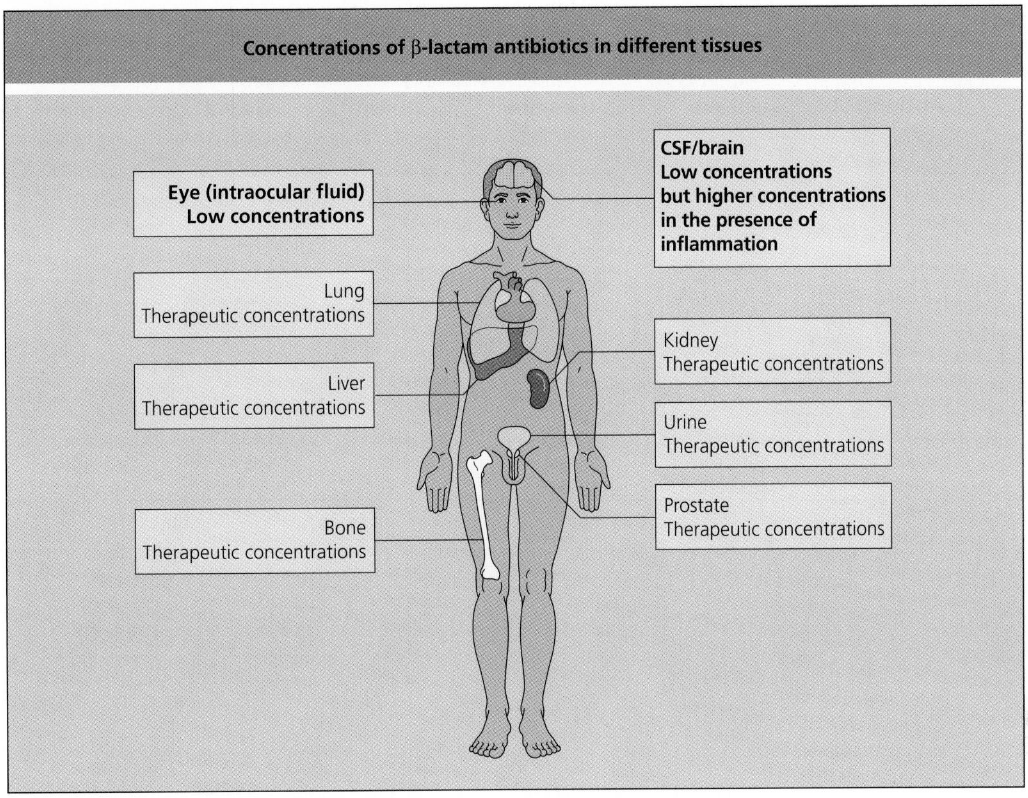

Concentrations of β-lactam antibiotics in different tissues

Eye (intraocular fluid)
Low concentrations

CSF/brain
Low concentrations
but higher concentrations
in the presence of
inflammation

Lung
Therapeutic concentrations

Kidney
Therapeutic concentrations

Liver
Therapeutic concentrations

Urine
Therapeutic concentrations

Prostate
Therapeutic concentrations

Bone
Therapeutic concentrations

Fig. 134.1 Concentration of β-lactam antibiotics in different tissues.

peritoneal fluid and bile. The microenvironment that may be found in an abscess, including a low pH, the presence of neutrophils and associated proteins, and low oxygen tension, does not inhibit the function of β-lactam antibiotics. In general, β-lactams are considered to be unable to penetrate host cells and are therefore ineffective against intracellular organisms. However, these agents have been shown to be effective in infections due to *Listeria* and *Salmonella* that are considered to be successful intracellular pathogens. Low concentrations of β-lactams are found in prostatic secretions, brain tissue, intraocular fluid and cerebrospinal fluid (CSF; Fig. 134.1). In the presence of inflammation, however, concentrations in the CSF are much higher, accounting for the efficacy of some β-lactams in the treatment of meningitis.[34] The penicillins and cephalosporins can penetrate the aqueous humor of the eye, but do not reach therapeutic levels in the posterior chamber.

ROUTE OF ADMINISTRATION AND DOSAGE

β-Lactams are available for oral, intravenous and intramuscular use. Generic names, routes of administration and standard dosages for adult and pediatric patients with normal renal function are listed in Table 134.3. In dosing the β-lactam antibiotics, it is important to remember that:

- food can have an effect on oral absorption; and
- absorption of both cefuroxime and cefpodoxime are decreased by H_2 blockers or nonabsorbable antacids.[35]

Clinical experience has supported the general concept that high doses of β-lactam antibiotics should be used in patients who are neutropenic and for severe infections such as bacteremia and meningitis. Dosing of β-lactams is based on achieving plasma drug concentrations above the minimum inhibitory concentration (MIC) of the infecting bacteria for substantial periods of the dosing interval; this

is the critical pharmacodynamic relationship to consider in choosing a dose regimen. Many of these agents have short half-lives after intravenous dosing and therefore could be more optimally dosed if infused over several hours.

INDICATIONS

The β-lactam antibiotics can be effectively used for the treatment of a variety of infections. These agents are widely distributed following administration and are routinely used in the treatment of sinusitis, otitis, pharyngitis, epiglottitis, dental infections, bronchitis, pneumonia, meningitis, infections of the genitourinary tract (including cervicitis and urethritis caused by *Neisseria gonorrhoeae*), peritonitis, biliary and gastrointestinal infections, skin and soft tissue infections, osteomyelitis, septic arthritis and infection of prosthetic devices, including venous access catheters. The choice of antibiotic and recommended duration of therapy for these infections is discussed in the chapters on the specific diseases. The remainder of this section focuses on the use of the β-lactam antibiotics in special circumstances. Table 134.4 summarizes the relative susceptibilities of various micro-organisms to the β-lactam antibiotics.

Prophylaxis

Antimicrobial prophylaxis in surgery (see also Chapter 132)

β-Lactam antibiotics are commonly used to decrease the incidence of infection for selected surgical procedures.[38] Prior to widespread methicillin-resistance in *Staph. aureus* infections acquired in the hospital setting, a single dose of cefazolin had been shown to decrease the incidence of wound infection for selected 'clean' procedures. This approach is used

Table 134.3 β-Lactam antibiotics – spectrum of activity, generic names, routes of administration and dosages used in patients with normal renal function

Agent	Antimicrobial spectrum	Generic name	Route	Adult dose (pediatric dose)
Penicillins				
Natural penicillins	Gram-positives, anaerobes and some Gram-negatives	Penicillin V	po	250–500 mg q6–12h (6.25–12.5 mg/kg q8h)
		Penicillin G (benzathine)	im	1.2 million U every 3–4 weeks (25 000–50 000 U/kg every 3–4 weeks; or if <27 kg, 300 000–600 000 U and if >27 kg, 900 000 U)
		Penicillin G (procaine)	im	300 000–600 000 U q12h (25 000–50 000 U/kg q24h or 12 500–25 000 U/kg q12h)
		Penicillin G, sodium or potassium	iv	1–4 million U q4–6h (6250–100 000 U/kg q6h or 4166.6–66 666 U/kg q4h)
Penicillinase-resistant penicillins	Penicillin-resistant, methicillin-susceptible staphylococci and some streptococci	Cloxacillin	po	250–500 mg q6h
		Dicloxacillin	po	125–500 mg q8h (3.125–6.25 mg/kg q6h)
		Methicillin	im/iv	1–2 g q6h
		Nafcillin	im/iv	1–2 g q4h (12.5–25 mg/kg q6h or 8.3–33.3 mg/kg q4h)
		Oxacillin	iv	1–2 g q4h (12.5–25 mg/kg q6h or 8.3–33.3 mg/kg q4h)
Aminopenicillins	Same as penicillin G plus β-lactamase-negative Gram-negative bacilli and some Enterobacteriaceae	Amoxicillin	po	250–500 mg q8h or 875 mg q12h (12.5–25 mg/kg q8h or 7–13 mg/kg q8h)
		Ampicillin	im/iv	500 mg–2 g q4–6h (25–50 mg/kg q6h)
			po	250–500 mg q6h
		Bacampicillin	po	400–800 mg q12h (12.5 mg/kg q12h)
with a β-lactamase inhibitor	Expanded activity against β-lactamase-producing bacteria	Amoxicillin–clavulanic acid	po	250–500 mg q8h or 875 mg q12h (if >40 kg, dose as adult)
		Ampicillin–sulbactam	im/iv	1.5–3 g q6h (25–50 mg/kg q6h)
Carboxypenicillins	Some ampicillin-resistant Gram-negatives including *Pseudomonas aeruginosa* (at highest dose regimens)	Ticarcillin	im/iv	3 g q4–6h (if <60 kg, 50 mg/kg q4–6h)
with a β-lactamase inhibitor	Expands activity against β-lactamase-producing bacteria	Ticarcillin–clavulanic acid	iv	3.1 g q4–6h (if <60 kg, 50 mg/kg [based on ticarcillin component] q4–6h)
Ureidopenicillins	Similar to carboxypenicillins	Mezlocillin	im/iv	3–4 g q4–6h (50 mg/kg q4h)
		Piperacillin	im/iv	3 g q4–6h (50–75 mg/kg q6h or 33.3–50 mg/kg q4h)
with a β-lacatamase inhibitor	Expands activity against β-lactamase-producing bacteria	Piperacillin–tazobactam	iv	3.375 g q4–6h (80 mg/kg q8h) 4.5 g q6h (for nosomomial pneumonia)
Cephalosporins				
Referred to as 'first generation'	Methicillin-susceptible staphylococci, streptococci and some Gram-negative bacilli	Cefadroxil	po	500 mg–1 g q12h (15 mg/kg q12h)
		Cefazolin	im/iv	1–2 g q8h (16.6–33.3 mg/kg q8h)
		Cephalexin	po	250–500 mg q6h (6.25–12.5 mg/kg q6h or 8.0–16 mg/kg q8h)
		Cephalothin	im/iv	500 mg–2 g q4–6h (25 mg/kg q6h or 16.6 mg/kg q4h)
Referred to as 'second generation'	Greater activity than earlier agents against Gram-negative bacilli. Some anaerobes for specific agents (especially cefotetan, cefoxitin)	Cefaclor	po	250–500 mg q8h (10–20 mg/kg q12h or 6.6–13.3 mg/kg q8h)
		Cefotetan	im/iv	1–3 g q12h (20–40 mg/kg q12h)
		Cefoxitin	im/iv	1 g q8h to 2 g q8h (27–33 mg/kg q8h)
		Cefprozil	po	250 mg q4h or 500 mg q12–24h (15 mg/kg q12h)

Table 134.3 β-Lactam antibiotics – spectrum of activity, generic names, routes of administration and dosages used in patients with normal renal function—cont'd

Agent	Antimicrobial spectrum	Generic name	Route	Adult dose (pediatric dose)
		Cefuroxime (axetil)	po	125–500 mg q12h (10–15 mg/kg q12h)
		Cefuroxime	im/iv	750 mg–1.5 g q6–8h (25–50 mg/kg q8h)
		Loracarbef	po	200–400 mg q12h (7.5–15 mg/kg q12h)
Referred to as 'third generation'	Many β-lactamase positive Gram-negatives, some *P. aeruginosa* (especially cefoperazone, ceftazidime)	Cefditoren (pivoxil)	po	200–400 mg q12h
		Cefdinir	po	300 mg q12h or 600 mg q24h (7 mg/kg q12h or 14 mg/kg q24h)
		Cefixime	po	200 mg q12h or 400 mg q24h (8 mg/kg q24h or 4 mg/kg q12h)
		Cefoperazone	im/iv	1 g q12h to 2 g q4h (25–100 mg/kg q12h)
		Cefotaxime	im/iv	1 g q12h to 2 g q4h (8.3–33.3 mg/kg q4h or 16.6–66.6 mg/kg q6h)
		Cefpodoxime (proxetil)	po	100–400 mg q12h (5 mg/kg q12h)
		Ceftazidime	im/iv	1 g q12h to 2 g q8h (25–50 mg/kg q8h)
		Ceftibuten	po	400 mg q24h (9 mg/kg q24h)
		Ceftizoxime	im/iv	500 mg q12h to 4 g q8h (50 mg/kg q6–8h)
		Ceftriaxone	im/iv	1–2 g q24h (50–75 mg/kg q24h or 25–37.5 mg/kg q12h)
Referred to as 'fourth generation'	Similar to above	Cefepime	im/iv	1–2 g q8–12h (50 mg/kg q8–12h)
	Gram-positives including MRSA, and many β-lactamase-positive Gram-negatives, some *P. aeruginosa*	Ceftobiprole (medocaril)	iv	500 mg q8h
Monobactam				
	Gram-negatives	Aztreonam	im/iv	1–2 g q6–12h (30–40 mg/kg q6–8h)
Carbapenems				
	Gram-positives (except MRSA), many Gram-negatives (including ESBL-producers) and many *P. aeruginosa* (except ertapenem)	Doripenem	iv	500 mg q8h
		Ertapenem	im/iv	1 g q24h
		Imipenem–cilastin	im/iv	500 mg–1 g q6h (15–25 mg/kg q6h)
		Meropenem	iv	1 g q8h (20–40 mg/kg q8h)

Dosing guidance as per references 9–12,18,19.

commonly for cardiac, noncardiac thoracic, vascular, orthopedic, ophthalmic and neurosurgical procedures. With the emergence of MRSA, concern has been raised about the effectiveness of using β-lactams with no activity against MRSA, especially in centers where MRSA prevalence is high.

For 'clean–contaminated' procedures in which colonized mucosa is violated, such as head and neck surgery, abdominal surgery and gynecologic surgery, antibiotic prophylaxis may also be used. Cefazolin can be used before head and neck surgery. Similarly, patients undergoing biliary tract surgery who are at high risk of infection due to advanced age, acute cholecystitis, a nonfunctioning gallbladder, obstructive jaundice, or choledocholithiasis may benefit from preoperative cefazolin. In the setting of acute appendicitis, cefoxitin or ampicillin–sulbactam has been recommended. Women undergoing vaginal or abdominal hysterectomy, emergency Caesarian section or first trimester abortion may be candidates for antibiotic prophylaxis with cefazolin or other agents.

Antibiotics should be used not only as prophylaxis but also as treatment for 'dirty' surgical procedures in which the surgical site is obviously contaminated by bacteria (e.g. a perforated viscus). Antimicrobial prophylaxis in surgery is summarized periodically in the publication *The Medical Letter*.[38]

Endocarditis prophylaxis

Patients who have underlying cardiac or congenital valvular abnormalities are candidates for antibiotic prophylaxis when they undergo procedures that can cause transient bacteremia. Cardiac conditions that place a patient at increased risk of endocarditis include prosthetic valves, a previous history of endocarditis, most congenital cardiac abnormalities (except an isolated secundum atrial septal defect), rheumatic and other acquired valvular dysfunction, hypertrophic cardiomyopathy and mitral valve prolapse when accompanied by regurgitation.

Procedures that can cause transient bacteremia and may place a patient at risk of endocarditis include:

- dental procedures (including professional cleaning);
- tonsillectomy and/or adenoidectomy;
- surgical procedures involving intestinal or respiratory mucosa;
- rigid bronchoscopy;
- sclerotherapy for esophageal varices;
- esophageal dilatation;
- gallbladder surgery;
- cystoscopy;

Table 134.4 Susceptibilities of selected bacteria to β-lactam antibiotics

Generic name	Streptococci*	Oxacillin-susceptible, penicillinase-producing *S. aureus*†	Enterococci	Enteric Gram-negative bacilli‡	*Pseudomonas aeruginosa*	Anaerobes
Penicillins						
Amoxicillin	++	0	++	0	0	0
Amoxicillin–clavulanate	++	++	++	++	0	++
Ampicillin	++	0	++	0	0	0
Ampicillin–sulbactam	++	++	++	++	0	++
Carbenicillin	+	0	0	0	+	0
Cloxacillin	+	++	0	0	0	0
Dicloxacillin	+	++	0	0	0	0
Methicillin	+	++	0	0	0	0
Mezlocillin	+	0	+	+	+	+
Nafcillin	+	++	0	0	0	0
Oxacillin	+	++	0	0	0	0
Penicillin	++	0	++	0	0	0
Piperacillin	++	0	+	+	++	+
Piperacillin–tazobactam	++	++	+	++	++	++
Ticarcillin	++	0	0	+	+	+
Ticarcillin–clavulanate	++	++	0	++	+	++
Cephalosporins						
Cefaclor	+	+	0	+	0	+
Cefadroxil	+	+	0	0	0	0
Cefazolin	++	++	0	0	0	0
Cefdinir	++	+	0	+	0	0
Cefditoren	++	+	0	+	0	0
Cefepime	++	+	0	++	++	0
Cefixime	++	0	0	++	0	0
Cefoperazone	++	+	0	+	+	+
Cefotaxime	++	+	0	++	0	0
Cefotetan	+	0	0	+	0	+
Cefoxitin	+	0	0	+	0	++
Cefpodoxime	++	++	0	+	0	0
Cefprozil	++	+	0	+	0	0
Ceftazidime	+	0	0	++	++	0
Ceftibuten	+	0	0	+	0	0
Ceftizoxime	++	+	0	+	0	+
Ceftobiprole	++	++[b]	++	++	+	0
Ceftriaxone	++	+	0	++	0	0
Cefuroxime	++	+	0	+	0	+
Cephalexin	++	+	0	+	0	+
Cephalothin	++	++	0	+	0	+
Loracarbef	+	+	0	+	0	+
Monobactam						
Aztreonam	0	0	0	++	+	0
Carbapenems						
Doripenem	++	++	+	++	++	++
Ertapenem	++	++	0	++	0	++
Imipenem	++	++	++	++	++	++
Meropenem	++	++	+	++	++	++

Interpretations: 0, not active, 90% of the minimum inhibitory concentrations (MICs) are greater than resistance breakpoint; +, intermediate activity, approximately 90% of the MICs are greater than susceptible, but less than the resistant breakpoint; ++, clinically useful activity, generally with 90% of the MICs within the susceptible range, using interpretive criteria as defined by the Clinical and Laboratory Standards Institute (CLSI) or the Food and Drug Administration (FDA). Susceptibility data based on references 17,36,37.
*Non-meningitis isolates.
†Methicillin-susceptible *Staphylococcus aureus* and *S. epidermidis*. All methicillin-resistant *S. aureus* and *S. epidermidis* are resistant to all β-lactams, with the exception of ceftobiprole.
‡Primarily *Escherichia coli*, *Klebsiella pneumoniae*, *Enterobacter cloacae*, *Enterobacter aerogenes* and *Proteus mirabilis*.

- urethral dilatation;
- urethral catheterization and/or urinary tract surgery if there is infection;
- prostatic surgery; and
- incision and drainage of infected tissue.

Recommendations for using β-lactams to prophylax patients at risk for infective endocarditis have recently been updated by an American College of Cardiology/American Heart Association Task Force on Practice Guidelines.[39] In this update, prophylaxis is not recommended for patients undergoing nondental procedures and is no longer recommended for many patients that had been considered candidates for prophylaxis in the past (specifically, patients with mitral valve prolapse and mitral regurgitation). For at-risk patients undergoing dental procedures, the antibiotic of choice has remained constant for over two decades and is a single dose of amoxicillin 2 g (50 mg/kg for children) taken orally 30–60 minutes before the procedure. Alternatives exist for patients who are allergic to penicillins.[39] Guidelines posted by the National Institute for Health and Clinical Excellence (NICE)[40] and published by the British Society for Antimicrobial Chemotherapy[41] further underscore that past practices of using antibiotic prophylaxis in patients at risk for infective endocarditis need to be reconsidered (see Chapter 132 for detailed discussion on antimicrobial prophylaxis).

Rheumatic fever prophylaxis

Because patients who have had acute rheumatic fever are at risk of recurrent attacks if they have group A streptococcal infections, the American Heart Association (AHA) recommends prophylaxis with penicillin for these patients. The dose is either a single injection of benzathine penicillin G 1.2 million U intramuscularly every 4 weeks or penicillin V 250 mg orally q12h. It seems that prophylaxis can be safely discontinued in patients with a history of carditis after 10 years or at age 25. In patients without a history of carditis, prophylaxis can be stopped after 5 years or at age 18. The decision to stop prophylaxis, however, must be individualized because a patient who is at continued risk of streptococcal infection (e.g. teacher or pediatrician) may benefit from continued antibiotic prophylaxis (see also Chapter 48).[42]

Intrapartum prophylaxis

Penicillin G is the agent of choice for use in intrapartum prophylaxis for early onset group B streptococcal disease in newborns. Ampicillin is an acceptable alternative agent. These agents should be given to women in labor as soon as risk for intrapartum transmission of group B streptococcus is identified. Initial intravenous doses (5 million U penicillin G or 2 g ampicillin) should be followed with half doses every 4 hours until the newborn is delivered.

Pneumococcal infections

Penicillin and amoxicillin are the antibiotics of choice for infections (such as community-acquired pneumonia, bacteremia or meningitis) caused by penicillin-susceptible strains of *Streptococcus pneumoniae*. However, an increasing proportion of isolates of this pathogen are not susceptible to penicillin. For meningitic isolates and epidemiologic purposes, an interpretation of intermediate is defined as a strain with a penicillin MIC of 0.1–1 μg/ml and resistance is defined by a penicillin MIC of ≥2 μg/ml. However, recent revisions to the interpretive criteria define penicillin MICs >2 μg/ml for non-meningitis-related *Strep. pneumoniae* isolates as nonsusceptible. Although only about 5% of clinical isolates in the USA were not susceptible to penicillin in the early 1990s,[43] a study of isolates collected from hospitalized patients throughout the USA in 2007 indicated that 25.4% were intermediate and 11.1% were resistant to penicillin.[44] Because of the emergence of resistance, some suggest that suspected cases of pneumococcal pneumonia and meningitis should be treated with vancomycin and/or a third-generation cephalosporin or meropenem until susceptibilities are known. There have been reports of failure of third-generation cephalosporins such as cefotaxime or ceftriaxone in the treatment of penicillin-resistant pneumococcal meningitis, again suggesting that vancomycin or meropenem should be included until susceptibilities are known.[45]

Staphylococcal infections

Soon after the introduction of penicillin for the treatment of staphylococcal infections, penicillinase-producing strains became so common that this agent was no longer effective. Penicillinase-resistant penicillins (nafcillin, oxacillin, methicillin, dicloxacillin, cloxacillin, flucloxacillin) are often agents of choice for methicillin-susceptible strains of *Staph. aureus*. Other β-lactam antibiotics that are effective in the treatment of susceptible staphylococcal infections are:

- the aminopenicillins in combination with a β-lactamase inhibitor (ampicillin–sulbactam or amoxicillin–clavulanate);
- the antipseudomonal penicillins in combination with a β-lactamase inhibitor (ticarcillin–clavulanate, piperacillin–tazobactam); and
- the carbapenems (doripenem, ertapenem, imipenem and meropenem).

The first-generation cephalosporins, which are as effective as the penicillinase-resistant penicillins in the treatment of staphylococcal infections, require less frequent dosing and may be used in patients with a history of mild penicillin allergy.

Isolates of *Staph. aureus* or *Staph. epidermidis* that are resistant to methicillin should be considered to be resistant to all other β-lactams,[46] with the exception of ceftobiprole.[36] Ceftobiprole has received regulatory approval in Canada and some European countries for treating patients with complicated skin and skin-structure infections, including those caused by MRSA.[47,48]

Gram-positive bacilli

Penicillin G is the treatment of choice for:

- infections (oral–cervicofacial, thoracic, abdominal) due to actinomycosis;
- elimination of the carrier state of diphtheria;
- infections (pulmonary, cutaneous, gastrointestinal) due to anthrax, except for β-lactamase-producing strains;
- gas gangrene caused by species of *Clostridium* spp.; and
- erysipeloid caused by *Erysipelothrix rhusiopathiae*.

Either penicillin G or ampicillin may be used for infections caused by *Listeria monocytogenes*. No currently available cephalosporin has useful activity against *L. monocytogenes*.

Infections caused by Gram-negative organisms including *Pseudomonas aeruginosa*

β-Lactam antibiotics with *in-vitro* activity against *P. aeruginosa* are ticarcillin, carbenicillin, piperacillin, ceftazidime, cefoperazone, cefepime, ceftobiprole, aztreonam, imipenem, meropenem and doripenem. Of these agents, the carbapenems doripenem, imipenem and meropenem have the most consistent activity against pseudomonads. Because resistance to carbapenems, most evident with imipenem, has emerged in many areas, it is important to be aware of *P. aeruginosa* resistance patterns for a particular health-care facility. During treatment of pseudomonal infections, resistance to all β-lactam agents used as sole therapy has been observed.[49] For this reason, a suitable β-lactam antibiotic is often used in conjunction with a second agent, such as a fluoroquinolone or an aminoglycoside.

The antipseudomonal penicillins piperacillin and ticarcillin are often used in conjunction with a β-lactamase inhibitor. However, the inhibitor does not confer improved activity against many β-lactam-resistant *Pseudomonas* spp., because the mechanism of resistance is typically not due to β-lactamase production.[50]

The development of drug-resistant isolates of *P. aeruginosa* and other Gram-negative bacilli has emerged as a clinically important challenge, especially in considering treatment of patients with nosocomial infections. These pathogens are commonly found in intensive care units where patients have been exposed to broad-spectrum antibiotics for prolonged periods of time. Many organisms produce chromosomal β-lactamases that are intrinsic to that species, including *Citrobacter* spp., *Enterobacter* spp., *Serratia* spp., *Proteus* spp., *Providencia* spp., *P. aeruginosa* and *Acinetobacter* spp. Many Gram-negative bacteria, especially *Escherichia coli* and *Klebsiella* spp., may acquire extra DNA (e.g. a plasmid) that encodes for other types of β-lactamase, such as extended-spectrum β-lactamases (ESBLs). These bacteria may develop resistance to most β-lactams during therapy if they acquire an ESBL or hyperproduce chromosomal β-lactamases.[51] Older recommendations of concurrent use of an aminoglycoside in conjunction with a cephalosporin for the treatment of infections caused by these bacteria to prevent therapeutic failures have been challenged due to the realization that cross-resistance in ESBL-producing bacteria can occur due to the co-acquisition of modifying enzymes for both antibiotic classes.[52]

Among β-lactams, carbapenems have the broadest spectrum of activity against Gram-negative organisms resistant to other antibiotics. Given the emergence of resistance, especially resistance due to ESBL-producing bacteria, carbapenems have been used more frequently as empiric therapy in seriously ill patients, especially those at risk for being infected with Gram-negative pathogens. Although imipenem resistance in *P. aeruginosa* has risen in some centers to 10–15%, some of these isolates continue to be susceptible to meropenem and doripenem, carbapenems with more potent *in-vitro* activity against most Gram-negative bacteria.[53] Resistance to carbapenems is increasing in some centers due to the production of acquired carbapenem-hydrolyzing β-lactamases, including enzymes that require metal ions for hydrolysis. The metallo-β-lactamases confer resistance to all β-lactams except aztreonam, in contrast to other carbapenemases that generally are associated with resistance to all β-lactams.[54]

Among the cephalosporins, cefepime is effective in the treatment of severe infections due to a broad spectrum of pathogens that involve the lower respiratory and urinary tracts, the skin and soft tissue, and the female reproductive tract. It has been shown to be more effective than ceftazidime in the treatment of pneumonia in patients with cystic fibrosis where *P. aeruginosa* is a common pathogen.[55] In addition to having activity against strains of *P. aeruginosa* resistant to ceftazidime, cefepime has also shown activity against many Enterobacteriaceae, including *Enterobacter* spp., that are resistant to other cephalosporins.[56] However, cefepime is inactivated by many ESBLs. Although a recent meta-analysis suggested that a subset of seriously ill patients had higher mortality rates after treatment with cefepime compared with alternative agents,[57] a 2009 FDA analysis did not show a statistically significant increase in mortality in cefepime-treated patients.

Anaerobic infections

Anaerobic bacteria may play a significant role in brain abscess, dental infection, sinusitis, lung abscess, intra-abdominal abscess and bone and soft tissue infection. Although β-lactam antibiotics have been used extensively in the treatment of anaerobic infections, there is a trend for increased resistance of anaerobes to some β-lactam antibiotics due to production of β-lactamases.[58]

Most *Clostridium* strains, with the exception of some strains of *C. ramosum*, *C. clostridiforme* and *C. innocuum*, remain susceptible to penicillin. Penicillin resistance is increasingly seen in the genus *Fusobacterium*, most commonly in *F. varium* and *F. mortiferum*, and although generally still sensitive to penicillin, the MICs for *F. nucleatum* have increased. Penicillin resistance is a major problem encountered in the treatment of infections caused by β-lactamase-producing *B. fragilis* and other *Bacteroides* spp.[59]

Penicillin is slightly more active than nafcillin against anaerobes, although neither is considered to be a potent anti-anaerobic agent. Ticarcillin, mezlocillin and piperacillin also have excellent activity against

anaerobes, although there has been an increase in *B. fragilis* strains resistant to ticarcillin. Of the β-lactamase-stable cephalosporins, cefoxitin, cefotetan and ceftizoxime all show activity against anaerobes. Cefoxitin remains the most active cephalosporin against *B. fragilis*. Resistance to these cephalosporins is seen with some species of *Clostridium*, *Fusobacterium* and non-spore-forming Gram-positive rods. Cephalosporins such as ceftazidime and the first-generation agents cefazolin and cephalothin have poor activity against Gram-negative anaerobes whereas the broader spectrum cephalosporins cefotaxime, cefoperazone and ceftriaxone have modest activity (resistance seen in 30–60% of strains) and are therefore not the agents of choice for the empiric treatment of anaerobic infections. Cefotaxime generates a desacetyl metabolite that works synergistically with the parent compound in the treatment of some anaerobic species *in vitro*, but is still not a primary agent for anaerobic infections *in vivo*.

β-Lactamases in anaerobes include the typical cephalosporinases in the *B. fragilis* group and the penicillinases in *Clostridium* spp. and *F. nucleatum*. Virtually all *B. fragilis* isolates produce β-lactamases, including a subset of isolates that produce a broad-spectrum metallo-β-lactamase. β-Lactamase production has not been reported in strains of *Clostridium perfringens*.[59]

The addition of a β-lactamase inhibitor increases the activity of some penicillins against β-lactamase producing anaerobes, in particular *Bacteroides* spp., resulting in efficacy for the combinations of ticarcillin–clavulanate, piperacillin–tazobactam, amoxicillin–clavulanate and ampicillin–sulbactam. The most active β-lactam agents against anaerobic isolates in the USA are the carbapenems, imipenem, meropenem, ertapenem and doripenem. Aztreonam has no activity against anaerobes and must be used with other agents when treating mixed aerobic and anaerobic infections.[60]

Central nervous system infections (meningitis)

Certain β-lactam antibiotics are able to penetrate inflamed meninges and are commonly used to treat meningitis (e.g. penicillin G, ampicillin, nafcillin, oxacillin, cefotaxime, ceftizoxime, ceftriaxone, ceftazidime and meropenem). The most common pathogens in a series of adult patients with meningitis in descending order were *Strep. pneumoniae*, *Neisseria meningitidis* and *L. monocytogenes*.[61] With the widespread use of conjugate *Haemophilus influenzae* and *Strep. pneumoniae* vaccines, *N. meningitidis* has become the most important cause of bacterial meningitis in children in the USA. These bacteria have remained consistently susceptible to β-lactam antibiotics.

Because of the severity of infections in the central nervous system there is a need to start effective therapy before the identity and susceptibility of the bacteria causing infection is known. The activity of β-lactams against the leading causes of these infections makes them appropriate choices for initial therapy. Although penicillin G at a dose of 20–24 million U/day intravenously q4h is a treatment of choice for susceptible strains of *Strep. pneumoniae* and for nearly all *N. meningitidis*, due to the possibility of infection by penicillin-resistant pneumococci, β-lactamase producing *H. influenzae* and the rare β-lactamase-producing *N. meningitidis*, the use of ceftriaxone with vancomycin is generally considered the most appropriate β-lactam-containing regimen for use as empiric therapy for bacterial meningitis. β-Lactams are not sufficient to eliminate the carrier state of *N. meningitidis* that often occurs in patients recovering from bacterial meningitis. For this reason rifampin should be given at the completion of therapy. The agent of choice for the treatment of meningitis due to *L. monocytogenes* is ampicillin or penicillin alone or in combination with gentamicin.

In children, the preferred agents for the treatment of *H. influenzae* meningitis are the third-generation cephalosporins cefotaxime or ceftriaxone.[62] Cefuroxime is not considered an appropriate alternative to these newer agents because of failures of treatment as well as the development of meningitis during cefuroxime treatment. A randomized trial found that ceftriaxone resulted in less hearing impairment and sterilized the CSF earlier than cefuroxime when used as treatment for meningitis in children.[63]

Patients with staphylococcal meningitis (which is usually seen after trauma or neurosurgical procedures) are best treated with high doses of nafcillin or oxacillin if the organism is susceptible. *Pseudomonas aeruginosa* meningitis has been effectively managed with ceftazidime, although meropenem may prove to be an alternative.[64]

Corticosteroids have been shown to reduce the neurologic sequelae of meningitis. Clinical trial experience has shown that early adjunctive therapy with dexamethasone can improve the outcome of bacterial meningitis.[65]

Biliary system infections (cholangitis)

Infection of the biliary tract generally occurs if there is an abnormality such as gallstones, strictures or a stent. Infection rarely complicates malignant obstruction of the biliary tree. In the obstructed biliary tract, there is very little excretion of any antibiotic. The β-lactams that achieve significantly higher biliary than serum levels are nafcillin, mezlocillin, piperacillin, cefoperazone and ceftriaxone. Ampicillin achieves concentrations in the bile equal to or greater than those in serum. Interestingly, biliary levels are higher after oral amoxicillin or ampicillin than they are after intravenous administration. Biliary concentrations of ticarcillin, cefazolin, cefotaxime, ceftazidime and cefuroxime are all less than serum concentrations.[66]

Ureidopenicillins mezlocillin and piperacillin have been used in biliary tract infections as has cefoperazone. Cefoxitin, cefuroxime and ceftriaxone are also commonly used in conjunction with an aminoglycoside in patients with cholangitis.

In patients undergoing biliary surgery, adequate serum levels of antibiotic have been shown to be more important than biliary levels when the goal is to reduce postoperative infection.

Intra-abdominal infections (see Chapter 37)

Intra-abdominal infections, such as acute appendicitis, penetrating abdominal trauma and bowel perforation, are generally polymicrobial in nature and caused by a combination of aerobic, anaerobic and facultative anaerobic organisms. Clinical trials have confirmed the efficacy of β-lactam antibiotics alone or in combination with other agents for various intra-abdominal infections.[67] Cefoxitin, imipenem, cefotetan, piperacillin–tazobactam and ticarcillin–clavulanic acid have all been shown to be effective in treating intra-abdominal infections when used as monotherapy. Meropenem has been shown to have efficacy similar to that of imipenem for the treatment of intra-abdominal sepsis.[68] Ertapenem has similar efficacy in treating intra-abdominal infections as piperacillin–tazobactam.[69] Doripenem has been shown to have similar efficacy to meropenem in treating patients with complicated intra-abdominal infections.[70] The combination of clindamycin with either ceftazidime or aztreonam has been successful in the treatment of intra-abdominal infections. Failures of ampicillin–sulbactam have occurred when pseudomonal infections occur.

Although enterococci are commonly isolated from intra-abdominal infections (14–33%), many physicians do not include anti-enterococcal therapy in the initial treatment of these infections. 'Breakthrough' enterococcal infections occur in patients who have been hospitalized for long periods of time with persistent or recurrent intra-abdominal sepsis or who are immunosuppressed.[71]

Spontaneous bacterial peritonitis

Few studies have evaluated the efficacies of different antibiotics in the treatment of spontaneous bacterial peritonitis (SBP). The organisms that typically cause SBP are the Gram-negative bacilli (especially *E. coli* and *Klebsiella* spp.), Gram-positive cocci (including pneumococci, other streptococci, enterococci and staphylococci) and anaerobes. When used in conjunction with an aminoglycoside, ampicillin had a cure rate of 76% in one study. Cefotaxime was shown to be more effective (cure rate 85%) than ampicillin and tobramycin (cure rate 56%) in another study of severe infections in patients with cirrhosis,

of which approximately 75% were SBP. In another study, amoxicillin and clavulanic acid had a cure rate of 80% for SBP. Aztreonam monotherapy has been associated with Gram-positive superinfection. Therefore, if aztreonam is to be used for SBP, then an additional antibiotic providing Gram-positive coverage is needed.[72]

Pancreatitis and its complications (see Chapter 37)

The prophylactic use of antibiotics in uncomplicated acute pancreatitis is controversial. Early studies that used ampicillin, an antibiotic that does not achieve therapeutic levels in pancreatic tissue, showed no benefit. However, several recent studies have shown a potential benefit. Patients with acute necrotizing pancreatitis treated with imipenem for 14 days had a lower incidence of pancreatic sepsis than those not treated; however, a trend toward a decreased mortality rate was not statistically significant.[73] A study that used cefuroxime in patients with acute necrotizing pancreatitis found that rates of bacteremia and mortality were both lower than those of controls.[74]

It is clear that β-lactam antibiotics have a role in the management of infectious complications of pancreatitis such as abscess or infected pseudocyst. The agents commonly used in addition to cefuroxime and imipenem include ticarcillin–clavulanic acid, piperacillin–tazobactam, ampicillin–sulbactam and meropenem.

Endovascular infections (endocarditis) (see Chapter 47)

Updated statements regarding the treatment of endocarditis were published by the AHA in 2005[75] and the British Society for Antimicrobial Chemotherapy (BSAC) in 2004.[76] The drug of choice for the treatment of endocarditis caused by viridans streptococci is penicillin G. Depending upon the drug susceptibility of the organism, gentamicin can be added for part or all of a 2–6 week course. A 2-week course of combination ceftriaxone with an aminoglycoside may be sufficient as therapy for patients with uncomplicated endocarditis due to viridans streptococci. Alternatively, a 4-week course of ceftriaxone can be used.[77] Enterococcal endocarditis is best treated with ampicillin or penicillin in combination with an aminoglycoside for 4–6 weeks.

The treatment of choice for native-valve endocarditis caused by methicillin-susceptible *Staph. aureus* is nafcillin, flucloxacillin or oxacillin for 6 weeks. Gentamicin has been used for the first 3–5 days to decrease the number of days of bacteremia, but has not been shown to change the outcome.[78]

Intravenous drug users with right-sided staphylococcal endocarditis have been successfully treated with 2 weeks of nafcillin and tobramycin.[79] Prosthetic valve endocarditis with methicillin-susceptible *Staph. aureus* is optimally treated with nafcillin or oxacillin (if the organism is sensitive) in combination with rifampin and gentamicin (for the first 2 weeks) for at least 6 weeks.

Endocarditis caused by the slow-growing fastidious Gram-negative organisms *Haemophilus parainfluenzae*, *H. aphrophilus*, *Actinobacillus actinomycetemcomitans*, *Cardiobacterium hominis*, *Eikenella corrodens* and *Kingella kingae* (the HACEK group) can be treated with ampicillin and gentamicin for 4 weeks or ceftriaxone alone for 4 weeks.

Neutropenic fever

β-Lactam antibiotics have been used for many years in managing febrile patients with cancer and treatment-induced neutropenia. Because life-threatening infections can occur due to Gram-negative bacteria, especially *P. aeruginosa*, and resistance to β-lactams has continued to become more prevalent among Gram-negative enteric pathogens, using these agents as monotherapy may not be as effective as has been previously reported.[80] Combining a β-lactam with a second agent that has activity against a broad-spectrum of Gram-negative bacteria, typically an aminoglycoside, has been recommended in patients who present with high risk for rapidly progressing disease.[81] Most recently, the emergence of methicillin-resistant staphylococci as an important cause of disease in this patient population has further complicated using a β-lactam to provide reliable activity against Gram-positive bacteria in these patients.

Lyme disease

Early infection caused by *Borrelia burgdorferi* can be managed with either amoxicillin or doxycycline. Since co-infection with *Ehrlichia* or *Anaplasma* spp. is known to occur in many areas, many clinicians now prefer to use doxycycline. For later manifestations of Lyme disease, however, the β-lactams are the agents of choice. Lyme carditis can be successfully treated with either a 2-week course of ceftriaxone or intravenous penicillin G. Lyme meningitis and Lyme arthritis can also be treated with ceftriaxone or penicillin G, but for 2–4 weeks. A 30-day treatment course of amoxicillin and probenecid has been used for the treatment of Lyme arthritis. In pregnant women, doxycycline cannot be used, amoxicillin is used in early Lyme disease and intravenous penicillin G is used for disseminated early Lyme disease or any manifestation of late disease (see Chapter 43).[82]

Syphilis

Parenteral penicillin G is the preferred agent for treating all stages of syphilis and is the only therapy that has proved effective for neurosyphilis, syphilis in pregnancy and congenital syphilis.[83] Primary and secondary syphilis can be treated with a single dose of benzathine penicillin G (2.4 million U in adults, 50 000 U/kg intramuscularly in children up to the adult dose). Late latent syphilis is treated with benzathine penicillin G (2.4 million U intramuscularly every week for 3 weeks). Procaine penicillin can be used where benzathine penicillin is unavailable, and there are alternatives for patients who are allergic to penicillin (see Chapter 57).

It is important to remember that patients being treated for any of the spirochete diseases – syphilis, Lyme disease or borreliosis – may develop a Jarisch–Herxheimer reaction, which may produce fever, tachycardia, chills, headaches, sore throat, malaise, myalgias, arthralgias, rash and, rarely, hypotension. This reaction has been observed in approximately 50% of patients treated for primary syphilis and 75% of patients with secondary syphilis.[84] Generally, it occurs a few hours after the first dose of penicillin, lasts for only a few hours and does not occur with subsequent doses of the antibiotic. Pre-treatment of patients with louse-borne relapsing fever (caused by *Borrelia recurrentis*) with hydrocortisone or acetaminophen does not prevent the Jarisch–Herxheimer reaction.[85] It is important to distinguish the reaction from penicillin allergy so that appropriate treatment is not discontinued.

DOSAGE IN SPECIAL CIRCUMSTANCES

Renal impairment

The majority of the β-lactam antibiotics are excreted almost entirely via the renal route, and so dose adjustments are necessary in the presence of kidney disease. Failure to reduce the dose of penicillin in uremic patients has resulted in toxicity, most notably encephalopathy.[86] In patients with especially high glomerular filtration rates, rapid clearance of renally excreted antibiotics may result in a need to increase dosages in order to achieve therapeutic exposures.[87] As biliary secretion plays a major role in the excretion of ceftriaxone, cefoperazone, nafcillin and oxacillin, the doses of these antibiotics do not need to be adjusted in renal failure. Because biliary secretion plays a lesser, although significant role in the excretion of the ureidopenicillins, the dosages of these drugs do not have to be reduced as much as for the other penicillins. Some β-lactams must be redosed after peritoneal dialysis, which removes variable amounts of the drug. With the exception of ceftriaxone, mezlocillin, nafcillin,

dicloxacillin and oxacillin, the β-lactams must be re-dosed following hemodialysis. Specific dose adjustments are needed for patients with renal impairment and for patients on hemodialysis or peritoneal dialysis (Table 134.5).

Hepatic impairment

The dosages of some β-lactams must be adjusted in patients with severe hepatic disease. As a result of reduced desacetylation in patients with liver disease, the half-life of cefotaxime may increase slightly, but the half-life of cefoperazone may increase significantly and dosage reductions are required. Although biliary excretion plays a role in the excretion of ceftriaxone, no dose adjustment is needed in patients with liver disease.

Extremes of age

Dose reductions of the β-lactam antibiotics should be made in the elderly in the presence of renal dysfunction (see Table 134.5). Otherwise, elderly patients tolerate standard doses of the β-lactam antibiotics.

Because neonates do not have fully developed renal function, special modifications in dosage are necessary. In addition, because children have a high risk of cholestatic complications with ceftriaxone, another agent should be used when possible (see Adverse reactions and interactions, below). Ceftriaxone should not be used in neonates with hyperbilirubinemia.

β-Lactams in pregnancy

The penicillins, the β-lactamase inhibitors and the cephalosporins, aztreonam, meropenem, ertapenem and doripenem are considered category B in pregnancy (Table 134.6). This means that animal studies have shown no risk to the fetus, but adequate human studies have not been performed, or that animal studies have shown risk and human studies have shown no risk. When they are indicated, these antibiotics are commonly used in clinical practice in pregnant women.

Imipenem–cilastatin is pregnancy category C, meaning that animal studies show toxicity to the fetus and human studies are inadequate. However, the benefit of using these drugs may exceed the risk of not treating a serious infection in a pregnant woman when no alternatives exist.[93] Meropenem or doripenem, category B, may be a suitable alternative to imipenem, category C, for infections with resistant Gram-negative aerobic organisms.

β-Lactam antibiotics that are not protein bound are transported across the placenta and reach the drug levels that are present in maternal serum. β-Lactams that are highly protein-bound reach only low concentrations in amniotic fluid and the fetus.[94]

As a general principle, the β-lactam antibiotics have accelerated elimination and lowered plasma concentrations in pregnant women as compared with nonpregnant women. As a result, the dose or frequency of administration should be increased in pregnant women.[93]

ADVERSE REACTIONS AND INTERACTIONS

Adverse reactions that occur with the β-lactam antibiotics are summarized in Table 134.7.

Allergic reactions

The most common adverse event associated with the use of β-lactam antibiotics is an allergic reaction. The reported frequency of allergic reaction to penicillin varies from 0.7% to 10%. Anaphylaxis historically was documented to occur in 0.004–0.015% of patients.[95] A maculopapular rash occurs late in the treatment course of 2–3% of patients receiving a course of penicillin. Ampicillin and amoxicillin induce rashes in a higher percentage of patients treated (5.2–9.5%) than other β-lactams and almost invariably cause a rash when given

Table 134.5 Drug dosages in patients with renal failure

Generic name	Dose in normal renal function	Max. daily dose with normal renal function	Adjustment in dose (D) or interval (I)	GFR (ml/min) >50	GFR (ml/min) = 10–50	GFR (ml/min) <10	Supplement after HD	Supplement with PD	CVVHD
Penicillins									
Amoxicillin	250–500 mg q8h	2–3 g/q24h	I	q8h	q8–12h	q24h	Yes, 250–500 mg	250 mg q12h	500 mg q8–12h
Amoxicillin–clavulanate	250–500 mg q8h		I	q8h	q8–12h	q24h	Yes, 250–500 mg q24h	Usual regimen	
Ampicillin	250 mg–2 g q6h	2–4 g/q24h	I	q6h	q6–12h	q12–24h	Yes	250 mg q12h	1–2 g q6–12h
Ampicillin–sulbactam (AM–SB)	1–2 g AM–500 mg–1 g SB q6–8h	8 g AM–4 g SB/q24h	I	q6h	q8–12h	q24h	Yes	2 g AM–1 g SB/24h	3 g q8h
Dicloxacillin	125–500 mg q8h	2 g/q24h	D	100%	100%	100%	No	No	
Mezlocillin	1.5–4.0 g q4–6h	24 g/q24h	I	q4–6h	q6–8h	q8h	No	No	2 g q4–6h
Nafcillin	1–2 g q4–6h	12 g/q24h	D	100%	100%	100%	No	No	2 g q4–6h
Oxacillin	1–2 g q4–6h	12 g/q24h	D	100%	100%	100%	No	No	
Penicillin G	0.5–4 million U q4–6h	24 million U	D	100%	75%	20–50%	Yes	Dose for GFR <10	0.5–3 million U q6h
Penicillin V	250–500 mg q6h	3 g/q24h	D	100%	100%	100%	Yes	Dose for GFR <10	300 mg q6h
Piperacillin	3–4 g q4–6h	24 g/q24h	I	q4–6h	q6–8h	q8h	Yes	Dose for GFR <10	
Piperacillin–tazobactam	3.375 g q6h	13.5 g/q24h	D&I	3.375 g q6h	2.25 g q6h	2.25 g q8h	Dose for GFR <10 + 0.75 g	Dose for GFR <10	2.25–3.375 g q6h
Ticarcillin	3 g q4h	24 g/q24h	D&I	1–2 g q4h	1–2 g q8h	1–2 g q12h	Yes, extra 3 g	Dose for GFR <10	
Ticarcillin–clavulanate	3.1 g q4h	24 g/q24h	D&I	3.1 g q4h	3.1 g q8–12h	2 g q12h	Yes, extra 3.1 g	3.1 g q12h	3.1 g q6h
Cephalosporins									
Cefaclor	250–500 mg q8h	1.5 g/q24h	D	100%	50–100%	50%	Yes	Usual regimen	
Cefadroxil	500 mg–1 g q12h	2 g/q24h	I	q12h	q12–24h	q36h	Yes, extra 500 mg–1 g	Usual regimen	
Cefazolin	1–2 g q8h	12 g/q24h	I	q8h	q12h	q24–48h	Yes, extra 500 mg–1 g	500 mg q12h	2 g q12h
Cefditoren (pivoxil)	200–400 mg q12h	800 mg/q24h	D&I	100%	200 mg q12h	200 mg q24h	Dose for GFR <10	No data	
Cefdinir	300 mg q12h	600 mg/q24h	I	q12h	q24h	q48h	Yes	Dose for GFR <10	
Cefepime	250 mg–2 g q8–12h	6 g/q24h	D&I	100%	50–100% q24h	25–50% q24h	Yes, dose for GFR <10	Dose for GFR <10	2 g q12h
Cefixime	200 mg q12h or 400 mg q24h	400 mg/q24h	D	100%	75%	50%	Yes	Usual dose	
Cefoperazone	1–2 g q12h	12 g/q24h	D	100%	100%	100%	Yes, extra 1 g	No	1 g q12h
Cefotaxime	1–2 g q6–12h	12 g/q24h	I	q6h	q6–12h	q24h or 50%	Yes, extra 500 mg–2 g	1 g q24h	2 g q12h
Cefotetan	1–2g q12h	6g/q24h	I	100%	q24h	q48h	Yes, extra 1g	1g q24h	

(Continued)

Table 134.5 Drug dosages in patients with renal failure—cont'd

Generic name	Dose in normal renal function	Max. daily dose with normal renal function	Adjustment in dose (D) or interval (I)	GFR (ml/min) >50	GFR (ml/min) = 10-50	GFR (ml/min) <10	Supplement after HD	Supplement with PD	CVVHD
Cefoxitin	1–2 g q6–8h	12 g/q24h	I	q6–8h	q8–12h	q24–48h	Yes, extra 1 g	1 g q24h	
Cefpodoxime (proxetil)	100–400 mg q12h	800 mg/q24h	I	q12h	q24h	q24h	Yes	Dose for GFR <10	
Cefprozil	250–500 mg q12h	1 g/q24h	D	100%	50%	50%	Yes, extra 250 mg	Dose for GFR <10	
Ceftazidime	1–2 g q8h	8 g/q24h	I	q8–12h	q12–24h	q24–48h	Yes, extra 1 g	500 mg q24h	2 g q12h
Ceftibuten	400 mg q24h	400 mg	D	100%	25–50%	25–50%	Yes, extra 400 mg	100–200 mg q24h	
Ceftizoxime	1–2 g q8–12h	12 g/q24h	D&I	q8–12h	q12–24h	q24h	Yes, extra 1 g	500 mg–1 g q24h	
Ceftobiprole (medocaril)	500 mg q8h	1.5 g/q24h		100%	500 mg q12h (30–50 ml/min)	250 mg q12h (<30 ml/min)	No data	No data	
Ceftriaxone	1–2 g q24h	4 g/q24h	D	100%	100%	100%	No	Usual regimen	2 g q12–24h
Cefuroxime	250–500 mg q12h	1 g/q24h	D	100%	100%	100%	Yes	Dose for GFR <10	250–500 mg q12h
Cefuroxime (axetil)	750 mg–1.5 g q8h	6 g/q24h	I	q8h	q8–12h	q24h	Yes	Dose for GFR <10	
Cephalexin	250–500 mg q6h	4 g/q24h	I	q6–8h	q8–12h	q12–24h	Yes	Dose for GFR <10	250–500 mg q12h
Loracarbef	200–400 mg q12h	800 mg/q24h	I	q12h	q24h	q3–5d	Yes	Dose for GFR <10	
Monobactam									
Aztreonam	500 mg–2 g q8–12h	8 g/q24h	D	100%	50%	25%	Yes, extra 500 mg	Dose for GFR <10	2 g q12h
Carbapenems									
Doripenem	500 mg q8h	1.5 g/q24h	D&I	100%	250 mg q8h (30–50 ml/min)	250 mg q12h (<30 ml/min)	No data	No data	250 mg q6h, 500 mg q8h or 500 mg q6h
Ertapenem	1 g q24h	1 g/q24h	D	100%	100%	50%	Yes, extra 150 mg If dose given within 6h of HD	Dose for GFR <10	
Imipenem–cilastatin	250 mg–1 g q6h	4 g/q24h	D	100%	50%	25%	Yes	Dose for GFR <10	
Meropenem	1 g q8h	4 g/q24h	D&I	100%	50% q12h	50% q24h	Yes	Dose for GFR <10	1 g q12h

Dosing guidance as per references 9,10,18,88–92.
CVVHD, continuous venovenous hemodialysis. GFR, glomerular filtration rate; HD, hemodialysis; PD, peritoneal dialysis.
Absence of information is due to lack of published data.

Table 134.6 Pregnancy categories of the β-lactam antibiotics

Class of β-lactam	Pregnancy category
Penicillins – all	B
β-Lactamase inhibitors – all	B
Cephalosporins – all	B
Aztreonam	B
Doripenem	B
Ertapenem	B
Imipenem–cilastatin	C
Meropenem	B

Categories as of August 2008. Category B means that animal studies have shown no risk to the fetus, but adequate human studies have not been performed, or animal studies have shown risk and human studies have shown no risk. Category C means that animal studies show toxicity to the fetus and human studies are inadequate.

Table 134.7 Adverse reactions associated with β-lactam antibiotics

Reaction site/system	Examples
Local	Pain, induration, tenderness at site of intramuscular injection; burning during intravenous administration; phlebitis
Hypersensitivity	Rash, pruritus, urticaria, fever, chills, Stevens–Johnson syndrome, anaphylaxis
Gastrointestinal	Diarrhea, nausea, vomiting, abdominal pain, *Clostridium difficile*-associated diarrhea
Hematologic	Eosinophilia, leukopenia, anemia, positive Coombs' test, hemolytic anemia, neutropenia, lymphopenia; thrombocytosis, thrombocytopenia, elevated prothrombin time, bleeding, abnormal clotting time, abnormal platelet aggregation
Hepatic	Elevated serum transaminases (aspartate transaminase, alanine transaminase), hepatitis, elevated alkaline phosphatase, elevated bilirubin
Renal	Elevated blood urea nitrogen and creatinine, falsely elevated creatinine, casts in urine
Central nervous system	Headache, dizziness, somnolence, confusion, tremor, myoclonus, seizures, encephalopathy
Genitourinary	Vaginitis
Superinfection	Thrush, vaginal candidiasis, infection with resistant bacteria

during acute infectious mononucleosis (Epstein–Barr virus). Reactions to penicillins are characterized according to the time of onset following administration of the drug:

- immediate reactions occur in the first hour;
- accelerated reactions occur 1–72 hours after drug administration; and
- late reactions occur 72 hours or more after starting a course of the antibiotic.

Both immediate and accelerated reactions may result in urticaria and anaphylaxis.

Previous exposure to penicillin does not seem to increase the risk of penicillin allergy. However, it is clear that people who have had allergic reactions to penicillin have a higher risk of allergic reactions than people who have tolerated therapy in the past. In patients with a history of penicillin allergy, rechallenge with penicillin results in acute reactions in an estimated 65% of patients, anaphylaxis in 5–10% and fatal anaphylaxis in 0.2–0.5%.

Skin testing is a useful technique in the evaluation of patients with a history of penicillin allergy, but is not useful as a screening test for the general population because many skin test positive patients without a history of penicillin allergy can tolerate penicillin therapy. Skin testing is not useful for identifying non-IgE-mediated adverse drug reactions such as drug fever.

Although fatalities have occurred as a result of the skin test itself, the procedure is generally regarded as safe. A wide range in the incidence of positive skin tests in patients with a previous history of penicillin allergy has been noted (8.75–63%), and therefore a significant proportion of patients who give a history of penicillin allergy can tolerate the drug.[96] In one large study, penicillin skin testing allowed the safe use of penicillin in 90% of patients who gave a history of penicillin allergy.[97] Skin test reactivity declines with time in patients with a history of penicillin allergy. People with dermatitis and allergic rhinitis do not have an increased risk of penicillin allergy, but the risk may be increased for atopic individuals.[98]

Patients with a history of penicillin allergy are four times as likely to have a reaction to first-generation cephalosporins than patients without a history of allergy (8.1 vs 1.9%). Second- and third-generation cephalosporins have an incidence of skin reaction (rash) ranging from 1% to 3%, similar to the incidence of rash with penicillin. Anaphylaxis, however, is uncommon with cephalosporins. There seems to be a lower incidence of allergy to second- and third-generation cephalosporins in patients with a history of penicillin allergy. Patients with allergy to penicillins should be considered allergic to the carbapenems, but there seems to be no cross-reactivity with aztreonam. No major allergic reactions to aztreonam have been reported, but rarely patients will develop a rash. There is more allergic cross-reactivity among penicillin derivatives than among cephalosporin derivatives. However, allergic cross-reactivity between cephalosporin derivatives is greater than cross-reactivity between cephalosporins and penicillins.[99]

At times, it may be necessary to administer penicillin to patients with a previous severe reaction to the drug. For instance, penicillin is the only acceptable treatment for a pregnant woman with syphilis. Effective methods of desensitization have been described,[100] but adverse reactions are common and the patient should be in an intensive care unit for close monitoring.

Hematologic effects

Hematologic toxicity is rare, but leukopenia (occurring in 0.2% of patients on mezlocillin in one study) has been observed when the penicillins or cephalosporins are used at high doses,[101] and also rarely with imipenem. Counts return when the drug is discontinued, and lower dosages can often be tolerated without neutropenia. Isolated eosinophilia can occur in patients on cephalosporins (1–7%). A Coombs' positive hemolytic anemia is rarely observed with the penicillins and cephalosporins.[102]

Dose-dependent defects of platelet aggregation and a prolongation of the bleeding time can be seen with carbenicillin and ticarcillin, and can occur with all of the penicillins at high doses. Clinically significant bleeding can occur but is uncommon.[103]

Hypoprothrombinemia occurred frequently with cephalosporins that are no longer widely used. These agents all had a methylthiotetrazole (MTT) group (i.e. cefoperazone, cefotetan, cefmenoxime), which may interfere with the activation of factors II, VII, IX and X, and may also prevent the activation of vitamin K.[104] Patients with renal failure, malnutrition, intra-abdominal infection or recent gastrointestinal surgery seem to be at the highest risk and may benefit from weekly prophylaxis with vitamin K when being given one of these antibiotics. Isolated thrombocytopenia rarely complicates the use of the β-lactam antibiotics. An immune mechanism has been documented. Thrombocytopenia can occur as soon as 5 days after the initiation of the antibiotic and generally resolves when the agent is withdrawn.[105]

Renal effects

Interstitial nephritis, characterized by fever, rash, eosinophilia, proteinuria, hematuria, eosinophiluria and occasionally renal insufficiency can be seen with the penicillins.[106] β-Lactam antibiotics that exist as sodium salts, particularly carbenicillin and ticarcillin, can induce hypokalemia.[106] Cephalothin can cause renal damage that histopathologically resembles that of nafcillin.[107] The concurrent use of aminoglycosides may add to the nephrotoxicity of cephalosporins such as cephalothin. About 1% of patients on ceftazidime have elevated blood urea nitrogen or creatinine, but these are generally not clinically significant.[108] The sodium load of some penicillins can be high, most notably with ticarcillin (4.7 mEq/g), but also with ampicillin, methicillin, penicillin G, azlocillin, mezlocillin and piperacillin, thereby posing a problem for patients with congestive heart failure.

Neurologic effects

Many of the β-lactams can cause neurotoxicity and, in particular, seizures. Seizures have been reported following the use of penicillin, ampicillin, amoxicillin, oxacillin, nafcillin, carbenicillin, ticarcillin, piperacillin, cefazolin, cefonicid, cephalexin, ceftazidime, imipenem, meropenem, ertapenem and doripenem. Benzylpenicillin, cefazolin and imipenem have the highest neurotoxic potential of the β-lactam antibiotics. Seizures have been reported to occur in 0.4–1.5% of patients taking imipenem.

Several risk factors that may predispose a patient to neurotoxicity have been identified, for example:

- high doses;
- renal insufficiency;
- disruption of the blood–brain barrier;
- pre-existing central nervous system (CNS) disease;
- advanced age;
- concurrent administration of nephrotoxic drugs;
- concurrent drugs that may reduce the seizure threshold; and
- concurrent administration of other β-lactam antibiotics.[109]

Neurotoxicity of penicillins is clearly related to elevated CSF antibiotic levels, such as may occur when high doses are being used in patients with impaired renal function. Penicillin levels in CSF should not exceed 5 mg/l.

Gastrointestinal effects

Gastrointestinal upset and diarrhea are common side-effects of the β-lactams. Enterocolitis caused by *Clostridium difficile* may result from use of any of the β-lactams.

Hepatitis is a rare side-effect of penicillins such as mezlocillin and nafcillin, and resolves after discontinuation of therapy. Hepatitis as a result of intravenous oxacillin can occur as early as 2 days into treatment, is thought to result from a hypersensitivity reaction, does not appear to be dose related and is reversible on discontinuation of the drug.[110] Mild elevations in transaminases and alkaline phosphatase also occur with the cephalosporins and carbapenems, but the drug can usually be continued.[111] Serum transaminases become elevated in 2–4% of patients receiving aztreonam.

Gallbladder sludge formation[112] and cholelithiasis[113] have occurred in patients on ceftriaxone. Children, patients receiving prolonged or high doses, and patients on total parenteral nutrition appear to be at risk of this complication.

A disulfuram-like reaction has been associated with the cephalosporins with an MTT group.[114] Patients taking these agents and then ingesting alcohol have developed flushing, tachycardia, diaphoresis, headache, nausea, vomiting and dizziness.

Other reactions

Local side-effects of the β-lactam antibiotics are not uncommon. At the intramuscular injection site, patients may experience pain, tenderness and edema. Thrombophlebitis can occur in up to 5% of patients receiving parenteral therapy with some agents.

Other reactions to penicillin are less common. Serum sickness, consisting of fever, urticaria, joint pains and angioneurotic edema, can occur and, rarely, exfoliative dermatitis, the Stevens–Johnson syndrome and allergic vasculitis. Late-onset morbilliform rashes can develop as a result of penicillin therapy and may disappear, even if the penicillin is continued, but desquamation can occur.

Drug interactions

The most clinically important drug interaction with the β-lactam antibiotics occurs with probenecid, a uricosuric and renal tubular blocking agent. Probenecid causes a two- to fourfold increase in the peak serum concentration of the β-lactam antibiotics. It also prolongs serum levels for these antibiotics. It is used most often with penicillin (e.g. in the treatment of gonococcal infections), but can also be used with ampicillin, methicillin, oxacillin, cloxacillin and nafcillin. The recommended dose in adults is 2 g/day in divided doses, and in children a 25 mg/kg initial dose is followed by 40 mg/kg/day in four divided doses (adult dose used for children who weigh over 50 kg). The mechanism of action involves not only inhibition of renal tubular secretion of the β-lactams, but also a decrease in the apparent volume of distribution of the drug.[115] Probenecid has little effect on the serum levels of imipenem and aztreonam and has no effect on drug levels of ceftazidime. Adverse reactions, including anaphylaxis, can occur with probenecid and the clinician must also be aware that toxicity can result from supratherapeutic levels of the β-lactam antibiotics when used with probenecid.

As cephalosporins with the MTT side chain can interfere with hemostasis, in the rare circumstance where these agents might be used in modern clinical practice, care must be taken when using these antibiotics in patients taking warfarin.

Synergistic activity against various bacteria occurs when the penicillins, cephalosporins, carbapenems and monobactams are used in conjunction with aminoglycosides.[116] However, using two β-lactam antibiotics together may result in either synergy or antagonism.

The bactericidal effect of ampicillin may be reduced when other antibiotics (chloramphenicol, erythromycin, sulfa drugs and tetracycline) are used simultaneously. The clinical significance of this is unclear.

When ampicillin is used in patients who are taking oral contraceptive agents, breakthrough bleeding may occur and the contraceptive may be less effective.

Piperacillin and ticarcillin must be used cautiously in any patient on vecuronium because the neuromuscular blockade can be further prolonged. Piperacillin can also lower serum levels of tobramycin if the drugs are used together.

Fatal reactions associated with the appearance of precipitates of calcium and ceftriaxone have occurred in neonates; this has led to recommendations not to administer ceftriaxone within 48 hours of giving intravenous calcium-containing solutions.

REFERENCES

References for this chapter can be found online at http://www.expertconsult.com

Chapter | **135** | *André Bryskier*

Macrolides, ketolides, lincosamides and streptogramins

Macrolides and Ketolides

INTRODUCTION

Shortly after the beginning of the antimicrobial era, it became increasingly apparent that bacteria could rapidly evolve resistance to existing antibacterial agents. New agents would need to be developed to keep pace with the remarkable capacity of bacterial pathogens to genetically adapt to antimicrobial chemotherapy. Systematic screening was performed by many researchers for new compounds possessing antibacterial activity in general and antistaphylococcal activity in particular. Researchers at Eli Lilly first discovered the erythromycin complex in 1952.

Erythromycin A, the most active component of the erythromycin complex, was initially intended to provide an alternative therapy in response to the emergence of penicillinase-producing strains of *Staphylococcus aureus*. The discovery of vancomycin did not supplant the use of erythromycin because of its poor tolerance, but the semisynthetic penicillins (methicillin and oxacillin) and the first injectable cephalosporins (cephalothin and cephaloridine) led to a decline in the use of erythromycin A.

Two circumstances led to a revival of interest in the macrolides (the second wave of macrolides in early 1980s – roxithromycin, clarithromycin, azithromycin, dirithromycin, flurithromycin):
- the recognition of the pathogenic potential of *Chlamydia trachomatis*; and
- the outbreak of 'Legionnaires' disease'.

Legionella pneumophila is an intracellular pathogen: β-lactams do not accumulate in phagocytic cells, in contrast to the excellent activity of the macrolides, tetracyclines, fluoroquinolones and ansamycins against this pulmonary pathogen.

The third wave of macrolides (the ketolides – telithromycin, cethromycin, CEM 101, modithromycin) was in response to the emergence of erythromycin A-resistant strains among Gram-positive cocci and *Campylobacter* spp., *Helicobacter pylori*, *Mycobacterium avium* complex, etc.

DEFINITIONS

The macrolides are hydrophobic molecules having a central 14- to 16-membered-ring lactone with few or no double bonds and no nitrogen atom. Several amino or neutral sugars may be attached to the lactone nucleus.

The azalides, such as azithromycin or tulathromycin (a veterinary drug), are not included as they have an endolactone nitrogen atom. Nevertheless, they are semisynthetic derivatives of erythromycin A and due to their antibacterial spectrum belong to the macrolide family. Semisynthetic ketolides (such as telithromycin, cethromycin, CEM 101) were obtained by the removal of the neutral sugar (L-cladinose). The 3-OH group obtained was oxidized yielding a 3-carbonyl group, which characterizes the ketolides.

CLASSIFICATION

There are several classifications of macrolides: a chemical classification and a simplified classification that considers the lactone structure and the natural or semisynthetic origin of the molecule. The natural macrolides of importance in human pathology are 14- or 16-membered-ring macrolides and, in addition in the semisynthetic derivatives, the 15-membered-ring macrolides (azalides).

The 14-membered-ring macrolides are divided into two groups: those of natural origin such as erythromycin A (Fig. 135.1) and olean-

Erythromycin A

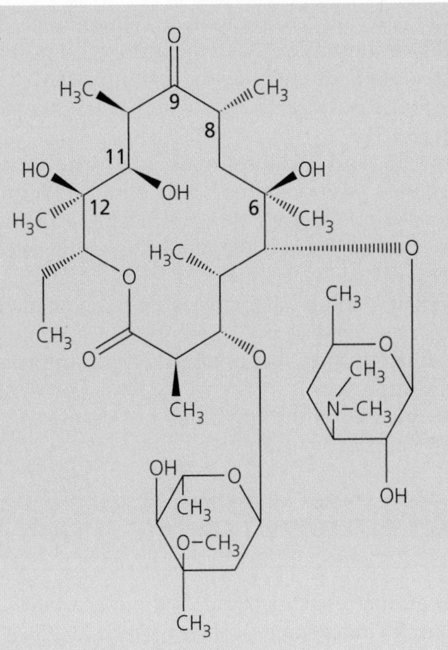

Fig. 135.1 Erythromycin A.

domycin, and the semisynthetic derivatives of erythromycin A. The latter may be separated into three subgroups:

- those with a modified substituent of the lactone nucleus, such as roxithromycin, clarithromycin, dirithromycin, flurithromycin and davercin (group II$_A$);
- those whose lactone nucleus has undergone modification, involving two subgroups, azalides (azithromycin, tulathromycin, gamithromycin) and oxolides (group II$_{B1}$ and II$_{B2}$); and
- those with a modification of the neutral sugar – ketolides (3-keto group) and acylide derivatives (alkyl or alkyl aryl 3-substituent) (group II$_C$) (Fig. 135.2).

Groups III and IV comprise, respectively, the 16-membered-ring natural molecules, such as josamycin, spiramycin and midecamycin, and the synthetic molecules such as miocamycin or rokitamycin.

Few specific macrolides are used in veterinary medicine but include tulathromycin (15-membered-ring derivative), tylosin and desmycosin (16-membered-ring macrolides). Some macrolides, such as spiramycin, are used in both animals and humans.

PHYSICOCHEMICAL CHARACTERISTICS

The main physicochemical properties of macrolides and ketolides are presented in Table 135.1.

Stability in acidic medium

Erythromycin A and, to a lesser extent, spiramycin and josamycin are unstable in an acidic medium. Erythromycin A is degraded by the formation of a hemiketal or a spiroketal form of erythronolide A (Fig. 135.3).

Josamycin (leucomycin A$_3$) may be converted in an acidic medium to isojosamycin, which has a hydroxyl group at C-13 because of the rearrangement of the dienole system of josamycin.

Spiramycin is a complex formed by three major components (I–III), which differ in the substituent at position 3 of the lactone nucleus: 3-OH (spiramycin I), 3-O-acetyl (spiramycin II) and 3-O-propionyl (spiramycin III). The spiramycins are much more stable than erythromycin A in an acidic medium.

Roxithromycin, clarithromycin and azithromycin are much more stable in an acidic medium than erythromycin A.

Roxithromycin is highly stable at pH 4.2 (Fig. 135.4) compared to erythromycin base and erythromycin A, 2'-propionate. Clarithromycin is 6-O-methylerythromycin A, and the hydroxyl at position 11 remains free. A degradation product devoid of antibacterial activity occurs under conditions of extreme acidity and is termed pseudoclarithromycin (Fig. 135.5).

Azithromycin and roxithromycin are hydrolyzed at the β-O-glycoside bond at position 3 in a highly acidic medium (pH 1.2). The resultant descladinose degradation product has a 3-hydroxyl group on the lactone nucleus. These compounds are highly stable in an acidic medium (Fig. 135.6).

The different ketolides are very stable in an acidic medium, even if the pH is 1.2 depending on the substituent fixed on aglycone. This stability is different from that obtained with clarithromycin, azithromycin or roxithromycin.

Ketolides such as telithromycin are not destroyed at pH 1.2 after more than 6 hours of exposure.

IN-VITRO ACTIVITY (SEE ALSO TABLE 135.2)

The natural antibacterial spectrum of the macrolides, irrespective of their structure, includes Gram-positive bacteria (e.g. *Staphylococcus* spp., *Streptococcus* spp., *Listeria* spp., *Erysipelothrix insidiosa*, *Corynebacterium* spp., *Lactobacilli* spp., *Leuconostoc* spp., *Pediococcus* spp.) and Gram-negative cocci along with fastidious Gram-negative bacilli (e.g. *Haemophilus*

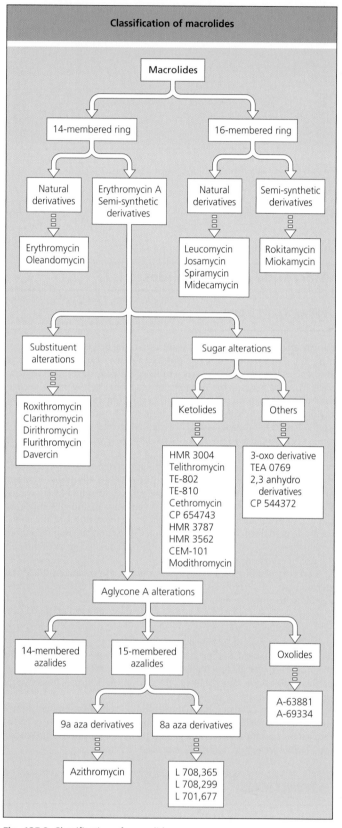

Fig. 135.2 Classification of macrolides.

influenzae, *Moraxella catarrhalis*, *Pasteurella* spp. and *Bordetella* spp.). Some anaerobic bacteria, intracellular bacteria, atypical bacteria such as mycoplasmas and related species are also susceptible to the macrolides. Some atypical mycobacteria, spirochetes, bacteria responsible for gastrointestinal infections (*Vibrio cholerae* and other *Vibrio* spp.,

Table 135.1 Main characteristic of macrolides and ketolides

	pK	Molecular weight
Erythromycin A	8.6	733.94
Oleandomycin	8.5	687.89
Clarithromycin	8.3	747.96
Roxithromycin	9.2	837.04
Dirithromycin	9.2	835
Erythromycylamine	8.9	734
Flurithromycin	–	751.95
Azithromycin	8.9–9.1	748.9
Josamycin	7.1	828.02
Midecamycin	6.9	813.99
Spiramycin I	7.7	843.06
Miocamycin	6.5	898.05
Rokitamycin	6.3	828
Telithromycin	8.7	812

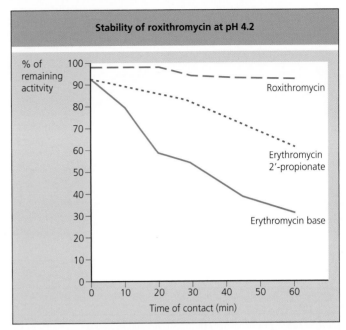

Fig. 135.4 Stability of roxithromycin at pH 4.2.

Campylobacter spp. and *H. pylori*) and *Treponema pallidum* remain susceptible to macrolides. They also display activity against *Leptospira*, *Borrelia* and *Bartonella* spp. However, these molecules are weakly active against enterococci and are moderately active against the viridans group of streptococci.

Erythromycin A overall is less active than clarithromycin but more active than azithromycin, roxithromycin and dirithromycin. Erythromycin A is the reference macrolide of natural origin. It is 10 times more active than oleandomycin, 2–10 times more active than josamycin, 2–12 times more active than spiramycin and up to 10 times more active than midecamycin.

The antibacterial spectrum of telithromycin, cethromycin and others encompasses that of the macrolides.

Telithromycin is more active *in vitro* than clarithromycin against Gram-positive and Gram-negative cocci, and also against erythromycin A-susceptible strains of Gram-positive bacilli. It is active against strains of Gram-positive cocci resistant to erythromycin A by an efflux or (inducible) MLS_B mechanism of resistance.

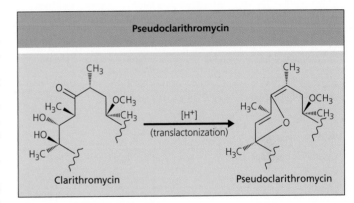

Fig. 135.5 Pseudoclarithromycin.

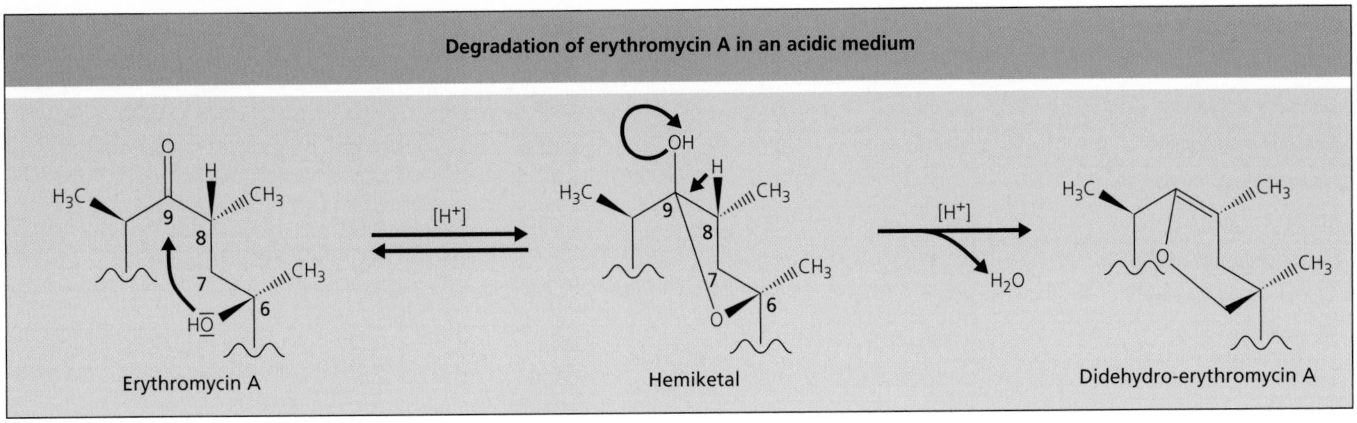

Degradation of erythromycin A in an acidic medium

Fig. 135.3 Degradation of erythromycin A in an acidic medium.

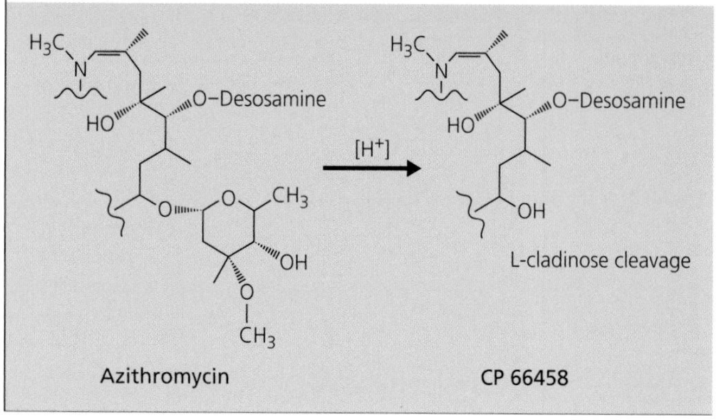

Fig. 135.6 Azithromycin: degradation in an acidic medium.

Telithromycin, like erythromycin A, is very active against β-hemolytic streptococci of Lancefield groups A, B, C and G when the strains are susceptible to erythromycin A. The *in-vitro* activity of telithromycin remains excellent against erythromycin A-resistant strains, particularly where an efflux mechanism is involved.

Ketolides remain highly susceptible against isolates of *Strep. pneumoniae* whatever their phenotype of resistance to erythromycin A.

Telithromycin displays a good activity against viridans group streptococci, irrespective of the resistance phenotype (erythromycin A-resistant, penicillin G-resistant). The Gram-positive bacilli comprise several bacterial genera and species, including *Listeria* spp., *Bacillus* spp., *Erysipelothrix rhusiopathiae*, coryneforms and lactic bacilli.

Diphtheria antibiotic treatment is based on penicillin G or erythromycin A. Rare erythromycin A-resistant strains have been described. Telithromycin is very active against *Corynebacterium diphtheriae*, whether or not the strain is toxigenic.

The *in-vitro* activity of macrolides and ketolides against *Listeria monocytogenes* and *Erysipelothrix rhusiopathiae* is good, and some reports have shown good *in-vitro* activity against *Bacillus anthracis*.

Table 135.2 *In-vitro* activity of macrolides and ketolides

	MIC$_{50}$ (mg/l)				
	ERY	**CLA**	**AZI**	**ROX**	**TEL**
Staph. aureus (methicillin sensitive)	0.25	0.25	1.0	0.5	0.06
Strep. pyogenes	0.06	0.015	0.06	0.12	≤0.008
Strep. agalactiae	0.06	0.015	0.06	0.12	0.008–0.12
Streptococcus groups C and G	0.06	0.03	0.12	0.12	≤0.008
Strep. pneumoniae	0.06	0.015	0.06	0.06	0.015
Enterococcus faecalis	4.0	4.0	8	8	0.12
Enterococcus faecium	>64	>64	>64	>64	2.0
Viridans streptococci	2.0	1.0	4.0	4.0	≤0.03–0.25
Listeria monocytogenes	0.25	0.06	0.5	0.25	0.03
Erysipelothrix rhusiopathiae	0.03	0.06	0.5	0.06	≤0.015
Corynebacterium diphtheriae	0.008	0.004	0.015	0.008	0.004
Nocardia spp.	16	16	>128	64	–
Pediococcus spp.	0.125	0.06	0.125	0.06	0.008
Lactobacillus spp.	0.06	0.015	0.06	0.06	≤0.03
Leuconostoc spp.	0.06	0.03	0.125	0.125	0.25
Corynebacterium jeikeium	>128	>128	>128	>128	0.06
Corynebacterium urealyticum	>64	>64	>64	>64	≤0.015
Rhodococcus equi	0.5	0.06	1.0	0.25	0.25
Gardnerella vaginalis	0.06	0.06	0.06	0.03	≤0.002
Neisseria meningitidis	0.12	0.015	0.015	0.06	0.0015–0.12
Neisseria gonorrhoeae	0.25	0.25	0.12	0.5	0.12
Moraxella catarrhalis	0.12	0.06	0.03	0.12	0.06
Haemophilus influenzae	4.0	4.0	1.0	8.0	1.0
Pasteurella multocida	4.0	2.0	1.0	4.0	1.0
Bordetella pertussis	0.06	0.015	0.03	0.12	0.01
Campylobacter jejunii	1.0	1.0	0.12	4.0	0.5–1.0
Haemophilus ducreyi	0.06	0.008	0.015	0.03	0.004

Table 135.2 *In-vitro* activity of macrolides and ketolides—cont'd

	MIC$_{50}$ (mg/l)				
	ERY	**CLA**	**AZI**	**ROX**	**TEL**
Helicobacter pylori	0.25	0.015	0.25	0.12	0.25
Mycoplasma pneumoniae	0.0039	0.019	0.0024	0.0039	0.00097
Legionella pneumophila	0.25	0.03	0.12	0.12	0.03
Chlamydophila pneumoniae	0.03	0.125	0.125	0.125	0.125
Borrelia spp.	0.015–0.03	0.0006–0.0025	0.002–0.008	0.0025–0.006	–
Bartonella spp.	0.06	0.03	0.03	–	0.006

ERY, erythromycin A; CLA, clarithromycin; AZI, azithromycin; ROX, roxithromycin; TEL, telithromycin.

The lactic bacilli form a complex group that includes *Lactobacillus*, *Leuconostoc*, *Pediococcus* and *Lactococcus* spp. against which telithromycin has shown a good *in-vitro* activity.

A number of coryneforms are involved in nosocomial infections, such as *Corynebacterium jeikeium* and *Corynebacterium urealyticum*. Macrolides are inactive against *C. jeikeium* and *C. urealyticum*; in contrast, telithromycin is very active against the majority of corynebacteria. Telithromycin activity against *C. jeikeium* is distributed in a bimodal population. There are discrepancies among authors with respect to the activity against *C. urealyticum*.

Macrolides are weakly active or inactive against enterococci; in contrast, telithromycin exhibits good activity against *Enterococcus faecalis*.

Neisseria meningitidis strains of reduced susceptibility to penicillin G have been described while rifampin (rifampicin)-resistant strains are increasingly common. Some erythromycin A or spiramycin-resistant strains have been observed which harbor an efflux mechanism of resistance mediated by Mtr (encoded by the *mtr* gene). The activity of telithromycin remains good.

Macrolides and ketolides are inactive against Enterobacteriaceae with few minor exceptions. Azithromycin exhibits a certain *in-vitro* activity against *Salmonella*, *Shigella* spp. and *Escherichia coli*.

Macrolides and ketolides are highly active against *Leptospira interrogans* whatever the serovar (minimum inhibitory concentrations (MICs) range from 0.01 to 0.04 mg/l) and *Bartonella* spp. (MICs 0.03–0.125 mg/l).

Lyme disease is caused by *Borrelia burgdorferi* which is divided into at least three subspecies which are responsible for different syndromes: rheumatismal (*B. burgdorferi sensu lato*), neurologic (*B. garinii*) and dermatologic (*B. afzelii*). Activity of macrolides/ketolides is species dependent.

Bacteria responsible for lower respiratory tract infections

Lower respiratory tract infections, whether parenchymatous (pneumonia) or nonparenchymatous (acute bronchitis or acute exacerbation of chronic bronchitis), are due to common respiratory pathogens or to intracellular or atypical bacteria.

The pathogens most commonly involved in lower respiratory tract infections are *Strep. pneumoniae*, *H. influenzae*, *Staph. aureus* and, more marginally, *Moraxella catarrhalis*.

The determination of the *in-vitro* activity of an antibacterial agent against *H. influenzae* is poorly standardized. Telithromycin has *in-vitro* activity similar to that of azithromycin against *H. influenzae* and greater than that of clarithromycin and roxithromycin which are poorly active. *Bordetella pertussis* is responsible for whooping cough. Macrolides remain the standard antibiotic treatment. Erythromycin

A-resistant strains are of rare occurrence. Activities of telithromycin and other macrolides are good.

Mycoplasma pneumoniae is susceptible to macrolides and ketolides and is also responsible for a so-called atypical pneumonia. Pneumonia due to *Chlamydophila pneumoniae* and *L. pneumophila* is highly susceptible to macrolides-ketolides.

In-vitro activities of macrolides and telithromycin against unusual bacteria involved in a pathologic process have been investigated.

Parachlamydia and *Simkania*

Trophozoites of *Acanthamoeba* hosting *Chlamydia*-like bacteria have been isolated from patients with fever associated with the use of humidifiers in Vermont (Hall's coccus strain) and from the nasal mucosa (strain Bn9). The use of antibiotics directed against *Parachlamydia* has been reported from patients suffering from community-acquired pneumonia. *Parachlamydia* does not grow on an acellular medium.

Tropheryma whipplei

T. whipplei is responsible for Whipple's disease, which is characterized by arthralgia and diarrhea.

The growth of *T. whipplei* in MRC5 cells is inhibited by macrolides/ketolides according to the method of quantification of the copies of DNA.

Bacteria involved in sexually transmitted diseases

Macrolides are highly active *in vitro* against *Neisseria gonorrhoeae*, irrespective of the resistance profile of the strain isolated (resistance to penicillin G, spectinomycin, tetracyclines, etc.), but the therapeutic activity is often disappointing.

Strains of *Treponema pallidum* resistant to erythromycin A and azithromycin have been reported.

Chancroid is caused by *Haemophilus ducreyi*. Macrolides represent the standard treatment; telithromycin is highly active against this bacterial species.

Chlamydia trachomatis is the causative agent of trachoma (ophthalmic disease) in endemic regions, nongonococcal urethritis and much pelvic inflammatory disease. The activity of macrolides/ketolides is good, with MICs ranging from 0.008 mg/l to 0.06 mg/l.

The *in-vitro* activity of macrolides/ketolides against *Ureaplasma urealyticum* is good, with MICs of 0.06 µg/ml.

Fourteen- and 15-membered-ring macrolides are inactive against *Mycoplasma hominis*, but 16-membered-ring macrolides exert good *in-vitro* activity; activity of ketolides is structure dependent.

Anaerobic bacteria

Macrolides exhibit variable activity against Gram-positive anaerobes and are poorly active against Gram-negative anaerobic bacilli. Telithromycin possesses excellent *in-vitro* activity against Gram-positive bacteria, moderate activity against Gram-negative bacilli of the *Bacteroides* group, good activity against *Porphyromonas* and *Prevotella* spp. and variable activity against *Fusobacterium* spp.

MECHANISM OF ACTION

The macrolides/ketolides inhibit protein synthesis by binding to the 50S subunit of the bacterial ribosomes. In the presence of macrolides/ketolides, peptidyl tRNA accumulates in the bacterial cell, causing depletion of the free transfer tRNA needed for activation of the α-amino acids. The presence of erythromycin A causes the release of a basic amino acid-rich peptide chain by transient inhibition of transpeptidation. Translocation is impaired by the nascent peptide, which adheres to the surface of the ribosome, generating friction forces. This phenomenon is optimal at certain chain lengths when it becomes a floating strip. What appears certain is that erythromycin A modifies the interaction between peptidyl tRNA and the peptidyltransferase donor site.

Intrabacterial penetration

Before reaching ribosomes, the molecule has to cross one (Gram-positive) or two (Gram-negative) barriers. Erythromycin A and its derivatives penetrate Gram-positive bacteria and also *H. influenzae* passively. The affinity for ribosomes is higher for ketolides than for erythromycin A.

Exit tunnel

The exit tunnel passes and spans through the middle of the 50S ribosomal subunit and is paved mainly by RNA loop. The tunnel accommodates a peptide of 25–40 amino acids of any sequence and any conformation, and is formed with proteins L22 and L4.

The binding site of macrolide, lincosamide and streptogramin B (MLSB) antibacterials is located in the entrance of the exit tunnel before the ribosomal proteins L4 and L22 constrict it, causing destabilization of peptidyl tRNA during translocation and inducing dissociation of peptidyl tRNA from the ribosomes during the elongation phase of protein synthesis.

Fourteen- and 15-membered-ring macrolides reduce the diameter of the tunnel entrance blocking the progression of the nascent peptide by steric hindrance.

Lincosamides and 16-membered-ring macrolides which possess an L-mycarose sugar inhibit the peptidyltransferase enzymatic activity. However, 14- and 15-membered-ring macrolides as well as streptogramin B analogues block the entrance of the exit channel of the 50S ribosomal subunit.

The translation reaction contains a peptidyl-tRNA hydrolase. This enzyme hydrolyzes peptidyl tRNAs that dissociate from the ribosome by drop off, but not those remaining bound to the ribosome. The length of the drop off nascent peptide is compound-dependent.

Peptidyltransferase center

The peptidyltransferase center consists of domains II and V, which formed a pocket with 5S rRNA. Macrolides and ketolides are fixed on domain V; ketolides are also fixed on domain II.

Cethromycin and telithromycin interact like erythromycin A with domain V through desosamine sugar and aglycone.

Ketolides are composed of two additional parts: C11–C12 carbamate residue and a long side chain either on the carbamate moiety for telithromycin or through the 6-hydroxyl group for cethromycin.

INTRACELLULAR CONCENTRATIONS

The macrolides penetrate and accumulate in phagocytic cells, thereby allowing the treatment of infections due to intracellular bacteria, such as *Chlamydia, Legionella, Rickettsia* spp. and *Francisella tularensis*.

The mean ratios of cell concentrations to those present in the extracellular medium are presented in Table 135.3.

Like azithromycin, telithromycin gradually accumulates in polymorphonuclear neutrophils, particularly in the granules (60%), and is eliminated progressively from the cell (efflux). Telithromycin uses a transport system to penetrate the phagocytic cell.

MECHANISM OF RESISTANCE

Epidemiology

Since the first report in the mid-1970s of *Strep. pneumoniae* multidrug-resistant strains in South Africa, the prevalence rate of erythromycin A resistance has increased worldwide. It is the same for *Strep. pyogenes* and other Gram-positive cocci. Surveillance programs such as Protek also include detection of phenotypes and genotypes of resistance. For 2004–2005, 116 centers were enrolled in 35 countries. The prevalence rate of erythromycin A resistance worldwide was 35%. The main mechanism of resistance was methylation (*erm B* gene) and represented about 66% of the resistant isolates. In the USA, the main mechanism of resistance was efflux (*mef A* gene) and represented about 80% of the resistant isolates.

In Europe, the highest rate of resistance was recorded in France, Spain and Italy where resistance rates were 52.5%, 32.2% and 33.5%, respectively, for *Strep. pneumoniae*. In Northern Europe except Belgium (31.8%), resistance rates were low.

Molecular mechanisms of resistance

There are currently four recognized mechanisms of resistance to erythromycin A:
- modifications in the ribosomal target;
- inactivation of the molecule;
- efflux; and
- mutations in the 23S ribosomal RNA and ribosomal proteins L4 and L22.

These resistance mechanisms are described in detail in Chapter 131.

Table 135.3 Accumulation ratio of the main macrolides (*in vitro*)

	Cells	C/E
Erythromycin A	PMN MA	4.4–18 18–38
Roxithromycin	PMN MA	14–100 61
Clarithromycin	PMN	9–16
Dirithromycin	PMN MA	7–60 668
Spiramycin	MA	20–35
Josamycin	PMN	16
Rokitamycin	PMN	30
Azithromycin	PMN	80–300
Telithromycin	PMN	250–300

C/E, accumulation ratio; MA, alveolar macrophages; PMN, neutrophils.

PHARMACODYNAMIC PROPERTIES

The thigh-infection models in neutropenic and normal mice have shown that macrolides/ketolides can be separated in two subgroups: those that are time dependent (T > MIC) such as erythromycin, roxithromycin, clarithromycin, and those that are concentration dependent such as azithromycin and dirithromycin.

The pharmacodynamics of telithromycin data indicates that there is a good correlation between efficacy and concentration, particularly the area under the curve (AUC).

PHARMACOKINETIC PROPERTIES

Adult volunteers

The absorption and bioavailability vary according to the molecule, partly explaining the difference in unit dosage and frequency of administration of the different macrolide or ketolide drugs.

Absorption can be rapid, with a lag time of 0.25 hours (roxithromycin, clarithromycin). The average peak serum concentration ranges from 0.4 mg/l (azithromycin 500 mg) to 11 mg/l (roxithromycin 300 mg). It is reached after a period of between 0.6 hour (rokitamycin) and 4.0 hours (dirithromycin) and is dose dependent. The relative bioavailability (AUC/F) ranges from 3.7 mg.h/l (rokitamycin) to 132 mg.h/l (roxithromycin 300 mg) and is dependent on the administered dose, but is not proportional to the dose for certain molecules with nonlinear pharmacokinetics. The apparent elimination half-life ranges from 0.1 hour (miocamycin) to 44 hours (dirithromycin). The absolute bioavailability of the different molecules ranges from 10% (dirithromycin) to about 50–60% for roxithromycin and clarithromycin. It is of the order of 37% for azithromycin and 14-hydroxyclarithromycin, the main metabolite of clarithromycin.

Plasma protein binding is mainly to the α_1-glycoproteins for macrolides, ranging from 15% (josamycin) to more than 90% (roxithromycin).

For telithromycin and cethromycin, peak plasma concentrations varied from 1.9 mg/l (telithromycin 800 mg) to 0.14–1.7 mg/l (cethromycin 100 mg and 1200 mg, respectively) and were reached 1.0 hour after administration and the apparent elimination half-life from 3.5–6.6 hours (cethromycin) to 7.16 hours (telithromycin 800 mg) (see Table 135.4).

Elderly subjects

In elderly patients with no liver abnormalities the pharmacokinetic profiles were similar to those of adults (Table 135.5). As macrolides are not eliminated via the kidney, there is no need to modify the daily dosing in renal insufficiency.

Table 135.4 Pharmacokinetics of macrolides and ketolides

	Dose (mg)	Compound or metabolite	C_{max} (µg/ml)	T_{max} (h)	AUC/F (µg/h/ml)	T½ β (h)
Azithromycin	500	–	0.35 ± 0.1	0.9 ± 0.9	3.58 ± 1.2	–
	500	–	0.59 ± 0.2	2.2 ± 0.02	3.35 ± 0.4	41.2 ± 4.3
Clarithromycin	100	C	0.35	1.46	1.67	2.27
	200	C	0.6	1.56	2.99	2.3
	–	OH-C	0.41	2.29	3.4	3.37
	400	C	0.13	1.86	8.55	3.6
	–	OH-C	0.78	2.11	7.52	3.89
	600	C	2.03	1.83	15.44	3.64
	–	OH-C	1.06	2.45	9.95	3.84
	800	C	2.63	2.67	24.73	4.25
	–	OH-C	1.02	2.72	10.72	5.09
	1200	C	3.97	2.2	44.6	5.98
	–	OH	1.54	2.61	23.9	9.19
	250	C	0.7–0.8	1.7 ± 1.9	4–4.2	2.6–2.8
	–	OH	0.6–0.7	2.2–2.3	4.6–4.9	3.9–5.1
	500	C	1.77–1.89	2.3	11.1–11.7	3.3–3.5
	–	OH	0.7–0.8	2.3–2.8	6.1–6.9	6.4–6.6
Dirithromycin	250	–	ND	–	–	–
	500	–	0.29 ± 0.2	4	0.86 ± 0.6	32.5
	750	–	0.64 ± 0.4	4	1.84 ± 1.2	30.6
	1000	–	0.41 ± 0.2	4	1.61 ± 1.1	31.9
Roxithromycin	150	–	7.9 ± 0.6	1.9	81 ± 10	10.5 ± 1.4
	300	–	10.8 ± 0.6	1.5	132 ± 17	11.9 ± 0.5
	450	–	12.2 ± 0.7	1.3	170 ± 20	13.8 ± 0.9
Flurithromycin	500	–	1 ± 0.7	0.92	0.4	3.54
	750	–	1.58 ± 0.3	0.72	3.52	2.8
	375	–	1.41 ± 0.5	1	4.41	3.94

(Continued)

Table 135.4 Pharmacokinetics of macrolides and ketolides—cont'd

	Dose (mg)	Compound or metabolite	C_{max} (μg/ml)	T_{max} (h)	AUC/F (μg/h/ml)	T½ β (h)
Oleandomycin	1000	–	2.8	2.6	10.8	3.4
Spiramycin	1000	–	0.96	3	5.43	5.37
	1500	–	1.53	3	9.8	5.52
	2000	–	1.65	4	11.26	6.23
	500	–	2.14	–	6.19	4.51
Josamycin	1000	–	2.74	0.75	4.2	1.5
Josamycin	400	–	0.33	0.77	0.91	1.51
	1000	–	2.41	0.75	4.9	2
Oleandomycin	1000	–	4	1	14	4.2
Midecamycin	400	–	0.25	0.5	0.34	1
Midecamycin	600	–	0.8	1	–	–
	1200	–	1.9	2	–	–
Rokitamycin	600	–	1.9	0.6	3.7	2
Miocamycin	600	–	3.01	2	3	1
	400	Mb12	0.6	0.48	0.73	1.24
	–	Mb6	0.17	0.6	0.28	1.47
	–	Mb9a	0.16	0.73	0.27	1.45
	800	Mb12	1.37	0.52	1.72	1.32
	–	Mb6	0.44	0.65	0.76	1.71
	–	Mb9a	0.4	0.83	1.46	2.34
	800	Mb12	1.73	0.79	2.59	1.31
	–	Mb6	0.66	0.83	1.46	2.34
	–	Mb9a	0.57	1.06	1.33	2.09
Telithromycin	800	–	1.90	1.0	8.25	7.16

C, parent compound; Mb, metabolite; OH-hydroxyl metabolite.

Table 135.5 Pharmacokinetics of macrolides in elderly patients

		Dose (mg)	Route	C_{max} (μg/ml)	T_{max} (h)	AUC$_{0-\infty}$ (μg/h/ml)	T½ (h)
Spiramycin adipate	Young	500	iv	2.14		6.7	4.5
	Elderly	500	iv	2.51		16.7	9.8
Josamycin	Young	1000	po			6.25	1.69
	Elderly	1000	po			6.25	3.4
Miocamycin (Mb12)	Young	800	po	1.34	0.67	1.92	1.24
	Elderly	800	po	1.15	0.58	2.52	2.36
Roxithromycin	Young	300	po	9.7	1.6	122.6	11.2
	Elderly	300	po	10.8	2.06	197.3	15.5
Dirithromycin	Young	500	po	0.34	3.90	0.91	
	Elderly	500	po	0.52	4.80	2.42	
Clarithromycin	Young	500	po	2.41		18.9	4.9
	Elderly	500	po	3.28		30.8	7.7
14-OH clarithromycin	Young	500	po	0.66			7.2
	Elderly	500	po	1.33			14.0
Azithromycin	Young	500	po	0.41	2.5	2.5	
	Elderly	500	po	0.38	3.8	3.0	
Telithromycin	Young	800	po	3.0	0.5	11.56	11.46
	Elderly	800	po	1.9	1.0	7.25	10.64

CLINICAL STUDIES

High concentrations in the tissues and biologic fluids of the main respiratory tract sites can be detected following single or multiple doses of macrolides (Table 135.6). For telithromycin, the concentrations in different part of the lung tissue after a single dose of 800 mg are summarized in Table 135.7.

TOLERANCE

Macrolides have the capacity to interfere with the metabolism and pharmacokinetics of other drugs (Table 135.8) and other drugs may produce adverse events when administered with macrolides (Table 135.9).

MACROLIDES/KETOLIDES VERSUS OTHER ANTIBACTERIALS: ADVANTAGES

Macrolides are considered safe drugs. They are mainly an alternative to β-lactam antibiotics when the latter are ineffective against main common pathogens or the patient is hypersensitive to β-lactams. However,

some primary indications remain for macrolides such as diphtheria, chancroid, *Helicobacter pylori* and *Mycobacterium avium*.

One of the major uses for macrolides is atypical and intracellular pathogenic infections such as *Chlamydia* and *Legionella* spp. in parenchymal lower respiratory tract infections or nongonococcal urethritis.

Oral antibacterials are mainly composed of β-lactams (penicillins, cephems), macrolides/ketolides, fluoroquinolones, cyclines, ansamycins and, where available, oral streptogramins.

One of the main advantages of macrolides compared to other compounds is their ability to be used during pregnancy, in the pediatric setting and in adult and elderly patients. Fluoroquinolones and tetracyclines are contraindicated during pregnancy and in pediatrics. However, since fluoroquinolones possess an oral and an intravenous formulation they may be useful in those patients in whom intravenous formulations of macrolides are not well tolerated.

Lincosamides

INTRODUCTION

Lincomycin was isolated in 1962 from fermentation of *Streptomyces lincolnensis* subsp. *lincolnensis*. Numerous analogues have been prepared from lincomycin by semisynthesis to enlarge the anti-

Table 135.6 Tissue distribution of macrolides (peak concentrations mg/kg and µg/ml)

	Dose (mg)	Serum (µg/ml)	RESPIRATORY TRACT		
			Bronchial mucosa	Bronchial secretions	Sinus
Erythromycin	500**	3.08	7.20	1.05	0.9–1.8
Oleandomycin	200*	6.26		3.77	2.68
Roxithromycin	150** / 500**	2.51 / 2.4		3.10	4.15 / 2.18
Spiramycin	2000**	0.39	13–36	7.3	2–8.8
Josamycin	1000**	2.3		1.60	2.8
Miocamycin	600**			5.16	
Azithromycin	500*		3.89	0.23	1.34
Dirithromycin	500**	0.22	1.9	1.3	

*Single dose;
**Multiple doses.

Table 135.7 Telithromycin concentration in lung tissues

Sampling time (h)	No.	Plasma concentration (mg/l)	CONCENTRATION OF TELITHROMYCIN		
			Bronchial mucosa (mg/kg)	ELF (mg/l)	Alveolar macrophages (mg/l)
1–3	5	1.07	0.68	5.4	65
6–8	6	0.61	2.2	4.2	100
24	6	0.07	3.5	1.17	41
48	6	ND	ND	ND	2.15

ELF, epithelial lining fluid; ND, not detectable.

Table 135.8 A selection of drugs whose metabolism may interfere with that of macrolides

- Alfentanil, sufentanil
- Antipyrine
- Astemizol
- Bromocriptine
- Carbamazepine
- Ciclosporin A
- Cimetidine
- Cisapride
- Clozapine
- Diltiazem
- Digoxin
- Dysopyramide
- Ergotamine
- Ethylestradiol
- Felodipine
- Glibenclamide
- Levodopa, carbidopa
- Lovastatin
- Methylprednisolone
- Phenytoin
- Rifampin (rifampicin), rifabutin
- Sodium valproate
- Theophylline
- Triazolam, midazolam
- Verapamil
- Warfarin
- Zidovudine

bacterial spectrum and enhance antibacterial activity. A series of 7-chlorolincomycin derivatives has been synthesized, yielding clindamycin. Two human drugs have been introduced in clinical practice, lincomycin and clindamycin; pirlimycin is used in veterinary medicine.

CHEMICAL STRUCTURES

The lincosamides consist of three components: an amino acid, a sugar and an amide bond connecting these two moieties to one another. The amino acid residue is a substituted L-proline. The sugar is lincosamine.

Clindamycin is the 7(S)-chlorodeoxylincomycin derivative. Pirlimycin is the 4-cis-ethyl-L-pipecolic derivative of clindamycin. For oral use, a palmitate salt of clindamycin hydrochlorine is available; for injection, clindamycin phosphate (1200 mg equivalent to 1000 mg clindamycin base) is available.

A number of compounds with which lincomycin is incompatible have been reported, including β-lactams (penicillin G, cloxacillin, methicillin, ampicillin, ticarcillin, cephalothin), novobiocin, hydrocortisone, streptomycin, vitamin B and potassium canrenoate. Compounds reported as being incompatible with clindamycin phosphate include ampicillin, calcium gluconate, magnesium sulfate, phenytoin, group B vitamins and barbiturates.

Solutions containing tobramycin sulfate and clindamycin phosphate are unstable.

ANTIBACTERIAL ACTIVITY

Lincosamides are antibiotics whose antibacterial spectrum includes Gram-positive cocci, anaerobic bacteria and certain so-called atypical bacteria. Enterobacteriaceae, *Pseudomonas* spp. and *Acinetobacter* spp. are excluded from the antibacterial spectrum of the lincosamides.

The lincosamides possess good antistaphylococcal activity. They are active against methicillin-susceptible *Staph. aureus* strains but not against methicillin-resistant strains (MIC >64 mg/l). They are active against coagulase-negative staphylococci, with the exception of *Staph. cohnii*, *Staph. sciuri* and *Staph. xylosus*, which have low-level resistance to lincomycin and to streptogramin B. The MICs of lincomycin are 4–8 mg/l, as opposed to 0.5–1 mg/l for susceptible strains. They are inactive against enterococci. They possess good activity against group A and B streptococci, viridans group streptococci and *Strep. pneumoniae*. These strains appear to be inhibited by concentrations of 0.4 mg/l. The lincosamides are active against *Corynebacterium diphtheriae*, *Nocardia* spp. and *Bacillus anthracis* but are inactive against *Listeria monocytogenes*.

Clindamycin is active against *Erysipelothrix rhusiopathiae*. They are inactive or weakly active against *Neisseria meningitidis* and *Neisseria gonorrhoeae*, *H. influenzae*, *Moraxella catarrhalis* and *Pasteurella* spp. Clindamycin is active against *Bordetella pertussis*, but lincomycin is inactive. Clindamycin is inactive against *Bordetella bronchiseptica*. Against *Campylobacter jejuni*, clindamycin possesses good activity (MIC$_{50}$ 0.4 mg/l), whereas lincomycin is inactive. The activity of clindamycin against *Helicobacter pylori* is good (MIC 1 mg/l).

The lincosamides are inactive against *Legionella pneumophila*. Clindamycin has activity against *Chlamydia trachomatis* (MIC 1.0 mg/l), whereas lincomycin is inactive (MIC 256 mg/l). In contrast to the 14-membered-ring macrolides, apart from certain ketolides, clindamycin is active against *Mycoplasma hominis* but is weakly active against *Mycoplasma pneumoniae* and *Ureaplasma urealyticum*. Clindamycin

Table 135.9 Drug interference by macrolides

	Theophylline	Carbamazepine	Ciclosporin A	Midazolam	Terfenadine
Erythromycin	+	+	+	+	+
Oleandomycin	+	+	+	+	NT
Azithromycin	–	–	NT	–	–
Clarithromycin	(+)	+	+	+	+
Dirithromycin	(+)	NT	+	NT	
Roxithromycin	(+)	–	(+)	+	+
Josamycin	+	–	+	NT	NT
Spiramycin	–	NT	–	NT	NT
Rokitamycin	(+)	NT	+	NT	NT
Midecamycin	–	NT	NT	NT	NT
Miocamycin	–	+	+	NT	NT
Flurithromycin	NT	+	NT	NT	NT

NT, not tested.

Table 135.10 *In-vitro* activity of clindamycin

Micro-organism(s)	MIC (mg/l) 50%	90%	Range
Staph. aureus Met^s	0.12	0.125	
Staph. aureus Met^r	1.0	>16	
Coagulase-negative staphylococci	0.25	>16	
Strep. pyogenes	0.03	0.06	
Strep. agalactiae	0.06	0.5	
Strep. pneumoniae Pen^s	0.125	0.25	
Strep. pneumoniae Pen^r	1.0	16	
Enterococcus spp.	>16	>16	
Viridans group streptococci	0.5	0.5	
Neisseria meningitidis			>5
Neisseria gonorrhoeae			2.0
Bordetella pertussis			0.25–>8
Bordetella bronchiseptica			≤32
Haemophilus influenzae			8.0
Mycoplasma pneumoniae			1.0
Mycoplasma hominis			0.03
Ureaplasma urealyticum			2.0
Chlamydia trachomatis			1.0
Campylobacter jejunii	0.4	0.8	0.1–>50
Helicobacter pylori	0.5	2.0	0.25–2.0
Gardnerella vaginalis	0.003	0.06	0.2–2.0
Nocardia spp.			0.78–0.25
Actinomyces spp.			0.03–0.25
Legionella pneumophila			12.5
Cornebacterium diphtheriae			≤0.2

Met^r, methicillin resistant; Met^s, methicillin sensitive; Pen^r, penicillin resistant; Pen^s, penicillin sensitive.

is active against *Gardnerella vaginalis*. Lincomycin is active against *Leptospira* spp. Clindamycin has good activity against anaerobes.

Among Gram-positive anaerobes, clindamycin exhibits good activity against *Clostridium perfringens*, *Clostridium tetani* and *Clostridium difficile*. Its activity against *Bifidobacterium*, *Propionibacterium* spp. and Gram-positive cocci is moderate. It exhibits good activity against *Eubacterium* spp.

Among Gram-negative anaerobes, clindamycin displays good activity against the *Bacteroides fragilis* group, with the exception of *Bacteroides thetaiotaomicron*, *Porphyromonas* spp. and *Prevotella* spp. Activity against *Veillonella* spp. is good (MIC >0.05 mg/l) (Table 135.10).

MODE OF ACTION AND RESISTANCE

The lincosamides act on the 50S ribosomal subunit of the bacterial ribosome. The binding sites are similar to those for erythromycin A. The lincosamides prevent transpeptidation during the formation of the nascent peptide chain by inhibiting peptidyltransferase.

The intrinsic resistance of Enterobacteriaceae, *Pseudomonas* spp. and *Acinetobacter* spp. is due to the relative impermeability of the bac-

terial outer membrane. In Gram-positive cocci, penetration is a passive phenomenon. The enterococci are resistant to the lincosamides. Acquired resistance to lincosamides may be due to at least three mechanisms: modification of the bacterial target, modification of the antibiotics and reduced permeability. The modification of the target is due to methylation of an adenine residue on the 23S rRNA of the 50S subunit by a bacterial methylase.

In the constitutive form of resistance in *Staph. aureus*, all macrolides, lincosamides and streptogramin B are also resistant (*erm* gene); conversely, when it is an inducible resistance, there is dissociation between the three families and the lincosamides remain active, even if the activity is reduced. In streptococci, in contrast to *Staph. aureus*, the lincosamides can induce resistance. Inducible resistance may be highlighted by the D-test in *Staph. aureus*.

A plasmid-mediated 3-lincomycin or 4-clindamycin-*O*-nucleotidyltransferase has been detected in *Staph. aureus*. There is high-level resistance to lincomycin and a reduction in susceptibility to clindamycin has been noted. In coagulase-negative staphylococci, the main mechanism of resistance is adenine methylation (MLS_B type) and is identical to that of *Staph. aureus*. These species possess more specific resistance mechanisms, such as a reduction in permeability to 14-membered-ring macrolides as has been described for *Staph. epidermidis*. The 14-membered-ring macrolides may also be inactivated enzymatically; this resistance phenotype has been described for *Staph. hominis*, *Staph. haemolyticus* and *Staph. saprophyticus*.

Like *Staph. aureus*, certain species may inactivate lincomycin or clindamycin by a plasmid-mediated enzyme: *O*-nucleotidyltransferase.

It has been shown that strains of *B. fragilis* are divided into three groups:

- those which are very susceptible to clindamycin (MIC ≤0.25 mg/l);
- those which are moderately susceptible (MIC 0.25–8 mg/l); and
- those which are resistant (MIC >16 mg/l).

Strains of *Strep. pneumoniae* and *Strep. pyogenes* susceptible to clindamycin and resistant to erythromycin A derivatives have been described. This dissociation is due to an efflux resistance mechanism (M phenotype).

Antiparasitic activity

In 1967, it was shown that clindamycin and its derivatives possessed good antiplasmodial activity. Several clinical studies have been conducted with clindamycin administered at a dose of 450 mg every 6 hours for 14 days to four patients to treat a *Plasmodium vivax* infection. A relapse occurred between 41 and 51 days after the end of treatment.

In nonimmune patients clindamycin (450 mg q6h for 3 days) was combined with quinine in the treatment of chloroquine-susceptible or chloroquine-resistant *P. falciparum* infections. A curative effect was obtained with the combination, but major gastrointestinal disorders were noted. Other studies have also been undertaken with various results obtained.

If clindamycin is used, it is recommended that a fast-acting schizonticide, such as quinine or amodiaquine, be administered first, followed by clindamycin, to avoid problems of gastrointestinal intolerance.

Activity against *Toxoplasma gondii*

Clindamycin has been proposed as alternative therapy in the treatment of encephalic toxoplasmosis in patients intolerant to sulfonamides.

There are contradictory studies on the *in-vitro* activity of clindamycin. Clindamycin exerts an inhibitory effect at 0.5 ng/ml and above, but the 90% inhibitory concentration is 100 mg/l. The discrepancy in the results between the different studies is probably due to slow inhibition of the growth of the parasite, which occurs after 24 hours.

It has been shown that clindamycin alone or in combination with pyrimethamine possesses curative activity in acute murine toxoplasmosis. Clindamycin exhibits protective activity against murine cerebral toxoplasmosis. Multicenter studies have shown beneficial effects of clindamycin combined with pyrimethamine in the treatment of acute cerebral toxoplasmosis. Clindamycin has also been proposed as treatment for toxoplasmic chorioretinitis.

PHARMACOKINETICS

Lincomycin

Lincomycin is presented in several pharmaceutical forms: oral, intravenous, intramuscular and rectal. *Micrococcus luteus* is used in the microbiologic assay and chromatographic methods have been described.

Oral form

After administration of 500 mg and 1000 mg, peak serum concentrations are reached in 2–4 hours and are 1.8–5.3 mg/l and 2.5–6.7 mg/l, respectively. The consumption of food affects the oral bioavailability. Concentrations in plasma are detectable for about 12 hours. Absorption of lincomycin represents about 20–35% of the administered dose. Fecal elimination is 30–40% of the administered dose over a period of 72 hours. The bioavailability of lincomycin after oral administration is not affected by celiac disease or colonic diverticulosis, but a reduction in the concentrations in plasma has been demonstrated in patients with Crohn's disease.

Intravenous form

After infusion over 1 hour, the concentrations obtained range from 9.1 mg/l (300 mg) to 36.2 mg/l (500 mg). The AUCs are proportional to the administered doses (300–1500 mg). The mean apparent elimination half-life is 5 hours and about 40% of the administered dose is eliminated in the urine.

Plasma protein binding, albumin, is dose dependent and ranges from 28% to 86%, depending on the dose and the method of determination. On average it is 75%.

Plasma clearance is dose dependent because of protein saturation and is 13.32 l/h. The clearance of the free fraction is between 28.6 l/h for 2400 mg intravenously and 36.4 l/h for 1200 mg intravenously. Renal clearance is weak – 43 ml/min (2.6 l/h). Urinary elimination ranged between 30% and 40%.

After an intravenous dose of 500 mg, fecal elimination of lincomycin is about 14% over 96 hours.

Intramuscular form

After a single intramuscular administration of 600 mg, the peak concentration in serum is between 7.2 and 18.5 mg/l and is reached after between 0.5 and 5 hours. After repeated doses of 600 mg, the residual concentration (8 hours) is 6.4 mg/l. After a daily dose of 500 mg, the residual concentration at 24 hours is 1.1 mg/l. The apparent elimination half-life range is 4–5 hours. The plasma clearance is dose dependent and is between 0.098 and 0.139 l/kg.

Urinary elimination is between 10% and 47%, depending on the study. Fecal elimination after a dose of 500 mg is 4–6% over a period of 48–72 hours.

The bioavailability after intramuscular administration appears to be absolute.

Rectal form

After administration of a 500 mg suppository of lincomycin, a peak concentration in serum of 1.1 mg/l is reached in 1.5 hours, with an AUC of 8.9 mg.h/l, compared to a peak of 2.8 mg/l and an AUC of 25.7 mg.h/l after administration of a rectal solution of lincomycin.

Specific underlying diseases

Renal impaired patients

After intramuscular administration of 600 mg of lincomycin, the apparent elimination half-life, the peak concentration in serum and the AUC are increased. Lincomycin is not dialyzable.

Hepatic impaired patients

After a single dose of 600 mg intramuscularly to patients with hepatic insufficiency, the apparent elimination half-life is increased (8.90 vs 4.85 hours) and the peak concentration in serum is decreased (9.2 vs 12.8 mg/l).

Metabolism

A small amount of lincomycin is inactivated in the liver. The metabolites have not been fully characterized and are devoid of antibacterial activity. Biliary elimination is extensive, ranging from 30% to 40% of the administered dose.

Clindamycin

Clindamycin is presented in the form of clindamycin phosphate for parenteral use and clindamycin hydrochloride for oral use. The assays are performed using a high-performance liquid chromatographic method or a microbiologic method using *Micrococcus luteus* as the test strain.

Intravenous form

Clindamycin phosphate is soluble in water. This solubility is pH dependent: at pH 7 the solubility is between 200 and 300 mg/ml, whereas at pH 4 it is 25 mg/ml. Clindamycin phosphate is administered in the form of an infusion over 10–45 minutes, depending on the dose to be administered. Clindamycin phosphate is slowly hydrolyzed to clindamycin, with a hydrolysis half-life of between 3 minutes (1200 mg) and 1 minute (300 mg). About 10% of the drug is present in the serum after 8 hours in the form of clindamycin phosphate. The peak concentration in serum of clindamycin appears about 3 hours after the end of the infusion and is between 5.4 mg/l (300 mg) and 15.87 mg/l (1200 mg). The apparent elimination half-life of clindamycin is 2–3 hours, whereas that of clindamycin phosphate is 0.04–0.16 hour. Plasma clearance is of the order of 0.18 l/h/kg for clindamycin and 0.40 l/h/kg for clindamycin phosphate. Clindamycin binding to α_1-glycoprotein ranges from 92% to 93%.

Clindamycin is mainly eliminated by the hepatobiliary route. The metabolites of clindamycin are found in the urine and stools, but about 28% of the parent compound is found in the urine.

Intramuscular form

After administration of single doses of 300, 450 or 600 mg of clindamycin phosphate, the peak concentrations in serum are between 3.17 and 6.56 mg/l and are reached in 1.5–3 hours. It is possible to detect clindamycin in the serum after 20 minutes. About 75% of the drug reaches the plasma in the form of clindamycin.

Oral form

After absorption, clindamycin palmitate (hydrochloride) is rapidly hydrolyzed in the intestinal lumen before being absorbed in the form of the hydrochloride and the palmitate is no longer detectable in the serum. The bioavailability is of the order of 80%. The degrees of absorption are identical after single and repeated doses. The bioavailability of clindamycin does not appear to be affected by the ingestion of food, although absorption is delayed by food consumption.

Clindamycin hydrochloride is poorly soluble in water and the solubility is pH dependent: when the pH is less than 6, the solubility is greater than 160 mg/ml, whereas between 7 and 8 the solubility is weak, of the order of 2.7 ± 1.0 mg/l.

After administration of a single dose of 150, 300 or 450 mg of clindamycin hydrochloride, the peak concentrations in serum are between 2.56 and 5.58 mg/l and are reached within 1 hour.

The dose eliminated in the urine ranges from 8% to 26%. A number of metabolites are eliminated in the urine. Traces of clindamycin hydrochloride are found there, in contrast to clindamycin phosphate, for which 1–2% of the administered dose is eliminated in this form.

Radiolabeled clindamycin hydrochloride (300 mg) was administered and the radioactivity was 61% and 28% over a period of 168 hours in feces and urine, respectively.

Metabolism

The free form of clindamycin is hydrolyzed in the liver. Seven metabolites have been described. Fecal and urinary elimination of the metabolites differ.

After a single dose of 300 mg of clindamycin hydrochloride, the compounds eliminated in the urine are distributed as follows: clindamycin 27%, clindamycin sulfoxide 37%, N-demethyl clindamycin 6% and clindamycin-N-demethyl sulfoxide 2%. A hydroxyl derivative and a carboxyl derivative, both incompletely identified, have been detected, and each accounts for about 15% of the compounds eliminated in the urine.

Patients with renal impairment

Clindamycin is mainly eliminated by the hepatobiliary route and metabolized in the liver. It is not significantly eliminated after hemodialysis or peritoneal dialysis.

It has been recommended that when the creatinine clearance is less than 10 ml/min the daily dosage be reduced by a half, as the apparent elimination half-life increases, with major interindividual variability (mean half-life of 5.28 hours compared to 2 hours).

In peritoneal fluid, about 3% of the dose of clindamycin phosphate is hydrolyzed to clindamycin in 2–4 hours. The peritoneal dialysis fluid must contain a concentration of 167 µg of clindamycin phosphate per ml to be certain of exerting therapeutic activity.

Elderly patients

After a single dose of 300 mg orally and intravenously the fractions absorbed were similar in young and elderly subjects (0.92 vs 0.85). The apparent elimination half-life and plasma clearance after intravenous administration did not differ significantly (2.46 vs 2.79 hours, 0.71 vs 0.75 l/kg, 3.36 vs 3.11 ml/min/kg, respectively). The dosage need not be modified in elderly subjects.

Patients with hepatic impairment

In patients with hepatic insufficiency, the apparent elimination half-life is prolonged from 5 to 15 hours compared to 2.5–3.6 hours in healthy volunteers. A reduction in the plasma clearance in cirrhotic patients has been demonstrated, with a reduction in protein binding to 79% (versus 93%).

Pregnancy

Clindamycin rapidly crosses the fetoplacental barrier. High concentrations of clindamycin have been detected in the liver, kidney and lungs, and low levels in cerebral tissue, bone or muscles of fetuses from spontaneous abortions occurring between the 10th and 22nd weeks of gestation.

Intraphagocytic concentration

The intracellular:extracellular concentration ratio in neutrophils is between 11 and 15, while in macrophages and monocytes it is 23. Inside the cell clindamycin is localized in the cytoplasm and granules. The ratio of intracellular:extracellular concentrations is of the order of 1.7:4.

Safety

The main side-effect of clindamycin is pseudomembranous colitis due to *Clostridium difficile*. Hypotension and even cardiorespiratory arrest have been reported at high intravenous doses of lincomycin, particularly after rapid administration. Skin rashes and drug fever have also been observed with clindamycin.

Streptogramins

INTRODUCTION

The streptogramins form a complex group of unique antibacterial agents. Pristinamycin (oral natural form) for historic reasons has limited clinical introduction, mainly in French-speaking countries. For the injectable form (dalfopristin–quinupristin) the clinical introduction is wide, including the USA. A new oral streptogramin – linopristin–flopristin (NXL 103, XRP 2868) – is currently in phase II clinical trials.

PROPERTIES OF NATURAL STREPTOGRAMINS

The streptogramins are composed of a mixture of two components: group A streptogramins and group B streptogramins These two components act synergistically at the microbiologic level. The two components are macrocyclic lactones and peptides, respectively.

Only two derivatives have been introduced in clinical practice: pristinamycin (Pyostacine) and virginiamycin (Staphylomycine). One injectable semisynthetic derivative has also been introduced in clinical practice, dalfopristin–quinupristin (Synercid), and one oral semisynthetic derivative is underdevelopment, linopristin–flopristin.

The ratios between the two groups of components are 30–40% for component I (group B) and 60–70% for component II (group A).

Antibacterial activities

These molecules exhibit different antibacterial activities, but their antibacterial spectra include Gram-positive cocci and bacilli, Gram-negative cocci and fastidious Gram-negative bacilli such as *Haemophilus*, *Moraxella*, *Bordetella* and certain intracellular bacteria (*Chlamydia* and *Rickettsia*).

Pristinamycin is active against Gram-positive cocci. It has good activity against methicillin-resistant or -susceptible strains and constitutive or inducible erythromycin A-resistant strains of *Staph. aureus* and against methicillin-resistant or -susceptible strains of *Staph. epidermidis*. Activities against common pathogens are given in Table 135.10 and those against other micro-organisms are given in Table 135.11. However, it is inactive against *Treponema pallidum* and *Brucella* spp.

Synergy between components A and B

The combination of the two components is synergistic in terms of activity against erythromycin A-susceptible or -resistant strains of *Staph. aureus*. This synergy is independent of the respective percentages of the two components within a large range of (20–80%) for each factor. However, *in vivo*, a higher quantity of pristinamycin II than pristinamycin I must be administered for this synergy to manifest itself in experimental *Staph. aureus* infections in the mouse because of the poor absorption of pristinamycin II$_A$.

Table 135.11 Antibacterial activity of streptogramins

Organism(s)	No.	LINOPRISTIN–FLOPRISTIN		PRISTINAMYCIN		DALFOPRISTIN–QUINUPRISTIN	
		50	90	50	90	50	90
Methicillin-sensitive *Staph. aureus*	16	0.12	0.12	0.25	0.50	0.25	0.50
Methicillin-resistant *Staph. aureus*	25	0.12	0.25	0.25	1.0	0.25	0.50
Glycopeptide intermediate-resistant *Staph. aureus*	3	0.12	–	0.25	–	0.12	–
Staph. aureus Lin^r	1	0.25	–	0.5	–	0.25	–
Strep. pyogenes	27	≤0.06	≤0.06	0.12	0.12	0.25	0.25
Strep. agalactiae	15	0.06	0.06	0.25	0.25	1.0	1.0
Group C and G streptococci	15	0.12	0.25	0.25	0.25	1.0	1.0
Viridans group streptococci	20	0.12	0.25	0.5	0.5	1.0	1.0
Strep. pneumoniae Ery^s	141	0.12	0.25	0.25	0.25	0.5	0.5
Strep. pneumoniae Ery^r	120	0.25	0.5	0.25	0.5	0.5	1.0
Staph. epidermidis	14	0.06	0.5	0.12	1.0	0.12	0.25
Enterococcus faecalis	21	1.0	2.0	2.0	8.0	8.0	16
Enterococcus faecalis Van^r	16	1.0	2.0	4.0	8.0	8.0	32
Enterococcus faecium	11	≤0.06	0.5	0.25	0.5	0.5	2.0
Enterococcus faecium VanA	12	0.12	0.25	0.25	0.5	0.5	1.0
Enterococcus faecium Lin^r	12	0.12	0.25	0.25	0.5	1.0	–
Enterococcus faecium Q/D^r	3	1.0	2.0	4.0	–	–	–
Enterococcus casseliflavus	15	0.5	0.5	1.0	1.0	2.0	4.0
Enterococcus gallinarum	15	0.25	0.5	0.5	0.5	2.0	2.0
Enterococcus avium	10	0.5	1.0	0.5	2.0	2.0	4.0
Enterococcus raffinosus	3	0.5	1.0	2.0	–	–	–
Corynebacterium jeikeium	10	≤0.03	0.25	0.12	0.5	0.25	0.5
Haemophilus influenzae β$^-$	50	0.25	0.5	1.0	2.0	2.0	4.0
Haemophilus influenzae β$^+$	79	0.25	1.0	1.0	2.0	4.0	4.0
Haemophilus influenzae^{BLNAR}	21	0.25	0.5	1.0	1.0	2.0	4.0

β$^-$, non-β-lactamase producing; β$^+$, β-lactamase producing; BLNAR, non-β-lactamase-producing strains; Ery^r, erythromycin resistant; Ery^s, erythromycin sensitive; Lin^r, lincomycin resistant; Q/D^r, quinupristin–dalfopristin resistant; VanA, vancomycin A phenotype; Van^r, vancomycin resistant.

Breakpoints

The French Antibiotic Sensitivity Test Committee has adopted a breakpoint of 2 mg/l for pristinamycin and virginiamycin. This corresponds to a diameter of ≥19 mm for a 15 μg disk.

Antibiotic combinations

The combinations of streptogramins plus aminoglycosides, rifampin or β-lactams are synergistic or additive. For staphylococci, pristinamycin combined with rifampin was bactericidal against 69% of the 16 tested strains responsible for septicemia; combination with an aminoglycoside induced bactericidal activity against 50% of the same strains.

Combination with fusidic acid or co-trimoxazole is synergistic, while the combination of pristinamycin and chloramphenicol is antagonistic.

PRISTINAMYCIN

Mechanism of action

Streptogramins inhibit bacterial protein synthesis by binding sequentially to the 50S ribosomal subunit. Pristinamycin II binds irreversibly, thus releasing a receptor site for pristinamycin I. Both streptogramins cross the bacterial cell wall by passive diffusion.

Pristinamycin II acts on the early stage of protein synthesis, especially on the elongation phase of translation. Pristinamycin I exerts inhibitory activity at the end of the process during extension of the peptide chain, causing premature detachment of the nascent peptide.

Resistance

Epidemiology

Until 1975 resistance to streptogramins was infrequent, of the order of 1–3%. In 1975 the first strain of *Staph. aureus* with plasmid-mediated pristinamycin I_A and II_A resistance was isolated in France. Outbreaks associated with this plasmid have been reported in many hospitals, with a prevalence of 4–5% of strains isolated. However, the level of resistance has remained low and affects about 1% of methicillin-susceptible strains of *Staph. aureus* (MSSA) and 10% of methicillin-resistant strains (MRSA).

In the Protek study conducted from 2000 to 2001, it was shown that less than 0.02% of *Strep. pneumoniae* strains are resistant to dalfopristin–quinupristin. For *Staph. aureus* resistant to linezolid (MIC >128 mg/l), the MIC of dalfopristin–quinupristin is ≤0.25 mg/l. For *Enterococcus faecium* resistant to linezolid, the MIC at which 50% and 90% of isolates are inhibited ($MIC_{50/90}$) for dalfopristin–quinupristin is ≤0.5/1 mg/l.

Mechanism

The antibacterial spectrum of the MLS_B group does not include Gram-negative bacilli such as Enterobacteriaceae, *Pseudomonas* spp. and other nonfermentative Gram-negative bacilli. Their intrinsic resistance is due to their outer membrane impermeability.

Acquired resistance of the MLS_B type is due to four mechanisms: modification of the antibiotic target, inactivation of the antibiotics, reduction of outer membrane permeability and efflux.

Many genes encode streptogramin resistance, a complex phenomenon which could be specific for each component.

MLS_B resistance in streptococci may be constitutive or inducible. Enterococci, *Strep. pneumoniae* and most viridans group streptococci have constitutive MLS_B resistance. Inducible expression occurs above all in group A, C, G and B streptococci and in certain viridans group streptococcal strains.

Enzymatic inactivation of pristinamycin or virginiamycin was described in 1975. Through a plasmid-mediated *O*-acetyltransferase, some strains of *Staph. aureus* are capable of acetylating the hydroxyl group at position 13, leading to a loss of ribosomal affinity and inactivating pristinamycin II. The macrolactone ring of pristinamycin I could be opened by a hydrolase which is carried by the same plasmid of *Staph. aureus*. The majority of these *Staph. aureus* strains have reduced susceptibility to lincosamides.

Pharmacokinetics

There are no published pharmacokinetic data for children, elderly subjects or patients with renal or hepatic insufficiency. In adults, pristinamycin and virginiamycin are not inactivated by gastric fluid. About 15–18% of pristinamycin II_A and virginiamycin M is absorbed in the ileojejunal section. There is also weak absorption of the I_A fraction.

After administration of 500 mg of pristinamycin or virginiamycin, the concentration in plasma is about 1 mg/l at 2 hours. Concentrations in plasma are minimal or nonexistent from 4 to 6 hours, depending on the subject.

The apparent elimination half-lives are 4–5 hours for pristinamycin I and virginiamycin M and 2.8–8 hours for pristinamycin II and virginiamycin S. After administration of ≤2 g orally, the peak plasma concentrations of drug for pristinamycins I and II are, respectively, 0.8 and 0.6 mg/l and are reached in about 3 hours. The apparent elimination half-lives are, respectively, 4 and 2.8 hours. The lag time is about 20 minutes. The AUCs are 2.2 and 1.2 mg.h/l. The global peak concentration in serum (pristinamycins I and II) is 1.34 ± 0.7 mg/l (mean ± standard deviation) and is reached in 3 hours. Plasma protein binding is 40–50% for pristinamycin I and 80–90% for pristinamycin II. Streptogramins are metabolized in the liver but this process has not been studied. Elimination occurs mainly in the bile and urinary elimination is weak (10% for pristinamycin I and 2% for pristinamycin II).

Drug interference

Pristinamycin does not interfere with cytochrome P450. There is the possibility of a metabolic interaction between pristinamycin and ciclosporin, which may be responsible for acute nephrotoxicity. It interferes with the metabolism of methotrexate.

DALFOPRISTIN–QUINUPRISTIN

Pristinamycin remains an antibacterial complex with good antistaphylococcal activity, particularly against methicillin- and erythromycin A-resistant strains. Its use in the hospital environment has been restricted by the absence of a parenteral formulation due to the poor water solubility of pristinamycin. The objective has been to prepare derivatives with the same antibacterial activity as pristinamycin but with greater hydrosolubility. One compound has been introduced in clinical practice, dalfopristin–quinupristin.

Semisynthesis from the isolated I_A and II_A components has yielded hydrosoluble derivatives. The semisynthetic derivative of pristinamycin I_A was obtained by introduction of an amino function at the 5δ position (5δ-thiomethylquinuclidine); the semisynthetic derivatives of pristinamycin II_A with an amino substituent at position 26 (diethylaminoethylsulfonyl) are soluble in water.

Antibacterial activity

Dalfopristin–quinupristin possesses the same antibacterial spectrum as pristinamycin and similar *in-vitro* activity.

The approved National Committee on Clinical Laboratory Standards (NCCLS) breakpoint is ≤1 μg/ml (diameter of zone of inhibition ≥18 mm) for a disk load at 7.5 μg (ratio 30:70).

Dalfopristin–quinupristin MICs ranged between 0.5 and 1.0 mg/l for glycopeptide-intermediate *Staph. aureus* (GISA) strains.

Pharmacokinetics

After repeated administrations to 10 young male volunteers of a dose of 7.5 mg of dalfopristin–quinupristin per kg for 5 days (q12h) and 4 days (q8h), there was no significant accumulation of either component. The accumulation ratio ranged between 1.16 and 1.43.

After an infusion over 1 hour, peak concentrations of dalfopristin–quinupristin were between 0.95 ± 0.22 mg/l (dose 1.4 mg/kg) and 24.20 ± 8.82 mg/l (dose 29.4 mg/kg). Quinupristin was rapidly converted to its active metabolite RP-12536. The activity of dalfopristin–quinupristin was detectable 6 hours after the end of the infusion.

Six volunteers received an infusion of a single dose of 12 mg of dalfopristin–quinupristin per kg (ratio 30:70) for 60 minutes. The peak concentrations in serum and suction blisters were, respectively, 8.65 ± 0.92 and 2.41 ± 0.75 mg/l. The AUCs were, respectively, 11.2 ± 1.45 mg.h/ml and 9.19 ± 2.02 mg.h/l. The apparent elimination half-life of dalfopristin–quinupristin was 1.48 ± 0.64 hours. The interindividual variabilities are 20–29% and 25–32% for quinupristin and dalfopristin, respectively.

Two other metabolites occur through a nonenzymatic process, similar to pristinamycin II: glutathione–quinupristin and cysteine–quinupristin.

The hepatic clearance and the fecal elimination are 74.7% and 77.5% for quinupristin and dalfopristin, respectively. Protein binding rates are 55–78% and 11–26% for quinupristin and dalfopristin, respectively.

FURTHER READING

Further reading for this chapter can be found online at http://www.expertconsult.com

James CM Brust
Franklin D Lowy

Chapter | **136** |

Oxazolidinones

The oxazolidinones are a family of bacteriostatic antimicrobials that are protein synthesis inhibitors. Because this new family works at the early stage of protein synthesis involving formation of the 70S initiation complex, there does not appear to be cross-resistance with other protein synthesis inhibitors. Originally developed for the treatment of bacterial and fungal infections of plants, these agents were subsequently found to have activity against Gram-positive bacteria. Upjohn originally developed two oxazolidinones, eperezolid and linezolid. Based on its more advantageous pharmacologic profile, linezolid was selected for further investigation. At present linezolid is the sole oxazolidinone available. The discussion below is therefore limited to this product. A number of comprehensive reviews of oxazolidinones and linezolid have recently been published.[1-5]

PHARMACOKINETICS AND DISTRIBUTION

Linezolid has similar pharmacokinetics whether administered parenterally or orally. It is completely absorbed following oral administration, achieving a bioavailability of 100%. Food causes a slight decrease in the rate of absorption but not in the overall amount absorbed. In normal volunteer studies peak plasma concentrations were achieved in 1–2 hours. Steady state concentrations were approximately 12 µg/ml and 18 µg/ml following oral doses of 375 mg and 625 mg twice daily, respectively. Following intravenous administration of 625 mg twice daily to volunteers for 7.5 days, the steady state level was 3.8 µg/ml.[6,7] The half-lives of oral and intravenously administered linezolid are 5.4 and 4.8 hours, respectively. The drug is excreted by both renal and nonrenal routes; 90% of circulating drug is not metabolized, but there are two inactive metabolites that are the result of oxidation of the morpholine ring. The P450 system does not appear to be involved in the metabolism of linezolid, thus limiting the number of possible drug–drug interactions.

Linezolid is 31% bound to plasma proteins. It has a relatively large volume of distribution of 40–50 l. Information on tissue penetration is still incomplete. However, linezolid appears to penetrate well into tissue blister fluid, pulmonary alveolar macrophages and sweat.[2,8] Preliminary studies suggest reasonable penetration of bone, fat and muscle. Mean ratios of linezolid in tissue fluid/plasma were 0.55, 1.2 and 0.71 for sweat, saliva and cerebrospinal fluid, respectively. There is little additional information at present on the tissue distribution of linezolid in humans.

ROUTE AND DOSAGE

As noted, linezolid can be administered orally or intravenously. Adjustment of dosage is not necessary when switching from one route to the other. The recommended dosage for serious infections such as nosocomial pneumonia or complicated skin and soft tissue infections is 600 mg q12h. For uncomplicated infections, including community-acquired pneumonias or uncomplicated cutaneous infections, 400 mg q12h is adequate.

In patients with mild-to-moderate renal impairment (creatinine clearance 10–79 ml/min), dosage adjustment is not necessary. However, with more severe forms of renal disease dosage adjustment may be necessary.

The pharmacokinetics of linezolid appears unaffected by age. Dosage adjustment for the elderly is unnecessary. The clearance of linezolid is more rapid in children than in adults. As a result, the dose recommended for infants and children is 10 mg/kg q8–12h. The only dosage schedule investigated to date in children has been q12h.

INDICATIONS

The oxazolidinones are primarily indicated for the treatment of bacterial infections caused by Gram-positive bacteria including staphylococci, streptococci and pneumococci, although their spectrum of antibacterial activity extends beyond these species. Linezolid has excellent *in-vitro* activity against staphylococcal species including methicillin-susceptible and resistant strains. There is little difference in the average minimal inhibitory concentrations (MICs) for methicillin-resistant and -susceptible staphylococcal isolates. Linezolid is also active against the recently described *Staphylococcus aureus* isolates that are intermediate in susceptibility to glycopeptides – *Staph. aureus* with intermediate susceptibility to vancomycin (VISA) or *Staph. aureus* with intermediate susceptibility to glycopeptides (GISA) isolates.

In contrast with the protein synthesis inhibitor combination dalfopristin–quinupristin, linezolid is active against all enterococci, including *Enterococcus faecalis* and *E. faecium*, as well as those enterococcal strains that are vancomycin resistant. It is also active against penicillin-susceptible and -resistant *Streptococcus pneumoniae*, again with comparable MIC values (Table 136.1). In addition to these common Gram-positive pathogens, linezolid also has activity (MIC = 4 µg/ml) against some of the less frequently encountered Gram-positive organisms such as *Corynebacterium* spp., *Bacillus* spp., *Listeria monocytogenes*, *Erysipelothrix rhusiopathiae* and *Rhodococcus equi*.

Linezolid is moderately active against some anaerobes including *Clostridium* spp., *Peptococcus* spp., *Bacteroides fragilis*, *Fusobacterium nucleatum* and *F. meningosepticum*. It has limited activity against some Gram-negative bacteria such as *Moraxella*, *Bordetella* and *Haemophilus* spp. and has no activity against Enterobacteriaceae or *Pseudomonas* spp. Linezolid also has activity against *Mycobacterium tuberculosis* and *M. avium* complex.

In animal studies linezolid has shown activity against methicillin-resistant *Staph. aureus* (MRSA) and vancomycin-resistant *E. faecium* in the endocarditis model.[9,10] In a rabbit model of penicillin-resistant

Table 136.1 *In-vitro* antimicrobial susceptibility for linezolid against common Gram-positive pathogens

Organism	MIC (µg/ml) 50%*	MIC (µg/ml) 90%	Overall (µg/ml)
Staph. aureus (n = 52 256)			
Oxacillin susceptible	1–4	1–4	0.5–8
Oxacillin resistant	1–4	1–4	0.5–8
Coagulase-negative staphylococci (n = 548)			
Oxacillin susceptible	0.5–2	1–4	0.25–4
Oxacillin resistant	0.5–2	1–2	0.5–4
β-Hemolytic streptococci (n = 547)	1–2	2–4	1–4
Strep. pneumoniae (n = 5454)			
Penicillin susceptible	0.5	1	<0.016–1
Penicillin resistant	0.5–1	1	0.06–4
Enterococcus spp. (n = 5980)			
Vancomycin susceptible	1–4	1–4	0.5–4
Vancomycin resistant	2–4	2–4	1–4

*Minimum concentration at which 50% of strains are inhibited.
Source: Adapted from ref 1 with original data in refs 26 and 31–36 from Diekema et al.

and -susceptible pneumococcal meningitis, meningeal penetration of linezolid was good (38% of serum levels); however, overall it was less effective than ceftriaxone.[11] In an experimental animal model of *Staph. aureus* osteomyelitis comparing cefazolin and linezolid, treatment outcome with linezolid was inferior to cefazolin and no better than in the untreated controls.[12]

At present linezolid is approved for the treatment of infections caused by vancomycin-resistant *E. faecium* with associated bacteremia; nosocomial infections caused by both MRSA, methicillin-susceptible *Staph. aureus* (MSSA) and multidrug-resistant strains of *Strep. pneumoniae*; complicated skin and soft tissue infections caused by MRSA, MSSA, *Strep. pyogenes* and *Strep. agalactiae*; and uncomplicated skin/soft tissue infections caused by MSSA and *Strep. pyogenes*.[13,14] It is also approved by the US Food and Drug Administration (FDA) for the treatment of community-acquired pneumonia due to *Strep. pneumoniae* (including multidrug-resistant strains) and MSSA (Table 136.2). Stevens et al.[15] recently reported that linezolid was comparable to vancomycin in the treatment of MRSA infections in a randomized open-label trial, primarily involving skin and soft tissue infections. A recent meta-analysis of randomized clinical trials compared linezolid with glycopeptides and β-lactams in the treatment of Gram-positive infections.[5] The authors found that, overall, linezolid was more effective in clearing skin and soft tissue infections and bacteremia than the comparator antibiotics, but there was no overall difference in mortality.

There is additional clinical and experimental experience with linezolid suggesting that it may have a broader therapeutic role although these other indications have not been FDA approved. These reports, while limited, include the successful treatment of enterococcal endocarditis and meningitis; MRSA prosthetic hip infections, osteomyelitis, endocarditis and meningitis; and central nervous system infections caused by *Nocardia* spp., *Capnocytophaga* spp. and *C. jeikeium*.[16–18] There is also increasing evidence that linezolid may have utility in mycobacterial infections, most notably in the treatment of multidrug-resistant tuberculosis and *M. avium* complex.[19] It is still not entirely clear how effective linezolid is in the treatment of infections such as endocarditis that require bactericidal activity, but it appears to be a useful alternative in subjects who cannot tolerate vancomycin.[17]

Resistance to linezolid is rare but has been reported in enterococci and staphylococci. To date it has occurred more commonly in enterococci, resulting from a specific mutation in the domain V region of the 23S rRNA coding region. Enterococci carry four copies of this gene and the degree of resistance appears to correlate with the number of mutant copies. There is a fitness cost to single mutants without a significant change in MIC, which may explain the rarity of spontaneous resistance or colonization with single-mutant variants. *In-vitro* studies have shown that the appearance of resistance is strongly dependent upon the exposure dose and duration.

Table 136.2 Clinical indications for the use of linezolid

FDA-approved indications Nature of infection	Potential pathogens
Skin and soft tissue (complicated)	MSSA, MRSA, *Streptococcus pyogenes*, *Strep. agalactiae*
Skin and soft tissue (uncomplicated)	MSSA, *Strep. pyogenes*
Infection with bacteremia	Vancomycin-resistant *Enterococcus faecium*
Nosocomial pneumonia	MRSA, MSSA, *Strep. pneumoniae* (including multidrug-resistant strains)
Community-acquired pneumonia	*Strep. pneumoniae* (including multidrug-resistant strains), MSSA

Non-FDA-approved (off-label) indications

Serious MRSA, VISA and VRSA infections or infections that are poorly responsive to vancomycin therapy
Infection with bacteremia caused by *Enterococcus faecalis* (including vancomycin-resistant strains)
Complicated infections requiring long-term oral therapy with an antistaphylococcal or enterococcal agent where β-lactams cannot be used (e.g. chronic osteomyelitis)*
Treatment of infections (e.g. nosocomial pneumonia, endocarditis, meningitis) caused by highly resistant (but linezolid susceptible) Gram-positive bacteria where alternative agents are not available or are contraindicated
Combination therapy for antimycobacterial infections where first- and second-line agents cannot be used

*Close monitoring for toxicity is required with prolonged linezolid therapy.
MRSA, methicillin-resistant *Staphylococcus aureus*; MSSA, methicillin-susceptible *Staph. aureus*; VISA, *Staph. aureus* with intermediate susceptibility to vancomycin; VRSA, vancomycin-resistant *Staph. aureus*.

Linezolid is an important addition to the Gram-positive armamentarium. It is an alternative agent for the treatment of resistant Gram-positive infections (see Table 136.2). It has an antibacterial spectrum that is similar to vancomycin with advantageous pharmacokinetics. The availability of an oral preparation allows completion of therapy with the same therapeutic agent and therefore may help reduce the duration of hospital stays.[20]

Dosage in special circumstances

As noted above, adjustment of dosage for moderate degrees of renal failure is not necessary. Because linezolid, as well as the linezolid metabolites, are cleared during hemodialysis, it is recommended that patients receive a supplemental dose following dialysis. For moderate degrees of hepatic disease dosage adjustment is not necessary.

ADVERSE REACTIONS AND INTERACTIONS

Linezolid has, in general, been well tolerated. The most common adverse events in the comparator-controlled trials were diarrhea (2.8–11%), nausea (3.4–9.6%) and headaches (0.5–11.3%).

Potentially the most serious adverse event, thrombocytopenia, was seen in 2.4% of patients. It was seen most often during prolonged therapy (longer than 2 weeks) and resolved upon completion of therapy. Others have reported a higher incidence of thrombocytopenia,[21,22] and there are reports of both anemia and leukopenia associated with linezolid therapy. As a result, hematologic monitoring of these parameters is recommended during prolonged therapy, especially for subjects who are already immunocompromised.

Now that linezolid has become much more widely used, several rare but important toxicities have emerged, including an irreversible peripheral neuropathy, a partially reversible optic neuropathy and severe lactic acidosis. Both the peripheral and optic neuropathies appear to occur after prolonged therapy (median 4 months and 10 months, respectively), whereas lactic acidosis has been reported after as little as 1 week of therapy.[23]

The oxazolidinones are monoamine oxidase (MAO) inhibitors. Linezolid appears to be a relatively weak MAO inhibitor and there are now more than a dozen reports of serotonin syndrome in patients treated with linezolid while also taking selective serotonin reuptake inhibitors (SSRIs). Recommendations on the co-administration of linezolid with SSRIs vary, with some authors advocating a full washout of the SSRI before starting linezolid and other authors simply advising close clinical follow-up.[23] Data on combination antibiotic therapy with linezolid are limited.

REFERENCES

References for this chapter can be found online at http://www.expertconsult.com

Richard H Drew

Chapter | 137 |

Aminoglycosides

INTRODUCTION

Introduced into clinical practice in the 1940s, aminoglycosides were often considered the mainstay in the treatment of many infections, most notably for serious Gram-negative infections. Currently, nine aminoglycosides (gentamicin, tobramycin, amikacin, streptomycin, neomycin, kanamycin, paromomycin, netilmicin and spectinomycin) are approved by the US Food and Drug Administration (FDA) for clinical use. A number of other aminoglycosides are in use throughout the world. Of these, gentamicin, tobramycin and amikacin are the most frequently prescribed for the treatment of severe Gram-negative infections and will be the focus of this chapter. Gentamicin and (less frequently) streptomycin are utilized as part of combination therapy for specific Gram-positive infections, while amikacin and streptomycin have also been used in the treatment of mycobacterial diseases. Use of paromomycin (for cryptosporidiosis), spectinomycin (for gonorrhea) and oral neomycin (for surgical prophylaxis) have largely been replaced by newer agents for these indications.

Popularity of the aminoglycosides declined considerably in the 1980s, due largely to concerns regarding their ototoxic and nephrotoxic potential, need for individualized dosing, serum concentration monitoring and the availability of safer therapeutic alternatives for many of their clinical indications. However, increasing Gram-negative drug resistance to β-lactams (including cephalosporins), fluoroquinolones and carbapenems, combined with a lack of development of new treatment options for serious Gram-negative infections, has resulted in a re-evaluation of the aminoglycoside class of antibiotics (most notably gentamicin, tobramycin and amikacin).

BACKGROUND

The aminoglycosides were discovered following systematic screening of soil actinomycetes for the production of substances with antimicrobial activity. These compounds exhibited particular activity *in vitro* against aerobic Gram-negative bacilli and Gram-positive cocci. Streptomycin, the first clinically useful aminoglycoside, was isolated from *Streptomyces griseus* in 1944.[1] Neomycin, kanamycin, tobramycin and paromomycin are also natural compounds that were subsequently isolated from various *Streptomyces* spp. and identified by the spelling 'mycin'. Gentamicin and sisomicin are natural products produced by *Micromonospora* spp. and are so designated by ending in 'micin'. Amikacin and netilmicin are semi-synthetic aminoglycosides derived from kanamycin and sisomicin, respectively.[1]

CHEMISTRY

The chemical structures of the aminoglycosides are shown in Figure 137.1. All aminoglycosides include a central six-membered ring containing amino groups termed an aminocyclitol, which is linked to two or more amino- or non-amino-containing sugars by glycosidic bonds.[1] Spectinomycin is a pure aminocyclitol and is often considered with the aminoglycosides, but is not strictly speaking an aminoglycoside because it contains neither aminosugars nor glycosidic bonds.[1] For this reason, the complete group of compounds is more accurately referred to as aminoglycoside–aminocyclitol antibiotics.

Microbiologic activity

Mechanism of activity

Aminoglycosides act by irreversibly binding to the bacterial 30S ribosomal subunit, resulting in disruption of peptide synthesis. Bactericidal activity against susceptible organisms is rapid, most notably in aerobic Gram-negative bacilli. Numerous conditions (either *in vitro* or *in vivo*) may influence this activity.[1-3] The rate of killing is generally enhanced at higher concentrations.[2] In contrast, the presence of divalent cations, increased osmolality, an acidic pH and an anaerobic environment can significantly reduce the *in vitro* activity of aminoglycosides.[1] This may be clinically relevant in tissues and fluids with low pH (such as lung and bronchial fluids) or in anaerobic environments (such as abscesses) where activity may be significantly reduced. The microbiologic effect of aminoglycosides is not significantly altered by low or high inocula of organisms.

Aminoglycosides exhibit a postantibiotic effect (PAE), which is the continued suppression of bacterial growth after antimicrobial exposure, against both Gram-positive and Gram-negative bacteria.[4,5] The duration of such an effect is highly variable (0.5–7.5 hours) and depends greatly on the test conditions, such as the organism, exposure duration and antimicrobial concentration.[4,5] In general, the PAE observed for Gram-positive organisms (<2 hours) is shorter than that observed for Gram-negatives (up to 7 hours).[4] Similar to the rate of bactericidal activity, the duration of PAE has been noted to increase with increasing aminoglycoside concentrations (such as those seen with consolidated dosing techniques discussed later in this chapter).[4,5]

While results vary with individual organisms and other test conditions, aminoglycosides generally exhibit indifferent, additive or synergistic effects *in vitro* against numerous aerobic Gram-negative bacilli when combined with several β-lactam antibiotics.[1] A similar effect is seen *in vitro* against Gram-positive cocci when combined with vancomycin, teicoplanin and daptomycin.[1,6] Such activity has contributed to the debate over the use of aminoglycosides as part of combination therapy for the treatment of various infections (see Clinical applications, below).

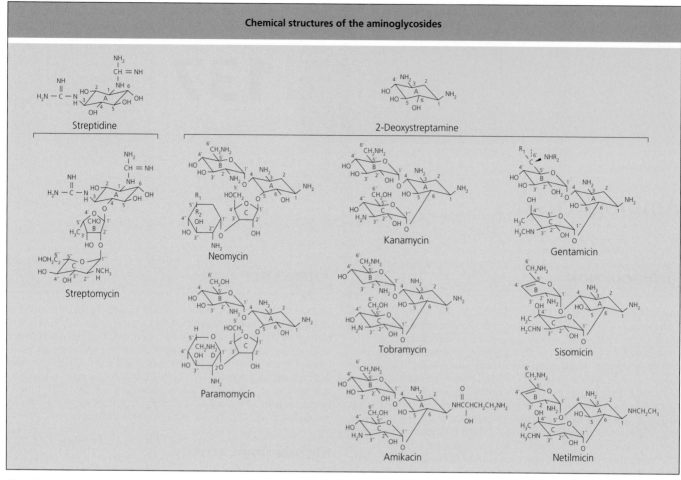

Fig. 137.1 Chemical structures of the aminoglycosides. All aminoglycosides include an aminocyclitol (a central six-membered ring containing amino groups), which is linked to two or more amino- or non-amino-containing sugars by glycosidic bonds. For streptomycin, the aminocyclitol ring is a streptidine, whereas for the remainder of the clinically available aminoglycosides it is 2-deoxystreptamine. Neomycin contains approximately equal amounts of neomycin B (R$_1$=H; R$_2$=CH$_2$NH$_2$) and neomycin C (R$_1$=CH$_2$NH$_2$; R$_2$=H). Kanamycin is principally kanamycin A, as shown. Gentamicin is gentamicin C complex with roughly equal amounts of C$_1$ (R$_1$=R$_2$=CH$_3$), C$_{1a}$ (R$_1$=R$_2$=H) and C$_2$ (R$_1$=CH$_3$; R$_2$=H). Courtesy of Richard Quintiliani Jr, Richard Quintiliani and Charles H Nightingale.

Spectrum of activity

In general, aminoglycosides demonstrate potent activity against a wide variety of aerobic Gram-positive and Gram-negative organisms. However, anaerobic bacteria are intrinsically resistant to aminoglycosides.

Gram-positive bacteria

Aminoglycosides generally demonstrate favorable activity *in vitro* against many species of staphylococci. Gentamicin, tobramycin and amikacin demonstrated activity *in vitro* against over 95% of methicillin-susceptible *Staphylococcus aureus* (MSSA).[7-9] Activity of coagulase-negative staphylococci exceeded 84% in one report.[8] Aminoglycosides also demonstrate a high degree of activity *in vitro* against methicillin-resistant *Staph. aureus* (MRSA), including community-associated strains (CA-MRSA).[10,11] However, significant geographic variability exists, and new clonal strains of CA-MRSA resistant to aminoglycosides have been reported throughout the world.[12] Despite their generally favorable activity *in vitro*, aminoglycosides are rarely used as monotherapy in the treatment of staphylococcal infections.

Aminoglycosides generally lack sufficient activity against pneumococci. While aminoglycosides alone are not active against enterococci and viridans group streptococci, they (most commonly gentamicin) are often used in the therapy of serious infections caused by these organisms (in the absence of high-level aminoglycoside resistance)

because of their frequent additive or synergistic effect when combined with other antibiotics (see Resistance, and Clinical applications, below). However, recent reports have highlighted growing concern regarding the increased incidence of high-level gentamicin resistance in enterococci.[13-15]

Gram-negative bacteria

Current clinical use of aminoglycosides is mainly due to their activity against a variety of Gram-negative pathogens. Gentamicin, tobramycin, netilmicin and amikacin often demonstrate favorable activity *in vitro* against *Acinetobacter* spp., *Citrobacter* spp., *Enterobacter* spp., *Escherichia coli*, *Klebsiella* spp., *Serratia* spp., *Proteus* spp., *Morganella* spp. and *Pseudomonas aeruginosa*.[8,16-19] However, there are differences in aminoglycoside *in-vitro* potencies against these pathogens. Among the Enterobacteriaceae, amikacin usually demonstrates the highest degree of activity (>90%), followed closely by gentamicin.[8,17] Relative to the Enterobacteriaceae, reduced activity is exhibited in the nonfermentative Gram-negative organisms *Acinetobacter* spp. and *P. aeruginosa* (including some multidrug-resistant strains).[18] Relative to gentamicin, tobramycin usually demonstrates superior activity *in vitro* against *P. aeruginosa* (ranging between 65% and 85% in most reports).[8,16] In contrast, gentamicin usually has superior activity *in vitro* against *Serratia* spp.[8]

Limited treatment options for specific multidrug-resistant organisms (most frequently *Klebsiella pneumoniae* and *E. coli*) producing extended-spectrum β-lactamases (ESBL) have renewed the interest in the potential use of aminoglycosides against such pathogens.[20–23] However, in-vitro activity of aminoglycosides against these pathogens is not predictable and is consistently inferior to that demonstrated by other agents (such as carbapenems and tigecycline).[24]

Despite possessing activity in vitro against Salmonella spp. and Shigella spp., and modest activity against Neisseria gonorrhoeae and Haemophilus influenzae, these agents are rarely used for such infections due to the availability of safer alternatives. In contrast, in-vitro activity against Burkholderia cepacia and Stenotrophomonas maltophilia[25] is poor.

Mycobacterium

Of the aminoglycosides, streptomycin and amikacin display favorable activity in vitro against a variety of mycobacteria.[26] Streptomycin is particularly active against Mycobacterium tuberculosis.[27] Against atypical strains, amikacin is generally the most active aminoglycoside against M. fortuitum, M. abscessus and M. chelonae.[26] While tobramycin has demonstrated activity in vitro against M. chelonae, it lacks activity against M. abscessus. Amikacin has also demonstrated activity in vitro against M. avium intracellulare.[26]

Resistance

Several mechanisms of resistance to aminoglycosides have been described in the literature (both intrinsic and acquired), including impaired drug uptake, efflux, ribosomal target modification and enzymatic drug modification with subsequent inactivation. Despite these mechanisms and years of clinical application, aminoglycosides have generally maintained favorable susceptibilities against a variety of pathogens.

Intrinsic resistance is often the consequence of impaired uptake, which generally has been associated with lower-level resistance (such as that exhibited by enterococci).[28] In such settings, gentamicin minimum inhibitory concentrations (MICs) of 8–64 μg/ml and streptomycin MICs of 64–512 μg/ml are not uncommon. In such circumstances, in-vitro synergy may be demonstrated when enterococci with low-level aminoglycoside resistance are exposed to an aminoglycoside in combination with cell wall-active agents, notably β-lactams.[28] Such potential for synergy, however, is generally lost in the setting of high-level gentamicin resistance (MIC >500 μg/ml).[28] In such cases, only streptomycin (in strains without high-level streptomycin resistance, defined as an MIC of 2000 μg/ml or more) can be used against enterococci and staphylococci highly resistant to gentamicin.[28] In contrast, Enterococcus faecium often demonstrates moderate resistance to tobramycin (MIC 64–1000 μg/ml) and therefore cannot be used for synergy.

Acquisition of transposon- and/or plasmid-encoded modifying enzymes is frequently the cause of acquired resistance. In Gram-negative pathogens, these most commonly include inactivating pathways (such as phosphorylation, adenylylation or acetylation) encoded by plasmids or associated with transposable elements, or decreased drug accumulation. In addition to these more common mechanisms, efflux of the drug has been reported in resistant forms of P. aeruginosa and would potentially confer resistance across the class.[29]

Treatment-emergent resistance (i.e. resistance developed during treatment of an initially susceptible Gram-negative organism) is infrequent.[1] In addition, cross-resistance among the members of the aminoglycoside class is generally incomplete (except as previously noted). For example, amikacin has generally maintained high levels of activity in vitro against specific pathogens exhibiting high rates of resistance to gentamicin and tobramycin.

PHARMACOKINETICS

The aminoglycosides exhibit characteristics of a three-compartmental pharmacokinetic model. An initial distribution (alpha) phase is followed by a rapid elimination (beta) phase and a slow elimination (gamma) phase. However, a one-compartment model is most often used clinically for calculating dosage regimens. Because they demonstrate linear pharmacokinetics, a direct relationship is seen between dose and area under the plasma concentration–time curve (AUC).

Absorption

Aminoglycosides undergo minimal absorption when given orally, topically or by rectal instillation. Nevertheless, in patients with hepatic encephalopathy and renal impairment, large and frequent doses of neomycin have been associated with sufficient absorption into the systemic circulation to produce deafness.[30] Detectable amounts of tobramycin following oral administration as part of a selective gut decontamination regimen have been reported in patients with significant renal impairment.[31] Similarly, detectable blood levels of aminoglycosides have been reported following topical use in burn patients with large areas of denuded skin.[32] Aminoglycosides penetrate extremely well into body spaces with large serosal surfaces (e.g. pleural space, peritoneal cavity, pericardial space, synovial fluid). Intraperitoneal doses may also result in significant systemic exposure.[33]

In addition to the parenteral route of administration, aminoglycosides (most notably tobramycin) have been administered via aerosols (see Clinical applications, below). Following endotracheal administration or aerosolization of aminoglycosides, systemic absorption is usually modest. For example, mean serum tobramycin concentrations 1 hour after inhalation in 258 cystic fibrosis patients receiving 300 mg twice daily were 0.95 ± 0.50 μg/ml.[34] The estimated systemic bioavailability in this study was 11.7%

Distribution

After an intravenous or intramuscular dose, peak aminoglycoside serum concentrations occur in 30–60 minutes and 45–90 minutes, respectively. In patients with poor vascular perfusion into soft tissue structures (such as those with diabetes mellitus), there may be a delay in the time to peak concentration. The low serum protein binding of aminoglycosides (approximately 10%) facilitates wide distribution into the extravascular space. Because aminoglycosides are highly water-soluble, their volume of distribution (Vd) is similar to that of the extravascular compartment. Studies performed in normal adult volunteers have reported volumes of distribution in the range of 0.2–0.3 l/kg. In patients with increased extravascular fluid (such as those with ascites, burns or pregnancy), the Vd is increased, whereas dehydrated patients may exhibit decreases in Vd.

Penetration of aminoglycosides has been reported in numerous body fluids and tissues. For example, in the unobstructed biliary tract, aminoglycoside concentrations approximate 30% of the simultaneous serum concentration.[35] Similar penetration has been reported in lung tissues and fluids.[36] Aminoglycosides penetrate poorly into the cornea and the aqueous and vitreous humors of the eye.[37] In patients with serious eye infections such as bacterial endophthalmitis, direct intravitreal injections are usually needed. In contrast, high concentrations are observed in specialized cells which have an active transport mechanism for aminoglycosides, such as the tubular cells of the renal cortex and the hair cells of the ear (see Ototoxicity and Nephrotoxicity, below). As a consequence, concentrations in these cells can exceed those of plasma or interstitial fluid. Aminoglycoside concentrations in the urine may exceed those of simultaneous serum concentrations by 25- to 100-fold. In addition, aminoglycoside concentrations can remain above therapeutic concentrations for extended periods of time (48–200 hours) as a result of renal tubular cell absorption and the prolonged release of aminoglycosides into urine.

The penetration of aminoglycosides into cerebrospinal fluid (CSF) is poor, both in the presence and absence of meningeal inflammation. Penetration of gentamicin into CSF was studied in 26 patients aged 6–20 years with mumps meningoencephalitis after administration of a single intramuscular dose of 1.2–4.0 mg/kg. Activity was found in only five of the 26 patients, with the highest level being 0.19 µg/ml. While use of intraventricular administration has been reported in the treatment of Gram-negative meningitis, such treatment is rarely employed.

Metabolism and elimination

After a rapid distributive phase of 15–30 minutes, the elimination phase begins. During eliminated by filtration, there is active reabsorption of aminoglycoside into the proximal renal tubular cells. A direct relationship exists between aminoglycoside clearance and glomerular filtration rate. Less than 1% of aminoglycoside is eliminated into feces, bile and saliva. Approximately 99% of the drug is excreted unchanged in the urine with a half-life of 1.5–3.5 hours in adult patients with normal renal function. In patients with increased extravascular fluid, the half-life can be prolonged. Impairment of renal function can result in considerable prolongation of the serum aminoglycoside half-life. In neonates less than 1 week of age or in small premature infants, the half-life is typically prolonged[38,39] (see Special populations, below).

Following the rapid elimination phase, there is a terminal elimination phase of 30–700 hours, secondary to prolonged release from the proximal renal tubules back into the urine. Because the amount of aminoglycoside eliminated is so low, it has no relevant effect on dosing.

PHARMACODYNAMICS

Numerous *in vitro* and animal model studies have been performed to characterize the exposure that best predicts outcome. For the aminoglycosides, the rate of bacterial eradication has been linked to both AUC/MIC and peak concentration/MIC ratios.[40] Increased rates of bactericidal activity have been noted with increasing concentrations (up to approximately 10–12 times above their MICs).

The concentration-dependent pharmacodynamic profile of aminoglycosides has stimulated *in vitro*, animal model and clinical investigations regarding the potential for consolidated dosing. In neutropenic and non-neutropenic animal models of infection, significantly more animals survive a potentially lethal challenge of bacteria if the animals are treated with a single large dose of an aminoglycoside than with the same dose divided on an 8-hour schedule.[2,41] However, the optimal exposure might be organism specific. For example, although divided doses were superior in one *in-vitro* model against *Staph. aureus*, this was not observed against *P. aeruginosa* in the same model.[42]

DOSAGE AND ADMINISTRATION

Individualized dosing of aminoglycosides is necessary to optimize the potential for favorable outcomes while minimizing the risks of treatment-related adverse effects.[40,43] Aminoglycosides are most commonly administered intravenously (over 0.5–2 hours depending upon the dose), but in specific cases may also be administered by intramuscular injection. Initial dosing should be based on indication, weight and estimates of renal function. Subsequent adjustments to the dose and/or frequency of administration should be based on results of serum concentration monitoring. Actual body weight is used in most patients to determine the initial dose. In obese patients, i.e. greater than 25% over ideal body weight (IBW), a dosing weight can be calculated using the following:

$$IBW + 0.4 \ (actual - ideal)$$

While estimates of creatinine clearance are most commonly performed using the Cockcroft–Gault equation,[44] disease states that limit the predictability of this equation (such as rapid changes in renal function, dialysis-dependent renal failure, liver disease and malnutrition)

should be considered. Creatinine clearance estimates can be used to determine the frequency of administration.

In general, two methods of dosing and administration are employed: divided daily dosing and consolidated dosing (used most frequently for gentamicin and tobramycin).

Divided daily dosing ('traditional dosing') of gentamicin and tobramycin in adults

In the divided dosing method, a loading dose is given and followed by maintenance doses. The loading dose is dependent on target serum concentrations (based on indication and/or infection site) but independent of renal function. Peak concentrations of 2–4 µg/ml are targeted for gentamicin and tobramycin in patients with uncomplicated lower urinary tract infection and synergy with β-lactams for serious Gram-positive infections. For these indications, loading doses of 0.6–1.2 mg/kg may be administered, although loading doses are not generally required when aminoglycosides are administered for synergy against Gram-positive pathogens. In patients with Gram-negative sepsis or other serious Gram-negative infections, gentamicin and tobramycin loading doses of 2.5 mg/kg are used to target peak serum concentrations of 6–8 µg/ml. Finally, in patients with Gram-negative pneumonia or acute life-threatening Gram-negative infection in a critically ill patient, loading doses of 3 mg/kg are used to target peak serum concentrations of 7–9 µg/ml.

Following administration of a loading dose, maintenance doses should be administered based on indication and renal function. In adult patients with normal renal function, this is usually 1.7–2 mg/kg q8h.

One method to determine initial maintenance doses of gentamicin and tobramycin is outlined in Table 137.1.

All patients should undergo steady-state serum concentration monitoring (generally between the second and third dose). Peak serum concentrations should be measured 30 minutes after the intravenous infusion or 60 minutes after the intramuscular dose. Trough concentrations are obtained within 30 minutes of drug administration. Sample times should be documented in all cases. Trough concentrations for gentamicin, tobramycin and netilmicin exceeding 2 µg/ml or excessive peak concentrations indicate the need for dosing adjustment. Serum creatinine concentration should be measured at baseline and daily thereafter for the first 3 days of therapy, then every 3–5 days thereafter. Weekly renal function monitoring can be used for prolonged therapy if renal function is stable. Significant increases in serum creatinine concentration would indicate the necessity to recalculate a new dosage regimen, repeat serum monitoring or consider an alternative therapy.

Table 137.1 Initial maintenance doses of gentamicin and tobramycin in adults

Creatinine clearance (ml/min)*	Percentage of loading dose†	Dose interval (hr)
≥90	84	8
80–89	80	8
70–79	76	8
60–69	84	12
50–59	79	12
40–49	72	12
30–39	86	24
20–29	75	24–36

*Estimated using the Cockcroft–Gault equation.
†Rounded to nearest 10 mg increment.

Consolidated dosing of gentamicin and tobramycin in adults

Considerable attention has been given to optimizing the concentration-dependent pharmacodynamic properties of aminoglycosides (notably gentamicin and tobramycin) by giving the entire daily dose consolidated into one dose. This strategy is also known as 'once-daily' or 'total daily dose'. The goal of such a strategy is to increase the probability that aminoglycoside concentrations will exceed the MIC approximately 10-fold and potentially extend the PAE[45] (Fig. 137.2).

Numerous reports have described the application of consolidated dosing of aminoglycosides in a variety of clinical settings. In the largest published outcome study in adults (n=2184) treated with consolidated gentamicin or tobramycin, nephrotoxicity (defined as an increase in serum creatinine concentration of 0.5 mg/dl or more over baseline during aminoglycoside therapy) was detected in only 1.2% (27 patients) and ototoxicity in 0.1% (three patients). The incidence of nephrotoxicity was significantly lower than the 3–5% observed from the same hospital when aminoglycosides were given by the conventional dosing technique. Other experience reported in immunocompetent adults (as summarized in a meta-analysis) has demonstrated that consolidated dosing was equivalent with regard to bacteriologic cure, but showed a trend towards reduced mortality rates and reduced toxicity.[46] In addition, pharmacoeconomic analyses of consolidated dosing report the potential for significant reductions in preparation, administration, monitoring and nephrotoxicity costs, while others have documented how consolidated dosing might help to facilitate transition to outpatient care.[47,48]

While different approaches have been used to administer consolidated aminoglycoside dosing, perhaps the most popular used by US hospitals has been modeled after the one developed at Hartford Hospital. For the treatment of serious Gram-negative infections in adults, a 7 mg/kg dose of gentamicin or tobramycin is administered to target a peak serum concentration of 20 µg/ml (Fig. 137.3). Based on simulations using a one-compartment intravenous model and a Vd of 0.3 l/kg in patients with normal renal function, serum concentrations typically fall below 0.5 µg/ml within 12 hours and then remain essentially undetectable for the remainder of the day (Fig. 137.3). Kinetic studies in humans have confirmed 7 mg/kg as a reasonable target dose

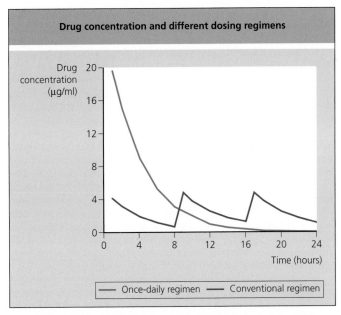

Fig. 137.3 Simulated concentration versus time profiles for once-daily (7 mg/kg q24h) and conventional (1.5 mg/kg q8h) gentamicin regimens in patients with normal renal function. Courtesy of Richard Quintiliani Jr, Richard Quintiliani and Charles H Nightingale.

in adults.[49] The drug-free interval is crucial for reduced toxicity as it facilitates increased aminoglycoside egress from the renal tubular and inner ear cells relative to that seen with the conventional intermittent dosing method.

Monitoring of patients on consolidated aminoglycoside therapy most frequently involves measuring a single random serum concentration 6–14 hours following the initial dose (Fig. 137.4). The resulting concentration is then plotted to determine the subsequent dosing interval (24, 36 or 48 hours) of the 7 mg/kg dose. If the concentration falls on the line of the nomogram that separates the dosing intervals, then the longer interval is chosen. Concentrations unable to be plotted using the nomogram due to excessive concentrations should result in suspension of therapy and serial serum concentration determinations. Patients suspected of having altered aminoglycoside pharmacokinetics (such as those with rapidly changing renal function) should be considered for more intensive monitoring.

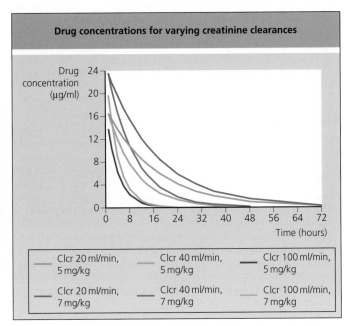

Fig. 137.2 Simulated concentration versus time profiles for once-daily 7 mg/kg and 5 mg/kg gentamicin regimens in patients with varying degrees of creatinine clearance (Clcr). Courtesy of Richard Quintiliani Jr, Richard Quintiliani and Charles H Nightingale.

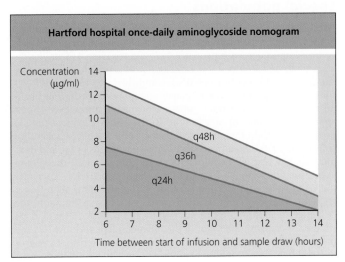

Fig. 137.4 Hartford Hospital once-daily aminoglycoside nomogram for gentamicin and tobramycin using the 7 mg/kg dose. Courtesy of Richard Quintiliani Jr, Richard Quintiliani and Charles H Nightingale.

Published experience with consolidated aminoglycoside dosing has focused on the use of either gentamicin or tobramycin. Relative to these agents, published experience with consolidated dosing of amikacin for the treatment of Gram-negative infections is limited. However, amikacin 15 mg/kg/day has been used with success.[50,51]

Similarly, netilmicin given as either 5 mg/kg q24h or 2 mg/kg q8h for 10 days was compared for the treatment of Gram-negative pyelonephritis in children in a prospective, randomized trial.[52] No difference in clinical efficacy, ototoxicity or nephrotoxicity was observed.

Published experience with consolidated aminoglycosides is expanding, including recent reports in patients with postpartum endometritis, mycobacterial infections, endocarditis,[53] osteomyelitis[54] and febrile neutropenia.[47,55] However, consolidated aminoglycoside dosing is not generally recommended for patients with severe renal insufficiency (including end-stage renal disease), pregnant women or those with major burns (>20%) or ascites due to the relative lack of data in these populations and the potential for altered pharmacokinetics. Alternative strategies for consolidated dosing are also required in the treatment of mycobacterial infections and when used for synergy (as part of combination therapy) (see Clinical applications, below).

Despite extensive published clinical experience with consolidated aminoglycoside dosing and wide acceptance in US hospitals, considerable debate persists regarding the appropriateness and optimal implementation of such therapy.[56] Alternative dosing regimens (ranging from 3 mg/kg to 7 mg/kg q24h of gentamicin or tobramycin) and dosing adjustment strategies have been advocated by some investigators. Dosing based on targeted AUC has also been proposed. For example, pharmacokinetic targets might be reached with 5 mg/kg if MIC ≤1, but higher (i.e. 7 mg/kg) if MIC ≥2.[40] However, it is uncertain which of these methods is superior.

Other aminoglycosides in adults

For amikacin and streptomycin, an initial dose of 7.5 mg/kg is administered, targeting peak concentrations of 15–30 µg/ml. Maintenance doses of amikacin are 15 mg/kg/day in divided doses q12h (for patients with normal renal function). Trough concentrations should be 5–10 µg/ml.

For netilmicin, a loading dose of 2 mg/kg is followed by 6 mg/kg/day (usually in divided doses q8h for patients with normal renal function). Similar to that previously described for gentamicin and tobramycin, maintenance doses and dosing intervals should be adjusted based on estimates of renal function. In all cases, serum concentration monitoring should be used to individualize the dose.

Special populations

The dosing of aminoglycosides should be modified in specific populations. The initial maintenance dosing to neonates and children should be based upon age, with neonates 0–7 days receiving 4–5 mg/kg/day and infants and children 5–7.5 mg/kg/day of gentamicin or tobramycin divided into two or three doses. Published experience with consolidated dosing in pediatric patients is growing, including use in neonates.[57,58] While similar pharmacodynamic principles should apply to the treatment of infections in the pediatric patient population, differences in the pharmacokinetic profile should be taken into consideration. For example, in children 6–12 months of age and those older than 1 year given a single intravenous dose of 20 mg/kg amikacin, the Vds were 0.5 l/kg and 0.33 l/kg, respectively.[59] Therefore, the Vd in children under 1 year of age is slightly higher than that of an adult, whereas that in children over 1 year of age is similar to that in adults. In addition, in this same study, the half-life in the younger children was longer than that in the older children and in adults, yet the peak and trough levels were similar. These observations suggest that children under 1 year of age may require a higher single dose (20 mg/kg) of amikacin than the dose (15 mg/kg) in older children and in adults. Other studies using a 20 mg/kg once-daily dose of amikacin in children undergoing bone marrow transplantation or with serious

Gram-negative bacterial sepsis have shown no differences in efficacy or toxicity compared with standard intermittent dosing.[59]

Patients undergoing dialysis require dosing modification based on the type and frequency of dialysis. Supplemental doses of 1–2 mg/kg gentamicin or tobramycin, 2 mg/kg netilmicin and 5–7 mg/kg amikacin may be required after each hemodialysis. Those undergoing continuous arteriovenous (AV) hemofiltration may be administered initial daily doses of 2.5 mg/kg gentamicin or tobramycin followed by serum concentration monitoring to ensure adequate peak and trough concentrations. Intraperitoneal administration of aminoglycosides (gentamicin, tobramycin or netilmicin 10 mg in 2 l dialysis fluid to four bags each day), with or without a traditional loading dose given intravenously, has been used in patients undergoing continuous ambulatory peritoneal dialysis (CAPD)-related peritonitis.[33] Alternatively, high concentrations (e.g. 40 mg gentamicin, tobramycin or netilmicin in 2 l dialysate) added to one exchange of dialysis fluid per day appear to have comparable efficacy.[33] Finally, patients undergoing continuous arteriovenous hemodialysis (CAVHD) and continuous venovenous hemodialysis (CVVHD) exhibit significant interpatient variability. Multiple serial aminoglycoside concentrations are generally necessary to determine optimal dosing in such patients.

In addition to these patient populations, other groups have been reported to demonstrate alterations in aminoglycoside pharmacokinetics requiring modification of the initial empiric recommendations. For example, initial empiric dosing of gentamicin and tobramycin in patients with cystic fibrosis should be 3.0–3.3 mg/kg q8h due to the increased volume of distribution and drug elimination demonstrated in this patient population. Higher doses of gentamicin and tobramycin (i.e. 7–9 mg/kg/day) may also be necessary in cystic fibrosis patients receiving consolidated dosing.[60] Similarly, larger volumes of distribution have been reported in patients with significant burns. Therefore, maintenance doses of gentamicin or tobramycin of up to 7–8 mg/kg/day (in divided doses) may be required to achieve target serum aminoglycoside concentrations. Increased dosing requirements have also been reported in burn patients receiving consolidated dosing of amikacin.[50]

Prophylaxis

Dosing of aminoglycosides for prophylaxis of infection secondary to surgery has been described in recent guidelines.[61,62] Patients receiving gentamicin (in combination with vancomycin) for cardiac surgery may be administered a single 4 mg/kg dose within 1 hour of the surgery.[61] For such an indication, re-dosing due to cardiopulmonary bypass is not necessary.[61] Patients receiving prophylaxis for colorectal or gynecologic surgery may receive gentamicin 1.5 mg/kg (as part of combination prophylaxis) within 1 hour of the incision.[62]

Coadministration with β-lactams

Although the aminoglycosides are often used in combination with β-lactams, the combination may lead to inactivation of both drugs. The reaction, which is time- and concentration-dependent, occurs by nucleophilic opening of the β-lactam ring and acylation of an amino group of the aminoglycoside, resulting in a biologically inactive amide.[63] Gentamicin and tobramycin appear to be more susceptible to inactivation than amikacin or netilmicin. This phenomenon is probably clinically meaningful only in patients with significant renal failure in whom β-lactams accumulate to very high concentrations.[63] As such, aminoglycosides should not be mixed with β-lactams before infusion or intraperitoneal instillation, and serum samples used for aminoglycoside assay should be run immediately or frozen until used.

Aerosol administration

As previously addressed, tobramycin has been administered via aerosol to patients with cystic fibrosis.[64] In this setting, 300 mg is administered twice daily.

Local administration

Aminoglycosides have been administered in a variety of novel (i.e. nonparenteral) forms, including bone cement, irrigation solutions, impregnated beads, antibiotic locks, intraventricular injections, etc. Such use is beyond the scope of this chapter.

CLINICAL APPLICATIONS

Aminoglycosides are used most frequently as part of combination therapy (usually with cell wall-active agents such as β-lactams) for the treatment of serious Gram-negative infections. Use as part of combination therapy for the treatment of Gram-positive infections (i.e. enterococci and staphylococci) is less common. Specific aminoglycosides have been employed for the treatment of *N. gonorrhoeae* (spectinomycin), mycobacterial (streptomycin, amikacin) and protozoal (paramomycin) infections.

Severe Gram-negative infections

With the increasing use of carbapenems (e.g. imipenem/cilastatin and meropenem) and fluoroquinolones (e.g. ciprofloxacin and levofloxacin), there has been a significant increase in the emergence of multidrug-resistant bacteria. Due predominantly to their broad spectrum of bactericidal activity against Enterobacteriaceae, *Acinetobacter* spp. and *P. aeruginosa*, gentamicin, tobramycin and amikacin have played a major role in the treatment of severe to life-threatening infections suspected or documented to be caused by Gram-negative bacteria.

Recent interest has focused on the potential application of aminoglycosides for the treatment of multidrug-resistant Gram-negative infections caused by organisms producing ESBLs.[65] Among the aminoglycosides, amikacin appears to be the most active *in vitro*. However, a marked increase in the incidence of aminoglycoside resistance is seen in ESBL producers (relative to nonproducers).

Infections treated with aminoglycosides as part of a combination therapy include (but are not limited to) empiric treatment of the febrile neutropenic patient,[66] sepsis,[67] nosocomial pneumonia[68,69] and intra-abdominal infections[70] (see Chapter 37). However, despite their favorable activity *in vitro*, there are concerns regarding treatment-related toxicity, need for serum concentration monitoring, availability of alternative therapies and the general lack of controlled clinical data to support their use as part of combination therapy. Such skepticism has been reflected in the general lack of support in recently published guidelines for their empiric use in clinically stable patients for many of these infections. In contrast, many of these recommend consideration of aminoglycoside-containing regimens (usually in combination with a β-lactam) in severe refractory infections or in patients with an increased risk of a multidrug-resistant pathogen (most notably *P. aeruginosa* and *Acinetobacter* spp.).

Gram-positive infections

Enterococci

Aminoglycosides (either gentamicin or streptomycin) may be combined with either a penicillin or vancomycin in an attempt to achieve a bactericidal effect for the treatment of specific, serious enterococcal infection (e.g. enterococcal endocarditis).[71] As previously discussed, all enterococci are resistant to aminoglycosides, based on achievable serum concentrations; however, in the absence of high-level resistance, the potential exists for synergistic activity with penicillins (usually ampicillin) or vancomycin.[28]

Enterococci with high-level resistance to gentamicin contain the bifunctional aminoglycoside-modifying enzyme acetyltransferase (AAC) (6′)-phosphotransferase (APH) (2′), which abolishes synergy with all aminoglycosides except streptomycin.[28] It is important to note that, although the bifunctional enzyme modifies amikacin and abolishes synergy with β-lactams and vancomycin, it does not lead to a resistant phenotype.[28] Therefore, amikacin should not be used against strains with high-level resistance to gentamicin, even in the absence of high-level resistance to amikacin. In the absence of high-level streptomycin resistance, this aminoglycoside remains the only alternative for strains with high-level resistance to gentamicin.[28]

In general, the use of aminoglycosides for the treatment of enterococcal infections is generally reserved for severe infections. For example, target peak and trough serum gentamicin concentrations are 3–4 µg/ml and <1 µg/ml, respectively, when 3 mg/kg/day is administered in three divided doses for the treatment of enterococcal endocarditis (as part of combination therapy) in the absence of evidence for high-level aminoglycoside resistance.[71] Since conflicting animal data exist, use of consolidated dosing for this indication is generally discouraged.[1]

Staphylococci

Because of alternative treatment options, aminoglycosides are rarely used as monotherapy for the treatment of staphylococcal infections.[6] However, the role for aminoglycosides (as part of combination therapy) for most staphylococcal infections is uncertain. In one study comparing nafcillin either alone or in combination with gentamicin for the treatment of *Staph. aureus* endocarditis (predominantly left-sided), the addition of the aminoglycoside reduced the duration of bacteremia by approximately 1 day, but otherwise did not improve outcome.[72] In contrast, an increase in aminoglycoside-associated nephrotoxicity was observed. The optimal dose of gentamicin for the treatment of staphylococcal infections is also unknown. In the setting of severe infections with MSSA (most notably endocarditis), gentamicin 3 mg/kg/day in divided doses (in combination with a β-lactam for MRSA) may be considered for a period of 3–5 days or up to 2 weeks in the setting of a prosthetic valve after susceptibilities have been confirmed.[71] Based on data from *in vitro* models, higher single doses may be more effective as part of combination therapy. In the absence of endocarditis, there is little support for the routine use of gentamicin in the treatment of staphylococcal infections.[73]

Streptococci

Similar to its roles in the treatment of enterococci and staphylococci, gentamicin (in combination with ceftriaxone) is included among the recommended options for the treatment of endocarditis due to viridans streptococci and *Streptococcus bovis*,[71] recently renamed *Strep. gallolyticus*. However, in contrast to these infections, a single daily dose of 3 mg/kg may be considered for native valve endocarditis with penicillin-sensitive viridans streptococci.[53,71]

Mycobacterial infections

The clinical role of streptomycin and amikacin as well as the other aminoglycosides in the treatment of mycobacterial infections is discussed in detail in Chapter 30.

Streptomycin has the greatest *in-vitro* activity among the aminoglycosides against *M. tuberculosis*. However, increasing streptomycin resistance (noted particularly in high-prevalence areas), combined with its toxicities, have made it a second-line agent in the treatment of tuberculosis.[27] Amikacin may be considered in specific cases of multidrug-resistant tuberculosis, since some streptomycin-resistant isolates may be susceptible *in vitro* to amikacin.[27,74] Streptomycin and amikacin are usually dosed in adults with normal renal function as a single daily injection of 15 mg/kg per day (maximum 1 g/day) five to seven times per week for 2–4 months, then two to three times weekly (depending upon response).[27] Children should receive streptomycin 20–40 mg/kg/day (maximum 1 g/day) or amikacin 15–30 mg/kg/day (maximum 1 g/day) as a single daily dose. Reduced doses (i.e. 10 mg/kg/day, maximum 750 mg/day) are administered to persons >60 years of age.[27]

The role of aminoglycosides in the treatment of atypical mycobacterial infections has been summarized elsewhere.[26] For *M. abscessus* and *M. fortuitum*, amikacin 15 mg/kg/day (once daily or in divided doses) or 25 mg/kg three times weekly can be considered. For *M. chelonae*, tobramycin is generally more active *in vitro* than amikacin. Streptomycin and amikacin may also have activity against specific strains of *M. kansasii*.[26] Three times weekly doses of amikacin or streptomycin 25 mg/kg have been employed in the treatment (as part of combination therapy) of select patients with *M. avium* complex, most often those with multilobar, cavitary pulmonary disease or those refractory to prior therapy.[26]

Other infections and indications

The principal uses of streptomycin as monotherapy have been for plague, tularemia and brucellosis (see Chapters 120, 121 and 123). Gentamicin therapy has also been used in such infections. However, streptomycin monotherapy has been associated with a high failure rate in patients with brucellosis, and is now used more commonly as part of a combination regimen.[75]

Because paromomycin is too toxic following intravenous administration and is not absorbed following oral administration, its use has been restricted to the treatment of intestinal infections, particularly cryptosporidiosis in patients who have AIDS.[76] However, the efficacy of this agent has been questioned in recent clinical trials, and the introduction of FDA-approved treatment options for this infection (i.e. nitazoxanide) will likely limit its use in the future.[76] For the treatment of intestinal amebiasis, the usual dose in adults and children is 25–35 mg/kg/day divided q8h with meals for 5–10 days. Historically, paromomycin has been used for treatment or prevention of travelers' diarrhea because it is also active against *E. coli* and *Salmonella* spp. However, such an indication has largely been replaced by newer, more widely available and better-tolerated agents.

Unlabeled uses of paromomycin include treatment of other parasitic infections such as *Dientamoeba fragilis* (25–30 mg/kg q8h for 7 days), *Diphyllobothrium latum*, *Taenia saginata*, *Taenia solium*, *Dipylidium caninum* (adult dose: 1 g every 15 minutes for four doses; pediatric dose: 11 mg/kg every 15 minutes for four doses) and *Hymenolepis nana* (45 mg/kg/day for 5–7 days).

Like paromomycin, neomycin is too toxic for systemic use. It has mainly been used by mouth as a prophylactic agent (along with erythromycin) in colonic surgery and in hepatic encephalopathy to reduce the number of aerobic enteric organisms. However, the availability of alternative prophylactic strategies has largely replaced neomycin for this indication.

In the treatment of hepatic encephalopathy, the usual dose in adults is 4–12 g/day in divided doses. Treatment is usually continued for 5–6 days. In patients with chronic hepatic insufficiency, neomycin may be required (in adults up to 4 g/day) indefinitely.

An infrequent use of gentamicin is to combine it with ampicillin in the therapy of infections due to *Listeria monocytogenes*.[77] In patients allergic to penicillin, trimethoprim–sulfamethoxazole (co-trimoxazole) can be used either alone or in combination with gentamicin.[77]

Although all aminoglycosides exhibit activity against *Neisseria* spp., only the aminocyclitol spectinomycin (not available in the USA) is used for gonococcal infection.[78] Use of aminoglycosides for such treatment, however, is very uncommon because most gonococci are susceptible to alternative therapies (such as third-generation cephalosporins). However, gentamicin (in combination with clindamycin) is considered a treatment option for pelvic inflammatory disease.[78]

Role in prophylaxis

The use of gentamicin (as part of a combination regimen) in the prophylaxis of infection has generally been restricted to colorectal or gynecologic procedures in patients at risk of Gram-negative infections unable to tolerate other options.[62] Aminoglycosides are no longer recommended for the prevention of infective endocarditis.[79] Their role as part of combination therapy (in addition to vancomycin in β-lactam allergic patients) for cardiac surgery is unclear.[61]

Aerosol therapy

Tobramycin has been administered by aerosol to patients with cystic fibrosis with the goal of providing high lung concentrations of antibiotic while minimizing systemic exposure. Data in this population have demonstrated the potential to decrease the density of *P. aeruginosa* in the sputum, thereby increasing pulmonary function and decreasing hospitalization.[64,80,81] However, its role in therapy is uncertain.

ADVERSE REACTIONS

The major adverse effects associated with aminoglycosides include neuromuscular blockade, nephrotoxicity and ototoxicity (auditory and vestibular). Aminoglycosides seldom produce hypersensitivity reactions, phlebitis, hematologic dyscrasias, hepatotoxicity, electrolyte disturbances (except those associated with renal dysfunction) or drug fevers.

Neuromuscular blockade

The neuromuscular blocking activity of aminoglycosides may manifest as weakness of the respiratory musculature, flaccid paralysis and dilated pupils. The true incidence of this reaction is unknown, but is thought to be infrequent. Risk factors include concomitant administration of drugs with neuromuscular blocking activity, rapid intravenous infusions and instillation of large concentrations into the peritoneal cavity. Infant botulism, myasthenia gravis, hypocalcemia and hypomagnesemia have also been associated with an increased risk for this adverse reaction. Consolidated dosing does not appear to increase the incidence of this reaction.[82]

Neuromuscular blockade was shown to be rapidly reversed by the administration of calcium gluconate in an animal model. With supportive care alone, in time, the blockade will resolve.

Nephrotoxicity

Except for spectinomycin, all aminoglycosides are capable of producing nephrotoxicity by interfering directly with renal tubular function and indirectly with glomerular filtration.[51] Clinical manifestations include a decreased urine concentrating ability, elevations in serum creatinine and polyuria. Because of excessive magnesium losses in the urine, hypomagnesemia may occur, which in turn can lead to secondary hypocalcemia and hypokalemia. Progression to anuric renal failure as a result of aminoglycoside nephrotoxicity is rare.

After discontinuing aminoglycoside therapy, evidence of nephrotoxicity usually disappears within several days in the absence of other causes of nephrotoxicity.[51]

Challenges exist in determining the incidence of nephrotoxicity secondary to aminoglycoside administration, including variations in study definitions and control of potential confounders. Using a definition of nephrotoxicity as a rise in serum creatinine concentration of 0.5 mg/dl above the baseline, approximately 5–20% of patients develop this adverse reaction using conventional dosing regimens. While previous clinical studies have compared the nephrotoxic potential of aminoglycosides, elements of their study design make definitive comparisons problematic. Based on animal model data, neomycin is generally considered the most nephrotoxic aminoglycoside: therefore, parenteral administration is avoided. Among the aminoglycosides most commonly prescribed (i.e. gentamicin, tobramycin, netilmicin and amikacin) there appear to be no clinically relevant differences in toxicity.

Risk factors for the development of aminoglycoside-induced nephrotoxicity include method of administration, underlying renal dysfunction, concomitant use of nephrotoxic agents, hypotension and duration of therapy.[1] Sustained elevated trough concentrations reflect impaired drug elimination and the need for dosing adjustment. Loop diuretics (such as ethacrynic acid and furosemide) may increase the risk of aminoglycoside renal toxicity through volume depletion. Concomitant use with vancomycin, *cis*-platinum, foscarnet, amphotericin B, methoxyflurane and intravenous radiocontrast agents has also been shown to increase the incidence of aminoglycoside-induced nephrotoxicity. Although elderly patients are traditionally considered to be at higher risk for aminoglycoside nephrotoxicity, they may actually not be if one adjusts for an age-related decrease in glomerular filtration rate.

The aminoglycoside enzyme transfer system has a finite (i.e. saturable) capacity for internalizing aminoglycosides within the proximal renal tubular cell. Therefore, the amount of aminoglycoside that enters the cell is the same over 24 hours whether the dose is given in divided fashion or as a single dose.[83] Because of low or undetectable levels of aminoglycosides for 10–12 hours during the 24-hour period with once-daily dosing, most of the previously internalized drug gets transported out of the cell, resulting in less accumulation. This would explain the observation (based on animal model data) that nephrotoxicity has been shown to be greatest when the daily dose is divided into multiple small doses rather than as the same dose given once. It may also help to explain why sustained trough concentrations above the therapeutic range also predispose the patient to an increased risk of nephrotoxicity. While few adequately controlled studies are available to validate this in humans, existing clinical data generally support the potential for reductions in nephrotoxicity when consolidated dosing is utilized.

Ototoxicity

The ototoxicity of aminoglycosides includes both auditory and vestibular components. Both auditory and vestibular toxicity can occur in the same patient either during or following therapy.

Auditory toxicity occurs as a result of the accumulation of aminoglycosides in the perilymph of the inner ear with subsequent damage of the sensory cells of the organ of Corti, while the target for vestibular toxicity is the sensory hair cells of the vestibular epithelia located at the summit of the ampullary cristae.[84,85] Serious damage to these cells typically results in a permanent deficit. Risk factors for ototoxicity include age (≥60 years), pre-existing ear disease, prolonged therapy, repeated treatment with aminoglycosides, and concomitant use of loop diuretics (e.g. ethacrynic acid) and other ototoxic drugs.[86] Since ototoxicity is rarely seen when given for less than 10 days, duration of therapy is likely to be the major determinant.

Symptoms of auditory toxicity include hearing loss, tinnitus and a sensation of fullness in the ear (most frequently bilateral).[85] The onset of symptoms may occur during or after cessation of treatment.

Cochlear toxicity is usually assessed by pure-tone audiometric testing, with earliest signs usually detected at frequencies above 8 kHz. Because perception of human speech occurs in the 0.3–3 kHz range, significant cochlear damage can occur before hearing loss is apparent.

Clinical studies show that the incidence of cochlear toxicity due to aminoglycoside use varies from approximately 5% to 15% with conventional dosing of aminoglycosides.[85] The frequency varies and depends upon the method of establishing toxicity. Data in humans are insufficient to address the comparative ototoxicity of aminoglycosides given by consolidated dosing. Similar to nephrotoxicity, there is controversy regarding the comparative potential for cochlear damage among the aminoglycosides. However, it appears that there is little, if any, clinically relevant difference between gentamicin, tobramycin, amikacin and netilmicin. Compared with these agents, neomycin has more often been associated with cochlear damage. The potential for ototoxicity in humans with topical preparations remains controversial. In a study of 44 children with chronic suppurative otitis media given topical preparations containing five different aminoglycosides (four neomycin; one gentamicin), there was no evidence of ototoxicity.[87]

Symptoms of vestibular toxicity include nausea, vomiting, vertigo, nystagmus, difficulty with gait and difficulty fixating on objects. Difficulty with gait is especially prominent in the dark because of the loss of sight, which compensates for vestibular dysfunction.

The frequency of vestibular toxicity is difficult to establish because vestibular function testing is poorly standardized. Of the aminoglycosides, streptomycin is more often associated with vestibular toxicity.

Acknowledgment

This chapter represents an edited and updated version of content previously written by Drs Richard Quintiliani Jr, Richard Quintiliani and Charles H Nightingale. Without their extensive contributions, this chapter would not be possible.

REFERENCES

 References for this chapter can be found online at http://www.expertconsult.com

Folate inhibitors

INTRODUCTION

Sulfonamides

Sulfonamides are competitive inhibitors of *para*-aminobenzoic acid (PABA), which is essential for folic acid synthesis in most bacteria, some protozoa and *Pneumocystis jirovecii* (formerly *P. carinii*) (Fig. 138.1).[1] A consequence of the mode of action is that sulfonamides lack activity against organisms for which PABA is not an essential metabolite (e.g. *Enterococcus* spp.). The eukaryotic cell does not use PABA and sulfonamides do not interfere with human folic acid synthesis.

Dihydrofolate reductase inhibitors

Dihydrofolate reductase is an enzyme common to mammals, bacteria and protozoa alike as part of the synthesis of tetrahydrofolate from folic acid. Trimethoprim is a diaminopyrimidine that competitively inhibits dihydrofolate reductase.[1,2] Compared with many other diaminopyrimidines with antimicrobial activity (e.g. pyrimethamine),

trimethoprim has a higher affinity for bacterial dihydrofolate reductase than for the human enzyme, thus reducing the risk of folic acid deficiency in the treated patient.[3] Pyrimethamine is also a competitive dihydrofolate reductase inhibitor. It has a high affinity for protozoal enzyme.

In addition to the above modes of action, it has been proposed that trimethoprim may inhibit the adhesion of bacteria to human mucosal cells.[4]

Combinations of sulfonamides and trimethoprim or pyrimethamine

Combinations of sulfonamides and trimethoprim or pyrimethamine interfere with two consecutive steps in the same metabolic chain in the micro-organism. This may lead to synergistic antimicrobial activity. The rationale for a fixed combination of trimethoprim and sulfamethoxazole is that, although both antibiotics alone are bacteriostatic, the combination may be bactericidal. The optimal trimethoprim–sulfamethoxazole (TMP–SMX) ratio for synergism inside a bacterium is 1:20. Based on the pharmacokinetics of the two agents, this ratio is obtained systemically with a 1:5 dosage combination.[5]

The clinical relevance of the synergism is difficult to prove in experimental infections and even more so in clinical trials. This has led to questioning of the clinical usefulness of the combination in comparison with trimethoprim alone for the treatment of bacterial infections.[6] An argument in favor of the combination is the possibility of the reduced risk of resistance; organisms initially susceptible to both sulfonamides and trimethoprim are less likely to develop resistance to combinations than to single drugs.

Folate inhibitor combinations are used for treating bacterial as well as fungal and protozoal infections. Because of the emergence of bacterial resistance and risks for adverse reactions, the sulfonamides have lost most of their usefulness as single agents. Emphasis will be put on combinations of sulfonamides and trimethoprim, especially the most widely used, namely TMP–SMX and pyrimethamine–sulfadoxine.

PHARMACOKINETICS

The sulfonamides are classically subdivided on the basis of their elimination time into short-acting (plasma half-life, $t_{1/2}$ <8 h), medium-acting ($t_{1/2}$=8–16 h), long-acting ($t_{1/2}$=17–48 h) and ultra-long-acting ($t_{1/2}$>48 h). Sulfonamides used as single agents today are short or medium acting.

Plasma kinetics

Currently used sulfonamides, as well as trimethoprim and pyrimethamine, are well absorbed after oral administration and have

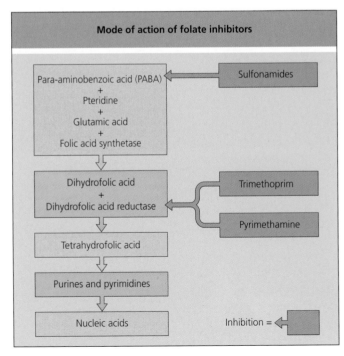

Fig. 138.1 Mode of action of folate inhibitors.

high bioavailability. Following an oral dose of 160 mg of trimethoprim and 800 mg of sulfamethoxazole, maximal plasma concentrations of 1.6–1.9 mg/l and 26–41 mg/l, respectively, are achieved.[7] After intravenous administration of 240 mg trimethoprim and 1200 mg sulfamethoxazole q12h, peak plasma concentrations in the steady state are about 6 mg/l for trimethoprim and 180 mg/l for sulfamethoxazole.[8] The protein binding of the sulfonamides varies from less than 50% for sulfadiazine to more than 90% for sulfadoxine. Importantly, sulfonamides bind firmly to albumin and may displace other compounds (e.g. bilirubin). In newborns this may lead to toxic levels of unbound bilirubin with a subsequent risk of 'kernicterus' (see Central nervous system reactions, below).

Distribution

Trimethoprim is lipid soluble at physiologic pH and has a large volume of distribution (100–120 l), whereas sulfamethoxazole is a weak acid with poor lipid solubility at pH values above 7, leading to a volume of distribution corresponding to that of the extracellular space (i.e. 12–18 l). In tissues concentrations similar to or higher than those in plasma are achieved with trimethoprim, whereas considerably lower levels of sulfamethoxazole reach peripheral compartments. Concentrations above the minimum inhibitory concentrations (MICs) of trimethoprim-susceptible strains are achieved in most tissues and tissue fluids. With sulfamethoxazole, the peripheral concentrations are sometimes so low that it should be questioned whether therapeutic levels are reached. All of the sulfonamides as well as trimethoprim achieve high urinary concentrations.

Elimination

The main routes of elimination of sulfonamides, trimethoprim and pyrimethamine are via liver metabolism and renal excretion.[9] In patients who have normal renal function, half-life varies from less than 6 hours for sulfisoxazole and sulfamethizole to 11–17 hours for sulfamethoxazole and sulfadiazine and more than 200 hours for sulfadoxine. Trimethoprim has a half-life of about 15 hours and pyrimethamine is eliminated slowly, with a half-life of about 100 hours.

Kinetics in children

The kinetics of both sulfamethoxazole and trimethoprim differ between children and adults (Table 138.1). Elimination is faster in children, who must be given relatively higher doses than adults.

ROUTE OF ADMINISTRATION AND DOSAGE

Most sulfonamides, trimethoprim and pyrimethamine are available for oral use. Trimethoprim, sulfamethoxazole and sulfadiazine are also used intravenously; intravenous use of TMP–SMX is recommended

Table 138.1 Comparative kinetics of trimethoprim (T) and sulfamethoxazole (S) in children and adults

Parameter	AGE (YEARS)			
	<1	1–9	10–19	20–63
T volume of distribution (l/kg)	2.0	1.6	1.5	1.4
S volume of distribution (l/kg)	0.5	0.5	0.4	0.4
T plasma half-life (h)	11	5.6	10	16
S plasma half-life (h)	7.5	9.8	10	15

Table 138.2 Adult dosages of some folate inhibitors*

Drug	Indication and recommended dose for adults
Pyrimethamine	Malaria prophylaxis (with sulfadoxine) 25 mg once weekly; malaria therapy (with sulfadoxine; Fansidar) 50–75 mg as single dose; toxoplasmosis encephalitis therapy (with sulfadiazine and calcium folinate) 75–200 mg loading dose, followed by 25–100 mg q24h for 3–6 weeks, followed by 25–50 mg q24h (maintenance therapy in AIDS); ocular toxoplasmosis (with sulfadiazine and calcium folinate) 100 mg loading dose q24h for 1–2 days followed by maintenance doses of 25–50 mg q24h
Sulfadiazine	Toxoplasmosis encephalitis therapy (with pyrimethamine and calcium folinate) 0.5–1.5 g q6h; ocular toxoplasmosis (with pyrimethamine and calcium folinate) 0.5–1 g q6h
Sulfadoxine	Malaria prophylaxis 500 mg once weekly (with pyrimethamine; Fansidar); malaria therapy 1–1.5 g (with pyrimethamine; Fansidar) as single dose
Co-trimoxazole (trimethoprim with sulfamethoxazole ratio 1 part to 5 parts)	UTI 1.92 g single dose or 480–960 mg q12h; systemic bacterial infections 960 mg q12h; pneumocystis pneumonia treatment 60 mg/kg q12h; pneumocystis pneumonia prophylaxis 960 mg thrice weekly or daily
Trimethoprim	UTI 100–200 mg q12h

*For pediatric doses, see the manufacturers' recommendations.

when patients are unable to take the drug orally. Dosages for some of the sulfonamides and for combinations of sulfonamides and dihydrofolic acid inhibitors are given in Table 138.2.

INDICATIONS

The activity of TMP–SMX against enterococci is controversial. There are reports in the literature of enterococcal bacteremia during treatment with TMP–SMX despite full in-vitro sensitivity pre-therapy, and of high failure rates and rapid emergence of resistance in enterococcal urinary tract infections (UTIs).[10]

Reduced susceptibility or resistance to penicillin G by *Streptococcus pneumoniae* seems to be coupled to resistance to TMP–SMX in a very high percentage of strains studied.[11,12] Overall, resistance to TMP–SMX in pneumococci is a rapidly increasing problem.[13]

Streptococcus pyogenes is normally sensitive to TMP–SMX, but resistance has been reported in macrolide-resistant isolates.[14] With regard to other Gram-positive organisms, *Listeria monocytogenes* is susceptible to the combination.[15]

Escherichia coli show marked variation in susceptibility to TMP–SMX, not only between but also within countries. However, there is a clear trend towards increasing frequencies of resistance and in most countries 12% or more of *E. coli* isolates are resistant to trimethoprim and TMP–SMX.[16,17]

Shigella and *Salmonella* spp. also show varying sensitivity to TMP–SMX, with frequencies of resistance ranging from less than 5% to over 50%.

Several studies have indicated a relatively high frequency of selection of resistance to TMP–SMX in Enterobacteriaceae when the antibiotic is used therapeutically or, in particular, prophylactically.[18]

Reduced rates of susceptibility of *Haemophilus influenzae* to TMP–SMX have also been reported.[13]

The spectrum of the folate inhibitors also includes micro-organisms other than bacteria. The treatment of choice for *Toxoplasma gondii* remains a combination of pyrimethamine and sulfadiazine. The combination of sulfadoxine and pyrimethamine is used for treatment but less often for prevention of falciparum malaria in areas with chloroquine resistance. However, unlike *T. gondii*, for which no resistance against pyrimethamine–sulfadiazine has yet been reported, resistance against pyrimethamine–sulfadoxine is not uncommon in *Plasmodium falciparum* and might become a problem with *Pneumocystis jirovecii*.[19,20]

Use of sulfonamides alone

Systemic sulfonamides have been used for the treatment of uncomplicated UTIs; however, this is no longer recommended.

Use of trimethoprim alone

In many European countries, trimethoprim is available as a single agent. Due to its better adverse reaction profile and avoidance of hypersensitivity reactions to sulfonamides, it is favored over TMP–SMX for some infections.

Urogenital infection

Whilst resistance can sometimes be a problem, trimethoprim is the first-line drug for the treatment of uncomplicated UTI in many European countries[21] at a dose of 200 mg orally twice daily for 3 days.

Respiratory tract infections

Trimethoprim has been shown comparable to TMP–SMX and doxycycline for the treatment of lower respiratory tract infections, although its first-line use is often hampered by emerging *Strep. pneumoniae* resistance.[22]

Use of trimethoprim–sulfamethoxazole

Trimethoprim–sulfamethoxazole has lost some of its usefulness through the emergence of resistance and increased awareness of the risk of adverse reactions, which may be serious or life-threatening.

Urogenital infections

Urogenital infections are the most common indications for TMP–SMX (Table 138.3); however, in some countries this has been replaced by the use of trimethoprim alone (see above). High frequencies of clinical and bacteriologic cure have been documented in women who have uncomplicated cystitis as well as in patients who have pyelonephritis, complicated UTI or prostatitis.

Importantly, the use of TMP–SMX is well documented for single-dose or short-term treatment of uncomplicated cystitis in women.[23] It is equally effective if given for 3 days compared with treatment for 5–10 days, and a single dose is only slightly less effective than 3-day treatment. For other types of UTI, longer treatment times are required. In countries where resistant uropathogens are uncommon, single-dose or short-term TMP–SMX is an inexpensive and effective treatment of cystitis in women. For other types of infection, where longer treatment times are required, the relatively high frequency of potentially serious adverse reactions must be taken into account, and in most adult patients alternative agents are now preferred.

Prostatitis is commonly treated with TMP–SMX and the few studies evaluating its use for this infection indicate a high degree of efficacy.[24]

Table 138.3 Clinical use of trimethoprim–sulfamethoxazole	
Type of infection	**Limitations**
Uncomplicated UTI	None for short-term therapy (single dose or 3 days)
Other types of UTI	Resistance, safety
Shigellosis	Resistance
Salmonellosis	Resistance
Enteric fever	Resistance
Travelers' diarrhea	Resistance, safety
Otitis media	Resistance
Community-acquired pneumonia	Resistance, safety
Melioidosis	Resistance, efficacy
Prophylaxis in immunocompromised patients	Resistance, safety, efficacy
Pneumocystis jirovecii pneumonia	None

For *Haemophilus ducreyi* infections 160 mg of trimethoprim plus 800 mg sulfamethoxazole q12h for 3 days has resulted in high cure rates, whereas shorter treatment times seem ineffective.[25]

Infections caused by *Chlamydia trachomatis* respond poorly to TMP–SMX.[25]

Enteric infections

These have been extensively treated with TMP–SMX because of its activity against *Salmonella* spp. (including *Salmonella typhi*), *Shigella* spp., *Vibrio cholerae* and enterotoxigenic *E. coli*. In a well-controlled trial in patients who had enteritis of verified etiology, the causative pathogens were eliminated on treatment day 2 in 41% of patients treated with TMP–SMX compared with 23% of those receiving placebo and 91% of patients on norfloxacin.[26]

A review of patients who had shigellosis showed that 97% of 149 patients treated with TMP–SMX responded clinically and 90% bacteriologically.[27] With the comparators (ampicillin, furazolidone or sulfadimidine) the clinical success rate was 78%. However, TMP–SMX may have lost some of its usefulness in shigellosis through the emergence of resistance.

Trimethoprim–sulfamethoxazole has been shown to be as effective as chloramphenicol for the treatment of enteric fever caused by susceptible strains of *S. typhi* and *S. paratyphi*.[28] However, the emergence of multidrug-resistant strains has limited their usefulness and other agents are now preferred.[29]

In salmonellosis TMP–SMX is effective for treatment of invasive infections caused by sensitive strains, but, like other antibiotics, it seems less effective in eliminating the carrier state of *Salmonella* spp.[30]

Treatment of cholera should be aimed mainly at rehydration of the patients. However, antibiotics may reduce symptoms and shorten the duration of the carrier state of *V. cholerae*, thereby reducing the risk of transmission. Trimethoprim–sulfamethoxazole has proved effective in patients who have cholera and one study showed that it was better than tetracycline or sulfamethoxazole alone.[31]

In several studies TMP–SMX has been shown to be effective in preventing travelers' diarrhea.[32] However, it has also been found to select for resistance which, along with serious adverse reactions, makes this type of prophylaxis of doubtful value.[33]

Respiratory tract infections

Due to adverse drug reactions and the emergence of resistance in *Strep. pneumoniae*, TMP–SMX is no longer considered first line for the treatment of lower and upper respiratory tract infections.

In pneumonia caused by *Burkholderia pseudomallei*, melioidosis, TMP–SMX remains a choice for oral long-term treatment after standard treatment with ceftazidime, although some doubt exists about its effectiveness.[34] Trimethoprim–sulfamethoxazole is the drug of choice for the treatment and prevention of *P. jirovecii* pneumonia in the immunosuppressed.[35]

Other infections

Both trimethoprim and sulfamethoxazole penetrate the blood–cerebrospinal fluid barrier and the combination has been found to be effective in experimental bacterial meningitis.[36] Trimethoprim–sulfamethoxazole has therefore been used as an alternative drug for the treatment of bacterial meningitis. Favorable clinical results have been reported in the treatment of meningitis caused by *L. monocytogenes* as well as other types of meningitis.[37]

Trimethoprim–sulfamethoxazole is considered a first-line drug in the treatment of health-care associated infections due to *Stenotrophomonas maltophila*. This relatively avirulent Gram-negative bacillus can cause infection in immunocompromised patients and is often a multidrug-resistant pathogen.

In patients who have brucellosis TMP–SMX can be considered a second-line drug.

Several studies have shown excellent clinical results with TMP–SMX, alone or in combination with aminoglycosides, in the treatment of actinomycosis or nocardiosis.[38,39]

Trimethoprim–sulfamethoxazole 160/800 mg twice daily for 6 weeks may be considered an alternative in the treatment of ocular toxoplasmosis.[40]

A controversial field for the use of TMP–SMX is prophylaxis in neutropenic patients. Early studies showed significant protection against bacterial infections but its role has generally been superseded by other classes (e.g. fluoroquinolones).

Pyrimethamine–sulfadiazine and pyrimethamine–sulfadoxine

Pyrimethamine–sulfadiazine remains the first-line drug combination for the treatment of toxoplasmosis.[41]

Pyrimethamine–sulfadoxine is an alternative for the treatment of *P. falciparum* malaria in areas with chloroquine resistance.[42] However, resistance to pyrimethamine–sulfadoxine is not uncommon and safety concerns reduce its usefulness for prophylaxis.

DOSAGE IN SPECIAL CIRCUMSTANCES

Renal impairment results in prolonged elimination times. Table 138.4 gives dosages of sulfamethoxazole and trimethoprim in patients who had decreased renal function. This includes patients of advanced age. As pointed out, the above doses used in children should be higher than those in adults because of different kinetic profiles (see Table 138.1). All sulfonamides should be avoided in patients aged less than 6 weeks because of the risk of cerebral accumulation of free bilirubin (kernicterus). There are no recommendations for reduced dosage of folate inhibitors in patients who have hepatic disease. Most of the folate inhibitors pass to breast milk but at concentrations that make any toxic effects on the child unlikely. During pregnancy, particularly in the first trimester, trimethoprim and pyrimethamine should be avoided because of the possible risk of altered folate metabolism in the fetus. Sulfonamides should not be given during the last trimester of the pregnancy because of the risk of kernicterus.

ADVERSE REACTIONS AND INTERACTIONS

A summary of the potential adverse effects of folate inhibitors is given in Table 138.5.

Table 138.4 Effect of renal function on dosage of TMP–SMX and trimethoprim[53]

Creatinine clearance	Co-trimoxazole (TMP–SMX)	Trimethoprim
>30–50 ml/min	Dose as in normal renal function	Dose as in normal renal function
15–30 ml/min	Normal dose for 3 days then use 50% of the normal dose as the normal frequency	Normal dose for 3 days then use 50% of the normal dose q18h
<15 ml/min	Normal dose for 3 days then use 50% of the normal dose as the normal frequency *Note*: High-dose treatment (60 mg/kg q12h) should only be given if hemodialysis facilities are available	Give 50% of the normal dose q24h

Table 138.5 Adverse actions of folate inhibitors in humans

Body system	Sulfonamides	Trimethoprim–pyrimethamine
Central nervous system	'Kernicterus' in newborns	Aseptic meningitis, especially in patients who have collagen diseases
Liver	Toxic hepatitis	Probably none
Lung	None	None
Kidney	Crystalluria	Increased serum creatinine (inhibition of creatinine excretion); increased potassium
Prostate/genitourinary	None	None

General safety profile

Since several studies have shown a correlation between the treatment time and the risk of adverse reactions to TMP–SMX when used for uncomplicated UTIs, short-course therapy (3 days) is encouraged.[23]

Hematologic reactions

The mode of action of trimethoprim has caused concerns over possible bone marrow toxicity. Studies in patients treated for 1 month or more with TMP–SMX have shown moderate folate deficiency.[43] The possibility of immune reactions causing hematologic adverse effects has been proposed.[44]

Serious and even fatal hematologic adverse reactions (usually cytopenias) to TMP–SMX have been reported. In a Swedish study of about 50 million daily doses an approximate frequency of fatal reactions to TMP–SMX was calculated to be 3.7/million treatments (data from SWEDIS, Medical Products Agency, Uppsala, Sweden). It was noteworthy that the mean age of the patients who died was 78 years (range 41–96 years) and that only three of 18 patients were below the age of 70. Taking into consideration the effect of aging on renal function, the doses of TMP–SMX were high. In addition, the treatment time was long (range 3–73 days, mean 17 days, median 12 days).

Pyrimethamine hematologic toxicity is less well described. Many use folinic acid to avoid folic acid deficiency. Support is lacking and hematologic reactions may very well be due to other mechanisms.

Skin, mucocutaneous and allergic reactions

These reactions may in some cases be serious, for example Stevens–Johnson syndrome or toxic epidermal necrolysis.[45] Such reactions seem to be related to the sulfonamide component rather than to trimethoprim.

It is worth noting that, in most reports on the safety of TMP–SMX or sulfonamides, skin reactions are only rarely reported in children. Possible explanations for this are the reduced risk for overdosing in children due to efficient elimination and less risk of sensitization to trimethoprim or sulfamethoxazole from previous exposures.

High numbers of serious cutaneous reactions have been reported following treatment with pyrimethamine–sulfadoxine.[46] Between 1974 and 1989, 126 cases of mucocutaneous syndromes were reported, giving an estimated risk of about 1.1/million treatments. This risk, which is most probably related to the sulfadoxine component, is considered to be high enough to discourage routine use of the combination for malaria prophylaxis.

Patients who have AIDS and *P. jirovecii* pneumonia and are treated with high doses of TMP–SMX have high frequencies of cutaneous reactions as well as other adverse reactions.[47,48] These reactions seem to be related to dose and treatment time, and many patients who have AIDS who have developed skin reactions later tolerate low-dose TMP–SMX prophylaxis against *P. jirovecii*.

Hepatic side-effects

Cases of severe hepatic reactions to TMP–SMX have been reported and are most likely to be caused by the sulfonamide component.[49]

Gastrointestinal adverse reactions

Like many other orally administered antibiotics, TMP–SMX causes upper gastrointestinal adverse effects in some patients. Because of its low activity on the intestinal anaerobic flora it causes diarrhea only infrequently.

Renal safety

Sulfonamides with poor solubility can cause crystalluria. With sulfamethoxazole this does not seem to be a problem but, with sulfadiazine in high doses, crystalluria has been reported in AIDS patients who had toxoplasmal encephalitis.[50]

Hyperkalemia and increased serum creatinine have been reported in patients treated with TMP–SMX; elevated serum levels of creatinine seems to be related to competitive inhibition of the renal excretion of creatinine by trimethoprim.[51]

Central nervous system reactions

Aseptic meningitis is related to trimethoprim therapy. Several cases have been reported in the literature with some over-representation of patients who have collagen vascular diseases (e.g. Sjögren's syndrome).[52] The pathogenesis remains obscure but seems to be of an allergic nature, with rapid onset and relapses after provocation.

Sulfonamides can cause central nervous system toxicity in newborns (kernicterus) because of displacement of bilirubin from albumin, resulting in toxic bilirubin concentrations in the brain.

Drug–drug interactions

The sulfonamides cause variable inhibition of the cytochrome P450 enzyme CYP2C9. Trimethoprim is a possible inhibitor of CYP2C8 and CYP2C9. Many of the resultant interactions (Table 138.6) are minor, with concurrent usage often only requiring increased monitoring. The major exception is with methotrexate where concurrent usage, especially of high-dosage regimens, has led to major morbidity.

Table 138.6 Interactions between trimethoprim (TMP), TMP–SMX and sulfonamides with other drugs

Drug	Folate inhibitor	Interaction	Suggested management
Angiotensin-converting enzyme (ACE) inhibitors	TMP (and TMP–SMX)	Rarely causes serious hyperkalemia in patients with concurrent renal impairment	Monitor potassium levels
Azathioprine	TMP (and TMP–SMX)	Increased risk of hematologic toxicity	If combination necessary, monitor for leucopenia
Ciclosporin A	TMP, TMP–SMX, many other sulfonamides	Not fully defined. Reversible decrease of renal function (TMP, TMP–SMX); risk of accumulation if function deteriorates. Possible reduction in ciclosporin levels with some sulphonamides.	Monitor levels if sulfonamides are added to ciclosporin
Dapsone	TMP (and TMP–SMX)	Reduced clearance of both dapsone and trimethoprim	Monitor patient; increased dapsone toxicity has occurred
Digoxin	TMP (and TMP–SMX)	Reduced tubular secretion of digoxin	Monitor for toxicity
Folate inhibitors	TMP–SMX, sulfonamides, pyrimethamine	Concurrent use of pyrimethamine with sulfonamides has led to folate deficiency, megaloblastic anemia and pancytopenia	Supplementation with calcium folinate reduces the risk of folate deficiency
Lithium	TMP (and TMP–SMX)	Possible increased lithium levels	If combination necessary, monitor levels

Table 138.6 Interactions between trimethoprim (TMP), TMP–SMX and sulfonamides with other drugs—cont'd

Drug	Folate inhibitor	Interaction	Suggested management
Methotrexate	TMP, TMP–SMX	Potential severe bone marrow depression and pancytopenia	Combination of low-dose methotrexate with low-dose prophylactic TMP–SMX is commonly used in well monitored patients without problems. Higher doses of either drug are likely to be more problematic and have led to major morbidity. Use only if absolutely necessary with close monitoring
Nucleoside reverse transcriptase inhibitors	TMP–SMX, TMP	Reduced urinary clearance of lamivudine, zalcitabine and zidovudine. Possible interaction between TMP and stavudine	Close monitoring advised if combinations used
Phenytoin	TMP (and TMP–SMX), sulfadiazine, sulfamethizole	Reduced metabolism of phenytoin	If combination necessary, monitor phenytoin levels
Procainamide	TMP (and TMP–SMX)	Reduced clearance of procainamide	Increased risk of toxicity; lower procainamide dose may be required
Repaglinide	TMP (and TMP–SMX)	Increased repaglinide levels likely to result in hypoglycemia	Avoid if possible; monitor closely if not
Sulphonylureas	TMP, some sulfonamides, TMP–SMX	Possible increased risk of hypoglycemia	Advise patients of risk
Warfarin	TMP–SMX, some other sulfonamides	Reduced metabolism of warfarin	Monitor international normalized ratio (INR) closely when initiating and stopping TMP–SMX

REFERENCES

References for this chapter can be found online at http://www.expertconsult.com

Quinolones

INTRODUCTION

The quinolones are a heterogeneous group of synthetic antimicrobial agents. Originally deriving from 1,8-naphthyridine compounds (e.g. nalidixic acid), modern quinolones have evolved as shown in Figure 139.1

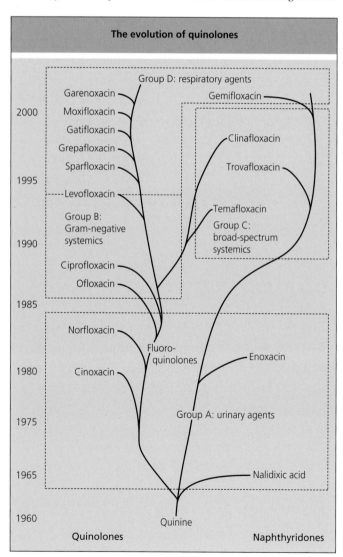

The evolution of quinolones

Group D: respiratory agents

Garenoxacin
Moxifloxacin
Gatifloxacin
Grepafloxacin
Sparfloxacin

Gemifloxacin

Clinafloxacin

Trovafloxacin

Levofloxacin

Group B:
Gram-negative
systemics

Temafloxacin

Group C:
broad-spectrum
systemics

Ciprofloxacin
Ofloxacin

Norfloxacin

Fluoro-
quinolones

Enoxacin

Cinoxacin

Group A: urinary agents

Nalidixic acid

Quinine

Quinolones

Naphthyridones

2000
1995
1990
1985
1980
1975
1965
1960

Fig. 139.1 The evolution of quinolones.

to give compounds initially with improved activity against Gram-negative bacteria (e.g. ciprofloxacin, ofloxacin) and more recently with greater activity against Gram-positives (e.g. gatifloxacin, moxifloxacin). A number of broader spectrum agents have been developed (e.g. clinafloxacin, trovafloxacin) but have had to be withdrawn due to problems with toxicity.

As quinolones have excellent tissue and tissue fluid penetration, they are suitable for infections in a wide range of organ systems. Adverse reactions are uncommon in marketed agents and relate mainly to the skin, the gastrointestinal system and central nervous system (CNS) and rarely warrant cessation of therapy. However, there are a number of potentially more serious adverse effects such as arthropathy, cardiotoxicity and phototoxicity. These occur as a class effect (although to different extents in different compounds) and have been a problem in drug development.

Modern fluoroquinolones are available in both intravenous and oral formulations. One of their major advantages has proved to be the ability to treat many serious infections with oral or intravenous–oral switch regimens, for example in the management of enteric fever, Gram-negative bacterial pyelonephritis, osteomyelitis, nosocomial pneumonia and severe exacerbations of both chronic bronchitis and cystic fibrosis. Many of the above previously demanded lengthy therapy with intravenous β-lactams, aminoglycosides or their combinations.

The activity of fluoroquinolones such as ciprofloxacin and ofloxacin in Gram-positive infections, notably those caused by pneumococci, has been disputed. Newer compounds, such as moxifloxacin, have markedly improved activity against Gram-positive pathogens and have found a place in the management of infections caused, for example, by penicillin-resistant pneumococci.

ANTIBACTERIAL SPECTRUM AND POTENCY

The antibacterial spectrum of quinolones is shown in Table 139.1. Quinolones are notable for the considerable knowledge that has been gained regarding structure–activity relationships.[1] The activity of the original naphthyridine and quinolone compounds (e.g. nalidixic acid) was limited to Gram-negative pathogens, primarily the Enterobacteriaceae, including Shigellae and Salmonellae. A major step forward in the development of the class was the addition of a fluorine at position 6, giving rise to the fluoroquinolones (Fig. 139.2). These agents are 10–100 times more active than their precursors against Gram-negative pathogens, including *Pseudomonas aeruginosa*, and have gained activity against the organisms causing atypical pneumonia. Potency, spectrum of activity and adverse effects/drug interactions are largely determined by substitutions at positions 1, 5, 6, 7 and 8:

- substitutions at position 1 (e.g. trovafloxacin) can alter potency (particularly against anaerobes) but may also affect interactions with theophyllines;
- substitutions at position 5 (e.g. grepafloxacin) can increase potency but may cause increased cardiotoxicity;

Table 139.1 Activity of quinolones against common pathogenic bacteria: MIC_{90} (mg/l)

Pathogen	Nalidixic acid	Norfloxacin	Ciprofloxacin	Ofloxacin	Levofloxacin	Grepafloxacin	Gemifloxacin	Gatifloxacin	Moxifloxacin	Garenoxacin
Streptococcus pneumoniae	>64	2–16	1–4	2–4	2	0.25	0.06	0.25	0.12	0.12
Staphylococcus aureus	>64	2	0.5–2	0.5–2	0.25	0.12	0.03	0.12	0.06	0.03
Enterococcus spp.	>64	8–16	1–8	2–8	2–8	1–16	0.25–>16	1–>16	0.5–4	0.5–8
β-Hemolytic streptococci	>64	4–8	2	4	1	0.25	0.03	0.5	0.25	0.12
Listeria spp.	NA	NA	1	2	1	NA	0.12	0.5	0.5	0.5
Haemophilus influenzae	1	0.25	0.03	0.03	0.03	0.016	0.015	0.03	0.06	0.03
Moraxella catarrhalis	4	0.25	0.06–0.25	0.12	0.06	0.015	0.03	0.12	0.12	0.03
Neisseria spp.	0.5	0.03	0.03	0.06	0.015	0.008	0.008	0.03	0.03	0.008
Escherichia coli	4–8	0.12–2	0.06–0.25	0.12–0.25	0.06–0.25	0.03	0.015	0.06–0.25	0.06	0.06–0.5
Klebsiella spp.	8–16	0.25–1	0.12–0.25	0.25–1	0.06–0.5	0.25–0.5	0.25	0.06–0.5	0.12–0.5	0.25–1
Enterobacter spp.	8–16	0.12–0.5	0.12–0.5	0.25–1	0.12–2	0.5–2	0.25–1	0.12–1	0.25	0.25–4
Salmonella spp.	2–4	0.25	0.12	0.25	0.25	0.015	0.06	0.06	0.25	0.12
Shigella spp.	8	0.25	0.12	0.25	0.03	0.008	0.008	0.03	0.06	0.03
Campylobacter spp.	8	0.25	0.12	0.25	0.12	NA	NA	0.12	0.06	0.12
Pseudomonas aeruginosa	>64	0.5–2	0.5–2	0.5–4	4	16	8	>4	8	16
Acinetobacter spp.	>64	>16	1–2	1–2	0.25–8	0.5–>16	0.5–>16	0.5–>16	0.25–16	0.12–8
Stenotrophomonas maltophilia	>64	NA	8	8	2–8	4	4	4	1	4
Bacteroides fragilis group	>64	16–32	4–16	8	2	8	1	1	0.5	0.5
Mycoplasma spp.	NA	4–16	1–2	1–2	0.5	0.12	0.12	0.12	0.12	0.06
Chlamydia spp.	NA	4–16	1–4	0.25–1	0.5	0.06	0.25	0.12	0.06	0.015
Legionella pneumophila	1	2	0.06	0.1	0.03	0.015	0.015	0.03	0.06	0.06
Mycobacterium tuberculosis	NA	2–8	1–4	0.5–2	1	NA	>4	0.25	0.12	2

NA, not available.

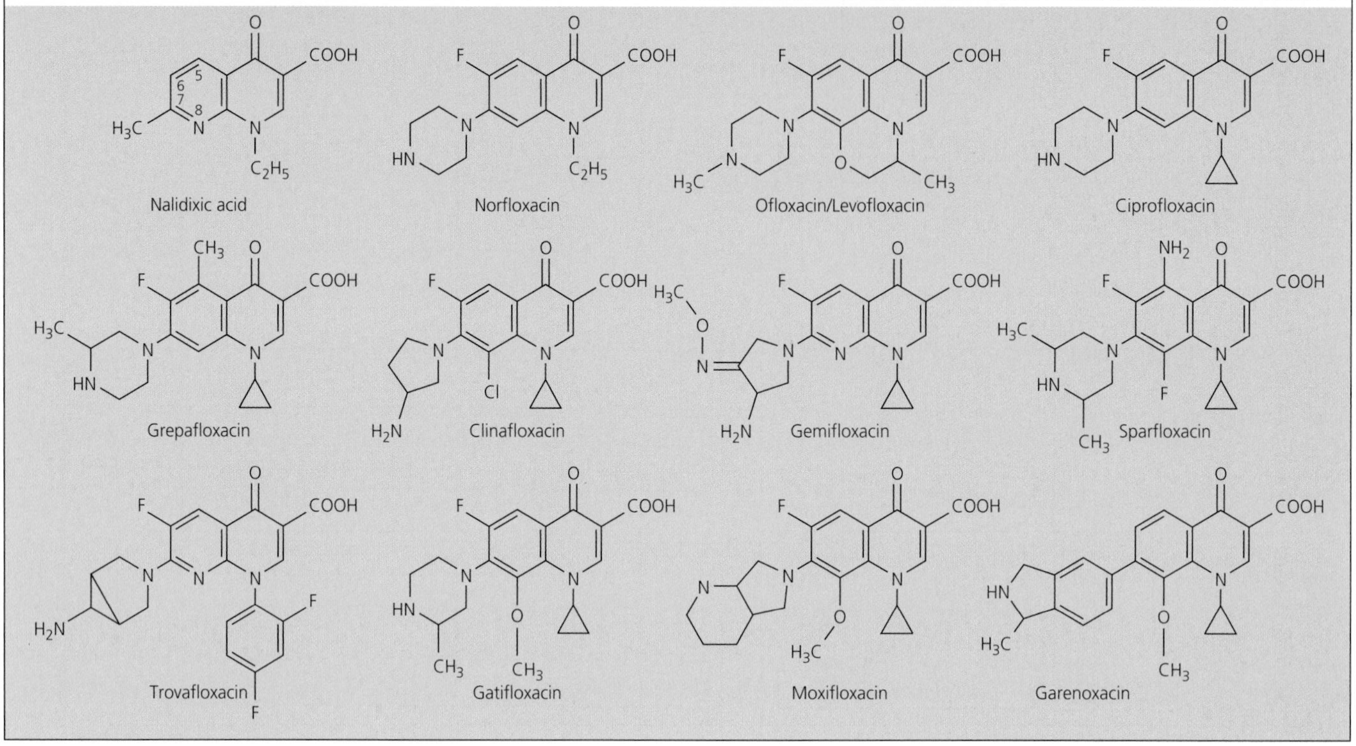

Fig. 139.2 Structure of quinolones.

- substitutions at position 7 (e.g. moxifloxacin, gemifloxacin, garenoxacin) can increase activity against Gram-positive organisms and increase the plasma half-life; and
- substitutions at position 8 (moxifloxacin, garenoxacin) can increase potency and reduce the rate of selection of resistant mutants but can be associated with increased phototoxicity (sparfloxacin).

Early representatives such as ciprofloxacin only have borderline activity against Gram-positive pathogens. However, developments such as the addition at position 7 of a five-membered ring (gemifloxacin) or an azabicyclo group (moxifloxacin, garenoxacin) have brought increased Gram-positive activity. Unfortunately, this has been partly at the expense of some activity against *P. aeruginosa*. Agents with good activity against both Gram-positive and Gram-negative bacteria have been developed (e.g. clinafloxacin) but have been withdrawn due to toxicity problems.

Fluoroquinolones have good activity *in vitro* against many intracellular pathogens such as *Legionella* spp., *Mycoplasma* spp., *Ureaplasma urealyticum*, *Chlamydia* spp., *Brucella* spp., *Salmonella typhi* and *Coxiella burnetii*. This may be enhanced by the concentration of fluoroquinolones within cells (see below). As shown in Table 139.1, *Mycobacterium tuberculosis* is susceptible to most of the fluoroquinolones with greater activity displayed by most of the newer agents (e.g. gatifloxacin and moxifloxacin). Fluoroquinolones should be used with caution in the treatment of pneumonia if there is a suspicion of tuberculosis, in order to avoid inadvertent monotherapy and the attendant risks of reduced diagnostic yield and selection of quinolone resistance. Of the other mycobacteria, *M. kansasii*, *M. marinum* and *M. fortuitum* tend to be fluoroquinolone susceptible, whereas *M. avium* complex, *M. chelonae* and *M. scrofulaceum* are more resistant.[2]

The quinolones are rapidly bactericidal against most susceptible species in a concentration-dependent manner and have a postantibiotic effect (PAE) of 2–4 hours. The pharmacodynamic determinants of efficacy are C_{max}/MIC (ratio of the maximum plasma concentration to minimum inhibitory concentration) and AUC_{0-24}/MIC (ratio of the area under the 24-hour drug concentration curve to MIC). Various groups have attempted to define the AUC_{0-24}/MIC ratio that would predict a successful outcome. It appears that the optimal ratio varies for different organisms so that a ratio of >125 has been proposed for infection caused by Gram-negative enteric pathogens and *P. aeruginosa*, but a much lower ratio of >34 is proposed for pneumococcal lower respiratory tract infections.[3,4] In addition to clinical efficacy, recent studies have focused on therapeutic strategies which may reduce the risk of fluoroquinolone resistance. The concept of the 'mutant selection window' has emerged, in which the survival of resistant organisms may be selectively encouraged by agents that only narrowly exceed the MIC of the organism. In accordance with this hypothesis, the use of the most potent agents may help to limit the risk of development of resistance by reducing the mutant selection window.[5]

MODE OF ACTION

Quinolones act by the rapid inhibition of bacterial DNA synthesis, leading to cell death. The primary targets are DNA gyrase and topoisomerase IV which are involved in the maintenance of the superhelical structure of DNA. Both enzymes are composed of two subunits that are homologous: DNA gyrase subunits encoded by *gyrA* and *gyrB*; topoisomerase IV encoded by *parC* (*grlA* in *Staphylococcus aureus*) and *parE* (*grlB* in *Staph. aureus*).

Although inhibition of these enzymes is the most important determinant of antibacterial activity, it appears that secondary activities may affect bactericidal activity. The addition of RNA and protein synthesis inhibitors or the use of high quinolone concentrations (which also inhibit RNA synthesis) can lead to a diminution in the cidality of some quinolones. Additional protein activity may be required to release the DNA ends from the DNA–gyrase–quinolone complex, with the release of free DNA ends resulting in bacterial apoptosis.[6]

BACTERIAL RESISTANCE

The major mechanism for acquired resistance to quinolones is by mutational modification of the antimicrobial target site. Mutations around the active site of *gyrA* have been identified in many strains of *Escherichia coli* and many other Gram-negative bacilli, giving rise to greater resistance to nalidixic acid than the fluoroquinolones. Alterations in *gyrB* are less common and cause lower levels of resistance.[7] The main site for resistance mutations in Gram-positive bacteria such as *Staph. aureus* and *Streptococcus pneumoniae* is the *parC* gene although mutations in *parE* have been described. In both Gram-negative and Gram-positive pathogens resistance develops in a stepwise fashion as mutations arise in one and then both targets. Following an initial mutation, the susceptibility to a quinolone will depend on the specificity of the agent for the alternative target. For example, in clinical practice it has been shown that an isolated *gyrA* mutation in *E. coli* will confer high-level resistance to nalidixic acid but only reduced susceptibility to ciprofloxacin. The acquisition of an additional *parC* mutation confers high-level resistance to ciprofloxacin.[8] For bacteria such as *P. aeruginosa* that inherently have less susceptibility to fluoroquinolones, a single mutation can give rise to clinically significant resistance.

Resistance to quinolones can also be achieved by active efflux of the drug from the bacterial cell. This has been best described in *P. aeruginosa* in which quinolone resistance has been associated with increased expression of the MexAB-OprM, MexCD-oprJ or MexEF-oprN efflux pumps.[9] In *E. coli* the pump is the acrAB-tolC system. Among Gram-positive pathogens, the *norA* pump has been described in *Staph. aureus* and the PmrA pump in *Strep. pneumoniae*.[10,11] On their own, efflux pumps will generally only cause low-level resistance and therefore may not be clinically important in inherently highly susceptible pathogens such as *E. coli*. However, the overexpression of efflux pumps becomes more significant in less susceptible organisms such as *P. aeruginosa*. The presence of efflux pumps may explain the reduced susceptibility of *Mycobacterium avium* when compared to other nontuberculous mycobacteria with similar susceptibility to gyrase inhibition.[12]

More recently, the spread of reduced susceptibility in Enterobacteriaceae by plasmid-mediated mechanisms such as Qnr proteins has been described. First discovered in the late 1990s, Qnr proteins protect gyrase and topoisomerase IV from quinolone inhibition. Despite a global distribution, Qnr proteins appear to be of low prevalence in most populations of Gram-negative bacteria. Qnr proteins confer low-level resistance which enhances the selection of resistant mutants *in vitro*, and may contribute to clinically significant levels of resistance by acting additively with other resistance mechanisms. The effect of *qnr* gene carriage on clinical outcome is as yet unknown. The aminoglycoside acetyltransferase, AAC(6′)-Ib-cr is another recently discovered mechanism for transferring low-level resistance on mobile elements. AAC(6′)-Ib-cr appears to act on piperazinyl-substituted quinolones such as ciprofloxacin.[13]

Resistance rates to quinolones continue to rise. In the UK, 2006 data from the Health Protection Agency reported that ciprofloxacin resistance among *E. coli* bacteremia isolates was 26%.[14] The increase in fluoroquinolone resistance across Europe is illustrated in Figure 139.3. Although methicillin-sensitive *Staph. aureus* is usually sensitive to fluoroquinolones, some clones of methicillin-resistant *Staph. aureus* (MRSA) – for example, epidemic MRSA (EMRSA)-16 seen in the UK – are resistant. Resistance among pneumococci remains uncommon, with most countries including the USA, Western Europe and Latin America reporting rates of resistance to levofloxacin below 1%,[15] although in some areas there is evidence that resistance is more common among penicillin-resistant pneumococci.[16]

Cross-resistance between the older fluoroquinolones is almost complete and minor differences in activity are not usually clinically exploitable. The mechanisms of resistance to antimicrobial agents are discussed in detail in Chapter 131.

PHARMACOKINETICS AND DISTRIBUTION

The quinolones are generally well absorbed and are widely distributed in body tissues and fluids, including the intracellular environment. They are excreted either by glomerular filtration or hepatic biotransformation, or a combination of these routes, and by biliary

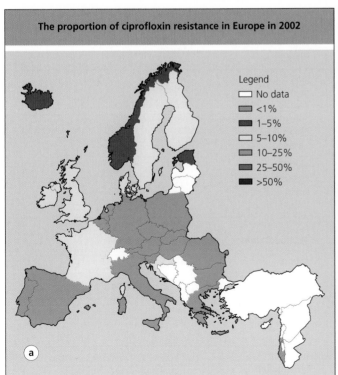

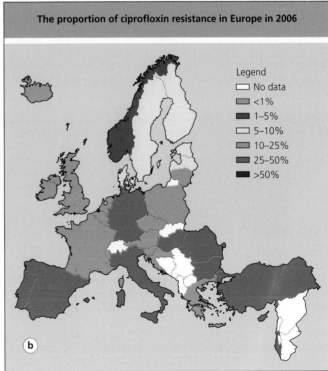

Fig. 139.3 The proportion of ciprofloxacin resistance in Europe.

Table 139.2 Basic pharmacokinetic parameters of quinolones

Agent	Dose (g)		C_{max} (mg/l)	AUC_{0-24} (mg/lh)	$t_{1/2}$ (h)	Protein binding %	% dose excreted unchanged in urine	Route
Nalidixic acid	1	QDS	V	V	1.5	90	<1	po
Norfloxacin	0.4	BD	2	12.5	3	15	25–40	po
Ciprofloxacin	0.75	BD	3	30	4	40	30–50	po/iv
Ofloxacin	0.4	BD	6	80	7	30	70–85	po/iv
Levofloxacin	0.5	OD	6.4	54	7	40	85–90	po/iv
Grepafloxacin	0.4	OD	2.2	14	14	50	<10	po
Gatifloxacin	0.4	OD	4.6	37	9	20	70–80	po/iv
Gemifloxacin	0.32	OD	1.8	9	7	65	30	po
Moxifloxacin	0.4	OD	4.5	44	13	50	20	po/iv
Garenoxacin	0.4	OD	6.5	84	12.5	80	40	po/iv

V, variable.

or transintestinal elimination. Bioavailability is high and protein binding usually low to intermediate. Fluoroquinolone kinetics are summarized in Table 139.2.

Absorption

Fluoroquinolones are well and rapidly absorbed after oral administration and exhibit linear absorption kinetics so that doubling the dose produces twice the plasma level.[12] Peak plasma concentrations are usually present 1–2 hours after an oral dose. Absorption may be delayed by food and is impaired by co-administration of antacids and ferrous iron, and possibly by zinc in multivitamin preparations.

Distribution

The fluoroquinolones are extensively distributed to the tissues as can be seen in Table 139.3. Apparent volumes of distribution are usually 2–3 l/kg, although values for precursor compounds are lower (e.g. 0.5 l/kg). Protein binding varies from 15% to 40% with norfloxacin, ofloxacin and ciprofloxacin[17] to 65% for gemifloxacin and higher still for garenoxacin and trovafloxacin (>80%).

Fluoroquinolones are concentrated approximately 10 times in polymorphoneutrophils (PMNs). Although it has been suggested that this may increase their *in vivo* efficacy against intracellular pathogens, there is evidence that the intracellular activity of different fluoroquinolones is variable, possibly related to where they are concentrated within the cell.[18] An additional result of the intracellular concentration of fluoroquinolones is that they may be transported by PMNs to a site of infection and then released.[19]

Elimination

Elimination half-lives vary from 1–2 hours for nalidixic acid to 3–5 hours for ciprofloxacin and 7–14 hours for newer agents.

Excretion of fluoroquinolones is primarily by renal glomerular filtration, hepatic metabolism and transintestinal elimination. The relative importance of glomerular filtration varies between agents and some compounds such as ofloxacin, levofloxacin and gatifloxacin exhibit minimal metabolism and are excreted largely unchanged in the urine. For these agents, renal clearance almost equals total clearance and dose modification is required in renal impairment.[17,20] Others, such as ciprofloxacin and moxifloxacin, have moderately extensive hepatic biotransformation (to oxo-, desethyl- and sulfo- derivatives,

subsequently partly eliminated as inactive glucuronides in the bile). For these compounds, renal clearance is half of the total clearance and dosage modification may not be required in renal impairment as long as other routes of elimination are intact.[21]

Table 139.3 Tissue distribution of fluoroquinolones

Tissue	Tissue: plasma ratio
Lung	
Bronchial mucosa	1.6
Epithelial lining fluid	2.1–8.7
Alveolar macrophages	11.8–21
CSF	
Uninflamed meninges	0.1
Inflamed meninges	0.3–0.5
Brain tissue	0.9
Skin/soft tissue	
Skin	1.8
Muscle	3.3
Subcutaneous tissue	~1
Blister fluid	~1
Sweat	2.5
Prostate	
Prostatic tissue	2.1–5.7
Prostatic fluid	0.25
Seminal fluid	6–8
Eye	
Aqueous humor	0.5
Kidney	
Kidney tissue	~6
Urine	~100
Liver	
Hepatic tissue	4
Bile	6
Heart	
Myocardium	2–4
Heart valves	~1

In hepatic impairment, the dosage of agents primarily cleared by the kidney (ciprofloxacin, ofloxacin and levofloxacin) rarely requires modification. However, for extensively metabolized drugs such as grepafloxacin, dose modification is necessary in patients with cirrhosis.

Fluoroquinolones that are not primarily eliminated by the kidney are present in significant quantities in the stool, partly by biliary excretion and, notably with ciprofloxacin, by transintestinal elimination. The majority is bound to ligands in the stool.

ROUTE OF ADMINISTRATION AND DOSAGE

Most agents are available in both oral and intravenous formulations. The high oral bioavailability of fluoroquinolones means that oral administration is adequate in most situations unless this route is unavailable. The manufacturers' dosage recommendations for quinolones are given in Table 139.4.

INDICATIONS

Early quinolones such as nalidixic acid were largely used for Gram-negative urinary tract infection (UTI) and shigellosis. The development and evolution of fluoroquinolones have led to a number of agents with differences in spectrum of activity and therefore indications. Some, such as norfloxacin, are used almost exclusively for UTI. Agents such as ciprofloxacin and ofloxacin have been used for a broad range of infective syndromes. Newer compounds, such as levofloxacin, moxifloxacin and gemifloxacin, have improved activity against Gram-positive pathogens and are more appropriate for respiratory tract infections.

Genitourinary tract infections

Uncomplicated lower urinary tract infection

Oral fluoroquinolone therapy is highly effective but to limit selection pressure for resistance should be used only when bacterial resistance precludes the use of other agents. Fluoroquinolones eradicate bowel reservoirs of uropathogenic E. coli and may reduce the incidence of early recurrence. Long-term suppression with low-dose norfloxacin or ciprofloxacin has been shown to be effective in preventing recurrent UTI in selected patients.[22,23]

Complicated ascending urinary tract infection

Fluoroquinolones given for 1–2 weeks are the recommended agents for the treatment of ascending or complicated UTI.[24] Oral ciprofloxacin has proved as efficacious as an intravenous regimen for initial empiric therapy.[25]

Prostatitis

Fluoroquinolones are concentrated in prostatic tissue and are recommended therapy for both acute and chronic bacterial prostatitis.[26] Ciprofloxacin for 28 days can give a clinical response of 98% in chronic bacterial prostatitis although relapse may occur in up to 40% of patients.[27]

Gonorrhea

The global prevalence of fluoroquinolone resistance continues to rise. In England and Wales the prevalence of ciprofloxacin resistance was 26.5% in 2006.[28] In the USA, the Centers for Disease Control and Prevention (CDC) treatment guidelines were updated in 2007 to recommend that fluoroquinolones should no longer be used to treat gonococcal infections in any patient group.[29]

Nongonococcal urethritis/cervicitis

The antichlamydial activity of fluoroquinolones varies and ofloxacin is the most potent of the established agents. A 7-day course of ofloxacin is as effective as doxycycline therapy.[30] Newer compounds such as moxifloxacin have excellent in vitro activity and may have a role in therapy.

Chancroid

A single dose or 3-day course of ciprofloxacin is a recommended treatment for chancroid. Despite reports of isolates with reduced susceptibility to quinolones, a study in Nairobi showed a 92% cure rate for single-dose ciprofloxacin, comparable to a 7-day course of erythromycin.[31]

Pelvic inflammatory disease

The ideal antimicrobial treatment for acute pelvic inflammatory disease has not been established by randomized clinical trials. In view of the high rates of resistance of Neisseria gonorrhoeae, fluoroquinolones are no longer included in recommended treatment regimens.[29]

Respiratory tract infections

The fluoroquinolones ciprofloxacin and ofloxacin have been used extensively for upper and lower respiratory tract infections. However, there have been concerns regarding their activity against Strep. pneumoniae. Newer agents, such as gemifloxacin, moxifloxacin and garenoxacin, have improved activity against pneumococci, including macrolide- and penicillin-resistant strains, and are often termed 'respiratory quinolones'.

Sinusitis

Oral fluoroquinolones have comparable efficacy to macrolides or cephalosporins and give cure rates of >85% in acute sinusitis.[32–34]

Ear infections

Topical preparations of ofloxacin or ciprofloxacin are effective for the treatment of acute otitis media in children with tympanostomy tubes and for chronic suppurative otitis media.[35] Clinical cure rates of >85% for otitis externa can be obtained with the topical preparations. Malignant otitis externa, which is usually caused by P. aeruginosa, can be treated with oral ciprofloxacin. A prolonged course is required (3 months) and gives cure rates in excess of 90%.[36]

Acute exacerbations of chronic bronchitis

Fluoroquinolones are among the agents of choice for the management of moderate to severe exacerbations of chronic bronchitis. They have equivalent efficacy to macrolides or β-lactam/β-lactamase inhibitor combinations and achieve cure rates of >90%.[37,38]

Community-acquired pneumonia

Older quinolones are not indicated for pneumococcal pneumonia when alternative antibiotics are available. However, results with ciprofloxacin and ofloxacin suggest clinical response and bacterial eradication rates of 90% or greater and, with levofloxacin, equivalence or superiority to ceftriaxone.[39] However, concerns have been raised regarding the efficacy of ciprofloxacin in severe pneumococcal pneumonia following reports of clinical failures.[40] Failures with levofloxacin have also been reported and in Europe it is suggested that it should be given at an increased dose of 500 mg twice daily or in combination with benzyl penicillin in cases of severe pneumonia.[41,42]

Table 139.4 Dosing recommendations for quinolones (from manufacturers' data sheets)

	Nalidixic acid	Norfloxacin	Ofloxacin	Ciprofloxacin		Levofloxacin	Gatifloxacin	Moxifloxacin
	po	po	po/iv	po	iv	po/iv	po/iv	po/iv
Urinary tract infection	500–1000 mg q6h	400 mg q12h (3–21 days)	200 mg q12h (3–10 days)	100–500 mg q12h (3–14 days)	200–400 mg q12h (7–14 days)	250 mg q24h (3–10 days)	200–400 mg q24h (3–10 days)	
Chronic bacterial prostatitis		400 mg q12h (28 days)	300 mg q12h (6 weeks)	500 mg q12h (28 days)	400 mg q12h (28 days)			
Acute sinusitis				500 mg q12h (10 days)	400 mg q12h (10 days)	500 mg q24h (10–14 days)	400 mg q24h (10 days)	400 mg q24h (10 days)
Acute bacterial exacerbation of chronic bronchitis			400 mg q12h (10 days)			500 mg q24h (7 days)	400 mg q24h (5 days)	400 mg q24h (5 days)
Community-acquired pneumonia			400 mg q12h (10 days)	500–750 mg q12h (7–14 days)	400 mg q8–12h (7–14 days)	500 mg q24h (7–14 days)	400 mg q24h (7–14 days)	400 mg q24h (7–14 days)
Skin and skin structure infection			400 mg q12h (10 days)	500–750 mg q12h (7–14 days)	400 mg q8–12h (7–14 days)	500–750 mg q24h (7–14 days)		400 mg q24h (7 days)
Bone and joint infection				500–750 mg q12h (≥4–6 weeks)	400 mg q8–12h (≥4–6 weeks)			
Intra-abdominal infection				500 mg q12h (7–14 days)	400 mg q12h (7–14 days)			
Infectious diarrhea				500 mg q12h (5–10 days)				
Uncomplicated urethral and cervical gonorrhea		800 mg single dose	400 mg single dose	250 mg single dose			400 mg single dose	
Nongonococcal cervicitis/urethritis			300 mg q12h (7 days)					
Pelvic inflammatory disease			400 mg q12h (10–14 days)					
Inhalational anthrax (postexposure)				500 mg q12h (60 days)	400 mg q12h (60 days)			

Newer agents such as gemifloxacin and moxifloxacin, which have improved activity against pneumococci and atypical pathogens, show promising results in clinical trials, with clinical cure rates in excess of 90%.[43] Additionally, *in vitro* tests suggest that the use of the most potent agents, or agents of intermediate potency with altered dose administration regimens, may reduce the emergence of resistance.

While high-level penicillin resistance was found to be associated with resistance to older quinolones such as ciprofloxacin, the newer agents have comparable MIC values for both penicillin-sensitive and penicillin-resistant pneumococci.[44]

Legionellosis can be successfully treated with quinolones such as ciprofloxacin, ofloxacin or levofloxacin. There are few clinical data to show whether or not they are superior to macrolides and often they are given in combination with a macrolide or rifampin (rifampicin)[45] (see also Chapter 27).

Nosocomial pneumonia

A large-scale study of ciprofloxacin showed equivalence with imipenem in moderately to severely ill patients, most of whom required ventilation and treatment in an intensive care unit.[46] In the 20–25% with infection caused by *P. aeruginosa*, the results with both regimens were less satisfactory, underlining the need for combination therapy. Newer fluoroquinolones such as gemifloxacin and moxifloxacin have reduced *in-vitro* potency against *P. aeruginosa* and will probably not have a role in the management of hospital-acquired pneumonia where *Pseudomonas* is a likely etiologic agent. A meta-analysis of efficacy in nosocomial pneumonia concluded that quinolones are an acceptable therapy and perform comparably to other standard regimes; the authors noted the importance of considering national and local antibiotic resistance trends when using fluoroquinolones (see Chapter 28).[47]

Cystic fibrosis

Oral ciprofloxacin is effective for exacerbations caused by *P. aeruginosa*, producing results equivalent to those of standard β-lactam and aminoglycoside therapy. In the UK a 3-week course of ciprofloxacin combined with colistin is recommended for the treatment of early pseudomonal infection.[48]

Mycobacterial infections

Older fluoroquinolones have only moderate activity against *Mycobacterium tuberculosis* and current evidence does not support the use of these agents in the treatment of drug-sensitive or resistant tuberculosis. Their role in therapy is currently limited to use in combination regimens for the treatment of multiply drug-resistant *M. tuberculosis* infection.[49] Newer agents such as moxifloxacin have enhanced antimycobacterial activity and animal studies suggest they may have a future role in antituberculous chemotherapy.[50]

As noted above, the susceptibility of nontuberculous mycobacteria to fluoroquinolones is variable. *Mycobacterium avium* complex is relatively resistant to quinolones. Nevertheless, the addition of ciprofloxacin to standard therapeutic combinations has been shown to be of benefit in HIV patients with disseminated disease.[51]

Skin and soft tissue infections

The fluoroquinolones give excellent results when compared with cephalosporins for the treatment of both uncomplicated and complicated skin and soft tissue infections.[52,53] However, more effective agents are routinely available for Gram-positive infections and usefulness in MRSA infections is limited by high rates of quinolone resistance.

Skeletal infections

Oral fluoroquinolones are highly effective for Gram-negative mixed acute (or chronic) contiguous osteomyelitis, giving cure rates of 80–90% after 3- to 6-month courses. They are also effective for post-surgical cases, *Salmonella* osteitis and in some cases of chronic *P. aeruginosa* osteomyelitis (ciprofloxacin), although resistance may emerge causing a failure of treatment or relapse.[54] In patients with orthopedic prostheses infected with staphylococci, ciprofloxacin or ofloxacin in combination with rifampin have been successfully used for conservative management (i.e. preserving the prosthesis).[55,56]

Gastrointestinal infections

Typhoid and paratyphoid fevers

Although fluoroquinolones are widely regarded as the agents of choice for typhoid and paratyphoid fevers,[57,58] a Cochrane systematic review in 2005 failed to find sufficient trial evidence regarding superiority of fluoroquinolones over first-line antibiotics in children and adults.[59] However, convalescent excretion states and long-term fecal carriage are rare after fluoroquinolone therapy, thereby reducing the human reservoir and possibly leading to a fall in incidence. Carriage states persisting after other antibiotic therapy may also respond to fluoroquinolones.

Decreased quinolone susceptibility has emerged in Asia over the last 10 years. Strains are typically resistant to nalidixic acid and have raised MICs of ciprofloxacin of 0.5–1 mg/l. These strains are ciprofloxacin susceptible by Clinical and Laboratory Standards Institute (CLSI) or British Society for Antimicrobial Chemotherapy (BSAC) criteria but the clinical response to fluoroquinolones in those infected by these stains is significantly worse than with nalidixic-acid sensitive strains, and longer courses or alternative agents are recommended.[58]

Salmonellosis

A 5- to 7-day course of oral fluoroquinolone is effective in reducing the duration and severity of severe salmonellosis.

Cholera

Three-day courses of oral fluoroquinolones are equal to standard trimethoprim–sulfamethoxazole or tetracycline regimens. A cure rate of >90% can be achieved with a single 1 g dose of ciprofloxacin.[60] Reports have emerged of strains of *Vibrio cholerae* 01 with reduced susceptibility to ciprofloxacin, resulting in clinical and bacteriologic treatment failure.[61]

Shigellosis

Fluoroquinolones are the drugs of choice for invasive shigellosis. A single oral dose (ciprofloxacin 1 g) is effective in adults. Rising levels of resistance to nalidixic acid have led to the abandonment of this agent as a first-line treatment for acute shigellosis in some countries.[62]

Campylobacter

Fluoroquinolones have been used for gastrointestinal *Campylobacter* infections. However, resistance levels are increasing and may be as high as 50% in some areas of the world.[63]

Travelers' diarrhea

Ciprofloxacin or norfloxacin in full oral dosage for 5 days is effective for 80% of unprotected subjects who develop profuse diarrhea (>3–5 watery stools/day).

Other treatment indications

Ocular infections

Topical fluoroquinolones are effective for the treatment of bacterial conjunctivitis and keratitis. Penetration of systemic quinolones into the vitreous is relatively good but may not exceed the MICs of all likely pathogens. Intravitreal ciprofloxacin has been used in the treatment of endophthalmitis.[64]

Infections associated with chronic ambulatory peritoneal dialysis

Ciprofloxacin and ofloxacin have been used with success both orally and intraperitoneally. However, the emergence of resistant staphylococcal infection has limited their usefulness as monotherapy.

Q fever

Fluoroquinolones are active against *Coxiella burnetii in vitro* and a combination of a fluoroquinolone (ofloxacin) with doxycycline has been suggested for Q fever endocarditis.[65]

Anthrax

A 60-day course of ciprofloxacin is recommended for postexposure prophylaxis against anthrax.[66] In patients with inhalational anthrax a combination of ciprofloxacin plus another active agent (e.g. doxycycline) is recommended.[67]

Meningitis

Fluoroquinolones have been successfully used for Gram-negative meningitis.[68] Newer agents such as moxifloxacin show promising results in animal models of pneumococcal meningitis.[69] Trovafloxacin had comparable efficacy to ceftriaxone in a trial of pediatric meningitis.[70]

Chemoprophylaxis

Meningococcal infection

Single-dose (500 mg) ciprofloxacin is effective in eradicating nasopharyngeal carriage in over 95% of subjects.[71]

Neutropenic patients

Norfloxacin, ofloxacin and ciprofloxacin have been widely used in the prophylaxis of opportunistic infection among neutropenic patients. Although prophylaxis has been shown to prevent febrile episodes of an infectious nature, current recommendations do not suggest their use due to concerns regarding the emergence and spread of antimicrobial resistance.[72]

Travelers' diarrhea

Once-daily prophylactic use of a fluoroquinolone (e.g. norfloxacin 400 mg or ciprofloxacin 500 mg) for the duration of potential exposure gives 75–90% protection from travelers' diarrhea caused by enterotoxigenic *E. coli* and other bacterial enteropathogens.

Surgical infections

Fluoroquinolones have been used effectively for the prevention of infection following transurethral prostatectomy and biliary surgery.

Pediatric use of fluoroquinolones

Pediatric use of fluoroquinolones has been limited by concerns regarding arthropathy observed in weight-bearing diarthrodial joints in juvenile dogs after prolonged high-dose administration. In the USA the only current licensed indications for fluoroquinolone use in patients under 18 years of age are complicated UTI, pyelonephritis and postexposure treatment for inhalational anthrax. Nevertheless, accumulated

experience has established other situations in which the benefits of fluoroquinolones outweigh potential risks. These include typhoid fever, cholera and shigellosis, complicated UTI due to multiresistant pathogens, chronic suppurative otitis media caused by *P. aeruginosa*, multiresistant Gram-negative sepsis (including osteomyelitis), prophylaxis of meningococcemia (single dose) and infection in neutropenia.

Treatment of pseudomonal infections in patients with cystic fibrosis is one of the commonest indications for the use of fluoroquinolones in children. Prolonged courses are often given but there has been little evidence of related arthropathy and fluoroquinolones continue to be widely used.

DOSAGE IN SPECIAL CIRCUMSTANCES

Renal impairment

The extent to which the dosage requires modification is dependent on the degree of renal elimination. Table 139.5 shows the manufacturer's recommendations for selected quinolones. Essentially, agents such as ofloxacin and levofloxacin that are extensively renally excreted have the dose reduced to one-quarter of the normal daily dose in severe renal impairment and most other agents have the dose halved. However, as noted above, there is evidence that ciprofloxacin may not require dose modification as long as alternative routes of elimination are intact.[16] Moxifloxacin, which has only 20% renal excretion, does not require dose modification.

Hepatic impairment

Apart for extensively metabolized quinolones, such as pefloxacin, dose modification is not necessary in patients with hepatic impairment. However, experience with newer agents such as moxifloxacin in patients with severe liver failure (Child–Pugh Class C) is limited.

Elderly patients

No specific changes in dosage are required for the elderly provided appropriate changes are made for reduced renal clearance.

Pediatrics

Optimal pediatric doses have not been established. Suggested doses of ciprofloxacin are 7.5–40 mg/kg/day (oral) or 5–10 mg/kg/day (intravenous), administered on an 8–12-hourly basis.

Pregnancy and lactation

Quinolones are not approved for use in pregnancy or during lactation.

ADVERSE REACTIONS AND INTERACTIONS

Adverse drug reactions

Fluoroquinolones are generally well tolerated although there are a number of potentially serious adverse effects that have been seen in some agents.[73] When adverse effects are reported, they are usually gastrointestinal (2–20%), dermatologic (0.5–3%) and CNS (0.5–2%) reactions which rarely necessitate withdrawal of therapy (1–3%). In most cases there are no specific age or racially related effects, but adverse drug reactions are more common in neutropenic patients and possibly in people who have AIDS.

Most fluoroquinolone adverse drug reactions are class effects, but incidence varies between compounds and can often be related to the specific structure of different agents. Certain group members have specific effects or more serious class effects that have led to restrictions on

Table 139.5 Manufacturers' dosage recommendations for patients with renal impairment

	RENAL IMPAIRMENT		Hemodialysis/CAPD
	Mild	**Moderate/severe**	
Ciprofloxacin (iv)		200–400 mg 18–24 hourly (CC = 5–29 ml/min)	
Ciprofloxacin (po)	250–500 mg q12h (CC = 30–50 ml/min)	250–500 mg 18 hourly (CC = 5–29 ml/min)	250–500 mg q24h after dialysis
Ofloxacin	400 mg q24h (CC = 20–50 ml/min)	200 mg q24h (CC <20 ml/min)	
Levofloxacin	250 mg q24h* (CC = 20–50 ml/min)	250 mg 48 hourly* (CC = 10–19 ml/min)	250 mg 48 hourly* (CC = 10–19 ml/min)
Norfloxacin		400 mg q24h (CC <30 ml/min)	
Gatifloxacin		200 mg q24h† (CC <40 ml/min)	200 mg q24h† (CC <40 ml/min)
Moxifloxacin	No adjustment required		

CC, creatinine clearance.
*Initial loading dose of 500 mg.
†Short courses up to 3 days do not require dosage alteration.

use or withdrawal. For example, the phototoxicity of sparfloxacin has restricted licensing by some registration authorities, and temafloxacin, which caused hemolytic–uremic syndrome and hypoglycemia, was withdrawn in 1992.

Gastrointestinal reactions

The usual reported symptoms are nausea, anorexia and dyspepsia. While diarrhea, abdominal pain and vomiting are less frequent, they are more likely to result in discontinuation of treatment. Antibiotic-associated diarrhea caused by *Clostridium difficile* is associated with fluoroquinolone use, and all of the available fluoroquinolones have been implicated in *C. difficile* outbreaks.[74] Liver enzyme abnormalities occur in 2–3% of patients receiving fluoroquinolones and are usually mild and reversible. However, more severe liver abnormalities have been seen with some agents which, in the case of trovafloxacin, led to its withdrawal

Dermatologic reactions

Although non-specific skin rashes, pruritus and urticaria have been reported, it is phototoxicity that has received most attention. This is a class effect and is thought to be related to the photodegradation of the fluoroquinolone and its ability to induce free radicals. The incidence and severity of phototoxicity differ between agents. Structurally, a fluorine moeity at position 8 causes more phototoxicity; sparfloxacin, which has this moiety, has caused a higher rate of phototoxicity. Phototoxic reactions are rare with ciprofloxacin, ofloxacin and levofloxacin. Gemifloxacin can cause a nonphototoxic rash which is seen particularly in female patients between the ages of 20 and 40 years, and postmenopausal women taking hormone replacement therapy; increased risk of rash was also associated with more than 7 days of therapy.[75]

Central nervous system reactions

These occur in less than 2% of patients with most fluoroquinolones and usually manifest as headache, dizziness, mild tremor or drowsiness. Convulsions occur rarely both as a primary effect and as a result of interactions with theophylline or nonsteroidal anti-inflammatory drugs (NSAIDs). Although the mechanism of quinolone toxicity has not been fully elucidated, it is believed to be due to inhibition of $GABA_A$ receptors.

Musculoskeletal effects

Fluoroquinolones as a class produce destructive arthropathy in weight-bearing, diarthrodial joints of juvenile animals, notably dogs, by production of cartilage erosions after prolonged high dosage. Some agents, notably precursors such as nalidixic acid, are considerably more likely to induce arthropathy. This effect has never been observed in human children. MRI follow-up and autopsy studies in children receiving both nalidixic acid and modern fluoroquinolones have revealed no evidence of joint damage.[76] Experience with ciprofloxacin in 1500 children noted reversible arthralgia in 3.2% of patients treated for pulmonary exacerbations of cystic fibrosis.[77] In a retrospective study of more 6000 fluoroquinolone-treated children, the incidence of tendon or joint disorders was <1% and comparable to the reference group of azithromycin-treated children.[78]

Tendinitis occurs rarely as a class effect although it may be more common with concomitant corticosteroid therapy. The Achilles tendon is most commonly affected and patients are usually >50 years of age. MRI can be useful for early detection of damage and discontinuation is recommended at the first sign of tendon pain or inflammation.

Cardiovascular effects

Cardiotoxicity is manifest as prolongation of the QT interval with the potential to cause ventricular arrhythmias. The significance of this effect varies between agents and appears to be affected by substitutions at position 5 (see Fig. 139.2).[79] Of the currently available fluoroquinolones, the risk of QT interval prolongation appears to be greatest with moxifloxacin and lowest with ciprofloxacin; grepafloxacin was withdrawn voluntarily following reports of seven cardiac-related fatalities. Although adverse effects due to cardiotoxicity are rare, the risk can be minimized by avoiding the use of multiple drugs that prolong the QT interval in high-risk patients, for example those with pre-existing cardiac disease or electrolyte disturbances.[80]

Dysglycemia

Two recent studies found gatifloxacin to be associated with an increased risk of both hypo- and hyperglycemia, probably due to the competing effects of the drug on both the beta cells and islet cells of the pancreas.[81] Gatifloxacin was removed from the market in 2006. In these studies levofloxacin therapy was found to be associated with a slightly increased risk of hypoglycemia, but no dysglycemic risk was noted with moxifloxacin or ciprofloxacin.

Other (rare) effects

Hypersensitivity occurs at a frequency of ~1%. Crystalluria and secondary interstitial nephritis are rare and relate to pH-associated solubility of fluoroquinolones in urine.

Interactions with other drugs

Interactions largely occur as a result of interference with fluoroquinolone absorption or by inhibition of biotransformation of unrelated drugs by the hepatic cytochrome P450 isoenzyme system. Central nervous system interactions due to GABA receptor inhibition occur with NSAIDs, notably fenbufen, and convulsions may follow, as reported with enoxacin.

Interactions affecting absorption of fluoroquinolones

The absorption of fluoroquinolones is reduced by up to 80% by co-administration of aluminum- and magnesium-containing antacids, probably by the formation of insoluble complexes and, to a lesser extent, by calcium antacids, sucralfate and ferrous iron preparations. H_2 antagonists have no effect.

Interactions affecting drug metabolism

Fluoroquinolones reduce the hepatic clearance of xanthines via the P450 cytochrome system. The effect is most marked with enoxacin and grepafloxacin, but ciprofloxacin and pefloxacin also reduce clearance of theophylline by 30% and co-administration may result in theophylline toxicity, usually nausea but possibly convulsions. Dosage of theophylline should be interrupted or reduced and serum levels monitored if enoxacin, pefloxacin or ciprofloxacin is to be administered.

A similar effect, induced by the same fluoroquinolones, is responsible for inhibition of caffeine metabolism and resultant insomnia. Metabolism of warfarin, cimetidine and ciclosporin is affected much less by P450 cytochrome inhibition and interaction may not be clinically significant.

REFERENCES

References for this chapter can be found online at http://www.expertconsult.com

Pamela A Moise
George Sakoulas

Chapter | **140**

Glycopeptides

Vancomycin

Vancomycin, a glycopeptide antibiotic that has been available clinically for half a century, has served as the primary therapy for Gram-positive infections due to methicillin-resistant *Staphylococcus aureus* (MRSA), other methicillin-resistant staphylococci, and ampicillin-resistant *Enterococcus* spp. Its use today is greater than any other point in its history, with the surge in the past two decades of infections caused by β-lactam-resistant staphylococci and enterococci. Vancomycin demonstrates activity against Gram-positive anaerobes, diphtheroids and *Clostridium* spp., including *C. difficile*.

Vancomycin is generally considered bactericidal antibiotic – minimum bactericidal concentration:minimum inhibitory concentration (MBC:MIC) <4 – except with enterococci, but vancomycin tolerance (MBC:MIC >32) has been increasingly documented among staphylococci as a precursor to reduced glycopeptide susceptibility. When tolerance has been demonstrated, many clinicians add a second antibiotic to the regimen in treating bacteremic disease with vancomycin. For example, vancomycin is frequently combined with gentamicin to treat bacteremia or endocarditis caused by vancomycin-susceptible strains of *Enterococcus* spp.

CLINICAL PHARMACOKINETICS

Several investigators have reported the pharmacokinetics of vancomycin in human pediatric, adult and geriatric patients (Table 140.1), and in various disease states.

Absorption

Vancomycin is administered intravenously or orally. The intramuscular route is not used because of severe discomfort and the possibility of tissue necrosis. It may be also given intraperitoneally and, based on limited data, via the intraventricular, intrathecal and intravitreal route. To treat systemic infections, vancomycin should be given intravenously, and is usually infused over 1 hour. Some recommend infusing at no more than 7.5–15 mg per minute.[6]

Oral administration of vancomycin is primarily used for the treatment of *C. difficile*-associated diarrhea (CDAD). When given orally, vancomycin is not appreciably absorbed in most patients (oral bioavailability <10%). Low concentrations of vancomycin may be found in the urine of patients with normal renal function, suggesting minimal absorption from the gastrointestinal tract. The oral administration of vancomycin does not usually result in measurable concentrations of the drug in serum, even in the presence of severely impaired renal function. However, therapeutic or potentially toxic concentrations of vancomycin have been documented in patients with impaired renal function who were administered oral vancomycin to treat CDAD.[7] Therefore, when using oral vancomycin to treat CDAD in patients with gut inflammation and renal dysfunction it may be prudent to monitor vancomycin serum concentrations.

Intraperitoneal vancomycin administration is used to treat peritonitis in patients receiving peritoneal dialysis (PD). Systemic absorption of vancomycin following intraperitoneal administration is 54–65% of a given dose in 6 hours and results in adequate serum concentrations. Peritonitis causes inflammation of the peritoneal membrane, which facilitates absorption of vancomycin from the peritoneal to plasma side of the peritoneum; however, it is poorly transferred in the opposite direction.[8] One dosing regimen[9] is to administer a loading intraperitoneal dose of 30 mg/kg followed by 1.5 mg/kg in each peritoneal exchange to yield vancomycin plasma concentrations of at least 10 mg/l at 180 hours in patients with chronic renal failure. Another dosing schedule is to administer 35 mg/kg intraperitoneally on day 1, followed by 15 mg/kg intraperitoneally once daily in automated peritoneal dialysis patients, in order to provide adequate concentrations for susceptible organisms over a 24-hour period.[8]

Intrathecal and intraventricular administration of vancomycin has been used for the treatment of central nervous system infections,[10] although systemic absorption of vancomycin following intrathecal or intraventricular administration has not been investigated. It is unlikely that intrathecal or intraventricular administration of vancomycin would achieve therapeutic or toxic serum concentrations, even in patients with impaired renal function, because the amounts of vancomycin administered by these routes are generally small (approximately 10–20 mg).

Intravitreal dosing of vancomycin has been administered for postoperative bacterial endophthalmitis.[5] As with intrathecal and intraventricular administration of vancomycin, the amounts of intravitreal vancomycin administered are small (~0.2–2 mg) so accumulation to appreciable serum concentrations is highly unlikely.

Distribution

Compared with aminoglycosides, the variability in the volume of distribution (Vd) of vancomycin is large, with a Vd ranging from 0.5 to 1.0 l/kg in non-obese adults with normal renal function (creatinine clearance >80 ml/min). In clinical practice, an average Vd of 0.7 l/kg is usually used. The Vd of vancomycin can be affected by factors such as age, gender and body weight. However, the Vd of vancomycin is far less dependent on patient fluid balance (underhydration or overhydration) than the Vd of aminoglycosides. Also, the Vd of vancomycin is not significantly correlated with creatinine clearance.

Peak serum concentrations of vancomycin are approximately proportional to the dose of drug infused. Administration of 500 mg, 1000 mg or 2000 mg of vancomycin to healthy volunteers resulted

Table 140.1 Vancomycin pharmacokinetics

Age	n	CL$_{cr}$ (ml/min)	t$_{1/2\alpha}$ (h)	t$_{1/2\beta}$ (h)	V$_c$ (l/kg)	V$_{ss}$ (l/kg)	Cl$_V$ (ml/min)	CL$_R$ (ml/min)
Premature neonates (30–34 weeks,* <1.2 kg)[1]	5	–	–	7.8 ± 3.0	–	0.47 ± 0.21	0.72 ± 0.23 ml/min/kg	–
Premature neonates (30–42 weeks,* ≥1.2 kg)[1]	6	–	–	3.8 ± 1.4	–	0.48 ± 0.13	1.58 ± 0.65 ml/min/kg	–
Premature neonates (>42 weeks,* >2.0 kg)[1]	2	–	–	2.1 ± 0.8	–	0.47 ± 0.06	2.82 ± 0.85 ml/min/kg	–
Premature neonates (26–45 weeks*)[2]	59	–	–	–	–	0.67	3.56 l/hr/kg	–
Neonates (26–42 weeks*)[3]	108	–	–	6.0	–	0.43 ± 0.01	0.95 ± 0.03 ml/min/kg	–
Children (0.01–18 years)[4]	78	138.6 ± 49.3	–	3.9	0.27 ± 0.07	0.43	1.72 ml/min/kg	–
Adults (46.3 ± 11.6 years)[5]	10	93.4 ± 28.3	0.40 ± 0.20	5.2 ± 2.6	0.21 ± 0.11	0.50 ± 0.20	98.4 ± 24.3	88.0 ± 33.6
Adults (49.5 ± 14.3 years)[5]	14	51.0 ± 8.3	0.49 ± 0.32	10.5 ± 3.6	0.21 ± 0.14	0.59 ± 0.27	52.6 ± 17.7	48.2 ± 10.8
Adults (61.6 ± 18.4 years)[5]	13	23.9 ± 8.2	1.51 ± 0.21	19.9 ± 10.2	0.24 ± 0.12	0.64 ± 0.18	31.3 ± 14.9	19.8 ± 7.9

CL$_{cr}$, creatinine clearance in ml/min/1.73 m^2 unless otherwise noted; t$_{1/2\alpha}$, distribution half-life; t$_{1/2\beta}$, elimination half-life; V$_c$, apparent distribution volume of the central compartment; V$_{ss}$, distribution volume at steady-state; CL$_V$, total body vancomycin clearance in ml/min/1.73 m^2 unless otherwise noted; CL$_R$, renal vancomycin clearance in ml/min/1.73 m^2 unless otherwise noted.
*Postconceptional age, i.e. sum of gestational age at birth and chronologic age.

in vancomycin serum concentrations of approximately 2–10 mg/l, 25 mg/l and 45 mg/l, respectively, 2 hours after the dose.[11]

The disposition of vancomycin after intravenous administration has been described with one-, two-, and three-compartment models. The half-life of the first distributive phase is short (approximately 0.4 hours), whereas the half-life of the terminal phase is dependent on the patient's renal function. The one-compartment model is most widely used by clinicians but its application requires postdistribution serum samples, which are often difficult to obtain accurately. The two-compartment model results in a significant improvement in both bias and precision in predicting vancomycin concentrations.

Investigations in health volunteers and patients with normal renal function have suggested that approximately 30–55% of vancomycin is bound to plasma proteins. Data concerning the penetration of vancomycin into various body fluids and body compartments are summarized in Table 140.2.

Metabolism

Approximately 80–90% of the intravenously administered vancomycin dose can be recovered unchanged in the urine in 24 hours, with very small amounts appearing in bile. By most authorities, the metabolism of the drug is not sufficiently altered in liver failure to warrant changes in vancomycin dosing. However, some suggest dose adjustments in patients with severe liver dysfunction.[19]

Excretion

The majority (80–90%) of an intravenous vancomycin dose can be recovered unchanged in the urine of adults with normal to moderately impaired renal function. Dosage adjustment is necessary in patients

with impaired renal function because elimination is primarily by glomerular filtration. The clearance of vancomycin approximates 65% of creatinine clearance. Differences between vancomycin and creatinine clearance suggests either renal tubular reabsorption or significant protein binding. Some investigators suggest that tubular secretion may be a significant component of vancomycin's net renal excretion.[20] Vancomycin clearance appears to correlate better with actual total body weight in obese patients.[21]

Creatinine clearance is often expressed as ml/kg/min and this value is multiplied by the patient's actual body weight (kg). However, it is important to exclude excessive third space fluid from the total body weight, since this weight would not be expected to be associated with an increase in the renal clearance of vancomycin. Creatinine clearance in ml/kg/min can be calculated by dividing the creatinine clearance by the patient's weight initially used to calculate the creatinine clearance.

Effects of disease states and conditions

Disease states and conditions that affect a patient's renal function will influence vancomycin elimination. In patients with normal renal function, the usual serum half-life of vancomycin is 6–10 hours, and in patients with end-stage renal disease, the half-life may approach 7 days.

The clearance rate for vancomycin increases in proportion to creatinine clearance. Patients with acute renal failure appear to eliminate vancomycin differently from patients with chronic renal failure. In patients with acute oliguric renal failure, substantial nonrenal clearance (approximately 16 ml/min; range 3.8–23.3 ml/min) of vancomycin appears to occur initially.[22] Then, as the duration of renal failure increases, the nonrenal clearance decreases, and eventually approaches the total clearance observed in patients with chronic renal failure (4–6 ml/min).

Table 140.2 Vancomycin penetration into various human body fluids and tissues following intravenous administration

Body fluid or tissue	Patient description	n	Tissue or fluid concentration range (mean), mg/l	Concomitant serum concentration range (mean), mg/l	% Tissue or fluid penetration
Cerebrospinal fluid[12]	Adults receiving ventriculoperitoneal shunts for hydrocephalus	25	0.1–1.5 (0.9)	9.1–38.7 (22.3)	4.6
Cerebrospinal fluid [13]	Hemodialysis adults with proved or suspected CNS infection	3*	<0.5–1.54 (0.92)	8.8–24.0 (15.8)	5.9
Cerebrospinal fluid [14]	Premature infants	3	2.2–5.6	–	26–68
Heart valve[15]	Adults undergoing open heart surgery	33	0–2h post-dose: 4.2 5–6h post-dose: 2.3	28.9 4.4	14.5 52.3
Pleural fluid[4]	Critically ill, ventilated patients	14	0.4–8.1 (4.5)	9–37.4 (24)	~18.8
Lung tissue[16]	Adults with normal kidney and liver function undergoing thoracotomy	26	6.9–40.6	2.4–9.6	24–41
Mammary tissue[17] aCapsular tissue bPericapsular tissue	Adult women undergoing reconstructive surgery	24	a2.0–7.7 (4.6) b2.3–18.1 (6.4)	3.1–38.8 (14.0)	a58 b74
Peritoneal dialysis fluid[18]	Adults with peritonitis and on chronic intermittent peritoneal dialysis	6	Undetectable to 22.5	–	0–96 (mean, 27)

% Penetration = fluid or tissue vancomycin concentration/serum vancomycin concentration × 100.
*Two CSF and two serum samples obtained during each episode of meningitis.

Major burn injuries (>30% body surface area) can cause significant increases in vancomycin clearance due to increases in the basal metabolic rate, with consequential increase in glomerular filtration rate and vancomycin clearance, that occurs within 72 hours of injury. The average half-life of vancomycin in burn patients is only 4 hours. Therefore, burn patients may require more frequent dosing of vancomycin (every 6–8 hours) to maintain therapeutic trough concentrations. Due to the variability in predicting creatinine clearance from serum creatinine data in burn patients, it may be prudent to measure creatinine clearance for all predictions of vancomycin pharmacokinetics.[21]

Intravenous drug abusers, critically ill patients and obese patients with normal serum creatinine concentrations (the last due to hyperfiltration) have considerably increased vancomycin clearance.[21]

Cardiac bypass appears to have no significant effect on the pharmacokinetics of vancomycin. A recent investigation found an abrupt decrease in vancomycin serum concentrations at the onset of cardiopulmonary bypass, followed by a moderate increase possibly secondary to redistribution from tissues.[23] This rebound in vancomycin serum concentration may occur at the time of reperfusion and warming. A significant relationship was found between the rebound in vancomycin concentration in serum and the length of time between unclamping the aorta and coming off cardiopulmonary bypass (r=0.94), as well as with the increase in temperature upon rewarming (r=0.92).[24] However, it appears that a 15 mg/kg intravenous dose of vancomycin administered 1 hour prior to bypass provides therapeutic serum concentrations for up to 6 hours.

The elimination half-life of vancomycin is significantly longer in elderly persons aged >65 years (12.1 hours) compared to younger subjects (7.2 hours).[25,26] Vancomycin dosing adjustments may be necessary in the elderly, even those with normal serum creatinine concentrations, due to the longer half-live of vancomycin in this patient population.

Effects of dialysis

An important element that needs to be taken in consideration in patients undergoing hemodialysis is the elimination of vancomycin in different types of membrane and with different dialysis techniques (intermittent and continuous). Although vancomycin is not significantly dialyzable when hemodialysis is performed using a low flux membrane, significant amounts of vancomycin are cleared in the dialysate with high-flux or high-efficiency hemodialysis using membranes such as polysulfone, polyacrylonitrile and polymethylmethacrylate (Table 140.3).[27–35] Early studies estimated that up to 30% of vancomycin is removed during high-flux hemodialysis. However, due to the unrecognized redistribution of vancomycin after completion of dialysis, a more recent report indicated that only approximately 17% of vancomycin is removed during high-flux hemodialysis.[32] It is important to note that high-flux membranes have largely replaced traditional low-flux membranes in hemodialysis and dosing of vancomycin needs to reflect this transition in order to maintain adequate vancomycin concentrations in these patients.

In patients undergoing continuous ambulatory peritoneal dialysis (CAPD), the small but continuous drug loss is significant. Vancomycin is often administered intravenously approximately every 3–5 days or administered directly into the peritoneal space to maintain desired plasma concentrations.[36]

PHARMACODYNAMICS

Clinical response

Data correlating pharmacodynamic indices with clinical response to vancomycin are summarized in Table 140.4. Studies suggest that vancomycin has concentration-independent cidal activity over Gram-positive

Table 140.3 Elimination of vancomycin in hemodialysis and hemofiltration

Investigator	n	Dialysis	Membrane	CL$_{HD}$ (ml/min)
Alwakeel et al.[27]	8	HD	Cuprophan	15
Lanese et al.[28]	6	HD	Cuprophan	9.6
Torras et al.[29]	8	HD	Cuprophan	9.7
Alwakeel et al.[27]	15	HD	Polyacrylonitrile	55
Torras et al.[29]	8	HD	Polyacrylonitrile	58.4
Zoer et al.[30]	7	HD	Polyacrylonitrile	45.7
Alwakeel et al.[27]	12	HD	Polysulfone	76
Foote et al.[31]	5	HD	Polysulfone	130.7
Lanese et al.[28]	6	HD	Polysulfone	44.7–85.2
Pollard et al.[32]	12	HD	Polysulfone	120
Touchette et al.[33]	8	HD	Polysulfone	108.5
Bellomo et al.[34]	16	CAVHDF	Polyacrylonitrile	6.9–15.4
Joy et al.[35]	5	CVVH	Polysulfone	5.2–22.1
Joy et al.[35]	5	CVVH	Polymethylmethacrylate	7.5–27
Joy et al.[35]	5	CVVH	Acrylonitrile	5.8–13.4

CAVHDF, continuous arteriovenous hemodiafiltration; CL$_{HD}$, hemodialysis clearance; CVVH, continuous venovenous hemofiltration; HD, hemodialysis.

Table 140.4 Vancomycin pharmacokinetic (PK) and pharmacodynamic (PD) data from select *in vitro*, animal and human studies predictive of success

Investigators	Organism	Model/patients	PK parameter or PD index and value
Larsson et al.[37]	*Staphylococcus aureus*	*In-vitro* PD model	T >MIC ≈100%
Duffull et al.[38]	*Staphylococcus aureus*	*In-vitro* PD model	T >MBC ≈100%
Ackerman et al.[39]	*Staphylococcus aureus* CONS	*In-vitro* model	No relationship between VAN concentration and killing curves
Knudsen et al.[40]	*Staphylococcus aureus* *Streptococcus pneumoniae*	Murine peritonitis	T >MIC, C_{max}:MIC, AUC_{24h}:MIC
Ahmed et al.[41]	*Streptococcus pneumoniae*	Rabbit meningitis model	CSF C_{max}:MBC ≥4
Lisby-Sutch & Nahata[1]	*Staphylococcus aureus* CONS *Enterococcus*, group D	Infants with a variety of infections	C_{max} 25–35 mg/l (SBT ≥1:8) C_{min} 5–10 mg/l (SBT 1:2 to 1:8)
Schaad et al.[25]	*Staphylococcus aureus* *Staphylococcus epidermidis*	Children with a variety of infections	C_{max} >25 mg/l (SBT ~1:16) C_{min} <12 mg/l (SBT ~1:4)
Louria et al.[42]	*Staphylococcus aureus*	Adults with a variety of infections	SBT ≥1:8
Sorrell et al.[43]	*Staphylococcus aureus*	Patients with bacteremia	MBC:MIC <32
Iwamoto et al.[44]	MRSA	Patients with pneumonia or bacteremia	C_{max} >25 mg/l C_{min} 10–15 mg/l
Moise et al.[45]	MRSA	Adults with lower respiratory tract infections	Clinical success: AUC_{24h}:MIC >345 Bacterial eradication: AUC_{24h}:MIC >428

CONS, coagulase-negative staphylococci; CSF, cerebrospinal fluid; MBC, minimum bactericidal concentration; MIC, minimum inhibitory concentration; MRSA, methicillin-resistant *Staphylococcus aureus*; SBT, serum bactericidal titers; UAC, area under the curve; VAN, vancomycin.

organisms, although some investigators propose the need to achieve certain peak and trough concentrations for optimal activity.[37,39,46,47] Once vancomycin concentrations exceed the MBC or four times MIC, vancomycin displays concentration-independent killing above which further increases in concentration do not increase the cidal activity according to *in-vitro* models and animal data.[41]

In-vitro pharmacodynamic models found vancomycin to display concentration-independent activity.[37,38] In one study, bolus doses achieving C_{max} values of 5, 10, 20 and 40 mg/l yielded similar time-kill curves against *S. aureus*. However, bactericidal activity was more efficient under aerobic conditions. The time to achieve a 3-log kill of bacteria was approximately twice as long in an anaerobic environment compared to an aerobic one.[48]

Ahmed and colleagues[41] reported the relationship between the bactericidal ratio of vancomycin in the cerebrospinal fluid (C_{max}:MBC ratio) and the rate of bacterial clearance of *Streptococcus pneumoniae* (vancomycin MBC = 0.5 mg/l) in a rabbit model of experimental meningitis. Animals were administered 80 mg/kg of vancomycin in two or four divided doses, with and without dexamethasone, over 36 hours. The concomitant administration of dexamethasone significantly reduced the penetration of vancomycin into the CSF from 20.1% to 14.3% ($p = 0.035$). Maximal cidal activity was achieved at concentrations fourfold greater than the MBC, above which no additional killing was observed.

A clinical investigation of *S. aureus* bacteremia[43] found an MBC:MIC ratio <32 to be predictive of successful response to vancomycin ($p = 0.04$). All 10 patients with an MBC:MIC ratio <32 experienced a vancomycin treatment success. However, only one of four infections with an MBC:MIC ratio >32 was considered a treatment success. All eight patients infected with *S. aureus* isolates having an MBC <32 mg/l were cured and three of six patients with an MBC >32 mg/l were cured of their infection. This difference was not statistically significant ($p = 0.11$). The investigators concluded that there is not a simple relationship between *in-vitro* tests and clinical response to vancomycin therapy, but tolerance was associated with poor therapeutic response. Several clinical investigators have demonstrated a relationship between successful response to vancomycin therapy and bactericidal serum titers of at least 1:8.[1,25,42]

A recent investigation[44] showed that vancomycin trough concentrations of 10–15 mg/l and peak concentrations >25 mg/l are optimal for MRSA-related pneumonia and bacteremia. Therapeutic failures have been reported in patients with endocarditis with vancomycin plasma trough concentrations <10 mg/l.[49] Small studies suggest that serum bactericidal titers of >1:8 are associated with vancomycin treatment successes.[1,25] These clinical investigations suggest that individualization of vancomycin dosage may be required for optimum therapy.

Adverse effects

Ototoxicity (<2%) and nephrotoxicity (5%) are well-recognized but relatively infrequent adverse events associated with vancomycin therapy and may be concentration related.[44,50] Attempts to relate serum concentrations of vancomycin to the development of nephrotoxicity have been difficult, although many studies suggest that the current preparations of vancomycin may have less potential for nephrotoxicity than earlier preparations. Farber and Moellering[50] reported a 5% incidence of nephrotoxicity in patients receiving vancomycin alone. In virtually all of the patients investigated, the renal function returned to baseline following discontinuation of vancomycin therapy. In contrast, when vancomycin was administered concomitantly with an aminoglycoside to adults, the incidence of nephrotoxicity was higher in some of the studies (range 22–35%).[50–53] Patients with neutropenia, peritonitis, increased age, liver disease, concurrent amphotericin B therapy and those of male gender may also have an increased risk of developing nephrotoxicity.[53]

While concerns regarding nephrotoxicity associated with vancomycin therapy have been mostly historical, their recent revival has been based on more aggressive dosing to treat *S. aureus* strains with increasing vancomycin MICs. Since it is accepted that the area under the concentration–time curve:minimum inhibitory concentration (AUC:MIC) is predictive of vancomycin treatment success in pneumonia, an increase in MIC of 0.5 mg/l to 2 mg/l would require a fourfold increase in patient exposure to the drug AUC to maintain the same ratio. If a 24-hour AUC:MIC of 400 is the target, then a 24-hour AUC of 800 would be required to treat an infection by an organism with a vancomycin MIC of 2 mg/l. This corresponds to mean serum concentrations of vancomycin of approximately 33 mg/l (peak serum concentration ~45 mg/l and trough ~25 mg/l). The doses required for such serum concentrations are frequently done with great hesitation, especially in light of some recent data suggesting potential nephrotoxicity associated with higher vancomycin doses.[54–56] While these studies are certainly not definitive in showing dose-related vancomycin nephrotoxicity, a more recent study was more definitive in associating nephrotoxicity with >4 g/day of vancomycin.[57] While this dose is higher than most clinicians are using, it is clear that these studies suggest an increasing awareness of this risk. A definitive study showing nephrotoxicity at <4 g/day may be difficult given the multitude of other causes of nephrotoxicity in the hospital environment.

Investigations on vancomycin-induced ototoxicity (hearing loss or tinnitus) have raised the possibility that ototoxicity may be related to excessively high serum concentrations (>80 mg/l), with recommendations to avoid serum vancomycin concentrations >50 mg/l.[50,58] A comparison of once- versus twice-daily vancomycin found no statistically different rates in ototoxicity rates.[59] Hearing loss developed in 1 of 31 (3.2%) and 5 of 32 (15.6%) in the once- and twice-daily groups, respectively. A recent case report has described a patient who developed ototoxicity after intrathecal administration of vancomycin,[60] although the relationship between intrathecal administration of vancomycin and ototoxicity requires further study.

A contemporary evaluation of vancomycin ototoxicity comparing baseline audiograms to audiograms after approximately 4 weeks of vancomycin therapy demonstrated 0% worsening in 32 patients aged <53 years but a 19% worsening in patients aged ≥53 years.[60A] The clinical significance and reversibility of these findings warrant a prospective clinical evaluation but they draw considerable attention to potential risks of vancomycin in older patients.

Nonconcentration-related toxicities have also been reported with vancomycin. Rapid intravenous infusion of vancomycin, >500 mg per 30 minutes in normal adults, may result in a non-IgE-mediated histamine reaction characterized by flushing, local pruritus, erythema of the neck and upper torso, tachycardia and/or hypotension.[61,62] This reaction, often referred to as 'red man syndrome', may occur at any point in the infusion and may occur for the first time after several doses or with slow infusion.[63] The effects of this reaction can be relieved by antihistamines.[64–66] The incidence of red man syndrome varies between 3.7% and 47% in infected patients,[67] and is between 30% and 90% in healthy volunteers.[62] It has been suggested that a relationship may exist between the area under the histamine concentration time curve and severity of the reaction.[68] It has been the authors' experience that some patients who experience flushing near the end of their infusion may have their symptoms relieved without discontinuation of the drug by administering the medication as a continuous infusion. It is important to realize that concomitant opiates for analgesia can potentiate the mast cell destabilization of vancomycin and patients receiving this class of medication may be at increased risk for red man syndrome.

Eosinophilia, neutropenia, rashes (including exfoliative dermatitis), Stevens–Johnson syndrome (infrequent), immune-mediated thrombocytopenia and drug fever also have been reported with vancomycin.

VANCOMYCIN RESISTANCE CONSIDERATIONS

The breakpoints of resistance to vancomycin in *S. aureus* are shown in Table 140.5. Unlike β-lactam antibiotics which bind to and interrupt the activity of penicillin-binding proteins, enzymes involved in cell

Table 140.5 Vancomycin susceptibility for *Staphylococcus aureus*

Vancomycin susceptibility	Abbreviation	MIC (μ/ml)
Susceptible	VSSA	≤2
Heteroresistant	hVISA	1–2*
Intermediate	VISA	4–8
Resistant	VRSA	≥16†

hVISA, heteroresistant vancomycin-intermediate *S. aureus*; VISA, vancomycin-intermediate *S. aureus*; VRSA, vancomycin-resistant *S. aureus*; VSSA, vancomycin-susceptible *S. aureus*.
*Consist of subpopulations (≤10⁻⁶) that may grow in media containing >2 μg/ml vancomycin.
†Requires back-up primary testing with 6 μg/ml vancomycin overnight plate.
Data from Clinical Laboratory Standards Institute. Performance standards for antimicrobial disc susceptibility tests; 16th informational supplement. Report M100-S16. Wayne, PA: National Committee for Clinical Laboratory Standards; 2006.

wall synthesis, vancomycin binds with high affinity to the D-alanyl-D-alanine (D-Ala-D-Ala) C-terminus of late peptidoglycan precursors and prevents reactions of cell wall synthesis utilizing these precursors in transglycosylase, transpeptidase and carboxypeptidase.[69] Resistance in vancomycin-resistant enterococci (VRE) and vancomycin-resistant *S. aureus* (VRSA) is due to the presence of operons that encode enzymes which produce the low affinity precursors D-Ala-D-lactate or D-Ala-D-serine and enzymes that eliminate competitive high-affinity peptidoglycan precursors that are normally produced.

In vancomycin-intermediate *S. aureus* (VISA) strains, altered cellular physiology results in cumulative effects of mutations and/or modulation of regulatory systems. This altered physiology appears to alter cell wall metabolism in such a way as to result in increased numbers of D-Ala-D-Ala target sites for vancomycin binding. This altered cell wall results in a reduced diffusion coefficient of vancomycin, sequestration of vancomycin within the cell wall by these false targets, and prevention of vancomycin reaching its site of action.[69] In addition, studies of *S. aureus* with reduced vancomycin susceptibility and isogenic vancomycin-susceptible progenitors showed cell walls with reduced peptidoglycan cross linking, reduced cell wall turnover and reduced autolysis that investigators suggested may be due to alterations in teichoic acid structure and metabolism.[70] These metabolic changes result in considerable morphologic cell wall thickening.[71]

The phenotype of many VISA strains is unstable, suggesting that the regulatory foci can be turned on or off depending on whether glycopeptide is present. Some of the genes whose expression has been found to be altered in glycopeptide-intermediate *S. aureus* (GISA) include *agr*, *pbp2*, *pbp4*, *pbpD*, *sigB*, *ddh*, *tcaA* and *vraSR*. However, what is now clear is that the end result of altered cell wall metabolism, rather than the specific genetic mechanisms achieving this altered metabolism, is of primary importance.[72]

While VISA and VRSA remain extremely rare, cases of glycopeptide treatment failure are common. Recent studies demonstrate increased clinical failure of vancomycin therapy in MRSA infections where the isolates have increased MICs that are still within the susceptible range. For example, comparing 51 patients with infections by MRSA with vancomycin MICs of 2 mg/l with 44 patients with MICs of <2 mg/l, response was significantly lower in the high MIC group (62% vs 85%, $p=0.02$), infection-related mortality was higher (24% vs 10%) and high MIC was an independent predictor of poor response in multivariate analysis.[54] The most recent study evaluating outcome and vancomycin MIC for susceptible MRSA showed a higher mortality when vancomycin was used empirically and the organism was found to have a vancomycin MIC of 2 mg/l by E-test with an odds ratio of 6.39 ($p<0.001$).[73] Clearly these results point to a need to re-evaluate the microbiologic breakpoint for vancomycin in *S. aureus* for bacteremia and pneumonia.

Why this discrepancy in clinical and microbiologic definitions for vancomycin? The answer is complex, but may relate to the heterogeneous resistance of staphylococci to glycopeptides, whereby small subpopulations, perhaps <1 in 10⁶, exist that can grow in higher concentrations of vancomycin than the MIC predicts. We refer to these strains as hetero-VISA (see Table 140.5). Such small populations may not be detected by low inocula testing used by standard microbiology laboratory methods, although these subpopulations may certainly exist *in vivo* in a pneumonia or an endocardial vegetation. The higher the vancomycin MIC, the more likely that these resistant subpopulations (hVISA) will be present[74] (see also Chapter 131).

CLINICAL APPLICATION OF PHARMACOKINETIC DATA AND DOSING CONSIDERATIONS

An understanding of the desired therapeutic range and pharmacokinetic parameters of vancomycin enables the clinician to select dosing strategies specific for the individual patient. Dosing nomograms for vancomycin are available, but due to the pharmacokinetic variability of vancomycin arising from nonrenal factors, it seems impractical to rely exclusively on nomograms that are based on renal function alone. In addition, studies have shown that the published nomograms may significantly underpredict vancomycin steady-state peak and/or trough concentrations. At this time, there appears to be no benefit in monitoring peak vancomycin serum concentrations. Trough concentrations are monitored before the fourth dose in patients whose creatinine clearance is in steady state, and then weekly for patients on vancomycin therapy for more than 2 weeks. Ideally, a baseline serum creatinine concentration and complete blood count are obtained before vancomycin therapy is initiated and then weekly thereafter. If the creatinine clearance is not in steady state or if the patient is receiving other nephrotoxic agents such as aminoglycosides or amphotericin B, serum creatinine and vancomycin serum troughs may need more frequent (two or three times per week) monitoring. Serum vancomycin trough concentrations are maintained at 10–20 mg/l, not necessarily for therapeutic benefit, but to prevent development of glycopeptide resistance.[48,75] If serum creatinine concentrations increase by more than 0.5 mg/dl over the baseline value (or more than 25–30% over baseline for serum creatinine values >2 mg/dl), and other causes of decrease in renal function are ruled out, alternatives for vancomycin may be warranted.

Ototoxicity is generally monitored at the same time intervals as serum creatinine determination. Instead of using audiometry, clinical signs and symptoms of auditory or vestibular ototoxicity are usually monitored in the clinical setting. Symptoms of auditory ototoxicity include decreased hearing acuity in conversational range, feeling of fullness or pressure in the ears and tinnitus. Symptoms of vestibular ototoxicity include loss of equilibrium, headache, nausea, vomiting, vertigo, nystagmus and/or ataxia.

As with all antibiotics, the development of resistance to the glycopeptides is inevitable and currently there is a growing understanding that what has been traditionally rendered a susceptible definition microbiologically may not necessarily correspond to successful treatment outcome, particularly with serious MRSA infections such as bacteremia, endocarditis and pneumonia. Therefore, emerging data appear to place vancomycin in a role analogous to that of penicillin for *Streptococcus pneumoniae* infections. This means that for the serious infections mentioned above, optimal empiric therapy may consist of the newer Gram-positive antimicrobials (e.g. linezolid for pneumonia, daptomycin for bacteremia), with 'de-escalation' to vancomycin once the vancomycin is confirmed at ≤1 mg/l. While it may seem intuitive to seek alternative therapies to glycopeptides for serious MRSA infections (i.e. pneumonia and bacteremia) when the organism has a vancomycin MIC of 2 mg/l, no study has been performed comparing vancomycin to daptomycin or linezolid under these microbiological circumstances. In addition, the role of combination therapy, for example with aminoglycosides or rifampin (rifampicin), also warrants further study. Readers should also be informed of the recent consensus statement on vancomycin administration published by leading authorities in this field during the production stages of this text.[75A]

Teicoplanin

Teicoplanin (formerly called teichomycin A) is a complex of five closely related glycopeptides that have the same heptapeptide base and an aglycone that contains aromatic amino acids, with D-mannose and N-acetyl-D-glucosamine as sugars, with a molecular weight of 1562–1891 Da. Teicoplanin is structurally similar to vancomycin. It is produced from the actinomycete *Actinoplanes teichomyceticus*.

Teicoplanin is similar but not identical to vancomycin in its spectrum of activity. The MICs for most Gram-positive bacteria and anaerobes are comparable, but teicoplanin is less active against some strains of *Staphylococcus haemolyticus* (MIC 16–64 mg/l compared to ≤4 mg/l for vancomycin). Its ease of administration and its low toxicity potential make it a suitable alternative to vancomycin for the treatment of Gram-positive aerobic and anaerobic bacteria in both the immunocompetent and the immunocompromised host. *In-vitro* activity against most Gram-positive organisms is equal to or greater than that of vancomycin.

In both open and comparative clinical trials, teicoplanin has been well tolerated, and adverse reactions have rarely prompted discontinuation of treatment. Nephrotoxicity caused by teicoplanin is uncommon, even when it is used concomitantly with aminoglycosides. Favorable pharmacokinetics allows for intramuscular administration as well as intravenous bolus dosing and, after appropriate loading doses, maintenance therapy may be given on a once-daily basis. The combination of all of these factors makes teicoplanin an effective, safe alternative to vancomycin in the treatment of Gram-positive infections. Although it is widely used in Europe, it is not approved by the Food and Drug Administration in the USA.

PHARMACOKINETICS AND DISTRIBUTION

Teicoplanin binds to the terminal D-Ala-D-Ala sequence of peptides that form the bacterial cell wall and, by sterically hindering the transpeptidase and transglycosylation reaction, inhibits the formation of peptidoglycan. Teicoplanin is a large polar molecule and, as it cannot penetrate the lipid membrane of Gram-negative bacteria, they are resistant to it (see Chapter 130). Enterococci expressing VanA (high-level) vancomycin resistance are also resistant to teicoplanin. Teicoplanin is not significantly absorbed from the gastrointestinal tract but it can be administered intravenously or intramuscularly, in a once-daily dosing schedule. It has a long half-life of approximately 47 hours, allowing for once-daily dosing once therapeutic serum levels are attained. In a study in which healthy volunteers were given intravenous injections of teicoplanin, doses of 3 mg/kg gave average peak plasma concentrations of 53.5 µg/ml and doses of 6 mg/kg gave average peak plasma concentrations of 111.8 µg/ml.[77] Bioavailability after intramuscular injection of teicoplanin is 90%, with peak plasma concentration occurring 2 hours after injection.[76]

Teicoplanin is approximately 90% protein-bound. It is more lipophilic than vancomycin and has excellent penetration into tissues and tissue fluids with a large volume of distribution after intravenous administration. High concentrations are achieved in peritoneal and blister fluid, bile, liver, pancreas, mucosa and bone.[77] Penetration into cerebrospinal fluid across uninflamed meninges is poor.

Teicoplanin does not undergo extensive metabolism and is excreted almost entirely by the kidneys.[78] As with vancomycin, its half-life is prolonged by renal failure.[79] Neither hemodialysis nor peritoneal dialysis significantly affects the clearance of teicoplanin.

ADMINISTRATION AND DOSAGE

Dosing recommendations for adults who have normal renal function have been based on both pharmacokinetic properties and results of open and comparative clinical trials. A single loading dose of 400 mg on the first day followed by maintenance doses of 200 mg/day (3 mg/kg/day for pediatric dose) appears adequate for the treatment of urinary tract infections, skin and soft tissue infections and lower respiratory tract infections. For serious infections, including endocarditis, osteomyelitis and sepsis, it is necessary to maintain serum concentrations of teicoplanin at 10 µg/ml or more.[80]

Treatment of endocarditis caused by *S. aureus* has been difficult with teicoplanin, especially when used as monotherapy.[80,81] In these cases, it is recommended that an aminoglycoside should be added and that teicoplanin trough levels should be maintained in the range of 20–60 µg/ml.

INDICATIONS

Indications for the use of teicoplanin are similar to those for vancomycin (Table 140.6). They include Gram-positive infections caused by strains that are resistant to penicillin, cephalosporin or methicillin, or Gram-positive infections in patients who are allergic to penicillin. In addition, teicoplanin may be used for subacute bacterial endocarditis or surgical prophylaxis, in patients who are allergic to β-lactam drugs and as an alternative to vancomycin or metronidazole in the treatment of pseudomembranous colitis caused by *C. difficile* (approved in Europe).

Teicoplanin, alone or in combination with other antibiotics, has proved effective in the treatment of various Gram-positive infections, including sepsis, endocarditis, skin and soft tissue infections, osteomyelitis and lower respiratory infections. It has also been found to be effective in both prophylaxis and treatment of Hickman catheter infections in immunocompromised patients.[82,83] Specially prepared catheters loaded with teicoplanin have been developed and tested *in vitro* and have been shown to prevent bacterial colonization for at least 48 hours, thus showing promise for inhibiting early-onset catheter infections.[84] Teicoplanin has also been used along with other antibiotics for empiric treatment of febrile neutropenic patients and in the treatment of documented Gram-positive infections in neutropenic patients.[85,86]

Table 140.6 Indications for the use of teicoplanin

Infections with:	*Staphylococcus* spp., including methicillin-resistant strains *Streptococcus* spp., *Streptococcus agalactiae*, *Streptococcus bovis* (recently renamed *Streptococcus gallolyticus*), *Streptococcus pneumoniae*, *Streptococcus pyogenes* and viridans streptococci Enterococci *Clostridium* spp., including *Clostridium difficile* *Corynebacterium* spp., including *Corynebacterium jeikeium*
The following types of infection with the above organisms	Sepsis Endocarditis Skin and soft tissue infections Osteomyelitis Lower respiratory tract infections Diarrhea associated with *Clostridium difficile* Nosocomial intravascular catheter infections (prophylaxis and treatment)

Courtesy of Jihad Slim & Leon Smith.

Oral teicoplanin is as effective as vancomycin in the treatment of diarrhea associated with *C. difficile*. A 10-day course or regimen of 100 mg oral teicoplanin q12h was found to be as effective as 500 mg oral vancomycin q6h.[87] Again, the risk of glycopeptide resistance development argues for the use of metronidazole for routine therapy for *C. difficile*-associated diarrhea.

DOSAGE IN SPECIAL CIRCUMSTANCES

A dosage nomogram for teicoplanin has been designed,[88] based on the relationship between teicoplanin clearance and creatinine clearance and an average desired steady-state concentration of 20 µg/ml. Although intravenous teicoplanin penetrates well into peritoneal fluid in normal patients, it does not penetrate well into the effluent of CAPD patients and is not recommended for the treatment of peritonitis in these patients. Intraperitoneal teicoplanin has been effective in CAPD patients who have Gram-positive peritonitis, however.

Another regimen for renal-impaired patients includes a normal loading dose followed by doubling the dosage interval for patients who have a creatinine clearance of 30–80 ml/minute and tripling the dosage interval for patients who have severe renal impairment (creatinine clearance <10 ml/minute).

ADVERSE REACTIONS AND INTERACTIONS

Teicoplanin is generally well tolerated at therapeutic dosages, with side-effects occurring in approximately 6–13% of the patients (Table 140.7).

Side-effects (including nephrotoxicity) with teicoplanin are consistently less common than with vancomycin, even when teicoplanin is used concomitantly with aminoglycosides.[83,85] The incidence of

Table 140.7 Adverse reactions to teicoplanin

Hypersensitivity	Skin rash Bronchospasm Anaphylaxis
Biochemical abnormalities	Increased liver function tests
Hematologic abnormalities	Eosinophilia
Local intolerance	Redness, pain (after intramuscular administration), phlebitis (after intravenous administration)
Nonspecific reactions	Nausea Diarrhea Dizziness Tremor

Courtesy of Jihad Slim & Leon Smith.

'red man syndrome' or anaphylactoid reactions caused by teicoplanin administration is exceptionally low.

The commonest side-effects were injection site intolerance, skin rash, bronchospasm and eosinophilia. Nephrotoxicity and ototoxicity are uncommon. Like vancomycin, teicoplanin is bound and inactivated by bile-binding resins such as colestyramine.[89]

Future Therapies in the Glycopeptide/Lipoglycopeptide Class

Oritavancin, telavancin and dalbavancin have each completed phase III trials for the management of Gram-positive infections. Dalbavancin is a semisynthetic lipoglycopeptide that inhibits cell wall synthesis. This investigational agent has a half-life of 6–10 days, which allows for once-weekly dosing. Dalbavancin 1 g given intravenously, followed by 500 mg given intravenously 8 days later, has been compared to linezolid in a randomized, double-blind trial for the management of skin and skin structure infections. At the time of writing, Pfizer globally withdrew all dalbavancin marketing applications for the treatment of skin and skin structure infections in the United States and Europe, and announced that an additional phase III study with dalbavancin is planned.

Telavancin is also a semisynthetic lipoglycopeptide with a dual mechanism; it inhibits cell wall synthesis and disrupts membrane barrier function. Telavancin has a 7–9-hour half-life and is dosed once a day (7.5–10 mg/kg/day). At the time of writing, the manufacturer of telavancin has completed phase III trials in patients with complicated skin and soft tissue infections, pneumonia and a phase II bacteremia study.

Oritavancin is a bactericidal intravenous semisynthetic glycopeptide that has a longer half-life (>10 days) than vancomycin, dalbavancin and telavancin and, thus, can potentially offer a shorter duration of treatment. However, the long half-life has also raised concerns with respect to drug accumulation and potential toxicity. Oritavancin also has a dual mechanism, inhibiting cell wall synthesis and disrupting cell wall membrane function. Currently, oritavancin has completed two phase III trials for the management of complicated skin and skin structure infections using oritavancin dosed at 200 mg daily, two phase II trials for the management of bacteremia, and one phase II study investigating a single dose and an infrequent dosing regimen (first dose on day 1 with an option for a second dose on day 5). The advent of investigational agents for clinical use could provide clinicians with a variety of options for the treatment of Gram-positive infections if approved.

REFERENCES

References for this chapter can be found online at http://www.expertconsult.com

Tetracyclines and chloramphenicol

Tetracyclines

INTRODUCTION

In 1948, Benjamin Duggar at the Lederle Laboratories isolated the first tetracycline, chlortetracycline, from a fungus producing a golden pigment. The fungus was therefore called *Streptomyces aureofaciens* and the antibiotic aureomycin. Interestingly, although 1948 is the acknowledged date for the discovery of the tetracyclines, it is likely that ancient civilizations were exploiting the therapeutic benefits of this class of antibiotic through consumption of beer contaminated with *S. aureofaciens*.

In 1950 oxytetracycline was isolated from a strain of *Streptomyces rimosus* by workers at Charles Pfizer & Co. and in 1953 tetracycline was produced semisynthetically from chlortetracycline. Demeclocycline, derived from a mutant strain of *S. aureofaciens*, was introduced in 1957 and in the following years the semisynthetic derivatives rolitetracycline and methacycline were also introduced. A so-called second generation of long-acting tetracyclines, doxycycline and minocycline, were synthesized in 1966 and 1972, respectively.

In response to the increasing incidence of bacterial resistance to first- and second-generation tetracyclines, a research program was initiated at Lederle Laboratories in the 1990s to seek new third-generation tetracycline analogues that would circumvent existing mechanisms of resistance. This led to the discovery of the glycylcyclines and the development of 9-(t-butylglycylamido)-minocycline (tigecycline) as a new therapeutic agent.

Chemically, the tetracyclines have the structure of a hydronaphthacene nucleus containing four fused rings. The specific analogues are obtained by substitutions on the fifth, sixth, seventh or ninth positions of the basic structure (Fig. 141.1).

Tetracyclines are mainly bacteriostatic and they act by binding to the 30S subunits of the ribosomes in susceptible micro-organisms, thereby inhibiting protein synthesis.

Tigecycline evades the major mechanisms responsible for resistance to earlier tetracyclines.

There are few reasons to use any of the older tetracyclines; however, amongst the older drugs doxycycline and to some extent minocycline should be preferred because they are better absorbed and distributed than other tetracyclines. However, one exception may be that dermatologists often seem to prefer tetracycline or another first-generation drug for the treatment of acne.

Tigecycline holds promise as a novel expanded-spectrum tetracycline and is approved for the treatment of complicated skin and soft tissue infections and complicated intra-abdominal infections. It is only available as an intravenous product. An oral formulation of the drug would expand the potential application of tigecycline in clinical practice.

ANTIMICROBIAL SPECTRUM

When they were introduced the tetracyclines were effective against a variety of Gram-positive bacteria and Gram-negative organisms within the Enterobacteriaceae group. Development of resistance has, however, led to restricted use of first- and second-generation tetracyclines for infections caused by streptococci, staphylococci, *Escherichia coli* or *Proteus* spp. However, first- and second-generation tetracyclines have retained good activity against *Mycoplasma*, *Chlamydia* and *Rickettsia* spp., *Borrelia* spp. (especially *Borrelia burgdorferi*) and *Propionibacterium acnes* (Table 141.1).[1] Tigecycline has a broad spectrum of *in-vitro* activity, including susceptible and multidrug-resistant Gram-positive and Gram-negative organisms, as well as anaerobes and atypical organisms (Table 141.1).[2,3] It is active against organisms displaying resistance to earlier tetracyclines mediated by ribosomal protection mechanisms or efflux systems belonging to the major facilitator superfamily (MFS).[4] Deficiencies in its spectrum include *Proteus* spp. and *Pseudomonas* spp. which are intrinsically resistant through expression of chromosomally encoded multidrug efflux pumps from the resistance–nodulation–division (RND) family.[5,6]

Doxycycline and minocycline often exhibit better activity *in vitro* than the other tetracyclines[7,8] but the differences are probably of little practical importance for clinical treatment.

Tigecycline exhibits antibacterial activity typical of earlier tetracyclines, but with potent activity against organisms resistant to first- and second-generation tetracyclines [2,3]

RESISTANCE

Oral therapy with earlier tetracyclines has a marked influence on the bowel flora and resistant strains may be quickly selected. This risk is somewhat reduced with doxycycline,[9] which is nearly completely absorbed.[10] Nevertheless, extensive use of first- and second-generation tetracyclines has led to widespread selection and dissemination amongst bacteria of genetic determinants encoding ribosomal protection and MFS-mediated resistance mechanisms (see also Chapter 131).[4] Most of these acquired tetracycline resistance genes reside on transposons, conjugative transposons and/or integrons which permit horizontal resistance transfer from one species to another and between unrelated genera.[4] Currently resistance to tigecycline in the clinical setting is rare.[11] However, in a recent report of treatment of two patients with tigecycline for other nosocomial infections, it appears that tigecycline-insusceptible *Acinetobacter baumannii* was selected, resulting in the development of bloodstream infections in both patients, one of whom died from the infection.[11]

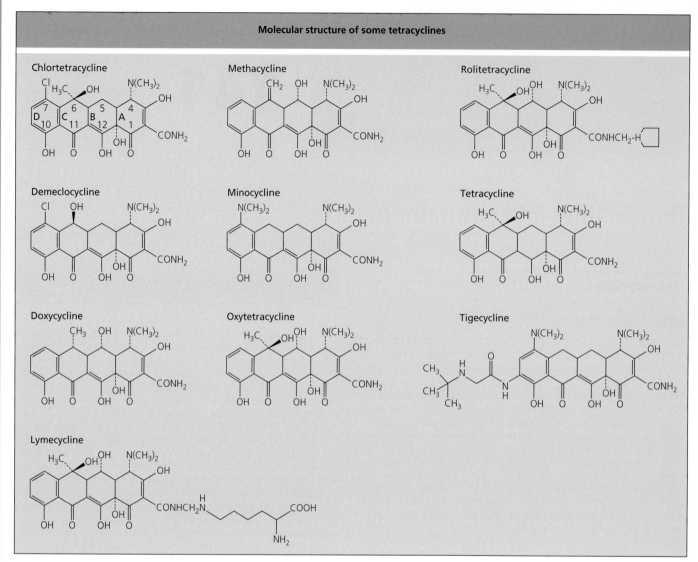

Fig. 141.1 Molecular structure of some tetracyclines.

Tetracyclines have been widely used in the veterinary field, not only to cure infections but also as a food additive to promote the growth of newborn animals. Tetracyclines are not now permitted as growth stimulators within the European Union but are still used in the USA.[4] In pigs, antibiotics promote an increase in weight of 8% and pigs are ready for slaughter 3 weeks earlier than animals that have not received antibiotics – an important economic advantage. This misuse of antibiotics is probably one important reason for the worldwide spread of tetracycline resistance within the Enterobacteriaceae group.[12–14]

Resistance to first- and second-generation tetracyclines is now common among bacteria causing respiratory tract infections such as pneumococci, *Haemophilus influenzae* and *Moraxella catarrhalis*.[15]

Obligatory intracellular pathogens such as *Chlamydia* and *Rickettsia* spp. have not yet acquired tetracycline resistance. Since these bacteria grow only inside mammalian cells, it would require that these cells be co-infected with two genera to allow gene exchange into the obligate intracellular pathogen.

PHARMACOKINETICS AND DISTRIBUTION

Clinical pharmacokinetics

After oral administration tetracyclines are absorbed from the stomach and the small intestine. Absorption is usually highest in the fasting state, but doxycycline and minocycline are also well absorbed with food. The degree of absorption and other pharmacokinetic parameters for some of the tetracyclines are shown in Table 141.2. The nearly complete absorption of doxycycline salts is reduced if the gastric pH is increased, as can occur in people who have atrophic gastritis or be caused by acid-reducing drugs. In some countries doxycycline is available in tablets bound to a polysaccharide, carragenate, which has been shown to increase absorption at higher pH.[16] There are also gelatin capsules available containing coated pellets of doxycycline hydrochloride that are resistant to gastric acid so that absorption will occur in the duodenum.[17]

Distribution

The tissue distribution of older tetracyclines is clearly related to their different lipid solubility, which is highest for doxycycline. Provided that tetracycline susceptible organisms are responsible for infection, doxycycline concentrations will be sufficient for treatment in the respiratory tract and lung tissue, the bile and the genital tract of both sexes.[18,19] Levels achieved in the central nervous system (CNS) are increased in chronic meningeal inflammation,[20] enabling treatment of neuroborreliosis.[21,22] Tigecycline has a large and variable volume of distribution.[2,23] It is concentrated in the gallbladder, lung and colon.[24] Tetracyclines, including tigecycline, cross the placenta and bind to metal ions in fetal bone and teeth. First- and second-generation tetracyclines are also known to be excreted in human breast milk. It is not known whether tigecycline is excreted in human breast milk; however,

Table 141.1 Susceptibility to first-, second- and third-generation (tigecycline) tetracyclines

	1st and 2nd generation	**Tigecycline**
Generally susceptible species	*Mycoplasma pneumoniae* *Ureaplasma urealyticum* *Chlamydia* spp. *Rickettsia* spp. *Brucella* spp. *Francisella tularensis* *Propionibacterium acnes* *Borrelia burgdorferi* *Yersinia* spp.	*Mycoplasma pneumoniae* *Ureaplasma urealyticum* *Chlamydia* spp. *Rickettsia* spp. *Brucella* spp. *Francisella tularensis* *Propionibacterium acnes* *Borrelia burgdorferi* *Yersinia* spp. Streptococci Enterococci Staphylococci Enterobacteriaceae *Haemophilus influenzae* Meningococci Gonococci *Serratia* spp.
Resistance common	Streptococci Staphylococci Enterobacteriaceae *Haemophilus influenzae* Meningococci Gonococci *Legionella pneumophila*	
Resistance usually found	Enterococci *Proteus* spp. *Pseudomonas* spp. *Serratia* spp. *Bacteroides* spp.	*Proteus* spp. *Pseudomonas* spp.

studies of radiolabeled drugs in rats indicate that tetracycline is readily excreted via the milk of lactating rats.[25]

Minocycline is even more lipid soluble than doxycycline. This may not be an advantage because side-effects such as vertigo and other CNS symptoms may be caused by increased drug concentrations in the cerebrosides of the brain.[26]

Elimination

Tetracyclines are metabolized in the liver in small amounts only, chlortetracycline being an exception with rapid metabolism. However, inducers of liver enzymes such as diphenylhydantoin may cause some metabolism of doxycycline. There is biliary excretion of older tetracyclines to a varying degree and possibly enterohepatic circulation. Biliary excretion is the primary route of elimination for tigecycline, with renal secretion as a secondary route.[27] Tetracyclines are partly excreted by glomerular filtration. For minocycline this excretion is less than 10% but it is more than 50% for tetracycline.

Incomplete absorption will contribute to high concentrations in feces for the older tetracyclines. Only a small fraction of doxycycline is found in active form in feces, the larger part being bound as chelate.

Doxycycline may be given in normal doses to patients who have renal insufficiency and to those undergoing hemodialysis as the reduced renal excretion is compensated for by intestinal excretion of bound substance.[28] For minocycline, caution is recommended because of a greater risk of side-effects.

No dosage adjustment of tigecycline is required in patients with renal impairment, or in patients undergoing hemodialysis.[27] Dosage adjustments are not required in patients with mild to moderate hepatic impairment, but patients with severe hepatic impairment should be treated cautiously and monitored for treatment response.

ROUTE OF ADMINISTRATION AND DOSAGE

Peak serum levels after an oral dose of 500 mg tetracycline or 200 mg of doxycycline or minocycline are usually 3–5 mg/l after 2 hours. Half-life in serum is longest for doxycycline (16–18 hours), followed by minocycline (11–13 hours) and tetracycline (8 hours). Doxycycline and minocycline can therefore be given orally once daily. For these older oral tetracyclines a higher starting dose on day 1 is recommended in order to achieve a steady-state level of the drug as soon as possible. Tigecycline is administered by intravenous infusion over 30–60 minutes. The initial dose is 100 mg followed by 50 mg every 12 hours. The peak serum level of tigecycline after a 30-minute infusion of 100 mg is approximately 1.5 mg/l. Dosages of several tetracyclines (including tigecycline) for adults are given in Table 141.3.

Doxycycline is also available for intravenous infusion but there is little difference in serum levels compared with oral administration. Tigecycline is only available for intravenous infusion.

DOSAGE IN SPECIAL CIRCUMSTANCES

In patients who have renal insufficiency or disease, doxycycline and tigecycline are the only tetracyclines that can be used safely without risk of accumulation and toxicity.

In patients who have hepatic disease, tetracyclines should generally be avoided. If treatment is important, liver tests should be performed repeatedly during treatment. However, toxicity has mostly been observed when older tetracyclines have been used at high doses or given during pregnancy.

Table 141.2 Pharmacokinetics of some tetracyclines in humans

	Tetracycline	**Doxycycline**	**Minocycline**	**Tigecycline**
Oral absorption in fasting state (%)	80	90–93	100	na
Serum half-life (h)	6–12	18–22	13	36
Serum protein binding (%)	24–65	80–90	55–75	68
Lipid solubility in comparison with tetracycline	1	5	10	nd
Excretion in urine (%) after: oral administration intravenous administration	20 na	35–40 nd	4–9 nd	na 15

na, not applicable; nd, not determined.

Table 141.3 Usual adult dosages for some tetracyclines*

General name	First dose	Common dosage
Oral preparations		
Tetracycline	500 mg	500 mg q6h
Oxytetracycline	500 mg	500 mg q6h
Doxycycline	200 mg	100 mg q24h
Minocycline	200 mg	100 mg q12h
Intravenous preparation		
Tigecycline	100 mg	50 mg q12h

*Doxycycline and minocycline may be given intravenously in the same doses. Higher doses of doxycycline are often used for sexually transmitted diseases and Lyme disease. Tigecycline is only available as an intravenous formulation.

During pregnancy tetracyclines should be avoided because of the depressive effect on the skeleton of the child. In lactating patients small amounts of older tetracyclines are excreted in breast milk but are harmless to the baby. Use of tigecycline in nursing women has not been adequately studied. It is not known whether tigecycline is excreted in human breast milk (but see section on 'Distribution' above).

In elderly patients kidney function is reduced according to age and the daily dose of a tetracycline should be reduced unless doxycycline or tigecycline is used.

In patients with severe hepatic impairment the initial dose of tigecycline should be 100 mg followed by a reduced dose of 25 mg q12 hours.[25]

INDICATIONS

Respiratory infections

Tetracyclines were first used for many types of respiratory tract infection. Because of increasing resistance in pneumococci and *H. influenzae*, they have been replaced in many areas by other antibiotics, mainly β-lactams.

Exacerbation of chronic bronchitis has been a classic indication for tetracyclines. Doxycycline has been found to be as effective as ampicillin. The advantage of one single dose per day may increase compliance in patients who have chronic respiratory diseases and many other medications (see Chapter 26).

Doxycycline is distributed to maxillary sinuses and can be used as a second-line drug in patients who have sinusitis and are allergic to β-lactams or in whom treatment with such drugs has failed.

Tetracyclines have good activity in pneumonias caused by *Mycoplasma pneumoniae*, *C. pneumoniae*, *C. psittaci* and *Coxiella burnetii*. Macrolides probably have an equal effect in infections caused by *M. pneumoniae* but clinical experience with the other infections is far greater with tetracyclines.

Tigecycline holds promise as a novel expanded-spectrum tetracycline, but is currently only approved for the treatment of complicated skin and soft tissue infections and complicated intra-abdominal infections.

Sexually transmitted diseases

Older tetracyclines are effective therapy for nongonococcal urethritis caused by *Chlamydia trachomatis* or *Ureaplasma urealyticum*. In an open evaluation of doxycycline in the treatment of urethritis and cervicitis caused by *C. trachomatis* the symptoms disappeared in 76% of cases.[28] Treatment should usually be given for 10 days and concurrent treatment of sexual partners is recommended (see Chapter 49).

First- and second-generation tetracyclines are usually effective for the treatment of lymphogranuloma venereum and granuloma inguinale. Nonpenicillinase-producing strains of gonococci are usually sensitive, which is an advantage in mixed infections with *C. trachomatis*.

Older tetracyclines can be used as alternative therapy for syphilis in penicillin-allergic patients. Treatment time is 15 days for early disease and 30 days for later stages of the disease.

Lyme disease and ehrlichiosis

Doxycycline can be used in penicillin-allergic patients to treat erythema migrans and is as effective as penicillin in a dose of 200 mg daily for 10 days. In erythema migrans with signs of dissemination such as multiple erythema and fever, doxycycline is often recommended as the primary drug. Treatment of neuroborreliosis with doxycycline 200 mg daily for 2 weeks has given similar results to those achieved with penicillin G (see Chapter 43).[29]

Doxycycline is also the preferred drug for infections due to *Ehrlichia* spp. (see Chapters 122 and 176).[30]

Other indications

First- and second-generation tetracyclines are very effective drugs for rickettsial infections (see Chapter 176). Doxycycline has been used for single-dose treatment of louse-borne typhus, but for other infections 7–10 days of treatment is usually needed. These infections can only be treated with tetracyclines or chloramphenicol. In children tetracyclines can often be given with minimal risk of staining the teeth if repeated treatments are avoided and the dose is kept as low as possible.

Doxycycline is also effective in a single dose for infections with *Borrelia recurrentis*. Tetracyclines are usually used in combination with other antibiotics such as streptomycin or rifampin (rifampicin) for brucellosis and tularemia.

For cholera in adults, tetracycline 500 mg q6h for 5 days or a single dose of 300 mg doxycycline have been recommended.[31]

Most of the older tetracyclines have been used for oral treatment of chronic acne. The drugs have an antibacterial effect on *P. acnes* as well as a general anti-inflammatory effect, which is probably of importance.[32] However, resistance of *P. acnes* to tetracyclines, including doxycycline, has been reported from England and the USA. Cross-resistance does not include minocycline, which may be used clinically.[33]

Doxycycline may also be used for malaria prophylaxis in areas where *Plasmodium falciparum* is resistant to other antimalarial drugs.[34]

ADVERSE REACTIONS AND INTERACTIONS

Adverse drug reactions

All oral preparations of tetracyclines can cause nausea and epigastric discomfort. It is usually an advantage if the drugs can be taken with food without decreasing absorption, as with doxycycline and minocycline. Diarrhea is less common but may occur, especially when tetracyclines with low absorption are used. Tigecycline is structurally related to other tetracyclines and therefore may share similar adverse effects to older tetracyclines.

Phototoxic reactions can occur with all tetracyclines.

Tetracyclines should not be used in children younger than 8 years because of the risk of enamel hypoplasia and tooth discoloration. They should also not be used during pregnancy. Tetracyclines, except doxycycline and tigecycline, are contraindicated in patients who have renal impairment.

Vertigo and dizziness are CNS symptoms that occur with minocycline.

Nausea, vomiting and headache are the most frequently reported adverse events associated with tigecycline therapy.

Hepatotoxicity and other severe organ reactions have occurred with older tetracyclines, mainly after parenteral therapy – often with high doses – and also when the drugs have had to be used during pregnancy.

Tigecycline is not recommended in patients under 18 years of age.

Drug–drug interactions

Tetracyclines form chelate complexes with many drugs containing metal ions (Table 141.4). When combined with diuretics the risk of accumulation of urea increases. Some drugs seem to stimulate liver enzymes, so increasing doxycycline metabolism and shortening its half-life. Tigecycline may decrease elimination of the anticoagulant warfarin, thereby increasing warfarin levels in the blood. The potential increased risk of bleeding should therefore be monitored.

In-vitro studies with human liver microsomes indicate that tigecycline does not inhibit metabolism mediated by the cytochrome P450 isoforms 1A2, 2C8, 2C9, 2C19, 2D6 or 3A4. Therefore tigecycline is not expected to alter the metabolism of drugs processed by these enzymes.[27]

Since tigecycline is not extensively metabolized, clearance of the antibiotic is not expected to be affected by drugs that induce or inhibit the activity of cytochrome P450 isoforms.[27]

Chloramphenicol

INTRODUCTION

Chloramphenicol was first isolated in 1947 from a sample of soil from Venezuela and the actinomycete was called *Streptomyces venezuelae*.

MODE OF ACTION AND SPECTRUM

Chloramphenicol inhibits protein synthesis by binding to the 50S subunit of the bacterial 70S ribosome. It is mainly a bacteriostatic agent. However, bactericidal activity on some bacteria, such as *H. influenzae*, *Streptococcus pneumoniae* and *Neisseria meningitidis*, has been reported.

Chloramphenicol has a very broad spectrum, similar to that of tetracyclines, and includes aerobic and anaerobic bacteria, spirochetes, *Rickettsia*, *Chlamydia* and *Mycoplasma* spp. It is very active against most anaerobic bacteria of clinical interest, including *Bacteroides fragilis*.

Chloramphenicol resistance can occur and is mediated by a bacterial enzyme, chloramphenicol acetyltransferase (CAT), which inactivates the drug. The gene that codes for CAT is carried on transmissible plasmids, and epidemics of chloramphenicol-resistant typhoid fever and *Shigella* infections have occurred.

Unrestricted use of chloramphenicol seems to have resulted in a resistance problem very similar to that observed with tetracyclines.

ROUTE OF ADMINISTRATION AND DOSAGE

Chloramphenicol is conjugated with glucuronic acid and is then excreted in active form by the kidneys. The metabolites are not toxic and dose reduction is not needed in renal insufficiency.

Chloramphenicol is a small lipophilic molecule and is well distributed in the body. The serum protein binding is about 44%. It reaches the CNS better than most other antibiotics and its concentration in the cerebrospinal fluid is often 30–50% of the serum concentration. Chloramphenicol also crosses the placenta and is found in breast milk.

Chloramphenicol is well absorbed (over 90%) after oral administration. Chloramphenicol 1 g gives a serum concentration of 10 mg/l and the half-life is 3–4 hours. It may also be given intravenously as a succinate ester but intramuscular injections should be avoided as absorption is unreliable.

INDICATIONS

Chloramphenicol is toxic and should therefore be used carefully in systemic infections, when other alternatives are lacking. It can be used instead of tetracyclines for the treatment of rickettsial infections and for bacterial meningitis in the few patients who have an allergy to β-lactam drugs, including third-generation cephalosporins and meropenem. It may also have a place as an oral alternative for CNS infections, especially brain abscesses.

Topical administration of chloramphenicol in drops or ointments is widely used for superficial bacterial infections of the eyes. Such treatment is still effective in comparison with the newer drugs such as quinolones or fusidic acid, which are also used locally for eye infections.[35,36]

ADVERSE REACTIONS AND INTERACTIONS

Adverse drug reactions

Neonates have a diminished ability to conjugate chloramphenicol and to excrete the active form in the urine. A dose of 25 mg/kg/day should not be exceeded[37] otherwise the 'gray baby syndrome' may develop, with severe cyanosis and circulatory collapse. Cranial and peripheral neuropathies and optic atrophy have also been reported rarely with chloramphenicol.

Dose-related reversible bone marrow depression can occur in adults given high doses of more than 4 g/day. The daily dose should not exceed 3 g, and when the accumulated dose exceeds 25 g reticulocytes should be checked regularly (e.g. twice weekly) until treatment is stopped.

A very severe reaction is aplastic anemia, which occurs with a frequency of 1/25 000–40 000 treatment courses.[38] No clear correlation to dose or duration of treatment has been observed and no route of administration is exempt from causing this catastrophic complication. There are also reports to indicate that the use of chloramphenicol may increase the risk of leukemia in children.[39]

Table 141.4 Drug interactions with tetracyclines*	
Interacting drug	**Effect**
Antacids with metal ions, calcium and iron supplements, magnesium salicylates, magnesium-containing laxatives, multivitamins	Chelate formation and impaired absorption
Diuretics	Risk of increased serum urea concentration – not with doxycycline
Rifampin (rifampicin), phenobarbital, phenytoin, carbamazepine	Half-life of doxycycline shortened

*There is a paucity of drug interaction data for tigecycline. However, at least some of the drug interactions that occur with earlier tetracyclines are also likely to occur with tigecycline.

Drug–drug interactions

As chloramphenicol is almost completely metabolized in the liver by cytochrome P450 enzymes, there is a possible risk of interactions with other drugs if they are metabolized by the same enzyme system. Chloramphenicol will decrease the rate of metabolism of tolbutamide, phenytoin, cyclophosphamide and warfarin. Rifampin may lower chloramphenicol concentrations by induced metabolism.

REFERENCES

References for this chapter can be found online at http://www.expertconsult.com

Nitroimidazoles: metronidazole, ornidazole and tinidazole

INTRODUCTION AND MODE OF ACTION

The nitroimidazoles, which include metronidazole, tinidazole and ornidazole, were initially introduced for the treatment of trichomonal vaginitis. They were subsequently recognized to be active against other protozoa as well as facultative anaerobes (*Helicobacter pylori* and *Gardnerella vaginalis*) and anaerobic bacteria, and are used on a worldwide basis for the treatment of infections caused by these organisms.

Once they have entered the cell by diffusion, the antimicrobial toxicity of the nitroimidazoles is dependent on reduction of the nitro moiety to the nitro anion radical and other highly active compounds, including nitroso and hydroxylamine derivatives.[1,2] These reduction products are damaging to macromolecules, and have been shown to cause DNA degradation and strand breakage.[1] The nitroimidazoles are selectively toxic for micro-organisms in which the redox potential of components of the electron transport chain are sufficiently negative to reduce the nitro group of metronidazole. Aerobic bacteria are therefore intrinsically resistant to these antibiotics since they are unable to attain the low intracellular redox environment required for drug activation. In susceptible organisms, the ongoing reduction of metronidazole maintains a favorable transmembrane metronidazole concentration gradient, facilitating further diffusion into the cell. In general, micro-organisms develop resistance to the nitroimidazoles by reducing or abolishing activity of elements of the electron transport reactions, with appropriate compensatory modifications of the normal fermentative pathway.[2-5] Resistance to metronidazole in *Bacteroides* spp. has been shown to be associated with specific nitroimidazole (*nim*) resistance genes that encode a 5-nitroimidazole reductase, which prevents the formation of the free radicals responsible for bactericidal activity.[6]

ROUTE OF ADMINISTRATION AND DOSAGE

The two most frequently used nitroimidazoles, metronidazole and tinidazole, have parenteral and oral formulations, and are also available as suppositories, as a gel for periodontitis and for vaginal administration. Dosing regimens of metronidazole are given in Table 142.1. The doses of tinidazole and ornidazole are similar but, because their half-lives are longer, these drugs can be administered at longer intervals. Recommendations in the USA for certain infections are for shorter dose intervals, although it is recognized that the half-life of the nitroimidazoles means that dose intervals shorter than 8 hours should not be needed and in most cases 12-hour regimens should be adequate.

PHARMACOKINETICS

Following oral administration, all nitroimidazoles are almost completely absorbed.[7] After rectal administration of metronidazole the bioavailability is approximately 60%, with considerable variability between individuals. When given vaginally the bioavailability of metronidazole is 20% or less. Following a 400 mg oral dose of metronidazole or tinidazole, peak plasma concentrations of about 10 mg/l are achieved after 3–5 hours. Dose proportional kinetics have been seen for doses up to 2 g. The concentrations after normal oral doses are well above the minimum inhibitory concentrations (MICs) for anaerobes but are borderline for *G. vaginalis*. The nitroimidazoles are well distributed to peripheral compartments, including brain tissue and cerebrospinal fluid,[7] but concentrations in subcutaneous fat are low (15% or less of concurrent serum levels).[8] Nitroimidazoles are metabolized mainly by the liver and excreted in the urine. The plasma half-life is about 8 hours for metronidazole and 12–13 hours for tinidazole. Metronidazole is partly metabolized to hydroxymetronidazole, which has a half-life of 10–13 hours.

Metronidazole elimination is prolonged in premature newborns and in patients with impaired liver function, and dose reduction is necessary in these groups. Although dose adjustment is not normally required in patients with renal impairment, the hydroxymetronidazole metabolite may accumulate in patients with end-stage disease and dose reduction may be necessary. Hemodialysis increases the clearance of metronidazole, shortening the half-life to 2–3 hours.

INDICATIONS

Bacterial infections

Nitroimidazoles are the most active antibiotics for the treatment and prevention of infections caused by anaerobic bacteria (Table 142.2) and resistance in these organisms is rare.[11] Nitroimidazoles are therefore important in the treatment of intra-abdominal and gynecologic sepsis, abscesses and tetanus. They are also an important component of prophylactic regimens for surgical procedures where contamination with anaerobic flora is likely. Nitroimidazoles are used to treat bacterial vaginosis (frequently associated with *G. vaginalis*) and dental infections, including acute necrotizing ulcerative gingivitis (Vincent's angina). Metronidazole continues to be first-line treatment for mild/moderate antibiotic-associated diarrhea caused by *Clostridium difficile* but is inferior to vancomycin in patients with severe, recurrent, complicated or fulminant disease (see also Chapter 35).[12] Nitroimidazoles are also a component of modern triple eradication regimens for *H. pylori*, although resistance may affect 10–50% of strains isolated in developed countries and virtually all strains from developing countries.[13]

Table 142.1 Dosages of metronidazole

Type of infection	Adult dose	Child dose*	Duration of treatment	Notes
Trichomoniasis	2 g	Not applicable	Single dose	Or 400 mg q12h for 5–7 days (250–500 mg q8h)[†]
Giardiasis	400 mg q8h (250 mg q12h or q8h)	15 mg/kg q12h	5–7 days	Or 2 g q24h for 3 days
Amebic dysentery	800 mg q8h (500–750 mg q8h)	20 mg/kg q12h	5–10 days	
Amebic abscess	800 mg q8h (500–750 mg q8h)	20 mg/kg q12h	10 days	
Bacterial vaginosis	400 mg q12h (500 mg q12h)	Not applicable	5–7 days	Or 2 g as a single dose
Helicobacter pylori	400 mg q8h (250 mg q8h)	Not applicable	7–14 days	
Clostridium difficile	800 mg then 400 mg q8h (250 mg q6h or 500 mg q8h)	7.5 mg/kg q12h	10–14 days	
Anaerobic infection (treatment)	800 mg then 400 mg q8h (500 mg q12h–q6h)	7.5 mg/kg q8h	7–10 days	
Anaerobic infection (prophylaxis)	400 mg (15 mg/kg then 7.5 mg/kg 6 and 12 h after initial dose)	7.5 mg/kg	Single dose	Repeat every 3 h for prolonged procedures

*Child dose is for children aged 8 weeks or more.
[†]US dosages in parentheses.

Table 142.2 Activity of metronidazole against anaerobic bacteria

Organism	Metronidazole MIC (mg/l) for 90% isolates	Percent sensitive (NCCLS)
Bacteroides fragilis	1–4	100
Prevotella spp.	4	100
Fusobacterium nucleatum	0.25–2	100
Fusobacterium spp.	0.25–4	100
Peptostreptococcus spp.	0.5–4	100
Propionibacterium acnes	>1.0	0
Clostridium difficile	0.5–4	100
Clostridium spp.	2–16	95

NCCLS, National Committee for Clinical Laboratory Standards.
Data from Wexler et al.[9] and Spangler et al.[10]

Protozoal infections

The nitroimidazoles are highly active against protozoa and provide the first-line treatment for giardiasis, amebiasis and trichomonal vaginitis. Although resistant strains of *Entamoeba histolytica* and *Trichomonas vaginalis* are rarely encountered, up to 20% of *Giardia lamblia* isolates may be resistant in general clinical practice.

Other

Topical metronidazole is used to reduce the odor produced by anaerobic bacteria in fungating cutaneous lesions and has also been used in the management of acne rosacea. Metronidazole may be beneficial for the treatment of diarrhea and perianal involvement in patients with active Crohn's disease.

ADVERSE REACTIONS AND INTERACTIONS

The most common side-effects of the nitroimidazoles are gastrointestinal (including nausea and diarrhea) and a metallic taste, especially when high doses are used. A reversible peripheral neuropathy may occur in patients receiving high doses for prolonged periods. Severe central nervous system effects have also been reported and the drug should be discontinued if any abnormal neurologic symptoms are reported. If combined with alcohol, metronidazole may cause a disulfiram-like reaction, with nausea, vomiting, flushing of the skin, tachycardia, hypotension and palpitations.

Although nitroimidazoles have been found to be mutagenic and carcinogenic in animal studies, there is a lack of evidence that they are carcinogenic to humans.[14] Although theoretical concerns of teratogenicity have not been confirmed,[15,16] it seems prudent that metronidazole should only be used in pregnancy when the benefits outweigh the risks, and should be avoided altogether in the first trimester. Because the concentrations of metronidazole in breast milk are similar to those in serum, a risk assessment should be performed before using this drug in lactating mothers.

REFERENCES

References for this chapter can be found online at http://www.expertconsult.com

Antituberculosis agents

INTRODUCTION

The discovery of the tubercle bacillus by Robert Koch in 1882 raised hopes that an effective remedy for tuberculosis would soon be found and many workers attempted to develop immunotherapeutic agents. The best known of these attempts was that of Koch himself who advocated injections of old tuberculin. Old tuberculin was later shown to be useless as a therapeutic, but priceless as a diagnostic test. The British bacteriologist Sir Almroth Wright also conducted extensive studies, which are immortalized in George Bernard Shaw's play *The Doctor's Dilemma*.

It was, however, the discovery of streptomycin in 1944 by Albert Schatz and Selman Waksman in the USA that opened the door to effective therapy and led to the belief that the disease would soon be conquered. Early jubilation turned to disappointment when it was found that patients treated with streptomycin often made an initial improvement but soon relapsed because their tubercle bacilli became resistant to this agent. Fortunately, other active antituberculosis agents were soon discovered and, as a result of extensive trials initiated by Sir John Crofton in the UK, multidrug regimens that cured patients and prevented the emergence of drug resistance were developed.[1]

Therapy of tuberculosis with these early drug regimens, usually consisting of streptomycin, isoniazid and *para*-aminosalicylic acid, was beset with problems. Streptomycin had to be given by injection and *para*-aminosalicylic acid caused such severe gastrointestinal effects that patients often failed to comply with therapy. In addition, it was necessary to treat patients for 18–24 months in order to achieve a cure.

The second therapeutic revolution came in the early 1970s when regimens containing rifampin (rifampicin) were developed. The introduction of this drug had three major effects on the treatment of tuberculosis. First, the duration of therapy could be reduced to only 6 months so that the era of 'short course' therapy had arrived. Secondly, regimens could be entirely by the oral route and thirdly, as a consequence, hospitalization was often unnecessary.

Modern short-course therapy, properly used, can achieve a cure in around 98% of patients and is among the most effective and cost-effective of all therapeutic interventions for a chronic disease.[2] Far from being conquered, however, tuberculosis remains one of the most prevalent causes of mortality and morbidity worldwide. It is responsible for one in seven deaths among young adults and it was declared a global emergency by the World Health Organization (WHO) in 1993. The problem is currently exacerbated by the HIV pandemic, the increasing prevalence of multidrug-resistant tuberculosis (MDRTB), defined as resistance to at least rifampin and isoniazid among the first-line drugs, and the more recent emergence of extremely drug-resistant tuberculosis (XDRTB), as defined below. There is therefore an urgent need to develop new therapies and to use the available therapies in a much more responsible manner.

CLASSIFICATION

Antituberculous agents can be classified in several ways (Table 143.1). They can be divided into:
- those that are synthetic molecules and those that are antibiotics or semisynthetic antibiotic derivatives;
- agents with a broad spectrum of activity and those only active against mycobacteria or, specifically, members of the *Mycobacterium tuberculosis* complex;
- first-line drugs that form the basis of the modern short-course regimens advocated by the WHO and second-line drugs that are used in cases of drug resistance and when toxic reactions prevent the use of one or more first-line drugs; and
- bacteriostatic and bactericidal agents, with a clinically important distinction of the latter between those that are bactericidal *in vitro* and those that are able to sterilize lesions of tubercle bacilli *in vivo* (Table 143.2).

MODE OF ACTION AND PHARMACOKINETICS

The sequencing of the genome of *M. tuberculosis*[3] has led to considerable advances in our understanding of the genetic basis of action of the drugs used for treating mycobacterial disease as well as the delineation of metabolic pathways that could serve as targets for novel drugs.

The targets of streptomycin and other aminoglycosides, rifamycins and fluoroquinolones are the same in mycobacteria as in other bacterial genera, and resistance is due to single amino acid substitutions in the target proteins. The targets of many important antituberculosis agents, notably isoniazid, pyrazinamide, ethambutol, ethionamide and prothionamide, are components of the complex and lipid-rich mycobacterial cell wall. The mode of action and target genes are discussed under the individual drug headings below and are summarized in Table 143.3; the targets are shown in Figure 143.1. Most of the antituberculosis agents are readily absorbed from the gastrointestinal tract. Exceptions are streptomycin and other aminoglycosides, capreomycin and viomycin, which must therefore be given parenterally. Binding to serum proteins varies from agent to agent, as does entry into the cerebrospinal fluid (CSF). Agents that enter into the CSF poorly in health often pass the inflamed meninges so that therapeutically useful levels are achieved in cases of tuberculous meningitis. The pharmacokinetics of the conventional antimycobacterial drugs, their principal metabolites and routes of excretion are summarized in Tables 143.4 and 143.5.

Table 143.1 Spectrum of activity, class of compound and cross-resistances of the antituberculosis agents*

Agent	Class of compound	Spectrum of activity	Cross-resistance to other antituberculosis agents
First-line agents			
Rifampin (rifampicin)	Antibiotic	Broad	Other rifamycins
Isoniazid	Synthetic	Tubercle bacilli	None
Pyrazinamide	Synthetic	Tubercle bacilli	None
Ethambutol	Synthetic	Tubercle bacilli	None
Streptomycin	Antibiotic	Broad	Other aminoglycosides, viomycin, capreomycin
Second-line agents			
Thiacetazone	Synthetic	Tubercle bacilli	Ethionamide and prothionamide
Para-aminosalicylic acid	Synthetic	Tubercle bacilli	None
Ethionamide and prothionamide	Synthetic	Tubercle bacilli	Thiacetazone
Capreomycin	Antibiotic	Tubercle bacilli	Aminoglycosides, viomycin
Viomycin	Antibiotic	Tubercle bacilli	Aminoglycosides, capreomycin
Cycloserine	Synthetic	Broad	None
Ofloxacin	Antibiotic	Broad	None

*Agents that are active against tubercle bacilli (*Mycobacterium tuberculosis* complex) may also show activity against some other species of mycobacteria. Strains of *Mycobacterium bovis* are naturally resistant to pyrazinamide. There are only limited data on other activities of capreomycin and viomycin.

Table 143.2 Efficacy of antituberculosis agents*

Agent	Early bactericidal activity	Sterilizing activity	Prevention of emergence of drug resistance
Rifampin (rifampicin)	Fair	Good	Good
Pyrazinamide	Poor	Good	Poor
Isoniazid	Good	Fair	Good
Ethambutol	Fair	Poor	Fair
Streptomycin	Poor	Poor	Fair
Thiacetazone	Poor	Poor	Poor

*In sterilizing lesions, reducing viable bacterial population rapidly and preventing the emergence of drug resistance.

Table 143.3 Antituberculosis agents: targets and genes for resistance

Agent	Target	Gene(s) encoding target(s) or those in which mutations conferring resistance occur
Isoniazid	Mycolic acid synthesis	*inhA, katG, KasA, oxyR-ahpC*
Rifampin (rifampicin)	DNA-dependent RNA polymerase	*rpoB*
Pyrazinamide	Fatty acid synthetase-1	*pncA*
Ethambutol	Arabinosyl transferase, involved in cell wall arabinogalactan synthesis	*embA, embB and embC*
Streptomycin	30S ribosomal subunit	*rspL* (encodes for ribosomal protein S12)
Other aminoglycosides	30S ribosomal subunit	Genes encoding 16S-rRNA (and possibly *aac(2')* encoding aminoglycoside acetyltransferase)

Table 143.3 Antituberculosis agents: targets and genes for resistance—cont'd

Agent	Target	Gene(s) encoding target(s) or those in which mutations conferring resistance occur
Thiacetazone	Mycolic acid synthesis	Unknown
Para-aminosalicylic acid	Mycobactin synthesis (?)	Unknown
Ethionamide and prothionamide	Mycolic acid synthesis	*inhA*
Fluoroquinolones	Inhibition of bacterial DNA gyrase topoisomerase IV	*gyrA* and *gyrB* (gyrase) *parC* and *parD* (topoisomerase IV)
Capreomycin and viomycin	50S or 30S ribosomal subunit	*vicA* (50S) or *vicB* (30S)
Clofazimine	Unknown; possibly RNA polymerase	–
Cycloserine	Peptidoglycan	*alrA*

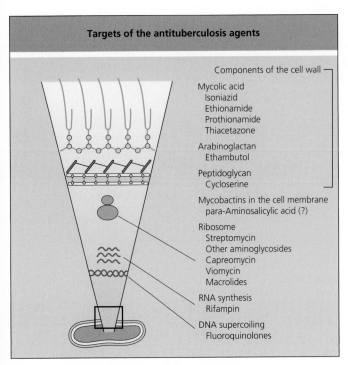

Targets of the antituberculosis agents

Components of the cell wall

Mycolic acid
Isoniazid
Ethionamide
Prothionamide
Thiacetazone

Arabinoglactan
Ethambutol

Peptidoglycan
Cycloserine

Mycobactins in the cell membrane
para-Aminosalicylic acid (?)

Ribosome
Streptomycin
Other aminoglycosides
Capreomycin
Viomycin
Macrolides

RNA synthesis
Rifampin

DNA supercoiling
Fluoroquinolones

Fig. 143.1 Targets of the antituberculosis agents.

DRUG TOXICITY

Although all antituberculosis drugs have some untoward side-effects, drug toxicity is, in general, not a serious problem in modern short-course chemotherapy based on the WHO-recommended first-line agents and is a small price to pay for the very real curative benefits. The major side-effects are hepatotoxicity, peripheral neuropathy, mental disturbances, skin reactions (Figs 143.2–143.4) and fevers. Side-effects are particularly likely to occur in HIV-positive patients and, of these, skin reactions due to thiacetazone are particularly serious and may be fatal.

The principal drugs used in modern short-course regimens – isoniazid, rifampin, pyrazinamide and ethambutol – are all potentially hepatotoxic, but this is seldom a problem in clinical practice. Some physicians, however, advocate regular liver function tests during therapy.[4] The adverse effects of the various drugs are discussed under the individual headings below and are summarized in Table 143.6.

FIRST-LINE DRUGS

Isoniazid (isonicotinic acid hydrazide)

This is included in all modern regimens and is also used as preventive monotherapy for infected (tuberculin-positive, without clinical disease; also known as latent tuberculosis) persons, particularly in the USA.

It has a powerful bactericidal action against actively replicating tubercle bacilli and thus rapidly reduces infectiousness by reducing the number of viable bacilli in cavities. It has little or no activity against slowly replicating bacilli but is included in the continuation phase of modern short-course therapy to kill any rifampin-resistant mutants that commence replication. It inhibits the synthesis of mycolic acids – long-chain fatty acids that form an important part of the mycobacterial cell wall. Although mycolic acids are common to all mycobacteria, and similar molecules occur in the genera *Nocardia* and *Corynebacterium*, susceptibility to isoniazid is essentially restricted to the *M. tuberculosis* complex and some strains of *M. xenopi* and *M. kansasii*. Isoniazid is a prodrug requiring oxidative activation by the mycobacterial catalase-peroxidase enzyme KatG and the commonest causes of isoniazid resistance are point mutations in, or deletion of, the *katG* gene that encodes this enzyme. Less frequent resistance-determining mutations are in the *inhA* locus (or in its promoter region) which codes for an NADH-dependent enoyl-acyl carrier protein reductase involved in mycolic acid synthesis and the *oxyR–ahpC* locus which, like the *katG* locus, is involved in protection against oxidative stress.[5] The predominant mutations conferring resistance to isoniazid differ between the various lineages of *M. tuberculosis* and therefore show geographic variations in their distribution.[6]

Isoniazid is readily absorbed from the gastrointestinal tract and is converted to inactive metabolites, principally by acetylation, the rate of which is genetically determined. Thus, patients can be divided into rapid acetylators and slow acetylators, in whom the elimination half-lives of the drug are 0.5–1.5 hours and 2–4 hours, respectively. About half of Caucasian and black patients but over 80% of Chinese and Japanese patients are rapid acetylators. If administered regularly, response to therapy is unaffected by acetylator status.

Owing to its widespread use since the 1950s, resistance to isoniazid is common and many strains that are resistant to other antituberculosis drugs, particularly to rifampin, are also resistant to isoniazid.

Adverse events are usually mild and are more likely to occur in slow acetylators. They include several neurologic effects, including insomnia, restlessness, peripheral neuropathy, optic neuritis and mild psychiatric disturbances. More serious, but less common, neurologic effects include severe psychiatric disturbance and encephalopathy. The latter is particularly likely to occur in renal dialysis patients.[7]

Table 143.4 Pharmacokinetics of the antituberculosis agents

Agent	Binding to serum proteins	Absorption from gastrointestinal tract (time to reach peak serum level)	Entry into CSF (with healthy meninges)
Isoniazid	Very low	Very rapid (30–60 minutes)	Good
Rifampin (rifampicin)	High (up to 95%)	Rapid (2 hours)	Poor
Pyrazinamide	Very low	Rapid (1–2 hours)	Good
Ethambutol	Binds to erythrocytes	Rapid (2 hours); 80% of dose absorbed	Poor
Streptomycin	Moderate (30–35%)	Not absorbed	Poor
Thiacetazone	Not bound	Rapid (2 hours)	Limited data
Para-aminosalicylic acid	High (60–65%)	Very rapid	Poor
Ethionamide and prothionamide	Limited data	Very rapid (30 minutes)	Good
Capreomycin	Limited data	Not absorbed	Poor
Viomycin	Limited data	Not absorbed	Poor
Clofazimine	Limited data	Slow (8–12 hours)	Limited data
Cycloserine	Not bound	Rapid (3 hours)	Good
Ofloxacin	Low	Rapid (1–1.5 hours)	Moderate

Table 143.5 Principal metabolic products and excretion of the antituberculosis agents

Agent	Principal metabolic products	Excretion
Isoniazid	Acetyl derivatives: rate of acetylation is genetically controlled	Unchanged and as acetyl derivatives in urine (ratio depends on rate of acetylation)
Rifampin (rifampicin)	Desacetyl derivative	As desacetylrifampin in bile
Pyrazinamide	Pyrazinoic acid	Mostly as pyrazinoic acid in urine
Ethambutol	Oxidation products and aldehydes	Mostly unchanged in urine; about 15% as metabolites
Streptomycin	None	Unchanged in urine
Other aminoglycosides	None	Unchanged in urine
Thiacetazone	Unknown	20% eliminated in urine, fate of remainder unknown
Para-aminosalicylic acid	Acetylation products and glycine conjugates	About 80% in the urine, mostly in the acetylated form
Ethionamide and prothionamide	Sulfoxide (biologically active) and methyl derivatives	Less than 1% unchanged in urine
Capreomycin	None	Unchanged in urine
Viomycin	None	Unchanged in urine
Clofazimine	Very small amounts of unidentified metabolites	Unchanged in urine and feces
Cycloserine	Up to 35% converted to unidentified metabolites	Varying amounts unchanged in urine
Ofloxacin	5% metabolized to oxides and dimethyl derivatives	70–95% unchanged in urine, small amounts in bile

Other adverse effects include hepatitis, particularly in patients aged over 35 years, arthralgia, fever and skin rashes. Very rare complications include hyperglycemia and agranulocytosis.

Adverse effects, particularly neurologic ones, are usually preventable by administration of pyridoxine (vitamin B6) 10 mg daily. In particular, pyridoxine should be given to patients who have liver disease, pregnant women, alcoholics, renal dialysis patients, HIV-positive patients, the malnourished and the elderly. Encephalopathy in renal dialysis patients may not respond to pyridoxine but usually resolves when isoniazid is withdrawn.[7]

Rifampin (rifampicin)

This is one of the rifamycins, semisynthetic derivatives of rifamycin S, a metabolite of *Amycolatopsis* (*Streptomyces*) *mediterranei*. Rifampin inhibits protein synthesis by a very specific inhibition of bacterial DNA-dependent RNA polymerase, thereby blocking the synthesis of mRNA. The corresponding mammalian enzyme is inhibited only by very high concentrations of rifampin. Resistance is due to single amino acid mutational changes in the *rpoB* gene, which encodes for the β subunit of the polymerase. Rifampin is a particularly effective drug because

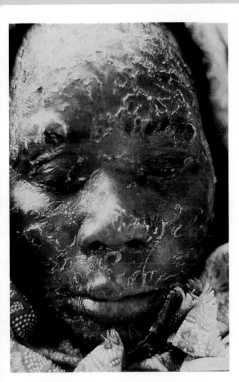

Fig. 143.2 Severe dermal reaction to isoniazid. Courtesy of Dr P Mwaba, Zambia.

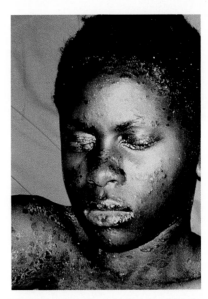

Fig. 143.4 Stevens–Johnson syndrome induced by thiacetazone. Courtesy of Dr P Mwaba, Zambia.

Rifampin may cause an influenza-like syndrome, which, paradoxically, occurs less often if the drug is given daily rather than intermittently. It causes transient abnormalities in liver function and, occasionally, clinically evident cholestatic hepatitis, although this is usually mild. Other adverse effects include gastrointestinal disturbances, skin rashes and antibody-mediated thrombocytopenia.

Acute renal failure is a rare complication, although in some regions it is more frequent; in one center in India it accounted for 11 of 607 (1.8%) admissions for acute renal failure.[8] The renal prognosis is usually favorable. It typically occurs after re-introduction of rifampin and intermittent therapy is a risk factor.

Although the evidence that rifampin is teratogenic is very limited, it is best avoided if possible during the first 3 months of pregnancy. For the same reason, women receiving rifampin should avoid becoming pregnant. In this respect it is important to note that this drug interferes with the action of oral contraceptives, and women of childbearing age should be advised to use another form of birth control while receiving rifampin.

Pyrazinamide (pyrazinoic acid amide)

This is regularly included in the initial intensive phase of short-course chemotherapy because it has the important property of killing intracellular tubercle bacilli and, possibly, extracellular bacilli in anoxic, acidic inflamed lesions. It is inactive in neutral or alkaline microenvironments. The mode of action of pyrazinoic acid is poorly understood but the available evidence suggests that it disrupts bacterial membrane function. There is also evidence that it inhibits the mycobacterial fatty acid synthase (FAS)-1 enzyme.[9] Pyrazinamide requires conversion to pyrazinoic acid by mycobacterial pyrazinamidase enzymes encoded for by the 600 base-pair *pncA* gene. Resistance is usually associated with a wide range of point mutations in this gene, which are detectable by various techniques including microarrays.[10] Pyrazinamidase activity is not detectable in most pyrazinamide-resistant mutants of *M. tuberculosis* or in strains of *M. bovis*, which are naturally resistant to this agent. A few pyrazinamide-resistant strains, however, lack mutations in the *pncA* gene, suggesting alternative mechanisms for resistance to this agent, including defects in transportation of the agent into the bacterial cell.[11]

Pyrazinamide is readily absorbed from the gastrointestinal tract and freely enters the CSF, in which levels similar to those in plasma are found. It is metabolized in the liver; the metabolites, mostly pyrazinoic acid, are excreted in the urine.

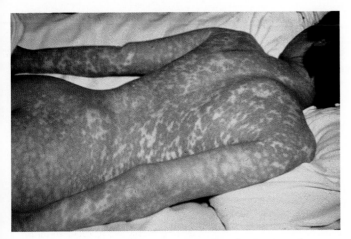

Fig. 143.3 Erythema multiforme reaction to rifampin. Courtesy of Dr P Mwaba, Zambia.

it kills both rapidly dividing bacilli and those that exhibit only occasional short bursts of metabolism. Ideally, therefore, it is given throughout the course of therapy. It is also used in the treatment of leprosy and for some other mycobacterial diseases.

Rifampin is rapidly absorbed from the gastrointestinal tract, although absorption is delayed if it is given with food, and it is widely distributed in the internal organs. Only small amounts enter the CSF in health but much more enters when the meninges are inflamed. Rifampin enters cells and is therefore active against intracellular mycobacteria. It is metabolized by hepatic microsomal enzymes to the desacetyl derivative, which is excreted in the bile. As this enzymatic activity is inducible, the rate of plasma clearance of rifampin increases as treatment proceeds. Although principally excreted in the bile, some rifampin and the desacetyl derivative enter the urine and impart an orange-red color to it. It also enters saliva and lachrymal secretions and may cause pink staining of soft contact lenses. The induction of microsomal enzymes may have clinically significant effects on the metabolism of several other drugs (see below).

Table 143.6 Adverse reactions to the antituberculosis agents

Agent	Adverse reactions
Isoniazid	
Uncommon reactions	Hepatitis, cutaneous hypersensitivity reactions including erythema multiforme, peripheral neuropathy
Rare reactions	Vertigo; convulsions; optic neuritis and atrophy; psychiatric disturbance; hemolytic anemia; aplastic anemia; dermal reactions including pellagra, purpura and lupoid syndrome; gynecomastia, hyperglycemia, arthralgia
Rifampin (rifampicin)	
Uncommon reactions	Hepatitis, flushing, itching with or without a rash, gastrointestinal upsets, 'flu-like syndrome', headache
Rare reactions (usually associated with intermittent therapy)	Dyspnea, hypotension with or without shock, Addisonian crisis, hemolytic anemia, acute renal failure, thrombocytopenia with or without purpura, transient leukopenia or eosinophilia, menstrual disturbances, muscular weakness, pseudomembranous colitis
Pyrazinamide	
Common reactions	Anorexia
Uncommon reactions	Hepatitis, nausea and vomiting, urticaria, nausea, arthralgia
Rare reactions	Sideroblastic anemia, photosensitization, gout, dysuria, aggravation of peptic ulcer
Ethambutol	
Uncommon reactions	Optic neuritis, arthralgia
Rare reactions	Hepatitis, cutaneous hypersensitivity including pruritus and urticaria, photosensitive lichenoid eruptions, paresthesia of the extremities, interstitial nephritis
Streptomycin	
Uncommon reactions	Vertigo, ataxia, deafness, tinnitus, cutaneous hypersensitivity
Rare reactions	Renal damage, aplastic anemia, agranulocytosis, peripheral neuropathy, optic neuritis with scotoma, severe bleeding due to antagonism of factor V, neuromuscular blockade in patients receiving muscle relaxants and in those with myasthenia gravis
Other aminoglycosides	
Uncommon reactions	Cutaneous hypersensitivity, vertigo, deafness
Rare reactions	Renal damage, hypoglycemia, hypokalemia
Thiacetazone	
Common reactions	Gastrointestinal upsets, cutaneous hypersensitivity, vertigo, conjunctivitis
Uncommon reactions	Hepatitis, erythema multiforme, exfoliative dermatitis, hemolytic anemia
Rare reactions	Agranulocytosis
***Para*-aminosalicylic acid**	
Common reactions	Gastrointestinal upsets
Uncommon reactions	Cutaneous hypersensitivity, hepatitis, hypokalemia
Rare reactions	Acute renal failure, hemolytic anemia, thrombocytopenia, hypothyroidism
Ethionamide and prothionamide	
Common reactions	Gastrointestinal upsets, salivation, metallic taste
Uncommon reactions	Cutaneous hypersensitivity, hepatitis
Rare reactions	Alopecia, convulsions, deafness, diplopia, gynecomastia, hypotension, impotence, psychiatric disturbance, menstrual irregularity, hypoglycemia, peripheral neuropathy
Capreomycin and viomycin	
Common reactions	Eosinophilia (with capreomycin), pain and induration at injection site
Uncommon reactions	Loss of hearing, vertigo, tinnitus, electrolyte disturbances including hypokalemia, leukopenia or leukocytosis
Rare reactions	Renal impairment, hepatitis, thrombocytopenia

Table 143.6 Adverse reactions to the antituberculosis agents—cont'd

Agent	Adverse reactions
Clofazimine	
Common reactions	Discoloration of skin and body fluids, nausea, vomiting, abdominal pain, diarrhea
Uncommon reactions	Dryness of skin, ichthyosis, photosensitivity
Rare reactions	Intestinal obstruction
Cycloserine	
Common reactions (especially with daily doses exceeding 500 mg)	Convulsions, drowsiness, sleep disturbance, headache, tremor, vertigo, confusion, irritability, aggression and other personality changes, psychosis (sometimes with suicidal tendencies)
Uncommon reactions	Cutaneous hypersensitivity, hepatitis, megaloblastic anemia
Rare reactions	Congestive heart failure
Fluoroquinolones	
Uncommon reactions	Gastrointestinal upsets, headache, dizziness, insomnia, cutaneous hypersensitivity reactions
Rare reactions	Restlessness; convulsions; psychiatric disturbances including psychotic reactions and hallucinations; edema of face, tongue and epiglottis; disturbance of taste and smell; anaphylactoid reactions

Adverse effects are uncommon. It causes raised serum transaminase levels but overt hepatotoxicity, contrary to earlier reports, is uncommon. It should be used with caution in alcoholics and in patients who have pre-existing hepatic disease, who should have regular liver function tests. Other adverse effects include anorexia, nausea, photosensitization of the skin,[12] arthralgia and gout caused by the inhibition of the excretion of uric acid by pyrazinoic acid.

Ethambutol

Ethambutol (S,S'-2,2'-(ethylenediimino)di-1-butanol) is included in the initial 2-month intensive phase of the WHO-recommended short-course antituberculosis regimens and also in some regimens for disease caused by other slowly growing mycobacteria, particularly members of the *M. avium* complex (MAC), *M. kansasii*, *M. xenopi* and *M. malmoense*. By inhibiting the enzyme arabinosyl transferase, ethambutol blocks the synthesis of the polysaccharide arabinogalactan, a macromolecule essential for the structural integrity of the mycobacterial cell wall. Resistance is associated with mutations in the *embA*, *embB* and *embC* cluster of genes (principally *embB*), which code for this enzyme.[13]

There is conflicting evidence on its effect on resistance to other antituberculosis agents. Thus there is evidence that it may enhance the activity of some of the other drugs by affecting cell-wall permeability, particularly in the MAC but possibly also in multidrug-resistant strains of *M. tuberculosis*.[14] There is also evidence that, in addition to determining resistance to ethambutol, a mutation in codon 306 of the *embB* gene predisposes *M. tuberculosis* to the development of resistance to a range of antituberculosis agents and transmission of such mutants has resulted in clusters of cases of drug-resistant tuberculosis.[15]

About 80% of the dose of ethambutol is absorbed from the gastrointestinal tract. Absorption is inhibited by antacids containing aluminum hydroxide. It does not cross the healthy meninges but up to 40% of the plasma level is found in the CSF in cases of tuberculous meningitis. It is mostly excreted unchanged in the urine but up to 15% is excreted as metabolites.

The principal side-effect is optic neuritis which may have an irreversible effect on vision, but this is rare if the drug is given for no longer than 2 months at a daily dose of 25 mg/kg, or for longer at a dose not exceeding 15 mg/kg. Nevertheless, care should be observed in the use of this drug, its recommended dose and duration of therapy should never be exceeded, and the patient should be informed of the risk of visual impairment and advised to discontinue the drug if such impairment occurs. Loss of color discrimination is the first sign of visual toxicity. Where facilities are available, visual acuity should be assessed before therapy and at intervals during it.

Most guidelines recommend that the drug should not be given to children under the age of 5 years because their visual acuity cannot be readily assessed, even though ocular complications in such young children are extremely rare.

Other side-effects of ethambutol include skin rashes, arthralgia, peripheral neuritis, hyperuricemia and, rarely, jaundice and thrombocytopenia.

Streptomycin

This was the first of the antituberculosis drugs to be discovered and it still has an important role in the treatment of tuberculosis. It inhibits protein synthesis by binding to the 30S subunit of the bacterial ribosome. It is active in neutral or alkaline environments such as the cavity wall but not in the more acidic environment of the closed, inflammatory foci and is therefore not a good sterilizing drug. It is very poorly absorbed from the gastrointestinal tract and must be given parenterally.

Streptomycin is toxic for the eighth cranial nerve (vestibular > cochlear), including that of the fetus, and its use should therefore be avoided in pregnancy. Other adverse reactions include impairment of renal function (uncommon) and hypersensitivity reactions – usually mild skin rashes or fever but occasionally anaphylactic reactions or exfoliative dermatitis.

SECOND-LINE DRUGS

There are, in addition to some agents used on anecdotal evidence of efficacy, six classes of second-line antituberculosis agents; namely, aminoglycosides, polypeptides, thioamides, fluoroquinolones, cycloserine and *para*-aminosalicylic acid.

Aminoglycosides

In addition to streptomycin, the aminoglycosides kanamycin, amikacin and aminosidine (paromomycin) have activity against *M. tuberculosis*.

Cross-resistance with streptomycin is usual. Kanamycin or amikacin is included in some regimens for the treatment of MDRTB and amikacin in some regimens for the treatment of disease due to the MAC, particularly in HIV-positive patients. In common with streptomycin, these aminoglycosides are not absorbed from the gastrointestinal tract and must therefore be given parenterally. Nephrotoxicity and ototoxicity are the major toxicities.

Polypeptides – capreomycin and viomycin

In common with the aminoglycosides, these structurally closely related, cyclic polypeptides inhibit protein synthesis by blocking ribosomal function and must be given by intramuscular injection. They are completely cross-resistant and highly resistant mutants are cross-resistant to the aminoglycosides. They do not readily enter cells or the CSF and are mostly excreted unchanged in the urine. Adverse effects include ototoxicity, nephrotoxicity and pain, bleeding and induration at the injection site. There is some evidence that capreomycin is active against dormant or nonreplicating cells of *M. tuberculosis*.[16] Viomycin is rarely used and is seldom available.

Thioamides – ethionamide and prothionamide

Ethionamide (ethylthioisonicotinamide) and prothionamide (propylthioisonicotinamide) are closely related drugs that are structurally similar to isoniazid; in common with isoniazid they inhibit the synthesis of mycobacterial mycolic acids by targeting the same molecule – enoyl-acyl carrier protein reductase encoded by the *inhA* gene.[17] Thus, in common with isoniazid, resistance is often associated with mutations in the *inhA* gene but, surprisingly, complete cross-resistance to isoniazid does not develop and partial cross-resistance is uncommon. Also in common with isoniazid, these agents are prodrugs that require activation by an enzyme encoded by the *ethA* locus but less than half the mutations conferring resistance to this agent occur in this locus.[18]

These two agents are degraded into several metabolites in the liver and less than 1% is excreted unchanged in the urine. The common occurrence of gastrointestinal irritation with these agents, even when they are given as enteric-coated tablets, limits their use in the treatment of tuberculosis. Prothionamide is slightly better tolerated and is used in some regimens for leprosy. Other adverse effects include skin reactions, hepatitis, impotence and gynecomastia in male patients, menstrual irregularities and various neurologic complications such as convulsions, mental disturbance and peripheral neuropathy.

Fluoroquinolones

These agents inhibit the enzyme DNA gyrase encoded by the *gyrA* and *gyrB* genes, and DNA topoisomerase IV encoded by the *parC* and *parD* genes involved in the regulation of DNA supercoiling. Several fluoroquinolones have early bactericidal activities approaching those of isoniazid, and although results of clinical trials have been rather variable,[19] there is evidence that the addition of ofloxacin to the standard regimen of isoniazid, rifampin and pyrazinamide enables the duration of therapy to be reduced by 1–2 months.[20]

Fluoroquinolones are readily absorbed from the gastrointestinal tract and enter tissues and fluids, including the CSF. Although metabolized to some extent by the liver, they are largely excreted unchanged in the urine. Doses therefore require modification in patients who have renal failure. Adverse effects include nausea and abdominal pain and various neurologic abnormalities including headache, vertigo, insomnia, restlessness, epileptiform attacks and psychiatric disturbances. They should be used with care in epileptic patients.

Cycloserine

This D-alanine analogue, a cyclic derivative of serine hydroxamic acid, inhibits synthesis of peptidoglycan. A related agent, terizidone, is a condensation product containing two cycloserine molecules. Cycloserine is bacteriostatic and thus of limited efficacy, although it is used in some cases of MDRTB. Psychiatric symptoms, including acute psychotic episodes, occur commonly and further limit the usefulness of this drug, although the risk may to some extent be reduced by giving pyridoxine. Allergic skin rashes are rare.

Para-aminosalicylic acid

The mode of action of this bacteriostatic drug is poorly understood although there is some evidence that it inhibits the salicylate-dependent synthesis of the mycobactins – a class of iron-chelating lipids unique to the mycobacteria. It is readily absorbed from the intestine and rapidly acetylated in the liver. About 80% is excreted in the urine, mostly in the acetylated form.

It is rarely used as adverse effects are common. Gastrointestinal effects, including nausea, abdominal pain and diarrhea, occur in up to 30% of patients. Other adverse effects include thyroid dysfunction, crystalluria, blood dyscrasias and, rarely, Löffier syndrome and encephalitis.

Other antituberculosis agents

In common with isoniazid, thiacetazone (acetylaminobenzaldehyde thiosemicarbazone) inhibits the synthesis of mycolic acid, but by a poorly understood mechanism. It is readily absorbed from the gastrointestinal tract. About 20% is eliminated in the urine but the fate of the remainder is unknown. Resistance develops readily and adverse effects, particularly skin reactions, are common. Less frequent adverse effects include gastrointestinal upsets, hepatitis, hemolytic anemia and, rarely, agranulocytosis. A very high incidence of severe, sometimes fatal, skin reactions – exfoliative dermatitis and Stevens–Johnson syndrome – occurs in HIV-positive tuberculosis patients. For this reason, and in view of its limited bacteriostatic activity, the WHO has advised that thiacetazone should no longer be used.

Rifabutin and rifapentine are closely related to rifampin, being semisynthetic derivatives of rifamycin S. Although rifabutin (ansamycin) is considerably more active than rifampin *in vitro*, its *in-vivo* action against *M. tuberculosis* is similar to that of rifampin. Cross-resistance between the rifamycins is usual, so the place for rifabutin in the treatment of MDRTB is limited except in patients receiving antiretroviral therapy (see Chapter 91).

Macrolides are broad-spectrum antibiotics that inhibit protein synthesis by binding to the ribosomal 50S subunit. The newer macrolides – clarithromycin, azithromycin and roxithromycin – are included in regimens used to treat disease due to MAC and other slowly growing mycobacteria including *M. kansasii* and *M. xenopi*. They have only partial *in-vitro* activity against *M. tuberculosis* and evidence for their clinical usefulness is limited. They are well absorbed from the gastrointestinal tract and are excreted in urine. Adverse effects include gastrointestinal upsets with occasional cases of pseudomembranous colitis and various psychiatric disorders, including rare episodes of acute mania.

Certain agents usually used for other infections may have useful activity against *M. tuberculosis*. For example, a combination of amoxicillin and clavulanic acid has *in-vitro* activity against *M. tuberculosis* and there is anecdotal evidence of a beneficial effect against MDRTB.[21]

EXPERIMENTAL ANTITUBERCULOSIS AGENTS

Very little research into new antituberculosis agents was undertaken for around three decades after the discovery of rifampin as it was considered that sales of novel agents would not cover the financial outlay required for their development. In October 2000, however, the Global

Table 143.7 Principal novel antituberculosis agents under investigation in the year 2007

Agent	Mode of action	Investigational status
Moxifloxacin	DNA gyrase and topoisomerase inhibition	Phase III clinical trials
Nitroimidazoles	Dual action: inhibition of protein synthesis and cell wall lipid synthesis	Phase I clinical trials
Pleuromutilins	Interaction with bacterial 50S ribosome subunit to block protein synthesis	*In-vitro* studies
InhA inhibitors	Direct inhibition of InhA, the target of isoniazid but avoiding metabolism by KatG and therefore not being cross-resistant with isoniazid	Identification of agents
Bacterial topoisomerase inhibitors	Similar to fluoroquinolones but binding outside the gyrase region responsible for resistance to fluoroquinolones	Lead identification
Electron transport inhibitors	Disrupt bacterial cell membrane energy functions	Lead identification
Peptide deformylase inhibitors	Inhibit protein maturation	Lead identification

Alliance for TB Drug Development was founded and includes various governmental and nongovernmental organizations, funding agencies and pharmaceutical companies.[22,23] This led to a resurgence of activity and several agents are now in various stages of evaluation. The stages of development of these agents are reported in the Global Alliance annual reports and updated on the alliance website.[23] The principal agents under investigation in 2007 were new quinolones, notably moxifloxacin, and quinolizinones, riminophenazines (related to clofazimine), rifamycins and ethambutol analogues. Compounds with novel modes of activity and those undergoing clinical trials are listed in Table 143.7.

Attempts to treat tuberculosis by enhancing or modifying immune defense mechanisms have been made with reported success.[24] In view of the increasing prevalence of MDRTB, and especially XDRTB, further extensive clinical studies are urgently required.

THE BASIS AND DESIGN OF THERAPEUTIC REGIMENS

The aims of modern chemotherapeutic regimens are:
- to cure the patient;
- to reduce infectivity as rapidly as possible; and
- to prevent the emergence of drug resistance.

In order to cure patients, it is necessary to destroy all the tubercle bacilli in the tissues; if even a few survive there is a high chance of relapse. In this respect, drugs that are bactericidal *in vitro* may not effectively sterilize the tissues *in vivo*.[25] This difference occurs because tubercle bacilli *in vivo* are in a number of different physiologic states or 'compartments':
- freely dividing extracellular bacilli, found mainly in the cavity walls;
- slowly dividing bacilli, found within macrophages and in acidic, inflammatory lesions; and
- dormant and near-dormant bacilli, within cells and in firm caseous material.

The antituberculosis drugs vary in their ability to destroy bacilli in these compartments and in preventing the emergence of resistance to a second drug.

During chemotherapy with modern short-course regimens, freely replicating bacilli in the walls of the cavities are rapidly killed; this is termed the early bactericidal effect. Subsequently, the slowly replicating and near-dormant bacilli are destroyed, but at a much slower rate.

Isoniazid plays a key role in achieving the early bactericidal effect because it is particularly effective in destroying the freely multiply-ing extracellular bacilli, particularly those in the walls of cavities. It has little or no effect on near-dormant bacilli and is therefore not a good sterilizing drug. Rifampin also contributes to the early bactericidal effect.

Ethambutol has bactericidal activity in the early stage of therapy but is not a sterilizing drug. Streptomycin is bactericidal in the slightly alkaline cavity walls but is likewise not a sterilizing agent because it is ineffective in the acidic environment within cells and caseous lesions. By contrast, pyrazinamide is effective within macrophages and acidic, anoxic inflammatory lesions, but not in the neutral or alkaline environment.

Thus, modern regimens commence with an intensive phase of therapy, usually lasting for 2 months, to optimize the early bactericidal effect, thereby eliminating most of the bacilli and rendering the patient noninfectious.[26] The principal drugs used are:
- isoniazid (active against bacilli in the cavity walls);
- pyrazinamide (active against bacilli in acidic closed lesions);
- rifampin (active against both); and
- ethambutol (active in the early stage of therapy and included as a fourth drug as drug resistance is increasingly prevalent).

The daily drug doses are listed in Table 143.8 and the intermittent doses in Table 143.9.

The intensive phase is followed by a continuation phase, usually lasting 4 months, in which any remaining dormant or near-dormant bacilli are destroyed. For this purpose, rifampin is the most powerful sterilizing drug. Although isoniazid is not a sterilizing drug, it is, by its potent activity against replicating bacilli, very good at preventing the emergence of rifampin-resistant mutants. It is thus given together with rifampin throughout the regimen.

Accordingly, the most effective and widely used modern short-course regimens are based on a 2-month phase of rifampin, isoniazid, pyrazinamide and ethambutol, followed by a 4-month phase of rifampin and isoniazid. The WHO has issued clear recommendations on drug regimens for the four categories of tuberculosis seen in clinical practice (Table 143.10).[26]

In most regimens drugs are given daily but, provided that therapy is closely supervised so that all doses are taken, they may be given three times weekly during the continuation phase or, in some regimens, throughout. Intermittent therapy renders the direct administration of the drugs less of a burden for both patients and supervisors.

There is general agreement, supported by clinical trials, that the modern chemotherapeutic regimens discussed above are suitable for the treatment of all types of tuberculosis. Some physicians, however, continue therapy for up to 12 months as a precautionary measure for some extrapulmonary forms of tuberculosis; particularly tuberculous meningitis in which a relapse would be particularly devastating.

Table 143.8 Daily doses of the antituberculosis agents

Agent	DAILY DOSE	
	Adults	**Children**
Rifampin (rifampicin)	450 mg if body weight <50 kg 600 mg if body weight ≥50 kg	10 mg/kg to maximum of 600 mg
Isoniazid	200–300 mg	5 mg/kg
Pyrazinamide	1.5 g if body weight <50 kg 2.0 g if body weight ≥50 kg	25 mg/kg
Ethambutol	15 mg/kg	
Streptomycin	750 mg if body weight <50 kg 1 g if body weight ≥50 kg 750 mg if age ≥40 years 500 mg if age ≥60 years	15 mg/kg to maximum of 0.75 g
Thiacetazone	150 mg	50 mg
Para-aminosalicylic acid	10–12 g	300 mg/kg
Ethionamide and prothionamide	500 mg if body weight <50 kg 750 mg if body weight ≥50 kg	15–20 mg/kg
Capreomycin	1 g	Avoid
Viomycin	1 g	Avoid
Cycloserine	500 mg if body weight <50 kg 750 mg if body weight ≥50 kg	Avoid
Ofloxacin	800 mg	Avoid

Table 143.9 Doses of the first-line antituberculosis agents in three times weekly intermittent therapy

Agent	Dose (adults and children) (mg/kg)	Maximum dose
Isoniazid	15	750 mg
Rifampin (rifampicin)	15	600 mg
Pyrazinamide	50	2.0 g if body weight <50 kg 2.5 g if body weight ≥50 kg
Ethambutol	30	1.8 g
Streptomycin	15–30	750 mg if body weight <50 kg 1 g if body weight ≥50 kg

DRUG-RESISTANT TUBERCULOSIS

Resistance to any given anti-infective agent occurs by mutation at a low but constant rate, so that treatment with a single drug, however powerful, will inevitably lead to selection of resistant mutants. This is largely, but not entirely, avoided by the use of multidrug regimens. Under ideal conditions and in the absence of drug resistance, relapses after completion of a modern short-course chemotherapeutic regimen are uncommon and are mostly due to drug-susceptible bacilli. Unfortunately, ideal treatment conditions have long been the exception rather than the rule and many deficiencies in the use of multidrug regimens has led to the increasing emergence of strains resistant to one or more drugs.[27]

Although resistance to isoniazid is common, patients whose disease is caused by such resistant strains usually respond to short-course chemotherapy. Resistance to rifampin is much more serious in view of the unique ability of this drug to eliminate near-dormant persisting bacilli. Many strains resistant to rifampin are also resistant to isoniazid and, because these drugs are the principal components of modern regimens, this combination renders such regimens ineffective. Thus, the term multidrug resistance has been adopted by the WHO to refer to strains that are resistant to these two drugs, with or without resistance to additional drugs.[28]

A combined initiative by the WHO and the International Union Against Tuberculosis and Lung Disease was launched in 1994 to perform a global survey of resistance to first-line antituberculosis drugs. The first report, published in 1997 and covering 35 countries, showed that resistance to these drugs was more widespread than was previously recognized and revealed certain 'hotspot' areas with a very high incidence, including Estonia, Latvia, Argentina, the Dominican Republic, Côte d'Ivoire and parts of China and Russia.[29] The second report was published in 2000, the third in 2004 and the fourth, covering 138 geographic settings in 114 countries and two special administrative regions (SARs) of China, in 2008, and confirmed the widespread occurrence of MDRTB.[30] The incidence of resistance to any drug and multidrug resistance in new and previously treated patients is summarized in Table 143.11. The range of all types of drug resistance varied enormously from setting to setting, being low in most Western European countries but high in some countries of the former Soviet Union and some SARs of China. According to WHO estimates, almost 490 000 cases of MDRTB emerged worldwide in 2006, 4.8% of the estimated total number of new cases of tuberculosis.[30]

Table 143.10 Principal antituberculosis regimens recommended by the World Health Organization

Diagnostic category	Characteristics of patients	Initial phase	Continuation phase
I	New smear-positive pulmonary TB; new smear-negative pulmonary TB with extensive parenchymal involvement; concomitant HIV disease or severe forms of extrapulmonary TB	*Preferred* 2 HRZE *Optional* 2 (HRZE)$_3$ *or* 2 HRZE	4 HR *or* 4 (HR)$_3$ 4 (HR)$_3$ *or* 6 HE
II	Previously treated sputum smear-positive pulmonary TB: relapse or treatment after default	*Preferred* 2 HRZES/1 HRZE *Optional* 2 (HRZES)$_3$/1 (HRZE)$_3$	5 HRE 5 (H RE)$_3$
	Treatment failure of category I in settings with adequate program performance; representative DRS data showing high rates of MDRTB and/or capacity for DST if cases and availability of category IV regimens	Specially designed standardized or individualized regimens	
	In settings where representative DRS data show low rates of MDRTB or individualized DST shows drug-susceptible disease, or in settings of poor programme performance; absence of representative DRS data insufficient resources to implement category IV treatment	*Preferred* 2 HRZES/1 HRZE *Optional* 2 (HRZES)$_3$/1 (HRZE)$_3$	5 HRE 5 (HRE)$_3$
III	New smear-negative pulmonary TB (other than category I); less severe forms of extrapulmonary TB	*Preferred* 2 HRZE *Optional* 2 (HRZE)$_3$ *or* 2 HRZE	4 HR, 4 (HR)$_3$ 4 (HR)$_3$ *or* 6 HE
IV	Chronic (still sputum-positive after supervised re-treatment); proven or likely MDRTB cases	Specially designed standardized or individualized regimens	

E, ethambutol; H, isoniazid; R, rifampin (rifampicin); S, streptomycin; Z, pyrazinamide. DRS, drug-resistance surveillance; MDRTB, multidrug-resistant tuberculosis. Prefixed numbers show duration of treatment in months. The subscripted figure 3 indicates thrice weekly intermittent dosing.

Extremely drug-resistant tuberculosis (XDRTB)

Tuberculosis resistant to many of the second-line, as well as first-line drugs, has been described in many countries and has been termed extremely drug-resistant tuberculosis (XDRTB). Although there was disagreement over the definition of XDRTB, at the WHO Emergency Global Task Force on XDRTB in October 2006 it was defined as resistance to at least rifampin and isoniazid among the first-line agents, to any fluoroquinolone and to at least one of the injectable second line agents (amikacin, kanamycin and capreomycin).[31]

There are few data on the global incidence and prevalence of XDRTB as a result of limited facilities for testing for susceptibility to a wide range of antituberculosis agents and technical difficulties in accurately determining resistance to the second-line agents. A total of 17 690 strains of *M. tuberculosis* from many countries, 11 939 of them from South Korea, isolated between 2001 and 2004, were subjected to extensive drug-susceptibility testing; 3520 were found to be multidrug resistant (MDR).[32] Of these, 347 (10%) were extremely resistant (XDR). The proportion of MDR strains being XDR was highest in South Korea (15%) and Eastern Europe/Western Asia (14%). Cases of XDRTB were found throughout the world, including industrialized countries, and the proportion of MDR strains being XDR rose over the study period in most regions, from an average of 5% to 7%.

The serious threat posed by XDRTB is illustrated by an outbreak in the Kwazulu-Natal province of South Africa where, between January 2005 and March 2006, 221 of 1539 patients had MDRTB and 53 of these had XDRTB. These included 44 patients who were tested for HIV infection and all were positive. Despite antituberculosis and antiretroviral therapy, all except one with XDRTB died, and among 42 whose date of death was recorded, the median survival was only 16 days after diagnosis.[33]

Causes of antituberculosis drug resistance

Two forms of drug resistance are encountered – acquired and primary (or initial):

- acquired resistance is the result of suboptimal therapy that encourages selective growth of mutants resistant to one or more drugs; and
- primary resistance is due to infection from a source case who has drug-resistant disease.

In practice, it is difficult to be sure that a patient with apparent primary resistant tuberculosis has, in fact, not received any antituberculosis therapy, and some workers therefore prefer the term initial resistance. The division of resistance into acquired and primary forms is of epidemiologic value because an increasing incidence of the former indicates that drug regimens or the supervision of therapy are suboptimal, whereas the continuing occurrence of primary resistance indicates that the transmission of the disease in the community is not being adequately controlled.

The development of drug resistance is due to many avoidable failures in the management of the disease (Table 143.12).

The traditional explanation for treatment failure is noncompliance or nonadherence to therapy and, though there will always be a small number of patients who will default on treatment in any situation, there is ample evidence that it is more often the health services

Table 143.11 Global prevalence of resistance to antituberculosis agents

Any drug resistance – new cases	
Weighted mean*	17.0% (95% CI 13.6–20.4)
Range	0–85.9%
Settings with over 30% resistance	13
Settings with very high prevalence of resistance	4
Multidrug resistance – new cases	
Weighted mean	2.9% (95% CI 2.2–3.6)
Range	0–22.3%
Settings with over 5% resistance	14
Any drug resistance – previously treated cases	
Weighted mean	35.0% (95% CI 24.1–45.8)
Range	0–85.9%
Settings with over 50% resistance	16
Multidrug resistance – previously treated cases	
Weighted mean	15.3% (95% CI 9.6–21)
Range	0–60%

*Means weighted for size of populations surveyed.

Table 143.12 Factors leading to suboptimal therapy and the emergence of drug and multidrug resistance

- Intermittent drug supplies
- Use of time-expired drugs
- Unavailability of combination preparations
- Use of poorly formulated combination preparations
- Prescription of inappropriate drug regimens
- Unregulated over-the-counter sale of drugs, including cough mixtures containing isoniazid
- Addition of single drugs to failing regimens in the absence of bacteriologic control
- Poor supervision of therapy
- Unacceptably high cost to patient in respect of the drugs, travel to the clinic and time off work

than the patient that are at fault. In order to enhance effective tuberculosis control, the WHO Global Plan to Stop Tuberculosis program has widely advocated the DOTS strategy.[34] Originally DOTS was an acronym for directly observed therapy short-course but it is now the 'brand name' for a control strategy with five components:

- government commitment to tuberculosis control;
- provision of a regular supply of good-quality drugs free at the point of delivery;
- passive case finding by sputum microscopy;
- directly observed therapy; and
- regular evaluation of the efficacy of the control program.

Combination drug preparations have been used to prevent patients from receiving monotherapy, but irregular and intermittent use of such preparations has led to drug and multidrug resistance.[30] In addition, the use of poorly formulated combination preparations has led to reduced bioavailability of the constituent agents and the risk of development of drug resistance.

There is no doubt that the blind addition of drugs to a failing regimen is likely to generate multidrug resistance. Unfortunately, the determination of drug resistance is far from easy and most parts of the world lack the facilities for conducting drug susceptibility tests under good quality control. Errors are not uncommon even in the most sophisticated centers in the developed world and may be noticed only when laboratory reports are considered in the light of clinical data. The presence of HIV infection does not by itself lead to an upsurge of MDRTB. Despite the increase in HIV-associated tuberculosis seen in most African countries, such an upsurge has not been the usual finding. On the other hand, several well-documented epidemics of MDRTB have occurred in institutions such as hospitals, prisons or common lodging facilities where immunocompromised HIV-infected persons are crowded together and exposed to an infectious source case.[35,36]

Ethnic minority communities, originating in countries where drug resistance is common, often have higher levels of drug resistance than the majority populations.[37]

The incidence of single-drug-resistant tuberculosis in a community can be reduced by establishment of good disease control programs.[34] This raises the question of whether the implementation of the WHO DOTS strategy would also reduce the incidence of MDRTB in a region. According to one mathematical model,[38] it would have such an effect, but the model assumes that multidrug-resistant strains of *M. tuberculosis* are less virulent than their drug-susceptible counterparts. Since the publication of this model, it has been established that strains of *M. tuberculosis* are divisible into several lineages that differ in their virulence, immunogenicity and ability to retain virulence on mutation to drug or multidrug resistance.[39] In a recently evolved sublineage of the Beijing or W-Beijing lineage, multidrug-resistant strains appear able to retain high virulence and to cause spreading epidemics of multidrug-resistant tuberculosis in certain geographic regions.[40] Further studies are therefore required in order to determine and predict the likely epidemiologic patterns of MDRTB and XDRTB and to take the necessary control measures.

Therapy of multidrug-resistant tuberculosis

Tuberculosis due to bacilli resistant to isoniazid alone usually responds to short-course drug regimens based on four drugs during the intensive phase but, by contrast, resistance to both isoniazid and rifampin (i.e. multidrug resistance) requires prolonged treatment with drugs that are much more costly, less effective and more toxic. The cost of such therapy is high; in the USA it can exceed $US250 000, compared with the cost of $US2000 for treating a patient who has drug-susceptible disease. The prognosis for patients who have MDRTB has improved considerably and, provided that the patient is diagnosed before severe lung damage has occurred and that the best supervised therapy and laboratory support is available, the outlook is good in the majority of cases. Under these optimal conditions, cure rates of 96% have been achieved.

The successful management of MDRTB requires laboratory support and a team of dedicated supervisors of therapy, the so-called 'DOTS-plus' strategy.[41] Ideally regimens should be designed for each patient on the basis of *in-vitro* susceptibility. Various regimens have been used and there have been few comparisons between them. Currently used regimens are usually based on a fluoroquinolone with at least two other drugs to which the strain is susceptible, such as kanamycin and ethionamide (or prothionamide).[42,43] Other agents include rifabutin, amikacin, capreomycin, clofazimine, cycloserine and *para*-aminosalicylic acid. Great care and dedication are required for the successful management of MDRTB (Table 143.13).

Treatment outcomes of patients with MDRTB and XDRTB were assessed in Latvia and the USA and were significantly less favorable in the latter.[32] Alternative forms of treatment, including immunotherapy, are therefore urgently required.

Table 143.13 Principles for management of multidrug-resistant tuberculosis

- Single agents should never be blindly added to failing regimens
- Before drug susceptibility tests become available, patients should be started on three agents that they have never received before
- All therapy should be fully supervised (use of an injectable agent enhances adherence to therapy)
- Therapy should last at least 24 months and should be continued for at least 18 months after bacteriologic conversion
- Drug susceptibility tests should be repeated if cultures remain positive after 3 months of therapy

TREATMENT OF PATIENTS IN SPECIAL CIRCUMSTANCES

Patients who have renal or hepatic disease

Modification of drug regimens and dosages may be required when there is substantial renal impairment or liver disease. The first-line drugs (rifampin, isoniazid, pyrazinamide) and also ethionamide and prothionamide are either completely metabolized or eliminated in the bile. They may therefore be used safely at normal doses in patients who have renal impairment. Isoniazid occasionally causes encephalopathy in patients who have renal failure and in those on dialysis but the risk is reduced, although not eliminated, by administering pyridoxine.[7] Although ethambutol is mainly eliminated by the kidney it can be used in reduced doses in patients who have impaired renal function. Streptomycin and other aminoglycosides are eliminated entirely by the kidney; as they are potentially nephrotoxic, special care must be taken.

In severe renal failure the dose of isoniazid should be reduced to 200 mg once daily (ensuring that pyridoxine is given to prevent peripheral neuropathy). Streptomycin and ethambutol are excreted by the kidney and adjustment to doses is necessary in renal failure. Streptomycin levels must be monitored and doses and spacing adjusted to achieve a peak level of 40 µg/ml and a trough level of <5 µg/ml to avoid toxicity. For patients on dialysis, a supplemental streptomycin dose should be given at approximately 5 mg/kg after hemodialysis.

Ethambutol dosages are dependent on creatinine clearances. For patients who have creatinine clearances between 50 ml/min and 100 ml/min, the dose is 25 mg/kg three times weekly; at 30–50 ml/min, the dose is 25 mg/kg twice a week; and at 10–25 ml/min the dose is 15 mg/kg at 2-day intervals. Patients on hemodialysis may be given 25 mg/kg ethambutol 6 hours before the procedure.

The catabolism of immunosuppressive agents administered to renal transplant patients, including azathioprine, corticosteroids, ciclosporin, sirolimus and tacrolimus, is increased by rifampin and dose adjustments may be required.[44] Streptomycin should be avoided in transplant patients as it increases the available level of ciclosporin, resulting in nephrotoxicity.

There is no clear evidence that the potentially hepatotoxic drugs rifampin and pyrazinamide are any more toxic in patients who have impaired hepatic function. Nevertheless, if they are used, hepatic function should be carefully and regularly monitored during therapy. Some physicians avoid them and treat such patients with isoniazid and ethambutol for 1 year, with the addition of streptomycin for the first 2–3 months. An alternative is to use a fluoroquinolone such as ofloxacin instead of rifampin.[45]

If rifampin is used, it should be used with caution; doses should be reduced in patients who have bilirubin concentrations exceeding 50 mmol/l. Liver function should be regularly monitored, where possible, in alcoholics, the elderly, malnourished children and children under 2 years of age.

If jaundice develops during antituberculosis therapy, treatment should be stopped until the jaundice resolves. In many cases resumption of treatment does not cause a recurrence of the jaundice. If the patient is seriously ill with tuberculosis, he or she may be treated with streptomycin and ethambutol even in the presence of jaundice.

HIV-positive patients who have tuberculosis

The treatment of tuberculosis in HIV-positive patients (see also Chapter 93) follows the same well-established principles used in the treatment of non-HIV-infected patients.[46] Despite a good bacteriologic response to treatment, patients who have HIV-related tuberculosis in Africa who are not receiving antiretroviral therapy have an extremely poor prognosis. They are almost four times as likely to die within 13 months of diagnosis as HIV-negative patients, with most deaths occurring during the first month of treatment.[47] This is largely due to other opportunistic infections but may also, in part, be due to an apparent synergistic immunosuppressive action of HIV infection and active tuberculosis. For this reason, prevention of tuberculosis is preferable to attempts to treat tuberculosis in HIV-positive persons. Drug reactions tend to be more severe in HIV-positive patients than in HIV-negative patients. In particular, thiacetazone often causes severe dermal reactions, with some patients developing fulminant and potentially fatal exfoliative dermatitis.

Pregnancy and the postpartum period

There is general agreement that the management of tuberculosis in pregnancy and in the postpartum period should be similar to that in other patients, although some advocate avoiding pyrazinamide. Short-course regimens seem to have a minimal risk of causing fetal abnormalities, and side-effects in the pregnant woman are no higher than in those who are not pregnant.[48] Opinions concerning the safety of pyrazinamide differ because there are limited experimental data on its effect on the fetus. Nonetheless, it is often used, particularly in regions where drug resistance is common. Streptomycin is avoided owing to its ototoxic properties. The treatment of drug-resistant tuberculosis, especially MDRTB, during pregnancy and the management of the neonate requires careful consideration, and experience is very limited.[49] Expert clinical and laboratory guidance, if available, is required.

An increased incidence of isoniazid-related epileptiform attacks and other neurologic symptoms has been reported in pregnant women but these are preventable by the prescription of pyridoxine 10 mg daily. Mothers taking antituberculosis drugs at the time of birth can care for their infants with little risk, unless the mother's disease is drug resistant or not responding to therapy. Likewise, although some of the drugs enter the milk in small concentrations, breast-feeding has no adverse effects on the infant.[50]

Adjunct corticosteroid therapy in tuberculosis

It has been postulated that corticosteroids, by reducing the host's immune response, would allow dormant bacilli to replicate freely and thereby facilitate killing by the drugs. There is little evidence to support this, and their use has not been shown to affect the outcome of modern short-course chemotherapy. On the other hand, in some forms of tuberculosis corticosteroids aid recovery and reduce long-term sequelae by suppressing inflammatory reactions and limiting subsequent scar formation (see also Chapter 30).

Chemoprophylaxis and preventive therapy of tuberculosis

Chemoprophylaxis is defined as the prescription of antituberculosis drugs for uninfected persons who are exposed to a risk of infection; preventive therapy refers to the treatment of persons who have already been infected with tubercle bacilli (as indicated by tuberculin testing) but who show no clinical or radiologic evidence of active disease. Chemoprophylaxis is principally used to protect children who are at risk of infections, particularly those under the age of 3 years, who are prone to develop serious extrapulmonary forms of tuberculosis, including meningitis.

Preventive drug therapy for those infected by *M. tuberculosis* (i.e. tuberculin reactors) is used in some countries, notably the USA, where tuberculosis is uncommon and where bacille Calmette–Guérin (BCG) is not used. Although highly efficacious, it is not without its problems. Isoniazid monotherapy, for up to 1 year, is the most widely used form of preventive therapy, although 6-month regimens are becoming more common. Although there is a theoretic risk of generating isoniazid resistance, this does not seem to happen in practice, probably because there are so few bacilli present. Hepatic toxicity has given cause for concern, particularly in older adults, and so such preventive therapy is generally not recommended for those aged over 35 years.[51]

Policies for the use of preventive therapy vary from country to country. National guidelines should be consulted for indications for such therapy and for the recommended drug regimens. In general, preventive therapy in tuberculosis control in regions with a high incidence of tuberculosis has, in view of problems of compliance and organization, not played a major role in tuberculosis control programs.

Transplant recipients receiving corticosteroids and other immunosuppressive drugs are at risk of developing tuberculosis. It has been suggested that such patients should be given isoniazid 300 mg and pyridoxine 25–50 mg daily if they have one or more of the following:[52]

- history of inadequately treated tuberculosis;
- an abnormal chest radiograph compatible with antecedent infection with tuberculosis;
- positive tuberculin test of more than 10 mm in diameter; and
- recent contact with a case of active tuberculosis.

Prophylaxis of tuberculosis in HIV-infected patients

In view of the very high risk of an HIV-infected person developing active tuberculosis, and the adverse effect of this disease on the immune status and survival of the patient, there is a very good theoretical case for provision of preventive therapy for those at risk. Several placebo-controlled studies of isoniazid monotherapy in patients co-infected with *M. tuberculosis* and HIV have shown that such preventive therapy is effective.[53] In practice, serious problems have been encountered in diagnosing dual infection, ruling out active tuberculosis and ensuring compliance with therapy without breach of confidence or enhancement of stigma. Studies of varying design from Haiti, Zambia and Uganda have shown that preventive therapy in HIV-infected adults significantly reduced the incidence of tuberculosis. The questions of how long the protection lasts, whether prophylactic treatment is safe and whether it can lead to the emergence of drug-resistant strains of tuberculosis require attention.

Although preventive therapy leads to a reduction of the risk of tuberculosis by around 60% in tuberculin-skin-test-positive adults who have HIV infection, identifying HIV-infected individuals is difficult in resource-poor settings. A major problem is ensuring compliance with therapy. It is important to ensure that HIV-positive persons receiving preventive therapy do not have active tuberculosis or there is a strong risk of masking the disease and encouraging the emergence of drug resistance. It is also necessary to supervise the therapy, and this adds another burden to stretched tuberculosis control services.

Isoniazid monotherapy for 9 months is suitable for preventive therapy in HIV-positive persons; continuation of therapy to 12 months adds very little. Shorter prophylactic regimens, such as rifampin with pyrazinamide for 2 months, have also been evaluated. These include a 3-month course of a rifamycin (rifampin or rifabutin) plus isoniazid, and a 2-month course of a rifamycin plus pyrazinamide. Although completion of treatment is significantly higher with the shorter regimens, the incidence of hepatic toxicity is much higher,[54] and as there

have been some deaths due to liver failure such short courses of preventive therapy should only be used where there are facilities for regular assessment of hepatic function. The relatively short-term benefit of preventive therapy is a further problem. By 18 months, the incidence of tuberculosis in those who receive such therapy is similar to that in those not receiving such therapy, indicating the need to consider repeated courses or, perhaps, lifelong preventive therapy.[55] As a general rule, prevention is more effective in those who have relatively limited immunosuppression (positive tuberculin tests, high lymphocyte counts and high hemoglobin levels). This, together with the difficulty in detecting co-infection, has led to the current recommendation to restrict preventive therapy to tuberculin-positive, HIV-positive persons (see Chapter 93 for further discussion).

Another problem with preventive therapy is the high incidence of multidrug-resistant tuberculosis in some regions, against which isoniazid monotherapy would afford no protection. It is understandable that health care staff are anxious about the risk to their health if reliance is placed on chemoprophylaxis rather than BCG vaccination. In general, in view of problems of compliance and organization, preventive therapy has not played a major role in tuberculosis control.[56]

DRUG INTERACTIONS

Clinically significant interactions between the first-line antituberculosis drugs themselves have been described but are uncommon;[57] however, such reactions could well occur when more complex regimens are used to treat MDRTB and XDRTB. Antituberculosis drugs may interact with drugs used to treat unrelated conditions (Table 143.14). Rifampin is the most important in this respect because it is a potent inducer of cytochrome isoenzymes involved in the metabolism of many drugs. The increased metabolism and clearance of these drugs may lead to therapeutic failure unless levels are adjusted and then readjusted when rifampin therapy ceases. Patients on oral contraceptives should be advised to use alternative forms of birth control.

Rifampin reduces the plasma concentrations and half-lives of the imidazole and triazole antifungals and these agents reduce plasma levels of rifampin. Because some patients, notably those who are HIV positive, may also require antifungal therapy, these interactions, which may lead to treatment failure, are of increasing importance. Patients who are HIV positive may also be receiving trimethoprim–sulfamethoxazole for prevention or treatment of *Pneumocystis jirovecii* (formerly *P. carinii*) infection. This agent significantly increases the serum levels and half-life of rifampin, leading to an increased incidence of adverse effects, including hepatotoxicity.[58]

Drug interactions with isoniazid are more pronounced in slow acetylators. The effects of isoniazid are potentiated by insulin and opposed by prednisone (prednisolone); its absorption from the intestine, and that of ethambutol and the quinolones, is inhibited by antacids containing aluminum hydroxide. The effects of carbamazepine and phenytoin are potentiated by isoniazid and those of enflurane are opposed.

Drug interactions with antiretroviral agents

The available antiretroviral agents all interact with rifampin, but this is most marked with protease inhibitors such as saquinavir, ritonavir, indinavir and nelfinavir.[59] Rifampin accelerates the metabolism of protease inhibitors (through induction of hepatic P450 cytochrome), resulting in subtherapeutic levels of these agents and thereby increasing the risk of the development of viral resistance. In addition, protease inhibitors retard the metabolism of rifampin, resulting in increased serum levels and the likelihood of increased drug toxicity (see Chapter 93).

When prescribing antiretrovirals with antituberculosis drugs, it is important to refer to the latest guidelines on the subject since these are updated frequently. As new antiretroviral agents are being discovered and used, new interactions with antituberculosis drugs are being discovered. Updates on these periodically appear on the US Centers for Disease Control and Prevention website – http://www.cdc.gov/mmwr.

Table 143.14 Clinically significant drug interactions with antituberculosis agents

Effects opposed by rifampin (rifampicin)

Antiretroviral agents	Opioids
Azathioprine	Oral contraceptives
Corticosteroids	Phenytoin
Ciclosporin	Propranolol
Diazepam	Quinidine
Digoxin	Theophylline
Haloperidol	Tolbutamide
Imidazoles	Warfarin

Potentiates the effects of rifampin (rifampicin)

Trimethoprim–sulfamethoxazole

Effects potentiated by isoniazid

Phenytoin
Carbamazepine

Potentiates the effects of isoniazid

Insulin

Effects opposed by isoniazid

Enflurane

Opposes the effects of isoniazid

Prednisone
Antacids (inhibit absorption)

Effects potentiated by streptomycin

Neuromuscular blocking agents

Effects potentiated by quinolones

Aminophylline and theophylline

Potentiates the effects of quinolones

Cimetidine

Opposes the effects of quinolones

Antacids, iron preparations, sucralfate, didanosine (all inhibit absorption)

The timing of antiretroviral therapy (ART) in HIV-infected patients receiving antituberculosis therapy has been the subject of some controversy. The priority is to treat tuberculosis and while it is desirable to treat the HIV also without delay, complicating factors including the possible development of the immune reconstitution inflammatory syndrome (IRIS)[60] make it safer to delay ART. In 2006, the WHO recommended that ART should be delayed for 2–8 weeks in those with CD4+ counts of <200 cells/mm³ and in those whose CD4+ counts are unknown, and for 8 weeks in those with CD4+ counts of 200–350 cells/mm³. Those with counts of >350 cells/mm³ should be evaluated after 8 weeks and, unless their clinical condition is deteriorating, ART can be withheld until the course of treatment for tuberculosis has been completed.[61]

Regimens not containing a rifamycin are much less effective than those that are rifamycin based for treatment of HIV-infected patients. Thus, except in cases of resistance or intolerance to these agents, regimens containing a rifamycin throughout should be used and any interactions between these and the antiretroviral agents should be managed appropriately. Whenever possible, rifampin should be replaced by rifabutin, a much less powerful inducer of cytochrome enzymes, and to commence or continue with the antiretroviral drugs.[62] The clinical experience of antiretroviral regimens based on a non-nucleoside reverse-transcriptase inhibitor such as efavirenz plus two nucleoside analogues with rifampin-based antituberculosis treatment regimens in terms of tolerance and impact on both tuberculosis and HIV disease has been very favorable.[63,64]

DRUG SUSCEPTIBILITY TESTING

The purpose of drug susceptibility testing is not to detect small numbers of drug-resistant mutants, which will inevitably be present in every patient who has tuberculosis and in every culture, but rather to determine whether the great majority of the bacilli are susceptible to levels of the drugs that are achieved clinically. In the developed nations with the requisite facilities, and particularly where MDRTB is common, susceptibility testing of all clinical isolates is definitely indicated. In most developing countries, facilities for conducting drug susceptibility tests are very limited.

Drug susceptibility testing is of epidemiologic importance in monitoring the global incidence and distribution of acquired and primary drug resistance. Unfortunately, susceptibility testing is expensive and time-consuming and requires good laboratory facilities, a high level of technical expertise and rigid quality-control procedures. There is no point in doing such testing unless high standards of accuracy can be maintained because much harm may be done by modifying regimens to include less effective and more toxic drugs on the basis of false reports of resistance.

Global surveys on drug resistance have been compromised by the variety of methods used for surveillance and for drug susceptibility testing and the lack of standardization of the methods. The WHO has therefore prepared guidelines for standardized surveillance techniques and has established a network of supranational reference laboratories to co-ordinate surveillance and to provide technical guidance and assistance.[65]

Methods of drug susceptibility testing

Methods for drug susceptibility testing can be divided into:
- those that are based on inhibition of bacterial growth on drug-containing standard media;
- those that detect growth inhibition by automated systems;
- those that use biologic indicators of bacterial viability, such as enzyme activity and bacteriophage replication; and
- those that use nucleic-acid-based technology to detect mutations in genes determining susceptibility to drugs.

Methods for drug susceptibility testing based on growth on conventional media are well established but have the great disadvantage that there is a long delay before results are available. Four methods are currently in use (Table 143.15).

In an (unpublished) investigation carried out by members of the European Society of Mycobacteriologists, there were only minor discrepancies between results obtained by different workers using the first three of the methods listed in Table 143.15. All these methods may be used either for direct susceptibility tests on smear-positive sputum or for indirect susceptibility tests on cultures. The relative merits and usefulness of these methods in differing circumstances have been reviewed.[66]

Conventional tests for susceptibility to pyrazinamide pose particular problems because the drug acts only in acidic environments in which bacterial growth is poor. Thus, the tests require careful standardization and interpretation.

Automated techniques are widely used in developed countries. They are more costly than the conventional methods but the rapidity of the results justifies the extra cost, especially where multidrug resistance is common. Susceptibility to all antituberculosis drugs, including pyrazinamide, can be determined by these methods. Although radiometric systems were used originally,[67] these have been largely replaced by nonradiometric systems, principally based on the unquenching of a fluorescent dye when oxygen is consumed by mycobacterial metabolism or on color changes in dyes when carbon dioxide is liberated from nutrients in the medium.[68]

Several rapid methods for the detection of mutations in the *rpoB* gene conferring resistance to rifampin have been described; one of these, based on a number of DNA probes for wild-type and mutated regions of the gene (line hybridization assay), is obtainable in a commercially available kit form. The sites of mutations responsible for resistance to some other antituberculosis drugs, including streptomycin, pyrazinamide, isoniazid and ethionamide, are also known, and so

Table 143.15 Techniques used to determine susceptibility to antituberculosis agents *in vitro*

Technique	Where technique is used	Description of technique
Proportion method	USA and some European countries	Drug-free and drug-containing media are inoculated with test strains and the colony counts are compared; strains are reported as resistant if the colony count on the drug-containing medium is over 1% of that on the drug-free medium
Absolute concentration method	Some parts of Europe	Based on growth on media containing doubling dilutions of a known concentration of drug, so that the minimal bactericidal concentrations of drugs may be determined
Resistance ratio method	UK and those countries influenced by British bacteriologists	Similar to the absolute concentration method except that results are expressed as the ratio of the drug concentration inhibiting the test and drug susceptible control strains, rather than as the actual inhibiting concentration
Disk diffusion method	Rarely used	Similar to absolute concentration method and resistance ratio method but technically simpler, as disks containing the drugs are placed on the solid media, thereby avoiding the need to prepare batches of media containing the various drugs

commercially available kits for rapid detection of resistance to these and other drugs may soon be obtainable.[69]

Bacteriophages have been used to detect bacterial viability in the presence of antituberculosis agents.[70]

CONCLUSIONS

Chemotherapy is the mainstay of tuberculosis control and modern short-course regimens are among the most effective and cost-effective of all therapeutic interventions for any human disease. Sadly, this potent intervention has been so badly used that tuberculosis remains the leading infectious cause of death worldwide and control of the disease is now seriously threatened by the emergence of multidrug resistance. Although recent advances in immunology and molecular biology may eventually yield novel preventive and therapeutic agents, the overwhelming need at the present time is ensure that the available disease control tools are universally deployed and used in the most effective ways possible.

REFERENCES

References for this chapter can be found online at http://www.expertconsult.com

Miscellaneous agents: fusidic acid, nitrofurantoin and spectinomycin

This chapter deals with three antibiotics that are chemically different and have different antibacterial spectra and clinical uses.

Fusidic Acid

Fusidic acid has a steroidal chemical structure.

MECHANISM OF ACTION

It inhibits protein synthesis by interfering with elongation factor G preventing the release of energy required for the translocation of peptidyl tRNA from the A site to the P site.

SPECTRUM OF ACTIVITY

Fusidic acid has a narrow spectrum of activity. It exhibits good activity against the staphylococci including both methicillin-sensitive and methicillin-resistant strains of *Staphylococcus aureus* (MSSA and MRSA), as well as coagulase-negative staphylococci, but activity against other Gram-positive cocci is poor. In addition, fusidic acid has anaerobic activity, with the exception of *Fusobacterium* spp., has been found to be active against some mycobacteria and has limited activity against the Gram-negative bacteria *Neisseria* spp. and *Legionella pneumophila*.[1]

MECHANISMS OF RESISTANCE

The most clearly described resistance in *Staph. aureus* is conferred through single point mutations at various points of the *fusA* gene, leading to amino acid changes in the elongation factor G protein structure.[2] Other described mechanisms are altered cell permeability, binding by chloramphenicol acetyltransferase type 1 and enhanced drug efflux.

PHARMACOKINETICS, ROUTE OF ADMINISTRATION AND DOSAGE

Fusidic acid is available for intravenous, oral or topical administration. The bioavailability after oral administration is 75–90% with tablets but only about 23% in children given a suspension.[3] After an oral dose of 500 mg given as tablets, the initial plasma concentration is approximately 30 µg/ml and in steady state the concentration is about 100 µg/ml after a dosage of 500 mg q8h. The protein binding is about 97%.

Fusidic acid is lipid soluble and is efficiently distributed to peripheral compartments, including brain tissue, but excluding cerebrospinal fluid.[4] The elimination half-life is about 9 hours. Fusidic acid is eliminated mainly by conjugation to glucuronide in the liver and subsequent biliary excretion.

The normal dosage is:
- adults 500 mg (as sodium fusidate tablets) q8h orally or intravenously;
- neonates 50 mg/kg (as fusidic acid suspension) in three divided doses;
- child 1 month–1 year, 15 mg/kg q8h;
- child 1–5 years, 250 mg q8h;
- child 5–12 years, 500 mg q8h;
- child 12–18 years, 750 mg q8h.

Doses should be reduced in patients who have hepatic disease, particularly biliary obstruction. Full doses can be given to patients who have renal insufficiency and to the elderly. Because of the high protein binding, administration of fusidic acid should be avoided during the last trimester of pregnancy and to newborn children (risk for accumulation of bilirubin in the central nervous system – 'kernicterus').

INDICATIONS

Fusidic acid is mainly used as an antistaphylococcal agent but has to be used in combination with other antibiotics to prevent the emergence of resistance during treatment. In experimental staphylococcal endocarditis it was shown that, when fusidic acid was used as a single agent, resistance emerged in five of 12 animals, whereas no resistance was seen in animals treated with vancomycin plus fusidic acid.[5] Resistance has also emerged as a problem clinically when it has been used as a single agent topically for skin infections; a number of clonal outbreaks of childhood impetigo due to fusidic acid-resistant MSSA in Scandinavian and European countries have been associated with the use of topical preparations of fusidic acid.[6,7]

Both *in-vivo* and *in-vitro* studies have shown that the antibacterial activity of the combination of fusidic acid with other antibiotics is unpredictable so that synergistic, antagonist, additive or indifferent effects have all been described.[8,9] For example, in a clinical study of 104 consecutive cases of *Staph. aureus* meningitis, a better outcome was demonstrated in those treated with fusidic acid in combination with another antistaphylococcal agent (mainly a penicillinase-stable penicillin, e.g. methicillin) than those treated with other regimens including methicillin alone.[10] However, in an experimental model of *Staph. aureus* meningitis, antagonism between methicillin and fusidic acid was observed.[11]

Fusidic acid is widely used for the treatment of bone and joint infections due to *Staph. aureus* as high bactericidal levels are achieved in infected joints and bone, including sequestra. It is usually combined with a penicillinase-stable penicillin (e.g. flucloxacillin) to prevent the emergence of resistance, although there are no formal studies showing that the combination is better than a penicillinase-stable penicillin alone.

The spectrum of fusidic acid makes it one of the few antibiotics that can be used for the oral treatment of methicillin-resistant staphylococci. It should then preferably be combined with another antibiotic to avoid the emergence of resistance. The combination of oral rifampin (rifampicin) with fusidic acid has been used successfully for the decolonization of respiratory tract carriage of MRSA and follow-on oral treatment of vancomycin-intermediate *Staph. aureus* (VISA) infections, but monitoring of liver function is advisable as hepatic failure has been described on this combination.[12,13]

ADVERSE REACTIONS AND INTERACTIONS

Table 144.1 lists the most important adverse reactions to fusidic acid. Most common adverse reactions are minor (diarrhea, abdominal discomfort, contact dermatitis with topical therapy). Intravenous fusidic acid causes local irritation and thrombophlebitis in about 15% of patients treated, and hemolysis may occur following rapid infusion (normal infusion time is 2 hours or more). Additionally, intravenous use appears to increase the risk of jaundice and liver impairment. In a cohort study including 131 patients with staphylococcal bacteremia treated with fusidic acid, reversible jaundice occurred in 48% of those treated intravenously compared to 13% treated orally (and 2% with other therapies).[14] These, along with sodium fusidate's high oral bioavailability, favor the oral route. In newborns fusidic acid may cause kernicterus. Fusidic acid may interact with coumarin derivatives and oral contraceptives, reducing the bioavailability of these drugs through interference with the fecal flora.

Nitrofurantoin

Nitrofurantoin has the structure 1-{[[(5-nitro-2-furanyl)methylene] amino}-2,4-imidazolidinedione and is the only compound of the nitrofuran class that has been used widely; the active component is the 5-nitro structure.

MECHANISM OF ACTION

Although this is not fully understood, it is known that the active form is produced intracellularly by reduction of the nitro group by cellular nitroreductases, which produce highly active intermediate metabolites that have been shown to bind to bacterial ribosomes, halting protein synthesis, and are thought to result in damage of bacterial DNA.

Table 144.1 Serious adverse reactions to fusidic acid	
Adverse reaction	**Risk factor**
Thrombophlebitis	Use of intravenous preparation for more than 24 h
Jaundice, liver impairment	Intravenous preparation, abnormal liver function

SPECTRUM OF ACTIVITY

Nitrofurantoin has broad-spectrum activity against Gram-negative and Gram-positive bacteria, including enterococci but excluding *Pseudomonas aeruginosa* and the Proteae (e.g. *Proteus, Morganella* and *Providencia* spp.) and some limited activity against *Bacteroides* spp.[15] Resistance is still rare in *Escherichia coli* and other extended-spectrum β-lactamase (ESBL)-producing Enterobacteriaceae.[16,17] As nitrofurantoin loses most of its antibacterial activity in alkaline pH, it is not active against the Proteae, even if susceptibility testing shows sensitivity.

MECHANISMS OF RESISTANCE

Acquisition of resistance is rare and the mechanism has not been fully elucidated. It is thought to be due to loss of nitroreductase activity or prevention of adequate intracellular concentrations of the drug being reached.

PHARMACOKINETICS, ROUTE OF ADMINISTRATION AND DOSAGE

Nitrofurantoin is administered orally as a microcrystalline or macrocrystalline formulation, of which the latter has a slower absorption rate. Absorption is almost complete, with 2–4% of the dose being recovered from the feces.[18] Serum concentrations are not measurable, except in patients who have severe renal failure. This is because of destruction of nitrofurantoin in the tissues and, in particular, a very rapid renal elimination by glomerular filtration (20%) and tubular secretion, resulting in a serum half-life of only 20 minutes in patients who have normal renal function.[18] Excretion is complete within 6 hours after intake and urine concentrations of 200–400 mg/l are achieved after a dose of 100 mg q8h. In patients who have renal failure – who should not be given nitrofurantoin – there are measurable but still very low serum and urine concentrations.[19]

Therapeutic doses of nitrofurantoin are 50–100 mg q8h or q6h for adults and 3 mg/kg/day q12h or q8h for children. Prophylactically, the adult dose is 50–100 mg and the pediatric dose 1–2 mg/kg at bedtime. The duration of treatment when nitrofurantoin is used therapeutically should be 5–7 days. Dosages are not affected by liver function.

INDICATIONS

Nitrofurantoin should only be used for the treatment and prevention of bacterial cystitis.

In a study comparing 3-day treatment regimens of trimethoprim–sulfamethoxazole 160–800 mg q12h, cefadroxil 500 mg q12h, amoxicillin 500 mg q8h and nitrofurantoin 100 mg q6h for the treatment of uncomplicated cystitis in women, significantly better results were obtained with trimethoprim–sulfamethoxazole than with the other three regimens, which did not differ from each other.[20]

However, similar efficacy results have been reported for trimethoprim–sulfamethoxazole and nitrofurantoin when they are used for 7 days. Despite these findings, nitrofurantoin has a place in the therapy of cystitis, and use is currently increasing with the emergent problem of multiresistant ESBL-positive *E. coli* and other enteric Gram-negative bacilli isolates which are resistant to the usual first-line oral therapies.

The use of a single dose of nitrofurantoin at night to prevent cystitis has been shown to be well tolerated with no emergence of nitrofurantoin-resistant organisms in the fecal flora.[21] Use in most stages of pregnancy appears to be safe. However, some authorities advise avoidance in pregnant women at term (38–42 weeks gestation) when labor is imminent due to the possible risk of hemolytic anemia in the newborn.[22]

ADVERSE REACTIONS

Table 144.2 lists the most important adverse reactions to nitrofurantoin. They occur at low frequencies (<0.5%).[23] The risk for these reactions can be markedly reduced by:

- avoiding long-term (>7 days) treatment, especially in the elderly;
- avoiding daily doses higher than 300 mg in adults; and
- reducing the dosage for elderly patients and patients who have renal impairment.

Nitrofurantoin should not be used for patients who have renal failure because the urine levels are too low and there is an increased risk of adverse reactions. Upper gastrointestinal adverse reactions (nausea, vomiting, anorexia) may occur and seem to be more common with the historical microcrystalline formulation than with the macrocrystalline one now in use.

Spectinomycin

Spectinomycin is an aminocyclitol antibiotic with a chemical structure similar to that of the aminoglycosides.

MECHANISM OF ACTION

Spectinomycin acts by inhibiting bacterial protein synthesis at the 30S ribosomal level.[24]

Table 144.2 Serious adverse reactions to nitrofurantoin

Adverse reaction	Risk factor
Eosinophilic lung infiltrates, fever	Prolonged treatment time, high doses
Pulmonary fibrosis	Elderly female patients, high doses
Polyneuropathy	High dose relative to renal function
Hepatitis	Long treatment time
Hemolytic anemia	Hereditary glucose-6-phosphate dehydrogenase deficiency

SPECTRUM OF ACTIVITY

Spectinomycin is most active against *Neisseria gonorrhoeae* where resistance is uncommon.[25,26] It is also active against various Gram-negative Enterobacteriaceae including *Escherichia coli*, *Klebsiella*, *Enterobacter* and some *Serratia* spp.[27] Activity against Gram-positive bacteria is more limited, with some strains of *Streptococcus pyogenes*, *Strep. pneumoniae* and *Staphylococcus* sensitive.

MECHANISMS OF RESISTANCE

Resistance is conferred through enzymic adenylylation via aminoglycoside adenylyltransferase.

PHARMACOKINETICS, ROUTE OF ADMINISTRATION AND DOSAGE

Spectinomycin is always given intramuscularly. It is rapidly and completely absorbed and a concentration of about 80 mg/l is achieved after a dose of 2 g.[28] Its protein binding is low (<5%) and it has an apparent volume of distribution of 0.3 l/kg. Elimination is renal, with a half-life of about 1 hour. It has no reported effects per se on any organ system.

Spectinomycin is given as a single intramuscular dose of 2 g for gonococcal urethritis and at a dose of 2 g q12h for 3 days for disseminated gonococcal infection. Dose reductions are not necessary in any patient category.

INDICATIONS AND ADVERSE REACTIONS

Spectinomycin is indicated in the treatment of gonococcal infection of the cervix, urethra or rectum. Although not normally used as first-line therapy, it should be considered as an alternative when the patient is allergic to cephalosporins.[29]

REFERENCES

References for this chapter can be found online at http://www.expertconsult.com

Chapter | **145** | *Christine J Kubin*
Scott M Hammer

Antiretroviral agents

INTRODUCTION

The field of antiretroviral therapy is well into its third decade. It began shortly after the discovery of HIV-1 in 1983, following which *in-vitro* cultivation of the virus permitted the screening of agents for antiviral activity. The first antiretroviral agent approved was zidovudine, a nucleoside analogue reverse transcriptase inhibitor, in 1987. The identification of viral-specific targets and a selected host target (Fig. 145.1) has facilitated high throughput screening and rational drug design efforts, which resulted in the availability of 25 US Food and Drug Administration (FDA)-approved agents by early 2009 (Table 145.1). Potent combination therapy, commonly referred to as highly active antiretroviral therapy (HAART), has led to dramatic reductions in morbidity and mortality in the developed world and has begun to demonstrate similar benefits in the developing world as a result of large-scale rollout efforts.[1] The availability of simpler, less toxic initial regimens and the recognition of the importance of 'non-AIDS' events linked to uncontrolled viremia have moved the pendulum to initiating therapy earlier. In parallel, the approval of a number of new agents in the past few years with activity against drug-resistant strains of HIV-1 has changed the perspective on the management of highly treatment experienced patients with multidrug resistance in resource-rich settings, permitting the goal of therapy to be complete viral suppression in all patients.[2,3]

Despite these advances, the challenges of adherence, toxicities and drug resistance have placed recognizable limits on the currently available agents. Thus, continued drug development is a necessity if further progress is to be made. The clinical use of antiretroviral agents involves a pathogenesis-based, combination treatment approach. The principles and approach to antiretroviral therapy and clinical monitoring tools are addressed in Chapters 99 and 100. The reader is also referred to published antiretroviral therapy guidelines from the Department of Health and Human Services,[2] the International AIDS Society–USA,[3] and the European AIDS Clinical Society.[4] This chapter will review approved antiretroviral agents. Selected investigational agents in advanced phase clinical testing are discussed in the web version.

NUCLEOSIDE ANALOGUE REVERSE TRANSCRIPTASE INHIBITORS

Nucleoside reverse transcriptase inhibitors (NRTIs) were the first class of antiretroviral agents developed (Fig. 145.2). These drugs share a common mechanism of action. As purine or pyrimidine analogues, they require intracellular anabolic phosphorylation to triphosphate forms to be active inhibitors of the HIV reverse transcriptase. The NRTI triphosphates act as competitive inhibitors of the normal nucleotides and act as chain terminators during proviral DNA synthesis.

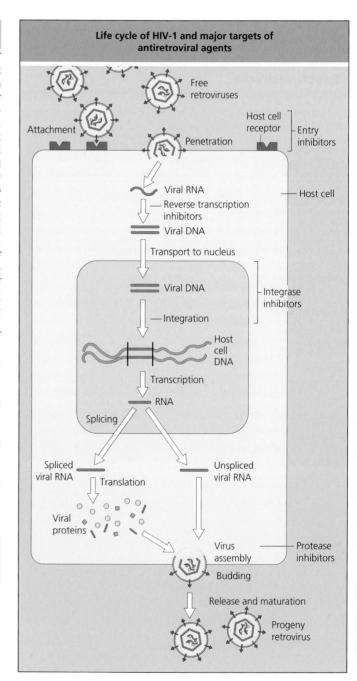

Fig. 145.1 Life cycle of HIV-1 and major targets of antiretroviral agents.

Table 145.1 List of FDA-approved agents*†

Nucleoside/nucleotide reverse transcriptase inhibitors	Non-nucleoside reverse transcriptase inhibitors	Protease inhibitors	Entry inhibitors	Integrase inhibitors
Zidovudine (Retrovir)	Nevirapine (Virammune)	Saquinavir (Invirase)	Enfuvirtide (Fuzeon)	Raltegravir (Isentress)
Didanosine (Videx, Videx EC)	Delavirdine (Rescriptor)	Indinavir (Crixivan)	Maraviroc (Selzentry, Celsentri)	
Stavudine (Zerit)	Efavirenz (Sustiva, Stocrin)	Ritonavir (Norvir)		
Lamivudine (Epivir)	Etravirine (Intelence)	Nelfinavir (Viracept)		
Abacavir (Ziagen)		Lopinavir/ritonavir (Kaletra, Aluvia)		
Emtricitabine (Emtriva)		Atazanavir (Reyataz)		
Tenofovir disoproxil fumarate (Viread)		Fosamprenavir (Lexiva, Telzir)		
		Tipranavir (Aptivus)		
		Darunavir (Prezista)		

*Includes US and non-US brand names.
†Combination products are not listed; please refer to text.

Zidovudine

Description

Zidovudine – 3′-azido-,3′-deoxythymidine (AZT, ZDV; see Fig. 145.2) – is converted to ZDV triphosphate sequentially by cellular thymidine kinase, thymidylate kinase and nucleoside diphosphate kinase. Zidovudine triphosphate possesses a 100-fold greater selectivity for the HIV-1 reverse transcriptase than for the cellular DNA polymerase alpha, thus accounting for its viral specificity. The drug is active against HIV-1, HIV-2 and human T-cell lymphotropic virus type 1 (HTLV-1).

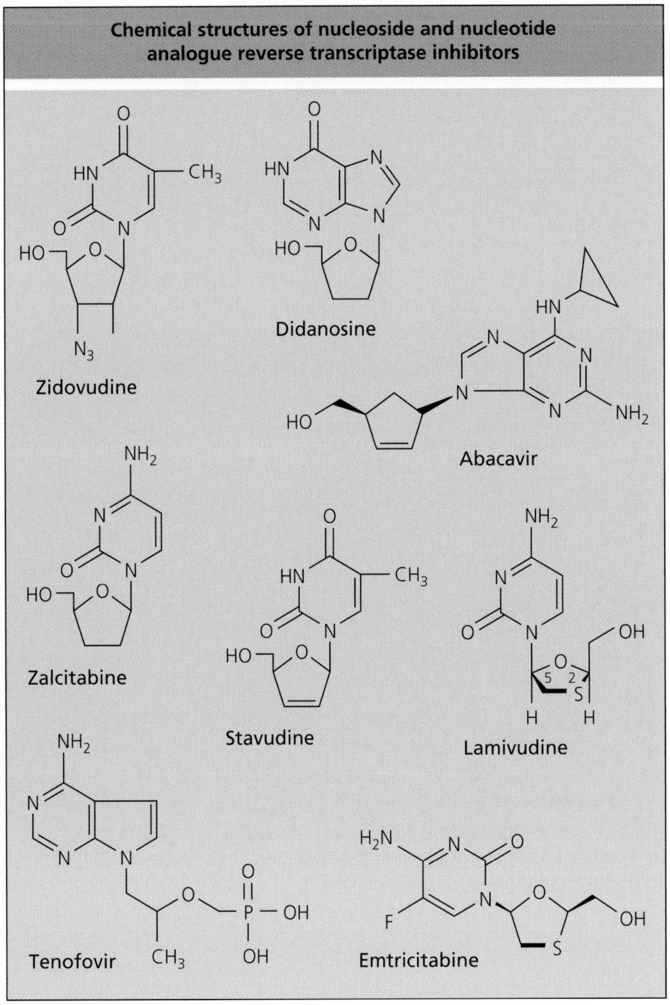

Pharmacokinetics and distribution

Zidovudine is rapidly and well absorbed following oral administration, but exhibits a mean systemic bioavailability of about 64% due to significant first-pass metabolism. Peak plasma concentrations of intravenous and orally administered zidovudine range from 1.5 to 18 µmol/l with single and multiple doses of 1–10 mg/kg. Zidovudine is highly lipophilic and widely distributed throughout the body. Concentrations in the cerebrospinal fluid (CSF) in adults have ranged from 15% to 135% of plasma concentrations. Zidovudine is approximately 25% protein-bound and is primarily metabolized by hepatic 5′-glucuronidation followed by renal excretion.[5] The serum half-life of ZDV is approximately 1 hour, but the intracellular half-life of zidovudine 5′-triphosphate is approximately 3 hours.

Use

The usual adult therapeutic dosage of zidovudine is 300 mg q12h. Typically, it is paired with another NRTI to form a dual nucleoside component of a three- or four-drug regimen. The second NRTI is most commonly lamivudine or emtricitabine but should never be stavudine because of demonstrated antagonism.[6] In antiretroviral-naive patients, these dual nucleoside components need to be prescribed with a ritonavir-boosted protease inhibitor (PI) or a non-nucleoside reverse transcriptase inhibitor (NNRTI) to form a combination regimen capable of suppressing plasma HIV-1 RNA to less than 50 copies/ml. Zidovudine is less frequently used than tenofovir or abacavir as part of the dual nucleoside or nucleotide–nucleoside component of initial regimens because of its toxicity profile. The use of zidovudine in treatment-experienced patients should be guided by the previous treatment history and the results of drug resistance testing. The presence of NRTI class cross-resistance often limits the efficacy of zidovudine in second- and third-line regimens.

Resistance

The mechanism of resistance[7] is thought to be mediated by pyrophosphorolysis, which facilitates the removal of zidovudine after its incorporation into the proviral DNA chain. Resistance to zidovudine is conferred primarily by six mutations, which include M41L, D67N, K70R, L210W, T215F/Y and K219Q/E. High-level zidovudine resistance requires the accumulation of three to four mutations. These zidovudine-associated mutations are referred to as thymidine or nucleoside–nucleotide analogue-associated mutations (TAMs, NAMs) because of the increasing recognition of their role in cross-resistance to other members of the NRTI class (Fig. 145.3). Resistance to zidovudine

Fig. 145.2 Chemical structures of nucleoside and nucleotide analogue reverse transcriptase inhibitors.

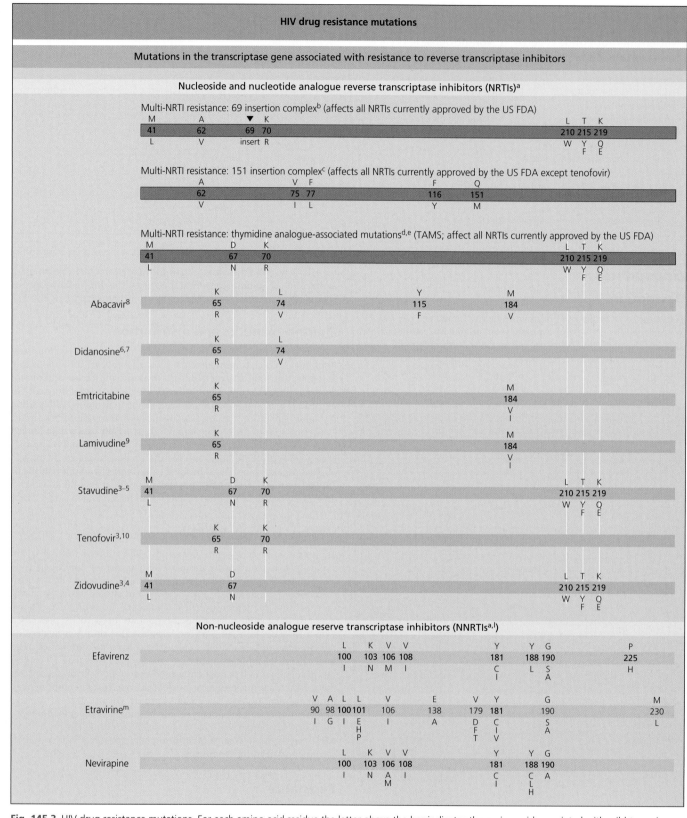

Fig. 145.3 HIV drug resistance mutations. For each amino acid residue the letter above the bar indicates the amino acid associated with wild-type virus and the letter(s) below indicate the substitution(s) that confer viral resistance. The number shows the position of the mutation in the protein. HR1, first heptad repeat. Courtesy of International AIDS Society–USA (for full details and footnotes see http://www.iasusa.org).

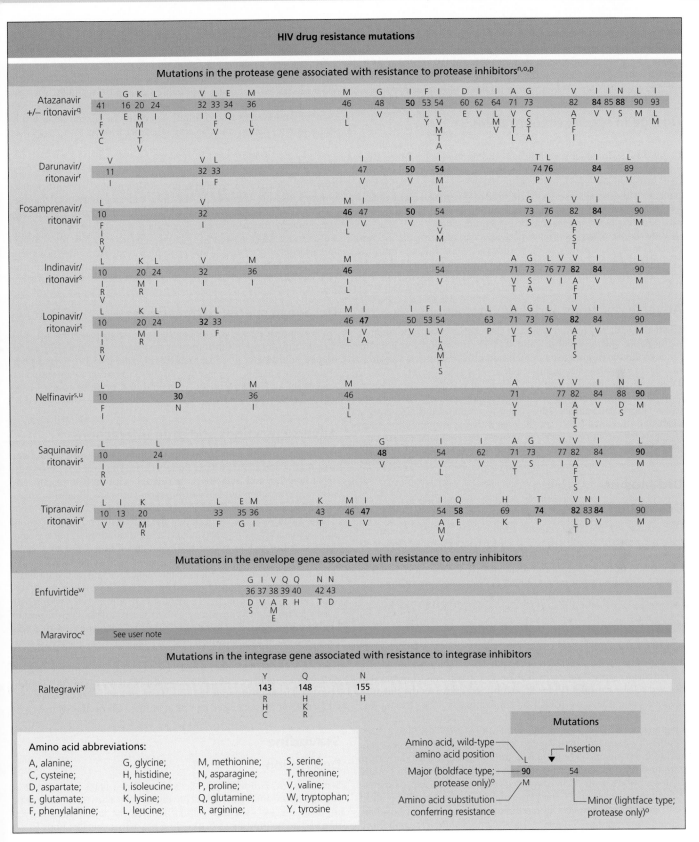

HIV drug resistance mutations

Mutations in the protease gene associated with resistance to protease inhibitors[n,o,p]

Fig. 145.3—cont'd.

can also be conferred by two multi-nucleoside resistance complexes: the Q151M complex (A62V, V75I, F116Y, Q151M) and a T69S 6 bp insertion in the presence of NAMs (see Fig. 145.3). Mutations in the RNase H (Q509L) and connection (N348I, A371V) domains of the reverse transcriptase increase the degree of zidovudine resistance in the presence of TAMs, probably by facilitating zidovudine excision.[8]

Dosage in special circumstances

Dosage adjustment is necessary in patients with severe renal disease (Table 145.2). In patients with hepatic dysfunction, zidovudine clearance is reduced and dosage modification is recommended. Limited data are available regarding specific dosage recommendations for patients with liver disease. Based on limited pharmacokinetic data in 14 patients with liver cirrhosis, a zidovudine dose reduction by 50% or a doubling of the interval has been recommended.[5]

Zidovudine crosses the placenta with concentrations in the fetal circulation approximately 85% of maternal plasma concentrations. Teratogenic effects with zidovudine have only been reported in rodents when exposed to lethal maternal doses (pregnancy category C).[9]

Adverse reactions and drug interactions

The major toxicities of zidovudine include nausea, headache, anemia, neutropenia and myopathy (Table 145.3). The myopathy is manifested by myalgias, muscle tenderness and proximal muscle weakness, mainly in the lower extremities. NRTI class toxicities are listed in Table 145.4. Clinically significant drug interactions are minimal because zidovudine is predominantly renally excreted; however, the use of zidovudine with stavudine is not recommended due to antagonism, and the concomitant use of drugs with myelosuppressive effects (e.g. ganciclovir, flucytosine) may increase the potential for hematologic adverse effects.

Didanosine

Description

Didanosine – 2′,3′-dideoxyinosine (ddI; see Fig. 145.2) – is sequentially converted intracellularly to 2′,3′-dideoxyinosine monophosphate by 5′-nucleotidase, and to 2′,3′-dideoxyadenosine monophosphate by adenylosuccinate synthetase and adenylosuccinate lyase. It is then converted to the ddA-triphosphate, which is the active form of the drug, possessing activity against HIV-1 and HIV-2.

Pharmacokinetics and distribution

Didanosine bioavailability varies from 21% to 54% following oral administration in adults. It is recommended that didanosine be administered on an empty stomach to increase absorption. Administration of delayed release capsules (Videx EC) with food decreases the didanosine area-under-the-curve (AUC) by approximately 19%. Didanosine exhibits linear pharmacokinetics with peak plasma concentrations ranging from 0.52 to 2.79 mg/l after oral doses of 125–375 mg q12h.[10] Results of pharmacokinetic studies suggest similar AUC values comparing the standard twice-daily regimen to the same total daily dose administered once daily.[11] Didanosine is less than 5% protein-bound. Concentrations in the CSF have been reported to be approximately 21% of those in plasma.[10] The plasma half-life of didanosine is short (<2 hours), but the *in-vitro* intracellular half-life of the triphosphate appears prolonged (>25 hours).[12] Didanosine is partially metabolized to ddATP or uric acid, or enters the purine metabolic pool.

Use

In adults, the usual dosage of didanosine is 400 mg q24h for those weighing over 60 kg and 250 mg q24h for those under 60 kg. It is typically prescribed as part of the dual nucleoside component of three- or four-drug combination regimens. It is most commonly paired with zidovudine or abacavir. It should not be prescribed with stavudine because of the risk of metabolic toxicities including lipodystrophy and lactic acidosis. Didanosine-containing dual NRTI components must be used with an agent or agents from another major antiretroviral drug class or classes to provide a potent combination regimen. The drug can be used in both treatment-naive and experienced patients but is generally reserved as a second-line agent. Its use should be driven by the treatment history and the drug resistance profile.

Resistance

Low-fold changes in susceptibility to didanosine are sufficient to compromise the response to the drug and this must be recognized to properly interpret phenotypic resistance results. Genotypically, the signature mutation conferring didanosine resistance is L74V but K65R and M184V have also been associated with low-fold changes in susceptibility. The Q151M complex, the T69S insertions and multiple NAMs also confer diminished susceptibility to didanosine (see Fig. 145.3).

Dosage in special circumstances

Didanosine clearance is significantly reduced in patients with renal disease and dosage modification is necessary (see Table 145.2). No dosage adjustment is recommended in patients with liver disease. Didanosine crosses the placenta. Studies evaluating long-term carcinogenicity and teratogenicity have produced negative results (pregnancy category B).[9]

Adverse reactions and drug interactions

The major toxicities of didanosine include pancreatitis, peripheral neuropathy and diarrhea (see Table 145.3). The drug can also cause hepatotoxicity and has been associated with hepatotoxicity and lactic acidosis when used in combination with stavudine in pregnant women (for NRTI class toxicities, see Table 145.4).

The didanosine oral solution has the potential for drug interactions with agents affected by concomitant antacid administration and with any agents that require gastric acidity for absorption. Clinically significant drug interactions have been reported between didanosine formulations and tenofovir disoproxil fumarate (tenofovir DF), delavirdine and indinavir. Administration of once-daily didanosine enteric-coated capsules (Videx EC) 2 hours before tenofovir DF administered with a light meal resulted in an approximate 48% increase in didanosine exposure. The administration of both of these agents simultaneously with a light meal resulted in an approximate 60% increase in didanosine exposure. There appears to be no effect of didanosine on the levels of tenofovir DF. If didanosine and tenofovir are used concomitantly, the dosage of didanosine should be reduced to 250 mg q24h (≥ 60 kg) or 200 mg q24h (<60 kg). Debate surrounds the use of the combination of didanosine and tenofovir DF because of reports of blunted CD4 cell responses.[13,14]

Stavudine

Description

Stavudine – 2′,3′-didehydro-3′-deoxythymidine (d4T; see Fig. 145.2) – is a thymidine analogue that is converted to the active form, stavudine triphosphate, by a series of cellular kinases; the initial phosphorylation is the rate limiting step. The drug has activity against both HIV-1 and HIV-2.

Pharmacokinetics and distribution

Stavudine is rapidly absorbed and exhibits linear pharmacokinetics. Peak concentrations of about 0.9 μg/ml are achieved within 2 hours. The oral bioavailability is 82–86%. The mean serum half-life is short

Table 145.2 Nucleoside and nucleotide dosage modifications in patients with renal dysfunction and with dialysis

Drug		Usual adult dose CrCL >50 ml/min	CrCL 30–50 ml/min	CrCL 10–30 ml/min	CrCL <10 ml/min	Hemodialysis*	Peritoneal dialysis	Continuous renal replacement therapy
Abacavir (po)		300 mg q12h or 600 mg q24h	300 mg q12h or 600 mg q24h	300 mg q12h or 600 mg q24h	300 mg q12h or 600 mg q24h	300 mg q12h or 600 mg q24h	300 mg q12h or 600 mg q24h	300 mg q12h or 600 mg q24h
Didanosine (po)	≥60 kg <60 kg	400 mg q24h 250 mg q24h	200 mg q24h 125 mg q24h	125 mg q24h 125 mg q24h	125 mg q24h 75 mg q24h	125 mg q24h 75 mg q24h	125 mg q24h 75 mg q24h	125 mg q24h 125 mg q24h
Emtricitabine (po)	Capsule Oral solution	200 mg q24h 240 mg q24h	200 mg q48h 120 mg q24h	200 mg q72h 80 mg q24h	200 mg q96h 60 mg q24h	200 mg q96h 60 mg q24h	200 mg q96h 60 mg q24h	200 mg q48–72h 80–120 mg q24h
Lamivudine (po)		150 mg q12h or 300 mg q24h	150 mg q24h	150 mg x1, then 100 mg q24h	150 mg x1, then 50 mg q24h	150 mg x1, then 25–50 mg q24h	150 mg x1, then 25–50 mg q24h	150 mg q24h
Stavudine (po)	≥60 kg <60 kg	40 mg q12h 30 mg q12h	20 mg q12h 15 mg q12h	20 mg q24h 15 mg q24h	20 mg q24h 15 mg q24h	20 mg q24h 15 mg q24h	20 mg q24h 15 mg q24h	N/A N/A
Tenofovir DF (po)		300 mg q24h	300 mg q48h	300 mg q72–96h	300 mg every 7 days	300 mg every 7 days	300 mg every 7 days	N/A
Zidovudine (po)		300 mg q12h	300 mg q12h	300 mg q12h	100 mg q8h	100 mg q8h	100 mg q8h	100 mg q8h

CrCL, creatinine clearance; N/A, specific dosing recommendations not available.
*Drug should be administered after the hemodialysis session.

Table 145.3 List of nucleoside and nucleotide reverse transcriptase inhibitor-specific toxicities

Zidovudine	Didanosine	Stavudine	Lamivudine	Abacavir	Emtricitabine	Tenofovir DF
Anemia or neutropenia Anorexia Bone marrow suppression Headache Insomnia Malaise Nausea Vomiting	Diarrhea Nausea Pancreatitis Peripheral neuropathy	Pancreatitis Peripheral neuropathy	Diarrhea Headache Insomnia Nausea Neuropathy Pancreatitis	Headache Hypersensitivity reaction* Malaise/fatigue Nausea Vomiting	Abdominal pain Asthenia Depression Diarrhea Dizziness Fatigue Headache Insomnia Nausea Skin hyperpigmentation	↓ Bone mineral density Asthenia Diarrhea Headache Nausea New onset/worsening renal impairment

*Hypersensitivity reaction can be fatal: symptoms may include fever, rash, nausea, vomiting, malaise, fatigue, loss of appetite, respiratory symptoms such as pharyngitis, dyspnea or cough.

Table 145.4 List of nucleoside reverse transcriptase inhibitor and protease inhibitor class toxicities

Nucleoside reverse transcriptase inhibitors	Protease inhibitors
Hepatomegaly with steatosis Lactic acidosis Lipoatrophy Mitochondrial toxicity	Cardiovascular effects (myocardial infarction, cerebrovascular accident) Fat redistribution Gastrointestinal intolerance Hepatitis Hyperglycemia (insulin resistance/diabetes mellitus) Hyperlipidemia (except atazanavir) Possible increased bleeding episodes in patients with hemophilia

(1–1.67 hours), with an intracellular half-life of about 3–4 hours. Protein binding is minimal. Stavudine penetrates into the CSF, achieving levels approximately 40% of plasma levels.[15] Stavudine is excreted by renal and nonrenal routes with approximately 50% of a dose excreted unchanged in the urine.[16]

Use

For adults weighing over 60 kg, the dose is 40 mg q12h; for those under 60 kg, the dose is 30 mg q12h. Like zidovudine, stavudine is used as part of a dual NRTI component, most commonly with lamivudine. These are then typically combined with a ritonavir-boosted PI or an NNRTI to form potent combination regimens. Stavudine can be used in treatment-naive patients or as an alternative to zidovudine in those patients who exhibit intolerance to zidovudine in the first few weeks after initiation of therapy. The association of stavudine with peripheral neuropathy, lipoatrophy, mitochondrial toxicity and lactic acidosis has led to a much diminished role for stavudine. The drug's use in treatment-experienced persons should be dictated by the treatment history and the results of drug resistance testing.

Resistance

Low-fold changes in susceptibility can impair the response to stavudine *in vivo* and this is important to keep in mind in the interpretation of phenotypic resistance testing. Genotypically, the V75T has been thought to be a signature mutation for stavudine resistance

but this mutation is only rarely seen in clinical isolates. Recent data suggest that stavudine and stavudine–didanosine can select for zidovudine-associated mutations (TAMs, NAMs) and the Q151M complex. Zidovudine and stavudine share cross-resistance at both the virion and enzyme levels. Zidovudine-resistant isolates should be considered resistant to stavudine (see Fig. 145.3).

Dosage in special circumstances

Stavudine requires dose adjustment in patients with renal disease (see Table 145.2). No dosage modification is recommended in patients with liver disease.

Stavudine crosses the placenta and teratogenicity studies in rodents were negative with a decrease in sternal calcium noted at high doses (pregnancy category C).[9]

Adverse reactions and drug interactions

The major toxicity of stavudine is peripheral neuropathy and the drug has been strongly implicated in lipoatrophic and mitochondrial dysfunction syndromes as noted above (see Table 145.3). Clinically significant drug interactions are minimal. The combination of stavudine and didanosine should not be used due to the increased risk for peripheral neuropathy and lactic acidosis.

Lamivudine

Description

Lamivudine – (−)2′,3′-dideoxy-3′-thiacytidine (3TC; see Fig. 145.2) – is the (−) enantiomer of a sulfur-containing cytidine analogue. This enantiomer was chosen on the basis of its potency and cytotoxicity profile. It is phosphorylated to its active form, lamivudine triphosphate, by cellular kinases. The drug is active against HIV-1, HIV-2 and hepatitis B virus (HBV).

Pharmacokinetics and distribution

Lamivudine is well absorbed following oral administration with a mean bioavailability of over 80% in adults. Systemic drug exposure is not influenced by administration with food. Peak and trough concentrations of approximately 2 µg/ml and 0.33 µg/ml, respectively, have been achieved following oral administration of 150 mg q12h.[17] The mean serum half-life is approximately 4–6 hours, with the intracellular half-life ranging from 10.5 to 15.5 hours.[18] Lamivudine is less than 36% protein-bound. It penetrates the CSF, but the CSF to serum ratio is lower than that of other nucleoside analogues. Lamivudine is not significantly metabolized and is eliminated primarily unchanged via the kidney.

Use

The usual adult dosage is 150 mg q12h or 300 mg q24h. Lamivudine is one of the cornerstones of current antiretroviral therapeutics given its potency and excellent tolerability. It is commonly prescribed as part of the nucleoside component of initial regimens, typically paired with zidovudine, tenofovir or stavudine. When combined with a ritonavir-boosted PI or an NNRTI, this NRTI combination creates a potent regimen for treatment-naive patients. In treatment-experienced patients, the M184V mutation is commonly present. This mutation confers high-level resistance to lamivudine (see below) but resensitizes virus to zidovudine and tenofovir. Thus, this well-tolerated drug is often continued in treatment-experienced patients with multidrug-resistant virus to try to maximize the activity of the nucleoside/nucleotide component of the regimen. Lamivudine is widely used as part of maternal therapies and as part of maternal–fetal transmission interruption regimens.

Resistance

High-level phenotypic resistance (>500-fold change in susceptibility) quickly and nearly uniformly develops in patients treated with partially suppressive regimens containing lamivudine (e.g. dual nucleoside regimens). This is mediated through the lamivudine signature mutation, M184V. The latter has also been reported to increase the fidelity of the HIV reverse transcriptase and to decrease replicative fitness. The M184V mutation can delay the emergence of zidovudine resistance and reverse zidovudine resistance when the T215F/Y mutation is present. However, high-level zidovudine–lamivudine co-resistance can develop when multiple zidovudine-associated mutations (TAMs) and the M184V are present. This mutation can also partially reverse the resistance to tenofovir conferred by the K65R mutation.[19]

The Q151M complex and the T69S insertions also confer lamivudine resistance. Multiple TAMs alone, however, do not reduce susceptibility to lamivudine. This distinguishes lamivudine from the other approved NRTIs (see Fig. 145.3).

Dosage in special circumstances

Dosage adjustment is required in patients with renal disease (see Table 145.2). No dosage adjustment is necessary in patients with liver disease. Lamivudine crosses the placenta. No carcinogenicity or teratogenicity has been observed in long-term animal studies (pregnancy category C).

Adverse reactions and drug interactions

Lamivudine is generally very well tolerated. Insomnia, headache, pancreatitis and peripheral neuropathy can occur (see Table 145.3). Clinically significant drug interactions are minimal. Hepatitis and pancreatitis have been described in children.

Abacavir

Description

Abacavir sulfate – (1S, 4R)-4-[2-amino-6-(cyclopropylamino)-9H-purin-9-yl]-2-cyclo pentene-1-methanol (ABC; see Fig. 145.2) – is converted to carbovir intracellularly. Adenosine phosphotransferase catalyzes the first phosphorylation step. A cytosolic 5′-nucleotidase then converts abacavir monophosphate to carbovir monophosphate. Cellular kinases then complete the di- and triphosphorylation steps. Carbovir triphosphate is active against HIV-1 and HIV-2.

Pharmacokinetics and distribution

Abacavir is rapidly and well absorbed with a reported absolute oral bioavailability of approximately 83%. Administration with food does not significantly affect the oral bioavailability. Peak concentrations achieved following multiple dose administration of 300 mg q12h are approximately 2.2 µg/ml.[20] The mean plasma half-life of abacavir is less than 2 hours, but the intracellular half-life of the active carbovir triphosphate is approximately 20 hours. Abacavir is 50% protein-bound. It is highly lipophilic and penetrates into the CSF, with concentrations approximately 30% of plasma levels.[21] Abacavir undergoes extensive hepatic metabolism by alcohol dehydrogenase and glucuronosyl transferase.

Use

The usual adult dosage is 600 mg q24h or 300 mg q12h. In treatment-naive individuals it is usually prescribed as part of a dual nucleoside combination with lamivudine along with a ritonavir-boosted PI or an NNRTI. Abacavir–lamivudine has been reported to be inferior to tenofovir–emtricitabine when combined with efavirenz or atazanavir–ritonavir in patients with baseline plasma HIV-1 RNA levels >100 000 copies/ml although debate concerning this point continues. The triple nucleoside combination of abacavir–zidovudine–lamivudine has been shown to be virologically inferior to efavirenz-containing regimens and is best avoided.[22] In treatment-experienced patients, abacavir's usefulness depends on the degree of cross-resistance that may have been conferred by previous NRTI therapy (see below).

Resistance

Changes in susceptibility of eightfold or greater compromise the clinical efficacy of abacavir. A number of mutations confer resistance to abacavir. The M184V mutation alone confers a twofold change in abacavir susceptibility and the drug should still be useful in this situation. However, the M184V mutation in the presence of multiple TAMs and/or L74V and K65R will confer higher level abacavir resistance and compromise the drug's efficacy. The Q151M complex and the T69S insertion also confer abacavir resistance (see Fig. 145.3).

Dosage in special circumstances

Dosage adjustment is not necessary in patients with renal disease. No specific dosage modification is recommended in patients with liver disease. Abacavir crosses the placenta. Developmental toxicity secondary to abacavir has been observed in rats (pregnancy category C).[21]

Adverse reactions and drug interactions

The major abacavir toxicity of concern is the idiosyncratic hypersensitivity reaction, which has at least a 5% incidence and can be fatal (see Table 145.3). Abacavir hypersensitivity has been linked to the HLA B*5701 genotype and screening for this HLA haplotype is recommended prior to initiating abacavir.[23,24] Abacavir may increase the risk for myocardial infarction but conflicting data on this question exist.[25,26]

Emtricitabine

Description

Emtricitabine – 5-fluoro-1-[(2R,5S)-2-(hydroxymethyl)-1,3-oxathiolan-5-yl]cytosine (FTC; see Fig. 145.2) – is a cytidine analogue with activity against HIV-1, HIV-2 and HBV.

Pharmacokinetics and distribution

Emtricitabine is rapidly and almost completely absorbed with bioavailabilities of 93% and 75% for the oral capsules and oral solution, respectively. Following multiple dose oral administration, a mean peak concentration of approximately 1.8 µg/ml is achieved. Protein binding of emtricitabine is negligible (<4%). The plasma half-life is approximately 10 hours, but the intracellular half-life of the triphosphate form is longer, 29 hours, allowing once-daily administration.[27] Emtricitabine is not significantly metabolized (13%) and is eliminated primarily unchanged via the kidney.

Use

The usual adult dose is 200 mg once daily for the capsules and 240 mg once daily for the oral solution. The clinical applications of emtricitabine are essentially the same as lamivudine. Most commonly, it is used in combination with tenofovir as a dual nucleoside/nucleotide component of ritonavir-boosted PI- or NNRTI-based regimens in treatment-naive individuals. The availability of the fixed-dose combination of emtricitabine, tenofovir and efavirenz permits a single pill, once-daily potent regimen that is the benchmark for simplicity and potency.

Resistance

The M184V mutation confers high-level resistance to emtricitabine and is the most commonly selected mutation in patients failing emtricitabine-containing regimens. Clinical trial data suggest that the rate of emergence of the M184V mutation with emtricitabine–tenofovir is lower than that seen with lamivudine–zidovudine in potent combination regimens. K65R, the Q151M complex and the T69S insertions also confer resistance to emtricitabine.

Dosage in special circumstances

Dosage adjustment is required in patients with renal disease (see Table 145.2). No dosage adjustment is necessary in patients with liver disease. In animal studies emtricitabine was not associated with fetal variations or malformations in mice and rabbits at drug levels 60- and 120-fold higher than used in humans. Emtricitabine is classified as pregnancy category B.

Adverse reactions and drug interactions

Emtricitabine is generally well tolerated. The most frequently reported adverse effects are mild to moderate headache, nausea, diarrhea, skin discoloration (hyperpigmentation on palms and soles) and skin rash (see Table 145.3).

NUCLEOTIDE ANALOGUE REVERSE TRANSCRIPTASE INHIBITOR

Tenofovir disoproxil fumarate (DF)

Description

Tenofovir DF – (R)-9-(2-phosphonomethoxypropyl) adenine (TDF; see Fig. 145.2) – is a prodrug of the nucleoside phosphonate 9-R-(2-phosphonomethoxypropyl)adenine (PMPA). Tenofovir DF is the first nucleotide reverse transcriptase inhibitor (NtRTI) approved for the treatment of HIV infection. These drugs differ from the nucleoside RTIs by having a phosphate group in the parent molecule. They thus require only diphosphorylation to be converted to their active compounds. Tenofovir DF is converted to tenofovir by serum esterases. Tenofovir is then activated by phosphorylation by cellular kinases. The drug is active against HIV-1, HIV-2 and HBV.

Pharmacokinetics and distribution

Tenofovir is administered orally as a prodrug, tenofovir DF. The oral bioavailability of tenofovir is approximately 25% and 40% in the fasting and fed state, respectively, as compared with 1 mg/kg intravenous dosing. Oral dosing of tenofovir DF at 300 mg q24h results in steady state peak concentrations of 303 ng/ml with an estimated half-life of

approximately 14 hours.[28] The intracellular half-life of tenofovir diphosphate ranges from 12 to 50 hours.[29] Tenofovir is primarily eliminated renally (70–80%) via a combination of glomerular filtration and active tubular secretion.

Use

The usual adult dosage is 300 mg q24h. The major use of tenofovir DF is as part of initial regimens in treatment-naive persons because of its potency, safety profile and convenience.[30–34] The combination of tenofovir with abacavir–lamivudine or didanosine–lamivudine results in an unacceptably high rate of early virologic failure associated with the emergence of K65R and M184I/V mutations, and should be avoided.

In HIV–HBV co-infected patients, the combination of tenofovir–emtricitabine or tenofovir–lamivudine (when used in combination with a PI or NNRTI) provides three active drugs versus HIV and two active drugs versus HBV. This approach is often used to try to treat both infections effectively while avoiding the emergence of drug resistance in either pathogen (see Practice Point 44).

Resistance

A phenotypic change in susceptibility of over four-fold compromises the virologic response to tenofovir DF. The K65R is a signature mutation for tenofovir DF but its appearance in patients treated with tenofovir DF is relatively infrequent. Four or more TAMs (especially M41L and L210W) and the T69S insertion also confer resistance to tenofovir DF. Tenofovir retains activity against viruses harboring the Q151M mutational complex. Interestingly, the M184V mutation enhances susceptibility to tenofovir DF.[19]

Dosage in special circumstances

Dosage adjustment and monitoring for drug toxicity are necessary in patients with renal disease (see Table 145.2). Dose adjustment is necessary in patients with creatinine clearance <50 ml/min; such recommendations are based not on safety and effectiveness, but rather on single-dose pharmacokinetic data in this population. The presence of hepatic insufficiency is likely to have a limited effect on tenofovir pharmacokinetics and no specific dosage modifications are recommended in this population. Tenofovir is classified as pregnancy category B. In rats and rabbits, studies have found no evidence of impaired fertility or teratogenicity.

Adverse reactions and drug interactions

Neutropenia, headache, fatigue, pancreatitis, elevated creatinine and hypophosphatemia have been reported (see Table 145.3). Tenofovir has been associated with reductions in bone mineral density and osteomalacia.[35] Concomitant use of tenofovir DF with didanosine increases exposure to didanosine and increases the potential for drug toxicity. The combination may also result in early virologic failure and a blunted CD4 cell response.[13,14]

NON-NUCLEOSIDE REVERSE TRANSCRIPTASE INHIBITORS

The NNRTI class of antiretroviral agents is a chemically heterogeneous group of compounds that share a common mechanism of action. These agents differ from the NRTIs in that the parent compound is active and no intracellular metabolism is necessary. The drugs in this class allosterically bind in a noncompetitive fashion to a hydrophobic pocket near the active site of the reverse transcriptase and 'lock' the enzyme into an inactive state. The agents in this class also differ from NRTIs in that they are active against HIV-1 except for subtype O and are inactive against HIV-2 strains.

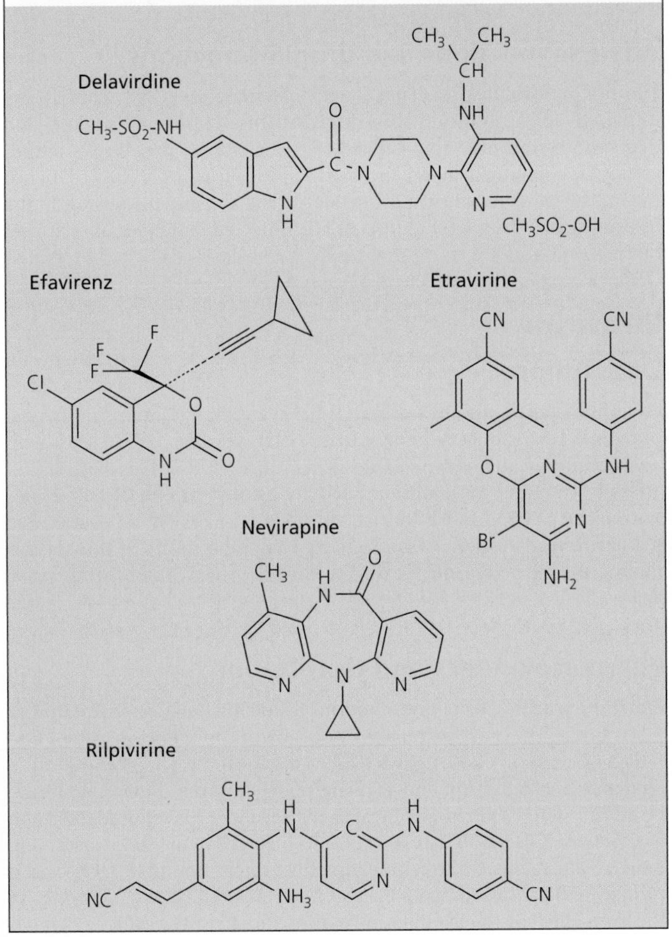

Fig. 145.4 Chemical structures of non-nucleoside reverse transcriptase inhibitors.

Nevirapine

Description

Nevirapine – 11-cyclopropyl-5,11-dihydro-4-methyl-6H-dipyrido [3,2-b:2′,3′-][1,4]diazepin-6-one (NVP; Fig. 145.4) – is the lead compound in this class and was the first NNRTI approved in the USA.

Pharmacokinetics and distribution

Nevirapine is well absorbed with an oral bioavailability of 90%. Absorption does not appear to be affected by co-administration with food or antacids. Maximum concentrations are achieved approximately 2 hours after an oral dose with a second peak occurring approximately 14 hours after a dose, presumably due to enterohepatic recycling.[36] Nevirapine exhibits linear pharmacokinetics. Following administration of a single 200 mg dose, a peak concentration of 7.5 μmol/l is achieved. Following 200 mg daily, average steady state plasma concentrations of peak and trough concentrations are 27.1 μmol/l and 15–17 μmol/l respectively. Nevirapine is very lipophilic and widely distributed throughout the body.[37] It is approximately 60% protein-bound. Concentrations in the CSF are approximately 45% of those achieved in plasma.[37] Nevirapine is primarily metabolized by the CYP3A4 and CYP2B6 isoenzymes to hydroxy-nevirapine metabolites and induces both of these enzyme systems.[38] Autoinduction of its own metabolism has been demonstrated. The half-life of nevirapine is approximately 25–30 hours.

Use

The usual adult dosage is 200 mg q24h for 14 days followed by 200 mg q12h. This dose escalation regimen is recommended to reduce the incidence and severity of rash during treatment initiation.

Due to the vulnerability of nevirapine to single-step, high-level resistance (i.e. a low genetic barrier to resistance), it needs to be used in potent combination regimens designed to suppress plasma HIV-1 RNA levels to less than 50 copies/ml. Partially suppressive regimens or poor drug adherence carry a high risk of engendering nevirapine resistance.

In individuals intolerant to the central nervous system (CNS) side-effects of efavirenz or in women of child-bearing age for whom access to effective contraception is problematic, nevirapine is an appropriate alternative to efavirenz. In previously naive persons who are virologically suppressed on a PI-containing regimen, a switch of the PI to nevirapine can maintain virologic suppression and improve serum lipid abnormalities.

Nevirapine has assumed an important role in the prevention of maternal–fetal HIV transmission in the developing world[39] (see Chapter 98).

In the prophylaxis of accidental needlestick exposure in health-care workers, the use of nevirapine should be avoided given the reports of severe hepatotoxicity when used in this setting.

Resistance

Low-level changes in susceptibility to nevirapine (and other NNRTIs), of the order of 2.5- to 10-fold, are the result of natural polymorphisms in wild-type strains and do not affect the response to these agents. Higher level resistance compromises or eliminates the virologic response to nevirapine. The signature mutation for nevirapine is Y181C, but other nevirapine-associated mutations include L100I, K103N, V106A/M, V108I, Y188C/L/H and G190A (see Fig. 145.3). Drug class cross-resistance among the first generation of approved NNRTIs (nevirapine, delavirdine, efavirenz) is nearly complete.

Dosage in special circumstances

Dosage modification is not required for patients with renal dysfunction. Limited data are available in patients with hepatic impairment and no specific dosage modification is currently recommended. Nevirapine is not associated with teratogenicity in rabbits or rats (pregnancy category C).[9] It rapidly crosses the placenta.

Adverse reactions and drug interactions

The major toxicities associated with nevirapine are rash and hepatotoxicity (Table 145.5). The risk of hepatotoxicity, which can be fatal, appears higher in women and in those with higher CD4 cell counts, namely >250 cells/μl in women and >400 cells/μl in men. Nevirapine is a moderate inducer of CYP3A4. Further discussion of the importance of drug interactions in HIV-infected patients can be found in Practice Point 45.

Table 145.5 List of non-nucleoside reverse transcriptase inhibitor specific toxicities

Nevirapine	Delavirdine	Efavirenz	Etravirine
Hepatotoxicity	Diarrhea	CNS symptoms*	Nausea
Hyperlipidemia	Fatigue	Hepatotoxicity	Rash
Rash	Nausea	Hyperlipidemia	
	Rash	Rash	

*CNS symptoms may include dizziness, insomnia, impaired concentration, somnolence, abnormal dreams, euphoria, confusion, agitation, hallucinations.

Delavirdine

Description

Delavirdine – 1-(5-methanesulfonoamido-1H-indol-2-ylcarbonyl)-4-[3-(1-methylethylamino)pyridinyl]piperazine (DLV; see Fig. 145.4) – was the second NNRTI approved in the USA.

Its use in clinical practice has been very restricted because of the high pill burden, the reluctance to use this agent if a severe reaction to nevirapine or efavirenz has occurred and the cross-resistance within this class of agents.

Efavirenz

Description

Efavirenz – (S)-6-chloro-4-(cyclopropylethynyl)-1,4-dihydro-4-(trifluoromethyl)-2H-3,1-benzoxazin-2-one (EFV; see Fig. 145.4) – is one of the most widely prescribed NNRTIs because of its potency, once-daily administration and lower incidence of rash compared to nevirapine.

Pharmacokinetics and distribution

Efavirenz is well absorbed with peak concentrations achieved 5 hours after oral administration. Absorption appears unaffected by administration with meals containing a moderate fat content. When administered with high-fat meals, a mean increase in AUC of 50% has been shown, and concomitant administration with high-fat meals is not recommended. Efavirenz exhibits linear pharmacokinetics. Average steady state plasma C_{min} and C_{max} following oral administration of 600 mg daily are approximately 6 µmol/l and 13 µmol/l, respectively.[37] Efavirenz is over 99% bound to plasma proteins, predominantly albumin, which limits crossing the blood–brain barrier, with CSF concentrations on average 0.69% of total plasma concentrations.[40] Efavirenz is metabolized in the liver, predominantly to inactive metabolites by CYP3A4 and CYP2B6. After multiple-dose oral administration, the half-life of efavirenz is approximately 40–55 hours. Efavirenz induces CYP3A4 *in vivo*, but has also been shown to inhibit CYP3A4, CYP2C9 and CYP2C19 *in vitro*.[41]

Use

Efavirenz is administered orally. The usual adult dosage is 600 mg q24h, which is available in a single tablet formulation and in a fixed-dose combination with tenofovir–emtricitabine.

Efavirenz plays a major role in the initial treatment of antiretroviral-naive patients and, in combination with tenofovir–emtricitabine, is a standard-of-care regimen for treatment-naive patients. The drug should be avoided in patients with a history of significant psychiatric illness because of its CNS side-effect profile. It is also contraindicated in the first trimester of pregnancy because of demonstrated teratogenicity.

Resistance

The most common mutation encountered clinically is K103N, which confers cross-resistance to efavirenz and delavirdine. Other clinically relevant mutations are L100I, V106M, V108I, Y181C, Y188L, G190S/A and P225H. High-level resistance is seen with the double mutations K103N+V108I and L100I+K103N (see Fig. 145.3).

Dosage in special circumstances

No dosage adjustment is required in patients with renal disease. Following a single-dose study in patients with chronic liver disease, efavirenz C_{max} was reduced and the half-life increased with no significant change in AUC compared to healthy volunteers.[37] Administration of the standard dose with close monitoring for toxicity is recommended in patients with liver disease.

Efavirenz crosses the placenta. Teratogenicity has been noted in primates and humans and administration to pregnant women should be avoided (pregnancy category D).[9]

Adverse reactions and drug interactions

The major toxicities associated with efavirenz are CNS related (e.g. impaired concentration, abnormal dreams, euphoria, anxiety and depression) and rash (see Table 145.5). As above, the drug is teratogenic. Efavirenz acts as an inducer or inhibitor of CYP3A4 depending on the concomitantly administered drug. Further discussion of the importance of drug interactions in HIV-infected patients can be found in Practice Point 45.

Etravirine

Description

Etravirine – 4-[[6-amino-5-bromo-2-[(4-cyanophenyl)amino]-4-pyrimidinyl]oxy]-3,5-dimethylbenzonitrile (ETR; see Fig. 145.4) – is a diarylpyrimidine analogue, 'second-generation' NNRTI. This designation arises from etravirine's antiviral activity against strains of HIV-1 harboring the K103N and a limited number of other NNRTI-associated resistance mutations.[42,43] This activity may be a result of the conformational and positional flexibility of etravirine. Etravirine is active against HIV-1 only.

Pharmacokinetics and distribution

Etravirine reaches peak concentrations following oral administration in 2.5–4 hours. The oral bioavailability of etravirine is unknown. After 1 and 8 days of etravirine 200 mg twice daily, the mean peak concentration of etravirine is 125.8 ng/ml and 451.3 ng/ml, respectively. Etravirine should be administered following a meal as the mean C_{max} is reduced 44% and the mean AUC is reduced 51% when administered in the fasted state compared to after a meal.[44] Etravirine is highly protein-bound (99.9%) and is primarily metabolized by CYP3A4, CYP2C9 and CYP2C19 enzymes in the liver. The half-life of etravirine is approximately 41 hours.

Use

Etravirine is administered orally as a tablet formulation. The usual adult dosage is 200 mg twice daily following a meal. Etravirine is indicated in individuals harboring multidrug-resistant virus who have experienced virologic failure on a first-generation NNRTI (e.g. efavirenz, nevirapine). Etravirine's clinical efficacy was demonstrated in trials which enrolled patients with virologic failure and multidrug-resistant virus.[45] The greatest experience with etravirine is in combination with darunavir–ritonavir so caution needs to be exercised when combining the drug with other PIs.

Resistance

Etravirine's activity is unaffected by the K103N mutation and good virologic responses are seen when there are fewer than three other NNRTI-associated mutations at baseline. Virologic response is diminished when three or more of the following mutations are present: V90I, A98G, L100I, K101E/P, V106I, V179D/F/T, Y181C/I/V and G190S/A. In patients who have experienced virologic failure on an NNRTI-based initial regimen and exhibit only the K103N mutation on resistance testing, etravirine should be combined with at least two other fully active agents as other NNRTI mutations may exist at low frequency and be undetected by routine resistance testing.

Dosage in special circumstances

Etravirine does not require dosage adjustment in patients with renal dysfunction. The pharmacokinetics of etravirine are not affected by mild-to-moderate liver disease (Child-Pugh Class A or B). Due to the lack of data, it is not recommended to use etravirine in patients with severe liver disease (Child-Pugh Class C).

Etravirine appears safe in pregnant animal models, but no adequate studies in pregnant women have been conducted. Etravirine is classified as pregnancy category B.

Adverse reactions and drug interactions

The most common adverse reactions associated with etravirine are rash, including Stevens–Johnson syndrome, and nausea (see Table 145.5). Etravirine is an inducer of CYP3A4 and inhibitor of CYP2C9 and CYP2C19, and has the potential for serious drug interactions and toxicity. Etravirine should not be co-administered with other NNRTIs, all unboosted PIs, or ritonavir-boosted tipranavir or fosamprenavir. It can be co-administered with darunavir–ritonavir, lopinavir–ritonavir (limited data), raltegravir and maraviroc (with dose adjustment of maraviroc). Further discussion of the importance of drug interactions in HIV-infected patients can be found in Practice Point 45.

PROTEASE INHIBITORS

Mature HIV virions are produced as the virus buds off the cell surface and gag and gag–pol polyprotein precursors are cleaved by a virally encoded aspartyl protease. Successful inhibition of this enzyme marked a revolution in antiretroviral therapy starting in 1996. The nine currently approved PIs all bind to the active site of the protease enzyme and inhibit both HIV-1 and HIV-2.

Saquinavir

Description

Saquinavir – N-tert-butyldecahydro-2-[2(R)-hydroxy-4-phenyl-3-(S)-[[N-(2-quinolylcarbonyl)-l-asparaginyl]-amino]butyl](4aS,8aS)-iso-quinoline-3(S)-carboxamide (SQV; see Fig. 145.5) – was the first PI approved in the USA.

Pharmacokinetics and distribution

Saquinavir-hard gel capsule (hgc) is poorly absorbed, with the mean absolute bioavailability of a 600 mg oral dose administered with food averaging only 4%. This is presumed to be due to limited absorption and extensive first-pass metabolism.[46] Absorption is improved upon administration with food or up to 2 hours after a meal. Saquinavir is approximately 98% bound to plasma proteins and is extensively hepatically metabolized to mono- and di-hydroxylated inactive compounds, primarily by CYP3A4 (>90%).[46] It is also a substrate of P-glycoprotein. The half-life following intravenous administration is approximately 7 hours.

Use

Saquinavir is administered orally. Given its poor oral bioavailability, the hgc formulation should only be prescribed with low-dose ritonavir enhancement. The dose of saquinavir-hgc is 1000 mg twice daily, always with ritonavir 100 mg twice daily. Saquinavir is used with low-dose ritonavir enhancement and for initial therapy is typically combined with two NRTIs. In patients with treatment failure on an NNRTI-based regimen, saquinavir–ritonavir can be a useful component of the second-line regimen. In the case of treatment failure in the presence of PI-associated resistance mutations, lopinavir–ritonavir, tipranavir–ritonavir or darunavir–ritonavir are, in general, better options for the alternative PI component of the new regimen, taking into account the specific resistance testing results.

Resistance

Resistance to saquinavir–ritonavir is mediated principally by the L90M mutation and to a lesser extent the G48V mutation. Other codon alterations that can contribute to saquinavir resistance include L10I/R/V, L24I, I54V/L, I62V, A71V/T, G73S, V77I, V82A/F/T/S and I84V (see Fig. 145.3). L90M is one of the major PI mutations associated with drug class cross-resistance.

Dosage in special circumstances

Saquinavir does not require dosage adjustment in patients with renal disease. Saquinavir pharmacokinetics has not been studied in patients with liver disease. No specific dosage recommendations are available in this patient population.

Saquinavir only minimally crosses the placenta. Animal studies have shown no mutagenicity or teratogenicity at 40–50% of AUC values achieved in humans (pregnancy category B).[9]

Adverse reactions and drug interactions

The major toxicity associated with saquinavir is gastrointestinal side-effects (Table 145.6), including diarrhea, abdominal discomfort and nausea. For PI class toxicities, see Table 145.4. Saquinavir (in the absence of ritonavir) is a weak inhibitor of CYP3A4. Further discussion of the importance of drug interactions in HIV-infected patients can be found in Practice Point 45.

Ritonavir

Description

Ritonavir: 10-hydroxy-2-methyl-5-(1-methylethyl)-1-[2-(1-methylethyl)-4-thiazolyl]-3,6-dioxo-8,11-bis(phenylmethyl)-2,4,7,12-tetraaza-tridecan-13-oic-acid, 5-thiazolyl-methyl ester [5S-(5R*, 8R*, 10R*, 11R*)] (RTV; see Fig. 145.5). Its intolerability at full therapeutic doses and its potent CYP3A4 inhibitory activity have combined to position this drug exclusively as a pharmacoenhancer of other PIs.

Pharmacokinetics and distribution

Ritonavir's oral bioavailability is estimated to range from 60% to 80%.[47] Relative to the fasting state, the AUC of ritonavir from the capsule formulation is approximately 15% higher when administered with food. For the oral solution, the AUC is decreased 7% when administered with food.[47] Following oral administration of ritonavir 600 mg q12h, the C_{max} and C_{min} are 11 mg/l and 4 mg/l, respectively. Ritonavir is greater than 98% protein-bound, both to albumin and α_1-acid glycoprotein. CSF concentrations are low and reported to be less than 0.05 mg/l.[47] Ritonavir is extensively metabolized, primarily by CYP3A4 isoenzymes, with the CYP2D6 isoenzyme also contributing to the production of the isopropylthiazolyl oxidation metabolite.[47] The half-life of ritonavir ranges from 3 to 5 hours.

Use

When administered as the sole PI, the adult dose of ritonavir is 600 mg q12h. However, ritonavir's major role is now as a pharmacoenhancer of other PIs. Pharmacoenhancement doses depend upon the co-administered PI(s) and whether an inducer of CYP3A4, such as efavirenz or nevirapine, is also included in the regimen. Most typically, ritonavir doses of 100–200 mg once or twice daily are used in pharmacoenhanced regimens.

Resistance

The major mutations conferring resistance to ritonavir are V82A/F/T/S and I84V. When used in low dose as a pharmacoenhancer of a second

Chemical structures of approved protease inhibitors

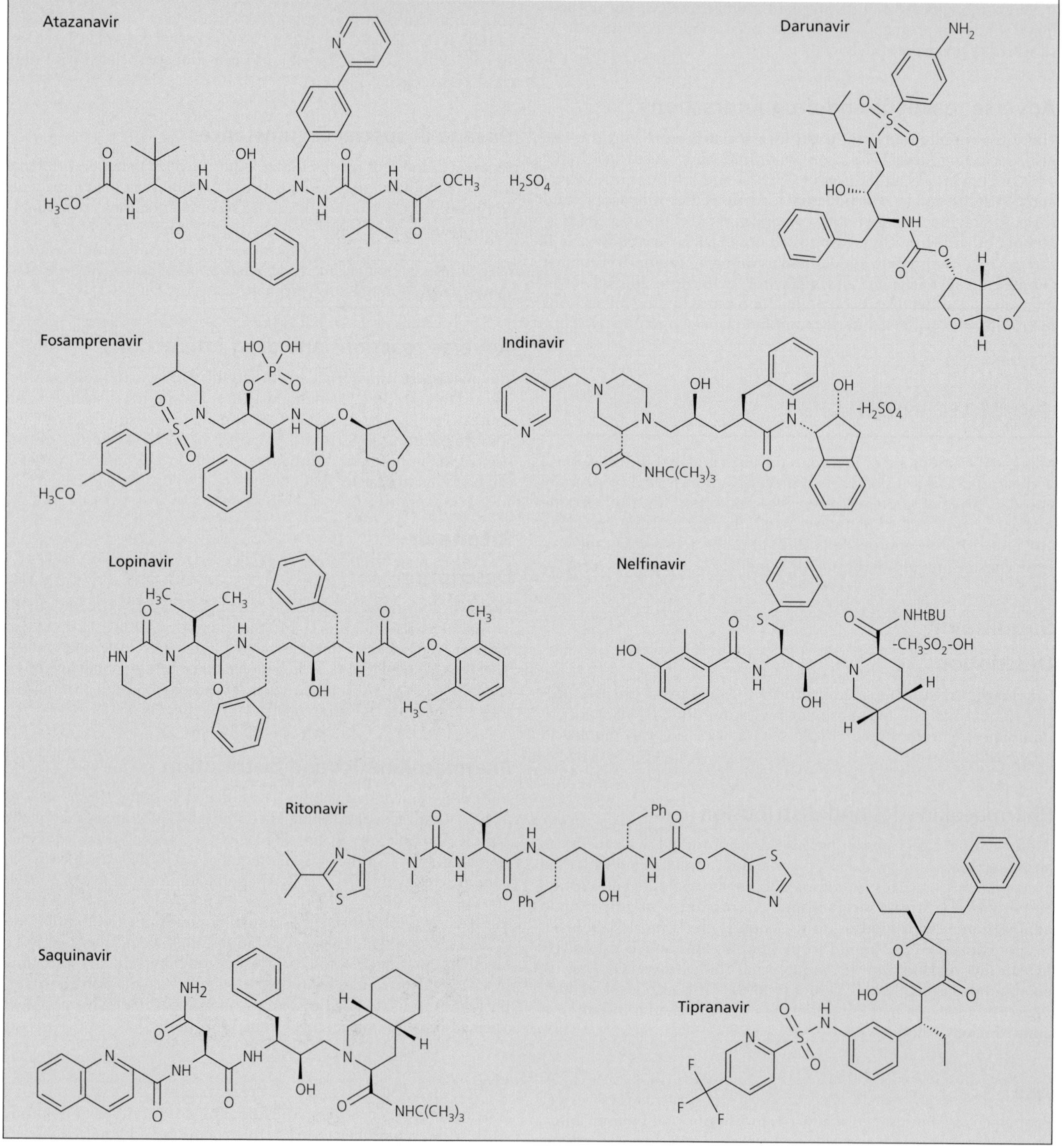

Fig. 145.5 Chemical structures of approved protease inhibitors.

PI, the pattern of mutations that emerges with virologic failure may be influenced by the presence of ritonavir.

Dosage in special circumstances

Renal disease is expected to have little effect on ritonavir pharmacokinetics and no dosage modification is necessary. In patients with mild-to-moderate hepatic insufficiency, the ritonavir pharmacokinetics vary little compared to patients with normal hepatic function when the dosage is reduced by 20%.[47] In addition, the elimination half-life increases from 4.6 hours in patients with normal hepatic function to 6.3 hours in patients with moderate hepatic disease. No specific dosage recommendations are available for patients with liver disease.

Table 145.6 List of protease inhibitor-specific toxicities

Saquinavir	Indinavir	Ritonavir	Nelfinavir	Lopinavir/r	Atazanavir	Fosamprenavir	Tipranavir	Darunavir
Nausea Diarrhea Headache	Nephrolithiasis Nausea Indirect hyperbilirubinemia Headache Asthenia Dizziness Rash Alopecia Hemolytic anemia	Nausea Vomiting Diarrhea Paresthesias (circumoral and extremities) Asthenia Taste perversion	Diarrhea	Nausea Vomiting Diarrhea Asthenia	Indirect hyperbilirubinemia Prolonged PR interval Nephrolithiasis	Rash Diarrhea Nausea Vomiting Headache	Rash Intracranial hemorrhage	Rash Diarrhea Nausea

Less than 10% of ritonavir appears to cross the placenta. Ritonavir is not mutagenic in bacteria or mammalian cells and teratogenicity has only been seen in rats at maternally toxic doses (pregnancy category B).[9]

Adverse reactions and drug interactions

The major toxicities associated with ritonavir are headache, diarrhea, altered taste, circumoral and peripheral paresthesias and hyperlipidemia (see Table 145.6). For PI class toxicities, see Table 145.4. Ritonavir is the most potent inhibitor of the cytochrome P450 system of all the PIs. Ritonavir inhibits CYP3A4 and CYP2D6 and also increases glucuronosyl transferase activity. Ritonavir also induces CYP3A4 activity and has been shown to induce its own metabolism. Further discussion of the importance of drug interactions in HIV-infected patients can be found in Practice Point 45.

Indinavir

Description

Indinavir – N-(2(R)-hydroxy-1(S)-indanyl)-2(R)-(phenylmethyl)-4(S)-hydroxy-5-[1-[4-(3-pyridylmethyl)-2(S)-(N-tert-butylcarbamoyl)piperazinyl]]pentanamide (IDV; see Fig. 145.5) – was the third PI approved in the USA but is infrequently used in current antiretroviral therapy because of its complex pharmacology and side-effects.

Nelfinavir

Description

Nelfinavir – [3S-(3R*, 4aR*, 8aR*, 29S*, 39S*)]-2-[2'-hydroxy-3'-phenylthiomethyl-4'-aza-5'-oxo-5'-(2''-methyl-3''-hydroxyphenyl)pentyl]decahydroisoquinoline-3-N-t-butyl-carboxamide (NFV; see Fig. 145.5) – was the mainstay of antiretroviral regimens for several years but has now been largely replaced by more potent, ritonavir-boosted, protease inhibitors.[48]

Lopinavir (co-formulated with ritonavir)

Description

Lopinavir – [1S-[1R*, (R*), 3R*, 4R*]]-N-[4-[[2,6-dimethylphenoxy)acetyl]amino]-3-hydroxy-5-phenyl-1-(phenylmethyl)pentyl] tetrahydro-alpha-(1-methylethyl)-2-oxo-1(2H)-pyrimidineacetamide (LPV; see Fig. 145.5) – is co-formulated with ritonavir (lopinavir–ritonavir).

Pharmacokinetics and distribution

Lopinavir is poorly bioavailable because it is rapidly metabolized by NADPH and cytochrome P450 3A4/5-dependent enzyme systems; thus, the rationale for co-formulation with ritonavir. Ritonavir's inhibition of the metabolism of lopinavir results in an over 100-fold increase in lopinavir AUC.[49] Concentrations achieved following administration of lopinavir–ritonavir tablets are not affected by food, but administration with food increases the AUC by 80% for liquid formulations. Therefore, the tablets can be administered with or without food, while the oral solution should be administered with food. Lopinavir is 98–99% protein-bound, both to albumin and alpha-1-acid glycoprotein. At steady state, lopinavir peak and trough concentrations are 9.6 µg/ml and 5.5 µg/ml, respectively, following twice-daily lopinavir–ritonavir 400/100 mg.[49] Lopinavir undergoes extensive oxidative metabolism via CYP3A. The half-life of lopinavir–ritonavir is approximately 6 hours.

Use

Lopinavir–ritonavir tablets contain 200 mg of lopinavir and 50 mg of ritonavir or 100 mg of lopinavir and 25 mg of ritonavir. The usual adult dosage is lopinavir–ritonavir 400 mg/100 mg (two tablets) q12h. This total daily dose may be administered once daily in treatment-naive patients, but not in patients also receiving efavirenz, nevirapine, fosamprenavir or nelfinavir. In patients taking these concomitant antiretrovirals, the lopinavir–ritonavir dosage should be increased to 500 mg/125 mg q12h.

In antiretroviral-naive patients, lopinavir–ritonavir in combination with two NRTIs is an effective regimen.[48] Lopinavir–ritonavir is also effective in constructing regimens for treatment-experienced patients, particularly those who have experienced virologic failure on their initial, NNRTI-based regimen, or those with a limited number of protease inhibitor-associated resistance mutations. Treatment history and the results of drug-resistance assays should guide whether lopinavir–ritonavir should be used for treatment-experienced patients with virologic failure.

Resistance

The major mutations conferring lopinavir–ritonavir resistance are V32I, I47V/A, V82A/F/T/S, L10F/I/R/V, K20M/R, L24I, L33F, M46I/L, I50V, F53L, I54V/L/A/M/T/S, L63P, A71V/T, G73S, I84V and L90M (see Fig. 145.3). The pharmacoenhancement of lopinavir by ritonavir permits the drug to be active against viruses with up to 10- and possibly 40-fold changes in susceptibility to lopinavir.

Dosage in special circumstances

Dosage adjustment is not necessary in patients with renal disease. In patients with mild-to-moderate hepatic impairment, the AUC of lopinavir is increased 30% compared to patients with normal hepatic function. Close monitoring is advised in patients with liver disease. No specific dosage recommendations are available for this patient population.

Lopinavir has been shown to cross the placenta in rats with resulting developmental toxicities (decreased fetal viability, decreased fetal body weight, skeletal variations) at maternally toxic doses. No embryonic or fetal developmental toxicities have been seen in rabbits. Lopinavir–ritonavir is classified as pregnancy category C.[9]

Adverse reactions and drug interactions

The principal toxicities associated with lopinavir–ritonavir include gastrointestinal side-effects, hyperlipidemia and liver enzyme abnormalities (see Table 145.6). Lopinavir is a moderate inhibitor of CYP3A4 and the combination of lopinavir with ritonavir (a potent CYP3A4 inhibitor) has a number of significant drug interactions. Further discussion of the importance of drug interactions in HIV-infected patients can be found in Practice Point 45.

Atazanavir

Description

Atazanavir sulfate – dimethyl (3S, 8S, 9S, 12S)-9-benzyl-3,12,di-tert-butyl-8-hydroxy-4,11-dioxo-6-(p-2pyridylbenzyl)-2,5,6,10,13-pentaazatetradecanedioate sulfate (ATV; see Fig. 145.5) – is an azapeptide PI whose advantage is once-daily administration and the relative lack of induction of hyperlipidemia.

Pharmacokinetics and distribution

Atazanavir is rapidly absorbed and requires an acidic environment for adequate absorption. The mean C_{max} at steady state is 5.35 µg/ml at a median time of 2.5 hours following the administration of 400 mg once daily. The co-administration of ritonavir increases the atazanavir AUC 2.4-fold and the C_{min} 10.9-fold.[50] Atazanavir administration with a light meal or a high-fat meal increased the AUC by 70% and 35%, respectively, compared to the fasted state. Co-administration with ritonavir in similar situations decreases the pharmacokinetic variability. Atazanavir is 86% protein-bound, both to alpha-1-acid glycoprotein and albumin, and CSF to plasma ratios are reported to be between 0.0021 and 0.0226. Atazanavir is extensively metabolized in the liver, primarily by the CYP3A4 isoenzyme. The mean half-life of atazanavir is approximately 7 hours.

Use

Atazanavir is administered orally with or without ritonavir boosting. The usual dose of atazanavir in adults is 400 mg once daily or atazanavir 300 mg with ritonavir 100 mg once daily.

Atazanavir's once-daily administration, efficacy and lesser tendency to induce hyperlipidemia have made atazanavir–ritonavir one of the preferred choices for initial therapy. In patients with treatment experience, unboosted atazanavir should not be used. Atazanavir–ritonavir is useful in patients in whom an NNRTI-based initial regimen has failed but in patients who have PI-associated mutations, atazanavir–ritonavir is generally not as efficacious as tipranavir–ritonavir or darunavir–ritonavir.[51,52]

Resistance

The major mutations conferring resistance to atazanavir or atazanavir–ritonavir are I50L, I84V and N88S. Twenty-one minor mutations have been reported to contribute to atazanavir or atazanavir–ritonavir resistance (see Fig. 145.3).

Dosage in special circumstances

No dosage adjustment is necessary in patients with renal dysfunction. A dosage reduction to 300 mg once daily when prescribed without ritonavir boosting is recommended in patients with moderate hepatic impairment (Child-Pugh Class B) and the drug is not recommended in patients with severe hepatic impairment (Child-Pugh Class C).

Atazanavir is classified as pregnancy category B. Cases of lactic acidosis have been reported in pregnant women taking atazanavir with nucleoside analogues. Hyperbilirubinemia has also been reported. No adverse fetal effects or teratogenicity have been reported in animal reproductive and developmental studies.

Adverse reactions and drug interactions

In general, atazanavir has been well tolerated with the relative absence of hyperlipidemia a notable feature. When the drug is combined with low-dose ritonavir, some lipidogenic effect of ritonavir can be seen. The most common adverse effects are gastrointestinal complaints. Unconjugated, benign, reversible hyperbilirubinemia is the most frequent laboratory abnormality noted and may be associated with scleral icterus or clinical jaundice, but rarely requires treatment discontinuation. Atazanavir competitively inhibits UGT1A1 in the liver which is responsible for bilirubin glucuronidation and the proportion of patients with hyperbilirubinemia varies with distinct UGT1A1 genotypes.[53] Atazanavir can prolong the PR interval and must be used with caution in patients with pre-existing conduction system disease and with other drugs that may prolong the PR interval. Nephrolithiasis has also been reported with atazanavir.

Atazanavir is an inhibitor of CYP3A and UGT1A1, and a weak inhibitor of CYP2C8. Further discussion of the importance of drug interactions in HIV-infected patients can be found in Practice Point 45. Atazanavir plasma concentrations are expected to be reduced when co-administered with proton-pump inhibitors, antacids, buffered medications or H_2-receptor antagonists.

Amprenavir–fosamprenavir

Description

Amprenavir–(3S)-tetrahydro-3-furyl-N-[(1S, 2R)-3-(4-amino-N-isobutyl-benzenesulfonamido)-1-benzyl-2-hydroxypropyl] carbamate (APV; see Fig. 145.5). Fosamprenavir (FPV) is the prodrug of amprenavir and is now the marketed drug as it has improved the bioavailability and lowered the pill burden of amprenavir. It is rapidly hydrolyzed to amprenavir and inorganic phosphate by cellular phosphatases in the gut epithelium.

Pharmacokinetics and distribution

Fosamprenavir is rapidly absorbed following oral administration. The peak concentration of amprenavir is approximately 4.82 µg/ml and is achieved within 1–2 hours following administration of 1400 mg q12h. When fosamprenavir 1400 mg is co-administered with ritonavir 100 mg, both once daily, the peak concentration of amprenavir is approximately 7.93 µg/ml. The relative bioavailability of amprenavir oral solution is 14% less than amprenavir oral capsules. Administration of a single 1400 mg dose of fosamprenavir as the oral solution in the fed state was associated with a 46% reduction in C_{max}, a delayed T_{max} and a 28% reduction in amprenavir AUC. Amprenavir is approximately 90% protein-bound, predominantly to alpha-1-acid glycoprotein. Amprenavir is hepatically metabolized by CYP3A4. The plasma half-life of amprenavir is about 7.7 hours.

Use

The dosage in therapy-naive adults without ritonavir enhancement is 1400 mg q12h. With ritonavir, the dosage is fosamprenavir 1400 mg with ritonavir 100 mg or 200 mg once daily, or fosamprenavir 700 mg with ritonavir 100 mg twice daily. In treatment-experienced patients, the twice daily regimen with ritonavir is recommended.

Fosamprenavir–ritonavir is primarily used as an alternative PI for initial treatment. For treatment-experienced persons, fosamprenavir–ritonavir can be used as part of a new regimen following failure on an NNRTI-based regimen and in those patients with limited PI experience.

In patients with greater treatment experience and multiple PI-associated mutations, tipranavir–ritonavir or darunavir–ritonavir generally has greater utility if a PI is chosen to be part of the next regimen.

Resistance

The major mutations conferring resistance to fosamprenavir–ritonavir are I50V and I84V. Viral isolates resistant to the other, earlier approved PIs may remain susceptible to amprenavir. The major mutations conferring amprenavir resistance are I50V (a signature mutation) and I84V. Other important mutations include L10F/I/R/V, V32I, M46I/L, I47V, I54L/V/M, G73S, L76S, V82A/F/S/T and L90M (see Fig. 145.3).

Dosage in special circumstances

Data on the effects of renal disease on amprenavir pharmacokinetics are limited and no dosage modification is necessary. The AUC of amprenavir in patients with moderate and severe cirrhosis is significantly greater than in patients with normal hepatic function.

Fosamprenavir is classified as pregnancy category C.

Adverse reactions and drug interactions

The major toxicities associated with fosamprenavir include gastrointestinal symptomatology (diarrhea, nausea, vomiting) and rash (see Table 145.6). Amprenavir is a moderate inhibitor of CYP3A4. Further discussion of the importance of drug interactions in HIV-infected patients can be found in Practice Point 45.

Tipranavir
Description

Tipranavir disodium – [R-(R*, R*)]-N-[3-[1-[5,6-dihydro-4-hydroxy-2-oxo-6-(2-phenylethyl)-6-propyl-2H-pyran-3-yl]propyl]phenyl]5-(trifluoromethyl)-2-pyridinesulfonamide disodium salt (TPV; see Fig. 145.5) – is a dihydropyrone, nonpeptidic PI whose molecular advantage is the flexibility of binding to the active site of the HIV protease, thus retaining activity against viral strains with diminished susceptibility to other approved PIs.[54]

Pharmacokinetics and distribution

Tipranavir's bioavailability has not been quantified but a high-fat meal enhances its absorption. Co-administration with aluminum- or magnesium-based liquid antacids decreases the tipranavir AUC by 25%. Tipranavir is always co-administered with ritonavir as ritonavir increases tipranavir exposure by 24- to 70-fold; tipranavir is a substrate and inducer of P-glycoprotein and may initially induce its own metabolism. Tipranavir 500 mg with ritonavir 200 mg administered twice daily results in a tipranavir mean C_{max} of 94.8 μM and 77.6 μM in females and males, respectively. Tipranavir is highly protein-bound (>99.9%) to both albumin and alpha-1-acid glycoprotein. Tipranavir is hepatically metabolized predominantly by CYP3A4. The half-life of tipranavir is approximately 5–6 hours.

Use

Tipranavir is always administered with ritonavir. The usual adult dosage is 500 mg tipranavir with ritonavir 200 mg administered twice daily with food. Tipranavir contains a sulfonamide moiety and the potential for cross-sensitivity in patients with a sulfa allergy is unknown.

Tipranavir–ritonavir is useful in the setting of substantial PI resistance and its use is generally reserved for this circumstance.[55]

Resistance

The major mutations conferring tipranavir–ritonavir resistance are L33F, I47V, Q58E, Y74P, V82L/T and I84V. At least 11 minor

mutations, which can contribute to tipranavir resistance, have been described (see Fig. 145.3).

Dosage in special circumstances

No dosage adjustment of tipranavir–ritonavir is necessary in patients with renal dysfunction. Effects of moderate or severe hepatic impairment have not been evaluated and usage is not recommended. No dosage adjustment is necessary in patients with mild hepatic impairment.

Tipranavir is classified as pregnancy category C.

Adverse reactions and drug interactions

The most frequent adverse effects associated with tipranavir–ritonavir are diarrhea, nausea and vomiting (see Table 145.6). Elevations in hepatic transaminases and deaths due to hepatitis and liver decompensation have been reported, especially in patients with concomitant hepatitis B or C. Rash may occur in patients with or without history of sulfa allergy. Tipranavir–ritonavir has been associated with reports of both fatal and nonfatal intracranial hemorrhage. Many of these cases occurred in patients with contributing factors for intracranial hemorrhage. Tipranavir inhibits platelet aggregation and must be used cautiously in patients who may be at increased risk of bleeding. The drug interaction profile of tipranavir–ritonavir is complex. Tipranavir is both an inducer and inhibitor of the hepatic CYP3A4 isoenzyme. When co-administered with ritonavir, the net effect is inhibition. Tipranavir is also a potent inducer of P-glycoprotein and a weak P-glycoprotein inhibitor, while ritonavir is a P-glycoprotein inhibitor. When co-administered, the net effect on P-glycoprotein is induction. Further discussion of the importance of drug interactions in HIV-infected patients can be found in Practice Point 45.

Darunavir
Description

Darunavir – [(1S,2R)-3-[[(4-aminophenyl)sulfonyl](2-methylpropyl)amino]-2-hydroxy-1-(phenylmethyl)propyl]-carbamicacid(3R,3aS,6aR)-hexahydrofuro[2,3-b]furan-3-yl ester monoethanolate (DRV; see Fig. 145.5) – is another protease inhibitor with excellent activity against HIV-1 strains resistant to other PIs. It is a synthetic nonpeptide analogue of amprenavir, with a critical change at the terminal tetrahydrofuran group (THF), namely two THF groups forming a bis-THF moiety. This structure increases interactions with the protease enzyme and increases the binding energy.[56]

Pharmacokinetics and distribution

Darunavir is administered orally. Its absolute oral bioavailability following a single 600 mg dose increases from 37% to 82% after co-administration with ritonavir 100 mg twice daily. Peak darunavir concentrations of approximately 11.2–14.9 μg/ml (co-administered with ritonavir) are achieved within 2.5–4 hours. When administered with food, the C_{max} and AUC of darunavir co-administered with ritonavir are increased 30% compared to the fasting state. Darunavir is highly protein-bound (95%) primarily to alpha-1-acid glycoprotein. Darunavir is extensively liver metabolized to oxidative metabolites, primarily by the CYP3A isoenzymes. The half-life is approximately 15 hours when co-administered with ritonavir.

Use

Darunavir is always co-administered with ritonavir. The usual adult dose and frequency of administration are dependent on the treatment history of the patient, namely 800 mg with ritonavir 200 mg once daily with food in treatment-naive patients and 600 mg with ritonavir 100 mg twice daily with food in treatment-experienced patients.

Darunavir/ritonavir has proven most useful in highly treatment-experienced persons with multidrug-resistant virus.

Resistance

The major mutations conferring resistance to darunavir–ritonavir are I50V, I54M/L, L76V and I84V. Other mutations which contribute to darunavir–ritonavir resistance are V11I, V32I, L33F, I47V, L74P and L89V (see Fig. 145.3).

Dosage in special circumstances

No dosage adjustment is necessary in patients with renal dysfunction as darunavir is extensively metabolized in the liver. No dosage adjustment is necessary in patients with mild-to-moderate hepatic dysfunction (Child-Pugh Class A and B), but no pharmacokinetic or safety data are available for patients with severe liver disease.

Darunavir is classified as pregnancy category C.

Adverse reactions and drug interactions

The most common adverse effects associated with darunavir–ritonavir are gastrointestinal symptoms, nausea and headache. Drug-induced hepatitis and rash, including Stevens–Johnson syndrome, have also been reported. Given the sulfa moiety in darunavir, it is unclear if the rash is associated with the presence of a sulfa allergy. Darunavir–ritonavir is an inhibitor of CYP3A and CYP2D6 isoenzymes. Further discussion of the importance of drug interactions in HIV-infected patients can be found in Practice Point 45.

ENTRY INHIBITORS

Remarkable advances have been made in the past several years in our understanding of the HIV entry process. Specifically, the identification of HIV co-receptors (e.g. CCR5 and CXCR4) and the understanding of the events involved in fusion of the viral envelope with the cell membrane have created new therapeutic targets. Entry inhibitors can be divided into three subcategories: attachment inhibitors, chemokine receptor antagonists and fusion inhibitors.[57,58]

Enfuvirtide

Description

Enfuvirtide – $C_{204}H_{301}N_{51}O_{64}$, T-20 – is a 36-amino acid peptide derived from the HR2 region of HIV-1$_{LAI}$, which binds to the HR1 region of the HIV gp41 fusion peptide and prevents the coil–coil zipping reaction, which leads to six-helix bundle formation and eventual viral–host membrane fusion (Fig. 145.6). Enfuvirtide is active against both

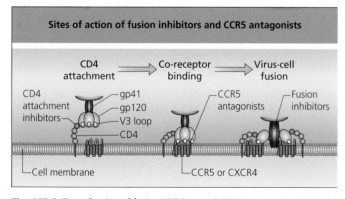

Fig. 145.6 Sites of action of fusion inhibitors and CCR5 antagonists. (Adapted from Moore JP, et al. Proc Natl Acad Sci USA 2003; 100; 10598–602.)

CCR5-using (R5) and CXCR4-using (X4) viral strains with susceptibility influenced by the time that the gp41 HR1 target is exposed to the drug as the viral entry process proceeds. Co-receptor density and affinity may influence the susceptibility of HIV strains to enfuvirtide.

Pharmacokinetics and distribution

Enfuvirtide is rapidly digested by peptidases in the gastrointestinal tract and consequently is not orally bioavailable. Following subcutaneous dosing of enfuvirtide, the mean C_{max} and C_{min} at steady state were reported as 2626 ng/ml and 972 ng/ml, respectively, at 50 mg q12h, and 4725 ng/ml and 1774 ng/ml, respectively, at 100 mg q12h.[59] The time to maximal concentrations was approximately 4 hours. The serum half-life of enfuvirtide after intravenous administration has been reported as approximately 2 hours, but more sustained concentrations throughout the 12-hour dosing interval have been reported following subcutaneous administration.

Use

Enfuvirtide is administered by subcutaneous injection. The adult dosage is 90 mg q12h.

Given the parenteral nature of the drug and its activity against drug-resistant virus, its role lies in the management of patients with treatment failure in whom other options are constrained. It is important to try to have at least two (and preferably more) other active drugs to administer with enfuvirtide so that enfuvirtide-resistant virus does not quickly emerge.

Resistance

Resistance to enfuvirtide has been documented to occur *in vivo* with most mutations mapping to positions 36–45 of the amino terminal (HR1 region) of gp41. The most commonly described mutations are G36D/S, I37V, V38A/M/E, Q39R, N42T and N43D (see Fig. 145.3). Interestingly, enfuvirtide-resistant viruses may be less fit than wild-type isolates. Thus an immunologic (and presumably clinical) benefit may persist beyond the point of virologic failure, similar to what has been described for PIs.

Dosage in special circumstances

The dose of the drug should not be influenced by renal or hepatic dysfunction given its peptide nature.

Adverse reactions and drug interactions

The major toxicity of enfuvirtide is injection site reaction, which occurs in a large proportion of patients to varying degrees. Painful, erythematous, indurated nodules have been reported in up to 98% of patients, but uncommonly require drug discontinuation. Rare cases of hypersensitivity have been reported.

Maraviroc

Description

Maraviroc – 4,4-difluoro-N-[(1R)-3-[(1S,5R)-3-(3-methyl-5-propan-2-yl-1,2,4-triazol-4-yl)-8-azabicyclo[3.2.1]octan-8-yl]-1-phenylpropyl]cyclohexane-1-carboxamide (MVC; see Fig. 145.7) – is the first in a new class of agents called CC chemokine receptor 5 (CCR5) antagonists. Chemokine receptors, namely CCR5 and the CXCR4, play a critical role in the entry of HIV into the CD4$^+$ cell as they serve as co-receptors following the binding of the virus to the primary receptor, the CD4 molecule (see Fig. 145.6). HIV-1 strains that exclusively use CCR5 for cell entry are termed R5-tropic, and strains that exclusively use CXCR4 are termed X4-tropic. Strains that are able to use both receptors for cell entry are termed R5/X4-dual tropic. Mixed populations of

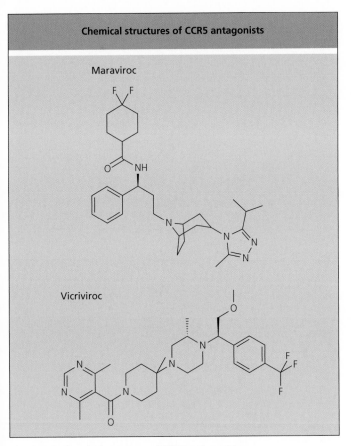

Chemical structures of CCR5 antagonists

Maraviroc

Vicriviroc

Fig. 145.7 Chemical structures of CCR5 antagonists.

R5 and X4 virus are termed R5/X4-mixed tropic. Maraviroc is a selective, reversible (noncompetitive) antagonist of the binding between human CCR5 and HIV-1 gp120 required for cell entry, thereby resulting in blocking of CCR5-tropic virus entry into cells. It represents a watershed in antiretroviral drug development because it is the first approved antiretroviral agent which targets a host cell molecule.

Pharmacokinetics and distribution

Maraviroc is administered orally with an absolute bioavailability of 23% and 33% (predicted) after a 100 mg and a 300 mg dose, respectively. Peak concentrations of 266–888 ng/ml have been reported in patients administered 300 mg twice daily, with peak concentrations achieved within 0.5–4 hours following a dose. Maraviroc is 76% protein-bound to both albumin and alpha-1-acid glycoprotein. It is primarily metabolized in the liver by CYP3A isoenzymes with a half-life of 14–18 hours.

Use

Maraviroc is available as an oral tablet formulation. The dosage regimen depends on the co-administration of other drugs that may inhibit or induce CYP3A. The usual adult dose with NRTIs, tipranavir–ritonavir, nevirapine, and drugs devoid of inhibition or induction of CYP3A4 is 300 mg twice daily. In the presence of potent CYP3A inhibitors, the dosage must be reduced to 150 mg twice daily. When co-administered with potent CYP3A4 inducers, the dosage must be increased to 600 mg twice daily.

Maraviroc has proven efficacy in the setting of multidrug-resistant virus when combined with an optimized background regimen.[60] In general, patients with more advanced or longer-standing HIV disease

have increasingly detectable proportions of X4 or dual–mixed tropic virus on tropism testing. Thus, the key to using maraviroc efficiently is to determine at what level of treatment failure to introduce the drug.

Resistance

Resistance to maraviroc appears to occur primarily via two mechanisms. The first, and most frequent, is the outgrowth of X4 virus subpopulations which existed but were undetected at baseline. The selective pressure of maraviroc on the R5 majority population allows the X4 virus to proliferate. The second is the result of mutations in the HIV-1 gp120 region which binds the CCR5 receptor which permit the virus to bind to the co-receptor and enter the cell despite the presence of bound maraviroc.[61-63] Early concerns that maraviroc would induce co-receptor switching on individual CD4+ cells have not been borne out.

Dosage in special circumstances

No dosage adjustment of maraviroc is necessary in patients with renal dysfunction or mild to moderate liver disease. No pharmacokinetic data are available in patients with severe hepatic impairment (Child-Pugh Class C).

Animal studies have not demonstrated increased pregnancy-related concerns with maraviroc. No adequate or well-controlled studies have been performed in pregnant women (pregnancy category B).

Adverse reactions and drug interactions

Maraviroc is generally very well tolerated. The most common adverse effects reported are upper respiratory tract infections, cough, pyrexia, rash and dizziness.

INTEGRASE INHIBITORS

HIV integrase is essential for viral replication and has been an attractive target since the early 1990s. However, it took the recognition of the key function of the HIV-1 integrase enzyme, the proviral DNA strand-transfer reaction, to develop true integrase inhibitors with clinical effectiveness.[64-66] Figure 145.8 illustrates the function of the HIV-1 integrase enzyme and the point at which integrase strand transfer inhibitors block virus replication.

Raltegravir

Description

Raltegravir – N-[(4-Fluorophenyl)methyl]-1,6-dihydro-5-hydroxy-1-methyl-2-{1-methyl-1-[[(5-methyl-1,3,4-oxadiazol-2-yl)carbonyl]amino]ethyl}-6-oxo-4-pyrimidinecarboxamide monopotassium salt (RAL; see Fig. 145.9) – is the lead drug in a new and important class of antiretrovirals called integrase inhibitors. Raltegravir binds to divalent cations in the catalytic core of integrase, preventing the formation of covalent bonds between integrase and host DNA. Three classes of integrase inhibitors have been identified: diketoacids, hydroxyquinolones and polyphenols. Raltegravir is a member of the diketoacid class.[66,67]

Pharmacokinetics and distribution

Raltegravir is administered orally with a mean peak concentration of 4.5 μmol/l achieved approximately 3 hours after dosing. It may be administered without regard to food, but a high-fat meal has been shown to increase the AUC by about 20% and slow the rate of absorption. Approximately 83% of raltegravir is protein-bound.

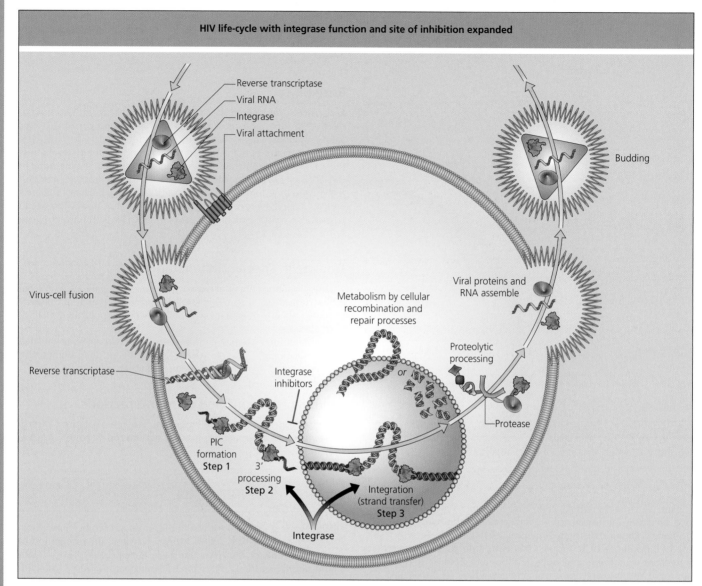

HIV life-cycle with integrase function and site of inhibition expanded

Fig. 145.8 HIV life-cycle with integrase function and site of inhibition expanded. (Courtesy, Dara Hazuda, Merck Research Laboratories.)

Raltegravir is metabolized by uridine diphosphate-glucuronosyl-transferase (UGT) to a glucuronide metabolite, mainly by UGT1A1. The dose is eliminated in both the urine (32%) and feces (51%), with metabolite accounting for 23% and 0% in the urine and feces, respectively. The half-life of raltegravir is approximately 9 hours.

Use

The usual adult dosage is 400 mg twice daily.

Raltegravir is primarily used in combination with other antiretroviral agents in persons with treatment-experience and multidrug-resistant virus. Raltegravir's approval was based on the results of two phase III studies which demonstrated clear superiority when raltegravir was added to an optimized background antiretroviral regimen compared to optimized background alone.[68,69]

Raltegravir has also demonstrated powerful, rapid, and durable antiretroviral activity in treatment-naive patients and studies are ongoing to determine what this agent's role might be in first-line therapy.[3,70,71]

Resistance

Raltegravir resistance is associated with mutations in HIV-1 integrase and evolves along one of three mutational pathways. The signature mutations for these pathways are Y143R/H/C, Q148H/K/R and N155H (see Fig. 145.3). Q148H+G140S is the most common pathway described thus far. Additional mutations seen are L74M+E138A and E138K. Additional mutations in the N155H pathway include L74M, E92Q, T97A, Y143H, G163K/R, V151I and D232N. The Y143R/H/C mutational pathway appears to be uncommon.[68]

Dosage in special circumstances

No dosage adjustment is necessary in patients with renal dysfunction. Raltegravir pharmacokinetics have not been studied in patients with severe hepatic dysfunction, but no dosage adjustment is necessary in patients with mild-to-moderate hepatic impairment.

Developmental and reproductive toxicity animal studies suggest possible fetal toxicity and therefore raltegravir is classified as pregnancy category C.

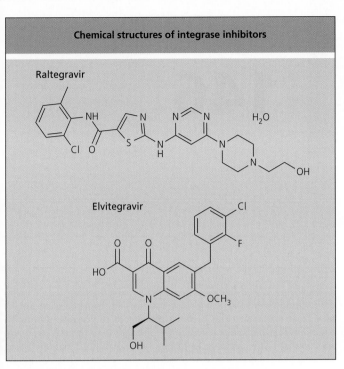

Chemical structures of integrase inhibitors

Raltegravir

Elvitegravir

Fig. 145.9 Chemical structures of integrase inhibitors.

Adverse reactions and drug interactions

Raltegravir is generally well tolerated. The most commonly associated adverse effects reported with raltegravir are nausea, headache and diarrhea. Raltegravir is not a CYP450 substrate, inducer or inhibitor and therefore is not expected to interact with drugs metabolized by CYP450 enzymes. As raltegravir is metabolized by UGT1A1, strong inducers of UGT1A1 such as rifampin (rifampicin) are expected to significantly decrease raltegravir concentrations and must be used with caution. Less strong inducers and inhibitors such as atazanavir have not been shown to significantly decrease raltegravir concentrations or increase toxicity, respectively.

CONCLUSION

The field of antiretroviral therapy has shown dramatic growth over the past 22 years with 25 agents in seven drug classes/subclasses approved over this time period. Clinicians and patients now have numerous choices for initial and subsequent therapy such that long-term viral suppression, immunologic preservation and clinical health should be achievable in most patients. The challenges of long-term adherence, toxicities and emerging drug resistance remain, however, such that the drug development pipeline needs to remain robust. In addition, and most critically, the advances in the developed world must continue to be translated into public health approaches for resource-limited settings where 90% of individuals with HIV infection live (see also Chapter 96).

REFERENCES

🖱 References for this chapter can be found online at http://www.expertconsult.com

Drugs for herpesvirus infections

DRUGS FOR TREATMENT OF HSV AND VZV INFECTIONS

Aciclovir and valaciclovir

Mechanism of action and *in-vitro* activity

Aciclovir, an acyclic analogue of guanosine, is a selective inhibitor of the replication of herpes simplex virus (HSV) types 1 and 2 and varicella-zoster virus (VZV). Valaciclovir is an orally administered prodrug of aciclovir with improved pharmacokinetic properties. Aciclovir is converted to its monophosphate derivative by virus-encoded thymidine kinase (TK), a reaction that does not occur to any significant extent in uninfected cells (Fig. 146.1). Subsequent diphosphorylation and triphosphorylation steps are catalyzed by cellular kinases, producing high concentrations of aciclovir triphosphate within HSV- or VZV-infected cells. Aciclovir triphosphate inhibits viral DNA synthesis by competing with deoxyguanosine triphosphate as a substrate for viral DNA polymerase. Since aciclovir triphosphate lacks the 3′-hydroxyl group required for further DNA chain elongation, incorporation into viral DNA results in obligate chain termination. Viral DNA polymerase has much higher affinity for aciclovir triphosphate than does cellular DNA polymerase, resulting in little incorporation of aciclovir into cellular DNA. Aciclovir exhibits good *in-vitro* activity against HSV-1, HSV-2 and VZV, with median inhibitory concentrations (IC_{50}) of 0.04, 0.10 and 0.50 µg/ml, respectively. Human cytomegalovirus (CMV) is not inhibited by aciclovir at clinically achievable concentrations.

Pharmacokinetics and distribution

Following oral administration, aciclovir is slowly and incompletely absorbed, with bioavailability of about 15–30%. After oral doses of 200 mg or 800 mg of aciclovir, mean plasma peak concentrations (C_{max}) at steady state are about 0.66 µg/ml and 1.6 µg/ml, respectively. Steady-state peak plasma aciclovir concentrations after intravenous doses of 5 mg/kg or 10 mg/kg of body weight every 8 hours are about 10 µg/ml and 20 µg/ml, respectively. Plasma protein binding is less than 20%. Aciclovir penetrates well into most tissues, including the central nervous system (Table 146.1). The CSF aciclovir area under the concentration–time curve (AUC) is about 20% of the serum AUC. In non-inflamed eyes, the mean vitreous-to-serum concentration ratio for aciclovir is about 24%. Significant concentrations of aciclovir (up to 300% of the serum concentration) can be found in breast milk. Aciclovir is minimally metabolized and about 85% of an administered dose is excreted unchanged in the urine via glomerular filtration and renal tubular secretion. The terminal plasma half-life of acyclovir is 2–3 hours in adults and 3–4 hours in neonates with normal renal function, but is extended to about 20 hours in anuric subjects.

Valaciclovir is an orally administered prodrug of aciclovir designed to overcome the problem of poor oral bioavailability. Valaciclovir, the L-valine ester of aciclovir, is well absorbed from the gastrointestinal tract via a stereospecific transporter and undergoes essentially complete first pass conversion in the gut and liver to yield aciclovir and L-valine. This prodrug improves bioavailability to about 54%, yielding peak plasma aciclovir levels that are three- to fivefold higher than those achieved with oral aciclovir. Oral doses of 500 mg or 1000 mg of valaciclovir produce peak plasma aciclovir concentrations of 3.3 µg/ml and 5–6 µg/ml, respectively. After administration of valaciclovir at a dose of 2 g orally four times daily, plasma aciclovir AUC values approximate those produced by aciclovir given intravenously at a dose of 10 mg/kg every 8 hours. Following enzymatic conversion of valaciclovir to aciclovir, the antiviral spectrum of activity, pharmacokinetic properties and excretion are the same as those described above.

Route of administration and dosage

Aciclovir is available in topical, oral and intravenous formulations. Outside of the USA, aciclovir is also available as a 3% preparation for ophthalmologic use. The dermatologic preparations consist of 5% aciclovir in a polyethylene glycol ointment or propylene glycol cream base. Oral aciclovir products include a 200 mg capsule, 400 mg and 800 mg

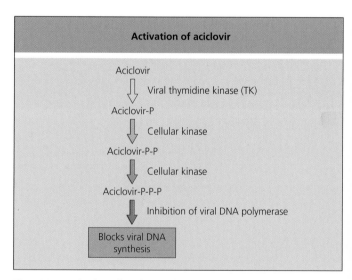

Fig. 146.1 Activation of aciclovir is dependent on monophosphorylation via viral thymidine kinase (TK). Aciclovir triphosphate inhibits the activity of viral DNA polymerase, thus blocking viral replication. Penciclovir and ganciclovir are activated by similar mechanisms.

Table 146.1 Tissue distribution of aciclovir*

	CSF/CNS	Lung	Liver	Kidney	Breast milk	Amniotic fluid	Heart
Aciclovir concentration (µg/ml)	10	26.7	26.7	206	66.7	<0.1–2.6	26.7

*Based on a steady-state plasma concentration (20.6µg/ml) after intravenous aciclovir dosing of 15mg/kg q8h.

tablets, and a liquid suspension (200mg/5ml). Aciclovir sodium for intravenous infusion is supplied as a sterile water-soluble powder that must be reconstituted and diluted to a concentration of 50mg/ml.

The recommended dose of aciclovir will vary with the specific indication (Table 146.2). Because of the greater intrinsic resistance of VZV to aciclovir, the doses required for treating VZV infections are higher than those used for HSV infections. In adults with normal renal function, oral aciclovir is given at a dose of 200mg (for HSV) to 800mg (for VZV) five times daily. The recommended dose of intravenous aciclovir is 5mg/kg every 8 hours for HSV infections and 10mg/kg every 8 hours for VZV infections, although higher doses (12–15mg/kg every 8 hours) are sometimes used for life-threatening infections, especially in immunocompromised patients.

Valaciclovir is available as 500mg and 1000mg tablets. The recommended doses are 500mg every 12 hours for episodic treatment of recurrent genital HSV infections and 1000mg every 8 hours for treatment of herpes zoster. A suspension preparation is not available.

Indications

HSV infections

Aciclovir and valaciclovir are effective for treatment of initial and recurrent episodes of genital herpes as well as for suppressive therapy (see Table 146.3).[1,2] There is no evidence of cumulative toxicity or emergence of drug-resistant HSV in immunocompetent patients even after years of suppressive therapy.[3] Suppression with aciclovir or valaciclovir will also significantly reduce (but not eliminate) the frequency of asymptomatic viral shedding and reduce the risk of transmission of genital herpes to an uninfected partner.[4,5]

Antiviral prophylaxis with aciclovir or valaciclovir can significantly reduce the necessity for Caesarian section due to active genital HSV lesions present at the onset of labor.[6] For babies that develop neonatal herpes, intravenous aciclovir therapy can significantly reduce both morbidity and mortality.

Valaciclovir (2g every 12 hours for 1 day) has been shown to reduce the duration of an episode of recurrent herpes labialis by 1.1 days.[7] Suppressive therapy with valaciclovir (1g daily) can reduce the frequency of clinical recurrences by about 50%.[8] Combination therapy with an antiviral drug (such as aciclovir or valaciclovir) plus corticosteroids is widely used for treatment of Bell's palsy, but the demonstrated benefit from the antiviral therapy has varied among clinical trials.[9] Oral aciclovir and valaciclovir have both been used successfully for treatment and prophylaxis of herpetic keratitis.

Aciclovir or valaciclovir prophylaxis of HSV infections is highly effective in severely immunocompromised patients, particularly those undergoing induction chemotherapy or organ transplantation. Clinical experience suggests that intravenous aciclovir (10mg/kg every 8 hours) is the treatment of choice for disseminated or visceral HSV infection (e.g. pneumonitis, hepatitis, esophagitis, etc.) in immunocompromised patients, although data from controlled clinical trials are lacking. Aciclovir is the drug of choice for HSV encephalitis and should be given intravenously at a dose of 10–15mg/kg every 8 hours for 14–21 days.

VZV infections

Oral aciclovir therapy (20mg/kg, up to a maximum of 800mg, every 6 hours) is effective for immunocompetent children with chickenpox, but the benefits are modest and many pediatricians consider antiviral treatment of chickenpox to be optional. Adolescents and adults are

at greater risk for varicella complications; aciclovir therapy (800mg orally five times daily for 7 days) is recommended for those who present within 24–48 hours of disease onset. Valaciclovir is also likely to be effective in this setting, but data from controlled clinical trials are lacking. Immunocompromised patients with chickenpox should receive intravenous aciclovir (10mg/kg or 500mg/m² every 8 hours for 7–10 days). Clinical experience suggests that intravenous aciclovir is the treatment of choice for patients with VZV infections complicated by visceral involvement (e.g. pneumonitis, encephalitis, etc.).

Both aciclovir and valaciclovir are effective for treatment of localized herpes zoster in immunocompetent patients if therapy is initiated within 48–72 hours of rash onset. Valaciclovir has the advantage of a simpler dosing regimen. Severely immunocompromised patients (e.g. bone marrow transplant, cancer chemotherapy, etc.) with herpes zoster are at high risk for disseminated VZV infection and should be treated with intravenous aciclovir (10mg/kg every 8 hours).

Other viral infections

While aciclovir is ineffective for established CMV infections, high-dose oral aciclovir or valaciclovir may have value for CMV prophylaxis in high-risk populations such as organ transplant recipients.[10] Aciclovir or valaciclovir can induce regression of Epstein–Barr virus (EBV)-associated oral hairy leukoplakia in HIV-infected patients. Aciclovir is considered the drug of choice for therapy of rare human infections

Table 146.2 Indications for aciclovir therapy

Infection	Route and dosage*
Genital HSV Initial episode	200mg po 5 times/d (or 400mg q8h) × 10 days
   Initial episode with complications	5mg/kg iv q8h × 5–7 days
Recurrent episodes	200mg po 5 times/d (or 400mg q8h) × 5 days
Suppression	400mg po q12h daily
Mucocutaneous HSV in immunocompromised patient	400mg po 5 times/d × 10–14 days, or 5mg/kg iv q8h × 10 days
Disseminated or visceral HSV (including encephalitis)	10–15mg/kg iv q8h × 14–21 days
Neonatal HSV	10–15mg/kg iv q8h × 14–21 days
Varicella (chickenpox) Normal host	20mg/kg (max. 800mg) po 4–5 times/d × 5 days
Immunocompromised patient	10–15mg/kg iv q8h × 7–10 days

Herpes zoster (shingles)
  Normal host
  Immunocompromised patient (disseminated or visceral VZV)
	800mg po 5 times/d × 7–10 days
	10–15mg/kg iv q8h × 7–10 days

*Given doses are indicated for patients with normal renal function.

Table 146.3 Oral antiviral therapy for genital herpes*

Drugs	Initial episode	Episodic therapy	Suppressive therapy
Aciclovir	200 mg q5h × 7–10 days *Alternative dose:* 400 mg q8h × 7–10 days	200 mg q5h × 5 days *Alternative doses:* 400 mg q8h × 5 days 800 mg q12h × 5 days 800 mg q8h × 2 days	400 mg q12h daily
Famciclovir	250 mg q8h × 7–10 days	125 mg q12h × 5 days *Alternative dose:* 1000 mg q12h × 1 day	250 mg q12h daily
Valaciclovir	1000 mg q12h × 7–10 days	500 mg q8h × 3 days *Alternative dose:* 1000 mg q24h × 5 days	500 mg once daily *Alternative doses:* 1000 mg q24h daily 500 mg q12h daily

*Recommended doses for immunocompetent adults with normal renal function.[1,50]

caused by cercopithecine herpesvirus-1 (B virus). Aciclovir is not directly active against HIV; however, studies of HIV/HSV-2 co-infected men have shown significant reductions in HIV plasma levels in those patients receiving valaciclovir.[11]

Dosage in special circumstances

Aciclovir is cleared primarily by renal mechanisms and dosage modification of aciclovir and valaciclovir is required for patients with significant renal dysfunction (Tables 146.3, 146.4). The mean elimination half-life of aciclovir after a single 1 g dose of valaciclovir is about 14 hours in patients with end-stage renal disease. No specific dosage modification is required for patients with hepatic impairment. Aciclovir and valaciclovir are not approved for use in pregnancy, but have been widely used to treat HSV and VZV infections in pregnant women without evidence of maternal or fetal toxicity.

In a study of pediatric cancer patients, the bioavailability of aciclovir after valaciclovir dosing was 64%. Aciclovir AUC values after oral valaciclovir dosing are slightly higher in elderly individuals when compared with younger control groups, due to age-related decline in renal function. Because no liquid valaciclovir preparation is available, experience with this drug in very young children is limited.

Adverse reactions

Aciclovir and valaciclovir are extremely well-tolerated drugs with few significant adverse effects. Allergic reactions to aciclovir or valaciclovir have been reported, but are very uncommon. With intravenous aciclovir therapy, inflammation and phlebitis may occur following localized drug extravasation. Renal dysfunction (including cases of acute renal failure) resulting from accumulation of aciclovir crystals in the kidneys has been observed following administration of large doses of aciclovir by rapid intravenous infusion, but is uncommon and usually reversible.

The risk of nephrotoxicity can be minimized by administering aciclovir by slow infusion (over 1 hour) and ensuring adequate hydration. Rarely, nephrotoxicity has been observed following oral dosing of aciclovir or valaciclovir. Risk factors for aciclovir-induced

Table 146.4 Aciclovir dosage modification for renal impairment

	ADJUSTED DOSAGE REGIMEN		
Normal dosage regimen	**CrCl (ml/min/1.73 m²)**	**Dose**	**Dosing interval (hr)**
Aciclovir 200 mg po q4h	>10 0–10	200 mg 200 mg	4 (5 times/day) 12
Aciclovir 400 mg po q12h	>10 0–10	400 mg 200 mg	12 12
Aciclovir 800 mg po q4h	>25 10–25 0–10	800 mg 800 mg 800 mg	4 (5 times/day) 8 12
Aciclovir 5 mg/kg iv q8h	>50 25–50 10–25 0–10	5 mg/kg 5 mg/kg 5 mg/kg 2.5 mg/kg	8 12 24 24
Aciclovir 10 mg/kg iv q8h	>50 25–50 10–25 0–10	10 mg/kg 10 mg/kg 10 mg/kg 5 mg/kg	8 12 24 24

CrCl, creatinine clearance.

nephropathy include pre-existing renal dysfunction and concomitant use of other nephrotoxic drugs.

Reports have linked administration of aciclovir with CNS disturbances, including agitation, hallucination, disorientation, tremors, clonus and seizures. Neurotoxicity has most often been recognized in elderly patients with underlying CNS abnormalities and renal insufficiency. Elevated concentrations of the main aciclovir metabolite, 9-carboxymethoxymethylguanine (CMMG), have been detected in serum and CSF of patients who developed neuropsychiatric symptoms while receiving aciclovir or valaciclovir and could play an etiologic role.[12] Aciclovir-induced neurologic toxicity has been successfully treated by emergent hemodialysis.

Patients receiving oral aciclovir or valaciclovir therapy occasionally complain of nausea, diarrhea, rash or headache, but at rates that do not differ from the placebo recipients. The safety of oral aciclovir and valaciclovir for long-term administration has been confirmed in patients receiving the drug for over 5 years for suppression of recurrent genital herpes.[3]

A syndrome of thrombotic microangiopathy (TMA) was described in HIV-infected patients receiving investigational high-dose valaciclovir (8 g/day) for prevention of CMV disease. A causal relationship between high-dose valaciclovir and TMA has not been proven. The TMA-like syndrome, which is characterized by fever, microangiopathic hemolytic anemia, thrombocytopenia and renal dysfunction, has not been observed in immunocompetent patients receiving valaciclovir at approved doses (up to 3 g/day). There is no contraindication to using valaciclovir at standard doses in HIV-infected patients and it has proven safe in wide clinical experience.[13]

Significant interactions between aciclovir and other drugs are extremely uncommon. Probenecid decreases the renal clearance of aciclovir and can prolong the plasma excretion half-life. Additive aciclovir-induced nephrotoxicity in patients receiving concomitant ciclosporin A therapy has been suggested. Lethargy has been reported in a few patients receiving both aciclovir and zidovudine, but a causative role for aciclovir has not been established. Concomitant administration of cimetidine and probenecid reduces the rate of valaciclovir conversion to aciclovir, but the effect is not clinically significant.

Resistance

Herpes simplex virus resistance to aciclovir can develop through mutation of the viral genes encoding thymidine kinase or DNA polymerase.[14] Most aciclovir-resistant clinical HSV isolates are TK deficient and are, therefore, unable to phosphorylate aciclovir. Consequently, these isolates will also be resistant to valaciclovir, penciclovir, famciclovir and ganciclovir, all of which have the same mechanism of action and require viral TK for activation.

Disease caused by aciclovir-resistant HSV isolates occurs almost exclusively in immunocompromised patients. The most common clinical presentation of infection caused by aciclovir-resistant HSV is chronic, progressive mucocutaneous ulcerations. Approximately 5–6% of HSV isolates recovered from HIV-seropositive patients are aciclovir-resistant ($IC_{50} > 2.0 \mu g/ml$).[15] Aciclovir-resistant VZV isolates (which are less frequently encountered than resistant HSV isolates) are occasionally recovered from AIDS patients. Clinical disease caused by aciclovir-resistant VZV has usually been limited to cutaneous involvement, often characterized by atypical lesions. The options for treatment of aciclovir-resistant HSV or VZV disease are foscarnet and cidofovir.

Penciclovir and famciclovir

Mechanism of action and *in-vitro* activity

Penciclovir is an acyclic guanine derivative that is similar to aciclovir in structure, mechanism of action and spectrum of antiviral activity. In HSV- or VZV-infected cells, penciclovir is first monophosphorylated by virally encoded TK and then further phosphorylated to the triphosphate moiety by cellular enzymes. Penciclovir triphosphate blocks viral DNA synthesis through competitive inhibition of viral DNA polymerase. Unlike aciclovir triphosphate, penciclovir triphosphate is not an obligate chain terminator and can be incorporated into the extending DNA chain. Compared with aciclovir triphosphate, intracellular concentrations of penciclovir triphosphate are much higher. For example, the half-life values for penciclovir triphosphate and aciclovir triphosphate in HSV-1-infected cells are 10 hours and 0.7 hour, respectively. However, this potential advantage is offset by a much lower affinity of penciclovir triphosphate for viral DNA polymerase. The *in-vitro* activities of penciclovir against HSV-1, HSV-2 and VZV are similar to those of aciclovir, with median IC_{50} values of 0.4, 1.5 and 4.0 μg/ml, respectively, in MRC-5 cells.

Just as valaciclovir is a prodrug of aciclovir, famciclovir is a prodrug of penciclovir. Because penciclovir is very poorly absorbed, famciclovir (the diacetyl ester of 6-deoxy-penciclovir) was developed as the oral formulation. The first acetyl side chain of famciclovir is cleaved by esterases found in the intestinal wall. On first pass through the liver, the second acetyl group is removed and oxidation catalyzed by aldehyde oxidase occurs at the 6 position, yielding penciclovir, the active antiviral compound.

Pharmacokinetics and distribution

Intravenous infusion of penciclovir at 10 mg/kg over 1 hour yields a peak plasma concentration of 12.1 μg/ml. Plasma protein binding of penciclovir is <20%. The drug is cleared by renal tubular secretion and passive filtration. The plasma elimination half-life of penciclovir is about 2 hours and approximately 70% is recovered unchanged in the urine.

When administered as the famciclovir prodrug, the bioavailability of penciclovir is about 77%. Following a single oral dose of 250 mg or 500 mg of famciclovir, peak plasma penciclovir concentrations of 1.9 μg/ml and 3.5 μg/ml, respectively, are achieved at 1 hour. The pharmacokinetics of penciclovir are linear and dose independent over a famciclovir dosing range of 125–750 mg. Food slows famciclovir absorption and lowers the peak plasma penciclovir concentration, but does not alter the AUC value.

Route of administration and dosage

Famciclovir is available as 125 mg, 250 mg and 500 mg tablets. Recommended dosages will vary with the indication. The usual dose of famciclovir is 125 mg every 12 hours for episodic therapy of recurrent genital herpes and 500 mg every 8 hours for herpes zoster. The intravenous preparation of penciclovir has not been commercially released. A topical preparation of penciclovir is available as a 1% cream for treatment of HSV labialis.

Indications

Genital HSV infections

Famciclovir is effective for initial and recurrent genital herpes and also provides effective suppressive therapy[1,16,17] (see Table 146.3). Famciclovir suppressive therapy reduces mucosal viral shedding from HSV-2 infected persons,[18] but its effect on virus transmission has not been studied. Famciclovir is also effective for suppression and treatment of recurrent mucocutaneous (orolabial and anogenital) infections in HIV-infected patients.

Three drugs (aciclovir, valaciclovir and famciclovir) with proven efficacy for long-term suppression of recurrent genital herpes are currently available. Direct comparative trials are not available to select the most effective treatment.[19] All three compounds are safe and well tolerated. Considerations in selecting the appropriate drug may include cost and dosing convenience. For any patient, the goal is to establish a suppressive regimen that is effective, economical and convenient. For these drugs, a dose–response relationship exists, meaning that higher total daily doses generally produce more complete suppression. Dose titration of the selected drug will be needed to identify optimal treatment for an individual patient (see Table 146.3).

Herpes labialis

Topical 1% penciclovir cream (applied every 2 hours while awake) and oral famciclovir (1500 mg) have demonstrated efficacy for treatment of herpes labialis.[20]

Herpes zoster

Famciclovir accelerated cutaneous healing and reduced the duration of viral shedding and postherpetic neuralgia in immunocompetent patients with dermatomal herpes zoster.[21] Famciclovir was proven effective for herpes zoster therapy in bone marrow transplant, cancer and HIV-seropositive patients. In the USA, the recommended dose of famciclovir for uncomplicated herpes zoster is 500 mg three times daily. Doses of 250 mg three times daily and 750 mg once daily are approved in Europe and the UK.

Three drugs (aciclovir, valaciclovir and famciclovir) are currently available in the USA for treatment of uncomplicated herpes zoster in immunocompetent patients (a fourth drug, brivudin, is available in some countries and is discussed below) (Table 146.5). All three drugs are well tolerated and appear to be comparable in clinical efficacy. In a large randomized clinical trial, valaciclovir and famciclovir were shown to be therapeutically equivalent for treatment of herpes zoster.[22] Because of their improved pharmacokinetic profiles and simpler dosing regimens, valaciclovir and famciclovir are preferred over aciclovir for this indication.

Other viral infections

Famciclovir suppresses hepatitis B virus (HBV) replication by targeting the viral polymerase, but treatment of hepatitis B using famciclovir monotherapy resulted in rapid emergence of HBV resistance. Case reports have suggested that famciclovir is effective for treatment of EBV-induced oral hairy leukoplakia in HIV-infected patients.

Dosage in special circumstances

Penciclovir is cleared predominantly by renal mechanisms, so adjustments of famciclovir dosing are required in patients with advanced renal insufficiency. In patients with hepatic insufficiency, the rate of conversion of famciclovir to penciclovir is decreased, but the plasma AUC value for penciclovir is not significantly changed; no famciclovir dosage modification is necessary. Plasma penciclovir concentrations are slightly higher in elderly patients treated with famciclovir due to age-related reduction in glomerular filtration rates, but dosage modifications are not required. Absorption after topical application is minimal and no dosage modifications are required for use of penciclovir 1% cream. No liquid preparation of famciclovir is currently available and few data regarding use in small children are available. Famciclovir has not been approved for use during pregnancy.

Adverse reactions

Safety data collected from over 3000 patients given famciclovir have shown the drug to be very safe and well tolerated. The most frequently reported adverse experiences have included occasional headache, nausea and diarrhea.

No clinically significant drug interactions have been noted with famciclovir. Co-administration of famciclovir with cimetidine or theophylline will increase the penciclovir AUC by about 20%.

Co-administration of famciclovir and digoxin results in a 19% increase in the peak digoxin concentration, but no change in the AUC.

Resistance

The majority of clinically encountered aciclovir-resistant HSV and VZV isolates are TK deficient and thus will generally be resistant to penciclovir and famciclovir, which also require viral TK for activation. However, some HSV strains that are aciclovir resistant by virtue of altered TK or DNA polymerase mutations may retain susceptibility to penciclovir.

Brivudin

Brivudin is a highly potent antiviral agent selectively active against VZV and HSV-1 with therapeutic equivalence to aciclovir. Because of concerns about potential toxicity, commercial development of brivudin has halted in many countries (including the USA), but the drug is widely available in Europe.

Mechanism of action and in-vitro activity

Brivudin, a 5′-halogenated thymidine nucleoside analogue, is sequentially phosphorylated by viral TK and cellular kinases to form BVDU triphosphate, a competitive inhibitor of viral DNA polymerase and an alternative substrate for incorporation in viral DNA. The intracellular half-life in virus-infected cells is about 10 hours. The drug is highly active against VZV, with IC_{50} values 28–1100-fold lower than those of aciclovir. Brivudin is active against HSV-1, but not against HSV-2. Thus, the clinical development of the drug has focused on its role for herpes zoster therapy.

Pharmacokinetics and distribution

Brivudin is well absorbed after oral administration and absorption is not affected by food. There is high first-pass metabolism in the liver to bromovinyluracil, which lacks antiviral activity. At steady state (brivudin 125 mg daily for 5 days), the C_{max} and C_{min} are 1.7 µg/ml (at 1 hour) and 0.06 µg/ml, respectively. The plasma terminal elimination half-life is approximately 16 hours; metabolites are excreted in urine (65%) and plasma (21%). Brivudin is highly protein-bound (>95%).[23]

Route of administration and dosage

Brivudin is available as a 125 mg tablet and as a 0.1% ointment for ophthalmologic use. The standard dose for herpes zoster is 125 mg orally once daily for 7 days.

Indications

In randomized clinical trials, brivudin has been compared with aciclovir and famciclovir in immunocompetent patients with herpes zoster and was equivalent to the comparator drugs for end points of zoster lesion healing and pain resolution.[24] With its once-daily dosing, brivudin offers a potential advantage of convenience and improved patient adherence.

Dosage in special circumstances

The pharmacokinetic properties of brivudin in elderly patients or in patients with renal or hepatic failure are not significantly changed from those seen in healthy volunteers.

Adverse reactions

In clinical trials with brivudin, the most commonly observed adverse effects were nausea (2.1%), abdominal pain (0.8%), vomiting (0.5%) and headache (1%) and did not differ significantly from adverse

---

Table 146.5 Oral antiviral therapy for herpes zoster*

Treatment options
- Aciclovir 800 mg q4h for 7–10 days
- Famciclovir 500 mg q8h for 7 days
- Valaciclovir 1000 mg q8 for 7 days
- Brivudin 125 mg q24h for 7 days

*Recommended doses for immunocompetent adults with normal renal function.

effects reported with aciclovir or famciclovir. Hypersensitivity reactions to brivudin are rare.

Brivudin has a critically important drug interaction that has been an obstacle to its regulatory approval in some countries. Bromovinyluracil (the primary metabolite of brivudin) irreversibly inhibits dihydropyrimidine dehydrogenase (DPD), an enzyme that regulates nucleoside metabolism.[25] Co-administration of brivudin with 5-fluorouracil (5-FU, a cancer chemotherapeutic agent) results in a 15-fold increase in systemic exposure to 5-FU, causing potentially lethal bone marrow suppression and gastrointestinal toxicity. Full recovery of DPD activity requires at least 18 days after brivudin dosing. Potential interactions with brivudin may also occur with other fluoropyrimidines such as flucytosine (5-FC), tegafur, floxuridine and capecitabine. Brivudin should be used with extreme caution in cancer patients to avoid concomitant dosing with 5-FU.

Other drugs

Vidarabine

Vidarabine was the first intravenous antiviral drug accepted for widespread clinical use, but has now been replaced by more potent antiviral drugs. Vidarabine 3% ophthalmic ointment is used for treatment of HSV keratoconjunctivitis.

Trifluridine

Trifluridine, a fluorinated pyrimidine nucleoside with good *in-vitro* activity against HSV, is a competitive inhibitor of HSV DNA polymerase. Trifluridine is widely used as a 1% ophthalmic solution for topical therapy of HSV keratitis. Topical trifluridine has also been used with moderate success for treatment of aciclovir-resistant mucocutaneous infections in AIDS patients.

Idoxuridine

Idoxuridine is an iodinated thymidine derivative with activity against HSV. Use of idoxuridine has been limited to topical application, since systemic administration is associated with significant myelosuppression. Idoxuridine (in topical 1% solution and 0.5% ointment formulations) has been used successfully for treatment of HSV keratitis, but has largely been replaced by topical trifluridine and aciclovir for this indication. Topical application of 15% idoxuridine in dimethyl sulfoxide was shown to shorten the course of herpes labialis in a placebo-controlled trial.

n-Docosanol

n-Docosanol is a 22-carbon fatty alcohol with *in-vitro* activity against several enveloped viruses, including HSV-1 and HSV-2. The drug acts by interfering with viral entry into target cells. n-Docosanol is available over the counter in a 2 g tube of 10% cream and is indicated for recurrences of herpes labialis.

DRUGS FOR TREATMENT OF CYTOMEGALOVIRUS INFECTIONS

Ganciclovir and valganciclovir

Mechanism of action and *in-vitro* activity

Ganciclovir is a nucleoside analogue that is structurally similar to aciclovir, but has a hydroxymethyl group at the 3′ position of the acyclic side chain. This relatively minor structural modification accounts for enhanced activity of ganciclovir against human CMV and also for the drug's greater toxicity. Ganciclovir triphosphate is a potent inhibitor of herpesvirus DNA replication, acting as both an inhibitor of and a substrate for viral DNA polymerase.[26]

In HSV- or VZV-infected cells, monophosphorylation of ganciclovir is induced by viral TK, as also occurs with aciclovir. In CMV-infected cells, ganciclovir monophosphorylation is carried out by a protein kinase encoded by the UL97 gene. The di- and tri-phosphorylation steps are mediated by cellular kinases. On a molar basis, aciclovir triphosphate is actually a more potent inhibitor of CMV than is ganciclovir triphosphate. However, aciclovir is a poor substrate for phosphorylation by the UL97 gene product; consequently, the concentration of ganciclovir triphosphate in CMV-infected cells is 10-fold higher than that of aciclovir triphosphate. Furthermore, the half-life of ganciclovir triphosphate in CMV-infected cells is 16.5 hours, compared with 2.5 hours for aciclovir triphosphate. Ganciclovir triphosphate does not function as a chain terminator, and can be incorporated into elongating viral DNA (and, to a much lesser extent, human DNA) where it functions to slow DNA chain extension.

Ganciclovir and aciclovir have similar *in-vitro* activity against HSV-1, HSV-2 and VZV. However, ganciclovir is much more active against CMV, with IC_{50} values of 0.1–1.8 µg/ml against clinical isolates.

Pharmacokinetics and distribution

Intravenous infusion of ganciclovir at a dose of 5 mg/kg yields peak and trough plasma levels of approximately 8 µg/ml and 1 µg/ml, respectively. Plasma protein binding is 1–2%. Reported plasma-to-CSF ratios for ganciclovir have ranged from 24% to 70%. Ganciclovir is not metabolized and is cleared by renal mechanisms, with an elimination half-life of about 3 hours. Ganciclovir is poorly absorbed after oral administration, with bioavailability of only 5–9%. Following oral dosing of ganciclovir at 1000 mg every 8 hours, steady-state plasma peak and trough concentrations of 1.2 µg/ml and 0.2 µg/ml, respectively, are achieved.

To overcome the limited oral bioavailability of ganciclovir, a prodrug called valganciclovir has been developed.[27] Valganciclovir, the L-valyl ester of ganciclovir, is rapidly and completely hydrolyzed to ganciclovir in the liver and intestinal wall. Bioavailability of ganciclovir is about 60% from the prodrug formulation and is significantly increased with food administration. Maximum plasma ganciclovir concentrations are four- to fivefold higher than those achieved after oral dosing with the parent drug. Oral valganciclovir doses of 450 mg and 875 mg once daily for 3 days produced peak plasma ganciclovir concentrations of 3.3 µg/ml and 6.1 µg/ml, respectively. The AUC of ganciclovir after administration of 900 mg valganciclovir is about 26 µg/ml/h, which is comparable to the AUC following administration of ganciclovir dosed at 5 mg/kg intravenously.

Route of administration and dosage

Ganciclovir is available as an oral capsule, an intravenous formulation and a delayed-release intraocular implant device. Recommended doses will vary with the indication. For treatment of acute CMV disease, the usual dose of intravenous ganciclovir is 5 mg/kg every 12 hours. Oral ganciclovir, supplied as 250 mg capsules, can be used for maintenance therapy of CMV disease at a dosage of 1000–2000 mg every 8 hours, but has largely been replaced by oral valganciclovir.[28,29]

Valganciclovir is available as a 450 mg tablet. The recommended dose for induction therapy of acute CMV retinitis is 900 mg orally every 12 hours for a total of 21 days, followed by maintenance therapy of 900 mg orally once daily. The dosage recommended for prophylaxis of CMV disease in kidney, heart and kidney–pancreas transplant recipients is 900 mg orally once daily. All dosages should be administered with food.

Indications

Treatment of CMV disease

Intravenous ganciclovir is used for therapy of serious CMV infections in immunocompromised patients, including CMV retinitis, pneumonitis, encephalitis and gastrointestinal disease. The usual dose of

Table 146.6 Systemic antiviral therapy for CMV retinitis*

Drugs	Induction therapy*	Maintenance therapy†
Ganciclovir	5 mg/kg iv q12h × 4–21 days	5 mg/kg iv daily, or 1000–2000 mg po q8h daily
Valganciclovir	900 mg po q12h × 14–21 days	900 mg po daily
Foscarnet	90 mg/kg iv q12h (or 60 mg/kg iv q8h) × 14–21 days	90–120 mg/kg iv daily
Cidofovir	5 mg/kg iv weekly × 2–3 weeks	5 mg/kg iv every other week

*Recommended doses for adults with normal renal function.
†Other therapeutic options include intraocular drug implants or intravitreal drug injections.

ganciclovir for induction therapy is 5 mg/kg given intravenously every 12 hours for 14–21 days, followed by a maintenance regimen (5 mg/kg once daily).

Intravitreal injections of ganciclovir have been used effectively for treatment of CMV retinitis, although ganciclovir intraocular implants are a better option for patients who cannot tolerate systemic ganciclovir therapy.

Ganciclovir, valganciclovir, foscarnet and cidofovir (see below) are all effective for initial and maintenance therapy of CMV retinitis in AIDS patients (Table 146.6). All of these drugs are associated with significant toxicity; drug selection in an individual patient hinges, to some extent, on which adverse effects would be most tolerable. Ganciclovir is primarily myelosuppressive, while foscarnet and cidofovir are nephrotoxic. Ganciclovir would be preferred in a patient who has baseline renal dysfunction or who requires therapy with other nephrotoxic drugs. Conversely, foscarnet might be a better choice in a patient with significant baseline neutropenia. Despite the survival benefits shown for foscarnet therapy in some studies, most clinicians use ganciclovir or valganciclovir for initial therapy on the basis of more predictable adverse effects. Combination therapy (e.g. ganciclovir plus foscarnet) may be more effective for CMV disease in selected patients.

Prophylaxis of CMV disease

Benefits of intravenous and oral prophylaxis of CMV infection in solid-organ transplant recipients have varied with the transplant type, immunosuppressive regimen and CMV serologic status of the donor and recipient.[30] Prophylaxis with intravenous ganciclovir or oral valganciclovir significantly reduces the incidence of CMV disease in high-risk immunocompromised patients, but is often complicated by drug-induced neutropenia. An alternative scheme is to withhold ganciclovir until there is early laboratory evidence (e.g. by polymerase chain reaction or antigenemia assay) of CMV activation. This pre-emptive therapy approach permits initiation of antiviral treatment before CMV disease becomes symptomatic, while avoiding the risk of neutropenia associated with long-term ganciclovir administration.[31–38]

Dosage in special circumstances

Because ganciclovir is cleared by renal mechanisms, dosage reduction is necessary in patients with creatinine clearance of <70 ml/min (Table 146.7). About 50% of an administered dose is removed during 4 hours of hemodialysis and dosing after dialysis is recommended. Valganciclovir dosage adjustment is required for patients with creatinine clearance <60 ml/min; the drug is not recommended for patients on hemodialysis. No dosage adjustment for hepatic impairment is necessary.

Ganciclovir is mutagenic, carcinogenic and causes reproductive toxicity in animal models. Use of ganciclovir or valganciclovir in pregnant or nursing women is not recommended without careful consideration of the risk–benefit ratio. Data on ganciclovir or valganciclovir use in children are currently limited. High inter- and intrapatient variability in ganciclovir levels was observed in kidney, bone marrow and pediatric liver and kidney transplant recipients.[39] Oral solution valganciclovir given to neonates with symptomatic congenital CMV disease resulted in plasma levels comparable to administration of intravenous ganciclovir;[40] however, valganciclovir is not commercially available in this formulation.

Adverse reactions

The most important adverse effects of ganciclovir noted in AIDS patients being treated for CMV retinitis were neutropenia and thrombocytopenia. About 40% developed granulocytopenia (absolute neutrophil count <1000/mm³) and 15% had thrombocytopenia (platelet count <50 000/mm³). Hematologic toxicity is also seen, although less commonly, in organ transplant recipients. Neutropenia and thrombocytopenia are usually reversible when ganciclovir therapy is discontinued. In many patients requiring ganciclovir therapy, neutropenia can be prevented or treated by co-administration of granulocyte colony-stimulating factor. Renal dysfunction has been reported in up to 20% of transplant recipients receiving ganciclovir prophylaxis, although this may be related to co-administration of other nephrotoxic drugs. In animal models, ganciclovir produces significant reproductive toxicity, especially azoospermia.

Valganciclovir appears to have hematologic toxicity similar to intravenous ganciclovir. Pooled data from two different studies indicated that 50% of patients developed granulocytopenia (absolute neutrophil count <1000/mm³), 35% experienced anemia (hemoglobin <9.5 g/dl) and 23% developed thrombocytopenia (platelets <100 000/µl). Gastrointestinal complaints were also common; 41% reported diarrhea, 30% nausea, 21% vomiting and 15% abdominal pain. In a study of valganciclovir 450 mg twice daily in kidney transplant recipients to prevent CMV disease, 5.7% (four patients) developed agranulocytosis (neutrophil count <500 cells/mm³) an average of 74 days after transplantation. Onset was abrupt and asymptomatic, with all patients recovering after discontinuation of valganciclovir.

In vitro, ganciclovir and zidovudine have mutually antagonistic antiviral activity, but this observation has not been shown to be clinically significant. Ganciclovir should be used with caution in combination with other myelosuppressive drugs such as zidovudine because of the risk of additive hematologic toxicity. When co-administered with didanosine, ganciclovir increases the AUC of didanosine from 50% to 114%; thus patients should be monitored for didanosine toxicity when these two drugs are administered together. Probenecid can reduce renal clearance of ganciclovir, resulting in clinically significant increases in ganciclovir AUC. Seizures have been reported in patients receiving concomitant therapy with ganciclovir and imipenem.

Resistance

HSV and VZV isolates that are TK deficient and aciclovir resistant will also be cross-resistant to ganciclovir. Ganciclovir resistance *in vitro* is defined as an IC$_{50}$ >6 µM (1.5 µg/ml). In a study of 72 AIDS patients treated with ganciclovir, 5 of 13 culture-positive patients treated for >3 months excreted resistant virus. Ganciclovir-resistant CMV has been identified as a cause of retinitis, encephalitis and polyradiculopathy in AIDS patients and enteritis and viremia among solid-organ transplant patients. Among solid-organ transplant recipients, resistance rates of

Table 146.7 Ganciclovir and valganciclovir dosage modification for renal impairment

Normal dosage regimen	ADJUSTED DOSAGE REGIMEN		
	CrCl (ml/min)	Dose	Dosing interval (hr)
Ganciclovir 5 mg/kg iv q12h	≥70 50–69 25–49 10–24	5 mg/kg 2.5 mg/kg 2.5 mg/kg 1.25 mg/kg	12 12 24 24
Ganciclovir 5 mg/kg iv q24h	≥70 50–69 25–49 10–24 HD	5 mg/kg 2.5 mg/kg 1.25 mg/kg 0.625 mg/kg 0.625 mg/kg	24 24 24 24 Post-HD (TIW)
Ganciclovir 1000 mg po q8h	≥70 50–69 25–49 HD	1000 mg 500 mg 500 mg 500 mg	8 8 24 Post-HD (TIW)
Valganciclovir 900 mg po q12h	>60 40–59 25–39 10–24 HD	900 mg 450 mg 450 mg 450 mg NR	12 12 24 48 –
Valganciclovir 900 mg po q24h	>60 40–59 25–39 10–24 HD	900 mg 450 mg 450 mg 450 mg NR	24 24 48 Twice weekly –

CrCl, creatinine clearance; HD, hemodialysis; NR, not recommended; post-HD, after each dialysis; TIW, three times weekly.

1.5–14% have been reported.[41,42] CMV resistance to ganciclovir is usually secondary to mutations in the UL97 gene, although alterations in the DNA polymerase gene have also been described. UL97 mutants remain susceptible to foscarnet, although polymerase mutants cross-resistant to both ganciclovir and foscarnet have been identified. Foscarnet and cidofovir are therapeutic alternatives for treatment of disease caused by ganciclovir-resistant CMV.

Foscarnet

Mechanism of action and *in-vitro* activity

Foscarnet is an analogue of inorganic pyrophosphate that functions as a noncompetitive inhibitor of herpesvirus DNA polymerase.[43] Foscarnet blocks the pyrophosphate binding site, preventing cleavage of pyrophosphate from deoxynucleotide triphosphates. Viral DNA polymerase is inhibited at foscarnet concentrations 100-fold lower than those required to inhibit cellular DNA polymerase. Unlike the aciclovir-like drugs discussed above, foscarnet is not a nucleoside analogue, does not require intracellular activation by viral kinase, and is not incorporated into the viral DNA chain. Therefore, TK-deficient HSV and VZV isolates that are resistant to aciclovir will remain susceptible to foscarnet. Foscarnet has *in-vitro* activity against HSV, VZV, CMV, EBV and human herpesvirus 6 (HHV-6). The IC$_{50}$ for most clinical isolates of CMV is in the range of 100–300 μM, but varies considerably with the experimental conditions. Foscarnet can also inhibit viral reverse transcriptase and has *in-vitro* activity against hepatitis B virus and HIV.

Pharmacokinetics and distribution

Foscarnet has low oral bioavailability (approximately 17%) and is administered only by the intravenous route. Peak plasma concentrations after steady-state dosing at 60 mg/kg every 8 hours or 90 mg/kg every 12 hours are about 500 μM and 700 μM, respectively. Plasma protein binding is about 15%. CSF foscarnet levels demonstrate wide interpatient variability, but average about 66% of plasma levels at steady state. Foscarnet is not metabolized and about 80% of an administered dose is excreted unchanged in the urine by glomerular filtration and tubular secretion within 36 hours. About 20% of the foscarnet dose is retained in bone, presumably due to the drug's structural similarity to inorganic phosphate. This results in a complex pattern of drug disposition, in which the initial elimination half-life is about 4.5 hours, followed by a prolonged terminal half-life of about 88 hours as drug is released from bone. Plasma foscarnet levels are reduced about 50% following hemodialysis; dosing after dialysis is recommended.

Route of administration and dosage

Foscarnet is available only as an intravenous formulation. The usual dose for induction therapy of CMV retinitis is 90 mg/kg every 12 hours, with a maintenance dose of 90–120 mg/kg every 24 hours. For aciclovir-resistant HSV, the usual dose of foscarnet is 40 mg/kg every 8–12 hours. When given via a central venous catheter, the drug can be diluted to 24 mg/ml; for infusion through peripheral vein catheters, foscarnet must be diluted to 12 mg/ml to avoid local phlebitis. The foscarnet dose must be administered over at least 1 hour using an intravenous infusion pump; bolus infusion can result in severe toxicity.

Indications

Intravenous foscarnet is used primarily to treat diseases caused by drug-resistant strains of HSV, VZV or CMV, or to treat patients who are intolerant of first-line antiviral therapy. Use of foscarnet for prophylaxis is limited by toxicity.[44,45]

Dosage in special circumstances

Foscarnet is excreted by renal mechanisms and dosage adjustment is required even for minor degrees of renal insufficiency. Serum creatinine should be monitored at least every other day during foscarnet therapy to assess the need for further dose adjustment. Dosage modification in hepatic impairment is not required. The safety of foscarnet during pregnancy has not been adequately evaluated and use is not recommended unless no other alternative therapy is available. Little information has been published regarding foscarnet safety and tolerance in neonates and children.

Adverse reactions

The most important adverse effect caused by foscarnet is nephrotoxicity. Dose-limiting renal toxicity occurs in at least 15–20% of patients treated with foscarnet for CMV retinitis. The primary mechanism of renal toxicity appears to be acute tubular necrosis, although interstitial nephritis and crystalline nephropathy have also been described. Loading the patient with intravenous saline prior to foscarnet infusion can help reduce the risk of nephrotoxicity. In most cases, the renal dysfunction is reversible and serum creatinine will return to normal within 2–4 weeks after foscarnet therapy is discontinued. However, irreversible renal failure may occur in patients who are volume depleted or who receive concomitant therapy with other nephrotoxic medications.

Foscarnet can induce a variety of electrolyte and metabolic abnormalities, most notably hypocalcemia. Hypercalcemia, hypomagnesemia, hypokalemia and hypo- and hyperphosphatemia have also been reported. The acute decline in ionized serum calcium that can occur with foscarnet infusion may be due to formation of a complex between foscarnet and free calcium. Further depletion of total serum calcium seen with long-term drug administration may be caused by renal calcium wasting, abnormal bone metabolism, concurrent hypomagnesemia, or some combination of these factors. Foscarnet-induced electrolyte disturbances can predispose the patient to cardiac arrhythmias, tetany, altered mental status or seizures. It is mandatory that serum creatinine and electrolyte levels be closely monitored during foscarnet therapy.

Foscarnet is much less myelosuppressive than ganciclovir, but anemia was reported in 10–50% of AIDS patients receiving foscarnet. Patients, especially uncircumcised males, may develop genital ulcerations due to local toxicity of high foscarnet concentrations in urine. Nausea and vomiting has been reported by 20–30% of patients receiving foscarnet. Other infrequent adverse effects include headache, diarrhea and abnormal liver function tests. When possible, foscarnet should be administered through a central venous line to avoid peripheral thrombophlebitis.

Specific drug interactions with foscarnet have not been described, although there is significant potential for additive toxicity. Concurrent therapy with foscarnet and intravenous pentamidine can result in severe and potentially fatal hypocalcemia. Concomitant administration of foscarnet with other potentially nephrotoxic drugs (such as amphotericin B or aminoglycosides) can compound the risk of serious nephrotoxicity. Foscarnet can be safely administered to patients receiving zidovudine, although there may be an increased risk of anemia. Due to foscarnet's chelating properties, a number of drugs may precipitate when administered through the same intravenous catheter. Thus, review of the package insert is recommended for dosing recommendations and drug incompatibilities prior to administration.

Resistance

Although uncommon, foscarnet-resistant isolates of CMV, VZV and HSV have been encountered in AIDS patients receiving foscarnet therapy. Resistance is due to a mutation in the DNA polymerase gene, which means that, in some circumstances, the foscarnet-resistant isolate may remain susceptible to aciclovir or ganciclovir. However, CMV isolates cross-resistant to both ganciclovir and foscarnet (containing both polymerase and UL97 mutations) have been recovered. Cidofovir may be an effective alternative drug in this setting, but in-vitro antiviral susceptibility testing is necessary to guide drug selection.

Cidofovir

Mechanism of action and *in-vitro* activity

Cidofovir is a nucleotide analogue of cytosine monophosphate with potent broad-spectrum antiviral activity.[46] Unlike aciclovir and other nucleoside analogues which require monophosphorylation by viral kinases for activation, cidofovir already carries a phosphonate group and does not require viral enzymes for conversion to cidofovir diphosphate, the active antiviral compound. Cidofovir diphosphate competitively inhibits the DNA polymerases of herpesviruses, thereby blocking DNA synthesis and viral replication. Cidofovir diphosphate inhibits viral DNA polymerases at concentrations much lower than those required to inhibit cellular DNA polymerases, accounting for its selectivity of action.

Cidofovir has potent *in-vitro* activity against human CMV, with IC_{50} values in the range of 0.1–0.9 µg/ml. Cidofovir retains activity against most CMV clinical isolates that are resistant to ganciclovir. Cidofovir also demonstrates *in-vitro* activity against HSV and VZV (including TK-deficient, aciclovir-resistant isolates), adenovirus, poxvirus (including variola or smallpox virus) and human papillomavirus.

Pharmacokinetics and distribution

Serum cidofovir concentrations are dose proportional over a dosing range of 1.0–10.0 mg/kg. Intravenous infusion of cidofovir at a dosage of 5 mg/kg produces peak plasma concentrations of about 11 µg/ml. The terminal half-life is 2.6 hours. Approximately 90% of the intravenous cidofovir dose is excreted by the kidneys within 24 hours, with clearance involving both glomerular filtration and tubular secretion. At cidofovir doses higher than 3 mg/kg, concomitant administration of probenecid can block tubular secretion of cidofovir and reduce its renal clearance. Cidofovir diphosphate and its metabolites have prolonged intracellular half-lives, which permit cidofovir to be effectively administered at extended dosing intervals.

Route of administration and dosage

Cidofovir for intravenous administration is supplied as 375 mg of an aqueous solution (75 mg/ml). The selected dose is diluted in 100 ml of normal saline prior to administration. For induction therapy, the usual dose of cidofovir is 5 mg/kg infused over 1 hour once weekly for 2 weeks. The dose for maintenance therapy for CMV disease is 5 mg/kg administered once every 2 weeks. To minimize nephrotoxicity, patients should receive 1 liter of normal saline intravenously over 1–2 hours immediately prior to cidofovir dose and an additional 1 liter of normal saline immediately following the cidofovir dose. Probenecid is given at a dose of 2 g orally 3 hours before the cidofovir dose, then 1 g doses at 2 hours and 8 hours after completion of the cidofovir infusion, for a total probenecid dose of 4 g.

Indications

Cidofovir is used primarily to treat diseases caused by drug-resistant strains of HSV, VZV or CMV, or to treat patients who are intolerant of first-line antiviral therapy.[47,48] Use of cidofovir for prophylaxis or pre-emptive therapy is limited by toxicity.

Dosage in special circumstances

Because intravenous cidofovir can cause significant nephrotoxicity, initiation of therapy in patients with pre-existing renal dysfunction – serum creatinine >1.5 mg/dl, calculated creatinine clearance <55 ml/min or proteinuria >100 mg/dl (>2+) – is not recommended. Declining renal function during cidofovir therapy mandates dosage adjustment. If the serum creatinine increases by 0.3–0.4 mg/dl above baseline, the cidofovir dose should be reduced from 5 mg/kg to 3 mg/kg. If the serum creatinine increases >0.5 mg/dl above baseline or if proteinuria >3+ develops, cidofovir therapy should be discontinued. Dosage adjustment in patients with hepatic impairment is not required. Cidofovir is embryotoxic in animals and the drug should not be used during pregnancy unless there are no other therapeutic options. In small studies of pediatric patients, cidofovir toxicity was similar to that seen in adults,[47] although large randomized trials are lacking.

Adverse reactions

The most important safety concern with cidofovir therapy is nephrotoxicity. Pretreatment with intravenous hydration and probenecid (which blocks cidofovir tubular secretion) reduces the incidence of nephrotoxicity. In a clinical trial using cidofovir 5 mg/kg plus probenecid, proteinuria occurred in 5 of 41 patients (12%) and elevated serum creatinine levels in 2 of 41 patients (5%). Neutropenia (ANC <750 WBC/mm³) was observed in 15% of cidofovir recipients. Anemia, thrombocytopenia and hepatotoxicity have not been observed with cidofovir therapy. Ocular complications (including iritis, anterior uveitis and hypotony) have been described following intravenous or intravitreal cidofovir administration.

Probenecid, a benzoic acid derivative with a sulfa moiety, can cause allergic symptoms (e.g. fever, chills, rash) in patients allergic to sulfonamides. Patients with a history of severe sulfa hypersensitivity should not be treated with probenecid and, consequently, should not receive systemic cidofovir. Other probenecid-related adverse effects include headache, nausea and vomiting, which can be minimized by administering the drug on a full stomach. In a CMV retinitis trial, probenecid-related adverse effects occurred in 23 of 41 patients (56%) and were dose limiting in three patients (7%).

Cidofovir injections in rats were associated with mammary adenocarcinomas, but surveillance studies in treated patients have not demonstrated any excess frequency of tumors. Cidofovir administration causes embryotoxicity and impaired spermatogenesis in animals; male and female patients are advised to use adequate birth control during and for 3 months after completion of cidofovir therapy.

No specific drug interactions with cidofovir have been described, although concomitant therapy with other nephrotoxic drugs may result in additive toxicity. Probenecid, however, is known to alter the renal excretion of a wide variety of drugs. The dose of zidovudine should be reduced to 50% on days when probenecid administration is planned.

Resistance

Instances of clinical failure of cidofovir therapy due to drug resistance have been reported. CMV resistance to cidofovir results from a mutation in the viral polymerase gene and resistant isolates may exhibit cross-resistance to ganciclovir and/or foscarnet. *In-vitro* susceptibility testing is necessary in this circumstance to guide appropriate drug selection.

Fomivirsen

Mechanism of action and *in-vitro* activity

Fomivirsen is a 21-nucleotide phosphorothioate oligonucleotide designed as an antisense molecule with activity against CMV.[49] The oligonucleotide is complementary to mRNA from the immediate-early region 2 of CMV. Antisense inhibition of target gene expression, while necessary for optimal antiviral activity, only partially explains the activity of fomivirsen against CMV. Nonspecific interactions between the oligonucleotide and virus particles may prevent adsorption or lead to inhibition of enzymes required for viral DNA synthesis. Fomivirsen has activity against clinical CMV isolates, including isolates resistant to conventional antiviral drugs, with a median IC_{50} of 0.37 μM in tissue culture.

Phamacokinetics and distribution

When cynomolgus monkeys were given 11, 57 or 115 μg of fomivirsen intravitreally, maximum vitreal concentrations (ranging from 0.11 to 1.28 μM) were achieved 2 days after injection of all doses. For the same dosages, retinal concentrations increased in a logarithmic pattern, with maximal concentration obtained 2 days after injection for all doses, ranging from 0.12 to 0.88 μM. For the 115 μg dose, the vitreal and retinal half-lives were 22 hours and 78 hours, respectively. Electrophoretic analyses of retina and vitreous specimens indicate that the oligonucleotide is metabolized by exonucleolytic cleavage. Both intact drug and its metabolic products diffuse from the vitreous humor to the retina and it is hypothesized that active metabolism occurs in both compartments.

Route of administration and dosage

Fomivirsen is supplied in single use vials containing 0.25 ml of 6.6 mg/ml solution. Dosage for induction therapy of CMV retinitis is 330 μg given intravitreally every other week for two doses. Maintenance therapy is 330 μg given intravitreally every 4 weeks.

Indications

Fomivirsen is indicated for treatment of CMV retinitis in AIDS patients who have failed or are intolerant of other CMV therapies, including those with CMV that is resistant to ganciclovir and foscarnet. It is not recommended for use in patients who have received intravitreal or intravenous cidofovir. Fomivirsen is not indicated for systemic CMV therapy and will not protect the contralateral eye from involvement.

Dosage in special circumstances

As there is little systemic exposure to fomivirsen after intravitreal injection, no dose adjustments are required. This drug has not been studied in pregnant or lactating women, or in pediatric or geriatric populations.

Adverse reactions

The most common adverse reactions reported were increased intraocular pressure and mild to moderate intraocular inflammation of the anterior and posterior chambers. The combined incidence of ocular reactions was 10–12% of patients treated every other week and 20% in patients treated weekly. Other adverse reactions reported in 5–20% patients included abnormal or blurred vision, conjunctival hemorrhage, retinal detachment and retinal edema. Topical steroids have been used with success to ameliorate some of these effects.

Resistance

A fomivirsen-resistant CMV isolate has been developed by exposing a laboratory strain to increasing concentrations of the drug. This resistant virus did not prove to have mutations which would have altered specificity for the fomivirsen target sequence, supporting the hypothesis that both antisense-specific and nonspecific mechanisms are involved in the drug's activity against CMV. There have been no reports of fomivirsen-resistant CMV isolates recovered from patients.

REFERENCES

References for this chapter can be found online at http://www.expertconsult.com

Chapter | **147** | *Michael G Ison*

Antiviral agents against respiratory viruses

M2 Inhibitors

Introduction and mechanism of action

Amantadine (Symmetrel) and rimantadine (Flumadine) are symmetric tricyclic amines that specifically inhibit the replication of influenza A viruses at low concentrations (<1.0 µg/ml) by blocking the action of the M2 protein. M2, an acid-activated ion channel found only in influenza A viruses, is a membrane protein required for efficient nucleocapsid release after viral fusion with the endosomal membrane (Fig. 147.1). Unfortunately, widespread resistance to all M2 inhibitors has been documented in circulating H3N2 strains. As a result, this class of agents is not currently recommended for the prevention or treatment of influenza unless the strain is known to be H1N1.

Amantadine and rimantadine share two concentration-dependent mechanisms of antiviral action.[1,2] Low concentrations of the drugs inhibit the ion channel function of the M2 protein, which inhibits viral uncoating or disassembly of the virion during endocytosis and, in H7 subtypes, alters hemagglutinin (HA) maturation during viral assembly. Amantadine and rimantadine also increase the lysosomal pH, which in turn may inhibit virus-induced membrane fusion events for several enveloped viruses. However, such effects are generally not seen at drug concentrations observed in humans and clinically relevant antiviral activity is confined to influenza A viruses, although studies in chronic hepatitis C are in progress.

Pharmacokinetics

Amantadine is rapidly absorbed, with a 53–100% bioavailability, and reaches peak plasma levels of 475 µg/l within 4.5 hours after 100 mg doses in healthy adults.[3] The drug is predominately excreted unchanged in the urine by glomerular filtration and tubular secretion. The plasma elimination half-life is about 11–15 hours in persons with normal renal function. Elimination is markedly prolonged in patients with renal impairment and decreases about twofold in the elderly so that dose adjustments are required (Table 147.1). Amantadine is widely distributed, with salivary levels equivalent to those of blood and nasal mucus comparable to plasma at 8 hours after dosing.[5,6] Amantadine crosses the placenta and blood–brain barrier, with cerebrospinal fluid (CSF) levels equal to 56–96% of serum levels, and distributes in breast milk (Table 147.2).

In experimental human influenza infection, a trough concentration at steady state of 300 µg/l, which corresponds to that observed after 200 mg/day dosing, was associated with lower infection rate than placebo.[6] Adverse events are dose related, and daily doses >200 mg in young adults and 100 mg in the elderly are associated with excess CNS adverse effects.[3]

Rimantadine has nearly complete oral bioavailability and achieves maximal plasma concentration 3–5 hours after ingestion. Peak concentrations average 416 µg/l after a 200 mg oral dose. Rimantadine levels in nasal secretions average 1.5 times those of plasma levels. The plasma half-life is long and ranges from 24 to 36 hours. Rimantadine undergoes extensive metabolism, including hydroxylation, conjugation and glucuronidation in the liver before being excreted in the urine. Only 25% of the parent drug is excreted unchanged in the urine. Dose adjustments are recommended for advanced renal or hepatic failure and older age (see Table 147.1).

Resistance

Resistance to the two agents occurs as the result of amino acid substitutions in the transmembrane portion of the M2 protein. Although resistant wild-type virus is uncommonly found (<1%),[9] it may rapidly emerge within 2–4 days after the start of therapy in up to 30% of patients.[10] Emergence of resistant virus does not appear to cause a rebound in illness in immunocompetent adults but may be associated with protracted illness and shedding in immunocompromised hosts.[11] Importantly, resistant virus can be spread to others and has caused failures of antiviral prophylaxis under close contact conditions, as in nursing homes and households.[10] The resistant virus appears to retain wild-type pathogenicity and causes an influenza illness indistinguishable from susceptible strains. Cross-resistance occurs to all M2 inhibitors without affecting susceptibility to the neuraminidase inhibitors and ribavirin. Recently, most circulating H3N2 viruses have been documented to be resistant to the M2 inhibitors; resistance among H1N1 viruses is increasing as well.[12] Among H5N1 viruses, resistance is commonly seen with clade 1 and clade 2 subclade 1 viruses; current susceptibility data should be obtained from reference viral isolation laboratories if M2 inhibitor therapy is being considered. The novel swine-origin 2009 H1N1 viruses are all currently resistant to the M2 inhibitors as well.

Indications

Amantadine and rimantadine are indicated for the prevention and treatment of influenza A virus illness; given significant resistance, these agents are not currently recommended for the prevention or treatment of influenza unless the susceptibility of circulating strains of H1N1 are known. In the majority placebo-controlled studies of these drugs in the management of influenza, most have been conducted in previously healthy persons.[6]

Prophylaxis

Prophylaxis with amantadine or rimantadine is approximately 70–90% effective in preventing symptomatic influenza A infections.[13] Administration is advised for postexposure prophylaxis in

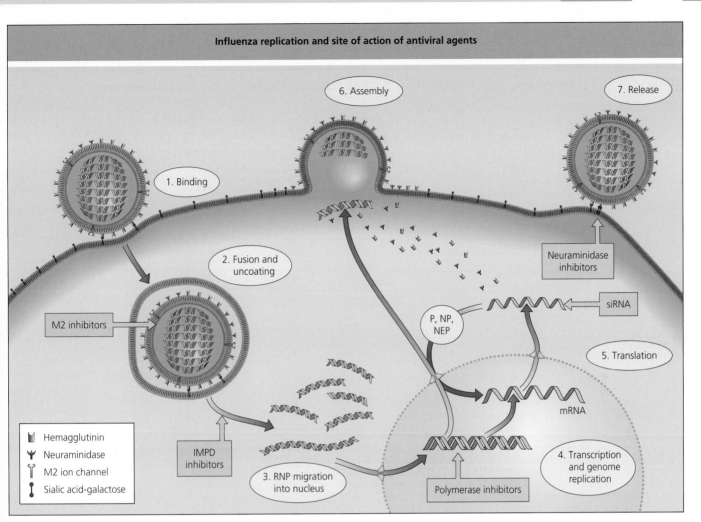

Fig. 147.1 Influenza replication and site of action of antiviral agents. IMPD, inosine monophosphate dehydrogenase; NEP, nuclear export protein; NP, nucleoprotein; P, polymerase; RNP, ribonuclear protein; siRNA-small inhibitory ribonucleic acid. From Beigel J, Bray M. Current and future antiviral therapy of severe seasonal and avian influenza. Antiviral Res 2008;78:91–102.

nursing home populations at 100 mg/day for 14 days or for at least 7 days after the last culture-confirmed illness in the ward or building; this regimen should be given with concomitant influenza vaccination for those not previously provided.[4] Rimantadine is better tolerated in this population.[14] Seasonal prophylaxis, during the 4–8 weeks of peak influenza virus circulation within the community, can be used for protection of high-risk patients who cannot tolerate immunization, who do not develop an adequate immune response to vaccine or when the strain circulating in the community does not match the vaccine strain. Postexposure prophylaxis in households appears protective when not used in conjunction with treatment of an ill index case.

Treatment

Amantadine or rimantadine therapy reduces duration of fever and symptoms in patients with documented influenza by about 1 day compared to placebo, when the medication is initiated within 48 hours of symptom onset.[15] Treatment is also associated with more rapid functional recovery[15] and resolution of small airways functional abnormalities. Studies comparing the therapeutic activity of amantadine and rimantadine are few but generally show comparability.[15] Amantadine appears safe and efficacious in reducing length of fever and illness in children older than 2 years of age.[15] Pediatric studies have found variable clinical benefits relative to acetaminophen controls and document the frequent emergence of drug-resistant variants.[15]

Controlled data to support the use of M2 inhibitors in treating severe influenza or in preventing complications is lacking; one retrospective study found no important differences in duration of illness or hospitalization between the amantadine-treated and untreated patients hospitalized with influenza.[16] In hematopoietic stem cell transplant and acute leukemia patients who received therapy with one of the M2 inhibitors, a reduced risk of progression to pneumonia (35% vs 76%) was found compared to no treatment.[17] However, resistance emergence is common in such patients.[11] One retrospective study of nursing home residents suggested that early treatment might reduce lower respiratory complications.[18] Amantadine is ineffective for treating influenza B or C infections.

Dosage and special consideration

Amantadine and rimantadine come as 100 mg tablets and a syrup formulation (50 mg/5 ml). In adults, the usual dose for treatment or prevention of influenza A infection is 100 mg q12h for both drugs (see Table 147.1).

Dosing of amantadine and rimantadine should be adjusted in the setting of renal failure (see Table 147.1). Neither M2 inhibitor is cleared by hemodialysis. Patients who are over 65 years of age should have the dose of both medications reduced to 100 mg once daily to avoid side-effects. Rimantadine needs dose adjustment to 100 mg/day for serious hepatic insufficiency. Amantadine and rimantadine are embryotoxic and teratogenic in preclinical tests and amantadine may be associated with birth defects. As a result, neither drug should be used in pregnant

Table 147.1 Agents used to prevent and treat influenza[4]

Drug	USUAL ADULT DOSAGE[#] Prophylaxis	Treatment	Dose adjustment state	Suggested dosage
Amantadine	100 mg q12h	100 mg q12h	Age 1–9 years	5 mg/kg to max of 150 mg in two divided doses
			CrCl 30–50 ml/min	100 mg q24h
			CrCl 15–30 ml/min	100 mg q24h
			CrCl 10–15 ml/min	100 mg q week
			CrCl 10 ml/min	100 mg q week
			Age ≥65 years	100 mg q24h
Rimantadine	100 mg q12h	100 mg q12h	Age 1–9 years*	5 mg/kg to max of 150 mg in two divided doses
			CrCl <10 ml/min	100 mg q24h
			Severe hepatic dysfunction	100 mg q24h
			Age ≥65 years	100 mg q24h
Zanamivir[†]	2 puffs	2 puffs	No dose adjustment needed	
Oseltamivir[‡]	75 mg q24h	75 mg q12h	CrCl <30 ml/min[§]	Treatment: 75 mg q24h Prophylaxis: 75 mg every other day
			≤15 kg	30 mg q12h (2.5 ml[¶])
			15–23 kg	45 mg q12h (3.8 ml[¶])
			23–40 kg	60 mg q12h (5 ml[¶])
			>40 kg	75 mg q12h (6.2 ml[¶])

Recommendations based on those provided by the Advisory Committee on Immunization Practices.[4]
*Investigational: not approved for treatment of children by the US Food and Drug Administration.
[†]Zanamivir is indicated for prophylaxis in children ≥5 years old and for treatment in children ≥7 years old.
[‡]Oseltamivir is indicated for prophylaxis and treatment in children ≥1 year old.
[§]No treatment or prophylaxis dosing recommendations are available for patients undergoing renal dialysis.
[¶]Volume of suspension.
[#]Duration of treatment is usually 5 days. Duration of prophylaxis depends on clinical setting.

Table 147.2 Pharmacokinetic properties of antivirals with activity against influenza[5–8]

Drug	Dose	Route	C_{max} (µg/l)	T_{max} (h)	$AUC_{0-12 h}$ (µg/ml•h)	$T_{1/2}$ (h)	Bioavailability (oral, %)	Protein binding (%)
Amantadine[5,6]*	200 mg	Oral (young)	510 (140)	2.1 (1)	10.2 (3.4)	14.4 (6)	62–93	67
	200 mg	Oral (elderly)	800 (200)	2.2 (2.1)	17.6 (6.5)	19 (9.1)	54–100	
Rimantadine[5,6]*	200 mg	Oral (young)	240 (70)	4.6 (2.1)	9.8 (4.5)	36.5 (17.3)	75–93	40
	200 mg	Oral (elderly)	250 (50)	4.0 (2.4)	11.5 (3.0)	36.5 (14.5)	NA	
Zanamivir[7†]	16 mg	Inhaled	29 (23–69)	0.75 (0.08–2)	0.03 (0.02–0.06)	3.6 (2.2–9.4)	4–17	10
	16 mg	Inhaled	54 (34–96)	0.75 (0.25–1)	0.16 (0.02–0.32)	—	4–17	
Oseltamivir[8]*	100 mg q12h	Oral (18–55 years)	439 (40.8)	3.5 (1)	3.85 (0.6)	6–10	79	42
	100 mg q12h	Oral (≥65 years)	575 (83.8)	3.5 (1.4)	4.94 (1.0)	—	—	

C_{max}, maximum serum drug concentration; T_{max}, time to C_{max}; $T_{1/2}$, serum elimination half-life; AUC, area under the serum drug concentration versus time for the dose interval; bioavailability, percentage of intravenous C_{max}.
*Values are mean (SD); [†]Values are median (range).

women unless the benefits of therapy clearly outweigh the potential risks (pregnancy category C). The recommended pediatric dosage of both amantadine and rimantadine is 5 mg/kg/day to a maximum of 150 mg/day in two divided doses in children younger than 10.[4]

Safety issues

The most common side-effects of the M2 inhibitors are minor central nervous system (CNS) complaints (anxiety, difficulty concentrating, insomnia, dizziness, headache and jitteriness) and gastrointestinal upset. Patients who receive amantadine may develop antimuscarinic effects, orthostatic hypotension and congestive heart failure at low frequencies. Particularly in the elderly or those with renal failure, serious CNS side-effects due to amantadine and less often rimantadine, include confusion, disorientation, mood alterations, memory disturbances, delusions, nightmares, ataxia, tremors, seizures, coma, acute psychosis, slurred speech, visual disturbances, delirium, oculogyric episodes and hallucinations.[6] Amantadine causes CNS side-effects in about 15–30% of persons, as well as dose-related abnormalities in psychomotor testing.[6] The incidence and severity of CNS adverse effects are less common with rimantadine.[14]

Concomitant ingestion of antihistamines or anticholinergic drugs increases the CNS effects of amantadine. Trimethoprim–sulfamethoxazole and triamterene–hydrochlorothiazide decrease the renal clearance of amantadine, which enhances the risk of CNS toxicity. Quinine and quinidine likewise reduce the clearance of amantadine. Co-administration with monoamine oxidase inhibitors may precipitate life-threatening hypertension. The drug does not appear to interact with the cytochrome P450 system. Cimetidine is associated with 15–20% increases and aspirin or acetaminophen with 10% decreases in plasma rimantadine concentrations; however, such changes are unlikely to be of clinical significance.[19] Patients receiving either amantadine or rimantadine along with drugs affecting CNS function, such as antihistamines, antidepressants and minor tranquilizers, should be monitored closely.

Conclusions

Given the emergence of resistance among influenza A/H3N2 virus, the M2 inhibitors, as a class, are not recommended for the prevention or treatment of influenza when significant resistance is present in circulating strains. They may have a role in the management of patients with susceptible H1N1 and H5N1 viruses; current recommendations of the Centers for Disease Control and Prevention (CDC) and the World Health Organization (WHO) should be consulted before using this class clinically.

Neuraminidase Inhibitors

Introduction and mechanism of action

Influenza A and B viruses possess a surface glycoprotein with neuraminidase activity whereas influenza C viruses do not (see Fig. 147.1). This enzyme cleaves terminal sialic acid residues and destroys the receptors recognized by viral hemagglutinin. This activity is essential for release of virus from infected cells, for prevention of viral aggregates, and for viral spread within the respiratory tract.[20] Zanamivir (Relenza) and oseltamivir (Tamiflu, a prodrug of the active carboxylate) are sialic acid analogues that potently and specifically inhibit influenza A and B neuraminidases by competitively and reversibly interacting with the active enzyme site.[21] These drugs are active against all nine neuraminidase subtypes in nature including most of the avian strains of influenza A H5N1 and H9N2 that infect humans.

Resistance

Zanamivir and oseltamivir carboxylate resistance in-vitro results from mutations in the viral hemagglutinin and/or neuraminidase.[22,23] In the hemagglutinin variants, mutations in or near the receptor binding site make the virus less dependent on neuraminidase action, whereas neuraminidase mutations directly affect interaction with the inhibitors. The altered neuraminidases typically show reduced activity or stability, and the mutated viruses usually have decreased infectivity in animals.[24] The particular neuraminidase mutation determines the degree of resistance and cross-resistance (i.e. R229K and H274Y cause high-level resistance to oseltamivir but not zanamivir).[22] One combined hemagglutinin and neuraminidase mutant has been recovered from an immunocompromised child with prolonged virus excretion despite receiving nebulized zanamivir.[25] Oseltamivir-resistant variants have been recovered from <1% of treated adults and about 4% of treated children.[21] The possible clinical and epidemiologic significance of such variants requires study and a global Neuraminidase Inhibitor Susceptibility Network has been established to address these concerns.[23] Unfortunately, resistance to oseltamivir among H1N1 strains (with H274Y change in the NA gene) has been described globally.[26] The impact and persistence of these resistant variants are still under investigation. Although resistance has been rarely documented, most novel swine-orgin 2009 H1N1 viruses are susceptible to oseltamivir.

ZANAMIVIR

Pharmacokinetics

The oral bioavailability of zanamivir is low (<5%) and most clinical trials have used intranasal or dry powder inhalation delivery. The current dry powder formulation is mixed with lactose (5 mg zanamivir per 20 mg lactose). Following inhalation of the dry powder, approximately 7–21% is deposited in the lower respiratory tract and the remainder in the oropharynx.[7,27] Median zanamivir concentrations are above 1000 ng/ml in induced sputum 6 hours after inhalation and remain detectable up to 24 hours. The peak plasma concentration averages 46 µg/l after a single 16 mg inhalation of zanamivir. The proprietary inhaler device for delivering zanamivir is breath-actuated and requires a cooperative patient.[28]

In both experimental and natural influenza, once-daily dosing appears protective.[29] Twice-daily administration is therapeutically active but increasing the dose frequency to four times per day does not appear to increase efficacy in treating natural influenza.[29] Intranasal dosing is protective against experimental infection but not natural infection and does not substantially increase the overall therapeutic response to inhaled zanamivir.

Indications

Prophylaxis

Zanamivir is indicated as once-daily inhalations for the prevention of influenza in patients more than 5 years old. Once-daily inhaled zanamivir for 4 weeks was 84% efficacious in preventing laboratory-confirmed illness with fever and 31% effective in preventing influenza infections, irrespective of symptoms.[29] When used for postexposure prophylaxis, inhaled zanamivir for 10 days reduced the risk of secondary influenza illness by 79% in households.[29] In nursing homes experiencing influenza outbreaks, inhaled zanamivir was more effective for prevention of influenza A illness than oral rimantadine, in part because of frequent resistance emergence to the M2 inhibitor.[29]

Treatment

In the USA, zanamivir is indicated for the treatment of uncomplicated acute illness due to influenza A and B virus in adults and pediatric patients 7 years and older who have been symptomatic for no more than 2 days. Inhaled zanamivir in adults has consistently shown at least one less day of disabling influenza symptoms, and most studies have found a reduction in the number of nights of disturbed sleep, in time to resumption of normal activities, and in the use of symptom relief medications.[29,30] Similar therapeutic benefits have also been shown in children aged 5–12 years old.[31] Greatest benefit was noted in patients who were febrile at the time of enrollment, those started on therapy within 30 hours after the onset of symptoms, and in adults aged 50 years and older.[29] Zanamivir has also been associated with a 40% reduction in lower respiratory tract complications of influenza leading to antibiotics, particularly bronchitis and pneumonia.[32] Zanamivir appears generally well tolerated and effective in treating influenza in patients with mild to moderate asthma or, less often, chronic obstructive pulmonary disease.[30,32]

An uncontrolled study found zanamivir to be safe and possibly effective in allogeneic stem cell transplant recipients, although viral shedding persisted an average of 2 weeks on therapy.[24] Further studies are needed in immunocompromised populations. Likewise, there may be benefit to using neuraminidase inhibitors beyond the initial 48 hours of symptoms in patients with severe illness, particularly if the patients are ill enough to warrant hospital admission (see oseltamivir treatment section for more details).

Dosage and special consideration

Zanamivir is delivered by inhalation with a proprietary breath-activated device (Diskhaler). The usual adult treatment dose is two inhalations (10 mg) twice a day for 5 days. Although the plasma elimination half-life increases with creatinine clearance ≤70 ml/min, drug accumulation is negligible after inhalation and dose adjustment is not necessary for renal or hepatic dysfunction. Certain populations, particularly very young, frail or cognitively impaired patients, may have difficulty using the drug delivery system.[28]

Safety issues

Topically applied zanamivir is generally well tolerated in controlled studies, including those involving patients with asthma and chronic obstructive pulmonary disease.[30] No difference in adverse events between zanamivir and placebo (lactose) recipients have been found.[30] Less than 5% zanamivir recipients have reported diarrhea, nausea, sinusitis, nasal signs and symptoms, bronchitis, cough, headache, dizziness, and ear, nose and throat infections. Postmarketing reports indicate that bronchospasm may be an uncommon but potentially severe problem, particularly in patients with acute influenza and underlying reactive airway disease.[33] Anecdotal reports of hospitalization and fatality indicate that inhaled zanamivir should be used cautiously in such patients. Current guidelines advise against the use of zanamivir in patients with underlying airway disease, unless the patient is closely monitored and has a fast-acting inhaled bronchodilator available when inhaling zanamivir.[4]

Low bioavailability is associated with low exposure to circulating zanamivir, and no clinically significant drug interactions have been recognized. In-vitro studies suggest that zanamivir does not inhibit or induce cytochrome P450 enzymes. The drug does not affect the immunogenicity of concomitant immunization with inactivated virus vaccines. It is uncertain whether inhaled zanamivir might reduce the immunogenicity of intranasal, live-attenuated vaccine if administered concurrently. Although not associated with teratogenic effects in preclinical studies, zanamivir should only be used in pregnancy when the potential benefit justifies the potential risk to the fetus (category C).

OSELTAMIVIR

Pharmacokinetics and distribution

Oral oseltamivir ethyl ester is well absorbed and rapidly cleaved by esterases in the gastrointestinal tract, liver or blood. The bioavailability of the active metabolite, oseltamivir carboxylate, is estimated to be ~80% in previously healthy persons.[8] Mean peak oseltamivir carboxylate concentrations of 456 µg/l are reached at 5 hours after oral administration of 150 mg doses in healthy adults, and the plasma elimination half-life is 6–10 hours. Although drug concentrations over time are 25–35% higher in the elderly at steady state, no dose adjustments are deemed necessary. Administration with food appears to decrease the risk of gastrointestinal upset without decreasing bioavailability. Both the prodrug and parent are eliminated primarily unchanged through the kidney by glomerular filtration and anionic tubular secretion. The dose should be reduced by half for patients with a creatinine clearance less than 30 ml/min.[34] Distribution is not well characterized in humans, but peak bronchoalveolar lavage levels are similar to plasma levels in animals.[8] Drug levels in middle ear fluid and sinus aspirates are similar to those in blood.[8]

There is no clear association between the area under the serum concentration versus time curve (AUC) for the oseltamivir carboxylate drug and viral titer after experimental infection; early therapy of experimental infection is associated with reduced median nasal lavage concentrations of interleukin 6 (IL-6), tumor necrosis factor and interferon gamma (IFN-γ) as compared to placebo.[8] In natural influenza, once-daily dosing appears as effective as twice daily dosing for prevention of influenza illness.[8] Doses of 75 mg and 150 mg twice daily provide comparable antiviral and clinical effects in the treatment of acute influenza A illness[8] and of experimental influenza B in adults.

Indications

Prophylaxis

Oseltamivir is indicated for the prevention of influenza infection in patients ≥1 year, with dosing once a day. The efficacy of once-daily oseltamivir 75 mg for 6 weeks in preventing influenza illness in healthy, nonimmunized adults was 84% and in preventing influenza infection irrespective of symptoms was 50%.[8] In immunized nursing home residents, the efficacy of prophylaxis was 92% against illness compared to placebo.[8] Similar efficacy was seen in a household-contact prophylaxis study,[8] and protection against influenza has been shown in children.[8] A small observational study among stem cell transplant recipients also documented that oseltamivir, when taken as directed, was highly effective in preventing infection. A prospective study among immunocompromised patients is currently underway to determine the safety and efficacy of long-term prophylaxis in these populations.

Treatment

Oseltamivir 75 mg twice daily for 5 days when started within the first 2 days of symptoms was associated with a shorter time to alleviation of illness (29–35 hours shorter) and with reductions in severity of illness, duration of fever, time to return to normal activity, quantity of viral shedding, duration of impaired activity, and complications leading to antibiotic use, particularly bronchitis, compared to placebo in previously healthy adults.[8] Preliminary analyses indicate that early treatment can reduce hospitalizations. In a pediatric study enrolling children between the ages of 1 and 12 years, oseltamivir 2 mg/kg every 12 hours for 5 days significantly reduced illness duration and severity, time to resumption of full activities, and the occurrence of complications leading to antibiotic use, particularly acute otitis media.[35] Little published information is available about therapeutic efficacy in elderly or high-risk persons, including those with underlying cardiopulmonary conditions or immunodeficiency. A recent observational study among hospitalized patients with influenza who were treated, irrespective of the duration of clinical symptoms, found that antiviral therapy (typically with oseltamivir) was associated with a significant reduction in mortality (OR 0.21, 95% confidence interval 0.06–0.80; $p < 0.03$). Based on these data, antiviral therapy should be considered, irrespective of time since symptom onset, in patients with severe disease or who warrant hospital admission, if viral replication is documented.[36]

Dosage and special consideration

Oseltamivir comes as 75 mg tablets and as a white tutti-frutti-flavored suspension. The suspension comes in bottles containing 25 ml of suspension after constitution equivalent to 300 mg oseltamivir base. The typical adult dose for treatment is 75 mg twice daily for 5 days and for prophylaxis is 75 mg once daily. Pediatric dosing is based on weight and is outlined in Table 147.1. Oseltamivir dose should be reduced to 75 mg once a day for treatment and 75 mg every other day or 30 mg of suspension daily for prophylaxis when a patient has a creatinine clearance of <30 ml/min. Doses of oseltamivir should be given after hemodialysis. The safety and pharmacokinetics in patients with hepatic impairment have not been evaluated. No clinical studies have been conducted to assess the safety of neuraminidase inhibitors in pregnancy. Despite this, current CDC guidelines state that 'pregnancy should not be considered a contraindication to oseltamivir or zanamivir use. Because of its systemic activity, oseltamivir is preferred for treatment of pregnant women.' The recommended pediatric dosage is listed in Table 147.1.

Safety issues

Oral oseltamivir is generally well tolerated and no serious end-organ toxicity has been found in controlled clinical trials. Oseltamivir is associated with nausea, discomfort and, less often, emesis in a minority of treated patients. Nausea and vomiting occur at approximately 10–15% excess in oseltamivir recipients. Gastrointestinal complaints are usually mild-to-moderate in intensity, usually resolve despite continued dosing, and are ameliorated by administration with food.[37] Clinical studies comparing 75 mg and 150 mg twice daily found similar frequencies of adverse events with the two doses. Other infrequent possible adverse events include insomnia, vertigo and fever. Postmarketing reports suggest that oseltamivir may be associated rarely with skin rash, hepatic dysfunction or thrombocytopenia. Additionally, there have been reports of abnormal neurologic and behavioral symptoms which have rarely resulted in deaths among mostly children; most of these reports have come from Japan. It is unclear if this unusual behavior is secondary to oseltamivir or the result of their influenza illness. It is currently recommended that patients be monitored closely for behavioral abnormalities.[37]

No clinically significant drug interactions have been recognized. However, probenecid blocks tubular secretion and doubles the half-life of oseltamivir. Studies with amoxicillin, aspirin and acetaminophen have found no clinically important interactions. No interactions with the cytochrome P450 enzymes occur *in vitro*. Protein binding is below 10%. Oseltamivir should not affect the immunogenicity of concomitant vaccination with inactivated virus but might impair the immunogenicity of concurrent live-attenuated intranasal influenza vaccine.

Conclusions

The neuraminidase inhibitors are currently the preferred agents for the prevention and treatment of influenza infection. Recently, low level, clonal resistance to oseltamivir in influenza A/H1N1 strains globally has been described. It is unclear if these viruses will be persistent and what their impact will be globally; the CDC and WHO influenza guidance programs should be consulted regularly in order to stay up to date with the current prevention and treatment recommendations.

Ribavirin

Introduction and mechanism of action

Ribavirin (Virazole, Rebetol) is a guanosine analogue with a wide range of antiviral activity including influenza viruses, respiratory syncytial virus (RSV) and parainfluenza viruses. Ribavirin is rapidly phosphorylated by intracellular enzymes and the triphosphate inhibits influenza virus RNA polymerase activity and competitively inhibits the guanosine triphosphate-dependent 5'-capping of influenza viral messenger RNA. In addition, ribavirin depletes cellular guanine pools.[38,39] Ribavirin also shows antiproliferative and immunomodulatory effects.

Pharmacokinetics

Oral ribavirin has a bioavailability of 33–45% in adults and children and achieves peak plasma concentration of 0.6 µg/ml 1–2 hours after ingestion of a 400 mg dose in adults. Ribavirin has a short initial (0.3–0.7 hour) and a long terminal (18–36 hours) phase half-life and is eliminated by hepatic metabolism and renal clearance.[40–43] After aerosol administration, plasma levels increase with exposure and range from 0.2 to 1 µg/ml. Respiratory secretions have levels up to 1000 µg/ml, which decline with a half-life of 1.4–2.5 hours.

Indications

Ribavirin aerosol is currently indicated for the treatment of severe RSV in children. Oral ribavirin is indicated in combination with interferon-α or pegylated interferon for the treatment of chronic hepatitis C (see Chapter 148). Trials of aerosolized ribavirin for the treatment of severe RSV infection in infants have shown no consistent effect on duration of hospitalization time or mortality.[44] Earlier studies were confounded by the use of water aerosol as placebo which may induce bronchospasm. Long-term follow-up of ribavirin recipients has likewise found no consistent benefits on pulmonary function.[44] Current guidelines recommend that aerosolized ribavirin be considered in the treatment of high-risk infants and young children, as defined by congenital heart disease, chronic lung disease, immunodeficiency states, prematurity and age <6 weeks, as well as for those hospitalized with severe illness.[44,45] Administration of a more concentrated aerosol solution (60 mg/ml) over 2 hours q8h appears well tolerated and easier to administer.[46] Aerosolized ribavirin has shown minimal efficacy in treating immunocompetent hospitalized children.[47]

Ribavirin has also been studied for the treatment of RSV and parainfluenza virus infections in immunocompromised patients. Intravenous ribavirin appears to be ineffective in reducing RSV-associated mortality in hematopoietic stem cell transplant (HSCT) patients with RSV pneumonia; there may be benefit among lung transplant recipients.[48] Aerosolized ribavirin may provide benefit in selected patient groups with less severe RSV disease. Survival was improved when treatment was started before respiratory failure or when infection was limited to the upper respiratory tract.[48] Although there have not been any reported prospective studies of aerosolized ribavirin versus combined ribavirin–antibody therapy (either intravenous immunoglobulin, RespiGam or palivizumab), combination therapy appears more effective, particularly when started before severe respiratory distress.[48] Oral ribavirin has been tried in the management of RSV with variable success. Systemic therapy is associated with a higher risk of adverse effects, particularly hemolytic anemia.[48] In the management of parainfluenza virus in bone marrow transplant recipients, two case series found that aerosolized ribavirin failed to improve 30-day mortality or reduce the duration of viral replication relative to no treatment.[48,49]

Dosage and special consideration

Ribavirin comes in three formulations: oral, intravenous (investigational in USA) and aerosol. Ribavirin for aerosolization is available as a 6 g/100 ml solution which is diluted to a final concentration of 20 mg/ml and delivered by small particle aerosol for 12–18 hours with a proprietary device (SPAG-2 nebulizer). A higher concentration of aerosol solution (60 mg/ml) has been given over 2 hours three times daily in some studies and appears well tolerated. Ribavirin also comes in 200 mg tablets and sterile solution for injection.

Systemic ribavirin is contraindicated in patients with creatinine clearance <50 ml/min and the dose should be reduced by one-third for patients under 10 years of age. Dose adjustment is needed if there is a substantial decline in hematocrit and the drug should be discontinued if the hemoglobin drops below 8.5 g/dl.

Safety issues

Systemic ribavirin can cause a dose-related extravascular hemolytic anemia and, at higher doses, suppression of bone marrow release of erythroid elements. Severe anemia may require dose adjustment or cessation or use of erythropoietin. Aerosolized ribavirin can cause bronchospasm, mild conjunctival irritation, rash, psychological distress if administered in an oxygen tent, and rarely acute water intoxication. Bolus intravenous administration may cause rigors. Antagonism of both drugs may occur when ribavirin is combined with zidovudine. Ribavirin is contraindicated in pregnant women and in male partners of women who are pregnant because of teratogenicity of the drug. Pregnancy should be avoided during therapy and for 6 months after completion of therapy in both female patients and in female partners of male patients taking ribavirin (pregnancy category X).

REFERENCES

References for this chapter can be found online at http://www.expertconsult.com

Kristen M Marks
Marshall J Glesby

Chapter | **148**

Drugs to treat viral hepatitis

INTRODUCTION

Tremendous progress in the treatment of viral hepatitis has been made over the past two decades, and with many new drug classes in development, the next 20 years hold similar promise. This chapter describes the mechanism of action, pharmacokinetics, indications and safety of the drugs used for the treatment of chronic hepatitis B and C infections and highlights some of the agents in development. The diagnosis and management of hepatitis B and C are covered in Chapter 38. Vaccination and prevention strategies are discussed in Chapters 38 and 154. Chronic hepatitis C infection is treated with pegylated interferon and ribavirin, while oral nucleoside or nucleotide analogue therapy represents standard initial treatment for chronic hepatitis B infection. The response to the drugs described in this chapter is affected by both host (e.g. age, gender, race, co-morbid conditions such as HIV, stage of illness, immune response) and viral factors (e.g. genotype, RNA/DNA level, resistance mutations). Therefore, the choice of the drug, dose and duration must take these factors into consideration. As no targeted treatments exist for hepatitis A or E infections, they will not be discussed.

INTERFERONS

Interferons (IFNs) are a family of naturally occurring proteins produced by eukaryotic cells that function as cytokines in an early response to viral infection. Interferons do not have direct antiviral activity, but instead induce an antiviral state in exposed cells and activate other immune functions.

Interferons are broadly characterized as type I (IFN-α and -β) and type II (IFN-γ). Interferon-α and -β have primary antiviral activity while IFN-γ has more potent immunoregulatory functions.

Interferons act through cell surface receptors to induce a complex series of intracellular events, with inhibition of viral protein production appearing to be the primary target.[1] A variety of purified and recombinant IFN-α preparations is available for clinical use. The pharmaceuticals are termed 'IFN-alfa' to distinguish them from naturally occurring IFN-α.

Recently, pegylated ('peg') varieties of IFN have become available, and their usage in hepatitis C virus (HCV) treatment has for the most part replaced standard interferon. Pegylation involves the addition of a polyethylene glycol side chain to the protein molecule, which extends the half-life significantly. Two formulations are currently available, pegIFN alfa-2a and pegIFN alfa-2b. PegIFN alfa-2a has a larger branched peg molecule of about 40 kDa attached at several sites. PegIFN alfa-2b has a smaller, linear peg molecule of about 12 kDa attached at several sites. Their proposed mechanism of action is similar to that of standard IFNs.[2]

Pharmacokinetics and distribution

Standard pharmacokinetic measurements may not be relevant for IFN therapy. In healthy male volunteers, maximum serum levels of IFN alfa-2b occur 3–12 hours after subcutaneous administration, and serum concentrations are undetectable after 16 hours. IFN alfa is filtered through the glomeruli and then undergoes rapid proteolytic degradation during tubular resorption. Negligible amounts of IFN are excreted in the urine. A small percentage of the administered dose undergoes hepatic metabolism and biliary excretion. PegIFN alfa-2b reaches maximum concentrations by 20 hours and has a half-life of 40 hours. PegIFN alfa-2a reaches maximum concentrations by 72–96 hours and has a longer $t_{1/2}$ of 80 hours compared to pegIFN alfa-2b.

Indications

Chronic hepatitis B virus infection

IFN alfa-2b and pegIFN alfa-2a are approved for the treatment of chronic hepatitis B virus (HBV) infection. A response to IFN therapy is judged by a loss of HBV DNA and hepatitis B e antigen (HBeAg) from the plasma (in eAg-positive patients), along with biochemical and histologic improvements. A meta-analysis of 16 randomized trials examining standard IFN versus control in HBeAg-positive patients found that loss of HBeAg occurred in 33% of patients while clearance of HBV DNA occurred in 37% of patients (although the DNA assays used in these studies were less sensitive than current methods).[3] Control patients experienced these outcomes in only 12% and 17% of cases, respectively. Clinical predictors of response to IFN in patients infected with HBV include low level of HBV DNA, elevated serum transaminases and evidence of active hepatic inflammation.[4]

PegIFN is thought to result in similar or slightly superior outcomes than standard IFN, although limited data exist from head-to-head comparisons. In HBeAg-positive patients, 48 weeks of pegIFN alfa-2a therapy was associated with loss of eAg in 30% and seroconversion in 27%, with persistence of these finding 24 weeks after discontinuation of therapy.[5] However, only 25% of patients achieved undetectable levels of HBV DNA. Studies of pegIFN alfa-2b yielded similar results.[6] In contrast, IFN and pegIFN treatment in HBeAg-negative patients results in high rates of HBV viral suppression; however, the response is generally not durable after treatment discontinuation.[7]

Recent years have seen a variety of new and effective oral medications for the treatment of HBV infection with improved rates of HBV DNA suppression. Oral agents have more favorable side-effect profiles compared to IFN, but HBeAg seroconversion rates are not as high. As a result of these therapies, IFN is no longer considered first-line treatment for HBV infection in most circumstances (see also Chapter 38).

Hepatitis C virus infection

Interferon treatment of acute HCV infection is currently recommended, yet proper timing of treatment, regimen and duration remain uncertain. A landmark study reported a 98% sustained virologic response rate with 24 weeks of IFN monotherapy; however, the study had no control group and some patients experience spontaneous resolution if left untreated.[8] As additional data have accumulated, the use of pegIFN has been advocated in the treatment of acute HCV, although the need for combination therapy with ribavirin remains controversial.

Treatment of chronic HCV infection is generally recommended in patients experiencing detectable HCV RNA levels and evidence of fibrosis on liver biopsy. A sustained virologic response (SVR) of HCV to therapy is defined as an HCV RNA assay below the limit of assay detection (using an assay with a cutoff of 50 IU/ml or lower) at 24 weeks after completion of therapy.[9] Over the past 10 years, it has been established that pegIFN plus ribavirin combination therapy is superior to combination therapy with standard interferon or pegIFN monotherapy and is now considered the standard of care.

Hepatitis C virus has a half-life of about 3 hours and infection results in the production of about 12 billion virions daily. The frequent dosing and pharmacokinetics of standard IFN result in wide variations in serum IFN levels and fluctuating antiviral activity. Standard IFN monotherapy results in SVR rates of less than 10% after 24 weeks of treatment and SVR rates of less than 20% after 48 weeks of therapy.[10] Pegylation of the IFN molecule maintains rapid absorption and rapid time to peak drug level, while providing a dramatically lengthened half-life. Studies show that the pegIFNs provide significantly improved response rates over standard IFNs. Monotherapy with pegIFNs yields SVR rates of 25–39% in treatment-naive patients with HCV infection.[11] These improved results over standard IFN apply to both pegIFN alfa-2a as well as pegIFN alfa-2b.

Route of administration and dosing

Interferons are administered subcutaneously for the treatment of chronic viral hepatitis. Dosages vary considerably according to the specific preparation and indication (Table 148.1). Guidelines for adjusting IFN dosage in patients who have renal insufficiency are poorly defined. Only limited data are available regarding administration to patients who have decompensated liver disease, but IFN may be poorly tolerated in this population and its use is generally not advised. In pregnant monkeys, IFN has abortifacient effects and should not be used in pregnant women unless the potential benefits clearly outweigh the potential risks to the fetus.

Table 148.1 Medication dosage regimens for adults. Preferred initial regimens are shown in bold

Disease	Therapy	Route	Dose	Duration
Chronic hepatitis B	IFN alfa-2b*	sc	5 × 10⁶ IU/day or 10 × 10⁶ IU three times/week	HBeAg-positive: 16–24 weeks[†] HBeAg-negative: 12+ months[†]
	PegIFN alfa-2a	sc	180 μg/week	48 weeks[†]
	Lamivudine	po	100 mg q24h	Optimal duration unknown
	Adefovir dipivoxil	po	10 mg q24h	Optimal duration unknown
	Entecavir	**po**	**0.5 mg q24h (lamivudine-inexperienced)** or 1.0 mg (lamivudine-experienced)	**Optimal duration unknown**
	Telbivudine	po	600 mg q24h	Optimal duration unknown
	Tenofovir[‡]	**po**	**300 mg q24h**	**Optimal duration unknown**
	Emtricitabine[§]	po	200 mg q24h	Optimal duration unknown
Chronic hepatitis C	IFN alfa-2a*	sc	3 × 10⁶ IU three times/week	24–48 weeks[¶]
	IFN alfa-2b*	sc	3 × 10⁶ IU three times/week	24–48 weeks[#]
	IFN alfacon*	sc	9 μg three times/week**	24-48 weeks[¶]
	PegIFN alfa-2a	**sc**	**180 μg/week**	**24 weeks genotype 2,3[††] 48 weeks genotype 1,4**
	PegIFN alfa-2b	**sc**	**1.5 μg/kg/week[††]** (or 1.0 μg/kg/week)[‡‡]	**24 weeks genotype 2,3** ** **48 weeks genotype 1,4**
	Ribavirin	**po**	**800–1400 mg/day divided in two doses[§§]**	**Co-administer with IFN or pegIFN for entire duration**

*The use of standard interferon has been replaced for the most part by the use of pegylated interferon for reasons of efficacy and convenience. Standard interferon may be used in certain situations (e.g. prior to liver transplant) when a shorter half-life is preferred.
[†]Optimal dosing and duration of interferons is unclear for HBV. Whether lower dose or shorter treatment of pegIFN may suffice for HBeAg-positive and whether longer treatment will improve response for HBeAg-negative patients is not known.
[‡]First-line therapy for HIV-infected patients who also require HIV treatment, usually in combination with lamivudine or emtricitabine as part of a combination antiretroviral regimen.
[§] FDA-approved for treatment of HIV infection but not HBV monoinfection.
[¶]Optimal duration of IFN therapy with these agents is based on genotype and what has become standard of care may vary from the package inserts.
[#]Dosing of 15 μg sc three times/week is recommended for **nonresponders** to prior treatment or **relapsers**. Daily dosing has also been studied and may be appropriate in certain circumstances.
**For HIV-infected patients, duration of treatment is extended to 48 weeks.
[††]Dual therapy with ribavirin.
[‡‡]Monotherapy.
[§§]Optimal dose of ribavirin varies with the co-administration of IFN products as well as patient weight and HCV genotype. Readers should refer to specific package inserts and practice guidelines.

Adverse reactions

Interferon therapy is associated with an extensive list of toxicities (see Fig. 148.1). Most patients receiving standard IFN doses of over one million units experience an 'influenza-like' syndrome characterized by fever, chills, headache, myalgias and arthralgias. These symptoms appear a few hours after the IFN injection, and usually resolve within 12 hours. The symptoms can often be prevented by premedication with antipyretics. Tolerance develops in many patients with continued therapy. The most frequent dose-limiting adverse effects are leukopenia and thrombocytopenia. Before beginning IFN therapy, a baseline complete blood count, liver function profile, urinalysis, antinuclear antibody screen and thyroid function tests should be obtained.

The adverse events seen with pegIFN are similar to those seen with standard IFN. The most common hematologic toxicity associated with pegIFNs is neutropenia with as many as 18% of patients requiring dose adjustments as a result.[12] Dose reduction or use of hematopoietic growth factors is often helpful in patients experiencing significant generalized or hematologic toxicity, respectively. The pegylated IFNs are also associated with psychiatric disturbances including depression, irritability, insomnia and suicidal ideation. Caution is warranted when using IFNs and pegIFNs in patients with a history of a psychiatric disorder.

RIBAVIRIN (SEE ALSO CHAPTER 147)

Ribavirin is a guanosine analogue that has broad-spectrum antiviral activity. Its mechanism of action is not clearly defined, but it is believed to act against HCV by one or more of the following mechanisms:
- enhancing T-cell mediated immune responses to HCV by shifting the balance towards a T-helper-1 response;
- inhibiting cellular inosine monophosphate dehydrogenase, thereby decreasing the intracellular guanosine triphosphate pool needed for viral RNA replication;
- directly inhibiting HCV polymerase; and
- acting as an RNA virus mutagen, thereby reducing viral fitness.[13]

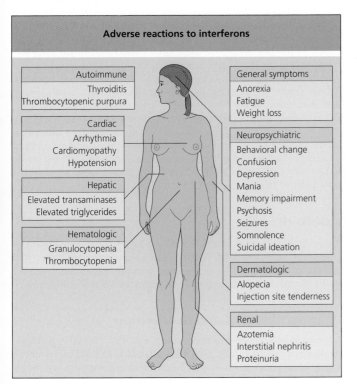

Adverse reactions to interferons

| Autoimmune |
| Thyroiditis |
| Thrombocytopenic purpura |

| Cardiac |
| Arrhythmia |
| Cardiomyopathy |
| Hypotension |

| Hepatic |
| Elevated transaminases |
| Elevated triglycerides |

| Hematologic |
| Granulocytopenia |
| Thrombocytopenia |

| General symptoms |
| Anorexia |
| Fatigue |
| Weight loss |

| Neuropsychiatric |
| Behavioral change |
| Confusion |
| Depression |
| Mania |
| Memory impairment |
| Psychosis |
| Seizures |
| Somnolence |
| Suicidal ideation |

| Dermatologic |
| Alopecia |
| Injection site tenderness |

| Renal |
| Azotemia |
| Interstitial nephritis |
| Proteinuria |

Fig. 148.1 Adverse reactions to interferons.

Pharmacokinetics

Ribavirin is well absorbed after oral administration, with bioavailability ranging from 33% to 69% of the dose and about 40% of the drug being eliminated via the kidneys.

Indications

Hepatitis C virus infection

Ribavirin is used in combination with IFN or pegIFN for the treatment of chronic HCV infection. As the benefits of ribavirin monotherapy in HCV infection disappear rapidly when the treatment is discontinued, monotherapy is not recommended.

Route of administration and dosing

Ribavirin is administered orally for the treatment of hepatitis C. The recommended dose of ribavirin varies by weight and HCV genotype (see Table 148.1). Retrospective analysis of phase III studies of pegIFN plus ribavirin revealed that response is inversely correlated with the patient's body weight. In the study by Manns *et al.*, patients receiving at least 10.6 mg/kg of ribavirin had significantly better response rates for the same doses of pegIFN.[12] A randomized clinical trial confirmed that weight-based dosing of ribavirin improves sustained virologic response rates in patients with genotype 1 infection.[14]

Adverse reactions and interactions

The major side-effect of ribavirin is hemolytic anemia, which may necessitate discontinuation of therapy. Ribavirin is highly teratogenic and birth control is required if the drug is used by women of childbearing age or their partners. In HIV-infected individuals, ribavirin should not be co-administered with didanosine because of excess toxicity, and co-administration with zidovudine should be avoided due to potentiation of anemia (see also Practice Point 46).

COMBINATION THERAPY FOR HEPATITIS C VIRUS INFECTION

Ribavirin given in combination with IFN has been shown to be more effective than the use of IFN alone for the treatment of HCV.[15] An SVR may occur in up to 40% of patients treated with combination therapy compared with approximately 20% of patients treated with standard IFN alone. Studies combining pegIFN alfa-2b with ribavirin had a 54% SVR compared to a 47% SVR with standard IFN alfa-2b plus ribavirin.[12] The SVR in patients infected with HCV genotype 1, which is associated with a poorer response to therapy, was also improved (42% vs. 33%). Trials of pegIFN alfa-2a plus ribavirin also demonstrate improved responses overall and for genotype 1 when compared to pegIFN alone (46% vs. 21% for genotype 1) and standard IFN plus RBV (46% vs. 36% for genotype 1).[11] A randomized trial of treatment-naive, HCV genotype 1 patients comparing the two available preparations of pegIFN (pegIFN alfa-2a and pegIFN alfa-2b) given in combination with weight-based ribavirin dosing demonstrated no significant difference in sustained virologic response for the two combinations. In patients with HIV/HCV co-infection, combination therapy with pegIFN and ribavirin for HCV has also been shown to be superior to pegIFN monotherapy or combination therapy using standard IFN[16-18] (see Practice Point 46).

As data on the use of these drugs have accumulated, refinements in the recommended ribavirin dose and total treatment duration have been made based on HCV genotype and HIV co-infection status (see Table 148.1). In addition, validated criteria for stopping treatment have been developed based on lack of response at 12 and 24 weeks. The rapidity of treatment response has also been explored as a rationale for foreshortening or extending the duration of therapy, but the usefulness of this approach has not been clearly demonstrated. In practice, many physicians extend the treatment duration in genotype 1 patients who take 24 weeks to achieve undetectable HCV RNA.

THERAPIES IN DEVELOPMENT FOR HEPATITIS C

Hepatitis C virus is a single-stranded (ss) RNA virus of about 9.4 kb in length. It is translated into a single polypeptide precursor, which is cleaved into several functional gene products, including structural proteins, RNA polymerase, helicase and serine protease.[19] Many drugs are in preclinical and clinical development to target key components of the viral life cycle, including inhibitors of viral entry, RNA polymerase activity (e.g. nucleoside and non-nucleoside inhibitors), protein translation, polyprotein processing (e.g. serine protease inhibitors) and viral assembly and release (Fig. 148.2).

Telaprevir, a protease inhibitor, is the agent furthest along in clinical development. Telaprevir given in combination with pegIFN and ribavirin was recently shown in phase II studies to achieve superior SVR rates over pegIFN plus ribavirin.[20,21] Similarly, the combination of pegIFN and ribavirin with bocepravir, another HCV protease inhibitor in clinical development, resulted in significantly higher SVR rates than pegIFN and ribavirin in phase II studies. Since monotherapy with telaprevir, bocepravir, and similar agents results in unacceptable rates of resistance, strategies for the use of newer agents typically involve co-administration with pegIFN and ribavirin. Nitazoxanide, an approved antiparasitic agent, has also been shown to possess antiviral properties and its use in combination with pegIFN and ribavirin is being studied.

In addition to novel strategies, longer acting and oral forms of interferon as well as analogues of ribavirin are also being investigated. Therapies targeted at preventing fibrosis are also in development.

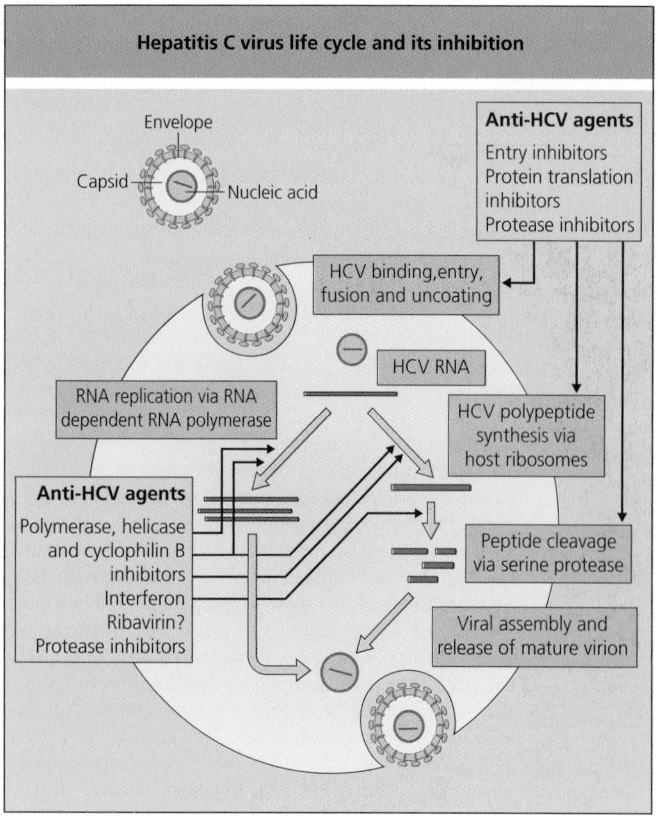

Fig. 148.2 Hepatitis C virus life cycle and its inhibition.

Disappointingly, a recent randomized clinical trial designed to investigate the long-term use of pegIFN maintenance therapy as an antifibrotic over a 4-year period did not show benefit in terms of fibrosis.[22]

NUCLEOSIDE AND NUCLEOTIDE ANALOGUES

Nucleoside and nucleotide analogues have been developed for use in the treatment of several viral pathogens and function either as nucleic acid chain terminators or as inhibitors of polymerase enzymes. A nucleotide differs from a nucleoside by the presence of one or more phosphate groups covalently bound to the molecule's sugar group. Intracellular phosphorylation is required before incorporation into the elongating nucleic acid chain. Nucleoside analogues include lamivudine, emtricitabine, entecavir and telbivudine, while nucleotide analogues are represented by adefovir and tenofovir. These drugs inhibit a critical step in the HBV life cycle where the reverse transcriptase activity of its DNA polymerase catalyzes the conversion of RNA to DNA. Resistance to nucleoside(tide) analogues can be caused by mutations in the active site of the DNA polymerase enzyme, including the highly conserved amino acid motif YMDD which confers resistance to lamivudine and emtricitabine.[23]

Nucleoside(tide) analogue therapy is generally indicated for patients with hepatitis B who have evidence of active viral replication and either persistent elevations in transaminases or histologically active disease (see Chapter 38). Based on the need for long-term treatment and their higher barrier to resistance, entecavir and tenofovir represent the currently preferred first-line monotherapy choices. The other available agents are no longer felt to be suitable for monotherapy in most circumstances due to unacceptably high rates of resistance. Viral breakthrough due to the development of resistance or discontinuation of this drug class may be associated with severe exacerbations of hepatitis.

Lamivudine (3TC)

Lamivudine was the first nucleoside analogue approved for HBV infection. It is also used for the treatment of HIV infection. Detailed pharmacokinetic and distribution data are provided in Chapter 145. The dose used for HBV (100 mg q24h) is lower than that used for HIV. Lamivudine therapy is associated with a significant improvement in hepatic histology, normalization of hepatic enzymes and suppression of plasma HBV DNA.[24] In most patients, however, values return to baseline levels when lamivudine is discontinued. Furthermore, the emergence of drug-resistant HBV limits the value of lamivudine for long-term therapy and may be associated with hepatitis flares.[25] Regimens combining lamivudine with other active compounds to enhance efficacy and limit the development of resistance are under investigation. Lamivudine (300 mg dose) is also available as a co-formulation with other drugs used in the treatment of HIV.

Adefovir

Adefovir is an approved nucleotide analogue for the treatment of HBV infection. Originally developed as an antiretroviral agent, it is associated with significant renal toxicity at the higher doses needed to inhibit HIV replication and is not approved for that indication.

Pharmacokinetics and distribution

Adefovir is administered as the prodrug adefovir dipivoxil. Unaffected by food, it achieves 60% oral bioavailability. Its half-life is about 12–30 hours and it undergoes renal excretion without significant observed metabolites. It does not substantially affect the cytochrome P450 system.

Indications

Chronic hepatitis B virus infection

Adefovir is highly active against HBV, producing reductions of HBV DNA of >3.5 logs. A phase III study in HBeAg-positive, treatment-naive patients randomized patients to adefovir 10 mg, 30 mg or placebo; HBV viral load reduction, histologic improvement and HBeAg seroconversion rates were superior in the adefovir arms.[26] The drug does not exhibit cross-resistance with lamivudine and is effective in the treatment of lamivudine-resistant HBV. As mutations associated with adefovir resistance emerge in 15% of patients by 96 weeks,[27] its use as first line-therapy is largely being supplanted by entecavir and tenofovir. Its role in combination therapy is also being explored.

Route of administration and dosing

Adefovir is approved for oral use only. The drug displays anti-HBV activity at doses above 5 mg/day. It is approved for use at 10 mg/day for HBV infection.

Adverse reactions and interactions

Adefovir appears well tolerated at the 10 mg dose. Renal impairment becomes significant, however, at the 30 mg dosage which is not used for the treatment of HBV.[25] Dose adjustment is recommended for patients with creatinine clearances (CrCl) <50 ml/min. The most common adverse reactions are headache, gastrointestinal upset and elevated transaminases. No significant drug interactions have been documented.

Tenofovir disoproxil fumarate (TDF)

Tenofovir is an orally bioavailable, nucleotide analogue approved for treatment of HIV and recently approved for treatment of chronic hepatitis B. Detailed pharmacokinetic and safety data are given in Chapter 145. Tenofovir exhibits potent viral suppression, with 93% and 76% of HBeAg-negative and HBeAg-positive patients having undetectable HBV DNA, respectively, at 1 year.[28] No patients in these studies exhibited genotypic resistance, and only case reports of drug resistance have been described to date.

Tenofovir has activity against lamivudine- and adefovir-resistant HBV isolates, and its efficacy has been shown in clinical trials of lamivudine- and adefovir-experienced patients. Tenofovir (usually in combination with lamivudine or emtricitabine) is the HBV treatment of choice for patients who require concomitant treatment of HIV infection (see Practice Point 44). It is available as a co-formulation with emtricitabine or with emtricitabine and efavirenz.

Emtricitabine (FTC)

Emtricitabine is an orally bioavailable, cytosine nucleoside analogue approved for treatment of HIV infection with efficacy against HBV. Because of its structural similarity to lamivudine, it shares a common resistance profile and its use in the treatment of HIV is felt to be interchangeable with lamivudine. Detailed pharmacokinetic and safety data are given in Chapter 145. In a study of both HBeAg-positive and HBeAg-negative patients, the 200 mg dose of emtricitabine was associated with viral suppression in 54% compared to 2% of placebo-treated patients at 48 weeks.[29] As with lamivudine, resistance with monotherapy is unacceptably high, with emtricitabine resistance mutations detected in 13% of patients in this study. It is available as a co-formulation with tenofovir or with tenofovir and efavirenz.

Entecavir

Entecavir is an orally bioavailable guanosine nucleoside analogue that functionally inhibits all three activities of the HBV DNA polymerase: base priming, reverse transcription of the negative strand and synthesis of the positive strand.

Pharmacokinetics and distribution

Entecavir's active phosphorylated form has a half-life of 15 hours. Entecavir is cleared by the kidneys primarily, and dose adjustment is recommended for patients with CrCl <50 ml/min.

Indications

Chronic hepatitis B virus infection

A dose-ranging study of entecavir at 0.01 mg, 0.1 mg and 0.5 mg versus lamivudine demonstrated reductions in HBV DNA of 2.4, 4.3 and 4.7 logs at each entecavir dose, respectively, compared with a 3.4 log reduction with lamivudine.[30] In studies of lamivudine-naive, HBeAg-positive subjects comparing entecavir and lamivudine, entecavir was associated with superior rates of virologic suppression at 48 weeks compared to lamivudine (67% vs. 36% <300 copies/ml); however, rates of eAg loss were similar.[31] In lamivudine-naive HBeAg-negative patients, entecavir was also shown to achieve superior rates of virologic suppression at 48 weeks.[32] Longer term treatment shows continued high rates of suppression through 4–5 years.

The presence of resistance mutations associated with lamivudine and telbivudine predisposes to the development of entecavir resistance, and its efficacy is reduced in the setting of prior lamivudine failure (e.g. cumulative development of resistance was 43% in lamivudine-refractory, compared to 1.2% in lamivudine-naive, subjects at 4 years).[33] An increased dose is recommended for patients with probable or known lamivudine resistance; however, use of alternative drugs without cross-resistance may be preferable. Because it is capable of inducing mutations in HIV reverse transcriptase associated with lamivudine resistance,[34,35] it should not be used in HBV/HIV co-infected patients who are not receiving antiretroviral therapy (see Practice Point 44).

Route of administration and dosing

Entecavir is approved for oral use only. The dose is 0.5 mg once daily except for patients with probable or known lamivudine resistance for whom the recommended dose is 1.0 mg daily. As its absorption is decreased by food, it is recommended that entecavir be administered on an empty stomach (at least 2 hours before or after a meal).

Adverse reactions and interactions

In studies, safety was similar between entecavir and lamivudine or entecavir and placebo. The most commonly observed adverse events that were possibly related to entecavir included headache, fatigue, dizziness and nausea.

Telbivudine (LdT)

Telbivudine is an oral thymidine nucleoside analogue with activity against HBV on both first and second strand synthesis.

Pharmacokinetics and distribution

Telbivudine distributes widely into the tissues and is excreted primarily by the kidneys. Dose adjustments are recommended for CrCl <50 ml/min. There are no significant known drug interactions.

Route of administration and dosing

Telbivudine is administered orally as 600 mg once daily with or without food as its absorption is not affected by food.

Indications

Chronic hepatitis B virus infection

Telbivudine showed superior rates of HBV DNA viral suppression when compared to lamivudine for both HBeAg-positive and

HBeAg-negative patients.[36] However, at 2 years, the development of genotypic resistance occurred in 21.6% and 8.6%, respectively.[37] The most commonly observed resistance mutation during treatment with telbivudine (M204I) confers cross-resistance to lamivudine. For these reasons, as with lamivudine, telbivudine monotherapy for HBV should generally be avoided. Telbivudine's use has not been investigated in patients with HIV co-infection.

Adverse reactions and interactions

Telbivudine was tolerated similar to lamivudine in studies comparing the two drugs except that grade 3–4 creatine kinase elevations were observed more frequently with telbivudine (9% vs. 3%). Myopathy with associated muscle weakness was rare (<1%).[37]

THERAPIES IN DEVELOPMENT FOR HEPATITIS B

Clevudine is an oral, once-daily nucleoside analogue which is approved for use in Korea. In phase III studies comparing clevudine with placebo, 24 weeks of treatment with clevudine resulted in HBV DNA suppression in 59% of HBeAg-positive and 92% of HBeAg-negative patients during treatment, and a higher than expected median DNA suppression 24 weeks after discontinuation of treatment.[38,39] Phase III studies are ongoing in the USA and Europe.

COMBINATION THERAPY FOR HEPATITIS B VIRUS INFECTION

Studies of combination therapy involving nucleoside analogues plus IFN demonstrated that while combination therapy could enhance viral suppression, post-treatment end points such as HBeAg seroconversion were not affected.[5,7] Combination studies involving use of two nucleoside(tide) analogues to date have provided signals that combination therapy may enhance viral suppression and increase the barrier to resistance but have yet to establish superiority of combination therapy compared to potent monotherapy. Thus, ongoing studies involving more potent combinations compared to potent monotherapy must be completed to determine whether particular combinations can be recommended definitively. For HIV/HBV co-infected patients who require combination therapy for the treatment of HIV, the use of the combination of tenofovir plus emtricitabine (available as a co-formulation) or tenofovir plus lamivudine is recommended as part of the regimen.

REFERENCES

References for this chapter can be found online at http://www.expertconsult.com

Shmuel Shoham
Andreas H Groll
Thomas J Walsh

Chapter | **149** |

Antifungal agents

Invasive fungal infections have emerged as important causes of morbidity and mortality in patients with severe underlying diseases. For more than three decades, treatment had been limited to amphotericin B deoxycholate with or without flucytosine. Therapeutic options only emerged with the clinical development of fluconazole and itraconazole in the late 1980s. The past 15 years, however, have witnessed a major expansion in our antifungal armamentarium through the introduction of less toxic formulations of amphotericin B, the development of improved antifungal triazoles and the advent of the echinocandin lipopeptides, a new class of antifungal agents that target the fungal cell wall. This chapter reviews the clinical pharmacology of approved and investigational antifungal agents for treatment of invasive fungal infections.

POLYENE ANTIFUNGAL AGENTS

Amphotericin B deoxycholate

Amphotericin B (AmB) is a natural polyene macrolide antibiotic and consists of seven conjugated double bonds, an internal ester, a free carboxyl group and a glycoside side chain with a primary amino group (Fig. 149.1). It is amphoteric, virtually insoluble in water, and not orally or intramuscularly absorbed. For parenteral use, AmB has been solubilized with deoxycholate as micellar suspension, and this formulation has now been available for more than 40 years.

Mechanism of action

Amphotericin B primarily acts by binding to ergosterol, the principal sterol in the cell membrane of most fungi, leading to the formation of ion channels and concentration-dependent cell death (Fig. 149.2). These pores, composed of AmB multimers, form most readily when ergosterol is present in the cell membrane.[1,2] With less avidity, the compound also binds to cholesterol, the main sterol of mammalian cell membranes, which is believed to account for most of its adverse effects. Amphotericin B may also induce cell damage through a cascade of oxidative reactions with formation of free radicals or an increase in membrane permeability.[3-5]

Antifungal activity

Amphotericin B has broad-spectrum antifungal activity that includes most pathogenic fungi. Primary resistance has been associated with qualitative or quantitative variations in membrane sterols, but may also be related to increased catalase activity with decreased susceptibility to oxidative damage. Resistance remains uncommon in *Cryptococcus neoformans* and *Candida* spp. although AmB appears

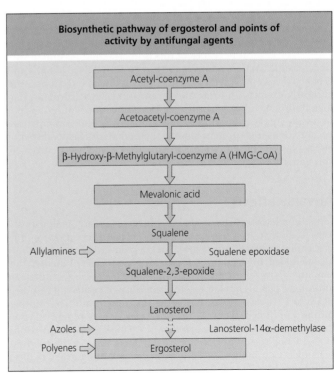

Fig. **149.2** Biosynthetic pathway of ergosterol and points of activity by antifungal agents.

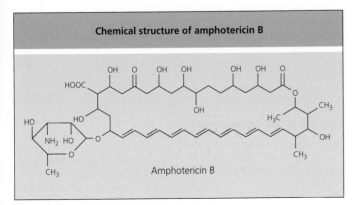

Fig. **149.1** Chemical structure of the polyene antifungal agents.

somewhat less active against *C. guilliermondii*, *C. parapsilosis* and *C. tropicalis*. *Candida lusitaniae* isolates are often resistant to AmB, and this resistance can develop during treatment.[6] *Aspergillus* spp. and other opportunistic molds, but not the dimorphic molds, tend to have more variable susceptibility. *Aspergillus terreus*, *Fusarium* spp., *Pseudallescheria boydii*, *Scedosporium prolificans*, certain other dematiaceous fungi and *Trichosporon* spp. can be resistant to AmB at concentrations safely achievable in patients.[6–8] Acquisition of secondary resistance has been anecdotally reported but its clinical role has not been fully defined.

Pharmacodynamics

AmB displays concentration-dependent fungicidal activity against susceptible *Candida albicans*, *Cr. neoformans* and *Aspergillus fumigatus* in time-kill assays and exhibits a postantifungal effect of up to 12 hours' duration against *C. albicans* and *Cr. neoformans in vitro*.[9–11] Studies in laboratory animals with disseminated candidiasis suggest that peak serum level/minimum inhibitory concentration (MIC) correlates best with efficacy *in vivo*. AmB may have immune stimulatory properties that enhance phagocyte responses to *Aspergillus* and *Fusarium* spp.[12,13]

Antifungal activity in biofilms has gained increasing attention. Biofilm-associated candidiasis typically occurs with infection of biomedical devices. Compared to planktonic yeast cells, biofilm-associated sessile cells show decreased susceptibility to AmB deoxycholate. By contrast, lipid formulations of AmB may remain active against sessile yeast.[14] Animal models suggest a role for AmB lipid formulations as antibiotic lock therapy in catheter-associated candidiasis.[15]

Pharmacokinetics

After intravenous administration, AmB dissociates from its vehicle and becomes highly protein-bound before distributing predominantly into liver, spleen, bone marrow, kidney and lung. A unique property of AmB is that protein binding in plasma is enhanced with increasing drug concentration.[16] Clearance from plasma is slow with a terminal half-life of 5 days and longer.[17] Concentrations in body fluids other than plasma may vary greatly between patients and are substantially lower than serum drug levels.[18,19] The clinical relevance of this is unclear and despite mostly undetectable concentrations in the cerebrospinal fluid (CSF), AmB is effective in central nervous system (CNS) fungal infections. AmB is mostly excreted in urine and feces as unchanged drug and no metabolites have been identified.[17] Dose adjustment of AmB is not necessary in patients with unrelated renal or hepatic dysfunction. Because of its high protein binding, hemodialysis usually does not affect plasma concentrations. Plasma drug clearance is inversely correlated with age.

Adverse effects

Infusion-related reactions and nephrotoxicity are major problems and often limit therapy. Infusion-related reactions (fever, rigors, chills, myalgias, arthralgias, nausea, vomiting and headaches) are mediated by cytokine release from monocytes. Whether this immune activation contributes to the effectiveness of AmB as an antifungal agent is not known. Infusion-related events can be noted in up to 73% of patients during the first dose, but often improve during continued therapy.[20] Slowing the infusion rate or premedication with acetaminophen (10–15 mg/kg), hydrocortisone (0.5–1.0 mg/kg) or meperidine (0.2–0.5 mg/kg) can blunt these reactions. Continuous 24-hour infusion of AmB further reduces symptoms, but data on the antifungal efficacy of this dosing strategy are limited.[21] Cardiac arrhythmias and cardiac arrest due to acute potassium release may occur with rapid infusion (<60 min),

especially if there is pre-existing hyperkalemia and/or renal impairment. True allergic reactions are rare.[22]

AmB-associated nephrotoxicity occurs due to alterations of membrane permeability in renal tubular and vascular smooth muscle cells. Tubular transport defects and decreased glomerular filtration rate (GFR) due to vasoconstriction are responsible for potassium and magnesium wasting, tubular acidosis, impaired urinary concentrating ability and azotemia. Decreased renal blood flow and recurrent ischemia may lead to permanent structural nephrotoxic effects.[3] Hypokalemia can be refractory to replacement until hypomagnesemia is corrected. Tubular acidosis and impaired urinary concentrating ability are rarely of clinical significance. Azotemia is common. In a large prospective clinical trial, baseline serum creatinine rose by more than double in over one-third of patients receiving AmB.[20] Renal toxicity is related to dose and duration of therapy, concomitant use of nephrotoxic agents and pre-existing renal dysfunction. AmB has the potential to lead to renal failure and dialysis. Often, however, azotemia stabilizes on therapy and is usually reversible after discontinuation of the drug. Avoiding concomitant nephrotoxic agents, and normal saline loading (10–15 ml 0.9% NaCl/kg/day) may lessen azotemia.

Amphotericin B may also cause hypotension, hypertension, flushing, vestibular disturbances and a normocytic, normochromic anemia after chronic administration.[15] As AmB deoxycholate is topically irritating, a central line should be used for infusion. Local instillation, including intrathecal administration, can cause focal areas of necrosis and requires expert consultation.[23]

Drug interactions

In rats, AmB decreases the concentration of hepatic microsomal cytochrome P450 and inhibits propafenone metabolism.[24] Drug interactions due to shared metabolic pathways have not been described in humans. Hypokalemia may be aggravated by corticosteroids, and hypomagnesemia may become especially profound in cancer patients with platinum-associated nephropathy. Amphotericin B may enhance plasma levels and toxicity of renally cleared drugs, including aminoglycosides, vancomycin, flucytosine and ciclosporin. Simultaneous infusion of granulocytes has been associated with acute pulmonary reactions and should be used with extreme caution.

Indications and dosing

Despite its toxicity profile, AmB deoxycholate remains an important option for initial treatment of many life-threatening fungal infections. Depending on the type of infection and the host, recommended daily dosages range from 0.5 mg/kg/day to 1.5 mg/kg/day administered over 2–4 hours as tolerated; the standard dosage for empiric therapy in persistently febrile neutropenic patients is 0.5–0.6 mg/kg/day.[22] Continuous infusion of AmB deoxycholate is counterintuitive to the concentration-dependent pharmacodynamics of AmB and is not recommended. Whether the enhanced plasma clearance in infants and young children has implications for dosing remains unknown. Currently, dosage recommendations for all pediatric age groups do not differ from those in adults. Treatment should be started at the full target dosage with careful bedside monitoring during the first infusion to allow for prompt intervention for infusion-related reactions.

Therapeutic monitoring

Historically, 1-hour postinfusion plasma concentrations of twice the MIC of the fungal isolate have been proposed as a target for the treatment of yeast infections.[25] However, monitoring of AmB concentrations in plasma or CSF appears of little value, since relationships between plasma and tissue concentrations and clinical efficacy or toxicity have not been adequately characterized.[10]

Amphotericin B lipid formulations

Three lipid formulations of AmB have been approved in the USA and most of Europe:

- AmB colloidal dispersion (ABCD, Amphocil or Amphotec);
- AmB lipid complex (ABLC or Abelcet); and
- a small unilamellar vesicle (SUV) liposomal formulation (L-AmB, AmBisome).

Because of their reduced nephrotoxicity in comparison to AmB deoxycholate, these compounds allow for the delivery of higher dosages of AmB. However, data from animal models also suggest that higher dosages are required for equivalent antifungal efficacy.

Physicochemical properties and pharmacokinetics

Each of the lipid formulations confers distinct plasma pharmacokinetic properties to AmB. All three formulations preferentially distribute to organs of the mononuclear phagocytic system (MPS); sequester lipid-associated drug within deep tissues and functionally spare the kidney. L-AmB, the only truly liposomal AmB, is composed of small spherical unilamellar lipid vesicles averaging 60–70 nm in size. This preparation has a prolonged circulation time in plasma, achieves strikingly high peak plasma concentrations and AUC values and is only slowly taken up by the MPS. However, most of the AmB in plasma remains liposome associated and free unbound drug concentrations are low.[16,17] ABLC is composed of ribbon-like lipid aggregates. It is efficiently opsonized by plasma proteins and rapidly taken up by the MPS to achieve high concentrations in cellular components of blood, liver, lung and spleen. ABLC exists as a depot in these tissues and free AmB is slowly released. Fungal and inflammatory cell lipases at the site of infection act to release AmB from the lipid carrier.[26] ABCD, a colloidal dispersion of microscopic disc-shaped particles, also preferentially collects in tissues of the MPS and free drug is slowly released over time. Drug levels in the plasma and kidney are low and terminal elimination half-life is long (Table 149.1). Whether these distinct pharmacokinetic features translate into different pharmacodynamic properties is largely unknown. Comparisons of all four formulations of AmB against defined infections suggest potentially important differences in efficacy depending on agent, dose, type and site of infection.[7]

Safety and antifungal efficacy

Safety and efficacy of the lipid formulations have been demonstrated in phase I/II studies in immunocompromised patients with a wide spectrum of underlying disorders.[27–29] The overall response rates in these trials ranged from 53% to 84% for invasive candidiasis and 34% to 5%, respectively, in probable or documented invasive aspergillosis. Clinical and microbiologic responses were observed even when lipid formulations were used after failure of conventional AmB deoxycholate. Patients with neutropenia responded to therapy with lipid formulations; however, as with other antifungal agents, outcomes were dependent on host factors. Several randomized controlled trials have compared lipid formulations with AmB deoxycholate. These studies have consistently shown at least equivalent efficacy and reduced nephrotoxicity in comparison to AmB deoxycholate. A meta-analysis of 1149 neutropenic patients from three trials found that prophylactic or empiric use of L-AmB tended to be more effective than AmB deoxycholate in preventing breakthrough fungal infections, was associated with less nephrotoxicity but did not alter survival.[30] Infusion-related side-effects are less frequent with L-AmB but may be increased with ABCD.[20,31,32] Substernal chest discomfort, respiratory distress and sharp flank pain have been noted during infusion of L-AmB. Hypoxic episodes associated with fever and chills are more frequent with ABCD than AmB deoxycholate.[22] Mild increases in serum bilirubin and alkaline phosphatases have been observed with lipid formulations. Generally mild increases in serum transaminases and pancreatic enzymes have been observed with L-AmB.

Indications and dosing

The lipid formulations are indicated for the treatment of patients with AmB-susceptible invasive mycoses who are refractory to, or intolerant of, AmB deoxycholate and are limited to L-AmB for empiric therapy of persistently neutropenic patients. Preliminary pediatric pharmacokinetic and safety data indicate no fundamental differences in comparison to adults. The optimal dosages of each formulation for the various types and sites of invasive fungal infection remain to be defined. Based on animal data and the few randomized studies that have used AmB deoxycholate as comparator,[33] the authors and most other experts in the field consider a dose of 5 mg/kg/day of ABCD, ABLC and

Table 149.1 Amphotericin B formulations: physicochemical properties and pharmacokinetic parameters

	DAMB	ABCD	ABLC	LAMB
Lipids (molar ratio)	Deoxycholate	Cholesterylsulfate	DMPC/DMPG (7:3)	HPC/CHOL/DSPG (2:1:0.8)
Mol% drug	34	50	50	10
Lipid configuration	Micelles	Micelles	Membrane-like	SUVs
Particle diameter (μm)	0.05	0.12–0.14	1.6–11	0.08
Dosage (mg/kg)	1	5	5	5
C_{max} (μg/ml)	2.9	3.1	1.7	58
$AUC_{0-\infty}$ (μg/ml.h)	36	43	14	713
VD_{ss} (l/kg)	1.1	4.3	131	0.22
Cl (l/h/kg)	0.028	0.117	0.476	0.017
Half-life (h)	39	28	6–18	7–10

DAMB, amphotericin B deoxycholate; ABCD, amphotericin B colloidal dispersion; ABLC, amphotericin B lipid complex; LAMB, liposomal amphotericin B; DMPC, dimiristoyl phosphatidylcholine; DMPG, dimiristoyl phosphatidylglycerol; HPC, hydrogenated phosphatidylcholine; CHOL, cholesterol; DSPG, disteaoryl phosphatidylglycerol; SUVs, small unilamellar vesicles (liposomes); C_{max}, peak plasma concentration; $AUC_{0-\infty}$, area under the concentration vs time curve from time zero to infinity; VD_{ss}, apparent volume of distribution at steady state; Cl, plasma clearance; Half-life, apparent plasma half-life during the dosing interval of 24 hours. Data represent mean values, stem from adult patients and were obtained after different rates of infusion. Modified from Groll et al.[52]

L-AmB equivalent to a dosage of 1 mg/kg/day of AmB deoxycholate. Accordingly, an initial dosage of 5 mg/kg/d of ABCD, ABLC or L-AmB is recommended for suspected or documented life-threatening infections, and 3 mg/kg/day when L-AmB is selected for empiric antifungal therapy in persistently febrile neutropenic patients; 3 mg/kg/day may be effective in histoplasmosis and selected patients with candidiasis.[34] Some clinicians have successfully used L-AmB at 10 mg/kg/day and 15 mg/kg/day in patients with recalcitrant invasive fungal infections. However, such doses may provide no additional efficacy and more nephrotoxicity.[35]

Use of the lipid formulations has been limited by their higher costs. Comprehensive analyses that include hospital and societal costs due to excess nephrotoxicity relating to the use of conventional AmB deoxycholate are indicating that the higher cost of lipid formulations of AmB may be supplanted by the even greater cost of AmB deoxycholate-induced nephrotoxicity. Among patients receiving AmB, even slight decreases in renal function are associated with longer hospitalizations and severe nephrotoxicity is a significant predictor of death.[36] At an increasing number of centers the current practice is to limit use of AmB deoxycholate to patients having the lowest risk for nephrotoxicity and to switch to a lipid formulation with decreasing renal function.

Aerosolized amphotericin B

Nebulized AmB is increasingly used as antimold prophylaxis in lung transplant and neutropenic patients. All four AmB formulations can be aerosolized. This approach appears promising in animal studies and early clinical trials.[37,38] Aerosol size and uniformity vary with AmB formulation and nebulizer technique.[39] These variables may impact delivered drug dose to the lung. Furthermore, within individual patients, delivered dose may be suboptimal in some lung segments.[33]

Current protocols employ varying doses, regimens and delivery systems. When tolerated, as in lung transplant recipients, aerosolized AmB is effective at preventing aspergillosis. Common side-effects are cough, adverse taste and nausea.[40,41] Tolerability remains a major drawback in very fragile and weak patients. Cough and inability to use an aerosol delivery system are common limitations.[37]

FLUCYTOSINE

Flucytosine (5-fluorocytosine; 5-FC) is a low molecular weight water-soluble synthetic fluorinated analogue of cytosine (Fig. 149.3). It has no antifungal activity of its own. It is taken up by the fungus-specific enzyme cytosine permease and converted in the cytoplasm by cytosine deaminase to 5-fluorouracil which causes RNA miscoding and inhibits DNA synthesis.[42,43] Although it was originally synthesized as a potential anti-tumor agent, 5-FC is relatively nontoxic to mammalian cells.

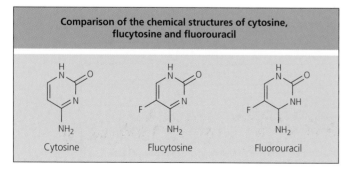

Comparison of the chemical structures of cytosine, flucytosine and fluorouracil

Cytosine Flucytosine Fluorouracil

Fig. 149.3 Comparison of the chemical structures of cytosine, flucytosine and fluorouracil.

Antifungal activity

The antifungal spectrum of 5-FC *in vitro* encompasses *Candida* spp., *Cr. neoformans*, *Saccharomyces cerevisiae* and selected dematiaceous molds; 5-FC has little to no activity against *Aspergillus* spp. and other hyaline molds.[43] Synergistic or additive effects in combination with AmB have been observed against *Candida* spp. and in combination with AmB, fluconazole or posaconazole against *Cr. neoformans*.[44,45] With the exception of *Candida krusei*, primary resistance occurs very rarely in *Candida* spp.[46] Resistance (MIC ≥32 µg/ml) has been observed in 1.6–2.2% of *Cr. neoformans* isolates.[47] In contrast to primary resistance, secondary resistance, which occurs predominantly by selection of resistant clones, can evolve rapidly and appears to result from a single point mutation. In *Cr. neoformans* resistance has been observed in 30–40% of isolates from patients with meningitis who relapsed following monotherapy. Resistance in susceptible fungi may involve either mutations in the enzymes necessary for cellular uptake, transport or metabolism, or competitive upregulation of pyrimidine synthesis.[42] As a consequence, 5-FC is rarely given alone but in combination with AmB or, more recently, fluconazole.

Pharmacodynamics

Flucytosine has demonstrated predominantly concentration-independent fungistatic (99% reduction in CFU) activity against *Candida* spp. and *Cr. neoformans* in time-kill assays and prolonged concentration- and exposure-dependent postantifungal effects of up to 10 hours.[48,49] Pharmacodynamic studies in mice with disseminated candidiasis indicate that time above the MIC and AUC/MIC are the most important parameters in predicting efficacy. The C_{max}/MIC ratio was the least important parameter and maximum efficacy was observed when levels exceeded the MIC for only 20–25% of the 24-hour dosing interval.[50] Thus, lower dosages or less frequent dosing may yield identical efficacy while reducing the mostly dose-dependent toxicities.

Pharmacokinetics

Oral 5-FC is readily absorbed from the gastrointestinal tract, has negligible protein binding and distributes evenly into tissues and body fluids, including the CSF, peritoneal fluid, inflamed joints and the eye. Intravenous 5-FC results in significantly higher serum drug levels, but the clinical or microbiologic implications of this are unknown.[51] At usual dosages, the drug undergoes little hepatic metabolism and is eliminated predominantly in active form by glomerular filtration into the urine with a half-life in plasma of 3–6 hours. Individual dosage adjustment is necessary in patients with impaired renal function and those undergoing hemofiltration. In patients undergoing hemodialysis, a dose of 37.5 mg/kg is recommended following dialysis; in peritoneal dialysis, 5-FC can be administered systemically or intraperitoneally.[42] Impaired liver function does not appear to alter 5-FC disposition.[52] As the pharmacokinetics of 5-FC in children have not been formally characterized, uniform dosing recommendations cannot be made.

Adverse effects

Common adverse effects of 5-FC include gastrointestinal intolerance and reversible elevations of hepatic transaminases and alkaline phosphatase. More rare are rashes, ulcerative colitis and bowel perforation, eosinophilia and crystalluria.[52] Hematologic adverse effects may include neutropenia, thrombocytopenia or pancytopenia. Among 202 AIDS patients receiving combination therapy with AmB and 5-FC for cryptococcal meningitis, the drug toxicity withdrawal rate of 3% was similar to those receiving AmB monotherapy.[53] Although adverse affects are usually reversible following discontinuation of the drug or dosage reduction, fatal outcomes have been reported. Some adverse effects may be due to conversion of 5-FC to 5-fluorouracil by gastrointestinal bacteria and toxic effects of endogenous metabolites.[42]

In patients treated with intravenous 5-FC, in whom the drug presumably did not undergo metabolism by intestinal microflora, 5-fluorouracil levels were not detected, but some toxicity was still observed. Hematologic adverse effects are less frequent if plasma levels do not exceed 100 μg/ml.[52]

Drug interactions

Orally administered, nonresorbable antibiotics and aluminum/magnesium hydroxide-based antacids may delay oral 5-FC absorption.[52] Flucytosine is not known to interfere with the CYP450 enzyme system. However, drugs causing reduction in the GFR may increase 5-FC serum levels. Cytosine arabinoside competitively inhibits 5-FC and both drugs should not be given concomitantly.

Indications and dosing

Due to the propensity for secondary resistance, 5-FC is generally not administered alone. An established indication for its use in combination with AmB deoxycholate is for induction therapy of cryptococcal meningitis.[53] In cryptococcosis, sterilization of CSF is significantly faster when AmB is used in combination with 5-FC.[55] This combination can also be recommended for deep tissue candidiasis, particularly in critically ill patients and when non-*albicans Candida* spp. are involved. This includes meningitis, endophthalmitis, endocarditis, vasculitis and peritonitis, as well as osteoarticular, renal and chronic disseminated candidiasis.[52] Flucytosine may delay hematopoietic recovery after cytotoxic chemotherapy and is not recommended as part of empiric therapy of persistently febrile neutropenic patients. Flucytosine with fluconazole may be used for cryptococcal meningitis, when treatment with AmB is not feasible. This combination may also be useful as second-line therapy for individual patients with invasive *Candida* infections involving aqueous body compartments. We recommend a starting dosage for both adults and children of 100 mg/kg/day

divided into three or four doses. However, when used in combination with AmB for disseminated candidiasis, 5-FC dosage of 25 mg/kg/day in four divided doses may suffice.[56]

Therapeutic monitoring

Monitoring of plasma concentrations is essential to adjust dosage to changing renal function and to avoid toxicity. Most patients have levels outside the expected therapeutic range and high levels are particularly common in neonates. In one report, nearly 10% of patients had potentially toxic levels (>100 μg/ml).[57] Following oral administration, near peak levels 2 hours post dosing overlap with trough levels as patients reach steady state and are thus sufficient for therapeutic monitoring. Peak plasma levels between 40 μg/ml and 60 μg/ml correlate with antifungal efficacy and are seldom associated with hematologic adverse effects.[54] The need for monitoring plasma concentrations has limited the use of 5-FC as this test is often restricted to referral laboratories.

ANTIFUNGAL TRIAZOLES

The antifungal azoles are a class of synthetic compounds that have one or more azole rings and – attached to one of the nitrogen atoms – a more or less complex side chain. The imidazoles miconazole and ketoconazole were the first azoles developed for systemic treatment of human mycoses. Severe toxicities associated with the drug carrier (miconazole), erratic absorption and significant interference with the human cytochrome P450 system (ketoconazole) have limited their clinical usefulness.[52] The subsequently developed triazoles (Fig. 149.4), however, have become extremely useful agents. They possess an expanded spectrum of activity and greater target specificity, and are overall well tolerated.

Chemical structures of fluconazole, itraconazole, voriconazole, posaconazole and ravuconazole

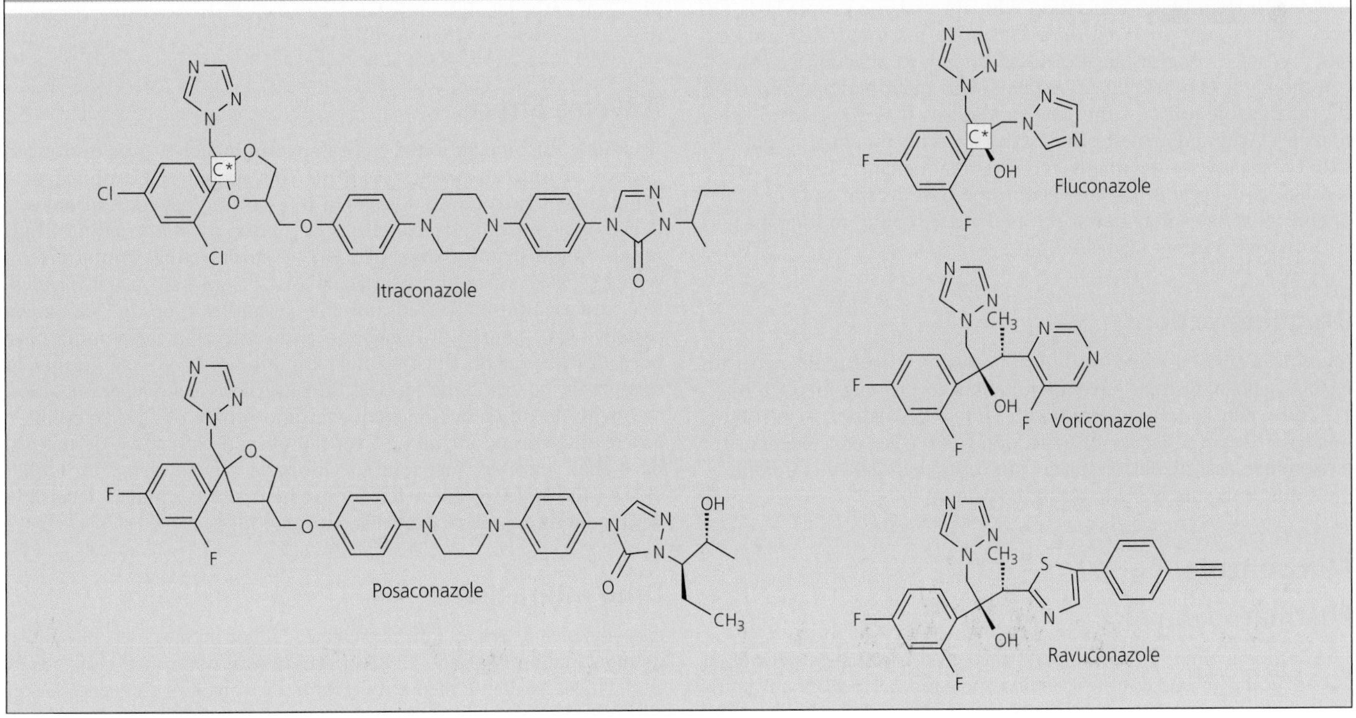

Fig. 149.4 Chemical structures of fluconazole, itraconazole, voriconazole, posaconazole and ravuconazole.

Mechanism of action

The antifungal azoles target ergosterol biosynthesis by inhibiting the fungal cytochrome P450-dependent enzyme lanosterol 14-α-demethylase. This inhibition interrupts the conversion of lanosterol to ergosterol, which leads to accumulation of aberrant 14-α-methylsterols and depletion of ergosterol in the fungal cell membrane (see Fig. 149.2). This alters cell membrane physiology and, depending on organism and compound, may lead to cell death or inhibition of cell growth and replication. The azoles also inhibit cytochrome P450-dependent enzymes of the fungal respiration chain.[52]

Antifungal activity

Fluconazole and itraconazole are principally active against dermatophytes, *Candida* spp., *Cr. neoformans*, *Trichosporon* spp. and some other uncommon yeast-like organisms, and against dimorphic fungi such as *Histoplasma capsulatum*, *Coccidioides immitis*, *Blastomyces dermatitidis*, *Paracoccidioides brasiliensis* and *Sporothrix schenkii*.[52] These azoles have less activity against *Candida glabrata* and almost none against *C. krusei*.[58] Itraconazole is active against *Aspergillus* spp. and dematiaceous molds. Neither is active against *Fusarium* spp. and the zygomycetes.[52] The second-generation triazoles, voriconazole and posaconazole, are active against *C. albicans* and *C. krusei*, *Aspergillus* spp. and some *Fusarium* spp. Posaconazole is also active against zygomycetes.[59]

Resistance

Selection and nosocomial spread of azole-resistant *Candida* spp. is a matter of increasing concern. Resistance in *Candida* is encountered most commonly in the form of a primarily resistant species or through selection of resistant subclones during exposure to azoles. Several mechanisms have been identified, including alterations at the target binding site, increased target expression and induction of cellular efflux pumps. *Candida* in biofilm is significantly less susceptible to fluconazole, voriconazole and posaconazole.[28] This is at least partly mediated by expression of efflux pumps and alteration in sterol composition.[60]

Azole-resistant oropharyngeal and esophageal candidiasis remains a challenge in some AIDS patients.[61] Emergence of *C. glabrata* and *C. krusei* infections in association with fluconazole prophylaxis has been sporadically observed in several bone marrow transplant centers.[62] While cross-resistance of *Candida* spp. to antifungal azoles is common,[63] it is not obligate: patients with microbiologic and clinical fluconazole-resistant mucosal candidiasis may respond to other triazoles. Acquired azole resistance has been documented in patients with *Cr. neoformans* meningitis receiving maintenance therapy. Azole-resistant *A. fumigatus* has emerged in the past decade and up to 6% of clinical isolates may have decreased susceptibility to itraconazole, voriconazole and posaconazole.[64]

Drug interactions

Caution is advised when antifungal azoles are co-administered with CYP3A4 substrates that have the potential to prolong the QTc interval and when co-administered with HMG-CoA reductase inhibitors that have the potential to cause rhabdomyolysis. The concurrent use of terfenadine, astemizole, cisapride, pimozide, halofantrine, dofetilide, quinidine and vincristine is contraindicated.

Fluconazole

Pharmacodynamics

Conventional time-kill assays performed over incubation periods of 24–48 hours in susceptible *Candida* spp. and *Cr. neoformans* show fungistatic activity of fluconazole with variable concentration-related growth effects.[65,66] However, with extended incubation of up to 14 days and under nonproliferating growth conditions, fungicidal activity has been observed against *C. albicans*.[67] In serum-free growth media, fluconazole displays no measurable postantifungal effect (PAFE) against *C. albicans* and *Cr. neoformans*, but concentration-dependent PAFEs of 1–3.6 hours were observed in the presence of fresh serum.[10] Clinical data and pharmacodynamic studies in murine models of disseminated *C. albicans* infection collectively suggest that the AUC/MIC ratio is the most predictive pharmacodynamic parameter of fluconazole.[68,69] Overall, the dose-independent pharmacokinetics and the available experimental and clinical data are in support of once-daily dosing regimens.

Pharmacokinetics

Fluconazole is available for oral and parenteral use, and exhibits linear plasma pharmacokinetics that are independent of route and formulation. Steady state is generally reached within 4–7 days following once-daily dosing, but can be rapidly achieved by doubling the dose on the first day. Bioavailability may vary greatly among critically ill surgical patients.[70] Protein binding is low, and the drug distributes evenly into virtually all tissue sites and body fluids, including the CSF, brain tissue and the eye. More than 90% of a dose is renally excreted, with approximately 80% recovered as unchanged active drug and 11% recovered as inactive metabolites. In patients with a creatinine clearance of ≤50 ml/min, a 50% reduction in dosage is required, and below 21 ml/min, a 75% reduction is needed. The initial loading dose need not be adjusted. Fluconazole is dialyzable; in patients undergoing hemodialysis, 100% of the target dose is given after each dialysis session. In continuous hemofiltration, clearance may be faster, requiring therapy at maximum approved dosages; in patients undergoing peritoneal dialysis, the compound can be administered either systemically or intraperitoneally. Hepatic insufficiency does not require dose adjustments, but careful monitoring of additional hepatic toxicity is warranted.[52]

The pharmacokinetics in children reflect developmental changes characteristic for a water-soluble drug with minor metabolism and predominantly renal elimination. Except for premature neonates, where clearance is initially decreased, children tend to have an increased weight-normalized clearance rate from plasma that leads to a shorter half-life in comparison to adults. As serum levels in neonates depend upon both gestational age at birth and postnatal age,[71] dosages at the high end of the recommended dosage range are necessary for the treatment of invasive mycoses in children.

Adverse effects

In adults, fluconazole has been safely administered over prolonged periods of time at dosages of up to 1600 mg/day.[72] Compiled data from adults who received dosages of 100–400 mg/day indicate an incidence of significant adverse effects or laboratory abnormalities leading to drug discontinuation of 2.8%. Gastrointestinal symptoms are seen in <5%, rashes and headaches in <2% and are usually reversible, and asymptomatic transaminase elevations in up to 7% of adult patients. QT segment prolongation and ventricular tachycardia have been described with fluconazole.[73] In children of all age groups, at dosages of up to 12 mg/kg/day, fluconazole is generally well tolerated with no differences in frequency and profile of adverse events.[29] Severe side-effects, including liver failure and exfoliative dermatitis, have been reported anecdotally.[52] Alopecia can be seen with higher doses (400 mg/day) given for 2 months or longer and is reversible with reduced dosage or drug discontinuation.[74]

Drug interactions

Fluconazole undergoes minimal CYP-mediated metabolism, but inhibits intestinal and hepatic CYP3A4 and several other CYP isoforms *in vitro*. Fluconazole interacts with enzymes involved in glucuronidation and is a substrate of the drug transporter P-glycoprotein, leading to a number of significant drug interactions (Table 149.2). Interactions

Table 149.2 Drug–drug interactions of fluconazole and itraconazole

Mechanism and drug involved	Triazole involved	Comment
Decreased plasma concentration of triazole		
Decreased absorption of triazole • Antacids, H$_2$ antagonists • Omeprazole, sucralfate • Didanosine, grapefruit juice	Itra**	Take antacids and antifungal agent at least 2 hours apart
Increased metabolism of triazole • Isoniazid, rifampin (rifampicin) • Rifabutin, phenytoin • Phenobarbital, carbamazepine	Itra**, flu	Potential for therapy failure; increased potential for hepatotoxicity
Increased concentration of co-administered drug through inhibition of its metabolism by triazole		
Terfenadine, astemizole, cisapride	Flu‡, Itra‡	Concom. use prohibited
Lovastatin, simvastatin, atorvastatin	Itra‡, Flu‡	Concom. use prohibited
Phenytoin	Flu*, Itra*	Monitor levels
Benzodiazepines	Flu†, Itra†	Monitor closely
Carbamazepine	Flu†	Monitor closely
Haloperidol	Itra†	Monitor closely
Rifampin (rifampicin), rifabutin	Flu†, Itra†	Monitor closely
Clarithromycin	Itra†	Monitor closely
Indinavir, ritonavir	Itra†	Monitor closely
Vincristine, vinblastine, vindesine	Itra*	Avoid concom. use
Busulfan	Itra†	Avoid concom. use
All-trans retinoic acid	Flu†	Monitor closely
Nifedipine, felodipine	Itra†, Flu†	Monitor closely
Ciclosporin A, tacrolimus	Flu†, Itra†	Monitor serum level
Sulfonylurea drugs, warfarin, prednisolone	Flu†, Itra†	Monitor closely
Digoxin, quinidine	Itra†	Monitor levels (digoxin)
Zidovudine, theophyllin	Flu†	Monitor closely

Flu, fluconazole; Itra, itraconazole.
*Major significance; †moderate significance; ‡contraindicated.
Modified from Groll et al.[52]

with other CYP3A4 substrates, including calcineurin inhibitors, may be more pronounced with oral fluconazole.[75] On the other hand, drugs notorious for hepatic enzyme induction – for example, rifampin (rifampicin) – may decrease fluconazole levels.[52] Altogether, the number of relevant drug interactions is lower than with ketoconazole and itraconazole.

Indications and dosing

Fluconazole is highly effective for treatment of superficial and invasive candidiasis, including infections in neutropenic patients.[76] However, in unstable patients and in recipients of azole prophylaxis, an alternative therapy should be considered. Other indications for fluconazole include consolidation therapy for chronic disseminated candidiasis, cryptococcal meningitis and infections by *Trichosporon* spp. Fluconazole is the drug of choice for treatment of coccidioidal meningitis and has effectiveness in nonmeningeal coccidioidal infections;[77,78] against paracoccidioidomycosis, blastomycosis, histoplasmosis and sporotrichosis, fluconazole is less active than itraconazole.[79–82] In the prophylactic setting, fluconazole has proven efficacy for primary prevention of invasive candidiasis in high-risk patients with acute leukemia, bone marrow and liver transplantation, for primary prevention of cryptococcosis and histoplasmosis in advanced AIDS and for secondary prevention of cryptococcosis and coccidioidomycosis in AIDS.[83,84]

In adults, the recommended dosage range for treatment of invasive infections is 400–800 mg/day and 100–400 mg/day in the preventive setting. In children, the recommended dosage range is 6–12 mg/kg/day. In view of the faster clearance rate, the larger volume of distribution

and its safety profile, 12 mg/kg/day may be more appropriate for serious infections in term neonates, infants and children. Given the extreme variability in extravascular water content and renal function, particularly in very low birth weight preterm infants, predictably effective and safe treatment with fluconazole may not be possible during the first days of life.

Itraconazole

Pharmacodynamics

Itraconazole (ITC) exerts species- and strain-dependent fungistatic or fungicidal pharmacodynamics *in vitro*. Time-kill experiments have demonstrated concentration-independent, fungistatic activity of ITC against *Candida* spp. and *Cr. neoformans*.[10] Against *Aspergillus* spp., however, ITC displayed time- and concentration-dependent fungicidal activity with >87% to >97% killing within 24 hours of drug exposure.[85] Persistent effects have not been reported thus far, and it remains to be determined which pharmacodynamic parameter best predicts antifungal efficacy *in vivo*.[10]

Pharmacokinetics

Itraconazole is a high-molecular weight, highly lipophilic bis-triazole. It is available as capsules and as an oral solution in hydroxypropyl-β-cyclodextrin (HP-β-CD). Absorption from the capsule form is dependent on a low intragastric pH and is compromised in the fasting state, and thus is unpredictable in granulocytopenic cancer patients and in patients with hypochlorhydria. Absorption is improved when the capsules are taken with food or an acidic cola beverage. Itraconazole oral solution in HP-β-CD provides better oral bioavailability that is further enhanced in the fasting state.[86]

Following oral administration, peak plasma concentrations occur within 1–4 hours; systemic absorption of the cyclodextrin carrier is negligible. With once-daily dosing, steady state is achieved after 7–14 days, but can be reached more rapidly by doubling the dose over the first 2–3 days. Itraconazole is highly protein-bound and is extensively distributed throughout the body. Although concentrations in nonproteinaceous body fluids are negligible, tissue concentrations in many organs, including the brain, exceed corresponding plasma levels by 2–10 times.[86]

Itraconazole is extensively metabolized in the liver and excreted in metabolized form into bile and urine. The major metabolite, hydroxy-itraconazole (OH-ITC), possesses antifungal activity similar to ITC.[52] The elimination of ITC from plasma follows a biphasic pattern; in comparison to single dosing, the elimination half-life at steady state is about twice as long, reflecting saturable excretion mechanisms.[52]

The dosage of oral ITC does not need to be adjusted with renal insufficiency or dialysis. In patients with severe hepatic insufficiency, the elimination half-life of ITC can be prolonged and additional hepatic toxicity or possible drug interactions should be carefully monitored.[86] The pharmacokinetics of oral HP-β-CD ITC in pediatric patients beyond the neonatal period appear similar to that of adults.[87–89]

Adverse effects

Itraconazole is usually well tolerated, with a similar spectrum and frequency of adverse effects as fluconazole. Adverse events leading to the discontinuation of ITC occur in approximately 4% of patients treated for systemic fungal infections at dosages of up to 400 mg/day. Most observed reactions are transient, and include nausea and vomiting (<10%), hypertriglyceridemia (9%), hypokalemia (6%), elevated hepatic transaminases (5%), rash and/or pruritus (2%), headaches or dizziness (<2%) and pedal edema (1%).[90] Gastrointestinal intolerance is frequent with oral HP-β-CD ITC at dosages exceeding 400 mg/day. Only a few cases of more severe hepatic injury or hepatitis have been described. Itraconazole can have negative inotropic effects; because of a possible risk of cardiac toxicity, ITC should not be administered to patients with ventricular dysfunction.[91]

Oral HP-β-CD ITC was safe and well tolerated in pharmacokinetic studies in pediatric patients.[92] Vomiting (12%), abnormal liver function tests (5%) and abdominal pain (3%) were the most common adverse effects in 103 neutropenic pediatric cancer patients who received the drug at 5 mg/kg/day or 2.5 mg/kg q12h for antifungal prophylaxis; 18% of patients withdrew from the study because of adverse events.[93]

Drug interactions

In comparison to fluconazole, both propensity and extent of drug–drug interactions are greater (see Table 149.2). Itraconazole is a substrate of CYP3A4, but also interacts with the heme moiety of CYP3A, resulting in noncompetitive inhibition of oxidative metabolism of many CYP3A substrates and increased and potentially toxic concentrations of co-administered drugs. Increased metabolism of ITC resulting in decreased plasma levels can result from co-administration of inducers of hepatic enzymes. Finally, the systemic availability of ITC depends in part on the activity of intestinal CYP3A4 and P-glycoprotein, which contributes to its variable bioavailability after oral administration.

Indications and dosing

Itraconazole is useful for dermatophytic infections, pityriasis versicolor and all forms of cutaneous and mucosal candidiasis; however, its clinical efficacy in invasive candidiasis has not been evaluated. Itraconazole has been successful for consolidation and maintenance treatment of cryptococcosis in the setting of HIV infection.[94]

Itraconazole is approved as a second-line agent for treatment of invasive aspergillosis; few data exist on its use for first-line treatment in neutropenic patients.[97] Itraconazole may be useful in the management of infections by certain dematiaceous molds, but is inactive against zygomycosis and fusariosis. Itraconazole is the current treatment of choice for lymphocutaneous sporotrichosis and non-life-threatening, nonmeningeal paracoccidioidomycosis, blastomycosis and histoplasmosis. In progressive nonmeningeal coccidioidomycosis, ITC appears at least as active as fluconazole.[77] However, AmB remains the treatment of choice for most immunocompromised patients and for life-threatening infection.

Itraconazole has been successful as antifungal prophylaxis in patients undergoing stem cell transplantation or intensive chemotherapy.[93] HP-β-CD ITC may reduce the incidence of proven or suspected invasive fungal infections in neutropenic patients with hematologic malignancies.[96] Itraconazole was at least as effective as conventional AmB and less toxic as empiric therapy in persistently febrile, neutropenic patients,[97] which has led to the approval of this indication by the US Food and Drug Administration (FDA).

The recommended dosage range of oral itraconazole is 100–400 mg/day (capsules) and 2.5 mg/kg q12h (HP-β-CD solution). For life-threatening infections, higher doses may be necessary. For such conditions, we recommend a loading dose of 600–800 mg/day for 3–5 days, followed by a maintenance dose of 400–600 mg/day, and monitoring of serum levels. Itraconazole is not approved for patients <18 years of age; based on the available pharmacokinetic data, a starting dosage of 2.5 mg/kg q12h of oral HP-β-CD ITC can be advocated. The recommended dosage range for the capsule formulation is 5–8 mg/kg/day with a loading dose of 4 mg/kg q8h for the first 3 days.

Therapeutic monitoring

Data from a large cohort of patients with acute leukemia receiving ITC have demonstrated an association of trough concentrations <0.5 μg/ml with occurrence of invasive fungal infections. We therefore recommend rapid achievement and maintenance of trough levels of ≥0.5 μg/ml when ITC is given for prevention or treatment of invasive fungal infections.

Second-generation antifungal triazoles

Further improvements in the structure–activity relationship of antifungal triazoles have led to a new group of synthetic compounds that are collectively known as second-generation triazoles, comprising voriconazole, posaconazole, ravuconazole and isavuconazole. Voriconazole and posaconazole are approved for clinical use. Ravuconazole (BMS-207147 and its prodrug BMS 292655; Eisai Inc., Woodcliff Lake, New Jersey) and isavuconazole (BAL8557; Basilea Pharmaceutica Ltd, Basel, Switzerland) are currently in clinical development. Ravuconazole and voriconazole are structurally related to fluconazole, and posaconazole is similar in structure to itraconazole.

Pharmacodynamics

The second-generation triazoles possess enhanced target activity and specificity. They are active against a wide spectrum of clinically important fungi, including *Candida* spp., *Trichosporon* spp., *Cr. neoformans*, *Aspergillus* spp., *Fusarium* spp. and other hyaline molds, and dematiaceous as well as dimorphic molds. They have demonstrated efficacy in animal models of invasive fungal infections. Similar to itraconazole, these novel triazoles exert fungistatic activity against susceptible yeast-like organisms and strain-dependent fungicidal activity against susceptible filamentous fungi. Fundamental differences in potency, spectrum and antifungal efficacy between posa-, isavu-, ravu- and voriconazole have not surfaced, but posaconazole appears to have the best activity against zygomycetes. In *Candida* spp. and *Cr. neoformans* voriconazole exhibits nonconcentration-dependent pharmacodynamics. Near-maximal fungistatic activity is achieved at a drug concentration of approximately three times the MIC.[98] A postantifungal effect of up to 4 hours has been observed with *C. albicans*.[99] Voriconazole also has immunomodulatory properties that may enhance the immune response to *A. fumigatus*.[100]

Voriconazole

Pharmacokinetics

Voriconazole is available as a tablet and parenteral solution that uses sulfobutyl ether-β-cyclodextrin (SE-β-CD) as a solubilizer. In tablet form, voriconazole is rapidly absorbed from the gastrointestinal tract. Although bioavailability is near 100%, steady-state plasma concentrations are achieved more rapidly with an intravenous loading dose. Multiple enzymes of the cytochrome P450 system including CYP2C19, which exhibits genetic polymorphism in certain racial groups, metabolize voriconazole. Drug levels in poor metabolizers, which may include up to 20% of Asian populations, can be significantly elevated. Plasma levels in extensive or ultrarapid metabolizers may be much lower.[101] In adults, voriconazole exhibits nonlinear pharmacokinetics, possibly due to saturable metabolism and systemic clearance.[102] In contrast, elimination of voriconazole in children is linear and higher relative dosages may be required to achieve exposures consistent with those in adults.[103] Given the multiplicity of factors that may impact voriconazole pharmacokinetics, therapeutic drug monitoring is increasingly used and may improve outcomes.[104]

Voriconazole has been used successfully in patients with central nervous system mycoses. Cerebrospinal fluid concentrations vary greatly, but are generally approximately half the serum concentration and have a linear relationship to dose.[105] Voriconazole has been evaluated in ocular infections, and concentrations in the vitreous and aqueous are 38% and 53% of serum levels, respectively.[106] The addition of a 1% topical voriconazole solution can further increase vitreous and aqueous levels and therapeutic concentrations against many pathogenic fungi may be achieved with topical therapy alone.[107,108] Voriconazole may also be injected directly into the cornea, the anterior chamber and the vitreous in cases of invasive fungal keratitis and endophthalmitis.

Following its metabolism in the liver, the drug is mostly excreted in urine. The pharmacokinetics are unaffected by renal function. Concern has arisen regarding the potential for accumulation of the renally metabolized, and potentially nephrotoxic, intravenous carrier solution SE-β-CD in patients with renal impairment. Whether accumulation of SE-β-CD in such patients is clinically relevant is unclear.[109,110]

Drug interactions

In addition to undergoing metabolism by the P450 system, voriconazole inhibits several CYP enzymes, leading to extensive potential for drug–drug interactions. Extreme care must be taken when co-administering voriconazole with agents metabolized through the P450 system, particularly with drugs having narrow therapeutic windows such as calcineurin inhibitors and sirolimus.

Adverse affects

Mild and reversible visual disturbances occur in approximately 30% of patients. This may manifest as altered color perception, photophobia or blurred vision. The mechanism is unknown, but is thought to be retinal. Other common adverse reactions include rashes and phototoxicity, gastrointestinal disturbances and hepatic abnormalities. Visual and/or auditory hallucinations occur in up to 16.6% of patients, may be related to higher serum drug levels and are particularly associated with intravenously administered voriconazole.[111]

Clinical studies

Voriconazole is indicated for primary treatment of aspergillosis and candidemia, as well as for salvage therapy for fusariosis and scedosporiosis.

In a randomized, open label trial of patients with invasive aspergillosis, initial therapy with voriconazole led to a significantly greater response rate, improved survival and less toxicity than the standard approach of initial therapy with AmB deoxycholate.[112] Voriconazole also has been used successfully in the treatment of invasive fungal infections including aspergillosis in children who were refractory to, or intolerant of, conventional antifungal therapy.[113] It has also been shown to be effective in oropharyngeal and esophageal candidiasis in immunocompromised patients and as primary therapy for candidemia in non-neutropenic patients.[114,115] A large, randomized, multicenter trial has been completed that compared 12-hourly administration of voriconazole (3 mg/kg intravenously or 200 mg orally) with liposomal AmB (3 mg/kg intravenously) for empiric antifungal therapy. This study showed comparable composite success rates, but less proven and probable breakthrough infections, infusion-related toxicity and nephrotoxicity in the voriconazole-treated cohort. However, patients receiving voriconazole had significantly more frequent episodes of transient visual disturbances and hallucinations.[116]

For treatment of invasive fungal infections in adults, an intravenous loading dose of 6 mg/kg q12h on day 1 followed by 4 mg/kg q12h thereafter is employed. For children, a dosage of 7 mg/kg intravenously q12h is used. Voriconazole by the oral route is administered at 200 mg q12h in adults. As SE-β-CD clearance is related to GFR, oral voriconazole should be used, when feasible, in patients whose creatinine clearances is <50 ml/min. In patients with mild to moderate hepatic cirrhosis, the standard loading dose is recommended, but the maintenance dose should be halved.

Posaconazole

Pharmacokinetics

At present, posaconazole is available as an oral suspension only and achieves optimal exposure when administered in two to four divided doses given with food or a nutritional supplement. The compound has dose-proportional pharmacokinetics in the 50–800 mg dose range, with saturation of absorption occurring above 800 mg. Following repeat dosing, steady state is achieved after 7–10 days with a six- to eight-fold accumulation of plasma concentrations.[117] Posaconazole has a large volume of distribution on the order of 5 l/kg and a prolonged elimination half-life of approximately 20 hours. It is not significantly metabolized through the cytochrome P450 enzyme system but primarily excreted unchanged in the feces. Approximately 10% of the compound is metabolized through glucuronidation.

Adverse effects

The safety profile of posaconazole appears to be comparable to that of fluconazole or itraconazole.[118,119] The overall safety of posaconazole has been assessed in more than 400 patients with invasive fungal infections from two open label clinical trials who received posaconazole suspension (800 mg/day in divided doses).[120,121] Treatment-related adverse events occurred in 38% of patients (164/428); the most common were nausea (8%), vomiting (6%), headache (5%), abdominal pain (4%) and diarrhea (4%). Treatment-related abnormal liver function test results were observed in up to 3% of patients. The most common severe adverse events were altered drug levels, increased hepatic enzymes, nausea, rash, and vomiting (1% each).

Drug interactions

Posaconazole is not significantly metabolized through the cytochrome P450 enzyme system, but inhibits cytochrome P3A4; it has no effect on 1A2, 2C8, 2C9, 2D6 and 2E1 isoenzymes.[122-125] As such, monitoring of ciclosporin, tacrolimus and sirolimus blood concentrations is mandatory, and dose adjustments should be made accordingly.

Indications and dosing

Posaconazole is indicated for treatment of aspergillosis, fusariosis, chromoblastomycosis and coccidioidomycosis in patients who are refractory to, or intolerant of, standard therapies. It is also indicated for prophylaxis of invasive *Candida* and *Aspergillus* infections in high-risk patients ≥13 years of age with allogeneic hematopoietic stem cell transplantation and graft-versus-host disease or those with hematologic malignancies and prolonged neutropenia. In a large phase II study including 330 patients with invasive fungal infections mostly refractory to standard therapies, the rates of successful outcome were 42% for aspergillosis (107 patients),[126] 39% for fusariosis (18 patients), 69% (16 patients) for coccidioidomycosis and 81% for chromoblastomycosis (11 patients).[127] Efficacy has also been found against other invasive fungal infections, including zygomycosis, candidiasis, cryptococcosis and refractory oropharyngeal candidiasis.[128–133] Two studies demonstrated the preventive efficacy of posaconazole, in particular against invasive *Aspergillus* infections in high-risk patients, including a statistically significant survival benefit in patients with acute myeloid leukemia/myelodysplastic syndrome undergoing remission induction chemotherapy.[118,119]

The recommended daily dosage for salvage treatment is 400 mg q12h given with food; for patients not tolerating solid food, a dosage of 200 mg q6h is recommended, preferably together with a nutritional supplement. The dosage for primary treatment of oropharyngeal candidiasis is 100 mg/day (day 1: 100 mg q12h) and 400 mg q12h for refractory disease; for prophylaxis of invasive *Candida* and *Aspergillus* infections, the recommended dosage is 200 mg q8h. The pharmacokinetics of posaconazole in pediatric patients (<18 years of age) have not been adequately studied.[134]

ECHINOCANDIN LIPOPEPTIDES

Anidulafungin, caspofungin, micafungin

The echinocandins are a novel class of semisynthetic amphiphilic lipopeptides composed of a cyclic hexapeptide core linked to a variably configured lipid side chain. The echinocandins act by noncompetitive inhibition of the synthesis of 1,3-β-glucan, a polysaccharide in the cell wall of many pathogenic fungi (Fig. 149.5). Together with chitin, the rope-like glucan fibrils are responsible for the cell wall's strength and shape. They are important in maintaining the osmotic integrity of the fungal cell and play a key role in cell division and cell growth. The structures of caspofungin, anidulafungin and micafungin are shown in (Fig. 149.6).

Antifungal activity

The current echinocandins appear to possess very similar pharmacologic properties. All three have potent and broad-spectrum fungicidal *in-vitro* activity against *Candida* species and potent inhibitory activity against *Aspergillus* spp.; their antifungal efficacy against these organisms *in vivo* has been demonstrated in various animal models. While still generally susceptible, *C. parapsilosis* isolates generally show elevated MICs for the echinocandins.

The current echinocandins have variable activity against dematiaceous and endemic molds, and are inactive against most hyalohyphomycetes, *Cr. neoformans* and *Trichosporon* spp. In *vitro*, echinocandins have limited activity against zygomycetes,[135] but animal models of zygomycosis and clinical experience suggest a role for echinocandins when combined with AmB.[136,137] *In-vitro* resistance has been observed in fungal isolates overexpressing a gene encoding for a Golgi protein involved in the transport of cell wall components.[138] The MIC breakpoint for echinocandin susceptibility is 2 μg/ml.

Primary resistance to echinocandins in otherwise susceptible fungal yeast species is rare and resistance induction studies have demonstrated a low potential for secondary resistance in *Candida* spp.[139] The frequency of primary echinocandin resistance among clinical isolates of *Aspergillus* spp. is unknown, but induction of secondary resistance has been achieved *in vitro*.[140]

Pharmacodynamics

The echinocandins demonstrate a species-dependent mode of antifungal activity. They have fungicidal activity against most *Candida* spp. but not against *Aspergillus* spp. In *Aspergillus* spp., microscopic examination of exposed hyphae show a dose-dependent formation of microcolonies with progressively truncated, swollen hyphal elements that appear to be cell-wall deficient, but that can regain their cell walls upon subculture in the absence of drug. In a process akin to pruning, caspofungin preferentially kills cells at active centers of cell wall synthesis within *A. fumigatus* hyphae.[141] These observations indicate differences in functional target sensitivity in both species that are not fully understood. *In-vitro* pharmacodynamic studies in *Candida* spp. have shown predominantly concentration-dependent

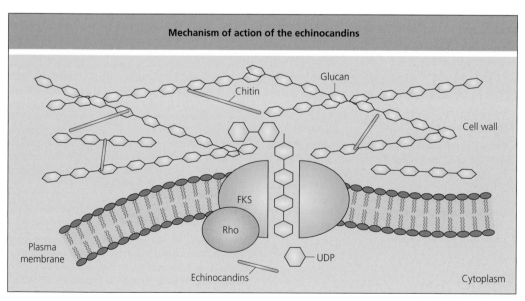

Fig. 149.5 Mechanism of action of the echinocandins.

Structures of echinocandins currently in clinical practice or in clinical trials

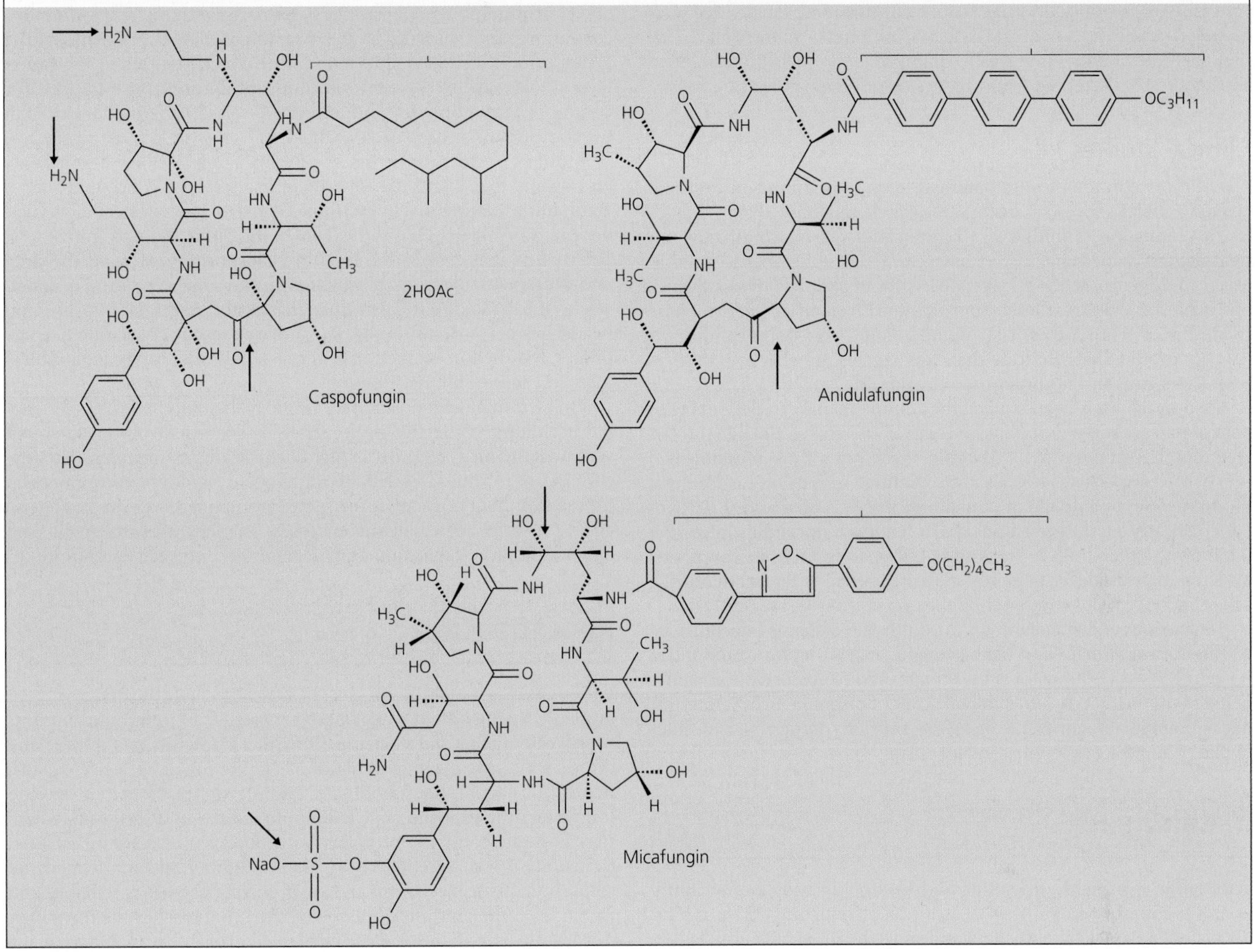

Fig. 149.6 Structures of echinocandins currently in clinical trials.

(≥99.9% reduction in CFU) fungicidal activity and rate of kill, and concentration-dependent prolonged postantifungal effects of up to 12 hours' duration.[9,142] Animal studies suggest similar concentration-dependent activity of the current echinocandins.

The echinocandins may have a role in biofilm-associated candidiasis. Therapeutic concentrations of echinocandins display potent in-vitro activity against C. albicans in biofilms.[143] When used as catheter lock solutions, echinocandins may effectively reduce or control fungal biofilms.[144] Combined systemic and catheter intraluminal lock therapy was highly effective in rabbits with venous catheter C. albicans infection.[145] Clinical studies are needed to define the role of the echinocandins in biofilms.

Data have emerged regarding interactions between echinocandins and phagocytic cells. Echinocandins alone do not completely inhibit in-vitro growth of A. fumigatus, but a powerful antifungal effect is seen in combination with phagocytes. Echinocandins enhance neutrophil activity against mold hyphae by unmasking β-glucans and activating host antifungal pathways via the Dectin-1 receptor.[146,147]

Pharmacokinetics

All current echinocandins are only available intravenously. They exhibit dose-proportional plasma pharmacokinetics with a β-half-life of 10–15 hours that allows for once-daily dosing. Echinocandins are >95% protein-bound and distribute into all major organ sites including the brain; however, concentrations in uninfected CSF are low. The echinocandins are hepatically metabolized and slowly excreted into urine and feces; only small fractions are excreted into urine in unchanged form.[148] The pharmacokinetic parameters are generally lower in children than in adults. Drug levels are especially low in smaller, younger children. The β-half-life in children is reduced by over one-third relative to adults.

Adverse effects and drug interactions

At the currently investigated dosages, all echinocandins are generally well tolerated. Only a small fraction of patients enrolled in clinical trials (<5%) discontinued therapy due to drug-related adverse events. The most frequently reported adverse effects include increased liver transaminases, gastrointestinal upset and headaches. Like other basic polypeptides, the echinocandins have the potential to cause histamine release; however, histamine-mediated symptoms have been observed in isolated cases only.

The current echinocandins appear to have no significant potential for drug interactions mediated by the CYP450 enzyme system. Caspofungin reduces the AUC of tacrolimus by approximately 20%

but has no effect on ciclosporin levels. However, ciclosporin increases the AUC of caspofungin by approximately 35%; because of transient elevations of hepatic transaminases in single-dose interaction studies, concomitant use of both drugs is not recommended. Finally, inducers of drug clearance and/or mixed inducers/inhibitors – namely efavirenz, nelfinavir, nevirapine, phenytoin, rifampin (rifampicin), dexamethasone and carbamazepine – may reduce caspofungin concentrations.

Clinical studies

The clinical efficacy of anidulafungin, caspofungin and micafungin against *Candida* spp. has been investigated in phase II or III studies of esophageal candidiasis.[149] Echinocandins are also effective for treatment of azole-refractory esophageal and oropharyngeal candidiasis.[150] All agents were well tolerated without serious adverse events, and achieved efficacy at least comparable with standard agents. Phase III studies of echinocandins for initial therapy of invasive candidiasis (mostly candidemia) indicate that these agents are effective, but less toxic than AmB and noninferior to fluconazole.[151–153]

Caspofungin has been studied for empiric therapy in patients with persistent fever and neutropenia and was as effective as and better tolerated than liposomal AmB.[154] The role of echinocandins in established invasive aspergillosis is less clear. In a salvage trial using caspofungin monotherapy, a complete or partial response was observed in 45% of patients. Early data suggest a possible role for echinocandins in combination with other drugs active against *Aspergillus* spp. and this approach is increasingly used.[155–157] Clinical trials are needed to further define the safety and efficacy of combination therapy in invasive aspergillosis.

The recommended daily doses in adults with systemic infections are 100 mg for micafungin and anidulafungin, and 50 mg for caspofungin. A loading does of 200 mg for anidulafungin and 70 mg for caspofungin is required on the first day. In children, doses of caspofungin at 50 mg/m²/day and anidulafungin at 1.5 mg/kg/day provide comparable exposures to that of adults treated with standard dosing.[158,159]

TERBINAFINE

Terbinafine is a highly lipophilic and keratophilic allylamine inhibitor of ergosterol biosynthesis. It is a potent noncompetitive inhibitor of fungal squalene epoxidase and prevents squalene epoxidation, an important early step in the synthesis of ergosterol. Treated fungi accumulate squalene and become deficient in ergosterol. Cell death is associated with the development of high intracellular squalene concentrations, which interfere with fungal membrane function and cell wall synthesis. In addition to its antifungal properties, terbinafine is also anti-inflammatory and can act as a free radical scavenger.

Terbinafine is active *in vitro* against a wide range of pathogenic fungi, including dermatophytes, molds, dimorphic fungi, *Cr. neoformans* and some but not all *Candida* and *Aspergillus* spp.[160] In-vitro studies with *Aspergillus* have shown terbinafine and amphotericin to have additive to synergistic interactions depending on the isolate. In combination with itraconazole or voriconazole, terbinafine displays potent synergistic interactions against *Aspergillus*. Fluconazole also increases the activity of terbinafine in an additive to synergistic fashion.[161] In-vitro combinations of terbinafine with voriconazole can overcome azole resistance in *Candida* spp. Terbinafine in combination with AmB or voriconazole is synergistic against some zygomycete isolates. Resistance to terbinafine has been observed following a single gene mutation in *Aspergillus*.[162] In *Candida*, cross-resistance following treatment with fluconazole can occur due to upregulation of target enzymes. Multidrug efflux pumps may also reduce susceptibility.[163]

Oral terbinafine is rapidly absorbed, with peak concentration occurring at 60–90 minutes post dose. It is quickly converted to multiple metabolites, which co-exist in plasma with the parent compound. Drug is delivered to peripheral tissues via sebum and by direct diffusion through the dermal layers. It is detected in sebum and hair within the first week of administration and by week 3 in stratum corneum and nail samples. The terminal half-life is approximately 3 weeks and fungicidal concentrations persist in peripheral tissues for weeks to months after administration of the last dose. Increasing age and concomitant hypertension are associated with higher plasma concentrations and smokers have lower levels than do nonsmokers.[164] When given as a 1% cream, terbinafine concentrations in the horny layer of skin far exceed the minimum inhibitory concentrations for common dermatophytes and effective levels of drug remain in skin well beyond discontinuation of therapy.[165]

Multiple cytochrome P450 enzymes metabolize terbinafine, and agents that affect this system may alter drug concentrations.[166] Terbinafine competitively inhibits CYP2D6 and elevated levels of desipramine have been observed when the drugs are co-administered. Terbinafine may reduce the level of ciclosporin A. Most of the drug and drug metabolites are eliminated in the urine. The drug is generally well tolerated, but gastrointestinal disturbances, skin rashes and headaches occur occasionally. Rare adverse reactions include hepatobiliary dysfunction, induction and exacerbation of lupus, agranulocytosis and severe skin reactions.

Oral terbinafine at doses of 250 mg/day in adults and 62.5–250 mg/day in children is effective and generally safe for cutaneous mycoses that warrant systemic therapy. It is highly efficacious as treatment for onychomycosis. At this time, however, this agent cannot be recommended for the treatment of systemic mycoses. Terbinafine 1% cream is effective against a variety of cutaneous mycoses. The length of treatment with either topical or oral formulation depends on the specific infection.

GRISEOFULVIN

Griseofulvin, a metabolic product of *Penicillium*, was the first oral agent available for treatment of dermatomycoses. This compound inhibits fungal cell mitosis and nucleic acid synthesis and disrupts spindle and cytoplasmic microtubule function.[167] Griseofulvin is active against many, but not all, dermatophytes. High-level resistance can develop following drug exposure and a multiple-layered thick cell wall, which may limit griseofulvin entry, has been observed in resistant isolates. Griseofulvin has extremely low water solubility and moderate lipid solubility. Absorption from the gastrointestinal tract is variable and depends on the amount of dissolved drug that reaches the intestines. Absorption is enhanced by a fatty meal. The bioavailability of the ultra-microsize formulation is higher compared to the microsize formulation. Once absorbed, the drug is highly protein-bound.

Griseofulvin is detected in the outer layer of the stratum corneum soon after it is ingested and is diffused from the extracellular fluid and sweat. Deposition of drug in growing cells may account for entry into hair and nails.[167] Concentration in plasma peaks at 3–4 hours and in skin blister fluid at 6 hours. The terminal half-life in plasma and in skin blisters is approximately 9–10 hours. During chronic administration, plasma and skin blister levels equilibrate. Griseofulvin is largely metabolized in the liver and degradation metabolites are excreted in the urine. Griseofulvin is also effective in several inflammatory skin conditions, possibly due to anti-inflammatory properties mediated by modulation of the expression of cell adhesion molecules on leukocytes and vascular endothelial cells.[168]

Adverse effects include gastrointestinal disturbances, headaches, hepatitis and rashes. Liver and thyroid neoplasia, abnormal germ cell maturation, teratogenicity and embryotoxicity have been observed in animal studies. The reproductive toxicity as well as the induction of chromosome aberrations in somatic cells may result from disturbance of microtubule formation. Griseofulvin also induces accumulation of porphyrins and formation of Mallory bodies in hepatocytes. These may represent additional carcinogenic mechanisms. Less common adverse events include exacerbation of lupus, porphyrias and blood dyscrasias. Drug interactions are related to induction of hepatic enzymes and include phenobarbital, oral anticoagulants and oral contraceptives.

For onychomycosis, griseofulvin has been largely supplanted by newer antifungals. Currently, its main indication is for the treatment of tinea capitis and other cutaneous mycoses. Doses of 500–1000 mg/day in adults and 15–20 mg/kg/day in children have been used successfully. Length of treatment depends on the site and type of infection.

AMOROLFINE

The morpholine derivative amorolfine is currently only used as a topical agent. This compound interferes with ergosterol biosynthesis and leads to the depletion of ergosterol and the subsequent accumulation of sterol precursors within the cell membrane. Amorolfine also weakly inhibits the fungal enzyme squalene epoxidase. *In-vitro* amorolfine has a broad spectrum of activity that includes dermatophytes, dimorphic, dematiaceous and filamentous fungi, and yeasts.[169] In patients, amorolfine has eradicated infections due to both *C. albicans* and a broad range of dermatophytes. In a murine model of dermatophytosis the combinations of amorolfine with griseofulvin, terbinafine, itraconazole and fluconazole were synergistic, but 5-FC appears to be antagonistic in some fungal isolates.

Amorolfine has been formulated as 0.125%, 0.25% and 0.5% creams and as a 5% lacquer. Following application, the amorolfine penetrates the nails rapidly and within 24 hours of contact exceeds the MIC of most fungi that cause onychomycosis. Following topical application, an active concentration of amorolfine is retained in the skin for several days. In experimental models of systemic mycosis amorolfine shows no significant activity, which may be due to strong protein binding and/or rapid metabolism. The bioavailability of topical amorolfine is 4–10% and drug is excreted in urine and feces.

Treatment-related adverse events are generally limited to burning, itching, erythema, skin dryness and scaling. Topical amorolfine has been used successfully in a variety of dermatomycoses and for the treatment of onychomycosis. Combination therapy with oral itraconazole or terbinafine may be a promising option for patients with severe disease.[170]

CICLOPIROX

Ciclopirox is a poorly absorbable, synthetic hydroxypyridone antifungal agent. The mechanism of action is related to its affinity for trivalent cations. By chelating essential metal co-factors ciclopirox inhibits fungal enzymes that are responsible for diverse metabolic processes and ultimately causes membrane and cytoplasmic disruption.[171] Ciclopirox at subinhibitory concentrations impairs candidal adherence to mucosal surfaces. This agent has potent antifungal activity against a broad range of dermatophytic and nondermatophytic fungi.

Ciclopirox is available in a variety of topical formulations including a 0.77% gel and 8% nail lacquer. It readily penetrates the skin via the epidermis and the hair follicles and achieves the highest concentration in the horny layer. When used as 8% nail lacquer, the drug achieves uniform distribution within the nail plate after daily use for 1 week, reaching a maximum at 3–4 weeks with uniform distribution to all nail layers.[172] Within the nail the drug achieves concentrations in excess of inhibitory and fungicidal concentrations for most pathogens. The bioavailability of topical ciclopirox is 2–5% and absorbed drug is mainly metabolized by glucuronidation. Excretion is predominantly renal with an elimination half-life of approximately 2 hours.[172]

Treatment-related adverse events are uncommon, but local reactions such as pruritus and burning sensation can occur. Ciclopirox has been used successfully for a variety of cutaneous mycotic infections, mucosal candidiasis, seborrheic dermatitis and as treatment for onychomycosis.

FUTURE DIRECTIONS

The past decade has seen a considerable expansion in antifungal drug research and the clinical development of several new compounds targeted against invasive fungal infections. Major progress has been made in defining paradigms for antifungal intervention and in designing and implementing clinical trials. Several novel and promising antifungal compounds are currently in early stages of preclinical investigation and the pursuit of novel biochemical and molecular targets will result in further candidate drugs. Cognizant of past and present epidemiologic trends, invasive fungal infections will likely remain a frequent and important complication in immunocompromised patients. An expanded drug arsenal, elucidation of resistance mechanisms, integration of pharmacokinetic and pharmacodynamic relationships, and combination therapies offer hope for further substantial progress in prevention and treatment.

REFERENCES

References for this chapter can be found online at http://www.expertconsult.com

Antiparasitic agents

INTRODUCTION

Antiparasitic agents are used to treat infestations caused by a diverse and complex group of organisms encompassing the unicellular protozoa, which have intricate life cycles often involving more than one host, as well as the helminths, which have highly developed organ systems. Many antiparasitic agents are old drugs that have never been subjected to the rigorous testing of efficacy and safety currently required by agencies in various countries, such as the US Food and Drug Administration.

The treatment options by organism or disease entity, along with the recommended adult and pediatric dosages, are listed in Table 150.1. Agents that are not readily available in the USA are listed in Table 150.2. Few of the antiparasitic agents have been extensively studied in pregnancy. Table 150.3 divides the drugs into those that are probably safe on the basis of clinical experience, those that are possibly safe on the basis of anecdotal experience or are safe during certain trimesters, and those that are known to be hazardous or for which too little information is known to make a recommendation. In general, however, the decision to use of any of these agents in a pregnant patient must be made on an individual basis, weighing the severity of the illness and the benefit of treatment to the mother against the potential toxicity to the fetus.

Antiprotozoal Agents

AMODIAQUINE

Amodiaquine is a 4-aminoquinoline with antimalarial activity and a mechanism of action similar to that of chloroquine.[6,7] The side-effect profile is also similar to that of chloroquine but agranulocytosis and severe hepatitis have been reported with long-term use (as chemoprophylaxis). The activity of amodiaquine against some chloroquine-resistant strains of *Plasmodium falciparum* has led to a revival in its use, particularly as part of combination therapy with artesunate.[8] While resistance to amodiaquine in certain parts of Africa may limit the usefulness of this combination in those regions, the artesunate–amodiaquine combination has proved very effective in areas where responses to amodiaquine alone exceed 80%.[9,10]

AMPHOTERICIN B

Amphotericin B, a polyene antifungal agent, is the drug of choice for primary amebic meningoencephalitis caused by *Naegleria* spp.[11] (see Chapter 182), and is used for the treatment of visceral leishmaniasis (see Chapter 117).[12,13] Its pharmacokinetics and side-effects are detailed in Chapter 149. Lipid-associated formulations of amphotericin B are effective in the treatment of visceral leishmaniasis, and in one study in India single-dose therapy with liposomal amphotericin B gave cure rates of more than 92% with minimal toxicity.[12,13]

ANTIFOLATE AGENTS

Antifolate agents act at various steps in the folic acid cycle. For *Plasmodium* spp., *Toxoplasma* spp. and other sensitive parasites, reduced folic acid derivatives are essential for de-novo pyrimidine synthesis. Unlike mammalian cells, these parasites cannot use preformed pyrimidines. Antifolate agents are most commonly used in combination to block sequential steps in the folic acid metabolic pathway (see Chapter 138).

Pyrimethamine

Pyrimethamine is a diaminopyrimidine that inhibits plasmodial dihydrofolate reductase at a concentration that is 1000 times less than that required to inhibit the mammalian enzyme.[6,7] It is effective against the erythrocytic stages of all *Plasmodium* spp. that are pathogenic for humans, but resistance has significantly limited its usefulness as a single agent.[14] In combination with sulfadiazine, clindamycin or atovaquone, it is used for the treatment of *Toxoplasma gondii*.[15,16] Pyrimethamine also has activity against *Isospora belli*.[17] The drug is available in oral form; it is slowly but completely absorbed, is 85% protein-bound and is extensively metabolized by the liver (<3% is excreted unchanged). The half-life is 4–6 days.

Although pyrimethamine is available as 25 mg tablets, it is almost exclusively used in combination with a sulfonamide (sulfadiazine, sulfadoxine) or a sulfone (dapsone; see below). The dosage for toxoplasmosis is listed in Table 150.1. Some clinicians give an initial pyrimethamine loading dose of 200 mg. In patients who cannot tolerate sulfonamides, clindamycin (1.8–2.4 g/day in divided doses) or atovaquone (1.5 g q12h) may be substituted. Side-effects of pyrimethamine include blood dyscrasias, rash and, very rarely, seizures or shock. At high doses, pyrimethamine causes bone marrow suppression, which can be prevented by concurrent administration of folinic acid. Sulfadoxine–pyrimethamine as 25 mg pyrimethamine and 500 mg sulfadoxine is used in combination with artesunate for the treatment of *P. falciparum* malaria in areas where susceptibility to sulfadoxine and pyrimethamine remains high (South America, the Middle East, South Asia).[9]

Table 150.1 Antiparasitic agents and dosages (Organism or disease entity is listed alphabetically. Both adult and pediatric dosages are indicated)

Infection	Drug	Adult dosage (po unless otherwise indicated)	Pediatric dosage (po unless otherwise indicated)
Acanthamoeba (keratitis)			
	Polyhexamethylene biguanide 0.02% plus 0.1% propamidine isethionate (topical)		
Amebiasis (*Entamoeba histolytica*)			
Asymptomatic or following metronidazole or tinidazole therapy	Paromomycin	25–35 mg/kg/day in three doses for 7 days	25–35 mg/kg/day in three doses for 7 days
Alternatives	Diloxanide furoate	500 mg q8h for 10 days	20 mg/kg/day in three doses for 10 days
OR	Iodoquinol	650 mg q8h for 20 days	30–40 mg/kg/day (maximum 2 g) in three doses for 20 days
Mild-to-moderate intestinal disease			
	Metronidazole	500–750 mg q8h for 5–10 days	35–50 mg/kg/day in three doses for 10 days
OR	Tinidazole	2 g/day for 3 days	≧3 years: 50 mg/kg (maximum 2 g) per day for 3 days
Severe intestinal disease and extraintestinal disease			
	Metronidazole	750 mg q8h for 5–10 days	35–50 mg/kg/day in three doses for 10 days
OR	Tinidazole	2 g/day for 5 days	≧3 years: 50 mg/kg or 60 mg/kg (maximum 2 g) per day for 5 days
Amebic meningoencephalitis (primary or granulomatous amoebic encephalitis)			
***Naegleria* spp.**			
	Amphotericin B	1.5 mg/kg/day iv, uncertain duration	1 mg/kg/day iv, uncertain duration
Acanthamoeba* spp.			
	Pentamidine, ketoconazole, flucytosine, uncertain duration		
Balamuthia mandrillaris			
	Clarithromycin	500 mg q8h, uncertain duration	
	Fluconazole	400 mg q24h, uncertain duration	
	Sulfadiazine	1.5 g q6h, uncertain duration	
	Flucytosine	1.5 g q6h, uncertain duration	
Sappinia diploides			
	Azithromycin	250 mg q24h, uncertain duration	
	Pentamidine	300 mg iv q24h, uncertain duration	
	Itraconazole	200 mg q12h, uncertain duration	
	Flucytosine	2.75 g q6h, uncertain duration	
***Ancylostoma caninum* (eosinophilic enterocolitis)**			
	Mebendazole	100 mg q12h for 3 days	100 mg q12h for 3 days
OR	Pyrantel pamoate	11 mg/kg (maximum 1 g) for 3 days	11 mg/kg (maximum 1 g) for 3 days
OR	Albendazole	400 mg, single dose	400 mg, single dose
Angiostrongyliasis			
Angiostrongylus cantonensis			
	Mebendazole	100 mg q12h for 5 days	100 mg q12h for 5 days
Angiostrongylus costaricensis			
	Mebendazole	200–400 mg q8h for 10 days	200–400 mg q8h for 10 days
Alternative	Thiabendazole	75 mg/kg/day in three doses for 3 days (maximum 3 g/day)	75 mg/kg/day in three doses for 3 days (maximum 3 g/day)
Anisakiasis (*Anisakis* spp.)			
Treatment of choice		Surgical or endoscopic removal	
Ascariasis (*Ascaris lumbricoides*, roundworm)			
	Mebendazole	100 mg q12h for 3 days or 500 mg, single dose	100 mg q12h for 3 days or 500 mg, single dose
OR	Pyrantel pamoate	11 mg/kg, single dose (maximum 1 g)	11 mg/kg, single dose (maximum 1 g)
OR	Albendazole	400 mg, single dose	400 mg, single dose

(Continued)

Table 150.1 Antiparasitic agents and dosages (Organism or disease entity is listed alphabetically. Both adult and pediatric dosages are indicated)—cont'd

Infection	Drug	Adult dosage (po unless otherwise indicated)	Pediatric dosage (po unless otherwise indicated)
Babesiosis (*Babesia* spp.)			
The recommendations below are for normal hosts. Immunocompromised individuals may require more prolonged (6 weeks or more) courses of therapy to achieve cure (see Krause *et al.*, Clin Infect Dis 2008;46:370–6).			
	Clindamycin	1.2 g q12h iv or 600 mg q8h po for 7 days	20–40 mg/kg/day po in three doses for 7 days
PLUS	Quinine	650 mg q8h for 7 days	25 mg/kg/day in three doses for 7 days
OR	Atovaquone	750 mg q12h for 7–10 days	20 mg/kg q12h for 7–10 days
PLUS	Azithromycin	600 mg q24h for 7–10 days	12 mg/kg q24h for 7–10 days
Balantidiasis (*Balantidium coli*)			
	Tetracycline	500 mg q6h for 10 days	40 mg/kg/day (maximum 2 g) in four doses for 10 days
Alternatives	Iodoquinol	650 mg q8h fro 20 days	40 mg/kg/day in three doses for 20 days
	Metronidazole	750 mg q8h for 5 days	35–50 mg/kg/day in three doses for 5 days
Baylisascariasis (*Baylisascaris procyonis*)			
	No drug proven effective – albendazole 25 mg/kg/d for 20 days recommended for known exposure to raccoon feces		
***Blastocystis hominis* (clinical significance controversial)**			
	Metronidazole	750 mg q8h for 5–10 days	
OR	Iodoquinol	650 mg q8h for 20 days	
Capillariasis (*Capillaria philippinensis*)			
	Mebendazole	200 mg q12h for 20 days	200 mg q12h for 20 days
Alternative	Albendazole	400 mg/day for 10 days	400 mg/day for 10 days
Cryptosporidiosis (*Cryptosporidium parvum*)			
No agent has yet been conclusively proven to be effective in AIDS patients. Nitazoxanide, in the doses listed below, showed efficacy in clearing infection from immunocompetent individuals.			
	Nitazoxanide	500 mg q12h for 3 days	1–3 years: 100 mg q12h for 3 days 4–11 years: 200 mg q12h for 3 days
Cutaneous larva migrans (creeping eruption, dog and cat hookworm)			
	Thiabendazole	Topical administration	Topical administration
OR	Ivermectin	150–200 μg/kg, single dose	150–200 μg/kg, single dose
OR	Albendazole	400 mg/day for 3 days	400 mg/day for 3 days
Cyclosporiasis (*Cyclospora cayetanensis*)			
	TMP–SMX	TMP 160 mg, SMX 800 mg q12h for 7–10 days	TMP 5 mg/kg, SMX 25 mg/kg q12h for 7–10 days
Dientamoeba fragilis			
	Iodoquinol	650 mg q8h for 20 days	40 mg/kg/day (maximum 2 g) in three doses for 20 days
OR	Paromomycin	25–30 mg/kg/day in three doses for 7 days	25–30 mg/kg/day in three doses for 7 days
OR	Tetracycline	500 mg q6h for 10 days	10 mg/kg q6h (maximum 2 g) for 10 days
Dracunculiasis (*Dracunculus medinensis*, guinea worm)			
	Physical removal of worm		
Entamoeba polecki			
	Metronidazole	750 mg q8h for 10 days	35–50 mg/kg/day in three doses for 10 days
Enterobiasis (*Enterobius vermicularis*, pinworm)			
	Pyrantel pamoate	11 mg/kg, single dose (maximum 1 g); repeat in 2 weeks	11 mg/kg, single dose (maximum 1 g); repeat in 2 weeks
OR	Mebendazole	100 mg, single dose; repeat in 2 weeks	100 mg, single dose; repeat in 2 weeks
OR	Albendazole	400 mg, single dose; repeat in 2 weeks	400 mg, single dose; repeat in 2 weeks
Filariasis			
Wuchereria bancrofti, Brugia malayi			
	Diethylcarbamazine	Day 1: 50 mg after food Day 2: 50 mg q8h Day 3: 100 mg q8h Days 4–14: 6 mg/kg/day in three doses	Day 1: 1 mg/kg after food Day 2: 1 mg/kg q8h Day 3: 1–2 mg/kg q8h Days 4–14: 6 mg/kg/day in three doses

Table 150.1 Antiparasitic agents and dosages (Organism or disease entity is listed alphabetically. Both adult and pediatric dosages are indicated)—cont'd

Infection	Drug	Adult dosage (po unless otherwise indicated)	Pediatric dosage (po unless otherwise indicated)
Loa loa			
	Diethylcarbamazine	Day 1: 50 mg after food Day 2: 50 mg q8h Day 3: 100 mg q8h Days 4–21: 9 mg/kg/day in three doses	Day 1: 1 mg/kg after food Day 2: 1 mg/kg q8h Day 3: 1–2 mg/kg q8h Days 4–21: 9 mg/kg/day in three doses
Mansonella ozzardi			
	Ivermectin	200 µg/kg single dose	
Mansonella perstans			
	Mebendazole	100 mg q12h for 30 days	
OR	Albendazole	400 mg q12h for 10 days	
Mansonella streptocerca			
	Ivermectin	150 µg/kg, single dose	
OR	Diethylcarbamazine	6 mg/kg/day for 14 days	
Tropical pulmonary eosinophilia			
	Diethylcarbamazine	6 mg/kg/day in three doses for 14 days	6 mg/kg/day in three doses for 14 days
***Onchocerca volvulus* (river blindness)**			
	Ivermectin	150 µg/kg, single dose, repeated every 6–12 months	150 µg/kg, single dose, repeated every 6–12 months
Fluke (hermaphroditic) infection			
***Clonorchis sinensis* (Chinese liver fluke)**			
	Praziquantel	75 mg/kg/day in three doses for 1 day	75 mg/kg/day in three doses for 1 day
OR	Albendazole	10 mg/kg for 7 days	
***Fasciola hepatica* (sheep liver fluke)**			
	Triclabendazole	10 mg/kg, single dose	
Alternative	Bithionol	30–50 mg/kg on alternate days for 10–15 doses	30–50 mg/kg on alternate days for 10–15 doses
***Fasciolopsis buski, Heterophyes heterophyes, Metagonimus yokogawai* (intestinal flukes)**			
	Praziquantel	75 mg/kg/day in three doses for 1 day	75 mg/kg/day in three doses for 1 day
***Metorchis conjunctus* (North American liver fluke)**			
	Praziquantel	75 mg/kg/day in three doses for 1 day	75 mg/kg/day in three doses for 1 day
Nanophyetus salmincola			
	Praziquantel	60 mg/kg/day in three doses for 1 day	60 mg/kg/day in three doses for 1 day
***Opisthorchis viverrini* (South East Asian liver fluke)**			
	Praziquantel	75 mg/kg/day in three doses for 1 day	75 mg/kg/day in three doses for 1 day
***Paragonimus westermani* (lung fluke)**			
	Praziquantel	75 mg/kg/day in three doses for 2 days	75 mg/kg/day in three doses for 2 days
Alternative	Bithionol	30–50 mg/kg on alternate for 10–15 doses	30–50 mg/kg on alternate for 10–15 doses
Giardiasis (*Giardia lamblia*)			
	Metronidazole	250 mg q8h for 5 days	15 mg/kg/day in three doses for 5 days
OR	Tinidazole	2 g, single dose	50 mg/kg, single dose (maximum 2 g)
Alternatives	Nitazoxanide	500 mg q12h for 3 days	1–3 years: 100 mg q12h for 3 days 4–11 years: 200 mg q12h for 3 days
OR	Furazolidone	100 mg q6h for 7–10 days	6 mg/kg/day q6h for 7–10 days
OR	Paromomycin	25–35 mg/kg/day in three doses for 7 days	
OR	Quinacrine	100 mg q8h for 5 days (maximum 300 mg/day)	2 mg/kg q8h for 5 days (maximum 300 mg/day)
Gnathostomiasis (*Gnathostoma spinigerum*)			
Treatment of choice		Surgical removal	
OR	Ivermectin	200 µg/kg/day for 2 days	200 µg/kg/day for 2 days
OR	Albendazole	400 mg q12h for 21 days	400 mg q12h for 21 days
Hookworm infection (*Ancylostoma duodenale, Necator americanus*)			
	Mebendazole	100 mg q12h for 2 days or 500 mg, single dose	100 mg q12h for 2 days or 500 mg, single dose
OR	Pyrantel pamoate	11 mg/kg (maximum 1 g) for 3 days	11 mg/kg (maximum 1 g) for 3 days
OR	Albendazole	400 mg, single dose	400 mg, single dose

(Continued)

Table 150.1 Antiparasitic agents and dosages (Organism or disease entity is listed alphabetically. Both adult and pediatric dosages are indicated)—cont'd

Infection	Drug	Adult dosage (po unless otherwise indicated)	Pediatric dosage (po unless otherwise indicated)
Isosporiasis (*Isospora belli*)			
	TMP—SMX	160 mg TMP, 800 mg SMX q6h for 10 days, then q12h for 3 weeks	
Leishmaniasis (*Leishmania mexicana, Leismania tropica, Leishmania major, Leishmania braziliensis, Leishmania donovani* (kala-azar), *Leishmania infantum*)‡			
Visceral or mucosal disease			
	Lipid-encapsulated amphotericin B	15–20 mg/kg (total dose over 5 days or longer)	15–20 mg/kg (total dose over 5 days or longer)
OR	Sodium stibogluconate	20 mg Sb/kg/day iv or im for 20–28 days	20 mg Sb/kg/day iv or im for 20–28 days
OR	Meglumine antimonate	20 mg Sb/kg/day for 20–28 days	20 mg Sb/kg/day for 20–28 days
OR	Miltefosine	2.5 mg/kg/day (maximum 150 mg per day) for 28 days	2.5 mg/kg/day (maximum 150 mg per day) for 28 days
Alternatives	Amphotericin B	0.5–1 mg/kg by slow infusion daily or every 2 days for up to 8 weeks	0.5–1 mg/kg by slow infusion daily or every 2 days for up to 8 weeks
OR	Paromomycin	15 mg/kg/day for 21 days	15 mg/kg/day for 21 days
Cutaneous disease			
	Sodium stibogluconate	20 mg Sb/kg/day iv or im for 20–28 days	20 mg Sb/kg/day iv or im for 20–28 days
OR	Meglumine antimonate	20 mg Sb/kg/day iv or im for 20–28 days	20 mg Sb/kg/day iv or im for 20–28 days
OR	Paromomycin	Topically q12h for 10–20 days	Topically q12h for 10–20 days
OR	Pentamidine	2–3 mg/kg iv or im q24h or qod for 4–7 doses	2–3 mg/kg iv or im q24h or qod for 4–7 doses
Malaria treatment (*Plasmodium falciparum, Plasmodium ovale, Plasmodium vivax, Plasmodium malariae*)			
Chloroqine-resistant *Plasmodium falciparum* (oral regimens)			
	Atovaquone/proguanil	Two adult tablets (250 mg atovaquone/100 mg proguanil) q12h for 3 days or four adult tablets q24h for 3 days	5–8 kg: two peds tablets/day (62.5 mg atovaquone/25 mg proguanil) for 3 days 9–10 kg: three peds tablets/day for 3 days 11–20 kg: one adult tablet/day for 3 days 21–30 kg: two adult tablets/day for 3 days 30–40 kg: 3 adult tablets/day for 3 days >40 kg: adult dose
OR	Quinine sulfate	650 mg q8h for 3–7 days	25 mg/kg/day q8h for 3–7 days
PLUS	Doxycycline	100 mg q12h for 7 days	2 mg/kg/day for 7 days
OR PLUS	Clindamycin	900 mg q8h for 5 days	20–40 mg/kg/day q8h for 5 days
Alternatives	Mefloquine	750 mg followed by 500 mg 12h later	15 mg/kg, single dose (if body weight <45 kg), followed by 10 mg/kg 12h later
OR	Artesunate†	4 mg/kg/day for 3 days	
PLUS	Mefloquine	750 mg followed by 500 mg 12h later	15 mg/kg, single dose (if body weight <45 kg), followed by 10 mg/kg 12h later
OR	Artemether/lumefantrine	Four tablets/dose administered at 0, 8, 24, 36, 48 and 60 hours	<15 kg: one tablet/dose at same intervals as adults 15–25 kg: two tablets/dose at same intervals 24–35 kg: three tablets/dose at same intervals >35 kg: same as adult dosage
Chloroquine-resistant *Plasmodium vivax*			
	Atovaquone/proguanil	Two adult tablets (250 mg atovaquone/100 mg proguanil) q12h for 3 days or four adult tablets/day for 3 days	5–8 kg: two peds tablets/day (62.5 mg atovaquone/25 mg proguanil) for 3 days 9–10 kg: three peds tablets/day for 3 days 11–20 kg: one adult tablet/day for 3 days 21–30 kg: two adult tablets/day for 3 days 30–40 kg: three adult tablets/day for 3 days >40 kg: adult dose
OR	Mefloquine	750 mg followed by 500 mg 12h later	15 mg/kg, single dose (if body weight <45 kg), followed by 10 mg/kg 12h later
Alternative	Quinine sulfate	650 mg q8h for 3–7 days	25 mg/kg/day in three doses for 3–7 days
PLUS	Doxycycline	100 mg q12h for 7 days	2 mg/kg/day for 7 days
All regimens followed by:			
	Primaquine phosphate	26.3 mg (15 mg base)/day for 14 days or 79 mg (45 mg base)/week for 8 weeks	0.3 mg base/kg/day for 14 days

Table 150.1 Antiparasitic agents and dosages (Organism or disease entity is listed alphabetically. Both adult and pediatric dosages are indicated)—cont'd

Infection	Drug	Adult dosage (po unless otherwise indicated)	Pediatric dosage (po unless otherwise indicated)
All *Plasmodium spp.* except chloroquine-resistant *Plasmodium falciparum* and chloroquine-resistant *Plasmodium vivax*			
	Chloroquine phosphate	1 g (600 mg base), then 500 mg (300 mg base) 6h later, then 500 mg (300 mg base) at 24h and 48h	10 mg base/kg (maximum 600 mg base), then 5 mg base/kg 6h later, then 5 mg base/kg at 24h and 48h
All *Plasmodium* spp. (parenteral regimens)			
	Quinidine gluconate	10 mg/kg iv loading dose (maximum 600 mg) in normal saline slowly over 1–2h, followed by continuous infusion of 0.02 mg/kg/min until oral therapy can be started	10 mg/kg iv loading dose (maximum 600 mg) in normal saline slowly over 1–2h, followed by continuous infusion of 0.02 mg/kg/min until oral therapy can be started
OR	Quinine dihydrochloride	20 mg/kg iv loading dose in 5% dextrose over 4h, followed by 10 mg/kg over 2–4h, q8h (maximum 1800 mg/day) until oral therapy can be started	20 mg/kg iv loading dose in 5% dextrose over 4h, followed by 10 mg/kg over 2–4h, q8h (maximum 1800 mg/day) until oral therapy can be started
Alternatives	Artemether†	3.2 mg/kg im, then 1.6 mg/kg q24h	3.2 mg/kg im, then 1.6 mg/kg q24h
	Artesunate†	2.4 mg/kg/dose iv for 3 days with doses at 0, 12, 24, 48 and 72 hours	2.4 mg/kg/dose iv for 3 days with doses at 0, 12, 24, 48 and 72 hours
Prevention of relapses (*Plasmodium vivax* and *Plasmodium ovale* only)			
	Primaquine phosphate	26.3 mg (15 mg base)/day for 14 days or 79 mg (45 mg base)/week for 8 weeks	0.3 mg base/kg/day for 14 days
Malaria prevention			
Chloroquine-sensitive areas			
	Chloroquine phosphate	500 mg (300 mg base) once per week	5 mg/kg base once per week, up to adult dose of 300 mg base
Chloroquine-resistant area			
	Atovaquone/proguanil	One adult tablet/day	5–8 kg: ½ ped tablet/day 9–10 kg: ¾ ped tablet/day 11–20 kg: one ped tablet/day 21–30 kg: two ped tablets/day 31–40 kg: three ped tablets/day >40 kg: adult dose
OR	Mefloquine	250 mg once per week	Weight <5 kg, no data; weight 5–9 kg, 1/8 tablet; weight 10–19 kg, ¼ tablet; weight 20–30 kg, ½ tablet; weight 31–45 kg ¾ tablet; weight >45 kg, one tablet
OR	Doxycycline	100 mg/day	2 mg/kg/day, up to 100 mg/day
Alternatives	Primaquine	0.5 mg/kg base/day	0.5 mg/kg base/day
Microsporidiosis			
Ocular microsporidiosis (*Encephalitozoon hellem, Encephalitozoon cuniculi, Vittaforma corneae (Nosema corneum)*)**			
	Albendazole	400 mg q12h	
PLUS	Fumagillin eye drops		
Intestinal microsporidiosis (*Enterocytozoon bieneusi, Encephalitozoon (Septata) intestinalis*)			
	Albendazole	400 mg q12h	
OR	Fumagillin	60 mg q24h for 14 days	
Disseminated microsporidiosis (*Enterocytozoon hellem, Enterocytozoon cuniculi, Enterocytozoon intestinalis, Pleistophora* ssp.)			
	Albendazole	400 mg q12h	
Moniliformis moniliformis			
	Pyrantel pamoate	11 mg/kg, single dose, repeat twice 2 weeks apart	11 mg/kg, single dose, repeat twice 2 weeks apart
Oesophagostomum bifurcum			
	Albendazole or pyrantel pamoate		
Schistosomiasis (bilharziasis)			
Schistosoma haematobium			
	Praziquantel	40 mg/kg/day in two doses for 1 day	40 mg/kg/day in two doses for 1 day
Schistosoma japonicum			
	Praziquantel	60 mg/kg/day in three doses for 1 day	60 mg/kg/day in three doses for 1 day

(Continued)

Table 150.1 Antiparasitic agents and dosages (Organism or disease entity is listed alphabetically. Both adult and pediatric dosages are indicated)—cont'd

Infection	Drug	Adult dosage (po unless otherwise indicated)	Pediatric dosage (po unless otherwise indicated)
Schistosoma mansoni			
	Praziquantel	40 mg/kg/day in two doses for 1 day	40 mg/kg/day in two doses for 1 day
Alternative	Oxamniquine	15 mg/kg, single dose	20 mg/kg/day in two doses for 1 day
Schistosoma mekongi			
	Praziquantel	60 mg/kg/day in three doses for 1 day	60 mg/kg/day in three doses for 1 day
Strongyloidiasis (Strongyloides stercoralis, threadworm)			
	Ivermectin	20 µg/kg/day for 1–2 days	200 µg/kg/day for 1–2 days
Alternative	Thiabendazole	50 mg/kg/day in two doses (maximum 3 g/day) for 2 days	50 mg/kg/day in two doses (maximum 3 g/day) for 2 days
Tapeworm infection (adult (intestinal stage))			
Diphyllobothrium latum (fish), Taenia saginata (beef), Taenia solium (pork), Dipylidium caninum (dog)			
	Praziquantel	5–10 mg/kg, single dose	5–10 mg/kg, single dose
Alternative	Niclosamide	2 g single dose	50 mg/kg, single dose
Hymenolepis nana (dwarf tapeworm)			
	Praziquantel	20 mg/kg, single dose	25 mg/kg, single dose
Tapeworm infection (larval (tissue stage))			
Echinococcus granulosus (hydatid cyst)			
	Albendazole	400 mg q12h for 28 days, repeated as necessary	15 mg/kg/day for 28 days, repeated as necessary
Echinococcus multilocularis			
Treatment of choice		Surgical excision	
Cysticercus cellulosa (cysticercosis)			
	Albendazole	400 mg q12h for 8–30 days, repeated as necessary	15 mg/kg/day (maximum 800 mg) in two doses for 8–30 days, repeated as necessary
OR	Praziquantel	50 mg/kg/day in three doses for 15 days	50 mg/kg/day in three doses for 15 days
Alternative	Surgery		
Toxoplasmosis (Toxoplasma gondii)			
	Pyrimethamine	25–100 mg/day for 3–4 weeks	2 mg/kg/day for 3 days, then 1 mg/kg/day (maximum 25 mg/day) for 4 weeks
PLUS	Sulfadiazine	1–1.5 g q6h for 3–4 weeks	100–200 mg/kg/day for 3–4 weeks
Alternative	Spiramycin	3–4 g/day	50–100 mg/kg/day for 3–4 weeks
Trichinosis (Trichinella spiralis)			
	Corticosteroids for severe symptoms		
PLUS	Mebendazole	200–400 mg q8h for 3 days, then 400–500 mg q8h for 10 days	
Trichomoniasis (Trichomonas vaginalis)			
	Metronidazole	2 g, single dose or 500 mg q12h for 7 days	15 mg/kg/day in three doses for 7 days
OR	Tinidazole	2 g, single dose	50 mg/kg, single dose (maximum 2 g)
Trichostrongyliasis (Trichostrongylus spp.)			
	Pyrantel pamoate	11 mg/kg, single dose (maximum 1 g)	11 mg/kg, single dose (maximum 1 g)
Alternative	Mebendazole	100 mg q12h for 3 days	100 mg q12h for 3 days
OR	Albendazole	400 mg, single dose	400 mg, single dose
Trichuriasis (Trichuris trichiura, whipworm)			
	Mebendazole	100 mg q12h for 3 days or 500 mg, single dose	100 mg q12h for 3 days or 500 mg, single dose
Alternative	Albendazole	400 mg, single dose	400 mg, single dose
Trypanosomiasis			
Trypanosoma cruzi (American trypanosomiasis, Chagas disease)			
	Nifurtimox	8–10 mg/kg/day in three or four doses for 90–120 days	1–10 years: 15–20 mg/kg/day in four doses for 90 days 11–16 years: 12.5–15 mg/kg/day in four doses for 90 days
OR	Benznidazole	5–7 mg/kg/day for 30–90 days	≤12 years: 10 mg/kg/day in two doses for 30–90 days

Table 150.1 Antiparasitic agents and dosages (Organism or disease entity is listed alphabetically. Both adult and pediatric dosages are indicated)—cont'd

Infection		Drug	Adult dosage (po unless otherwise indicated)	Pediatric dosage (po unless otherwise indicated)
Trypanosoma brucei gambiense (West African trypanosomiasis) – hemolymphatic stage				
		Difluoromethylornithine (eflornithine)	400 mg/kg/day iv in four divided doses for 14 days	
	OR	Pentamidine isethionate	4 mg/kg/day im for 10 days	4 mg/kg/day im for 10 days
Alternative		Suramin	100–200 mg (test dose) iv, then 1 g on days 1, 3, 7, 14 and 21	20 mg/kg in on days 1, 3, 7, 14 and 21
Trypanosoma brucei rhodesiense (East African trypanosomiasis) – hemolymphatic stage				
		Suramin	100–200 mg (test dose) iv, then 1 g on days 1, 3, 7, 14 and 21	20 mg/kg iv on days 1, 3, 7, 14 and 21
Late disease with central nervous system involvement, both *T. brucei gambiense* and *T. brucei rhodesiense*				
		Melarsoprol	2–3.6 mg/kg/day iv for 3 days; after 1 week 3.6 mg/kg/day iv for 3 days; repeat again after 10–21 days	18–25 mg/kg over 1 month; initial dose of 0.36 mg/kg iv, increasing gradually to maximum 3.6 mg/kg at intervals of 1–5 days for a total of 9–10 doses
	OR	Difluoromethylornithine	400 mg/kg/day iv in four divided doses for 14 days	
Visceral larva migrans (toxocariasis)				
		Albendazole	400 mg q12h for 3–5 days	400 mg q12h for 3–5 days
	OR	Mebendazole	100–200 mg q12h for 5 days	100–200 mg q12h for 5 days

Sb, antimony; SMX, sulfamethoxazole; TMP, trimethoprim.
*These recommendations are based on a handful of cases for each type of infection as summarized in Visvesvara *et al*.[2]
†Artesunate, artemether and other artemenisin derivatives should be paired with another antimalarial to avoid high rates of recrudescence (see text).
‡There appears to be significant variation in the susceptibility of *Leishmania* spp. to different agents, hence the choice of therapies should reflect the known sensitivities of organisms within the region where disease was acquired.
Data modified from Med Lett Drugs Ther 2007;(5):11.[1]

Trimethoprim

Trimethoprim (TMP) is another diaminopyrimidine that inhibits microbial dihydrofolate reductase. It has activity against:
- a variety of bacteria (see Chapter 138);
- *Pneumocystis jirovecii* (see Chapter 91); and
- the parasites *Isospora belli* and *Cyclospora cayetanensis* (see Chapter 180).[17]

Trimethoprim is readily absorbed, widely distributed and 50% protein-bound. Less than 20% is hepatically metabolized to inactive metabolites and the drug is excreted both in the urine and bile. The half-life is 9–11 hours.

For parasitic infections, TMP is used in fixed combination with sulfamethoxazole (SMX; see below). Side-effects include rashes, pruritus, nausea, vomiting, glossitis, elevated liver enzymes, cytopenias, megaloblastic anemia, fever, aseptic meningitis and impaired renal function.

Sulfonamides

Sulfonamides, which are derivatives of sulfanilamide, interfere with microbial folic acid synthesis by competitively inhibiting the enzyme dihydropteroate synthase.[6,7] This enzyme is involved in the step in folic acid synthesis that precedes the step blocked by pyrimethamine and TMP. Sulfonamides are separated into four groups:
- short- and intermediate-acting agents;
- long-acting agents;
- agents that are limited to the bowel lumen; and
- topical agents.

Only agents from the first two of these categories are used to treat parasitic diseases; these are generally combined with either pyrimethamine or TMP.

Sulfamethoxazole

Sulfamethoxazole is an intermediate-acting sulfonamide. It is rapidly absorbed, widely distributed, 50–70% protein-bound, hepatically metabolized and renally excreted. The half-life is 7–12 hours. It is available in a fixed combination with TMP (see below) for numerous indications.

Sulfadiazine

Sulfadiazine, another intermediate-acting sulfonamide, is also rapidly absorbed, widely distributed (including within the cerebrospinal fluid), 45–55% protein-bound, hepatically metabolized and renally excreted. The half-life is 12 hours. It is used with pyrimethamine in the treatment of toxoplasmosis, as detailed above.

Sulfadoxine

Sulfadoxine, a long-acting sulfonamide, is rapidly absorbed but slowly eliminated and has a half-life of 7–9 days. It is available in a fixed combination with pyrimethamine for the treatment of malaria (see pyrimethamine above).

Side-effects of sulfonamides

Side-effects of sulfonamides are numerous. Nausea, vomiting and anorexia occur in 1–2% of patients. Hypersensitivity reactions include:
- drug eruptions (ranging from morbilliform rash to severe exfoliation);
- fever;
- serum sickness; and
- hepatocellular dysfunction and necrosis.

Table 150.2 Availability* of antiparasitic agents

Agent	Trade name	Manufacturer
Available from the drug service provided by the US Centers for Disease Control and Prevention (CDC)		
Artesunate		Walter Reed Army Institute of Research
Bithionol	Bitin	Tanabe (Japan)
Diethylcarbamazine		CDC
Melarsoprol	Arsobal	Rhône-Poulenc Rorer
Nifurtimox	Lampit	Bayer
Sodium stibogluconate	Pentostam	Wellcome Foundation
Suramin	Germanin	Parke–Davis
Commercially available only outside the USA		
Amodiaquine	Camoquin Flavoquine	Parke–Davis Aventis
Artemether	Artenam	Arenco (Belgium)
Benznidazole	Rochagan	Roche
Diloxanide furoate	Furamide	Boots (UK)
Fumagillin	Flisinit	Sanofi-aventis (France)
Meglumine antimonate	Glucantime	Aventis
Niclosamide	Yomesan	Bayer
Ornidazole	Tiberal	Roche
Oxamniquine	Vansil	Pfizer
Proguanil	Paludrine	AstraZeneca (UK)
Quinacrine	Atabrine	Sanofi
Quinine dihydrochloride	(Generic)	ACF Chemiefarma NV (The Netherlands)
Spiramycin	Rovamycine	Aventis
Triclabendazole	Egaten	Novartis

*It is often difficult to obtain antiparasitic agents in the USA. This is not a comprehensive list; many drugs have multiple trade names and manufacturers, only some of which are included. Agents are divided into those available from the drug service provided by the Centers for Disease Control and Prevention (call 404-639-3670 during business hours, 404-639-2888 at other times) and those that are commercially available only outside the USA. Some of the latter may be available through compounding pharmacies within the USA. These include: Panorama Compounding Pharmacy, 6744 Balboa Blvd, Lake Balboa, CA 91406. Tel: (800) 247-9767, http://www.uniquerx.com; Medical Center Pharmacy, 800 Howard Avenue, New Haven, CT 06511. Tel. 203-688-6816. The National Association of Compounding Pharmacies (800-687-7850) and the Professional Compounding Centers of America (800-331-2498) can provide the names of additional compounding pharmacies.

Table 150.3 Safety of antiparasitic agents in pregnancy*

Category 1 drugs: probably safe	Category 3 drugs: insufficient data or established as unsafe (contraindicated)
Amphotericin B Azithromycin Chloroquine Clindamycin Niclosamide Paromomycin Praziquantel Pyrantel pamoate Proguanil Spiramycin	Albendazole – highest risk in first trimester Artemisinin and derivatives Atovaquone Benznidazole – contraindicated Bithionol Diethylcarbamazine Difluoromethylornithine – contraindicated Diloxanide furoate Doxycycline – contraindicated Fumagillin Furazolidone – contraindicated at term Iodoquinol
Category 2 drugs: possibly safe or safe during certain trimesters	Ivermectin Melarsoprol Miltefosine – contraindicated Nifurtimox Nitazoxanide Oxamniquine – contraindicated Pentamidine isethionate
Dapsone Mebendazole Mefloquine Metrifonate Metronidazole Piperazine Pyrimethamine – contraindicated in first trimester Sulfonamides – contraindicated at term Trimethoprim – contraindicated at term	Primaquine Quinacrine Quinidine-large doses contraindicated Quinine Sodium stibogluconate Suramin Tetracycline Thiabendazole Triclabendazole

*There are no well-controlled studies proving the safety of any of these antiparasitic agents in pregnancy. Category 1 drugs are those for which extensive clinical experience has demonstrated safety in pregnancy. Category 2 drugs are those that have been reported as safe only anecdotally or those that have been used safely in certain trimesters only. Category 3 drugs fall into two categories: those that should not be used because inadequate information makes risk assessment difficult, or those that are contraindicated because of documented fetal harm. Drugs in this group should be used only when there is a strong clinical indication for immediate treatment, there are no safer alternatives available, and the benefit of treatment to the mother outweighs the potential or known risks to the fetus.[3–5]

Acute hemolytic anemia, agranulocytosis and aplastic anemia are rare. Reversible bone marrow suppression is not uncommon in immunocompromised patients, particularly those who have AIDS. Crystalluria can occur with sulfadiazine and can be avoided by increasing fluid intake or alkalinizing the urine.

Trimethoprim–sulfamethoxazole

Trimethoprim–sulfamethoxazole (TMP–SMX) is a combination used to treat bacterial infections (see Chapter 138), P. jirovecii (see Chapter 91)

and the parasites I. belli and C. cayetanensis.[17] This combination also has some efficacy against P. falciparum, but resistance to the TMP component limits its use.[18] It is available as single-strength tablets (80 mg TMP and 400 mg SMX) and as double-strength tablets (160 mg TMP and 800 mg SMX). An oral suspension (40 mg TMP and 200 mg SMX per 5 ml) and an intravenous formulation (80 mg TMP and 400 mg SMX per 5 ml vial) are available as well.

The dose for isosporiasis is one double-strength tablet orally q6h for 10 days, followed by one double-strength tablet q12h for 3 weeks. Immunocompromised patients usually require maintenance therapy of one double-strength tablet daily or three times weekly. For cyclosporiasis, one double-strength tablet q12h for 7–10 days is generally used, but some clinicians extend treatment to 14 days. Immunocompromised patients sometimes require four tablets per day and usually need maintenance therapy as well.

Side-effects of TMP–SMX include those listed for each of the two component drugs, as detailed above. Dermatologic reactions (3–4%) and gastrointestinal disturbances (3–4%) are the most common side-effects in nonimmunocompromised patients. For unclear reasons, patients who have AIDS have a much higher rate of complications, ranging in different series from 45% to 90%.

Trimetrexate

Trimetrexate is a lipid-soluble dihydrofolate reductase inhibitor that was originally developed as a myelosuppressive agent, but was found to have antiparasitic activity against *P. jirovecii* and *T. gondii*.[15] It is available for intravenous injection only. Adverse effects include rash, leukopenia, elevated liver enzymes and a reversible peripheral neuropathy. Folinic acid is administered concurrently to diminish the incidence of bone marrow suppression.

Proguanil

Proguanil is a biguanide that inhibits plasmodial dihydrofolate reductase.[6,7] Although it is seldom used for monotherapy because of its slow action, in combination with atovaquone it is effective in the prevention and treatment of *P. falciparum* malaria (see below, under Atovaquone).[19-21]

Proguanil is slowly absorbed after oral administration, is 75% protein-bound, is metabolized to the active triazine metabolite cycloguanil, and is excreted in urine (40–60%) and feces (10%). The drug is safe and well tolerated. Pancytopenia has been rarely reported. Nausea, vomiting, abdominal pain, diarrhea and hematuria are associated with the use of high doses.

ARTEMISININ AND ITS DERIVATIVES

A major change in malaria therapy over the past 5 years has been the growing use of combination therapy for chloroquine-resistant *Plasmodium falciparum* infections. Artemisinin-based combination treatments (ACTs) have become a foundation of this effort.[9] Artemisinin, or qinghaosu, is a sesquiterpene lactone derived from the leaves of the sweet wormwood *Artemisia annua*.[7,9,22,23] It has been used for centuries in traditional Chinese medicine and is now known to be active against intraerythrocytic forms of *P. falciparum* and *P. vivax*, *Schistosoma mansoni*, *Schistosoma japonicum*, *Clonorchis sinensis* and *Naegleria fowleri*. Its main clinical use is the treatment of drug-resistant *P. falciparum* infections.

Route of administration and dosage

Artemisinin and its derivatives, the water-soluble hemisuccinate artesunate, the oil-soluble derivatives artemether and artemotil, and the active metabolite dihydroartemisinin are the most rapidly acting of known antimalarials and appear to be quite safe. These compounds can be given by several routes:

- artemisinin is available in oral and suppository forms;
- artesunate is available in oral, intravenous and intramuscular forms;
- artemether is available in oral and intramuscular forms;
- artemotil is available for intramuscular injection; and
- dihydroartemisinin is available in oral form.

They are rapidly absorbed and eliminated, with half-lives ranging from minutes (artesunate) to hours (artemether). The parent drug and derivatives are hepatically hydrolyzed to the active metabolite, dihydroartemisinin. These compounds are believed to act by disrupting parasite protein synthesis via the production of oxygen free radicals.

Artemisinin and its derivatives are best administered in conjunction with a longer acting antimalarial (e.g. mefloquine, lumefantrine, amodiaquine, sulfadoxine–pyrimethamine) to decrease the emergence of resistance and enhance efficacy. Recrudescence is a significant problem when artemisinin compounds are used as single agents. Artesunate (4 mg/kg orally) is usually given q24h for 3 days and is followed by a course of mefloquine. A fixed combination of artesunate (200 mg) and mefloquine (400 mg) base dosed at mefloquine 8 mg/kg/day for 3 days has been used with good success and, as noted above, the combination of artesunate and amodiaquine has been effective in certain regions.[9,10,24] Artemether can be given at a dose

of 3.2 mg/kg intramuscularly initially, followed by 1.6 mg/kg q24h. It is available orally in combination with lumefantrine (artemether 80 mg/lumefantrine 480 mg) as a six-dose regimen. This has been used effectively and is well tolerated, but requires twice daily dosing and co-administration of fat for optimal absorption.[9,25] The fixed dose combination of dihydroartemisinin (40 mg) and piperaquine (a 4-aminoquinolone related to chloroquine) (320 mg) has been used successfully to treat *P. falciparum* infections in Asia and Africa.[9,26]

Adverse reactions

Adverse events from artemisinin and its derivates include diarrhea, abdominal pain, transient first-degree heart block and reversible mild decreases in reticulocyte and neutrophil counts. Neurotoxicity has been described in animals but not with clinical use in humans. Resistance to artemisinin has occurred in murine malaria, and the resistant parasites also developed cross-resistance to chloroquine, quinine and mefloquine. In the USA the only artemisinin derivative currently available is the intravenous form of artesunate, which must be obtained from the US Centers for Disease Control and Prevention (www.cdc.gov/malaria/features/astesunate_now_available) and is currently released only for patients that cannot receive or tolerate quinidine.[20]

ATOVAQUONE AND ATOVAQUONE–PROGUANIL

Atovaquone, a synthetic hydroxynaphthoquinone derivative, has activity against *P. jirovecii* (see Chapter 91), *P. falciparum*, *T. gondii* and *Babesia microti*.[16,20,21,27] It interferes with pyrimidine synthesis by uncoupling mitochondrial electron transport. Because of its erratic absorption it is usually administered with a fatty meal. It is hepatically metabolized and excreted in the bile and urine. Atovaquone is an alternative oral agent for the treatment of mild to moderate *P. jirovecii* pneumonia in those who are intolerant of TMP–SMX, and experimental data indicate that it is synergistic with pyrimethamine or sulfadiazine for *T. gondii* infection. Atovaquone has also been used with azithromycin in the treatment of babesiosis.

The combination of atovaquone and proguanil has become a treatment of choice for *P. falciparum* malaria contracted in areas where chloroquine resistance is present (most of the malarious world with the exception of Central America west of the Panama Canal, Mexico, Hispaniola, parts of China and the Middle East)[20] and the combination pill containing atovaquone 250 mg and proguanil 100 mg has rapidly become a leading drug for malaria prophylaxis in travelers.[20,21,28,29] A randomized controlled trial comparing mefloquine and atovaquone–proguanil for malaria prophylaxis in nonimmune travelers found equivalent efficacy for the two agents, with a similar number of adverse events, but fewer adverse effects of moderate or severe intensity were reported in the atovaquone–proguanil group.[29] The adult dosage for prophylaxis is one tablet q24h (250 mg atovaquone/100 mg proguanil), beginning 1–2 days prior to arrival in the malarious area and continuing for 1 week after return. Side-effects include rash, nausea, vomiting, diarrhea, headache, fever, anemia, elevated liver function tests, hyponatremia and hyperglycemia. *P. falciparum* strains resistant to atovaquone–proguanil resulting in treatment failures have now been identified, with most strains showing mutations in the parasite cytochrome b gene.[30] Combination therapy of artesunate with atovaquone–proguanil has been tested and found to be well tolerated and highly effective in limited trials.[31]

BENZNIDAZOLE

Benznidazole is a nitroimidazole derivative that is active against both the trypomastigote and amastigote forms of *Trypanosoma cruzi*.[6,7,32] It is available in oral form and has a half-life of 12 hours. Side-effects include malaise, nausea, photosensitivity rash, peripheral neuropathy, bone marrow suppression and psychiatric disturbances.

CHLOROQUINE

Chloroquine, a 4-aminoquinoline that was first synthesized in 1934 but did not become popular until the end of the Second World War, has been the agent most widely used for treating the erythrocytic stage of uncomplicated malaria caused by *P. vivax*, *P. ovale*, *P. malariae* and chloroquine-sensitive *P. falciparum*.[6,7,20,21] Its precise mechanism of action has not been delineated, but chloroquine and its metabolites inhibit the ability of the parasite to polymerize the heme moiety of hemoglobin, resulting in toxic levels of free heme.

Pharmacokinetics and distribution

Absorption after oral ingestion is excellent (90%), and the volume of distribution is large owing to its extensive tissue sequestration, particularly in the liver, spleen, kidneys and erythrocytes. It is approximately 50% bound to plasma proteins and is eliminated slowly. Its half-life of 4–6 days permits weekly dosing for prophylaxis. Chloroquine is metabolized by the liver to the active metabolite desethylchloroquine, but 50% is cleared by the kidneys unchanged. Thus, dosing need not be altered for abnormal renal function, but caution must be exercised in patients who have hepatic, gastrointestinal, neurologic or hematologic disorders.

Route of administration and dosage

The drug is formulated as a phosphate, sulfate or hydrochloride salt and is dosed by base content. It can be administered orally or rectally or by intravenous, intramuscular or subcutaneous injection. In the USA, chloroquine is marketed as Aralen phosphate in 500 mg salt tablets (equal to 300 mg base). The dosage for the treatment and prophylaxis of malaria is given in Table 150.1. If chloroquine hydrochloride is given intravenously, it must be administered by slow, constant infusion to avoid respiratory depression, hypotension, heart block, cardiac arrest and seizures that may occur with transient toxic levels. A dose of 300 mg base q8–12h may be given by intramuscular injection.

Adverse reactions

Reversible side-effects include headache, gastrointestinal disturbances, blurred vision, dizziness, fatigue and pruritus. Rarer side-effects include hair depigmentation, weight loss, myalgias, leukopenia and eczematous eruptions. Very rarely, acute psychosis may occur. Permanent retinal damage has been observed with long-term (longer than 5 years) prophylactic use. The drug is contraindicated in patients who have retinal disease, psoriasis and porphyria. An oral dose of 5 g is fatal without immediate mechanical ventilation, adrenaline (epinephrine) and diazepam.

Resistance of *Plasmodium falciparum* to chloroquine

Resistance of *P. falciparum* to chloroquine is ubiquitous in regions where malarial transmission occurs with the exception of Central America west of the Canal Zone, Mexico, Haiti, the Dominican Republic and much of the Middle East (although there are reports of resistance from Yemen, Oman and Iran).[20] There is a report that withdrawal of chloroquine as preferred treatment from a region can, after an 8-year period, result in the re-emergence of chloroquine-sensitive *P. falciparum*.[33] Resistance to chloroquine among *P. vivax* isolates has been reported in Brazil, Colombia, India, Myanmar, Papua New Guinea and Indonesia.[20,34,35] A single oral dose of mefloquine (15 mg base/kg) has been used successfully in such cases.

CLINDAMYCIN

Clindamycin, a lincosamide antibiotic, is active against bacteria (see Chapter 135), *P. falciparum*, *T. gondii* and *Babesia* spp.[15,36,37] It is well absorbed after oral administration and is 90% protein-bound and widely distributed. It is hepatically metabolized and excreted in the urine and bile; its half-life is 2.5–3 hours.

Dosages for malaria and babesiosis are listed in Table 150.1. For cerebral toxoplasmosis in the case of sulfonamide hypersensitivity, 1.8–2.4 g divided into three daily doses is combined with a course of pyrimethamine. Clindamycin has been used in combination with quinine for short-course (3-day) treatment of travelers who have *P. falciparum* malaria, with excellent results.[38] Side-effects include rash, diarrhea, nausea, vomiting, abdominal pain, pseudomembranous colitis, hepatotoxicity and cytopenias.

DIFLUOROMETHYLORNITHINE

Difluoromethylornithine is an ornithine decarboxylase inhibitor that is effective in the treatment of both early and late sleeping sickness caused by *Trypanosoma brucei gambiense*.[7,39,40] It has variable efficacy against *T. brucei rhodesiense* because many strains are resistant. Difluoromethylornithine inhibits ornithine decarboxylase, an enzyme involved in the first step in polyamine synthesis. It is available as the hydrochloride salt for both oral and intravenous administration. It has a half-life of approximately 3 hours, and 80% of the drug is excreted unchanged by the kidneys.

Side-effects of difluoromethylornithine include anemia, thrombocytopenia, leukopenia, abdominal pain, nausea, vomiting, weight loss, arthralgias, seizures, hearing loss and alopecia. Overall, difluoromethylornithine is less toxic than other available antitrypanosomal agents, but it has not seen widespread use because of its high cost.

DILOXANIDE FUROATE

Diloxanide furoate is a dichloroacetamide derivative that is a luminally active agent used to eradicate cysts of *E. histolytica* in asymptomatic carriers and in those who have mild, noninvasive disease, as well as after treatment with metronidazole in those who have invasive amebiasis.[6,41] It is not useful in extraintestinal disease. After oral administration, diloxanide furoate is hydrolyzed by intestinal esterases, thus releasing diloxanide, the absorbable component, and the ester furoic acid, which is not well absorbed and thus attains higher intraluminal concentrations in the colon. Both compounds are amebicidal, but the mechanism of action is not known. The drug has a half-life of 6 hours, is hepatically conjugated to form a glucuronide and is 60–90% excreted in the urine.

Side-effects are mild; they include flatulence and, less commonly, nausea, vomiting, diarrhea, pruritus and urticaria. Because it is relatively inexpensive, diloxanide furoate is an attractive agent for use in developing countries.

FUMAGILLIN

Fumagillin, a water-insoluble antibiotic derived from *Aspergillus fumigatus*, was discovered in 1949 and originally used in humans as an amebicide. Fumagillin is an inhibitor of parasite RNA synthesis, but may also act by inhibiting a key proteinase, type 2 methionine aminopeptidase.[42] A water-soluble preparation (Fumidil B) is used to control nosematosis, a disease of honey bees that results from infection with microsporidian *Nosema apis*. Topical fumagillin has been used to treat microsporidial keratoconjunctivitis caused by *Encephalitozoon hellem, Encephalitozoon cuniculi, Encephalitozoon (Septata) intestinalis* and, with less success, *Vittaforma corneae (Nosema corneum)* in AIDS patients.[43] Studies of oral fumagillin for intestinal microsporidiosis have provided promising results.[44]

FURAZOLIDONE

Furazolidone is a nitrofuran derivative that is commonly used to treat giardiasis in children because of its availability in a liquid form for oral use.[6,45] Furazolidone also has activity against *I. belli* and *Trichomonas vaginalis* as well as many enteropathogenic bacteria, and is also used for treatment of *Helicobacter pylori* infections. The mechanism of action involves damage to DNA. It is well absorbed and is excreted mainly in the urine.

Adverse reactions include diarrhea, fever, nausea and vomiting. Urticaria, serum sickness, hypoglycemia and orthostatic hypotension occur rarely. Furazolidone has disulfiram-like properties and patients should therefore be warned to avoid alcohol. Furazolidone has monoamine oxidase inhibitor activity, but hypertensive crises have not been reported in association with this agent. Furazolidone may cause hemolysis in patients who have glucose-6-phosphate dehydrogenase (G6PD) deficiency.

HALOFANTRINE

Halofantrine is an oral synthetic 9-phenanthrene methanol with activity against the intraerythrocytic stages of chloroquine-sensitive and chloroquine-resistant *P. falciparum* and *P. vivax*.[6,7,21,46] It is more active and generally better tolerated than mefloquine, but is poorly absorbed. Ingestion with fatty meals increases absorption. Halofantrine is hepatically metabolized and excreted in feces, with a half-life of 1–2 days for the parent compound and 3–5 days for the active metabolite. Its mechanism of action is poorly understood.

There is some evidence of cross-resistance with mefloquine; therefore halofantrine may not be useful for those patients in areas with mefloquine resistance. Its side-effects include prolongation of the PR and QT_c intervals on the electrocardiogram, diarrhea, abdominal pain, pruritus and rash. Because of reports of sudden death associated with halofantrine therapy, it is absolutely contraindicated in individuals with a history of congenital QT prolongation, other conduction defects or anyone taking medications known to prolong the QT interval.

IODOQUINOL

Iodoquinol, a halogenated hydroxyquinoline, is a luminal amebicide used to eradicate cysts in patients who have asymptomatic *E. histolytica* infection.[6,41] It is also given after metronidazole therapy to eradicate cysts in patients who have invasive disease. Iodoquinol is the drug of choice for *Dientamoeba fragilis* infection and is an alternative for *Balantidium coli*.[47] It has been used to treat *Blastocystis hominis*, but the pathogenicity of this protozoan and its need for treatment are controversial.[48] Iodoquinol also has activity against *Giardia lamblia* and *T. vaginalis*, but other agents are typically employed. The mechanism of action of iodoquinol is uncertain. It is available in oral form, but is poorly absorbed and should be given with meals. Side-effects include nausea, vomiting, diarrhea, abdominal pain, headache, fever, seizures and encephalopathy.

Iodochlorhydroxyquin, a related compound, is better absorbed than iodoquinol, but is rarely used because of the high incidence of subacute myelo-optic neuropathy described with its use in Japan in the early 1970s. Because iodoquinol may rarely cause this syndrome when given at high dose or for prolonged periods, treatment recommendations should not be exceeded. For this reason many clinicians prefer alternative agents such as paromomycin or diloxanide furoate for these indications.

LUMEFANTRINE

Lumefantrine is an aryl amino alcohol compound that is structurally related to mefloquine and halofantrine. It is active against all *Plasmodium* spp. that infect humans.[9] As noted above, a fixed tablet combination of lumefantrine and artemether has proven to be highly effective in the treatment of multidrug-resistant *P. falciparum* infection.[9]

MACROLIDE ANTIBIOTICS

Spiramycin

Spiramycin is used in Europe to prevent the transmission of *T. gondii* from mother to fetus.[15] The drug is concentrated in the placenta and has been shown to reduce transmission by 60%. It is given at a dose of 1 g orally q8h on an empty stomach. If fetal infection has not occurred (as assessed by amniotic fluid polymerase chain reaction testing for *T. gondii*), spiramycin is continued until delivery. Because spiramycin does not cross the placenta well, it cannot be used to treat fetal toxoplasmosis; pyrimethamine and sulfadiazine are recommended in this situation. Oral spiramycin is generally well tolerated; gastrointestinal distress is the main side-effect.

Azithromycin

Azithromycin (see Chapter 135), both alone and in combination with pyrimethamine, has been shown to be effective in cerebral toxoplasmosis in AIDS patients.[15] It is considered relatively safe in pregnancy, but has not been extensively studied in preventing the vertical transmission of *T. gondii*. Azithromycin has also been used with both quinine and atovaquone for babesiosis.[36] Azithromycin has activity against *Plasmodium* spp., and is being evaluated as a component of combination therapy for *P. falciparum* paired with pyrimethamine–sulfadoxine, artesunate or quinine.[49]

MEFLOQUINE

Mefloquine is a fluorinated 4-quinoline methanol derivative of quinine. It is an oral formulation that was developed as part of a search for new antimalarials.[6,7,20,21,23] It is a blood schizonticide effective against all *Plasmodium* spp. that infect humans, including *P. falciparum* isolates that are resistant to chloroquine and pyrimethamine–sulfadoxine. It is ineffective against exoerythrocytic forms and gametocytes. The mechanism of action is unknown, but mefloquine may interfere with the function of *Plasmodium* food vacuoles or inhibit the polymerization of heme. The drug is slowly absorbed, has a bioavailability of 85% and is almost completely protein-bound in plasma. The long elimination half-life of 2–3 weeks allows for weekly prophylaxis. Mefloquine is extensively metabolized and is excreted in bile and feces.

Common side-effects at therapeutic doses include nausea, vomiting, dizziness, weakness and dysphoria.[29,50] Neuropsychiatric reactions, including acute psychosis, sleep disturbances and seizures, have been documented in approximately 0.5% of patients taking therapeutic doses and in less than 0.5% of those taking prophylactic doses. Thus, the drug is not recommended for those who have a history of seizures or psychiatric disorders. Judicious use is suggested for those whose occupations require spatial discrimination and fine motor coordination. Cardiac rhythm and conduction abnormalities and at least one instance of nonfatal cardiac arrest have occurred in patients on β-adrenergic blockers who took mefloquine; caution should be exercised in any patient who has cardiac disease. Mefloquine should not be co-administered with quinine, quinidine or halofantrine owing to potentially fatal prolongation of the QT_c interval. Mefloquine may also decrease the response to the live *Salmonella typhi* oral vaccine, and thus the vaccine series should be completed at least 3 days before beginning mefloquine prophylaxis.

Mefloquine resistance in *P. falciparum* isolates has been increasing along the Thailand–Myanmar and Thailand–Cambodia borders, in western Africa and in the Amazon region. In these areas, doxycycline at a dose of 100 mg/day or atovaquone–proguanil may be used for prophylaxis. Even the combination of mefloquine and artesunate may no longer be effective for treatment of acute falciparum malaria in those regions.[24,51] Treatment options include:

- quinine plus tetracycline or doxycycline for 7 days;[52]
- lumefantrine and artemether;[9]
- doxycycline plus artesunate;[53]
- atovaquone–proguanil and artesunate;[31]
- quinine plus clindamycin;[37] and
- dihydroartemisinin and piperaquine.[9]

MELARSOPROL

Melarsoprol is a trivalent arsenical compound introduced in 1949 and used for the treatment of late-stage African trypanosomiasis caused by either *T. brucei gambiense* or *T. brucei rhodesiense*.[6,7,40] It is also effective in treating the early or hemolymphatic stage of infection, but its toxicity prohibits routine use for this stage and it should be used only in patients who have failed to respond to suramin and pentamidine.

Melarsoprol acts by interacting with protein sulfhydryl groups and subsequently inactivating enzymes, a nonspecific action that is also responsible for the toxicity of the drug. Melarsoprol, formulated as a 3.6% weight per volume solution in propylene glycol, is given intravenously. A small, but adequate amount of the drug penetrates the cerebrospinal fluid, where it is taken up and concentrated by susceptible trypanosomes. Resistant organisms appear to concentrate the drug poorly. Melarsoprol is rapidly excreted in the urine.

Melarsoprol is highly toxic. It is irritating to tissues and care must be taken to prevent extravasation. Fever is commonly seen. Reactive encephalopathy occurs in up to 18% of patients and may be fatal; it usually occurs during the first 3–4 days of therapy.[54] It is manifested by headache, confusion, dizziness, mental slowing and ataxia, with seizures and a progressive decline in mental status, and it is felt to be an immunologic reaction to parasite antigens released during therapy. Corticosteroids have been used to treat the encephalopathy with some success. Very rarely, a hemorrhagic encephalopathy, which is almost always fatal, may occur. Arthralgias, rash, hypertension, proteinuria and hepatic dysfunction have been seen. Abdominal pain and vomiting may be minimized by slow administration of the drug to a patient who is supine and fasting. Erythema nodosum leprosum may be precipitated in patients who have leprosy. Hemolysis may be seen in G6PD-deficient patients.

MILTEFOSINE

Miltefosine, an alkyl phospholipids compound, was developed as an anticancer agent, but had dose-limiting gastrointestinal toxicity that outweighed its clinical benefits. However, it was discovered to have excellent antileishmanial activity and has become an important oral drug in the treatment of visceral leishmaniasis.[55,56] Its mechanism of action remains unknown, but parasite death appears to occur via apoptosis.[57] A 21-day course of miltefosine has proven safe and effective in the treatment of adults with visceral leishmaniasis in India.[58] It has also been studied in the treatment of cutaneous leishmaniasis in the Americas where it showed variable efficacy depending on the region and parasite strain.[59] Gastrointestinal side-effects including nausea, vomiting and diarrhea are frequent, occurring in roughly one-third of subjects. Elevations in transaminases may be seen in 15% of recipients, and increases in serum creatinine in 10%; both tend to normalize during treatment.

NIFURTIMOX

Nifurtimox, an oral nitrofuran, is used to treat acute Chagas disease (American trypanosomiasis), although benznidazole is gaining favor as a first-line agent in some regions with endemic Chagas disease (see Chapter 118).[6,7,32] Nifurtimox has also been used against resistant strains of *T. brucei gambiense*.[39] It acts by inhibiting nucleic acid synthesis by oxygen free radical formation. It is rapidly absorbed, has a half-life of approximately 3 hours, is extensively metabolized by the liver by a first-pass effect that results in low serum and tissue levels, and is excreted by the kidneys. There is considerable geographic variation in responsiveness to nifurtimox; better results are obtained in Argentina and Chile than in Brazil and other countries. Effectiveness in indeterminate-phase and chronic-phase infection is variable and organ damage is not reversible.

Gastrointestinal side-effects including nausea, vomiting, anorexia and abdominal pain; weight loss may occur. Neurologic side-effects include headache, restlessness, insomnia, disorientation, paresthesias, polyneuritis, weakness and seizures. Rash, decreased sperm counts and neutropenia have also been described. Adherence to a full 4 months of therapy is often poor, and better agents are needed.

NITAZOXANIDE

Nitazoxanide is a nitrothiazole benzamide derivative with *in-vitro* activity against a wide variety of bacterial, protozoal and helminthic pathogens. In randomized, double-blind, placebo-controlled clinical trials it showed efficacy comparable to metronidazole in the treatment of giardiasis and amebiasis, and was very successful in eradicating helminths from individuals in Egypt and Mexico.[60] Healthy adults treated with nitazoxanide cleared cryptosporidia from their stool more rapidly than did placebo controls, but the efficacy of nitazoxanide in AIDS patients remains to be established.[60]

NITROIMIDAZOLE DERIVATIVES

Metronidazole

Metronidazole (see Chapter 142) has activity against many anaerobic parasites. It is the drug of choice for the treatment of:

- invasive enterocolitis and liver abscess caused by *E. histolytica* and the rarely reported *Entamoeba polecki*;[6,7,41]
- vaginitis caused by *T. vaginalis*;[61] and
- enteritis caused by *G. lamblia*.[45]

It has been used to treat *Blastocystis hominis* in the stool (although its efficacy remains unproven) and is considered an alternative agent for *Balantidium coli* infection. Metronidazole is also used in the treatment of infections with the guinea worm, *Dracunculus medinensis*; it decreases inflammation and facilitates worm removal, but has no direct toxic effect on the worm itself.

Metronidazole acts as an electron sink under anaerobic or microaerophilic conditions, depriving the parasite of necessary reducing equivalents such as nicotinamide adenine dinucleotide phosphate, reduced form (NADPH). Reduced metronidazole (i.e. drug molecules that have gained electrons) causes a loss of the helical structure of DNA and strand breakage.

Metronidazole is available for oral and intravenous use. It is rapidly and almost completely absorbed orally, has limited protein binding and is widely distributed throughout the body. The half-life is 6–11 hours and metabolism is hepatic. Although excretion is mainly by the kidney, dosage adjustments are seldom needed in renal failure because the metabolites are less active compounds. However, the dosage should be modified in patients who have liver failure.

The most common side-effects are headache, metallic taste, dry mouth and nausea. Less frequent are urticaria, pruritus, urethral burning, reversible neutropenia, and vaginal and oral candidiasis. Rarely, patients may experience central nervous system toxicity, including dizziness, vertigo, ataxia, encephalopathy and seizures, as well as peripheral neuropathy. Acute pancreatitis has been reported. Patients should be advised to avoid consuming alcohol because of the disulfiram-like effects of metronidazole, including headache, flushing, abdominal pain and vomiting. Some patients may experience a red–brown discoloration of the urine owing to the presence of metabolites of metronidazole.

Tinidazole and ornidazole

Tinidazole and ornidazole are two other nitroimidazole derivatives (see Chapter 142). Their antimicrobial spectrum is similar to that of metronidazole,[6,7,41] and tinidazole has been used successfully for single-dose therapy of amebic liver abscess.[62] Tinidazole has also been used to treat metronidazole-resistant *Trichomonas* spp. and may show greater efficacy in the treatment of bacterial and trichomonal vaginitis.[61] These compounds are well absorbed orally and are widely distributed. Tinidazole has a half-life of 14 hours and ornidazole has a half-life of 12–13 hours; both compounds are probably hepatically metabolized and are excreted primarily in the urine. Generally, these drugs are better tolerated than metronidazole; the main side-effects are headache, dizziness and anorexia.

PAROMOMYCIN

Paromomycin (also known as aminosidine) is a nonabsorbable aminoglycoside antibiotic (see Chapter 137) that is concentrated in the lumen of the colon. It is active against *E. histolytica*, *D. fragilis* and *G. lamblia* as well as the cestodes *Taenia saginata*, *Taenia solium*, *Diphyllobothrium latum*, *Dipylidium caninum* and *Hymenolepis nana*.[6,41,45,47] Paromomycin with methylbenzethonium chloride has been used topically in the treatment of cutaneous leishmaniasis and systemically for visceral leishmaniasis.[39,63] Paromomycin is available as the sulfate salt for oral administration.

The dose is 25–35 mg/kg/day in three divided doses for 7 days. Side-effects include cramps, nausea, vomiting, diarrhea, rash, headache and vertigo. Burning may occur with topical preparations.

PENTAMIDINE ISETHIONATE

Pentamidine isethionate, an aromatic diamidine derivative, is effective in the treatment of the early or hemolymphatic stages of sleeping sickness caused by *T. brucei gambiense*, some forms of leishmaniasis and *P. jirovecii* pneumonia (see Chapters 105 and 117).[6,7,39] It is less effective against *T. brucei rhodesiense*. It has also been used in the treatment of disseminated *Acanthamoeba* spp. infections and babesiosis.[64,65] The mechanism of action of pentamidine is unclear, but it may involve the binding of DNA and the interruption of DNA replication. The drug is available for parenteral and inhalational use; the latter mode is used only in the prophylaxis and treatment of *P. jirovecii* pneumonia because little of the inhaled drug is absorbed systemically. Parenterally administered pentamidine isethionate penetrates extensively and is excreted slowly from tissues such as liver, spleen, kidneys and adrenal glands. Very little crosses the blood–brain barrier, accounting for the lack of utility of pentamidine in late-stage trypanosomiasis.

Route of administration and dosage

There are different recommendations for dosing pentamidine isethionate. For early *T. brucei gambiense* infection, the CDC recommends 4 mg/kg/day for 10 days. The World Health Organization (WHO) recommends 3–4 mg/kg/day or every other day for 7–10 doses. Because of the rapidity with which *T. brucei rhodesiense* invades the central nervous system, this drug is generally not used for this organism.

Pentamidine has also been used for prophylaxis against infection with *T. brucei gambiense* at a dose of 4 mg/kg (to a maximum of 300 mg) given every 3–6 months.

For leishmaniasis, the CDC recommends 2–4 mg/kg/day or every other day for 12–15 doses; a second course is sometimes given after an interval of 1–2 weeks. Alternatively, the WHO recommends 4 mg/kg three times a week for 5–25 weeks or longer. The dosage regimen varies slightly depending on the species of *Leishmania* and the region of the body affected. A study of 315 patients in Surinam found good results in the treatment of cutaneous leishmaniasis with a single dose weekly for 3 weeks.[66]

Adverse reactions

Pentamidine isethionate may cause toxicity in 50% of patients. Precipitous hypotension with dizziness, dyspnea, tachycardia, headache, vomiting and syncope can occur with rapid intravenous infusion. Intramuscular administration may result in sterile abscesses. Hypoglycemia, which may be life threatening, pancreatitis, hyperglycemia and diabetes mellitus probably result from a direct toxic effect of pentamidine on pancreatic β cells. Reversible renal failure occurs in up to 25% of patients. Other side-effects include fever, arrhythmias (particularly torsades de pointes), hypocalcemia, confusion, hallucinations, leukopenia, thrombocytopenia and elevated transaminases.

PENTAVALENT ANTIMONIAL COMPOUNDS

The pentavalent antimonial compounds remain a mainstay of therapy for leishmaniasis and are less toxic than the older trivalent compounds.[6,7,39,67] Sodium stibogluconate has been the most extensively studied and is the only pentavalent antimonial available in the USA. Meglumine antimonate is used largely in French-speaking countries and parts of Latin America. These compounds appear to inhibit bioenergetic pathways such as glycolysis and fatty acid oxidation in *Leishmania* amastigotes. *Leishmania* strains resistant to pentavalent antimony compounds are becoming more common, especially in India, and this has led to treatment failures and the need for alternative agents.[68]

These compounds are available as aqueous solutions for intravenous or intramuscular use only. Each milliliter of sodium stibogluconate contains the equivalent of 100 mg of pentavalent antimony, whereas each milliliter of meglumine antimonate contains 85 mg. They are rapidly absorbed and are eliminated in two phases. The first has a half-life of 2 hours, but the second is longer, with a half-life of between 33 hours (after intravenous administration) and 76 hours (after intramuscular administration). This slow terminal elimination may result from a conversion to trivalent antimony, which thus may be responsible for the toxicity seen with long-term therapy. Excretion is primarily renal.

Pentavalent antimonials are relatively well tolerated, but malaise, nausea, vomiting, abdominal pain, headache, arthralgias, myalgias, fever, rash, elevated transaminases, nephrotoxicity and pancreatitis may be seen. Dose-related electrocardiographic changes include T-wave flattening and inversion and QT_c-interval prolongation. Arrhythmias and sudden death have been described with high-dose therapy.

PIPERAQUINE

Piperaquine phosphate is a bisquinolone antimalarial drug that is structurally related to chloroquine and has activity against *P. vivax* and *P. falciparum*. Piperaquine is used in combination with dihydroartemisinin for the treatment of chloroquine-resistant *P. falciparum*. The drug is generally well tolerated, with relatively few adverse events noted to date.[69]

PRIMAQUINE

Primaquine, an 8-aminoquinoline active against hypnozoites of *P. vivax* and *P. ovale* in the liver, is the only agent with the potential for yielding complete resolution of malaria caused by these organisms.[6,7,20,21] Primaquine combined with clindamycin is also effective in the treatment of *P. jirovecii* pneumonia (see Chapter 91). Recently, primaquine in a dose of 30 mg/day showed efficacy as prophylaxis against *P. falciparum* (88% protection) and *P. vivax* (92% protection) malaria.[70] Primaquine acts by interfering with plasmodial mitochondrial function, possibly through its effects on the electron transport chain and pyrimidine biosynthesis. Primaquine phosphate, which is available only in oral form, is rapidly absorbed (bioavailability 96%), widely distributed and hepatically converted to three metabolites, yielding an elimination half-life of 6–7 hours. It is unclear whether the parent compound or the metabolites possess the antimalarial activity.

Primaquine phosphate is formulated in tablets containing 26.3 mg of the salt, equivalent to 15 mg of the base. Dosages are given in Table 150.1. Relapse of *P. vivax* after conventional primaquine treatment has been described in up to 30% of cases in Papua New Guinea, the Solomon Islands, Thailand and other parts of South East Asia.[71] Therefore, for cases acquired in South East Asia or Oceania, the dose should be increased to 22.5 mg base per day.

The principal toxicity of primaquine is hemolysis in patients who are G6PD-deficient, and thus G6PD levels should be measured before therapy is begun. Headache, nausea, vomiting and abdominal cramps have been reported. At higher doses, mild anemia, cyanosis (due to methemoglobinemia) and leukopenia may occur. Rarely, neurotoxicity, arrhythmias, hypertension and agranulocytosis occur.

QUINACRINE

Quinacrine is an acridine dye derivative that is effective against *G. lamblia*.[6,45] It has recently been used as combination therapy with metronidazole for individuals who failed therapy with metronidazole alone.[72] It also has activity against adult cestodes, but for this indication it has been supplanted by less toxic alternatives. In the Second World War, quinacrine was used for malaria prophylaxis and treatment. The mechanism of antiparasitic action is unclear, but the drug has been shown to intercalate with DNA and inhibit nucleic acid synthesis. Quinacrine is available in an oral formulation and is well absorbed and widely distributed. It has extensive tissue binding and has been detected in the urine 2 months after stopping therapy. Its metabolic fate is poorly understood.

The dosage in giardiasis is 100 mg q8h for 5–7 days. A second treatment course may be given 2 weeks later. The drug has a bitter taste and may induce nausea and vomiting. Dizziness and headache are also common. Reversible yellow skin discoloration (with spared sclerae) is seen in 4–5% of those treated with quinacrine for giardiasis. Under Wood's light, a bright yellow–green fluorescence distinguishes this side-effect from hyperbilirubinemia. Toxic psychosis may occur in 0.1–1.5% of patients. Other rare side-effects include blood dyscrasias, ocular toxicity and urticaria. Patients who have psoriasis may experience exfoliative dermatitis. Quinacrine has a disulfiram-like effect, and thus patients should be advised to avoid alcohol consumption while taking it. It also interferes with the metabolism of primaquine, and toxic levels of primaquine can result from co-administration of quinacrine with primaquine.

QUINIDINE

Quinidine is the dextrostereoisomer of quinine. It is a blood schizonticide and is the parenteral therapy of choice for chloroquine-resistant *P. falciparum* as a result of its wide availability as an antiarrhythmic.[6,7,20,21] It is supplied as the gluconate salt for intravenous use,

with a half-life of 6–8 hours. It is 80–90% protein-bound, hepatically metabolized and renally excreted.

During treatment, continuous electrocardiographic and blood-pressure monitoring are recommended. Widening of the QRS complex and prolongation of the QT_c interval may be seen, and hypotension may ensue if the drug is infused rapidly. Other side-effects are similar to those of quinine.

QUININE

Quinine is an alkaloid derived from the bark of the South American cinchona tree. It has been used as an antimalarial for over 350 years.[6,7,20,21] It is effective against the asexual blood stages of all four *Plasmodium* spp. that cause malaria in humans, and is used for chloroquine-resistant *P. falciparum* infections. Quinine is also used with clindamycin in the treatment of *Babesia microti* infection.[36] The basis for the antimalarial activity of quinine is unclear, but three mechanisms have been proposed:

- intercalation with parasite DNA, interrupting replication and transcription;
- interaction with erythrocyte fatty acids, promoting hemolysis and preventing schizont maturation; and
- alkalinization of parasite digestive vacuoles, interfering with hemoglobin degradation.

Pharmacokinetics and distribution

Quinine is available as the sulfate, bisulfate, hydrochloride, dihydrochloride, hydrobromide and ethylcarbonate salts for oral administration and as the dihydrochloride salt for parenteral use. It is rapidly absorbed after oral administration (bioavailability 80%), extensively protein-bound (90%), hepatically metabolized (80%) and renally excreted. The therapeutic range in plasma is 8–15 mg/l, which is achieved within 1–3 hours after a single oral dose. The half-life is approximately 11 hours. In cases of severe illness, the volume of distribution decreases, clearance is reduced and the half-life is prolonged. Thus, on a given dosage schedule, plasma quinine concentrations are elevated with acute illness and decrease as the patient improves. Monitoring blood levels is recommended in those who have renal or hepatic dysfunction; dosage reduction is needed with severe renal failure.

Route of administration and dosage

The oral dose of quinine sulfate (unlike other antimalarial agents, it is dosed by weight of salt) is 650 mg salt q8h for 3–7 days. A longer course is preferred for those in areas where *P. falciparum* is less sensitive to quinine, including South East Asia and western Africa.[73]

Intravenous quinine dihydrochloride may be used for severe infections. A 20 mg salt/kg loading dose in 5% dextrose is given over 4 hours, followed by 10 mg salt/kg over 2–4 hours q8h (maximum 1800 mg salt/day) until oral therapy can be given. The loading dose should be omitted in those who have received oral quinine, quinidine or mefloquine during the previous 24 hours. Intravenous quinidine gluconate has become the parenteral therapy of choice worldwide (see above).

Adverse reactions

The term cinchonism refers to a cluster of dose-related and reversible side-effects of quinine, including tinnitus, decreased hearing, headache, nausea, vomiting, dysphoria and visual disturbances. Hypoglycemia can occur secondary to quinine stimulation of insulin release in conjunction with parasite consumption of glucose. Skin rashes (urticaria, flushing), pruritus, hepatitis, thrombocytopenia, agranulocytosis and massive hemolysis with hemoglobinuria (with resultant bilirubinuria, termed blackwater fever) occur rarely. Quinine can cause respiratory depression in patients who have myasthenia gravis and hemolysis in those who have

G6PD deficiency. Myocardial depression, vasodilatation and shock may result from rapid intravenous infusion. Overdose can result in delirium, seizures, coma, respiratory depression, cortical blindness, shock and death. An oral quinine dose of 2–8 g may be fatal for adults.

SURAMIN

Suramin is a sulfated naphthylamine introduced in 1920 and is used in the treatment of the early or hemolymphatic stage of African trypanosomiasis.[6,7,39] It is more effective against *T. brucei rhodesiense* than against *T. brucei gambiense*, for which pentamidine is often used for early disease. Suramin has also been used for prophylaxis in those who have intense exposure. Additionally, suramin is active against the adult forms of *Onchocerca volvulus*, but is rarely used for this infection because of its toxicity.

The mechanism of action of suramin is unclear; it is a polyanion that inhibits many cellular enzymes. Notably, its antitrypanosomal activity correlates with inhibition of glycerol-3-phosphate oxidase and dehydrogenase, enzymes involved in energy metabolism.

Pharmacokinetics and distribution

Suramin is 99% protein-bound and persists at low levels in plasma for 3 months, which supports its use in prophylaxis. It is not metabolized and is excreted mainly by the kidneys. The large, polar, polyanionic structure affords poor cellular penetration. Very little drug penetrates into the cerebrospinal fluid, accounting for the lack of efficacy of suramin in late-stage disease.

Route of administration and adverse reactions

Suramin is available only for intravenous use. The dosage for trypanosomiasis is given in Table 150.1 Suramin has a variety of side-effects, which are generally more severe in malnourished patients. Immediate reactions include malaise, nausea, vomiting, fatigue, fever, urticaria, shock, loss of consciousness and, rarely, death. Late reactions include fever, rash, stomatitis, exfoliative dermatitis, lacrimation, photophobia, headache and hyperesthesia. Renal dysfunction (hematuria, proteinuria, casts and elevated creatinine), hepatic dysfunction (elevated transaminases and bilirubin), diarrhea, thrombocytopenia and agranulocytosis may occur. Additional side-effects during treatment for onchocerciasis include pruritus, dermal edema, papular eruptions, palmoplantar paresthesias and iridocyclitis.

TETRACYCLINES

Tetracycline (see Chapter 141) is used in combination with quinine in the treatment of drug-resistant *P. falciparum* in South East Asia, where resistance to chloroquine, Fansidar and quinine is common.[6,7,20,21,52] Doxycycline, a longer-acting derivative, is used for malaria prophylaxis in this area, and worldwide in individuals unable to tolerate mefloquine, although atovaquone–proguanil is now preferred for this indication.[20,21,74] Tetracycline is also the drug of choice for infection with the ciliate, *Balantidium coli*.

Tetracyclines are well absorbed after oral administration and are probably active against parasite protein synthesis. Side-effects include gastrointestinal distress, photosensitivity and vaginal candidiasis.

TRYPARSAMIDE

Tryparsamide, a pentavalent arsenical first described in 1919, is used primarily for the treatment of advanced *T. brucei gambiense* infections resistant to other therapy.[6,7] It has poor efficacy against *T. brucei*

rhodesiense. Side-effects of tryparsamide include fever, rash, abdominal pain, vomiting, tinnitus, optic atrophy and blindness, and encephalopathy.

Anthelmintic Agents

ALBENDAZOLE

Albendazole is a benzimidazole carbamate that has a broad spectrum of anthelmintic activity, including against *Ascaris lumbricoides*, *Enterobius vermicularis*, *Ancylostoma duodenale*, *Necator americanus*, *Strongyloides stercoralis*, *Echinococcus* spp. and *T. solium* cysticerci.[6,7,75–78] The drug has also been used to treat eosinophilic enterocolitis caused by *Ancylostoma caninum*, *Capillaria philippinensis*, cutaneous and visceral larva migrans, *C. sinensis*, *Gnathostoma spinigerum*, *Oesophagostomum bifurcum* and *Trichostrongylus* spp. It is also used in combination with diethylcarbamazine or ivermectin for mass treatment of lymphatic filariasis (*Brugia malayi* and *Wuchereria bancrofti*).[79] Additionally, it has variable efficacy in the treatment of microsporidiosis caused by *Encephalitozoon hellem*, *E. cuniculi*, *E. intestinalis*, *E. bieneusi* and *Vittaforma corneae*.[80] Albendazole has some activity against *G. lamblia*.[45]

The mechanism of action is similar to that of mebendazole with blockade of parasite microtubule assembly. Albendazole is poorly soluble in water and should be taken with a fatty meal to enhance absorption. It undergoes extensive first-pass metabolism in the liver, and albendazole sulfoxide is responsible for most of the systemic anthelmintic effects. This metabolite has a half-life of 9–15 hours and is mostly excreted renally.

Single doses of albendazole are generally well tolerated; abdominal discomfort, diarrhea or migration of *Ascaris* into the mouth and nose occur infrequently. Prolonged, high-dose treatment can be associated with reversible aminotransferase elevations, bone marrow suppression and alopecia.

BITHIONOL

Bithionol is a chlorinated bisphenol that is used for infections with *Fasciola hepatica*, but may have been supplanted by triclabendazole. Bithionol is also an alternative agent against *Paragonimus* spp.[6,7] It has activity against many other flukes, but has been replaced by praziquantel. Its mechanism of action is poorly understood.

Side-effects include anorexia, abdominal pain, nausea, vomiting, headache, dizziness, diarrhea, urticaria and proteinuria, some of which may be allergic responses to liberated fluke antigens.

DIETHYLCARBAMAZINE

Diethylcarbamazine is a piperazine derivative used in the treatment of filariasis. It is microfilaricidal for *W. bancrofti*, *B. malayi* and *B. timori*.[6,7,75,81,82] It appears to be macrofilaricidal for these species as well (i.e. it kills adult worms) and is considered to be the drug of choice for these three infections. Diethylcarbamazine is a key component of mass chemotherapy approaches for the eradication of lymphatic filariasis.[79] It has been used as a sole agent for single-dose therapy, administered long term as diethylcarbamazine-fortified dietary salt, and as a component of combination single-dose regimens with ivermectin or albendazole. Diethylcarbamazine is also the mainstay of therapy against *Loa loa* and *Mansonella streptocerca*. It has been used to treat tropical pulmonary eosinophilia, supporting the contention that the pulmonary infiltrates in this disorder are due to migrating microfilariae. It has also been used for visceral larva migrans.

Diethylcarbamazine is effective in eliminating microfilariae of *O. volvulus* in the skin and eye, but the resulting inflammation can cause permanent ocular damage, including uveitis, punctate keratitis and retinal pigment epithelium atrophy. Adult *Onchocerca* worms are not killed, however, and the infection may return once treatment has stopped. Ivermectin has largely replaced diethylcarbamazine for ocular onchocerciasis. Diethylcarbamazine also has activity against *A. lumbricoides*.

The mechanism of action of diethylcarbamazine involves two processes:

- first, filarial muscular activity decreases, probably secondary to hyperpolarization of membranes by the piperazine moiety of diethylcarbamazine; and
- second, microfilarial surface membranes are altered by making them more susceptible to host defenses.

Diethylcarbamazine is available as the citrate salt in 50 mg tablets. It is rapidly absorbed, widely distributed in the body, hepatically metabolized and renally eliminated. It has a half-life of approximately 10 hours.

Side-effects, although common, are usually mild and transient; they include headache, malaise, arthralgias, anorexia, nausea and vomiting. Toxicity can result from the destruction of organisms and release of antigens which provoke an inflammatory response. This reaction is most severe in patients who are heavily infected with *O. volvulus*. This is termed the Mazzotti reaction and consists of severe pruritus, edema, rash, arthralgias, lymphadenopathy, fever, hypotension, increased eosinophilia, proteinuria and splenomegaly. These symptoms persist for 3–7 days. Nodular swellings along lymphatics and lymphadenitis may occur with *W. bancrofti* and *B. malayi* infections. Patients heavily infected with *L. loa* may experience encephalopathy and other neurologic complications.[83] Pre-treatment with corticosteroids may lessen the severity of these inflammatory responses.

FLUBENDAZOLE

Flubendazole is a fluorine analogue of mebendazole and the two drugs have similar spectra of activity.[6,7] Flubendazole is poorly absorbed after oral administration. It has been used against many of the common intestinal helminths and, with limited success, in the treatment of neurocysticercosis.

IVERMECTIN

Ivermectin is a derivative of avermectin B1, a type of macrocyclic lactone that was discovered in the 1970s as a product of the actinomycete *Streptomyces avermitilis*.[6,7,76,84] Ivermectin is used as a broad-spectrum veterinary agent for infections with helminths and arthropods. Since the 1980s, it has become the drug of choice for onchocerciasis because it kills microfilariae in the skin and the eye while provoking much less inflammation than diethylcarbamazine. The response to ivermectin is rapid and can last for 6–12 months. Adult worms appear to be unaffected by ivermectin, but the drug seems to prevent developing larvae from leaving the uterus. The drug also has activity against *W. bancrofti*, *B. malayi*, *B. timori*, *L. loa*, *Mansonella ozzardi* and *Mansonella streptocerca*, and is being used as a component of mass chemotherapy for lymphatic filariasis.[79] Ivermectin is effective against *S. stercoralis* and is active against *E. vermicularis*, *A. lumbricoides* and *Trichuris trichiura*. Ivermectin causes tonic paralysis of the helminth musculature, but the mechanism of action is poorly understood, although it is known to include γ-aminobutyric acid (GABA) blockade.

Ivermectin is available as 6 mg tablets. It is highly protein-bound, has an elimination half-life of 50–60 hours, is concentrated in liver and adipose tissue, and is almost entirely excreted in the feces (only 1–2% appears in the urine). Side-effects include headache, fever, pruritus, lymphadenopathy, myalgias, arthralgias and, less commonly, orthostatic hypotension.

MEBENDAZOLE

Mebendazole is a benzimidazole carbamate with a broad range of anthelmintic activity.[6,7,75,76] It is active against the larvae and adults of *E. vermicularis*, *A. lumbricoides*, *T. trichiura*, *N. americanus* and *A. duodenale*. It is ovicidal for *Ascaris* and *Trichuris* spp. It is less effective than thiabendazole against *S. stercoralis*. Mebendazole has been used at high doses and for long periods in the treatment of *C. philippinensis*. It can also be used for infections caused by *Angiostrongylus cantonensis*, *Angiostrongylus costaricensis*, *Toxocara canis* and *Trichostrongylus* spp. The drug has activity against adult *Trichinella spiralis*, with some activity against larval forms, and it is currently recommended in the treatment of trichinosis.

Mebendazole is also effective in the treatment of certain types of filariasis; it is considered the drug of choice against *Mansonella perstans* (diethylcarbamazine is ineffective) and has been shown to have efficacy against *L. loa*, *O. volvulus* and *Dracunculus medinensis* infections. The drug has activity against *T. saginata*, *T. solium* and *Hymenolepis nana*, although praziquantel is more effective. Although mebendazole does not eradicate echinococcal infection, the drug prevents progression of existing cysts and the development of new cysts when administered in high dose for a prolonged period. Mebendazole has largely been replaced by albendazole for echinococcosis.

Mebendazole acts by binding parasite tubulin, thus blocking microtubule assembly and interfering with glucose absorption. Susceptible helminths become paralyzed and depleted of energy stores, but death and clearance of the worms from the gastrointestinal tract can take days. Mebendazole, formulated as 100 mg tablets, has low water solubility and is poorly absorbed. It is 95% protein-bound in plasma and undergoes rapid and extensive first-pass metabolism in the liver. Thus, systemic bioavailability is low, accounting not only for its poor tissue levels and relative lack of usefulness in extraintestinal infections, but also for its low rate of side-effects.

Abdominal pain and diarrhea may occur after mebendazole administration. The drug also has been reported to prompt the migration of adult *Ascaris* spp. into the mouth and nose. At high doses, reversible bone marrow suppression with neutropenia, alopecia, allergic skin reactions, hepatitis, vertigo and oligospermia occur rarely.

METRIFONATE

Metrifonate is an organophosphate inhibitor of acetylcholinesterase that was originally developed as an insecticide. It has activity against *Schistosoma haematobium*[6,7,85] but has largely been replaced by praziquantel as primary therapy.

The dosage is 7.5–10 mg/kg orally once every 2 weeks for three cycles. Side-effects include nausea, vomiting, vertigo and lethargy. Patients receiving metrifonate should neither be exposed to other insecticides nor receive neuromuscular blocking agents in the 2 days before or after taking metrifonate.

NICLOSAMIDE

Niclosamide is a salicylamide derivative that is active against the cestodes *Diphyllobothrium latum*, *D. caninum*, *H. nana*, *T. saginata* and *T. solium*, as well as the trematodes *Echinostoma* spp., *Fasciolopsis buski* and *Heterophyes heterophyes*.[6] It acts by interfering with oxidative phosphorylation and production of adenosine triphosphate. Treatment failures of *Taenia* spp. with niclosamide have been reported, and praziquantel has been used successfully in these cases.[86]

Niclosamide is supplied as 500 mg tablets that should be chewed thoroughly because of its very poor absorption. The dosage is 2 g as a single dose (or 1 g and 1 g, given 1 hour apart), except for *H. nana* infection, which requires 2 g then 1 g q24h for 6 days. Side-effects include gastrointestinal distress, dizziness and rash.

OXAMNIQUINE

Oxamniquine is a tetrahydroquinoline that is effective in *S. mansoni* infections.[6,7,85] Its mechanism of action is unclear, but it causes adult worms to become paralyzed and dislodged from the veins they inhabit, resulting in subsequent killing by host defenses. The drug is available in 250 mg capsules that are rapidly absorbed and extensively metabolized in the liver. The half-life is approximately 2 hours, and 70% of the drug is excreted by the kidneys. Side-effects include drowsiness, dizziness, orange–red discoloration of the urine and, rarely, seizures. The drug should be given cautiously to patients who have a history of seizures.

PIPERAZINE

Piperazine has activity against *A. lumbricoides* and *E. vermicularis*.[6,7,74] In many parts of the world it has been replaced by less toxic agents such as mebendazole. However, because of its lower cost, piperazine is still frequently used. Piperazine blocks the helminth muscle response to acetylcholine by altering membrane ion permeability and causing hyperpolarization and decreased action potentials. Flaccid paralysis ensues and the worms are eliminated in the stool.

Piperazine is available as the citrate salt in 250 mg tablets. There is good oral absorption and a small amount of hepatic metabolism; 60% of the drug is excreted in the urine unmodified. Different dosage schedules exist, but a single dose of 75 mg/kg (maximum 4 g) per day for 2 days is effective for ascariasis, and a single dose of 65 mg/kg/day for 7 days is used for enterobiasis.

Side-effects include gastrointestinal disturbances, headache, dizziness and urticaria. Seizures occur rarely, and piperazine is contraindicated in patients who have a history of a seizure disorder. Piperazine and pyrantel pamoate are antagonistic and should not be co-administered.

PRAZIQUANTEL

Praziquantel, a pyrazinoisoquinoline derivative developed in the early 1970s, has broad activity against trematodes and cestodes but not nematodes.[6,7,75,85] All *Schistosoma* spp. that infect humans are susceptible. The drug also has activity against the trematodes *C. sinensis*, *Dicrocoelium dendriticum*, *Echinostoma* spp., *F. buski*, *H. heterophyes*, *Metagonimus yokogawai*, *Metorchis conjunctus*, *Nanophyetus salmincola*, *Opisthorchis viverrini* and *Paragonimus westermani* and other *Paragonimus* spp. *Fasciola hepatica* does not appear to be adequately treated with praziquantel; bithionol is used instead. Praziquantel is effective in treating adult cestodes, including *D. latum* and other *Diphyllobothrium* spp., *D. caninum*, *H. nana*, *Hymenolepis diminuta*, *T. saginata* and *T. solium*. It has been used successfully to treat neurocysticercosis (larval *T. solium*), but it is not useful in echinococcosis. The drug has several actions, including promoting calcium influx and parasite muscle contraction and causing vacuolization and bleb formation in the helminth tegument, thereby activating host defenses.

Praziquantel is available as 600 mg tablets that are nearly insoluble in water. There is good oral absorption, 80% protein binding and rapid first-pass metabolism. The half-life is 1.5 hours. About 80% of the drug is excreted in the urine. Side-effects are common but transient and include headache, dizziness, nausea, vomiting and abdominal pain. Fever and rashes are occasionally seen.

PYRANTEL PAMOATE

Pyrantel pamoate, a tetrahydropyrimidine that was originally developed as a veterinary anthelmintic, has a broad range of activity in humans.[6,7,75,76] It is considered by many to be the treatment of choice for *E. vermicularis*. It is also effective for *A. lumbricoides*, eosinophilic enterocolitis caused by *Ancylostoma caninum*, hookworm, the acanthocephalan *Moniliformis moniliformis* and *Trichostrongylus* spp. It does not have activity against *T. trichiura*. Oxantel pamoate, an *m*-oxyphenol derivative, can be given in a single dose for *Trichuris* spp. Pyrantel pamoate and its analogues act by causing depolarizing neuromuscular blockade and by blocking acetylcholinesterase, which result in spastic paralysis and muscle contracture, respectively, and allow expulsion of the worms.

Pyrantel pamoate is available as an oral suspension of 250 mg of pyrantel base per 5 ml. It is poorly absorbed. Less than 15% is excreted in the urine and most remains in the feces unmodified. Side-effects include headache, dizziness, insomnia, nausea, vomiting, anorexia and abdominal pain. Pyrantel pamoate, which causes depolarization and increased spike frequency in worm muscle cells, should not be given with piperazine, which causes hyperpolarization and a reduction in spike frequency.

THIABENDAZOLE

Thiabendazole is a substituted benzimidazole compound that has better activity against *S. stercoralis* and *Strongyloides fuelleborni* than mebendazole.[6,7,75,76,85] It is active against *A. costaricensis*, *C. philippinensis*, *D. medinensis*, *Trichostrongylus* spp. and *T. spiralis*. In trichinosis, however, larval stages are often resistant to thiabendazole. The drug is also used in the treatment of both cutaneous and visceral larva migrans. Thiabendazole has some activity against *A. lumbricoides*, hookworm, *E. vermicularis* and *T. trichiura*, but mebendazole is less toxic and is thus preferred. The drug acts by inhibiting parasite fumarate reductase, and it may bind tubulin as well.

Thiabendazole is available in tablet and liquid form and, in contrast to other benzimidazole derivatives, is rapidly absorbed. It is extensively metabolized by the liver, has a half-life of 1 hour and is mainly excreted by the kidneys.

Side-effects are frequent; they include nausea, vomiting, anorexia and dizziness. Pruritus, epigastric pain, headache, drowsiness, giddiness and diarrhea are less common. Rarer still are tinnitus, hallucinations, numbness, seizures, altered olfaction, altered color perception, hypotension, bradycardia, crystalluria, leukopenia, elevated liver enzymes and intrahepatic cholestasis. Allergic manifestations, including fever, angioneurotic edema, erythema multiforme and Stevens–Johnson syndrome, have been described and may result from the release of parasite antigens during treatment. Increased theophylline levels and consequent nausea and vomiting may result from the co-administration of theophylline and thiabendazole.

TRICLABENDAZOLE

Triclabendazole, a benzimidazole derivative used as a veterinary fasciolicide, has been used safely and successfully in cases of human chronic hepatic fascioliasis.[87,88] It is now considered the drug of choice for human hepatic fascioliasis, but in the USA it is available only through compounding pharmacies.

REFERENCES

References for this chapter can be found online at http://www.expertconsult.com

Section | 8 |

Andy IM Hoepelman & Timothy E Kiehn

Clinical Microbiology

Arturo S Gastañaduy
Rodolfo E Bégué

Chapter | **151**

Acute gastroenteritis viruses

Acute gastroenteritis is a major cause of morbidity and mortality worldwide, most commonly affecting children both in developing and developed countries. Its importance was clearly defined in the 1980s and 1990s (Table 151.1).[1–4] Recent studies indicate that it continues to be a significant burden for human health.[5,6] While fewer than 5% of stool samples in patients with diarrhea show a bacterial or parasite pathogen,[7] recent technology allows for identifying an increasing number of viral etiologies.

APPROACH TO MANAGEMENT

No specific antiviral exists for any of the gastroenteritis viruses. Primary objectives of management are prevention and treatment of dehydration and malnutrition.[8] Most patients will improve with the administration of oral rehydration solutions (ORS) and continuous feeding with their regular diet. Rarely, intravenous fluids may be needed for severe dehydration, intractable vomiting or very high stool output. Although lactose malabsorption develops frequently during acute gastroenteritis, most children can be fed their usual lactose-containing formulas in small frequent feeds. Human milk has high lactose content, yet it reduces stool output and provides excellent nutrients and anti-infectious factors; therefore, breast-feeding should be continued. Moderate to severe malnourished children with diarrhea present a special problem. Malnutrition causes total body sodium excess, potassium and micronutrient deficiencies and increased energy requirements. ReSoMal is recommended for these patients. It is a specially formulated ORS that provides less sodium and more potassium and glucose. Magnesium, zinc and copper are added to ReSoMal.[9]

APPROACH TO PREVENTION

Viruses that cause gastroenteritis are transmitted mainly by the fecal–oral route, through direct person-to-person contact or contaminated food, water and fomites. Aerosol transmission from respiratory secretions or vomit occurs rarely. Hygienic measures decrease person-to-person spread. However, because these measures are difficult to enforce, particularly in young children, and because some viruses are resistant to commonly used disinfectants, transmission of the disease continues even in developed countries. Outbreaks require isolating ill personnel, thoroughly cooking food, disinfecting the environment and proper handling of food, water and sanitation. Careful hand washing cannot be overemphasized, especially among food handlers and personnel from hospitals, schools and day-care centers. Hospitalized or other institutionalized patients should have universal precautions and contact isolation until 48–72 hours after symptom resolution. The best preventive method will be effective, safe and affordable vaccines. Currently, such a vaccine is commercially available only for rotavirus.[10]

APPROACH TO DIAGNOSIS

An etiologic diagnosis is not necessary for the management of most cases of acute gastroenteritis. For viral gastroenteritis, an etiologic diagnosis may be desired in specific clinical circumstances or for epidemiologic and research purposes. Detection of viral antigens by immunoassays (IAs) is the method of choice. IAs are simple and rapid, have good sensitivity and specificity, and are practical

Table 151.1 Morbidity and mortality rates of diarrheal diseases in children*

	DEVELOPING COUNTRIES			USA–CANADA
	Snyder & Merson (1982)[1]	Claeson & Merson (1990)[2]	Bern et al. (1992)[3]	Glass et al. (1991)[4]
No. of studies evaluated	24	276	22	4
Diarrheal episodes/year (millions)	1000	1500	1000	21–37
Episodes/child/year (median)	2.2–3.0	3.3	2.6	1.3–2.5
No. of diarrheal deaths/year	4.6 million	4.0 million	3.3 million	325–425

*Estimates from longitudinal, prospective, community-based studies in developing and developed countries.

for testing large numbers of samples. IAs are commercially available for rotaviruses, adenoviruses and astroviruses. Reverse transcriptase polymerase chain reaction (RT-PCR) techniques have been developed for many gastroenteritis viruses. Because they are more sensitive than IAs, they allow viral detection not only in clinical specimens (stools, vomitus) but also in contaminated food, water and fomites. These techniques are most useful for caliciviruses. Electron microscopy (EM) and immune electron microscopy (IEM) identify viruses of distinct morphology and excreted in large numbers (>10[6] virions/ml of stools), such as rotavirus or astrovirus. However, these techniques are not suitable for a large number of samples or routine laboratory diagnosis. Viral culture is essential for virus characterization, the study of their pathogenesis and the production of diagnostic reagents but is slow and cumbersome. Not all gastroenteritis viruses can be cultured.

VIRAL AGENTS OF GASTROENTERITIS

The morphologic, epidemiologic and clinical characteristics of the main gastroenteritis viruses are presented in Tables 151.2–151.4. Most cases of acute gastroenteritis worldwide are caused by caliciviruses in all age groups and rotaviruses in children; all the other viruses are responsible for approximately 10% of cases.

Caliciviruses (Norovirus, Sapovirus)

In 1972, Kapikian *et al.*, investigating a gastroenteritis outbreak in Norwalk, Ohio, visualized 27 nm particles in a stool filtrate and noted that infected individuals developed a specific antibody response against the particles. This was the first confirmation of a virus as an etiologic agent of gastroenteritis.[11] The virus was named Norwalk virus (NV) and was believed to belong to the Picornaviridae family. Similar viruses were named by the location where they were first identified (Hawaii, Sapporo, etc.) and, as a group, were known as Norwalk-like viruses or small round structured viruses (SRSVs). Soon, it became evident that the SRSVs were different from the picornaviruses in structure, mode of replication and other characteristics. Cloning of the NV genome[12] led to the classification of these viruses within the Caliciviridae family.

NATURE

Caliciviruses are small (27–40 nm), nonenveloped viruses with a single-stranded, positive-sense RNA genome.[13] They have an icosahedral capsid with cup-like depressions on the viral surface (*calici* is derived from the Latin word *calyx*, which means cup) (Fig. 151.1).

Four genera have been identified in the Caliciviridae family: Lagovirus, Vesivirus, Norovirus (NoV) and Sapovirus (SaV). Lagovirus and Vesivirus only infect animals. Norovirus and Sapovirus have human and animal strains and are further classified into genogroups and genetic clusters (Table 151.5).

The calicivirus genomes are about 7.3–8.5 kb in length and organized in two or three open reading frames (ORFs). In the genera with three ORFs, Norovirus and Vesivirus, the first ORF (ORF1) encodes for a large protein that by proteolytic cleavage produces the nonstructural proteins. ORF2 encodes for the single major structural protein (viral protein 1, VP1) and ORF3 encodes for a minor structural protein (viral protein 2, VP2). Sapovirus and Lagovirus have only two ORFs. In these viruses, VP1 and VP2 are encoded in ORF1 and ORF2, respectively.[14]

The molecular weight of VP1 is approximately 60 kDa. Ninety VP1 dimers form the capsid with 90 arch-like protruding capsomers arranged in such a way as to leave 32 calices on the viral surface. VP1 has two major domains: the shell (S) domain and the protruding (P) domain. The S domain forms the inner part of the capsid. It has 225 amino acids (aa), including aa 10–49 corresponding to the *N*-terminal region of the protein (N subdomain), which faces the interior of the capsid. The P domain includes amino acids 226–520 and is subdivided into subdomains P1 and P2. The P1 subdomain (aa 226–278 and 406–520) forms the sides of the capsomers, whereas the P2 subdomain (aa 279–405) forms the most protruding part of the capsomer arches (see Fig. 151.1). VP1 self-assembles into virus-like particles (VLPs) without RNA or VP2 participation. The VLPs are morphologically and antigenically similar to natural virions.[15]

Each virion has only one or two copies of VP2 (12–29 kDa). The function of VP2 is unknown; however, in feline caliciviruses, intact VP2 is needed to produce infection. A third structural protein, VPg, is also present as one or two copies per virion. It is linked to the genomic or subgenomic RNA and may function as a nonstructural protein during replication.[14]

The caliciviruses have seven nonstructural proteins (NSP1–NSP7). The function of some of them has been inferred based on similar sequences in picornavirus proteins. NSP3 is a nucleoside triphosphatase,

Table 151.2 Structure and morphological characteristics of gastroenteritis viruses

Characteristics	Norovirus	Sapovirus	Rotavirus	Astrovirus	Enteric adenovirus
Family	*Caliciviridae*	*Caliciviridae*	*Reoviridae*	*Astroviridae*	*Adenoviridae*
Virion size (nm)	27–35	27–40	70–75	41	70–80
Envelop	Non-enveloped	Non-enveloped	Non-enveloped	Non-enveloped	Non-enveloped
Capsid	Icosahedral	Icosahedral	Triple shelled	Icosahedral	Icosahedral
Genome type	Positive sense ssRNA	Positive sense ssRNA	Segmented dsRNA	Positive sense ssRNA	dsDNA
Morphology on electron microscopy	Round surface, cup-shaped indentations	Round surface, cup-shaped indentations	Wheel-like capsid with radiating spokes	Round, 28–30 nm, 5–6-pointed star shape	Fiber-like projections from vertices
Electron micrograph					

ds, double-stranded; ss, single-stranded.
Norovirus and sapovirus electron micrographs courtesy of C Humphrey (CDC); rotavirus, astrovirus and enteric adenovirus electron micrographs courtesy of S Spangenberger.

Table 151.3 Epidemiological characteristics of gastroenteritis viruses

Characteristic	Norovirus	Sapovirus	Rotavirus	Astrovirus	Enteric adenovirus
Age group	All ages	Children	6–24 months	<7 years, elderly	<4 years
Seasonality	No	No	Winter	Winter	Summer
Disease pattern	Outbreaks, endemic	Endemic, outbreaks	Endemic, annual epidemics	Endemic, nosocomial outbreaks	Endemic
Transmission	Person-to-person, water, food, shellfish	Person-to-person, water, cold foods, shellfish	Person-to-person, food, water	Person-to-person, food, water	Person-to-person
Fecal excretion (days)	7–13	–	10	–	Persistent, months
Outpatient prevalence (%)	Endemic: 10–25 Outbreaks: 90	1–10	5–10	7–8	4–8
Inpatient prevalence (%)	Rare	3–5	35–40	3–5	5–20

Table 151.4 Usual clinical characteristics of gastroenteritis virus infections

Signs and symptoms	Norovirus	Sapovirus	Rotavirus	Astrovirus	Enteric adenovirus
Prodrome (days)	1–2	1–3	1–3	3–4	8–10
Diarrhea: watery	66–95% 4–8/day Adults >children	88–95% Mild	96–100% 10–20/day	72–100% 2–4/day	97% 1/3 >14 days
Vomitus	57–95% Children >adults	44–65%	80–90% Early	20–50% 1/day	79% Early
Fever	24–48% Low grade	18–34%	60–65% Moderate	20% Low grade	Occasionally Low grade
Abdominal pain	11–91% Cramps	–	Colicky	50%	–
Dehydration	~1%	Infrequent	Frequent in young children	Infrequent	Infrequent
Other symptoms	Myalgia 26%, headache 22%	Respiratory 22%, myalgia, headache	Respiratory 22–52%	Malaise, respiratory	Respiratory occasionally
Duration of illness (days)	0.5–2.5	4	3–8	2–3	5–12

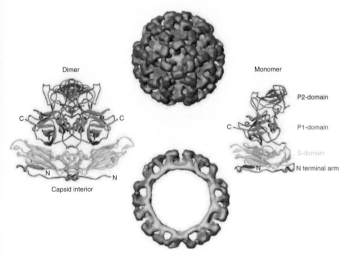

Fig. 151.1 Norwalk virus-like particle. Adapted from Hutson *et al.* Trends Microbiol 2004;12:279–87, with permission.

NSP6 is a proteinase and NSP7 is an RNA-dependent RNA polymerase. While the function of the other NSPs is unknown, they may play a role in the replication process.[14]

EPIDEMIOLOGY

Human caliciviruses (HuCV) have worldwide distribution. Noroviruses infect persons of all ages, both in developed and developing countries. They are the most common cause of gastroenteritis outbreaks and are also recognized as the most common cause of viral gastroenteritis in community-based studies.[16] Studies show an increasing prevalence of specific antibodies since infancy, reaching 80–90% in young adults.[17] The prevalence of specific antibodies rises faster in developing countries, indicating early infections.[18] Genogroups I and II produce the majority of community infections. Most infections are caused by a single circulating strain. For example, Genogroup II.4 became the most common cause of outbreaks around the world in the 1990s. Co-infections occur, giving the opportunity for the exchange of genetic material between strains and the generation of new virus strains.[19] Outbreaks occur mainly in

Table 151.5 Taxonomy of the Caliciviridae family

Genus	Genogroups	Genetic clusters	Representative species	Representative strain*
Norovirus (Nov)	I	1–8	Norwalk virus	Hu/NoV/GI.1/Norwalk/1968/US
	II	1–19	Hawaii norovirus	Hu/Nov/GII.1/Hawaii/1971/US
	III	1–2	Bovine norovirus	Bo/NoV/GIII.1/Jena/1980/DE
	IV	1	Alphatron virus	Hu/Nov/GIV.1/Alphatron98-2/1998/NL
	V	1	Murine norovirus	M/NoV/GV.1/MNV-1/2003/US
Sapovirus (SaV)	I	1–3	Sapporo virus	Hu/SaV/G1.1/Sapporo/1982/JP
	II	1–3	London sapovirus	Hu/SaV/GII.1/London/1992/UK
	III	1	Swine sapovirus	Sw/SaV/GIII.1/PEC-Cowden/1980/US
	IV	1	Houston sapovirus	Hu/SaV/GIV.1/Hou7-1181/1990/US
	V	1	Argentina sapovirus	Hu/Sav/GV.1/Argentina 39/AR
Lagovirus (LaV)			Rabbit hemorrhagic disease virus	Ra/LaV/RHDV/GH/1988/DE
			European brown hare syndrome virus	Ha/LaV/EBHSV/GD/1989/FR
Vesivirus (VeV)			Vesicular exanthema of swine virus	SW/VeV/VESV/A48/1948/US
			Feline calicivirus	Fe/VeV/FCV/F9/1958/US

Host species abbreviations: Hu, human; Bo, bovine; M, murine; Sw, swine; Ra, rabbit; Ha, hare; Fe, feline. **Country abbreviations**: US, United States; DE, Germany; NL, Netherlands; JP, Japan; UK, United Kingdom; AR, Argentina; FR, France.
*Host species/genus/species or genogroup/strain name/year of occurrence/country of origin.
Adapted with permission from Green et al.[13]

day-care centers, schools, colleges, hospitals, nursing homes, military personnel, restaurants, vacation facilities and cruise ships. Noroviruses also cause travelers' diarrhea. They were the only pathogens isolated from Hurricane Katrina evacuees with gastroenteritis in a large shelter in Houston, Texas.[20] Noroviruses can spread internationally through contaminated food or beverages.[21] A study of 8271 food-borne outbreaks of gastroenteritis reported to the US Centers for Disease Control and Prevention (CDC) shows a median of affected persons of 25 vs 10 for the bacterial outbreaks. Ten percent of the individuals required medical care and 1% were hospitalized.[22]

Caliciviruses are ubiquitous and stable in the environment, providing a persistent source of infection. Noroviruses survive freezing, heating to 140°F (60°C) for 30 minutes and are stable in water chlorinated to 6.25 mg/l; most municipal water systems contain <5 mg/l of chlorine. The virus is also acid-resistant and ether-stable.[23,24]

PATHOGENICITY

Caliciviruses are transmitted mainly by the fecal–oral route, but airborne transmission has also been reported.[25,26] The infectious dose has been estimated at less than 10 virions.[16] The incubation period ranges from 10 to 51 hours with a mean of 24 hours.[23,27] Norovirus infection mainly affects the proximal portions of the small intestine with broadening and blunting of the villi, crypt cell hyperplasia, cytoplasm vacuolization and mononuclear cell infiltration in the lamina propria. There is malabsorption of D-xylose, lactose and fat, and a decrease in brush border enzymes.[28,29] Pathologic changes are transient and resolve within 2 weeks. No histologic lesions are seen in the gastric or rectal mucosa, and the secretion of hydrochloric acid, pepsin and intrinsic factor remain normal.[30] Gastric emptying is markedly delayed, which could explain the frequent occurrence of nausea and vomiting; however, the degree of delay does not correlate with the severity of vomiting.[31] Virus excretion in the stool may begin during the prodrome stage,[32] last 7–13 days,[33] and persist for several weeks after resolution of symptoms, especially in infants,[34] and for months to years in immunocompromised patients.[35]

The cell and tissue tropism of HuCV are largely unknown. Calicivirus replication may be similar to that of other positive-strand RNA viruses. Following attachment to specific receptors, the virus enters the cell and is uncoated, and ORF1 produces the NSPs. Synthesis of negative-strand RNA begins. This serves as a template for positive-strand genomic and subgenomic RNA, which will serve as a template for the synthesis of VP1 and VP2. It is known that VP1 can self-assemble to form the capsid, but the process of packing of the viral RNA within the capsid, maturation and release of the virions is poorly understood.[14] It is assumed that replication occurs in the epithelial cells of the upper gastrointestinal tract; however, no viral particles have been observed by EM of the jejunal mucosa. While there is no animal model for the human caliciviruses, it has been shown that radiolabeled Norwalk VLPs bind and, in some cases, enter various cell lines.[36] The development of a human cell line for norovirus and a murine norovirus model will advance the study of norovirus pathogenesis.[37,38]

Susceptibility to NV infection is peculiar. Some individuals have natural resistance to the infection. They lack virus receptors; repeated challenges with the virus fail to produce illness or antibody response. The virus receptors are histo-blood group antigens (HBGAs). These are membrane carbohydrates present on the surface of red blood cells, enterocytes and other mucosal cells. The carbohydrates have an $\alpha 1,2$-linked fucose in common, e.g. Fucoα2Galβ3GlcNac. The protruding domain of VP1 of NV VLPs attaches to this trisaccharide or similar molecules, allowing binding and subsequent internalization of the VLPs. The receptors are host and viral-strain specific. Receptor production is genetically controlled by alleles at the ABO, FUT2 and FUT3 loci. Individuals with O blood group are more easily infected, while B blood group individuals have decreased risk. Individuals with the FUT2 –/– genotype are highly resistant to NV infections and represent about 20% of the European population.[39,40]

Acquired immunity is mostly short term and type specific. Challenges with the virus produce illness and specific antibody response. Although re-exposure to the same virus strain within 6–14 weeks does not result in illness, a re-challenge 27–42 weeks later results in disease and serum antibody response.[23,41,42] Serum or local jejunal antibodies do not correlate with resistance in volunteer studies.[33,43,44]

On the other hand, a rapid mucosal IgA response, associated with resistance to illness, has been shown in volunteers.[40] Cell-mediated immune responses have been observed in volunteers immunized with Norwalk VLPs.

PREVENTION

To date, no commercially available vaccine exists against HuCV. Vaccine development has been hampered by the following factors:
- partial understanding of HuCV immunogenicity;
- multiple virus types and infrequent cross immunity;
- inability to culture the virus; and
- lack of a small animal model for human caliciviruses.[45]

Nevertheless, rNV VLPs given orally to mice and human volunteers are safe and induce IgG$_1$ and IgA antibody responses.[46] While waiting for the vaccine, preventive measures should follow the procedures mentioned above. Contaminated water supplies can be treated with chlorine concentrations >10 mg/l.

DIAGNOSTIC MICROBIOLOGY

RT-PCR is the most widely used technique. It is very sensitive and allows virus detection in clinical specimens and the environment. Primer selection is important as genetically diverse strains may not be detected; RT-PCR with multiple primers identified Norwalk-like viruses as the etiologic agent of 96% of gastroenteritis outbreaks.[14,16,47] Immunoassays to detect viral antigens in stools are less sensitive; however, IAs to detect antibodies to the viruses have been very useful in sero-epidemiologic and vaccine development studies.

CLINICAL MANIFESTATIONS

The usual clinical characteristics of norovirus and sapovirus infections are presented in Table 151.4. Most of the time, infections are acute, short lived or asymptomatic; however, severe illness, including disseminated intravascular coagulation, has been described in healthy soldiers under severe environmental conditions.[48]

MANAGEMENT

No specific therapy exists for HuCV infections. Treatment is supportive with oral or intravenous rehydration. Bismuth subsalicylate reduces severity and duration of illness in experimental infections in adults,[49] but the use of symptomatic medications for the management of acute gastroenteritis in children is not recommended by the American Academy of Pediatrics.[50]

Rotaviruses

First described in 1973 by Bishop *et al.*,[51] human rotaviruses (RVs) represent the main agent of acute gastroenteritis in infants and young children.

NATURE

Rotaviruses belong to the family Reoviridae.[52] Intact 75 nm particles have a triple-layered capsid with core, inner and outer layers. Sixty spike-like structures (capsomers) radiating from the inner to the outer layer give the virus its characteristic wheel-like appearance. The core

capsid encloses the viral genome, consisting of 11 segments of double-stranded RNA. Each segment encodes for one protein, except segment 11 which encodes for two. Six proteins (VP1–VP4, VP6–VP7) form the virion structure, and six nonstructural proteins (NSP1–NSP6) are expressed only in the infected cell (Fig. 151.2, Table 151.6).[53,54] The core is made of VP1, VP2 (its major contituent) and VP3. VP6 is the sole component of the inner capsid. The outer capsid is composed of VP7 (90%) and VP4, which forms the capsomers.

VP6 defines seven antigenic groups (A–G), with group A rotaviruses causing most human infections. The outer capsid proteins VP4 and VP7 determine the serotypes. Those defined by VP7 are called G (for glycoprotein) serotypes, and those defined by VP4 are called P (for protease-sensitive protein) serotypes. There is full concordance between VP7 serotypes and genotypes; there are at least 15 G serotypes designated G1–G15. The concordance between VP4 serotypes and genotypes is poor. There are 14 VP4 serotypes (P1–P14) and 26 genotypes (1–26). P1 and P5 include subtypes A and B; P2 includes subtypes A, B and C; Genotype 5 has a 5A subtype. Rotaviruses are formally designated using the G and P letters followed by the serotype number; a second number in parentheses after the P indicates the genotype. For example, the human RV strain Wa is designated G1P1A[8].

EPIDEMIOLOGY

Transmission of RVs is mainly person to person by the fecal–oral route. Fecal excretion starts immediately before the onset of symptoms and lasts for 5–7 days. Spread is favored by the large number of virions excreted in feces (1 trillion per ml) and the low infective dose (10 RV particles). Contamination of food and water has been implicated in some outbreaks. Since RVs can survive for 60 days on environmental surfaces at different temperatures (39.2–68°F/4–20°C) and humidities (50–90%), fomites may play a role in such settings as day-care centers and nurseries.[55] Respiratory transmission has been suspected in a few outbreaks and is supported by the way the annual RV epidemic spreads in North America. However, attempts to isolate RV from respiratory secretions have been mostly unsuccessful.

Rotaviruses are the most commonly identified viral enteropathogens of infants and young children. The proportion of diarrhea cases caused by RVs increases from community to clinic to hospital populations, reflecting the tendency of the virus to produce dehydration. In the USA, RVs cause 5–10% of all diarrheal episodes and 30–50% of severe diarrhea in children under 5 years of age, resulting in 3.5 million cases, 55 000 hospitalizations, 20–40 deaths and costs in excess of one billion dollars.[56] Worldwide, the estimates are 111 million episodes, 2 million hospitalizations and 600 000 deaths annually. RVs account for a larger proportion of cases in developed countries than in developing ones (38–89% vs 20–46%, respectively) and in high-income groups than in low-income ones (60% vs 4–30%, respectively).[57]

Incidence rates peak at age 6–24 months. Neonates are affected infrequently. Adults exposed to infected children become infected frequently (11–70%) but rarely develop clinical disease.[58,59] Outbreaks have been described in nursing homes for the elderly, hospital wards and military bases. RVs have been detected in as many as 20% of cases of travelers' diarrhea. Asymptomatic shedding of RVs occurs in 10–15% of individuals.

In temperate climates, RVs appear in characteristic and predictable winter epidemics. In North America, the epidemic starts in late fall in Mexico and the southwestern USA, spreads in a northeast direction and ends in the spring in the northeastern USA and the Maritime provinces of Canada.[60] The reasons for this spread pattern are not clear; climate, virus characteristics or other factors may play a role. In tropical climates, RVs are endemic throughout the year, with some clustering in the cooler, drier months. Globally, group A serotypes G1–G4, in conjunction with P[8] or P[4], constitute most human infections. However, there is much geographic and temporal variability, with G9, G8, G5 and others emerging as prevalent in some parts of the world.[53,61] Multiple serotypes can co-circulate during a specific year.

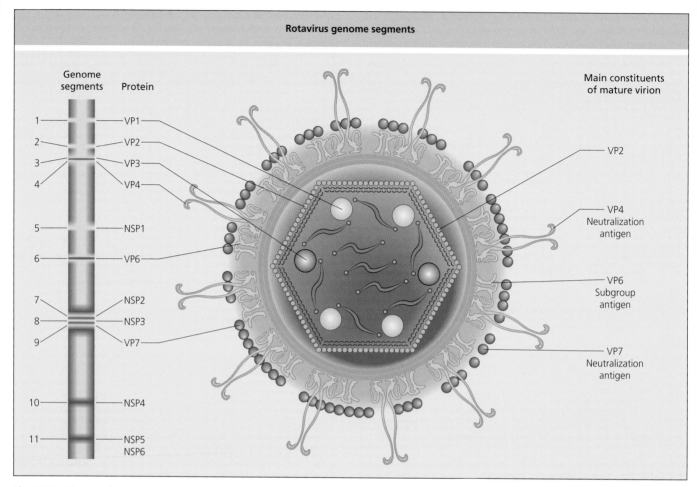

Rotavirus genome segments

Genome segments | Protein

1 — VP1
2 — VP2
3 — VP3
4 — VP4
5 — NSP1
6 — VP6
7 — NSP2
8 — NSP3
9 — VP7
10 — NSP4
11 — NSP5 NSP6

Main constituents of mature virion

VP2
VP4 Neutralization antigen
VP6 Subgroup antigen
VP7 Neutralization antigen

Fig. 151.2 Diagram showing rotavirus genome segments, protein products and their location in the viral particle. Adapted with permission from Gentsch *et al.*[53]

Group B RVs have been associated with epidemics of diarrhea among adults in China, and group C RVs have been identified in Central and South America, Europe, Australia and Asia.

PATHOGENICITY

Rotaviruses preferentially infect the mature enterocytes of the small intestine. Infected cells change from columnar to cuboidal, with enlarged cisternae of the endoplasmic reticulum and fewer and shorter microvilli. The cells are eventually killed and sloughed off and, with denudation of the tip cells, the villi become shortened. Mononuclear leukocyte infiltration is minimal. These changes occur within 24 hours of infection, start proximally and progress caudally.[51,62] Recently, RV RNA has been detected in blood and cerebrospinal fluid, suggesting that RV may represent a systemic infection.[63] Diarrhea results from decreased absorption of salt and water secondary to enterocyte damage and replacement of absorptive intestinal cells by secreting cells from the crypts. Loss of disaccharidases at the damaged brush border results in carbohydrate malabsorption and osmotic diarrhea. NSP4, the first described viral enterotoxin, increases plasma membrane chloride permeability, leading to chloride secretion and secretory diarrhea.[64]

The replication cycle of RV has been reviewed elsewhere.[54] Some key points are noted here. The nature of the receptors on the host cell remains elusive. On the virus side, VP4 mediates attachment, and its cleavage into VP5* and VP8* by proteases-like trypsin is essential for cell penetration. Cell penetration also requires VP7. The virus enters the cell either by direct membrane penetration or by receptor-mediated endocytosis; intracellular levels of Ca^{2+} trigger virus uncoating. RNA synthesis occurs in the core of the virion, mediated by an endogenous RNA-dependent RNA polymerase. The RNA transcripts encode the RV proteins, which are translated by the cellular translational machinery. The initial steps of virus replication occur in cytoplasmic inclusions called viroplasms. The viral subparticles bud through the membrane of the endoplasmic reticulum and become mature particles. NSP4 plays a key role in the assembly process, which is Ca^{2+} dependent. Lastly, mature virus particles are released by cell lysis in nonpolarized cells or by nonclassic vesicular transport in polarized epithelial cells.

Immunity against RV infection and illness are not completely understood.[65] Clinical protection may involve local (mucosal) and systemic (serum) antibodies as well as cellular immunity. VP7- and VP4-induced serum-neutralizing antibodies against the infecting serotype (homotypic) appear within 2 weeks of infection. Heterotypic antibodies against different serotypes also occur, but mostly among adults, and vary with the infecting strain. There is a correlation between the presence of homotypic neutralizing antibodies and protection.[58] The duration of homotypic protection is probably longer than that of heterotypic but is both incomplete and short lived, as shown by the occurrence of re-infections with the same serotype. Antibody levels are high at birth, decline by 3–6 months, rise to a peak at 2–3 years and remain elevated throughout life (this is probably because of repeated, mostly asymptomatic infections).[66] Serum antibodies do not always prevent the infection. Mucosal immunity may be more important than systemic immunity. It develops 4 weeks after the illness and persists for several months, eventually decreasing with advancing age.[67]

Passively acquired mucosal immunity by breast-feeding or orally administered immune globulins has conferred protection to high-risk individuals. Cell-mediated immunity also seems to be important.

Table 151.6 Rotavirus genome segments and their corresponding viral proteins

Genome segment (size, bp)	Protein product (MW, kDa)	Location in virus particles	Function
1 (3302)	VP1 (125)	Core capsid	RNA-dependent RNA polymerase, complex with VP3
2 (2729)	VP2 (94)	Core capsid	Main constituent of core, RNA binding
3 (2591)	VP3 (88)	Core capsid	Complex with VP1, guanylyl and methyl transferase, synthesis of capped mRNA transcripts
4 (2359)	VP4 (86.7)	Outer capsid	Hemagglutinin, cell attachment, neutralization antigen, determines P serotypes, cleaved by trypsin into VP5* (52.9) and VP8* (24.7), virulence
5 (1566)	NSP1 (58.6)	Nonstructural	Basic protein, RNA binding
6 (1356)	VP6 (44.8)	Inner capsid	Main constituent of inner capsid, determines group specificity, protection, required for transcription
7 (1074)	NSP3 (34.6)	Nonstructural	Acidic protein, RNA binding, inhibits host cell translation
8 (1059)	NSP2 (36.7)	Nonstructural	Basic protein, RNA binding, forms viroplasms with NSP5
9 (1062)	VP7 (37.4)	Outer capsid	Glycoprotein, major constituent of outer capsid, determines G serotypes
10 (750)	NSP4 (20.2)	Nonstructural	Role in morphogenesis, interacts with viroplasms, modulates intracellular Ca^{2+} and RNA replication, enterotoxin, virulence
11 (664)	NSP5 (21.7)	Nonstructural	Role in morphogenesis, forms viroplasms with NSP2, interacts with VP2 and NSP6
11 (664)	NSP6 (12)	Nonstructural	Interacts with NSP5, present in viroplasms

bp, base pairs; MW, molecular weight.
Adapted with permission from Estes & Kapikian.[54]

In mice, RV-specific cytotoxic T cells appear in the intestinal mucosa soon after infection. Mice with severe combined immmunodeficiency are able to clear RV infection when reconstituted with CD8 T cells, despite their lack of antibodies against the virus.[68] Recent experimental data suggest a role for non-neutralizing anti-VP6 antibodies in protection, though its significance in human infection is still unclear.[69]

PREVENTION

Breast-feeding reduces the overall incidence of diarrhea. For RVs, however, the effect of breast-feeding may be not so much in reducing incidence as in reducing the severity and duration of illness.[70]

Careful hand washing is important to reduce virus transmission. Fecal contamination of surfaces and objects occurs frequently, and RVs can survive in the environment for weeks.[71] Effective disinfectants are 6% hydrogen peroxide, 2500 ppm chlorine, 80% ethanol, ethanophenolic disinfectants, ultraviolet radiation and heat; drying and phenolic disinfectants are not effective;[72] hypochlorites are inactivated by fecal organic matter. Nondisposable objects are better cleaned by washing at 176°F (80°C) for at least 1 minute. Household laundry should be washed with detergent and bleach, followed by a drying cycle.

The first commercial RV vaccine, RotaShield by Wyeth-Ayerst Laboratories, was licensed in the USA in 1998. It was a rhesus–human reassortant live vaccine containing strains with specificities for G1–G4 serotypes. Three doses given orally at 2, 4 and 6 months of age were 49% effective for all RV diarrhea and 80% effective for severe RV diarrhea, thereby decreasing physician intervention by 73% and basically eliminating all cases of RV dehydration.[73] The vaccine was suspended less than 1 year later due to an association with intussusception, estimated as one additional case/10 000 infants vaccinated.[74]

More recently a new vaccine, RotaTeq, has been licensed in the USA (Table 151.7). This is also a live reassortant vaccine but of bovine–human origin and containing five strains of G1–G4 and P1[8] specificities. Three doses of the vaccine administered at 2, 4 and 6 months of age have demonstrated 74% efficacy to prevent any RV disease and 98% efficacy for severe disease with no detected association to intussusception.[75] A second RV vaccine, Rotarix (Table 151.7), also prevents any (73%) or severe (85%) RV disease without association to intussusception.[76] Rotarix is a live monovalent vaccine derived of a human attenuated strain of G1P[8]; two doses at 2 and 4 months are recommended. It is licensed in Latin America, Europe and recently in the US. Both vaccines decrease the overall burden of diarrhea hospitalization by ~50%, which may significantly improve the worldwide health of children. Both vaccines are recommended for universal immunization of children in the US.

DIAGNOSTIC MICROBIOLOGY

Various antigen detection kits based on enzyme immunoassays (EIAs) and the latex agglutination test are commercially available and represent the tests of choice for most clinical circumstances. They are relatively inexpensive and permit rapid diagnosis with high sensitivity and specificity (70–100%). Newborns and breast-feeding children might have higher false-positive results. Samples should be obtained during the symptomatic period to optimize the performance of the test. If samples are not to be processed immediately, they can be stored at 39.2°F (4°C) or frozen. In special situations, other tests can be considered, such as EM, gel electrophoresis of viral RNA, hybridization of radiolabeled nucleic acid probes to the viral RNA, amplification by RT-PCR and viral culture. Serologic tests are rarely used. Neutralizing antibodies can be detected by plaque reduction or cytopathic effect inhibition.

Table 151.7 Comparison of two licensed rotavirus vaccines		
Name	RotaTeq®	Rotarix™
Producer	Merck & Co., Inc	GlaxoSmithKline
Vaccine type	Live, bovine–human reassortant	Live-attenuated human RV strain (RIX4414)
Serotypes	Pentavalent: G1, G2, G3, G4, P1[8]	Monovalent G1P[8]
Dose	>2 × 10⁶ infective doses, each	>1 × 10⁶ infective doses
Administration	Oral, three doses at 2, 4 and 6 months of age	Oral, two doses at 2 and 4 months of age
Intussusception risk*	1.6 (0.4–6.4)	0.85 (0.30–2.42)
Efficacy:†		
RV GE, any severity	74 (67–80)	73 (27–91)
RV GE, severe	98 (88–100)	85 (72–92)
All diarrhea hospitalization	59 (52–65)	42 (29–53)
Virus shedding	9%	50–80%

*Odds ratio vaccine vs placebo (95% CI).
†Percent decrease vaccine vs placebo (95% CI).
GE, gastroenteritis; RV, rotavirus.

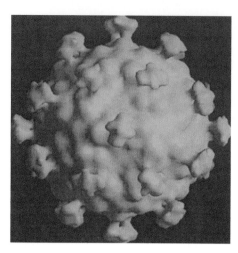

Fig. 151.3 Three-dimensional reconstruction of cryoelectron microscopy image of human astrovirus. Reproduced with permission from Mendez & Arias.[85]

CLINICAL MANIFESTATIONS

The clinical spectrum of RV infections ranges from asymptomatic to severe disease with dehydration and death. The usual clinical picture is presented in Table 151.4. The disease is self-limiting; chronic infection has not been described in the normal host.[66] Neonatal RV infections are symptomatic in <10–20% of cases, and usually mild. Severe infections may occur among premature infants and in special care units.

MANAGEMENT

Rehydration and appropriate feeding are the main therapies for RV diarrhea. Oral immune globulin and colostrum or human milk containing RV antibodies have been used in the treatment of RV diarrhea with good results.[77] The anti-RV titer is low in human preparations but higher in colostrum from cows immunized against RV. This form of therapy might prove useful for immunocompromised patients and those with chronic or severe disease. Also, formulas supplemented with *Bifidobacterium bifidum* and *Streptococcus thermophilus* reduce the incidence of diarrhea and RV shedding in infected children.[78] Interference with the overgrowth of bacteria and promotion of the intestinal immune response to RV have been suggested as possible mechanisms. Recently, nitazoxanide (a broad-spectrum anti-infective) has been reported to decrease the duration of severe RV diarrhea.[79]

Astroviruses

Astroviruses belong to the family Astroviridae. In 1975, they were described by Madeley & Cosgrove as small (28 nm) particles with a five- or six-pointed star appearance by EM.[80] Later studies showed an icosahedral, 41 nm morphology with well-defined spikes (Fig. 151.3). If the viruses are subjected to high pH, they transform to the previously described star.[81] The virus is nonenveloped, with a single-stranded, positive-sense RNA genome that contains three ORFs. ORF1a and ORF1b encode viral protease and polymerase, respectively. ORF2 encodes a protein capsid precursor, which gives rise to VP32, VP29 and VP26 (structural capsid proteins). VP26 and VP29 appear to be responsible for antigenic variation.[82] Eight serotypes have been described (HAstV-1 to HAstV-8).

Human astrovirus are responsible for 2–4% of endemic diarrhea in children worldwide; HAstV-1 is the most prevalent.[83,84] Astroviruses are the 'second or third most common cause of viral diarrhea in young children'.[85] They have been associated with outbreaks in day-care centers, schools and pediatric wards. Infection confers protective antibodies, which become more prevalent with increasing age. More than 80% of adults have antibodies against the virus. Immunocompromised subjects and the elderly are also affected.

Astrovirus pathogenesis is not completely understood. Histopathologic studies in an immunocompromised patient show infection in mature epithelial cells of the small intestine,[86] without inflammatory response. Mild crypt cell hyperplasia, also without inflammation, has been observed in turkeys.

Prevention or control of outbreaks can be accomplished by following the procedures mentioned above. The virus is inactivated by methanol 70–90% and heating at 140°F (60°C) for 10 minutes; however, it is resistant to chloroform and ethanol. As yet there is no vaccine.

Diagnosis can be made by commercial IAs with good sensitivity and specificity when compared with EM and RT-PCR.[84] The clinical characteristics of astrovirus infection are presented in Table 151.4. Symptoms are similar to those of RV infection but less severe. Management is supportive.

Enteric Adenoviruses

The Adenoviridae family has 51 human adenovirus serotypes, which are divided into six species or groups (A–F). Described in 1975,[87] enteric adenoviruses belong to species F and comprise serotypes 40 and 41. Other serotypes have also been associated with gastroenteritis, but their significance is less clear.

Adenoviruses are nonenveloped, with a dsDNA genome surrounded by an icosahedral capsid with fiber-like projections from each of the 12 vertices. Morphologic characteristics are presented in Table 151.2. Each virion contains 240 hexons (major surface protein) and 12 pentons. Each penton consists of a base and a fiber. Genus-specific antigens are located in the hexon. Type-specific antigens are located in the hexon and the fiber, which are in the virion surface and give rise to serum neutralizing antibodies.

The fiber protein of most adenoviruses binds to the coxsackie–adenovirus receptor (CAR) of epithelial cells and the penton base mediates internalization of the virus. Infected cells degenerate in typical ways. The process is related to the E3 virus proteins.[88] No specific receptors to explain species tissue tropism have been identified. The pathogenesis of gastroenteritis produced by serotypes 40 and 41 remains elusive.

Enteric adenoviruses have worldwide distribution, mainly affecting young children, and are responsible for 4% of acute gastroenteritis episodes seen in outpatient clinics and 2–22% seen in hospitalized children.[89] Outbreaks lasting 7–44 days have occurred in hospitals and day-care centers; approximately 40% of children were infected, half of them asymptomatically.[90]

Transmission is person to person by the fecal–oral route. Infected persons developed group- and type-specific antibodies. The latter are needed for long-term immunity and can be measured by neutralization or hemagglutination inhibition (HAI) tests. Stool excretion of adenoviruses lasts 10–14 days, from 2 days before and 5 days after diarrhea. Asymptomatic excretion may last months to years; thus, their isolation in diarrheic stools does not necessarily mean acute infection.

Outbreak control can be accomplished following the procedures mentioned above. Adenoviruses are less resistant than RVs and are rapidly inactivated at 133°F (56°C) and by exposure to ultraviolet light or formalin. No vaccine is under development.

Viral antigen detection by immunoassay is the diagnostic test of choice. IAs are simple, quick and inexpensive; sensitivity and specificity are 98% when compared with EM; however, real-time RT-PCR has proven superior to IAs and EM.[91] Enteric adenoviruses do not grow in routine tissue culture.

The clinical manifestations of enteric adenoviruses are presented in Table 151.4. In general, the disease is milder but more prolonged than that with RV. Treatment is supportive. Cidofovir alone or with ribavirin have been used for immunocompromised patients.

Other Viruses

Cases of human gastroenteritis have been associated with picornaviruses (Aichi virus) coronaviruses, parvoviruses, pestiviruses, toroviruses, picobirnaviruses, Breda viruses and others, but their role as agents of gastroenteritis is under study.

REFERENCES

 References for this chapter can be found online at http://www.expertconsult.com

Measles, mumps and rubella viruses

INTRODUCTION

The epidemiology of the viruses discussed in this chapter (measles, rubella and mumps) has changed dramatically since the successful introduction of live attenuated vaccines. As infections such as measles and rubella become less frequent, clinicians are less familiar with their clinical presentations and surveillance based solely on clinical recognition is not always sufficiently accurate. Laboratory confirmation of suspected clinical cases is essential and should be complemented by genotyping of circulating viral strains for effective surveillance.[1]

Measles

NATURE

Measles (rubeola) was first identified over 2000 years ago, although its infectious nature was not recognized until the mid 19th century when epidemics in island communities were described. It is one of the infectious diseases targeted by the World Health Organization (WHO).

Measles virus is a member of the *Morbillivirus* genus of the Paramyxoviridae and was first isolated in cell culture in 1954; the first live attenuated vaccine became available in 1963. It is pleomorphic, with a diameter of 150 nm or more. Single-stranded RNA is enclosed in a capsid of helical symmetry of 18 nm. This is enclosed within an envelope, the surface of which carries the hemagglutinin and fusion proteins. Replication is mainly cytoplasmic; however, there is some nuclear involvement. Although there is only one measles virus serotype, 23 genotypes of measles virus have been described, which are organized in eight clades (A–H).[2]

EPIDEMIOLOGY

Measles is endemic worldwide except in those countries in which complete control has been achieved by immunization (Fig. 152.1). Infection in childhood before the impact of immunization is almost 100%, confirming measles as one of the most infectious of microbial pathogens. Epidemics occur every 2–3 years, but are less defined in the tropics.

The epidemiology of measles has been profoundly modified by immunization strategies, with a 74% reduction in measles death globally from 757 000 in 2000 to 197 000 in 2007. The target set by the global immunization vision and strategy program developed by the WHO and UNICEF is to reduce mortality due to measles by 90% by 2010.[3]

Despite efforts to eradicate measles, outbreaks continued to occur in Europe during 2006 and 2007 and the number of measles cases reported to the Centers for Disease Control and Prevention (CDC) in the first half of 2008 was the highest year-to-date figure since 1996.[4,5] Most measles cases were reported in unvaccinated children and suboptimum vaccine uptake due to parenteral concerns and/or religious reasons remains a major obstacle towards achieving elimination of the disease in Europe.

PATHOGENICITY

Infection is spread by droplet from person to person. The incubation period to onset of rash is about 14 days, with prodromal symptoms starting 1–3 days earlier. Maximum infectivity is during the prodrome, although patients are considered to be infective from 4 days before to 4 days after onset of the rash.

After infection, initial replication occurs in the respiratory epithelium with local spread by lymphatics and a primary viremia 2–3 days after infection. A secondary viremia occurs 3–4 days later and lasts for up to 7 days. The peak viremia coincides with the prodromal symptoms. The rash results from the immunologic reaction between the virus antigens and host antibody, with involvement of capillary walls. Intrauterine infection has not been convincingly reported.

PREVENTION

Live attenuated measles vaccine became available in 1963 based on the Edmonston strain, but those in current use such as Schwarz and Moraten strains are further attenuated. The measles vaccine is available in monovalent form, as well as combined with mumps and rubella vaccine (MMR). Two doses of the vaccine are necessary to achieve high levels of immunity (>98% efficacy). They are included in the routine childhood immunization scheme at age 12–15 months and at school entry (4–6 years). Administration before 12 months can result in lower protection because of interference by residual maternal antibody. This is especially problematic for developing countries, where many cases of measles occur in infants under 12 months of age. For most developing countries, the WHO recommends immunization at 9 months of age.[3]

In HIV-infected children the vaccine is less effective but protective antibody levels can be achieved in HIV-infected children on highly active retroviral therapy (HAART) with immune recovery.[6] Measles vaccine is contraindicated in pregnancy and in those with impaired cell-mediated immunity because measles-specific complications, as well as potential side-effects, such as localized pain and tenderness, mild fever (about 10%) and transient rashes (about 5%), may occur.

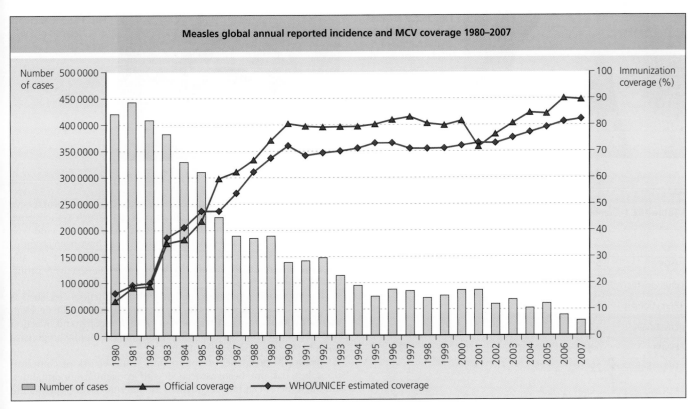

Measles global annual reported incidence and MCV coverage 1980–2007

Fig. 152.1 Measles global annual reported incidence and measles-containing vaccine coverage 1980–2007.

Encephalitis has been reported in one in a million doses, but its causal relationship with the vaccine is uncertain. Anxieties had been expressed as to whether MMR immunization may lead to inflammatory bowel disease and autism,[7] but strong evidence has been published since then against an association of autism with MMR vaccine exposure.[8,9]

DIAGNOSTIC MICROBIOLOGY

Virus isolation may be attempted from throat swabs, conjunctival swabs, nasopharyngeal aspirates (NPAs) and sedimented cells from urine, but is technically demanding and unreliable. The cell line used in global reference laboratories for the isolation of measles virus is a Vero/SLAM cell line – a Vero cell line transfected with a plasmid encoding human SLAM (signaling lymphocyte-activation molecule) which is a cellular receptor for the measles virus. The cytopathic effect after inoculation is not immediately apparent as multinucleated giant cells can take up to 15 days to develop. Measles virus can also be detected by hemadsorption (monkey, human or guinea-pig red blood cells) and isolation can be confirmed by specific neutralization of the hemadsorption or by immunofluorescence.

Immunofluorescent antigen detection in NPA cells may be performed and is particularly useful for diagnosing atypical cases or infection in the immunocompromised host. The measles virus genome, amplified from cells obtained by throat swab or NPA by reverse transcriptase polymerase chain reaction (RT-PCR) can be used for genetic characterization and to determine the geographic origin of the infecting strain.[2]

As RT-PCR can detect the viral genome without viable virus being present, a diagnosis can be made up to several weeks after rash onset. Serologic diagnosis is dependent on demonstrating seroconversion, rising antibody titer or detecting specific IgM. Hemagglutination inhibition and complement fixation testing (CFT) have been the established methods in the past, but are now being replaced by immunoglobulin-specific enzyme immunoassays (EIAs). Serum-based IgM EIAs are currently recommended for the rapid laboratory detection of measles. IgM assays are available in the format of IgM capture assays or as indirect assays. False-negative IgM assays can occur if serum is collected within 3 days of rash onset.[10]

IgG assays require the collection of two serum specimens about 10–30 days apart. A fourfold rise in the IgG titer is considered to be significant. IgG assays are not routinely used for the diagnosis of acute measles virus infection. They are used for the clarification of equivocal IgM results and in seroprevalence studies.[1] Simultaneous detection of IgM and viral RNA from dried blood specimens or from oral fluid sampling are possible alternatives for diagnosis and surveillance of measles, especially in countries where specimen transport or refrigeration is challenging.

Subacute sclerosing panencephalitis may be diagnosed by detection of the genome or isolation of virus by co-cultivation from brain tissue. A more usual approach, however, is the detection of elevated concentrations of measles antibody in serum and concentrations indicating intrathecal synthesis in cerebrospinal fluid (CSF) by CFT.

CLINICAL MANIFESTATIONS

Toward the end of the incubation period, the prodromal symptoms of fever and malaise appear and persist for up to 4 days before the rash appears. Pyrexia may rise to 103–104°F (39.4–40°C) and is often accompanied by conjunctivitis, cough and coryza (the three 'C's of measles). Koplik's spots are a pathognomonic feature of measles, and can be seen for up to 2 days before rash onset as punctate white spots on an erythematous background on the buccal mucosa.

The rash usually begins on the face and neck, and evolves to the body and limbs (Fig. 152.2). Although lesions are usually discrete, they can coalesce, and desquamation may occur. The rash usually

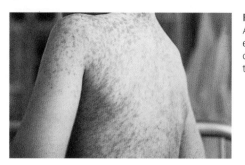

Fig. 152.2 Measles. A disseminated erythematous rash can be seen over the trunk and arms.

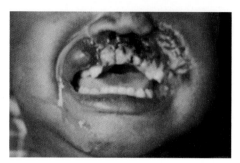

Fig. 152.3 Cancrum oris. Necrosis of the upper lip.

Table 152.1 Complications of measles (% of cases)

	USA			UK
Age	**5 years**	**5–19 years**	**>20 years**	**All ages**
Otitis media	14	2	2	5
Pneumonia	9	2	7	4
Encephalitis	0.2	0.1	0.3	0.1
Death	0.3	0.2	0.3	0.25
Hospitalization	25	8	24	1

USA data are broken down into three age groups, whereas UK data are not; however, UK data primarily reflect infection in early childhood.[11,12]

persists for 5–6 days. Generalized lymphadenopathy and diarrhea are common.

Complications are most common in younger and older patients (Table 152.1) and those with underlying malnutrition, particularly vitamin A deficiency. Pneumonia, either viral or, more usually, secondary bacterial, occurs in up to 4% of patients. Neurologic complications include convulsions, in up to 1% of cases, and encephalitis, which has been reported in 1/1000 cases with a reported mortality rate of 15% and residual neurologic deficit rate of 25%. Overall, estimates of the mortality rate for measles are 1 per 1000 patients in developed countries but higher in the developing world.

Subacute sclerosing panencephalitis (SSPE) manifests from months to years after the initial natural measles or measles immunization; the mean interval is 7 years after natural measles and 3.3 years after immunization. The risk is less after measles immunization (1:1 million) than after natural infection (1:100 000), and is three times more common in boys than in girls. Specific risk factors for the development of SSPE have not been identified. SSPE is a progressively fatal degenerative disease of the central nervous system, manifests itself as a progressive intellectual impairment, which may not be noticed initially and moves to convulsions, motor abnormalities and coma; death is inevitable after a progressive deterioration over months or years. Its pathogenesis is not well understood, but persistent infection of the central nervous system with a genetic variant of measles virus may be involved. SSPE virus has unique phenotypic features that are different from those of wild-type measles virus, which are referred to as nonmutated measles. For example, some SSPE virus strains are highly neuropathogenic in hamsters, mice and other rodents. Also, SSPE virus produces few infectious virus particles, if any, and thus its spread from infected to uninfected cells is almost completely dependent on cell-to-cell infection. This defective feature is thought to be caused by a variety of mutations affecting primarily the viral matrix (M) protein and the cytoplasmic tail of the fusion (F) glycoprotein. This results in the lack of functional M protein and is thought to be responsible, at least partly, for the viral inability to produce virus particles and for chronic progressive neuropathogenicity in the host. Other viral genes, such as the F gene, also undergo unique mutations that are not found in the wild-type measles virus. These viral genetic mutations must have been accumulated during viral persistence over a long period of time, especially after the onset of SSPE symptoms, when the virus is actively proliferating in the brain.[13]

The immunocompromised patient with T-cell deficiencies, such as those who have leukemia or HIV, is at particular risk for the development of complications. A typical rash is often missing and infection persists, manifesting as a giant cell pneumonitis or rapidly progressive encephalitis; the fatality rate is high.[14]

Measles in pregnancy seems to carry a higher risk of complications but has not been associated with congenital abnormalities, although there is an increased risk of intrauterine death or premature delivery.[15]

Measles presents special problems in developing countries, where case fatality rates of up to 25% have been described. The high mortality rate is associated with malnutrition and, in particular, vitamin A deficiency.[16] Death usually results from bacterial superinfection, such as pneumonia, or diarrheal illness, although cancrum oris, a progressive oral necrosis, is also seen (Fig. 152.3).

MANAGEMENT

Postexposure prophylaxis with human normal immunoglobulin is indicated for those who are susceptible and who would be at risk from complications, in particular immunocompromised children and pregnant women. In outbreak situations and in immunocompetent persons administration of measles vaccine within 3 days of contact can provide protection.

Uncomplicated measles is managed symptomatically, with vitamin A supplementation for malnourished children. Antimicrobial therapy active against *Streptococcus pneumoniae* and *Haemophilus influenzae* is indicated for presumed bacterial superinfection. In those with major complications, such as pneumonitis in immunocompromised patients, specific antiviral treatment with ribavirin may be of benefit;[17] however, such treatment is of no value in SSPE.

Rubella

NATURE

Although rubella had been recognized as a distinct clinical illness since the 18th century, it was not until 1941 that Sir Norman Gregg, an Australian ophthalmologist, made the association between rubella in early pregnancy and congenital abnormalities.[18] In 1962 the causative virus was isolated, leading to techniques for specific diagnosis and the development of attenuated live vaccines.

Rubella is a single-stranded RNA virus, with an icosahedral nucleocapsid surrounded by an envelope. Replication occurs in the cytoplasm of infected cells. It is the sole member of the genus *Rubivirus* within the family Togaviridae. There are three major virus polypeptides: C, E_1 and E_2. Polypeptide E_1 is present in the envelope and has hemagglutinating properties. Only one serotype of the virus is recognized, but phylogenetic analysis of the coding region of E_1 revealed at least seven distinct genotypes grouped in two clades [19] and natural infection of species other than humans has not been shown.

EPIDEMIOLOGY

Rubella is a mild disease presenting with fever and rash. Existing vaccines, single or in combination with measles and/or mumps, have been proven to be highly efficacious. Rubella elimination is one of the primary targets of the WHO as infection during the early months of pregnancy can lead to fetal death or serious congenital birth defects (congenital rubella syndrome, CRS). It is estimated that more than 100 000 infants are born with CRS each year, the majority occurring in countries without an effective rubella vaccination program.[20]

PATHOGENICITY

Infection is transmitted by the airborne route, by direct contact or indirectly through fomites. Patients are potentially infective from 1 week before to 1 week after the onset of rash. After replication in the upper respiratory tract and local lymph nodes, a viremia infects target organs such as skin, joints and placenta. Similarly to measles, the rash is immunologically mediated and marks the production of specific antibodies.

If the patient is pregnant, placental infection can occur; transmission to the fetus is possible but not inevitable.[21] Confirmed rubella during the first trimester of pregnancy resulted in damage to 50–90% of fetuses (see Table 152.2).[22]

PREVENTION

Passive prophylaxis with human normal immunoglobulin has not been demonstrated to reduce the risk of rubella after contact, although it may attenuate the illness. Control of rubella has resided in using the live attenuated vaccines available since the early 1970s. The vaccine strain RA27/3 induces seroconversion in over 95% of susceptible vaccinees, and protection persists for at least 15–20 years.[23] Vaccine virus can be isolated from the throat of vaccinees, but transmission to susceptible contacts has not been demonstrated. A mild, transient rubelliform rash illness with arthralgia can occur 2–3 weeks after immunization, but chronic joint problems have not been associated with administration of the vaccine. If vaccine virus is inadvertently administered to pregnant women, fetal infection occurs in approximately 1% of cases, but extensive postvaccine surveillance did not detect any fetal damage.[24] Rubella immunization presents no significant risk to the individual who has HIV infection.

With rubella being a mild illness, control has focused on preventing infection in pregnant women. Two approaches have been used. First, as exemplified in the UK until 1988, rubella vaccine was targeted at adolescent girls and susceptible women, with rubella remaining endemic in children and men. Although cases of congenital rubella were markedly reduced, there were still 2–3% of women susceptible and at risk of rubella in pregnancy. The alternative approach, as used in the USA and in the UK from 1988, was to combine rubella vaccine with measles and mumps vaccines (MMR), and offer it to all children in the second year of life to eradicate rubella from the community. This policy was supported by identifying and immunizing susceptible women. If uptake rates of more than 90% can be obtained, control of endemic rubella is achievable (Fig. 152.4). Elimination of the congenital rubella syndrome has been accomplished in the USA and in other developed countries although sub-Saharan Africa still remains a problem.[25]

DIAGNOSTIC MICROBIOLOGY

With the clinical diagnosis of rubella being unreliable, laboratory confirmation of infection is required. In pregnancy it is imperative to

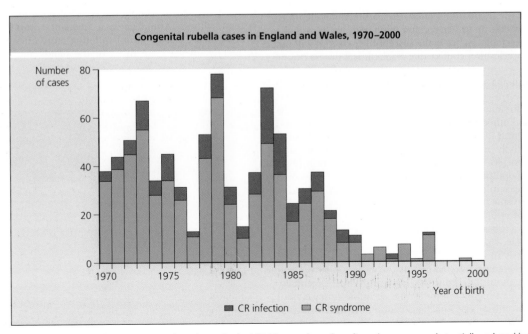

Fig. 152.4 Cases of congenital rubella (CR) infection and syndrome in the UK. The number of confirmed cases was substantially reduced by the introduction of MMR vaccine in 1988. Data from National Congenital Rubella Surveillance Programme and the PHLS Communicable Disease Surveillance Centre.

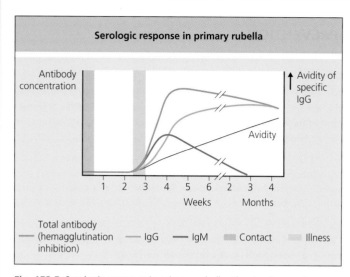

Serologic response in primary rubella

Fig. 152.5 Serologic response in primary rubella. The development of specific IgG and IgM and the increasing avidity of specific IgG are illustrated.

investigate both a rash illness and contact with a rash illness because subclinical rubella may occur, and this has been proven to be a risk to the fetus.[26] It is debatable whether such investigation of contacts should be pursued if there is a documented history of past detection of rubella antibody or vaccine. However, vaccine is not 100% effective in inducing protection, and if there has been only one previous detection of rubella antibody, there is a remote possibility that a laboratory error may have occurred.

The diagnosis of postnatal rubella infection is made by serology and the serologic response is detailed in Figure 152.5; tests for total rubella antibody (such as hemagglutination inhibition) have been progressively replaced with tests specific for IgG and IgM, particularly EIAs. Serum should be obtained as soon as possible after onset of illness or after contact. Detection of rubella-specific IgG, but failure to demonstrate specific IgM, indicates immunity to rubella and that the illness being investigated is not rubella. If neither rubella-specific IgG nor specific IgM are detected, repeat testing of a later serum is needed. The incubation period after contact may be up to 21 days, and it may take up to 10 days after onset of illness for rubella antibody to be detectable. Hence in the susceptible person it will not be until about 4 weeks after contact that a subclinical illness can be excluded.

Detection of rubella-specific IgM indicates recent primary rubella infection, but care is needed in interpretation. Rubella-specific IgM reactivity persists for about 1–3 months and false-positive IgM results occur in a range of other infections such as parvovirus B19 infection and Epstein–Barr virus infection (infectious mononucleosis). Rubella-specific IgM reactivity may also be nonspecific and may occur in rubella re-infection (see below). In the first 2 days after rash onset RT-PCR testing of oral fluid specimens can identify more cases than IgM testing.[27] Other serologic approaches, such as determining specific IgG avidity, are of value in confirming primary rubella,[28] with specific IgG early after infection being less tightly bound to antigen (low avidity) than the antibody found in the mature antibody response (high avidity; see Fig. 152.5).

For the diagnosis of congenital rubella isolation of virus in cell culture is of value because infected infants can excrete high titers of virus in the throat and urine during the first year of life; congenitally infected infants can be highly infectious to susceptible contacts until approximately 6 months of age. Rubella isolation can be performed in many cell culture lines, but a cytopathic effect is only produced in a few of them, for example RK 13. Immunofluorescence is probably the best method for detecting virus growth.

Congenital rubella is routinely diagnosed by detecting specific IgM; all congenitally infected infants are positive for the first 3 months of life and most for the first 6 months. As passively transmitted maternal IgG antibodies have declined by 6 months of age, persistence of IgG antibodies beyond this time period indicates fetal infection as well.

Occasionally there may be problems with diagnosis or management of rubella in pregnancy and intrauterine diagnosis may be considered. Approaches used, but of limited availability, have included virus isolation and genome detection from amniotic fluid or trophoblast, and detection of specific IgM in fetal blood; this latter method is unreliable before 24 weeks' gestation, however, because the infected fetus may not be capable of an IgM response until that age.

Oral fluid samples can be used both for detection of antibodies and for amplification of the viral genome by RT-PCR. Detection of IgM in saliva is especially helpful for clarifying the etiology of rashes in childhood because they are noninvasive and more acceptable for infant sampling.

The majority of developed countries have programs in place to identify susceptible women of child-bearing age and offer immunization. Tests for specific IgG are many and include EIAs and latex agglutination. An area of contention is the concentration of rubella-specific IgG taken to indicate protection (or, more correctly, as not necessitating immunization), with opinions varying from any confirmed antibody (possibly as low as 3–5 IU) up to 15 IU; 10 IU has been recommended in the USA.[29]

CLINICAL MANIFESTATIONS

In childhood, primary rubella is subclinical in approximately 50% of patients, but in adolescence or older it is usually (90% or more) clinically apparent. After an incubation period of up to 21 days (usually 15–17 days) a pinkish-red maculopapular rash develops, starting on the face and neck and rapidly spreading over body and limbs (Fig. 152.6). Individual spots may coalesce but the rash usually clears in 3–4 days. Nonspecific symptoms, such as fever, malaise and upper respiratory tract symptoms, may precede and accompany the rash. In childhood the illness is benign and may have no systemic impact. Lymphadenopathy commonly occurs, the suboccipital nodes being frequently involved.

In adolescence and adulthood, rubella is often far more severe, not only because of complications but also because of a more severe systemic illness. Arthralgia is a frequent complication in adults, with women (30% or more) suffering more often than men. Joints frequently involved are those of the hands and wrists; resolution

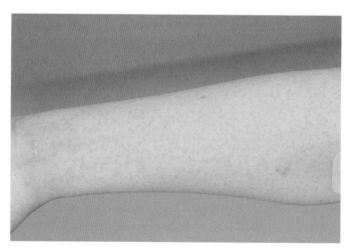

Fig. 152.6 Rubella. A pink macular rash can be seen on the forearm.

Table 152.2 Features of congenital rubella

Cardiovascular defects
    Persistent ductus arteriosus
    Pulmonary artery stenosis
    Myocarditis

Ocular defects
    Cataracts (unilateral or bilateral)
    Pigmentary retinopathy
    Micro-ophthalmus
    Glaucoma
    Iris hypoplasia

Auditory defects
    Sensorineural deafness (unilateral or bilateral)

Central nervous system
    Microcephaly
    Psychomotor retardation
    Meningoencephalitis
    Behavioral disorders
    Speech disorders

Intrauterine growth retardation

Hepatitis/hepatosplenomegaly

Thrombocytopenia, with purpura

Bone 'lesions'

Pneumonitis *

Diabetes mellitus *

Thyroid disorders *

Progressive rubella panencephalitis *

*These disorders become apparent in infancy or later.

usually occurs in 2–4 weeks but can persist for some months or even years. Thrombocytopenia and postinfectious encephalitis are rare complications, occurring in less than 1/5000–10 000 patients, with fatal outcome virtually unknown. Even in patients with HIV infection and other immunocompromised patients, rubella rarely carries any additional risk.[30]

Primary rubella infection in the first 16 weeks of pregnancy presents major risks to the fetus. Consequences for the fetus and the pregnancy include abortion, miscarriage or stillbirth or multiple birth defects (Table 152.2). The congenital rubella triad comprises cardiac, ophthalmic and auditory lesions, but purpura, intrauterine growth and neurologic problems are also frequent.

The gestation at which the mother suffers her rubella infection is critical for the outcome. Onset of rubella before conception carries little, if any, risk,[31] whereas from conception to the 12th week the risk is about 90%.[23] Between 12 and 16 weeks' gestation the risk falls to about 20%, with sensorineural deafness being the only consequence. Beyond 16 weeks' any risk is minimal, with only rare cases of sensorineural deafness.

It has been established for many years that re-infections can occur in those with a past history of natural rubella or successful immunization. Such re-infections are rarely clinically apparent and are usually identified by a serologic response after exposure, which is usually to a close contact such as the patient's own child. Fetal infection and damage can occur after maternal re-infection, but this is rare, with the fetal risk probably being less than 5%.[32] Because of the difference in risk to the fetus, it is critical to distinguish between subclinical primary rubella and re-infection in early pregnancy. This may be difficult in the absence of past rubella-specific IgG test results because a specific IgM response can occur in both; IgG avidity testing will usually resolve the problem because re-infection would be characterized by the presence of high avidity IgG.

MANAGEMENT

Rubella is a self-limiting illness that usually runs a benign course. Supportive and symptom-relieving therapy is indicated for complications such as arthralgia, and the patient can be reassured as to the unlikely occurrence of symptoms persisting beyond a few months.

Management of rubella in pregnancy is first dependent on achieving a correct diagnosis. A serum sample must be taken as soon as possible after contact or onset of illness, and the testing laboratory given full details of past testing and/or vaccination. On the basis of results and the clinical details, the laboratory will advise on diagnosis and any further testing required. If primary rubella or re-infection in the first 16 weeks of pregnancy is diagnosed, further management will have to take into account social, legal and religious perspectives because in many countries the risk to the fetus is sufficient to justify consideration of termination of pregnancy.

Mumps

NATURE

Mumps was first identified as a distinct clinical illness by Hippocrates in the 5th century BC, but has only attracted attention in the past two to three centuries, particularly because of the impact of outbreaks in the armed forces. Natural infection is limited to humans and is endemic worldwide.

Mumps virus is a member of the *Paramyxovirus* genus of the Paramyxoviridae family. It was first isolated in the chick embryo in 1945, with the first live attenuated vaccine being licensed in 1967. On electron microscopy it is pleomorphic (Fig. 152.7) and varies in size from 80 to 350 nm, although it is usually approximately 200 nm. The envelope is studded with projections containing hemagglutinin/neuraminidase or fusion proteins. Within the envelope the nucleoprotein has helical symmetry with a diameter

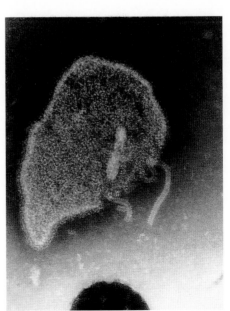

Fig. 152.7 Electron micrograph of mumps virus. Courtesy of Dr A Curry.

of 15–19 nm. The RNA is single stranded and of negative sense; the nucleocapsid contains an RNA-dependent RNA polymerase. This enzyme enables replication of the RNA in the cytoplasm once the cell has been penetrated. Mature virions are released from the cell by budding.

Twelve mumps virus genotypes (A–L) with different geographic distribution have been described. There is only one serologic type although studies suggest that cross-neutralization between genotypes might not be complete.[33]

EPIDEMIOLOGY

Mumps is endemic worldwide, with epidemics occurring every 2–3 years in populations not influenced by widespread use of mumps vaccine. In the prevaccine era 50% of children aged 4–6 years and 90% of children aged 14–15 years had positive serology for mumps.[34] With the introduction of mumps vaccines the epidemiology of the disease shifted, depending on the number of vaccine doses, age at vaccination and vaccine uptake. Mumps outbreaks are not uncommon in countries with routine mumps vaccination; in 2004/2005 the UK experienced a large scale outbreak[35] and in 2006 more than 5800 cases of mumps were reported in the USA.[36] In both countries the majority of infections occurred in young adults attending college. Although the majority of college students in the USA had been MMR vaccinated, suboptimal vaccine effectiveness and insufficient vaccine uptake allowed transmission in this population.[36] In addition, whereas natural infection seems to result in lifelong immunity, immunity induced by vaccination can decrease.[37]

PATHOGENICITY

Infection is acquired by droplet spread, direct contact or contaminated fomites. Replication in the upper respiratory epithelium is followed by spread to local lymph nodes and subsequent primary viremia, with seeding of target organs such as parotid glands, central nervous system and genital organs. A secondary viremia occurs at the onset of symptoms.

The incubation period is usually 16–18 days, with infectivity commencing 2 days before onset of symptoms and persisting for 5–7 days after onset. Both in the health-care setting and in the community patients with mumps should be isolated with droplet and contact precautions for a 5-day period after onset of parotitis.[38] Intrauterine infection has been reported only rarely.

PREVENTION

Two live attenuated vaccine strains have been mainly used since 1967: Jeryl Lynn and Urabe strain vaccines. Both are produced in chick embryo cell culture and are available in monovalent form or combined with measles and rubella vaccine (MMR). The vaccine is usually administered as MMR at 12–15 months of age, with second doses being given later in childhood. The protective efficacy is 75–85%, with clinically apparent mumps in immunized individuals being well documented. Minor complications of mumps vaccine include mild parotitis, fever and, very rarely, orchitis. Although Urabe strain vaccines were withdrawn in some countries in the 1990s due to higher rates of aseptic meningitis occurring with this vaccine strain, the WHO justifies the use of the Urabe strain in national vaccination programs as aseptic meningitis postvaccination is generally benign and the Urabe strain seems to be more immunogenic and is cheaper.[39]

Mumps vaccine is contraindicated in those with previous anaphylaxis to egg and in pregnancy, although adverse implications for the fetus have not been reported. It should also not be given to immunocompromised patients, with the exception of children with HIV infection, in whom no adverse consequences have been seen.

DIAGNOSTIC MICROBIOLOGY

Virus isolation may be achieved from throat swabs, saliva, CSF and possibly urine. Mumps virus is readily isolated in either Vero cells (African green monkey kidney) or Caco-2 (human colorectal adenocarcinoma epithelium). Although cytopathic effect may sometimes be observed (multinucleated giant cells), isolation is usually confirmed by immunofluorescence staining. RT-PCR is performed directly on the clinical specimen and sequencing of the amplified product can be used to identify individual genotypes. RT-PCR was found to be more sensitive than culture methods in detecting virus in cerebrospinal and oral fluid.[40]

Serologic diagnosis is usually achieved by detection of virus-specific IgM antibody by direct or indirect enzyme-linked immunosorbent assay (ELISA). False-negative IgM results can occur for serum collected before day 4 of clinical presentation.[41] A fourfold rise of IgG titer between acute and convalescent serum is considered diagnostic as well. Although ELISA is routinely used for the diagnosis of infection, it can give false-positive results in assessing immunity. Serologic testing can also be performed on CSF specimens in patients with mumps, meningitis or encephalitis. Saliva specimens can be used for specific IgM detection and are valuable for surveillance of mumps-like illness in the community.[34]

CLINICAL MANIFESTATIONS

Towards the end of the incubation period of 16–18 days prodromal symptoms such as pyrexia and malaise develop, which is followed by the characteristic tender swelling of the parotid glands. There is often accompanying headache and earache. Recovery is usually complete within 4–5 days. Asymptomatic mumps is common and occurs in about one-third of infections. Parotitis is present in 95% of symptomatic infections and is unilateral in about one-quarter; other salivary glands are involved in about 10% of patients. Parotitis similar to that seen with mumps may also be found in other virus infections, for example coxsackievirus and Epstein–Barr virus B infection.

Complications are common;[39] the risk is the same at all ages except for orchitis and oophoritis, which are virtually limited to post puberty. Orchitis generally arises a few days after parotitis. The risk of orchitis in the adolescent or adult male is about 35%, with bilateral involvement in one-third of these. There may be some persisting testicular atrophy, but sterility is remarkably uncommon, despite public perceptions. Oophoritis is only observed in about 5% of mumps in adult women and causes lower abdominal pain; it is uncertain whether there may be long-term consequences.

Meningeal involvement, as shown by CSF pleocytosis, occurs in about 50% of patients, with signs of meningitis or meningeal irritation in about 1–10%. Up to 50% of meningitis cases occur without concomitant parotitis.

Mumps virus may also cause encephalitis, presenting as impaired level of consciousness, seizures, aphasia, etc. Mumps meningitis is, in general, a benign disease; persistent sequelae are found in a small percentage of encephalitis and are more common in adults.

The incidence of encephalitis is about 1/6000 patients, with a mortality rate of 1.4%. Transient hearing impairment as a result of a labyrinthitis is not uncommon, with persisting deafness occurring in about 1/20000 patients. Other complications include pancreatitis, which is usually mild, arthritis, mastitis, thyroiditis and myocarditis. Investigation of renal function will often demonstrate kidney involvement, but there are no clinical consequences.

Mumps in immunocompromised patients seems to carry no undue risk and persistent infection has not been described.

Infection in the first trimester can lead to spontaneous abortion, but infection later in pregnancy carries no increased risk, and congenital infection and damage have not been convincingly shown.

MANAGEMENT

Postexposure prophylaxis with normal immunoglobulin is of no benefit, and specific mumps immunoglobulin is no longer available, although it may have reduced the risk of orchitis in adult men. Mumps vaccine administered as postexposure prophylaxis is of no benefit.

There is no specific antiviral treatment available for mothers and management of infection is symptomatic, with the patient being reassured that recovery occurs in a few days, even when complications are present.

REFERENCES

References for this chapter can be found online at http://www.expertconsult.com

Chapter | 153

Gustavo Palacios
Inmaculada Casas
Gloria Trallero

Human enteroviruses

The Viruses

DISCOVERING THE ENTEROVIRUSES

History

The history of enteroviruses is the history of poliovirus. The first known clinical description of poliomyelitis is attributed to Michael Underwood, a British physician, who in 1789 reported an illness which appeared to target primarily children with paralysis and fever. In 1840, von Heine published a monograph describing the clinical symptoms. Later, the Swedish physician Medin contributed to the descriptions. The syndrome was named Heine–Medin disease. However, it was not until the early 20th century that the number of paralytic poliomyelitis cases began to reach epidemic proportions. Poliovirus was discovered to be the causative agent of poliomyelitis in 1908 by Viennese investigators Landsteiner and Popper who successfully transmitted the clinical disease and its pathology to monkeys using a filtrate from paralytic patients. Prevention of infantile paralysis and control of poliovirus spread was attempted by the use of two vaccines, one inactivated (Salk; intramuscular route) and one attenuated (Sabin; oral route). The real impact of those early studies is demonstrated by the ongoing success of the global poliovirus eradication program.

In addition to polioviruses, during these initial studies on poliomyelitis, other enteric viruses (thus named enteroviruses) were discovered. In 1948, an antigenically distant virus to poliovirus was isolated from the feces of a paralytic child in Coxsackie, New York, during a poliomyelitis epidemic. It was aptly termed Coxsackie virus. Later, when a second diverse virus was isolated in the same area from cases of aseptic meningitis, the first virus become the first member of the Coxsackie A virus group, while the second formed the Coxsackie B virus group. Finally, in 1951 from the stool of asymptomatic individuals, several antigenically independent viruses were isolated. They were named echoviruses, corresponding to *e*nteric isolates, *c*ytopathogenic in tissue culture, isolated from *h*umans and *o*rphans (no association with known clinical disease). After 1969, new serotypes were numbered sequentially.

Physical and chemical properties

The pathology, transmission and general epidemiology of enteroviruses are all shaped by their biophysical properties (Table 153.1). Their structural stability and their resistance are key factors in their mechanism of transmission. They may also explain their cytolytic life cycle and their singular characteristics within the Picornaviridae family.

Table 153.1 Physical and chemical properties of enterovirus particles

Characteristic	Properties
Sedimentation	Constant buoyant density in cesium chloride (irrespective of pH or time of centrifugation)
Stability	Stable in weak acid, retain the infectivity at pH values up to 3.0 (allow replication in the alimentary tract)
Structural stability	Insensitive to lipid solvents (ether and chloroform) Stable in many detergents at ambient temperature Relatively resistant to laboratory disinfectants (70% ethanol, isopropanol, lysol, quaternary ammonium compounds)
Inactivation	Chemical: formaldehyde, glutaraldehyde, strong acid, sodium hypochlorite, free residual chlorine Environmental: temperatures higher than 42°C, ultraviolet light, drying on surfaces

Classification

Members of the family Picornaviridae are small, single-stranded RNA viruses (ssRNA). The family is subdivided into nine genera: Enterovirus, Rhinovirus, Cardiovirus, Aphthovirus, Hepatovirus, Parechovirus, Erbovirus, Kobuvirus and Teschovirus. The genus Enterovirus can be further grouped into eight species, four of them infecting humans, each with a variable number of serotypes (Table 153.2).

The original classification was based on the clinical manifestations observed in human infections as well as on the pathogenesis in intracranially and subcutaneously inoculated experimental suckling mice. This classification defines the following homogeneous antigenic groups:

- polioviruses, which cause flaccid paralysis (poliomyelitis) in humans;
- Coxsackie A viruses (CAV), which are linked to human central nervous system (CNS) disease and herpangina, as well as acute flaccid paralysis in suckling mice;
- Coxsackie B viruses (CBV), associated with ailments of the human cardiac and central nervous systems, necrosis of the fat pads between the shoulders, focal lesions in skeletal muscle, brain and spinal cord, as well as spastic paralysis in the suckling mouse experimental model; and
- echoviruses, which were not originally associated with human disease or with paralysis in mice.

Table 153.2 Classification of enterovirus species and serotypes

Species	Serotypes
Human enterovirus A	CVA2–8, CVA10, CVA12, CVA14, CVA16, HEV71, HEV76, HEV89–91 (contains most of the old Coxsackie A virus group)
Human enterovirus B	CVA9, CVB1–6, E1–7, E9, E11–21, E24–27, E29–33, EV69, EV73–75, EV77–88, EV93, EV97, EV98, EV100, EV101 (contains all Coxsackie B virus group and all echoviruses of the old nomenclature)
Human enterovirus C	CVA1, CVA11, CVA13, CVA15, CVA17–22, CVA24, PV1–3, EV95, EV96, EV99, EV102, EV104 (contains the remainder of the Coxsackie A virus group and the poliovirus)
Human enterovirus D	EV68, EV70, EV94

Since 1969, new enterovirus types have been assigned type numbers, starting with 68 and today reaching 101.

The introduction of molecular typing methods is the basis for the modern classification scheme. Under the new genetic scheme, human enteroviruses are subdivided into four species of human enterovirus A to D supported by genome organization, sequence similarity and biologic properties. Incorporation of polioviruses into the human enterovirus C species is pending approval by the International Committee on Taxonomy of Viruses (ICTV) (http://www.picornastudygroup.com).[1] Nowadays, new enteroviruses are being phylogenetically grouped into their species[2–8] instead of being antigenically characterized. The ICTV has proposed genetic criteria for inclusion of a new enterovirus in one concrete species. Similarly, criteria to define new serotypes are under discussion (Table 153.3).

Table 153.3 Criteria for species and serotype classification

Taxonomic level	Criteria
Enterovirus species (ICTV)	Members of a species of the genus Enterovirus: • Share greater than 70% aa identity in P1 • Share greater than 70% aa identity in the nonstructural proteins 2C+3CD • Share a limited range of host cell receptors • Share a limited natural host range • Have a genome base composition (G+C) which varies by no more than 2.5% • Share a significant degree of compatibility in proteolytic processing, replication, encapsidation and genetic recombination
Enterovirus serotype (proposed)	Members of a serotype of the a species of Enterovirus: • Share greater than 75% nucleotide similarity in the VP1-coding sequence • Share greater than 85% amino acid similarity in the VP1-coding sequence Members of different serotypes of species of Enterovirus: • Share less than 70% nucleotide similarity in the VP1-coding sequence • Share less than 85% amino acid similarity in the VP1-coding sequence

Structure and genome organization

The structure of poliovirus 1 was determined by X-ray crystallography in 1985.[9] Virions are spherical with a diameter of about 30 nm. The naked RNA genome is surrounded by proteins without a lipid envelope and its infectivity is not affected by organic solvents. The capsid is composed of four structural proteins – VP1, VP2, VP3 and VP4 – which are arranged with icosahedral symmetry (20 triangular faces and 12 vertices). A total of 60 structural proteins are involved. One copy of each of the four proteins builds the capsid promoter. VP1, VP2 and VP3 have no sequence homology but have the same topology. The internal VP4 is essential for the stability of the virion.

The three-dimensional structure of the poliovirus particle was solved as a star-shaped plateau (mesa) at the fivefold axis of symmetry surrounded by a deep depression (canyon) which is proposed as the receptor-binding site. The connecting loops and the C-terminus of the capsid proteins are located in the outer surface of the virion and determine the viral serotype since this area contains the major neutralization antigenic sites. The RNA genome stabilizes the capsid by interactions with conserved residues of VP4.

The genome of the enteroviruses is a single, positive-stranded RNA molecule. The genome varies in length from 7209 nt to 8450 nt and consists of three distinct regions: the 5' nontranslated region (NTR), a single open reading frame (ORF) and the 3' NTR (Fig. 153.1).

Infection by Enterovirus

PATHOGENICITY

Viral cycle

The picornavirus cycle of replication occurs, in general, in the cell cytoplasm. The cycle can be divided into:

* adsorption;
* penetration and uncoating;
* synthesis of virus-specific protein and RNA; and
* virus assembly and release from the infected host cell.

Again, the cycle of polioviruses is the most studied and best characterized.

Adsorption

Enterovirus adsorption at the cell surface is regulated by binding to cell-specific receptors. Its mechanism of pathogenesis appears to be mainly determined by cell tropism which depends on the specific recognition of the virus by receptors on the surface of susceptible cells (Table 153.4).

The poliovirus receptor (PVR, CD155) – a glycosylated, three-domain membrane protein that appears in different isoforms (molecular weight 67–80 kDa) – was identified by DNA transformation. Briefly, it was known that although mouse cells were permissive to poliovirus replication, they were not susceptible to poliovirus infection.[10] Thus, poliovirus-susceptible mouse cells were generated by introducing human genomic DNA into mouse cells. Later, these findings were confirmed *in vivo* using transgenic mice.[11] Although PVR transgenic mice are not susceptible to infection by the oral route they have proved to be a valuable model for studying the pathogenesis of poliomyelitis.[12] The poliovirus receptor presents three extracellular immunoglobulin-like domains: a membrane-distal V-type domain followed by two C2-type domains. The first domain contains the site that binds poliovirus.

Some species C enteroviruses use intercellular adhesion molecule-1 (ICAM-1, CD54) as their receptor. Their physiologic ligand is the lymphocyte function-associated molecule-1 (LFA-1), at the surface of leukocytes. The binding site is located in the first immunoglobulin-like domain. The superfamily of integrins also contains other enterovirus receptors: Decay-accelerating factor (DAF, CD55), vitronectin ($\alpha_v\beta3$) and very late-activating antigen-2 (VLA-2).

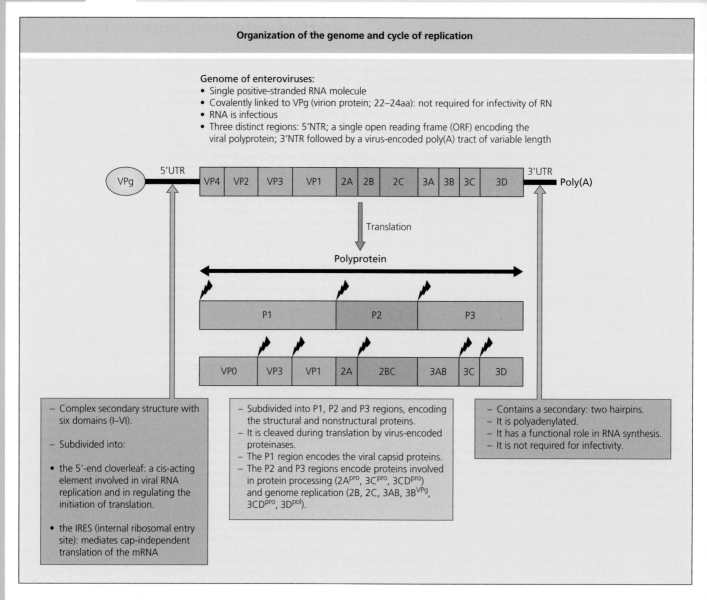

Organization of the genome and cycle of replication

Genome of enteroviruses:
- Single positive-stranded RNA molecule
- Covalently linked to VPg (virion protein; 22–24aa): not required for infectivity of RN
- RNA is infectious
- Three distinct regions: 5'NTR; a single open reading frame (ORF) encoding the viral polyprotein; 3'NTR followed by a virus-encoded poly(A) tract of variable length

VPg — 5'UTR — VP4 | VP2 | VP3 | VP1 | 2A | 2B | 2C | 3A | 3B | 3C | 3D — 3'UTR — Poly(A)

Translation

Polyprotein

P1 | P2 | P3

VP0 | VP3 | VP1 | 2A | 2BC | 3AB | 3C | 3D

– Complex secondary structure with six domains (I–VI).

– Subdivided into:

- the 5'-end cloverleaf: a cis-acting element involved in viral RNA replication and in regulating the initiation of translation.

- the IRES (internal ribosomal entry site): mediates cap-independent translation of the mRNA

– Subdivided into P1, P2 and P3 regions, encoding the structural and nonstructural proteins.
– It is cleaved during translation by virus-encoded proteinases.
– The P1 region encodes the viral capsid proteins.
– The P2 and P3 regions encode proteins involved in protein processing ($2A^{pro}$, $3C^{pro}$, $3CD^{pro}$) and genome replication (2B, 2C, 3AB, $3B^{VPg}$, $3CD^{pro}$, $3D^{pol}$).

– Contains a secondary: two hairpins.
– It is polyadenylated.
– It has a functional role in RNA synthesis.
– It is not required for infectivity.

Fig. 153.1 Organization of the genome and cycle of replication. NTR, nontranslated region; UTR, untranslated region.

Table 153.4 Cell receptors for enterovirus

Virus	Receptor	Co-receptor
PV1, PV2, PV3	PVR	
CAV13, CAV18, CAV21	ICAM-1	
CAV21	Decay-accelerating factor (CD55)	ICAM-1
CAV9	$\alpha_v\beta_3$, $\alpha_v\beta_6$	
CBV1–6	Coxsackievirus–adenovirus receptor	
CBV1, CBV3, CBV5	Decay-accelerating factor (CD55)	$\alpha_v\beta_6$-integrin
E1, E8	$\alpha_v\beta_1$-integrin (VLA-2)	β_2-microglobulin
E3, E6, E7, E11–13, E20, E21, E24, E29, E33	Decay-accelerating factor (CD55)	β_2-microglobulin
EV70	Decay-accelerating factor (CD55)	
EV68	Sialic acid	

The receptor for coxsackievirus B is a 46 kDa glycoprotein that is also used as a receptor by human adenoviruses 2 and 5; thus, it is named the coxsackievirus and adenovirus receptor (CAR). For most enteroviruses, however, interaction with the receptor is not sufficient for infection as they require a second molecule, named co-receptor, for viral entry.

In general, the canyons of poliovirus and coxsackievirus are the sites of interaction with cell receptors as demonstrated by mutation analysis.

Penetration and uncoating

A series of conformational changes occur during virus entry. The interaction of poliovirus with its receptor, PVR, leads to major structural changes in the virus. The *N*-terminus of the capsid protein VP1 becomes accessible after release of the internal capsid protein VP4. These altered particles, known as A-particles, play a significant role in the more widely accepted hypothesis on poliovirus entry. The exposed *N*-terminal VP1 domain inserts into the cell membrane, forming a pore though which the viral RNA can travel to the cytoplasm. This role has been questioned by the finding that poliovirus can replicate at 25°C without formation of A-particles.

Synthesis of virus-specific protein and RNA

After the virus has been uncoated, the viral parental positive-stranded RNA serves as a template for synthesis of viral protein and RNA. After release of the VPg, viral protein synthesis takes place at the rough endoplasmic reticulum. Enteroviral mRNA has no m7G cap group. Initiation of viral protein synthesis takes place in the 5′ NTR, which houses the internal ribosome entry site (IRES). Following translation of mRNA, the viral proteins are originated by proteolytic cleavage. The first cleavage of the polyprotein is catalyzed by the 2A protease at a tyrosine–glycine dipeptide and results in release of the P1 structural segment of the genome. Subsequent cleavages of the P1 precursor into VP0, VP3 and VP1 are mediated by the 3CD protease. The cleavage of P2 and P3 precursors into stable end products is catalyzed by the 3Cpro/3CDpro at glutamine–glycine dipeptides.

The replication of viral RNA takes place at the smooth endoplasmic reticulum using intermediate negative-stranded RNA copies of the viral genome. The mature RNA polymerase 3D regulates viral transcription by interaction with viral and cellular factors through secondary structural motifs in the nontranslated regions of positive- and negative-stranded RNAs.

Virus assembly and release

Virus morphogenesis is characterized by intermediate assembly steps of the virus capsid via precursors and a procapsid. At the final stage, one molecule of positive-stranded RNA is encapsidated in the provirus and a final proteolytic cleavage of the precursor protein VP0 into VP2 and VP4 finalizes the virus maturation.

Cytopathic effects

The reproduction cycle of poliovirus is 6–8 hours. Infected cells are rounded and contain cytoplasmic protrusions. The nucleus is pyknotic and the chromatin is condensed. During the early stage of the cycle, mitosis is enhanced; at later stages, mitosis is arrested at metaphase. Two hours after infection, poliovirus shuts down synthesis of cellular protein, RNA and DNA. Cellular protein synthesis inhibition is caused by proteolytic cleavage of the cellular protein p220, the eukaryotic initiation factor eIF-4G. Analysis by scanning electron microscopy reveals that the first changes in the cell surface can be observed as early as 3 hours after infection. Eight hours after infection the changes are characterized by condensation of collapsed microvilli, formation of elongated filopodia and 'rounding up' of the cell. At this time, up to 10 000 virus particles have been synthesized in a single cell.

EPIDEMIOLOGY

Hosts

The natural host of enteroviruses is the human. Some animals are susceptible to experimental infection with human enteroviruses: nonhuman primates and CD155 transgenic mice for poliovirus; mice and some species of monkeys for coxsackievirus A and B and echovirus.

Coxsackievirus B5 is an interesting case. It is antigenically and genetically (50% homology) related to a porcine enterovirus (swine vesicular disease virus). Epidemiologic studies from outbreaks of this disease suggest that CBV5 was introduced into swine decades ago and led to establishment in this new host.[13]

The routes of enterovirus transmission are summarized in Table 153.5.

Immune response

Innate immune system

The major factor affecting the outcome of an enteroviral infection is the efficacy of the immune response. The role of the innate immune system is especially important as an early determinant of pathogenesis and

Table 153.5 Routes of transmission of enterovirus

Type	Route
Individual	• Fecal–oral route (associated with poor sanitary conditions). Except EV70, and possible EV68, all EV can be transmitted by fecal–oral route • Respiratory route (EV70 and possibly EV68) • Other proven routes of transmission: – Human breast milk – Environmental sources – Contaminated sources of water (swimming pools) – EV have been isolated from mollusks and crustaceans, demonstrating stability in sea salt waters – EV70 and CAV24 (causing hemorrhagic conjunctivitis) can be isolated from eye secretions; those causing vesicular exanthema can be spread by direct and indirect vesicular fluid. In both cases, common routes for infection are hand contact with secretions, and autoinoculation of mouth, nose and eyes
Groups	• Enterovirus household transmission • Familial outbreaks • Schools • Nosocomial transmission

as a regulator of the adaptive immune response. Studies of poliovirus in wild-type CD155 transgenic mice demonstrate that the interferon response is an important determinant of tissue tropism and pathogenicity.[14] Interferons stimulate many genes that induce an antiviral state. Protection against poliovirus infection is mediated by interferon alpha (IFN-α)-induced 2′,5′-oligoadenylate synthetases and ribonuclease (RNase) L, and interferon gamma (IFN-γ)-induced double-stranded RNA (dsRNA)-dependent RNA-activated protein kinase (PKR) in coxsackievirus B-infected pancreatic islet cells.[15] Nuclear factor kappa B (NF-κB), a regulator that activates interferon beta (IFN-β) and initiates the cascade of proinflammatory cytokines, has been shown to be activated early after poliovirus infection. On the other hand, IFN-stimulated gene effects may be complex, and reductions in inflammation have been associated with a slight increase in survival in animal transgenic models.[16]

The role of innate lymphocytes and natural killer (NK) cells has been less studied and these cells may play a role, not only in protection, but also in mediating disease.

B-cell response

The key role of the humoral immune response is demonstrated by the following facts:

- high level of poliovirus neutralizing antibodies following natural infection or vaccination protect against disease, although there is no sterilizing immunity (e.g. infection of the gut can occur);
- high frequency of persistent infections in agammaglobulinemics; and
- increased susceptibility to enteroviral infection as well as increased severity of disease among neonates and infants.

The neutralization sites are generally conformational antigenic sites that correspond to exposed loops of the capsid proteins, although some regions that are internally located in the native virion can also function as neutralization sites. Only a limited number of studies have been performed to identify neutralization sites of nonpolio enterovirus; however, the results suggest similarities in the location of their antigenic sites to those found with poliovirus.

Circulation and geographic spread

Enteroviruses have a worldwide distribution. Within a given geographic locality, some serotypes may be endemic, with little or only gradual change in the range of serotypes present from year to year. In contrast, other serotypes may be introduced periodically, causing epidemics, with very few viral isolations reported in previous years. Since warm weather favors their spread, enteroviruses are more prevalent in temperate climates and in the tropics.

CLINICAL MANIFESTATIONS

Asymptomatic infections

Most enterovirus infections are silent, mild or subclinical. Since the cells of the gut epithelia normally have a high rate of turnover, it has been hypothesized that enterovirus passage through the gut may be the reason for the high incidence of inapparent infections.

Clinical syndromes
Nonpolio enterovirus

Enterovirus are implicated in a wide variety of clinical syndromes ranging from neurologic (aseptic meningitis, paralysis, encephalitis, ataxia and Guillain-Barré syndrome), muscular (pleurodynia, acute and chronic inflammatory muscle disease), respiratory infections, exanthema, herpangina and hand, foot and mouth disease (HFMD), acute hemorrhagic conjunctivitis, myocarditis and pericarditis, diabetes and pancreatitis, and neonatal sepsis-like infections (Table 153.6).

Among the nonpolio enteroviruses, two serotypes seem to be associated with particular severity of disease – enteroviruses 70 and 71 (EV70 and EV71).

EV71 is one of two serotypes most often associated with large outbreaks of HFMD and may also cause a variety of neurologic diseases, including aseptic meningitis, encephalitis and poliomyelitis-like paralysis. EV71 has caused epidemics of severe neurologic disease in Australia, Europe, Asia and the USA. Most recently, it was associated with fatal cases of brain stem encephalitis during large HFMD

Table 153.6 Clinical manifestations of enterovirus infections

Clinical disorders	Enterovirus serotypes	Characteristics
Paralysis	PV1–3 (severe paralysis) CVA4, 7, 9 E4–6 EV71 EV70	Transient mild paresis with aseptic meningitis may occur Younger children have milder disease
Aseptic meningitis	CVA2, 4, 7, 9, 10, 12, 16 CVB1–6 PV1–3 E4, 6, 7, 9, 11, 30 EV71	Benign in infants and children May involve rash or encephalitis Virus isolated from the throat, stool or cerebrospinal fluid
Acute hemorrhagic conjunctivitis	EV70 CVA24 variant	Rarely accompanied by transient radiculomyelopathy or poliomyelitis-like paralysis May produce subconjunctival hemorrhage and keratitis Pain, blurred vision, aversion to light, discharge from the eye
Hand, foot and mouth disease	CVA10, 16 (rarely CVA4, 5, 9) EV71	Vesicular exanthem, usually brief and benign, initially as a sore throat involving the tongue, followed by a rash on the hands and sometimes the feet The rash often forms small blisters, which lead to ulcers Symptoms generally resolve within a week
Rash and exanthema with fever	CVA2, 4–6, 9, 16 CVB1, 3, 4, 5 E2, 4, 9, 11, 14, 16, 19, 25	Nonpruritic, does not desquamate, on the face, neck, chest and extremities. Maculopapular, morbilliform; occasionally hemorrhagic, petechial or vesicular Summer and fall rashes in children
Respiratory disease	E4, 8, 9, 11, 20 CVA2, 10, 21, 24 CVB1–6	Fever, coryza, pharyngitis; in some patients vomiting and diarrhea Bronchitis and interstitial pneumonia are seen occasionally
Herpangina	CVA1–6, 8–10, 16, 21, 22	Palatal and pharyngeal lesions particularly severe, multiple ulcers in the throat. Swallowing becomes very painful; symptoms can persist for several weeks
Myocarditis	CVB1–6 CVA4, 16 E9	Newborns infected after birth or rarely in utero can present with sepsis with fever, lethargy, disseminated intravascular coagulation, bleeding and multiple organ failure; death may occur from circulatory collapse or hepatic failure Older children or adults may make a complete recovery
Diabetes and pancreatitis	CVB1–5 CVA9	Juvenile onset of IDDM 30% of children with IDDM have IgM antibodies to coxsackie B viruses
Chronic fatigue syndrome (myalgic encephalomyelitis)	CVBs	Persistent infection with high prevalence of antibodies against coxsackie B viruses

IDDM, insulin-dependent diabetes mellitus.

outbreaks in Malaysia in 1997 and in Taiwan in 1998. Like poliovirus, EV71 displays an affinity for anterior horn cells.

EV70 was first isolated in 1971 associated with a newly described pandemic acute hemorrhagic conjunctivitis (AHC). The epidemic of AHC had begun in 1969 in Ghana and spread across Africa to India and the Far East, with small outbreaks in Europe. It subsided, only to reappear in India in 1979, with subsequent spread to South America and the Caribbean, with isolated cases in the southern United States.

In the postpolio age, the more important causes of morbidity of enterovirus infections are the neurologic manifestations. Aseptic meningitis is a nonbacterial inflammation of the meninges associated with fever, headache, photophobia and meningeal signs in the absence of signs of brain parenchymal involvement. Meningitis and mild paresis can be induced by most nonpolio enteroviruses. Early symptoms are fever, malaise, headache, nausea and abdominal pain; these are followed by meningeal irritation with neck or back stiffness and vomiting before the onset of meningitis and mild paresis. Aseptic meningitis is very often accompanied by a rash. The manifestation of the CNS disease is usually milder and patients nearly always recover from paresis. Enteroviruses are the more frequent cause of aseptic meningitis in both children and adults in developed countries.

Encephalitis, ataxia and Guillain–Barré syndrome have been attributed to enterovirus infections. Encephalitis signifies that the brain parenchyma is infected and is not infrequently associated with a disturbed state of consciousness, focal neurologic signs and seizures, and sometimes with aseptic meningitis, resulting in meningoencephalitis. The frequency of diagnosis of viral encephalitis is low, although enteroviruses rank second to herpes simplex infection as a recognized cause of encephalitis in the USA.

Polio and acute flaccid paralysis

The infection route of polioviruses is the best understood of all enteroviruses. Following ingestion, poliovirus replicates locally at the initial virus implantation sites (e.g. tonsils, intestinal M cells, ileal Peyer's patches and the mesenteric lymph nodes) and occasionally enters the bloodstream and infects other tissues, including motor neurons.

Only a small proportion (<1%) of poliovirus infections in susceptible individuals result in paralytic poliomyelitis. Most infections are asymptomatic, although some people experience minor illness such as fever, headache and malaise or, in some cases, aseptic meningitis. Paralytic polio is preceded by 1–3 days of minor illness and a symptom-free interval, followed by the acute onset of flaccid paralysis with fever. Paralysis, usually asymmetric, progresses within a few days, and may affect skeletal muscles (spinal poliomyelitis), respiratory systems (bulbar poliomyelitis), or both (bulbospinal poliomyelitis). The loss of motor neurons is permanent and the denervated muscles atrophy.

Poliomyelitis is highly contagious and, in the past, wild viruses in endemic areas infected virtually the entire population. Paralytic attack rates vary by serotype. A small number of infected people developed recrudescence of paralysis and muscle atrophy several decades after paralytic poliomyelitis. However, postpoliomyelitis muscle atrophy cannot be assigned to persistent virus infection but results from the additive effects of physiologic aging and the prolonged loss of neuromuscular function from the earlier infection.

CONTROL OF INFECTION

Vaccines

Two different vaccines have been developed for poliovirus: Salk and Youngner's inactivated poliovirus vaccine (IPV)[17] and Sabin's attenuated oral poliovirus vaccine (OPV)[18] (Table 153.7). Both contain the three serotypes and induce humoral immunity with circulating antibodies. Both are safe and effective, each with particular advantages and disadvantages,[19] and both have played an important role in disease control.[20]

Eradication of poliomyelitis

The global effort to eradicate poliomyelitis is the largest public health initiative in history. The objectives of the Global Polio Eradication Initiative are to:

- interrupt transmission of the wild poliovirus;
- achieve certification of global polio eradication; and
- contribute to health systems development and surveillance for communicable diseases in a systematic way.

Four eradication strategies are recommended by the WHO:

- high routine infant immunization coverage with at least three doses of OPV plus a dose at birth in polio-endemic countries;
- national immunization days (NIDs) targeting all children <5 years;
- acute flaccid paralysis (AFP) surveillance and laboratory investigations; and
- mop-up immunization campaigns to interrupt the final transmission chains.

Overall, since launch of the Global Polio Eradication Initiative, the number of cases has fallen by over 99%, from an estimate of more than 350 000 cases in 1988 to 1997 reported cases in 2006. Widely endemic on five continents (125 countries) in 1988, polio is now found only in parts of Africa and South Asia (four countries: Afghanistan, India, Nigeria and Pakistan). In 1994, the WHO Region of the Americas with 36 countries (last indigenous case: Peru, 1991) was certified polio free, followed by the Western Pacific Region with 37 countries including China (last indigenous case: Cambodia, 1997) in 2000 and the European Region with 51 countries (last indigenous case: Turkey, 1998) in 2002.

The impact of the global initiative can also be monitored by the declining genetic diversity of wild poliovirus genotypes and lineages. Wild poliovirus type 2 has probably been eradicated, as it was last detected in October 1999 in Uttar Pradesh, India.[21] Wild poliovirus

Table 153.7 Characteristics of poliovirus vaccines

Properties	Inactivated poliovirus vaccine	Oral poliovirus vaccine
Antigen	Three wild reference strains: PV1 Mahoney; PV2 MEF-1 and PV3 Sauckett	Three attenuated
Administration	Injection	Orally
Induces	Circulating antibodies	Circulating antibodies and local immune response in intestinal lining
Protection	Protects individual against spread of the virus to central nervous system	Protects individual against infection and passive immunization of close contacts (risk for revertants)
Local immunity	Very low levels of local immunity (in the gut)	Induces intestinal local immunity
Viral circulation	Cannot spread poliovirus circulation	Interrupts wild poliovirus transmission

type 3 survives by steadily diminishing the chains of transmission, and in 2004 was endemic partially in five countries (India, Niger, Nigeria, Pakistan and Sudan). Wild poliovirus type 1 is highly localized in Afghanistan, Egypt, India and Pakistan, but remains more widespread in West and Central Africa following outbreaks in 2003–2004 from northern Nigeria.[22]

The endgame of poliovirus vaccination

Although OPV is safe and effective, in extremely rare cases (approximately 1 in every 2.5 million vaccine doses) the live attenuated vaccine virus in OPV can cause paralysis, either in the vaccinated child or in a close contact. Immune deficiency of the recipient may be among the possible causes. The possibility of genetic exchanges between the Sabin OPV strains and closely related enteroviruses has also come under study. Indeed, numerous vaccine-associated paralysis cases secondary to circulation of vaccine-derived poliovirus in poorly immunized communities has been documented.[23]

The recent roadblocks in India and Nigeria have led to a debate about the most appropriate vaccination protocol to achieve the goal of eradication.[24–26] In industrialized countries with no incidence of wild-type poliovirus-associated paralytic poliomyelitis, use of the OPV is avoided in favor of the safer IPV. In developing countries, however, the use of the more expensive IPV presents many logistic problems that are compounded by the fact that IPV is thought to be ineffective at producing immunity at the gut mucosal surface. As a result, it provides individual protection against polio paralysis but, unlike OPV, is less effective in preventing the spread of wild-type circulating poliovirus.

In light of these events, there is renewed interest to develop new or improved poliovirus vaccines. Three approaches have recently been proposed: attenuated vaccines where viral RNA translation efficiency is compromised by the introduction of synonymous rare codons,[27] where the 5′ IRES structure is modified to stabilize attenuation determinants[28] and where the replication fidelity is controlled by the use of a high-fidelity polymerase.[29]

Treatment

Infections caused by nonpolio enteroviruses cannot be prevented by vaccination. There are, however, several therapies (e.g. interferon and antiviral antibodies) that target early stages in the virus life cycle.[30] Pooled immunoglobulin was used with some success in enterovirus-induced CNS infections in immunocompromised patients and neonates.[31] Oral administration of WIN 54954 significantly decreased the number of upper respiratory infections. More recently, other WIN-type compounds (Pleconaril, VP63843, licensed to Schering-Plough) showed broad in-vitro inhibitory activity against 95% of the 215 nonpolio human and animal enteroviruses tested.[32] A clinical study – Pleconaril Enteroviral Sepsis Syndrome – is currently (2008) recruiting. All other antiviral compounds to date have been proven to show antiviral activity only in cell culture systems.[33]

DIAGNOSIS

A key factor to understanding the epidemiology of the enteroviruses, their diversity, frequent silent infections and variable clinical manifestations is virus identification and characterization. Effective diagnostic virology depends on adequate timing, collection of appropriate clinical specimens and optimal transport.

Specimens for diagnosis

For viral diagnosis, the specimens of choice will depend on the clinical manifestations observed and the type of assay available (classic or molecular), usually stool, rectal or throat swabs and cerebrospinal fluid (CSF) samples. Stool is generally the best specimen for enteroviral

detection, since virus concentrations are the highest relative to the other sources (see Fig. 153.3). However, the detection of enteroviruses in stool or throat swabs might be misleading in terms of causality of the disease due to asymptomatic viral shedding. Generally, etiologic association of enterovirus with disease requires virus isolation from fluids or tissues manifesting lesions.

Thus, stools and rectal swabs are the specimens of choice for poliovirus diagnosis and AFP surveillance, CSF for neurologic disease and throat swabs for respiratory illness, together with sites of vesicular fluid for vesicular rashes, ocular secretions for hemorrhagic conjunctivitis, and tissue material from heart, muscle or brain for myocarditis, myositis or encephalitis, respectively.

Classic techniques

These involve direct detection, virus isolation, seroneutralization and serology.

Nonmolecular direct detection

Direct enterovirus detection by techniques such as immunofluorescence (IF), agglutination or ELISA are not useful due to virus antigenic diversity and the relatively low viral burden in most specimens. Electron microscopy had been used to visualize virus directly in specialized laboratories (Fig. 153.2).

Enterovirus isolation

Most enteroviruses will show a characteristic cytopathic effect (CPE) – rounded and refractile, with cell detachment in tissue culture (Fig. 153.3). It is common to use several cell lines to increase sensitivity. Viral propagation is usually attempted in Buffalo green monkey kidney (BGM) and human cell lines: rhabdomyosarcoma (RD), lung carcinoma (A-549) and embryonic fibroblasts (HEF). WHO recommends inoculation into L20B cells (a genetically engineered mouse cell line expressing PVR) for all specimens suspected to contain polioviruses. In the presence of CPE, identification of enterovirus should be done by IF.

Serotyping of enterovirus isolates

Traditional nonpolio enterovirus typing depends on neutralization with specific or pools of antisera. A standardized hyperimmune equine antiserum developed by Lim and Benyesh-Melnick (LBM) is used to identify 42 common enterovirus serotypes.[34] It consists

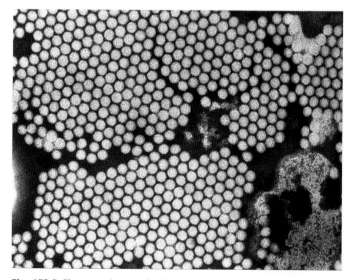

Fig. 153.2 Electron micrograph showing poliovirus particles negatively stained with 2% phosphotungstic acid.

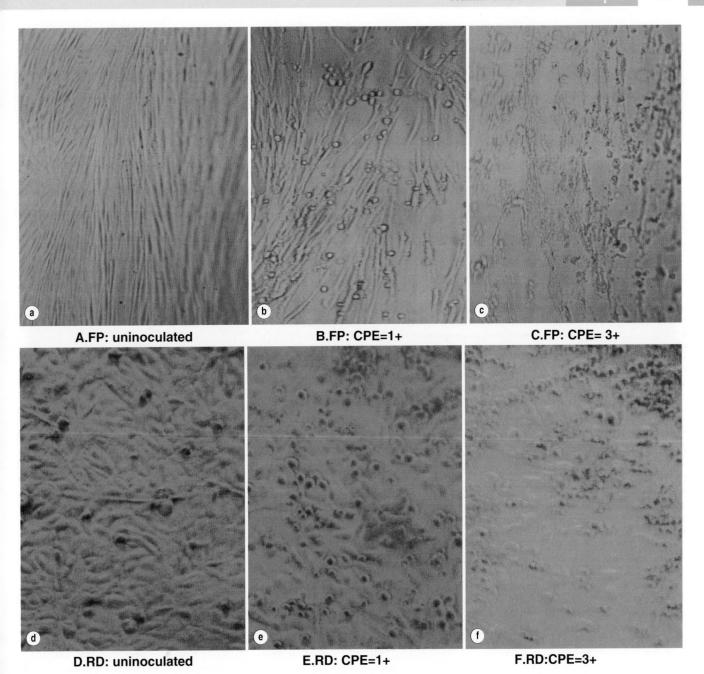

A.FP: uninoculated   **B.FP: CPE=1+**   **C.FP: CPE= 3+**

D.RD: uninoculated   **E.RD: CPE=1+**   **F.RD:CPE=3+**

Fig. 153.3 Enterovirus (EV) cytopathic effect (CPE). Rhabdomyosarcoma (RD) cells and lung fibroblasts (FP) in culture: normal and EV infected, neither fixed nor stained. (a) Uninoculated FP monolayer. (b) FP showing typical early stage CPE by EV (25% CPE), especially rounding, indicating virus multiplication (1+). (c) FP illustrating more advanced CPE (3+); almost 100% of the cells are affected. Most of the cell sheet has come loose from the culture tube wall. The same occurs in (d), (e) and (f) with RD cells.

of a panel of eight combined pools (A–H). Enterovirus isolates are identified by their neutralization pattern against these pools (Fig. 153.4). A second panel of antisera was prepared by the National Institute of Public Health and the Environment (RIVM, Bilthoven, The Netherlands) to identify 19 coxsackievirus A serotypes.[35] After identification with these pools, further confirmation is needed by repeating the neutralization with the specific serotype antiserum. However, since such broad collections of specific reagents are rarely available in diagnostic and reference laboratories, this last step is normally ignored.

Polioviruses could be serotyped by IF with a panel of monoclonal antibodies (Chemicon, USA) or by neutralization with polyclonal antisera (RIVM). Differentiation between wild-type and Sabin vaccine-like strains is made by neutralization with monoclonal antibodies against

wild-type and vaccine-like viruses or by ELISA using cross-adsorbed rabbit antisera. The latter is recommended by WHO for single serotype isolates.

Despite the use of all these techniques, some enteroviral isolates will remain unidentified because of:

- representing an untypable strain or mixture;
- problems with virus aggregation;
- extreme antigenic drift;
- microbial contamination of clinical samples, particularly throat swabs; and
- low infective viral load, thus precluding cell culture propagation.

In spite of all these drawbacks and the labor intensity of the techniques involved, it is still important to attempt the traditional methods;

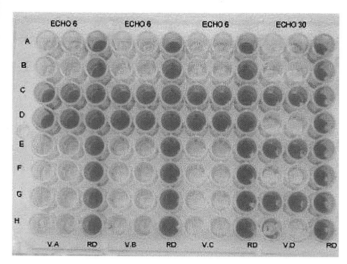

Fig. 153.4 Typing of enterovirus by seroneutralization. Rhabdomyosarcoma-stained microplate showing neutralization patterns of A, B, C and D virus with Lim Benyesh-Melnick antiserum pools (A–H). Viruses A, B and C are considered E6 as a result of neutralization with C and D pools containing specific antisera. Virus D is neutralized by C, E and G pools; thus, it is considered an E30.

pathogenesis and epidemiologic studies are often hampered by the lack of a viral specimen to continue its virulence characterization.

Serologic analysis

Several methods such as complement fixation, ELISA and immunoblotting are used to screen and detect enterovirus group-specific antibodies. However, the use of serologic techniques for primary diagnosis of suspected enteroviral illness is impractical due to virus diversity. On the other hand, these methods are useful to confirm poliovirus infection and immunization. Serologic diagnosis is performed by comparing titers in paired acute and convalescent serum specimens, in order to detect a significant fourfold antibody titer increase.

Many studies have examined the prevalence of antibodies to enteroviruses in specific populations.[36–43] The number of persons who show neutralizing antibody to any given enterovirus is large, indicating a high incidence of past infection. A high incidence of recent infection is also suggested by immunoglobulin M (IgM) surveys, which typically show 4–6% positivity. Infections with one serotype of enterovirus can boost the antibody titers to other enterovirus serotypes. The pattern of the heterotypic response varies by serotype and among individuals, and the pattern of serotype antibody prevalence varies by geographic location, by time and by age. Thus prevalence data from different years and locations are not directly comparable. These general characteristics must be considered when interpreting the findings of serologic studies of associations between enterovirus infection and disease.

Molecular techniques

Detection and typing

Application of molecular biology techniques to clinical virology has introduced significant changes in enteroviral diagnosis. Reliability has increased significantly. In addition, molecular techniques provide short detection times and diagnosis of isolates that do not readily grow in cell culture, and allow typing of enteroviruses that are difficult or impossible to identify by traditional techniques.[44]

Nucleic acid probe hybridization tests were the first application of molecular techniques to detect enteroviruses, but have been replaced by the polymerase chain reaction (PCR). In general, diagnostic assays for enterovirus are targeted to amplify conserved fragments of the 5′ NTR of the virus genome.[45]

The availability of sequence data for all members of the Enterovirus genus has enabled differentiation of viruses based on the nucleic acid sequence encoding the VP1 capsid protein.[46] Molecular identification can be performed using sequences of the reverse transcriptase PCR (RT-PCR) amplification products obtained directly from clinical specimens[47,48] or virus isolates.[48–54] Sequences surrounding the VP4–VP2 junction have also been used for molecular typing,[55–57] but this region does not always provide a reliable identification.[58] Only VP1 capsid sequence correlates with serotype, due to the high frequency of interspecies recombination among co-circulating enteroviruses (e.g. within HEV-B).[6,59–63] Several new enteroviruses, including EV73,[2,64] EV74,[3,6] EV75,[6] EV77 and EV78,[65] EV79–88, EV97, EV100 and EV101,[5] have been detected and characterized using molecular typing systems and sequencing (Fig. 153.5).

Phylogenetic studies of clinical isolates are useful in examining enteroviral evolution and to characterize enterovirus molecular epidemiology[66] (Fig. 153.6). There are two major patterns of enterovirus prevalence: endemic and epidemic.[67] The epidemic pattern is characterized by sharp peaks in numbers of isolations followed by periods with few isolations.[66,68,69] In contrast, the endemic pattern corresponds to serotypes that are isolated in about the same numbers every year, with rare peaks.[70]

Intratypic characterization of polioviruses

Differentiation between wild-type and Sabin vaccine-like strains could be performed by several molecular techniques:

- amplification of viral genomes by RT-PCR followed by restriction enzyme analysis;
- nucleic acid probe hybridization methods use digoxygenin-labeled Sabin and wild type-specific virus genotype-specific probes; or
- poliovirus Sabin strain-specific RT-PCR.

New strategies for enterovirus discovery and typing

The majority of molecular typing techniques today rely on the sequencing of partial fragments in the capsid region of the enterovirus genome. Reliability issues arise, however, when attempting to sequence samples directly without cell isolation which underestimate the circulation of enteroviruses that grow poorly or do not grow at all in cell culture.[71] As early as in 2001[48] and recently,[72] a number of strategies had been proposed to increase sensitivity via nested or seminested PCR. Despite moderate success, inherent limitations exist with nested PCR assays, including carry-over contamination and potential for misclassification. Since the method ability to adequately discriminate partially sequenced fragments for all enterovirus serotypes relies on the database of sequences behind it, the fact that different methods work in different regions of the genome makes comparison and sharing of the results impossible. Finally, these current typing methods do not offer the ability to detect recombination events in the enterovirus genome.

Ideally, future enterovirus typing should attempt to examine the viral genome as a whole. This would allow for greater insight into the recombination events that occur throughout the enterovirus genome, as well as provide the potential to attribute sequence information to virulence of the different serotypes. One particular platform that can be implemented for the broad interrogation of the viral genomes is DNA microarray technology. The multiplex capabilities of the DNA chip platform could expand the ability to characterize enterovirus genomes by investigating not only the capsid region, but also the noncapsid, nonstructural and untranslated regions as well. By screening the different regions of the enterovirus genome, it would be possible to observe the various enterovirus types as a whole without the need for full-length genome sequencing.

Phylogenetic analysis of VP1 for typing purposes

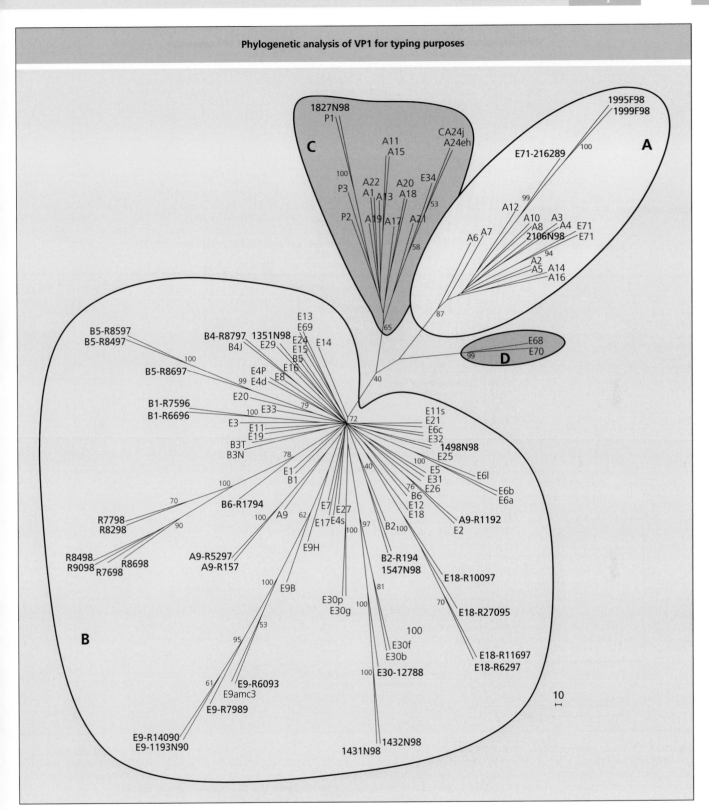

Fig. 153.5 Phylogenetic analysis of VP1 for typing purposes.

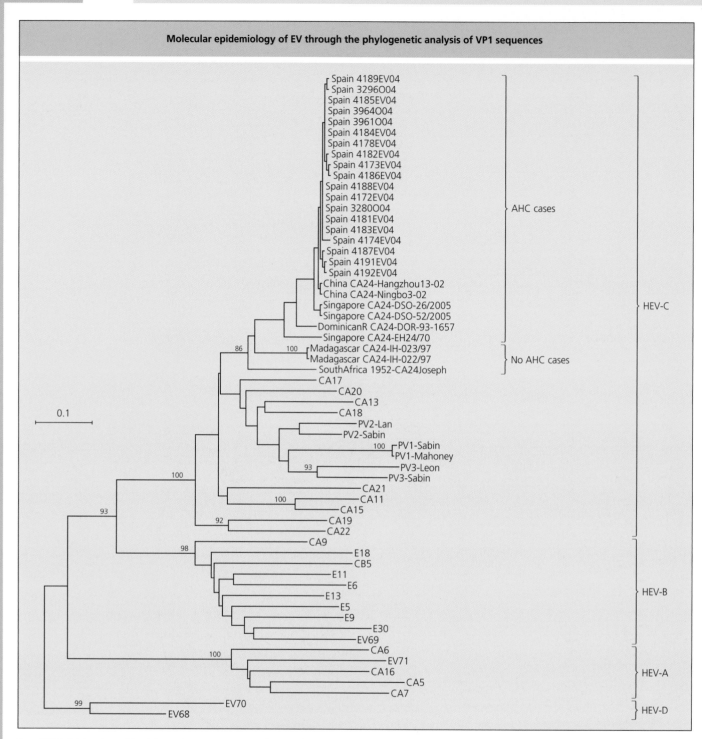

Molecular epidemiology of EV through the phylogenetic analysis of VP1 sequences

Fig. 153.6 Molecular epidemiology of enterovirus though the phylogenetic analysis of VP1 sequences. Phylogenetic tree with 28 CV-A24 sequences and other reference strains of species HEV-A to D based on 415 nucleotides within the 3′-VP1 region. HEV-D was used to root the dendrogram. The dendrograms were constructed by the neighbor-joining method, with 1000 bootstrap pseudoreplicates. Only bootstrap values >70% are shown at nodes. Genetic distances were calculated with Tamura-Nei's evolution model, and the horizontal branch lengths are drawn to scale.

REFERENCES

References for this chapter can be found online at http://www.expertconsult.com

Hepatitis viruses

INTRODUCTION

Viral hepatitis is a major public health problem throughout the world that affects several hundreds of millions of people. Viral hepatitis is a cause of considerable morbidity and mortality, both from acute infection and from chronic sequelae. In the case of infection with hepatitis B virus (HBV), hepatitis D virus (HDV) and hepatitis C virus (HCV), these chronic sequelae include chronic active hepatitis, cirrhosis and primary liver cancer.

There are five recognized pathogens, A–E; additionally the so-called non-A–E hepatitis viruses also exist, which include a range of unrelated and often unusual human pathogens (Table 154.1).

Hepatitis A Virus

Outbreaks of jaundice have been described frequently in many centuries and the term infectious hepatitis was coined in 1912 to describe the epidemic form of the disease. Hepatitis A virus (HAV) is spread by the fecal–oral route. It continues to be endemic throughout the world and hyperendemic in areas with poor standards of sanitation and hygiene.

NATURE

Classification

Electron microscopy examination of concentrates of filtered fecal extracts from patients in the early stages of infection reveals 27 nm particles typical of the Picornaviridae (Fig. 154.1). Hepatitis A virus (HAV) is a small, unenveloped, symmetric RNA virus. After the determination of the entire nucleotide sequence of the viral genome, comparison with other picornavirus sequences revealed limited homology to the enteroviruses and also to the rhinoviruses. Although the structure and genome organization is typical of the Picornaviridae, hepatitis A virus has been placed as hepatovirus within the heparnavirus genus.

Organization of the hepatitis A virus genome

The HAV genome comprises about 7500 nucleotides of positive-sense RNA. The RNA is polyadenylated at the 3′ end and has a viral polypeptide (VPg) attached to the 5′ end. A single, large open reading frame (ORF) occupies most of the genome and encodes a polyprotein with a theoretic molecular mass of M_r 252 000. An untranslated region of

around 735 nucleotides precedes the ORF. Secondary structure within this region of the genome may be important for efficient translation of the RNA. There is also a short untranslated region at the 3′ end of the HAV genome (for further details see the web version of this chapter).

Hepatitis A virus is stable at low pH and is resistant to degradation by environmental conditions.

EPIDEMIOLOGY

Viral hepatitis type A (infectious or epidemic hepatitis) occurs endemically in all parts of the world, with frequent reports of minor and major outbreaks.[1] The exact incidence is difficult to determine because of the high proportion of subclinical infections and infections without jaundice, because of differences in surveillance and because of differing patterns of disease. The degree of underreporting is very high.

Specific serologic tests for hepatitis A have shown that infections with HAV are widespread and endemic in all parts of the world, that chronic excretion of HAV does not occur and that the infection is rarely transmitted by blood transfusion, although transmission by blood coagulation products has been reported. There is no evidence of progression to chronic liver disease.

The seroprevalence of antibodies to HAV has declined since the Second World War in many countries, and infection results most commonly from person-to-person contact, but large epidemics do occur. For example, an outbreak of hepatitis A in Shanghai in 1988 associated with the consumption of clams resulted in almost 300 000 cases.

PATHOGENICITY

The incubation period of hepatitis A is 3–5 weeks (Fig. 154.2), with a mean of 28 days. Subclinical and anicteric cases are common and, although the disease generally has a low mortality rate, patients may be incapacitated for many weeks. There is no evidence of progression to chronic liver damage.

Hepatitis A virus is spread by the fecal–oral route, most commonly by person-to-person contact; infection occurs readily under conditions of poor sanitation and overcrowding. Common source outbreaks are initiated most frequently by fecal contamination of water and food, but water-borne transmission is not a major factor in maintaining this infection in industrialized communities. On the other hand, many outbreaks related to food have been reported. This can be attributed to the shedding of large quantities of virus in the feces by infected food handlers during the incubation period of the illness – the source of the outbreak can often be traced to uncooked food or food that has been handled after cooking. Although hepatitis A remains endemic and common in developed countries, the infection occurs mainly in small clusters, often with only a few identified cases.

Table 154.1 The hepatitis viruses

Virus	Description	Viral group	Mode of transmission
Hepatitis A virus	Small unenveloped symmetric RNA virus	Hepatovirus, in heparnavirus genus	Fecal–oral
Hepatitis B virus	Enveloped double-stranded DNA virus	Hepadnavirus	Blood–blood Sexual
Hepatitis C virus	Enveloped single-stranded RNA virus	Related to flavivirus	Blood–blood
Hepatitis D virus	Circular single-stranded RNA virus	Related to plant viral satellites and viroids	Blood–blood
Hepatitis E virus	Unenveloped single-stranded RNA virus	Related to caliciviruses; closely resembles rubella virus and a plant virus (beet necrotic yellow vein virus)	Fecal contamination of water Food-borne

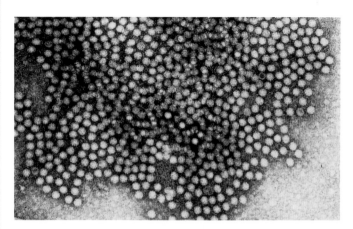

Fig. 154.1 Hepatitis A virus. Note the vast number of virus particles present in a fecal extract.

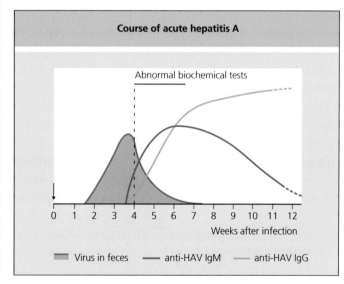

Fig. 154.2 Course of acute hepatitis A.

Course of acute hepatitis A

Abnormal biochemical tests

0 1 2 3 4 5 6 7 8 9 10 11 12
Weeks after infection

Virus in feces   — anti-HAV IgM   — anti-HAV IgG

The clinical expression of infection with HAV varies considerably, ranging from subclinical, anicteric, mild illnesses in young children to the full range of symptoms with jaundice in adolescents and adults. The ratio of anicteric to icteric illnesses varies widely, both in individual cases and during outbreaks.

Hepatitis A virus enters the body by ingestion. The virus then spreads, probably by the bloodstream, to the liver, the target organ. Large numbers of virus particles are detectable in feces during the incubation period, beginning as early as 10–14 days after exposure and continuing, in general, until peak elevation of serum aminotransferases. Virus is also detected in feces early in the acute phase of illness but relatively infrequently after the onset of clinical jaundice. Immunoglobulin G antibody to HAV persists and is also detectable late in the incubation period, coinciding approximately with the onset of biochemical evidence of liver damage.

Hepatitis A viral antigen has been localized by immunofluorescence in the cytoplasm of hepatocytes after experimental transmission to chimpanzees. The antigen has not been found in any tissue other than the liver following experimental intravenous inoculation in susceptible nonhuman primates.

Pathologic changes induced by HAV appear only in the liver (Fig. 154.3). These include marked focal activation of sinusoidal lining cells; accumulation of lymphocytes and histiocytes in the parenchyma – these cells often replace hepatocytes that have been lost by cytolytic necrosis, especially in the periportal areas; occasional coagulative necrosis resulting in the formation of acidophilic bodies; and focal degeneration.

PREVENTION

In areas of high prevalence, most children are infected early in life, and such infections are generally asymptomatic. The later in life that infection occurs, the greater the clinical severity – fewer than 10% of cases of acute hepatitis A in children up to the age of 6 years are icteric, but this increases to 40–50% in the 6- to 14-year-age group, and to 70–80% in adults. Of 115 551 cases of hepatitis A in the USA between 1983 and 1987, only 9% of the cases, but more than 70% of the fatalities, were in those aged over 49 years. It is important, therefore, to protect those at risk because of personal contact with infected people or because of travel to a highly endemic area. Other groups at risk of hepatitis A infection include staff and residents of institutions for the mentally handicapped and day-care centers for children, sexually active male homosexuals, intravenous drug users, sewage workers, certain groups of health-care workers such as medical students on elective

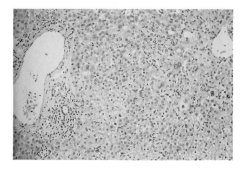

Fig. 154.3 Histologic changes in the liver of a patient with acute hepatitis A.

studies in countries where hepatitis A is common, military personnel and certain low socioeconomic groups in defined community settings. Patients with hemophilia and other blood-clotting disorders should be immunized.

Patients with chronic liver disease, especially if visiting an endemic area, should be immunized against HAV. In some developing countries, the incidence of clinical hepatitis A is increasing as improvements in socioeconomic conditions result in infection later in life, and strategies for immunization are yet to be agreed,[2] although active immunization for travelers, particularly to hyperendemic regions, is strongly recommended.

Passive immunization

Control of HAV infection is difficult. Because fecal shedding of the virus is at its highest during the late incubation period and the prodromal phase of the illness, strict isolation of cases is not a useful control measure. Spread of HAV is reduced by simple hygienic measures and the sanitary disposal of excreta.

Prevention or attenuation of a clinical illness can be achieved by the intramuscular administration of normal human immunoglobulin that contains at least 100 IU/ml of hepatitis A antibody. The dosage should be at least 2 IU of hepatitis A antibody per kilo of body weight; however, in pregnancy or in patients with liver disease, this dosage may be doubled (Table 154.2). Immunoglobulin does not always prevent excretion of HAV. The efficacy of passive immunization is based on the presence of hepatitis A antibody in normal human immunoglobulin, and the minimum titer of antibody required for protection is believed to be about 10 IU/l.

Titers of HAV antibody vary among batches of pooled normal human immunoglobulin and the titers are decreasing in batches obtained from pooled plasma of donors in industrialized countries, resulting in clinical cases despite prophylaxis with immunoglobulin. Immunoglobulin is used most commonly for close personal contacts of patients with hepatitis A and for those exposed to contaminated food. Immunoglobulin has also been used effectively for controlling outbreaks in institutions such as homes for the mentally handicapped and nursery schools. Prophylaxis with immunoglobulin is recommended for people without HAV antibody who are visiting highly endemic areas, but active immunization is recommended, particularly for travelers and for controlling outbreaks, especially if vaccine is given to all contacts immediately.

Active immunization against hepatitis A

Killed hepatitis A vaccines

The foundations for a hepatitis A vaccine were laid in 1975 by the demonstration that formalin-inactivated virus extracted from the liver of infected marmosets induced protective antibodies in susceptible marmosets on challenge with live virus. Subsequently, HAV was cultivated,

Table 154.2 Passive immunization with normal human immunoglobulin for travelers to highly endemic areas

Body weight	Period of stay less than 3 months	Period of stay longer than 3 months
≤55 lb (<25 kg)	50 IU anti-HAV (0.5 ml)	100 IU anti-HAV (1.0 ml)
55–66 lb (25–30 kg)	100 IU anti-HAV (1.0 ml)	250 IU anti-HAV (2.5 ml)
≥110 lb (>50 kg)	200 IU anti-HAV (2.0 ml)	500 IU anti-HAV (5.0 ml)

after serial passage in marmosets, in a cloned line of fetal rhesus monkey kidney cells, thereby opening the way to the production of hepatitis A vaccines. Several formalin-inactivated hepatitis A vaccines are available, including combined vaccines with hepatitis B vaccine and with typhoid vaccine; other polyvalent vaccines are under development.

Live attenuated hepatitis A vaccines

The major advantages of live attenuated vaccines include ease of oral administration, relatively low cost because the virus vaccine strain replicates in the gut, production of both local immunity in the gut and humoral immunity, thereby mimicking natural infection, and the longer term protection afforded. Disadvantages include the potential of reversion toward virulence, interference with the vaccine strain by other viruses in the gut, relative instability of the vaccine and shedding of the virus strain in the feces for prolonged periods.

As with vaccine strains of polioviruses, attenuation may be associated with mutations in the 5' noncoding region of the genome, and this affects the secondary structure of the protein compounds. There is also evidence that mutations in the region of the genome encoding the nonstructural polypeptides may be important for adaptation to cell culture and attenuation. However, markers of attenuation of HAV have not been identified and reversion to virulence may be a problem. On the other hand, there is also concern that 'over-attenuated' viruses may not be sufficiently immunogenic. Attenuated vaccines are available so far only in China, using the H2 and L-A-1 strains.

DIAGNOSTIC VIROLOGY

Various serologic tests are available for HAV, including immune electron microscopy, immune adherence hemagglutination, radioimmunoassay and enzyme immunoassay. Immune adherence hemagglutination, which has been used widely, is moderately specific and sensitive. Radioimmunoassay has been largely replaced by sensitive enzyme immunoassay techniques.

Only one serotype of HAV has been identified in volunteers infected experimentally with the MS-1 strain of hepatitis A, in patients from different outbreaks of hepatitis in different geographic regions and in random cases of hepatitis A. Seven genotypes of the virus are recognized.

Isolation of virus in tissue culture requires prolonged adaptation and it is therefore not suitable for diagnosis.

CLINICAL MANIFESTATIONS

The following description of the acute disease applies to all types of viral hepatitis. Prodromal nonspecific symptoms such as fever, chills, headache, fatigue, malaise and aches and pains are followed a few days later by anorexia, nausea, vomiting and right upper quadrant abdominal pain followed by the passage of dark urine and clay-colored stools. Jaundice of the sclera and skin develops. With the appearance of jaundice, there is usually a rapid subjective improvement of symptoms. The jaundice usually deepens for a few days and persists for 1–2 weeks. The feces then darken and the jaundice diminishes over a period of about 2 weeks. Convalescence may be prolonged (see Chapter 38).

Hepatitis E Virus

Retrospective testing of serum samples from patients involved in epidemics of hepatitis associated with fecal contamination of water supplies has indicated that an agent other than HAV or HBV was involved. Epidemics of enterically transmitted non-A, non-B hepatitis in the Indian subcontinent were first reported in 1980, but outbreaks involving tens of thousands of cases have also been documented in the former Soviet Union, South East Asia, northern Africa, Mexico and elsewhere. A huge outbreak occurred in New Delhi in 1956–7, but tests for HAV or HBV were not available then. Infection has been reported in returning travelers, and sporadic infections have also been identified in patients who had not traveled abroad.

NATURE

Hepatitis E virus (HEV) is a nonenveloped single-stranded RNA virus that shares many biophysical and biochemical features with caliciviruses.

Morphologically the virus is spherical and unenveloped, measuring 32–34 nm in diameter with spikes and indentations visible on the surface of the particle. Confirmation that the virus has been propagated in cell culture is awaited. The virus appears similar to the caliciviruses. However, detailed morphologic studies and the lack of similarities in genome sequence between HEV and recognized caliciviruses suggest that HEV is a single member of a novel virus genus. However, HEV resembles most closely the sequences of rubella virus and a plant virus, beet necrotic yellow vein virus. These three viruses have been placed in separate but related families.

Genomic organization

Hepatitis E virus was cloned in 1991 and the entire 7.5 kb sequence is known. The genome is a single-stranded, positive-sense, polyadenylated RNA molecule, with three overlapping ORFs.

Recent studies indicate that HEV may be distributed into at least nine different groups based on sequencing.

EPIDEMIOLOGY

The epidemiologic features of the infection resemble those of hepatitis A. The highest attack rates are found in young adults and high mortality rates of 10–40% (and occasionally higher) have been reported in women infected during the third trimester of pregnancy.

All epidemics of hepatitis E reported to date have been associated with fecal contamination of water, with the exception of a number of food-borne outbreaks in China. Sporadic hepatitis E has been associated with the consumption of uncooked shellfish and has been seen in travelers returning from endemic areas. Hepatitis E virus is an important cause of large epidemics of acute hepatitis, and these, together with a high prevalence of antibody determined by serologic tests, have occurred in the subcontinent of India, South East and central Asia, the Middle East, and northern and western Africa. There have also been outbreaks in eastern Africa and Mexico.[3]

Unexpectedly, the highest prevalence of antibody to HEV is found in young adults and not in infants and children.

Hepatitis E virus has also been isolated from patients with sporadic acute hepatitis in countries not considered to be endemic for HEV such as the USA, Italy and other European countries and in individuals who had not traveled abroad. There is now evidence that HEV may have an animal reservoir and there are HEV isolates from swine with high sequence identity to human HEV strains isolated from pigs in areas without HEV epidemics. There is recent evidence of a higher prevalence of HEV antibodies among swine farmers, particularly in those with an occupational history of cleaning barns or assisting sows at birth, and also a history of drinking raw milk. Zoonotic spread of HEV may also occur from rodents.

PATHOGENICITY

Virus-like particles have been detected in the feces of infected people by immune electron microscopy using convalescent serum. Cross-reaction studies between sera and virus in feces associated with a variety of

epidemics in several different countries suggest that a single serotype of virus is involved, although two distinct isolates have been recognized and designated as the Burma (B) strain and the Mexico (M) strain.

The average incubation period is slightly longer than for HAV, with a mean of 6 weeks.

The clinical spectrum of infection with HEV is similar to that caused by the other hepatitis viruses, although cholestatic features are common. Hepatitis E does not progress to chronic liver disease and persistent infection does not occur.

Infection with HEV is associated with a relatively high mortality of 1–4% of patients admitted to hospital, and fulminant hepatitis during pregnancy may lead to a mortality rate of 10–40%. Premature delivery and infant mortality of up to 33% have been recorded.

PREVENTION

The provision of safe and chlorinated public water supplies, public sanitation and hygiene, safe disposal of feces and raw sewage (including safeguarding the water supply from animal waste from farm animals) and personal hygiene are essential measures.

Passive protection with immunoglobulin prepared from pooled plasma obtained from blood donors living in endemic countries is not effective.

Several recombinant and subunit HEV vaccines have been developed and are undergoing clinical trials. A purified polypeptide vaccine preparation which was produced in *Spodoptera frugiperda* cells with recombinant baculovirus containing a truncated HEV genomic sequence encoding the capsid antigen was found to be safe and effective in the prevention of hepatitis E in a high-risk population in Nepal.[4]

DIAGNOSTIC VIROLOGY

Serologic tests are necessary to establish the diagnosis. The tests commercially available at present detect anti-HEV IgM in up to 90% of acute infections if serum is obtained 1–4 weeks after the onset of illness, with IgM remaining detectable for about 12 weeks. Anti-HEV IgG appears early and reaches a maximum titer 4 weeks after the onset of illness, falling rapidly thereafter.

Tests for HEV RNA by the polymerase chain reaction (PCR) are available in specialized laboratories.

CLINICAL MANIFESTATIONS

Individual cases cannot be differentiated on the basis of clinical features from other cases of hepatitis. In epidemics, most clinical cases will have anorexia, jaundice and hepatomegaly. Serologic tests indicate, however, that clinically inapparent cases occur (see Chapter 38).

Hepatitis B Virus

Hepatitis B virus was recognized originally as the agent responsible for 'serum hepatitis', an important and frequent cause of acute and chronic infection of the liver including up to 80% of cases of primary hepatocellular carcinoma.

NATURE

Hepatitis B virus is a member of the hepadnavirus group, which contains double-stranded DNA viruses that replicate by reverse transcription. Hepatitis B virus is endemic in the human population and hyperendemic in many parts of the world. The virus is transmitted essentially by blood–blood contact and by the sexual route. Mutations of the surface coat protein of the virus and of the core and other proteins have been identified in recent years.[5-7] Natural hepadnavirus infections also occur in other animals, including woodchucks, beechy ground squirrels and ducks.

Structure and organization of the virus

The hepatitis B virion is a 42 nm particle comprising an electron-dense core (nucleocapsid), which is 27 nm in diameter, and an outer envelope of the surface protein (hepatitis B surface antigen, HBsAg) embedded in membranous lipid derived from the host cell (Fig. 154.4). The surface antigen, originally referred to as Australia antigen, is produced in excess by the infected hepatocytes and is secreted in the form of 22 nm particles and tubular structures of the same diameter.

The 22 nm particles are composed of the major surface protein in both nonglycosylated (p4) and glycosylated (gp27) form in approximately equimolar amounts, together with a minority component of the so-called middle proteins (gp33 and gp36) which contain the pre-S2 domain, a glycosylated 55 amino acid amino-terminal extension. The surface of the virion has a similar composition but also contains the large surface proteins (gp39 and gp42) which include both the pre-S1 and pre-S2 regions. These large surface proteins are not found in the 22 nm spherical particles (but may be present in the tubular forms in highly viremic people) and their detection in serum correlates with viremia. The domain that binds to the specific HBV receptor on the hepatocyte is believed to reside within the pre-S1 region.

The nucleocapsid of the virion consists of the viral genome surrounded by the core antigen (HBcAg). The genome, which is approximately 3.2 kb in length, has an unusual structure and is composed of two linear strands of DNA held in a circular configuration by base-pairing at the 5′ ends (for further details, see the web version of this chapter).

There are nine subtypes of HBV, with a common main antigenic determinant, *a*. The nine subtypes described, *ayw*1–*ayw*4, *ayr*, *adw*2, *adw*4, *adrq*⁻ and *adrq*⁺, differ in their geographic distribution. Subtyping is employed for epidemiologic studies and to trace nosocomial infection. Traditional subtyping is complemented by classification of different HBV strains into genotypes A–G.

EPIDEMIOLOGY

More than a third of the world's population has been infected with HBV, and the World Health Organization estimates that HBV results in 1 000 000–2 000 000 deaths every year.

The virus persists in approximately 5–10% of immunocompetent adults and in as many as 90% of infants infected perinatally. Persistent carriage of HBV, defined by the presence of HBsAg in the serum for more than 6 months, has been estimated to affect about 350 000 000 people worldwide.

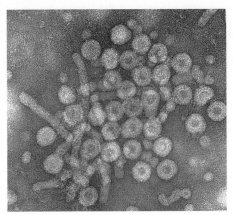

Fig. 154.4 Serum from a patient with hepatitis B. The double-shelled particle is the complete virion. Tubular structures and 22 nm HBsAg particles are present in small numbers.

Although various body fluids (blood, saliva, menstrual and vaginal discharges, serous exudates, seminal fluid and breast milk) have been implicated in the spread of infection, infectivity appears to be especially related to blood and to body fluids contaminated with blood. The epidemiologic propensities of this infection are therefore wide; they include infection by inadequately sterilized syringes and instruments, and transmission by unscreened blood transfusion and blood products, by close contact and by sexual contact. Transmission of HBV from mother to child may take place – antenatal transmission is rare but perinatal transmission occurs frequently; in some parts of the world (South East Asia and Japan) perinatal transmission is very common. Clustering of hepatitis B may occur within family groups, but it is not related to genetic factors and does not reflect maternal or sexual transmission. The mode of intrafamilial spread of HBV is not known.

PATHOGENICITY

The incubation period of hepatitis B is variable, with a range of 1–6 months.

As mentioned above, about 350 million people are carriers of HBV. The pathology is mediated by the cellular immune response of the host to the infected hepatocytes. Long-term continuing virus replication may lead to progression to chronic liver disease, cirrhosis and hepatocellular carcinoma (Fig. 154.5).

In the first phase of chronicity, virus replication continues in the liver and replicative intermediates of the viral genome may be detected in DNA extracted from liver biopsies. Markers of virus replication in serum include HBV DNA, the surface proteins (HBsAg) and a soluble antigen, HBeAg, which is secreted by infected hepatocytes. In those infected at a very young age this phase may persist for life but, more usually, virus levels decline over time. Eventually, in most infected people, there is immune clearance of infected hepatocytes associated with seroconversion from HBeAg to anti-HBe.

During the period of replication, the viral genome may integrate into the chromosomal DNA of some hepatocytes and these cells may persist and expand clonally. Rarely, seroconversion to anti-HBs follows clearance of virus replication but, more frequently, HBsAg persists during a second phase of chronicity as a result of the expression of integrated viral DNA.

Immune responses

Antibody and cell-mediated immune responses to various types of antigen are induced during the infection; however, not all of these are protective and in some instances they may cause autoimmune phenomena that contribute to disease pathogenesis. The immune response to infection with HBV is directed toward at least three antigens: HBsAg, the core antigen and the e antigen. Evidence suggests that the pathogenesis of liver damage in the course of HBV infection is related to the immune response by the host.

The surface antigen appears in the serum of most patients during the incubation period, 2–8 weeks before biochemical evidence of liver damage or onset of jaundice. The antigen persists during the acute illness and usually clears from the circulation during convalescence. Next to appear in the circulation is the virus-associated DNA polymerase activity, which correlates in time with damage to liver cells as indicated by elevated serum transaminases. The polymerase activity persists for days or weeks in acute cases and for months or years in some persistent carriers. Antibody of the IgM class to the core antigen is found in the serum 2–10 weeks after the surface antigen appears and persists during replication of the virus. Core antibody of the IgG class is detectable for many years after recovery. Finally, antibody to the surface antigen component, anti-HBs, appears.

During the incubation period and during the acute phase of the illness, surface antigen–antibody complexes may be found in the serum of some patients. Immune complexes have been found by electron microscopy in the serum of all patients with fulminant hepatitis but are seen only infrequently in nonfulminant infection.

Fig. 154.5 Possible consequences of hepatitis B virus infection in an adult.

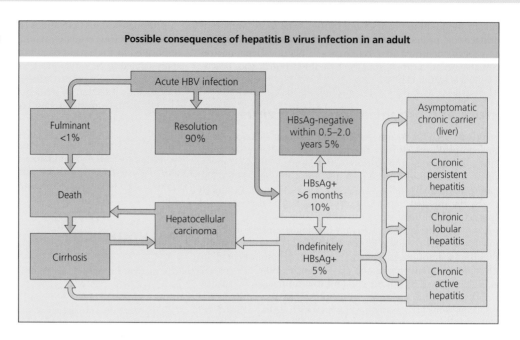

Possible consequences of hepatitis B virus infection in an adult

Acute HBV infection

Fulminant <1%

Resolution 90%

HBsAg-negative within 0.5–2.0 years 5%

Asymptomatic chronic carrier (liver)

Death

Chronic persistent hepatitis

Hepatocellular carcinoma

HBsAg+ >6 months 10%

Chronic lobular hepatitis

Cirrhosis

Indefinitely HBsAg+ 5%

Chronic active hepatitis

Immune complexes have been identified in variable proportions of patients with virtually all the recognized chronic sequelae of acute hepatitis B. Deposits of such immune complexes have also been demonstrated in the cytoplasm and plasma membrane of hepatocytes and on or in the nuclei; the reason why only a small proportion of patients with circulating complexes develop vasculitis or polyarteritis is, however, not clear. Perhaps complexes are critical pathogenic factors only if they are of a particular size and of a certain antigen–antibody ratio.

Cellular immune responses are known to be particularly important in determining the clinical features and course of viral infections. The occurrence of cell-mediated immunity to HBV antigens has been demonstrated in most patients during the acute phase of hepatitis B and in a significant proportion of patients with surface-antigen-positive chronic active hepatitis, but not in asymptomatic persistent HBV carriers. These observations suggest that cell-mediated immunity may be important in terminating the infection and, in certain circumstances, in promoting liver damage and in the genesis of autoimmunity. Evidence also suggests that progressive liver damage may result from an autoimmune reaction directed against hepatocyte membrane antigens, initiated in many cases by infection with HBV.

Hepatitis B virus and hepatocellular carcinoma

When tests for HBsAg became widely available, regions of the world where the chronic carrier state is common were found to be coincident with those where there is a high prevalence of primary liver cancer (Fig. 154.6). Furthermore, in these areas, patients with this tumor are almost invariably seropositive for HBsAg. A prospective study in

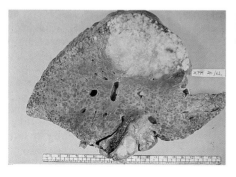

Fig. 154.6 Hepatocellular carcinoma.

Taiwan revealed that 184 cases of hepatocellular carcinoma occurred in 3454 carriers of HBsAg at the start of the study, but only 10 such tumors arose in the 19 253 control males who were HBsAg negative.[8]

Other case-control and cohort studies and laboratory investigations indicate that there is a consistent and specific causal association between HBV and hepatocellular carcinoma, and that up to 80% of such cancers are attributable to this virus. Hepatitis B is thus second only to tobacco among the known human carcinogens. Primary liver cancer is the seventh most common cancer in males and the ninth most common in females. Hepatocellular carcinoma is one of the three most common causes of cancer deaths in males in east and South East Asia, the Pacific Basin and sub-Saharan Africa.

Southern hybridization of tumor DNA yields evidence of chromosomal integration of viral sequences in at least 80% of hepatocellular carcinomas from HBsAg carriers. There is no similarity in the pattern of integration between different tumors, and variation is seen both in the integration sites and in the number of copies or partial copies of the viral genome. Sequence analysis of the integrants reveals that the direct repeats in the viral genome often lie close to the virus–cell junctions, suggesting that sequences around the ends of the viral genome may be involved in recombination with host DNA. Integration seems to involve microdeletion of host sequences, and rearrangements and deletions of part of the viral genome also may occur. When an intact surface gene is present, the tumor cells may produce and secrete HBsAg in the form of 22 nm particles. Production of HBcAg by tumors is rare, however, and the core ORF is often incomplete; modifications such as methylation may also modulate its expression. Cytotoxic T lymphocytes targeted against core gene products on the hepatocyte surface seem to be the major mechanism of clearance of infected cells from the liver. Thus, there may be immune selection of cells with integrated viral DNA that are incapable of expressing HBcAg.

The mechanisms of oncogenesis by HBV remain uncertain. Hepatitis B virus may act nonspecifically by stimulating active regeneration and cirrhosis, which may be associated with chronicity. However, HBV-associated tumors arise occasionally in the absence of cirrhosis, and such hypotheses do not explain the frequent finding of integrated viral DNA in tumors. In rare instances, the viral genome has been found to be integrated into cellular genes such as cyclin A and a retinoic acid receptor. Translocations and other chromosomal rearrangements have also been observed. Although insertional mutagenesis of HBV remains an attractive hypothesis to explain its oncogenicity, there is insufficient supportive evidence. Transactivation by the X-gene is another possible mechanism.

Like many other cancers, the development of hepatocellular carcinoma is likely to be a multifactorial process. The clonal expansion of cells with integrated viral DNA seems to be an early stage in this process and such clones may accumulate in the liver throughout the period of active virus replication. In areas where the prevalence of primary liver cancer is high, virus infection usually occurs at an early age and virus replication may be prolonged, although the peak incidence of tumor is many years after the initial infection.

PREVENTION

The discovery of variation in the epitopes presented on the surface of the virions and subviral particles identified several subtypes of HBV, which differ in their geographic distribution. All isolates of the virus share a common epitope – a. This epitope is a domain of the major surface protein, which is believed to protrude as a double loop from the surface of the particle. Two other pairs of mutually exclusive antigenic determinants – d or y and w or r – are also present on the major surface protein. These variations have been correlated with single nucleotide changes in the surface ORF, which lead to variation in single amino acids in the protein. Four principal subtypes of HBV are recognized: adw, adr, ayw and ayr. Subtype adw predominates in northern Europe, the Americas and Australasia, and is also found in Africa and Asia. Subtype ayw is found in the Mediterranean region, eastern Europe, northern and western Africa, the Middle East and the Indian subcontinent. In the Far East, subtype adr predominates, but the rarer subtype ayr is occasionally found in Japan and Papua New Guinea.

Passive immunization

Hepatitis B immunoglobulin (HBIG) is prepared specifically from pooled plasma with a high titer of hepatitis B surface antibody and may confer temporary passive immunity under certain defined conditions. The major indication for the administration of HBIG is a single acute exposure to HBV, such as occurs when blood containing surface antigen is inoculated, ingested or splashed on mucous membranes and the conjunctiva. The optimal dose has not been established but doses in the range of 250–500 IU have been used effectively. It should be administered as early as possible after exposure and preferably within 48 hours. The dose is usually 3 ml (200 IU/ml) in adults. The first dose should not be administered more than 7 days following exposure. It is generally recommended that two doses of HBIG should be given 30 days apart.

Results with the use of HBIG for prophylaxis in neonates at risk of infection with HBV are encouraging if the immunoglobulin is given as soon as possible after birth or within 12 hours of birth, and the chance of the baby developing the persistent carrier state is reduced by about 70%. More recent studies using combined passive and active immunization indicate an efficacy approaching 90%. The dose of HBIG recommended in the newborn is 1–2 ml (200 IU/ml).

Active immunization

The major response of recipients of hepatitis B vaccine is to the common a epitope with consequent protection against all subtypes of the virus. First-generation vaccines were prepared from 22 nm HBsAg particles purified from plasma donations from chronic carriers. These preparations are safe and immunogenic but have been superseded in most countries by recombinant vaccines produced by the expression of HBsAg in yeast cells. The expression plasmid contains only the 3′ portion of the HBV surface ORF, and only the major surface protein, without pre-S epitopes, is produced. Vaccines containing pre-S2 and pre-S1, as well as the major surface proteins expressed by recombinant DNA technology, are undergoing clinical trials.

In many areas of the world with a high prevalence of HBsAg carriage, such as China and South East Asia, the predominant route of transmission is perinatal. Although HBV does not usually cross the placenta, the infants of viremic mothers have a very high risk of infection at the time of birth.

Administration of a course of vaccine with the first dose immediately after birth is effective in preventing transmission from an HBeAg-positive mother in approximately 70% of cases and this protective efficacy rate may be increased to greater than 90% if the vaccine is accompanied by the simultaneous administration of HBIG.

Immunization against HBV is now recognized as a high priority in all countries. Universal vaccination of infants and adolescents is under examination as a possible strategy to control the transmission of this infection. More than 168 countries now offer universal hepatitis B vaccine, including the USA, Canada and most western European countries.[9]

In a number of countries with a low prevalence of hepatitis B, immunization against HBV is recommended only to groups that are at an increased risk of acquiring this infection. These groups include people requiring repeated transfusions of blood or blood products, people undergoing prolonged inpatient treatment, patients who require frequent tissue penetration or need repeated circulatory access, patients with natural or acquired immune deficiency, and patients with malignant diseases. Viral hepatitis is an occupational hazard among health-care personnel and the staff of institutions for the mentally retarded and some semiclosed institutions. High rates of infection with HBV occur in narcotic drug addicts and intravenous drug users, sexually active male homosexuals and prostitutes. People working in highly endemic areas are at an increased risk of infection and should be immunized. Young infants, children and susceptible people (including travelers) living in certain tropical and subtropical areas where socioeconomic conditions are poor and the prevalence of hepatitis B is high should also be immunized. It should be noted that, in about 30% of patients with hepatitis B, the mode of infection is not known – this is a powerful argument in favor of universal immunization.

Site of injection for vaccination and antibody response

Hepatitis B vaccination should be given in the upper arm or the anterolateral aspect of the thigh and not in the buttock. There are over 100 reports of unexpectedly low antibody seroconversion rates after hepatitis B vaccination using injection into the buttock. In one center in the USA a low antibody response was noted in 54% of healthy adult health-care personnel. Many studies have since shown that the antibody response rate is significantly higher in centers using deltoid injection than centers using the buttock. On the basis of antibody tests after vaccination, the Advisory Committee on Immunization Practices of the Centers for Disease Control and Prevention in the USA recommended that the arm be used as the site for hepatitis B vaccination in adults, as has the Department of Health in the UK.

These observations have important public health implications, well illustrated by the estimate that about 20% of the 60 000 people immunized against HBV in the buttock in the USA by March 1985 had failed to attain a minimum level of antibody of 10 IU/l and were therefore not protected.

Hepatitis B surface antibody titers should be measured in all people who have been immunized against HBV by injection in the buttock, and when this is not possible a complete course of three injections of vaccine should be administered into the deltoid muscle or the anterolateral aspect of the thigh, the only acceptable sites for HBV immunization.

Apart from the site of injection there are several other factors that are associated with a poor antibody response or no antibody response to currently licensed vaccines. Indeed, all studies of antibody response to plasma-derived HBV vaccines and HBV vaccines prepared by recombinant DNA technology have shown that 5–10% or more of healthy immunocompetent subjects do not mount an antibody response (anti-HBs) to the surface antigen component (HBsAg) present in these preparations (i.e. they are nonresponders) or that they respond poorly (i.e. they are hyporesponders). The exact proportions of each group depend partly on the definition of nonresponsiveness and hyporesponsiveness; the usual definitions are a level of less than 10 IU/l for nonresponders and 100 IU/l for hyporesponders, measured against an international antibody standard.

Hepatitis B surface antigen mutants

Production of antibodies to the group antigenic determinant *a* mediates cross-protection against all subtypes, as has been demonstrated by challenge with a second subtype of the virus following recovery from an initial experimental infection. The epitope *a* is located in the region of amino acids 124–148 of the major surface protein and appears to have a double-loop conformation. A monoclonal antibody that recognizes a region within this *a* epitope is capable of neutralizing the infectivity of HBV for chimpanzees, and competitive inhibition assays using the same monoclonal antibody demonstrate that equivalent antibodies are present in the sera of subjects immunized with either plasma-derived or recombinant HBV vaccine.

During a study of the immunogenicity and efficacy of HBV vaccines in Italy, a number of people who had apparently mounted a successful immune response and became anti-HBs positive, later became infected with HBV. These cases were characterized by the co-existence of noncomplexed anti-HBs and HBsAg, and in 32 of 44 vaccinated subjects there were other markers of HBV infection.

Furthermore, analysis of the antigen using monoclonal antibodies suggested that the *a* epitope was either absent or masked by antibody. Subsequent sequence analysis of the virus from one of these cases revealed a mutation in the nucleotide sequence encoding the *a* epitope, the consequence of which was a substitution of arginine for glycine at amino acid position 145.

There is now considerable evidence for a wide geographic distribution of the point mutation in HBV from guanosine to adenosine at position 587, resulting in an amino acid substitution at position 145 from glycine to arginine in the highly antigenic group determinant *a* of the surface antigen. This is a stable mutation that has been found in viral isolates from children and adults. It has been described in Italy, Singapore, Japan, Brunei, Taiwan, Hong Kong, India, Germany and the USA; from liver transplant recipients with hepatitis B in the USA, Germany and the UK who had been treated with specific hepatitis B immunoglobulin or humanized hepatitis B monoclonal antibody; and in patients with chronic hepatitis in Japan and elsewhere.[6–8,10]

The region in which this mutation occurs is an important virus epitope to which vaccine-induced neutralizing antibody binds, as discussed above, and the mutant virus is not neutralized by antibody to this specificity. It can replicate as a competent virus, implying that the amino acid substitution does not alter the attachment of the virus to the liver cell. Variants of HBV with altered antigenicity of the envelope protein show that HBV is not as antigenically singular as believed previously and that escape mutation can occur *in vivo*. This finding gives rise to two causes for concern: failure to detect HBsAg may lead to transmission through donated blood or organs, and HBV may infect people who are anti-HBs positive after immunization. Variation in the second loop of the *a* determinant seems especially important.

Hepatitis B virus precore mutants

The nucleotide sequence of the genome of a strain of HBV cloned from the serum of a naturally infected chimpanzee showed a point mutation in the penultimate codon of the precore region, which changed the tryptophan codon (TGG) to an amber termination codon (TAG). The nucleotide sequence of the HBV precore region from a number of anti-HBe-positive Greek patients was investigated by direct sequencing PCR-amplified HBV DNA from serum. An identical mutation of the penultimate codon of the precore region to a termination codon was found in seven of eight anti-HBe-positive patients who were positive for HBV DNA in serum by hybridization. In most cases there was an additional mutation in the preceding codon.

Similar variants were found by amplification of HBV DNA from serum from anti-HBe-positive patients in Italy and Greece. These variants are not confined to the Mediterranean region; the same nonsense mutation (without a second mutation in the adjacent codon) has been observed in patients from Japan and elsewhere, along with rarer examples of defective precore regions caused by frameshifts or loss of the initiation codon for the precore region.

Some precore variants may be more pathogenic than the wild-type virus because in many patients with severe chronic liver disease precore variants are found.

DIAGNOSTIC VIROLOGY

Direct demonstration of virus in serum samples is feasible by electron microscopy, by detecting virus-associated DNA polymerase, by assay of viral DNA and by amplification of viral DNA by various techniques. All these direct techniques are often impractical in the general diagnostic laboratory and specific diagnosis must therefore rely on serologic tests (Table 154.3).

Hepatitis B surface antigen appears first during the late stages of the incubation period and is easily detectable by radioimmunoassay or enzyme immunoassay. Enzyme immunoassay is specific and highly

Table 154.3 Interpretation of results of serologic tests for hepatitis B virus

HBsAg	HBeAg	Anti-HBe	Anti-HBC IgM	Anti-HBC IgG	Anti-HBs	Interpretation
+	+	–	–	–	–	Incubation period
+	+	–	+	+	–	Acute hepatitis B or persistent carrier state
+	+	–	–	+	–	Persistent carrier state
+	–	+	±	+	–	Persistent carrier state
–	–	+	±	+	+	Convalescence
–	–	–	–	+	+	Recovery
–	–	–	+	–	–	Infection with HBV without detectable HBsAg
–	–	–	–	+	–	Recovery with loss of detectable anti-HBs
–	–	–	–	–	+	Immunization without or recovery from infection with loss of detectable anti-HBc

sensitive and is used widely in preference to radioisotope methods. The antigen persists during the acute phase of the disease and sharply decreases when antibody to the surface antigen becomes detectable. Antibody of the IgM class to the core antigen is found in the serum after the onset of the clinical symptoms and slowly declines after recovery. Its persistence at high titer suggests continuation of the infection. Core antibody of the IgG class persists for many years and provides evidence of past infection.

CLINICAL MANIFESTATIONS

The clinical features of acute infection resemble those of the other viral hepatitides. Acute hepatitis B is frequently anicteric and asymptomatic, although a severe illness with jaundice can occur and occasionally acute liver failure may develop. Hepatitis B, with or without its satellite hepatitis D, may be associated with persistent infection, a prolonged carrier state and progression to chronic liver disease, which may be severe. There is an etiologic association between hepatitis B and hepatocellular carcinoma (see Chapter 38).

Hepatitis D Virus

This virus requires hepadnavirus helper functions for propagation in hepatocytes and is an important cause of acute and severe chronic liver damage in some regions of the world.

NATURE

Hepatitis D virus (HDV) is an unusual single-stranded circular RNA virus with a number of similarities to certain plant viral satellites and viroids.[11]

Delta hepatitis was first recognized following detection of a novel protein, δ-antigen (hepatitis D antigen, HDAg), by immunofluorescent staining in the nuclei of hepatocytes from patients with chronic active hepatitis B. Hepatitis D virus is now known to require a helper function of HBV for its transmission. The virus is coated with HBsAg, which is needed for release of the HDV from the host hepatocyte and for entry in the next round of infection.

Two forms of HDV infection are known. In the first form, a susceptible person is co-infected with HBV and HDV, often leading to a more severe form of acute hepatitis caused by HBV. In the second form, a person who is chronically infected with HBV becomes superinfected with HDV. This may cause a second episode of clinical hepatitis and accelerate the course of the chronic liver disease, or cause overt disease in asymptomatic HBsAg carriers. Hepatitis D virus itself seems to be cytopathic and HDAg may be directly cytotoxic.

The HDV particle is approximately 36 nm in diameter. It is composed of an RNA genome associated with HDAg, surrounded by an envelope of HBsAg. The HDV genome is a closed circular RNA molecule of 1679 nucleotides and resembles those of the satellite viroids and virusoids of plants, and similarly seems to be replicated by the host RNA polymerase II with autocatalytic cleavage and circularization of the progeny genomes by way of transesterification reactions (ribozyme activity). Consensus sequences of viroids that are believed to be involved in these processes are also conserved in HDV.

EPIDEMIOLOGY

Hepatitis D is common in some areas of the world with a high prevalence of HBV infection, particularly Italy and other countries bordering the Mediterranean; eastern Europe, particularly Romania; the Middle East; the former Soviet Union; South America, particularly the Amazon basin, Venezuela, Columbia (hepatitis de Sierra Nevada

de Santa Marta), Brazil (labrea black fever) and Peru; and parts of Africa, particularly western Africa. Antibody to HDV has been found in most countries, commonly among intravenous drug users, patients with hemophilia and those requiring treatment with blood and blood products. It has been estimated that 5% of HBsAg carriers worldwide (approximately 18 000 000 people) are infected with HDV. In areas of low prevalence of HBV, those at risk of hepatitis B, particularly intravenous drug abusers, are also at risk of hepatitis D.

The ratio of clinical to subclinical cases of HDV and superinfection is not known. However, the general severity of both forms of infection suggests that most cases are clinically significant. A low persistence of infection occurs in 1–3% of acute infections and in 80% or more of cases of superinfection in chronic HBV carriers. The mortality rate is high, particularly in the case of superinfection, and ranges from 2% to 20%.

PATHOGENICITY

Hepatitis B virus provides a helper function to HDV, which is a defective virus. The histopathologic pattern in the liver is suggestive of a direct cytopathic effect.

Pathologic changes are limited to the liver and histologic changes are those of acute and chronic hepatitis with no particular distinguishing features apart from severity and, in tropical areas in particular, microvesicular steatosis. It should be noted, however, that the virus was discovered by specific nuclear fluorescence in hepatocytes of patients with chronic hepatitis B.

The modes of transmission are similar to the parenteral transmission of HBV.[11]

PREVENTION

Prevention and control for HDV are similar to those for HBV. Immunization against HBV protects against HDV. The difficulty is protection against superinfection of the many millions of established carriers of HBV. Studies are in progress to determine whether specific immunization against HDV based on HDAg is feasible.

DIAGNOSTIC VIROLOGY

Laboratory diagnosis in acute infection is based on specific serologic tests for anti-HDV IgM or HDV RNA or HDAg in serum. Acute infection is usually self-limiting and markers of HDV infection often disappear within a few weeks.[11]

Superinfection with HDV in chronic hepatitis B may lead to suppression of HBV markers during the acute phase. Chronic infection with HDV (and HBV) is the usual outcome in nonfulminant disease.

CLINICAL MANIFESTATIONS

The clinical features of hepatitis D are identical to those of hepatitis A (for further details, see Chapter 38).

Hepatitis C Virus

NATURE

Hepatitis C virus (HCV) is an enveloped single-stranded RNA virus that appears to be distantly related (possibly in its evolution) to flaviviruses, although HCV is not transmitted by arthropod vectors.

Hepatitis C virus is unusual because it was identified using molecular methods rather than a conventional virologic approach.

Transmission studies in chimpanzees established that the main agent of parenterally acquired non-A, non-B hepatitis was likely to be an enveloped virus some 30–60 nm in diameter. Using infected chimpanzee plasma as a starting point, complementary DNA was used to create a library which was screened using serum from a patient with chronic non-A, non-B hepatitis. This approach led to the detection of a clone that was found to bind to antibodies present in the serum of several patients infected with non-A, non-B hepatitis. Eventually, clones covering the entire viral genome were assembled and the complete nucleotide sequence determined.[12]

Properties of hepatitis C virus

The genome of HCV resembles those of the pestiviruses and flaviviruses in that it comprises around 10 000 nucleotides of positive-sense RNA, lacks a 3′ poly-A tract and has a similar gene organization. It has been proposed that HCV should be the prototype of a third genus in the family Flaviviridae. All these genomes contain a single large ORF, which is translated to yield a polyprotein (of around 3000 amino acids in the case of HCV) from which the viral proteins are derived by post-translational cleavage and other modifications (for further details, see the web version of this chapter).

Hepatitis C virus consists of a family of highly related but nevertheless distinct genotypes – presently numbering six – and various subtypes with differing geographic distribution and a complex nomenclature. The C, NS3 and NS4 domains are the most highly conserved regions of the genome and therefore these proteins are the most suitable for use as capture antigens for broadly reactive tests for antibodies to HCV. The sequence differences observed between HCV groups suggest that virus–host interactions may be different, which could result in differences in pathogenicity and in response to antiviral therapy.

It is important, therefore, to develop group-specific and virus-specific tests. The degree of divergence that is apparent within the viral envelope proteins implies the absence of a broad cross-neutralizing antibody response to infection by viruses of different groups.

In addition to the sequence diversity observed between HCV groups, there is considerable sequence heterogeneity among almost all HCV isolates in the amino-terminal region of E2–NS1, implying that this region may be under strong immune selection. Indeed, sequence changes within this region may occur during the evolution of disease in individual patients and may play an important role in progression to chronicity.[12,13]

EPIDEMIOLOGY

Infection with HCV occurs throughout the world, and it is estimated that at present 170 million people are infected. Much of the seroprevalence data are based on blood donors, who represent a carefully selected population. The prevalence of antibodies to HCV in blood donors varies from 0.02% to 1.25% in different countries. Higher rates have been found in southern Italy, Spain, central Europe, Japan and parts of the Middle East, with as many as 19% in Egyptian blood donors. Until screening of blood donors was introduced, hepatitis C accounted for the vast majority of non-A, non-B post-transfusion hepatitis. However, it is clear that, although blood transfusion and the transfusion of blood products are efficient routes of transmission of HCV, these represent a small proportion of cases of acute clinical hepatitis in the USA and a number of other countries (with the exception of patients with hemophilia). Current data indicate that in some 50% of patients in industrialized countries, the source of infection cannot be identified, although 35% of patients have a history of intravenous drug use, and occupational exposure in the health care setting accounts for about 2% of cases. Household contact and sexual exposure do not appear to be major factors in the epidemiology of this common infection. Transmission of HCV from mother to infant occurs in about 10% of viremic mothers and the risk appears to be related to the level of viremia. The possibility of transmission in utero is also being investigated.[12,13]

PREVENTION

Difficulties in vaccine development include the sequence diversity between viral genotypes and the substantial sequence heterogeneity among isolates in the amino-terminal region of E2–NS1. Neutralizing antibodies have not been clearly defined. The virus has not been cultivated *in vitro* to permit the development of inactivated or attenuated vaccines (compared with yellow fever vaccines). Much work is in progress employing recombinant DNA techniques.[12–14]

DIAGNOSTIC VIROLOGY

Successful cloning of portions of the viral genome has permitted the development of new diagnostic tests for infection by the virus. Because the antigen was originally detected by antibodies in the serum of an infected patient it was an obvious candidate as the basis of an enzyme-linked immunosorbent assay (ELISA) to detect anti-HCV antibodies. A larger clone, C100, was assembled from a number of overlapping clones and expressed in yeast as a fusion protein using human superoxide dismutase sequences to facilitate expression. This fusion protein formed the basis of first-generation tests for HCV infection.

It is now known that antibodies to C100 are detected relatively late after acute infection. Furthermore, the first-generation ELISAs were associated with a high rate of false-positive reactions when applied to low-incidence populations and there were further problems with some retrospective studies on stored sera. Second-generation tests include antigens from the nucleocapsid and nonstructural regions of the genome. The former antigen (C22) is particularly useful and antibodies to the HCV core protein appear relatively early in the course of infection.

Positive reactions by ELISA require confirmation by supplementary testing using, for example, a recombinant immunoblot assay. Nevertheless, indeterminate results obtained by ELISA represent a significant problem that needs resolution. It should also be noted that the time for seroconversion is variable; when it can be measured more precisely (e.g. after transfusion) it is generally 7–31 weeks.

The presence of antibodies to specific antigen components is variable and may or may not reflect viremia and, in the case of interferon treatment, a correlation between response and loss of specific antibodies to the E2 component.

Detection and monitoring of viremia are important for management and treatment. Sensitive techniques are available for the measurement of HCV RNA based on reverse transcription (RT)-PCR amplification, nested PCR, signal amplification using branched DNA analytes and others.

The identification of specific types and subtypes is important, with observations suggesting that there is an association between response to interferon and particular genotypes and that different types may differ in their pathogenicity.

CLINICAL MANIFESTATIONS

Most acute infections are asymptomatic and about 20% of acute infections cause jaundice. Fulminant hepatitis has been described. Extrahepatic manifestations include mixed cryoglobulinemia, membranous proliferative glomerulonephritis and porphyria cutanea tarda (see Chapter 38).

Current data suggest that about 60–80% of infections with HCV progress to chronicity. Histologic examination of liver biopsies from asymptomatic HCV carriers (among blood donors) has revealed none with normal histology; indeed up to 70% have been found to have chronic active hepatitis, cirrhosis, or both (Figs 154.7, 154.8). Whether the virus is cytopathic or whether there is an immunopathologic element remains unclear. Infection with HCV is also associated

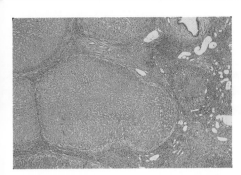

Fig. 154.7 Hepatitis C virus active cirrhosis.

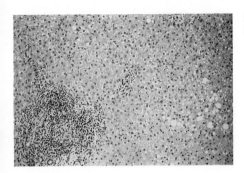

Fig. 154.8 Acute hepatitis C.

with progression to primary liver cancer. For example, in Japan, where the incidence of hepatocellular carcinoma has been increasing despite a decrease in the prevalence of HBsAg, HCV is now believed to be a major risk factor.[13]

Other Hepatitis Viruses

About 30–40 years ago, a series of transmission studies of human viral hepatitis were initiated in small South American tamarins or marmosets, which were chosen because their very limited contact with humans implied that they were unlikely to have been infected with human viruses.

Serum obtained on the third day of jaundice from a young surgeon (GB) induced hepatitis in each of four inoculated marmosets and was passaged serially in these animals. These important observations remained controversial until the recent application of modern molecular virologic techniques. Preliminary results indicate the identification of two independent viruses, GB virus A (GBV-A) and GB virus B (GBV-B), in the infectious plasma of tamarins inoculated with GB.[15]

GB virus A does not replicate in the liver of tamarins, whereas GBV-B causes hepatitis. Cross-challenge experiments showed that infection with the original infectious tamarin inoculum conferred protection from re-infection with GBV-B but not GBV-A. A third virus, GBV-C, was subsequently isolated from a human specimen that was immunoreactive with a GBV-B protein. GB virus C RNA was found in several patients with clinical hepatitis and was shown to have substantial sequence identity to GBV-A.

A series of studies, including phylogenetic analysis of genomic sequences, showed that GBV-A, GBV-B and GBV-C are not genotypes of HCV and that GBV-A and GBV-C are closely related. GBV-A–GBV-C, GBV-B and HCV are members of distinct viral groups. The organization of the genes of the GBV-A, GBV-B and GBV-C genomes shows that they are related to other positive-strand RNA viruses with local regions of sequence identity with various flaviviruses. The three GB viruses and HCV share only limited overall amino acid sequence identity.

Serologic reagents were prepared with recombinant antigens and limited testing for antibodies and by RT-PCR for specific RNA was carried out in groups of patients, blood donors and other selected people – patients with non-A,B,C,D,E hepatitis, multitransfused patients, intravenous drug users and other populations with a high incidence of viral hepatitis. Preliminary studies indicated the presence of antibody to each of the GB viruses in 3–14% of these people. The development and availability of specific diagnostic reagents will establish the epidemiology of these newly identified viruses, their pathogenic significance in humans, and their clinical and public health importance. It should be noted that the virus identified more recently as hepatitis G (HGV) as a new transfusion-transmitted agent is now believed to be identical to GBV-C.[16,17]

The blood-borne nature of GBV-C has been clearly demonstrated and there is evidence that the virus persists. The association of the virus with liver damage is illustrated by raised levels of alanine transaminase and detectable GBV-C RNA in a number of patients. However, 40–90% of viremic subjects have normal alanine transaminase levels. In a significant proportion of patients there is co-infection with HBV, HCV, or both. The primary manifestations of GBV-C infection may be extrahepatic or hepatic and these may be the result of co-infection with the hepatitis viruses or a (as yet unidentified) hepatotropic agent. At present, GBV-C appears to be a virus in search of a disease.[17]

A novel human virus was isolated in Japan in 1997 from the serum of a patient with post-transfusion hepatitis and was designated TT virus (TTV) after the initials of the patient (TTV is not an acronym for transfusion-transmitted virus as has been assumed and perpetuated in numerous publications). The virus has a circular single strand DNA, nonenveloped, of negative polarity and is 3965 nucleotides in length. There is 30% diversity in the coding region accounting for numerous genotypes believed to result mainly from recombination. The virus replicates in many tissues, particularly the liver, and is shed into the blood and feces. TT virus DNA is found in saliva (78%), breast milk, semen (60%), cervical swabs and other body fluids of infected persons. The virus is ubiquitous and is found in 20% to more than 90% of the general population and healthy blood donors. There is no evidence of involvement of TTV in acute or chronic liver disease. TT virus is found in farm animals, including chickens (19%), cows (25%), pigs (20%) and sheep (30%), and in other mammals including nonhuman primates.

TTV-like mini virus (TLMV) and several related viruses such as SANBAN, YONBAN and others have been described, but without any disease association in humans. These different viruses have been divided into at least 29 genotypes with sequence divergence of more than 30% from each other and placed into four phylogenetic groups. Since 1999, much attention has been devoted to the SEN virus (again the initials of a patient infected with a virus possibly related to TTV). The SEN virus (SENV) was isolated from an immunocompromised HIV patient with post-transfusion hepatitis of unknown etiology. Eight genotypes of this virus have been described (SENV-A to SENV-H), each differing by at least 25% in nucleotide sequence. SENV-C, SENV-D and SENV-H are supposedly associated with transfusion hepatitis and, although the prevalence of these viruses is common in patients with non-A–E liver disease, a causal association has not been demonstrated and these should not be considered as candidate hepatitis viruses.[18]

REFERENCES

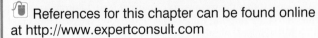

References for this chapter can be found online at http://www.expertconsult.com

Chapter | **155** | *Paul E Klapper*
Anton M van Loon

Herpesviruses

NATURE

Taxonomy

The herpesviruses are double-stranded DNA viruses belonging to Herpesvirales order.[1] More than 150 individual viruses have been described that have been found in almost all the species (both vertebrate and invertebrate) in which they have been actively sought. Their widespread occurrence suggests that they first colonized animal species at an early stage of evolution[2] and this ancient colonization has led to adaptation to their natural host so that they are generally highly host specific. This adaption is exemplified by their high rates of infection, the generally mild symptoms associated with primary infection, and their strategy for maintaining themselves in a population with a high level of immunity by establishing a latent infection.

Genetic analysis shows that the Herpesvirales fall into three distinct families.[1] The family containing the human herpesviruses, the Herpesviridae, is subdivided into three subfamilies – the Alphaherpesvirinae, the Betaherpesvirinae and the Gammaherpesvirinae based upon the biologic properties of the viruses (Table 155.1).

At present eight herpesviruses are known to infect man (Table 155.2). A further primate virus, B virus (Macacine herpesvirus 1), a virus belonging to the Simplexvirus genus of the Alphaherpesvirus subfamily, can also cause severe and sometimes fatal infections in humans.[3] The virus is enzootic among old world macaques and usually causes minimal or no morbidity in its natural host.

Structure

Herpesviruses are morphologically distinct from all other viruses. The virion often has a pleomorphic appearance when visualized by transmission electron microscopy (Fig. 155.1). Examination of herpes simplex virus type 1 (HSV-1) using the technique of cryoelectron tomography (Fig. 155.2) which permits three-dimensional visualization of the virion[4] shows that the virion has a bilayer membrane with an average diameter of 186 nm. An array of spikes protrudes from each virion, making the full diameter, approximately 225 nm.[4]

Between the capsid and envelope is the tegument. Studies with HSV-1 suggest that the tegument contains at least 20 proteins that are believed to have important functions in the early stages of virus replication following penetration of the host cell by the virion.

Physical properties

Herpesviruses are thermolabile. In cell culture media their half-life at 86°F (30°C) is between 1.5 and 14 hours. Drying in air leads to desiccation of the viral envelope and loss of infectivity. Ether in water (20%) and other lipid solvents such as 70% alcohol or chloroform rapidly and completely inactivate herpesviruses.

DNA

The genetic information of the virus is encoded by a linear molecule of double-stranded (ds)DNA and the size of this molecule varies for different herpesviruses, from approximately 80 000 to 150 000 kDa (125–245 kbp). The G+C composition of individual herpesvirus DNAs ranges from 31% to 75% and for human herpesviruses between 36% and 69%. The complete sequence of each of the human herpesviruses is known (Table 155.3) and the phylogenetic relationships of the human herpesviruses are shown in Figure 155.3.

Virion polypeptides

Herpes simplex virus type 1 virions contain about 33 virus-specific proteins, but more than double this number are found within an infected cell. The transcription of mRNAs from the genome proceeds from both strands of the genome, in either direction, with evidence of overlapping transcription and of splicing of genes and gene products.[5] Three rounds of transcription and translation are observed, the so-called:

- α phase (resulting in the production of 'immediate-early proteins');
- β phase (proteins responsible mainly for DNA metabolism); and
- γ phase (principally structural proteins).

Replication

The replicative cycle of the virus is illustrated schematically in Figure 155.4. The initial attachment of a herpesvirus to a host cell is mediated by a glycoprotein or a complex of glycoproteins projecting from the virus envelope interacting with its specific receptor on the host cell.[6]

Initial contact of the herpesviruses with the cell is usually made by low-affinity binding to glycosaminoglycans, preferentially heparan sulphate, on the cell surface. In this way viruses are concentrated at the cell surface, facilitating subsequent binding to a specific receptor. The major pathway for virus entry is fusion of the envelope with the plasma membrane, introduction of tegument proteins and viral nucleocapsid into the cell cytoplasm, and transport of the released nucleocapsid to the nuclear pore. Alternate ancillary pathways have also been identified in cell culture, including fusion within an acidic endosome and fusion within a neutral endosome.[7]

Table 155.1 Biologic properties of Herpesviridae

Common properties	Spherical enveloped virions, 150–200 nm in diameter Large, linear, dsDNA genome of 125–290 kbp contained within a T = 16 icosahedral capsid, which is surrounded by a proteinaceous matrix named the tegument and then by a lipid envelope containing membrane-associated proteins Synthesis of DNA and assembly of capsid within the nucleus, acquire envelope by budding through host cell membranes Specify a large array of enzymes involved in nucleic acid metabolism and synthesis Production of progeny virus results in destruction of the host cell Establish latency in their natural host
Alphaherpesvirinae	Variable host range Short reproductive cycle Rapid spread in cell culture Efficient destruction of infected cells Establish latency primarily but not exclusively in sensory ganglia
Betaherpesvirinae	Restricted host range (a nonexclusive property of this subfamily) Long reproductive cycle Infection progresses slowly in culture, frequently forming enlarged (cytomegalic) cells Latency in secretory glands, lymphoreticular cells, kidneys and other tissues
Gammaherpesvirinae	Experimental host range limited to family or order of natural host *In-vitro* replication in lymphoblastoid cells *In-vivo* replication and latency in either T or B cells

Table 155.2 Human herpesviruses

ICTV* name	Common name†	Subfamily	Genus
Human herpesvirus 1	Herpes simplex virus type 1	Alphaherpesvirinae	Simplexvirus
Human herpesvirus 2	Herpes simplex virus type 2	Alphaherpesvirinae	Simplexvirus
Human herpesvirus 3	Varicella-zoster virus	Alphaherpesvirinae	Varicellovirus
Human herpesvirus 4	Epstein–Barr virus	Gammaherpesvirinae	Lymphocryptovirus
Human herpesvirus 5	Human cytomegalovirus	Betaherpesvirinae	Cytomegalovirus
Human herpesvirus 6	Human herpesvirus 6	Betaherpesvirinae	Roseolovirus
Human herpesvirus 7	Human herpesvirus 7	Betaherpesvirinae	Roseolovirus
Human herpesvirus 8	Kaposi's sarcoma-associated herpesvirus	Gammaherpesvirinae	Rhadinovirus

Two variants, 'a' and 'b', of human herpesvirus 4 and human herpesvirus 6 are known.
*The International Committee on Taxonomy of Viruses (ICTV) classification scheme names the herpesviruses according to the taxon of the host that (in its natural setting) harbors the virus.[1]
†As many viruses have acquired commonly used names – for example, human herpesvirus 1 is commonly known as herpes simplex virus (HSV) type 1 – the classification is not yet rigorously applied. However, newly discovered viruses are now named in accordance with this classification scheme, for example human herpesviruses-6, -7 and -8.

The tegument proteins serve to both 'disable' the host cell and initiate viral replication. Soon after virus entry, host cell DNA synthesis is shut off, host cell protein synthesis declines rapidly and glycosylation of host cell proteins ceases. In this way the virus ensures that the metabolic machinery of the cell is fully available for virus replication. At the same time the virion nucleocapsid is transported via microtubules of the cell cytoskeleton to a nuclear pore. At the nuclear pore the viral nucleocapsid breaks down, releasing its DNA into the cell nucleus where the linear DNA molecule immediately circularizes.

Transcription of viral DNA takes place within the host cell nucleus. The first sets of viral genes to be transcribed are the immediate-early or α genes; these produce control proteins that stimulate and regulate all the subsequent steps in the replicative cycle. Their production is essential to stimulate the production of β polypeptides, which

are the enzymes and other proteins involved in viral nucleic acid reproduction (e.g. DNA-dependent DNA polymerase, which reproduces the viral genome). Products of α and β genes transactivate the translation of the γ genes, which produce the late or γ proteins, the structural proteins for the virion including the viral capsid and glycoproteins.

The synthesis of nucleocapsid and all other structural proteins occurs when γ gene expression is induced by β gene products. Nucleocapsids are assembled around viral scaffolding proteins in the nucleus. Other viral proteins then interact with replicated viral DNA to allow DNA encapsidation. The DNA-filled capsids proceed to associate with tegument (matrix) proteins near the nuclear membrane. Three different models for the release of mature nucleocapsids from cells have been proposed (see Fig. 155.4). Whichever method the viruses use for their release, productive infection is fatal for the

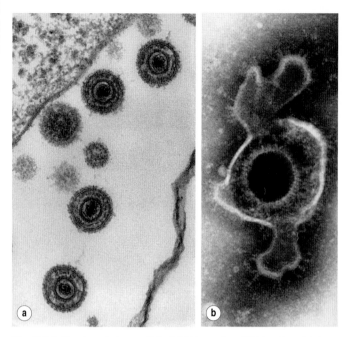

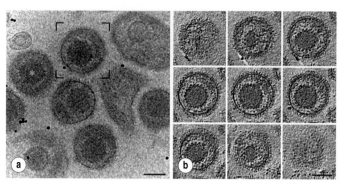

Fig. 155.2 Herpes simplex virus type 1 cryoelectron tomography. Tomographic reconstruction of HSV-1 virions in vitreous ice. (a) Zero-tilt projection from a tilt series. Black dots are 10-nm gold particles used as fiducial markers. (b) Gallery of parallel slices, 15.5 nm apart and 5.2 nm thick, through the virion framed in (a). Each slice represents the average over seven planes. Red arrowheads mark filaments in the tegument. Scale bars, 100 nm. Reproduced with permission from Grünewald, et al.[4]

Fig. 155.1 Enveloped virus particle. (a) Thin section. (b) Negative staining. These electron microscopic views show HSV. The DNA is surrounded by a nucleocapsid comprised of 162 individual protein subunits (150 hexavalent capsomers and 12 pentavalent capsomers) arranged in the form of an icosahedron. The nucleocapsid is in turn enclosed by the tegument and virus envelope bearing glycoprotein spikes. Courtesy of Hans Gelderblom.

host cell because in the process of viral DNA replication host cell chromosomes are degraded. In addition host cell metabolism is irreversibly damaged.

Latency

During the course of a primary infection a latent infection is established, with the exact site(s) of latency varying for each subfamily of herpesvirus (Table 155.4). No virions can be detected within the latently infected cell. In the latent state the virus is believed to exist as extrachromosomal circularized DNA (analogous to plasmids). The host immune response to infection rapidly eliminates virus and

virus-infected cells from peripheral sites, but does not recognize latently infected cells as harboring virus since no viral antigens are expressed on the cell surface.

This establishment of latency is central to the success of herpesviruses as a pathogen, allowing the virus to persist to cause lifelong infection in the presence of a fully developed immune response. Through periodic reactivation of latent virus and the production of recurrent infection, virus shedding occurs at intervals throughout life, allowing the virus to be spread to new susceptible hosts. In order to avoid elimination by the host immune system, each herpesvirus encodes multiple proteins that combat virtually every aspect of immune recognition.[8–11] A key mechanism is to reduce or prevent expression of virus-specific peptide-MHC class I complexes at the cellular membrane, thus preventing recognition by cytotoxic T cells that would kill the infected cell.

Cell transformation

Human herpesviruses can induce mutations in host cell DNA and some human herpesviruses – HSV-1, HSV-2 and cytomegalovirus (CMV) – can transform cells in culture, albeit at a very low frequency.

Table 155.3 Properties of the human herpesviruses

Virus	Site of latency	G+C (moles %)	Genome (kb pairs)	Sequence*
HHV-1	Sensory nerve ganglia	68	152	X14112
HHV-2	Sensory nerve ganglia	69	154	Z86099
HHV-3	Sensory nerve ganglia	46	125	X04370
HHV-4	Leukocytes, epithelial cells	60	172	V01555
HHV-5	B lymphocytes	57	229	X17403
HHV-6A	T lymphocytes (CD4+), epithelial cells	43	159	X83413
HHV-6B	T lymphocytes (CD4+), epithelial cells	43	162	AF157706
HHV-7	T lymphocytes (CD4+)	36	153	AF037218
HHV-8	B lymphocytes, epithelial cells	59	170	AF402655

*European Molecular Biology Laboratory Accession Numbers (http://www.embl-heidelberg.de).

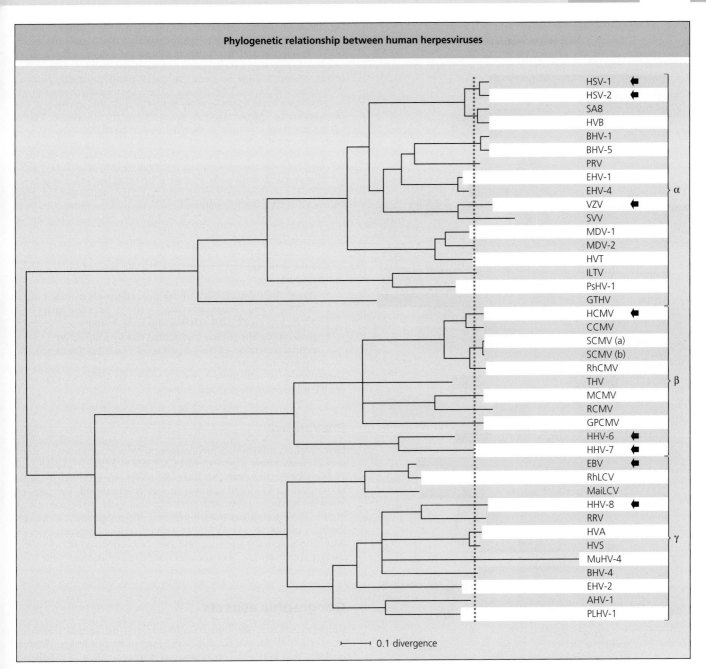

Phylogenetic relationship between human herpesviruses

—— 0.1 divergence

Fig. 155.3 Phylogenetic relationship between the human herpesviruses. The tree was constructed based on an alignment of amino acid sequences for six genes of HSV-1: UL15, UL19, UL27, UL28, UL29 and UL30. Reproduced with permission from McGeoch, *et al.*[5]

These viruses can also amplify persisting genomes of small tumor viruses. CMV, for example, permits the replication of the polyomavirus JC when co-transfected in human fibroblasts, providing an indirect means by which human herpesviruses could contribute to human carcinogenesis.[12] Greater oncogenic potential can be demonstrated for the human gammaherpesvirinae Epstein–Barr virus (EBV)[13] and human herpesvirus (HHV)-8.[14] EBV-infected human lymphocytes can be transformed into lymphoblast cell lines. All cells that carry the EBV genome express virus-specific nuclear antigens (EBNAs), regardless of whether mature virus is released. There are also clear epidemiologic links to several types of tumor: Burkitt's lymphoma, infectious mononucleosis that progresses to fatal B-cell lymphoma in boys with an X-linked immunodeficiency, nasopharyngeal carcinoma and

post-transplant lymphoproliferative disease in immunosuppressed solid-organ transplant recipients.[13] HHV-8 similarly has strong epidemiologic links to Kaposi's sarcoma (KS) and primary effusion lymphoma. HHV-8 DNA is found in all forms of KS and infection rates are high in groups in which KS is frequent and low in groups in which KS is rare.[14]

The ubiquitous nature of herpesvirus infections and their establishment of lifelong infections make it difficult to interpret their association with tumor cells. Because of the relatively low efficiencies of transformation *in vitro* it seems likely that herpesvirus infection represents only one part of a complex sequence of events (perhaps involving a genetic predisposition and/or environmental co-factors) that ultimately leads to neoplasia.

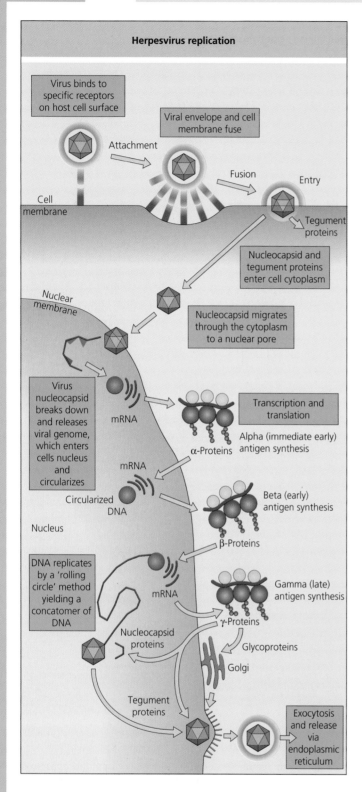

Herpesvirus replication

Virus binds to specific receptors on host cell surface

Attachment

Viral envelope and cell membrane fuse

Fusion

Entry

Cell membrane

Tegument proteins

Nucleocapsid and tegument proteins enter cell cytoplasm

Nuclear membrane

Nucleocapsid migrates through the cytoplasm to a nuclear pore

Virus nucleocapsid breaks down and releases viral genome, which enters cells nucleus and circularizes

mRNA

Transcription and translation

α-Proteins

Alpha (immediate early) antigen synthesis

mRNA

Circularized DNA

Nucleus

Beta (early) antigen synthesis

β-Proteins

DNA replicates by a 'rolling circle' method yielding a concatomer of DNA

mRNA

Gamma (late) antigen synthesis

γ-Proteins

Nucleocapsid proteins

Glycoproteins

Golgi

Tegument proteins

Exocytosis and release via endoplasmic reticulum

Fig. 155.4 Herpesvirus replication. The tegument proteins effect the shut-down of host cell metabolism. On entry to the nucleus the DNA circularizes and binds a tegument protein and cellular factors to initiate transcription. Transcription and translation occur in three phases: immediate-early, early and late. Capsid proteins migrate into the nucleus and the viral DNA is encapsidated. The viral glycoproteins are extensively modified post-translationally by transit through the Golgi apparatus. The glycoproteins diffuse to the nuclear envelope. The nucleocapsids are enveloped at the inner nuclear membrane and are either transported within vesicles that fuse with the plasma membrane to release the enveloped capsids into the extracellular milieu, or undergo de-envelopment at the outer nuclear membrane and re-envelopment at cytoplasmic membranes. Alternatively, nuclear pores become enlarged sufficiently to allow egress of naked capsids and the capsids then become enveloped at cytoplasmic membranes.

and moist mucosal layers. Two broad groupings of virus can be distinguished:

- those where virus is transmitted most effectively by oral secretions and nongenital contact – HSV-1, varicella-zoster virus (VZV), EBV, CMV, HHV-6 and HHV-7; and
- those where the virus is transmitted most effectively by genital secretions – HSV-2 and Kaposi's sarcoma-associated herpesvirus (HHV-8).

These modes of transmission have a profound influence upon the epidemiology of the individual viruses.

Prevalence

Herpesviruses transmitted predominantly by oral secretions or nongenital contact have a peak incidence of infection in early childhood (Table 155.5). The peak incidence for infections acquired by genital transmission is in adolescence and early adulthood. The rates of infection by viruses transmitted by the genital route are not usually as high as those for viruses transmitted by a nongenital route. However, for both groups there is a further distinct relation between rates of acquisition, sexual preference and the socioeconomic status of the study population (i.e. low socioeconomic status equates with high seroprevalence).

Geographic aspects

Herpesviruses are distributed worldwide and no animal reservoirs of infection are known for any of the human herpesviruses. There is evidence that in tropical areas varicella is less prevalent in childhood than in temperate climatic areas and is more common in adults.[15] Possible explanations for this include the relative isolation of clusters of population in rural areas, epidemiologic 'interference' through infections caused by other viruses, and perhaps decreased efficiency of transmission as a result of the lability of VZV in areas where there is a high ambient temperature. Other complications of herpesvirus infection such as Burkitt's lymphoma, which is associated with EBV infection, are endemic only in tropical Africa.[13] Nasopharyngeal carcinoma is also associated with EBV infection and is endemic in Japan and Southern China.[16] A sporadic, non-HIV-associated Kaposi's sarcoma is found predominantly in countries bordering the Mediterranean and in Central Africa.[14]

Periodicity

The human herpesviruses are endemic in human populations as a result of their strategy of establishing latent infections. In addition, because of their modes of transmission there is no seasonal variation in the efficiency of transmission. For infections for which

EPIDEMIOLOGY

Transmission pathways

Herpesviruses are relatively fragile in that they require a lipid envelope to achieve attachment to, and penetration of, the host cell. As a consequence these viruses transmit most easily on contact of warm

Table 155.4 Principal sites of latency for herpesviruses

Virus	Established (most probable) sites of latency	Other possible sites of latency
HSV-1	Neurons (trigeminal ganglia)	Other sensory nerve ganglia, brain, eye
HSV-2	Neurons (sacral ganglia)	Other sensory ganglia
VZV	Neurons (dorsal, thoracic and trigeminal ganglia)	Brain, other sensory ganglia
EBV	B cells (epithelial cells of nasopharynx and submandibular salivary glands)	–
CMV	Monocytes, lymphocytes, epithelial cells	Salivary glands, renal tubule cells
HHV-6, HHV-7	T cells	Bone marrow progenitors, monocytic/macrophage cells
HHV-8	Not firmly established	B cells

Table 155.5 Features of herpesvirus infections

Virus	PEAK INCIDENCE OF PRIMARY INFECTION		Adult seroprevalence (%)	Principal route(s) of transmission	Notes
	Childhood	Adolescence			
HSV-1	+++	+	75–95+	Oral secretions, close contact	Overall seroprevalence predominantly determined by socioeconomic status
HSV-2	–	+++	4–95	Genital secretions, close contact	Lifetime number of sex partners is predominant influence on rates of seropositivity
VZV	+++	+	90–95	Aerosol, close contact	Epidemic spread in childhood, in tropics relatively more common in adults than children
CMV	++	++	40–95+	Oral secretions, genital secretions	Infection common in infancy, but a significant proportion of women of childbearing age are susceptible; overall seroprevalence predominantly determined by socioeconomic status
EBV	++	++	70–95	Oral secretions	Second peak of incidence in early adolescence (glandular fever)
HHV-6	+++	–	>85	Oral secretions	Infection common in infancy – peak age of acquisition 2 years
HHV-7	+++	–	>85	Oral secretions	Infection common in infancy – peak age of acquisition 3 years
HHV-8	–	+++	10–25	Oral secretions, genital secretions	Homosexual men who have AIDS have highest seroprevalence

CMV, cytomegalovirus; EBV, Epstein–Barr virus; HHV, human herpesvirus; HSV, herpes simplex virus; VZV, varicella-zoster virus.

reactivation is infrequent (e.g. VZV infection) there may be 'outbreaks' of infection (mini-epidemics) when infection spreads rapidly through a nonimmune population. Outbreaks can also occur if large numbers of susceptible individuals are brought together (e.g. infectious mononucleosis among military recruits or college students).[17]

Determinants of infection

Early acquisition of infection is common for all herpesviruses transmitted by the nongenital route (see Table 155.5). In a classic study of HSV infection, Burnet & Williams[18] showed that there was a clear relationship between the age of acquisition of the virus and socioeconomic status. Populations associated with a low socioeconomic environment collectively showed earlier acquisition of HSV infection than more affluent populations, although in both groups, infection rates of 90–95% were observed by early adulthood. Primary HSV-1 infection was rare in those over 30 years of age. In recent years several seroepidemiologic studies have shown a general decrease in the overall prevalence of HSV-1 antibody in developed countries.[19,20] However, even within individual countries there are variations in seroprevalence; for example, the seroprevalence rates are generally higher among inner city residents than among those from rural areas. Here, the major factor determining the seroprevalence is the frequency of direct person-to-person contact rather than the socioeconomic status of the individual populations.

If infection does not occur in infancy, transmission routes other than direct oral contact can constitute important risk factors. An example is found in the acquisition of CMV. Although most CMV infections occur in infancy a significant proportion (40–50% in developed countries) of women of child-bearing age are still susceptible to infection and may acquire the infection during pregnancy. Sexual transmission of infection then becomes an important mode of acquisition of infection for these women. In addition, contact with young children of less than 24 months of age is a further important risk factor.

Viruses such as HSV-2, for which the principal mode of transmission is sexual, are generally not acquired until the onset of sexual activity in adolescence and early adulthood. HSV-2 prevalence, overall and by age, varies markedly by country, region within country, population subgroup and in populations with higher risk sexual behavior.[21]

The seroprevalence of HHV-8 infection is low (<5%) in most northern, western and central European countries except for parts of Italy, Greece and to a lesser extent Spain. It is also low in the USA (0–5%). In many African countries, particularly sub-Saharan Africa, rates of 40–60% are found in adults and adolescents. In accordance with the high rates of Kaposi's sarcoma seen in HIV-infected homosexual and bisexual men, HHV-8 antibodies are more common in these groups than in the general population of the same country.

PATHOGENICITY

Molecular and cellular basis of pathogenicity

The combination of virion surface glycoproteins and the distribution of cellular receptors provide a partial explanation of the cell- and tissue-specific tropism of members of the human herpesviruses. After primary infection, herpesviruses persist in their host by a combination of lytic infectious processes (cellular persistence) and latent infections in other sites or tissues. Latent infections are characterized by restriction of viral gene expression to those required for maintenance of the latent infection and by the absence of expression of genes required for lytic infection (e.g. DNA replication and production of structural proteins). In response to various stimuli, latent virus can be reactivated to a lytic state. Virus produced during the reactivated lytic state can cause disease and provide a source of virus for transmission to susceptible individuals. In individuals who have deficits in cell-mediated immunity (CMI), infection is more poorly controlled than in those who have intact CMI. Primary infection is in consequence more severe, and reactivation of latent infection is more likely to result in asymptomatic disease.

Herpes simplex virus

In vitro, HSV can infect most types of human cells and even cells of other species, but *in vivo* it is host specific. It causes lytic infection of fibroblasts and epithelial cells, and establishes latent infection in neurons. The two biotypes of HSV, HSV-1 and HSV-2, show some predilection for infecting defined anatomic sites – oropharyngeal and genital, respectively. Both viruses are capable of infecting and producing latent infection at either site, but HSV-2 reactivation 'above the waist' and HSV-1 reactivation 'below the waist' are infrequent compared with HSV-1 reactivation 'above the waist' and HSV-2 reactivation 'below the waist', respectively.[22]

Varicella-zoster virus

Primary VZV infection begins in the mucosa of the respiratory tract and progresses via the blood and lymphatic system to cells of the reticuloendothelial system. A secondary viremia at 11–13 days disseminates virus to the skin where the characteristic vesicular lesions of 'chickenpox' are produced. The virus establishes latent infection in the cranial, dorsal root and autonomic nervous system ganglia during this viremic phase. The molecular basis of latency and reactivation is poorly understood. In contrast to studies in neurons latently infected with HSV-1 (where only the LAT transcript is found) neurons latently infected with VZV have four transcripts corresponding to VZV genes 21, 29, 62 and 63.[23]

Epstein–Barr virus

During primary infection EBV establishes a productive infection in the epithelial cells of the oropharynx. Virus is shed in the saliva and gains access to B cells in lymphatic tissue and the blood.[13] A lytic infection leads to the production of infectious virus with EBV proteins, including the early antigens, viral capsid antigen and the glycoproteins of the membrane antigen being produced by the infected cell (Fig. 155.5). Epstein–Barr virus is a B-cell mitogen, stimulating the growth and immortalization of B cells by preventing apoptosis. In EBV-immortalized cells the genome is maintained as a circular episome which is replicated by cellular DNA polymerase and is equally distributed to daughter cells when EBV-infected cells divide. The resting cell contains nine latent proteins and several noncoding

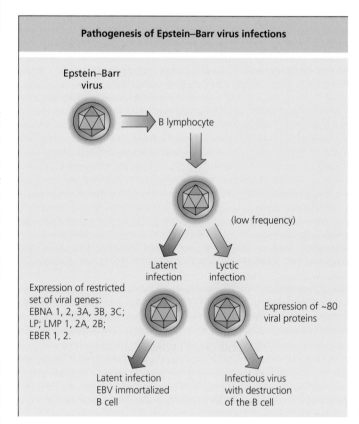

Fig. 155.5 Pathogenesis of Epstein–Barr virus (EBV) infections. Infection may result in lytic infection of the cell or cell immortalization, which can be distinguished by the production of virus and the expression of different viral proteins and antigens. T cells limit the outgrowth of EBV-infected cells. EBER, Epstein–Barr encoded small RNA; EBNA, Epstein–Barr nuclear antigen; LMP, latent membrane protein; LP, EBNA leader protein.

RNAs that are under the master control of EBNA2. These co-operate to drive the cell to resemble an antigen-activated lymphoblast. EBV-transformed proliferating lymphocytes are constantly held in check by the immune response.[8] By promoting cell growth and preventing apoptosis, the latency program of EBV is believed to assume the prime role in oncogenesis. By contrast the lytic program is not thought to be involved in oncogenesis because cells that enter a lytic program invariably die.

Cytomegalovirus

Cytomegalovirus is capable of producing lytic, productive, infection of epithelial, endothelial, smooth muscle, stromal, fibroblast and neuronal cells *in vivo*. However, viral latency only appears to occur in a restricted subpopulation of cells.[24] Hematopoietic cell precursors (CD34[+]) are a common precursor of both lymphoid and myeloid cells. Cells of the monocyte/myeloid lineage have been shown to become latently infected by as yet undefined mechanisms.[25] In the latently infected cell there is absence of lytic gene transcription although transcripts of the major immediate early gene (IE) region of the CMV genome can be detected. The major IE transcripts IE72 and IE86 are not, however, expressed in latently infected cells. Between two and 10 copies of the CMV genome are carried in an episomal form in mononuclear cells of healthy seropositive individuals. It is presently unknown how the viral genome is maintained in dividing progenitor cells.

Human herpesviruses 6 and 7

Human herpesvirus 6 was originally isolated from T-cell cultures derived from the blood of patients who had AIDS[26] and HHV-7 was isolated from the CD4[+] T cells of a healthy individual. Both viruses infect and kill CD4[+] T cells, just like HIV, yet the outcome of infection is markedly different. In contrast to HIV infection, infection by HHV-6 or HHV-7 is rapidly controlled by the host immune response, and the virus establishes a state of latency. HHV-6 and HHV-7 establish chronic persistent infection with low-level replication in salivary, submandibular and parotid glands. Candidate sites for true latency are found in monocytes and early bone marrow progenitor cells. In HHV-6, the product of gene U94 has been shown to enable establishment and/or maintenance of latent infection in these cells.[27]

HHV-6 exists as two closely related variants: HHV-6A and HHV-6B. Although closely related, consistent differences have been observed in their biologic, immunologic, epidemiologic and molecular properties. HHV-6B is the primary etiologic agent of exanthema subitum, whereas no single disease has been definitively associated with HHV-6A. HHV-7 is responsible for a subset of exanthema subitum and other exanthema cases but like HHV-6A also remains an 'orphan' virus with no firm disease association.[28]

Human herpesvirus 8

Using representational difference analysis[29] HHV-8 was initially identified in 90% of AIDS-related Kaposi's sarcoma (KS) lesions and in 15% of non-KS tissues from people who had HIV infection. Following these observations HHV-8 sequences were identified using polymerase chain reaction (PCR) in all forms of KS, including KS from different geographic locations in individuals who had and did not have HIV infection.[14] Most KS spindle cells can be shown to be latently infected; only a small proportion (1–3%) show lytic, replicative, markers. Although HHV-8 can infect many cell types *in vitro* it is only infection of primary epithelial cell cultures that results in changes in morphology and growth. Once latency is established in these cells, dramatic elongation occurs to produce spindle-like cells. The changes can be traced to changes in the organization of the actin cytoskeleton and are related to the expression of a single viral gene – V-FLIP.[14] The modifications are not, however, related to cell immortalization and this marks a clear difference between the latency program of HHV-8 and that of

EBV. A series of six proteins are known to be expressed in the latently infected KS cell; latency associated antigen (LANA), v-cyclin, v-FLIP and kaposin proteins A, B and C.

PREVENTION

In a well-controlled environment, such as that of a hospital, prevention of host-to-host transmission for most human herpesviruses is achieved by simple hygiene. In the home or other social situations prevention of transmission by avoiding contact with a person who has evidence of recurrent infection is only partially effective. This is because infectious virus is often excreted before the appearance of overt symptoms of recurrent infection and 'silent' recurrent infections also occur.

Herpesviruses are readily inactivated by a variety of physical and chemical agents (see Physical properties, above) and standard methods of sterilization, including autoclaving, dry heat, ultraviolet or gamma irradiation, and ethylene oxide sterilization are adequate for decontaminating medical equipment. Most common disinfectants (5% phenol, formaldehyde, glutaraldehyde, 1:10 000 quaternary ammonium compounds and 0.3 ppm hypochlorites) rapidly inactivate virus. Other virucidal compounds include detergents, chlorhexidine, Merthiolate, sodium azide, β-propiolactone, ethylene oxide and some proteolytic enzymes. Ultraviolet and X-ray or gamma irradiation also inactivate herpesviruses.

Active immunization

Except for VZV infection (for which a live attenuated vaccine is available) there are currently no licensed vaccines available to prevent herpesvirus infections. Varicella-zoster virus infection causes particular problems in immunosuppressed children. Primary infection in immunosuppressed patients can result in a fulminant, generalized infection or severe respiratory disease. A live attenuated VZV vaccine has been licensed for use and is administered using the same schedule as the measles, mumps and rubella vaccine. The vaccine has an excellent safety record and although breakthrough infections can occur, they usually result in mild illness. In the USA the vaccine is recommended for use for all children over 12 months of age and susceptible healthy adolescents and adults. In most other countries vaccination is only recommended for patients who are immunosuppressed or immunodeficient and who have never had chickenpox. A single dose is 80–85% effective in preventing disease of any severity and >95% effective in preventing severe varicella.[30]

Studies of the Oka-derived strain of VZV vaccines showed that these can elicit a significant increase in VZV cell-mediated immunity (CMI) in immunocompetent older adults. This led to a study of immunization of older adults with live attenuated Oka VZV vaccine (at 14 times the minimum potency of the standard vaccine) to boost their waning VZV CMI. The vaccine significantly reduced the morbidity of herpes zoster (by 61.1%) and the incidence of postherpetic neuralgia, the most common debilitating complication of herpes zoster, by 66.5%.[31]

Research on the production of effective vaccines against HSV has been actively pursued since the 1920s. A very wide range of vaccines have been explored. Two HSV-2 glycoprotein adjuvant vaccines (gB2 + gD2 and gD2) have reached phase III clinical evaluation. The overall protection rates were not significant. A gD2 vaccine formulated with an adjuvant alum and 3-deacetylated monophosphoryl lipid A showed a 73–74% protection from disease – but not infection – in women seronegative to HSV-1 and HSV-2. Gender differences and preexisting HSV-1 serologic status influence vaccine efficacy in these trials.[32]

For CMV a candidate vaccine was developed by Plotkin in the 1970s.[33] The vaccine was prepared using an isolate from a congenitally infected child (the Towne strain) after serial passage in human embryonic fibroblasts. In early studies seroconversion was seen in nearly 100% of volunteers, as well as a protective effect against a low-dose challenge with CMV. However, the vaccine failed to prevent infection of mothers in contact with CMV-excreting children, and therefore failed its primary objective: the prevention of primary infection in pregnancy. Later efforts have focused on the development of recombinant subunits, dense bodies (enveloped, replication-defective particles), peptide-based vaccines and DNA vaccines, so far with little success.[34]

Attempts to develop a prophylactic EBV vaccine have focused on the gp350 and EBNA3 antigens. Immunization with gp350 antigen has been shown to prevent infectious mononucleosis but not EBV infection in seronegative young adults.[35] Synthetic peptides based on the EBNA3 latent antigen have been the subject of small scale clinical trials. The latent antigen epitopes restricted through common MHC class I alleles can induce CD8+ T-cell responses in the vaccinee. The value of this approach has been underscored by studies which show that autologous CD8+ cells against EBNA3 propagated *in vivo* and then given to immunosuppressed patients at risk of post-transplant lymphoproliferative disease (PTLD), can prevent PTLD and in some cases cause regression of PTLD.[36]

Passive immunization

Varicella-zoster virus hyperimmune globulin (VZVIG) is an effective prophylaxis for babies born to mothers who develop varicella (but not herpes zoster) in the period 7 days before to 7 days after delivery.[37] VZVIG is also recommended for VZ antibody-negative infants exposed to chickenpox or herpes zoster (other than in the mother) in the first 7 days of life and VZ antibody-negative infants of any age exposed to chickenpox or herpes zoster while still requiring intensive or prolonged special care nursing. It is also given to VZ antibody-negative pregnant women exposed at any stage of pregnancy, providing VZVIG can be given within 10 days of contact. The rationale for the use of VZVIG prophylaxis in this situation is twofold: reduction in severity of maternal disease and reduction of risk of fetal infection for women contracting varicella in the first 20 weeks of pregnancy. The risk of fatal varicella is estimated to be about five times higher in pregnant than nonpregnant adults with fatal cases concentrated late in the second or early in the third trimester. Prophylactic use of VZVIG is also appropriate to control infection in pediatric units caring for immunocompromised children.

Adoptive immunotherapy

Infectious complications of human herpesvirus infection are common in immunocompromised individuals. Particular problems are found in recipients of hematopoietic stem cell transplants (HSCT) and in solid-organ transplant recipients (SOT) where conditioning regimens can ablate the recipient's immune system. In HSCT the recipient's immune system can recover after engraftment and expansion of the recipient immune system *in vivo*. In SOT the recipient's immune system never recovers its full potential because immunosuppression must be maintained life long. A process in which donor CD4+ and CD8+ cells are cultured *in vitro* in the presence of virus or peptides representing the virus and the stimulated cells are clonally expanded using mitogen stimulation, results in a population of cytotoxic T lymphocytes (CTLs). These may be infused into the recipient to provide virus-specific cytotoxicity that provides for prophylaxis and/or treatment of herpesvirus infection in the recipient. Successful procedures for CMV and EBV adoptive immunotherapy have been described and developments of the technique promise to accelerate the preparation of therapeutic solutions by direct selection of virus-specific CTLs from donor lymphocytes.[38]

Antiviral prophylaxis

A number of specific antiviral compounds are available for the treatment of herpesvirus infection (Table 155.6) and prophylactic use of antiviral chemotherapy to control infection is well established.

Most antiherpetic drugs are nucleoside analogues that inhibit virus-specified DNA polymerases and terminate DNA chain elongation. The first generation of these drugs – idoxuridine, vidarabine and trifluridine – had only a limited selectivity for the viral DNA polymerase due to the interaction of the phosphorylated form of these drugs with cellular DNA polymerases. The use of these compounds was associated with severe adverse effects.

Aciclovir is the prototype of the present generation of antiviral drugs (see Chapter 146). Its high specificity and therefore safety is based on its specific interaction with viral and not cellular enzymes. It is an acyclic analogue of guanosine that is activated by the viral and not the cellular thymidine kinase to serve as substrate for the viral DNA polymerase. Aciclovir is a safe, relatively nontoxic drug and is effective for therapeutic use as well as long-term suppressive treatment.

The oral bioavailability of aciclovir is relatively low and for this reason a prodrug – the L-valyl ester of aciclovir, valaciclovir – was developed. Valaciclovir hydrochloride is rapidly absorbed from the gastrointestinal tract and rapidly and almost completely converted to aciclovir and L-valine by first-pass intestinal and/or hepatic metabolism. The mode of action, safety profile and clinical spectrum of activity of valaciclovir are believed to be identical to that of aciclovir.

Penciclovir is a further acyclic nucleoside analogue whose mode of action and safety profile is essentially identical to that of aciclovir. The drugs differ in their rate of cellular uptake, phosphorylation rate, stability of the intracellular triphosphate and inhibitory concentration for HSV DNA polymerase (100-fold higher for penciclovir triphosphate than for aciclovir triphosphate). The intracellular half-life of the active antiviral (penciclovir triphosphate) is substantially longer (7–20 hours) than that of aciclovir triphosphate (0.7–1 hour) which compensates for the slightly lower activity of the drug.

Table 155.6 Currently used antiherpesvirus drugs

Antiviral drug	Chemical class	Mechanisms of action	Target virus
Aciclovir	Guanosine analogue	Virus-activated DNA polymerase inhibitor	HSV-1, HSV-2, VZV
Valaciclovir	Guanosine analogue	Virus-activated DNA polymerase inhibitor	HSV-1, HSV-2, VZV
Penciclovir	Guanosine analogue	Virus-activated DNA polymerase inhibitor	HSV-1, HSV-2, VZV
Famciclovir	Guanosine analogue	Virus-activated DNA polymerase inhibitor	HSV-1, HSV-2, VZV
Cidofovir	Cytidylic acid analogue	DNA polymerase inhibitor	CMV, HSV-1, HSV-2
Foscarnet	Pyrophosphate analogue	DNA polymerase inhibitor	CMV, HSV-1, HSV-2
Ganciclovir	Guanosine analogue	Virus-activated DNA polymerase inhibitor	CMV (HSV-1, HSV-2)
Maribavir*	Benzimidazole riboside	Inhibits UL 97 kinase	CMV, EBV

CMV, cytomegalovirus; EBV, Epstein–Barr virus; HSV, herpes simplex virus; VZV, varicella-zoster virus.
*Scheduled to become available in 2009.

Famciclovir is the diacetyl 6-deoxy prodrug of penciclovir. Famciclovir achieves high levels of systemic bioavailability following oral administration. Following administration the drug is deacetylated and oxidized to form penciclovir. The mode of action and clinical spectrum of activity is thus identical to that of penciclovir.

The alternate antiherpetic drugs, ganciclovir (and its prodrug valganciclovir), foscarnet and cidofovir have similar mechanisms of action (i.e. inhibition of the viral DNA polymerase), but generally have a higher toxicity profile, including neutropenia and thrombocytopenia for ganciclovir, and nephrotoxicity for foscarnet and cidofovir. The newest antiviral maribavir[39] directly inhibits UL97 kinase, an early gene involved in viral DNA elongation, DNA packaging and egress of viral capsids from the cell nucleus. Maribavir does not cause nephrotoxicity or hematologic toxicity and has activity against ganciclovir-resistant CMV. The susceptibility of different herpesviruses to the various antiviral drugs is shown in Table 155.7.

Antiviral resistance has been described for all of the antiherpes compounds mentioned, particularly when antivirals are administered to immunocompromised patients over extended periods of time. Studies in these patients have shown resistance to aciclovir in 5% and to ganciclovir in 7% of patients. Antiviral resistance is due to mutations in the viral thymidine kinase or in the DNA polymerase. Resistant viruses, however, appear to be less virulent. Significant circulation in the general population has not yet been found. Because of their similar mechanisms of action, cross-resistance frequently occurs (e.g. between aciclovir, famciclovir and valaciclovir).

The nucleoside analogues are virostatic and it is thus of crucial importance that therapy is initiated very early in infection, even before laboratory confirmation of the clinical diagnosis (Table 155.8). Antiviral drug therapy is probably only effective when the disease is due to a viral rather than an immunopathologic process.

Table 155.7 Comparative susceptibility of herpesviruses to antiviral drugs

Antiviral drug	Viral susceptibility					Main target agents*
	HSV-1	**HSV-2**	**VZV**	**CMV**	**EBV**	
Aciclovir, valaciclovir	+++	+++	++	–	+	HSV-1, HSV-2, VZV
Penciclovir, famciclovir	+++	+++	++	–	+	HSV-1, HSV-2, VZV
Cidofovir	+	+	++	+++	+	CMV, resistant HSV
Foscarnet	++	++	+	++	+	CMV, resistant HSV, VZV, CMV
Ganciclovir, valganciclovir	+	+	+	+++	+	CMV
Maribavir	–	–	–	+++	+++	CMV, resistant CMV

CMV, cytomegalovirus; EBV, Epstein–Barr virus; HSV, herpes simplex virus; VZV, varicella-zoster virus.
*Ganciclovir and foscarnet have *in-vitro* activity against HHV-6 and HHV-8 and have been used on a compassionate basis in severe disease associated with these agents.

Table 155.8 Indications for antiherpesvirus drug treatment

Antiviral drug	Target virus	Infections	Possible side-effects
Aciclovir, valaciclovir, famciclovir	HSV-1,2	Severe and/or frequent mucocutaneous HSV infection, including genital herpes; herpes encephalitis, herpes keratitis	Headache, nausea, diarrhea
	VZV	Severe cases of varicella, varicella in patients at risk for complications (immunocompromised, adolescents, adults) Severe cases of herpes zoster, including those at risk of developing postherpetic neuralgia, herpes zoster ophthalmicus, oticus	Headache, nausea, diarrhea
Cidofovir	CMV	CMV retinitis	Severe nephrotoxicity
Foscarnet	CMV, HSV-1, HSV-2, VZV; severe disease due to aciclovir-, valaciclovir- and famciclovir-resistant HSV or VZV strains	Severe CMV disease refractory to ganciclovir treatment	Nephrotoxicity, crystalluria
Ganciclovir	CMV	Severe CMV disease in immunocompromised host (e.g. retinitis, esophagitis, colitis, pneumonia, encephalitis)	Neutropenia, thrombocytopenia

CMV, cytomegalovirus; HSV, herpes simplex virus; VZV, varicella-zoster virus.

EBV and HHV-6 have shown *in-vitro* susceptibility to various antiherpesvirus drugs such as aciclovir, ganciclovir and cidofovir. However, apart from aciclovir treatment of oral hairy leukoplakia in patients who have AIDS, no significant clinical benefit has so far been demonstrated. Anecdotal use of ganciclovir or foscarnet for HHV-6, HHV-7 and HHV-8 infections has been reported. However, so far no data from well-designed clinical studies have been reported to show the effectiveness of these drugs in the treatment of these infections.

DIAGNOSTIC VIROLOGY

A key feature of the herpesviruses is their close adaption to their host. In general, primary infection is usually asymptomatic or is accompanied by nonspecific mild signs and symptoms. Consequently, most primary infections and many recurrent infections are not recognized as herpesvirus infections. Where symptoms are observed, speed in using diagnostic procedures is important because the peak of virus replication and shedding is likely to precede the appearance of symptoms. The diagnostic method chosen (Table 155.9) varies for different herpesviruses and also depends upon the type of infection (whether primary or recurrent), duration of symptoms and clinical manifestations.

Test specimens

If there are visible lesions (HSV-1, HSV-2, VZV) the base of the lesion may be sampled with a dry cotton-tipped swab, which should be placed in virus transport medium and transported to the virus laboratory as quickly as possible. If there are vesicles, vesicle fluid can be aspirated using a fine (intradermal) needle. The fluid should then be transported directly to the laboratory for virus detection by PCR testing, electron microscopy, direct immunofluorescent antibody staining or culture.

Viruria and viremia are common during both primary infection and recurrent infection with CMV, EBV, HHV-6, HHV-7 and HHV-8. Urine collected in urine transport medium is a useful specimen for detection of CMV. Blood collected in anticoagulant (EDTA) can be used in direct detection of virus. In neurologic disease, cerebrospinal fluid (CSF) and a clotted peripheral blood specimen (for CSF and blood serology) are essential. Clotted blood specimens should be collected during the acute stages of illness and again after 10–14 days.

Virus culture

While the use of virus culture has declined in many diagnostic virus laboratories it remains an essential tool in reference laboratories when live virus is required for detailed analysis. The fragility of the viral envelope presents a problem if virus is to be cultured. Collection of specimens into appropriate viral transport medium and rapid transportation of specimens to the diagnostic laboratory is essential for successful isolation in cell culture systems. Virus culture is only usually attempted for HSV-1, HSV-2, VZV and CMV.

Electron microscopy

Transmission electron microscopic examination of negatively stained vesicle fluid presents one of the most rapid methods for detection of VZV or HSV. Although now only available in few diagnostic laboratories, this procedure can be very helpful in establishing a rapid, early diagnosis. Collection of specimens for electron microscopy is a skilled procedure and several methods are available.[40] The technique is relatively insensitive and a specimen must contain at least 10^6 or more particles per milliliter to allow detection of virus.

Antigen detection

Antigen detection has a limited but important role to play in the diagnosis of most herpesvirus infections. In general, specimens may contain too little virus to allow reliable detection of antigen. Nevertheless, in a case of vesicular eruption, vesicle fluid (air dried and fixed in cold acetone) can be stained with monoclonal antibodies tagged with fluorescein isothiocyanate to provide a rapid specific diagnosis of infection. A variety of rapid immunoassay tests have also been developed

Table 155.9 Laboratory diagnosis of herpesvirus infections

Virus	Disease manifestation	Virus culture	Serology	Antigen detection	DNA amplification
HSV-1	Skin lesions	++	+	+	+++
	CNS infection	–	++	–	+++
HSV-2	Genital lesions	++	+	+	+++
	CNS infection	–	+	–	+++
VZV	Skin lesions	+	++	++	+++
	CNS infection	–	+	–	+++
CMV	Mononucleosis-like illness	–	+++	–	–
	Neonatal disease	++	++	–	+++
	Systemic infection in immunocompromised	+	+	++	+++
	CNS disease	–	+	–	+++
EBV	Mononucleosis-like illness	–	+++	–	–
	Systemic infection in immunocompromised	–	+	+	+++
	CNS disease	–	+	–	+++
HHV-6	Exanthema subitum	+	+++	–	–
	CNS disease	–	++	–	+++
HHV-8	Kaposi's sarcoma	–	+	–	+++

CMV, cytomegalovirus; EBV, Epstein–Barr virus; HHV, human herpesvirus; HSV, herpes simplex virus; VZV, varicella–zoster virus.

for 'within the office' testing for HSV. However, the sensitivity and specificity of these tests are too low to allow their use in diagnosis for hospitalized patients. As with virus cultures, these approaches are now being replaced by rapid molecular diagnostic techniques.

Nucleic acid amplification

A number of alternative nucleic acid amplification or signal amplification techniques have been applied to the diagnosis of herpesvirus infections but it is nucleic acid amplification, in particular PCR, that is most widely applied. A wide variety of PCR techniques have been used, including single, semi-nested and nested, with product detection via gel electrophoresis, Southern blotting, ELISA-like hybridization, microarray or bead-based arrays such as the 'Luminex' procedure. 'Real-time' PCR is now the most commonly used procedure; this offers testing of high sensitivity, reduced risk of intralaboratory cross-contamination of samples from amplicon release and reduces test turnaround times by combining the detection of amplification within the thermal amplification process. The test allows direct detection of the products of amplification in 'real time', is quantitative, and can allow, for example, typing of HSV-1 and HSV-2 within the same test. Multitarget or 'multiplex' PCR procedures are also available in both real-time and conventional PCR formats. Careful optimization of these test procedures is necessary to ensure that the sensitivity of detection of each of the individual target viruses within the test is maintained when targets are combined.

Many types of clinical sample contain substances that prove inhibitory to the polymerase chain reaction which, if not efficiently removed, will result in the production of false-negative test results. The use of internal control molecules within PCR tests is used to monitor for test failure through test sample inhibition. Where internal molecules are not available the same check may be performed by 'spiking' a sample with a known amount of virus or by checking for an alternate human gene always expected to be present within a clinical sample.

Nucleic acid amplification techniques are now considered obligatory for the diagnosis of herpesvirus infections, particularly for example in HSV infection of the CNS[41] or in the diagnosis of the acute retinal necrosis syndrome.[42] Determination of the viral load in blood is an indispensable tool for the early detection, monitoring and medical management of CMV, EBV, HHV-6, and HHV-8 infections in HSTC and SOT patients.[43] Rigorous quality control and attention to detail is of course essential for routine application of any PCR technique, but in the latter application of quantitative PCR, standardization of variables through parallel comparative and proficiency testing, development of standards and of uniform units for expressing results, have all become essential to allow clinical correlation with the results of these molecular assays.

Genotypic analyses

Sequencing of products of PCR is a useful method for the comparison of strains of virus detected. For example, sequencing of viruses obtained from different bodily sites or from different persons provides a more rapid method for epidemiologic and population diversity investigation[44] than the technically demanding restriction-fragment polymorphic analyses previously applied in such studies. The widespread use of ganciclovir (GCV) to treat CMV infections in immunosuppressed patients has led to the development of drug resistance. Phenotypic assays for CMV drug resistance are presently too time-consuming to be therapeutically useful and this has led to the development of genotypic assays for GCV resistance.[45] For other human herpesviruses the genomic mutations resulting in antiviral drug resistance have not all been identified. Phenotypic tests are easier to interpret and may detect resistance that genotypic analysis cannot yet discriminate. Maintenance of the capability of cell culture in diagnostic laboratories is thus important.

Virus serology

Complement fixation and indirect immunofluorescence tests are still used in many viral diagnostic laboratories. However, their use is declining in favor of more reproducible and sensitive enzyme-linked immunosorbent assay (ELISA) methodologies. Neutralizing antibody tests for herpesvirus antibodies are not routinely performed in diagnostic laboratories and none of these viruses has hemagglutinating capability.

Immunoassays are available for the detection of IgM or IgG antibodies to HHV-1 to HHV-8. As IgM antibody is the first antibody to be produced in response to infection it is by nature a broadly reactive antibody, and cross-reactions with other viral antigens and false-positive reactions may occur. IgM antibody is also produced during both acute (primary) infection and recurrent disease (although the amount produced is generally higher during primary infection). Quantitation of virus-specific IgG antibody in serial samples (10 or more days apart) often provides a more reliable diagnostic procedure. Determination of the avidity of IgG can provide valuable information when only a single, acute phase, sample of blood is available. IgG antibody avidity matures with time after onset of infection, thus detection of IgG antibody of low avidity provides evidence of recent (primary) infection; detection of high avidity IgG antibody allows differentiation of recurrent infection from primary infection.[46]

CLINICAL MANIFESTATIONS

With the exception of VZV, primary herpesvirus infections in the immunocompetent host are usually asymptomatic or are associated with a minor illness only, with no specific symptoms. As a consequence, primary herpesvirus infections may not be recognized. When symptoms do occur, herpesvirus infections in the immunocompetent host are normally self-limiting and require only symptomatic treatment. Antiviral therapy is available for a number of herpesviruses, but is usually only indicated for those patients who have more severe disease manifestations or when it is appropriate to minimize the likelihood of complications. Herpesvirus infections in the immunocompromised host are frequently severe and sometimes life threatening. Antiviral drug therapy is required for these patients to control the infection (see Table 155.7).

Herpes simplex viruses

Oropharyngeal infection

Primary oropharyngeal HSV-1 infection usually occurs in childhood and is often asymptomatic. In symptomatic infections acute gingivostomatitis is seen accompanied by fever and submandibular lymphadenopathy. The incubation period varies from 2 to 12 days (mean 4 days). The duration of clinical illness may extend from 2 to 3 weeks, with virus excretion from the oropharynx for an average of 7–10 days.

The severity and duration of clinical illness in recurrent infection is considerably less than in primary HSV infection. Recurrent orolabial lesions ('cold sores') are heralded by a prodrome of pain, burning, itching or tingling for several hours before the development of the characteristic vesicles. The vesicular stage persists for less than 48 hours and progresses to the ulcerative and crusting stage within 3–4 days. Pain resolves quickly during the same period, and healing is generally complete within 8–10 days. Systemic illness is usually absent in recurrent infection. Recurrence rates are highly variable and the precipitating factors involved are not well defined, but include the type of HSV (HSV-1 is more likely to recur than HSV-2), fever, stress, exposure to ultraviolet light and impaired CMI in the host.

Genital infections

Primary genital herpes usually occurs in adolescents and young adults. During the last decade 40% to more than 60% of isolates of HSV from first-episode genital herpes have been found to be due to HSV-1 in studies of populations with a high socioeconomic status from the UK, Scandinavia and the USA.[21] A similar change has not been observed in populations of low socioeconomic status.

Primary genital herpes is, in the majority of cases (50–70%), asymptomatic or so mild that the infection is not recognized. Where lesions are observed the disease is characterized by the appearance of vesicular lesions – in males usually on the glans penis, on the penile shaft or in the perianal region, and in women involving the vulva, vagina, cervix and perineum. Extragenital lesions (on the buttocks and thighs) occur in 10–20% of patients (see Chapter 58)

The recurrence rate of genital HSV-2 infections is 10 times higher than that of genital HSV-1 infections. The signs and symptoms of recurrent genital herpes are usually restricted to the genital region and are relatively mild and of shorter duration than for primary disease. As for primary disease, recurrent lesions in women are more often painful and of longer duration than in men (60–90% vs 30–70%, and mean 5.9 vs 3.9 days, respectively).

Other manifestations

A wide variety of other manifestations of infection are known (Fig. 155.6) including herpes simplex virus encephalitis, neonatal herpes and keratoconjunctivitis.[21] Patients compromised by immunosuppressive therapy (e.g. organ transplant recipients) or patients who have immunodeficiency are at risk of developing a severe primary infection and more severe and frequent recurrent disease. Disease severity is directly related to the degree of immunosuppression or immunodeficiency.

Varicella-zoster virus

Varicella (chickenpox) and herpes zoster (shingles) are due to infection with the same virus, VZV. Varicella is the usual manifestation of primary infection, herpes zoster the most usual manifestation of recurrent infection.

Varicella (see Chapter 8)

Varicella is a common childhood exanthematous disease, usually affecting children in their early school years. The incubation period is 14–15 days (range 10–20 days). The rash is characterized by maculopapular lesions that vesiculate in about 3–4 days before crusting and scab formation. Scabs may remain *in situ* for up to 3 weeks. The exanthem is centripetal rather than centrifugal, with most lesions being present on the trunk and proximal extremities. Secondary bacterial infection of the lesions as a result of scratching is the most frequent complication. Occasionally cerebellar ataxia, transverse myelitis or Reye's syndrome may complicate the infection. Primary VZV infection occurring in adolescence and adult life is often associated with more severe disease including visceral complications such as pneumonitis, encephalitis and hepatitis.

Primary VZV infection may have a more aggressive course in pregnant women. This frequently includes visceral complications, notably pneumonitis. The fetus is at risk of infection and there is a low risk of severe fetal abnormalities ranging from long-lasting rash, limb or dermatomal scarring, to severe neurologic damage.[47] Severe neonatal varicella may occur when maternal varicella presents within 5 days of delivery.

As for other herpesvirus infections, primary VZV infection of immunocompromised patients such as children undergoing cancer chemotherapy or corticosteroid treatment usually has a more severe protracted course with an increased rate of complications, particularly pneumonitis.

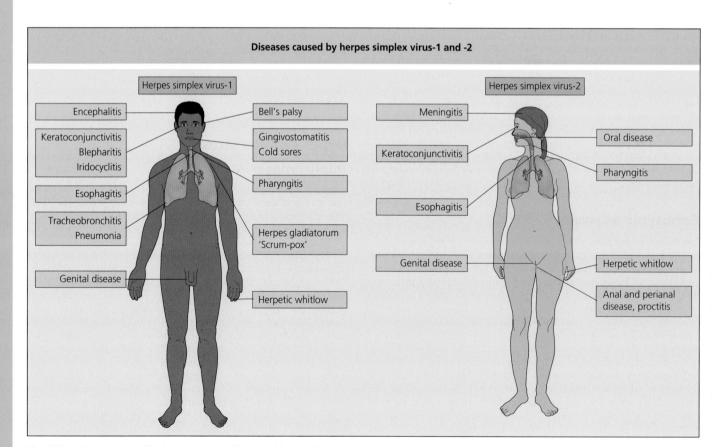

Fig. 155.6 Diseases caused by herpes simplex virus-1 and herpes simplex virus-2.

Herpes zoster

Herpes zoster is typically a disease of the elderly. Usually there is a prodrome of pain followed within a few days by the development of a unilateral vesicular rash within the dermatome served by the sensory nerve from the affected ganglion. The sites most commonly affected by herpes zoster are the dermatomes T3 through L3, often the same as those that were most affected during chickenpox. New lesions form over 2–5 days and the rash then pustulates and scabs over 2–3 weeks.

Complications including motor weakness and visceral manifestations may occur, but are unusual. However, in up to 50% of patients where herpes zoster involves the trigeminal nerve, ocular manifestations such as conjunctivitis, ulcerative keratitis, uveitis and iridocyclitis occur. Ocular complications are particularly common when the zosteriform lesions extend to the tip of the nose. Herpes zoster oticus, also called the Ramsay Hunt syndrome, consists of lesions on the ear or within the auditory canal, which are sometimes barely visible, and can result in hearing loss and facial paralysis. Persisting pain, known as postherpetic neuralgia, is the most common complication of herpes zoster. It can be severe and last for several months. The rate, severity and duration of postherpetic neuralgia are directly related to age. It is uncommon in patients under 50 years of age, but occurs in over 40% of those over 60 years of age.

Herpes zoster is frequently observed in patients who are immunocompromised. Chronic cutaneous lesions and disseminated infections have been described, particularly in patients who have HIV infection. Meningoencephalitis, pneumonitis or hepatitis can also occur in immunocompromised patients, but are rare.

Cytomegalovirus

CMV is an uncommon cause of disease in people who are immunocompetent. Primary infection may occasionally cause a glandular fever-type illness resembling EBV mononucleosis. In such patients persistent fever, myalgia and asthenia accompanied by atypical lymphocytosis and elevated liver transaminases are common signs and symptoms. Occasionally hepatitis is the presenting symptom. The presence of fever and atypical lymphocytes distinguishes CMV mononucleosis with liver involvement from infections by the usual hepatitis viruses.

Congenital and perinatal infections

CMV infections are the most common cause of congenital viral infections.[48] Both primary and recurrent infection in a pregnant woman can cause congenital and perinatal disease, but the frequency of severe disease is at least 10-fold higher after primary maternal infection. Overt clinical symptoms occur in 5–10% of cases of intrauterine CMV infection and include growth retardation, hepatosplenomegaly and thrombocytopenic purpura, and less frequently jaundice, microcephaly and chorioretinitis. The prognosis is poor for these infants. Another 10–15% of cases are neonates who are asymptomatic at birth and develop late sequelae, particularly mental retardation and sensorineural hearing loss.

Perinatal infections are nearly always asymptomatic, but neonates occasionally develop CMV pneumonitis, particularly when born prematurely. Severe disseminated disease may follow transfusion of CMV-infected blood products to premature neonates who have CMV-seronegative mothers.

Immunocompromised patients

The pathogenesis and clinical spectrum of CMV disease in patients who are immunocompromised depend upon the cause and degree of immunosuppression.[49] Treatment regimens must take into account the fact that the disease manifestations may have an immunopathologic or viral etiology.

Persistent intermittent fever is often the presenting symptom of CMV infection in patients who have had a transplant (see also Chapter 74). The infection may progress to cause pneumonitis, gastrointestinal disease, hepatitis and retinitis. In recipients of a solid-organ transplant, CMV disease most frequently occurs when the donor is CMV seropositive and the recipient is CMV seronegative. In bone marrow transplant patients, however, CMV disease most commonly results from reactivation of latent virus in the recipient, usually 20–90 days after the transplant. The most frequent manifestation is CMV pneumonitis. Unless treated very early, preferably before the appearance of respiratory symptoms, pneumonitis in these patients is often fatal.

Reactivation of latent CMV is usually the cause of CMV disease in patients who have HIV infection, frequently occurring in the later stages of the HIV infection when CD4+ T-cell counts are less than 50/ mm3. The most frequent manifestation is CMV retinitis presenting with blurred vision and decreased acuity (see Chapter 91).

Gastrointestinal disease, hepatitis, encephalitis and pneumonia also occur in patients who have HIV infection. Gastrointestinal disease includes esophagitis, gastritis, enteritis and colitis and is usually associated with fever and weight loss. Although CMV is often detected in respiratory specimens from patients with AIDS who have pneumonitis, the pulmonary process is usually caused by other pathogens, particularly *Pneumocystis jirovecii*.

Epstein–Barr virus

In most individuals EBV infection does not cause overt disease.[13] Primary infections in adolescents can, however, result in infectious mononucleosis. As for CMV infection, immunocompromised hosts may develop severe manifestations during both primary and recurrent EBV infection. Such severity is exemplified by the role of EBV infection in the causation of lymphoproliferative disease.

Immunocompetent host

Infectious mononucleosis (glandular fever) usually presents as fever, fatigue and malaise accompanied by a sore throat, cervical lymphadenopathy, hepatomegaly and splenomegaly. A rash may develop, particularly in those treated with ampicillin. Disease manifestations, especially fatigue and malaise, can persist for several weeks. Relapses and a chronic course have been described but the relationship to EBV infection is uncertain (see Chapter 70).

Immunocompromised host

Immunocompromised patients are at risk of developing lymphoproliferative disorders following EBV infection. The polyclonal B lymphocyte proliferation is often associated with fever, lymphadenopathy and hepatosplenomegaly and is frequently life threatening in severely immunocompromised patients, such as bone marrow transplant patients.

Patients who have AIDS may develop oral hairy leukoplakia, which is characterized by white plaques on the lateral margin of the tongue. EBV is associated with lymphocytic interstitial pneumonia (which is common in pediatric patients who have AIDS) and a rapidly progressing, diffuse encephalitis.

Human herpesvirus 6

HHV-6, variant B, is the cause of exanthema subitum (roseola infantum) in young children. Symptomatic infection is characterized by a high fever, often associated with inflammation of tympanic membranes and sometimes associated with a mild respiratory illness and lymphadenopathy. This is followed by the appearance of a fine maculopapular rash spreading from the trunk to the extremities. Only a small proportion of these (<10%) develop exanthema subitum.[27] Recovery is usually rapid and uneventful, although a more protracted and severe course characterized by severe meningoencephalitis, fulminant hepatitis or fatal pancytopenia has been described. In adolescents and adults primary HHV-6 infection can cause a mononucleosis-like illness.

In severely immunocompromised patients, such as those who have AIDS or who have received a bone marrow transplant, reactivation of HHV-6 infection has an immunosuppressive effect, subsequent to which other pathogens may cause severe disease. In bone marrow transplant patients HHV-6 reactivation is associated with bone marrow suppression, probably as the result of viral replication in particular progenitor cells.[27] HHV-6 has also been associated with interstitial pneumonia and encephalitis in these patients.

Human herpesvirus 7

Although some cases of exanthema subitum appear to be due to HHV-7, a causal association between human disease and HHV-7 infection has not yet been established. HHV-7 has been associated with infant febrile illness as well as subsequent CNS complications. In renal transplant patients evidence has been obtained that HHV-7 may be a co-factor in the development of CMV disease.

Human herpesvirus 8

No association has been recognized between primary HHV-8 infection and specific clinical disease, but it is now generally accepted that HHV-8 has a causal role in KS, primary effusion lymphoma and multicentric Castleman's disease.[14]

Herpes B virus

Macacine herpesvirus 1 (herpes B virus) causes a benign latent infection in macaques that is analogous to HSV infection in humans. The infection is infrequently transmitted to humans. After an incubation period varying from 3 days to 3 weeks there may be localized pain, redness and vesicular skin lesions near the site of the viral inoculation, followed by localized neurologic symptoms. Encephalopathy is common and fatal in up to 70% of patients. The virus is susceptible to aciclovir and early treatment can be life saving.[49]

MANAGEMENT

As most herpesvirus infections in the immunocompetent host are self-limiting, patients usually only require supportive care. The type of supportive treatment required varies for different disease manifestations and may consist of rest, hydration, the appropriate use of antipyretics and analgesics, and treatment to soothe skin lesions and prevent secondary bacterial infection. Effective antiviral therapy is available for more severe cases of infection caused by HSV, VZV or CMV. It is stressed, however, that although antiviral drugs can help to control a herpesvirus infection they cannot eliminate the infection (see Table 155.8 and Chapter 146).

REFERENCES

References for this chapter can be found online at http://www.expertconsult.com

Papillomaviruses

NATURE

The papillomaviruses are now considered to be in a distinct taxonomic family, Papillomaviridae, and unrelated to the polyomaviruses. Papillomaviruses are widely distributed in nature; among mammals they infect humans, cattle, dogs, rabbits, monkeys and other species. Some animal papillomaviruses affect both epithelial and fibroblastic tissues and produce fibropapillomas, but human papillomaviruses (HPVs) are strictly epitheliotropic and infect the skin or the mucous membranes. Papillomaviruses cannot be propagated in cell culture. Therefore, rapid advances in the knowledge about papillomaviruses date from the 1970s, when molecular cloning of the viral genomes allowed comparisons between viruses from different species and from different sites of the same species. The cloned genomes provided reagents for examination of affected tissues for viral sequences.

The papillomavirus particle (Fig. 156.1) is about 55 nm in diameter and has a double-stranded, covalently closed, circular genome of about 8000 bp. All of the genomic information is located on one strand. The genome is divided into an early region that has eight open reading frames (ORFs E1–E8), a late region that has two ORFs (L1 and L2) and a noncoding long control region (LCR), which contains regulatory elements for viral DNA replication and transcription. The L1 ORF codes for the major L1 capsid protein, which accounts for most of the virion mass and mediates viral attachment. The L1 protein displays immunodominant type-specific neutralizing epitopes.[1] The currently available prophylactic HPV vaccines are based on the use of the L1 protein expressed by recombinant DNA technology and self-assembled as virus-like particles (VLPs). Experimental vaccines based on the minor L2 capsid protein, which displays a subdominant cross neutralizing epitope, may provide cross protection against related HPV genotypes.[2] The early region genes E6 and E7 of high-risk HPVs code for the transforming proteins of the virus that mediate the oncogenic properties of the virus. The E1 gene is required for viral DNA replication and the E2 gene modulates viral transcription. The E5 gene is a membrane protein that interacts with growth factor receptors; it is the main transforming gene for bovine papillomaviruses but not for HPVs. The E4 gene, although it is located in the early region, is expressed late in the virus cycle; it disrupts cytokeratins and probably facilitates virus exit from infected cells. The functions of E3 and E8 ORFs are not known.

EPIDEMIOLOGY

More than 100 individual HPV types have been described to date.[3] They naturally fall into two groups, mucosal HPVs and cutaneous HPVs.

Mucosal human papillomaviruses

The genital tract is the reservoir for mucosal HPVs, except for two HPV types (HPV-13 and HPV-32) which infect the oral cavity. About 40 HPV types infect the genital tract. Genital HPV infections are the most prevalent sexually transmitted pathogens. As many as 30–40% of sexually active young women may have an HPV infection of the genital tract, as determined by sensitive DNA detection techniques. A history of multiple sexual partners, and having a male sexual partner who has many sexual partners, are the main risk factors for a woman for the acquisition of HPVs. Circumcision may decrease the risk of HPV acquisition in the male. The HPV prevalence reaches its peak in young adults and declines at older ages. HPV infections are largely asymptomatic and of 1–2 years' duration. Infection probably confers partial immunity to re-infection with the same type. The course of HPV infection is altered profoundly by HIV-induced immunosuppression.[4]

HPV-6 and HPV-11 are the etiologic agents of genital warts (condylomas), which occur in sexually active individuals, and also of recurrent respiratory papillomatosis (RRP), which may have onset in childhood or in adult life. HPV-16, -18, -31, -45 and some other types account for nearly all cervical cancers, as described in later sections of this chapter. HPV-13 and HPV-32 cause focal epithelial hyperplasia in the oral cavity. This condition is found frequently in indigenous populations, but rarely in other groups. How they are transmitted from person to person is unclear.

Cutaneous human papillomaviruses

Skin warts are transmitted by direct contact with an infected tissue or indirectly by contact with virus-contaminated objects. There is some specificity between HPV type, and site and morphology of the warts; plantar warts most often yield HPV-1, common warts HPV-2 and flat warts HPV-3 and HPV-10.

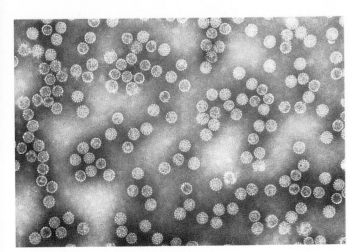

Fig. 156.1 Human papillomavirus particles. The particles are nonenveloped, have icosahedral capsids and are 55 nm in diameter. Courtesy of Dr M Reissig.

Epidermodysplasia verruciformis is a rare condition in which an extensive lifelong wart virus infection of the skin is never resolved.[5] The disease may be familial. The warts may be flat or they may be in the form of reddish-brown macular plaques. In about one-third of these patients, malignant transformation occurs in the reddish-brown plaques in areas exposed to sunlight. The epidermodysplasia verruciformis lesions contain a large number of HPV types. Types most commonly associated with skin cancers in epidermodysplasia verruciformis patients are HPV-5 and HPV-8. Low levels of HPV DNA sequences of a number of HPV types, including several novel types, have been recovered from nonmelanoma skin cancers (NMSC). HPV sequences are also found in plucked hair roots of healthy skin. It is not clear if HPVs play a role in the development of nonmelanoma skin cancers.[6] Ultraviolet (UV) light is considered the most significant risk factor of NMSCs. Cutaneous HPVs through the anti-apoptotic activity of their E6 gene may act as co-carcinogens by preventing elimination of cells with UV-induced DNA damage.

PATHOGENICITY

Papillomaviruses have a high degree of species and tissue specificity. Genital HPVs are rarely detected on skin other than that of the genital tract, but they can infect other mucosal sites in the body such as the aerodigestive tract. Cutaneous HPVs are almost never encountered in the genital tract. Papillomaviruses cannot be grown in monolayer cell cultures to yield virus particles. Full epithelial differentiation is required for the production of infectious particles.

Nearly all cervical cancers originate in the 'transformation zone', located at the lower end of the cervix, where the stratified squamous epithelium of the vagina forms a junction with the columnar cells of the endocervix. The cells in the transformation zone of the cervix must be highly susceptible to the oncogenic effects of HPVs, because cancers arise much less frequently at other sites in the genital tract (vulva, vagina, penis) that are infected with HPVs as frequently as the cervix but do not have an area similar to the transformation zone. Invasive cervical cancer is preceded by a progressive spectrum of cytologic abnormalities, classified as atypical squamous cells of undetermined significance (ASCUS), low-grade squamous intraepithelial lesions (LSILs) and high-grade squamous intraepithelial lesions (HSILs). The progression from initial HPV infection to invasive cancer may take 15–20 years.

Although almost all squamous cell abnormalities of the cervix including cervical cancer are the result of HPV infections, the probability of any one HPV infection progressing to cervical cancer is quite small (for review see[7]). Most HPV infections produce only transient cytologic abnormalities and are resolved completely without a trace. Cytologic abnormalities are seen in only about 10% of women who are positive for HPV DNA in the genital tract. A large majority of LSILs regress completely. In the USA, annually, there are tens of millions of HPV infections but only about 15 000 cases of invasive cancer. The relatively small number of cases is partly the result of treatment of LSILs and HSILs identified from Pap smear screening programs, but it is also, in a large measure, because most HPV infections do not result in significant cervical disease. In countries that have no effective Pap smear screening programs, the number of cases of cervical cancer is still a small fraction of the number of HPV infections in women.

HPVs are found in nearly all lesions spanning the entire spectrum of cytologic abnormalities from a LSIL to invasive cancer. The distribution of HPV types changes markedly with increasing severity of disease.[8] Almost all genital HPV types are represented in HPV DNA-positive cytologically normal specimens and in ASCUS and LSIL cases, but only about a dozen HPV types are found in invasive cervical cancer. Of these, four HPV types, HPV-16, -18, -45 and -31, account for nearly 80% of invasive cancers (Fig. 156.2). The genital HPV types have therefore been categorized as high-risk, intermediate-risk or low-risk types (Table 156.1) on the basis of their prevalence in invasive cervical cancer.

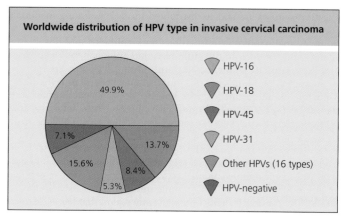

Fig. 156.2 Worldwide distribution of HPV type in invasive cervical carcinoma. The data are based on tests of over 900 cancers from different countries.[27]

Table 156.1 Major clinical associations of HPV infections

Disease	HPV types	Transmission

Cervical cancer
  High risk
  Intermediate risk
  Low risk
	HPV-16, -18, -45, -31
	HPV-33, -35, -39, -51, -52, -56, -59, -68, -73
	HPV-6, -11, -26, -42, -43, -44, -53, -54, -55, -62, -66
		Sexual

Cancer of vulva, vagina, anal canal, penis	HPV-16	Sexual
Oropharyngeal cancer	HPV-16	Sexual
Anogenital warts	HPV-6, -11	Sexual
Juvenile-onset RRP	HPV-6, -11	Mother–child, at birth
Adult-onset RRP	HPV-6, -11	Unclear
Cutaneous warts	HPV-1, -2, -3, -4, -10	Nonsexual contact
Epidermodysplasia verruciformis (EV)	HPV-5, -8, -9, -12, -14, -15, -17, -19, -25, -36, -38, -47, -50	Nonsexual contact
Nonmelanoma skin cancer	EV HPVs and novel HPVs	Unclear
Focal epithelial hyperplasia of the oral cavity	HPV-13, -32	Nonsexual contact

RRP, recurrent respiratory papillomatosis.

The oncogenic potential of HPVs is mediated by the E6 and E7 proteins of high-risk HPVs. In laboratory studies, E6 and E7 of high-risk HPVs can each transform mouse 3T3 cells and, together, can immortalize human keratinocytes. Viral constructs containing E6 and E7 genes of high-risk HPVs produce HSIL-like lesions in organotypic cervical epithelium. The E6 and E7 genes are invariably expressed in cells of HPV-associated cervical cancers. The viral genome of HPVs remains episomal in infections that are not associated with cervical cytopathology, as well as in cases of LSIL and in most instances of HSIL. However, in most invasive cancers the viral genome is integrated into the cellular DNA. Integration requires linearization of the circular viral genome, which almost always occurs by a break in the E2 region of the genome. The E6 and E7 genes not only remain intact after integration, but they are released from the inhibitory effect of the E2 protein, and are expressed at high levels in invasive cancers. High levels of antibodies to E6 and E7 proteins are markers for invasive cancer.[9]

The molecular mechanisms of cellular transformation by E6 and E7 genes of high-risk HPVs are well understood and are described in detail in excellent reviews.[10] Briefly, the E6 protein complexes with tumor suppressor protein p53 and targets it for destruction via the ubiquitin pathway. The E7 protein complexes with tumor suppressor protein Rb, thereby releasing the transcription factor E2F from its complex with Rb. The E2F activates expression of *myc* and other genes that activate the cell cycle. In the normal cell cycle, tumor suppressor proteins p53 and Rb inhibit cellular proliferation. The functional inactivation of both of these cellular tumor suppressor proteins by the HPV oncoproteins results in continued cell proliferation without time for repair of DNA damage (Fig. 156.3). This leads to genetic instability and accumulation of additional cellular mutations and chromosomal changes. Thus, infections with high-risk HPVs prepare the ground for the cellular genetic alterations that underlie cervical cancer. For example, gain of 3q chromosome was found to be consistently associated with the early stages of invasive cervical carcinoma (Fig. 156.4).[11]

PREVENTION

HPV-related diseases for which preventive strategies are being investigated are cervical and other lower genital tract cancers, tonsillar/oropharyngeal cancers, genital warts and recurrent respiratory papillomatosis.

Improved screening for cervical cancer

Implementation of Pap smear screening and treatment of cervical cancer precursor lesions identified by follow-up investigation of abnormal Pap smears have resulted in a marked reduction in the incidence of cervical cancers in the industrialized world but it has been difficult to establish effective Pap smear screening programs in the developing world. Primary cervical cancer screening by examination of cervical scrapes for DNAs of high-risk HPVs has been shown to have a sensitivity greater than that of Pap smears for the detection of HSIL and cancer.[12] Furthermore, adequate genital tract specimens can be self-collected by the women themselves, thus making it possible to avoid a pelvic examination. Assays for genital tract HPV DNAs are useful in the clinical management of mild cervical cytologic abnormalities.[13] Visual inspection of the cervix after acetic acid application (VIA) combined with treatment (if necessary) at the same visit has also been proposed as a screening method for developing countries.

Prophylactic vaccines

Virus-like particles (VLPs) that self-assemble from the L1 capsid protein when it is expressed by baculovirus or yeast recombinant DNA vectors have provided the immunogen for prophylactic vaccines. The VLPs are free of viral DNA and possess conformational epitopes of authentic virions. Immunization with VLPs of an HPV type leads to very high titers of virus neutralizing antibodies and to nearly 100% protection against subsequent HPV infection by that type.[14] Gardasil

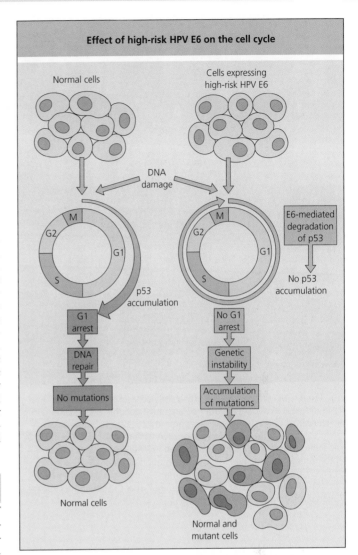

Effect of high-risk HPV E6 on the cell cycle

Fig. 156.3 Effect of high-risk HPV E6 on the cell cycle. In normal cells (left), DNA damage results in increased p53 production, which leads to arrest of cell cycle in G1 phase, allowing the cell time to repair DNA damage. In cells infected with high-risk HPVs (right), the HPV E6 mediates degradation of p53, so there is no accumulation of p53, no cell-cycle arrest, and continued cell multiplication. This leads to genetic instability and accumulation of cellular mutations. Courtesy of Dr TD Kessis.

from Merck is a quadrivalent vaccine that has VLPs of high-risk HPV-16 and HPV-18 (which account for about 70% of invasive cervical cancers) and of low-risk HPV-6 and HPV-11 (which are responsible for 90% of genital warts and 100% of recurrent respiratory papillomas). Cervarix from GlaxoSmithKline is a bivalent vaccine with VLPs of HPV-16 and HPV-18. The vaccines largely provide immunity only to the VLP types included in the vaccine preparation.[15] Gardasil is commercially available in the USA and is recommended for young girls prior to sexual debut. It is not yet known if the vaccines will be effective in preventing infections in men.

Therapeutic vaccines

Several strategies are also being tried for therapeutic immunization, aimed at destroying established lesions of HSIL and invasive cancer.[16] For this purpose, the objective is to generate cytotoxic T cells directed against cells expressing the E6 and E7 proteins of high-risk HPVs.[17] Chimeric vaccines which may have both prophylactic and therapeutic properties are also under investigation.

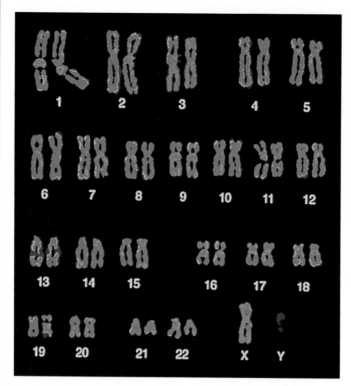

Fig. 156.4 Gain of chromosome 3q in early cervical carcinoma. The figure displays a ratio image after comparative genome hybridization, in which normal reference metaphase chromosomes are hybridized with a mixture of differentially labeled tumor DNA (green label) and normal DNA (red label). The chromosomes are ordered in a karyogram-like fashion. Chromosome 3q is gained (over-representation of green label) and chromosomal band 13q21 is lost (over-representation of red label) in this carcinoma. With permission from Heselmeyer et al.;[11] copyright (1996) National Academy of Sciences, USA.

DIAGNOSTIC MICROBIOLOGY

Hybridization assays

The presence of HPV in a tissue is ascertained by nucleic acid hybridization assays. The most widely used methods, especially in epidemiologic investigations, are those based on polymerase chain reaction (PCR) amplification.[18,19] Typically, consensus primers are employed to target conserved regions of the viral genome so that a large number of HPVs are amplified in a single amplification reaction. The PCR products are then screened for different HPVs by hybridization with type-specific oligonucleotide probes and by a 'generic' probe (a mixture of probes of several HPVs) that would detect many HPVs. The methods have high analytic sensitivity and a high specificity. In a modification of this assay, type-specific hybridizations are performed in a single step as line blots against probes immobilized on a strip.[20] Hybrid Capture is a signal amplification-based hybridization assay approved by the US Food and Drug Administration (FDA). In this assay, genital tract specimens are screened for HPVs in an enzyme-linked immunosorbent assay (ELISA)-type format with two pools of HPV probes, one pool consisting of high-risk HPVs and the other of low-risk HPVs.[21] This test has been found to be useful in 'triaging' women with abnormal Pap smears for colposcopy.[13]

Immunologic assays

Immunologic assays are rarely used for type-specific HPV diagnosis. In most HPV infections, viral particles and capsid proteins are present in very small amounts and so are difficult to detect with antiviral serum. Also, as cervical SILs progress toward higher grade disease and cervical cancer, synthesis of capsid proteins and infectious particles is completely shut down. Type-specific antiserum is not available for any HPV type.

Antibody response to HPVs may be measured using ELISA with VLPs.[22] Antibody response to HPV infections is low-titered and detectable in only about 40–50% of infected individuals. The proportion of infected individuals who are antibody positive increases with increased duration of infection and with greater viral load in the genital tract specimens.[23] Antibodies to E6 and E7 proteins are markers of HPV-associated invasive cancer. These antibodies may be detected by peptide-based ELISA or by radioimmunoprecipitation assays with *in vitro* synthesized full length E6 and E7 proteins. Elevated levels of E6 or E7 antibodies are found in about 70% of patients who have invasive cancer but in less than 5% of controls.[9]

CLINICAL MANIFESTATIONS

The major clinical associations of HPVs are listed in Table 156.1. Aspects not covered in the earlier sections of this chapter are discussed below. Clinical features of these infections are also discussed in Chapter 59.

Cervical cancer

Cervical cancer is the most common female malignancy in the developing world. Approximately 500 000 cases of cervical cancer occur worldwide per year. The incidence of cervical cancer varies widely in different countries. Cervical cancer has long been known to have all the epidemiologic characteristics of a sexually transmitted disease. Observations from field, clinical and laboratory studies are mutually corroborative in building a compelling case for the HPV etiology of cervical cancer (Table 156.2), making it the first major human cancer with a single infectious etiology. The sexual behavior of the female,

Table 156.2 Evidence linking HPVs with invasive cervical cancer

Field	Evidence
Epidemiology	• HPVs present in nearly 100% of cancers in low- and high-incidence areas • HPV infection precedes cancer • HPV epidemiology and cervical cancer screening practices account for differences in worldwide incidence of cervical cancer
Pathogenesis	• HPV genome present in every cancer cell • HPV associated with entire spectrum of cervical neoplasia, from low-grade cytologic abnormalities to invasive cancer • HPV types most frequent in cancers are the most oncogenic in laboratory assays • HPV oncogenes E6 and E7 invariably expressed in cancers • HPV genome is episomal in preinvasive disease and integrates into cellular DNA in invasive cancers
Molecular mechanisms	• E6 and E7 proteins of high-risk HPV types distort cell cycle and promote genetic instability by degradation of tumor suppressor protein p53 and inactivation of tumor suppressor protein Rb • Integration of viral genome into cellular DNA enhances E6 and E7 expression

the sexual behavior of her male partners and the availability of an effective Pap smear screening program explain the wide differences in cervical cancer incidence in different countries.[24] In many high-incidence areas, male sexual behavior is the key factor for the high cervical cancer rates among relatively monogamous women.

HPV etiology of cervical cancer was proposed in 1976 and HPV vaccines which can prevent cervical cancer became available in 2006. Understanding the cause of a major human cancer and development of practical means to prevent it over a 30-year span is widely regarded as a major achievement in public health and cancer control.

Other anogenital cancers

HPV infections are responsible for the basaloid or warty vulvar cancers that occur in younger women but are not related to the more common typical keratinizing squamous cell carcinomas that occur in older women. They are strongly associated with cancers of the anal canal, vagina and penis.

Oropharyngeal/tonsillar cancer

A subset of oropharyngeal/tonsillar cancer is etiologically linked to high-risk HPVs, especially HPV-16.[25] Virologically, these tumors have a transcriptionally active HPV genome localized to tumor cell nuclei. HPV-16 accounts for more than 90% of the HPV-associated cancers at this site. As compared to other patients with head and neck cancers, these patients are less likely to have a history of alcohol and tobacco exposure, more likely to have a history of multiple sexual partners and of oral sex, and a significantly better prognosis. A majority of the estimated 51 000 annual cases of oropharyngeal cancers worldwide are due to HPV infection and are very likely vaccine-preventable.

Genital warts

Although they are benign, genital warts (condylomas) are a significant problem in sexually active populations and especially in immuno-compromised individuals. Vaccines which contain HPV-6 and HPV-11 VLPs are likely to prevent a large majority of genital warts.

Recurrent respiratory papillomatosis (RRP)

This results from the transmission of HPV-6 and HPV-11 infections from the genital tract to the respiratory tract. For juvenile-onset disease, a large majority of the transmissions occur at birth, during passage of the fetus through an infected birth canal (for review of the clinical spectrum of juvenile-onset RRP, see[26]). Some reports suggest occasional intrauterine transmission. About 25% of the cases occur in the first year of life and most of these in the second 6 months. There are progressively fewer cases in each year thereafter.

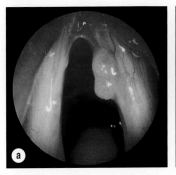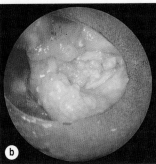

Fig. 156.5 RRP of juvenile onset. (a) A respiratory papilloma on the vocal cord of a child. (b) Papilloma obstructing the respiratory tract. Courtesy of Dr H Kashima.

The most common site of the papilloma is in the larynx on the vocal cords (Fig. 156.5). The tumors are benign but may threaten life if they grow and obstruct respiration. The tumors tend to recur after surgical removal, and in the worst cases operations may be required every few weeks. Operative procedures, especially tracheotomy, may spread the tumor by inadvertently transplanting tumor cells to other sites. Rarely, the tumor may undergo malignant transformation. Caesarian delivery when there is an active infection of the maternal genital tract will reduce the risk of juvenile-onset disease in the child. Mothers who have been immunized with HPV vaccines which have HPV-6 and HPV-11 VLPs are probably protected against having a child with juvenile-onset RRP.

MANAGEMENT

The clinical conditions associated with HPV infections are very diverse. Regular Pap smear screening and follow-up of women who have Pap smear abnormalities would greatly decrease the risk of cervical cancer. The preinvasive cervical disease is readily treated with greater than 90% cure rates. Genital and skin warts may regress spontaneously or may be treated with caustic agents (podophyllin), cryotherapy, application of an immunomodulating agent (imiquimod) or by surgical removal. Intralesional or parenteral administration of interferon has been successful in the treatment of refractory genital warts (see Chapter 59 for additional information).

REFERENCES

References for this chapter can be found online at http://www.expertconsult.com

Polyomaviruses

NATURE

Polyomaviruses are small, nonenveloped viruses, which are widespread in nature. Although previously grouped with papillomaviruses in a single family, the International Committee on Taxonomy of viruses has now recognized polyomaviruses as an independent family, the Polyomaviridae. They are highly adapted to grow in the species and the tissue they infect. The first human polyomaviruses were isolated in 1971 from immunocompromised patients. JC virus (JCV) was isolated from the brain of a patient with Hodgkin's disease who died of progressive multifocal leukoencephalopathy (PML), a demyelinating disease of the central nervous system.[1] BK virus (BKV) was isolated from the urine of a renal transplant patient who developed ureteral stenosis.[2]

In 2007, genomes of two new human polyomaviruses, KI virus and WU virus, were independently detected in respiratory tract secretions of children by use of molecular techniques.[3,4] These two viruses share ~65–70% amino acid similarity with each other, but only ~15–50% similarity with JCV and BKV. The prevalence, biology and pathogenicity of these viruses are currently unknown. The viruses have been detected in respiratory specimens in the presence of other recognized respiratory pathogens and thus their role in disease is unclear. Very recently, another new human polyomavirus, Merkel cell virus (MCV), was detected by employing mass sequencing of a messenger RNA library of tumor cells and bioinformatics analysis of the data to identify nonhuman sequences with homology to known infectious agents. The viral genome was shown to be integrated within the genome of cells of a rare human skin cancer, Merkel cell carcinoma.[5] MCV is distantly related to the other known human polyomaviruses (Fig. 157.1). The prevalence of the virus in human populations is unknown and the precise role of the virus in the etiology of Merkel cell carcinoma remains to be established.

Polyomavirus virions are about 44 nm in diameter, have icosahedral symmetry and are composed of 72 capsomeres. The viral genome is a circular, covalently closed, supercoiled, double-stranded DNA of about 5000 bp. The viral genome is organized into three functional regions, the early and late coding regions and a regulatory region. The early region encodes the two viral regulatory proteins, the large T and small t antigens. The large T antigen regulates viral transcription and initiates viral DNA replication. Additionally, the large T antigen can interact with cellular proteins. Among the known properties of large T antigen is the ability to inactivate host cell tumor suppressor proteins, which contributes to the oncogenic potential of polyomaviruses. The late region codes for the major structural protein, VP1, and the two minor structural proteins, VP2 and VP3. The structural proteins assemble into capsomeres composed of five VP1 molecules and a single VP2 or VP3 molecule, which then form capsids from 72 capsomeres. The viral regulatory region spans 300–500 bp and contains elements for viral DNA replication, binding sites for cellular transcription factors,

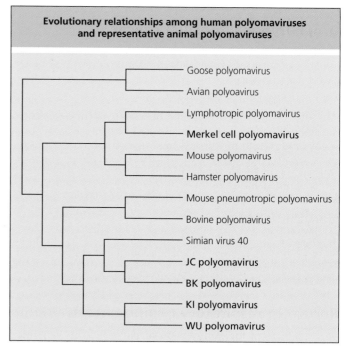

Evolutionary relationships among human polyomaviruses and representative animal polyomaviruses

- Goose polyomavirus
- Avian polyoavirus
- Lymphotropic polyomavirus
- **Merkel cell polyomavirus**
- Mouse polyomavirus
- Hamster polyomavirus
- Mouse pneumotropic polyomavirus
- Bovine polyomavirus
- Simian virus 40
- **JC polyomavirus**
- **BK polyomavirus**
- **KI polyomavirus**
- **WU polyomavirus**

Fig. 157.1 Evolutionary relationships among human polyomaviruses and representative animal polyomaviruses. BKV and JCV are closely related to each other and to the rhesus macaque polyomavirus (SV40). KI and WU form a separate evolutionary group, which is nevertheless related to the BKV/JCV/SV40 group. The Merkel cell virus is very distantly related to the other human polyomaviruses but is closely related to a polyomavirus whose natural host is believed to be the African green monkey (lymphotropic polyomavirus).

and promoters for transcription of early and late genes. The regulatory region contains repeat elements which are subject to deletions, insertions and rearrangements. As compared to strains excreted in the urine, polyomaviruses detected in nonurinary specimens often have regulatory region rearrangements, which may confer increased viral fitness in the host cell environment. Infection of cells is initiated by adsorption of virions to the cell surface by interaction with cell surface sialic acids. The protein component of the cellular receptor for BKV is unknown; however, that for JCV is the serotonin receptor $5HT_{2A}$.[6] Polyomaviruses enter the cell cytoplasm by endocytosis and are transported to the nucleus via the cytoskeleton transport machinery. Within the nucleus, viral DNA replication and formation of progeny virions takes place. New virions are thought to be released by either lysis of host cells or secretion from the plasma membrane.

EPIDEMIOLOGY

Both BKV and JCV infections occur in childhood, but BKV occurs at an earlier age than JCV. BKV seropositivity increases rapidly with age and reaches 98% at 7–9 years of age. JCV seropositivity increases more slowly with increasing age, reaching 50% among children aged 9–11 years and 60–70% by adulthood.[7] The most likely mode of transmission of BKV and JCV is via the respiratory tract. No serologic assays are available for the new human polyomaviruses, KI, WU and Merkel cell polyomavirus, and thus the prevalence of these viruses in human populations is unknown.

PATHOGENICITY

Primary BKV and JCV infections are either entirely asymptomatic or may be associated with nonspecific flu-like symptoms. The viruses probably multiply at the site of entry, and then reach the kidney, the main target organ, by viremia. They undergo further multiplication in the kidney and produce transient viruria. After primary infection, the viruses remain latent in the kidney for an indefinite period of time. The viruses may activate periodically and be associated with asymptomatic shedding of virus in the urine. BKV DNA can be detected in the urine of ~0–1% of healthy persons and JCV DNA can be found in ~35% of healthy individuals, with a higher incidence of JCV shedding in older individuals.[8] After primary infection the viruses also persist in B lymphocytes and JCV has been reported to persist as a latent infection of the brain.[9] Nearly all significant illnesses due to BKV and JCV occur in immunocompromised hosts, mostly as a result of reactivation of latent virus but sometimes as a primary infection in an immunocompromised host. Conditions in which viruses are reactivated include pregnancy, diabetes, organ transplantation, anti-tumor therapy, and AIDS and other immunodeficiency diseases.

PREVENTION

No attempt has been made to prevent primary BKV or JCV infection since infection is harmless in immunocompetent individuals and disease is uncommon even in immunocompromised individuals.

DIAGNOSTIC MICROBIOLOGY

BKV can be cultivated in several cell lines of human origin. JCV grows best in human fetal glial cultures. Isolation of BKV and JCV in cell culture is rarely attempted because it is inefficient and cumbersome and the needed cell types are not readily available. It is not known if WU, KI or Merkel cell polyomaviruses can be propagated in cell cultures. Cells and tissue infected with BKV and JCV can be identified by immunoperoxidase and immunofluorescence staining with antiviral antiserum. Immunization of rabbits with disrupted viral capsids or VP1 protein produces a broadly cross-reactive antiserum.

BKV and JCV DNA, as well as WU and KI virus DNA, can be readily identified by polymerase chain reaction (PCR) assays. Efforts to standardize these assays and prepare international reference samples are ongoing. Serologic diagnosis of BKV and JCV infection can be made by hemagglutination-inhibition assays or by enzyme-linked immunosorbent assays (ELISA) which use virus-like particles formed by self-assembly of VP1 protein produced in eukaryotic expression systems. Because BKV and JCV infections occur early in life and are very common,[10] serologic assays have limited utility for clinical diagnosis.

CLINICAL MANIFESTATIONS

Progressive multifocal leukoencephalopathy

Progressive multifocal leukoencephalopathy (PML) is a fatal, subacute demyelinating disease of the central nervous system that results from JCV infection of oligodendrocytes in the brain. It occurs as a complication of conditions associated with T-cell deficiency, including lymphoproliferative disorders, primary immunodeficiency diseases, prolonged immunosuppressive therapy and secondary immunodeficiency disorders such as human immunodeficiency virus (HIV) infection. Until the advent of HIV/AIDS, PML was a rare disease with onset typically in middle age or later life. At present, HIV is estimated to be the underlying cause of immunosuppression in 55–85% of cases of PML, and PML is diagnosed in approximately 5% of AIDS cases.[11] In 2006, three patients with multiple sclerosis or Crohn's disease developed PML in association with administration of natalizumab, a monoclonal antibody to alpha-4 integrin that prevents entry of inflammatory cells into brain and other tissues.[12] Why natalizumab would uniquely predispose persons to the development of PML remains unexplained.

Progressive multifocal leukoencephalopathy has an insidious onset. Early signs are impairment of speech and vision and mental deterioration. Paralysis of limbs, cortical blindness and sensory impairment occur in later stages of the disease. Patients remain afebrile and headache is uncommon. Typically, the disease is progressive, resulting in death within 3–6 months after onset. The introduction of highly active antiretroviral therapy (HAART) for HIV/AIDS has had only a modest effect on the incidence of PML, but prognosis is improved.[13] At disease onset, factors associated with better survival include higher CD4 cell count, lower JCV viral load, prior exposure to HAART, elevated myoinositol in PML lesions on MRI and higher levels of macrophage chemoattractant protein (MCP)-1 in cerebrospinal fluid (CSF).

The diagnosis of PML is established conclusively by pathologic examination of biopsy tissue. The brain shows foci of demyelination, most frequently found in subcortical white matter. Microscopically, the presence of enlarged nuclei of oligodendrocytes is the pathognomonic lesion of PML. These altered nuclei contain abundant numbers of JCV viral particles. Noninvasive techniques, particularly MRI of the brain, provide an effective means for diagnosis of PML. MRI scans are nearly always abnormal in association with PML.[14] The typical abnormalities are localized to subcortical white matter and are characterized by increased T2 signal and little contrast enhancement after gadolinium administration. CSF analysis typically shows minimal pleocytosis and modestly elevated protein. PCR of CSF for JCV DNA is the best noninvasive test for diagnosis of PML. Sensitivity of PCR is ~80% and specificity is 100%.[15]

BK virus nephropathy in kidney transplant recipients

BK virus nephropathy (BKVN), also designated polyomavirus-associated nephropathy (PVAN), has recently been recognized as an important cause of graft dysfunction and graft loss in patients with renal allografts. The incidence of BKVN is 1–10% and graft loss occurs in from 10% to 80% of cases.[16] The majority of cases occur in the first year post transplantation (Fig. 157.2). The variable incidence and outcome of BKVN most likely reflect differences across renal transplant centers in diagnostic criteria for BKVN, patient populations, immunosuppressive regimens and management strategies. The emergence of BKVN has coincided with the expanding use of tacrolimus and mycophenolate mofetil in immunosuppressive regimens to control graft-versus-host disease.

The intensity of immunosuppression appears to be a more important factor in disease than a specific drug. Bolus therapy with corticosteroids also may be a risk factor for BKVN. Host factors such as

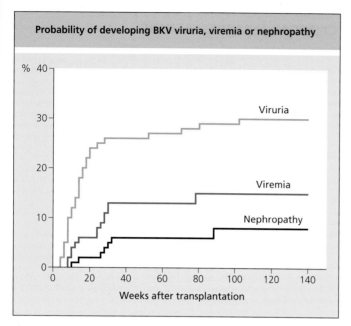

Probability of developing BKV viruria, viremia or nephropathy

Viruria

Viremia

Nephropathy

Weeks after transplantation

Fig. 157.2 Probability of developing BKV viruria, viremia or nephropathy in the weeks following renal transplantation. Adapted from Hirsch et al.[16]

age greater than 50 years, male gender, white ethnicity and underlying diabetes mellitus, and allograft factors such as number of human leukocyte antigen (HLA) mismatches between donor and recipient and prior tubular injury to the graft can increase the risk of BKVN. Apart from donor BKV seropositivity and recipient seronegativity, there is no convincing evidence that viral factors play a role in the risk of BKVN.

The definitive diagnosis of BKVN requires a renal biopsy showing polyomavirus-induced cytopathic changes in tubular or glomerular epithelial cells. Enlarged nuclei with basophilic inclusions in the tubular epithelium are the pathognomonic lesion of BKVN. Depending on the stage of disease, necrosis of cells of the tubules and collecting ducts and varying degrees of interstitial inflammation can also be observed.[17] Noninvasive diagnostic techniques can be used to screen for BKV replication and to make an early diagnosis of BKVN. Polyomavirus-bearing 'decoy cells' can easily be detected in urine with a Papanicolaou-stained cytology preparation. The positive predictive value for BKVN of the detection of decoy cells is 25–30%. BKV DNA can be detected in urine and plasma by PCR. Because of the high rate of excretion of BKV in urine of renal transplant recipients, the finding of BKV DNA by PCR in urine is of limited clinical value for diagnosis of BKVN. On the other hand, detection of BKV DNA in plasma by PCR has been shown to have a sensitivity of 100% and a specificity of ~85% for biopsy-confirmed BKVN.[18]

Hemorrhagic cystitis in bone marrow transplant recipients

BK viruria occurs in ~50% of patients after bone marrow transplantation (BMT). Hemorrhagic cystitis is the most prevalent and serious clinical manifestation of BKV infection in BMT recipients, with an incidence of 10–25%.[19] Less common clinical manifestations of BKV infection in BMT include ureteral stenosis and interstitial nephritis. Patients with hemorrhagic cystitis experience urgency, frequency of urination, dysuria, suprapubic pain and variable degrees of hematuria. BKV-associated hemorrhagic cystitis must be distinguished from noninfectious hemorrhagic cystitis resulting from direct cytotoxic effects of antineoplastic treatment. Typically, BKV infection is associated with late onset hemorrhagic cystitis and drug toxicity with early onset disease. Potential risk factors for BKV-associated hemorrhagic cystitis include acute graft-versus-host disease, intensive immunosuppressive conditional regimens, allogeneic transplant and magnitude of BKV urine viral load. BKV DNA can be detected by PCR in urine of patients with BKV-associated hemorrhagic cystitis; however, detection of BKV DNA does not have high specificity. A high urine viral load or viremia has greater specificity.

Role of polyomaviruses in human malignancies

JCV and BKV are oncogenic for laboratory animals and they transform cultured cells.[20] These viruses, therefore, have been investigated for their role in human malignancies. There are reports of finding JCV DNA in brain and colon tumors and BKV DNA in prostate, bladder and brain tumors, as well as neuroblastomas and insulinomas. However, a reproducible and consistent etiologic association of JCV or BKV with any human malignancy has not been demonstrated.

The recently described Merkel cell polyomavirus provides a more convincing example of a polyomavirus-induced human malignancy since the viral genome was found to be integrated into cellular DNA, a key event in experimental polyomavirus-induced animal tumors.[5] Additionally, the observation of integration at different chromosomal sites in virus-positive tumors suggests that viral infection precedes clonal expansion of Merkel carcinoma tumor cells.

MANAGEMENT

The majority of patients with BKV and JCV infections are asymptomatic and do not require treatment. There are no antiviral drugs with proven clinical efficacy against human polyomaviruses. The mainstay of treatment for BKV nephropathy is the reduction, change in drugs or discontinuation of immunosuppressive therapy.[21] Historically, the prognosis for PML was poor with death occurring within 3–4 months of diagnosis. However, for HIV patients, the introduction of HAART has improved survival of patients with PML. Paradoxically, in some patients with PML on HAART, a successful response to HAART is associated with an intense inflammatory response and a poor PML outcome.

REFERENCES

References for this chapter can be found online at http://www.expertconsult.com

Parvoviruses

NATURE

The family Parvoviridae consists of remarkably small (*parvus* in Latin), nonenveloped, single-stranded DNA viruses of animals, divided into the subfamilies Parvovirinae of vertebrates and Densovirinae of arthropods. The Parvovirinae subfamily is further divided into five genuses: *Parvovirus, Erythrovirus, Dependovirus, Amdovirus* and *Bocavirus.* The genus *Parvovirus* consists of a large number of nonhuman mammalian viruses, including minute virus of mice, feline panleukopenia virus, Kilham rat virus and bovine, porcine, canine, goose and feline parvoviruses. The genus *Erythrovirus* consist of primate parvoviruses with the unique property of requiring erythroid precursor cells for productive infection. The important human pathogenic B19 virus belongs to this genus. Dependoviruses consist of mammalian parvoviruses that require a helper virus for replication. The typical helper virus is adenovirus, hence the name adeno-associated virus (AAV). Human AAVs are candidate gene therapy vectors because they can infect many cell types but do not replicate and are considered nonpathogenic. The *Amdovirus* genus has recently been defined to accommodate Aleutian mink disease virus, hence the name, when it appeared to differ essentially from *Parvovirus* members. Finally, there is the genus *Bocavirus*, named after the bovine and canine minute parvoviruses which share several properties. A human virus was described in 2005 with features that fit well in this genus. Since then, this human bocavirus has been confirmed to occur worldwide and to be associated with respiratory disease.

The other subfamily of the Parvoviridae, Densovirinae, infects arthropods: some species in this large and diverse group have economic importance, such as those affecting silk production.

Therefore, at this moment, two viruses belonging to the Parvoviridae are known as human pathogens, B19 virus and human bocavirus. The latter has only recently been discovered and definitive conclusions on its precise clinical significance are not yet possible. Nonetheless, as it is clear that this virus differs essentially from B19 virus, it will be dealt with separately at the end of the chapter.

Further details will now be given of the virus which is known as human parvovirus B19. With the description of another human pathogenic virus in the family, the use of the extension 'B19' has become more important and the name of the virus should preferably be abbreviated as B19 virus (B19V). This remarkable name does not refer to any systematic nomenclature but has been assigned by Yvonne Cossart, who in 1974 detected an immunoreactive antigen in human serum obtained from a donor referred to as B19. This antigen was subsequently determined to be a previously unrecognized small icosahedral viral particle on electron microscopy, with parvovirus-like features.[1] The corresponding antibodies were widely present in the human population and appeared to be increasing with age but it took some time before several important disease associations were revealed. First, infection with this virus was associated with aplastic crisis among persons with sickle cell disease,[2] subsequently with the frequent childhood exanthema known as erythema infectiosum[3] and finally with a serious complication during pregnancy, hydrops fetalis.[4] These three clinical entities are still the most relevant consequences of infection by parvovirus B19, although a number of other possible presentations have been added since then.[5]

The B19 virus appeared a typical member of the Parvoviridae family: a small (23 nm) viral particle, with a small (5.6 kb) genome consisting of single-stranded DNA (Fig. 158.1). The DNA has palindromic hairpin structures at either end and encodes only three major viral proteins, the viral capsid proteins VP1 and VP2 and one nonstructural protein, NS1, in addition to two smaller products of unknown significance. Replication of this virus is limited to human erythroid precursor cells, likely related to the presence of the cellular receptor P-antigen or globoside.

Progeny virus is assembled in the nucleus and may be observed as intranuclear inclusions. Equal numbers of B19 positive- and negative-sense DNA strands are encapsidated. The VP1 and VP2 proteins are overlapping, with the VP2 (58 kDa) fully contained in the VP1 (84 kDa) sequence. VP2 is the major constituent of the viral capsid (96%). NS1 has helicase activity and is involved in viral DNA transcription and replication. In addition, this protein has effects on the host cell,

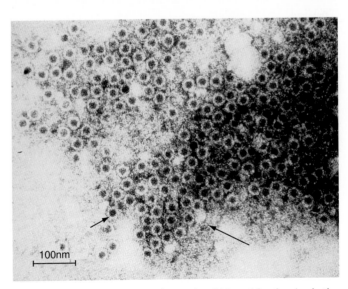

100nm

Fig. 158.1 Electron micrograph of parvovirus B19 particles showing both full particles (short arrow) and empty capsids (long arrow). Courtesy of Stanley Naides, MD.

causing cell cycle arrest and apoptosis. All further functional requirements for viral replication are derived from the host cell. Although the B19 genome is generally highly conserved, three clades are known to circulate.[6] No clear correlations are present between these three genotypes and distinctive pathologic and clinical manifestations.[7]

EPIDEMIOLOGY

Parvovirus B19 is found worldwide and infections occur in all seasons. In addition, two patterns can be recognized with regard to the occurrence of infections in time: a yearly peak in late winter and early spring in most moderate climates and a peak occurring in an approximate 4-yearly interval. This latter phenomenon of a cyclic pattern has been observed with other childhood exanthems, at least before vaccination intervened, and is related to the proportion of susceptible hosts in the population. Transmission of B19 virus occurs via nasopharyngeal secretions. Populations of children acquire B19 antibodies in an age-dependent fashion, beginning with entry into schools. Most surveys indicate that 50–70% of adults are anti-B19 virus IgG seropositive, indicating past infection and immunity. Clinical signs of infection occur after an incubation period of 7–18 days,[8] while infectivity is already present before this time. B19 virus may resist current methods of blood decontamination and therefore pooled blood products may contain infectious B19 virus.[9]

PATHOGENICITY

The particular tropism of parvovirus B19 for erythroid precursor cells plays a central role in the understanding of the pathogenesis of associated diseases. About 7–8 days after exposure to the virus, local replication in the bone marrow leads to a brisk viremia of 10^{11} or more viral particles/ml. In this same phase, the virus becomes detectable in respiratory secretions, leading to further spread. Viral replication causes maturation arrest at the giant pronormoblast stage of erythroid development, likely through viral induction of apoptosis.[10] Nonerythroid lineages may be affected as well, although these are less efficient in supporting B19 viral replication. Interestingly, in all infected individuals a temporary total disappearance of reticulocytes is observed, reflecting an arrest of erythropoiesis, which is usually too short in duration to lead to a relevant effect on hemoglobin levels. However, in individuals with shortened erythrocyte survival, as in those with hemolytic anemias, this period of areticulocytosis is extended and will often lead to severe anemia.

In recipients of recent stem cell transplantation, parvovirus B19 infection may lead to an aplastic crisis. Most likely, these complications arise as a consequence of the inability to recruit new erythroid progenitors in time, in situations of pre-existing hematopoietic stress. This also applies to the expanding hematopoietic system of the fetus, which would explain the observation of extreme fetal anemia with associated hydrops fetalis which may follow maternal infection. A few days after the peak of viremia, septic antibodies appear. In this phase the clinical signs of erythema infectiosum may develop, characteristically consisting of a skin rash and arthralgia. This temporal association is a clear indication of the likely immunopathogenetic origin of these signs.

Modern techniques have shown that there is a strong decrease in viral titers in the blood in this period which does not always immediately lead to viral clearance. Virus may remain detectable in the blood at a low level for an extended period in some hosts, possibly reflecting some steady state level of viral clearance and replication.[11] Ultimately, in normal hosts the virus will be cleared from the blood but a failure to produce sufficient antibody responses may result in persistent or recurrent viremia and chronic or recurrent bone marrow suppression.[12]

The described pathogenesis results in two clinical phases of illness, as observed in experimental infections,[8] but these may overlap

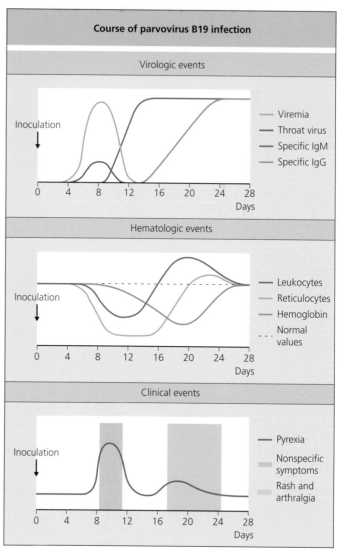

Fig. 158.2 Course of parvovirus B19 infection. Volunteers were inoculated nasally with viremic serum and virologic, hematologic and clinical events observed. Courtesy of Stanley Naides, MD.

in natural infections (Fig. 158.2). In the first phase, mild fever, malaise and myalgia may occur during the viremia, with associated areticulocytosis, leukopenia and thrombocytopenia. In the second phase, the appearance of antiviral IgM is associated with a rash and arthralgia. In an infected pregnant woman, the virus may cross the placenta, most likely during the initial extreme peak of viremia.[13] Fetal infection without an effective immune response results in a persistent arrest of erythroid maturation with a deep anemia and a high-output congestive heart failure presenting as hydrops fetalis. Theoretically, myocardial expression of the P-antigen could imply an additional role of viral myocarditis as a cause of cardiac failure but this has not been firmly established.

PREVENTION

Infected patients shed virus in nasopharyngeal secretions, at the time of, or even before, the typical signs of erythema infectiosum are apparent. This severely limits the effects of measures based on the recognition of this disease. Hygiene regarding contact with secretions as well as precautions against the spread of infectious droplets are warranted if susceptible persons are involved. Patients should be considered infectious until 1 or 2 days after onset of rash.[14] Generally, attention is focused on pregnant women who have been in contact with (preferably proven) cases of erythema infectiosum. In these cases, it is important to determine potential susceptibility by testing for B19 virus-specific antibodies. Nonimmune exposed pregnant women should be offered further monitoring to enable a timely diagnosis of potential maternal and eventually fetal infection, which could necessitate an intrauterine transfusion.[15] No vaccine is available and there is no experience with the prophylactic administration of immunoglobulins.

DIAGNOSTIC MICROBIOLOGY

The antibody response against the virus is highly useful for diagnostic purposes. An acute infection can be confirmed by testing for IgM antibodies against B19 virus and immunity is demonstrated by the presence of IgG antibodies. Antibody determination employs recombinant capsid antigens, as the virus itself cannot be readily grown in tissue culture. The B19 virus can be demonstrated by testing for viral DNA, usually by amplification techniques, although the extreme values during the initial peak in blood also allow detection by less sensitive hybridization techniques.

Viral detection by polymerase chain reaction (PCR) is extremely useful in cases of suspected fetal infections. Maternal serology is unable to confirm such infections: maternal IgM would support the presence of this complication but may also notoriously be lacking in cases of established B19 virus-associated hydrops fetalis. Viral DNA can then be detected, often at extremely high levels, in amniotic fluid as well as umbilical cord blood samples obtained before intrauterine transfusions are given.[15] Recent experiences with the quantitative results of viral DNA detection suggested that these may provide useful additional information on the stage of the infection.[13,16–18] Maternal blood levels of viral DNA correlate with fetal viral loads but are consistently lower, suggesting a fetal origin of the extended viremia.

Detection of viral DNA is also important in the diagnosis of persisting infections in immunocompromised individuals, who may have chronic or recurrent viremia accompanied by poor IgM or IgG responses.[19] The extreme sensitivity of DNA-based techniques makes it possible to make a diagnosis in outbreak settings if minute samples are used, as obtained by finger pricks.[20]

CLINICAL MANIFESTATIONS

Although asymptomatic infections occur in an unknown but likely substantial proportion of infections, the most frequently observed clinical consequence is classic erythema infectiosum or 'fifth disease', characterized by a fairly typical exanthema described as 'slapped cheek' (Fig. 158.3). The macular or maculopapular rash spreads to trunk and extremities and may be recurrently present for some time with conditions increasing skin perfusion. The rash as a clinical presentation is not highly specific and may be easily confused with several other conditions; serologic confirmation is therefore advised to make a diagnosis.

Accompanying joint symptoms are rare in children but may be severe in adults, more often in women. These consist of an acute, symmetric, rheumatoid-like polyarthritis which usually improves within 2 weeks but occasionally may persist for months.

In individuals with chronic hemolytic anemia, such as sickle cell disease or hereditary spherocytosis, a transient aplastic crisis may develop as a consequence of parvovirus B19 infection, which may be severe.[21] Although the erythroid precursors are most severely affected, in some cases thrombocytopenia or pancytopenia may occur, rarely even without an underlying hematologic disorder. Failure to clear parvovirus B19 effectively after infection in immunocompromised hosts may lead to a chronic suppression of erythropoiesis. Persistent B19 virus infection should be suspected in cases of transplant recipients[19,22] or untreated HIV infections[23] presenting with chronic anemia. B19 virus could also complicate recovery after chemotherapy for leukemia.[24] As a consequence of infection during pregnancy, infection of

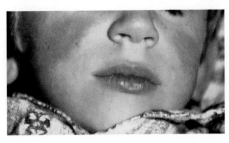

Fig. 158.3 Classic 'slapped cheeks' of a child with erythema infectiosum, or fifth disease, caused by parvovirus B19. A lacy macular erythematous eruption is also present on the trunk but not shown. Courtesy of Dr K Motton.

the unborn child occurs in up to half of the cases. This may lead to the development of hydrops fetalis, again as a consequence of erythroid suppression. Affected fetuses present with extremely low hemoglobin values; if untreated, fetal death is often the consequence, although spontaneous recovery may occur.

A number of other conditions have more rarely been associated with a concomitant parvovirus B19 infection. These include hepatitis, myocarditis and a variety of neurologic complications, notably brachial plexus neuritis, and these associations are reasonably well documented. Myocarditis was recently proposed as an additional consequence of infection.[25] In general, it is difficult to provide definitive proof of the relationship between a specific clinical condition and the occurrence of this frequent infection, with a sometimes longlasting presence of IgM antibodies and viral DNA. However, it is clear that some individuals react in less typical ways to this infection. Exanthema, arthralgia and hematologic disturbances, including hydrops fetalis, remain the most relevant manifestations of parvovirus B19 infection.

MANAGEMENT

No specific antiviral therapy is available. In immunocompromised patients with persistent B19 virus infection and anemia, intravenous immunoglobulin may allow clearance of the infection and resolution of bone marrow suppression.[22,23] Patients with transient aplastic crisis may require blood transfusions. B19 virus-associated fetal hydrops requires urgent intrauterine transfusion to correct the severe anemia present with this condition and to prevent fetal death.[15] Although B19 virus in general is not considered a cause of congenital anomalies, it appeared that this correction of the anemia did not prevent some neurodevelopmental delay in these children.[26]

HUMAN BOCAVIRUS AND POSSIBLE ADDITIONAL HUMAN PARVOVIRUSES

The discovery of an additional human virus belonging to the Parvoviridae family, in specimens obtained from children with respiratory tract disease,[27,28] was followed by confirmation of the worldwide occurrence of this virus in such conditions. The delineation of associated clinical conditions is still preliminary but this virus appeared indeed to be correlated with respiratory tract disease and also with systemic infections (see also Chapter 162).

The human bocavirus was discovered as a result of random genome amplification and after sequence analysis provisionally classified the isolate in the *Bocavirus* genus of the Parvovirinae subfamily, originally only consisting of a bovine and a canine virus, hence the name. Shortly after the description of this virus, it became clear that the virus could often be detected in respiratory secretions obtained from young children, with relatively high prevalence rates of between 1% and 19%. Although in a large proportion of the cases other respiratory pathogens were also present, there clearly were cases of lower respiratory tract disease with bocavirus as the single potential pathogen.[29] Typically, in such cases the quantity of viral DNA often appeared higher, suggesting that more common lower viral loads resulted from viral persistence for longer periods. In addition, it has been established that some infections are readily detectable in blood and therefore likely systemic in nature.[30]

Respiratory symptoms in cases of bocavirus infection are largely nonspecific, and include not only fever, cough, bronchitis, bronchiolitis and acute wheezing, but also pneumonia. Preliminary serologic findings confirmed that in particular bocavirus infections with high respiratory viral loads and viremia correlated with immune responses.[31] The virus is often detected in fecal samples but its status as a gastrointestinal pathogen is still unclear. Proper interpretation of bocavirus findings would benefit from including quantitative information or viral detection in blood to identify those infections more likely to be of clinical relevance.[32]

Another new virus belonging to the Parvoviridae was found in patients with a less clearly defined viral syndrome and has been indicated as PARV4.[33] However, in subsequent studies, no clear clinical correlates associated with detection of this virus could be defined.

REFERENCES

References for this chapter can be found online at http://www.expertconsult.com

Poxviruses

NATURE

Virion morphology, structure and biochemistry

Poxviruses are the largest of all animal viruses and can be visualized under the light microscope, although the details of the virion structure remain obscure. Using negative-staining electron microscopy and/or cryoelectron microscopy, parapoxvirus virions appear ovoid with long and short axes of approximately 260 and 160 nm, respectively, whereas all other poxviruses are 'brick'-shaped, with dimensions of 350 × 250 nm on average. In clinical specimens two forms of virion have been identified: the intact 'M' (mulberry; Fig. 159.1) form is found mainly in the vesicular fluid, and the 'C' (capsule) form, which appears to be a degenerative 'M' form, is associated with dried scabs.

Electron micrographs of thin sections of poxvirus-infected tissue culture cells have revealed at least three infectious forms of the virion: intracellular mature virions, extracellular enveloped virions and occluded virus in A-type inclusion body.[1]

It has been proposed that the intracellular mature virions form from the membrane structures of the intermediate compartment, and can acquire an additional two membranes from the Golgi, one of which is lost on egress at the plasma membrane. These extracellular enveloped virions are thought to be most important in cell-to-cell spread and systemic disease. In certain poxvirus species the intracellular mature virion can also occlude in a dense protein matrix within the cytoplasm to form an acidophilic inclusion body (A-type inclusion or Downie body), which is thought to protect the virion from the

environment.[2] All vertebrate poxviruses have cytoplasmic basophilic (B-type) inclusion bodies, which represent areas of the infected cells that contain large amounts of virus DNA and protein.

Depending on the poxvirus, the genome can range from 130 kbp for the parapoxviruses to 300 kbp for the avipoxviruses, which is sufficient to encode more than 140 proteins. A schematic intracellular replication cycle based on the poxvirus vaccinia is presented in Figure 159.2 and described in more detail by Moss.[1] The poxvirus virion is notoriously stable in the environment, and this stability is increased by its association with the A-type inclusion bodies or scab material. Thus for poxviruses, fomites must be considered in disease transmission.

Poxviruses pathogenic for humans

Ten poxviruses infect humans (Table 159.1).[2] Except for the 'extinct' variola virus and the increasingly important molluscum contagiosum virus, the poxvirus diseases are zoonoses. With rare exception these zoonotic poxviruses fail to establish a human chain of transmission. Most human poxvirus infections occur through minor abrasions in the skin. Orf, molluscum contagiosum and monkeypox viruses cause the most frequent poxvirus infections worldwide; the incidence of molluscum contagiosum and monkeypox virus infections is on the rise, the former as an opportunistic infection in late-stage AIDS and the latter as a zoonotic infection in central Africa. Individuals with atopic dermatitis may be predisposed to poxvirus infections such as molluscum contagiosum, orf or cowpox.

PREVENTION

Because most poxvirus infections are rare zoonoses or, as in molluscum contagiosum virus, cause only superficial, 'nuisance' skin lesions in immunocompetent individuals, there are no recommended prevention strategies other than education of patients and various types of workers as to how the diseases are spread.

Molluscum Contagiosum Virus

EPIDEMIOLOGY

Geographic range

Molluscum contagiosum virus has a worldwide distribution. Restriction endonuclease analysis of genomic DNA from molluscum contagiosum virus isolates has revealed the existence of at least four virus

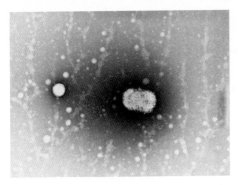

Fig. 159.1 A negative-stained M form of molluscum contagiosum virus. Molluscum contagiosum virus from lesion material.

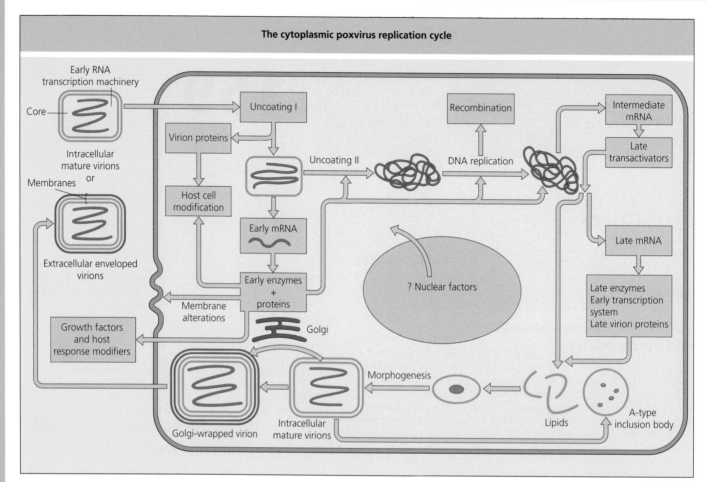

The cytoplasmic poxvirus replication cycle

Fig. 159.2 The cytoplasmic poxvirus replication cycle. Poxvirus virions containing early RNA transcription machinery attach to, and fuse with, the plasma membrane (uncoating I). Early genes are expressed that code for a variety of functions that modify the host cell for optimal virus replication, attentuate the host response to infection and mediate virus synthetic processes. After further uncoating (II), the virus genome is replicated via concatamers, late transcription factors are expressed from intermediate genes and late gene RNA is synthesized. Late genes encode the early transcription system, enzymes and structural proteins necessary for virion assembly, which commences with the formation of membrane structures in the intermediate compartment and the packaging of resolved unit length genomic DNA. The intracellular mature virion has one membrane derived from the intermediate compartment. It may remain in the cytoplasm or (in certain virus species) become occluded in an A-type inclusion body or become wrapped by a further two membranes in the Golgi and exported from the cell with the loss of one membrane (extracellular enveloped virions). The extracellular enveloped virions are thought to be most important in cell-to-cell spread and systemic disease. This replication scheme is based on the study of the prototypic poxvirus vaccinia.[1] Other poxvirus species probably vary from this model mainly in the types of growth factors and host response modifiers encoded by the virus and the amounts of extracellular enveloped virions produced. Adapted from Moss.[1]

subtypes or strains, and one recent study suggests the distribution of subtypes can vary geographically.[3]

Prevalence and incidence

For nonsexually transmitted molluscum contagiosum, the disease is more prevalent in the tropics than in Europe. For example, molluscum contagiosum was diagnosed in 1.2% of outpatients in Aberdeen, UK between 1956 and 1963, the mean age of infection was between 10 and 12 years and spread within households and schools was infrequent. On the other hand, in Fiji in 1966, 4.5% of an entire village had the disease, mean age of infection was between 2 and 3 years and 25% of households harbored more than one case.[4,5] Prevalence of infection in New Guinea was greater than 50% in many villages. In England between 1971 and 1985 there was a 400% increase in cases of genital molluscum contagiosum; the majority of patients were aged 15–24 years, with affected women being younger than affected men.[5] In the USA between 1966 and 1983 there was a 10-fold increase in cases in patients aged 25–29 years.[5] Molluscum contagiosum is a common and

sometimes severely disfiguring opportunistic infection of between 5% and 18% of patients with HIV infection, especially those with severely depressed CD4+ T-cell numbers.[6] In one study 24% of patients were also diagnosed with atopic dermatitits.[7]

PATHOGENICITY

Transmission

Molluscum contagiosum is observed in children and adults, with spread within this latter group governed in part by sexual practices. Nonsexual transmission is a consequence of infection by direct contact or through fomites. Case histories have suggested transmission from surgeons' fingers, swimming pools, bath towels in gymnasia, contact between wrestlers and as a result of tattooing.[4] Transmission between persons in the absence of fomites requires fairly close contact. Lesions can be commonly observed on opposing surfaces and the virus can be further spread on the person by autoinoculation.

Table 159.1 Poxviruses pathogenic for humans. *Presented by genus in order of importance for human disease.*

Genus/species	Hosts	Geographic distribution	Disease
Molluscipoxvirus Molluscum contagiosum virus	Humans*	Worldwide	Molluscum contagiosum, single or multiple skin nodules
Parapoxvirus Orf virus (contagious pustular dermatitis virus or contagious ecthyma virus)	Sheep*, goats, dogs, bighorn sheep, thinhorn sheep, Rocky Mountain goat, chamois, reindeer, musk-ox, Himalayan tahr, Steenbok, alpaca	Worldwide	Orf, localized skin lesions
Pseudocowpox virus (milkers' nodule or paravaccinia)	European cattle*	Worldwide	Milkers' nodule, localized skin lesions
Bovine papular stomatitis virus	European cattle*	Worldwide	Localized skin lesions
Orthopoxvirus Cowpox virus	Rodents*, cats, cows, zoo animals	Europe, western Asia	Cowpox, localized pustular lesions
Monkeypox virus	Squirrels*, monkeys	Western and central Africa	Monkeypox, rash, generalized disease
Vaccinia virus	Natural host unknown (buffalo[†] and cattle)	Asia, India, Brazil and laboratory	Buffalopox, localized pustular lesions
Variola virus	Eradicated from humans in 1977	Was worldwide	Smallpox, rash, generalized disease
Yatapoxvirus Tanapoxvirus	Monkeys? Rodents?	Eastern and central Africa	Tanapox, localized nodular skin lesions
Yaba monkey tumor poxvirus	Monkeys?	Western Africa	Localized nodular skin lesions

*Natural reservoir.
[†]During the smallpox eradication program, water buffalo in India and cattle in Brazil were infected with the local vaccine strain of vaccinia virus, which apparently persists in these animals and occasionally infects humans.
?Putative host.

Lesion histopathology

Molluscum contagiosum virus has one of the narrowest cell tropisms of any virus, replicating only in the human keratinocyte of the epidermis.[8] As the virus-infected cell approaches the surface of the skin, the accumulation of progeny virions in a granular matrix in the cytoplasm forces the cell organelles, including the nucleus, to the periphery of the cell. Under light microscopy these cells stain as hyaline acidophilic masses, are referred to as molluscum or Henderson–Patterson bodies and are pathognomonic for disease (Fig. 159.3). Higher magnifications of molluscum bodies reveal them to be entirely filled with virions, partial virions and debris.

CLINICAL MANIFESTATIONS

Signs, symptoms and severity

Molluscum contagiosum manifests as small clusters of lesions in immunocompetent individuals. The lesions are generally painless; they appear on the trunk and limbs (rarely palms and soles) in the nonsexually transmitted disease. In children, the virus can also be fairly common in the skin of the eyelids, with solitary or multiple lesions, and can be complicated by chronic follicular conjunctivitis and later by a superficial punctate keratitis.[9] There may be an associated erythema 1–11 months after the appearance of the lesion, with no correlation to a history of allergy or eczema.[10] Lesions can persist for as little as 2 weeks or as long as 2 years. Re-infections can be common. As a sexually transmitted disease in teenagers and adults, the

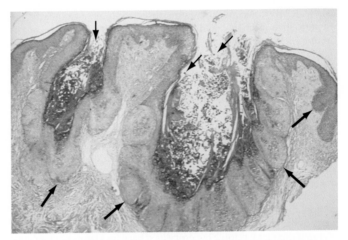

Fig. 159.3 Molluscum contagiosum lesion. In this lesion a major and minor umbilicus has formed as a result of the hypertrophy of infected cells and hyperplasia of the basal cells, which caused a severe invagination of the epidermis but no loss of integrity of the basement membrane. The molluscum bodies stain as pink to purple acidophilic hyaline masses up to 37 × 27 µm in size. Small arrows: molluscum bodies. Large arrows: epidermis–dermis boundary. (H & E.)

lesions are mostly on the lower abdominal wall, pubis, inner thighs and genitalia. As yet there is no solid correlation of virion DNA type with specific pathology or location of lesions (i.e. genital versus nongenital).[11]

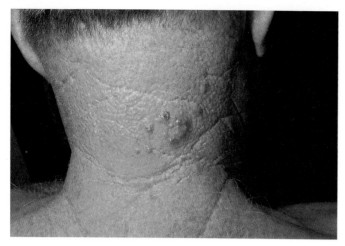

Fig. 159.4 Molluscum contagiosum lesions. These are the more typical, but still large, lesions of molluscum contagiosum. Courtesy of J Burnett.

In immunocompromised individuals (especially those with HIV infection), the infection is not self-limiting, with more frequent and larger lesions present especially on the face, neck, scalp and upper body. Multiple adjacent lesions sometimes become confluent. Molluscum contagiosum can be considered a cutaneous marker of severe immunodeficiency.

Gross lesion pathology

In immunocompetent patients, molluscum contagiosum virus lesions are epidermal, flesh-colored, raised nodules of 2–5 mm in diameter. Occasionally the gross lesions may have a hypopigmented or erythematous halo. Rarely they will present as a large lesion called giant molluscum (>5 mm in diameter). Both types of lesion usually have an umbilicated center (Fig. 159.4). Although giant molluscum lesions have been reported frequently in severely immunodeficient individuals with HIV infection, they were observed in New Guinea before the introduction of HIV, and therefore may not be a consequence of immunodeficiency.[6,12]

DIAGNOSIS AND DIFFERENTIAL DIAGNOSIS

The diagnosis is usually made clinically based on the gross appearance of the lesions and their chronic nature. Confirmation is easily obtained through the detection of molluscum bodies by hematoxylin and eosin staining of a biopsy or a squash preparation of expressed material from the lesion.

Molluscum contagiosum (especially giant molluscum) can be confused with a number of other disorders such as keratoacanthoma, warty dyskeratoma, syringomas, hidrocystomas, basal cell epithelioma, trichoepithelioma, ectopic hyperplastic sebaceous glands or giant condylomata acuminata, chalazion, sebaceous cysts, verrucas, milia, lid abscess or granuloma on eyelids.[13–15] In immunodeficient patients, disseminated cutaneous cryptococcosis and cutaneous histoplasmosis can resemble typical molluscum contagiosum.[12,13] An inflamed molluscum lesion without the association of typical lesions can be mistaken for a bacterial infection.

Parapoxviruses

The parapoxviruses orf, bovine stomatitis and pseudocowpox generally cause occupational infections of humans, with orf infections being the most common. Because of the clinical similarity of the diseases caused by these agents, they have been referred to collectively as 'farmyard-pox' diseases. No human-to-human transmission of parapoxvirus infections has been reported.

EPIDEMIOLOGY

Geographic range

Orf in sheep and goat populations has been reported in Canada, the USA, Europe, Japan, New Zealand and Africa. Pseudocowpox virus and bovine papular stomatitis virus are both maintained in European-derived dairy herds in all parts of the world.

Prevalence and incidence

In a 1-year New Zealand study 500 meat workers out of a population of 20 000 at risk were infected with orf; those involved in the initial stunning, killing and hanging of the sheep had the highest risk (4%) of infection.[16] Serologic surveys of orf-infected sheep and goat herds yielded orf antibody prevalences of up to 90%. The high seroprevalence of orf antibody in herds is likely attributable to the highly stable nature of the orf virion, which contaminates the pasture.

Pseudocowpox virus and bovine papular stomatitis are probably endemic in all European-derived dairy herds.

PATHOGENICITY

Transmission

Direct transmission of orf virus has been observed as a consequence of bottle-feeding lambs, from animal bites to the hand and contact with sheep and goat products during slaughter. Fomites such as splinters, barbed wire or farmyard surfaces, including soil, feeding troughs or barn beams, have been implicated as sources of virus.

Pseudocowpox virus from lesions on teats of cows is a major source of virus for milkers' nodule of the hand.

Bovine papular stomatitis virus infection of humans occurs generally from lesions confined to the mouth, tongue, lips or nares and occasionally from the teats of infected cattle.

Lesion histopathology

Epidermis

The most striking change in the epidermis is hyperplasia in which strands of epidermal keratinocytes penetrate the dermis.[17] Generally, a mild to moderate degree of acanthosis is detected, and parakeratosis is a common feature. Cytoplasmic vacuolation, nuclear vacuolation and deeply eosinophilic, homogeneous cytoplasmic inclusion bodies often surrounded by a pale halo are also characteristic of the infection. An intense infiltrate of lymphocytes, polymorphs or eosinophils frequently involves the epidermis.

Dermis

A dense, predominantly lymphohistiocytic inflammatory cell infiltrate is present in all cases with marked edema. The most striking feature of the dermis is the massive capillary proliferation and dilatation.

CLINICAL MANIFESTATIONS

Signs, symptoms and severity

The clinical presentation of orf is usually 3–4 weeks after infection. The disease involves the appearance of single or multiple nodules (diameters of 6–27 mm),[17] which are sometimes painful, usually on the hands and, less frequently, on the head or neck. Orf infection can also be associated with a low-grade fever, swelling of the lymph nodes and/or erythema multiforme bullosum. Resolution of the disease occurs over 4–6 weeks, usually without complication; however, autoinoculations of the eye can lead to serious sequelae, and enlarged lesions can arise in humans suffering from immunosuppressive conditions, burns or atopic dermatitis.[18] Lesion healing can be complicated by bullous pemphigoid.[19] Re-infections have been documented.[16]

Pseudocowpox virus lesions usually appear on the hands and are relatively painless, but may itch. The draining lymph node may be enlarged. The nodules are gradually absorbed and disappear in 4–6 weeks.[20]

In bovine papular stomatitis, lesions occur on the hands, diminish after 14 days and are no longer evident 3–4 weeks after onset.[21]

Gross lesion pathology

The orf lesion characteristically goes through a maculopapular target stage in which a red center is surrounded by a white ring of cells which is surrounded by a red halo of inflammation (approximately 1–2 weeks after infection); however, patients usually present later when the lesion is at the granulomatous or papillomatous stages.[18]

In pseudocowpox virus infection, milkers' nodules are first observed as round, cherry-red papules; these develop into purple, smooth nodules of up to 2 cm in diameter and may be umbilicated. The lesions rarely ulcerate.[20]

The lesions of bovine papular stomatitis appear as circumscribed wart-like nodules that gradually enlarge until they are 3–8 mm in diameter.[21]

DIAGNOSIS AND DIFFERENTIAL DIAGNOSIS

Parapoxvirus disease diagnosis is by clinical (lesion morphology) and epidemiologic (recent contact with cattle or sheep) evidence, and electron microscopy of negative-stained lesion material (presence of ovoid particles).[17]

Without knowing the animal source of the infection, orf cannot easily be differentiated from milkers' nodule on the basis of clinical finding, histology or electron microscopy (i.e. disease acquired from sheep is orf and from cattle is milkers' nodule or possibly bovine papular stomatitis).[17] Atypical giant orf lesions in patients who are immunocompromised or suffering from burns or atopic dermatitis may be confused with pyogenic granuloma.[18,22] Orf can also be misdiagnosed as inflammatory vascular neoplasms.

Orthopoxviruses

Although four orthopoxviruses have been shown to cause disease in humans, only two still cause significant human infections. With the global eradication of the disease smallpox in 1977, the causative agent variola virus no longer circulates in human populations, but there is concern that it may be used as a biologic weapon by terrorist groups or rogue nations (see Chapter 71).[23]

In nature, vaccinia virus infections are limited to exposure to a vaccinia-like virus infecting milking buffalos and dairy cattle in Asia and Africa (called buffalopox) and cattle in Brazil (Cantagalo virus). Vaccinia virus (smallpox vaccine) is used also in the immunization of personnel in the laboratory, but is not recommended at this time for the general population due to the occurrence of frequent and sometimes severe complications.[23] Currently only monkeypox and cowpox viruses cause significant human infections, and the incidence of human monkeypox is increasing.

EPIDEMIOLOGY

Geographic range

Traditionally monkeypox virus is found in the tropical rain forests of countries in western and central Africa, most notably the Democratic Republic of the Congo, but its range may be expanding. In 2003 monkeypox virus was imported into the USA in a shipment of rodents destined for the pet trade, and in 2005 an outbreak was recorded in southern Sudan.[24] The reservoir of monkeypox virus in nature is most likely the African arboreal squirrels (*Funisciurus* and *Heliosciurus* spp.), other rodents and perhaps monkeys.[24] Cowpox virus is endemic in Europe and some western states of the former Soviet Union. Rodents (voles, wood mice and rats) have been implicated as reservoirs of cowpox virus; cows, zoo animals and cats are incidental hosts.[24]

Prevalence and incidence

Intensive surveillance between 1981 and 1986 in Zaire by the World Health Organization confirmed 338 cases of human monkeypox, with the greatest risk of infection to inhabitants of small villages within 100 m of tropical rain forests.[25] In recent years there has been an increase in the frequency of human monkeypox in central Africa, perhaps due in part to the cessation of vaccination for smallpox.[24]

Although humans have been infected by cows and rodents, the domestic cat is responsible for the majority of human cowpox infections. Between 1969 and 1993 there were approximately 45 human cowpox cases in the UK, three published case histories from Germany and two each from Belgium, Sweden and France.[26]

PATHOGENICITY

Transmission

The exact mode of transmission of monkeypox virus from an animal source to humans is not known but may be via the oropharynx or nasopharynx or through abrasions of the skin or oral cavity. Person-to-person transmission (like eradicated smallpox) is believed to be by the upper respiratory tract, with virus released in oropharyngeal secretions of patients who have a rash.[25] Unlike smallpox, monkeypox person-to-person transmission is very inefficient and rarely surpasses three generations.[25]

Cowpox virus is acquired usually by direct introduction of the virus from an animal source into minor abrasions in the skin; however, 30% of infections show no known risk factor.[26]

Lesion histopathology

Orthopoxvirus lesions are characterized by epidermal hyperplasia, with infected cells becoming swollen, vacuolated and undergoing 'ballooning degeneration'.[26]

CLINICAL MANIFESTATIONS

Signs, symptoms and severity

Approximately 12 days after infection with monkeypox virus, fever and headache occur. This is followed 1–3 days later by a rash and generalized lymphadenopathy. The rash (the number of lesions is variable) appears first on the face and generally has a centrifugal distribution. The illness lasts 2–4 weeks, depending on its severity. The case fatality rate is approximately 12%.[25]

With cowpox virus infection, a lesion, usually solitary, appears on the hands or face; this can be extremely painful, and the patient can present with systemic symptoms, including pyrexia, malaise, lethargy, sore throat and local lymphadenopathy. Complete recovery takes between 3 and 8 weeks. Person-to-person transmission has not been reported. Complications can include ocular or generalized infections; the latter occurs in patients who have atopic dermatitis, allergic asthma or atopic eczema and in one case was associated with death.[26]

Gross lesion pathology

The monkeypox virus skin lesions begin as macules but rapidly progress to pustules. About 8 or 9 days after the onset of rash the pustules become umbilicated and dry up; by 14–16 days after the onset of the rash a crust has formed. Most skin lesions are about 0.5 cm in diameter.[25]

The cowpox lesion appears as an inflamed macule, progresses through an increasingly hemorrhagic vesicle stage to a pustule that ulcerates and crusts over by the end of the second week to become a deep-seated, hard black eschar 1–3 cm in diameter.[26]

DIAGNOSIS AND DIFFERENTIAL DIAGNOSIS

The diagnosis of monkeypox infection requires clinical (rash), epidemiologic (equatorial Africa) and laboratory (brick-shaped virion in scab material) findings. Although the rash with associated lymphadenopathy is usually pathognomonic, the sporadic nature of the disease makes it difficult to arrive at an accurate diagnosis solely on clinical grounds.[25]

Diagnosis of cowpox virus infection is rarely made on clinical findings (lesion morphology and systemic illness) and usually requires laboratory results (brick-shaped virion in scab material). Cowpox should be considered in patients who have had contact with cats and who present in July to October with a painful hemorrhagic vesicle or black eschar, with or without erythema, accompanied by lymphadenopathy and a systemic illness.[26]

Monkeypox can be confused with a number of other conditions that result in a rash:

- chickenpox, although its varicella-zoster lesions are more superficial, appear in crops and have a centripetal distribution;
- tanapox, except the tanapox lesions evolve slowly, are nodular and large, without pustulation; and
- syphilis, although the secondary rash of syphilis does not evolve past the papular stage.[25]

Generalized cowpox can be misdiagnosed as eczema herpeticum, whereas localized cowpox is most frequently misdiagnosed as:

- orf or milkers' nodules, although the parapoxvirus lesion is clinically distinct, and there are often no systemic disease symptoms;
- herpes virus reactivation, even though herpes lesions are not usually hemorrhagic or erythematous and the scab is not so deep-seated and of lighter color; and
- anthrax, although the anthrax lesion is painless and rapidly progresses to the eschar stage (5–6 days).[26]

DIAGNOSTIC MICROBIOLOGY

The appropriate biosafety level precautions must be taken for the handling, transport and processing of infected lesion material.[27]

Molluscum contagiosum virus

For a squash preparation the keratotic dome-shaped molluscum lesion is placed on a regular slide and under a coverslip or second slide.

The lesion is flattened and can be examined using light microscopy either directly or after staining with Wright's or methylene blue stains. Round to ovoid molluscum bodies up to 37 × 27 μm are diagnostic of molluscum contagiosum.[4]

For histopathologic analysis, a biopsy specimen is fixed in 10% formal saline and submitted for wax embedding, sectioning at 5 μm and staining with hematoxylin and eosin. Microscopic examination should provide a field of view similar to that shown in Figure 159.3.

Parapoxvirus, orthopoxvirus and yatapoxvirus

Orthopoxvirus (brick-shaped), parapoxvirus (ovoid) and tanapox virus (enveloped brick-shaped) virions can be differentiated from one another by an experienced electron microscopist. Scab material or fluid from the vesicle should be processed by standard methods for negative-staining electron microscopy.[27] Polymerase chain reaction is rapidly becoming the assay of choice for laboratory diagnosis of poxvirus infections.[28]

MANAGEMENT

The management of parapoxvirus, orthopoxvirus and yatapoxvirus infections is supportive. Although at this time there are no approved systemic or topical chemotherapeutic agents commercially available for the treatment of poxvirus infections, it is anticipated that cidofovir or related compounds will be approved to treat orf virus, molluscum contagiosum virus and orthopoxvirus infections.[29,30] One new compound, ST-246, an orthopoxvirus egress inhibitor, is a promising candidate for early treatment of othopoxvirus infections.[31] Prevention of secondary bacterial infections through the use of antibiotic ointments is an option. In the case of cowpox, corticosteroids are contraindicated and may exacerbate the illness.[26] Because of the chronic nature of molluscum contagiosum lesions, one can consider curettage and cryotherapy of lesions. Removal of giant molluscum lesions, but not regular lesions, usually results in scar formation. Molluscum lesions may remit when HIV infection is controlled with anti-HIV therapy.

CURETTAGE WITH AN ANALGESIC

With children, pretreatment of molluscum lesions with lidocaine (lignocaine)–prilocaine for between 1 and 30 hours under plastic occlusion resulted in a decrease in the reported pain on lesion removal with a comedo extractor or curette.

CRYOTHERAPY

Molluscum lesions are treated for 6–30 seconds with a cotton-tipped applicator dipped in liquid nitrogen; this is repeated at 3-week intervals as needed. Cryotherapy is relatively painless, cost-effective and yields good cosmetic results. For patients with HIV infection, this treatment has the added advantage of mitigating the risk of disease transmission to medical personnel.

REFERENCES

References for this chapter can be found online at http://www.expertconsult.com

Mary J Warrell
David A Warrell

Chapter | **160**

Rabies and rabies-related viruses

INTRODUCTION

Rabies is a zoonosis of dogs and other mammals that is occasionally transmitted to humans, causing fatal encephalomyelitis. Dog rabies virus is universally fatal in humans and is the cause of more than 95% of human rabies deaths. However, prophylaxis can be 100% effective, so all human deaths are due to a failure of prevention.

Classic rabies virus is genotype 1 of the lyssaviruses, and genotypes 2–7 are rabies related-viruses, which may also cause fatal human infections[1] (see end of chapter). They are members of the large Rhabdoviridae family of animals and plants.

STRUCTURE

The bullet-shaped virions contain a nonsegmented negative strand of rabies RNA encoding five proteins. The RNA is coiled with a nucleoprotein, a phosphoprotein and an RNA-dependent RNA polymerase to form a helical ribonucleoprotein complex or nucleocapsid. This is covered by a matrix protein. An outer coat studded with the virus-coded, glycoprotein-bearing, club-shaped projections is acquired by budding through a host cell lipid membrane. Rabies virus strains from different vector species and geographic areas are distinguished by nucleotide sequencing and monoclonal antibody typing.

EPIDEMIOLOGY

Animal rabies

Rabies is enzootic in most parts of the world. Globally, the domestic dog is the most important reservoir species and is the dominant vector in Asia, Africa and urban areas of Latin America. Separate reservoirs of enzootic infection occur in certain wild mammalian species (Table 160.1). The sylvatic pattern of infection predominates in North America,[2,3] Europe, parts of southern Africa[4] and the Caribbean.[1] All mammals are potentially susceptible, and infection may be transmitted to other species, including domestic animals, especially cats, and to humans. Lyssaviruses have not been reported from a few areas including Iceland, Norway, Sweden, Finland, Italy, Greece, Cyprus, some other Mediterranean islands, Singapore, Sabah, Sarawak, New Guinea, New Zealand, Antarctica, Oceania, Hong Kong islands, Japan, Taiwan and some Caribbean islands. Although these countries have no apparent indigenous rabies, infected animals cross national boundaries and so infection may be imported. Genotype 1 (classic rabies) infects terrestrial mammalian reservoir species and bats in the American. Western Europe and Australia are free of genotype 1 rabies, but rabies-related lyssaviruses are found in bats (see Table 160.1). As the epizootiology changes constantly, up-to-date local advice should be sought for detailed information.

Human rabies

Estimates of human rabies mortality are notoriously unreliable in tropical areas where about 99% of the deaths occur. In Asia and Africa, 55 000 deaths annually are estimated. However, it is suspected that only 3% of cases are recorded, and the rate of underreporting may be 20 times in Asia and 160 times in Africa. Areas of high incidence include India, Bangladesh and Pakistan. There is very little surveillance in Africa.

In Europe, 5–10 deaths are reported annually, usually in Eastern Europe or in cases imported from Asia or Africa. In the USA, an average of three cases were diagnosed annually from 2000 to 2006. Up to 80% of cases are indigenous, and 90% are associated with insectivorous bat rabies virus. Although few (39%) patients remember a bat bite, possible bat contact is more often reported.

PATHOGENICITY

Transmission

Human infection is usually the result of a bite by a rabid dog or other mammal. Virus in saliva can penetrate broken skin or intact mucous membranes, and so scratches or licks by a rabid animal may cause infection.

On two occasions, human rabies may have resulted from inhalation of virus in caves in Texas that were densely populated by insectivorous bats,[5] and after laboratory accidents with aerosols of virus. The saliva, respiratory secretions and tears of rabies patients contain virus,[6] which could infect another person, but the only documented instances of human-to-human transmission have been through human tissue transplants from donors in whom rabies had not been suspected. Eight cases of infection by corneal graft have been reported. In the USA and Germany, two donors transmitted rabies to seven recipients of solid-organ transplants (kidney, liver, lung, pancreas) and one patient received only a segment of artery.[7] Several women with rabies encephalitis have delivered healthy infants. Only one case of neonatal rabies has been reported, although vertical transmission is well documented in animals.

Pathogenesis[8,9] (Fig. 160.1)

Rabies virus will attach to a variety of cellular receptors, but in a bite wound, competitive binding to acetylcholine receptors at neuromuscular junctions is a possible route of entry into the nervous system.

Table 160.1 Distribution of rabies reservoir species

Africa	Domestic dog (*Canis familiaris*) Black-backed jackals (*Canis mesomelas*) Yellow mongoose (*Cynictis penicillata*) Bat-eared fox (*Otocyon megalotis*) Frugivorous and insectivorous bats (bat lyssaviruses; see Table 160.3)	Widespread dominant reservoir Southern Africa Southern Africa Southern Africa
Asia	Domestic dog (*Canis familiaris*) Wolf (*Lupus lupus*)	Widespread dominant reservoir Middle East
Americas	Arctic fox (*Alopex lagopus*) Red fox (*Vulpes fulva*) Gray fox (*Urocyon cinereoargenteus*) Striped skunk (*Mephitis* spp.) Raccoon (*Procyon lotor*) Frugivorous bats Insectivorous bats Vampire bat (*Desmodus* spp.) Mongoose (*Herpestes* spp.) Domestic dog (*Canis familiaris*)	Alaska, North-west Canada Western Canada and north-east USA Texas, Arizona Texas, Central USA, California Eastern USA, south-east Canada South America Very widespread Mexico, Trinidad, Tobago, Isla de Margarita, northern South America Puerto Rico Mexico, parts of central and South America
Australia	Flying foxes or fruit bats (*Pteropus* spp.) Insectivorous bats (Australian bat lyssavirus; see Table 160.3)	Eastern coastal area
Europe	Red fox (*Vulpes vulpes*) Arctic fox (*Alopex lagopus*) Raccoon dog (*Nyctereutes procyonoides*) Wolf (*Lupus lupus*) Domestic dog (*Canis familiaris*) Insectivorous bats (European bat lyssaviruses; see Table 160.3)	Eastern Europe, Russian Federation Northern Russia Eastern Europe Eastern Europe, Russian Federation Turkey (act as vectors in Eastern Europe and Russian Federation) Widespread

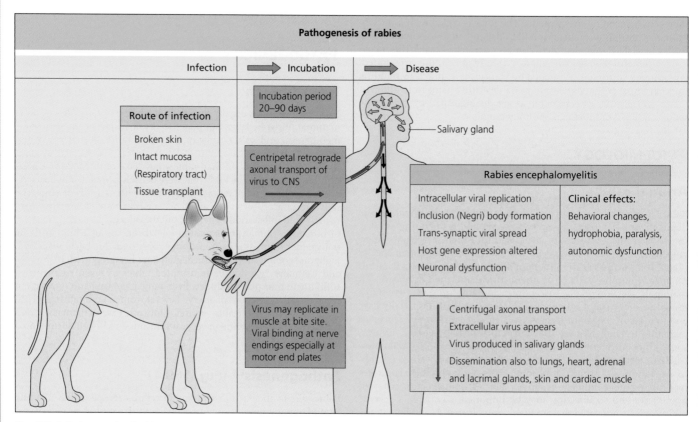

Fig. 160.1 Pathogenesis of rabies.

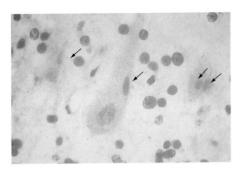

Fig. 160.2 Negri bodies in cerebellar Purkinje cells in a human victim of rabies encephalitis. The intracytoplasmic, dark-staining Negri bodies are marked with arrows. Courtesy of Armed Forces Institute of Pathology, Bethesda, USA.

During the incubation period, the virus or viral components travel to the central nervous system by retrograde axonal transport. Infection can be halted by sectioning the nerve or by disrupting microtubular function. It is presumed that viral proteins are carried by microtubule motor molecules, particularly dynein, but the means of attachment is still unknown, possibly because there is more than one mechanism.

When the virus reaches the brain, replication proceeds in neurons by budding from intracellular membranes and accumulations of viral proteins form inclusions, large examples of which are the classic Negri bodies (Fig. 160.2). The virus spreads trans-synaptically and remains intraneuronal and hidden from immune recognition. The viral glycoprotein is essential for transfer to adjacent cells.

Disruption of neuronal physiology has been observed experimentally, including neurotransmitter activity, electroencephalograph patterns and ion-channel function. The demonstrated viral effects on host gene expression are either upregulation of genes which could enhance viral spread and replication, and downregulation of genes related to cell protein synthesis. The latter will impair cell metabolism and probably contributes to the widespread dysfunction of apparently intact neurons. Viral pathogenicity correlates with low levels of rabies glycoprotein expression, inhibition of host protein synthesis, a minimal inflammatory response and little if any apoptosis. Pathologic features of diffuse encephalomyelitis may be minimal or even absent in humans.

The virus progresses centrifugally, again via peripheral nerves, to many tissues including the salivary and lachrymal glands, where replication produces extracellular rabies virus, which may initiate an immune response (see Fig. 160.1).

Immunology

Following infection, rabies virus evades the immune system[10] and no immunologic response can be detected in unvaccinated patients before signs of encephalitis develop. Rabies antibody does not appear until 1–2 weeks after the onset of symptoms, if at all, and later in the cerebrospinal fluid (CSF). Rabies-specific IgM is not detectable any earlier than IgG. The presence of antibody is diagnostic in unvaccinated patients. Specific transformation of peripheral blood lymphocytes has been found in a few patients with furious rabies, but not in paralytic cases. The reverse is found experimentally in rabid mice. The virus is immunosuppressive, which is reflected in the minimal histopathologic changes in the brain. Interferon (IFN) production in humans is very low, and high levels of IFN-α and IFN-β in animal brains do not protect animals against death. T lymphocytes are not efficient in combating rabies and, surprisingly, apoptosis of immune reactive CD3+ T cells has been observed in mouse brains.[10] Clearance of a lethal virus from the brain and recovery in rodents is associated with early induction of neutralizing antibody, increased expression of viral genes, a greater inflammatory response, early appearance of IFN-γ and neuronal apoptosis. The result is limitation of viral spread, as well as an inevitable loss of neuronal tissue.[10]

CONTROL

The elimination of rabies virus from domestic dogs would prevent more than 95% of human rabies deaths, without any need of expensive prophylaxis. This has been achieved, for example, in Western Europe, North America, Japan, several urban areas of Latin America[11] and even one in India.[12] Mass killing is ineffective, but campaigns of dog vaccination and population control can be successful, if accompanied by enthusiastic education, publicity and adequate funding. Although oral vaccination of dogs is possible, it remains impracticable.

Appropriate rabies control strategies are based on surveillance to determine the principal domestic or wild reservoir species, with laboratory diagnosis to confirm the local prevalence of infection.

Sylvatic rabies has been eliminated in the red fox *Vulpes vulpes* in Western Europe by distributing oral vaccine in suitable baits around the countryside. Repeated campaigns of oral vaccination with either a live attenuated rabies virus or a vaccinia-recombinant vaccine expressing rabies glycoprotein are needed over many years. In North America, raccoons and foxes have been similarly immunized,[3] as well as jackals in southern Africa. Vaccines for skunks and mongooses are being developed. Control of vampire bat rabies,[11] which causes many deaths in cattle in Latin America, is attempted by treating cattle with small doses of anticoagulant in order to poison the bats. Vaccination of cattle is possible but expensive. No active measures are taken to control rabies in insectivorous or fruit bats in the Americas, Europe, Africa or Australia, but instructions are issued to encourage people to avoid direct contact with these animals.

CLINICAL FEATURES

The incubation period (bite to first symptom) ranges from 4 days to at least 19 years, but in about 75% of cases it is between 20 and 90 days. The only prodromal symptoms that are reasonably suggestive of rabies are itching, pain or paresthesiae, either at the site of the causative bite or radiating proximally from it. After 1–7 days of generally nonspecific symptoms, features of either furious or paralytic (dumb) rabies develop.

The pathognomonic symptom of furious rabies is hydrophobia[13] or aerophobia. Jerky and violent contractions of the diaphragm and accessory muscles of inspiration are associated with an inexplicable terror. This reflex can be provoked by attempts to drink liquid or by a draught of air on the skin. The hydrophobic spasm may end with the patient in opisthotonos, having generalized convulsions and in cardiac or respiratory arrest. Other features of furious rabies are periods of excitement, sometimes with hallucinations or aggression, interspersed with lucid intervals; fever; tachycardia and other arrhythmias; hypersalivation; lacrimation; sweating; and fluctuating temperature and blood pressure. All these features are suggestive of stimulation of the autonomic nervous system as seen in severe tetanus. Conventional neurologic examination may prove surprisingly normal, unless hydrophobia is provoked, but meningism, cranial nerve lesions, upper motor neuron lesions, fasciculation and involuntary movements are sometimes detected. Without intensive care, patients usually die, often during a hydrophobic spasm, in the first few days of their encephalitic symptoms.

Paralytic or dumb rabies is probably underdiagnosed but was recognized during an epidemic of rabies transmitted by vampire bats in Trinidad in the 1920s and 1930s. Although associated particularly with vampire bat rabies and other genotype 1 bat infections (i.e. in the Americas), it is also seen in patients bitten by dogs. After the prodromal symptoms described above, together with headache, local paresthesiae and flaccid paralysis develop, usually in the bitten limb, and ascend symmetrically or asymmetrically. There is accompanying pain and fasciculation in the affected muscles and mild objective sensory disturbances. Death follows paralysis of the muscles of deglutition and respiration; there is usually no evidence of hydrophobia or aerophobia.

Patients with rabies whose lives are prolonged by intensive care may develop a variety of respiratory, cardiovascular, neurologic and gastrointestinal complications including fatal cardiac arrhythmias, pneumothorax, cerebral edema, diabetes insipidus, inappropriate antidiuretic hormone secretion, hypo- or hyperpyrexia, diffuse axonal neuropathy and hematemesis.

Differential diagnosis

Severe and unusual neurologic symptoms, whether encephalitic or paralytic, should suggest the possibility of rabies in any unimmunized person who has had contact with mammals in a rabies-endemic area. However, children may not report animal contact and rabies patients infected by bats in the USA usually deny any exposure to a bat.

Furious rabies can be mimicked by the pharyngeal form of cephalic tetanus ('hydrophobic tetanus'); however, severe tetanus usually has a shorter incubation period than rabies and there is sustained muscle rigidity, often associated with trismus. Delirium tremens and the excitatory effects of some plant toxins and recreational drugs[7] have been confused with rabies. Paralytic rabies is indistinguishable from many other causes of an ascending paralysis, including postvaccinal encephalomyelitis complicating the use of obsolete nervous tissue rabies vaccines still used in Asia, Africa and Latin America.

Prognosis and recovery

Patients with furious rabies encephalitis usually die within 2 weeks, but some patients with paralytic rabies have survived for as long as 1 month, even without intensive care.

Only six documented cases of recovery from rabies, or survival for more than 2 years, have been reported during the virologic era.[14] No rabies virus or antigen was detected in any of them and all were diagnosed serologically. Two patients were treated after exposure with nervous tissue vaccines and recovered. The diagnosis of one of these was doubtful and the second was a 6-year-old boy bitten by a bat in Ohio, USA,[15] who began having duck embryo rabies vaccine 4 days later. He recovered completely from an encephalitic illness and lives a normal life.

Three other patients, given only pre-exposure nervous tissue vaccine or postexposure tissue culture vaccine, were left with profound neurologic deficits.

The first unvaccinated patient known to survive is a 15-year-old girl in Wisconsin, USA, bitten by a bat.[16] She developed paresthesiae of the bitten hand and features of paralytic rabies, including progressive cranial nerve paralyses and leg weakness, with fever and hypersalivation. Rabies antibody had appeared unusually early, by the sixth day after the onset of symptoms, but no virus or antigen was detected. Her intensive treatment included ketamine-induced coma and the antiviral agents ribavirin and amantadine. She has made a slow recovery over 3 years, with only minor residual neurologic deficits, and has graduated from high school. This case has features similar to the boy in Ohio. It is likely that they both had rabies antibody present at, or soon after, the onset of symptoms and had no damaging hydrophobic spasms. They are the only reported 'survivors' who were infected by an American bat virus, genotype 1, which has a different pattern of infection from the dog rabies strains experimentally. It is slower to evolve and progress and there is relatively little neuronal apoptosis. However, the treatment protocol that was apparently effective in the Wisconsin girl has not proved effective in several other patients infected by bats or dogs.[17]

DIAGNOSIS

Confirmation of the diagnosis of rabies encephalitis should be possible within a day, if ideal samples are supplied to a specialist laboratory (Table 160.2). Rapid identification of antigen can be followed by virus isolation and, in unvaccinated patients, by detecting antibody.[18]

Table 160.2 Diagnostic methods

Diagnostic sample	Aim	Method
Full thickness **skin**[†] punch biopsy	Antigen detection	IFA test on frozen section / RT-PCR
Saliva Tears CSF	Virus isolation and antigen detection	Tissue culture / Mouse inoculation test / RT-PCR
Serum	Antibody test	Detectable antibody is diagnostic in unvaccinated patients / Save sample for comparison later if vaccinated previously
CSF	Antibody test	Test in parallel with serum
REPEAT skin and saliva samples daily until a diagnosis is confirmed		
Brain post-mortem: needle biopsy[‡] or autopsy sample brain stem and cerebellum	Virus isolation and antigen detection	Tissue culture / Mouse inoculation test / IFA test on impression smear / RT-PCR

[†]Bold = most important, potentially helpful, samples
[‡]See text for details.

Skin, saliva, respiratory secretions, CSF, tears and brain are all suitable samples, but a full-thickness skin biopsy is the most likely to yield a rapid result. A punch biopsy is taken from a hairy area, usually at the nape of the neck. Frozen sections show the characteristic immunofluorescent staining of rabies antigen visible in nervous tissue around the base of hair follicles. With controls to ensure specificity and examination of many sections, sensitivity is 60–100%.[19] False-positive results have not been reported, whereas the corneal impression test is insensitive and false-positive results do occur. Reverse transcriptase polymerase chain reaction (RT-PCR) can be performed on the samples mentioned, although skin and saliva are the most likely to be positive. Viral isolation in suckling mice or tissue culture is the ideal method of diagnosis. Genetic analysis will indicate the likely reservoir species and geographic origin of the virus. Tests should be repeated until the diagnosis of rabies is excluded.

In unvaccinated patients, diagnostic seroconversion usually occurs in the second week of illness.[20] In vaccinated patients, very high levels of antibody both in the serum and in the CSF have been used to make a diagnosis.[15]

Post-mortem brain samples should be cultured, but antigen can be detected by immunofluorescent staining of impression smears, enzyme immunoassay or RT-PCR. A needle necropsy of brain can be taken without a full autopsy by inserting a Vim-Silverman needle via the medial canthus of the eye through the superior orbital fissure, via the foramen magnum, or via the nose and ethmoid sinus.

MANAGEMENT

No antiviral or ancillary treatments have proved effective in animal models and human rabies of canine origin remains 100% fatal. Patients should be admitted to hospital so that their agonizing symptoms can be palliated with adequate doses of analgesic and sedative drugs.[21] Friends, family and medical staff in close contact with the patient should be given postexposure vaccination as reassurance, even though such person-to-person transmission has not been documented.

Intensive care may be appropriate for patients infected by an American bat, who present early and are already seropositive. New antiviral methods may yet be discovered against rabies, perhaps combined with an immunologic approach (e.g. IFN-γ). Until a treatment has proved effective experimentally, intensive care therapy is usually inappropriate, especially in developing countries.

PREVENTION

Postexposure prophylaxis[3,22–24]

In a rabies-endemic area, the risk of infection, and hence the decision to give postexposure prophylaxis, depends on the species of animal, its behavior and the circumstances of contact. An unprovoked attack by a known local vector suggests a high risk of exposure to rabies, especially if the animal is unvaccinated, is unusually excitable or is partially paralyzed, or if a wild animal is unusually tame. Vaccinated animals have, however, transmitted rabies. The virus gains access through any bite, scratch or contamination of broken skin or mucous membrane, but intact skin is an adequate barrier against infection. Bites or scratches by bats may pass unnoticed. The risk of infection is greatest from bites on the head, neck and hands, and multiple bites carry a higher risk than single bites.[25] Before vaccines were available, the mortality from all proven rabid dog bites in India was 35–57%.

Strenuous efforts should be made to have the biting animal tested for rabies. The routine immunofluorescent test for antigen may give a false-negative result in 1–2% of rabies cases. In addition, as the test is unreliable for rabies-related viruses, the result of viral culture is important in highly suspicious cases. Specific treatment should not await laboratory results and it should always be started immediately, irrespective of the time since the bite.

Postexposure prophylaxis aims to inactivate rabies virus in a wound and to stimulate immunity to kill the virus before it enters the nervous system, where it is protected from immune attack. Postexposure therapy includes urgent wound treatment, active prophylaxis with vaccine and passive immunization with rabies immune globulin (RIG). The complete therapy is very effective, and failures of optimal treatment started on the day of exposure are rare. Seven cases have been reported following high-risk exposure. However, many deaths occur because treatment is often delayed, unaffordable, inadequate or incomplete.

Treatment of mammal bites, scratches or licks

The treatment can be summarized as follows:
1. Scrub vigorously with soap or detergent and water, reaching the depth of the wound, and remove foreign material. Local or even general anesthesia may be necessary to allow effective wound cleaning and debridement, especially for children.
2. Swab with a virucidal agent: povidone iodine or 40–70% ethanol. (The virucidal effect of quaternary ammonium compounds is neutralized by soap, and so they are not recommended.)
3. Suturing of wounds should be avoided or delayed.
4. Tetanus prophylaxis (tetanus immune globulin or toxoid booster plus metronidazole) must not be forgotten. Antibiotic prophylaxis against other potential wound pathogens is recommended only in the case of bites on the hands.
5. If there is a risk of rabies, give specific therapy immediately.

Rabies vaccines

Vaccines of nervous tissue origin

All human rabies vaccines contain killed virus. Those produced from infected sheep or goat brain (Semple vaccines) and suckling mouse brain (SMB) are still used in Asia and Africa. SMB vaccine is also used in parts of South America. These are weak antigens and neurologic reactions still occur (1:200 Semple vaccinees).[14]

Purified tissue culture vaccines

Tissue culture-grown vaccines are used exclusively in North America, Europe, China, Thailand, Sri Lanka, India, Nepal and the Philippines and increasingly in other countries. The use of the original expensive human diploid cell vaccine (HDCV) is giving way to cheaper vaccines of equivalent efficacy and safety, including German and Indian purified chick embryo cell vaccines (PCECV) and a French purified Vero cell vaccine (PVRV), which are now widely distributed in endemic areas.

Immunologic response to vaccination

The presence of serum-neutralizing antibody is the best available indicator of protection against rabies, and it appears 7–14 days after starting a primary course of a modern rabies vaccine. A level of 0.5 IU/ml is considered satisfactory, although the protective level cannot be ascertained in humans. Only the viral surface glycoprotein molecules induce neutralizing antibody. They also stimulate helper and cytotoxic T-lymphocyte responses.

The speed and degree of the antibody response to vaccine varies, probably under genetic influence. A relatively delayed, lower level of antibody is found in about 3% of people receiving vaccine. Increasing age and immunosuppression, for example by HIV infection, also impair the response.

The induction of neutralizing antibody can be enhanced by increasing the amount of antigen (within limits) or by dividing the dose between multiple sites and injecting it intradermally.

Postexposure vaccine regimens

Intramuscular vaccine regimens

The standard regimen is one dose of tissue culture vaccine (1 ml or 0.5 ml, depending on the product) intramuscularly into the deltoid on days 0, 3, 7, 14 and 28.

Intradermal vaccine regimens

The five-dose intramuscular regimen is unaffordable by the vast majority of patients in developing countries, but other more economic regimens are as immunogenic as the standard method[26] and have proved effective. The World Health Organization recommends multiple-site intradermal (ID) economical regimens using specified vaccines – PVRV, PCECV and HDCV.[22,24] The manufacturers' instructions must be used for all other vaccines.

An eight-site regimen[22,24,27] consists of:
- Day 0: eight ID injections of 0.1 ml using a whole vial divided between the deltoids, thighs and suprascapular and lower abdominal areas
- Day 7: four doses of 0.1 ml over the deltoids and thighs
- Day 28: two 0.1 ml doses over the deltoids.

Human diploid cell vaccine or PCECV can be used, as the ampoule contains 1 ml, but it is not economic using PVRV with an ampoule of 0.5 ml. The eight-site regimen has a wide margin of safety because an adequate antibody response has been achieved with only four of the eight initial ID doses. Only three visits are needed. Patients who are anxious about the risk of rabies do not object to the method.

A two-site regimen[22,24] consists of:

- Days 0, 3, 7 and 28: two ID doses (0.1 or 0.2 ml depending on whether the intramuscular vaccine dose is 0.5 or 1.0 ml) over the deltoids.

Although it can be used economically with all three vaccines, ampoules of vaccine must be shared at each of four or five visits. The two-site regimen has proved effective in thousands of patients who usually also received RIG treatment in Thailand, the Philippines and Sri Lanka.

The eight-site regimen has induced higher levels of antibody than the two-site regimen from the earliest sample on day 7, onwards.[28] All the ID regimens require a similar amount of vaccine, less than two intramuscular doses, a saving of 60%. When one ampoule is shared between several patients, a new syringe and needle must be used for each. Diluted vaccine must be stored in a refrigerator and used within 8 hours.

These economic regimens are used in a few areas in Asia, but hardly at all in Africa due to practical and pharmaceutical difficulties. A new, simplified four-site ID regimen overcomes many of the problems, is immunogenic and can be used with vaccines of any ampoule size. It has all the advantages of the eight-site method, including the need for only three visits.[26]

A four-site regimen consists of:

- Day 0: four ID injections using a whole vial divided between the deltoid and thigh areas
- Day 7: two doses (0.1 or 0.2 ml depending on whether the vial contains 0.5 or 1.0 ml) over the deltoids
- Day 28: one dose over the deltoids.

This economical regimen is now the method of choice.

Passive immunization with rabies immune globulin

Every primary postexposure vaccine course should be accompanied by RIG to cover the first 7–10 days before vaccine-induced immunity appears. Rabies immune globulin treatment is especially important after bites on the head, neck or hands, or multiple bites. A single dose of 20 IU/kg of human RIG or 40 IU/kg of equine RIG is given at the same time as the first dose of vaccine. As much as possible is infiltrated into and around the wound, but care is needed when injecting into fingers or other tight tissue compartments. Any remaining vaccine is injected intramuscularly distant from the vaccine site. Increasing the dose of RIG may impair the response to vaccine, but if the volume is insufficient for infiltration, it can be diluted in saline two- or threefold in order to infiltrate all wounds. Skin testing with equine RIG does not predict most early (anaphylactic) reactions and is no longer recommended.[24] Adrenaline (epinephrine) should always be ready in case of very rare anaphylaxis. Reactions occur in 1.8% of equine RIG recipients and serum sickness is seen in 0.7%, but not after human RIG therapy.[29]

Postexposure treatment of previously vaccinated patients

Treatment is always urgent, but, provided that the patient has previously had a complete pre-exposure or postexposure course of tissue culture vaccine or if a neutralizing antibody level >0.5 IU/ml has been recorded at some time, only two doses of intramuscular vaccine are needed on days 0 and 3. Rabies immune globulin treatment is unnecessary.

Side-effects of tissue culture vaccines[30]

The incidence of minor symptoms is very variable. Local pain or erythema occurs in about 15% of people vaccinated and irritation is more common following intradermal injections. Generalized nonspecific symptoms are reported by about 7% of patients and transient maculopapular and urticarial rashes are occasionally seen. In the USA, 6% of late pre-exposure booster injections of HDCV have been accompanied

by a mild immune complex-like disease between 3 and 13 days later. All of these patients responded to symptomatic treatment. Neurologic symptoms,[14] either Guillain–Barré-like or local limb weakness, are extremely rare, and the incidence following treatment is no greater than those following other routine vaccines. No complications have been observed in pregnancy.

Pre-exposure prophylaxis

Pre-exposure vaccination is recommended for anyone at risk of exposure to rabies virus, particularly veterinary surgeons, animal handlers, zoologists, all bat handlers, laboratory staff working with rabies, wildlife officers and people living in or traveling to rabies-endemic areas where dogs are the dominant vector species. A total of three doses of cell culture vaccine are needed on days 0 and 7 and on day 28.[22–24] The last dose can be advanced towards day 21 if time is short,[24] but the antibody level may fall more rapidly. The dose can be intramuscular or 0.1 ml ID.[22,24] Families or student groups who cannot afford intramuscular vaccine can share ampoules economically if inoculated the same day. Malarial prophylaxis with chloroquine inhibits the antibody response to this course given intradermally, so anyone on antimalarial therapy must have intramuscular injections.[31] A booster dose after 1 or 2 years prolongs the antibody response, which usually lasts 5–10 years.[32] Unnecessary boosters can be avoided if antibody is detected. As booster doses induce a reliable, prompt secondary immune response, repeated boosters are not needed for travelers who will have access to vaccine if exposed; otherwise boost after 3–5 years. Serologic testing is useful to determine the need for booster injections and is necessary if immunosuppression is suspected.

RABIES-RELATED VIRUSES

The rabies-related lyssaviruses, genotypes 2–7, are continent-specific in Europe, Australasia and Africa, and are viruses of bats (with one exception).[1] All but one, genotype 2 Lagos bat virus, have caused fatal human disease (Table 160.3). New unclassified lyssaviruses are emerging.

Africa[4,25]

Genotype 3, Mokola virus, is genetically separate from the others; it has been identified occasionally in shrews and rodents but never in bats. Clinical rabies encephalitis is not seen in humans, but Mokola virus has been associated with two doubtful infections in Nigerian children (see Table 160.3). Genotype 4, Duvenhage virus, is found rarely in bats and has caused a rabies-like encephalitis in three patients.[4,33,34] The true prevalence of these African infections is uncertain as the diagnosis of human rabies is normally made on clinical grounds and rabies-related viruses may give a weak or negative result with the routine diagnostic rabies immunofluorescent test.

Europe

There are two genotypes of European bat lyssaviruses (EBLVs):[1] genotype 5, EBLV type 1, is widely distributed in insectivorous bats across Europe and genotype 6, EBLV type 2, which is very rare. There are five reports of fatal rabies-like encephalitis following bat bites in Europe (see Table 160.3).[35–37]

Australia

Genotype 7, Australian bat lyssavirus,[38] was identified in 1996 in flying foxes (*Pteropus* spp.) and other bats, and has caused two fatal human infections indistinguishable from rabies encephalitis.[39] Lyssavirus seropositive bats have also been found in the Philippines, Thailand, Cambodia and Bangladesh.

Table 160.3 Rabies-related lyassaviruses

Genotype	Virus found*	Animal reservoirs (potential vectors)	Disease in humans
3 Mokola	South Africa, Nigeria, Cameroon, Ethiopia (rare)	Shrews, rodents (cat, dog)	• Child febrile convulsion;[†] recovered[1,25] • Child encephalitic signs;[‡] died[1,25] • Vaccinated laboratory worker, mild illness; recovered.
4 Duvenhage	South Africa, Zimbabwe, Kenya (very rarely identified)	Insectivorous/fruit bats (cats)	• Man bitten by a bat, signs of typical furious rabies; died[1,25] • Man scratched by a bat, signs of classic rabies encephalitis; died[33] • Woman scratched by a bat, signs of rabies encephalitis; died[34]

5 European bat lyssavirus (EBLV)
  EBLV type 1a
  EBLV type 1b
	Northern and Eastern Europe
	Western Europe
		Insectivorous bats	• Girl had bat bite, had acute ascending paralysis and encephalitis; died (clinical diagnosis only)
			• Girl had bat bite, signs of furious rabies; died of EBLV 1a[35]
			• Man had bat bite, signs of furious rabies; died (clinical diagnosis only)

6 European bat lyssavirus
 	
  EBLV type 2a
  EBLV type 2b
	
	Netherlands, UK
	Switzerland (very rare)
		Insectivorous bats (*Myotis* spp.)	• Bat conservationist bitten by bats, signs of classic rabies encephalitis; died of EBLV 2a[36]
			• Zoologist bitten by sick bat, signs of furious rabies; died of EBLV 2b[37]

7 Australian bat lyssavirus	Australia	Fruit bats (*Pteropus* spp.), insectivorous bats	• Woman bat carer, scratched by bats, signs of classic rabies encephalitis; died • Woman, bitten by a fruit bat, signs of paralytic rabies; died[39]

*There is serologic evidence of lyssavirus infection of bats in the Philippines, Cambodia, Thailand, Bangladesh and China.
[†]Doubtful diagnosis;
[‡]Alternative diagnosis possible.

REFERENCES

References for this chapter can be found online at http://www.expertconsult.com

Chapter | **161** | Cillian F De Gascun
Michael J Carr
William W Hall

Influenza viruses

INTRODUCTION

Influenza is a seasonal respiratory viral infection that results in some 250 000–500 000 deaths globally each year.[1] The illness is characterized by a sudden onset of high temperature and debilitating systemic symptoms. In healthy individuals, infection is typically self-limited; however, complications often occur in certain high-risk groups such as the elderly or the immunocompromised. Despite the availability of preventive vaccines and anti-influenza therapeutics, seasonal influenza remains a major global health problem. Moreover, as well as direct medical costs, the indirect social and economic costs remain significant.

In addition to the seasonal influenza epidemics which usually occur annually in the autumn and winter, global pandemics also occur, albeit much more infrequently. At the time of writing, the world is in the midst of the first influenza pandemic of the 21st century. The virus involved is a novel H1N1 virus of swine origin that originated in Mexico in the spring of 2009 and has now spread globally. To date, there have been more than 145 000 reported cases worldwide with over 1000 deaths. The emergence of this new pandemic serves to secure influenza's place in history as 'the last great uncontrolled plague of mankind'.[2]

NATURE

Virus structure

Influenza viruses are enveloped, single-stranded, negative-sense RNA viruses of the family Orthomyxoviridae, and there are three major antigenic types, A, B and C. These can be differentiated not only on the basis of antigenic differences in their nucleocapsid and matrix proteins, but also with respect to the number of gene segments and viral proteins, host range and capacity to cause disease.[3]

Influenza viruses possess segmented genomes: influenza A and B contain eight RNA segments and influenza C seven. Influenza A, the predominant pathogen in seasonal influenza and the cause of pandemic influenza, will provide the main focus for the remainder of this section. The influenza A genome encodes 11 viral proteins:

- haemagglutinin (HA), which is divided into two domains or subunits (HA1 and HA2);
- neuraminidase (NA);
- two matrix proteins (M1 and M2);
- the heterotrimeric RNA-dependent RNA polymerase, composed of one polymerase acidic (PA) and two polymerase

basic (PB1 and PB2) subunits and the alternatively transcribed proapoptotic peptide, PB1-F2;
- nucleoprotein (NP); and
- two nonstructural proteins (NS1 and NS2; NS2 is also known as NEP, or nuclear export protein).[3–5]

The virus particle (virion) has an irregular spherical shape with a lipid envelope, approximately 80–120 nm in diameter. The surface is covered with spike-like projections composed of the two primary viral glycoproteins, HA and NA, which are involved in host cell attachment and host cell exit, respectively. In addition, M2 (a transmembrane ion channel) is also present on the external surface of the virus. M1 is found within the lipid bilayer, which surrounds the virus core. The core is a ribonucleoprotein (RNP) complex which consists of the viral RNA segments and the NP and the RNA polymerase (Fig. 161.1). Influenza A is currently classified on the composition of the HA and NA proteins. At present, 16 different HA (H1–H16) and 9 different NA (N1–N9) molecules are known to exist.[5]

Virus replication

At the initiation of human infection, the HA binds to receptors on the host cell surface that contain α2,6-linked sialic acid residues, and virion entry occurs via receptor-mediated endocytosis. In the host cell cytoplasm, the vesicle containing the virus undergoes an acidification process through fusion with intracellular endosomes. This triggers a conformational change in the HA, exposing a fusion peptide and permitting exit from the endosome; in addition, hydrogen ions are pumped from the endosome through the M2 ion channel into the virus particle. This allows the viral RNPs to be released, and they are then actively transported into the nucleus through the nuclear pore complex.[3] The M2 inhibitor class of antiviral agents, the adamantanes, inhibits this acidification process.

Transcription of the influenza viral genomic RNA (vRNA) into messenger RNA (mRNA) takes place in the nucleus. Following transcription, viral mRNA strands are exported to the cytoplasm where new viral proteins are synthesized. Newly synthesized viral RNAs are exported via a vRNP–M1–NEP protein complex. Packaging of progeny virions occurs at the host cell surface where the RNP–M1–NEP complex assembles at the cytoplasmic membrane under regions containing viral glycoproteins. As the new viruses bud and are released from the host cell, the NA is responsible for cleaving sialic acid residues that would cause the virus to remain bound to either the cell surface or other viral particles (Fig. 161.2). The neuraminidase inhibitor class of antiviral agents prevents this cleavage process and thereby the release of virus and subsequent infection of new host cells.

Structure of the influenza virion

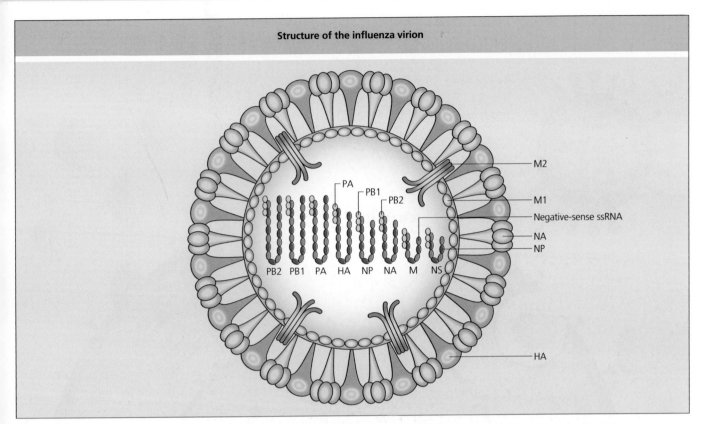

Fig. 161.1 Structure of the influenza virion. The genome of the influenza A virus is composed of eight genomic segments and each segment contains a region that encodes one or two proteins. In all, the eight segments encode 11 proteins. Details of the proteins, their biologic functions and their roles in virus replication are summarized in the text. Reproduced with permission from Nelson & Holmes.[6]

EPIDEMIOLOGY

Natural reservoirs of influenza viruses

Wild aquatic birds are the natural reservoir of all influenza A viruses.[7,8] Influenza A viruses in humans are maintained by human-to-human transmission during acute infection; however, other animals including primates, swine, ferrets, horses, seals, whales and mink can also become infected.

Antigenic variation – antigenic drift and shift

The influenza A viruses evolve rapidly primarily because of the absence of a proofreading mechanism during the copying of the vRNA to mRNA. The antigenic variation in influenza viruses occurs as a result of small changes, *antigenic drift*s, over time within the RNA segments encoding the surface glycoproteins NA and, in particular, HA. Antigenic drift leads to positive selection of these escape mutants from neutralizing antibody responses elicited by previous exposure(s) to wild-type viruses.

Human influenza virus HA molecules preferentially bind α2,6-linked sialic acid expressed on respiratory epithelia, whereas the HA of avian viruses binds predominantly α2,3-linked sialic acid receptors. Reassortment of influenza vRNA segments can occur if different viruses infect a single cell at the same time, allowing RNA exchange. This can result in the production of a novel progeny virus and is known as *antigenic shift*. Reassortment may occur in an intermediate host species such as swine (the mixing vessel hypothesis) which can be infected with both human and avian viruses as swine epithelia possess both α2,3- and α2,6-linked sialic acid receptors. Antigenic shift can lead to the introduction of a new influenza subtype into an immunologically naive population, and has the potential for pandemic spread.

Influenza pandemics

During influenza pandemics, virus spreads rapidly, resulting in significant morbidity and mortality. The 'Spanish influenza' pandemic of 1918–19 was caused by a highly virulent influenza A, subtype H1N1 virus that infected approximately one-third of the human population, leading to the deaths of more than 50 million people.[9,10] One striking feature of the 1918–19 pandemic was the disproportionately high numbers of healthy young individuals who succumbed to infection that has been attributed to an uncontrolled immune response with hyperproduction of proinflammatory cytokines, the so-called 'cytokine storm'. In 1957–58, the 'Asian' influenza pandemic arose after genetic shift of the circulating H1N1 virus to an H2N2 subtype.

The H2N2 viruses were subsequently supplanted by the H3N2 'Hong Kong' influenza pandemic of 1968. Lindstrom and co-workers performed a whole genome phylogenetic analysis of human influenza H2N2 viruses isolated from 1957 to 1968 and human H3N2 viruses isolated from 1968 to 1972.[11] The data suggest that H2N2 viruses continued to circulate for some time after 1968 and that the subsequent establishment of human H3N2 was associated with multiple reassortment events that increased the genetic diversity. In 1977 an outbreak of H1N1 occurred by an unknown mechanism involving a virus which was identical to that circulating in humans in the 1950s. Since then, seasonal influenza outbreaks have involved two main subtypes, H1N1 and H3N2, and these viruses continue to undergo antigenic drift.

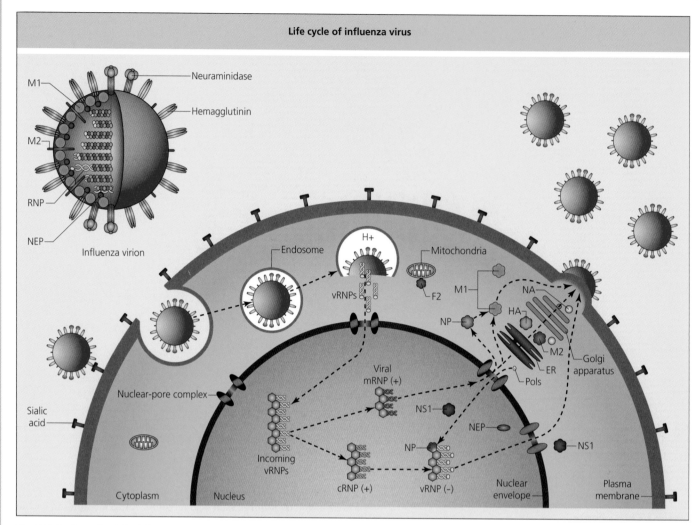

Fig. 161.2 Life cycle of the influenza virus. Virus particles initially associate with the host cell by binding to sialic acid-containing receptors on the cell surface. The bound virus is endocytosed, with the eventual release of the uncoated viral ribonucleoprotein (vRNP) complex into the cytoplasm. The ribonucleoprotein complex is transported through the nuclear pore complex into the nucleus. The incoming viral RNA (vRNA) is transcribed into messenger RNA (mRNA). The viral proteins are expressed and processed and eventually assemble with vRNAs at budding sites within the host cell membrane. The viral protein complexes and ribonucleoproteins are assembled into viral particles that bud from the host cell. Further details are provided in the text. Reproduced with permission from http://www.reactome.org.

Transmission of avian influenza to humans

Until 1997, the difference in HA receptor-binding specificities was thought to provide a host range barrier such that direct infection of humans by an avian-origin virus seemed highly unlikely. However, in 1997 avian influenza A, subtype H5N1 virus was transmitted to humans from infected chickens in poultry markets in Hong Kong, resulting in the deaths of 6 of the 18 patients infected.[12] The high case fatality rate and the subsequent global spread of highly pathogenic H5N1 in birds raised the possibility of a significant future pandemic. The cumulative number of confirmed human cases from 2003 to 2009 has been reported as 423 with 258 deaths, a 61% case fatality rate.[13] In most cases, infected individuals have had close contact with infected poultry. On rare occasions human-to-human transmission has been reported in Thailand, China, Vietnam, Indonesia and Azerbaijan; however, fortunately, there has been no sustained human-to-human transmission.[14–20] In March 1999, influenza A, subtype H9N2 viruses infected two children in Hong Kong; however, these two cases were mild and self-limiting.[21] Subsequently, an outbreak of highly pathogenic avian influenza A H7N7 occurred in early 2003 in commercial poultry farms in the Netherlands which resulted in 89 human infections of whom 83 developed conjunctivitis. Notably, one fatality occurred in a veterinarian who developed acute respiratory distress and fatal pneumonia.[22]

Swine influenza (H1N1v) pandemic 2009

In March 2009, public health authorities in Mexico City observed a large increase in the number of patients presenting with influenza-like illness. Subsequent testing in Canada and the USA confirmed that a previously undescribed influenza A virus was responsible. In April 2009, a novel swine-origin influenza A virus (H1N1v) infection was reported to the World Health Organization (WHO) by the Centers for Disease Control and Prevention (CDC) in Atlanta in two children presenting with a febrile respiratory illness from neighboring counties in southern California.[23] These cases were not epidemiologically linked and neither child had exposure to swine. Phylogenetic characterization of the virus from the US index case (A/California/04/2009) showed that the virus had a unique gene constellation not previously seen in humans or other animal reservoirs. Six genes (PB2, PB1, PA, HA, NP and NS) were similar to viruses previously identified in triple-reassortment swine influenza viruses in North American pigs and the remaining two gene segments (NA and M) were derived from Eurasian swine influenza viruses (Fig. 161.3).[25,26]

By the end of May 2009, Mexico had documented 4910 laboratory-confirmed cases with 85 deaths.[27] At the time of writing, Mexico has also reported the largest number of cases with severe clinical presentations, in contrast to other countries which have reported

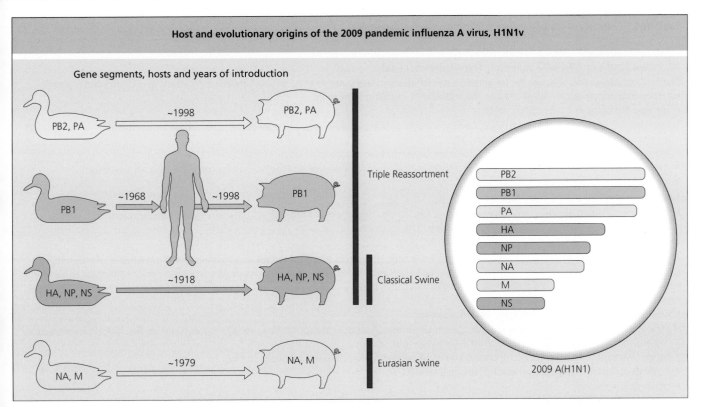

Fig. 161.3 Host and evolutionary origins of the 2009 pandemic influenza A virus, H1N1v. Host and lineage origins for the gene segments of the 2009 A (H1N1) virus: PB2, polymerase basic 2; PB1, polymerase basic 1; PA, polymerase acidic; HA, hemagglutinin; NP, nucleoprotein; NA, neuraminidase; M, matrix gene; NS, nonstructural gene. Color of gene segment in circle indicates host. Reproduced with permission from Garten *et al.*[24]

predominantly mild cases of a self-limiting influenza-like illness. However, deaths have occurred in individuals with underlying medical conditions. Since the original identification of H1N1v, sustained human-to-human transmission has occurred globally and on June 11, 2009, the WHO declared the first pandemic of the 21st century. In addition to the rapid global spread, a major concern is the continued co-circulation – and potential reassortment – of the novel H1N1v with seasonal H1N1 (which has acquired oseltamivir resistance approaching 100%) and the highly pathogenic H5N1 avian virus.

PATHOGENESIS

Influenza virus is classically acquired by the inhalation of infectious droplets. However, transmission by airborne droplet nuclei, small-particle aerosols, or self-inoculation (via virus-contaminated hands or fomites) may also occur. Following inhalation, the virus attaches to specific α2,6-linked sialic acid receptors expressed on respiratory epithelial cells. Although these receptors are widespread, the virus attaches preferentially to tracheal and bronchial epithelium.[28] In contrast, human infection by avian influenza viruses preferentially involves the distal airways.[29]

In uncomplicated influenza, histologic examination reveals diffuse mucosal inflammation with edema of the upper airways: epithelial cells become vacuolated and edematous and lose their cilia; this is accompanied by hyperemia and infiltration with primarily lymphocytes and histiocytes. Virus replication peaks at about 48 hours and the level of viral shedding correlates directly with severity of symptoms.[3] In the more severe primary viral pneumonia, the pathologic process extends distally to the lung causing an interstitial pneumonitis. Damage to the alveoli with formation of hyaline membranes allows exudates and hemorrhage from alveolar capillaries into the alveolar lumina, resulting in impaired gas exchange and severe respiratory dysfunction.

The host immune response against influenza virus is complex. Following infection of the respiratory epithelial cells, proinflammatory cytokines – primarily interleukin (IL)-6 and interferon alpha (IFN-α) – are produced by, and secreted from, infected cells. Cytokine production typically peaks by day 2 after infection, and corresponds with the peak of systemic symptoms.[30] In addition to cytokines, neutralizing antibodies (predominantly of the IgA subclass) are also produced at the site of infection. However, it is serum antibody levels (to HA and NA) that correlate with resistance to illness and with restriction of infection. Serum antibodies (IgM, IgG and IgA) are present within 1 week of the onset of illness, and may provide immunity and protection against re-infection by homotypic viruses for many years.[31] Cell-mediated immune responses are detectable before humoral responses and involve the activity of both CD8+ cytotoxic T cells and CD4+ helper T cells. Although these two classes of T cells closely interact, animal models have demonstrated that the response of either alone is capable of clearing infection.[32]

PREVENTION

Vaccination

Vaccination remains the cornerstone of the prevention of seasonal influenza. Indeed, some 80% of the population in the USA are now included in groups for whom seasonal influenza vaccination is recommended by the Advisory Committee for Immunization Practices (ACIP) (Table 161.1).[33]

As a result of antigenic drift, the process of candidate vaccine selection is complex. The WHO is responsible for decisions as to which influenza strains should be included in the vaccine, and separate recommendations are made annually to regional health authorities in the Northern and Southern hemispheres. The WHO conducts global surveillance programs through a network of national and regional

---

Table 161.1 Summary of seasonal influenza vaccination recommendations

Children and adolescents aged 6 months to 18 years

All children aged 6 months to 18 years should be vaccinated annually.

Children and adolescents at higher risk for influenza complications should continue to be a focus of vaccination efforts as providers and programs transition to routinely vaccinating all children and adolescents, including those who:

- are aged 6 months to 4 years (59 months);
- have chronic pulmonary (including asthma), cardiovascular (except hypertension), renal, hepatic, cognitive, neurologic/neuromuscular, hematologic or metabolic disorders (including diabetes mellitus);
- are immunosuppressed (including immunosuppression caused by medications or by HIV);
- are receiving long-term aspirin therapy and therefore might be at risk for experiencing Reye's syndrome after influenza virus infection;
- are residents of long-term care facilities; and
- will be pregnant during the influenza season.

Note: Children aged <6 months cannot receive influenza vaccination. Household and other close contacts (e.g. day-care providers) of children <6 months, including older children and adolescents, should be vaccinated.

Adults

Annual vaccination against influenza is recommended for any adult who wants to reduce the risk of becoming ill with influenza or of transmitting it to others. Vaccination is recommended for all adults without contraindications in the following groups, because these persons either are at higher risk for influenza complications or are close contacts of persons at higher risk:

- persons aged ≥50 years;
- women who will be pregnant during the influenza season;
- persons who have chronic pulmonary (including asthma), cardiovascular (except hypertension), renal, hepatic, cognitive, neurologic/neuromuscular, hematologic or metabolic disorders (including diabetes mellitus);
- persons who are immunosuppressed (including immunosuppression caused by medications or by HIV);
- residents of nursing homes and other long-term care facilities;
- health-care personnel;
- household contacts and caregivers of children aged <5 years and adults ≥50 years, with particular emphasis on vaccinating contacts of children <6 months; and
- household contacts and caregivers of persons with medical conditions that put them at higher risk for severe complications from influenza.

From Advisory Committee for Immunization Practices[33]

---

virology reference laboratories which provide information on circulating viruses. In parallel, serologic surveys are performed on recipients of the previous year's vaccine to evaluate immune responses to the emerging strains of the current season.[34]

Since 1977, seasonal influenza has been caused by two co-circulating influenza A viruses (H1N1 and H3N2) and influenza B, and all three viruses are included in seasonal vaccines. During influenza outbreaks where a close match exists between circulating virus strains and those in the vaccine, efficacy has been estimated at 80%. In seasons with a poor match, this can fall to as low as 50%.[35]

Seasonal influenza vaccines may comprise either inactivated virus particles or live attenuated virus. Both vaccine formulations have been shown to be safe and efficacious in healthy children and adults, although, in general, the immune responses tend to be poorer among the elderly and young children. Live attenuated influenza virus vaccine (LAIV) is presently only licensed for use in healthy children aged 2 years and older, and in healthy nonpregnant adults through the age of 49 years. Trivalent inactivated influenza vaccine (TIV) is licensed for use in all ages and all high-risk groups. Studies have shown that both vaccine types have equivalent efficacy.[35]

Seasonal influenza vaccination is both clinically and cost-effective. It results in lower rates of laboratory-confirmed influenza cases; lower rates of clinical influenza-like illness; reduced numbers of physician visits, days of illness, days of work loss, hospitalization rates and mortality. From a logistics perspective, LAIV has the advantage of intranasal administration, thus avoiding the need for injections. As patient surveys have indicated a preference for intranasal immunization over parenteral, more widespread use of the former would be expected to lead to an increased uptake of seasonal vaccine.[34]

In general, vaccination is well tolerated. Local reactions to TIV (discomfort, erythema and swelling) are typically mild. Systemic symptoms, which include fever, malaise and myalgia, may also occur.

Despite widespread concern following an association between swine influenza vaccine and Guillain–Barré syndrome (GBS) in the USA in 1976, no definitive association between seasonal influenza vaccination and GBS has been demonstrated.[36]

Chemoprophylaxis

According to the Infectious Diseases Society of America, 'influenza vaccination is the primary tool to prevent influenza and antiviral chemoprophylaxis is not a substitute for vaccination'.[37] However, antiviral chemoprophylaxis is effective and should be considered in the following groups:

- high-risk individuals within 2 weeks of influenza vaccination (before an adequate immune response develops);
- high-risk individuals for whom vaccination is contraindicated, unavailable or expected to have low effectiveness (significantly immunocompromised);
- high-risk individuals who have not yet been vaccinated (influenza vaccine should be also administered);
- those who are in close contact with people at high risk of developing influenza complications; and
- all residents (vaccinated and unvaccinated) of institutions experiencing influenza outbreaks.

The adamantane M2 inhibitors amantadine and rimantadine, and the neuraminidase inhibitors oseltamivir and zanamivir, are recommended for the chemoprophylaxis of influenza A virus infections; only the neuraminidase inhibitors are recommended for chemoprophylaxis of influenza B.[37] Chemoprophylaxis is estimated to be 70–90% effective in preventing illness in healthy adults. However, decisions regarding choice of antiviral should take into account drug resistance in circulating influenza viruses. Thus, oseltamivir is no longer appropriate for seasonal H1N1 chemoprophylaxis and the adamantanes should not be used for H3N2 chemoprophylaxis.[37] In a situation where influenza A virus infection has been diagnosed but subtype information is not available, then either zanamivir or a combination of oseltamivir and rimantadine should be employed. In hospital or residential institution settings, strategies for the prevention of nosocomial transmission of influenza should be implemented. These include staff and patient vaccination programs, chemoprophylaxis if appropriate, and compliance with droplet isolation precautions.

DIAGNOSTIC MICROBIOLOGY

Laboratory diagnosis plays a crucial role in the management of influenza. The development of highly sensitive and specific methods for virus detection allows the laboratory to provide a rapid definitive diagnosis, enabling clinicians to initiate prompt and appropriate management.

Virus isolation in culture

Influenza viruses can be isolated in culture from a range of specimens taken from the upper and lower respiratory tract; preferred specimen types are nasopharyngeal or nasal swabs and nasal washes or aspirates. Recently, the capital costs and longer turnaround times of culture compared to other more rapid detection systems have called into question the relevance of culture isolation methods.[38] However, it is clear that virus isolation remains essential for phenotypic antiviral susceptibility testing. In addition, the isolation process can be accelerated using centrifugation-enhanced ('shell vial') techniques.[39]

Serology

Serologic assays, such as hemagglutinin inhibition and complement fixation, require an acute-phase serum to be collected within 7 days of the onset of symptoms and compared to a convalescent serum specimen taken 14–21 days later to demonstrate a greater than fourfold rise in strain-specific, antibody titer. Because of this time frame, serology is of little use for the diagnosis of acute influenza; however, it remains important in basic research, epidemiologic investigations and the evaluation of antibody responses to vaccination.[40]

Rapid antigen testing

Rapid antigen or point-of-care (POC) testing has become increasingly important as timely results can lead to the prompt initiation of antiviral therapy, implementation of outbreak control measures and a reduction of inappropriate antibiotic usage.[41] The POC testing devices are simple to use and easily interpretable. However, whilst they have high specificities for virus detection, they have a lower sensitivity than 'gold standard' methods such as virus culture and reverse transcriptase polymerase chain reaction (RT-PCR).[42–46] In general, the sensitivity of POC tests in adults is lower than in pediatric patient populations, attributable to the higher viral loads and antigen shedding in younger age groups.[47] Thus, a negative test may not definitively exclude a positive diagnosis.

Immunofluorescence microscopy

The detection of influenza virus by direct fluorescent antibody (DFA) or immunofluorescent antibody (IFA) testing is extremely rapid and employs specific monoclonal antibodies to influenza virus antigens and visualization by fluorescence microscopy. The specificity and the sensitivity of this approach depend on sample collection and the presence of infected cells in the specimens. This is widely employed and is an excellent first-line choice for clinicians requesting a laboratory confirmation of POC positives already identified in the clinical setting.

Molecular detection

Molecular diagnostic approaches are increasingly replacing virus isolation and to a lesser extent immunofluorescence and rapid antigen testing for the detection of influenza due to their rapidity, cost-effectiveness and standardization. Molecular detection of nucleic acids extracted from respiratory specimens, employing real-time RT-PCR, is the method of choice. In addition, multiplex PCRs have been developed for the identification of multiple viral and bacterial respiratory pathogens, and are being incorporated into diagnostic algorithms for the differential diagnosis of respiratory tract infections.[48–50] Rapid real-time influenza subtyping approaches have also been developed and these can be employed downstream of universal influenza molecular detection assays, allowing the differentiation of seasonal human influenza, H1N1 and H3N2, avian H5N1 subtypes and novel swine H1N1v.[51] With the spread worldwide of seasonal human influenza A H1N1 with oseltamivir resistance (the H275Y mutation in the NA protein), several molecular methods have been developed to detect the single nucleotide polymorphism underlying resistance.[52,53] More recently, pyrosequencing ('sequencing by synthesis') has also been applied for the detection of drug resistance.[54]

CLINICAL MANIFESTATIONS

Seasonal influenza

Influenza A and B cause primarily an acute respiratory illness, with fever, cough, coryza and headache. However, it is the associated systemic symptoms that distinguish influenza from other respiratory virus infections, such as rhinovirus or respiratory syncytial virus. The incubation period for influenza infection averages 2 days (range 1–4 days). The classic illness has an abrupt onset with headache, high-grade fever, chills, dry cough, myalgia and malaise. Rhinorrhea, nasal congestion and pharyngitis may also be present. Fever typically peaks within the first 24 hours of illness. It begins to decline on the second or third day and is usually resolved by day 6; however, fever may be continuous or intermittent. Systemic symptoms usually resolve within a similar timescale. Weakness and fatigue, which on occasions can be accompanied by cough, can persist for an additional 1–2 weeks. Influenza attack rates are higher in children compared to adults, with fever, cervical lymphadenopathy, nausea and vomiting being frequent manifestations; bronchiolitis and croup (laryngotracheitis) may also occur.

Subclinical or asymptomatic infection can also occur, particularly in individuals with pre-existing immunity to the circulating strains of virus. In contrast to influenza A and B, influenza C typically causes only a sporadic and usually afebrile upper respiratory tract illness.

Complications

Complications occur not infrequently. Whilst the most common complications are bronchitis in adults and otitis media in children, exacerbations of pre-existing chronic medical conditions, such as asthma, chronic obstructive pulmonary disease and congestive heart failure, have been well described.

Pulmonary

Three distinct syndromes of severe pneumonia can occur after influenza infection in children or adults:

- primary viral pneumonia;
- combined viral–bacterial pneumonia; and
- secondary bacterial pneumonia.

Pneumonia complicates influenza predominantly in the elderly, patients with chronic cardiopulmonary disease, pregnant women and immunocompromised individuals.

Primary influenza virus pneumonia develops abruptly after the onset of symptoms and progresses within 24 hours to a clinical picture resembling severe acute respiratory distress syndrome (ARDS) associated with hypotension, hypoxia and cyanosis. Fatality rates are as high as 50%, with death typically occurring within 4 days.

Combined viral–bacterial pneumonia is more common than primary viral pneumonia, with *Streptococcus pneumoniae*, *Staphylococcus aureus* and *Haemophilus influenzae* being predominantly involved. The clinical syndrome is indistinguishable from primary viral pneumonia. However, the later onset and the detection of both virus and bacteria in clinical samples confirm the diagnosis. The case fatality rate for combined pneumonia is some 10%, although this is frequently higher in cases of *Staph. aureus* co-infection.

Secondary bacterial pneumonia typically manifests after the patient has started to improve clinically from the original influenza illness. The onset of new respiratory symptoms is accompanied by localized clinical and radiologic findings. Bacteria may be isolated from clinical specimens, but usually virus is no longer detectable. The case fatality for this group of patients has been reported at around 7%.

Extrapulmonary

A variety of extrapulmonary manifestations has been described. Central nervous system (CNS) involvement, ranging from irritability and drowsiness to seizures and coma has been reported, although the pathogenesis remains unclear. Influenza-associated acute encephalopathy (IAAE), which is associated histologically with diffuse cerebral congestion and edema, is a recognized, uncommon, but potentially fatal neurologic syndrome generally occurring in children and adolescents and typically presenting during the early phase of infection.[55] A post-influenza encephalitis may also occur (albeit rarely) 2–3 weeks following recovery from the acute illness; fortunately, recovery occurs in the majority of cases. Reye's syndrome has also been reported following influenza (B more frequently than A) infection. Though the etiology is unknown, the risk of Reye's appears to be increased by the administration of therapeutic doses of salicylates and their use is now contraindicated in influenza infection.

Myocarditis has also been reported but the pathogenesis is poorly understood and is probably due to a combination of viral and host factors. Clinically, myocarditis may be associated with heart failure, pericardial effusion or conduction system disorders. Myositis or myopathy has also been described. While most cases recover, this may be so severe that acute renal failure secondary to myoglobinuria can occur. Toxic shock syndrome may also present in the context of influenza virus infection. It is believed that this is the consequence of bacterial exotoxin (TSST-1) secreted by colonizing or co-infecting *Staph. aureus* strains.

Infection in specific groups

In the immunocompromised host, influenza virus infection is associated with an increased risk of complications, hospitalizations and death. While the observed illness typically reflects that seen in the healthy individual, the clinical presentation may be atypical in the elderly (e.g. confusion, lethargy, low-grade fever) or in the transplant population (e.g. pneumonia, rejection). A prolonged disease course with viral shedding and the rapid emergence of antiviral resistance are also features of influenza in the immunocompromised.

Pregnant women in the second or third trimester have an increased risk of mortality from influenza. Although this is more commonly seen in the pandemic setting, it is also a feature of seasonal influenza, and the cause of death is usually overwhelming pulmonary disease. There are no clear explanations for the increased risk of pulmonary disease in pregnancy; however, it has been postulated that the increased pulmonary blood flow in pregnancy may predispose to pulmonary edema when alveoli are damaged.[56] Although maternal influenza infection has been associated with an increased risk of congenital anomalies and fetal loss, no specific teratogenic effect has been attributed to influenza virus.

Avian influenza (H5N1)

H5N1 avian influenza, in contrast to seasonal influenza and H1N1v, is highly pathogenic in humans with high morbidity and mortality.

Although a definitive explanation for the severity of H5N1 infection remains to be established, much is known.[57] The virus is capable of infecting pulmonary epithelial cells, thereby causing diffuse alveolar damage and hemorrhage (this process is not dissimilar to primary viral pneumonia as described above). In addition, H5N1 (unlike seasonal influenza) disseminates beyond the respiratory tract during infection. The virus also has the capacity to impair cytotoxic T-cell activity *in vitro*, thereby reducing the capacity of the host to clear infection. Studies indicate that aberrant production of proinflammatory cytokines may also contribute to the pathogenesis of H5N1 influenza.

Pandemic influenza (H1N1v)

In general, the clinical presentation of pandemic influenza is similar to that described above, although some symptoms atypical for seasonal influenza may be more prominent. This is the case in the present H1N1v pandemic with diarrhea and/or vomiting being reported in some 38% of patients. At the time of writing (July 2009), and it should be stressed that this situation may change over time, 'this pandemic has been characterized by the mildness of symptoms in the overwhelming majority of patients'.[58] However, despite mild disease, the hospitalization rate is significant, and recent reports from Australia have indicated this may be in the region of 10% of 'laboratory-confirmed' cases.[59] Furthermore, severe respiratory disease and death have been reported, both in previously healthy individuals and those with underlying chronic disease.[27] Pregnant women, those with a body mass index (BMI) of >40 and those with pre-existing pulmonary disease may be particularly at risk of severe respiratory distress following H1N1v infection.[60,61] Notably, initial serologic studies suggest that a degree of pre-existing immunity to H1N1v exists in adults >60 years.[62]

MANAGEMENT

The majority of individuals infected with influenza virus have a self-limited, uncomplicated illness. However, in those patients with severe illness, early treatment with antiviral therapy may reduce the severity and duration of symptoms, the number of hospitalizations, the incidence of complications, the use of outpatient facilities, and in some cases the inappropriate use of antibiotics.[37]

Antiviral therapy for influenza has been covered in detail elsewhere in this text. However, in brief, there are two classes of agents with anti-influenza activity: the adamantane M2 inhibitors (amantadine and rimantadine) and the neuraminidase inhibitors (oseltamivir and zanamivir). All four agents are licensed for the treatment of influenza A, while the latter two are licensed for influenza B. Three of the four are administered orally, whereas zanamivir is delivered by inhalation. To be effective, antiviral therapy must be administered within 24–48 hours of the onset of symptoms. In general, both classes of agents are well tolerated, although minor CNS complaints are not uncommon in the case of the M2 inhibitors. With regard to the neuraminidase inhibitors, behavioral abnormalities have been described in children following oseltamivir administration. This has been reported primarily from Japan and may well reflect a genetic predisposition; however, patients should be advised accordingly. Zanamivir-induced severe bronchospasm has also been described, particularly in individuals with a history of asthma.

In recent years, antiviral drug resistance has become prevalent for both classes of antivirals and therefore local resistance data should inform their use. With regard to the two current co-circulating human seasonal influenza viruses, widespread resistance to the M2 inhibitors has been documented in the H3N2 virus, and therefore these should not be used to treat influenza unless the virus has been definitively identified as H1N1. Conversely, the prevalence of oseltamivir resistance in the H1N1 virus is now greater than 90%, and this should only be used to treat H3N2 virus infection.[37]

At the time of writing, rare oseltamivir resistance (H275Y mutation in NA) has been reported by the WHO in novel H1N1v from treated patients but also notably in one case without exposure to the drug; furthermore, resistance to the adamantanes has been reported in all H1N1v viruses studied to date. However, the virus remains sensitive to zanamivir.

The following groups should be considered for antiviral therapy if influenza virus infection is documented: unvaccinated infants aged 12–24 months and individuals with any of the following: chronic pulmonary disease; hemodynamically significant cardiac disease; HIV infection; sickle cell anemia or other hemoglobinopathies; disease requiring long-term aspirin therapy; chronic renal dysfunction; cancer; chronic metabolic conditions; neuromuscular disorders; and seizure disorders. In addition, all adults over 65 years of age and all residents of nursing homes (or other long-term care facilities) should be considered for treatment.[37]

REFERENCES

 References for this chapter can be found online at http://www.expertconsult.com

Respiratory viruses

INTRODUCTION

Respiratory viral infections are among the most common diseases of humans. These illnesses are caused by a heterogeneous group of viruses commonly known as human respiratory viruses (RVs). Over the last decade new molecular diagnostics have expanded the range of viruses detected in respiratory samples and several novel RVs have been identified. Real-time polymerase chain reaction (PCR) has been established as a powerful tool to diagnose and quantify RVs. The characteristic illnesses associated with the different respiratory viruses and the populations at higher risk are presented in Table 162.1. Other viruses, such as some of the enteroviruses, influenza viruses and herpesviruses, can also cause respiratory disease but they are discussed in separate chapters.

Respiratory viral infections are largely benign and self-limited, although newer studies using molecular amplification approaches have highlighted the importance of respiratory viruses as common pathogens in adults with pneumonia. They can exacerbate underlying chronic cardiopulmonary diseases, increase visits to health-care providers and result in unnecessary prescription of antibiotics. Among patients at the extremes of age with underlying cardiopulmonary diseases or those with primary or secondary immunodeficiencies, these illnesses can be associated with serious, potentially fatal complications.

The most common methods for the laboratory diagnosis of viral respiratory infections are summarized in Table 162.2 and Figures 162.1–162.5.

ADENOVIRUS

Nature

Adenoviruses were first isolated in the 1950s from human adenoids and later from respiratory secretions of military recruits with acute febrile respiratory illnesses. Human adenoviruses belong to the family Adenoviridae. More than 50 serotypes have been described and are being grouped into six species (A–F). Approximately one-half of these serotypes are known human pathogens. Virions are non-enveloped icosahedral particles measuring 80–100 nm in diameter and containing a linear double-stranded DNA genome. The capsid consists of 252 capsomers, of which 240 are hexons and 12 are pentons (at the vertices). A fiber with a knob at the end projects from every penton.

Epidemiology

Although epidemiologic characteristics of the adenoviruses vary by type, the route of transmission is either via the respiratory route, fecal–oral or water-borne. Infections are most common during early childhood and nearly 100% of adults have serum antibodies against multiple serotypes. Adenoviruses have been found to account for 3–5% of acute respiratory infections in children and up to 2% in adults. Close contact in crowded institutions increases the risk for adenovirus infections and outbreaks have been described in day-care centers, hospitals, shipyards and military quarters. Adenovirus infections can occur throughout the year but outbreaks of adenovirus-associated respiratory disease have been more common in the late winter, spring and early summer.

Pathogenesis

Adenoviruses causing respiratory disease can be spread via contact transmission (direct or indirect) and droplet transmission. Droplet transmission occurs when droplets containing infectious viral particles generated from the infected person are propelled a short distance (<1 meter) and deposited on the host's conjunctivae, nasal mucosa or mouth. Droplet particles (>5 µm diameter) are produced during coughing, sneezing or talking and during the performance of certain procedures such as suctioning and bronchoscopy.

Virions attach to human cells via interaction of the fibers with the CAR receptor (coxsackievirus and adenovirus receptor) on the cell surface and enter the cell via endocytosis. Virus uncoating occurs in the cytoplasm and the virus core is imported into the nucleus. The transcription of viral DNA depends in part on host cell machinery.

The replicative cycle in the host cells may be lytic or may result in the establishment of a latent infection, primarily in lymphoid tissue. The symptoms of adenovirus disease are due to the lysis of infected epithelial cells and the resulting inflammatory response. The initial immune response is probably the recognition of infected cells by natural killer cells and monocytes, which evokes a cytokine response, followed by induction of cytotoxic T cells and B cells. Prolonged shedding of adenoviruses in stools has been recognized even in immunocompetent individuals. Some adenovirus serotypes (especially 12, 18 and 31) can induce oncogenic transformation in cultured cell lines. In recent years, intensive research has focused on the use of adenoviruses as gene vectors.[1]

Prevention

An effective oral enteric-coated vaccine has been used to prevent adenovirus serotypes 4 and 7 infections in military recruits; however, this vaccine is not used in the general population. Contact and droplet precautions are indicated for controlling nosocomial transmission of adenovirus infection. Contact precautions include the isolation or cohorting of infected patients, the use of personal protective equipment (gloves, gowns), hand washing and the use of dedicated patient

Table 162.1 Human respiratory viruses: characteristic illnesses and populations at higher risk

Virus	Associated illnesses [most common virus subtype]	Patient population at higher risk
Adenovirus	URI [1–3, 5–7] Pharyngoconjunctival fever [3, 7, 14] URI, pneumonia [3, 4, 7, 14, 21] Pertussis-like syndrome [5] Pneumonia [1, 2, 3, 4, 7]	Infants, young children School-aged children Military recruits Infants, young children Infants, young children, immunocompromised
Coronavirus	Common cold Otitis Pneumonia Exacerbation of asthma-COPD Severe acute respiratory syndrome	All ages Children Military recruits, elderly, immunocompromised Persons with asthma-COPD All ages
Reovirus	Common cold (?) Enteritis (?)	All ages Children
Rhinovirus	Common cold URI Exacerbation of asthma-COPD Pneumonia	All ages All ages Persons with asthma-COPD Infants, young children, elderly, immunocompromised
Respiratory syncytial virus	URI Pneumonia Bronchiolitis Otitis	All ages Infants, young children, elderly, immunocompromised Infants, young children Children
Parainfluenza virus	URI Croup Otitis media Pneumonia	All ages Children Children Children, immunocompromised
Metapneumovirus	URI Pneumonia Bronchiolitis	All ages Infants, young children, elderly, immunocompromised Infants, young children
Human bocavirus	URI (?) Pneumonia (?)	Children Children

COPD, chronic obstructive pulmonary disease; URI, upper respiratory tract infection.

Table 162.2 Human respiratory viruses

Most common methods for laboratory diagnosis: culture, direct assay and serology

Virus	Culture cell lines	Characteristic findings	Direct assay	Serology
Adenovirus	Primary human embryonic kidney (HEK) and the human lung carcinoma (A549) cell lines are sensitive for a broad range of adenoviruses. Some adenoviruses may require up to 28 days to grow. The continuous epithelial lines, such as Hep-2 and HeLa, are sensitive but more difficult to maintain for a long period of time as required by some serotypes	Enlarged, refractile, rounded cells forming grape like clusters (Fig. 162.1), with some isolates forming a lattice-type arrangement of rounded cells	IF and EIA	Genus-specific EIA
Coronavirus	Culture not performed in most laboratories. SARS-CoV and HCoV-NL63 can be cultured in monkey epithelial cells	Cytocidal coronavirus infections may form multinucleated syncytia, lysis or both	EIA used in research settings	IF, EIA
Reovirus	Rarely isolated in the routine diagnostic setting. PRMK, LLC-MK2, HNK, HeLa, MDBK and H292 cell lines may support the growth of this virus	CPE is slow to develop. CPE may be nonspecific with increased granularity and progressive degeneration. HI and IFA can be used for typing	IF used in research settings	CF, NT, EIA used in research settings

(Continued)

Table 162.2 Human respiratory viruses—cont'd

Most common methods for laboratory diagnosis: culture, direct assay and serology

Virus	Culture cell lines	Characteristic findings	Direct assay	Serology
Rhinovirus	Human embryonic kidney and human fibroblast cell lines have been used most extensively: WI-38, HFF and MRC-5. HeLa is also sensitive	CPE is usually detected within the first week. CPE consists of rounded, highly refractile cells in loose clusters (Fig. 162.2). CPE permits a presumptive diagnosis of picornavirus infection. Demonstration of lability at pH 3 is used for differentiation from enteroviruses	EIA used in research settings	NT, CF, EIA used in research settings
Respiratory syncytial virus	Hep-2 is the preferred cell line. Alternatives include HeLa, A549, MRC-5, RhMK and Vero. Calcium and glutamine in the culture medium are important for optimal replication and cytopathic effect	CPE requires 3–7 days or more. Syncytia develop along with nonspecific granular degeneration (Fig. 162.3). Confirmation by means of IF (Fig. 162.3) or EIA	IF (Fig. 162.3), EIA, IP	CF, IF, EIA, NT
Parainfluenza virus	PRMK or MDCK are the preferred cell lines. LLC-MK2, a rhesus kidney heteroploid cell line and NCI_H292, a human lung carcinoma line, are also sensitive	CPE is variable and nonspecific. HPIV-2 and HPIV-3 may induce syncytia formation. Growth may be detected by means of HAd (Fig. 162.4) with confirmation and typing (Fig. 162.5), EIA, HAdI or HI	IF, EIA	HI, CF, EIA, NT
Metapneumovirus	Many strains replicate in tertiary monkey kidney cells/LLCMK-2 cells. Vero cell clone 118 seems to be permissible for all four lineages	CPE usually occurs after 10–21 days as syncytia formation or rounding of cells	IF	EIA
Human bocavirus	No cell culture model available	–	–	–

CF, complement fixation; CPE, cytopathic effect; EIA, enzyme immunoassay; HAd, hemadsorption inhibition; HAdI, hemadsorption assay; HI, hemagglutination inhibition; IF, immunofluorescence; IP, immunoperoxidase staining; LA, latex agglutination; NT, neutralization test; SARS, severe acute respiratory syndrome; PRMK, primary rhesus monkey kidney.

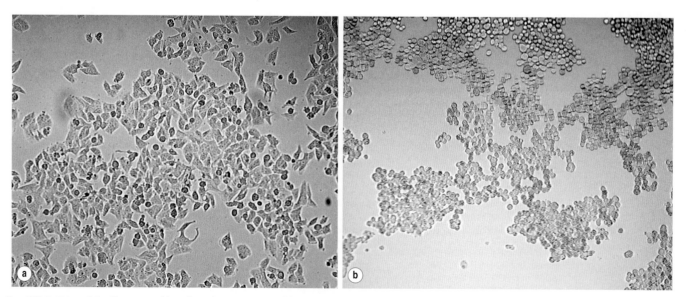

Fig. 162.1 Cytopathic effect caused by adenovirus on Hep-2 cell line culture. (a) Uninoculated cell line. (b) Enlarged, refractile, rounded cells forming grape-like clusters.

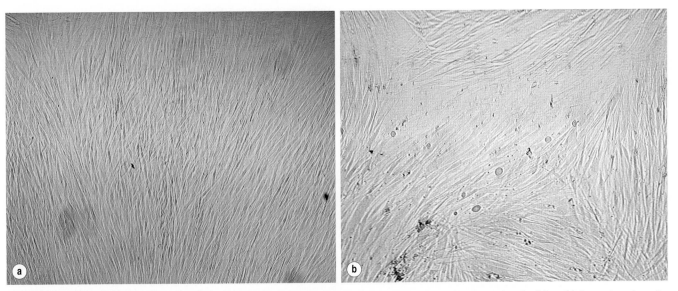

Fig. 162.2 Cytopathic effect caused by rhinovirus on human foreskin fibroblasts (HFF) cell line culture. (a) Uninoculated cell line. (b) Formation of small teardrop- to oval-shaped highly refractile cells.

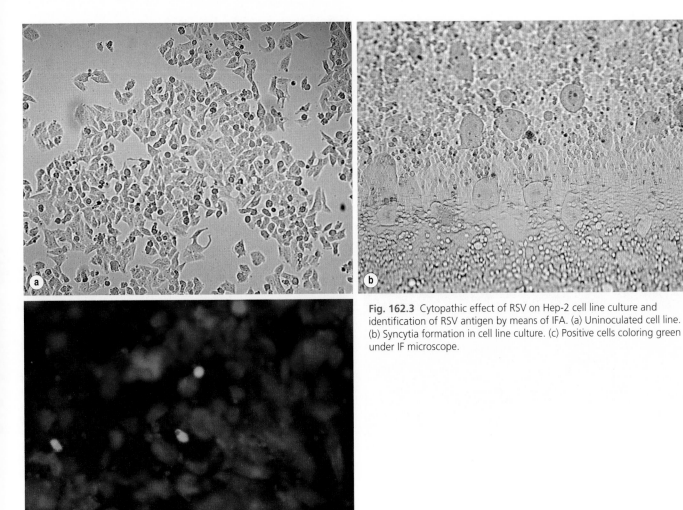

Fig. 162.3 Cytopathic effect of RSV on Hep-2 cell line culture and identification of RSV antigen by means of IFA. (a) Uninoculated cell line. (b) Syncytia formation in cell line culture. (c) Positive cells coloring green under IF microscope.

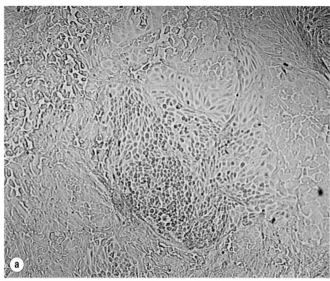
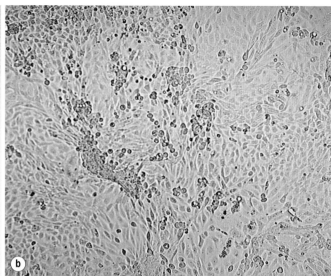
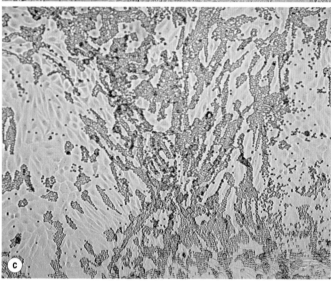

Fig. 162.4 Identification of hemadsorbing viruses. (a) Uninoculated primary rhesus monkey kidney (PRMK) cell line. (b) Nonspecific rounding or clumping of PRMK cells. (c) Positive hemadsorption of guinea-pig red blood cells.

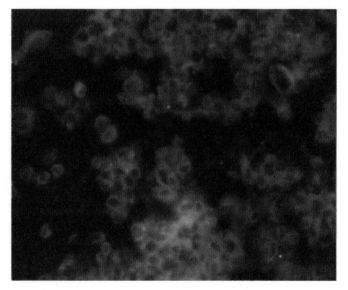

Fig. 162.5 Differentiation of hemadsorbing viruses by means of IFA. Negative control.

care equipment when possible. Droplet precautions include the additional use of masks by health-care workers within the patient's room and the use of masks by the patient when outside the room. Maintaining adequate levels of chlorination is necessary to prevent swimming pool-associated outbreaks of adenovirus conjunctivitis.

Diagnostic microbiology

Virus isolation, antigen detection, PCR assay and serology can be used to identify adenovirus infections. Adenovirus serotyping is usually accomplished by hemagglutination inhibition and/or neutralization with type-specific antisera. The isolation of adenoviruses from body secretions is not sufficient to establish a diagnosis of adenovirus disease as prolonged asymptomatic shedding of adenoviruses can occur. New molecular diagnostics such as quantitative PCR have improved the rapid diagnosis of adenovirus infections and monitoring of viral loads in blood has been shown to correlate with clinical progression of disease.[2]

Clinical manifestations

Respiratory illnesses associated with adenovirus infections include undifferentiated upper respiratory illness, pharyngoconjunctival fever, pertussis-like syndrome and pneumonia. The various adenovirus serotypes associated with respiratory disease are shown in Table 162.1. In addition, adenoviruses may also cause gastroenteritis, keratoconjunctivitis, cystitis, meningoencephalitis and hepatitis, depending on the serotype. The incubation period for the endemic serotypes ranges from 5 to 10 days and the symptoms last approximately 1 week. Chronic lung damage in the form of bronchiolitis obliterans has been reported after infections with serotypes 1, 3, 4, 7 and 21.

The incidence of severe adenovirus disease is increasing with the rising number of immunomodulatory treatments used in modern medicine. Pediatric patients are more susceptible to adenovirus infection and disease than adults, probably due to the higher rate of primary infections occurring among children. However, cases of severe adenovirus disease have also been reported in apparently normal hosts. Immunocompromised patients, particularly hematopoietic stem cell transplant (HSCT) and solid-organ transplant recipients, are susceptible to severe and potentially fatal adenovirus disease,[3–5] such as protracted hemorrhagic cystitis, encephalitis, nephritis, hepatitis, enteritis, pneumonia or a combination of these illnesses (disseminated disease).

Management

Most infections are mild and require only symptomatic treatment. Ribavirin has *in-vitro* activity against several adenovirus serotypes but the clinical experience in immunocompromised individuals has produced conflicting results (see Chapter 147).

CORONAVIRUS

Nature

Human coronavirus (HCoV) was first isolated in 1965 from a patient with symptoms of the common cold. Three new coronaviruses have been detected since 2001: the severe acute respiratory syndrome (SARS)-associated coronavirus in 2003, coronavirus NL63 in 2004 and coronavirus HKU1 in 2005. Coronaviruses are classified into three groups: group 1 consists of HCoV-229E and HCoV-NL63, group 2 harbors HCoV-OC43 and HCoV-HKU1, and SARS-CoV is classified independently and is thought to be of animal origin.[6] Virions are pleomorphic and measure 80–200 nm in diameter. The outer envelope bears distinctive 'club-shaped' peplomers that correspond to the S (long spike) glycoprotein. The resulting 'crown-like' appearance under electron microscopy gives the family its name. The S glycoprotein is involved in receptor binding and cell fusion and is a major target for neutralizing antibodies. Other structural proteins include the M (matrix) protein, the E (envelope) protein and the N (nucleocapsid) phosphoprotein. In some types, there is also a glycoprotein HE (hemagglutinin-esterase, short spike). Entry occurs via endocytosis and membrane fusion. Replication of the linear single-stranded positive-sense RNA genome takes place in the cytoplasm.

Epidemiology

HCoVs are ubiquitous. Serologic studies with the initial two coronaviruses OC43 and 229E have suggested that these viruses are a major cause of respiratory disease and account for 10–30% of all common colds. Serologic studies have also suggested that one-half of the infections with coronaviruses are asymptomatic.[7] The identification of a coronavirus as the underlying pathogen for SARS was published in 2003 and this was the first time that a coronavirus was definitely demonstrated to cause severe human disease.[8,9] The SARS epidemic was contained through global infection control efforts organized by the World Health Organization (WHO) and currently there is no evidence that SARS coronavirus is active in human populations. More than 8000 cases were reported in the course of the SARS epidemic in 29 affected countries, leading to more than 800 deaths worldwide.[10] Since the discovery of SARS two newer coronaviruses HKU1 and NL63

have been identified. These HCoVs are similar to their older cousins in being mostly associated with common cold symptoms but severe clinical disease can be caused in young children, the elderly and in immunocompromised patients.[11]

Pathogenesis

Intranasal inoculation of volunteers with these viruses results in common colds with disruption of the ciliated epithelium and ciliary dyskinesia.[12] Aminopeptidase N (APN), the receptor for HCoV-229E, is expressed on the apical surfaces of respiratory and intestinal epithelium, myelocytic cells, kidney tubular epithelium and synaptic junctions. HCoV-OC43 binds to cells by means of the HE glycoprotein or the viral S glycoprotein, which can recognize 9-O-acetylated sialic acid on the cell surface.

Prevention

No specific antiviral drugs or vaccines are currently available. The major transmission modes for SARS are the contact and/or droplet route, although airborne transmission over a limited distance had been suggested.[13] The outbreak of SARS was successfully controlled through early detection of cases by screening of persons with symptoms of a respiratory infection and implementing strict contact and droplet precautions. The Centers for Disease Control and Prevention (CDC) currently recommends contact precautions and airborne precautions with N95 or higher respirator masks[13] although in Hong Kong the use of contact and droplet precautions alone was sufficient to protect health-care workers.[14]

Diagnostic microbiology

Diagnosis of infection is achieved by nucleic acid extraction, reverse transcription and PCR. Coronaviruses are included in multiplex assays that have been developed for the diagnosis of respiratory viral infections. Some of the coronaviruses can be cultured in monkey epithelial cells (SARS-CoV and NL63). Most of the population studies of HCoVs have used serologic methods, including complement fixation, hemagglutination inhibition (OC43 only) and recently enzyme immunoassay (EIA).

Clinical manifestations

Apart from SARS-HCoV, HCoVs are predominantly associated with mild upper respiratory tract infections and occasionally severe disease is observed in immunocompromised patients. In a study of adult volunteers the mean incubation period was 3.3 days, with a range of 2–4 days. The symptoms lasted for a mean of 7 days, with a range of 3–18 days.[15] In contrast, SARS-HCoV was capable of causing a multisystem disease with infection of the gastrointestinal tract, liver, kidney and brain.[16]

The clinical course is mainly characterized by fever, dyspnea, lymphopenia and lower respiratory tract infection; 30–40% of patients had diarrhea.[10] Compared to the other coronaviruses SARS was causing a much more severe disease with a mortality rate of nearly 10%.[17] Coronavirus particles have also been seen (via electron microscopy) in the stools of children and adults with diarrhea and gastroenteritis. Earlier speculations that coronavirus could participate in the etiology of multiple sclerosis were not confirmed.[10] However, the importance of human coronaviruses as a cause of diseases outside the respiratory tract remains to be determined.

Management

No effective antiviral therapy against coronaviruses, including SARS, has been found so far. *In-vitro* ribavirin is capable of inhibiting viral replication but there are no *in-vivo* data supporting its therapeutic efficacy.[10] Steroids were used to treat SARS-infected patients with the aim of modulating cytokine levels. Interferons were found to possess antiviral activity *in vitro* and in animal models.[10] A protective vaccine against SARS has not yet been generated.

REOVIRUS

Nature

Isolation of the first reovirus was made in 1951, but it was in 1959 that Sabin coined the term reovirus to emphasize the fact that these viruses were isolated from the respiratory and enteric tracts and that they were not associated with any known human disease (Respiratory Enteric Orphan viruses). Reoviruses are nonenveloped viruses of about 65–75 nm in diameter. Viruses of the genus *Orthoreovirus* are composed of two concentric icosahedrically symmetric protein capsids, containing 10 discrete segments of genomic double-stranded RNA. Orthoreoviruses have been isolated from a wide variety of mammalian, avian and reptilian hosts, and over recent years several previously unknown reoviruses (especially of bat origin) have been reported.[18]

Epidemiology

A study using enzyme linked immunosorbent assay (ELISA) as the diagnostic method showed that the prevalence of antibodies against reoviruses increased steadily throughout life from about 35% in infants to 60% in teenagers and to more than 85% among those older than 60 years of age.[19]

Diagnostic microbiology

Trying to diagnose reovirus infection on a routine basis is not recommended. In the research setting, a variety of techniques are available.

Clinical manifestations

In a study of adult volunteers, intranasal inoculation of reovirus was followed by an increase in serotype-specific antibodies, enteric virus isolation and development of respiratory illness in a third of the individuals infected with reovirus T1L.[20] Two newer reoviruses, Melaka virus and Kampar virus, were isolated from patients with acute respiratory tract disease, raising the possibility that the clinical importance of this group of viruses was underestimated in the past.

RHINOVIRUS

Nature

Human rhinovirus (HRV) was first isolated in the 1950s from nasopharyngeal secretions of patients with the common cold. HRV belongs to the Picornaviridae family, which includes the genera *Enterovirus* and *Hepatovirus* (hepatitis A virus). Rhinoviruses are small (30 nm), nonenveloped particles that contain a linear single-stranded positive-sense RNA genome. The icosahedral capsid is composed of 60 subunits arranged as 12 pentameres. Each subunit is composed of one of each of four structural proteins (VP1 to VP4). VP1–3 have exterior projections that are major epitopes for neutralizing antibodies.

More than 100 serotypes have been identified to date. Phylogenetic analysis of genome sequences revealed two different species of rhinovirus A and B, HRV-A and HRV-B. Recently, a third genetic cluster was proposed (HRV-C) by analysis of viruses amplified from children with exacerbations of asthma.[21]

Epidemiology

Rhinoviruses are ubiquitous and infections occur in all age groups. They cause about half of all common colds and over the last few years an increasing number of publications have linked HRVs to more severe upper and lower respiratory tract infections in children, the elderly and immunocompromised patients.[22–24] HRV infections occur throughout the year, with peaks in the fall and spring, and with multiple serotypes circulating simultaneously in a given geographic location. Preschool children commonly introduce the virus to the rest of the family, with a secondary attack rate of about 50% after an interval of 2–5 days. Extensive studies in susceptible individuals have shown that 95% of challenged subjects become infected and about 75% of them become ill. The major factor determining the risk of illness is the prechallenge level of neutralizing antibodies.

Pathogenesis

In spite of the extensive literature on the transmission of rhinoviruses, controversy still exists about the predominant mode of transmission. Most data support the notion that contact transmission, primarily as hand shaking followed by inoculation of the nasal mucosa and lacrimal canals, is the most efficient mode of transmission. HRVs can survive from a few hours to as long as 4 days on nonporous surfaces and for over 2 hours on human skin. Although droplet or airborne transmission of rhinovirus infection is possible, prolonged and close exposure is apparently required. There is no convincing clinical evidence to support the common notion that exposure to cold plays a role in the genesis of HRV illness.

Rhinoviruses attach to respiratory epithelium and spread locally. The leukocyte binding protein CD54/intercellular adhesion molecule 1 (ICAM-1) is the receptor for the majority of rhinovirus serotypes. The receptor-binding site resides in a depression of the capsid surface that is not accessible to antibodies. After endocytosis, a conformational change of the capsid allows the release of the viral RNA into the host cell cytoplasm, where viral replication and assembly take place. A polyprotein precursor is processed mainly by two viral proteases designated 2A and 3C. The 2A protease makes the first cleavage between the structural and nonstructural proteins, while the 3C protease catalyzes most of the remaining internal cleavages.

Infection is followed by activation of several inflammatory mechanisms including the release of cytokines, particularly interleukin (IL)-8, bradykinins, prostaglandins and histamine, as well as stimulation of parasympathetic reflexes.

The resulting process includes vasodilatation of nasal blood vessels, transudation of plasma, glandular secretion and stimulation of nerve fibers, triggering sneeze and cough reflexes. Nasal mucociliary transport is reduced markedly during the illness and may be impaired for weeks. Immunity to individual rhinoviruses is type specific and not long lasting. Protection correlates more with the level of locally synthesized IgA antibodies, which decline within months of infection, rather than with IgG levels in serum, which may persist for a few years.

Prevention

Hand washing after personal contact with a symptomatic person or after touching potentially contaminated objects is strongly recommended. Alcohol-based antiseptics are also effective for this purpose. Symptomatic patients should be advised to wash hands frequently and to use disposable tissues. The CDC recommends droplet precautions for the prevention of nosocomial HRV infections.

The diversity of serotypes and the specificity of the immune response have precluded the development of an effective vaccine. A number of drugs have been studied for the prophylaxis of HRV infection, including interferon alpha (IFN-α), pirodavir and the recombinant soluble CD54/ICAM-1 molecule. However, the practical utility of these drugs remains to be demonstrated.

Diagnostic microbiology

In clinical practice HRV infections are diagnosed by viral RNA detection with RT-PCR. RT-PCR assays are more rapid and sensitive than isolation techniques for the detection of HRV RNA in clinical specimens. Historically, HRV infections have been detected by virus isolation in cell culture followed by acid lability testing to distinguish them from enterovirus infections. Virus isolation typically requires 2–14 days. Presumptive identification of a cell culture isolate as rhinovirus is based on a combination of enterovirus-like cytopathic effects and clinical information. Further differentiation from enteroviruses is based on the diminished replication of rhinoviruses at 98.6°F (37°C) compared to growth at 91.4°F (33°C) and at pH 3.0 compared with pH 7.0, respectively

ELISA has been developed for the detection of rhinovirus antigens. The use of serologic assays is limited by the diversity of serotypes and the lack of a group-specific antigen.

Clinical manifestations

Symptoms of the common cold include profuse watery rhinorrhea, nasal congestion, sneezing and quite often headache, sore throat and cough. The symptoms begin within 8–10 hours of infection and peak around 1–3 days. There is little or no fever. By days 3–5 of the illness, nasal discharge may become mucopurulent from polymorphonuclear leukocytes that have migrated to the infection site in response to IL-8. Resolution of symptoms generally occurs within a week. Complications include sinusitis, otitis media and exacerbation of asthma or chronic obstructive pulmonary disease (COPD). Secondary bacterial infections may also occur. Studies using CT of the sinuses have shown that HRV infections can cause the accumulation of secretions in the sinuses, possibly from the passage of nasal secretions into the sinuses during nose blowing.[25,26]

Recent published evidence has confirmed the association of HRVs with severe airway disease in immunocompromised patients, children and the elderly.[21,22] A novel HRV species (HRV-C) has been found in a significant proportion of children with exacerbations of asthma.

Management

Symptomatic treatment with decongestants, antihistamines and antitussives is currently the mainstay of therapy. The efficacy of zinc lozenges is controversial and their practical utility is limited because of their metallic taste. A variety of candidate drugs have been studied.[27]

Interferon alpha 2b has been found to be effective for the prevention of rhinovirus-associated colds but ineffective for the treatment of established colds.[28] Recent therapeutic advances include the development of protease 3C inhibitors, recombinant soluble ICAM-1 antagonist and capsid-function inhibitors (pleconaril), all of which exhibit potent antirhinoviral activity *in vitro* and varying activity in clinical trials.[27,29] Recombinant soluble ICAM-1 molecule (Tremacamra) has been found to be effective in reducing the symptoms of experimental common colds in randomized controlled trials when given either as a preventative or a therapeutic agent.[30]

Pleconaril binds to a hydrophobic pocket in the viral capsid, inducing conformational changes that lead to altered receptor binding and viral uncoating. Pleconaril is orally bioavailable and achieves serum concentrations in excess of those required to inhibit 90% of clinical rhino- and enteroviral isolates *in vitro*. In a placebo-controlled study of rhinovirus infections, pleconaril-treated patients had a 1.5-day reduction in time to resolution of symptoms, significant reduction in symptom severity within 12–24 hours after initiation of therapy and a significant reduction in median viral titers in nasal mucus.[31] The US FDA Advisory Committee has not yet recommended the approval of pleconaril for treatment of the common cold.

RESPIRATORY SYNCYTIAL VIRUS

Nature

Respiratory syncytial virus (RSV) was first isolated in the mid-1950s from a symptomatic laboratory chimpanzee during an outbreak of illness resembling the common cold. This virus derives its name from the characteristic formation of multinucleated giant cells in tissue culture.

RSV is a linear single-stranded, negative-sense genomic RNA of the Paramyxoviridae family of viruses. Virions are pleomorphic, with both spherical and filamentous forms averaging 120–300 nm in diameter. The envelope consists of host-derived plasma membrane and three virally encoded transmembrane surface glycoproteins: the attachment protein G, the fusion protein F and the small hydrophobic SH protein. The F protein can mediate fusion with neighboring cells to form syncytia. The G glycoprotein plays a major role in the process of attachment. Two major types of RSV – A and B – are distinguished serologically based on the antigenic characteristics of the surface glycoprotein G. Other viral proteins include the matrix proteins (M and M2), the major nucleocapsid (N) protein, a phosphoprotein (P) and the major polymerase (L).

Epidemiology

RSV is the most common cause of bronchiolitis and pneumonia among infants and young children worldwide.[32] Virtually all children are infected by the time they reach 3 years of age. Natural immunity is transient and re-infection is common. Crowding in households and day-care centers increases the attack rate of RSV. A large CDC-initiated study found that among children with acute respiratory infection admitted to hospital or attending outpatient services, 18% of specimens were positive for RSV.[33] Extrapolating this figure to the entire US population, 2 million children under 5 years of age would require medical attention due to RSV infection on a yearly basis.[33] In older children and immunocompetent adults, RSV infections are seldom severe and are usually manifested as upper respiratory infection (URI) or tracheobronchitis. Individuals at high risk for severe RSV infection include premature infants (particularly those born at less than 34 weeks of gestation), young infants with chronic lung disease or a hemodynamically significant congenital heart defect, elderly individuals and immunocompromised subjects. Recent studies indicate that the disease burden caused by RSV in elderly and high-risk adults had previously been underestimated and is currently thought to be similar to that of endemic influenza A.[34] Development of an effective RSV vaccine is therefore required for both young children and the elderly.

RSV activity follows a seasonal pattern in temperate zones of the world. In urban centers, annual outbreaks occur during the fall, winter and early spring. In the northern hemisphere most outbreaks peak in February or March. In tropical or subtropical areas, epidemics peak during the rainy season.

Pathogenesis

RSV is present in large numbers in the respiratory secretions of symptomatic infected persons and viral titers remain high for about 1 week, followed by a gradual decline over 3–4 weeks. The portal of entry is usually the conjunctiva or the nasal mucosa. Although transmission can occur via large droplets, contact transmission predominates.[35] Virus can be viable for approximately 30 minutes on impervious surfaces such as bed rails. Thus, caregivers can contaminate their hands during routine care and transmit the virus by contact to other patients. Neutralizing antibodies to the surface glycoproteins F and G correlate with resistance to re-infection, but protection is not complete and is of short duration.[36]

The pathology of RSV bronchiolitis is characterized by necrosis of ciliated bronchiolar epithelial cells, mononuclear infiltrates and edema of the peribronchial space. Bronchiolar obstruction from increased mucus production results in air trapping and total obstruction results in atelectasis. Pathologic examination of lungs from patients with RSV pneumonia has revealed marked interstitial inflammation and edema of the lung parenchyma, along with the findings of bronchiolitis.

Prevention

In the household setting, the transmission of RSV may be decreased by frequent hand washing and not sharing household items such as cups, glasses and utensils. The CDC recommends contact precautions for the prevention of nosocomial RSV infections. Some institutions also observe droplet isolation precautions. Implementation of multifaceted infection control strategies resulted in a reduction of the incidence of nosocomial RSV infections.[37] Passive immunoprophylaxis is indicated for high-risk children.

RSV intravenous immunoglobulin (RSV-IVIG, RespiGam) is a human polyclonal immunoglobulin with high RSV microneutralization titers. In placebo-controlled studies, monthly intravenous doses of 750 mg/kg during the RSV season significantly reduced the incidence of RSV hospitalizations and the severity of illness among premature infants and infants with bronchopulmonary dysplasia.[38,39] Palivizumab is a humanized monoclonal antibody that specifically inhibits an epitope at the A antigenic site of the F protein of RSV subtypes A and B. In a large multicenter placebo-controlled trial involving high-risk infants, palivizumab prophylaxis resulted in a 55% reduction in hospitalization rates and number of hospital days ascribed to RSV infection.[40] Both agents have been well tolerated, with few adverse effects; however, their high cost necessitates strict guidelines for their use. RSV-IVIG or palivizumab is indicated for the prophylaxis of RSV infections among infants with chronic lung disease (formerly designated bronchopulmonary dysplasia) and premature infants. In children with a hemodynamically significant congenital heart defect only palivizumab is indicated for prophylaxis.[41] Cost-saving benefit has not been observed uniformly,[42–46] perhaps as a result of major differences in the prevalence of RSV lower respiratory tract infections in different countries and regions, suggesting the need for locally adapted recommendations. Palivizumab is easier to administer and does not interfere with the measles, mumps, rubella (MMR) vaccine or varicella vaccine. RSV-IVIG, however, provides additional protection against other respiratory viral illnesses and may be preferred for children receiving replacement IVIG because of underlying immune deficiency.[40]

The role of passive immunoprophylaxis for the prevention of RSV infections in high-risk adults remains to be defined. Development of an RSV vaccine is ongoing but none is yet available.

Diagnostic microbiology

The gold standard diagnostic method is isolation of the virus from respiratory secretions, but increasingly nonculture diagnostic methods are used for RSV.

RSV was the first respiratory virus to be readily identified by means of rapid diagnostic tests based on antigen detection. Current methods for rapid detection of RSV antigen include EIA, immunoperoxidase staining, direct and indirect immunofluorescence tests and RT-PCR. Serologic diagnosis requires a convalescent-phase RSV IgG antibody titer at least four times higher than the acute-phase titer.

Clinical manifestations

The incubation period for RSV ranges from 2 to 8 days. Illness begins most frequently with rhinorrhea, sneezing and cough. When fever is present it is generally low grade. Most children experience recovery from illness after 8–15 days. During their first RSV infection, 25–40% of infected infants and young children have signs or symptoms of bronchiolitis or pneumonia and 0.5–2% require hospitalization.

In contrast, hospitalization will be required in up to 25% of high-risk children such as those with a history of prematurity or chronic lung disease. RSV bronchiolitis or pneumonia should be suspected when an infant or young child presents with progressive cough, wheezing and dyspnea during the RSV season.

Radiographic findings in patients with bronchiolitis include hyperlucency, diaphragmatic flattening and outward bowing on the intercostal spaces. Findings compatible with pneumonia include interstitial infiltrates and, less frequently, consolidation, particularly in the right upper and middle lobes.

In neonates, the clinical presentation may be atypical with lethargy, irritability or poor oral intake. RSV has been detected in lung tissue of infants with sudden death syndrome, but a causal relationship has not been confirmed. Prolonged pulmonary function deficit and airway hyperreactivity have been reported following RSV infection but it remains unclear whether these abnormalities were present before the infection.[47] Otitis media has also been associated with RSV infection.

Among immunocompetent adults, RSV infection usually manifests with rhinorrhea, pharyngitis, cough, bronchitis, headache, fatigue and fever. In older persons, particularly the institutionalized elderly and those with chronic cardiopulmonary illnesses, severe pneumonia may occur, leading to respiratory failure. Among immunocompromised individuals, RSV has been the most frequently isolated viral respiratory pathogen in surveillance studies performed at large cancer centers.[48] In this setting RSV infection typically begins as a URI and may evolve into lower respiratory tract disease in up to 50% of cases. A particularly high rate of progression to pneumonia (70–80%) has been reported among adult HSCT recipients developing RSV infection within the period prior to engraftment. In such settings RSV pneumonia resulted in 60–80% mortality, regardless of whether antiviral drugs were used for treatment.

Management

For patients with mild disease, only symptomatic treatment is necessary. Children with severe disease may require hospitalization for supplemental oxygen therapy, hydration and nutrition, or for mechanical ventilation. Improvements in supportive care have made a significant impact on the mortality from RSV bronchiolitis and pneumonia. The use of bronchodilators is likely beneficial for patients with significant bronchospasm. Corticosteroids are commonly used as anti-inflammatory therapy, although there is no supportive data demonstrating the benefits of such intervention. Aerosolized ribavirin (Virasole) was approved in 1986 for the treatment of infants and children with severe RSV disease. The treatment is cumbersome to deliver and its impact on mortality remains controversial.[49,50]

A combination of immune therapy and ribavirin has been reported to be well tolerated and to improve the outcome of severe RSV infection among bone marrow transplant recipients.[51,52] In one open trial the mortality was only 22% among nine adults with pneumonia in whom therapy was initiated prior to the onset of profound respiratory failure.[52] Pre-emptive treatment strategies are being investigated primarily in immunocompromised individuals. Delay of immunosuppressive chemotherapy should be considered when severely immunosuppressed individuals, such as HSCT recipients, develop acute RSV infection.

PARAINFLUENZA VIRUS

Nature

Human parainfluenza viruses (HPIVs) were first described in the 1950s, originally as croup-associated viruses; they belong to the Paramyxoviridae family.

The virions are pleomorphic and range in average diameter from 150 to 200 nm. They are enveloped particles with a linear singlestranded, negative-sense RNA genome. The HPIVs encode two surface glycoproteins: an attachment protein called HN (hemagglutinin-neuraminidase) that binds to sialic acid-containing receptors on host cell surfaces, and a fusion protein F that is involved in the fusion of the viral membrane with the cellular plasma membrane. The HN protein is a multifunctional molecule with binding activity (binding to sialic acid containing surface glycoproteins and glycolipids), neuraminidase activity and fusion promotion activity. The attachment activity can be measured by hemagglutination assay. The neuraminidase activity prevents aggregation of virus particles by removing sialic acid from the virion glycoproteins and facilitates infection in the respiratory tract by digesting the mucin coating of epithelial cells.

These viruses also encode three nucleocapsid associated proteins, NP, P and L, and the nonglycosylated internal protein M. The four HPIVs are segregated into two genera, the *Respirovirus* (HPIV-1 and HPIV-3) and the *Rubulavirus* (HPIV-2 and HPIV-4), based on antigenic and structural characteristics, including additional accessory proteins (V, D, W, I, X, C and SH).

Epidemiology

HPIVs are distributed worldwide. Each of the four HPIVs can cause a full spectrum of acute respiratory tract illnesses. HPIV-1 and HPIV-2 are the most common pathogens associated with croup or laryngotracheobronchitis.[53] HPIV-1, -2 and -3 are also important causes of bronchiolitis and pneumonia among infants and young children;[53,54] less is known about HPIV-4. Most children have serologic evidence of infection by 5 years of age. Most HPIV infections are detected during seasonal epidemics. In a study on an outpatient pediatric population,[55] HPIV-1 occurred in the fall of odd-numbered years, HPIV-2 was less predictable and HPIV-3 appeared yearly with peak activity in spring or summer.

Pathogenesis

Although droplet transmission can occur, contact is thought to be the primary mode of transmission of HPIV infection. This can be direct person-to-person contact or indirect through intermediate objects. Inoculation is via the nasopharyngeal or oral mucosa. The pathogenesis of the ensuing laryngotracheobronchitis and croup is not completely understood. The immune response after HPIV infection is complex and includes the production of serum-neutralizing antibodies directed towards epitopes of the HN and F proteins. The mucosal immune response plays an important role in the protection against HPIVs infection, primarily through the production of IgA antibodies. In animal model studies, CD8+ T cells were critical for virus clearance.

Prevention

The CDC recommends contact precautions for the prevention of nosocomial HPIV infections. Some institutions also observe droplet isolation precautions. No specific vaccine is yet available and no drugs have been tested for prophylactic use.

Diagnostic microbiology

Definite diagnosis relies on the isolation of the virus from respiratory secretions. Other diagnostic methods include detection of viral antigens or nucleic acid, and serologic analysis. Primary isolation and identification by hemadsorption assay can be followed by typing of the virus through immunofluorescence or hemadsorption inhibition. PCR assays are more sensitive than isolation and antigen detection methods.[56]

Clinical manifestations

Infection in children is associated with an acute febrile illness in up to 80% of cases. Initial symptoms include coryza, sore throat, hoarseness and dry cough. In croup, a brassy or barking cough may progress to stridor and occasionally to airway obstruction. The anteroposterior radiograph of the neck shows glottic and subglottic narrowing ('steeple sign') which differentiates croup from epiglottitis. In cases of bronchiolitis and pneumonia, progressive cough is accompanied by wheezing, tachypnea and hypoxemia. Chest X-ray examination may reveal air trapping and interstitial infiltrates. Otitis media is a common finding in patients with HPIV infections.

In older children and adults, HPIV infections tend to be milder and present as URI. However, HPIV-1 and -3 have been diagnosed by serology in a significant number of adults admitted with acute respiratory illness.[57] A few cases of HPIV meningitis have been described.[58] Immunocompromised pediatric and adult individuals such as HSCT,[59–64] lung[65] and renal[66] transplant recipients may develop severe HPIV infections with a high rate of progression to pneumonia. The use of corticosteroids was linked with a higher risk of HPIV-3 pneumonia among HSCT recipents.[61]

Management

Symptomatic treatment of croup usually includes humidification of air by ultrasonic nebulizer and inhalations of racemic adrenaline (epinephrine). Adrenaline (epinephrine) provides rapid but transient relief of the airway obstruction. The anti-inflammatory effect of systemic corticosteroids is advocated to prevent or shorten the period of intubation in severe croup. Patients with bronchiolitis are additionally treated with bronchodilators. Ribavirin has exhibited *in-vitro* activity against HPIVs[67] but data from controlled clinical trials are lacking.

HUMAN METAPNEUMOVIRUS

Nature

In June 2001, it was reported that a new respiratory virus had been isolated from nasopharyngeal aspirates of 28 young children in the Netherlands. Based on virologic data, sequence homology and gene constellation, the virus was classified as a member of the *Metapneumovirus* genus of the Paramyxoviridae family and was named human metapneumovirus (HMPV).[68] HMPV is the first known mammalian metapneumovirus causing disease. Serologic analysis detected antibodies against the virus being present in all individuals older than 8 years of age in specimens collected since 1958.[68]

The genome of HMPV consists of negative-sense, nonsegmented RNA. Similar to other paramyxoviruses, virions are pleomorphic with a mean diameter of 200 nm. The lipid envelope, which is derived from the plasma membrane of the host cell, contains three viral glycoproteins, the attachment (G), fusion (F) and small SH proteins. The functions of these proteins are similar to those of their counterparts found in other paramyxoviruses (see above). There are two major genotypes of HMPV, A and B.[69] Both of these major genetic lineages are further divided into two genetic subgroups termed A1 and A2 and B1 and B2. Current evidence suggests that the two genetic lineages are not distinct antigenic subtypes.[70] HMPV replicates slowly in cell culture with characteristic syncytia formation

Epidemiology

HMPV infections have been diagnosed worldwide in patients of all age groups with respiratory disease. In temperate climates the virus is predominantly transmitted in late winter and spring, whereas in the subtropics infections culminate in spring/summer. Infection rates peak at the same time or shortly after the RSV infection peak.[71] HPMV has been associated with upper and lower respiratory tract infections in young children and is the second most frequently isolated viral pathogen after RSV to cause bronchiolitis in early childhood.[72–75]

Pathogenesis

Transmission most likely occurs in a fashion similar to RSV via droplets and contaminated fomites; nosocomial transmission has been reported.[76] Human respiratory infection was associated with an increase of IL-8 in respiratory secretions and with chronic inflammatory changes in the airways. Levels of inflammatory cytokines (IL-12, tumor necrosis factor, IL-6, IL-1β) found in HMPV disease were lower than levels observed with RSV infection.[77]

Prevention

Both droplet precautions and direct contact precautions should be observed to prevent transmission in the health-care setting.

Diagnostic microbiology

The virus is difficult to grow in cell culture. Most strains show cytopathic effect in LLC-MK2 (tertiary monkey kidney) cells; recently a Vero cell clone was reported as being permissible for all four viral lineages.[70] Cytopathic effects usually occur after 10–21 days and vary from syncytia formation to rounding of cells. Direct immunofluorescence assays with commercially produced virus-specific antibodies are available, although they are probably less sensitive than RT-PCR for the detection of virus. Molecular methods have become the method of choice for the detection of the HMPV genome. Real-time RT-PCR targeting the N and/or L gene has been found to be sensitive, specific and rapid in detecting the virus in clinical specimens.[78] Serologic diagnosis can be achieved by ELISA methods demonstrating a fourfold increase in antibody titers or seroconversion.

Clinical manifestations

HMPV has been associated with respiratory tract infections in all age groups: severe lower respiratory tract infections have been observed in very young children, the elderly and immunocompromised patients. HMPV infection in adults usually presents with flu-like symptoms such as rhinorrhea, sore throat and cough. Children are at higher risk for the development of lower airway disease (bronchiolitis, pneumonia), especially infants younger than 2 years of age.[79] The severity varies from self-limiting mild respiratory illness to respiratory failure requiring mechanical ventilation. Clinical disease associated with HMPV is similar to RSV disease and 12% of outpatients with acute lower respiratory tract infections were harboring HMPV which was second only to RSV.[72] Heikkinen *et al.* reported that 60% of children less than 3 years of age developed acute otitis media due to HMPV infection.[79]

Management

Several vaccine candidates have shown promising results in animal models but their safety and efficacy in humans remains to be determined. Antiviral treatment strategies for severe disease are derived from experiences obtained with RSV infections. Ribavirin shows equivalent antiviral potential against HMPV[80] to that observed with RSV and

an HMPV-neutralizing monoclonal antibody for prophylaxis in high-risk infants (similar to palivizumab in RSV) is likely to be developed.

HUMAN BOCAVIRUS

Human bocavirus (HBoV) was identified in 2005 by random amplification and cloning of DNA followed by large scale sequencing and bioinformatic analysis.[81] By sequence analysis it has been provisionally classified as a parvovirus. Since then multiple studies have confirmed the worldwide presence of HBoV in the respiratory tract of children, usually under 2 years of age.[82] HBoV is often present as a co-infection with other respiratory viruses (such as RSV) raising the issue of disease association.

Determination of the pathogenicity of HBoV is complicated by the lack of an *in-vitro* culture system and a suitable animal model. High viral loads in respiratory specimens and detection of viral DNA in blood seem to be associated with respiratory tract symptoms, whereas the presence of low viral loads is of unclear significance.[83,84] The first serologic studies analyzing the antibody response in humans against HBoV structural proteins have now been published.[85,86] Antibodies against HBoV were detected in 71.1% of serum samples collected from people from infancy to 41 years in Japan.[85] High viral load in the nasopharynx and viremia correlated with a serologic diagnosis of primary infection (IgM antibodies and/or an increase in IgG antibody level).[86] Further studies are needed to clarify the pathogenesis and the natural course of infection of HBoV.

CONCLUSION

A better understanding of the profound impact that human respiratory viruses have on human morbidity and mortality has resulted in more resources being devoted to their study. More efficient diagnostic tools, new antiviral agents, the use of passive immunoprophylaxis, improvements in vaccination programs and in strategies to control the nosocomial transmission of these infections are among the most significant accomplishments.

Acknowledgment

Illustrations are contributed by Joseph Yarsa BS, MT(ASCP) and Xiang-Yang Han MD, PhD from the Microbiology Laboratory at The University of Texas MD Anderson Cancer Center, Houston, Texas, USA.

REFERENCES

References for this chapter can be found online at http://www.expertconsult.com

Retroviruses and retroviral infections

INTRODUCTION

The Retroviridae constitute a large family of viruses that predominantly infect both human and animal vertebrates. Retroviral infections can cause a wide spectrum of diseases ranging from malignancies to immune deficiencies and neurologic disorders. However, most retroviral infections occur without any detectable deleterious effect to the host. In spite of this diversity of associated pathology and the broad range of hosts, all retroviruses share a similar virion structure and genome organization and a common mode of replication.

This chapter discusses the general features of human retroviruses, such as virion structure and genome organization, as well as the procedures used in the laboratory for diagnosis and treatment evaluation. During the past decades, the AIDS pandemic has resulted in an upsurge of scientific interest in retroviral infections and related pathology in humans. Several human retroviruses have been identified, of which only the human immunodeficiency viruses (HIVs) and the human T-lymphocyte leukemia viruses (HTLVs) are known to cause clinical manifestations and are discussed in this chapter.

NATURE

The electron microscopic view of retroviral particles shows spherical particles approximately 100 nm in diameter with an electron-dense core (Fig. 163.1). Retroviruses are enveloped viruses (Fig. 163.2).

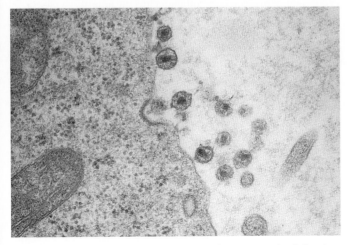

Fig. 163.1 Typical electron microscopic view of retroviruses (HIV) showing an electron-dense core. Courtesy of Dr Piet Joling.

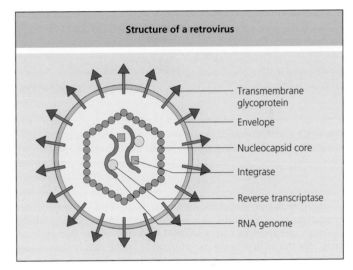

Structure of a retrovirus

- Transmembrane glycoprotein
- Envelope
- Nucleocapsid core
- Integrase
- Reverse transcriptase
- RNA genome

Fig. 163.2 Structure of a retrovirus.

The envelope consists of a phospholipid double layer derived from the plasma membrane of the host cell. Viral-encoded transmembrane glycoproteins are inserted into the envelope, enabling the virus to attach to the host cell. The envelope surrounds the nucleocapsid core, which contains the viral genome: two identical RNA molecules, having the same polarity as mRNA, with which an RNA-dependent DNA polymerase enzyme, reverse transcriptase (RT), is closely associated. Also present in the core is the integrase enzyme.

The genome of retroviruses is approximately 10 000 base pairs (bp) in length. Each end of the genome consists of repeating nucleotide sequences of 4–6 bp, called the long terminal repeats (LTRs). The LTRs flank the three genomic regions that encode for sets of structural genes:

- the group antigen (*gag*) region, which codes for the core antigens;
- the polymerase (*pol*) region, which codes for the enzymes protease, RT and integrase; and
- the envelope (*env*) region, which codes for glycoproteins of the envelope.

The structural genes always appear in the same order: *gag-pol-env* (Fig. 163.3).[1] The genomes of so-called simple retroviruses only contain a *gag*, *pol* and *env* gene. There are several retroviruses that contain additional genes that encode for viral proteins involved in the regulation of several processes in the replication cycle of the virus, such as the rate of transcription, the splicing of mRNA, the transport of mRNA from the nucleus to the cytoplasm and the release of progeny virus. Retroviruses that contain additional genes are called complex retroviruses; examples of these are the HIVs and the HTLVs.

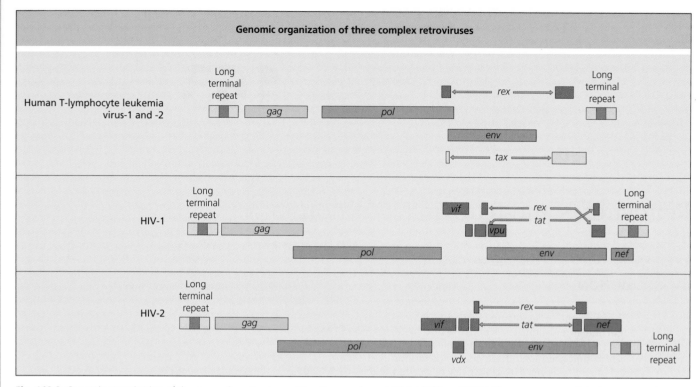

Fig. 163.3 Genomic organization of three complex retroviruses. The diagram shows HIV-1, HIV-2 and HTLV. The components of the long terminal repeats are shaded. The open reading frames that encode viral proteins are depicted by unshaded boxes. Adapted from Galasso *et al*.[1]

The first step in the replication cycle (Fig. 163.4) of retroviruses is attachment of the virus to a host cell through interaction of the envelope glycoprotein with a receptor molecule on the host cell surface. This interaction between virus and host cell largely determines the host range of the virus (i.e. which species or cell type the virus can infect). After attachment, fusion of the envelope membrane with the host cell membrane takes place and the nucleocapsid core is released into the cell. However, some retroviruses enter the cell by receptor-mediated endocytosis followed by fusion of the viral envelope with the endosomal membrane.[2]

Following the entry of the nucleocapsid core into the cytoplasm of the host cell, the viral RNA is transcribed into double-stranded DNA (dsDNA). This process is catalyzed by the viral enzyme RT. The viral dsDNA, in association with RT and the viral enzyme integrase, is transferred to the nucleus. Subsequently the dsDNA is integrated into the chromosomal DNA of the cell by the action of the viral enzyme integrase. Once integrated the viral DNA copy is called a provirus.

Using the proviral DNA as template, cellular DNA-dependent RNA polymerases synthesize viral mRNA molecules. Some of them are spliced and transported to the cytoplasm, where they are translated and yield full-length viral precursor polyproteins. These polyproteins, combined with two copies of genomic viral RNA, are then assembled into immature virus particles. By budding through the plasma membrane the immature particles acquire a bilipid layer envelope. Maturation into infectious and replication-competent virions is accomplished after release of the immature particles from the host cell; this process requires processing of the precursor polyproteins by the viral-encoded protease. Then, a new cycle of replication may start.

A particular feature of retroviruses is that the retroviral DNA becomes integrated in the host chromosomal DNA and can be inherited into the progeny of the infected cell. When retroviruses infect germline cells (sperm or egg cells) and the viral DNA is integrated into the chromosomal DNA of these cells, the retrovirus is passed from parent to offspring of the infected host. Such a virus is called an endogenous retrovirus. Most vertebrates carry the remnants of

retroviral DNA in their chromosomes as a result of common ancestors who were infected with endogenous retroviruses.

Retroviruses that are not integrated in germline cells of their host are called exogenous retroviruses. The transmission route of exogenous retroviruses is both horizontally and vertically via blood and saliva and by sexual intercourse.

HUMAN ENDOGENOUS RETROVIRUSES

Approximately 1% of the human genome consists of sequences of human endogenous retroviruses (HERVs).[3] Full-length HERVs contain sequences that are homologous to the *gag*, *pol* and *env* genes of infectious exogenous retroviruses. The biologic properties and functions of endogenous retroviruses are still under investigation.

Nine different HERV families have been described, some of which have as many as 50 copies in the human genome.[3] In general, HERVs are defective proviruses.[3,4] Expression of HERV mRNA and HERV proteins has been demonstrated in several normal and pathologic tissues, and HERV retroviral particles have been detected by electron microscopy in these tissues.

Because it was demonstrated that HERV mRNA and proteins can be expressed, it has been postulated that HERVs might be etiologically involved in human disease. The possible role of HERVs in human disease has been reviewed,[4] but more research is required to elucidate the general role of HERVs and their specific role in human disease.

Human Foamy Virus

In 1971, a human foamy virus (HFV) was the first human exogenous retrovirus to be successfully isolated from human tissue.[5] Human foamy virus is a member of the family of Spuma retroviruses. A clear relationship between HFV and human disease has never been established. These viruses have been associated with a variety of diseases, such as subacute

Replication cycle of retroviruses

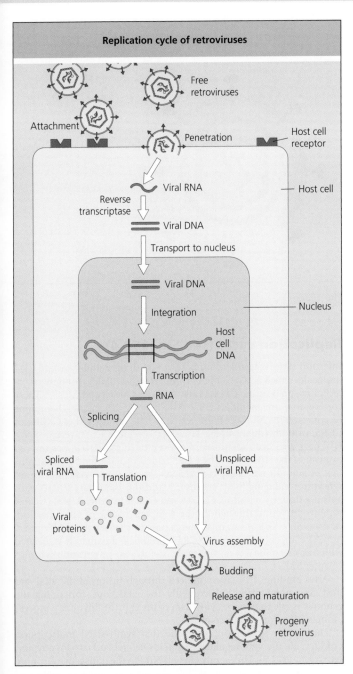

Fig. 163.4 Replication cycle of retroviruses.

thyroiditis, chronic fatigue syndrome, hemodialysis encephalopathy, multiple sclerosis, Guillain–Barré syndrome, amyotrophic lateral sclerosis and Kawasaki's disease. However, no definitive evidence has been found to support involvement of HFV in any of them.

Human T-Lymphocyte Leukemia Viruses

NATURE

Human T-lymphocyte leukemia virus-1 and HTLV-2 are complex retroviruses. In addition to a *gag*, *pol* and *env* gene, they contain four open reading frames in the pX region; these open reading frames have regulatory and accessory functions.[6,7] Two of these proteins, *rex* and *tax* (see Fig. 163.3), play an important role in regulation of viral replication. The *rex* protein is involved in the stabilization of viral mRNA

and the transport of viral mRNA from nucleus to cytoplasm. The *rex* protein also regulates the splicing and processing of viral mRNA. The *tax* protein is a transactivator protein; by acting on the LTR located 5′ to the viral *gag* gene, *tax* induces the transcription of viral mRNA and is also believed to play a role in oncogenesis.

EPIDEMIOLOGY

Seroepidemiologic studies have shown that the highest incidence of anti-HTLV-1 antibodies is found in south-western Japan, ranging from 5% to 35% in endemic areas. Other areas with high incidence are the Caribbean islands, some regions of South and Central America, the south-west Pacific and Papua New Guinea.[2] The general incidence in the USA and Europe is low (0.05%), although an increasing incidence has been reported among homosexuals and intravenous drug users.

The epidemiology of HTLV-2 has been less well studied. A high incidence of HTLV-2 has been found among native Americans in Panama and New Mexico and among intravenous drug users in the USA and Italy.

PATHOGENESIS

HTLV-1 is transmitted by infected lymphocytes and not as free virus in cell-free body fluids. Three transmission routes for HTLV-1 have been described.

- transmission of HTLV-infected lymphocytes via the placenta, during birth or after birth through the mother's milk;
- transmission from male to female during sexual intercourse; and
- blood transfusion.

Human T-lymphocyte leukemia virus-1 is a lymphotropic virus that preferentially infects CD4+ T cells. Usually, the leukemic cells in adult T-lymphocyte leukemia (ATL) have the following phenotype: CD2+, CD3+, CD5+, CD7−, CD4+ and CD8−; they also express the activation surface markers CD38 (the interleukin (IL)-2 receptor), CD30 and major histocompatibility complex class II.

The molecular mechanisms by which HTLV-1 is able to induce cell transformation have not been unraveled. Human T-lymphocyte leukemia virus does not contain a typical oncogene. Several hypothetical mechanisms of HTLV-induced oncogenesis have been formulated. However, these hypotheses do not explain why it takes an average incubation time of 20–30 years to develop ATL or why only a small number of HTLV-1-infected people develop clinical manifestations of ATL.

DIAGNOSTIC MICROBIOLOGY

Infection with HTLV-1 and HTLV-2 can be diagnosed using serologic assays (enzyme-linked immunosorbent assays and rapid tests) to detect antibodies against the virus. Confirmation and distinction between HTLV-1 and HTLV-2 can be done through polymerase chain reaction (PCR) detection of proviral DNA in lymphocytes.

CLINICAL FEATURES

Human T-lymphocyte leukemia virus-1

Adult T-lymphocyte leukemia

Several pieces of evidence established the causal relationship between HTLV-1 and ATL:[8]

- ATL has an identical geographic distribution to that of HTLV-1, having a high incidence in south-western Japan, as was shown in seroepidemiologic studies.

- All ATL tumor cells contain one or more copies of the HTLV-1 provirus in their genomic DNA.
- *In-vitro* infection of human T cells with HTLV-1 results in T-cell immortalization.
- HTLV-1 has been demonstrated to be oncogenic in animals.

The lifetime chance of an infected person developing ATL is very low (about 1%). The first clinical manifestations of ATL generally occur 20–30 years after infection with HTLV-1.[9] The median age of ATL onset is 52.7 years.

Tropical spastic paresis

Infections with HTLV-1 have also been associated with a neurologic syndrome affecting the pyrimidal tract called tropical spastic paresis or HTLV-1-associated myelopathy (HAM). This disorder is characterized by a slowly progressive symmetric myelopathy combined with high titers of antibodies to HTLV-1 in plasma and cerebrospinal fluid (CSF). The myelopathy primarily affects the pyramidal tract. The mechanism by which HTLV-1 infection causes HAM is unclear.

Ophthalmologic complications and arthopathy

Human T-lymphocyte leukemia virus-1 infections have also been associated with ophthalmologic complications and arthropathy.[2]

Human T-lymphocyte leukemia virus-2

Human T-lymphocyte leukemia virus-2 infections have been associated with T-cell malignancies, predominantly hairy T-lymphocytic leukemia and chronic lymphatic leukemia. Neurologic complications similar to those seen in tropical spastic paresis have been described.

Human Immunodeficiency Viruses

NATURE

The human immunodeficiency viruses HIV-1 and HIV-2 are members of the family of Lentiviruses. Both HIV-1 and HIV-2 are the causative agents of AIDS. For detailed information regarding the clinical manifestations of HIV infection and AIDS, see Chapters 84–99; antiretroviral therapy is discussed in Chapters 100 and 145. This chapter describes viral structure, replication, epidemiology and diagnostic procedures.

Virion structure

The electron microscopic view of human immunodeficiency retroviruses shows an electron-dense, cone-shaped core[10] (see Fig. 163.1). The viral p24 capsid protein functions as a shell for the condensed core, which contains the two identical genomic RNA strands in close association with RT (Fig. 163.5). The viral genome is approximately 9200 bases long and contains nine genes[11] (see Fig. 163.3). The viral proteins Vpr (in HIV-1) and Vpx (in HIV-2) and the p6 protein are found in the virion and outside the core. The Vif protein may also be present in the viral particle in close association with the viral core. The inner part of the viral membrane is covered with a myristylated p17 core protein, which provides the matrix for the viral structure. Glycoprotein spikes project from the virion surface and are anchored into an envelope that consists of a phospholipid bilayer derived from the host cell membrane. The spikes contain two viral glycoproteins (gp), gp120 and gp41. The gp41 acts as a transmembrane protein and its central portion binds to the external surface gp120. In addition to gp41 and gp120, the viral envelope can contain various proteins derived from the host cell.

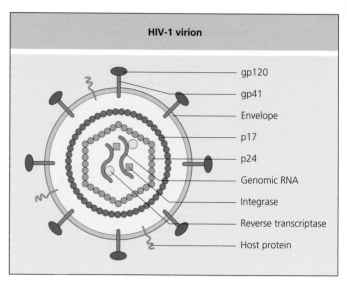

Fig. 163.5 HIV-1 virion.

Replication cycle (see Fig. 163.4)

Infection starts with the binding of gp120 to the cellular surface CD4 molecule, which acts as a high-affinity receptor. Two secondary or co-receptors can be used: CXCR4 (also known as fusin) and CCR5.[12] These co-receptors are members of a cellular transmembrane chemokine receptor family. All HIV strains tested to date can use either CXCR4 or CCR5, or both (dual tropic). However, several other co-receptors for HIV have also been identified. Co-receptor usage determines the cell tropism of the HIV strain. The CCR5 co-receptor is used by HIV strains that *in vitro* do not cause cell fusion (syncytia) in T-cell lines (non-syncytium-inducing (NSI) strains). Syncytium-inducing (SI) HIV variants use both co-receptors CXCR4 and CCR5. In general, NSI (CCR5) variants are found throughout the complete course of HIV infection, whereas SI (CXCR4) variants emerge only in a later stage of HIV infection. The appearance of SI (CXCR4) variants in a patient is associated with a more rapid CD4 decline and faster disease progression (see also Chapter 88).

After binding, HIV enters the cell through fusion of the viral and host cell membranes. Subsequently the viral core, containing the genome, is released in the cytoplasm of the cell; this involves a process of internalization and uncoating.

During the replication cycle, the first synthesized transcription products are the viral regulatory proteins *nef, tat* and *rev* (for a review see Greene *et al.*[13]). The *tat* protein will bind to the transactive response element region on the proviral DNA and, as a consequence, high-level expression of all viral genes occurs. The *nef* protein is required for high-level viral replication *in vivo* and it decreases CD4 on the cell membrane. The *nef* protein may also enhance the efficiency of reverse transcription.

Through the action of *rev* a switch may occur toward the synthesis of late regulatory and viral structural proteins. The *rev* protein facilitates the nuclear transport of unspliced and incompletely spliced RNA transcripts that contain the *rev*-responsive element, located in the *env* gene. In addition it promotes translation of messages containing the *rev*-responsive element. It remains unclear to what extent the relative amounts of each of these regulatory proteins and their interaction with cellular factors can determine whether the infection of a cell results in a productive cycle or merely a viral latent state.

The *gag* and the *pol* open reading frames (ORFs) overlap. The *pol* ORF is positioned in the −1 frame relative to the *gag* ORF. In the unspliced, full-length mRNA, both reading frames are present. Translation starts at the beginning of the *gag* ORF and continues in most cases until the end of the ORF, and a 55 kDa *gag* precursor protein (p55), containing p17, p24, p7, p2, p1 and p6, is made. During translation of full-length mRNA, approximately 5–10% of the ribosomes slip back one nucleotide (frame shift) and gain access to the *pol* ORF, and translation continues. A partial *gag* precursor protein is fused to the *pol* polyprotein, resulting in a *gag-pol* polyprotein. The *pol* gene encodes for three proteins: protease, RT and integrase. Cleavage of the *gag-pol* protein generates protease, RT and integrase. The 99-amino acid protease is coded for at the 5′ end of the *pol* gene. HIV protease is active only as homodimer, which is generated by an autolytic process. It is possible that aggregation of two *gag-pol* proteins is required to generate the active form, thereby limiting activation to the budding site. Both *gag* and *gag-pol* polyproteins are post-translationally modified by a covalent attachment of a lipophilic myristyl group onto their aminoterminal glycine by a host cell-derived myristyl transferase. Myristylation may be required for intracellular transport to the cell membrane because, in the absence of myristylation, no infectious particles are produced.

The *gag* precursor protein is cleaved by viral protease into four structural proteins (p17, p24, p7 and p6) and two smaller proteins (p2 and p1). The p2 protein may be important for proper assembly of the virions. The *gag* precursor protein may also play a role in the packaging of viral RNA into the virus particle, specifically through the action of the nucleic acid binding protein p7. This protein binds to a sequence at the 5′ end of the viral genome, possibly through the interaction of so-called cystine-histidine motifs. The p6 protein has been shown to be rich in proline, and through binding to p6, Vpr is incorporated in the viral particle. Viruses with a mutation in p6 are not released from the cell surface.

The accessory genes *vif*, *vpr* and *vpu/vpx* influence the viral assembly and budding process, and alterations in these genes lead to a decrease in infectivity. These proteins may be more important for replication in macrophages and primary lymphocytes than for T-cell lines. The protein Vpr can cause cell cycle arrest in the G2 phase, and it is as yet unclear whether this phenomenon plays a role in viral replication. The protein Vpu interacts with CD4 and may cause CD4 degradation.[2] The Vif protein is considered to enhance infectivity.

TRANSMISSION AND EPIDEMIOLOGY

A large variety of nonhuman primates in Africa have been reported to be infected with the retrovirus simian immunodeficiency virus (SIV). Two of these viruses are the cause of AIDS in humans. It has been estimated that they have been transmitted to humans on at least seven different occasions.[14]

Transmission

The three major routes of transmission of HIV are by sexual contact or blood or blood products or vertically through maternal-fetal transmission. The first step in infection is binding of the viral particles to submucosal dendritic cells. These cells, which normally process antigens and present them to immune cells, express a protein termed DC-SIGN. The viral gp120 binds to DC-SIGN with high affinity; subsequently the viral particles are internalized and presented again at the cell surface after the dendritic cells have migrated to the regional lymph tissues and present viral particles to the T cells (see Chapter 88).

The amount of infectious HIV in the inoculating material is the most important factor determining the risk of transmission. The amount of virus is, at least in the blood of the donor, determined by disease stage. The relation between the amount of HIV in semen and disease stage has not been fully explored. Individuals with a primary infection are extremely infectious, most likely because they have a very high amount of virus in their body fluids; given the recent infection most of the circulating viruses are closely related to the inoculating strain and therefore infectious themselves.

The risk of heterosexual transmission correlates to the HIV RNA concentration in the plasma of the positive partner and the stage of disease.[15,16] The rate of transmission may also be determined by biologic properties of the virus and the integrity of mucocutaneous membranes of the urogenital tract. Among heterosexual couples the risk of transmission increases when the negative partner has a genital infection.[16]

Studies addressing transmission from mother to baby have also shown that the risk of vertical transmission increases with a higher viral load in the mother at the time of delivery (as measured as by HIV p24 antigen, HIV-1 RNA, proviral DNA or peripheral blood mononuclear cell viral titer) and with lower CD4+ lymphocyte counts.[17] The current opinion is that the majority of infections of the child occur late during pregnancy and most commonly during delivery, because elective Caesarian section and antiretroviral treatment of the mother around the time of delivery lowers the transmission rate significantly.[17–19]

The global HIV-1 epidemic is seen as a composite of infections from at least nine genetically distinct subtypes or clades of virus, designated A to H.[20] Together they form the M group. Subtypes can be distinguished on the basis of sequence information (*env* and *gag* genes and RT). Two isolates that are highly divergent from group M have been fully sequenced. The results show that viruses from the new group O are almost as close to HIV-2 as to HIV-1. The distribution of certain HIV-1 subtypes is still geographically limited, but geographic dispersion will contribute to the growing pandemic (see Chapters 84 and 96). The distribution of subtypes within countries as well as throughout the world shows that there is no evidence for host specificity for certain subtypes. Dual infection with two subtypes and hybrids between two subtypes have been described in infected individuals.

Five distinct subgroups have been identified for HIV-2; in analogy with HIV-1 these were designated A to E. The observed viral variation has clear implications not only for vaccine development but also for drug development and treatment of patients.

The non-nucleoside reverse transcriptase inhibitors (NNRTIs) inhibit RT activity through binding various amino acids of RT, the most important amino acid being the tyrosine residue at codon 181 for HIV-1 RT. Selection of drug-resistant HIV-1 isolates both *in vitro* and *in vivo* results in a substitution at codon 181 of a cysteine. The cysteine substitution gives a considerable increase in the 50% inhibitory concentration for all NNRTIs. Sequence analysis of several HIV-2 RT genes has shown that at codon 181 the cysteine is normally present. The presence of the cysteine variant makes HIV-2 viruses naturally resistant to the NNRTIs.

The *env*-based classification of widely divergent HIV-1 strains into sequence subtypes is also supported by nucleotide sequence analysis of the *gag* genes. The distinction between SI and NSI viruses, conferred by gp120 described in clade B, is also present among other HIV-1 subtypes. Detailed information is available on the prevalence of the different subtypes for certain areas in the world. Information on the prevalence of different clades in a region may give interesting information on the spread of the infection and the possible transmission routes. For instance, in Thailand it has been shown that type A is mainly spreading through sexual intercourse, whereas type B is transmitted among intravenous drug users. Monitoring the prevalence of different clades around the world and searching for possible new clades is important for the use and development of diagnostic procedures. For instance, some screening assays for HIV antibodies have been shown to be relatively insensitive for clade O viruses. The use of diagnostic PCR procedures, especially in children born to mothers who have HIV infection, may be complicated by sequence variation in the region where the primers have to anneal to their substrate.

DEVELOPMENT OF RESISTANCE DUE TO ANTIRETROVIRAL THERAPY (SEE ALSO CHAPTERS 99 AND 100)

After the introduction of (partial active) monotherapy in the mid-1980s, drug-resistant viruses were selected in most treated patients. Initially a large pool of patients who failed therapy harbored nucleoside-resistant viruses. Some of these patients infected other individuals with these drug-resistant viruses. After the first report, it became apparant that transmission of resistant viruses was a relatively frequent event, occurring at 10–20% in the USA and Europe.[21–23] Subsequent introduction of the NNRTIs and the first generation of protease inhibitors (PIs) in these nucleoside analogue failing patient populations did not result in complete virus suppression in most patients; indeed, a second wave of viruses now also resistant to the NNRTIs and/or PIs were selected. These viruses were also transmitted, albeit with a lower frequency.

With the introduction of second-generation boosted PIs and the availability of novel classes of fusion inhibitors and integrase inhibitors it became possible to finally fully suppress virus replication in those patients previously failing. Moreover, these novel highly active retroviral therapy (HAART) regimens, when used as first-line regimens, rarely select for resistance virus. These developments will most likely significantly reduce the future rate of transmission of drug-resistant virus in the USA and Europe.

DIAGNOSTIC TOOLS FOR HIV

Serologic assays

Assays have been developed for detection of HIV antibodies in serum, whole blood, saliva, urine and dried blood collected on filter paper.

Enzyme-linked immunosorbent assay

Current antigen sandwich enzyme-linked immunosorbent assays (ELISAs) have a sensitivity and specificity that approach 100%. In contrast to earlier tests, which detected only IgG antibodies, third-generation HIV ELISAs detect all classes of anti-HIV antibodies, considerably shortening the time to diagnosis following acute infection. However, these assays may fail to detect antibodies to the highly divergent HIV-1 subtypes from groups N and O.

Circulating HIV-1 capsid (p24) antigen can be detected by qualitative or quantitative antigen-capture ELISA. Qualitative assays for p24 antigen are useful in diagnosing HIV-1 infection prior to seroconversion, but quantitative assays have been replaced by more sensitive viral RNA assays. The newer generations of ELISA combine detection of antibodies with the detection of antigen in the plasma. These ELISAs have shortened the window between the moment of infection and the first positive ELISA considerably because samples obtained early after infection (a couple of days) contain unbound HIV antigen while antibodies at that stage may not be present.

Rapid tests

Diagnostic tests based on red cell or particle agglutination as well as dot-blot assays have been developed that permit rapid diagnosis of HIV-1 infection. In laboratory comparisons, sensitivity and specificity are similar to those of the ELISA, but performance may be somewhat lower in the field. The simplicity and wide operating temperature of these tests make them suitable for use in resource-poor settings, for women during labor and delivery, and for source patients following an occupational needlestick injury.

Western blot

Despite a specificity of 99%, a reactive HIV ELISA has a relatively low positive predictive value when applied to populations at low risk for HIV infection. Thus, a confirmatory test is essential to exclude false-positive results. The Western blot (WB) method is currently the most widely used. In a WB, viral proteins are separated by polyacrylamide gel electrophoresis and transferred by blotting onto a nitrocellulose strip. The strips are then reacted with the test serum to determine which, if any, viral proteins are recognized by patient antibodies. Figure 163.6 shows a typical WB positive for HIV-1, with the different

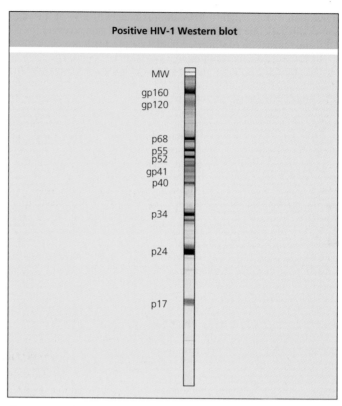

Positive HIV-1 Western blot

MW
gp160
gp120
p68
p55
p52
gp41
p40
p34
p24
p17

Fig. 163.6 Positive HIV-1 Western blot. The binding of the patient's antibodies to viral antigens coated on the strip is revealed by an enzyme-labeled antihuman globulin. gp160, gp120 and gp41 are *env* gene products. p55, p24 and p17 are *gag* gene products. p68, p52 and p34 are *pol* gene products. MW, molecular weight of the viral proteins.

reactive proteins, and in Figure 163.7 the pattern as observed in an HIV-1 seroconverter is shown. Serologic differentiation between HIV-1 and HIV-2 can be done using detection of specific antibodies against the HIV-2 transmembrane protein (gp36).

HIV isolation

HIV can be isolated from blood, plasma, CSF, genital secretions or tissue by co-culture with lymphocytes from a seronegative donor that

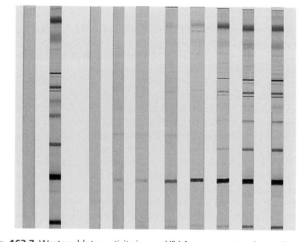

Fig. 163.7 Western blot reactivity in one HIV-1 seroconverter. Lanes 1 and 2, negative (NC) and positive controls (PC). Lanes 3–10, serial samples collected on days (D) 0, 2, 3, 5, 7, 12, 22 and 30. Day 0 corresponds to the first collected sample. Anti-p24 was the first antibody detected, rapidly followed by anti-gp160, p55, p40 and gp120. Later, gp41 and p18 are weakly reactive.

have been stimulated with phytohemagglutinin and interleukin-2 before use. Virus isolation is successful in more than 95% of individuals infected with HIV-1, but sensitivity is lower in patients with higher CD4 cell counts

Viral nucleic acid detection

HIV-1 DNA polymerase chain reaction

HIV-1 DNA PCR assays are used almost exclusively for early diagnosis of infection in neonates. These tests have limited utility in adults, but occasionally may be useful in resolving cases in which results of serologic tests are ambiguous.

Quantitative HIV-1 RNA assays

Use of these assays is now standard in the management of HIV-1-infected patients in the developed world. Several different assay formats have been developed for HIV-1 RNA quantification. In PCR-based assays HIV-1 RNA is converted into DNA by reverse transcription followed by PCR amplification of the DNA. The PCR product is detected by hybridization to an enzyme-conjugated probe specific for HIV-1, and quantified by reacting bound probe with a substrate that undergoes a color change, as in an ELISA. Branched DNA assay uses nonenzymatic means to amplify the signal from HIV RNA. In this assay, viral RNA is 'captured' by hybridization to complementary oligonucleotides that are bound to the wells of a microtiter plate. The captured viral RNA target is then hybridized to branched oligonucleotides (hence the name 'branched' DNA assay), which in turn are hybridized to enzyme-conjugated oligonucleotides that can be quantified as above. Performance characteristics of most commercially available assays are similar. Most assays have a lower limit of quantification of approximately 50–80 copies/ml. Assay sensitivity can be extended by concentrating plasma virus from larger sample volumes. Although detection limits of 3–5 copies/ml are achievable by such means, these assays are much less precise at plasma HIV-1 RNA titers below 200 copies/ml. Once infection becomes established, steady-state plasma virus levels are relatively stable, varying by 0.3–0.4 $\log_{10}$ copies/ml over weeks to months. Given these factors, changes of greater than 0.5–0.7 $\log_{10}$ (three- to fivefold) are likely to reflect significant changes in HIV-1 replication.[24]

Plasma HIV-1 RNA levels that appear to be lower than expected in a patient with advanced disease can be a clue to infection with a nonsubtype B strain. Incorporation of alternative primer sets in the latest versions of the HIV-1 molecular quantitative assays has improved the ability of these assays to detect diverse HIV-1 subtypes. The kinetics of viral markers as they occur during primary infection are shown in Figure 163.8.

Drug resistance assays

A variety of assays are available for assessing drug resistance which now has become routine practice in Europe and the USA[25,26] based on the results of clinical studies[27–29] including:

- genotypic assays, in which nucleotide sequencing of viral genetic material is used to detect the presence or absence of critical drug resistance mutations; and
- phenotypic assays, in which the concentration of drug necessary to inhibit virus replication *in vitro* is estimated in a drug susceptibility assay.

Each method has potential advantages and disadvantages. An important limitation of both approaches is that they provide a measure of the characteristics of the predominant viral species but do not indicate the presence of minor species that may emerge as resistant variants during subsequent treatment (Table 163.1).

Genotypic tests of HIV-1 drug resistance

Several approaches to genotyping are available, ranging from full-length sequencing of the target gene to point mutation assays, which

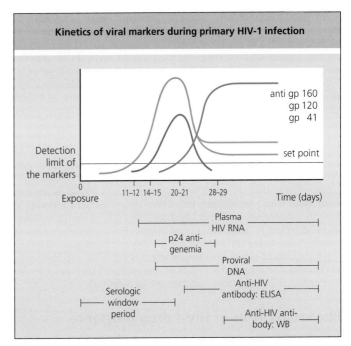

Fig. 163.8 Kinetics of viral markers during primary HIV-1 infection. The first positive viral marker is plasma RNA 11–12 days after infection. p24 Antigenemia is detectable on day 14 or 15. The first anti-HIV antibodies are detectable by third-generation ELISAs on days 20–21. (Pink, plasma HIV RNA; purple, p24 antigenemia; blue, anti-HIV antibody.)

Table 163.1 Comparison of genotypic and phenotypic drug resistance tests for HIV

Type of assay	Advantages	Disadvantages
Genotypic assays	Rapid turn-around time Appearance of resistance mutations may precede change in phenotype Widely available	Genotype may not correlate with phenotype Require expert/database interpretation Fail to detect minor species Unable to assess mutational interaction
Phenotypic assays	Direct measure of viral drug susceptibility Assess net effect of mutational interactions and cross-resistance patterns	Cost Longer turn-around time Fail to detect minor species

focus only on a particular mutation of interest. The most commonly used genotypic assays rely on automated DNA sequencing. Using this technique, the nucleotide sequence of some or all of the gene of interest (e.g. protease or reverse transcriptase or integrase) is obtained, then translated into the predicted amino acid sequence in order to determine whether specific mutations are present or absent. Automated sequencing offers the most complete data on viral genotype, but generates more information than is needed for most clinical purposes. For example, HIV-1 RT has 550 amino acids, but mutations at only a small number of these positions are implicated in drug resistance. Therefore, interpretation of the genotype is needed in order to help distinguish which changes are merely polymorphisms and which might be significantly associated with drug resistance.

In most commercially available genotypic tests, viral RNA is extracted from a sample of plasma and reverse transcribed into complementary DNA in the laboratory. The protease and RT or integrase coding regions of the cDNA are then amplified by PCR, and the nucleotide sequence of the PCR product is determined on an automated DNA sequencer. Some laboratories use specific diagnostic kits that provide standardized reagents needed for the RT-PCR and DNA sequencing steps. Generally, these kits are part of an HIV-genotyping system that includes equipment for running the sequencing assays and software for interpreting assay results.

The frequency of false-positive and false-negative results is 0.1% for genotypic assays when assessed using samples that carry predominantly mutant or predominantly wild-type virus populations. However, sensitivity for detecting presence of a mutation is variable when both wild-type and mutant viruses are present as a mixture. In general, mutant species must constitute 10–20% of the population to be detected by standard sequencing methods. Some mutations may go undetected unless they are present as the majority species. Interpretation of genotyping results requires expertise and the access to databases relating the presence of mutations to therapy outcome and drug activity (see Table 163.2 for useful websites).

Phenotypic tests of HIV-1 drug resistance

Drug susceptibility tests with HIV-1 are usually performed using a recombinant virus assay, in which the viral genes of interest (e.g. protease and reverse transcriptase) are introduced into a plasmid that carries all of the other viral genes needed for replication in cell culture (Fig. 163.9).[30,31] Modification of the assay allows introduction of the integrase (*in*) or envelope (*env*) genes in order to determine susceptibility to integrase inhibitors and entry inhibitors, respectively. Using these assays, small differences in susceptibility can be detected

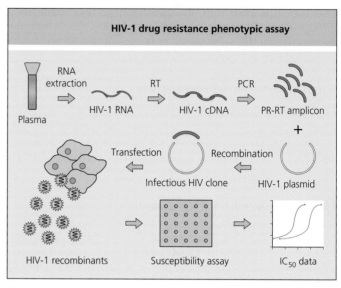

Fig. 163.9 HIV-1 drug resistance phenotypic assay. RT, reverse transcription reaction; cDNA, complementary DNA; PR-RT, protease and reverse transcriptase gene; IC$_{50}$, 50% inhibitory concentration.

(approximately two- to fourfold compared with control). Phenotypic assays are more complex and labor intensive than genotypic assays. Automation makes it possible to test many samples simultaneously, and allows for high throughput. However, the cost and complexity of the automation limit availability of these assays to a few reference laboratories.

REFERENCES

References for this chapter can be found online at http://www.expertconsult.com

Table 163.2 Useful websites for interpreting HIV-1 genotypic resistance tests	
International AIDS Society-USA	http://www.iasusa.org
Stanford HIV RT and Protease Sequence Database	http://hivdb.stanford.edu
Los Alamos National Laboratory	http://hiv-web.lanl.gov

David Brown
Graham Lloyd

Chapter | **164** |

Zoonotic viruses

INTRODUCTION

Zoonotic infections are infections of animals that can naturally infect humans. More than 400 viruses cause clinically important zoonoses and infection is acquired by several different routes. Humans can be infected directly from the host animal species, for example following the bite of a rabies-infected animal, through inhalation of rodent urine (hantavirus) or by direct contact with rodent urine (Lassa fever). However, the majority of zoonotic infections are spread by arthropod vectors and are classified as arboviruses.

The geographic distribution of the infections described in this chapter depends on many factors and changes over time. Recent examples include West Nile fever, which has recently spread to and become established across the USA. Nipah and Hendra viruses, newly recognized causes of encephalitis in humans, have been identified in Australia, Malaysia, Singapore and India. Congo-Crimean hemorrhagic fever has re-emerged in Kosovo, following social dislocation resulting from conflict. Other important zoonotic infections include DNA viruses, such as poxviruses and herpes B virus, and RNA viruses, such as rabies. A number of rare occupational viral zoonoses have been described, including foot and mouth disease, vesicular stomatitis virus and swine vesicular disease.[1,2]

ARBOVIRUSES

Over 400 viruses that cause human disease are classified as arboviruses. These are distributed worldwide because of their close association with lower vertebrates and insects and their wide host range. Most arbovirus infections are caused by RNA viruses and include members of the togaviruses, bunyaviruses and reoviruses.

Many arboviruses that infect humans cause nonspecific symptoms such as acute fever. Three broad clinical patterns are recognized with arbovirus infection:

- fever, rash and arthritis or retinitis;
- encephalitis; and
- viral hemorrhagic fevers (VHFs).

Several comprehensive reviews are available.[3,4]

Most arboviruses are maintained in complex life cycles that involve nonhuman vertebrate hosts with or without a primary vector. Mosquitoes are the most important arbovirus vector, followed by ticks, sandflies (*Phlebotomus* spp.) and midges (*Culicoides* spp.). These arbovirus life cycles only become evident when humans are bitten directly by the natural enzootic focus, or when they are exposed to a virus that has escaped the primary cycle via a secondary vector or vertebrate host. Many arboviruses have several vertebrate hosts and many can be transmitted by a number of vectors.

Viruses such as urban dengue, urban yellow fever and occasionally urban St Louis encephalitis cause significant viremia and represent the simplest form of epidemic transmission cycle, in which the virus is transmitted directly between mosquitoes and humans (see Fig. 164.1). In some cases the introduction of a secondary vector may allow the transmission of the virus to other nonhuman vertebrate reservoirs (sylvatic cycle), many of which can be regarded as blind-end hosts (Fig. 164.2). Prime examples of sylvatic cycles with multiple hosts are the encephalitides such as Western equine encephalitis, eastern encephalitis and St Louis encephalitis. Many arboviruses are maintained in arthropods, through transovarial transmission. Amplification of the cycle occurs by spread to and from small mammals (Fig. 164.3). The flavivirus infections are discussed in Chapter 18. The key features of the clinically important arboviruses transmitted to humans by hematophagous arthropod vectors, such as mosquitoes, ticks and *Phlebotomus* flies (sandfly), are given in Table 164.1. Yellow fever is an example of a mosquito-borne zoonotic virus infection.

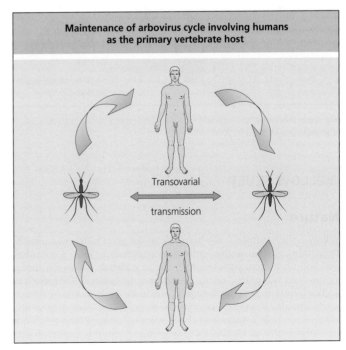

Maintenance of arbovirus cycle involving humans as the primary vertebrate host

Transovarial transmission

Fig. 164.1 Maintenance of arbovirus cycle involving humans as the primary vertebrate host (e.g. urban dengue and urban yellow fever).

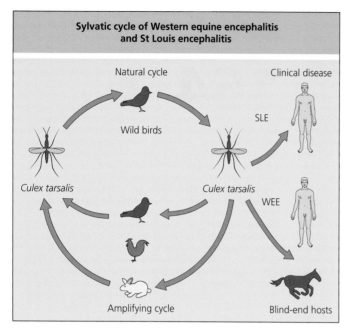

Fig. 164.2 Sylvatic cycle of Western equine encephalitis (WEE) and St Louis encephalitis (SLE).

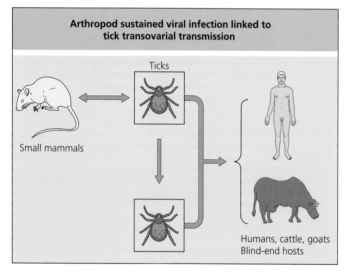

Fig. 164.3 Arthropod sustained viral infection linked to tick transovarial transmission.

YELLOW FEVER

Nature

Yellow fever has historically been one of the great killers of humans. Regrettably, this mosquito-borne virus continues to exact a considerable toll on human populations living in endemic areas even today. Yellow fever was principally responsible for the failure of the French to successfully complete the Panama Canal in the 1880s as the workforce was decimated by epidemics of yellow fever. Yellow fever was the first virus shown to be transmissible by a mosquito vector. Pioneering work by Carlos Finlay and Walter Reed are credited with this important discovery, which led to mosquito control efforts and dramatic reductions in the incidence of yellow fever. Yellow fever remains a considerable public health risk to travelers and inhabitants in endemic regions of South America and Africa.

Epidemiology

The World Health Organization (WHO) reported that between 1987 and 1991 there were 18 735 cases of yellow fever worldwide, with 4522 deaths.[5] This represented the greatest number of reported cases over a 5-year period since active reporting began in 1948. Yellow fever primarily occurs in jungle regions of the world and it is estimated that the incidence of yellow fever is grossly under-reported. The WHO estimates that perhaps as many as 200 000 cases of yellow fever occur annually.[6] Countries reporting active cases of yellow fever as of January of 1999 are indicated in Figure 164.4.[7] Yellow fever has caused significant outbreaks in recent years; in Guinea in 2000, Peru in 2001 and Senegal in 2002. The value of mass vaccination for controlling an outbreak was demonstrated in Guinea.[8]

There are two transmission cycles of yellow fever. The first and most common today is the jungle (or sylvatic) cycle of yellow fever. The jungle transmission cycle consists of a natural reservoir of disease in nonhuman primates with transmission by forest-dwelling mosquitoes. In South America the mosquito primarily responsible for yellow fever transmission to humans is the *Haemagogus* sp. mosquito. In sub-Saharan Africa yellow fever is transmitted in rural areas primarily by *Aedes africanus*. The urban (or epidemic) cycle of yellow fever is related to urban outbreaks transmitted by the human-adapted mosquito *Aedes aegypti*.

All susceptible populations appear to be equally at risk for disease yet most cases occur in children or young men (particularly those involved in the logging industry or construction in heavily forested areas). The increased incidence of yellow fever recently may reflect population expansion and economic development of rainforest areas and inadequate distribution of yellow fever vaccine in regions of the world where yellow fever remains endemic. Expanding commercial trade and international travel increases the risk of yellow fever outbreaks in nonendemic regions of the world in which the mosquito vector is found. Competent vectors for yellow fever are found in southern USA where the risk for yellow fever outbreaks remains a public health concern.[9]

Pathogenesis

Yellow fever is a prototypic mosquito-borne viral hemorrhagic fever. The virus is a 38 nm ssRNA virus with a genome of approximately 4×10^6 Da. The virus is injected into humans during the course of a mosquito bite as the salivary contents of the mosquito contaminate the bite site. Local replication of the virus takes place in human skin and regional lymph nodes, followed by viremia and dissemination to multiple organs of the body.

Major pathologic findings are found in the liver, kidney, heart and gastrointestinal tract. The virus infects the liver and causes massive hepatic necrosis. The characteristic pathologic finding is that of mid-zone necrosis with sparing of hepatocytes around the central vein and portal triads. Another characteristic finding is that of Councilman bodies within degenerating hepatocytes. Councilman bodies are acidophilic cytoplasmic deposits and not viral inclusion bodies. Diffuse areas of petechial hemorrhage are found throughout the body with the most marked changes found in the brain, kidney and gastrointestinal tract.

Prevention and control

Control of the mosquito vector population within yellow fever endemic areas is a key control measure. This can be accomplished by environmental control measures that remove mosquito habitats from areas of human habitation.

There is a highly effective preventive vaccine against yellow fever. This is a live attenuated vaccine using strain 17-D.[10] The vaccine is highly effective and one dose of 1000 mouse LD_{50} units results in immunity in >95% of recipients and neutralizing antibody that persists for >10 years. Adverse events following yellow fever vaccine are

Table 164.1 Important arbovirus infections that cause human disease

Genus	Virus	GEOGRAPHIC DISTRIBUTION								Main hosts	Clinical diseases
		Afr.	Asia	Aust.	Eur.	N. Am.	C. Am.	S. Am.	Pac.		
Mosquito vector											
Alphavirus	Western equine encephalitis	–	–	–	–	+	–	+	–	Rodents, birds, marsupials, equines	Encephalitis
	Eastern equine encephalitis	–	–	–	–	+	–	–	–	Wild birds, bats, rodents, equines, reptiles	Encephalitis
	Venezuelan equine encephalitis	–	–	–	–	–	+	+	–	Rodents, birds, marsupials, equines	Encephalitis
	Chikungunya	+	+	–	+	–	–	–	–	Primates, birds, bats, squirrels	Fever, rash, myalgia, polyarthritis
	Ross River	–	–	+	–	–	–	–	+	Large mammals, marsupials	Fever, rash, myalgia, arthralgia, hemorrhagic fever
Flavivirus	Dengue	+	+	+	–	–	+	+	+	Nonhuman primates	Encephalitis
	Japanese B encephalitis	–	+	+	–	–	–	–	–	Birds, pigs	Encephalitis
	St Louis encephalitis	–	–	–	–	+	–	+	–	Rodents, mammals	Encephalitis
	Murray Valley encephalitis	–	+	+	–	–	–	–	–	Birds	Encephalitis
	West Nile fever	+	+	–	+	+	+	+	–	Birds	Fever, rash, myalgia, polyarthritis, encephalitis
	Yellow fever	+	–	–	–	–	+	+	–	Primates, marsupials	Hemorrhagic fever
Phlebovirus	Rift Valley fever	+	–	–	–	–	–	–	–	Wild mammals, domestic livestock	Hemorrhagic fever, retinitis, encephalitis
Tick vector											
Flavivirus	Central European encephalitis	–	–	–	+	–	–	–	–	Rodents	Encephalitis
	Russian spring-summer encephalitis	–	–	–	+	–	–	–	–	Rodents	Encephalitis
	Omsk hemorrhagic fever	–	+	+	–	–	–	–	–	Water voles, muskrats	Encephalitis
	Powasson	–	–	–	–	+	–	–	–	Rodents	Encephalitis
Nairovirus	Crimean-Congo hemorrhagic fever	+	+	–	+	–	–	–	–	Wild and domestic mammals	Hemorrhagic fever
Coltivirus	Colorado tick fever virus	–	–	–	–	+	–	–	–		Febrile illness
Sandfly vector											
Phlebovirus	Sandfly fever Naples	+	+	–	+	–	–	–	–	Rodent	Febrile illness, myalgia, conjunctivitis
	Sandfly fever Sicilian	+	+	–	+	–	–	–	–	Rodent	Febrile illness, myalgia, conjunctivitis
	Toscana	–	–	–	+	–	–	–	–	Rodent	Febrile illness, myalgia, conjunctivitis

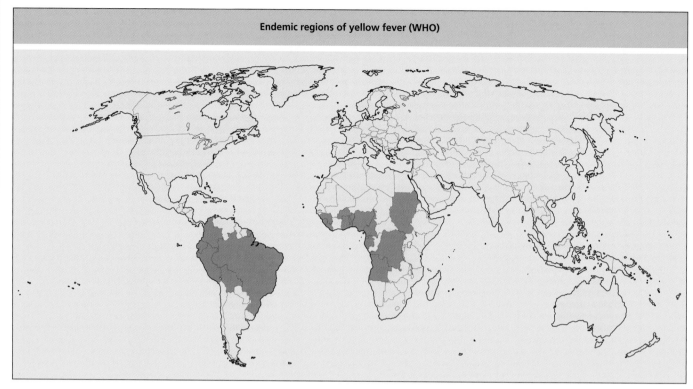

Endemic regions of yellow fever (WHO)

Fig. 164.4 Endemic regions of yellow fever (WHO), 1 January 1999. Dark purple areas show the worldwide distribution of reported cases.

generally mild. Recently, a new pattern of yellow fever vaccine-associated neurologic adverse disease (YEL-AND) has been recognized which resembles severe yellow fever. Risk is estimated to be 4 per million doses and is higher in recipients aged more than 60 years. Travelers to yellow fever endemic areas and residents within endemic areas should be considered for vaccination.[11,12]

Diagnostic microbiology

The virus can be isolated from a number of cell lines including Vero cells and AP-61 cells. Virus isolation represents an extreme biohazard and should only be attempted in specialized laboratory facilities. Serodiagnosis is possible within 1 week of onset of infection, with IgM antibodies detectable using enzyme-linked immunosorbent assay (ELISA), hemagglutination inhibition or plaque reduction neutralization tests. Virus detection can also be accomplished using reverse transcriptase semi-nested polymerase chain reactions (PCRs) from blood as well as tissue samples.[13]

Clinical manifestations

Human infection with yellow fever follows three discrete phases. The first phase of infection lasts approximately 72 hours and is initiated by headache, malaise, weakness, nausea and vomiting. The virus is replicating rapidly and high titers of infectious virus are found in the body fluids of patients at this point. This initial period of infection is followed by a brief period of remission where fever and symptoms remit. After 24–48 hours, symptoms recur and are dominated by symptoms of acute hepatic failure and renal failure. Patients develop jaundice and very high fever (hence the name yellow fever) and begin developing clinically overt signs of a hemorrhagic diathesis with petechiae, mucosal hemorrhages and gastrointestinal bleeding. A characteristic physical finding is marked bradycardia in the face of high fever (Fagetis' sign). Patients develop delirium, seizures, coma, acute renal failure and death within 7–10 days of illness. The mortality rate may be as high as 50% in some outbreaks and as low as 5% if optimal medical supportive care is available.[14]

Management

The management of yellow fever remains primarily supportive. Intravenous fluids, blood product support and management of hepatic and renal insufficiency are the mainstays of therapy. Ribavirin does not appear to be effective and no other antiviral agent has been shown to be useful to treat yellow fever thus far. Transmission to health-care workers, particularly after needlestick injuries, has been described. Patients should be isolated as their blood and body secretions may contain infectious virus.

WEST NILE VIRUS

Recently human and horse West Nile virus (WNV) infection have been identified in new temperate regions of Europe[15] and North America. Clinical presentation is variable, but severe infection is characterized by encephalitis and a significant mortality rate in humans and horses as well as certain domestic and wild birds. The virus was first isolated from the blood of a febrile women in the West Nile district of Uganda in 1937[16] and was subsequently isolated from patients, birds and mosquitoes in Egypt in the early 1950s.[17] The WNV was first recognized as a cause of human meningoencephalitis in Israel in 1957 and as a cause of equine disease in Egypt and France in the early 1960s.

Virology

The WNV is an RNA virus belonging to the family Flaviviridae (genus flavivirus). It is a member of the Japanese encephalitis complex, which also includes Kunjin, Murray Valley encephalitis and St Louis encephalitis. The WNV strains can be divided genetically into two lineages. Only members of lineage 1 have been associated with clinical human encephalitis. Lineage 1 has been isolated from Africa, India, Australia, Europe, Asia and North America. Among lineage 1 WNV causing the recent human and equine outbreaks throughout Europe and Asia are closely related to the WNV (strain ROM96) first isolated in Romania and subsequently in Kenya in 1998. The virus responsible for the outbreak in the USA (NY99) is genetically distinguishable from ROM96, but it is closely related to the virus circulating in Israel from 1997 to 2000 (Isi98). Only the USA and Israel have reported illness and death in humans and animals caused by the WNV strains Isi98 and NY99. The close relations between these strains suggest that the virus causing the outbreak in the USA was imported from the Middle East.

Epidemiology

Since the original isolation of WNV, outbreaks have occurred infrequently in humans, those in Israel (1951–4 and 1957) and South Africa (1974) being the most noticeable. Since the mid-1990s there have been three distinct epidemiologic trends.

First, there has been an increase in disease frequency in humans, notably in Romania,[18] the Czech Republic, Russia[19] and the USA.[20] Epizootics of disease in horses have occurred in Morocco where 42 of 94 affected horses died, Italy (14 cases in 1998, six died), USA (1999–2002) and the Camargue region of France (2003, 58 confirmed cases, 20 deaths).

Second, there has been a noticeable increase in severity of human disease, with large outbreaks with significant mortality rates, especially in temperate urban areas. They include Bucharest, Romania (1996, over 400 cases, 17 deaths); Volgograd, Russia (1999, over 800 human cases, 40 deaths); New York City (1999–2000, 83 human cases, nine deaths); and Israel (2000, over 300 human cases, 29 deaths).[21] Since the introduction of WNV into the USA in 1999[17] it has been responsible for the identification of an increased number of cases (1999–2001, 149 human cases, 18 deaths; during the first 9 months of 2002, 2369 human cases, 139 deaths). The WNV is responsible for the spread of human disease westward, found in all states of the USA in less than 6 years and reported as far south as Argentina.[22]

Finally, high avian death rates accompanying human outbreaks have been a significant feature of WNV outbreaks in the USA and Israel.

The principal vectors are mosquitoes, predominantly of the genus *Culex* (*C. pipiens* and *C. restuans*), and the principal amplifying hosts are wild birds. Humans and horses are considered 'end-hosts' or 'incidental hosts'. A striking feature of the initial human epidemic in New York City in 1999 was the high number of avian deaths among American crows (*Corvi brachrhyncos*) and other corvids.

Clinical manifestations

The incubation time in humans is reported to be 3–14 days. Symptoms generally last 3–6 days. Reports from earlier outbreaks describe a mild form of WNV infection presenting as a febrile influenza-like illness with sudden onset. This is often accompanied by malaise, anorexia, nausea, vomiting, rash, myalgia, lymphadenopathy and retro-orbital pain. A small proportion of cases (<1%) develop severe illness, such as acute encephalitis, aseptic meningitis or Guillain–Barré syndrome. In the recent outbreak in the USA those patients hospitalized with severe disease reported fever, weakness, gastrointestinal symptoms and flaccid paralysis. Persons of all ages appear to be equally susceptible to WNV infection, but it is reported that the incidence of neuroinvasive WNV disease and death increases with age, especially those between 60 and 89 years of age.[20] A minority of patients with severe disease develop a maculopapular rash or morbilliform rash involving the neck, trunk, arms or legs. Neurologic presentations include ataxia and extrapyramidal signs, cranial nerve abnormalities, myelitis, optical neuritis and seizures, and are more common in those over 50 years of age and in young children. New modes of transmission through blood donations, organ transplants and the intrauterine route have been reported in the USA[23,24] and Italy.[25]

Diagnostic microbiology

Diagnosis of patients with WNF encephalitis or meningitis is made by the detection of IgM antibody to WNV in serum or cerebrospinal fluid (CSF) collected within 8 days of illness using the IgM antibody capture ELISA (MAC-ELISA). As IgM does not cross the blood–brain barrier, IgM antibody in the CSF strongly suggests central nervous system (CNS) infection. Roehrig and colleagues described the long-term persistence of IgM antibody in patients with West Nile (WNV) infection. Care must therefore be taken since the IgM test cannot differentiate between recent and past infections.[26] As such, the laboratory diagnostic confirmation strategy involves the serologic detection of IgM or IgG ELISA in CSF and serum with subsequent plaque reduction neutralization test (PRNT) confirmation. In addition, highly sensitive reverse transcriptase (RT)-PCRs have been described. Virus isolation on acute CSF samples provides an alternative approach. Antigenic cross-reactivity with other closely related flaviviruses is a major problem in serologic testing, and this underlines the need for confirmation with PRNT. It should be noted that samples from patients recently vaccinated against or recently infected with related flaviviruses (e.g. yellow fever, Japanese encephalitis) may give positive WNV MAC-ELISA results.

Management

There is no specific therapy or vaccine available and management is supportive.[27]

ARENAVIRIDAE

Nature

Members of the Arenaviridae have been isolated from diverse species of rodents, which are their natural hosts, in a wide range of geographic locations. Two arenavirus complexes are recognized – the complex of lymphocytic choriomeningitis virus and Lassa virus (LCMV-LASV), or old world arenaviruses, and the Tacaribe complex, or new world arenaviruses.[28] This broad antigenic classification is supported by more detailed phylogenetic comparisons. A wide range of arenaviruses have been described in their host species; several cause human infection, of which the most important human pathogens are listed in Table 164.2.

Arenavirus virions range from spheric to pleomorphic and have a mean diameter of 110–130 nm. Particles are characterized by a variable number of electron-dense ribosomes (diameter 20–25 nm) within the virus particles. They have a lipid membrane with glycoprotein spikes that project 8–10 nm from the surface.

The genome consists of two ssRNA molecules, L (large) and S (small). The L and S RNAs of arenaviruses have an ambience coding arrangement; nucleocapsid (N) is encoded in the viral-complementary sequence corresponding to the 5′ half of segment S, whereas the viral glycoprotein precursor (GPC) is encoded in the viral-sense sequence corresponding to the 3′ half of S.[28]

The N protein, which is the most abundant polypeptide, is nonglycosylated and forms a ribonucleoprotein (RNP) complex with the genomic RNA. Two glycosylated proteins, GP-1 and GP-2, are derived by post-transitional cleavage from the GPC. The L segment codes for the L protein, which is an RNA polymerase, and the Z protein, a putative zinc binding protein. α-Dystoglycan has recently been identified as a receptor for LCMV and Lassa fever virus.[29] This belongs to a highly conserved family of proteins found in epithelial, muscle and neurologic cells in humans.

Pathogenesis

In their natural rodent hosts, arenavirus infections occur in two distinct patterns: during the neonatal period, a chronic viremic infection

Table 164.2 Arenaviruses known to cause human disease

Virus	Host in nature	Geographic distribution	Main features of human disease
Lymphocytic choriomeningitis virus (LCMV)	*Mus domesticus, Mus musculus*	Europe, Americas, perhaps elsewhere	Isolated 1933; causes lymphocytic choriomeningitis, which usually presents as an aseptic meningitis with a mortality rate <1%
Lassa fever	*Mastomys* spp.	West Africa	Isolated 1969; causes Lassa fever, a severe systemic illness; severe cases suffer shock and hemorrhages; mortality rate 16%
Junin virus	*Calomys musculinus*	Argentina	Isolated 1958; causes Argentine hemorrhagic fever (AHF), which causes a similar illness to Lassa but hemorrhage and CNS disease more frequent; mortality rate up to 30%
Machupo	*Calomys callosus*	Beni region of Bolivia	Isolated 1963; causes Bolivian hemorrhagic fever; similar clinical picture to AHF; mortality rate 25%
Guanarito virus	*Zygodontomys brevicauda: Sigmodon aistoni*	Venezuela	Isolated 1990; similar to AHF; mortality rate 25%
Sabia virus	Unknown	Brazil	Isolated 1990; only three human cases described, one fatal; clinical picture probably similar to AHF

is established; in adult rodents the infection is transient and self-limiting. This lifelong infection does not have major clinical sequelae for the infected rodent.[28]

In humans several arenavirus infections cause severe illness, including meningoencephalitis and hemorrhagic fever, with significant mortality rates. The pathogenesis is not fully understood, and microscopic changes found at autopsy are modest and do not account for the severity of illness. Petechial hemorrhages of the skin are found, and multiple hemorrhages and focal necrosis may be present in internal organs. Serous effusions and interstitial pneumonia have been described. Hemorrhages are more common with South American arenavirus infections. In contrast to these modest pathologic lesions, the physiologic changes are extensive. The state of shock characteristic of severe disease reflects an increase in vascular permeability. The mechanism involved is not fully understood, but may be an indirect effect of immune mediators on endothelial cells produced by infected macrophages and monocytes, rather than direct viral damage.

Epidemiology

The epidemiology of individual arenaviral disease in humans is dependent on the geographic distribution of infected rodents and the nature of their contacts with humans (Fig. 164.5).

Several distinct patterns are seen. In Lassa fever, which is a common human infection, the reservoir host is *Mastomys* spp., which is a peridomestic rodent found in sub-Saharan Africa. The rodents are persistently infected and contaminate the environment with the virus, which generates infectious aerosols on drying. Other routes of transmission include direct contact with rodent excretions during the capture and killing of these animals for consumption. The host of junin virus, the cause of Argentine hemorrhagic fever, is *Colomys musculinus*. The natural habitat of this rodent is the hedgerow and transmission occurs at harvest time, presumably because of aerosol transmission during mechanical harvesting.

Infection by LCMV is found worldwide, wherever its natural hosts *Mus domesticus* or *Mus musculus* are infected. The burden of disease is not well established, but LCMV infection is linked with up to 10% of CNS disease of suspected viral origin. Antibody studies show a prevalence of 5% in urban populations in the USA,[30] 9% in urban populations in Germany and 2.2% in Argentina. An increase in the number of cases is reported in the autumn, which may result from the reservoir host moving into homes for the winter. The potential for LCMV

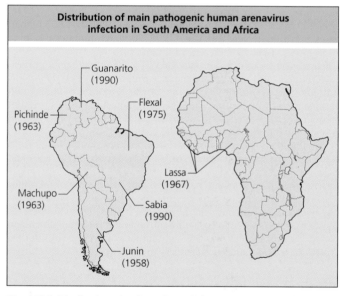

Fig. 164.5 Distribution of main pathogenic human arenavirus infection in South America and Africa, and year of first isolation of each virus.

to cause human disease was recently highlighted by a case linked to transplantation from an infected blood donor.[31]

Lassa fever is a serious public health problem in West Africa, in two distinct hyperendemic areas – Sierra Leone, Guinea and Liberia and Nigeria. Identification of a recent case in Côte d'Ivoire indicates that infection may be distributed more widely in West Africa.[32] Infections are found throughout the year, but a peak incidence is seen in the dry season. Lassa fever is a more common infection than previously thought, with estimates of up to 400 000 human cases annually and an overall mortality rate of 2%.[33] More severe hospitalized cases have a mortality rate of 16%.[34]

Several hundred cases of Argentine hemorrhagic fever are identified each year, and are associated with the harvest. Most cases occur in adult males.

Bolivian hemorrhagic fever was first identified in 1963–4, when it caused an extensive outbreak in San Joaquin that resulted in 113 deaths.[35] This followed the rodent host entering the small town,

However, the disease has since been uncommon, with occasional cases reported in rural communities in those more likely to come into contact with the infected rodent host.

Prevention

Two strategies have been proposed to prevent arenaviral disease in humans – rodent control and vaccination. Rodent control was important in controlling the Bolivian hemorrhagic fever outbreak, by the eradication of *Colomys callosus*. The house mouse, *Mus domesticus*, can be effectively eliminated from homes, thus reducing exposure to LCMV. However, its value in controlling other arenavirus infections has not been established. *Mastomys natalensis* is widespread and it has not proved practical to control rodent populations with living conditions found in West Africa. Both *C. callosus* and *C. musculinus* inhabit rural areas and control is not feasible.

A live, attenuated junin vaccine (Candid–1) has been developed and its efficacy demonstrated in a trial of 6500 volunteers.[36] It is now used for high-risk workers.

Lassa fever is the most important human arenavirus infection and vaccination seems to be the best hope for control. Killed and live vaccines have been developed and evaluated in animal models, and the most promising candidate vaccine is a vaccinia recombinant containing the Lassa virus glycoprotein gene. In challenge experiments this vaccine prevented death from Lassa challenge in guinea pigs and non-human primates. No human studies have been performed.[28]

Diagnostic microbiology

All arenavirus infections present similar diagnostic problems; the virus can be isolated early in the disease and this is followed by the later development of IgM and IgG antibody responses. There has been relatively little development of diagnostic assays for these agents because they are relatively rare and geographically localized.

Infection by LCMV is generally diagnosed by the detection of specific antibody. Usually immunofluorescence is used, but an ELISA test has been described. For virus isolation, blood and CSF samples are the most useful. Mice and guinea pigs are the most sensitive culture system, but isolation in Vero cells is more practical.

Lassa fever and several of the South American hemorrhagic fevers cause severe infections and can be transmitted by aerosol. Consequently, they have been classified as biohazard level 4 viruses and work on these agents is confined to the few high-containment laboratories worldwide.

The early clinical diagnosis of Lassa fever is difficult, and because ribavirin is an effective treatment if started early in the disease course, laboratory confirmation of infection is important. For rapid diagnosis either virus culture in Vero E6 cells or genome detection by RT-PCR is used on acute blood samples. Now RT-PCR is the first-line diagnostic test because it enables same-day diagnosis, and the use of guanadinium to extract RNA also inactivates viral infectivity, which makes the sample safe to work on outside the containment laboratory. In a recent study all Lassa fever patients were diagnosed by RT-PCR within 3 days of admission.[37] Detection of Lassa-specific antibody by immunofluorescence is widely used, but antibody rises late in clinical disease and is often not detectable until the second week of illness, which is often too late to effect patient management. Baculovirus-expressed nucleoprotein (NP) has been used for serologic diagnosis and avoids the need to culture virus. Quantitative real-time PCR has now been applied to the diagnosis of Lassa fever. The ability to quantify and monitor viral load may have prognostic value and help to guide treatment, but substantive studies are required.

The South American arenaviruses can be cultured from acute blood samples in newborn mice and hamsters or Vero cells. The detection of virus-specific IgG and IgM by immunofluorescence is widely used, and more recently ELISA using baculovirus-expressed viral proteins to detect antibody and RT-PCR tests have been described.

Clinical features

Arenavirus infections are often mild or subclinical. Even in severe infections, early illness is characterized by nonspecific symptoms, such as fever and myalgia, before the onset of severe systemic disease.

In LCMV infection headache, nausea or vomiting accompany the febrile prodrome. In the second week of illness CNS disease develops in a minority of cases and usually presents as an aseptic meningitis. In severe cases encephalitis can develop and this accounts for a significant minority of hospitalized cases. Full recovery is the most common outcome, but occasional deaths have been reported.

The incubation period of Lassa fever is about 10 days. It generally begins with a gradual onset of fever and malaise. As the disease progresses, abdominal pain, nausea and vomiting become more pronounced and an exudative pharyngitis and conjunctivitis are common. More pathognomonic signs and symptoms develop during the second week of illness, including facial edema, pleural edema, encephalopathy and shock. In severe cases illness is progressive, with shock followed by death. In survivors, defervescence is followed by recovery after 2–3 weeks. Hemorrhagic complications are not uncommon in severe cases and generally present with epistaxis, bruising and conjunctival hemorrhage. In the convalescent period pericarditis has been described. Deafness is now recognized as a late complication.[38] It can be unilateral or bilateral and is not related to the severity of disease; it may be immune mediated.

Argentine and Bolivian hemorrhagic fever present with a similar clinical picture. The progression of illness is more rapid than in Lassa fever, with severe prostration developing 3–4 days after onset. In more severe cases mucous membrane hemorrhage and bruising at intravenous injection sites are seen, which indicate a poor progress. In a few cases substantial neurologic involvement leads to convulsions. Recovery usually starts at the end of the second week of illness.

Management

Lassa fever has caused nosocomial infections in Africa and is the biohazard level 4 agent most commonly imported into nonendemic countries. Consequently, many countries have developed containment guidelines for the management of suspected Lassa fever cases to prevent secondary transmission.[39,40] Transmission is through direct contact with infected body fluids and little evidence suggests that airborne transmission is important. The guidelines follow a similar approach based on an initial patient risk assessment, which leads to different levels of investigation, containment and monitoring of close contacts, depending on risk (see also Chapter 126).

Ribavirin, a guanosine analogue, is effective *in vitro* against arenaviruses, but its mode of action is unknown. Ribavirin has been evaluated for the treatment of severe Lassa fever cases and dramatically reduces the mortality rate provided it is given early in the illness.[41] Its use for prophylaxis of contacts with Lassa fever cases and for the treatment of other arenavirus infections has been proposed, but no trial reports have been published to date.

Treatment of Argentine hemorrhagic fever infections with convalescent human plasma is effective in reducing the mortality rate from 15–30% to less than 2% if given during the first 8 days of illness. Convalescent plasma could potentially play a role in Lassa fever treatment, but this has not been established in practice. Patient management of arenaviral infections requires general supportive care, with particular attention to fluid balance.

HANTAVIRIDAE

Nature

Hantavirus is the most recently described genus in the Bunyaviridae family and comprises a growing number of isolated viruses, including those that cause hemorrhagic fever with renal syndrome (HFRS) and

Table 164.3 Characteristics of some known hantaviruses found in Europe, Asia, Russia and India

Species	Human illness	Pathology	Mortality rate (%)	Reservoir	Geographic virus distribution
Hantaan (HTN)	Severe: HFRS, EHF, KHF	Renal	5–15	*Apodemus agrarius* (striped field mouse)	China, Russia, Korea
Dobrava/Belgrade (DOB)	Severe: HFRS	Renal	5–15	*Apodemus flavicollis* (yellow neck mouse)	Balkans
Seoul (SEO)	Moderate: HFRS	Renal	1	*Rattus norvegicus* (Norway rat)	Worldwide
Puumala (PUU)	Mild; NE	Renal	1	*Clethrionomys glareolus* (bank vole)	Europe, Russia, Scandinavia
Khabarovsk (KHB)	?	?	?	*Microtus fortis* (reed mole)	Russia
Tula (TUL)	?	?	?	*Microtus arvalis* (European common vole)	Europe
Thailand (THAI)	?	?	?	*Bandicota indica* (bandicoot rat)	Thailand
Thottapalayan (TMP)	?	?	?	*Suncus murinus* (musk shrew)	India
Topografov (TOP)*	?	?	?	*Lemmus sibiricus* (Siberian lemming)	Siberia

EHF, epidemic hemorrhagic fever; HFRS, hemorrhagic fever with renal syndrome; KHF, Korean hemorrhagic fever; NE, nephropathia epidemica.
?Not yet documented.
*Virus not yet isolated/molecular analysis suggests they are probable hantavirus species.

hantavirus pulmonary syndrome (HPS).[42,43] Some recently recognized probable species that have been identified by molecular genetic analysis have not yet been isolated (Table 164.3). Hantaviruses contain a tripartite, single-stranded, negative-sense RNA genome. The three segments are designated as small (S), medium (M) and large (L), and encode for the nucleocapsid (N) protein of 50–53 kDa, the two envelope proteins (G1 and G2) of 65 and 74 kDa, respectively, and an associated virus of 200 kDa.[44]

Epidemiology

The epidemiology of hantavirus disease in humans is dependent on the geographic distribution of persistently infected rodent hosts.[45] The hantaviruses linked with HFRS are associated with specific rodent hosts, each named for the region in which they were first isolated:

- *Apodemus agrarius* (the striped field mouse) for the hantavirus;
- *Rattus norvegicus* (the Norway rat) and *Rattus rattus* (the black rat) for the Seoul virus; and
- *Apodemus flavicollus* (the yellow necked field mouse) for the Dobrava virus.

The hantavirus from Korea, Russia and China and the Dobrava virus (DOBV) from the Balkan countries of Europe (Bosnia, Croatia, Yugoslavia, Albania, Slovenia, Greece, Bulgaria and Russia) are associated with the severe form of HFRS, with an estimated mortality rate of 5–15% (see Table 164.3).[46,47] DOBV appears to be the most life-threatening hantavirus in Europe; a moderate form of HFRS is caused by the Seoul virus, which (along with its host) is found virtually worldwide. Serologic evidence for infection with Seoul-like hantaviruses has been found in rodents in major cities within the USA.

A mild form of HFRS, caused by the Puumala virus (PUUV), is responsible for nephropathia epidemica (NE) in Scandinavia, the European regions of the former USSR and south of this through much of Europe to France, Spain and Portugal.

The hantavirus associated with HPS, Sin Nombre virus (SNV), has been recognized throughout the USA since its discovery in 1993.[48] Molecular biologic studies have identified similar viruses – Black

Creek Canal (BCC), New York, Bayou (BAY) and Andes – that are also associated with HPS illness, that extend their geographic distribution from North America to Mexico and South America (Table 164.4). The distribution of specific host species throughout the Americas suggests a wider distribution of hantaviruses which potentially could cause further clinical cases. Recently, two novel hantaviruses, with unknown pathogenic potential, were found in Africa.[49–51]

All rodent hosts are persistently infected with specific hantavirus strains that apparently cause no illness. In wild rodent populations, most infections occur through age-dependent horizontal routes, predominately in mature males. Horizontal transmission among cage mates was experimentally demonstrated via the aerosol route at median infectious doses of 1.0 plague forming units (pfu) for each virus tested. However, although rodents are susceptible to hantavirus through the aerosol route, their susceptibility is increased by inoculation (median infectious doses 0.003–0.016 pfu). Vertical transmission from dam to pup has proved negligible or absent, both in wild and experimental settings.

Hantavirus disease, irrespective of strain, is a seasonal disease. This seasonality is associated with population dynamics of the rodent hosts that maintain each virus and their interaction with local human populations. Rodent population cycles vary according to climatic changes and interspecies competition. Rural-associated HFRS in Asia and Europe is linked to human rodent contact during the planting and harvesting of crops (late autumn and early winter). Similarly, in Scandinavia Puumala virus causes most cases of NE during the same period. Both Puumala outbreaks in Scandinavia and the original HPS outbreak in America were associated with increases in the natural rodent population followed by rodent migration from the fields to buildings in response to adverse weather conditions. Alternatively, in Greece, HFRS is observed predominately in the warmer months as a result of increased human outdoor activities, including camping. These cases point to higher risk being experienced by people such as forestry workers and shepherds. In China HFRS induced by Seoul virus appears to be most common in the spring.

The aerosol route of infection is regarded as the most common means of transmission among rodents and to humans. Rodent bites cannot be excluded as a way of maintaining the disease among

Table 164.4 Some known hantaviruses found in North and South America

Species	Human illness	Pathology	Mortality rate (%)	Reservoir	Geographic virus distribution
Sin Nombre virus (SNV)	Severe: HPS	Pulmonary	50	*Peromyscus maniculatus* (deer mouse)	USA, Canada, Mexico
New York (NY)	HPS	Pulmonary	Not recorded	*Peromyscus leucopus* (white-footed mouse)	USA
Black Creek Canal (BCC)	HPS	Pulmonary	Not recorded	*Sigmodon hispidus* (cotton rat)	USA
El Monro Canyon (ELMC)	?	?	?	*Reithrodontomys megalotis* (Western harvest mouse)	USA, Mexico
Bayou (BAY)*	HPS	Pulmonary/renal	?	*Oryzomys palustris* (rice rat)	USA
Andes (AND)*	HPS	Pulmonary	50	*Oligoryzomys longicaudatus* (long tailed pygmy rice rat)	Argentina
Unnamed*	HPS	Pulmonary	?	*Calomys laucha* (vesper mouse)	Paraguay
Rio Segundo (RIOS)*	?	?	?	*Reithrodontomys mexicanus* (Mexican harvest mouse)	Costa Rica
Rio Manore (RIOM)*	?	?	?	*Oligoryzomys microtis* (small-eared pygmy rice rat)	Bolivia
Isla Vista (ISLA)*	?	?	?	*Microtus californicus* (California vole)	USA
Bloodland Lake (BLL)*	?	?	?	*Microtus ochrogaster* (prairie vole)	USA

HPS, hantavirus pulmonary syndrome.
?Not yet documented.
*Virus not yet isolated/molecular analysis suggests they are unique hantavirus strains.

rodents or occasionally resulting in human infection. Epidemiologic investigations link virus exposure to farming activities, sleeping on the ground and military exercises. Indoor exposure has been linked to rodent infestation of homes during cold weather or to nesting rodents in or near dwellings. Many hantavirus infections are identified among people who live in poor housing conditions or in those who pursue recreational activities such as camping and various water sports. Human-to-human transmission is rare and consequently hantaviruses do not pose a risk to hospital workers. However, recent outbreaks of HPS in South America suggested that minimal exposure to body fluids of infected patients resulted in apparent person-to-person spread.

The annual incidence of HFRS involving hospitalization throughout the world is estimated to be between 150 000 and 200 000 cases. More than half these cases predominate in the endemic center of epidemic hemorrhagic fever in the Chinese provinces of Hubei, Heilongjiang, Jiangxi, Jilin and Shanxi. Annual incidence rates here range from 0.05 to 3.0/1000. Russia and Korea also report hundreds to thousands of cases of HFRS each year. Most of the remaining cases (a few hundred) are reported from Japan, Finland, Sweden, Belgium, The Netherlands, Greece, Hungary, France and the Balkan countries formally constituting Yugoslavia. Mortality rates range from less than 0.1% for HFRS caused by Puumala to approximately 5–10% for HFRS caused by hantavirus.

Several hundred cases of HPS have been reported throughout North and South America (see Table 164.4).[52] Most of the identified cases in America and Canada were caused by SNV. Cases of HPS in southwestern USA and South America are caused by molecularly identified strains that include BAY, BCC and Andes viruses.[53]

A number of hantavirus infections have caused several laboratory-associated outbreaks of HFRS, all of which were traced to persistently infected rodents obtained from breeders, to wild-caught naturally infected rodents or to experimentally infected rodents. No illness has been associated with laboratory workers using cell-culture adapted viruses, although asymptomatic seroconversions have been documented.

Pathogenesis

The process by which hantaviruses cause multisystem organ dysfunction syndrome is unclear. Thrombocytopenia, defects in platelet function, transient disseminated intravascular coagulation (DIC) and increased vascular fragility are all thought to play a key role in the early stages of the disease. Hantavirus disease is mainly microvascular in nature and endothelium is the predominant cell type involved. The presence of hantavirus antigen has been demonstrated by immunochemistry in vascular endothelial cells of fatal HFRS infections, experimentally infected rodents and endothelium of lung capillaries in the highly lethal form of HPS.[54] Endothelial damage or dysfunction leads to capillary engorgement, leakage of erythrocytes and increased permeability.

Recent studies implicated the disease process as being immunologically based, with lymphocytes playing a key role, especially T cells. The CD4:CD8 ratio is greatly decreased, although abundant CD4+ and CD8+ lymphocytes have been reported in the lung interstitium of HPS patients.[54] Lymphocyte induction of migrating macrophages and other inflammatory cells results in the production of cytokines, such as tumor necrosis factor (TNF), interleukin (IL)-1 and IL-2, and interferon gamma (IFN-γ), which in turn increases vascular permeability.

Prevention

Prevention of hantavirus infection is dependent upon reducing contact between humans and infected rodents. However, many rodent control programs in known highly endemic areas, such as China, have been ineffective. Guidelines in the USA to control HPS infections have been aimed at reducing rodent access to homes, clean-up recommendations of buildings with heavy rodent infestations, and precautions for workers exposed to rodents and for campers and hikers in infected areas.

Although a number of candidate (inactivated, recombinant) vaccines against hantaviruses are under development, none is currently available.

Both wild-caught rodents introduced into laboratories and laboratory-bred colonies have caused a number of laboratory-based infections. Current recommendations directed at the manipulation of hantaviruses call for handling at biosafety containment levels 2 and 3, dependent on the strain. Work with infected laboratory rodent colonies that may lead to the generation of infectious aerosols in urine or feces should be undertaken in facilities that have suitable room ventilation and high-efficiency particulate air (HEPA) filtration, primary containment of animals, and personal protective equipment at a minimum of biosafety containment level 3. Precautions should also ensure suitable decontamination of animal bedding, cages and animal waste.

It is prudent to introduce hantavirus screening of laboratory-bred and wild-caught rodents and cell lines that originate from rodent tissue before use. Such animals and cells should be segregated from other animals, with care being taken to prevent possible aerosolized spread of infectious virus.

Diagnostic microbiology

Diagnosis of hantavirus infection relies upon the recognition of characteristic clinical features, a history consistent with the epidemiology of the disease and serologic confirmation.[52]

Direct isolation of hantavirus from acutely ill patients is prolonged and often unsuccessful and consequently of little diagnostic value. Similarly, the success of antigen-capture ELISA or the application of RT-PCR on acute blood samples is of no practical value for the diagnosis of human infection.

Although the immunofluorescence assay is regarded as a useful diagnostic tool, the method of choice to diagnose acute hantavirus infection is an IgM antibody assay of high sensitivity and specificity.[55] Currently two alternatives are available:

* M antibody capture IgM enzyme immunoassay (EIA) based on the use of cell-culture grown hantavirus antigen; and
* M antibody capture IgM EIA based on baculovirus or *Escherichia coli* expressed full-length nucleocapsid protein.[56]

As IgG antibodies persist for life in both humans and rodents, the presence of IgG seropositivity may not reflect a recent infection. In addition, a rise in IgG has not always been observed in recent clinical cases. The IgG ELISA or immunofluorescent antibody (IFA) test is well suited for epidemiologic studies, whereas determination of the specific infecting virus is best achieved by focus reduction neutralization tests.

Other methods are also under development to investigate hantavirus:

* hantavirus recombinant immunoblot assay (RIBA), which uses recombinant and synthetic peptides; and
* application of RT-PCR and immunohistochemical staining of antigen contained in formalin-fixed autopsy tissues.[57]

Clinical manifestations

Although HFRS has been clinically recognized and reported in Asia, Russia and Scandinavia for the past century, the causative agent, hantavirus, was not isolated until 1978.[58] The HFRS complex comprises

Table 164.5 Main characteristics of the two severe forms of hantavirus disease

Characteristics	Hemorrhagic fever with renal syndrome	Hantavirus pulmonary syndrome
Primary target organ	Kidney	Lung
Acute phase	Febrile	Febrile 'prodrome'
Later phases	Shock, hemorrhage	Shock, pulmonary edema
Disease progression	Hypotensive, oliguric, diuresis, convalescence	Diuresis, convalescence
Other clinical and laboratory features	Thrombocytopenia, leukocytosis, proteinuria, hematuria, creatinine >100 mmol/l, hemoconcentration, raised transaminases	Thrombocytopenia, leukocytosis, hemoconcentration, shortness of breath, abnormal respiratory rate, lung infiltrates
Mortality rate (%)	1–15	≥50

three distant clinical diseases, each infection being caused by a specific hantavirus.[45,46] The spectrum of disease ranges from nonapparent infection to fulminant hemorrhagic fever with renal failure (sometimes having a fatal outcome). Depending on which hantavirus is responsible for the illness, HFRS can appear as a mild, moderate or severe disease. Fatality rates range from less than 1% for HRFS caused by Puumula virus to approximately 5–10% for HFRS caused by hantavirus (Table 164.5).

The clinical course of pathogenic hantavirus infection comprises an acute febrile illness characterized by variable degrees of hemorrhagic and renal dysfunction. More severe disease involves five overlapping stages – febrile, hypotensive, oliguric, diuretic and convalescent.

The onset of the disease is abrupt and characterized by high fever of 102.2–104°F (39–40°C), chills, intensive headache, malaise, myalgia, dizziness and anorexia. A petechial rash may also appear on the face, neck and trunk. The main laboratory findings include normal-to-elevated white blood count (WBC), decreasing platelets, rising hematocrit and rising proteinuria.

As the febrile phase ends, hypotension can abruptly develop and last for a few hours or days. Prominent features are tachycardia, falling arterial pressure and narrowing pulse pressure, and in severe cases classic shock. Laboratory findings include leukocytosis with a left shift, thrombocytopenia and prolonged bleeding times. Urinalysis shows heavy proteinuria, mild hematuria and hyposthenuria. About one-third of fatalities occur during this phase.

The oliguric phase lasts 3–7 days, during which blood pressure returns to normal or is slightly raised because of hypervolemia. Laboratory findings include normal WBC and platelet counts, initially normal and then depressed hematocrit, continual marked hematuria and elevated blood urea nitrogen and creatinine. Hyponatremia, hyperkalemia and hypocalcemia result from renal failure. Pulmonary edema may occur and fluid management should be handled with care. Almost half of the deaths occur during this phase, often from pulmonary edema or infection, electrolyte imbalance, late shock or hemorrhage into the brain.

Clinical recovery is signaled by the diuretic phase, with improved renal function and normal clotting. Diuresis over a few hours or days is evident, with an output of 3–6 liters. Fluid management must be maintained to prevent negative fluid balance that may lead to shock. The final (convalescent) phase can last weeks to months before recovery is complete.

Seoul virus infections (mild HFRS) are less severe than those caused by hantavirus. Typically the phases are shorter and difficult to recognize or even absent. The disease is characterized by fever, anorexia, chills and nausea, and vomiting. Palatal injection is common, although other hemorrhagic signs (epistaxis, melena, hematemesis) are observed in fewer than 30% of patients. Laboratory findings include lymphocytosis, thrombocytopenia, microscopic hematuria and proteinuria, and elevation of serum transaminase. Renal involvement is less severe and fatalities are uncommon.

Puumula virus infection (NE) is characterized by a sudden onset of fever accompanied by headache. Characteristically, by the fourth day of illness nausea, vomiting, petechiae in the throat and soft palate, and facial flush and petechial rash have occurred. A mild thrombocytopenia can be observed. Hypotension may be found, but evidence of shock is rare. Onset of oliguria or recognition of renal failure around the sixth day of disease is the main cause of hospital admission. Serum creatinine levels rise and dialysis may be required in 10% of cases. As with other hantavirus infections, the onset of polyuria indicates the recovery process.

First recognized as a severe, often fatal respiratory illness in adults, HPS was characterized as a severe, systemic illness with a nonspecific onset, fever, myalgia, cough or dyspnea, gastrointestinal symptoms and headache that typically lasted 3–5 days.[59,60] Rapid and abrupt onset of noncardiogenic edema, hypotension (systolic blood pressure ≤80 mmHg) then follow, resulting in shock and death in over half of the recognized cases (see Table 164.5). Laboratory findings indicate leukocytosis, an increase in polymorphonuclear leukocytes, left shift, increased hematocrit, thrombocytopenia, prolonged prothrombin and partial thromboplastin time, elevated serum lactate dehydrogenase, decreased serum protein concentrations and proteinuria. Increases in hematocrit and thromboplastin time are considered to be predictors of death. Radiographic examinations show bilateral pulmonary infiltrates and evidence of pleural effusions in the majority of hospitalized patients. Histopathologic features seen in lung tissue reveal mild-to-moderate interstitial pneumonitis with variable degrees of congestion, edema and mononuclear infiltrates. The virus has been identified extensively within endothelial cells of the pulmonary microvasculature, spleen and lymph nodes.

Current understanding of the disease indicates little evidence of renal damage as a feature of this hantavirus infection. The extensive pulmonary endothelial involvement and severe pulmonary edema make clinical management difficult.

Management

Effective management of HFRS and HPS requires early diagnosis, knowledge of disease course and prompt hospitalization. Aggressive clinical management is essential to improve survival. Care should be phase specific, with special attention given to fluid management. Ribavirin may be efficacious in the treatment of HFRS patients, but its treatment of HPS is not proved.

FILOVIRIDAE

Nature

The family Filoviridae consists of two distinctive species, Marburg and Ebola, which cause severe and often fatal hemorrhagic disease in humans and monkeys (see Chapter 126). The viruses have a distinctive filamentous morphology under the electron microscope with a genome that consists of a nonsegmented, negative stranded RNA approximately 19 kb in length. Several features of their molecular organization and structure have linked these viruses to members of the Paramyxoviridae and Rhabdoviridae under the taxonomic order Mononegavirales.[57] The virions are composed of a central core formed by an RNP complex, which is surrounded by a lipid envelope derived from the host cell plasma membrane. The RNP is composed of a genomic RNA molecule bound by the NP, virion structural protein 30 (VP30), VP35 and the L protein (RNA transcriptase polymerase). The three remaining structural proteins are membrane associated – GP, VP24 and VP40 are located on the inner side of the membrane. Among the newly isolated Ebola viruses are differences in molecular structure, pathogenicity and virulence in humans.[61]

Marburg and Ebola were first detected in 1967[62] and 1976,[63,64] respectively, although human infections since then have been rare. Fresh outbreaks of Ebola infections were identified in Côte d'Ivoire (1994, 1995), Republic of Congo (formerly Zaire; 1995, 2001, 2002, 2003, 2007),[65] Gabon (1994, 1996, 1997, 2001) and Uganda (2000, 2008).[66] In addition, importation of Ebola-infected monkeys into the USA (1989–1990, 1996) and Italy (1992) attracted extensive worldwide media coverage and raised public concerns about the potential public health threat of these pathogens through international travel and commerce.[67,68]

Pathogenesis

The precise mechanisms by which filoviruses cause the most severe forms of VHF are unclear, but there is marked hepatic involvement, DIC and shock, producing extremely high fatality rates (30–90%). In the early stages of infection laboratory findings, such as high aspartate transaminase/alanine transaminase (AST/ALT) ratios, and marked lymphopenia followed by a marked neutropenia with left shift, suggest other extrahepatic targets affected by the virus. As with other VHF infections (HFRS, Lassa, dengue) fluid imbalance and platelet abnormalities indicate endothelial cell and platelet damage or dysfunction. Human monocytes and/or macrophages, fibroblasts and endothelial cells support virus replication. Infected monocyte and/or macrophages have been shown in in-vitro models to secrete the cytokine TNF which has the ability to increase vascular endothelial cell damage.[69] The data currently available support mediator-induced vascular damage that leads to increased permeability and shock observed in severe cases. Hemorrhage is likely to be caused by reticuloendothelial system damage that cannot be repaired because of platelet and coagulation malfunctions.

Epidemiology

The natural history and reservoirs of filoviruses remain to be established, but recently the potential role of bats has been highlighted.[70] In 1967, a fulminating hemorrhagic fever, Marburg disease, occurred in Marburg and Frankfurt, Germany, and Bosnia, Croatia and Yugoslavia among laboratory workers handling blood and tissue from a shipment of African green monkeys (Cercopithecus aethiops) soon after being imported from Uganda via London. Among the 31 human cases, 25 of which were primary infections, there were seven (23%) deaths.[62] None of the secondary cases died. Since then, sporadic cases have been reported from South Africa and Kenya (Fig. 164.6). The geographic spread widened with a major outbreak of Marburg in the Uige Providence of Angola during 2004–5 where 252 cases were identified with 227 deaths (case fatality rate 90%).

In 1976, the first known cases of Ebola hemorrhagic fever were identified in southern Sudan (Table 164.6) and in a simultaneous outbreak in northern Republic of Congo (formerly Zaire), with fatality rates of about 60% and 90%, respectively.[63,64] A further smaller outbreak occurred in the same region of Sudan in 1979, when 22 (65%) of 34 infections proved fatal. Lack of community co-operation hampered control efforts and investigations during an outbreak of Ebola in the Republic of Congo during 2002. Recent instances of Ebola infection were the severe illness of a Swiss zoologist working with infected chimpanzees (Pan troglodytes verus) in the Taï National Park in Côte d'Ivoire, West Africa, in late 1994 and a major epidemic in Kikwit, Bandundu Province, Republic of Congo (formerly Zaire), in 1995. Of 315 recorded cases of Ebola hemorrhagic fever a total of 244 died (77% case fatality rate).[64] A further four outbreaks between 2001 and 2007 in the D.R Congo recorded over 499 cases where 387 died (77.5% case

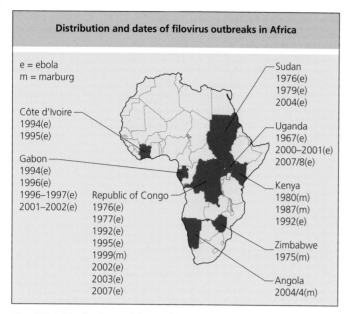

Distribution and dates of filovirus outbreaks in Africa

e = ebola
m = marburg

Côte d'Ivoire
1994(e)
1995(e)

Gabon
1994(e)
1996(e)
1996–1997(e)
2001–2002(e)

Republic of Congo
1976(e)
1977(e)
1992(e)
1995(e)
1999(m)
2002(e)
2003(e)
2007(e)

Sudan
1976(e)
1979(e)
2004(e)

Uganda
1967(e)
2000–2001(e)
2007/8(e)

Kenya
1980(m)
1987(m)
1992(e)

Zimbabwe
1975(m)

Angola
2004/4(m)

Fig. 164.6 Distribution and dates of filovirus outbreaks in Africa.

fatality rate). In the later part of 1995 further cases were identified in the Côte d'Ivoire among refugees who originated in Liberia. Finally, three reportedly independent human outbreaks of Ebola have occurred in the forested areas found in north-eastern Gabon (1994, February 1996, July 1996, December 2001). Subsequent investigations of the 2001–2 outbreak suggested that cases in villages north of Mekambo resulted from contact with a gorilla whose remains were found to be positive for Ebola virus. A severe outbreak occurred between August 2000 and January 2001 in Uganda (Gulu and Masindi districts) that recorded 425 cases with 224 fatalities.[69] A case from the 1996 infection was treated in South Africa and the source of a fatal nosocomial transmission to a health-care worker. All three outbreaks were associated with the deaths of chimpanzees, also thought to be from Ebola virus infection. In 2008, a newly discovered Ebola virus was found responsible for two cases in young men working lead and gold mines in Kamwenge District, Uganda.[70]

Hence, since 1994 West Africa has been considered to be part of the African filovirus map (see Fig. 164.6). Although filovirus outbreaks are rare events, the public health importance lies in their high mortality rate rather than the total number of infections in the 30 years since they were first identified (Tables 164.6 and 164.7).

Ebola virus has also appeared outside Africa, among shipments of imported cynomolgus monkeys in Reston, Philadelphia and Texas, USA, in 1989, 1990 and 1996, respectively, and Sienna, Italy, in 1992.[66] The monkeys involved in each epizootic event were imported from the Philippines and traced to the same handling facility, where the presence of the virus was also documented. The epizootics indicate that monkeys acutely infected with filoviruses present a major veterinary emergency and possibly could pose a serious hazard to other animals or humans if not recognized in the future. Although an Asian origin of these virus strains cannot be discounted, molecular biologic and serologic studies carried out to date suggest a close similarity with the original Ebola viruses isolated from the 1976 African outbreaks. Current interest in this strain of Ebola virus has increased with the description of Ebola-Reston in samples originating from domestic pigs originating in the Philippines.

Prevention

The imposition of ecologic controls to prevent outbreaks is impossible until the natural history of the viruses has been discovered. It is important that health-care workers in areas where hemorrhagic fever exists are aware of the high risk of nosocomial spread if patients are not recognized early and placed in complete isolation.[71] In nonendemic areas an awareness of the changing epidemiology associated with viral re-emergence or emergence should always be considered, bearing in mind the threat and consequences of importation.[72] High-risk patients are those who during the 3 weeks before illness had:

* traveled into areas where VHF occurred recently;
* been in contact with body fluids from a person with VHF; or
* worked in a laboratory environment handling the virus.

(See also Chapter 126.)

Importantly, filovirus illness is a rare event if patients do not meet any of these criteria.

As nonhuman primates are responsible for the introduction of Marburg into Europe, and of Ebola into the USA and Italy, the management of transportation, quarantine facilities and animal husbandry must ensure that personnel understand the hazards of handling nonhuman primates, and thus reduce the risks of future human outbreaks.[73]

Clinical manifestations

The incubation period for Ebola ranges from 4 to 10 days and for Marburg from 3 to 9 days.[62] The shorter times have been associated with exposure to contaminated needles.[74]

Filoviruses enter the host through close contact with contaminated body fluids. Epidemiologic studies in humans indicate that infection is not readily transmitted by the aerosol route. Although studies in nonhuman primates have established that aerosol transmission can cause infection,[75] extra care must be taken with contaminated body fluid, tissue, hospital material and waste.

Both Marburg and Ebola virus infections follow a similar pattern of illness. Following exposure, initial symptoms include an abrupt onset with fever, severe frontal headache, malaise and myalgia. Such symptoms are similar to those of many viral illnesses that originate locally and in tropical areas. The initial diagnosis of a filovirus infection is very difficult. Disease progression is characterized by pharyngitis, nausea, severe vomiting of blood and production of bloody stools. Uncontrolled bleeding follows, which can be seen from under the skin, from venepuncture sites and from other orifices of the body. A characteristic maculopapular rash occurs 7–10 days (range 1–21 days) after onset of the clinical disease. If fatal, death occurs 6–9 days after onset of the clinical disease and results from severe blood loss and shock. Convalescence is slow, taking many weeks, and is marked by weight loss, prostration and amnesia of the acute phase of illness.[76]

Clinical laboratory findings in the early acute phase include lymphopenia followed by neutrophilia, marked thrombocytopenia and abnormal platelet aggregation. Serum AST and ALT are elevated and characterized by an AST/ALT ratio of between 10 and 3:1.

Diagnostic microbiology

The clinical diagnosis of Ebola or Marburg should be considered in patients who show acute, febrile illness and have traveled in known epidemic or suspected endemic areas of rural sub-Saharan Africa and Asia, particularly when hemorrhagic signs are present. As the differential diagnosis in the early acute phase of illness is difficult, other causes (malaria, typhoid) should not be excluded and treatment delayed. Laboratory diagnosis carried out on patient specimens is undertaken by more than one procedure to guard against false-positives.

Care should be taken when drawing or handling blood specimens at the acute stage of illness because they contain large amounts of infectious virus – the virus is stable for long periods at room temperature at this stage.

Although their morphologic appearance is similar by electron microscopy, Marburg and Ebola are immunologically distinct. The basic diagnostic tool for filovirus infection and the only one to date that has widespread acceptance for the diagnosis of human filovirus disease is IFA, although some epidemiologic serology based on this

Table 164.6 Characteristics of some known filovirus infections in Africa

Date	Filovirus Infections	Documented fatalities/total cases	Main characteristics
Marburg			
1967	Marburg, Germany	5/23	Infected through contact with African green monkeys imported from Uganda
1967	Frankfurt, Germany	2/6	Infected through contact with African green monkeys imported from Uganda
1967	Belgrade, Yugoslavia	0/2	Infected through contact with African green monkeys imported from Uganda
1975	Zimbabwe	1/3	Contracted by travelers entering region – source unknown
1980	Mount Elgon, Kenya	1/2	Contracted by travelers entering region – source unknown
1987	Mount Elgon, Kenya	1/1	Contracted by travelers entering region – source unknown
1998–2000	D.R. Congo	128/154	Gold miners near Durba
2004–05	Angola	227/252	Outbreak started in Uige Province
2007	Uganda	1/2	Contracted infection in mine
2008	Netherlands	1/1	Contracted illness in Uganda
Total mortality rate		**367/446 (82.3%)**	
Ebola (Africa)			
1976	Yambuku, D.R. Congo	280/318	Virus when introduced into hospital amplified disease
1976	Maridi, Sudan	151/284	Virus when introduced into hospital amplified disease
1976	England	0/1	Laboratory acquired infection
1977–8	Tandala, D.R. Congo	1/1	Child infected
1979	Nzara and Yambio, Sudan	22/34	Amplified by nosocomial transmission in hospital
1994	Taï Forest, Côte d'Ivoire	0/1	Worker infected after autopsy of chimpanzee – repatriated to Switzerland
1994	Gabon	31/52	Origin gold mining camps at Mekokou and Andcock. Primarily reported as yellow fever
1995	Kikwit, D.R. Congo	250/315	Included laboratory confirmed cases. Rapid transmission among unprotected health-care workers
1995	Taï Forest, Côte d'Ivoire	0/1	Case originated in Liberia? four additional cases in Liberia
1996 (January-March)	Mayibout, Gabon	21/37	Contact with dead chimpanzees
1996 July & anuary 1997	Booué and Libreville, Gabon	45/60	Index case hunter living in forest area – infected chimpanzees identified
1996	South Africa	1/2	Epidemiologically linked with outbreak in Gabon. Fatal case – nosocomial infection of nurse by patient transferred from Gabon
2000–1	Uganda	224/425	Occurred in Gulu, Misindi and Mbarara districts of Uganda. Spread associated with attending funerals, community nursing and medical care without personal protective measures
2001–2	Gabon	53/65	Community outbreak evidence suggests contact with dead nonhuman primates (gorilla)
2001–2	D.R. Congo	43/57	Outbreak occurred over the border of Gabon with Republic of the Congo
2002–3	D.R. Congo	128/143	Outbreak in Mbomo and Kelle
2003	D.R Congo	29/35	Outbreak in Mbomo and Mbandza villages
2007	D.R. Congo	187/264	Outbreak in Kasai Province
2007–8	Uganda	37/149	Outbreak in Western Uganda
Total mortality rate		**1503/2244 (66.9%)**	

Table 164.7 Recorded filovirus (Ebola (Reston)) infections

Date	Filovirus infections	Documented fatalities/ total cases	Main characteristics
1989	Richmond, Virginia, USA	0/4	Reston strain isolated from monkeys imported from Philippines. Serologic evidence of asymptomatic infection among animal workers
1990	Manila, Philippines	0/12	Serologic evidence of asymptomatic infection among animal workers
1992	Siena, Italy	No cases	Reston strain isolated from monkeys imported from Philippines
1996 (April)	Alice Texas, USA	No cases	Reston strain in monkeys imported from Philippines
1996	Philippines	No cases	Virus identified in primate export facility
2008	Philippines	No cases	Virus identified in pigs
Total mortality rate		**0/16 (0%)**	

assay has been regarded as nonspecific and unreliable. A rising antibody in paired serum or a high IgG titer (>64) and the presence of IgM antibody together with clinical symptoms compatible with hemorrhagic fever are consistent with a diagnosis of filovirus infection.

Filoviruses can be readily isolated from fresh or stored (−94°F) specimens of blood or serum collected during the acute phase of illness. Vero cells (clone E6) and MA104 have proved the most sensitive for the propagation and assay of Marburg and Ebola viruses. As primary isolation using tissue culture rarely produces a specific cytopathic effect, evidence of infection is confirmed by immunofluorescence staining using antivirus-specific monoclonal or polyclonal antibodies. Some strains of Ebola, such as Ebola Sudan, proved difficult to grow in tissue culture and success was improved through interperitoneal inoculation of young guinea pigs. The resultant febrile response coincides with high levels of virus in the blood, which can be easily recovered by tissue culture or examined directly by electron microscopy. The isolation or propagation of filoviruses should not be attempted outside a biosafety containment level 4 laboratory.

During recent epizootic and human African outbreaks, early detection of filovirus infections was considerably improved by the development of an antigen-capture ELISA, amplification of filovirus RNA by RT-PCR, and immunohistochemistry identification of Ebola in skin biopsies. Skin biopsies fixed in formalin can be safely transported to reference facilities for confirmation without the need for low temperature preservation. Recent advances in molecular biology have expressed the NP gene of Ebola virus in a baculovirus expression system. The noninfectious N protein can replace the need for inactivation of infectious virus used in many serologic assays (IFA and ELISA). The diagnostic capabilities of such a system are currently being evaluated.

Management

No specific treatment is available. Treatment is limited to the provision of intensive nursing and effective control of blood volume and electrolyte balance. Shock, renal failure, depletion of blood clotting factors, severe bleeding and oxygen depletion must be managed. Human interferon and human convalescent plasma have been used to treat patients, but their efficacy is not proved. Ribavirin has no therapeutic value.

Patient management is further complicated by the need to isolate the patient and protect medical and nursing staff.[67,71] Use of patient isolators is a requirement in many countries, whereas strict barrier nursing techniques are acceptable in others. The latter can be supplemented using high efficiency particulate air filter respirators for protection against aerosols if considered feasible. Particular emphasis should be placed on ensuring that high-risk procedures (such as handling blood, secretions, catheters and introducing intravenous lines) are undertaken under barrier nursing conditions. It is recommended that patients who die from the disease should be buried or cremated promptly.

NIPAH AND HENDRA VIRUSES

Epidemiology

Both Hendra virus (HeV; formerly called equine morbillivirus) and Nipah virus (NiV) are newly recognized hazard group 4 zoonotic viruses.

Two outbreaks of a new zoonotic disease affecting horses and animals in Australia were reported within 1 month of each other in Brisbane (southeast Queensland) and Mackay (central Queensland) in 1994. A third event involving a single fatal equine case occurred near Cairns (North Queensland) in 1999. To date, two humans and 16 horses have died from this disease with acute respiratory failure.[77-79] Within the subfamily Paramyxovirinae, the extent of nucleotide homology in the N gene between different viruses in the same genus ranges from 56% to 78%, whereas the extent of nucleotide similarity between viruses from different genera is 39–78%. The N genes of HeV and NiV have 78% nucleotide homology, but the two viruses have no more than 49% similarity with any other members of the Paramyxovirinae.[80] Phylogenetic analysis of the N gene sequences show that HeV and NiV form a distinct cluster within the subfamily Paramyxovirinae. Both NiV and HeV are identified as henipaviruses, a new family of emerging paramyxoviruses.[80]

Another member of the Paramyxoviridae (NiV) was responsible for an outbreak of severe febrile encephalitis in humans in Malaysia in 1998–9. The outbreak was associated with respiratory illness in pigs and was initially considered to be Japanese encephalitis. Of a total of 256 cases, 105 were fatal. In March 1999, a cluster of 11 cases (one fatality) was described in Singapore in abattoir workers who handled pigs imported from the outbreak regions in Malaysia.[81] Measures to control the concurrent outbreak of respiratory disease in pigs resulted in the culling of over one million pigs (almost half the national pig herd) and had major domestic and international trade implications.

Seven outbreaks of NiV also occurred in Bangladesh between 2001 and 2008, the last outbreak affecting two villages in the Rajbari district,[82] 70 km west of the city of Dhaka. Of the 12 identified cases, there were 10 deaths, resulting in a case fatality rate of 83%.[83] The original outbreaks in 2001 and 2003 involved primary men and women more than 25 years of age; the last outbreak involved boys, 15 years of age. Further NiV infections were identified in Siliguri, West Bengal, India.[84]

The geographic distribution of both HeV and NiV is currently undefined although Australia and South East Asia are considered to be endemic areas on the basis of the known incidents reported in the literature. Fruit bats of the genus *Pteropus* are considered to be the reservoir hosts of HeV and NiV[85] and are found in north, east and southeast areas of Australia, Indonesia, Malaysia, Philippines, the Indian subcontinent and some of the Pacific Islands.[86] Pigs were the apparent source of infection among most human cases in the Malaysian outbreak of NiV, but other sources, such as infected dogs and cats, cannot be excluded.[87,88] Unpublished laboratory data from Bangladesh have not supported the presence of an intermediate or primary reservoir host other than *P. giganteus*. Available data suggest that direct transmission of NiV to humans is through contact with bat secretions (saliva, urine, guano, partially eaten fruit) during fruit-tree climbing.[89]

Virology

Nipah and Hendra are closely related and difficult to distinguish serologically, although they have a diverse geographic distribution.[79,90] Both NiV and HeV share a nonsegmented, negative-stranded RNA genome and similar genome organization, replication strategy and domain structure in the polymerase proteins to members of the Filoviridae, Paramyxoviridae, Rhabdoviridae and Bornaviridae. While being related to these families they are closely related to the Paramyxoviridae and more specifically the morbilliviruses. The genome organization of NiV and HeV is the same as for the rest of the Paramyxoviridae. There are a total of six transcription units encoding six structural proteins. These are the nucleocapsid protein (N), phosphoprotein (P), matrix protein (M), fusion protein (F), glycoprotein (G) or attachment protein, and large protein (L) or RNA polymerase. They are found on the genome in the order 39-N-P-M-F-G-L-59. Evidence suggests that NiV and HeV form a distinct group of viruses within the subfamily Paramyxovirinae.[90]

Clinical features

The emergence of NiV and HeV has raised clinical concerns in the management of individuals returning from Australia and South East Asia presenting with pyrexia and other nonspecific signs and symptoms. The incubation period for NiV and HeV is generally from 4 to 18 days. Onset of disease is usually influenza-like with high fever and myalgia. Sore throat, dizziness, and drowsiness and disorientation have been described. The case fatality rate for clinical cases is about 50% and subclinical infections may be common.[91]

Experimental studies have confirmed the possibility of transmission through close contact with infected body fluids and that aerosol transmission does not seem to be significant. Human-to-human transmission has been reported in a study within the Bangladesh community[92] and the risk of transmission from horse to human has not been established. The mode of transmission from animal to animal, and from animal to human is uncertain.

Laboratory diagnosis

Virus isolation has been an important primary diagnostic tool in early outbreaks.

Both NiV and HeV grow well in Vero cells. A cytopathic effect (CPE) usually develops within 3 days but two 5-day passages are recommended before virus isolation is considered to be unsuccessful. However, isolation should only be attempted in a containment level 4 laboratory.

Virus neutralization tests are considered to be the reference standard in the serologic identification of NiV and HeV infection. This procedure needs to be carried out at a containment level 4 laboratory. Sera are added into the media covering virus-inoculated Vero monolayers in a 96-well plate format. Positive results are demonstrated by the inhibition of CPE production by sera.[93]

To reduce the dependence on high containment facilities (CL4), both the indirect IgG and capture IgM ELISA NiV and HeV systems can use irradiated viral antigens purified from cell culture. The level of sample processing involved to make the antigen safe to use outside Advisory Committee on Dangerous Pathogens (ACDP) 4 containment reduces the specificity and sensitivity of the assay.

NiV-specific primers that amplify a 228 bp segment of the N gene region of the virus will form the basis of the RT-PCR detection system that has proven of diagnostic value when used in conjunction with specimens (sera, tissue from humans and animals) implicated in HeV and NiV outbreaks.[94] In addition, another published primer pair that amplifies a 200 bp region of the matrix (M) protein will form a proven alternative primer set for the RT-PCR detection of HeV originally designed by Halpin *et al.*[85]

Management

As there are neither vaccine nor antivirals for treatment and because the viruses are potentially able to transmit by the aerosol route,[95] both HeV and NiV have been classified as hazard group 4 agents. Working with these agents requires the use of ACDP containment level 4 laboratories. Therefore, with the increasing movement of horses and travelers to endemic areas, both clinicians and veterinarians have increasingly expressed a need to consider these infections as part of the current differential diagnosis. Care in the management of patients should be exercised as NiV has been isolated in the respiratory secretions and urine of patients identified as having Nipah virus encephalitis in Malaysia[94] and nosocomial risks identified in a Bangladesh hospital.[95]

REFERENCES

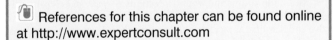 References for this chapter can be found online at http://www.expertconsult.com

Staphylococci and micrococci

GENERAL CLASSIFICATION

Classification

Historically, based on morphologic similarities, the genera *Staphylococcus, Micrococcus, Planococcus* and *Stomatococcus* were placed together in the family Micrococcaceae. More recently, however, based on DNA/rRNA analysis and guanine–cytosine (GC) content, the genus *Staphylococcus* has been classified together with the genera *Bacillus, Brochothrix, Gemella, Listeria* and *Planococcus*, in the family Bacillaceae of the broad *Bacillus–Lactobacillus–Streptococcus* cluster of Gram-positive bacteria with a low GC-content.

The genus *Micrococcus* currently contains three species, *M. luteus, M. lylae* and *M. antarcticus*,[1,2] and resides in the family Micrococcaceae of the order of the Actinomycetales;[3] a fourth species, *M. flavus*, has been proposed. *Stomatococcus mucilaginosus*, the sole species in the former genus *Stomatococcus*, was recently reclassified as a member of the genus *Rothia* (family of the Micrococcaceae) and renamed *Rothia mucilaginosa*;[4] *R. dentocariosa* is the only other *Rothia* spp. isolated from humans.

Staphylococci, in particular *Staphylococcus aureus*, are frequent causes of infection in humans. Next to *S. aureus*, the foremost pathogenic staphylococcal species are *S. lugdunensis, S. schleiferi, S. epidermidis, S. haemolyticus* and *S. saprophyticus. S. lugdunensis* and *S. schleiferi* may cause infections similar to those caused by *S. aureus*, including abscesses, endocarditis and wound infections. *S. epidermidis* is primarily responsible for foreign body infections, and both prosthetic and native valve endocarditis. *S. saprophyticus* is a cause of urinary tract infections. Multiple animal species can be colonized or infected by different staphylococcal species. *S. hyicus* is the main causative agent of infectious dermatitis and arthritis in swine, *S. aureus* causes bovine mastitis, and has also been reported in pigs, pigeons, cats and dogs. *S. intermedius* causes infections in dogs, foxes, mink, pigeons and horses.

This chapter will focus mainly on the staphylococci. *R. mucilaginosa* and *Micrococcus* spp. colonize humans but rarely cause disease; these bacteria will be briefly discussed. *R. dentocariosa* is discussed in Chapter 167.

Staphylococci

NATURE

History

The name 'staphylococcus' (derived from the Greek σταφυλη, a bunch of grapes) was introduced by Alexander Ogston, a Scottish surgeon who in 1881 described the presence of grape-like clusters of spherical micro-organisms in pus from abscesses.[5] In a series of laboratory experiments and clinical observations he subsequently described staphylococcal disease and its role in sepsis and abscess formation. The first to isolate and culture staphylococci was the German surgeon Friedrich Rosenbach. Rosenbach distinguished two different species of staphylococci based on colony color: a species with yellow/orange/golden colonies which he named *Staphylococcus aureus*, and a species with white colonies which he called *Staphylococcus albus* that was later renamed *Staphylococcus epidermidis*.

Staphylococcal infections appeared to play a major role in wound infections. As the cause of postinfluenza necrotizing pneumonias, *S. aureus* was considered responsible for many deaths during the Spanish influenza pandemic of 1917–1918. It is estimated that half of the casualties in the trenches of the First World War were due to septic wound infections with *S. aureus*. Such was the impact of *S. aureus* infections on military campaigns that during the Second World War the production process for penicillin (then still universally active against the bacterium) was considered a military secret by the allied forces. Even now, in the antibiotic era, *S. aureus* continues to be a major community-acquired pathogen and the single most relevant cause of nosocomial infections.

Other staphylococci, mainly *S. epidermidis*, are important pathogens in immunocompromised patients and patients with prosthetic materials and indwelling catheters.

Microbiology

Staphylococci are Gram-positive spherical bacteria about 1 micrometer in diameter, which divide in two planes and, therefore, grow in clusters; they are nonmotile, nonspore-forming, and have a genome size of between 2000 and 3000 kbp, with a 30–39% GC-content. In 2007, 39 species were recognized within the genus *Staphylococcus*, 17 of which were isolated from humans; new species continue to be discovered (http://www.bacterio.cict.fr) (Fig. 165.1). Most staphylococcal species demonstrate catalase activity and are facultatively anaerobes. Further characteristics of the genus include susceptibility to furazolidone, resistance to bacitracin, and production of acid from glucose under anaerobic conditions or in the presence of erythromycin.

The main constituents of the staphylococcal cell wall are peptidoglycan, which constitutes 50% of the dry cell mass (Fig. 165.2), and teichoic acid (40% of the dry cell mass). The glycan chains of the peptidoglycan layer are built with approximately 10 alternating subunits of *N*-acetylmuramic acid and *N*-acetylglycosamine. Pentapeptide side chains are attached to the *N*-acetylmuramic acid subunits; the glycan chains are then cross linked with peptide bridges between the side chains. The teichoic acids are macromolecules of phosphate containing polysaccharides (Fig. 165.3). Teichoic acid is bound both to the peptidoglycan layer and to the cytoplasmic membrane. The polysaccharides are species specific; ribitol teichoic acids are present in *S. aureus* cell walls and glycerol teichoic acids are present in *S. epidermidis*.

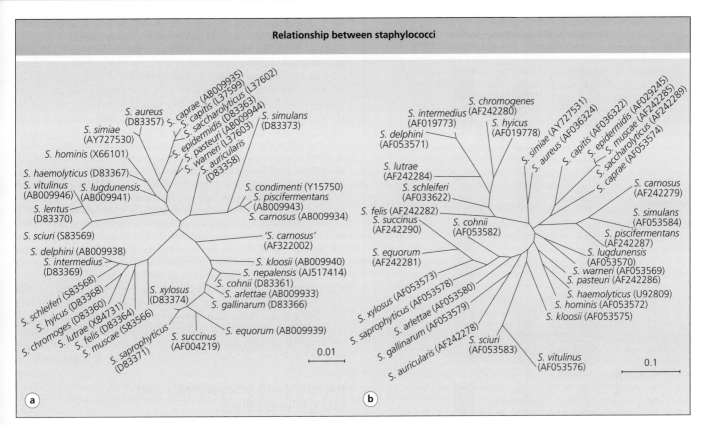

Relationship between staphylococci

Fig. 165.1 Unrooted phylogenetic trees constructed on the basis of 16S rRNA gene sequences, showing the relationship between staphylococci. The GenBank accession numbers of the sequences of the organisms used are shown in parentheses. Redrawn from Pantcek R, Sedlácek I, Petrás P, et al. *Staphylococcus simiae* sp. nov., isolated from South American squirrel monkeys. Int J Syst Evol Microbiol 2005;55:1953–8.

PATHOGENICITY OF *STAPHYLOCOCCUS AUREUS*

The broad spectrum of diseases caused by *S. aureus* is associated with its production of many surface-bound and extracellular virulence factors. The bacterium has a large variety of molecules that specifically counteract the host defense mechanisms, and it excretes a number of toxins with membrane damaging, pyrogenic or epidermolytic actions (Table 165.1).

Adherence to host cells and tissues

Staphylococcus aureus expresses a number of adhesion molecules that facilitate interactions with host cells and extracellular matrix (ECM) components allowing effective colonization. These 'microbial surface components recognizing adhesive matrix molecules' (MSCRAMMs) are surface-anchored molecules that bind host molecules like collagen, laminin, fibronectin, elastin, vitronectin and fibrinogen.[6] The collagen-binding adhesin, for instance, recognizes collagen type I and IV and was shown to play an important role in the pathogenesis of septic arthritis induced by *S. aureus*. MSCRAMMS are also involved in the attachment of *S. aureus* and *S. epidermidis* to foreign body materials and indwelling devices: coating of the biomaterials with a mixture of host proteins and platelets subsequently leads to biofilm formation[7] (Fig. 165.4).

Blocking host defenses

The immune response against *S. aureus* largely depends on the innate immune system: antimicrobial peptides, the complement system and

phagocytes. The bacterium, in response, produces highly specific, small, soluble proteins that enable it to suppress the innate immunity and survive in the human body.

Resistance to antimicrobial peptides

In response to infectious stimuli, skin keratinocytes, mucosal epithelial cells and neutrophils produce high levels of antimicrobial peptides (AMPs) known as cathelicidins (LL-37) and defensins. The *S. aureus* metalloproteinase aureolysin cleaves LL-37, while staphylokinase (SAK) inhibits the bactericidal effect of α-defensins.[8] Furthermore, modification of cell wall teichoic acids promotes *S. aureus* resistance to AMPs.[9]

Complement evasion

The complement cascade serves three major functions in innate immunity:

- to opsonize bacteria (through C3b) (Fig. 165.5);
- to attract phagocytes (through C3a and C5a); and
- to perturb bacterial membranes of Gram-negative bacteria (C5b–9, the membrane attack complex).[10,11]

Complement activation is initiated by three different pathways (classical, lectin or alternative) that result in the formation of C3 convertases, bimolecular enzymes that cleave the central complement protein C3 (Fig. 165. 6). The C3 cleavage product C3b covalently binds to the bacterial surface and is recognized by phagocytic cells expressing complement receptors. Furthermore, C3b associates with C3 convertases to form a C5 convertase that cleaves C5 into C5a (a potent chemoattractant) and C5b (part of the membrane attack complex). *S. aureus* produces a variety of molecules that interfere with the complement cascade:

- the secreted staphylococcal complement inhibitor (SCIN) blocks C3 convertases through stabilization of these complexes;[12]

Structure of the peptidoglycan layer

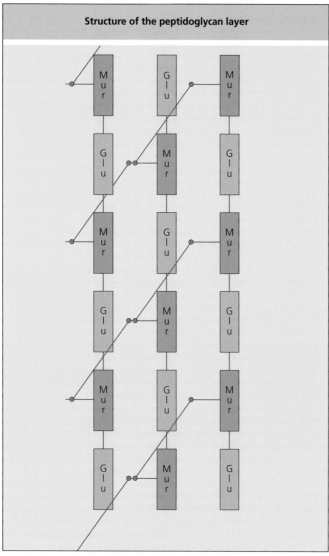

Fig. 165.2 Structure of the peptidoglycan layer. The peptidoglycan layer consists of three integral parts. The glycan chains are built with 10–12 alternating N-acetylglucosamine (Glu) and N-acetylmuramic acid (Mur) subunits jointed with β-1,4 glycosidic bonds. Vertical pentapeptide side chains are linked to the muramic acids subunits, and the side chains are in turn cross linked with diagonal intrapeptide bridges. For example, the glycan chains in *Staphylococcus aureus* are crosslinked with pentaglycine bridges attached to L-glycine in one pentapeptide chain and D-alanine in an adjacent chain. Courtesy of Jan Verhoef, Ad C Fluit and Franz-Josef Schmitz.

- extracellular fibrinogen binding protein (Efb) and extracellular complement binding protein (Ecb) target surface-bound C3b-containing convertases,[13] inhibiting C3b deposition via the alternative pathway and C5a formation via all pathways;
- the staphylococcal cell wall-associated protein Sbi has two extracellular complement-inhibitory domains that bind C3; and
- staphylococcal superantigen-like (SSL) protein 7 specifically binds to C5, preventing cleavage by C5 convertases and subsequent formation of C5a.[14]

Inhibition of neutrophil recruitment

Effective eradication of *S. aureus* depends on phagocytosis and intracellular killing by cells of the monocyte and granulocyte lineage, mainly neutrophils.[15] This critical role is reflected by the increased risk for *S. aureus* infections in patients with defects in granulocyte function, both inherited (e.g. chronic granulomatous disease, myeloperoxidase deficiency, leukocyte adhesion deficiencies) and acquired (e.g. diabetes mellitus, rheumatoid arthritis, HIV). During an infection, neutrophils are rapidly recruited from the circulation to sites of microbial invasion by host stimuli (complement fragments C3a and C5a, interleukin 8, leukotriene B4) and pathogen-derived stimuli (fMLP, phenol-soluble modulins).[16] These chemotactic factors activate neutrophils, increase vascular permeability and induce expression of adhesion molecules on endothelial cells. Neutrophils express selectins and integrins that bind these adhesion molecules; the cells start to roll on the endothelial lining and firmly adhere to it.[17] Subsequently, the neutrophils migrate through the endothelial cell layer (diapedesis) and move towards the site of infection under a gradient of chemoattractant substances, the foremost being C5a (chemotaxis).

The staphylococcal superantigen-like 5 (SSL5) inhibits the interaction between P-selectin on endothelial cells and P-selectin glycoprotein ligand-1 (PSGL-1) on neutrophils, thereby inhibiting neutrophil rolling on the endothelium.[18] Extracellular adherence protein (Eap) of *S. aureus* inhibits the next steps in neutrophil extravasation by its interactions with the intercellular adhesion molecule 1 (ICAM-1), fibrinogen or vitronectin.[19] Finally, *S. aureus* secretes two molecules that specifically block chemotactic movement of phagocytes: the chemotaxis inhibitory protein of *S. aureus* (CHIPS) which binds the formylated peptide receptor and the C5a receptor,[20] and the FPRL1 inhibitory protein (FLIPr) which binds the formylated peptide receptor-like 1.[21]

Resistance to phagocytosis and intracellular killing

Neutrophil ingestion of opsonized micro-organisms in phagosomes depends on the interaction between opsonic ligands on the bacterium and receptors on the phagocyte membrane. Upon bacterial uptake, the interaction of opsonic ligands with receptors triggers the release of oxidative products and granule contents (e.g. myeloperoxide, defensins) into the phagosome, destroying the ingested particle. *S. aureus* is most efficiently phagocytosed after opsonization by both complement and antibodies.

Staphylococci are often surrounded by a loose-fitting polysaccharide capsule (Fig. 165.7) that interferes with opsonization, either by shielding the cell wall from reacting with antibodies and complement, or by hindering the binding of surface-bound complement factors to phagocyte receptors. Effective opsonization of encapsulated *S. aureus* therefore requires anticapsular antibodies, largely directed against the O-acetyl group of the capsular polysaccharide. Eleven putative capsular serotypes have been proposed; expression of type 5 and type 8 capsules (75% of all capsulated strains) is associated with increased virulence in animal infection models.[22]

Staphylokinase (SAK), a plasminogen-activating molecule, generates surface-bound plasmin. This, in turn, cleaves the major opsonins IgG and C3b, preventing their recognition by phagocytes. The *S. aureus* surface protein A (SpA) binds the Fc terminal of human IgG, covering the bacterial surface with outward-facing IgG molecules that cannot be recognized by Fc receptors on phagocytes (Fig. 165.8). SSL7 interacts with human IgA1 and IgA2 to interfere with IgA-dependent cellular effector functions.[23]

Once phagocytosed, staphylococci may inhibit killing and travel through the bloodstream within neutrophils. The golden pigment (for which *S. aureus* is named) is a carotenoid molecule with antioxidant properties that scavenges free oxygen radicals.[24] Furthermore, *S. aureus* can resist oxidative stress by two superoxide dismutase enzymes that remove superoxide.

Cytolytic toxins

Cytotoxins secreted by *S. aureus* lyse host cells by forming β-barrel pores in cytoplasmic membranes of target cells. Well-known examples are α-toxin and the bi-component leukotoxins γ-toxin and the exfoliative toxins (ETA and ETB) that cause separation of the

Structure of teichoic acid

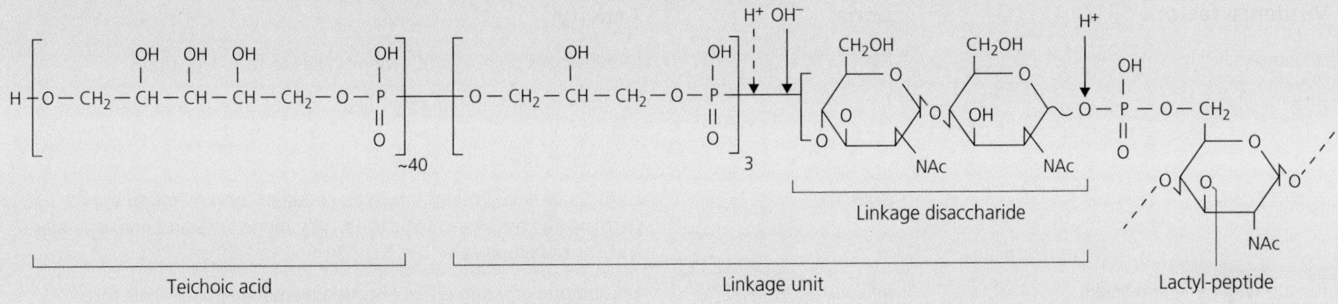

Fig. 165.3 Structure of teichoic acid and linkage unit attaching teichoic acid to peptidoglycan in *Staphylococcus aureus*. The C2 and C4 positions of the ribitol residues are substituted by D-alanyl and *N*-acetylglucosamine residues. Adapted with permission from Crossley KB, Archer GL, eds. The staphylococci in human disease. New York: Churchill Livingstone; 1997.

Table 165.1 Virulence factors of *Staphylococcus aureus*

Immune evasion mechanisms

Virulence factor	Acronym or gene	Activity
Clumping factor (bound coagulase)	ClfA, ClfB	Binds fibrinogen, coating the bacterial cell and inhibiting phagocytosis
Chemotaxis inhibitory protein of *S. aureus*	CHIPS	Downregulates the C5a receptor and the formylated peptide receptor (FPR) on neutrophils; inhibits chemotaxis
Extracellular adherence protein	EAP	Binds to ICAM-1, fibrinogen, vitronectin Blocks leukocyte adhesion, diapedesis and extravasation
Extracellular fibrinogen-binding protein/ extracellular complement binding protein	Efb/Ecb	Binds to the C3d part of C3 molecules, inhibiting C3b-containing convertases Efb also binds fibrinogen
Staphylococcal complement inhibitor	SCINSCIN-C	Binds and stabilizes C3 convertases, inhibiting C3b deposition and phagocytosis
Staphylokinase	SAK	Activates human plasminogen at the bacterial surface, leading to degradation of IgG and C3b; inhibits bactericidal effect of α-defensins
Polysaccharide capsule		Antiphagocytic function
FLPR1 inhibitory protein	FLIPr	Impairs neutrophil responses to formylated peptide receptor-like-1 agonists
Polysaccharide intercellular adhesin	PIA	Holds multilayered cell complexes that form biofilms together, decreases susceptibility to defensins
Catalase		Inhibits bacterial killing by inactivating hydrogen peroxidase and free radicals formed by the myeloperoxidase system within phagocytic cells
Protein A	SpA	Binds Fc part of human IgG and prevents phagocytic uptake by Fc receptors; stimulates B lymphocytes
Free coagulase	*coa*	Coats the bacterial cell with fibrinogen and inhibits phagocytosis
Staphylococcal superantigen-like 5	SSL5	Binds PSGL-1 and inhibits P-selectin-mediated neutrophil rolling
Staphylococcal superantigen-like 7	SSL7	Binds IgA and blocks FcαRI-mediated responses. Binds C5 and blocks C5 cleavage into C5a and C5b
Aureolysin		Metalloproteinase that cleaves LL-37
Staphylococcal immunoglobulin-binding protein	SBI	Binds IgG and C3. Blocks complement activity

(Continued)

Table 165.1 Virulence factors of *Staphylococcus aureus*—cont'd

Invasion mechanisms

Virulence factor	Gene	Activity
α-Hemolysin	*hla*	Multimerizes on eukaryotic membranes to form lytic pores
β-Hemolysin	*hlb*	Sphingomyelinase; damages eukaryotic cell membranes containing sphingomyelin by enzymatic alteration of their lipid content; causes lysis of sheep erythrocytes on blood agar
γ-Hemolysin	*hlgA, hlgB*	Consists of two proteins which assemble to form membrane-perforating complexes; toxic to PMNLs, monocytes and macrophages, lytic for red blood cells
Panton–Valentine leukocidin	*lukS (lukS-PV, lukF-PV)*	Homologue of γ-hemolysin encoded by mobile phage, lytic to leukocytes; associated with furunculosis and necrotizing pneumonia
Leukocidin E-D	*LukED*	Lytic to leukocytes
δ-Hemolysin	*hld*	Variety of attributed actions: multimerizes on eukaryotic membranes to form lytic pores; possible mediator of staphylococcal membranous enterocolitis; increases vascular permeability in guinea pig skin, inhibits water absorption and activates adenylate cyclase; activation of membrane phospholipase A_2 stimulation of prostaglandin synthesis, release of lysozyme and β-glucuronidase from PMNL granules, activation of the acetyltransferase
Exfoliative toxins	*eta, etb*	Toxins with protease activity, sequence similarity to serine protease of *S. aureus*; epidermolytic effect on stratum granulosum of the keratinized epidermis; causes staphylococcal scalded skin syndrome
Fibrinolysins		Break down fibrin clots
Hyaluronidase	*hysA*	Hydrolyzes intercellular matrix of mucopolysaccharides
DNAse/thermonuclease	*nuc*	Hydrolyzes RNA and DNA, frees nutrients
Lipase	*geh*	Facilitates spread in subcutaneous tissues; associated with furunculosis
Superantigens/pyrogenic exotoxins		Stimulate T cells nonspecifically to cytokine release
Enterotoxins A, B, C, D, E, G, H, K (and others)	*sea, seb, sec, sed, see, seg, seh, sek*	Cause staphylococcal food poisoning and half of the cases of nonmenstrual toxic shock syndrome (TSS)
Toxic shock syndrome toxin	TSST-1/*tst*	Responsible for about 75% of cases of TSS, including all cases of menstrual TSS

Microbial surface components recognizing adhesive matrix molecules

MSCRAMM	Gene	Activity
Fibronectin-binding protein	*fnbpA, fnbpB*	Binds fibronectin, fibrinogen and elastin
Collagen-binding protein	*cna*	Binds collagen/cartilage
Clumping factor	*clfA, clfB*	Binds fibrinogen

ICAM-1, intercellular adhesion molecule 1; PMNLs, polymorphonuclear leukocytes; PSGL-1, P-selectin glycoprotein ligand-1.

dermis at the granular cell layer resulting in extensive scalding (staphylococcal scalded skin syndrome).

Panton–Valentine leukocidin (PVL) is a cytotoxin associated with furunculosis and hemorrhagic pneumonia.[15] In the last decade community-acquired infections, mainly skin and soft tissue infections, have been increasingly caused by PVL-positive community-acquired methicillin-resistant *S. aureus* (MRSA) strains (CA-MRSA). Although PVL is found in 69–98% of CA-MRSA clinical isolates,[25] the exact role of PVL in the pathogenesis of these infections is not completely clear and studies of its pathogenicity in animal models have yielded conflicting results.

Phenol-soluble modulins are a class of secreted staphylococcal peptides that recruit, activate and subsequently lyse human neutrophils, thus eliminating the main cellular defense against *S. aureus* infection.

A recent study revealed a contribution of these factors to the virulence of CA-MRSA.[16]

Immunostimulatory molecules

Superantigens (or pyrogenic exotoxins) are the agents responsible for toxic shock syndrome (TSS) (Fig. 165.9). These extracellular proteins bind to the exterior surface of major histocompatibility complex (MHC) class II molecules on antigen-presenting cells (APCs), and link them to receptors on the surface of T-helper cells, activating them without the need for antigen presentation by the APCs. Up to a third of the T cells may be stimulated to proliferate and release cytokines. Due to this nonspecific activation of T cells, the immune response

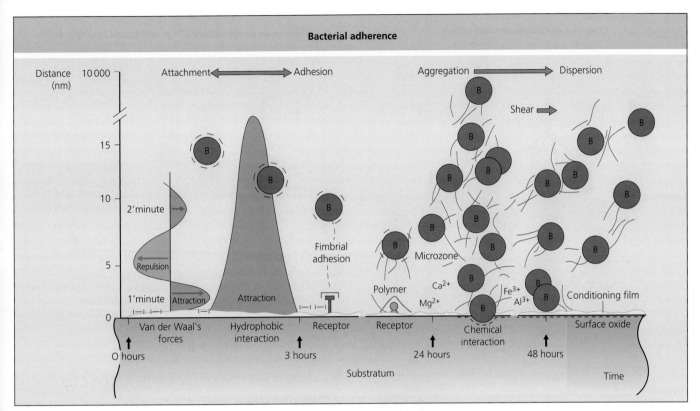

Fig. 165.4 Bacterial adherence. The figure illustrates the events associated with bacterial (B) adherence to a biomaterial in relation to time and the molecular sequence in bacterial attachment, adhesion, aggregation and dispersion at substratum surface. A number of possible interactions may occur depending on the specificities of the bacteria or substratum system, the distance from the biomaterial and the stage of adherence. The attachment stage is mediated by nonspecific forces. Adhesion is driven by specific adhesin–receptor interactions. The final aggregative step results in a bacterial macrocolony on the biomaterial surface in which the bacteria are firmly adherent to the biomaterial and each other. Bacterial exopolysaccharide blankets the macrocolony and may serve to improve the nutritional microenvironment and protect the bacteria from host defenses. In the dispersion phase, bacteria disaggregate, break loose from the macrocolony and drift free into the bloodstream. Adapted with permission from Gristina AG. Biomaterial centered infection: microbial adhesion versus tissue integration. Science 1987;237:1588.© 1987 American Association for the Advancement of Science.

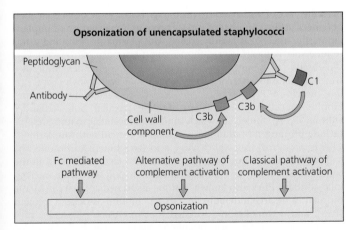

Fig. 165.5 Opsonization of unencapsulated staphylococci. Opsonization through complement activation is primarily a function of C3b and iC3b. When antibody (ab) molecules bind to antigen, the antigen–antibody complex activates the first complement component, C1. C1 is then converted into an esterase, initiating the classical pathway. Additionally, some cell-wall components can activate the alternative pathway. Courtesy of Jan Verhoef, Ad C Fluit and Franz-Josef Schmitz.

against superantigenic toxins is impaired and patients suffering TSS often lack specific antibodies against superantigens.[15]

Toxic shock syndrome toxin 1 (TSST-1) causes most cases of TSS, including all cases of tampon-associated TSS; approximately one-fourth of the cases are caused by enterotoxins. Apart from their superantigenic activity, when ingested orally the enterotoxins may also cause gastrointestinal disease (*S. aureus* food poisoning), characterized by emesis with or without diarrhea. The target responsible for initiating the emetic reflex is located in the abdominal viscera, where putative (unidentified) cellular receptors for the enterotoxins exist. Staphylococcal protein A (SpA) binds to the surface of B lymphocytes, where it also exerts a potent immunostimulatory activity.[26]

Interactions with the coagulation system

S. aureus produces extracellular coagulase which binds to prothrombin to form a complex called staphylothrombin, thereby activating the protease activity of thrombin. The activated thrombin converts fibrinogen to fibrin, causing localized clotting and shielding the bacteria from host defenses.[27] In addition, most strains express a fibrin/fibrinogen binding protein (clumping factor) which promotes attachment to blood clots and traumatized tissue.

Genetic location and regulation of virulence factors

S. aureus virulence factors can be chromosomally encoded and uniformly present, or located on mobile genetic elements such as insertion sequences, bacteriophages, plasmids, transposons and pathogenicity islands. The genes for exfoliative toxins A and B are located on a bacteriophage and a plasmid respectively, and have been demonstrated in 0–2% of strains. PVL is located on a bacteriophage and was present in only 2% of isolates. The pathogenicity island harboring TSST-1 is found in 14–24%. The immune modulators CHIPS, SCIN,

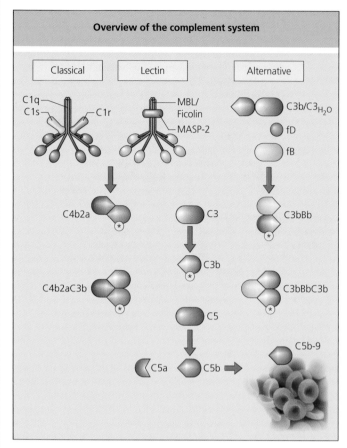

Fig. 165.6 Schematic overview of the complement system. Complement activation can occur via three different pathways. The antibody-dependent classical pathway starts when C1q in the C1q–C1r$_2$–C1s$_2$ complex recognizes antibodies that are bound to the microbial surface. In the lectin pathway, mannose binding lectin (MBL) and ficolins recognize microbial sugar patterns and activate the MBL-associated serine protease 2 (MASP-2). Both C1s and MASP-2 can cleave complement proteins C4 and C2 to generate the CP/LP C3 convertase, C4b2a. Within this complex, C4b is covalently (*) attached to the microbial surface. The alternative pathway C3 convertase (C3bBb) is generated after binding of factor B (fB) to surface-bound C3b or fluid-phase C3(H$_2$O). Factor B is subsequently cleaved by factor D (fD) to generate C3bBb. Both C3 convertases C4b2a and C3bBb cleave C3 into covalently bound C3b (*) and an anaphylatoxin C3a. C3b contributes to phagocytosis, antigen presentation and formation of C5 convertases, C4b2a3b and C3bBb3b. C5 convertases cleave C5 into an anaphylatoxin C5a and C5b, which forms a complex with complement proteins C6, C7, C8 and C9 to generate the membrane attack complex (MAC) and mediate microbial lysis.

SAK and SEA are clustered together on a β-hemolysin converting bacteriophage present in 90% of clinical *S. aureus* isolates.[20]

The expression of virulence factors in *S. aureus* is controlled by a complex system of regulatory mechanisms. A well-studied response regulator is the accessory gene regulator (*agr*), a two-component quorum sensing system which, through a positive feedback loop, switches from the preferential expression of surface adhesins during the exponential phase of growth to the expression of exoproteins during the postexponential and stationary growth phases.[28] When bacterial density increases above a certain level, *agr* drives the transcription of RNAIII, an RNA molecule that modulates virulence factor expression both at the transcriptional and translational levels. *Agr* downregulated gene products include protein A (*spa*) and fibronectin-binding protein (*fnb*); the hemolysins, enterotoxins, exfoliatins and phenol-soluble modulins are examples of virulence factors which are upregulated by *agr*. Most other currently known regulatory mechanisms interact at some level with *agr*, either synergistically or reciprocally.[29]

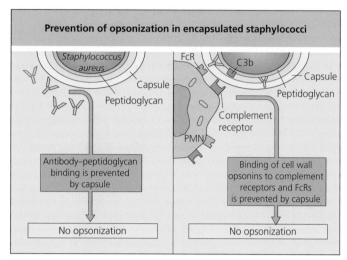

Fig. 165.7 Prevention of opsonization in encapsulated staphylococci. (Left) The capsule of *Staphylococcus aureus* prevents binding of antibodies to peptidoglycan: no opsonization. (Right) The capsule prevents binding of opsonins on the cell wall of *Staphylococcus aureus* to complement and Fc receptors on PMNLs. Courtesy of Jan Verhoef, Ad C Fluit and Franz-Josef Schmitz.

PATHOGENICITY OF *STAPHYLOCOCCUS EPIDERMIDIS*

Most of the pathogenicity studies in coagulase-negative staphylococci (CoNS) have focused on virulence factors involved in foreign-body infections by the most common and relevant species, *Staphylococcus epidermidis*. These infections are characterized by the formation of biofilms: first the bacteria adhere to the foreign body or indwelling device, followed by an accumulation phase in which the bacteria form multilayered cell clusters embedded in extracellular material.

Hydrophobic interactions and Van der Waal's forces play a role in initial adherence of the bacteria to the foreign body (more often than not a polymer), as do a number of surface proteins. On insertion or implantation, the material is rapidly coated with plasma proteins and extracellular matrix proteins (e.g. fibronectin, fibrinogen, vitronectin, von Willebrand factor), providing additional attachment sites. Molecules which mediate attachment to polymers include the staphylococcal surface proteins SSP-1 and SSP-2, the surface-associated autolysin AtlE, biofilm-associated protein (Bap) and the capsular polysaccharide/adhesin (PS/A). Molecules which bind to extracellular matrix proteins include fibrinogen-binding protein (Fbe, a protein with similarity to ClfA in *S. aureus*), cell-wall techoic acid (attachment to fibronectin) and AtlE (binds to vitronectin). A number of factors involved in the accumulation phase have been identified: the polysaccharide intercellular adhesin (PIA), also known as slime-associated antigen (SAA); the capsular polysaccharide/adhesin (PS/A); biofilm-associated protein (Bap); and accumulation-associated protein (AAP).[30] Elastases, proteases, lipases and fatty-acid modifying enzymes have been identified in *S. epidermidis* and are considered possible virulence factors.[30]

EPIDEMIOLOGY AND CLINICAL PRESENTATION OF *STAPHYLOCOCCUS AUREUS*

Epidemiology

In healthy humans, carriage (or colonization) of *S. aureus* may occur on multiple sites of the skin and mucosal surfaces (including the intestine and vagina), the main reservoir being the anterior nares (vestibulum

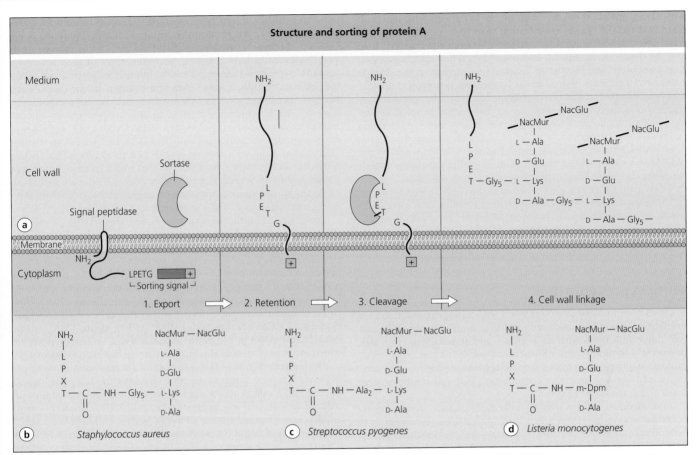

Fig. 165.8 Structure and sorting of protein A. Structure of the cell wall anchor of surface proteins in *Staphylococcus aureus* and other Gram-positive bacteria. (a) Cell wall sorting of surface proteins consists of four distinct steps, which lead to the proteolytic cleavage of the polypeptide chain between threonine (T) and glycine (G). The carboxyl of threonine is subsequently amide-linked to the free amino group in the pentaglycine cross-bridge of the staphylococcal cell wall. The cell wall linkage of surface proteins in *S. aureus* (b) is compared with that proposed for other Gram-positive bacteria such as *Streptococcus pyogenes* (c) and *Listeria monocytogenes* (d). NacGlu, *N*-acetylglucosamine; NacMur, *N*-acetylmuramic acid. Adapted with permission from Crossley KB, Archer GL, eds. The staphylococci in human disease. New York: Churchill Livingstone; 1997.

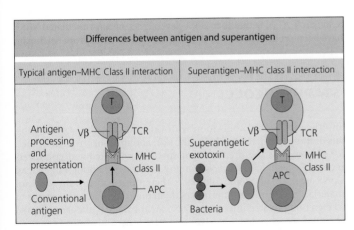

Fig. 165.9 Differences between antigen and superantigen. Staphylococcal enterotoxin and TSST-1 act as superantigens, binding directly to MHC class II and the Vb chains of the T-cell receptor (TCR) without the need for normal antigen processing. Courtesy of Jan Verhoef, Ad C Fluit and Franz-Josef Schmitz.

nasi/nostrils). Generally, the established flora of the nose prevents the acquisition of new strains. Person-to-person spread is believed to occur mainly by direct hand/skin contact, in a hospital setting primarily mediated by health-care workers. Furthermore, up to 10% of healthy *S. aureus* carriers disperse the bacterium into the air. Under

normal circumstances, when airborne dispersers are at rest, they are surrounded by 0.01–0.1 colony-forming units/m³ but up to 0.3 cfu/m³ in selected cases. However, the bacterial density may increase 40-fold with movement (due to release of bacteria from the clothing) and with respiratory tract infections. A number of outbreaks have been attributed to single airborne spreaders.[31] Although acquisition occurs primarily on the skin, *S. aureus* can only persist in the long term if the nares or perineum become colonized.

Cross-sectional prevalence rates of colonization among healthy subjects differ extensively; from as low as 14% in African American job applicants, to as high as 64% in UK hospital personnel.[32] Persons can be subdivided into 'persistent carriers', 'intermittent carriers' and 'non-carriers', based on the proportion of positive nasal swabs as well as the quantity of isolates. Based on different definitions and different populations of healthy individuals, 2–71% are considered non-carriers, 19–70% are considered intermittent carriers and 9–37% are considered persistent carriers.[32] Groups with documented increased risks of colonization include patients with type 1 diabetes, patients undergoing hemodialysis, surgical patients, intravenous drug users and HIV patients. Heavy antibiotic pressure may lower (detectable) colonization rates.

Nasal carriage of *S. aureus* is a risk factor for subsequent infection. Colonized surgical patients had an absolute risk of wound infection of roughly 5–15%, which was two to eight times the risk of control patients without *S. aureus* carriage preoperatively. A relation between colonization and (bacteremic) infection has also been demonstrated for continuous ambulatory peritoneal dialysis (CAPD) patients, hemodialysis patients, HIV patients and hospitalized patients colonized with MRSA. Infection risk was even higher in patients who had both nasal and rectal *S. aureus* colonization than in those who only had nasal colonization, suggesting a relation between the bacterial load and the chance of subsequent infection.[33] When linking *S. aureus* isolates from blood and previously obtained specimens from the anterior nares of 219 patients with *S. aureus* bacteremia, genotypical identity was demonstrated in 180 of 219 patients (82.2%).[34] In another study patients colonized with *S. aureus* in the nares upon hospital admission and subsequently developing nosocomial *S. aureus* bacteremia (with identical strains) had a lower mortality than those developing *S. aureus* bacteremia while not already being colonized when admitted.[35] It was suggested that colonization may offer protection against an overexaggerated inflammatory response during infection.

S. aureus has been reported to persist in dust and on fomites for up to 7 months. It has been isolated from door handles, desk tops, water bowls, computer keyboards, faucet handles and blood pressure cuffs. Although (methicillin-resistant) *S. aureus* was isolated from inanimate surfaces in several documented outbreaks, the role of environmental contamination or airborne transmission is controversial.

Clinical presentation

S. aureus is an invasive micro-organism with a propensity for abscess formation. Community-acquired infections mostly involve skin and soft tissue infections such as cellulitis and furunculosis, but also pneumonia (typically post-influenza), osteomyelitis and acute endocarditis. Staphylococcal toxins may be responsible for food poisoning, staphylococcal toxic shock syndrome (TSS) and staphylococcal scalded skin syndrome (SSSS).[36]

In nosocomial settings *S. aureus* is the main causative agent of postoperative wound infections, often leading to abscess formation. It is notorious for infecting prosthetic materials, such as prosthetic joints, prosthetic heart valves and internal pacemakers. Furthermore, it is one of the main causes of intravascular catheter-associated bloodstream infections, hospital-acquired pneumonia and ventilator-associated pneumonia. *S. aureus* bacteremia (SAB), although more a symptom than a disease, is often regarded as a specific clinical entity due to its associated mortality risk and high rate of relapses and complications.[37]

S. aureus infrequently causes urinary tract infections, predominantly in patients with recent urinary tract surgery or other manipulations, and in patients with urinary tract obstruction.[38]

EPIDEMIOLOGY OF ANTIBIOTIC RESISTANCE

Although penicillin was initially considered a miracle drug for *S. aureus*, the first cases of penicillin resistance, due to β-lactamase production, were reported as early as 1944. By 1950 approximately 80% of hospital-acquired infections were caused by these penicillinase producers. Shortly after the introduction of the β-lactamase-stable antibiotics (e.g. methicillin) in the early 1960s, the first reports of MRSA appeared. Methicillin resistance resulted from the production of an alternative penicillin-binding protein, PBP2A (or PBP2'), encoded by the *mecA* gene on the staphylococcal cassette chromosome mec (SCCmec), a mobile genetic element.[39]

In most countries colonization with MRSA is now endemic within hospital populations. In the USA, for instance, the proportion of MRSA infections among patients with nosocomial *S. aureus* bacteremia increased from 2.4% in 1975 to 29% in 1991, and in American intensive care units the proportion of MRSA infections had risen to nearly 60% by 2003.[40] A few countries, such as the Netherlands and the Scandinavian countries, have succeeded in containing the nosocomial spread of MRSA by using extensive infection control measures and restrictive antibiotic policies.

An epidemiologic characteristic of MRSA has been the almost complete absence of patient-to-patient transmission outside the hospital. Recently, though, MRSA strains with clear potential for transmission between healthy subjects have emerged. The most prominent example of these so-called community-acquired MRSA (CA-MRSA) is the USA300 genotype (based on pulsed-field gel electrophoresis analysis).[41] Outbreaks have occurred in communities of men who have sex with men, homeless populations, inmates in correctional facilities, military recruits, sports teams and children in day-care centers. Recently, percentages of CA-MRSA infections have been reported as high as 76% by different American health-care institutions. In contrast to hospital-acquired MRSA (HA-MRSA), young age and absence of co-morbidity are associated with CA-MRSA infections.[42] Apparently, USA300 has acquired a number mobile genetic elements that encode resistance and virulence determinants that could enhance fitness and pathogenicity. In several European countries, MRSA also appears to be widely spread among animals, such as pigs and calves, with subsequent transmission of MRSA to caretakers.

Based upon multilocus sequence typing (MLST) the population structure of MRSA is characterized by five major clonal complexes (CCs): CC5, CC8, CC22, CC30 and CC45. Within these five clonal complexes different SCCmec types are found, indicating that MRSA clones emerged by multiple independent introductions of the *mecA* gene.[43] Four of the five major CCs represent pandemic clones of HA-MRSA: CC5 (New York/Japan clone, pediatric clone), CC8 (Vienna clone, Brazilian, Portuguese, Irish-1 and Iberian clone), CC22 (Barnim clone) and CC45 (Berlin clone). USA300 belongs to CC8 and the nontypeable MRSA linked to the animal reservoir in Europe is ST398, which is not phylogenetically linked to any of the major MRSA CCs.

The high prevalence of MRSA in hospitals necessitated extensive use of the glycopeptide vancomycin, which has been the 'last resort' antibiotic for MRSA infections for many years. The first *S. aureus* strain with reduced vancomycin was isolated in Japan in 1997 (the Mu50 strain) and has now emerged among all five major hospital MRSA-lineages.[44] In 2005 0.2% of 240 000 *S. aureus* isolates in the Surveillance Network data from US laboratories were vancomycin-intermediate *S. aureus* (VISA), defined by a minimum inhibitory concentration (MIC) of >2 and ≤8 mg/l.[45] Intermediate resistance to glycopeptides is associated with thickening of the bacterial cell wall, but the exact mechanism remains to be elucidated. Unfortunately, reduced susceptibility to vancomycin appears to be associated with reduced susceptibility to new drugs such as linezolid and daptomycin.[46]

High-level vancomycin-resistant *S. aureus* (VRSA) (MIC ≥32 mg/l) can result from acquisition of the enterococcal *vanA* resistance gene by *S. aureus*.[47] As of September 2007, seven cases of *vanA*-mediated VRSA have been reported, all from the USA and five of them from Michigan.

EPIDEMIOLOGY OF COAGULASE-NEGATIVE STAPHYLOCOCCI

Shortly after birth colonization with CoNS occurs, the normal habitats of these staphylococci being the skin and the mucous membranes. *S. epidermidis* is the predominant species; other frequent colonizers include *S. hominis*, *S. haemolyticus* and *S. warneri*. Although in general CoNS are nonpathogenic colonizers, their propensity to adhere to biomaterials and form biofilms makes them important causative agents of foreign body-related infections. CoNS are the main pathogens isolated in catheter-associated bloodstream infections and drain-associated meningitis. They are amongst the foremost causes of prosthetic joint infections and prosthetic heart valve endocarditis, and they cause 7.8% of all cases of native valve endocarditis in patients without a history of intravenous drug use.[48] Furthermore, *S. saprophyticus* causes urinary tract infections (see Chapter 53) and *S. lugdunensis* and *S. schleiferi* may cause infections very similar to those of *S. aureus*.

The colonizing CoNS flora may be influenced by antibiotic therapy. In hematology and neonatology wards with high antibiotic pressure, a population of more resistant and/or more virulent CoNS strains may be selected and become epidemic among patients and health-care workers: multiple reports describe outbreaks of *S. epidermidis* clones causing intravascular catheter-related bloodstream infections.[49]

PREVENTION

Prevention of MRSA/spread

Several countries have implemented nationwide 'search-and-destroy policies' to limit the spread of MRSA within hospital settings. These strategies were implemented in the late 1980s, when carriage of MRSA among hospitalized patients was still extremely low. The cornerstone of the search-and-destroy policies is that colonized patients are treated in strict isolation; admitted patients with an increased risk of MRSA carriage are screened (see below) and isolated until culture results rule out MRSA carriage. Finally, contact patients and health-care workers are screened for MRSA carriage in case of unexpected detection of MRSA in a hospitalized patient.

More detailed information on infection control is provided in Chapter 6.

Prevention of hospital-acquired infections

Decolonization

Eradication of *S. aureus* carriage preoperatively has been evaluated in several studies. The use of oral rifampin (rifampicin), which appeared effective in a cohort of hemodialysis patients, has been largely abandoned, due to increasing rifampin resistance and associated toxic effects of this agent. Mupirocin is highly effective in short-term nasal eradication of carriers (87–94% of patients are negative after 1 week), but high recurrence rates after 6 months were found in one study. Two randomized placebo-controlled trials with 4030 and 614 surgical patients failed to demonstrate a statistically significant reduction in postoperative surgical site infections when using decolonization with mupirocin. However, in the larger of these trials, there was a significant difference in nosocomial *S. aureus* infections observed among *S. aureus* carriers (4% vs 7.7%).[50,51] In smaller populations, such as CAPD patients, hemodialysis patients and patients with recurrent skin infections, mupirocin treatment was associated with significant reductions in *S. aureus* infections.[52]

DIAGNOSTIC MICROBIOLOGY

Isolation and determination

Most staphylococcal lesions contain numerous polymorphonuclear leukocytes (PMNLs) and large numbers of *S. aureus*, which may readily be demonstrated by a direct Gram smear of pus (Fig. 165.10). Direct

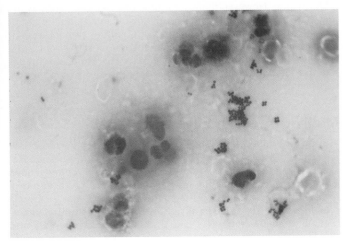

Fig. 165.10 *Staphylococcus aureus* in a Gram stain of pus. Courtesy of Jan Verhoef, Ad C Fluit and Franz-Josef Schmitz.

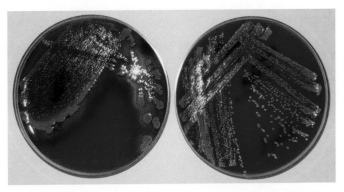

Fig. 165.11 Growth of *Staphylococcus aureus* (left) and *Staphylococcus epidermidis* (right) on trypticase soy agar with sheep blood.

Gram smears of sputum samples may also assist in rapid identification of staphylococcal pneumonia.

Staphylococci generally grow overnight on most conventional bacteriologic media. The preferential medium for isolation is (sheep) blood agar, on which they form colonies of 2 mm or more in diameter (Fig. 165.11). Blood cultures from untreated bacteremia patients are usually positive after overnight incubation. Staphylococci may grow at a temperature range of 15–45°C and at NaCl concentrations as high as 15%. Differentiation from other Gram-positive cocci may be aided by the determination of a couple of characteristics (Table 165.2). The fermentation of mannitol by *S. aureus* is used in mannitol salt agar to screen for this bacterium in clinical and environmental samples.[53]

S. aureus colonies on blood agar can be differentiated from other staphylococci by their yellowish (gold-colored) pigment. Confirmation tests include latex agglutination assays that detect protein A and clumping factor ('bound coagulase') on the cell surface of *S. aureus* (Fig. 165.12), testing for free coagulase and for DNAse/thermostable endonuclease. However, nonoptimal sensitivity of these tests has been reported, especially in identifying MRSA. Most CoNS species can be determined with carbohydrate utilization tests and enzyme tests (e.g. phosphatase, urease, nitrate reduction). *S. saprophyticus* from urine samples may be identified by demonstrating novobiocin resistance.

S. aureus can also be identified by molecular techniques demonstrating specific genes such as nuclease (*nuc*), coagulase (*coa*), protein A (*spa*), surface-associated fibrinogen-binding protein or the sa442 gene; however, none of these techniques is 100% sensitive or specific.

Susceptibility testing

S. aureus susceptibility testing can be performed by disc diffusion or E-test on several standard bacteriologic media, or by microbroth and macrobroth dilutions. Guidelines and breakpoints are available from the Clinical and Laboratory Standards Institute (CLSI), the European Committee on Antimicrobial Susceptibility Testing (EUCAST) and the International Organization for Standardization (ISO). A number of automated systems are available for broth dilution susceptibility testing. These tests are adequate for most antibiotics, but certain special considerations apply.

Clindamycin susceptibility testing

Methylation of the ribosomal target, usually encoded by *ermA* or *ermC*, is the main mechanism of resistance against clindamycin, and also results in cross-resistance to macrolides, lincosamide and streptogramin B (MLS$_B$).[54] The methylase genes are associated with clinical failure of clindamycin therapy, but as clindamycin does not induce expression of these genes *in vitro*, tested strains may wrongly appear susceptible to the antibiotic. Erythromycin *is* a potent inducer of methylases *in vitro*, and erythromycin resistance is an initial clue to MLS$_B$ resistance. An induction test (with an erythromycin and clindamycin

Table 165.2 Differentiation of staphylococci from other Gram-positive cocci

	Staphylococcus spp.	*Micrococcus* spp.	*Kocuria kristinae*	*Rothia mucilaginosa*
Gram stain	Gram-positive cocci, in clusters	Gram-positive cocci, in clusters	Gram-positive cocci in tetrads	Gram-positive cocci in pairs or clusters with capsules
Color	Cream colored to yellow/white	Cream colored to canary yellow	Cream colored to canary yellow	Clear to white
Mupirocin	Susceptible	Resistant	Resistant	–
Bacitracin	Resistant	Susceptible	Susceptible	Susceptible
Growth in 6.5% NaCl	Yes	Yes	Yes	No
Oxidase	Negative	Positive	Positive	Negative
Catalase	Positive	Positive	Positive	Weakly positive or negative

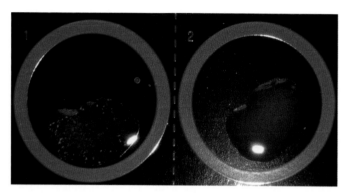

Fig. 165.12 Slide coagulase test. Latex particles coated with fibrinogen and IgG agglutinate when a colony of *Staphylococcus aureus* is suspended in the solution (left), and negative control (right).

disk placed 20–26 mm from each other) should, therefore, be performed on erythromycin-resistant *S. aureus* strains. After overnight incubation, MLS$_B$ resistance will be induced by erythromycin, creating a characteristic D-shaped inhibition zone around the clindamycin disk. Such strains should also be considered resistant to the streptogramin B antibiotic quinupristin–dalfopristin. Enzymatic inactivation of clindamycin is another potential resistance mechanism, but this occurs much less frequently.

Isoxazolyl penicillins

Identifying methicillin-resistant strains in the bacteriologic laboratory is challenging. The gold standard for identification of MRSA is the detection of the *mecA* gene, which encodes the altered penicillin-binding protein PBP2a. Although all MRSA strains harbor the *mecA* gene, in heterogeneous MRSA populations expression of PBP2a is suppressed in most colony-forming units and may not always be detected by disk diffusion with oxacillin or by automated (microbroth dilution) systems. A screening assay with 30 μg cefoxitin disks has the highest sensitivity for MRSA detection, with specificity being comparable to other susceptibility assays.[55] Rapid latex agglutination assays which react to PBP2A may confirm MRSA, but these tests are less sensitive than cefoxitin screening.[55]

Screening for MRSA colonization is performed on selective media (both liquid and solid) which contain either oxacillin or cefoxitin. Several rapid MRSA detection media are available (both commercially and in-house produced media) which contain an indicator agent to distinguish *S. aureus* from CoNS. Sensitivity and specificity of most of these tests are reported to be higher than 90–95%.[56]

Recently, rapid molecular detection tests for MRSA screening have been introduced. Polymerase chain reaction (PCR) targets are usually the *mecA* gene in combination with a specific *S. aureus* gene (e.g. the sa442 gene, the coagulase gene or the nuclease gene). PCR-based techniques detect MRSA in screening specimens within 4–6 hours and appear to be highly specific and sensitive.[57] However, performance may vary; depending on the primer set used, certain MRSA clones will not be detected. At present, cultures remain essential in MRSA screening, especially to confirm positive PCR results.

Typing methods

The epidemiology of (methicillin-resistant) *S. aureus* may be studied by typing the isolated strains. Numerous typing methods are available, differing in reproducibility, cost, ease, speed and discriminatory capacity. The currently most widely employed techniques are discussed below.

Pulsed field gel electrophoresis

Pulsed field gel electrophoresis (PGFE) is based on the digestion of bacterial DNA with restriction endonucleases (for MRSA usually *smaI*), generating large fragments of DNA (10–800 kb). A sharper resolution of the fragments is obtained by alternating the direction of the electric current on the separation gel. PFGE has a high discriminatory power and the results are highly reproducible.[58] As such, the technique has been proposed as the gold standard for MRSA typing. However, there are limitations to its use, such as the long time interval until the final results are obtained, and the cost of reagents and specialized equipment.[58] Furthermore, even though relatively few bands are generated, small differences in electrophoretic conditions can alter the distance traveled by each band and complicate the comparison between isolates submitted to electrophoresis in different gels.

Multilocus sequence typing

Multilocus sequence typing (MLST) characterizes bacterial isolates by using the sequences of internal fragments of seven housekeeping genes.[59] Every polymorphism of a housekeeping gene is assigned a number, yielding a code consisting of seven numbers for each bacterial isolate; subsequently, each new code receives a sequence type (ST) number. Advantages of MLST include its unambiguous nomenclature, easy global exchange of typing data and the possibility for population structure and evolutionary analyses. On the downside, MLST is less discriminatory than PFGE and quite expensive.

Spa typing

Spa typing is a single-locus sequence typing technique for *S. aureus*, based on the polymorphic region X of the protein A gene.[60] Spa typing is highly reproducible and easy to interpret. It has less discriminatory power than MLST and PFGE, but is less costly and easier to perform. A web-based reference database (http://www.spaserver.ridom.de), which uses a standardized spa-type nomenclature, permits global epidemiologic comparison of isolated MRSA strains.

MANAGEMENT OF *S. AUREUS* INFECTIONS

Management of *S. aureus* infections often includes the combined use of source control and antibiotic therapy. Uncomplicated wound or skin and soft tissue infections should be treated locally by drainage (after incision in case of abscess formation or necrotectomy in case of necrosis). Systemic antibiotics may be required if there is severe cellulitis or associated deep tissue infection.

β-Lactam antibiotics are the agents of first choice in the treatment of (severe) systemic methicillin-sensitive *S. aureus* (MSSA) infections. Comparative studies between different β-lactam antibiotics are lacking, as are studies evaluating different durations of treatment. Isoxazolyl penicillins (cloxacillin, dicloxacillin, flucloxacillin), penicillin/β-lactamase inhibitor combinations (amoxicillin–clavulanic acid, piperacillin–tazobactam), first- and second-generation cephalosporins and carbapenems are considered equally effective in the treatment of MSSA infections. Clinical experience with the isoxazolyl penicillins and their narrow spectrum of activity makes them the first choice of therapy. Vancomycin, a glycopeptide, is the antibiotic of choice for (severe) systemic infections with MRSA and in patients with β-lactam allergy. The glycopeptides are, however, significantly less active than the β-lactams.[61] CA-MRSA strains are mostly still susceptible to several antibiotic classes and can often be treated with co-trimoxazole (trimethoprim–sulfamethoxazole) or clindamycin (used especially in the treatment of abscesses, for its high tissue penetration). Other antibiotics with antistaphylococcal activity include the glycopeptide teicoplanin, the macrolides, the newer classes of the fluoroquinolones, rifampin, fusidic acid, tigecycline, linezolid and daptomycin.

Because of the severe complications of *S. aureus* bacteremia and its propensity to relapse,[37] treatment with systemic antibiotic therapy for a minimum of 2 weeks is recommended.[62] *In vitro*, aminoglycosides act synergistically in *S. aureus* killing, and the addition of an aminoglycoside (most often gentamicin) may shorten the duration of fever and bacteremia, although improved outcome with this combined therapy has not been demonstrated. In any case, because of nephrotoxic side-effects, it is advised to limit the duration of aminoglycoside therapy to 3–5 days. Because of the high a priori risk of endocarditis in patients with *S. aureus* bacteremia (12% in a large observational study[37]), transesophageal echocardiography should always be considered in these patients and is mandatory in all patients who fail to improve or maintain positive blood cultures under adequate antibiotic therapy.[62]

Intravascular catheters colonized with *S. aureus* are associated with a high risk of subsequent *S. aureus* bacteremic complications, even when there were no signs of catheter site infection at the time of line removal or negative blood cultures. Antistaphylococcal antibiotic therapy in such cases was associated with a markedly reduced incidence of complications and is, therefore, advised.[63]

Recently, several new antistaphylococcal drugs (linezolid, quinupristin–dalfopristin and daptomycin) have been approved. Televancin and dalbavancin, two lipoglycopeptides, are pending registration, and several cephalosporins and carbapenems with anti-MRSA activity are in phase III studies. Clinical trials evaluating new drugs are usually manufacturer-sponsored studies intended for registration, designed as non-inferiority studies, and underpowered to demonstrate superiority of new drugs when compared to standard therapy. Thus far, in randomized controlled trials, none of the new agents has been proven superior to standard therapy in regard to mortality and clinical cure, although trends towards superiority are sometimes observed, and meta-analysis may yield significant differences. At present there is clearly no such thing as the 'ideal anti-MRSA antibiotic'. Prolonged therapy with linezolid (one of the few new anti-MRSA drugs available in an oral formulation) may cause central (optic) neuropathy and bone marrow depression (especially thrombocytopenia) and it is therefore advised not to extend therapy beyond 28 days. Daptomycin is inhibited by pulmonary surfactant, and should not be used in case of a clinical suspicion of pneumonia.[64]

One thing that *has* become clear from all the clinical trials conducted to evaluate new antibiotics is that intravenous administration of vancomycin, the predominant comparator antibiotic for new anti-MRSA agents, is safe with limited nephrotoxic effects. The nephrotoxicity formerly attributed to vancomycin probably resulted from either contamination of previously used vancomycin formulations (these suspensions were known as 'Mississippi mud' for their turbid, dark brown appearance), the underlying illness of patients, or co-medication.[65] Vancomycin is believed to enhance aminoglycoside nephrotoxicity but the evidence for this effect is limited and contradictory.[66] Nevertheless, it seems prudent to avoid the combination of these drugs as much as possible, especially when longer treatment periods are indicated. Vancomycin trough levels should be monitored to ensure adequate (high enough) dosing in patients with severe infections, especially when patients fail to respond to treatment.

Rifampin and fusidic acid, both available in oral and parenteral formulations, are regularly used in combination therapy for particular *S. aureus* infections. Both agents are unsuitable as monotherapy due to the rapid development of resistance by *S. aureus*. Because of its penetration in biofilms and its activity on slowly dividing bacteria, rifampin is often part of an antibiotic regimen to treat foreign body infections (e.g. prosthetic joints) and endocarditis, in particular endocarditis involving prosthetic heart valves.[67] Fusidic acid is used in combination therapy for the treatment of MRSA infections, particularly bone and joint infections and in *S. aureus* endocarditis.[67] Unfortunately, clinical evidence regarding the use of these two drugs remains scarce, and further studies are needed to determine their exact place in clinical practice.

MANAGEMENT OF COAGULASE-NEGATIVE STAPHYLOCOCCAL INFECTIONS

Vancomycin is usually the agent of choice in the treatment of CoNS infections, but when thorough laboratory testing indicates that a CoNS is methicillin susceptible, the isoxazolyl penicillins or first-generation cephalosporins are preferred. Other antibiotics which may be considered include teicoplanin, linezolid, daptomycin, co-trimoxazole and quinupristin–dalfopristin. Since CoNS are often multiresistant, therapy should be guided by the susceptibility test results.

In intravascular catheter-associated bloodstream infections, removal of the intravascular catheter is the foremost part of the treatment, and this may even suffice (without antibiotic therapy) in patients who are not immunocompromised, do not have prosthetic implants, without underlying valvular heart disease and whose CoNS are not *S. lugdunensis* or *S. schleiferi*; no studies have been conducted which indicate that antibiotic treatment has additional value in these patients. Nonetheless, some experts advise a standard treatment of 5–7 days of systemic antibiotic therapy for all patients.[62] If removal of the intravascular catheter is not possible, systemic antibiotic therapy should be initiated, preferably in combination with antibiotic lock therapy.

The treatment of CoNS endocarditis does not differ in principle from the treatment of *S. aureus* endocarditis.[67]

Micrococci

Micrococci are human commensals that colonize the skin, mucosa and oropharynx. Based on phylogenetic and chemotaxonomic data, the genus *Micrococcus* was, in 1995, split into five separate genera: *Micrococcus*, *Kocuria*, *Nesterenkonia*, *Kytococcus* and *Dermacoccus*.[68] The only clinically relevant species within the genus *Micrococcus* is *M. luteus*, which occasionally may cause invasive disease, usually in neutropenic patients. Micrococci have occasionally been reported as the cause of pneumonia, meningitis associated with ventricular shunts, septic arthritis, bacteremia, catheter-associated bloodstream infection and endocarditis.

Other former micrococci which have been reported to cause (opportunistic) infections include *Kocuria rosea*, *Kocuria kristinae* and *Kytococcus schroeteri*.

DIAGNOSIS

Micrococci are catalase-positive, oxidase-positive, strictly aerobic Gram-positive cocci that grow in clusters. On sheep blood agar they form cream-colored to yellow colonies. Resistance to mupirocin and staphylolysin, and susceptibility to bacitracin and lysozyme differentiate them from the staphylococci. Micrococci isolated from clinical specimens usually represent contamination, either from the skin and mucous membranes or from the environment. *M. luteus* may be differentiated from *K. kristinae* and *K. rosea* by testing for carbohydrate usage. *Kytococcus* differs from micrococci by resistance to penicillin and methicillin and by arginine dihydrolase activity. *Kocuria* and *Kytococcus* spp. usually appear as tetrads in Gram smears.

MANAGEMENT

A study with 188 micrococci, identified only to the genus level, demonstrated MICs at achievable concentrations for most β-lactams, aminoglycosides, glycopeptides, clindamycin and the most active drug *in vitro*, rifampin. Fosfomycin, erythromycin and fusidic acid should be considered inactive.[69]

Clinical data on infections with micrococci are too scarce to formulate any clear therapeutic recommendations. In case of infections of prosthetic materials, combination therapy with rifampin should be considered. Three cases of prosthetic valve endocarditis with *K. schroeteri* were treated successfully with valve replacement and combination therapy of vancomycin, gentamicin and rifampin.

Rothia Mucilaginosa

Rothia mucilaginosa is a normal inhabitant of the human oral cavity and respiratory tract. It is an infrequent pathogen, mostly affecting severely immunocompromised patients.[70] Cases of bacteremia, endocarditis, catheter-associated bloodstream infection, central nervous system infections, endophthalmitis, spondylodiscitis, osteomyelitis, prosthetic joint infection, pneumonia, cholangitis and CAPD peritonitis have been described.

Obsolete names for *R. mucilaginosa* are *Staphylococcus salivarius*, *Micrococcus mucilaginosus* and *Stomatococcus mucilaginosus*.

DIAGNOSIS

Rothia mucilaginosa is a facultative anaerobe, oxidase-negative, catalase-variable Gram-positive coccus; in smears the bacterium appears in pairs or clusters. It grows well on most nonselective media and in standard blood culture systems. On sheep blood agar the bacterium forms clear to white, nonhemolytic, mucoid or sticky colonies that adhere to the agar surface. Further distinguishing characteristics include susceptibility to bacitracin, inability to grow on media containing 5% NaCl, and hydrolyzation of gelatin and esculin.

MANAGEMENT

In vitro, penicillin, ampicillin, second- and third-generation cephalosporins, imipenem, glycopeptides and rifampin have high activity against most *R. mucilaginosa* isolates; applying the non-species-specific breakpoints set by EUCAST (www.srga.org/eucastwt/MICTAB/index.html; no susceptibility cut-off points have been defined by the CLSI), the micro-organism may be considered susceptible to these agents. MICs for fluoroquinolones, aminoglycosides, co-trimoxazole, erythromycin, clindamycin and fosfomycin are generally higher,[69] suggesting that these drugs are less suitable as antibiotic therapy.

Clinical data are limited and mainly concern neutropenic patients. In case reports, vancomycin is mostly employed (sometimes intrathecally in case of meningitis); other drugs include piperacillin–tazobactam, meropenem and third-generation cephalosporins. Sometimes combination therapy is given, combining one of the former drugs with rifampin or an aminoglycoside. Treatment with penicillin and chloramphenicol has also been described.[70]

REFERENCES

References for this chapter can be found online at http://www.expertconsult.com

Ellen M Mascini
Rob JL Willems

Chapter | **166**

Streptococci, enterococci and other catalase-negative cocci

INTRODUCTION

The genus *Streptococcus* consists of round or slightly oval Gram-positive cocci with a diameter of <2 μm. The cocci are often in pairs or chains. The detection of cytochrome enzymes with the catalase test distinguishes members of the catalase-positive family of Micrococcaceae (see Chapter 165) from the members of the family of Streptococcaceae, which are catalase negative. Most of these micro-organisms are facultative anaerobes, but some need carbon dioxide for growth and others may be strictly anaerobic. The major representatives of the genus *Streptococcus* include *Streptococcus* and *Enterococcus*.[1] The further division of streptococci has been the topic of an extensive taxonomic re-evaluation and we still lack a complete picture of the genetic relationship between different subgenera and species. Some of the older classification systems are therefore still in use despite access to more accurate genetic taxonomic methods.

The traditional division of streptococci into α-streptococci, β-streptococci and γ-streptococci on the basis of the capacity of the bacterial colony to hemolyze erythrocytes in the blood agar medium is still considered the first step in the classification of streptococci. This allows separation of streptococci into 20 different serogroups (the Lancefield grouping system).[2] The clear zone produced by lysis of the erythrocytes around the colony is typical of the β-hemolytic streptococci, but the zone may vary considerably in size. Colonies of α-hemolytic streptococci are surrounded by a zone that is usually green, whereas no color changes (and no hemolysis) are seen around the colonies of γ-streptococci on blood agar plates. Optochin (ethylhydro-cupreinhydrochloride) inhibits the growth of most pneumococci, in contrast to other α-hemolytic streptococci, and is thus an easy method for distinguishing between these species.

Commercial kit systems in which group-specific antisera (usually containing A, B, C, D, F or G antibodies) are coupled to latex beads are now widely used for identification of β-hemolytic streptococci. Nonhemolytic streptococci do not possess Lancefield cell wall grouping antigens, but some strains may possess similar antigens that show cross-reaction with β-hemolytic streptococcal group-specific antisera.

The taxonomic classification of viridans streptococci has caused confusion for a long time but was substantially simplified by a scheme worked out by Facklam and Washington (Table 166.1).[3]

Five species or groups of species can be identified on the basis of various biochemical tests or fermentation capacities.[3]

The identification of these streptococci has long since been recognized as unsatisfactory, with the result that a significant proportion of these isolates remain misidentified or unidentified.[4] Therefore, a variety of molecular methods have been developed for correct identification of streptococci and related organisms. These methods include DNA–DNA and DNA–RNA hybridization, determination of tRNA intergenic length, arbitrarily primed polymerase chain reaction (PCR), restriction amplification of rRNA genes and sequencing of a large variety of targets,[5] such as 16S rRNA, *rnpB*, *sodA*, *tuf*, *groESL*, *rpoB* and the tRNA gene intergenic spacer. In general, sequencing will provide the highest discriminatory power but is limited by high costs and low speed. To overcome these disadvantages, pyrosequencing of the *rnpB* gene was recently proposed as an identification method of extreme high resolution, which is also relatively simple, fast and reproducible with lower costs than normal sequencing.[6] Oligonucleotide array-based identification has also been proposed as an alternative rapid and high-throughput system for identification of the genera *Abiotrophia*, *Enterococcus*, *Granulicatella* and *Streptococcus*.[7]

MOLECULAR BIOLOGY AND POPULATION STRUCTURE

Various methods are used to type streptococci and enterococci (Table 166.2). With the introduction of sequence-based typing methods such as multilocus sequence typing (MLST) it became possible to unambiguously assign names or codes to genotypes. This has improved worldwide tracking of clinically relevant (i.e. particularly virulent or resistant) circulating clones. MLST also allowed construction of web-based international databases of which three currently harbor MLST schemes for 42 bacterial species (http://www.mlst.net, http://pubmlst.org, http://mlst.ucc.ie), including schemes for *S. pyogenes*, *S. agalactiae*, *S. pneumoniae*, *E. faecalis* and *E. faecium*. In addition and also boosted by the rapid expansion in sequence capacity and reduction in sequencing costs, an increasing number of streptococcal genomes have been sequenced, providing data on strain variation and molecular correlates for disease specificity. At the moment whole genomes of 12 *S. pyogenes*, 6 *S. agalactiae*, 25 *S. pneumoniae*, 5 *E. faecalis* and 5 *E. faecium* strains are either completely or partially sequenced. Finally, numerous microarrays for the various *Streptococcus* and *Enterococcus* species have been developed, not only for comparative genomics but also for transcriptomics. A systems biology approach integrating comparative genome sequence, transcriptome, proteome, metabolome analysis and functional studies, including animal infection models and human patient studies, has given us insights in the population structure of streptococci and enterococci, revealed the extent of lateral gene transfer and identified particular clinically relevant genetic lineages. This is not only highly relevant for (molecular) epidemiologic research but also to link genetic differences to clinical behavior, to improve understanding of pathogenic behavior of particular clones and to identify novel targets for vaccines or immunotherapy.

Table 166.1 Biochemical identification of viridans group streptococci

Species or group	TEST					
	Mannitol	Sorbitol	Voges–Proskauer	Arginine	Esculin	Urease
S. mutans (includes S. cricetus, S. downei, S. ferus, S. macace, S. rattus (arginine positive), S. sobrinus)	1	1	1	2	1	2
S. salivarius (includes S. intestinalis, S. vestibularis)	2	2	1	2	1	6
S. sanguis (includes S. gordonii, groups H and W streptococci)	2	2 (1)	2	1	1	2
S. mitis (includes S. mitior, S. oralis, S. sanguis biotype II)	2	2	2	2	2	2
S. anginosus (includes S. intermedius, S. constellatus, S. milleri, DNA groups I and III)	2 (1)	2 (1)	1 (2)	1	1	2

1, positive reaction; 2, negative reaction; 6, some strains positive, other strains negative; 1 (2), usually positive but occasional exceptions; 2 (1), usually negative but occasional exceptions.
Data from Facklam & Washington.[3]

Table 166.2 Commonly used methods for typing streptococci

Serologic methods	M typing and T typing R typing OF typing (inhibition of the opacity reaction) group A streptococci Polysaccharide antigen typing combined with latex agglutination	
Molecular methods	DNA fingerprinting	• M genotyping • pulsed-field gel electrophoresis • amplified fragment length polymorphism
	Ribotyping DNA sequencing	Multilocus sequence typing (MLST) emm gene sequencing
	PCR-based	Multiple locus variable number of tandem repeat analysis (MLVA)
Other methods	Multilocus enzyme electrophoresis Whole cell protein analysis	
Rarely used methods	Bacteriophage typing Bacteriocin typing	

Group A streptococci

The cell wall proteins of group A streptococci that are used in strain typing include T protein and M protein. M antigen, a potent virulence factor, is the basis for the further serologic and genetic identification of more than 100 types. Using specific antisera against these M proteins and sequence typing, more than 90% of fresh isolates of group A streptococci can be typed. During the last two decades invasive infections with M1 group A streptococci have increased. MLST, genome sequencing, single nucleotide polymorphism (SNP) analysis, transcriptomics and proteome analysis have revealed the molecular events involved in the emergence of this highly successful clone of group A streptococci. These molecular processes included the acquisition of prophages encoding particular virulence genes, accumulation of a very limited number of mutations that enhance expression of chromosomally located genes, reciprocal recombination of a chromosomal segment harboring two extracellular toxins and acquisition through lateral gene transfer of a M12-like 26 kbp region.[8] Full genome comparison of 12 group A streptococcus genomes, including (in addition to M1 and M3) M4, M5, M6, M12, M18 and M28 strains, indicated that, in agreement to what has been reported for M1 and M3 strains, a large portion of the Streptococcus metagenome resides on exogenous genetic elements. Interestingly, these elements not only include prophages, as reported previously for M1 and M3 strains, but also integrated conjugative elements (ICE), such as conjugative transposons and plasmids, encoding antibiotic-resistance genes, bacteriocins, putative virulence encoding cell-surface proteins tentatively involved in adhesion and extracellular matrix binding.[9] The identification of large numbers of ICE substantiates that lateral gene transfer contributes to metagenome diversification in group A streptococci. Genetic diversification by recombination appeared to be more prevalent and the dominant mechanism in emm patterns D and E, accounting for more than 80% of emm types.

Group B streptococci (GBS)

Comparison of the complete sequence of three Streptococcus agalactiae strains and draft genome sequences of five additional strains revealed that although the core genome accounts for 80% of any single genome, it represents only a fraction of the pangenome.[10] The seemingly ultimate large pool of genes from which GBS strains may acquire genes, resembling an open pangenome, has obvious consequences for pathogenesis-related questions and vaccine design. MLST of a global GBS collection showed recombination at the capsular locus and the existence of a highly invasive neonatal lineage of GBS.[11]

Streptococcus pneumoniae

Although multiple S. pneumoniae strains have been sequenced, the complete genome sequence of only four isolates have been reported.[12,13] Genome comparisons of completely sequenced S. pneumoniae strains revealed extensive variation in gene content and confirmed that lateral gene transfer and recombination is the most important driving mechanism generating genetic diversity and mosaicism in the pneumococcal genome.[12] A remarkable feature of the *S. pneumoniae* genome is the presence of many insertion sequence (IS) elements and repeated sequences, which may have facilitated genome plasticity of this organism and the generation of pseudogenes. This extreme level of genetic diversity, most likely facilitated by genetic transformation, is also exemplified by the presence of over 90 distinct capsular serotypes. This, however, may not be true within all *S. pneumoniae* lineages since, despite its high potential of genetic variation, the genomes of strains R6 and D39 showed nearly 100% conserved gene synteny, suggesting that rearrangements and transpositions have not occurred frequently since R6 was separated from D36 several decades ago.[13] Frequent recombination, resulting in a panmictic rather than clonal population structure, was also inferred from MLST analysis of *S. pneumoniae*.[14]

Enterococcus

Extensive genetic variation driven by recombination has also been reported for *E. faecalis* and *E. faecium* when both enterococcal species MLST schemes were developed and applied to diverse strain collection from various ecologic sources and geographic locations.[15–17] In contrast to *S. pneumoniae*, horizontal gene transfer in enterococci is most likely the result of conjugation, involving conjugative plasmids and/or conjugative transposons. Enterococci have become especially notorious for their unprecedented abilities to acquire and disseminate antibiotic-resistance genes. As for group A streptococci and pneumococci, enterococcal intra- and interspecies genetic exchange facilitates rapid adaptation of enterococci to stringent and changing environmental conditions. This seems to be a repetitive theme for these low G+C Gram-positive organisms. The availability of the completely sequenced *Enterococcus* genome, *E. faecalis* V538,[18] underlined the enormous potential for genomic rearrangement, with more than 25% of the genome consisting of mobile or exogenously required genetic elements. Comparative genomic hybridization (CGH) of eight *E. faecalis* strains, representing different MLST-based genetic lineages, identified a core genome covering only 66% of the predicted open reading frames, which is more or less in line with the available genome information.[19] CGH, as well as MLST, also showed that virulence and antibiotic-resistance genes were distributed among multiple genetic lineages, but that in some lineage resistance, which could be designated as high-risk enterococcal clonal complexes (HiRECC), antibiotic-resistance and virulence genes converged, causing infections and outbreaks globally (Fig. 166.1).[19,20]

Surprisingly, no completely annotated *E. faecium* genome is yet available. Despite this, genotyping data, especially MLST, and CGH have provided ample information on the population structure of *E. faecium*. MLST identified a single genetic subpopulation responsible for 90% of the *E. faecium* hospital outbreaks and 70% of invasive infections occurring globally.[17] Based on MLST, this subpopulation was named CC17 after its presumed founder ST-17 (see Fig. 166.1).[17,20] Through CGH more than 100 genes that were more or less specific for CC17 were identified, including a putative pathogenicity island, genes encoding cell surface proteins and novel metabolic pathways, antibiotic-resistance genes and IS elements.[21]

EPIDEMIOLOGY

β-Hemolytic streptococci of groups A, C and G

β-Hemolytic streptococci of groups A, C and G are often found in the upper respiratory tract, especially in children aged between 5 and 15 years, although people of all ages may be infected. The frequency of streptococcal-induced upper respiratory tract infections and especially pharyngitis and tonsillitis is higher during the early autumn months and the spring. Spread among family members and in classrooms is a common finding. In residential schools and detention centers pharyngeal carriage rates approach 50%. Except in epidemics, skin carriage is not common. However, in certain geographic areas where streptococcal pyoderma is common, skin colonization rates may be as high as 40%. Colonization rates are higher in patients who have skin diseases, such as eczema and psoriasis, and wounds. Children who have streptococcal pharyngitis may excrete this organism in their feces or carry it in the perianal region, which may be the cause of widespread streptococcal infections in closed facilities.

Large numbers of pyogenic streptococci are shed in the immediate environment, where the bacteria may be cultivated from clothing as well as from sheets and mattresses belonging to the infected person. This is important, especially in the treatment of patients who have skin infections such as impetigo. Recurrent streptococcal throat or skin infection is a common finding within families or institutions. Generally, pets are not a common source of re-infection because group A streptococci are highly host specific. However, group C streptococcal infections can be acquired by close contact with infected horses and group G streptococci can be obtained from dogs, in which group G streptococci are the dominant cause of streptococcal pharyngitis.

In a given population only a limited number of M types are prevalent and the population gradually seems to acquire immunity to these. New types seem to enter the population when the immunity against these diminishes below a certain level.

Scarlet fever used to be a frightening disease, but during the past few decades it seems to have had a mild course in the Western world. However, since the mid-1980s a worldwide increase in the incidence of severe group A streptococcal disease has been reported, including rheumatic fever, cellulitis, necrotizing fasciitis and other invasive forms. These serious infections were reported as being associated with the reappearance of M1 and M3 strains and the production of pyrogenic exotoxins A and B, although subsequently other exotoxins have also been implicated.[22] The global burden of disease caused by group A streptococci is not known, but it is estimated that there are at least 517 000 deaths each year due to severe group A streptococcal disease, including rheumatic fever and invasive infections (Fig. 166.2).[23] Food-borne epidemics (especially carried by milk) were common before pasteurization and were usually caused by group A streptococci, but groups C and G streptococci were also implicated on occasion. Food-borne infection can cause epidemic outbreaks of streptococcal infections such as scarlet fever and pharyngitis.

Group B streptococci

Group B streptococci are less commonly found in the upper respiratory tract, but their presence in the vagina of women aged between 15 and 45 years is rather common. Their numbers fluctuate and are higher before the monthly menstrual period and in pregnancy. Isolation frequencies as high as 30–35% have been recorded in some surveys. During delivery, vaginal colonization causes transmission to the infant in 50–75% of cases. A small number of these infants will develop symptoms of disease (see Clinical manifestations, below).

Enterococci

Enterococci are the most prevalent aerobic cocci in the bowel. Resistance against glycopeptides has been emerging since 1990, especially in *E. faecium* isolated in intensive care units and nursing homes in the USA. This emergence can be attributed to epidemic spread of a single clonal lineage, CC17 (see above). CC17 is characterized by high-level ampicillin and quinolone resistance.[17,24] Ampicillin resistance preceded and may have facilitated the emergence of glycopeptide-resistant *E. faecium* in the USA. In Europe, prevalence of vancomycin-resistant enterococci (VRE) started to increase after the turn of the century, with prevalence rates

Population snapshot of 855 *E. faecium* isolates on the basis of MLST allelic profiles using the eBURST algorithm

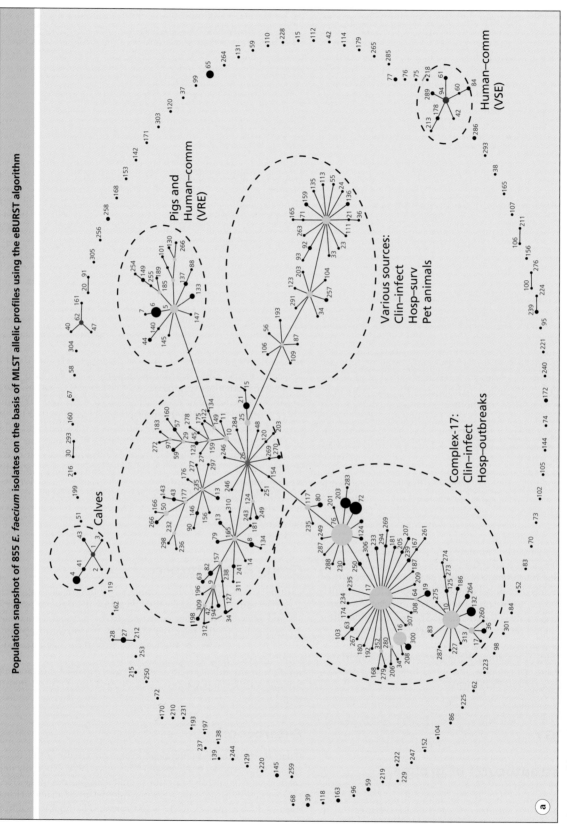

Fig. 166.1 (a) Population snapshot of 855 *E. faecium* isolates on the basis of MLST allelic profiles using the eBURST algorithm. CC17, the major subpopulation representing hospital outbreaks and clinical infections, is indicated, as well as the source of other major subgroups. Clin–infect, isolates from clinical sites (mainly blood) from hospitalized patients; Hosp–outbreaks, isolates from hospital outbreaks; Hosp–surv, feces isolated from hospitalized patients without an enterococcal infection and not associated with an enterococcal outbreak; Human–comm, feces isolated from human volunteers not connected to hospitals; VRE, vancomycin-resistant enterococci; VSE, vancomycin-susceptible enterococci. Copyright Elsevier 2006.

(Continued)

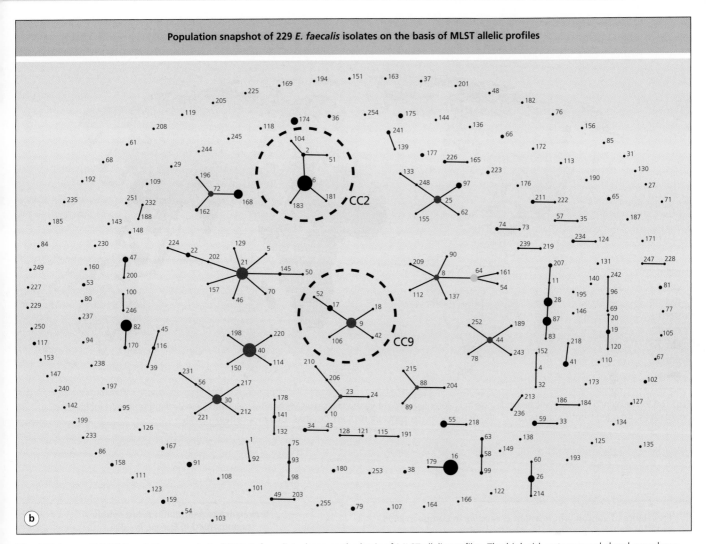

Population snapshot of 229 *E. faecalis* isolates on the basis of MLST allelic profiles

Fig. 166.1—cont'd (b) Population snapshot of 229 *E. faecalis* isolates on the basis of MLST allelic profiles. The high-risk enterococcal clonal complexes CC2 and CC9, exclusively containing hospital-related isolates, are indicated. These snapshots show all clonal complexes, singletons and patterns of evolutionary descent. The relative size of the circles indicates their prevalence. Numbers correspond to sequence types (STs) and lines connect single locus variants: STs that differ in only one of the seven housekeeping genes. Adapted from Leavis *et al.*[20] Copyright Elsevier 2006.

above 10% in countries such as Greece, Ireland, Israel, Italy, Portugal and the UK (Fig. 166.3). In other countries, such as the Netherlands, the prevalence of VRE has remained low but the number of ampicillin-resistant *E. faecium* has increased explosively during the past 10 years.[25]

Streptococcus pneumoniae

Streptococcus pneumoniae is an obligate parasite in humans, who may be colonized at a very early stage of life. The pneumococcus is a regular inhabitant of the nasopharynx in humans, especially among children, although adults are also frequently colonized. In certain populations carrier rates of 70% are found. In general, the rate of disease in a population depends on the frequency with which invasive serotypes are carried in the nasopharynx.[26] Nasopharyngeal carriage is often accompanied by the development of protection against infection by the same serotype. Carriage rates are inversely related to age and the levels of anticapsular antibody, and thus it is clear that the immune status of the host is an important determinant of the prevalence and longevity of carriage.[26] Of the 90 capsular types in the pneumococci, some seem to be more invasive than others (e.g. type 3 is among the most invasive strain types).[27] The capsular types 6a, 6b, 14, 19a, 19f and 23f are the dominant types found in pneumococcal infection during the first 2 years of life, whereas in adults these

types and the types 1, 3, 4, 7f, 8, 9, 10a, 11a, 12f, 14, 15b, 17f, 18c, 20 and 22f seem to cause the greatest number of bacteremic infections recorded in the USA.

A viral infection may predispose to a pneumococcal infection; this seems to be the case in children, who very often get pneumococcal otitis media 1–2 weeks after a virus infection.

Certain penicillin-resistant pneumococcal clones may have a strong epidemic potential owing to their relative resistance to penicillin and other commonly used antibiotics, showing a facilitated spread in subpopulations regularly exposed to both the pneumococcus and to numerous antibiotics.[28] Since the 1980s, the prevalence of penicillin-nonsusceptible pneumococci has been constantly increasing worldwide with alarming high prevalences in countries bordering the Mediterranean (Fig. 166.4).

Viridans group streptococci

Viridans group streptococci are fairly constant in the upper respiratory tract and dominate the aerobic normal flora in this region in the same way that enterococci dominate the aerobic normal flora in the gut. Viridans group streptococci are part of the normal flora of human mucous membranes in the mouth and upper respiratory tract as well as in stool samples.

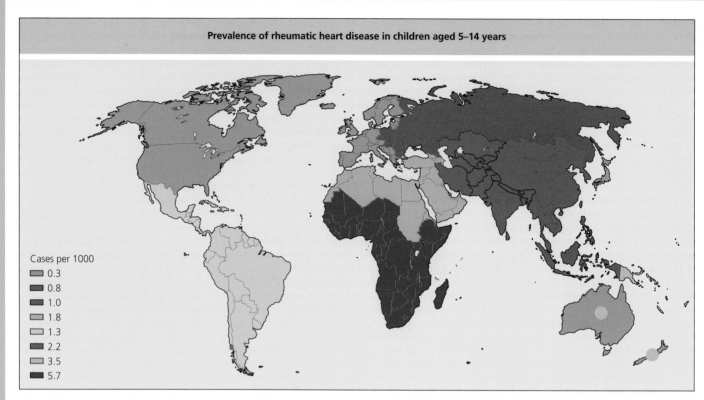

Fig. 166.2 Prevalence of rheumatic heart disease in children aged 5–14 years. The circles within Australia and New Zealand represent indigenous populations. Adapted from Carapetis *et al.*[23] Reprinted from The Lancet Infectious Diseases. Copyright Elsevier 2005.

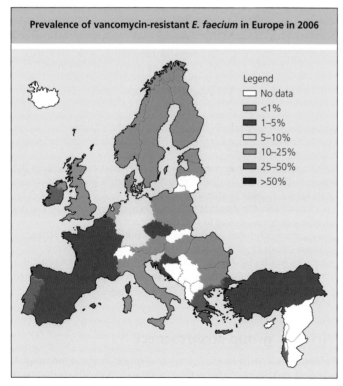

Fig. 166.3 Prevalence of vancomycin-resistant *E. faecium* in Europe in 2006 (see http://www.earss.rivm.nl).

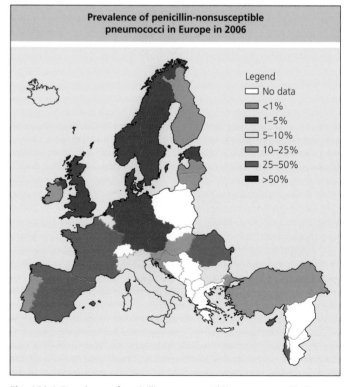

Fig. 166.4 Prevalence of penicillin-nonsusceptible pneumococci in Europe in 2006 (see http://www.earss.rivm.nl).

PATHOGENESIS

Group A streptococci (GAS)

The virulence factors of group A streptococci comprise both surface structures and proteins released from the cells during growth (Fig. 166.5).

Two-component regulatory systems

Two component regulatory systems in group A streptococci control co-ordinated expression of toxins, adhesins and other virulence-associated molecules that promote bacterial survival and pathogenesis in response to changing environmental conditions. Group A streptococci harbor 12 of these two-component systems and insertional activation followed by analysis in mouse infection models showed that these systems are involved in host–pathogen interactions (Fig. 166.6).[29,30] Co-ordinated regulation of virulence gene expression in response to different host environments is central to the success of group A streptococci. Mga is a virulence regulator that controls genes whose products are necessary for adherence, internalization and host immune evasion. Expression of the Mga regulon is influenced by conditions that signify favorable growth conditions, presumably allowing GAS to take advantage of promising new niches in the host.[31]

Cell wall antigens

The M protein is an α-helical structure similar to some muscle proteins such as myosin and tropomyosin and has also been shown to cross-react immunologically with these contractile proteins. It has been speculated whether this is of significance for the pathogenesis of rheumatic fever. A type-specific immunity is induced during the streptococcal infection and it has been shown in vaccination experiments that purified M protein can be used to induce immunity. Because these antibodies cross-react with human heart muscle proteins, there has been a reluctance to proceed with these experiments in humans. Lately it has been shown that M proteins may also function as superantigens and this has further emphasized that the proteins in the M-protein family may be important virulence factors.[32] M-negative streptococci are phagocytosed quickly in the serum milieu after being opsonized via the alternative complement pathway in the absence of antibodies against the M antigen, whereas M-positive streptococci resist phagocytosis in the absence of type-specific antibodies. The inability of M-positive streptococci to bind to phagocytosing cells efficiently indicates that C3b is not deposited on the surface of the streptococci or it is not accessible to the C3b receptor on the streptococci. The deposition of C3b is probably regulated by factor H, for which the M antigen has a high affinity.[32]

Several other M-like factors have been identified on the surface of group A streptococci. These have been shown to bind immunoglobulins such as IgG and IgA as well as several other serum proteins, including fibrinogen, plasmin, β_2 microglobulin and factor H. Binding of the M protein with the β_2 integrin adhesion molecule on the surface of neutrophils results in a massive inflammatory response which might be important in establishment of streptococcal toxic shock syndrome.[31] It has also been shown that some group A streptococcal strains have the ability to inhibit the activation of complement via the classic pathway by binding C4b to M protein-like structures. The way in which all these factors influence the virulence of the streptococci is not clear at present, but these factors can be seen as an expression of the complex interplay between the host and the micro-organism in group A streptococcal infections.[32]

One of the most the most exciting recent findings was the identification of pili in Gram-positive bacteria, including group A and group B streptococci, pneumococci and *E. faecalis*. In group A streptococci these pili are encoded by an 11 kb pathogenicity island and are involved in adherence and colonization of human tissue.[33]

Extracellular products, toxins and enzymes

Group A streptococci produce a great number of extracellular products (see Fig. 166.5). Streptolysin O is an oxygen-labile hemolysin that is biologically closely related to pneumolysin, tetanolysin and hemolysins from some other micro-organisms. Intravenous injections of this toxin in animals have demonstrated a cardiotoxic effect. It also inhibits chemotaxis, the mobility of neutrophils and phagocytosis by macrophages.

Streptokinase (fibrinolysin) is produced by groups A, C and G streptococci. Streptokinase binds to plasminogen in the blood, forming a complex that transforms plasminogen to plasmin, which has fibrinolytic activity. Purified streptokinase from group C streptococci is commonly used clinically to treat thrombosis in the coronary vessels and the deep veins of the leg. The plasmin formed by the plasminogen–streptokinase complex also activates complement via the alternative pathway.

The pyrogenic exotoxins (scarlatina toxins) have been proposed as being responsible for the scarlatina erythema. Numerous different toxins are produced; they are designated streptococcal pyrogenic exotoxin (Spe)A, SpeC, SpeF, SpeG, SpeH, SpeJ, SmeZ, mitogenic factor (MF) and streptococcal superantigen (Ssa). (SpeB is now known to be a constitutive cysteine protease and SpeE and MF have been shown to be identical.) Most group A strains produce more than one of these toxins. Several biologic effects have been attributed to the toxins, including pyrogenicity, a decrease in the blood–brain barrier permeability, cardiotoxic effect, T-cell activation and potentiation of the effects of endotoxin. The toxins may be responsible for the development of the shock syndrome that sometimes appears after streptococcal infections.[34] It has been suggested that this reaction, like many of the biologic effects, is induced by the release of cytokines because these toxins function as very active superantigens and thereby stimulate a high level of proliferation of T cells (Fig. 166.7). Patients who develop the toxic shock syndrome have been shown to have very low or undetectable levels of neutralizing antibodies against one or more of these toxins. Development of the streptococcal toxic shock syndrome might be hindered if toxin-neutralizing antibodies could be administered at a very early stage. Several of these extracellular products facilitate resistance of group A streptococci to killing by polymorphonuclear (PMN)-derived products.[35] In addition to evasion of neutrophil killing, group A streptococci are able to modulate PMN genes, resulting in apoptosis (Fig. 166.8).[29,35]

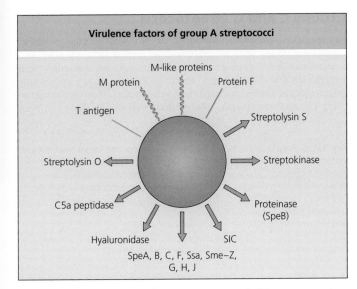

Fig. 166.5 Virulence factors of group A streptococci. SIC, streptococcal inhibitor of complement-mediated lysis; Spe, streptococcal pyrogenic exotoxins; Ssa, streptococcal superantigens.

SpeB and Sic (streptococcal inhibitor of complement), in combination with polypeptides involved in carbohydrate transport and metabolism, like the maltodextrin-binding protein MalE, as well as regulation, MalR, have also been implicated in prolonged survival in saliva, thereby promoting enhanced colonization and survival

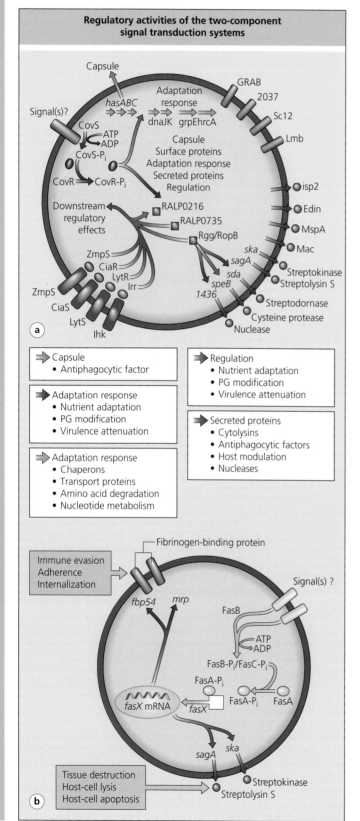

Regulatory activities of the two-component signal transduction systems

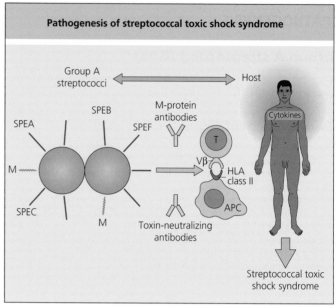

Pathogenesis of streptococcal toxic shock syndrome

Fig. 166.7 Pathogenesis of streptococcal toxic shock syndrome. In this model, patients who have opsonizing antibodies against the M antigen are protected against infection. In the absence of these antibodies, they may develop a serious infection if they are also lacking neutralizing antibodies against the streptococcal pyrogenic exotoxins which, as superantigens, may induce a cytokine cascade. This process will be hindered by the presence of toxin-neutralizing antibodies. The affinity of the toxins to the class II major histocompatibility complex of antigen-presenting cells (APC) and T-cell receptors of specific Vβ (variable region of β chain of the T-cell receptor) bearing T cells determines the outcome in each individual patient.

in the upper respiratory tract.[29,31] Furthermore, SpeB is also implicated in the transition from local to systemic infection of group A streptococci.

Group A streptococci also produce three distinct DNases, two of which are encoded by bacteriophages, which are crucial in avoiding neutrophil killing, thus facilitating normal progression of both pharyngitis and invasive infections.[31]

Groups C and G streptococci

The species *S. equisimilis* (a group C streptococcal species) produces streptolysin O as well as streptokinase, and *S. zooepidemicus* and *S. equi* (also group C streptococci) form hemolysins that differ from streptolysin S and O. Group C streptococci often have a very strong antiphagocytic hyaluronic capsule similar to that of group B streptococci. Group C streptococci, like group G streptococci, have not been

Fig. 166.6 Regulatory activities of the two-component signal transduction systems (TCSs) CsrRS/CovRS (a) and FasBCAX (b). (a) CsrRS/CovRS controls capsule expression, surface proteins, secreted proteins, other regulators (RofA-like protein (RALP) family and Rgg/RopB) and influences adaptive responses by transcriptional regulation of genes encoding chaperones, transport proteins and proteins associated with amino acid degradation and nucleotide metabolism. (b) Genes controlled by the FasBCAX system. This TCS appears to act on target genes through the action of a small putative regulatory RNA, FasX. TCSs are marked by rods and ovals (histidine kinases and response regulators, respectively), 'stand-alone' response regulators (RRs) by squares, secreted proteins by dots and surface proteins by rectangles. Red lines denote downregulation; green lines denote upregulation. Numbers denote SPy numbers assigned for serotype M1 group A streptococcus (GAS) strain SF370 ORFs. Adapted from Kreikemeyer et al.[30] Copyright Elsevier 2003.

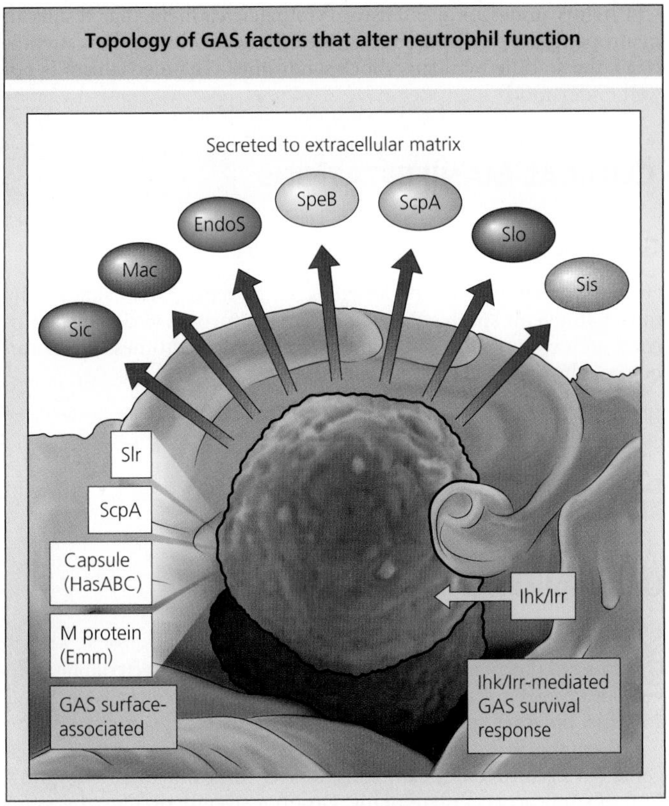

Topology of GAS factors that alter neutrophil function

Fig. 166.8 Topology of group A streptococcus (GAS) factors that alter neutrophil function. GAS (orange) produces several proteins (ovals) that are secreted to the extracellular matrix. Most of these proteins inhibit polymorphonuclear (PMN) phagocytosis. GAS also generates surface-bound molecules (white squares) that block phagocytosis. It is not clear how much capsule is shed from the GAS cell surface and therefore not surface-associated. Ihk/Irr (yellow box) is a gene-regulatory system directly linked to inhibition of human PMN function. Ihk/Irr expression is triggered by interaction with human PMNs (gray) and/or associated PMN microbicidal components. Adapted from Voyich *et al.*[35] Copyright Elsevier 2004.

isolated from patients who have rheumatic fever, but both can cause bacteremia and sepsis. Like the group A streptococci, they have an antiphagocytic M protein on their surface and form several enzymes. They should be regarded as pathogens.

Group B streptococci

Vaginal colonization with group B streptococci is common among adult women and transmission to the infant during childbirth occurs in 50–75% of cases. A small proportion of these infants will be infected. This indicates that particular strains or a defect in the immunity of the host play a role in the establishment of infection. It has long been known that antibodies against the capsular polysaccharide are a crucial factor for protection against group B streptococcal infections.[36] These polysaccharide types are designated 1a, 1b and 2–10. *In-vitro* studies indicate that phagocytosis and killing by polymorphonuclear leukocytes require the presence of both antibodies and complement. The capsular polysaccharide types 1a, 1b, 2 and 3 are clinically the most important as they are responsible for infections during the early weeks after birth. Nonencapsulated mutants of group B streptococci belonging to type 3 have been demonstrated to lack virulence in an experimental neonatal rat model. The significance of the capsular polysaccharide for the virulence of group B streptococci was further strengthened by the finding that transplacentally acquired maternal antibodies to the group B streptococcal polysaccharides conferred protection against infection of the baby. Consequently, human

experiments have been performed with polysaccharide–protein conjugate vaccines, which were capable of inducing opsonizing antibodies and killing group B streptococci.[37] The significance of sialic acid as part of the capsular polysaccharide in the inhibition of complement activation adds to the importance of the capsule in the pathogenesis of group B streptococcal disease.

Group B streptococci also produce other potential virulence factors, such as the CAMP factor, hemolysins, neuraminidase and surface proteins. Although these substances may contribute to pathogenesis, the exact role of some of these molecules awaits further studies. One class of surface proteins molecules comprises the α-like proteins or Alp family of proteins. Four members of the Alp protein family have been identified in group B streptococci: α, Rib, Alp2 and R28.[38] R28 was initially discovered in group A streptococci. Most, if not all, *S. agalactiae* strains express an Alp family protein and it has been suggested that these proteins may bind to human glycosaminoglycans, followed by human cell entry.[38] ScpB is a C5a peptidase that inactivates human C5a and inhibits recruitment of neutrophils. In addition, ScpB is able to bind fibronectin, which may promote adherence and/or invasion.[38] Of potential clinical importance is the fibrinogen-binding protein FbsA. It elicits a fibrinogen-dependent aggregation of platelets and may therefore may play an important role in *S. agalactiae*-induced endocarditis.[39]

As described above, pilus-like structures were also identified in group B streptococci.[40] These surface appendages confer adhesive properties, i.e. adhesion to human epithelial cells,[41] and contribute to adherence to and invasion of brain microvascular endothelial cells, which may facilitate penetration of group B streptococci through the blood–brain barrier.[42]

Enterococci

Although members of the genus *Enterococcus* cause many different infections in humans, little is known about the pathogenic mechanisms involved and the virulence factors carried by these microorganisms are less well understood than those of many other streptococci. It is clear, however, that infections caused by enterococci are often found in patients who have various types of immunodeficiency, in patients using mechanically compromising devices, such as intravascular lines and urinary catheters, and in seriously ill patients. The increasing importance of enterococci as nosocomial pathogens may in part be explained by their natural ability to acquire and exchange extrachromosomal elements encoding virulence traits or antibiotic resistance. Adhesion to extracellular matrix molecules and biofilm formation on indwelling medical devices leading to infections of artificial joints, implanted intravascular catheters, artificial hearts and artificial valves, stents and liquor shunt devices are often reported. A number of adhesins have been implicated in these processes including microbial surface components recognizing adhesive matrix molecules (MSCRAMMs) and the *E. faecalis* proteins Ace and Esp or Acm and Esp of *E. faecium*. The *bop* and *bee* loci, as well as two *sagA*-like genes, *salA* and *salB* of *E. faecalis*, appeared to be involved in biofilm formation.[43] Adherence to host tissue may also be mediated by enterococcal aggregation substance, fibronectin-binding protein and capsular polysaccharides in *E. faecalis*.[43,44] Furthermore, capsular polysaccharides mediate resistance to phagocytic killing of both *E. faecalis* and *E. faecium*.[44] Extracellular toxins such as cytolysin, gelatinase and a serine protease also contribute to *E. faecalis* pathogenesis.[44]

Pili were also discovered on the surface of *E. faecalis* and were demonstrated to be involved in biofilm formation and contributed to *E. faecalis* endocarditis in a rat endovascular infection model.[45]

Streptococcus pneumoniae

Pneumococci are a perfect example of the significance of the role that the mucous lining plays in the inhibition of potentially pathogenic micro-organisms. Thus, pneumococcal infections often occur after a respiratory tract viral infection that has damaged the epithelium, thereby helping the pneumococci to establish themselves in the mucous membranes. Factors that disrupt the normal clearing process in the airways predispose patients to pneumococcal infections in the lungs. Defects in systemic host defenses (i.e. HIV infection, asplenia, immunoglobulin deficiency) may also contribute to pneumococcal infections in the respiratory tract, sometimes causing invasive infections such as bacteremia, meningitis and endocarditis. However, the above may suggest a relatively passive role of *S. pneumoniae* in the pathogenesis of pneumococcal infections, waiting for defects in host defenses to seize its opportunity. Actually, *S. pneumoniae* is equipped with an impressive armory of virulence determinants, favoring mucosal adherence and sustained colonization, migration across the extracellular matrix and dissemination into host tissue. Following dissemination, *S. pneumoniae* has strategies to evade host immunity.

The initial event in pneumococcal colonization is adherence to the mucosal surface. Macromolecular structures, including surface-exposed adhesins such as pneumococcal pili and LPxTG-containing cell-surface protein, are implicated in this process. Pneumococcal pili, extending beyond the polysaccharide capsule, are encoded by the *rlrA* pathogenicity islet, which is present in a subset of clinical isolates.[46] Pneumococcal pili have been shown to be involved in pneumococcal adherence to lung epithelial cells and virulence in a mouse infection model.[46] Whether pneumococcal pili are pivotal in human pneumococcal disease remains to be seen since they are present in only a minority of strains and are associated with only certain serotypes.[47] PspC (also known as CbpA and SpsA) binds to the polymeric immunoglobulin receptor (pIgR), facilitating adhesion to mucosal epithelial cells.[48] PspC belongs to a large family of choline-binding proteins (CBPs) with adhesive properties and roles in transcytosis and immune evasion (Fig. 166.9). Another member of the CBP family, cholin-binding protein E (CBPE), is an important receptor for plasminogen/plasmin, leading to plasmin activation and migration across the extracellular matrix (ECM).[49] Activation of host proteases like the plasminogen–plasmin system results in proteolytic cleavage of the ECM, thereby increasing bacterial invasion and dissemination in host tissue. Other adhesins include the fibronectin binder PavA (pneumococcal adherence and virulence factor A) and the pneumococcal surface antigen A (PsaA), which is a metal binding lipoprotein implicated in binding to nasopharyngeal cells through an interaction with E-cadherin.[48]

Expression of a capsule, which is structurally distinct for each of the known 90 serotypes, is important for survival in blood and is strongly associated with the ability of *S. pneumoniae* to cause invasive disease. Thus, laboratory strains that have lost the ability to produce a capsule are nonpathogenic. Expression of capsule polysaccharide (CPS) is essential for virulence due to its antiphagocytic capsular properties.[50] As the virulence capacity of pneumococci is neutralized by complement-dependent opsonizing antibodies, polyvalent polysaccharide vaccines have been developed to confer protection against pneumococcal invasive disease in children and adults. Protection is afforded by type-specific antibodies with opsonizing capacity.[27,50]

Viridans group streptococci

Viridans group streptococci can be divided into those that have a tendency to induce endocarditis and those that do not. The endocarditis-related species usually produce dextrans and this is true for *S. mutans*, *S. sanguis* and *S. mitior*, as well as *S. bovis* (recently renamed *S. gallolyticus*). A prerequisite for the endocarditis-inducing capacity seems to be an ability to adhere to endothelial cells in the endocardium and this, in turn, is related to dextran production. In contrast, *S. salivarius* produces levan as its exopolysaccharide and is usually not related to endocarditis. Dextran production is probably not the only virulence factor because these micro-organisms can cause several other types of infection.

Patients undergoing intensive cytotoxic treatment that results in neutropenia are predisposed to severe infections with viridans streptococci, the so-called viridans shock syndrome.[51] The mechanism is not well understood.

CLINICAL MANIFESTATIONS

Groups A, C and G streptococci

Group A streptococcus, or *Streptococcus pyogenes*, is considered the most pathogenic species of β-hemolytic streptococci. Group A streptococci are involved in a wide variety of clinical syndromes, which can be roughly divided into:

- uncomplicated superficial infections;
- severe invasive infections; and
- postinfectious autoimmune sequelae.

Depending on climate and portal of entry, the infections are preferentially related to the upper airways or to the skin.

Uncomplicated infections

Uncomplicated respiratory infections

Group A streptococci are the most prevalent cause of bacterial pharyngitis and tonsillitis, especially in school children aged between 5 and 15 years; however, people of all ages can be affected.

When the infecting strain produces one of the so-called pyrogenic (or erythrogenic) exotoxins, scarlet fever may be a complication of streptococcal pharyngitis. Group A streptococci are the main causative agents in scarlet fever, but streptococci of groups C and G are isolated from a small number of patients. As well as the signs observed in pharyngitis, scarlet fever is characterized by a diffuse erythematous rash over the trunk, the neck and face, and the limbs. The area around the lips is generally free of erythema (circumoral palor). The rash is a diffuse light erythema that blanches on pressure. A white coating on the tongue develops and then resolves, leaving red swollen papillae, the so-called 'strawberry tongue'. Patients usually recover within about 5–7 days (see also Chapter 24).

Uncomplicated skin infections

Streptococci can cause skin infections of various forms and the clinical features are determined by which skin layers are infected:

- infections immediately below the stratum corneum result in impetigo;
- infections in the epidermis can give rise to ecthyma; and
- infections in the dermis give rise to erysipelas and cellulitis.

Clinical descriptions of these conditions can be found in Chapter 9.

Invasive infections

Invasive group A streptococcal infections occasionally occur. Examples are sepsis (including puerperal sepsis), pneumonia, septic arthritis, meningitis and lymphangitis.[52]

Remarkably, the most severe infections, such as necrotizing fasciitis with or without the toxic shock-like syndrome (TSS), have been increasingly seen since the mid-1980s.[34] The skin serves as the main portal of entry, followed by the mucous membranes of the throat, but in many cases the portal of entry is unknown. Early clinical features of group A streptococcal infections, before the development of toxic shock, may be flu-like in nature, with fever, sore throat, vomiting and diarrhea. Sometimes there is a history of blunt trauma. Necrotizing fasciitis is often difficult to diagnose; although redness and bullae may be visible, edema is sometimes the only superficial sign. Discrepancy between the unimpressive clinical observations and the extremely severe pain indicated by the patient is then the only clue to the correct diagnosis. Subsequent surgery may reveal massive

Functions of pneumococcal adherence molecules for pneumococcal colonization and invasive pneumococcal diseases

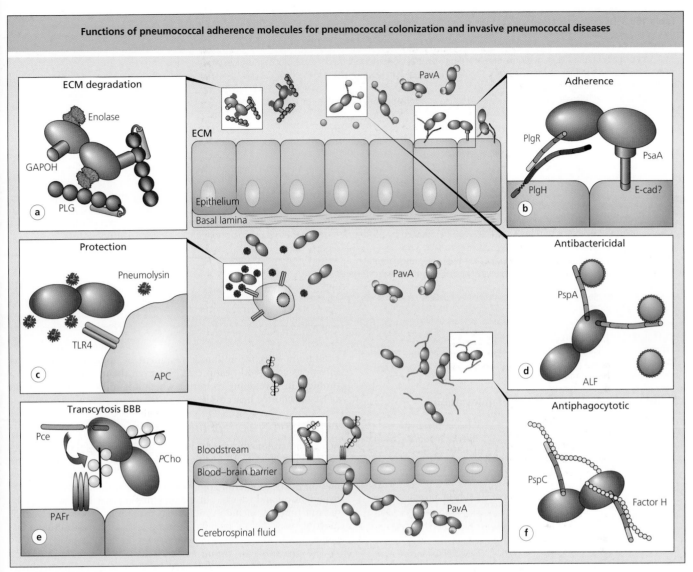

Fig. 166.9 Schematic representation highlighting functions of pneumococcal adherence molecules for pneumococcal colonization and invasive pneumococcal diseases. (a) The acquisition of plasmin(ogen) (PLG) by binding to surface-exposed GAPDH and enolase promotes degradation of the extracellular matrix (ECM). (b) The adhesins PspC and PsaA mediate adherence of pneumococci to epithelial cells. PspC binds to plgR and PsaA probably interacts with E-cadherin (E-cad). (d) Binding of ALF by PspA on mucosal surfaces protects against the bactericidal effect of ALF. (f) Within the blood, binding of factor H by PspC/Hic protects against complement-mediated phagocytosis and (c) pneumolysin functions as the pathogen-associated molecular pattern for Toll-like receptor 4 (TLR4) on antigen-presenting cells (APC). It is suggested that the pneumolysin–TLR4 interaction provides protection against the innate immune response of the host. (e) On stimulated cells, the PAFr is targeted by the PCho of pneumococci. This interaction is involved in transcytosis of pneumococci through the blood–brain barrier (BBB). The amount of PCho is modulated by another choline-binding protein, the Pce protein. PavA, a fibronectin-binding protein of pneumococci, has also been shown to have a crucial impact on pneumococcal adherence and invasive diseases including septicemia and meningitis. Adapted from Hammerschmidt.[48] Copyright Elsevier 2006.

tissue necrosis along the fascial planes. In the course of hours or days, toxic shock with hypotension and multiple organ failure may develop. Clinically this disease resembles the staphylococcal toxic shock syndrome (Table 166.3). Despite adequate antibiotic treatment and intensive care, these infections are characterized by a high mortality rate of between 30% and 80%, with up to 50% of the survivors having to have limbs amputated and requiring major debridement of tissue.

Autoimmune sequelae

In some cases, streptococcal disease is followed by autoimmune sequelae, either acute rheumatic fever or acute glomerulonephritis.

Rheumatic fever

Rheumatic fever, a delayed, nonsuppurative sequela of a pharyngeal infection due to the development of cross-reacting antibodies, is seen predominantly during fall and winter in children aged between 5 and 15 years, who also show the highest incidence of streptococcal pharyngitis.[53] Clinical manifestations may vary from mild to highly aggressive. The disease is largely self-limiting. Most patients give a history of preceding pharyngitis. Acute rheumatic fever is a clinical syndrome; there is no specific diagnostic test. Guidelines for the diagnosis of initial attacks of acute rheumatic fever are described in the Jones criteria (Table 166.4). Typically, patients present 10–25 days after the preceding streptococcal infection with fever, tachycardia and nonsuppurative inflammatory changes of the joints, heart, skin and subcutaneous tissue. Migratory arthritis is the

Table 166.3 Definition for streptococcal toxic shock-like syndrome

I. Isolation of GAS from:
  A. a normally sterile site (e.g. blood, cerebrospinal, pleural or peritoneal fluid, tissue biopsy, surgical wound, etc.)
  B. a nonsterile site (e.g. throat, sputum, vagina, superficial skin lesion, etc.)
II. Clinical signs of severity
  A. Hypotension: systolic blood pressure ≤90 mmHg in adults or <5th percentile for age in children

  and

  B. ≥2 of the following signs
  1. Renal impairment: creatinine ≥177 μM for adults or ≥2 × the upper limit of normal for age. In patients with pre-existing renal disease, a ≥2-fold elevation over the baseline level.
  2. Coagulopathy: platelets ≤100 × 10^9/l or disseminated intravascular coagulation defined by prolonged clotting times, low fibrinogen level and the presence of fibrin degradation products.
  3. Liver involvement: alanine aminotransferase, aspartate aminotransferase or total bilirubin levels ≥2 × the upper limit of normal for age. In patients with pre-existing liver disease, a ≥2-fold elevation over the baseline level.
  4. Adult respiratory distress syndrome defined by acute onset of diffuse pulmonary infiltrates and hypoxemia in the absence of cardiac failure or evidence of diffuse capillary leak manifested by acute onset of generalized edema or pleural or peritoneal effusions with hypoalbuminemia.
  5. Generalized erythematous macular rash that may desquamate.
  6. Soft tissue necrosis, including necrotizing fasciitis or myositis or gangrene.

An illness fulfilling criteria IA and II (A and B) is defined as a *definite* case; an illness fulfilling criteria IB and II (A and B) is defined as a *probable* case if no other etiology for the disease is identified.

Table 166.4 Revised Jones criteria for the diagnosis of poststreptococcal rheumatic fever

Major manifestations	Minor manifestations	
Carditis Polyarthritis Chorea Erythema marginatum Subcutaneous nodules Positive throat culture Increased titer(s) Recent scarlet fever	Clinical	Previous rheumatic fever or rheumatic heart disease Arthralgia Fever
	Laboratory	Acute phase reactants Leukocytosis Elevated erythrocyte sedimentation rate Elevated C-reactive protein Prolonged P–R interval on electrocardiogram
	Supporting evidence of streptococcal infection	

The presence of two major criteria or of one major and two minor criteria is highly suggestive of rheumatic fever, if supported by evidence of preceding group A streptococcal infection.

most common manifestation and can be diagnosed in 70% of patients; carditis is found in about 50% of patients. There is an inverse relationship between the severity of joint involvement and the risk of developing carditis. The carditis is a pancarditis, which means that the pericardium, the myocardium and the endocardium can all be affected.

Repetitive group A streptococcal infections tend to cause relapses in these patients, resulting in chronic progressive damage to the cardiac valves. Carditis is the only manifestation of rheumatic fever that has the potential to cause long-term disability or death.

Strains of certain M types are strongly associated with rheumatic fever, especially strains that appear mucoid on blood agar plates. Other equally prevalent serotypes fail to initiate the disease or even to reactivate it in susceptible hosts. Rheumatic fever is associated with pharyngeal strains carrying M proteins of types 1, 3, 4, 5, 6, 12, 14, 18, 19 and 24.

In the developed world, the incidence of rheumatic fever declined throughout the 20th century, probably owing to improved living conditions, effective antibiotic treatment of upper respiratory tract infections and good health care. However, rheumatic fever is still a problem in developing countries, where it is still the most common cause of acquired heart disease.[23]

Acute glomerulonephritis

Acute glomerulonephritis is diagnosed on the basis of the clinical presentation in combination with evidence of a recent infection (in the previous 1–3 weeks) with *S. pyogenes*. This syndrome of acute inflammation of the glomeruli comprises oliguria, hematuria, proteinuria, hypertension and edema, but the presentation may be mild. The laboratory findings include proteinuria, hematuria and reduced renal function as evidenced by renal function tests. Decreased serum complement is an important parameter to support the diagnosis.

The prognosis in young adults is usually favorable, but sporadically acute disease is followed by chronic glomerulonephritis and subsequent renal failure. The incidence of glomerulonephritis is lower in Western Europe than in the USA, as is the incidence of pyoderma. The attack rate varies within wide ranges but seems to decrease substantially in the developed world and many cases can only be detected by slight proteinuria and confirmed by renal biopsies.

Glomerulonephritis is observed more in connection with skin isolates of M types M2, M49, M55, M57, M59, M60 and M61, and throat isolates of M1, M4, M12 and M25. Although the incidence of rheumatic fever has declined dramatically in the developed world, it is still a major concern in developing countries.

Chorea and other neurologic syndromes

Sydenham's chorea (St Vitus' dance) is characterized by rapid involuntary movements, sometimes associated with emotional lability and other neuropsychiatric features.[54] Although it can occur in close association with acute rheumatic fever, in which case diagnosis is relatively easy, it may present many years later as a seemingly distinct clinical syndrome, making the association with past streptococcal infection in these cases very difficult.

More recently, a syndrome with the rather unwieldy title of 'poststreptococcal autoimmune neuropsychiatric disorder associated with streptococci' (PANDAS) has been described to encompass a range of neurologic conditions such as tics and obsessive compulsive disorder.[55] The precise relationship with streptococcal infection is still being investigated.

Group B streptococci

Neonatal disease

Group B streptococci (*Streptococcus agalactiae*) are a leading cause of bacteremia and meningitis in neonates.[56] Most group B streptococcal infections are thought to be transmitted to the infant from the maternal genital tract during delivery.

Early-onset group B streptococcal infection (up to 5 days of age) is associated with a high mortality rate and occurs predominantly in immature neonates whose deliveries have been characterized by complications predisposing to infection (premature onset of labor, rupture of membranes for more than 24 hours before delivery, maternal fever or anogenital colonization of the mother).[56]

With rapid diagnosis, including screening of pregnant women, and better supportive care, mortality has decreased and is now between 15% and 40%. A substantial proportion of children with group B streptococcal sepsis develop meningitis and lumbar punctures should therefore be performed in all infants with suspected sepsis. Pulmonary involvement occurs in 40% of neonates with group B streptococcal sepsis, which cannot be distinguished from hyaline membrane disease on the basis of clinical or radiologic findings.[56]

Late-onset disease (occurring at 7 days of age or older) is infrequently associated with obstetric complications, but is acquired from exogenous sources (e.g. the mother or another infant). Typically, septic patients present with fever, poor feeding and irritability; 80% have meningitis. Death rates are much lower than in early-onset disease, but survivors of meningitis may have permanent neurologic sequelae, including central diabetes insipidus, thermal dysregulation, cortical blindness, deafness, mental retardation and generalized spasticity.[56]

As with group A streptococci, a correlation has been found between certain clinical conditions and the streptococcal type causing the infection. In early-onset neonatal infections, all four of the first serotypes are isolated at about the same frequency, whereas in late-onset disease, type 3 streptococci are the most prevalent.

Adult disease

In recent years, group B streptococci have been recognized with increasing frequency as a substantial cause of morbidity and mortality among adults.[57] Two groups of adults are at increased risk of group B streptococcal infection: pregnant women and patients with serious underlying disease (e.g. diabetes mellitus, malignancy).[56,57] The spectrum of group B streptococcal disease in adults includes (among others) bacteremia with or without sepsis, cellulitis and other soft tissue infections, pneumonia, arthritis, meningitis, osteomyelitis, endocarditis and urinary tract infection.

Enterococci

Initially thought of as merely harmless commensals because of their low intrinsic virulence compared with other organisms such as group A streptococci, enterococci have become the third most common nosocomial pathogen overall. This appears to have been caused by selection of these organisms by the widespread use of broad-spectrum antibiotics, such as the cephalosporins, which lack enterococcal activity, and acquisition of new mechanisms of antibiotic resistance.[58]

Enterococci are commonly associated with urinary tract infections, particularly in patients who have indwelling catheters, and are recovered from abdominal and pelvic wound infections and abscesses. However, most clinical studies suggest that patients who have normal host defenses are resistant to enterococcal infections.[58] Furthermore, there is a low frequency of enterococcal bacteremia originating from an intra-abdominal source when antimicrobial agents that do not cover enterococci are used.[58] Enterococcal bacteremia in surgical patients is almost always associated with the ongoing or previous use of antimicrobial agents that are not specific for enterococci.

The most frequently seen infections are infections of the cardiovascular system, with bacteremia related to an intravascular catheter being the most common,[58] although endocarditis also occurs. Other types of infection caused by enterococci include intra-abdominal and deep surgical wound infections; bone and joint infections, especially in prosthetic joints; infections of the central nervous system (CNS) associated with shunts; and urinary tract infections.

Classically, enterococcal endocarditis is a disease of older people, with a male predominance as a result of obstructive urinary tract disease; it can also affect those who have prosthetic valves.

It has been reported that 60% of enterococcal infections are nosocomial, with half of them occurring in intensive care units. Originally, *E. faecalis* was responsible for 80–90% of enterococcal infections and *E. faecium* for 10–20%.[58] This ratio, however, has changed during the last decade in favor of *E. faecium*.

Streptococcus pneumoniae

Streptococcus pneumoniae is an important agent of human disease at the extremities of age and in those who have underlying disease. Pneumococcal disease is most commonly associated with an antecedent viral respiratory infection such as influenza or with chronic conditions such as chronic obstructive pulmonary disease, diabetes mellitus, congestive heart failure, renal failure, smoking and alcoholism. Immunodeficiency such as that caused by splenic dysfunction or splenectomy is an additional risk factor for the development of severe pneumococcal disease because of decreased bacterial clearance and defective production of antibodies.

Streptococcus pneumoniae is the causative agent of the majority of cases of community-acquired pneumonia and otitis media, one of the three most common pathogens in bacterial meningitis and an important cause of sepsis and sinusitis.[26,59] Bacteremia occurs in 10% of patients who have pneumococcal pneumonia and in more than 80% of patients who have pneumococcal meningitis. Children with sickle cell disease and individuals with hypogammaglobulinemia or who have had a splenectomy (especially in the first year) are at greatly increased risk of fulminating pneumococcal sepsis, which has a high mortality.

Pneumococcal pneumonia is discussed in Chapter 27 and pneumococcal meningitis in Chapter 18.

Viridans group streptococci

Viridans group streptococci are usually found as normal inhabitants of the oral cavity, the upper respiratory tract and the bowel.[60] When these organisms gain access to the bloodstream, people who have damaged heart valves are at increased risk of endocarditis. Infection is usually endogenous and is preceded by disease, dental extraction or trauma to a mucosal surface. It is often associated with an immunocompromised condition.[61] However, blood cultures that are positive for α-hemolytic streptococci or nonhemolytic streptococci have no clinical relevance in many cases. If the same strain is isolated from more than one blood culture bottle or is isolated on repeated occasions, the assumption of clinical relevance is strengthened.

Viridans group streptococci are the most frequent cause of native valve endocarditis and are generally associated with a better clinical outcome than endocarditis caused by staphylococci, enterococci or fungi. A special population prone to develop infections with viridans streptococci is those with hematologic malignancies who are treated with cytotoxic drugs with high cytotoxicity for mucosal surfaces. The course of infection in these patients may vary from mild to highly severe, with shock, adult respiratory distress syndrome and death.

Streptococcus milleri is a cause of abscesses in association with previous surgery, trauma, diabetes and immunodeficiency. The digestive tract has been recognized as the most likely portal of entry.[62] These bacteria are an infrequent cause of endocarditis and pharyngitis.

Streptococcus gallolyticus (previously *S. bovis*) can be isolated from patients who have endocarditis and bacteremia. There is a strong association between bacteremia caused by this micro-organism and adenocarcinoma of the colon, as well as neonatal sepsis and meningitis.[63]

MANAGEMENT

Groups A, B, C and G streptococci

Penicillin is the traditional first-choice therapy for infections caused by groups A, B, C or G streptococci. *Streptococcus pyogenes* is still extremely sensitive to penicillin and erythromycin is a good alternative in case of penicillin allergy. However, an increase in the prevalence of erythromycin-resistant group A streptococcal strains has been reported in several areas. Resistance occurs in relation to an increased macrolide consumption and may reach 40%.[64]

Persistent oropharyngeal carriage after a complete course of penicillin therapy can occur in up to 30% of patients. β-Lactamase production by pharyngeal flora as well as penicillin tolerance of group A streptococci have been suggested as causes of failure of penicillin in the eradication of group A streptococci.

The object of therapy in patients who have acute rheumatic fever is to reduce inflammation, decrease fever and toxicity, and control cardiac failure. Depending on the clinical condition of the patient, treatment varies from analgesia to anti-inflammatory drugs (aspirin-like agents or, in severe cases, corticosteroids). Antibiotic treatment of streptococcal infections effectively prevents development of acute rheumatic fever and minimizes the possibility of transmission of rheumatogenic streptococcal strains.[53]

In life-threatening infections such as necrotizing fasciitis and streptococcal toxic shock, rapid diagnosis immediately followed by adequate treatment is essential. Surgery (debridement of necrotic tissue or even amputation) is the key event in the treatment of necrotizing fasciitis.[34] The combination of penicillin and clindamycin is the therapy of choice. Preliminary data suggest that the addition of intravenous immunoglobulin may be efficacious, although convincing clinical trial data are lacking.[34] Supportive therapy in the intensive care unit, including fluid replacement, inotropics, hemodialysis and resuscitation, is also required.

Group B streptococci

Group B streptococci remain susceptible to penicillin G. However, the minimum inhibitory concentration (MIC) of penicillin G for group B streptococci is considerably higher (average 0.04 μg/ml) than that observed for group A streptococci.[56] Susceptibility to ampicillin and cephalosporins is also uniform, whereas resistance to erythromycin and clindamycin occurs in 15–20% of isolates and tetracycline resistance is seen in 85–92% of recent isolates.[57] Resistance to aminoglycosides is uniform, but the combination of penicillin and gentamicin has synergistic activity and accelerates the killing of group B streptococci *in vitro*.

Because of the inoculum-like effect and the direct relation between delayed sterilization of the CNS and the occurrence of neurologic sequelae, initial therapy of suspected group B streptococcal meningitis should include increased dosages of penicillin to ensure efficacy.

Enterococci

Antimicrobial therapy for enterococcal infections is complicated because most antibiotics are not bactericidal at clinically relevant concentrations. Combination therapy with a cell wall agent plus an aminoglycoside improves the outcome of enterococcal endocarditis and probably of enterococcal meningitis, but may not improve the outcome in bacteremia.[65] High-level aminoglycoside resistance, vancomycin resistance and high-level ampicillin resistance are increasing in prevalence.[25,58,65]

Enterococcus faecium is typically high-level penicillin and ampicillin resistant and this type of resistance has been reported as a significant predictor of lack of cure.[58,65] Therapy of enterococcal infections caused by vancomycin-resistant *E. faecium* is very difficult because these organisms are usually resistant to alternative antibiotics currently available.[58] The newly developed streptogramins (quinupristin and dalfopristin), oxazolidinones (linezolid), daptomycin and tigecycline appeared promising against vancomycin-resistant enterococci.[66] Nitrofurantoin is active against many strains of vancomycin-resistant enterococci and should be useful for urinary tract infections.[65]

Streptococcus gallolyticus should be differentiated from the enterococci because it is usually susceptible to penicillin alone, and both endocarditis and meningitis due to *S. gallolyticus* have a better prognosis.[63]

Streptococcus pneumoniae

Penicillin used to be the first-choice therapy for pneumococcal disease, and in penicillin-sensitive strains it still is. For patients who have penicillin allergy, cephalosporins and erythromycin are valuable alternatives.

Resistance to penicillin is increasing in many parts of the world and is associated with a decreased affinity of the antibiotic for penicillin-binding proteins present in the bacterial cell wall. At least 30% of the pneumococcal strains in the USA show intermediate resistance to penicillin (MIC 0.1–2.0 μg/ml). Except for meningitis patients, these are readily treatable with increased doses of penicillin. Of more concern is the appearance of pneumococcal isolates that are regarded as highly resistant to penicillin (MIC ≥2.0 μg/ml). Penicillin resistance is associated with a higher mortality rate than is penicillin susceptibility in hospitalized patients with pneumococcal pneumonia. If these strains are circulating, it might be more reliable to treat severe pneumococcal infections with vancomycin. International surveillance studies demonstrate a high global prevalence of macrolide resistance up to 30% among pneumococcal isolates obtained from patients with community-acquired respiratory tract infections.[67] Low-level resistance to macrolides (usually <16 μg/ml) is due to the *mefA* gene encoding an efflux pump. High antibiotic concentrations might overcome the pump and exert an antibacterial effect. High-level resistance is due to the *ermB* gene that encodes methylation of the 23S rRNA. In this case increasing the dose will exert little effect.

Remarkably, the rate of resistance to erythromycin, tetracycline and trimethoprim–sulfamethoxazole is much greater in penicillin-resistant strains than in penicillin-sensitive strains.[28,59]

Viridans group streptococci

Viridans group streptococci have long been considered uniformly susceptible to β-lactams, macrolides, lincosamines, rifampin (rifampicin) and vancomycin. Occasionally, however, mostly under the pressure of long-term penicillin therapy, serious infections due to penicillin-resistant or penicillin-tolerant strains have been reported.[68] In endocarditis, high-dose penicillin in combination with an aminoglycoside is recommended. If MIC values are below 0.12 μg/ml, the duration of this combination therapy may be limited to 14 days; alternatively, penicillin monotherapy can be given for 4 weeks. In cases of penicillin allergy, vancomycin is a good alternative.

Surgical drainage remains central to the management of abscesses (caused by *S. milleri*) and is often augmented by antibiotics.[62] The antibiotic of choice for infections caused by *S. milleri* is penicillin, to which all but a few strains are very sensitive.[60,62] Suitable alternatives include erythromycin, clindamycin and cephalosporins.[62]

Leuconostoc and *Pediococcus* spp. are vancomycin resistant but are generally susceptible to clindamycin, carbapenems and gentamicin, and most are susceptible to penicillin as well.

PREVENTION

Several of the infections caused by streptococci are followed by complications of such a serious nature that preventive measures should be instituted. Preventive measures can include:

- improved hygiene;
- antibiotic prophylaxis; and
- vaccination.

Group A streptococci

Carefully controlled trials in patients who have rheumatic fever have demonstrated convincingly that a monthly intramuscular dose of benzathine penicillin produces a statistically significant reduction in the frequency of recurrent streptococcal infections and subsequent attacks of rheumatic fever. The recommended dose is benzathine penicillin intramuscularly 1.2 million units every 4 weeks or penicillin V orally 250 mg q12h. It is not clear how long prophylaxis should be continued, but presumably it should be for life.[53]

In contrast, a favorable effect of penicillin prophylaxis in cases of glomerulonephritis has never been demonstrated, and relapses of glomerulonephritis occur at such a low frequency that prophylaxis is not warranted. For patients who have streptococcal cellulitis or erysipelas with frequent recurrences, prophylaxis with penicillin is warranted. Close contacts of severe invasive manifestations of group A streptococcal disease should be considered for prophylaxis.[69]

No vaccine is at present available for protection against group A streptococcal infections, but intensive research is ongoing.

Group B streptococci

Group B streptococci colonize the vagina, vulva and rectum of about 25% of fertile women. This micro-organism therefore represents a threat of bacterial sepsis to the newborn baby, especially in those cases where obstetric complications or prematurity are likely. Although the incidence of serious infections, such as septicemia and meningitis, is only around 1%, antibiotic prophylaxis has been recommended for patients who have obstetric complications, especially if earlier pregnancies have been complicated by group B streptococcal infections. Studies have clearly demonstrated that intrapartum administration of penicillin or ampicillin reduces the transmission of group B streptococci from the mother to the infant, and at least 80% of early-onset group B streptococcal disease can be prevented in this way.[70] Reverse vaccinology strategies resulted in the identification of new protein antigens that in animal models were shown to be promising potential vaccine candidates.[71]

Streptococcus pneumoniae

In order to control the spread of (penicillin-resistant) pneumococci, restrictive antibiotic policies, isolation facilities and vaccination are indispensable. The currently available polysaccharide pneumococcal vaccines are composed of a mixture of 23 pneumococcal capsular polysaccharides; antibodies against these polysaccharides are protective.[72] However, the 23 vaccine serotypes do not cover more than 63% of the streptococcal types responsible for pneumococcal infections in other parts of the world. The response rate in the healthy adult population is variable.[26] Although there have been some conflicting data, pneumococcal vaccination does not appear to protect against nonbacteremic pneumonia in adults. The poor immunogenicity of the polysaccharide vaccine in children younger than 2 years and people at risk for pneumococcal disease is a major problem; an insufficient response is observed in asplenic or elderly people. An answer to immunogenicity would be to include a protein in the antigen preparation, thereby generating a T-cell-dependent memory response.[59] A 7-valent conjugate vaccine has been licensed in the USA. Surveillance after the introduction of PCV7 to the standard childhood immunization schedule has shown that the vaccine is effective in preventing invasive pneumococcal disease (IPD) and providing herd immunity. However, surveillance of pneumococcal isolates in children with IPD indicates that, since the introduction of PCV7 to the routine childhood immunization schedule, there has been an increase in the proportion of cases of IPD caused by nonvaccine serotypes (e.g. replacement serotypes).[73]

Prevention of endocarditis

Recommendations for the routine use of antibiotics for the prevention of (mainly streptococcal) endocarditis have recently been the subject of substantial review and discussion (Table 166.5).[74,75] For a more detailed discussion see Chapter 47.

REFERENCES

References for this chapter can be found online at http://www.expertconsult.com

---

Table 166.5 Endocarditis prophylaxis

Patients at the highest risk	Prophylaxis was recommended only in those settings associated with the highest risk of developing an adverse outcome if infective endocarditis (IE) were to occur. Patients with the following cardiac conditions were considered to meet this criterion: • prosthetic heart valves, including bioprosthetic and homograft valves • a prior history of IE • unrepaired cyanotic congenital heart disease, including palliative shunts and conduits • completely repaired congenital heart defects with prosthetic material or device, whether placed by surgery or by catheter intervention, during the first 6 months after the procedure • repaired congenital heart disease with residual defects at the site or adjacent to the site of the prosthetic device • cardiac 'valvulopathy' in a transplanted heart (valvulopathy is defined as documentation of substantial leaflet pathology and regurgitation). Similar limited criteria for prophylaxis were proposed in 2006 by the Working Party of the British Society for Antimicrobial Chemotherapy. 'Valvulopathy' in a transplanted heart was not included, but these guidelines also included complex left ventricular outflow abnormalities including aortic stenosis and bicuspid aortic valves, or acquired valvulopathy or mitral valve prolapse with echocardiographic evidence of substantial leaflet pathology and regurgitation.
No longer indicated	Common valvular lesions for which antimicrobial prophylaxis is no longer recommended in the 2007 American Heart Association guidelines include bicuspid aortic valve, acquired aortic or mitral valve disease (including mitral valve prolapse with regurgitation and those who have undergone prior valve repair) and hypertrophic cardiomyopathy with latent or resting obstruction.

Reproduced from Wilson et al.[75]

Chapter | **167** | *Guy Prod'hom*
Jacques Bille

Aerobic Gram-positive bacilli

INTRODUCTION

The last 20 years have led to the description of an explosion of new bacterial species, and aerobic Gram-positive bacilli are not an exception. Although most of the new species have been recovered only occasionally from human material, the key representative species have enjoyed renewed interest, for very different reasons.

Listeria monocytogenes, feared for its high associated morbidity and mortality, has extended its clinical presentations from the classic invasive food-borne pathogen to a sporadic or epidemic gastroenteritis. *Bacillus anthracis*, once an occasional agent of cutaneous anthrax in exposed persons, is now the most studied agent of bioterrorism. *Corynebacterium* spp. also enjoy renewed attention with their propensity to colonize and infect foreign materials. Finally, *Nocardia* spp. are still a rare but classic finding in the growing population of severely immunosuppressed patients.

Thus, this chapter will essentially focus on the few pathogenic species that play a major role in infectious diseases. Practical algorithms will be proposed to speed up their preliminary identification (Fig. 167.1). The major emphasis is on the laboratory diagnosis of these bacteria; their associated clinical presentations are discussed elsewhere in this book.

If most of the aerobic Gram-positive rods have an irregular shape, the most important (*Listeria*, *Bacillus*, *Erysipelothrix*) have a regular one. Almost all are nonpigmented, except *Oerskovia*. All are nonspore forming except *Bacillus* spp. A few exhibit filamentous growth: *Nocardia*, *Gordonia*, *Rhodococcus*, *Tsukamurella* and *Streptomyces*.

Commonly found aerobic Gram-positive rods can be preliminarily differentiated by a few simple tests:

- *Listeria monocytogenes* is catalase positive, motile and β-hemolytic on blood agar plates;
- *Bacillus* spp. display spores;
- *Erysipelothrix* is catalase negative and produces H_2S in triple sugar iron (TSI) slants; and
- *Corynebacterium* spp. are catalase positive, club-shaped, nonbranching rods.

Listeria monocytogenes

NATURE

The genus *Listeria* comprises six species: *L. monocytogenes*, *L. ivanovii*, *L. seeligeri*, *L. innocua*, *L. welshimeri* and *L. grayi*. Only *L. monocytogenes* is regularly pathogenic for humans; *L. ivanovii* very rarely causes clinical disease but it is pathogenic for animals. The genus *Listeria* belongs

to the *Clostridium* subdivision of Gram-positive bacilli, where it forms a family with *Brochothrix* with a characteristic low G+C DNA content (<42%). The six *Listeria* species are separated into two lineages, one comprising *L. monocytogenes*, *L. innocua* and *L. ivanovii*, and the other *L. welshimeri*, *L. seeligeri* and *L. grayi*.[1]

Morphologically, *Listeria* colonies appear as nonspore forming, nonbranching, regular short (0.5–2 × 0.4–0.5 μm) Gram-positive rods occurring singly or in short chains. *Listeria* is motile at room temperature but not at 99°F (37°C). On blood agar plates, *Listeria* grows as smooth, gray, small colonies (1–2 mm in diameter after 1–2 days of incubation at 95°F/35°C). Its growth is optimal at 95–99°F (35–37°C) in an aerobic atmosphere, but occurs also at lower temperatures (including refrigerator temperature), in an anaerobic atmosphere, at low pH (≥4.5) and in a high salt concentration (up to 10% NaCl).

Listeria spp. produce catalase but not oxidase, and characteristically hydrolyze esculin. Indole reaction is negative and H_2S is not produced. Acid production from various sugars allows a differentiation within species. In addition, *L. monocytogenes* is β-hemolytic on blood agar plates, and can be differentiated from another β-hemolytic species, *L. ivanovii*, by the CAMP reaction (enhancement of β-hemolysis in the vicinity of *Staphylococcus aureus* streak culture).[2]

EPIDEMIOLOGY

Listeria spp. are widely distributed in the environment, and have been regularly recovered from soil, water, sewage, vegetables and animal feed.

Listeria monocytogenes has been isolated from a wide variety of food or food products such as milk products, raw or transformed meat, smoked fish, seafood and raw vegetables. It is a very robust organism, resisting many adverse conditions in the food processing chain or during storage.[3] *Listeria monocytogenes* colonizes or causes disease in many animals, mainly in bovines, ovines and caprines, but also in fish, crustaceans and birds. In humans, it can be carried asymptomatically and transiently in feces in up to 5% of the healthy population.

Listeria monocytogenes infections are almost all caused by the ingestion of contaminated food. They occur as sporadic cases or as outbreaks. Two major forms of clinical presentation can occur: the classic invasive disease causing bacteremia, meningitis or meningo-encephalitis or infection of the offspring in pregnant women, and the newly recognized, less severe gastroenteritis form.[4] Host factors and level of inoculum are the main determinants of these two presentations.

The annual incidence of invasive listeriosis varies between 3 and 15 cases per 10^6 population in countries with a surveillance system.

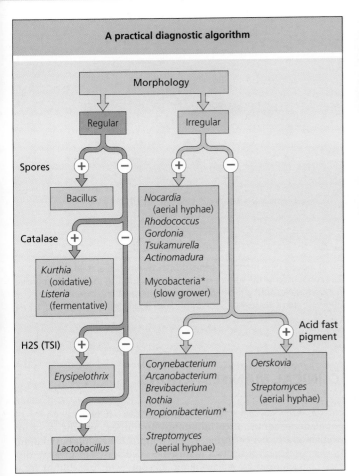

A practical diagnostic algorithm

Fig. 167.1 A practical diagnostic algorithm. * Not dealt with in this review.

Although much less common than *Salmonella* or *Campylobacter*, foodborne listeriosis is much more severe, with an associated hospitalization rate of more than 95%, and a mortality rate of 20–40%. At particular risk of developing an invasive disease are the populations at the two extremes of age, as well as some immunocompromised patients (renal transplant patients and those with HIV infection with a low CD4$^+$ cell count). Other predisposing conditions are diabetes, alcoholism, liver or renal insufficiency and a high gastric pH. During outbreaks, immunocompetent persons exposed to a high inoculum can develop invasive disease. Outbreaks of invasive cases have been ascribed to different food vehicles. Among them, milk products (in particular ripened cheese), raw or undercooked meat and smoked fish have been implicated. When known, the level of contamination has been as high as 10^5 to 10^6 cfu/g of food. In these outbreaks the proportion of the maternofetal versus nonpregnant adult cases has varied greatly, as well as the distribution between bacteremia, meningitis and meningoencephalitis cases.

Not all *L. monocytogenes* strains are able to cause an invasive disease or an outbreak. Whereas *L. monocytogenes* strains can be classified into three serogroups and 13 serotypes, only three usually cause invasive disease (serotypes 4b, 1/2a and 1/2b). Most of the outbreaks described between 1980 and 1995 were caused by *L. monocytogenes* serotype 4b and within this serotype by restricted clones defined by phage or various molecular typing methods. Recently it has been shown that only the isolates harboring an intact internalin sequence are associated with invasive disease.[5]

Outbreaks of gastroenteritis seem to be associated with different strains and particularly with a very high level of contamination

($>10^6$ cfu/g of food). Major vehicles have been milk-based beverages, various salads or cold prepared dishes served during hot weather.[6]

Small nosocomial outbreaks have occasionally occurred in neonatal wards.

PATHOGENICITY

The mechanisms of pathogenicity of *L. monocytogenes* from its ingestion to its multiplication in selected target organs are incompletely understood. The inoculum necessary to trigger an invasive infection is not known, but it probably varies according to the magnitude of defects in host defenses. Resistant to the pH of gastric fluid, *L. monocytogenes* cells first attach to epithelial cells of the intestinal mucosa. The initial event involves the bacterial surface protein internalin A (InlA), a potent virulence factor which attaches to E-cadherin, a transmembrane glycoprotein adhesin molecule at the surface of intestinal epithelial cells. E-cadherin interacts with actin which polymerizes. A second protein, internalin B (InlB), contributes to *Listeria* entry by a different mechanism.[7]

After entry into the cell, *Listeria* cells are able to escape from the internalization vacuole thanks to listeriolysin O (LLO), a pore-forming toxin. In the cytosol, *Listeria* replicates freely and moves by the recruitment and polymerization of actin at one pole of the bacterium, the surface protein Ac+A. Moving to the opposite surface of the cell, *Listeria* protrudes into the neighboring cell and, by cell-to-cell spread, is able to disseminate in tissues. Recent advances have been made in the understanding of the very peculiar tropism of *Listeria* for specialized tissues such as placenta or the central nervous system (CNS). Both have an E-cadherin at the surface of some specialized cells (syncytiotrophoblasts, choroid plexus epithelium), allowing attachment of the bacteria.

Acquired immunity after infection is mediated by phagocytosis (by macrophages and monocytes), followed by binding of the bacterial peptides to major histocompatibility complex (MHC) class I molecules. This complex is then recognized by CD8$^+$ cytotoxic T cells and by T-helper cells. Cytokines – interferon gamma (IFNγ), macrophage colony-stimulating factor (M-CSF) and tumor necrosis factor (TNF) – are produced which enhance host resistance. In the premature infant and the neonate, macrophage activation is delayed and the number of natural killer (NK) cells reduced, increasing the susceptibility to *Listeria*. Both antibodies against somatic (O) and flagellar (H) antigens are produced after infection, but their determination is too complex to be used for diagnosis. More recently, the detection of antibodies to listeriolysin O in the blood has been claimed to be both sensitive and specific, but has not yet been used extensively.

Diagnostic Microbiology

Direct examination

Gram staining of clinical material should be attempted, particularly in normally sterile samples such as cerebrospinal fluid (CSF), amniotic fluid or placenta. Small Gram-positive bacilli or coccobacilli are suggestive in an appropriate specimen.

Listeria may sometimes be confused with enterococci, streptococci or corynebacteria.

The sensitivity of Gram stain direct examination of CSF to detect *Listeria* is rather low (30–40%) due to the usual low number of organisms.[8] It is much higher in meconium or ear swab of the infected neonate.

Culture

Listeria monocytogenes is easy to isolate from normally sterile clinical samples such as blood, CSF, placenta or amniotic fluid. These

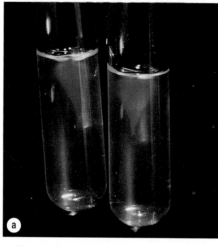
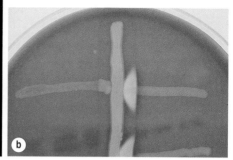

Fig. 167.2 Tests for the identification of *Listeria monocytogenes*. (a) Demonstration of motility of *L. monocytogenes* grown in semisolid agar at room temperature. Note that the migration of the organism from the central stab is more pronounced at the surface of the soft agar, forming the typical umbrella-shaped pattern in both tubes. (b) CAMP test. Enhanced hemolysis patterns of *L. monocytogenes* (left) and *Streptococcus agalactiae* (right) colonies are shown; these are growing adjacent to a streak of *Staphylococcus aureus* colonies in the center. Courtesy of Robert Bortolussi and Timothy Mailman.

specimens can be plated onto blood agar plates and blood inoculated in standard blood culture bottles.

Normally contaminated samples such as stool, genital swabs, gastric fluid and ear swab require the addition of selective solid or liquid media.

Food samples require special handling, with selective enrichment steps and indicator media.

On solid media, *L. monocytogenes* will grow in 18–24 hours as small grayish smooth colonies with a discrete β-hemolysis underneath the colonies.

Identification

Key characteristics to identify *L. monocytogenes* from colonies on agar media are the Gram stain morphology, tumbling motility in a wet mount or in semisolid agar slant (Fig. 167.2a), a positive catalase reaction and hydrolysis of esculin. A correct determination of hemolysis is essential to differentiate *L. monocytogenes* from other hemolytic or nonhemolytic *Listeria* spp. The CAMP test (for Christie, Atkins, Munch-Peterson) uses a strain of *S. aureus* producing a betalysin and a strain of *Rhodococcus equi* streaked in one direction on a sheep blood agar plate, and the *Listeria* spp. culture to test streaked at right angle (Fig. 167.2b).[1] *Staphylococcus aureus* betalysin enhances the hemolysis of *L. monocytogenes* whereas *R. equi* enhances the hemolysis of *L. ivanovii*.

Commercial kits allow the identification of *Listeria* to the genus level or to the species level (API-Listeria test, Vitek 2). A DNA probe assay performed on colonies provides rapid confirmation of *L. monocytogenes*.

Antimicrobial susceptibility testing is not mandatory for *L. monocytogenes*, the susceptibility pattern of which is rather predictable. Penicillin, aminoglycosides and trimethoprim–sulfamethoxazole are bactericidal. Cephalosporins are inactive *in vitro*, and should not be used when *Listeria* is among the suspected agents of CNS infection.

There is no currently commercially available serologic test to be recommended.

Several typing systems have been developed primarily for the investigation of food-borne outbreaks. Serotyping is still the reference phenotypic method whereas pulsed field gel electrophoresis is the most widely used for molecular typing. More recent methods (multilocus sequence typing, polymerase chain reaction (PCR)-based methods) are currently being evaluated.[9]

CLINICAL MANIFESTATIONS

Listeria monocytogenes causes invasive disease in two categories of populations: adults, often immunocompromised, and the pregnant woman and/or her offspring. In the nonpregnant adult population, *L. monocytogenes* causes two main types of disease: an invasive disease characterized by a bacteremic episode, with or without focal organ involvement (CNS, disseminated disease), and a febrile gastroenteritis.[4]

Invasive disease varies in presentation according to the age of the patient and the level of immunosuppression. Classically, one differentiates uncomplicated bacteremia without obvious organ involvement from bacteremia with CNS involvement. Several presentations of CNS disease can occur: meningitis, meningoencephalitis, rhombencephalitis and rarely brain abscesses.

Isolated bacteremia is the most frequent presentation of listeriosis, particularly among severely immunocompromised patients, representing about 40% of all cases of invasive diseases.

Associated clinical symptoms are rather nonspecific: fever, myalgias, nausea and diarrhea in a minority of patients. Focal infections following bacteremia are uncommon. The most frequently reported are liver abscess, cholecystitis, peritonitis, splenic abscess, joint infections and endophthalmitis. Endocarditis is rare and can occur both on native and prosthetic valves. *Listeria* endocarditis is a severe disease with a high rate of complications and a high mortality (>50%).

Central nervous system infections

Listeria display a particular tropism for CNS tissue, which has been recently explained at the molecular level. Following bacteremia, three main presentations may occur: meningitis, meningoencephalitis and brain abscess. A peculiar form of encephalitis involving the pons is classically described under the name of rhombencephalitis.

Meningitis due to *Listeria* ranks as number four or five, but as number one for mortality (≥20%). In neonates and patients older than 60 years, *Listeria* represents 20% of all bacterial etiologies of meningitis. In patients with lymphoma, solid-organ transplant or on steroid therapy, it ranks as number one. Almost all patients are either immunocompromised or older than 50 years, or both.

The clinical presentation is subacute to acute, nuchal rigidity is less common than with other etiologic agents, movement disorders can be seen in 15–20% of the cases, as well as seizures and fluctuation of mental status. The triad of fever, neck stiffness and alterations of mental status is present in less than 50% of cases.[8]

The diagnosis is based on blood cultures (positive in up to 75% of the cases) and CSF culture (40% of the cases have a low glucose level and a positive direct Gram stain). There is usually a moderate CSF pleocytosis; despite its name, listerial meningitis can be characterized by neutrophils rather than monocytes.

Listeria encephalitis, also named rhombencephalitis due to its similarity to the circling disease described in sheep, is more frequent in previously healthy adults than the meningitic form. It classically occurs in two phases, starting with an episode of fever, headaches, nausea and vomiting, followed 3–5 days later by the development of cranial nerve deficits, cerebellar signs or hemiparesis.[10,11] Nuchal rigidity is seen in about 50% of the cases and respiratory failure in 40%. Mortality is very high, in part due to the often delayed diagnosis and treatment. The microbiologic diagnosis of *Listeria* rhombencephalitis is sometimes particularly difficult because blood cultures are positive in only 60% of the cases and CSF culture in no more than 40%. MRI is more helpful than CT to document the lesions.

Brain abscess represents about 10% of CNS listerial infections, usually with a concomitant bacteremia, and in 25–40% of cases of concomitant meningitis. Typical locations are the thalamus, the pons and the medulla. Most occur as a single lesion. Associated mortality is high (40%), as well as the occurrence and severity of sequelae in surviving patients.[12]

In pregnant women, listeriosis presents classically in two phases. The first phase presents as an acute influenza-like illness with fever, chills, fatigue, myalgias and headaches, mostly in the second half of the pregnancy. When this episode is unnoticed and/or untreated, premature labor and delivery occur 2–14 days after the acute presentation. It is thus important to diagnose the first episode by blood culture. Early appropriate antibiotic treatment can prevent progression of the infection to the fetus. When the infection progresses (second phase), it can lead to death in utero or to the (premature) birth of an infected neonate. Neonatal mortality reaches 40–50%. The clinical manifestations of neonatal listeriosis differ greatly, as well as the mortality and the sensitivity of the diagnostic procedures according to the rapidity of disease onset at or after birth.[13]

Early-onset neonatal listeriosis is present at delivery or within the first 48 hours of life, and corresponds to an infection acquired in utero. The most common presentation is a pneumonia with or without sepsis (Table 167.1). The diagnosis is generally made by blood cultures or culture of meconium. Anemia and thrombocytopenia are common. The mortality of early-onset neonatal listeriosis is about 20%. Late-onset neonatal listeriosis develops generally after the first week of life

and corresponds to the acquisition of this pathogen during birth or shortly thereafter from an infected mother or from the environment. The main presentation is meningitis.

Interestingly, the proportion of fetomaternal listeriosis has diminished considerably during the last two decades, most probably reflecting a higher awareness among pregnant women to at-risk food. On the whole, the incidence of invasive listeriosis has also decreased in many developed countries, reflecting the positive impact of various measures taken at many steps during food production and among consumers.

Listeria gastroenteritis is a rather recently described entity, undisputedly documented in several large outbreaks involving numerous previously healthy subjects exposed to a highly contaminated food product, as for example, chocolate milk, rice or corn salad. Major symptoms have been fever, vomiting, abdominal cramps and diarrhea, abating after 48 hours. Very few patients develop bacteremia.[6]

TREATMENT

Listeria monocytogenes is almost uniformly susceptible to penicillins, aminoglycosides and trimethoprim–sulfamethoxazole. Based on animal studies showing synergism, the current recommendations for a severe infection is the combination of intravenous ampicillin (2 g q4h) and intravenous gentamicin (1.5–2 mg/kg q8h) for 2–4 weeks. Fewer cases have been successfully treated with intravenous trimethoprim–sulfamethoxazole (20 mg/kg q24h trimethoprim part divided into two to four doses) for 2–3 weeks. Carbapenems are alternative drugs. Bacteremia without distant focal infection can be treated by intravenous amoxicillin for 10–14 days. In the neonate, the combination of ampicillin (150 mg/kg q24h divided into three to four doses) and gentamicin (2.5 mg/kg q8h) is recommended.

Listeria gastroenteritis is usually not treated by antibiotics due to its benign and rapidly favorable course, and low risk of associated invasive disease. Oral ampicillin or trimethoprim–sulfamethoxazole may be considered in patients at risk.[6] In pregnant women with positive blood cultures, intravenous ampicillin (2 g q6h) should be administered.

PREVENTION

The great majority of *Listeria* infections are food-borne, occurring more often sporadically (>90%) than as an outbreak.[14]

Several measures have been, or should be, taken at various levels in the food chain:

- pathogen elimination at production level of ready-to-eat at-risk food (especially meat or poultry); and
- in the consumer kitchen, wash raw vegetables, keep refrigerator temperature below 5°C, keep raw food products separate, wash hands and kitchen instruments after use, and cook raw meat properly.

Individuals at risk, such as pregnant women and the immunocompromised, should not eat at-risk food products such as cold meat, refrigerated pates or meat spreads, unwashed salad, various soft cheese or smoked seafood.

Bacillus

NATURE

The genus *Bacillus* comprises more than 200 species of which two, *B. anthracis* and *B. cereus*, are especially important as agents of disease in humans. *Bacillus* spp. are ubiquitous Gram-positive bacilli. They

Table 167.1 Neonatal listeriosis		
	Early onset (1–2 days of life)	**Late onset (>7 days of life)**
Pneumonia	62%	
Meningitis	21%	94%
Anemia	62%	
Thrombocytopenia	35%	
Positive blood culture	73%	
Positive meconium stain and culture	69%	17%
Mortality (live-born)	20%	

are characterized by their production of resistant endospores in the presence of oxygen. They have a wide range of G+C content (from 32 to 69). Morphologically, *Bacillus* spp. cells appear as spore-forming, large (3–5 × 1 μm), Gram-positive aerobic or facultative anaerobic mesophilic rods occurring singly or in pairs. Some *Bacillus* spp. are motile, others are not. On agar media, *Bacillus* spp. usually grow as large, irregular colonies easy to recognize. Most are saprophytes widely distributed in the environment.[15]

Bacillus anthracis

EPIDEMIOLOGY

Known since 1877 when Robert Koch first cultivated *B. anthracis*, this agent received increased attention only after its use as a bioterrorism agent in 2001.[16]

Bacillus anthracis is ubiquitous and can be recovered worldwide as a saprophytic organism from soil, water and dust. It belongs to the normal intestinal flora of many mammals including humans. As a sporulating bacterium, *B. anthracis* can survive for decades in soil before being ingested, usually by herbivore animals in which it can transform into a vegetative form or is eliminated in feces. In animals, *B. anthracis* causes severe gastrointestinal damage and high losses, particularly in nonimmunized herds in developing countries. Major outbreaks involving thousands of bovines have been reported in Africa, whereas the incidence of animal anthrax is very low in the Western world, particularly for inhalation anthrax. In humans the most frequent presentation by far is cutaneous anthrax (>95% of the reported cases), with very few cases of inhalation anthrax or gastrointestinal anthrax, which is the most frequent form in ruminants. Accidental anthrax can occur in laboratory workers or in relation to a bioterrorism event, leading to pulmonary anthrax. Naturally acquired human infections occur by accident, when *B. anthracis* spores or cells enter the body, generally through an abrasion. It is mainly restricted to persons in contact with an infected animal (farmers or veterinarians) or with animal products (skin handlers).

There are no documented cases of human-to-human transmission. The incubation time can vary widely, from a few days (1–7) to months when few spores have been inhaled. The lethal dose is probably small (2500–50 000 spores), as suggested by the tragic episode in Russia (Sverdlovsk) in 1979, when an explosion in an arms manufacturing plant caused at least 66 deaths, some of them up to 60 km from the epicenter.[17]

PATHOGENICITY

The virulence of *B. anthracis* is mediated by a complex interplay of three thermolabile proteins under the control of two plasmids. In addition, a large capsule made of poly-D-glutamic acid contributes to the virulence.[18]

The three components of the toxins are a protective antigen (PA, 83 kDa), an edema factor (EF, 89 kDa) and a lethal factor (LF, 90 kDa). Individually, they have no harmful effect. PA binds to two cell surface receptors – the tumor endothelium marker 8 (TEM8) and the capillary morphogenesis protein 2 (CMG2) – and is subsequently cleaved by a cell protease.[19] The cleaved particle (PA 63) binds to the two other components and enters by endocytosis. EF activity depends on calcium; LF interferes with the protein kinase signal transduction pathway. When assembled, PA–EF and PA–LF kill the macrophages by proteolysis and induce a release of cytokines, particularly interleukin (IL)-1 and TNF, interfering with the coagulation system and causing edema (PA–EF).

The large capsule observed mostly *in vivo* in clinical specimens is made of linear polymer of glutamic acid, and is antiphagocytic and very weakly immunogenic. These virulence factors are under the control of two large interconnected plasmids, pX01 (controlling for toxin production and carrying a pathogenicity island) and pX02 (controlling for capsule production). The toxins are mainly produced during the multiplication of the vegetative form in host tissues. External factors such as the temperature and the sodium bicarbonate concentration act on regulatory plasmid genes. In addition to the capsule, *B. anthracis* possess another unique cell-wall structure named the S layer, which is made of glycoproteins and is responsible for the shape of the bacteria.

DIAGNOSTIC MICROBIOLOGY

Direct examination

Gram staining of appropriate clinical material (skin lesion or ulcer biopsy, blood, CSF, sputum, pleural fluid) shows large, encapsulated, box-shaped, Gram-positive bacilli without spores. The sensitivity of direct examination in skin material from cutaneous anthrax is rather low (<30%). A direct fluorescent antibody (DFA) stain using an antibody against the capsular glutamic acid or a special stain (McFadyean methylene blue) can enhance detection of the capsule.

Direct detection in clinical samples can also be attempted by *B. anthracis*-specific molecular amplification or by antigen detection.[20]

Culture

Bacillus anthracis grows rapidly on aerobic standard agar media as large, flat, spreading, nonhemolytic, white to gray sticky colonies, with a typical morphology called 'medusa-head'. Cells are catalase-positive, nonmotile and produce endospores but no capsule on solid media.

Identification

Key characteristics to identify *B. anthracis* from appropriate clinical material are the Gram staining morphology, a positive catalase reaction, and the absence of motility and of frank hemolysis on blood agar. Confirmation of identification can be achieved with species-specific PCR and/or by lysis of colonies by a specific phage (γ phage).[21] Growth on agar medium enriched in sodium bicarbonate (at 0.8%) and incubated under 5% CO_2 will favor the formation of a large capsule. DFA assay and a rapid immunochromatographic test targeting the S layer to be used with colonies are also available.

Antibiotic susceptibility testing is generally not attempted because *B. anthracis* wild strains are usually susceptible to penicillins, tetracyclines, quinolones, rifampin (rifampicin), vancomycin and clindamycin, and resistant to the cephalosporins and to trimethoprim–sulfamethoxazole.

CLINICAL MANIFESTATIONS

There are three clinical presentations due to *B. anthracis* directly related to the mode of infection: a cutaneous form by direct transdermal inoculation of spores, a respiratory form following spore inhalation and a digestive form following ingestion of spores. By number of cases the most important is the cutaneous form and by severity the respiratory form. The digestive form, predominant in ruminants, is exceedingly rare in humans. (For further discussion, see Chapter 128.)

Bacillus cereus

NATURE

Bacillus cereus is the second *Bacillus* species of interest in human diseases. It is ubiquitous in nature, and can easily contaminate various raw or processed foods or damaged human skin.

Bacillus cereus is a large Gram-positive bacillus with four major properties, differentiating it from *B. anthracis*: motility, hemolysis, absence of capsule and resistance to penicillin.

EPIDEMIOLOGY

Bacillus cereus represents a significant cause of food poisoning (variable incidence, usually 1–3%). It is widely present in various raw or processed food products such as rice, vegetables, turkey meat and spices. Spores usually naturally contaminate the food environment.

PATHOGENICITY

Bacillus cereus carries two toxins, one responsible for a diarrheal syndrome (enterotoxin) and one for an emetic syndrome. The enterotoxin is a 38–57 kDa thermolabile protein, preformed or produced in the small intestine, acting on adenylcyclase. The emetic toxin is a 10 kDa peptide which is highly thermostable and resistant to proteolytic degradation. Its effect is classically observed when rice or pasta meals are consumed cold after cooking. In both cases, spores of *B. cereus* resist the heating process, and germinate and multiply during storage of the leftover food.[22]

DIAGNOSTIC MICROBIOLOGY

In clinical material – particularly in tissue – *B. cereus* appears as a large bacillus with a central endospore. *Bacillus cereus* can be cultured easily from blood or tissue biopsies, and appears on blood agar as large, flat, granular to ground-glass, β-hemolytic colonies of variable shape (circular to irregular) (Fig. 167.3, lanes 6C and 6D). They can be easily taken up with a loop, as opposed to *B. anthracis* colonies which are sticky. Its isolation from contaminated material such as feces, vomitus or food items requires selective media usually containing mannitol, egg yolk and antibiotics. *Bacillus cereus* is facultative anaerobe and gives a positive lecithinase reaction on egg yolk medium.[15]

CLINICAL MANIFESTATIONS AND MANAGEMENT

The diarrheal syndrome caused by the enterotoxin is characterized by an episode of profuse diarrhea with abdominal pain and cramps, occurring 8–16 hours after ingestion of the contaminated food. Fever and vomiting occur rarely.

The other clinical syndrome is food poisoning. For an extensive clinical discussion, see Chapters 34 and 35.

As well as the classic gastrointestinal diseases, *B. cereus* also occasionally causes an array of focal or invasive diseases:

- in immunocompromised hosts, bacteremia, meningitis, endocarditis, brain abscess, pneumonia;
- in surgical patients, wound infections, after traffic accidents or burns;
- in neonates, infection of the umbilical cord; and
- in contact lens-wearing patients, keratitis or endophthalmitis.

It is important to consider the potential pathogenic role of *B. cereus* in these situations and not automatically disregard a positive culture for *Bacillus* considered as a simple contamination.

Bacillus cereus is resistant to penicillins and cephalosporins (due to the presence of a β-lactamase) but is usually susceptible to aminoglycosides, glycopeptides, clindamycin, ciprofloxacin and erythromycin. The recommended therapy for severe infection is the combination of vancomycin and an aminoglycoside, and clindamycin with gentamicin for ophthalmic infections. Ciprofloxacin has been used successfully to treat wound infections and bacteremia.

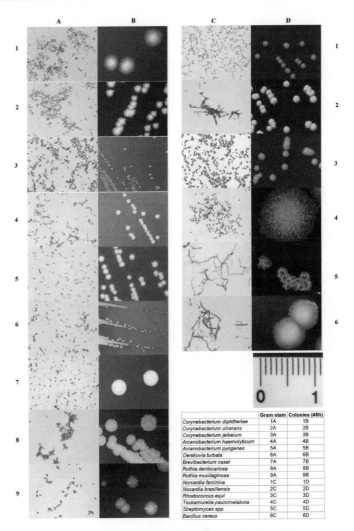

	Gram stain	Colonies (48h)
Corynebacterium diphtheriae	1A	1B
Corynebacterium ulcerans	2A	2B
Corynebacterium jeikeium	3A	3B
Arcanobacterium haemolyticum	4A	4B
Arcanobacterium pyogenes	5A	5B
Oerskovia turbata	6A	6B
Brevibacterium casei	7A	7B
Rothia dentocariosa	8A	8B
Rothia mucilaginosa	9A	9B
Norcardia farcinica	1C	1D
Nocardia brasiliensis	2C	2D
Rhodococcus equi	3C	3D
Tsukamurella paurometabola	4C	4D
Streptomyces spp.	5C	5D
Bacillus cereus	6C	6D

Fig. 167.3 Gram stain and colonies (48-hour incubation) of different Gram-positive bacilli.

Erysipelothrix

NATURE

Erysipelothrix rhusiopathiae is a small Gram-positive bacillus, widespread in nature, causing self-limited illnesses or systemic infections in various animals, swine in particular, and occasionally in humans. *Erysipelothrix rhusiopathiae* is a thin, elongated (0.2–0.4 × 0.8–2.5 μm) Gram-positive to gram-labile, aerobic to facultative anaerobic bacillus, nonmotile, nonsporulated and nonencapsulated, belonging to the clade of Gram-positive bacilli with a low G+C content (36–40%) (*Listeria*, *Lactobacillus*, *Kurthia*, *Brochothrix*).[23]

EPIDEMIOLOGY

Erysipelothrix rhusiopathiae is ubiquitous in nature, found on plants, in humid soil and used water, as well as in many animals as asymptomatic carriers. The major reservoir is the pig, where it is carried in the pharynx or digestive tract as a commensal. It can also cause a disease called swine erysipelas, presenting as skin infection, arthritis or septicemia.[24]

Humans usually develop a local infection through direct contact with an infected animal or animal product. At particular risk are butchers and fishermen handling crabs, but also farmers, abattoir workers and veterinarians. There is no documented human-to-human transmission.

PATHOGENICITY

Several components of *E. rhusiopathiae* are though to play a role in virulence: these include an antiphagocytic capsule, a surface protein (Spa A), the enzyme neuraminidase and the capacity to survive in macrophages. The exact mechanisms, however, are not firmly established.

DIAGNOSTIC MICROBIOLOGY

For localized erysipeloid lesion(s), the best clinical specimen is a deep tissue biopsy or liquid when present in vesicles. Swabs of the skin surface are to be discouraged. Blood cultures are taken for systemic disease.

The microscopy of a tissue biopsy is occasionally positive for thin Gram-positive bacilli. On blood agar, *E. rhusiopathiae* appears as punctiform colonies, α-hemolytic after 2 days, either as gray, translucent and regular S colonies (smooth variant) or as larger, opaque, irregular R colonies (rough variant). Growth is enhanced in 5–10% CO_2 at 91–99°F (33–37°C) and usually present in liquid media.

Preliminary identification relies on the pleomorphic Gram stain and cultural appearance of the colonies. *Erysipelothrix rhusiopathiae* is catalase-negative, nonmotile and non-β-hemolytic, but H_2S positive in 24–48 hours on TSI or Kligler slant agar.[2] There is an indirect immunofluorescence test, as well as a mouse inoculation test used in reference laboratories. There is no serologic test currently available.

Erysipelothrix rhusiopathiae isolates can be typed in two serogroups (A and B) and 23 serovars for epidemiologic purposes. *Erysipelothrix rhusiopathiae* is susceptible *in vitro* to penicillins, cephalosporins, clindamycin and erythromycin, more or less susceptible to tetracyclines and chloramphenicol, and resistant to vancomycin, aminoglycosides, sulfonamides and trimethoprim–sulfamethoxazole.[25]

CLINICAL MANIFESTATIONS AND MANAGEMENT

Erysipelothrix rhusiopathiae has three distinct clinical presentations, as follows.

- A cutaneous lesion called erysipeloid, localized to the upper extremities (generally the fingers) around an inoculation site, and characterized by a painful itching and burning erythematous, violaceous, well-demarcated lesion developing over 10 days after inoculation. Fever or arthralgias are uncommon, but localized lymphangitis (30%) and lymphadenopathy (30%) are frequent. In the absence of treatment, spontaneous healing generally occurs.
- A diffuse cutaneous disease with skin and soft tissue extension from the original inoculation site. This form is less frequent and is observed in some immunocompromised patients, in whom systemic manifestations (fever, arthralgia) are common.
- A disseminated disease, usually septicemia, often (up to 90%) complicated by an endocarditis on native valve. This form is usually a primary infection but can follow an erysipeloid lesion in about 40% of cases. The disease is often characterized by a long-lasting fever, with multiple cutaneous lesions on the trunk or the extremities. Classic underlying conditions are alcohol abuse and/or chronic liver disease, as well as corticosteroid use or chemotherapy. The associated mortality is rather high (38%).[26]

The treatment of uncomplicated erysipeloid skin lesions (with oral penicillin, 500 mg q6h, for 1 week or another active drug, such as another β-lactam, fluoroquinolones or clindamycin) will accelerate natural healing. For severe cutaneous disease or disseminated disease the recommended therapy is intravenous benzylpenicillin (2–4 million units q4h), ceftriaxone (2 g q24h) or ciprofloxacin (400 mg q12h) for 2–4 weeks.[24] As there are no human vaccines, the only form of disease prevention is to limit occupational exposure to the organism.

Corynebacterium diphtheriae and *C. ulcerans*

NATURE

Diphtheria is now a rare disease. This communicable infectious and vaccine-preventable disease may result in acute localized respiratory infection with typical 'croup' symptomatology due to the development of oropharyngeal adherent pseudomembranes. The mortality is due to airway obstruction or myocarditis caused by toxin production. *Corynebacterium diphtheriae* is a small, irregular, nonsporulated, Gram-positive bacillus with enlarged extremities and a typical 'club-shaped' morphology. A 'palisade' or 'V' arrangement or clusters with a so-called Chinese-letter appearance are observed in liquid media (Fig. 167.3, lanes 1A and 1B). *Corynebacterium* spp. belong to the broad class Actinobacteria. Phylogenetic studies show that *Corynebacterium* spp. are closely related to acid-fast bacilli such as *Mycobacterium*.

Corynebacterium ulcerans shares certain common features with *C. diphtheriae*. *Corynebacterium ulcerans* causes a rare oropharyngeal diphtheria-like illness, as well as extra pharyngeal infections due to the presence of a toxin similar to diphtheria toxin. Taxonomic studies show that *C. ulcerans* is closely related to *C. diphtheriae*.[27]

EPIDEMIOLOGY

Diphtheria remains endemic in numerous countries throughout the world – Eastern Europe, South East Asia, South America and the Indian subcontinent. In developed countries, diphtheria occurs sporadically and most cases are imported from areas of endemicity.[28]

During the 1990s, an important outbreak occurred in Russia and the newly independent states of the former Soviet Union, with more than 157 000 cases and 5000 deaths. Several factors may explain the re-emergence of epidemic diphtheria, notably the introduction of a toxigenic strain, insufficient coverage of vaccination of children and an increasing proportion of adults with waning vaccine-induced immunity. Contrary to the prevaccine era, where diphtheria was essentially a childhood disease, a shift in the age of patients was observed. The epidemic began in towns and in groups with close contacts (e.g. hospitals, military troops), before dissemination to socioeconomically disfavored groups (e.g. alcoholics).[29,30]

Achieving a high coverage (90–95%) of primary immunization is mandatory for diphtheria elimination and periodic booster doses for adults are necessary in regions at high risk of diphtheria. Control measures allow the control of epidemic diphtheria. In 1997, the World Health Organization (WHO) identified 10 countries with more than 10 cases for a total number of 15 839 cases reported, whereas in 2006 the number of reported cases decreased to 4000.

Humans represent the sole significant reservoir for *C. diphtheriae*. Acquisition occurs essentially through direct transmission (or via airborne droplet) with contaminated respiratory secretions or skin lesions.

In temperate climates, respiratory infections due to toxigenic strains predominate, while in the tropics, cutaneous diphtheria is more commonly caused by nontoxigenic strains. A peak incidence of respiratory infections is observed during the cold months.

In diphtheria endemic areas with high prevalence of cutaneous diphtheria, respiratory diphtheria is rare due to the high rate of natural immunity attained through exposure to cutaneous diphtheria. In most cases, transmission of *C. diphtheriae* to susceptible individuals results in transient pharyngeal carriage rather than in disease. Cutaneous diphtheria appears to be more contagious than the respiratory form of diphtheria and persists longer than *C. diphtheriae* infections of the tonsils or nose in a carrier state.

Corynebacterium ulcerans is a commensal of wild and domestic animals. Human *C. ulcerans* infection is considered a zoonosis, since human transmission occurs via manipulation of infected dairy animals or consumption of contaminated milk; however, these risk factors are absent in half of the cases. Global epidemiologic data on *C. ulcerans* infection are missing but *C. ulcerans* strains represent 58% of toxigenic *Corynebacterium* strains submitted to WHO reference laboratories.[31]

PATHOGENICITY

Corynebacterium diphtheriae contains pili or fimbriae involved in initial adhesion of the bacteria to host-cell receptors; the pili also promote the aggregation of other bacteria to ensure colonization. These structures contain subunits of pilin proteins, a backbone protein component (SpaA; Spa for sortase-mediated pilus assembly) and two ancillary proteins (SpaB, SpaC). The pili are covalently linked to the peptidoglycan structure of the bacterial cell wall. Minor pilins, SpaB and SpaC, are required for pharyngeal cell adhesion, the specific receptor being currently unknown.[32] This type of pilus is encoded on a pathogenicity island, probably acquired by recent horizontal transfer. *Corynebacterium diphtheriae* is responsible for a localized predominantly pharyngeal infection with the appearance of a so-called 'pseudomembrane' made of fibrin, neutrophilic inflammation and abundant colonies of *C. diphtheriae*. The major virulence factor is a 58 kDa exotoxin responsible for the systemic complications of diphtheria, notably for myocardial and neurologic toxicity.[33] This exotoxin is very effective, since one molecule introduced into a cell can kill it.

The exotoxin gene (*tox*) is present on a family of corynephages hosted by some *C. diphtheriae* strains. The expression of toxin is reliant on an iron-dependent regulatory element (*dtxR*). The presence of iron activates *dtxR* and blocks the transcription of *tox*. Under iron-limiting conditions, generally observed on the mucosal surface, *dtxR* is inactivated and diphtheria toxin is produced. The toxin is excreted through the bacterial cell and diffuses both locally and via the circulation to all organs, the myocardium and the peripheral nerves being the most affected. Diphtheria toxin has a complex activity, resulting in cytolysis through cell-protein inhibition.

Three distinct domains of diphtheria toxin have been described:

* the carboxyl-terminal R-domain (fragment B) which is responsible for binding to the heparin-binding epidermal-like growth factor, the specific receptor for the toxin;
* internalization into endocytic vesicles which is mediated by the central part of the toxin; and
* the amino-terminal C-domain (fragment A) which is delivered in the cytosol and is responsible for the inhibition of protein synthesis by inactivating the eukaryotic elongation factor 2 (eEF-2) through adenosine diphosphate (ADP) ribosylation of diphthamide residue[34] (Fig. 167.4).

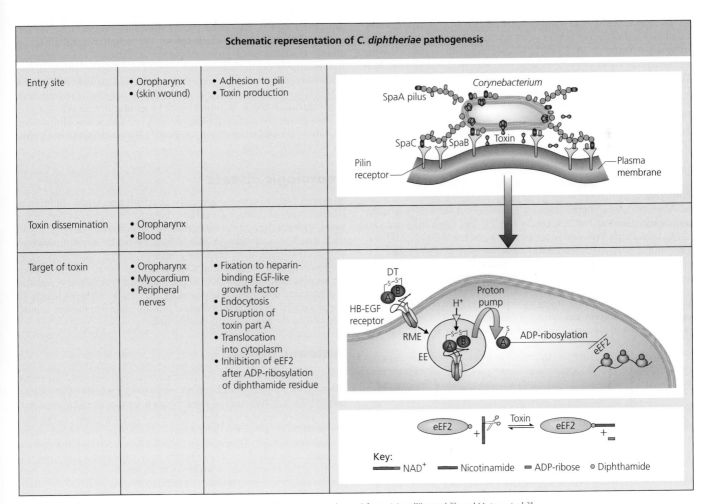

Fig. 167.4 Schematic representation of *C. diphtheriae* pathogenesis. Adapted from Mandlik et al.[32] and Yates et al.[34]

Histology of heart tissues shows necrosis associated with active inflammation in the interstitial space. Cardiac conduction tissue may also be affected. Diphtheria toxin may affect peripheral nerves, causing a demyelination localized around the nodes of Ranvier. In severe cases, axonal degeneration can occur.[35]

Corynebacterium ulcerans also carries a corynephage coding for the diphtheria toxin, and the *C. ulcerans tox* gene has 95% homology with *C. diphtheriae tox* gene. Most differences are located in the B fragment of the toxin in the translocation (T) region and in the receptor-binding (R) domain.[36]

DIAGNOSTIC MICROBIOLOGY

Due to the declining incidence of diphtheria the policy for screening throat swabs varies in different countries. In endemic regions, routine screening for *C. diphtheriae* in throat swabs is recommended since milder infections or atypical infections may be misdiagnosed. When diphtheria is suspected, clinicians should inform the laboratory.

Cotton or polyester-tipped swabs are appropriate for sampling. When membranes are removed, they should be sent to the laboratory for culture and a swab from areas under the membranes should be obtained. Standard Amies transport media ensure adequate maintenance of viability during transport to the laboratory. When molecular testing is available, Dacron polyester swabs are preferred for sampling. Suspected cases should have specimens taken from both the nose and the throat. For wound infections, swabs or aspirates of inflamed lesions are recommended.

For culture, selective media such as cysteine–tellurite blood agar or Tinsdale medium and nonselective sheep blood agar are recommended.[37] When selective media are not available, multiple colonies from sheep blood agar are picked and biochemically identified to rule out *C. diphtheriae*. Commercial biochemical tests accurately identify *C. diphtheriae* strains. *Corynebacterium diphtheriae* appear as small 0.5 mm up to 2 mm large colonies with a gray to white opaque surface (see Fig. 167.3, lanes 1A and 1B). Some strains (biotype intermedius) appear dysgonic on standard media, their colonies being enlarged on lipid-enriched media (lipophilism). Based on colony morphology and biochemical reactions, *C. diphtheriae* can be divided into four biotypes: *gravis, mitis, belfanti* and *intermedius*. However, biotyping is of limited use and is generally carried out only in reference laboratories.

Corynebacterium ulcerans grows on standard sheep blood agar media, but the use of selective media such as cysteine–tellurite blood agar or Tinsdale medium facilitates the isolation of pathogenic corynebacteria.

After 24 hours, 1 mm colonies are observed with a gray-white appearance (see Fig. 167.3, lanes 2A and 2B) and slight hemolysis on sheep blood agar. Presence of urease and a positive reverse CAMP test (inhibition reaction) differentiate *C. ulcerans* from *C. diphtheriae*.[38]

The detection of toxin is the most important test; molecular tests based on the amplification of the *tox* gene constitute an alternative to the classic Elek immunoprecipitation test. Recently, the direct detection of the *tox* gene from clinical specimens has been described; however, the amplification test cannot differentiate the *C. diphtheriae tox* gene from other toxin-producing corynebacteria such as *C. ulcerans* and *C. pseudotuberculosis*.[39]

Some toxigenic *C. ulcerans* strains show atypical results in real-time PCR for toxin detection. Specific amplification of the *C. ulcerans tox* gene have been described based on the polymorphic region of the *tox* gene.[40]

CLINICAL MANIFESTATIONS

Respiratory tract disease

Corynebacterium diphtheriae is responsible for localized infection of the upper respiratory tract. The oropharynx and rhinopharynx are most frequently affected. Symptoms generally occur 2–5 days after transmission,

the most common symptoms being a moderate fever and sore throat followed by weakness, painful swallowing and headaches. Classical adherent and gray pseudomembranes are not always present and their extent can vary from small patches on infected tonsils to an extensive involvement of the posterior oropharynx and larynx. A serous or serosanguinous discharge can be observed in nasal diphtheria which is often milder and chronic. Signs of toxicity may be present with edema of the neck, hoarseness and stridor and a marked local lymphadenopathy. In adults, atypical presentations are observed with oral lesions.[35]

Respiratory infections due to *C. ulcerans* are similar to infection due to *C. diphtheriae*.

Cutaneous disease

Cutaneous diphtheria appears usually as a chronic and nonspecific disease. In fact, *C. diphtheriae* may colonize any kind of primary cutaneous lesion. Superinfection with *C. diphtheriae* begins with vesicles or pustules evolving as skin ulcers, with edematous surrounding tissues. Dark pseudomembranes may be observed during the first 1–2 week(s). Their localization is predominantly on the legs and hands. Co-infection with other pathogens such as *S. aureus* and *Streptococcus pyogenes* is common. Systemic toxic manifestations of cutaneous diphtheria are rarely seen. Chronic cutaneous infections with gray membranes due to toxigenic *C. ulcerans* have been described.[41]

Infections due to *C. diphtheriae* and *C. ulcerans* are undoubtedly underreported since cutaneous manifestations may be mild and corynebacteria are often considered as contaminants.

Myocardial disease

Myocardial toxicity occurs in 10–20% of patients with respiratory diphtheria and is associated with a mortality rate of 40%. Its frequency depends on the extension of the oropharyngeal infection and on the delay until antitoxin therapy is started. Cardiac manifestations appear during the second week of the disease with a dilated cardiomyopathy and depressed left ventricular function. ECG shows anomalies of conduction and dysrhythmia may be observed with atrioventricular block, bundle branch block and hemiblock. Markers of poor prognosis and carditis in children are a high myoglobin level and an increased lactate dehydrogenase (LDH) isoenzyme level, with an LDH1/LDH2 ratio >1.[42]

Neurologic disease

Neuronal toxicity appears generally in severe respiratory diphtheria. Distinct types of damage are observed due to the regional effect of the toxin, with paralysis of the soft palate, of the posterior pharyngeal wall with dysphonia, dysphagia and defects of ocular accommodation; a delayed complication consisting of a peripheral neuritis affecting the limbs and/or the diaphragm can also occur up to 3 months later. Recovery is slow and only 20% of patients with diphtherial peripheral neurotoxicity were completely healthy after 1 year.[43] The incidence of severe paralysis seems reduced when prompt antitoxin therapy is initiated within the first 2–3 days of infection.

Systemic disease

Deep seated infections due to *C. diphtheriae* (e.g. endocarditis, septic arthritis, osteomyelitis and splenic abscesses) have also been documented. Risk factors such as intravenous drug use, homelessness and alcoholism have been identified. The portal of entry is likely to be skin colonization or skin infections with *C. diphtheriae*. Strains belonging to different biotypes (*gravis, mitis, belfanti*) have been isolated and are generally nontoxigenic.[44] These strains may represent a potential reservoir for the emergence of toxigenic *C. diphtheriae* strains since they possess the functional regulation machinery represented by the 'diphtheria toxin repressor (*dtxR*) genes' and thus could become toxigenic by acquiring the *tox* gene.[45]

MANAGEMENT

The management of respiratory tract diphtheria includes specific and nonspecific measures. Specific measures include the administration of diphtheria antitoxin and antibiotic treatment for *C. diphtheriae* eradication, whereas nonspecific measures are the surveillance and support of respiratory and cardiac functions. Neutralization of circulating toxin through diphtheria antitoxin represents the mainstay of diphtheria therapy. Since diphtheria antitoxin is prepared with horse hyperimmune serum, the sensitivity of the patient to horse serum should be tested before administration. According to the extent and duration of the illness, a variable dose of antitoxin is administered (Table 167.2).[46] Penicillin or erythromycin constitutes the standard antibiotic treatment. *In-vitro* resistance to penicillin has not yet been described but *in-vitro* penicillin tolerance has been documented and could explain some eradication failures.[47] Erythromycin is generally highly active *in vitro* but inducible resistance has been described.[48]

Antibiotics are used to reduce the carrier state and are combined with antitoxin to treat the disease. Erythromycin 40–50 mg/kg/day intravenously for 7–14 days is the treatment of choice, but oral penicillin (benzylpenicillin G 50 000 IU/kg/day for 5 days followed by penicillin V 50 mg/kg/day for 5 days) has been shown to be superior in a randomized trial.[48]

Testing for *C. diphtheriae* eradication is recommended at the end of treatment. Continue treatment for 10 days if culture remains positive.[46]

Close contacts should receive a single dose of penicillin or a 7-day course of erythromycin.[46]

PREVENTION

The following measures to control diphtheria have been proposed by international experts:

- primary prevention of disease based on a childhood immunization program;
- secondary prevention through rapid investigation of close contacts of index cases to prevent emergence of secondary cases, with investigation of carriage rate, clinical surveillance, penicillin prophylaxis and administration of a booster dose of diphtheria toxoid-containing vaccine; and
- tertiary prevention based on early diagnosis and proper management to prevent complications of suspected cases.[49]

Table 167.2 Dosage of antitoxin recommended for various types of diphtheria

Type of diphtheria	Dosage (units)	Route
Nasal	10 000–20 000	Intramuscular
Tonsillar	15 000–25 000	Intramuscular or intravenous
Pharyngeal or laryngeal	20 000–40 000	Intramuscular or intravenous
Combined types or delayed diagnosis	40 000–60 000	Intravenous
Severe diphtheria: extensive membrane and/or severe edema (bull-neck diphtheria)	40 000–100 000	Intravenous or part intravenous and part intramuscular

From Bonnet & Begg.[46]

Primary prevention with diphtheria toxoid obtained from formaldehyde-treated toxin is highly effective, providing high immunization rates. Recent epidemics have shown that more than 90% of children should be vaccinated to interrupt efficiently the transmission of epidemic clones.[50] The primary vaccination is based on a series of three doses started at 6 weeks of age and given at intervals of 4 weeks. Three doses induce the formation of protective toxin-neutralizing antibodies in 95.5% of children. This series is completed by at least one booster dose in the preschool period. The waning of adult immunity should be prevented with booster doses of diphtheria toxoid every 10 years throughout life. Recently, a new vaccine formulation called Tdap (for tetanus toxoid, reduced diphtheria toxoid and acellular pertussis vaccine) has been recommended for adults aged 19–64 years.[51] In endemic regions, booster doses are less necessary since natural boosting of immunity may occur through *C. diphtheriae* colonization.

Coryneforms

NATURE

The genus *Corynebacterium* contains more than 70 species, half of them being considered as pathogenic for humans in case reports or small series of cases. Taxonomic studies have shown that the genus is quite homogeneous except for a distinct subgroup formed by *Corynebacterium diphtheriae*, *C. kutscheri*, *C. pseudotuberculosis*, *C. vitarumen* and *C. ulcerans*.[27] Some *Corynebacterium* spp. have been reported as opportunist pathogens with some frequency, including *C. amycolatum*, *C. jeikeium* (formerly group JK) and *C. urealyticum*.

The so-called coryneforms represent a heterogeneous group of asporogenous, irregularly shaped, nonacid-fast, generally Gram-positive rods. This group contains the following genera representative species considered as human pathogens: *Arcanobacterium*, *Brevibacterium*, *Oerskovia* and *Rothia* (Tables 167.3, 167.4).

EPIDEMIOLOGY

For most *Corynebacterium* spp. and coryneforms, the reservoir and ecology are unknown. *Corynebacterium* spp. may be isolated from normal skin and mucous membranes, whereas *C. jeikeium* has also been isolated from inanimate hospital environments. *Arcanobacterium* may colonize mucous membranes from humans and farm animals. *Brevibacterium* can be isolated from dairy products (e.g. cheese) and *Oerskovia* from the inanimate environment. *Rothia* are members of the oropharyngeal microflora. Possible human-to-human or animal-to-human transmission may occur with *Arcanobacterium*.

PATHOGENICITY

Except for *Arcanobacterium*, most coryneforms and *Corynebacterium* spp. are opportunistic human pathogens. The major risk factors are immunosuppressive diseases such as malignancy, organ transplantation, iatrogenic manipulation (e.g. urinary tract instrumentation for *C. urealyticum*), breaks in the skin barrier (e.g. medical devices for *C. jeikeium*, *Brevibacterium* spp., *Oerskovia* spp., *Rothia* spp.) and therapy with broad-spectrum antibiotics (*C. jeikeium*, *C. urealyticum*, *C. amycolatum*).

DIAGNOSTIC MICROBIOLOGY

Several *Corynebacterium* spp. and coryneforms colonize the mucocutaneous epithelium and are part of the normal microflora. Their isolation from clinical specimens is difficult to interpret. Criteria have been proposed to help clinical microbiologists and clinicians to distinguish colonization from a possible role in infection (Table 167.5).

Table 167.3 Taxonomy of medically relevant Actinomycetales

Suborders	Families	Genera	Frequency	Practical classification
Actinomycineae	Actinomycetaceae	*Actinobaculum, Actinomyces, Arcanobacterium*, Mobiluncus*	+	Ac
Propionibacterineae	Propionibacteriaceae	*Propionibacterium*	+++	An
Micrococcineae	Micrococcaceae	*Arthrobacter, Micrococcus, Rothia**	+	Co
	Cellulomonadaceae	*Cellulomonas, Oerskovia*, Tropheryma†*	+	Co
	Dermatophilaceae	*Dermatophilus*	+	Aa
	Brevibacteriaceae	*Brevibacterium**	+	Co
	Dermabacteraceae	*Dermabacter*	+	Co
	Microbacteriaceae	*Microbacterium*	+	Co
Corynebacterineae	Corynebacteriaceae	*Corynebacterium*, Turicella*	+++	Co
	Mycobacteriaceae	*Mycobacterium†*	++	My
	Nocardiaceae	*Nocardia*, Rhodococcus**	+	Aa
	Gordoniaceae	*Gordonia**	+	Aa
	Tsukamurellaceae	*Tsukamurella**	+	Aa
	Dietziaceae	*Dietzia*	+	Aa
Streptomycineae	Streptomycetaceae	*Streptomyces**	+	Aa
Streptosporangineae	Nocardiopsaceae	*Nocardiopsis*	+	Aa
	Thermomonosporaceae	*Actinomadura**	+	Aa

Aa, aerobic actinomycetes; Ac, actinomycetes; An, anaerobic Gram-positive rods; Co, coryneforms; My, mycobacteria.
*Genera dealt with in this overview; †genera discussed in separate chapters.

With few exceptions, *Corynebacterium* spp. and coryneforms grow in 24–48 hours in aerobic conditions in standard liquid media (blood culture) or on solid media (blood-containing media). *Corynebacterium jeikeium* (see Fig. 167.3, lanes 3A and 3B) and *C. urealyticum* grow better in lipid-enriched media such as those containing Tween. Some morphologic or physiologic characteristics of colonies may help to differentiate them; for example:

- *C. amycolatum* produces dry colonies;
- β-hemolysis is observed around *Arcanobacterium* spp. colonies;
- *Brevibacterium* produces a cheese-like smell;
- *Oerskovia* colonies are pigmented in yellow to orange;
- white colonies with a 'spoked-wheel' aspect are observed in *Rothia dentocariosa*; and
- *R. mucilaginosa* produces mucoid colonies which adhere on agar (see Fig. 167.3, lanes 4–9A and 4–9B).

Antibiotic susceptibility testing is obtained generally by using E-test technology which allows the determination of the minimal inhibitory concentration on blood-containing agar. However, standardized interpretation criteria are lacking for these bacteria.

Corynebacterium jeikeium, C. urealyticum and *C. amycolatum* exhibit high levels of resistance to several antibiotics (including resistance to penicillins, cephalosporins, macrolides and aminoglycosides) but are uniformly susceptible to glycopeptides. Resistance to glycopeptides attributed to the presence of the *vanA* gene has been described in *Oerskovia turbata* and *Arcanobacterium haemolyticum* strains.[52]

CLINICAL MANIFESTATIONS AND MANAGEMENT

Corynebacterium spp. and coryneform bacteria have a low index of pathogenicity and are considered as opportunistic. Clinical syndromes that have been reported include bacteremia, endocarditis, infections of prosthetic joints, infections of the urinary tract and pneumonia in immunocompromised hosts.

For detailed discussions, see specific chapters and Table 167.4.

Aerobic Actinomycetes

NATURE

The term 'aerobic actinomycetes' helps clinical microbiologists to define noncoryneform Gram-positive rods which grow better under aerobic conditions. Table 167.6 shows the different genera belonging to this heterogeneous group. Only the most frequently encountered species in human pathology will be discussed. Important pathogens such as *Mycobacterium* and *Tropheryma* are covered elsewhere (see Chapters 30, 36 and 174).

EPIDEMIOLOGY

The prevalence of disease due to aerobic actinomycetes is not precisely established but remains rare. For nocardiosis, which represents the most frequently encountered disease in this group of micro-organisms, a frequency of about 2 per million cases annually has been proposed.[53,54] During the period prior to highly active antiretroviral therapy (HAART), the incidence of nocardiosis in AIDS patients with fewer than 100 CD4 cells/microliter was estimated to vary from 0.3% to 1.8% according to geographic differences, and predominated in rural environments.[55] In organ transplant recipients, nocardiosis was diagnosed in 0.6% of the patients in a recent case-control study. Independent risk factors were high-dose steroids, history of cytomegalovirus disease and high levels of calcineurin inhibitors.[56]

Rhodococcus equi, the second most frequent aerobic actinomycete, occurs in patients with the same predisposing factors. Rarely, infection may be observed in immunocompetent patients with a male-to-female ratio of 3:1 and a history of exposure to livestock.[57]

Table 167.4 Medically relevant *Corynebacterium* spp. and coryneform bacteria (all acid-fast stain negative)

Genera	Predominant species	Gram stain	Natural habitat	Site of infection	Risk factors, transmission	Diagnostic comments
Corynebacterium	*C. diphtheriae*	Club-shaped morphology, arrangement in liquid media: V forms, in palisades or in clusters with so-called Chinese letter appearance	Human	Upper respiratory tract, wound	No or insufficient vaccination, human-to-human transmission (close contact)	Four biotypes: *gravis, mitis, belfanti* and *intermedius* C. *diphtheriae* biotype intermedius: lipophilism (growth enhanced in presence of Tween 80)
	C. ulcerans		Cattle, domestic cats and dogs	Upper respiratory tract, wound	Contact with animals, rural setting, ingestion of unpasteurized dairy products	Small β-hemolytic colonies; reverse CAMP test with *S. aureus* positive; positive urease test
	C. jeikeium		Human skin (axillary, inguinal and perineal areas), mucous membranes (urinary tract), inanimate hospital environment	Bacteremia, endocarditis, foreign body infections, wound infections	Immunosuppression, medical devices, prolonged hospital stay, therapy with broad-spectrum antibiotics	Lipophilism; multiresistance to antibiotics
	C. amycolatum		Human skin	Bacteremia, endocarditis, foreign body infections, wound infections	Immunosuppression, underlying heart disease (endocarditis)	–
	C. urealyticum		Urinary tract, skin (axilla and groin of hospitalized patients)	Bacteremia, urinary tract infections, alkali-encrusted cystitis (struvite stones), wound infections	Immunosuppression (kidney transplant), urologic procedures	Lipophilism; strong positive urease test; multiresistance to antibiotics
Arcanobacterium	*A. haemolyticum*	Gram-positive rod (to gram-variable, with branching bacilli)	Oropharyngeal microflora	Pharyngitis (20% with morbilliform rash), soft tissue infections, sepsis (immunosuppression), endocarditis	Possible human-to-human transmission (pharyngitis in teenagers and young adults), immunosuppression	Small β-hemolytic colonies; reverse CAMP test with *S. aureus* positive
	A. pyogenes		Normal flora of farm ruminants and swine	Abdominal abscesses, soft tissue abscesses, bacteremia, endocarditis	Contacts with animals, rural setting	Small β-hemolytic colonies
Brevibacterium	*B. casei*	Small Gram-positive rods (coccoid forms – old colonies)	Dairy products/skin flora	Bacteremia, endocarditis	Immunosuppression, medical devices (intravascular catheter)	Nonhemolytic colonies; typical cheese-like smell
Oerskovia	*O. turbata*	Branching bacilli, coccoid forms (breaking up of mycelia)	Inanimate environment (soil)	Bacteremia, endocarditis	Immunosuppression, medical devices (intravascular catheter)	Yellow-orange pigmented colonies
Rothia	*R. dentocariosa*	Gram-positive rods	Oro-pharyngeal microflora	Bacteremia, endocarditis, meningitis	Immunosuppression, medical devices, underlying heart disease (endocarditis)	First isolation from carious lesions; nonhemolytic white colonies with a 'spoked-wheel' aspect
	R. mucilaginosa	Coccoid forms, encapsulated	Oro-pharyngeal microflora	Bacteremia, endocarditis, meningitis, lower respiratory tract infections	Immunosuppression, indwelling foreign material	Nonhemolytic white to gray mucoid colonies; adherence of older colonies to the agar surface

Table 167.5 Clinical conditions where precise identification of coryneform bacteria is recommended

- When isolated from an upper respiratory tract specimen, notably throat and nose swabs (*C. diphtheriae*)
- When isolated from a wound or skin specimen from a person having recently traveled abroad (*C. diphtheriae*)
- When isolated from normally sterile body fluids or if coccobacilli have been seen on Gram stain, notably when multiple specimens are positive for the same coryneforms
- When two or more blood cultures are positive for coryneforms
- When coryneform bacteria are seen on direct Gram stain associated with a strong leukocyte reaction, especially if other organisms recovered from the same specimen have a low pathogenicity
- When isolated from a urine specimen, if the organisms are the sole agent in counts of 10^4 cfu/ml or greater or if they are the predominant agent in counts of 10^5 cfu/ml or greater

Adapted from Efstratiou *et al.*[37] and Funke & Bernard.[38]

The reservoir of all aerobic actinomycetes is the soil environment where micro-organisms are implicated in decaying plant matter. *Rhodococcus equi* is found in high proportion in dung from horses and foals. Aerobic actinomycetes are thought to be acquired essentially by inhalation from the soil. Colonization or infections may also be acquired through a traumatic lesion contaminated with soil, wound infections or catheter colonization.

PATHOGENICITY

Few studies have investigated the virulence mechanisms of aerobic actinomycetes. The complete genome sequence of *Nocardia farcinica* has revealed the presence of potent virulence determinants such as mammalian cell entry (Mce) proteins with homology with *Mycobacterium tuberculosis* Mce proteins,[58] allowing mycobacteria to multiply in a mammalian host. Similar Mce genes have also been identified in *R. equi*[59] and *Streptomyces coelicolor*.[60]

Nocardia farcinica and *R. equi* also possess adherence factors with proteins belonging to fibronectin-binding protein families presenting a homology with antigen 85 of *M. tuberculosis*.[58,59]

Murine models have shown the importance of cell-mediated immunity in nocardiosis.[61] Studies with human monocytes show a resistance of *Nocardia* spp. to killing mechanisms of phagocytes by inhibition of phagosome–lysosome fusion and by bacterial detoxification enzymes (superoxide dismutase, catalase).[61] In-vitro studies have also demonstrated the induction of apoptosis related to caspase activation during contact of cells with *N. asteroides*.[62] This may play a role in the progression of nocardiosis.

Abscess formation with polymorphonuclear cell infiltration and later cell necrosis represents the hallmark of histologic lesions of both *Nocardia* and *Rhodococcus*. Malakoplakia is a granulomatous inflammation in which large macrophages have basophilic inclusions known as Michaelis–Gutmann bodies. This entity is observed in *R. equi* infection in HIV-infected patients.[63] The origin of Michaelis–Gutmann bodies is attributed to an abnormal degradation of bacteria by phagocytes.

DIAGNOSTIC MICROBIOLOGY

Microscopy and culture on appropriate media are critical for the precise clinical diagnosis of these infections, and contact with the laboratory is mandatory. Samples from the respiratory tract represent the majority of specimens, others being blood, cutaneous tissue, subcutaneous tissue biopsy and abscess collection from a large variety of organs. Multiple specimen examination is recommended, particularly from the respiratory tract.

Macroscopic examination of skin and soft tissue specimens is important to detect the presence of granules or concretions. These granules will be used selectively for microscopic examination since they represent masses of filaments embedded in necrotic tissue. Gram staining is preferred to modified acid-fast stain for visualization of this group of micro-organisms. However, determination of acid fastness is used as confirmatory staining. According to the species, the

microscopic appearances may vary from coccoid and diphtheroid bacteria seen for *Rhodococcus* spp. and *Gordonia* spp. to branched and filamentous Gram-positive bacilli for *Nocardia* spp. and *Streptomyces* spp. (see Table 167.6 and Fig. 167.3, lanes 1–5C and 1–5D).

Routine media are generally used for recovery of aerobic actinomycetes; for specimens containing surface or mixed flora, selective media with antibiotic cocktails such as buffered charcoal yeast extract (BCYE) agar is recommended, particularly for *Nocardia* and for respiratory tract specimens. Media appropriate for mycobacteria such as Löwenstein may also be used. The incubation period for bacterial growth is prolonged, up to 2–3 weeks. Conventional blood cultures may be used for the detection of bacteremia due to *Rhodococcus* or *Gordonia*, but prolonged incubation is mandatory. In a review of *Nocardia* bacteremia, the detection time ranged from 2 to 14 days with a median of 4 days.[64]

A minimum of 48–72 hours is necessary before colonies became visible on routine media. Phenotypic aspects such as pigmentation or aerial hyphae appear later (see Table 167.6). Aerial hyphae give a powdery aspect to most *Nocardia* and *Streptomyces* isolates; sparse aerial hyphae can be observed with *Actinomadura* isolates or rarely for *Rhodococcus* strains. Mucoid colonies are typically seen for *R. equi* strains and *Actinomadura*. Only a small fraction of bacteria appear acid fast, this property being enhanced in lipid-rich media such as Löwenstein.

Biochemical identification to species level is difficult since most commercial kits are not appropriate for aerobic actinomycete differentiation. Molecular techniques, notably sequencing of 16S rRNA, have now replaced biochemical identification.[65] Analysis of heat shock protein genes by PCR paired with restriction fragment length polymorphisms has also been described.[66]

The distinction of pattern of resistance to antimicrobial agents has been used to subtype *N. asteroides* complex into six different groups.[67] Species most frequently isolated in human specimens are *N. asteroides* sensu stricto type VI, *N. brasiliensis*, *N. farcinica* and *N. nova*, the proportion of each species varying according to the type of specimen and the geographic location.

Antibiotic susceptibility testing with broth microdilution is the recommended method.[68] The breakpoints for *Nocardia* and other aerobic actinomycetes are based on pharmacokinetic/pharmacodynamic (PK/PD) data. For clinical laboratories not performing these tests, collaboration with reference laboratories is important since these tests remain problematic due to the slow growth and the degradation of the antimicrobial agent.

CLINICAL MANIFESTATIONS AND MANAGEMENT

Pulmonary infections and disseminated infections

Nocardiosis

Pulmonary infections and disseminated infections represent the most frequent form of nocardiosis. The patients are generally severely immunocompromised due to advanced HIV infections with low (<100)

Table 167.6 Medically relevant aerobic Actinomycetes

Genera	Gram stain	Acid-fast stain	Predominant species	Natural habitat	Site of infection	Risk factors, transmission	Diagnostic comments
Nocardia	Branched filamentous Gram-positive bacilli, short rods (breaking up of mycelia)	Positive	*N. asteroides, N. brasiliensis, N. farcinica*	Inanimate environment (soil)	Soft tissue infection, nonmycetomic (mycetoma), respiratory and disseminated infection	Penetrating wound (occupational disease, male predominance, tropical and subtropical regions), immunosuppression (inhalation), underlying chronic lung disease	Presence of white to yellow intralesional grains (mycetoma); colonies white to red, superficially chalky appearance (powdery aerial hyphae); slow growth with aerial mycelium (3–7 days)
Rhodococcus	Coccoid forms to coccobacilli (may be dismissed as diphtheroids)	Weakly positive	*R. equi*	Inanimate environment (coprophilic soil – dung of horses)	Pulmonary (lung abscesses) and bacteremic infections, rare cutaneous infections (traumatic wounds)	Immunosuppression (AIDS, organ transplant recipients), contact with animals	Pink mucoid colonies (variant: yellow pigmentation, rough appearance)
Gordonia	Thin Gram-positive coccobacilli (may be dismissed as diphtheroids)	Weakly positive	*G. terrae*	Inanimate environment (soil)	Bacteremia, endocarditis	Immunosuppression, indwelling foreign material, wound infections	Dry, wrinkled beige to orange colonies
Tsukamurella	Gram-positive rods	Positive	*T. paurometabola*	Inanimate environment (soil)	Bacteremia, endocarditis	Immunosuppression, indwelling foreign material	Psychrophilic micro-organism (grows best at cooler temperatures); slow growth
Actinomadura	Branched filamentous Gram-positive bacilli with short chains of spores	Negative	*A. madurae, A. pelletieri*	Inanimate environment (soil)	Soft tissue infection (mycetoma), rare nonmycetomic disseminated infection, pneumonia (immunosuppression)	Penetrating wound (occupational disease, tropical and subtropical regions), inhalation (immunosuppression)	Colonies white to red, usually mucoid, molar tooth appearance after a few days of growth; aerial hyphae if present are sparse and appear later during growth incubation
Streptomyces	Filamentous Gram-positive bacilli	Negative	*Streptomyces somaliensis*	Inanimate environment (soil)	Soft tissue infection (mycetoma), perianal soft tissue infection	Penetrating wound (occupational disease, tropical and subtropical regions)	Presence of yellow to brown intralesional grains (mycetoma); smooth to rugous colonies, generally with powdery aerial hyphae

CD4 counts or are receiving chemotherapy with cytotoxic agents or immunosuppressive drugs. Pulmonary nocardiosis is also observed in patients with impaired local defenses due to chronic lung disease such as chronic obstructive pulmonary disease, bronchiectasis and chronic sarcoidosis.

Clinical presentation is subacute or chronic with cough, dyspnea, productive sputum, hemoptysis and systemic symptoms such as fever, weight loss and sweats. Lung infiltrates with and without abscess formation represent a frequent radiologic finding. Other findings are the presence of nodules, reticulonodular infiltrates, interstitial infiltrates and pleural effusions. Nocardial lesions are poorly localized and may extend to adjacent tissues with pleural effusion, pericarditis or mediastinitis. Misdiagnosis as malignancy or tuberculosis is frequent. In a recent observational study performed on adult patients diagnosed with pulmonary nocardiosis during a 13-year period, disseminated nocardiosis was observed in 30% of patients.[69] Any organ may be involved; however, a predilection for brain and cutaneous dissemination is frequently mentioned. In a review of 1050 cases in the literature, 44% of patients with systemic nocardiosis had cerebral infections, with pulmonary infection being the primary site.[61] Brain abscess may be an unapparent infection; in other cases seizures, headache or focal deficits predominate.

Pulmonary and disseminated nocardiosis treatment is based on antibiotic therapy. Standard treatment is co-trimoxazole for 3–6 months. Combination therapy with imipenem or a third-generation cephalosporin with or without amikacin is recommended for severely ill patients or for those with cerebral lesions.[70] There is, however, considerable debate over the extent to which *in-vitro* antibiotic susceptibility testing is helpful in guiding the choice of therapy.

Clinical management of nocardial brain abscess has been reviewed.[71] If the nocardial infection is not documented elsewhere, aspiration or biopsy is recommended. When the nocardial infection is already documented, medical management is feasible for a brain abscess smaller than 2 cm. Surgical intervention and aspiration are needed if the clinical condition deteriorates, if the lesion does not shrink within 1 month or if the lesion is larger than 2.5 cm.

Mortality of pulmonary nocardiosis remains high in spite of adequate therapy. In one recent series, the mortality from pulmonary nocardiosis was 39%, 64% in case of disseminated nocardiosis and 100% in case of cerebral abscess.[69] In another series of organ recipients, 89% of patients were cured including six of seven cases with disseminated disease.[56] The mortality rates may vary from series to series according to diagnostic procedure, optimization of treatment and the severity of the patient's immunosuppression.

Rhodococcus equi

The lung represents the primary site of infection due to *R. equi*. Inhalation is the portal of entry and severe immunosuppression is the major predisposing factor, in particular advanced HIV infection. In a large retrospective study in HIV patients, the lung was involved in more than 90% of cases.[72] The clinical presentation develops insidiously over days to weeks, with fever, nonproductive cough, dyspnea and pleuritic pain predominating. Lung infiltrates or nodules are observed on chest radiographs and pleural effusions may occur. Cavitation is seen in 63% of immunocompetent patients and in 41–77% of HIV-immunosuppressed patients.[57,73] Bacteremia is detected in more than 50% of cases and dissemination to the CNS, bone and soft tissue may occur.

Treatment of *R. equi* lung infection is based on antibiotic therapy. Surgical resection is considered for isolated lung abscesses and failure of medical treatment. *Rhodococcus equi* is usually susceptible *in vitro* to erythromycin, rifampin, fluoroquinolones, aminoglycosides, glycopeptides and imipenem. Several successful antibiotic regimens exist. A few principles guide the treatment:

- a combination regimen is necessary to avoid the appearance of resistance;
- prolonged therapy (2–6 months) is recommended to avoid frequently observed relapses;

- initial intravenous therapy with bactericidal agents such as imipenem and vancomycin is followed by oral therapy (e.g. macrolide plus quinolone);
- use antibiotics able to kill intramacrophagic micro-organisms; and
- initiate HAART in HIV patients to reduce mortality.[72]

Rhodococcus equi causes a serious disease with a high mortality rate. The outcome depends on predisposing factors. In the pre-HAART period, mortality was estimated to be greater than 50%. In an extensive series of *R. equi* infections in patients with HIV, HAART was the unique independent factor associated with reduced mortality.[72] In transplant recipients and immunocompetent patients, mortality is about 20%.[57,74]

Cutaneous and soft tissue infection

Nocardia spp., *Actinomadura*, *Streptomyces*

Cutaneous nocardiosis can be divided into two main groups: primary lesions observed generally in immunocompetent patients and secondary lesions observed following dissemination in immunosuppressed patients representing metastatic lesions due to a bacteremic episode. In primary cutaneous nocardiosis, infection results from inoculation of the micro-organism during skin trauma (outdoor activities) or following iatrogenic trauma such as surgery. Rarely, in immunosuppressed patients, primary cutaneous lesions may evolve in a disseminated disease.[75]

Clinical presentation of primary cutaneous lesions is as cellulitis or abscess, or in chronic state as mycetoma. *Nocardia braziliensis* is isolated in the majority of cases.[67] Mycetoma predominates in men living in rural and subtropical or tropical areas. Lesions are usually on the feet, legs, shoulders and back. Mycetoma is a general term for a chronic granulomatous infection of the subcutaneous tissue due to either aerobic actinomycetes (actinomycetoma) or filamentous fungi (eumycetoma) (see Chapter 179). In actinomycetoma the following etiologic agents predominate: *Nocardia*, *Streptomyces* and *Actinomadura*. Mycetoma begins as nodules which fistulate to the skin. Exudates contain granules corresponding to masses of bacteria embedded in necrotic tissue. The lesion is chronic, and pain or systemic manifestations are generally absent. In late-stage infection, deep soft tissue and bone are implicated. Superinfection with pyogenic bacteria is frequent. Identification of the etiologic agent is necessary to determine the appropriate antibiotic regimen. Co-trimoxazole prescribed for several months is the treatment of choice.[76] For treatment failure, amoxicillin–clavulanate is recommended.[77]

Bacteremia and catheter-related Infections

Nocardia

A positive blood culture for *Nocardia* is a rare event. In a large review, the incidence was estimated at 0.003%.[64] Secondary bacteremia associated with pulmonary infection and cutaneous infection predominates. In this series, less than 20% of *Nocardia* positive blood culture was attributed to contamination. Catheter-related nocardial infections are also rare and catheter removal is recommended.

Rhodococcus equi

Bacteremia due to *R. equi* represents a secondary bacteremia during disseminated or lung infection. In HIV co-infected patients, up to 50% with *R. equi* lung disease have bacteremia.[72]

Gordonia

Gordonia is a rarely isolated human pathogen and only case reports or small series have been published. Several of these infections were bacteremias associated with an intravenous catheter.[78] The propensity of *Gordonia* spp. to biodegrade rubber may contribute to the pathogenesis of these infections.[79] Infections generally resolved with catheter removal and an antibiotic regimen containing vancomycin.[80] *In vitro*, *Gordonia* strains are susceptible to imipenem and ciprofloxacin, frequently susceptible to gentamicin, vancomycin, azithromycin, ceftriaxone and ceftazidime (80–90% of isolates) and variably susceptible to doxycycline, trimethoprim–sulfamethoxazole, erythromycin, penicillin, ampicillin and rifampin (30–70% of isolates).[80]

Tsukamurella

Tsukamurella have also been isolated in relation to central venous catheter-related infection.[81] In a review published in 2004, fewer than 20 cases of *Tsukamurella* infections were identified, the majority being catheter related, generally in immunosuppressed patients.[82]

Management is based on medical device removal associated with an antibiotic regimen, generally with a β-lactam and an aminoglycoside.

REFERENCES

References for this chapter can be found online at http://www.expertconsult.com

Neisseria

INTRODUCTION

The genus *Neisseria* was named after Albert Neisser who observed gonococci (*Neisseria gonorrhoeae*) in leukocytes in urethral exudates from patients with gonorrhea in 1879. Eight years later Weichselbaum isolated the meningococcus (*Neisseria meningitidis*) from six of eight cases of primary sporadic community-acquired meningitis. The gonococcus and the meningococcus are exclusively human pathogens and the most studied species of the Neisseriaceae family.

Neisseria gonorrhoeae causes gonorrhea, a sexually transmitted disease. Gonorrhea was named by Galen in AD 130 after the Greek words *gonor* (seed) and *rhoia* (flow), suggesting that the disease was related to the flow of semen. In the 13th century Maimonides recognized that the urethral discharge of male gonorrhea patients was not semen, but a sexually transmitted disease. Gonorrhea was not clearly distinguished from syphilis until the 19th century. In 1885 Bumm proved gonococci as the cause of gonorrhea by inoculating human volunteers. Effective therapy became available in the 1930s when sulfonamides became available and in 1943 when penicillin was produced. Sulfonamide resistance occurred early and rapidly and the prevalence of strains resistant to penicillin and other antibiotics has risen steadily worldwide. Vaccine development is hampered by the multitude of gonococcal immune evasion strategies.

Neisseria meningitidis is a cause of endemic and epidemic meningitis and/or septicemia worldwide. Epidemic meningococcal meningitis was first described by Vieusseaux in 1805 in Geneva. Throughout the 19th century periodic epidemics occurred, involving mainly young children and adolescents including military recruits. In 1896 Kiefer described the nasopharyngeal meningococcal carrier state among healthy people. The outcome of meningococcal disease improved drastically by treatment with antibiotics. Selected meningococcal conjugate polysaccharides vaccines are now successfully used worldwide. A universal vaccine that protects against *N. meningitidis* serogroup B, which causes most cases of disease in temperate countries, is still under development. The absence of a serogroup B vaccine limits the effective control of meningococcal disease.

MICROBIOLOGY

Taxonomy

In the 2005 edition of *Bergey's Manual of Systemic Bacteriology* the family of the Neisseriaceae consists of the genus *Neisseria* as well as the heterogeneous genera (in order of decreasing relatedness to genus *Neisseria*) *Kingella, Eikenella, Alysiella, Simonsiella, Microvirgula, Laribacter, Vogesella, Vitreoscilla, Chromobacterium, Aquaspirillum,*

Prolinoborus, Formivibrio and *Iodobacter*.[1] The taxonomy of the family has been extensively revised over the past decades, mainly based on 16S rRNA sequence analysis, even though this methodology does not reflect all the complex levels of relationships between these heterogeneous entities.

The members of the amended family of Neisseriaceae typically are Gram-negative coccal or coccoid micro-organisms. Some species are rod shaped (*N. weaveri* and *N. elongata*) or exhibit a multicellular micro-morphology (*Simonsiella* spp. and *Alysiella* spp.). Several species possess capsules and are fimbriated (piliated). Endospores are not found and flagella are absent. Members of the genera *Simonsiella* and *Alysiella* show gliding motility. Some *Neisseria* spp., including *N. gonorrhoeae* and *N. meningitidis*, may show surface-bound twitching motility. All species are aerobic, but *Kingella* and *Eikenella* spp. also grow under anaerobic conditions. The G+C content of DNA ranges from 41 to 58 mol%.

Among the Neisseriaceae, *N. gonorrhoeae* and *N. meningitidis* are genetically very closely related human pathogens (Fig. 168.1). *Neisseria lactamica* and *N. cinerea* are related to *N. gonorrhoeae*, but frequently colonize the nasopharynx of children and adults. The saccharolytic Neisseriaceae (*N. polysacchareae, N. subflava, N. sicca* and *N. mucosa*) are more distantly related to the other Neisseriaceae and colonize humans less frequently. The species of animal origin are even more distantly related to the human pathogens. The *Kingella* spp. and *Eikenella corrodens* are commensals that are occasionally isolated from human infections. These species are discussed in Chapter 172.

Growth characteristics

The genus *Neisseria* is composed of 17 species that may be isolated from humans and six species that colonize various animals (Table 168.1).[1] *Neisseria* spp. grow best aerobically in an atmosphere containing 5–10% carbon dioxide at a temperature of 89.6–98.6°F (32–37°C) and a pH of 7–7.5. The micro-organisms typically appear in pairs (diplococci) and occasionally in tetrads or clusters. *Neisseria elongata* and *N. weaveri* are medium-to-large plump rods that sometimes occur in pairs or short chains. Diplococci have flattened opposing sides, imparting the characteristic kidney or coffee-bean appearance seen in stained smears. Cell size ranges from 0.6 to 1.5 mm depending upon the species source of the isolate and the age of the culture.

Neisseria spp. are fastidious. Blood agar and chocolate medium (blood heated at 176–194°F/80–90°C) are suitable growth media. Bacterial colonies usually appear after 24–48 hours of growth. Colonies of *N. gonorrhoeae* are 0.5–1 mm in size. Colonies of *N. meningitidis* are usually larger (1–2 mm) and flatter. Colonies of the nonpathogenic *Neisseria* spp. are similar in size, appearance and consistency, except for the saccharolytic *Neisseria* spp. (*N. subflava, N. sicca* and *N. mucosa*) that are larger (1–3 mm), more convex and smooth (*N. mucosa*). Colonies of *N. subflava* and *N. sicca* are opaque and have varying consistency. *Neisseria sicca* adhere to the agar surface and become wrinkled

Neisseria species as depicted by phylogenetic analysis of 16S rRNA gene sequences

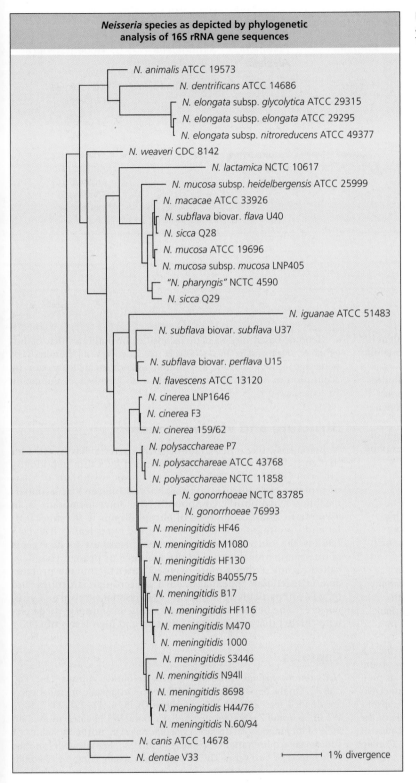

Fig. 168.1 *Neisseria* species as depicted by phylogenetic analysis of 16S rRNA gene sequences. Redrawn from Tønjum.[1]

with prolonged incubation. Some nonpathogenic *Neisseria* spp. form a yellow pigment (*N. flavescens*) or a greenish-yellow pigment (*N. mucosa, N. subflava*).

Neisseria spp. are oxidase positive and catalase positive, except *N. elongata*, which is catalase negative. All species produce acid from a few carbohydrates by oxidation. The ability to produce polysaccharide from sucrose, to produce catalase and deoxyribonuclease, to reduce nitrate and nitrite, and to oxidize the tributyrin fatty acid are also used to identify *Neisseria* spp.

Genome dynamics

The size of the *Neisseria* chromosome is approximately 2.2–2.3 Mb. The average G+C content is 48–56 mol%. *Neisseria meningitidis* and *N. gonorrhoeae* share about 95% of their gene content.[2] The vast majority of genes are also present in nonpathogenic *N. lactamica*, but gene regulation may be different in pathogenic and commensal strains.[3] Due to genetic instability, the *Neisseria* spp. have hyperdynamic genomes.[4] The genome plasticity contributes to the pathogenic

Table 168.1 Amended classification of micro-organisms within the family Neisseriaceae

Neisseria			Kingella	Eikenella, Alysiella	Simonsiella	Recent genera
Humans		Animals	Humans	Humans	Humans and animals	*Microvirgula Laribacter*
Urogenital tract	Oropharynx	Oropharynx	Oropharynx and urogenital tract	Oropharynx	Oral cavity	*Vogesella Vitreoscilla*
N. gonorrhoeae	*N. gonorrhoeae N. meningitidis N. lactamica N. sicca N. subflava N. flavescens N. mucosa N. cinerea N. polysaccharea N. elongata*	Dogs: *N. weaveri* Guinea-pigs: *N. animalis, N. denitrificans* Cows: *N. dentiae* Iguanas: *N. igaunae* Dolphins: *N. mucosa* Monkeys: *N. macacae*	*K. kingae K. denitrificans*	*E. corrodens A. filiformis*	*S. crassa*	Chromobacterium Aquaspirillum Prolinoborus Formivibrio Iodobacter

potential of *Neisseria* spp. and the development of hypervirulent lineages. The most important sources of neisserial genome instability (Fig. 168.2) are as follows.

- *Phase variation*, i.e. variable protein expression due to slipped-strand mispairing of nucleotide runs found within or close to the promoter region (affect transcription) or within open reading frames (affect translation).
- *Recombination*, i.e. the genetic exchange or rearrangement of DNA from external or internal sources. This may, for example, lead to the generation of millions of variants of pilin subunits.
- *Horizontal gene transfer*, i.e. the introduction of genes predominantly via natural transformation (the natural uptake of DNA) and integration into the chromosome by RecA-mediated homologous recombination. *Neisseria* spp. are naturally competent for transformation throughout their growth cycle.[6]
- *Hypermutation*, i.e. increased global mutation rates often associated with DNA repair deficiencies, replication infidelity or overexpression of DNA translesion polymerases. High mutation rates in specific loci (more than 100 phase-variable candidate genes in the pathogenic *Neisseria* spp.) result in rapid generation of variants.

The pathogenic *Neisseria* spp. share several genomic regions, including up to nine prophage and eight genetic islands, that are absent from *N. lactamica*.[7] There are no classic pathogenicity islands as present in many other bacterial species. *Neisseria meningitidis*-specific DNA sequences include the *cps* locus encoding the polysaccharide capsule, genes that encode the RTX family of toxins and an orthologue of the filamentous hemagglutinin of *Bordetella pertussis*. The genomes of disease and carriage isolates show no consistent differences. Certain hypervirulent lineages contain the filamentous prophage Nf1.[8] About 80% of the gonococcal clinical isolates and *N. meningitidis* strains of serogroups W135, H and Z contain the 'gonococcal genetic island' (GGI, 57 kb).[7] This is an often chromosomally integrated conjugative plasmid that encodes a type IV secretion system involved in DNA secretion. The genome of *Neisseria* spp. has a variable number of noncoding repeat arrays and insertion (IS) elements among which IS*1655* appears unique to *N. meningitidis*.

Most isolates of *N. gonorrhoeae* but not *N. meningitidis* carry plasmids.[9] Nearly all gonococcal strains carry a 4.2 kb cryptic plasmid of unknown function and many strains carry plasmids encoding β-lactamase causing resistance to penicillin. The conjugative plasmid TetM confers tetracycline resistance.

Genome-based phylogenetic reconstruction indicates that pathogenic *N. meningitidis* has relatively recently (several hundreds of years ago) emerged from a common unencapsulated ancestor by acquisition of capsule genes, probably from members of the family Pasteurellaceae.[10]

Structure and virulence factors

Neisseria spp., like other Gram-negative bacteria, have a cell wall that consists of two membranes separated by a thin peptidoglycan layer (Fig. 168.3). The inner cytoplasmic membrane consists of proteins embedded in a phospholipid bilayer that is impermeable for hydrophilic compounds. The outer membrane is an asymmetric bilayer composed of phospholipids in the inner leaflet and lipo-oligosaccharide (LOS) in the outer leaflet. The LOS renders the outer membrane relatively resistant to detergents and is semipermeable due to the presence of protein channels, called porins. Other surface-exposed outer membrane proteins and extracellular appendages such as capsular structures and type IV pili particularly contribute to neisserial survival and virulence.[12,13] The neisserial outer membrane continuously sheds vesicles (blebs) that contain DNA, protein and high levels of LOS.

Capsules

Neisseria meningitidis produces a polysaccharide capsule (see Fig. 168.3). On the basis of structural differences in capsule, meningococci are divided into at least 13 serogroups (A, B, C, D, 29E, H, I, K, L, W135, X, Y and Z). Serogroups A, B, C, Y and W135 cause more than 90% of meningococcal disease. Capsular types are normally stable but strains can acquire variant capsule gene alleles.[14] Serogroup B can thus switch to C or vice versa. The serogroup A capsule contains *N*-acetyl-mannosamine-1-phosphate. The capsules of the serogroups B, C, Y and W135 consist of polymers of *N*-acetylneuraminic (sialic) acid. The B polysaccharide resembles structures present in human neural tissues, limiting its immunogenicity and vaccine potential. The carbohydrates can be variably O-acetylated. The capsule polymers are anchored in the outer membrane through a 1,2-dipalmitoyl glycerol moiety. Capsule biosynthesis can vary and is subject to regulation. Isolates from healthy carriers are frequently unencapsulated due to reversible changes in capsule gene expression. A substantial proportion of meningococcal carrier isolates are incapable of capsule production due to deletions in or a lack of capsule genes. Isolates from the bloodstream or cerebrospinal fluid (CSF) are invariably encapsulated.

Mechanisms contributing to genetic instability of the *Neisseria* species

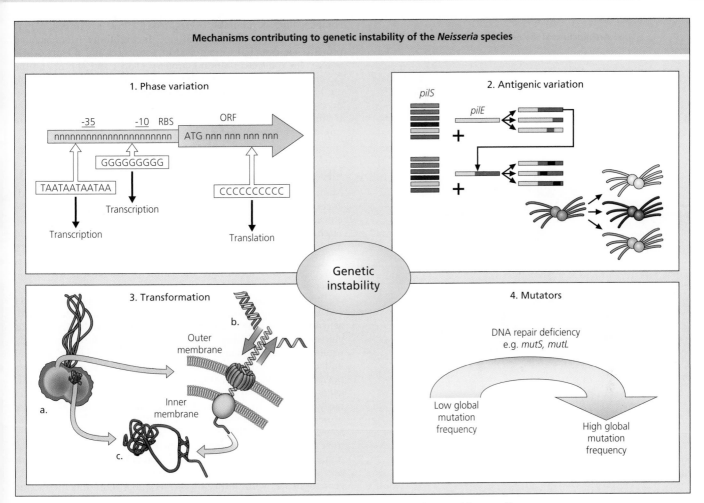

Fig. 168.2 Mechanisms contributing to genetic instability of the *Neisseria* species. Redrawn from Davidsen *et al.*[5]

Neisseria gonorrhoeae does not produce a polysaccharide capsule. However, both meningococci and gonococci are covered with a loosely adherent capsular-like structure containing high-molecular weight polyphosphate. This layer provides protection against environmental stress.

Pili

Pili are hair-like fibers consisting of thousands of protein subunits (pilin, 16–20 kDa).[15] Pathogenic *Neisseria* spp. have long pili (up to 4300 nm in length) termed type IV pili that protrude from the bacterial surface (see Fig. 168.3). Nonpathogenic *Neisseria* spp. may express both long and short pili (175–210 nm in length). Type IV pili confer bacterial cell-to-cell interactions and twitching motility – a form of locomotion that is powered by extension and retraction of the pilus filament. Pili are essential for adhesion to epithelial and endothelial cells and impart tissue tropism.[12,13] Expression of type IV pili is also required for efficient transformation of DNA.[6]

The main structural constituent of the type IV pilus fiber is the pilin subunit (PilE). During infection pilins undergo rapid phase shifts and antigenic variation. The single *pilE* expression locus is changed by unidirectional donation of coding sequences from multiple silent partial *pilS* genes in a process similar to gene conversion (see Fig. 168.2), producing an extensive repertoire of antigenic variants.[15] The frequency of antigenic pili variation may be as high as 10^3. Pilin can be post-translationally modified with phosphorylcholine, phosphoethanolamine and variable acetylated O-linked glycans.[16,17]

Neisseria gonorrhoeae produces one type of pili (class I). *Neisseria meningitidis* can express class I or class II pili which are antigenically and structurally distinct. Class II pili are encoded by a different *pilE* gene that has no silent cassette counterparts.

Surface proteins

The repertoire of the meningococcal and gonococcal surface proteins is very similar.[12,13] Trimeric protein channels (porins) confer transport of low-molecular nutrients across the outer membrane. The principal gonococcal porin is PorB (formerly protein I, 32–36 kDa). Gonococci express either of two PorB isotypes, termed PorB-IA and PorB-IB. The proteins are stably expressed but display interstrain variation due to amino acid differences in surface-exposed regions. The antigenic heterogeneity is the basis for PorB-based serologic typing. PorB-IA strains are resistant to normal human serum and can cause disseminated gonococcal infection. The gonococcal PorB porin is essential for bacterial survival.

Neisseria meningitidis can express two types of porin simultaneously: PorA and PorB. PorA (class 1 protein, 44–47 kDa) is variably expressed and PorA-negative variants can be isolated from patients. PorA antigenic differences serve as the basis for serologic subtyping of meningococci. Meningococcal PorB is equivalent to the gonococcal PorB protein and is present as either PorB-IA (class 2 protein, 40–42 kDa) or PorB-IB (class 3 protein, 37–39 kDa).[12,13] Serotyping of meningococci is based on antigenic differences in PorB. Expression of at least one of the porin types is required for meningococcal survival.

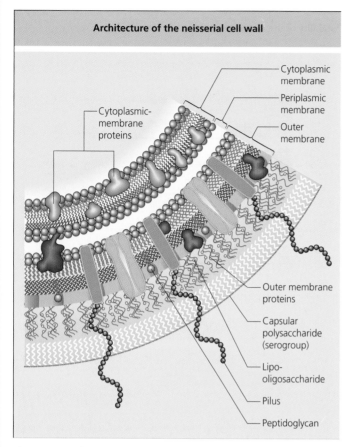

Architecture of the neisserial cell wall

Cytoplasmic membrane

Periplasmic membrane

Outer membrane

Cytoplasmic-membrane proteins

Outer membrane proteins

Capsular polysaccharide (serogroup)

Lipo-oligosaccharide

Pilus

Peptidoglycan

Fig. 168.3 Architecture of the neisserial cell wall. Redrawn from Stephens *et al.*[11]

The neisserial RmpM protein (formerly protein III or class 4 protein) is complexed to and likely stabilizes outer membrane protein complexes including porins. The protein is stably expressed by gonococci and meningococci. Its C-terminal periplasmic region resembles *Escherichia coli* OmpA domains and interacts with peptidoglycan. Rmp-specific antibodies may interfere with the bactericidal activity of antibodies directed to other surface antigens and increase the risk of infection.[18]

Both pathogenic *Neisseria* spp. can express different opacity (Opa) proteins (formerly protein II or class 5 proteins, 20–28 kDa).[12,13] Colonies of gonococci expressing Opa proteins often have a more opaque appearance. In meningococci colonial opacity is most evident at 88°F (31°C) when capsule production is low. Opa proteins are structurally very similar but display considerable intra- and interstrain variation in their surface-exposed regions. Antigenic variation occurs during natural infection due to selective immunologic pressure. Intrastrain variation results from intragenomic recombination and horizontal gene transfer. Opa proteins are variably expressed. The high-frequency phase variation is due to translational frame shifting caused by the presence of pentameric nucleotide repeats in each of the *opa* genes (see Fig. 168.2). The expression of each Opa protein can thus independently be switched on and off, enabling expressing of multiple proteins simultaneously.[13] The gonococcus contains up to 11 different *opa* genes. The meningococcal genome contains three to four *opa* genes. The proteins have an important role in neisserial adherence and invasion of eukaryotic cells. Their phase and antigenic variation limits their vaccine potential. Many meningococcal strains (~70%) express the Opc protein. This protein also confers colonial opacity and has functional similarity with Opa proteins. The Opc protein is absent in gonococci.

In addition to the aforementioned major outer membrane proteins, both pathogenic *Neisseria* spp. express more than 80 other outer membrane proteins, among which the pilus-related secretin

complex PilQ is naturally overexpressed. Protein expression may vary, depending on the bacterial growth conditions. Iron-regulated proteins are essential for survival of gonococci and meningococci *in vivo*. The transferrin-binding proteins (Tbp-1 and Tbp-2) and the lactoferrin-binding proteins (Lbp) are scavenger proteins that mediate internalization of iron into the bacterium. Conserved surface-exposed proteins such as OMP85, NspA, NadA, GNA1870 (factor H binding protein) and GNA2132 (hypothetical lipoprotein) are candidate vaccine antigens.

Lipo-oligosaccharide

Approximately half of the neisserial surface comprises lipid-anchored oligosaccharides (LOS) (see Fig. 168.3). The LOS lacks the repeating carbohydrate units (O chain) of enterobacterial lipopolysaccharide (LPS). Neisserial LOS is composed of hexa-acylated lipid A, two KDO molecules, and one or more carbohydrate chains of 8–12 saccharide units, the core oligosaccharide. Lipid A anchors LOS in the outer membrane and is one of the most potent bacterial endotoxins.

The core oligosaccharide of neisserial LOS is divided into an inner and an outer core region. The composition of the inner core is heterogeneous due to variable substitutions (phosphoethanolamine, glycine, glucose, O-acetyl groups).[19] This variation in glycoforms is partially regulated by environmental cues. The outer core is highly variable and undergoes high-frequency phase and antigenic variation due to frequent nucleotide mismatching during replication of LOS biosynthesis genes and horizontal gene transfer.[20] A single strain can simultaneously express up to six related LOS structures. The terminal structure of neisserial LOS is the target for sialylation by bacterial sialyltransferase. Gonococci utilize host sialic acid (CMP-NeuNAc) to modify their LOS. Meningococci produce their own CMP-NeuNAc. The terminal LOS of the pathogenic *Neisseria* spp. often shares epitopes with host glycolipids.[20] This molecular mimicry is exploited by the pathogens to interact with host cell lectin receptors and limits the vaccine potential of the LOS.

Peptidoglycan

Neisserial peptidoglycan consists of long chains of repeated disaccharide units cross linked via peptide bridges.[21] Covalent linkages of peptidoglycan to lipoproteins have not been found, unlike in *E. coli*. Peptidoglycan metabolism is a dynamic process involving co-ordinated activity of lytic and synthetic enzymes. The peptidoglycan is synthesized by up to four penicillin-binding proteins (PBPs). O-acetylation of peptidoglycan protects against autolysis by endogenous lytic transglycosyates and host lysozymes. Released peptidoglycan fragments activate the innate immune response and contribute to the inflammatory response.

Secreted factors

Meningococcal and gonococcal genome analyses predict the presence of autotransporter-, two-partner-, type I and type II secretion mechanisms.[22] The pathogenic *Neisseria* spp. secrete immunoglobulin A1 (IgA1) protease. This serine protease directs its own transport across the outer membrane and secretion into the environment. The enzyme cleaves in the hinge of IgA1 separating the Fab and Fc regions, making IgA ineffective. IgA protease also cleaves other proteins such as endosomal Lamp1 important for intracellular vesicle trafficking. The function of the other secreted proteins including the filamentous hemagglutinin (FHA)-like protein TpsA and FrpA/C is largely unknown. A subset (~80%) of gonococcal strains secrete DNA via a type IV secretion system.[23] The genes encoding this system are located on the gonococcal genetic island (GGI) that is acquired by horizontal gene transfer. *Neisseria* spp. lack a type III secretion mechanism which present in many other pathogens.

PATHOGENESIS

Gonorrhea

Neisseria gonorrhoeae infects the human urogenital epithelia. Other frequently infected anatomic niches are the rectum, oropharynx and conjunctiva.[24] Certain gonococcal strains may cause disseminated infection and/or arthritis.[25–27] All *N. gonorrhoeae* strains are considered to be pathogenic. The infective dose for the male urethra is as low as 250 gonococci; for the uterine cervix this ranges from 10^2 to more than 10^7 gonococci.

In males infection usually manifests after development of inflammation caused by local induction of cytokines and influx of polymorphonuclear cells (PMNs). Examination of male biopsies and exudates shows gonococci attached to and within the epithelial cells, development of (sub)mucosal microabscesses and exudation of pus with gonococci inside PMNs. Several weeks after the start of the infection gonococci can no longer be observed histologically or recovered by culture. Gonococcal infection in women is often asymptomatic (50–80%). The basis for this gender difference in host response may be niche-related differences in host receptors and/or innate host defense.[28]

At the cellular level, a large repertoire of often phase-variable adhesins and invasion-promoting surface factors enables gonococcal infection of different niches and cell tropism (Table 168.2).[12,13] The first step in gonococcal infection is the type IV pilus-mediated attachment to mucosal cells (Fig. 168.4). Once attached, PilT-mediated pilus retraction brings the bacteria into intimate contact with the cell surface and stimulates mechanosensitive host cell signaling pathways.[29] Shortly after initial attachment Opa proteins interact with CEACAM and/or heparan sulfate proteoglycan (HSPG) receptors.[29] Different Opa proteins bind to distinct receptors types. *In vitro* Opa-receptor interactions result in efficient internalization of the gonococci by host cells[12,13] (Fig. 168.4). PorB-IA expressing strains also efficiently invade cells in the absence of Opa proteins.[30] Distinct LOS variants may invade through binding of lectin receptors.[28] Sialylated LOS variants are impaired in invasion but more resistant to killing by complement, indicating the importance of the presence of variant phenotypes in the bacterial population. Gonococci induce recruitment and show intimate association with polymorphonuclear leukocytes (Fig. 168.4). Type IV pili and distinct Opa protein confer non-opsonophagocytosis by this cell type.[12,13] Part of the ingested gonococci resist killing by phagocytes.

In women gonococcal infection can ascend to the upper genital tract and selectively adhere to nonciliated cells of the fallopian tubes. Ciliated cells are lost through direct or indirect (tumor necrosis factor-mediated) cytotoxic effects of released peptidoglycan fragments and LOS. Gonococci do not produce exotoxins. Tissue invasion and the generated inflammatory response may manifest as pelvic inflammatory disease and lead to infertility.

The presence of *N. gonorrhoeae* is sensed by the host innate immune system. Neisserial LOS is recognized by the Toll-like receptor (TLR)4–MD2 complex. Porins interact with the TLR2 receptor complex. Peptidoglycan fragments activate the cytoplasmic Nod-1 receptors. These interactions induce the secretion of cytokines, chemokines and antimicrobial peptides.

Gonococcal infection elicits a strong humoral immune response, even though distinct Opa proteins that bind CEACAM1 suppress CD4$^+$ T-lymphocyte function.[31] Dominant antigens are PorB, Opa proteins, RmpM, LOS and iron-regulated proteins. Nevertheless, the antibodies provide limited protection due to bacterial surface variation and an array of bacterial immune evasion mechanisms (see Table 168.2). The extensive phenotype variation and immune escape mechanisms are major obstacles in the generation of a broadly protective gonococcal vaccine.

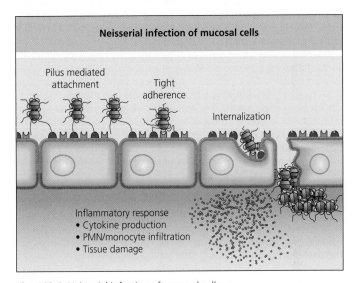

Fig. 168.4 Neisserial infection of mucosal cells.

Table 168.2 Neisserial virulence factors	
Virulence factor	**Function**
Lipopolysaccharide (LPS/LOS)	Lipo-oligosaccharide (LOS) has endotoxin activity and is released as bacterial outer membrane vesicles (blebs) or through cellular lysis. LOS is responsible for toxic damage to the human tissue, development of septic shock and disseminated intravascular coagulation (DIC) through interactions with Toll-like receptors (TLR4) and cytokine induction
Polysaccharide capsule (*N. meningitidis* only)	Polysaccharide surface component which works as a protective shell and blocks the insertion of the membrane attack complex of the complement system and protects the bacteria from phagocytosis. The capsule is the main component enabling bacterial survival in blood and resisting bactericidal antibodies. The serogroup B capsule can also mimic human antigens
Type IV pili	Major adhesins that mediate initial attachment to nonciliated human cells. Also required for efficient transformation of DNA
Outer membrane proteins (OMP)	Dominant antigens. Porin protein promotes intracellular survival. Opacity proteins mediate firm attachment to eukaryotic cells. RmpM protein may protect other antigens from bactericidal interactions with antibodies. Frequent antigenic variation makes it difficult for the host immune system to recognize the porin and opacity protein antigens
Iron-binding proteins	Transferrin-, lactoferrin- and hemoglobin-binding proteins. Pathogenic *Neisseria* spp. are dependent on a constant iron supply for growth
IgA1 protease	Destroys mucosal IgA which is a part of the local immune system
β-Lactamase	An enzyme that hydrolyzes the β-lactam ring of penicillin. Important for antibiotic resistance development in *Neisseria* spp.

Meningococcal disease

Infection due to *N. meningitidis* commonly results from asymptomatic oronasopharyngeal carriage.[32] At any time about 10% of the general population is colonized with meningococci. The carrier state may persist for many months. In children under 4 years of age the carriage rate is less than 1%, but this progressively increases with age to peak at about 20–25% in late teenage and early adult life. During carriage, nongroupable meningococci are most often isolated as the expression of capsule polysaccharide is absent or low. Meningococcal carriage may not be confined to the mucosal surface. Immunohistochemistry has demonstrated meningococci within the tonsilar tissues in 45% of patients undergoing tonsillectomy compared to a carriage rate of 10% determined by nasopharyngeal swabbing.[33]

Meningococcal carriage induces bactericidal antibodies within 1–2 weeks after colonization. Antibodies may last for several months after carriage. *Neisseria lactamica* carriage elicits bactericidal antibodies that cross-react with various meningococcal serogroups and serotypes. As carriage of *N. lactamica* is approximately 4% by 3 months of age and peaks at 21% by 18–24 months of age, this is much higher than carriage of *N. meningitidis* at this age.[32] *Neisseria lactamica* may contribute to protection against meningococcal disease. Development of invasive meningococcal disease correlates with the absence of bactericidal antibodies.[34]

Meningococcal colonization of the nasopharynx largely resembles the events following gonococcal infection (see above and Fig. 168.4). Type IV pili facilitate initial adherence, and opacity-associated proteins (Opa and Opc) and PorB trigger uptake of the bacteria into the cells largely via similar types of receptor (CEACAM, HSPG). Particular sets of Opa protein variants are found in hyperinvasive meningococcal lineages. Opa and Opc proteins that bind heparan sulfate and thus are able to recruit heparin-binding proteins such as vitronectin and fibronection enter cells via integrin receptors.[35] This is accompanied by a downregulation of pili and capsule, enabling optimal contact between bacterial adhesins and the host mucosa. Transferrin (TbpA, TbpB) and hemoglobin (Hbp) binding proteins recruit the iron sources required for growth.[36] Ciliated mucosal cells may be damaged by released peptidoglycan fragments and LOS. Meningococcal (and gonococcal) infection of the oropharynx is usually entirely asymptomatic, possibly because of the relatively high threshold for activation of an inflammatory response compared to more sterile anatomic niches such as the urethra.

The major difference in pathogenesis between gonococci and meningococci is the ability of distinct meningococcal lineages to survive in the bloodstream and to access the CSF (Fig. 168.5). The few phylogenetic groups of *N. meningitidis* that cause meningococcal disease often carry a filamentous prophage in their genome that is secreted from the bacteria via the type IV pilin secretin.[8] The prophage may promote the development of new epidemic clones. The mechanism of meningococcal penetration and passage of the mucosa is only partially understood.[12] Meningococci survive and multiply during epithelial cell traversal. The IgA1 protease and PorB may promote survival inside epithelial cells. Meningococci isolated from the bloodstream invariably produce polysaccharide capsule. The capsule protects the bacterium from phagocytosis and complement-mediated lysis by preventing insertion of the terminal complement attack complex. Invasive meningococci express sialylated LOS which influences binding of C4b, while the proteins PorA and GNA1870 recruit the negative regulators of complement activation C4BP and factor H.[37] Individuals with inherited deficiencies in the late complement components (C6–C9) have a high risk of developing meningococcal disease. Intriguingly, they acquire the infection at a much later age, have frequent recurrences, and the fatality rate is much lower than for normocomplementemic individuals.[37]

In the blood *N. meningitidis* replicates to high levels and sheds outer membrane vesicles (blebs). The blebs may subvert the complement system and high levels of circulating LOS overactivate the innate immune system. Circulating levels of proinflammatory mediators – tumor necrosis factor (TNF), interleukin (IL)-1 and interferon gamma (IFN-γ) – strongly correlate with development of lethal septic shock.[11]

Meningococci enter the CSF likely by the hematogenous route via the veins in the subarachnoidal space (the blood–CSF barrier) and the choroid plexi rather than through the brain parenchyma (blood–brain barrier). Encapsulated *N. meningitidis* invade the CSF probably via the transcellular route.[38] The absence of non-opsonophagocytosis in CSF enables uncontrolled bacterial growth and inflammation of the leptomeninges and subarachnoid space. In the CSF *N. meningitidis* produce polysaccharide capsule and pili and stimulate proinflammatory cytokine (IL-6, IL-8, MCP-1) and chemokine (RANTES, granulocyte–macrophage colony-stimulating factor) production in meningeal cells.[39] Attracted PMNs aggravate the inflammatory response and release cytotoxic mediators.

Immunity to invasive meningococcal disease depends upon the presence of bactericidal IgG antibodies directed against capsule (except serogroup B), PorA, PorB, Opa, LOS, iron-regulated proteins and minor surface proteins. Carriership and nonpathogenic *Neisseria* spp. (e.g. *N. lactamica*) in the nasopharynx elicit cross-reactive antibodies

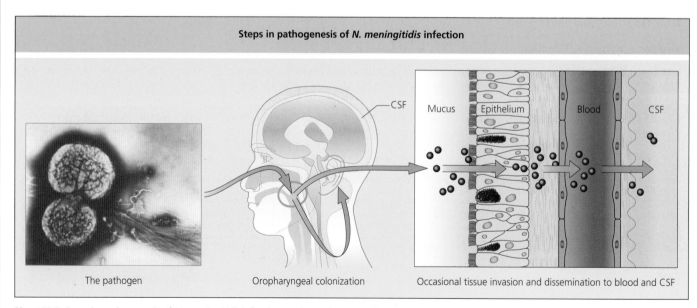

Steps in pathogenesis of *N. meningitidis* infection

The pathogen | Oropharyngeal colonization | Occasional tissue invasion and dissemination to blood and CSF

Fig. 168.5 Steps in pathogenesis of *N. meningitidis* infection. Redrawn from Davidsen *et al.*[5]

that contribute to development of immunity against *N. meningitidis*. *In vivo* phase and antigen variation of meningococcal surface antigens indicate selective immunologic pressure during natural infection.

EPIDEMIOLOGY

Gonorrhea

Gonorrhea is a common sexually transmitted disease worldwide. *Neisseria gonorrhoeae* infection is the second most common notifiable disease in the USA, with 358 366 cases reported in 2006.[40] Incidences in Europe and in the developing world are 10–30 and 4000–10 000 per 100 000 population, respectively.[41] The actual disease burden is probably higher due to underdiagnosis and underreporting. The highest attack rates occur in 15–25-year-old men and women. In regions where collected statistics include sexual orientation, rates of gonococcal infection more than tripled from 1995 to 2003 among homosexual men.

Gonococci are exclusive human pathogens. They cannot spontaneously infect animals. The risk of acquiring a urethral infection for men is approximately 20% after a single vaginal exposure to an infected woman, rising to 60–80% after four or more exposures. The transmission rate from male to female is approximately 50% per contact, rising to 90% after three exposures. Gonococci can be transmitted by orogenital contact or rectal intercourse. Perinatal transmission may also occur. Although gonococci can survive for brief periods outside the human reservoir, extracorporeal transmission is extremely rare.

The major reservoir for continued spread of gonorrhea is the asymptomatic patient. Among infected women, 30–50% are asymptomatic or show no symptoms associated with a sexually transmitted disease.[42] Among infected men, only 5–10% are asymptomatic. Asymptomatic women and men remain infectious for months. Maintenance and transmission of gonorrhea are also related to a social subset of 'core

transmitters' who have unprotected intercourse with multiple new partners and either are asymptomatic or choose to ignore symptoms.[43] The average incubation period for developing gonorrhea is 2–7 days but varies between 1 and 14 days.

Meningococcal disease

Meningococcal disease is a global major health problem (Fig. 168.6).[11,44] Disease patterns differ among populations and infecting strains and can be endemic, hyperendemic, epidemic and pandemic. In 2007, mortality from meningococcal disease worldwide was estimated at 170 000.[41] The case fatality rate is 5–10% in industrialized countries and 10–20% of survivors develop permanent sequelae. Transmission of meningococci occurs by respiratory droplets, requiring close contact. Invasive disease particularly occurs when bactericidal antibodies against the invading strain are lacking and in complement factor-deficient individuals.[34,44] Concurrent viral or mycoplasmal respiratory tract infections facilitate systemic invasion.

The major virulence factor of disease-associated meningococci is the polysaccharide capsule. Most infections are caused by strains belonging to serogroups A, B, C, Y and W135[11,44] (see Fig. 168.6). In Western Europe and the Americas, meningococcal disease is endemic and caused mainly by serogroups B or C with incidences of 1–3/100 000. Periodically, local hyperendemic outbreaks occur when new lineages spread through the population. A serogroup B infection has spread worldwide, culminating in outbreaks in Australia and New Zealand in 2001–2006.[11,44] In China, the Middle East and parts of Africa, serogroups A and C predominate. Large epidemics are attributed predominantly to serogroup A strains. In the African 'meningitis belt', major periodic epidemics of serogroup A disease occur every 5–12 years, with attack rates of 500/100 000 population or higher.[45] The emergence and global importance of serogroups W135, X and Y has been recognized only in the last 10 years. Serogroup W135 was identified in 2002–2003 as a major threat and the main pathogen during outbreaks in Africa.[41]

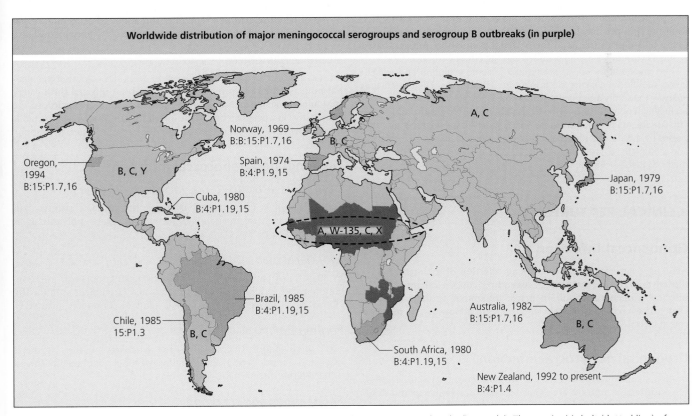

Fig. 168.6 Worldwide distribution of major meningococcal serogroups and serogroup B outbreaks (in purple). The meningitis belt (dotted line) of sub-Saharan Africa is shown. Redrawn from Stephens *et al.*[11]

An unprecedented incidence of serogroup X meningitis was observed in Niger in 2006.[46] Occasionally, particularly virulent strains arise that cause pandemic outbreaks across continents.[11] In the USA, Israel and Sweden, disease due to serogroup Y strains has increased.[47]

The occurrence of meningococcal disease varies with climate, age and social behavior. Serogroup A and C disease increases during the dry season in Africa. The number of serogroup B and C cases peaks during the winter months in the developed countries.[11,44] In the meningitis belt, young school-aged children represent the peak age group. In developed countries, children aged between 1 and 4 years account for the majority of cases with a second peak among teenagers.[11,44] Smoking young adults who socialize frequently at discos and parties may be particularly at risk. The attack rate among family members of a clinical case is 1000-fold higher than in the general population. The acquisition of meningococcal disease requires a combination of a pathogenic organism, a susceptible host, and possibly coincidental mucosal damage by other infections or low humidity. Hereditary factors such as late complement deficiencies and receptor polymorphisms may be additional predisposing factors.[11,37]

Molecular typing of *N. gonorrhoeae* and *N. meningitidis*

The classic methods of monitoring transmission of *N. gonorrhoeae* are auxotyping and serotyping.[48] Auxotyping is based on the different requirements of gonococcal strains for amino acids (proline, arginine) and nucleotides (hypoxanthine, uracil). *Neisseria gonorrhoeae* can be subdivided in 35 auxotypes. Gonococcal serotyping is based on a panel of monoclonal antibodies directed against variant epitopes on PorB-IA and PorB-IB. At least 55 serovars have been identified. These methods have, however, been replaced by DNA-based analysis such as multilocus sequence typing (MLST).[49,50]

Phenotypic classification of *N. meningitidis* is based on antigenic differences of the major surface antigens which provides information about the serogroup (capsule, e.g. B), serotype (PorB porin, e.g. 15), serosubtype (PorA porin, e.g. P1.7) and LOS immunotype (e.g. L3) of a particular strain. This results in the classification: B, 15, P1.7, L3. Multiple epitopes may be recognized depending upon the presence of phase or antigen variants in the bacterial population. Antigen-based typing is currently only relevant for vaccine efficacy studies.

For larger studies on *N. meningitidis* genome evolution and surveillance, multilocus enzyme electrophoresis (ET) typing, DNA restriction analysis, randomly amplified polymorphic DNA (RAPD), restriction fragment length polymorphism (RFLP) and ribotyping have been employed.[32] The current strain typing method, MLST, shows that epidemics are often caused by specific complexes of related hypervirulent lineages.[32,51] Targeted and complete genome sequencing is the next generation of typing methods that is being applied.[52]

CLINICAL FEATURES

Gonococcal infection

Neisseria gonorrhoeae usually causes an infection of the urethra (urethritis) and cervix (cervicitis).[53] Ascending gonococcal infection in infected women can result in pelvic inflammatory disease (PID). Dissemination to more distant sites occurs in about 0.5–3% of gonococcal infection.[24,25]

Urogenital gonococcal infection

In men, acute anterior urethritis is the most common manifestation of gonorrhea. Symptoms are a purulent urethral discharge and dysuria. Acute epididymitis is the most common local complication. In women, the endocervix is the primary site of infection. The infection is characterized by (muco)purulent discharge and intermen-strual bleeding, but is often asymptomatic. Urethral infection is present in 70–90% of women who have gonococcal cervicitis. Infection of the Bartholin's glands leads to abscess formation in about 35% of the patients.

Gonococcal infection in women may ascend to cause endometritis or acute salpingitis in 10–20% of the cases. Symptoms of the clinical syndrome of PID include lower abdominal pain, abnormal cervical discharge and bleeding, fever and peripheral leukocytosis. The onset of gonococcal salpingitis occurs early rather than late in infection and often during or shortly after menstruation. PID causes obstruction of the fallopian tubes and infertility in 10–20% of patients. In pregnant women gonorrhea is associated with an increased risk of spontaneous abortion, premature labor, early rupture of fetal membranes and perinatal infant mortality. PID is uncommon after the first trimester.[54,55]

Gonorrhea in children

Historically gonococcal infection in children included only ophthalmia neonatorum (acute gonococcal conjunctivitis).[56] However, children can acquire gonococcal infection by sexual contact with an infected person.[49,50] Such infection indicates sexual abuse. In girls the infection often produces a vulvovaginitis. Complications affecting the internal genital organs are rare.

Localized gonococcal infection outside the urogenital tract

Proctitis

Anorectal gonorrhea is present in up to 5% of women who have gonorrhea, although gonococci can be cultured from the anorectal region of 40% of women with gonorrhea. A similar proportion of homosexual men have positive rectal cultures for gonococci. Proctitis manifests as anal pruritus, tenesmus, purulent discharge or rectal bleeding.

Pharyngeal gonorrhea

Pharyngeal infection occurs in 10–20% of women who have gonorrhea, in 10–25% of homosexual men who have the infection and in 3–7% of heterosexual men. The infection is due to orogenital sexual exposure. Most cases are asymptomatic and resolve spontaneously.

Acute conjunctivitis

Ocular gonococcal infection is seen in neonates. Ophthalmia neonatorum is acquired during passage through an infected birth canal. In adults ocular infection usually results from autoinoculation of the conjunctiva in a person who has the infection. Gonococcal conjunctivitis is usually severe, with an overt purulent exudate and corneal ulceration.

Disseminated gonococcal infection

Dermatitis–arthritis–tenosynovitis syndrome

This infection is characterized by fever, hemorrhagic painful skin lesions, primarily on the hands or feet, tenosynovitis, polyarthralgias and frank arthritis.[27]

Monoarticular septic arthritis

In 30–40% of patients who have disseminated gonococcal infection, gonococci are localized in one joint and cause a purulent arthritis. The elbows, wrists, fingers and knee or ankle joints are commonly involved.[26]

Perihepatitis

Acute perihepatitis (Fitz-Hugh–Curtis syndrome) occurs by direct extension of gonococci from the fallopian tube, lymphangitic spread or bacteremic dissemination to the liver capsule.

Endocarditis and meningitis

These complications are reported in 1–2% of patients who have disseminated gonococcal infection.[53]

Meningococcal infection

The clinical spectrum of meningococcal disease includes meningo-encephalitis, meningococcemia without meningitis and bacteremia without septic complications.[44,47] On admission, 60% of cases have had symptoms for less than 24 hours and 12–20% for less than 2 days. These symptoms may occur discretely or may blend into one another during clinical disease progression. The disease usually begins abruptly with headache, meningeal signs including stiffness of the neck (Fig. 168.7a) and fever. However, classic signs of men-ingitis (e.g. confusion, headache, fever and nuchal rigidity) are seen in only about one-half of the patients. Very young children often have only nonspecific signs such as fever, abdominal pain and vom-iting. Other signs may be reduced consciousness and photophobia. Mortality approaches 100% in untreated cases, but is around 10% when appropriate antibiotic therapy is instituted. The incidence of neurologic sequelae is low, with hearing deficits, epilepsy and arthritis most commonly noted. These sequelae are most probably underreported.

Meningitis

The most frequent form of meningococcal infection is acute pyo-genic meningitis due to inflammation of the meninges. Meningitis may occur with or without meningococcemia. Among patients who have meningococcal disease, 75% have meningitis; 40% of them also have bacteremia.

Meningococcemia

Meningococcemia may be transient, occult or result in severe sep-sis. Bacteremia without meningitis occurs in 7–10% of patients. Meningococcemia can manifest as pink maculopapular petechial eruptions (Fig. 168.7b).[11] Rapidly progressive infections may result in purpuric/petechial or ecchymotic skin lesions that are hemorrhagic and necrotic (Fig. 168.7c,d). However, skin lesions may be atypical, evanescent or even entirely absent in patients who have blood cul-ture-positive meningococcal sepsis. Fulminant shock may dominate the clinical picture of acute meningococcal sepsis.[11,58] Sepsis may prog-ress to disseminated intravascular coagulation (DIC) characterized by increasing petechiae or purpura fulminans, resulting in extensive areas of tissue destruction secondary to coagulopathy, rapid onset of hypotension and adrenal hemorrhage (Waterhouse–Friderichsen syn-drome). Gangrenous cases in the extremities may occur due to periph-eral vasoconstriction and death may supervene as a result of DIC.

Other meningococcal infections

Persistent meningococcal bacteremia is associated with low-grade fever, rash and arthritis (arthritis–dermatitis syndrome). Meningococci are implicated as the etiologic agent in approximately 5–14% of patients who have community-acquired pneumonia. Pharyngitis is associated with recent contact with individuals who are colonized by meningo-cocci and is often a prior symptom and sign of serious meningococ-cal disease. Due to hematogenous spread meningococci may cause

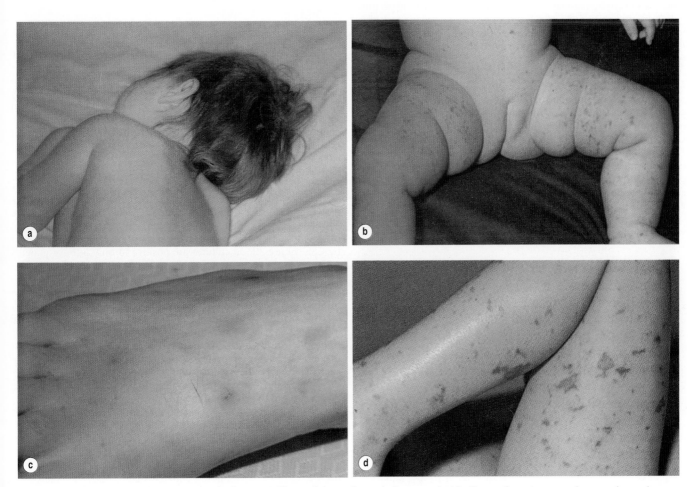

Fig. 168.7 Typical symptoms of meningococcal infection. Stiffness of the neck may indicate meningitis. Fine erythematous macules, maculopapular petechial eruptions and purpuric/petechial or ecchymotic skin lesions that are hemorrhagic and necrotic may accompany meningococcal sepsis. From Brandtzaeg et al.[57]

endocarditis, pericarditis, arthritis, endophthalmitis, osteomyelitis, conjunctivitis and peritonitis. Arthritis is particularly common with an incidence of 11% in adults and 5% in children.

LABORATORY DIAGNOSIS

Gonococcal infection

Diagnosis of gonococcal infection is made at two levels: presumptive and confirmed. Antimicrobial treatment must be started based on the results of the presumptive tests, but additional tests must be performed to yield a confirmatory diagnosis.

Collection of specimens for diagnosis depends on the clinical manifestations and the sites exposed. When appropriate, cultures from blood and biopsies from skin lesions and joint fluid aspirates are started. Male urethral exudates and female cervical swabs should be taken from all cases of suspected gonococcal infection for direct examination and culture. Neutrophils containing Gram-negative cocci in the Gram-stained smear are presumptive evidence of gonococcal infection (Fig. 168.8). Gram stain is highly sensitive and specific for diagnosing genital gonorrhea in men. Gram-stained smears from endocervix specimens of symptomatic women have a sensitivity of only 40–60% relative to culture, but have a high predictive value. In asymptomatic women, Gram stain has a low predictive value and is not useful.

Direct detection (i.e. without culture) of gonococci may also involve rapid and sensitive diagnostic nucleic acid amplification tests (NAATs) that simultaneously detect *N. gonorrhoeae* and *Chlamydia trachomatis*.[42] NAATs require only a freshly voided urine sample. Limitations are cost, risk of carryover contamination, inhibition and inability to provide antibiotic resistance data.[59] Frequent horizontal genetic exchange leading to commensal *Neisseria* spp. acquiring *N. gonorrhoeae* genes may give false-positive results. Furthermore, some *N. gonorrhoeae* subtypes may lack specific sequences targeted by a particular NAAT due to sequence variation in the dynamic gonococcal populations, leading to false-negative results.

Maximal recovery of gonococci requires immediate plating of the collected specimen.[1] If this is not possible, swabs can be transported in commercially available charcoal-containing transport media. Commonly used culture media are Thayer–Martin and Martin–Lewis. These media contain lysed or heated blood (chocolate agar) supplemented with growth factors and a variety of antimicrobials to suppress the growth of other bacteria and yeast. Specimens taken from sites that are normally sterile are cultured on antibiotic-free media to enable growth of occasional strains that are susceptible to the antibiotics added to the growth media. Growth is performed in an atmosphere with 5–10% carbon dioxide at 95–98.6°F (35–37°C) for 24–48 hours.

Isolates on primary culture media are predominantly of the P⁺ (piliated) colony type, being small, glistening and raised. After subculture, P⁻ (nonpiliated) colonies appear that are larger, smoother and flatter than P⁺ colonies. Smears are prepared from suspicious colonies and examined with Gram stain. Gram-negative diplococci with a positive oxidase and catalase test may be *N. gonorrhoeae*.

For confirmatory identification of gonococci, other types of *Neisseria* spp. as well *Moraxella* and *Kingella* spp. have to be considered.[1] Confirmatory identification includes carbohydrate utilization tests, monoclonal antibody fluorescence, chromogenic detection of specific enzyme activities and DNA-based culture confirmation tests. Gonococci oxidize glucose (but not maltose, sucrose or lactose). Serologic tests do not have sufficient sensitivity and specificity for clinical use.

Meningococcal infection

Cerebrospinal fluid, blood, skin biopsies, nasopharyngeal swabs and aspirates are relevant specimens for the diagnosis of meningococcal disease. Additionally, synovial fluid, sputum and conjunctival swabs may be cultured if clinically indicated. Because meningococci, like gonococci, are susceptible to desiccation and temperature extremes, collected specimens should be cultured as soon as possible.

For presumptive diagnosis specimens are examined by Gram stain. Gram-stained smears are made directly from CSF if the CSF is cloudy or after centrifugation if the CSF is clear. The majority of the smears will show Gram-negative diplococci inside and outside PMNs when the CSF bacterial count is >10⁵ ml. Smears from CSF containing <10³ ml of bacteria will be positive in only 25%; on average 60–90% of culture-positive CSF specimens are positive in the Gram stain. Gram-stained smears from petechial skin lesions due to meningococcemia may detect meningococci in more than 70% of cases.

Direct detection of meningococcal capsular polysaccharides in CSF is performed by latex agglutination and coagulation tests with polyclonal antibodies for serogroups A, B, C, Y and W135.[60] These methods can detect 0.02–0.05 mg of antigen per ml. Their sensitivity is only about 50% compared to 82–90% for direct detection of meningococci in CSF and blood by NAATs/PCR.[61] The latter tests are also useful in confirming the diagnosis in patients who had antibiotic treatment prior to collection of CSF and whose CSF Gram stain, antigen test and culture are negative.

The proportion of PMNs in CSF from patients who have meningitis ranges from 49% to 98% (mean of 86%). Other CSF abnormalities include low glucose and an elevated protein concentration. In patients partially treated with antibiotics, the CSF leukocyte count, glucose and protein concentration, and the antigen tests remain abnormal for several days, whereas bacteria might not be evident on smear or by CSF culture. Blood cultures are positive in only 50% of patients with meningococcal disease. In those who have received antibiotics prior to the collection of blood for culture, blood cultures are sterile. A nasopharyngeal swab from young children will provide valuable information in cases of suspected meningococcal disease.

For isolation of *N. meningitidis* the clinical specimen should be inoculated on selective and nonselective growth media (Table 168.3).[1] Appropriate nonselective media are 5% sheep blood agar (in contrast to gonococci, meningococci grow well on this medium) and chocolate agar. Selective media used to culture nasopharyngeal specimens are the same as those mentioned for gonococci. Most blood-containing media support the growth of meningococci. Meningococci are grown on agar media in a 5–10% carbon dioxide-enriched atmosphere with rather high humidity at 95–98.6°F (35–37°C). After 18–24 hours, flat, gray-brown, translucent, smooth, 1–3 mm in diameter colonies of *N. meningitidis* are present which can be analyzed by Gram stain.[1] The finding of oxidase- and catalase-positive Gram-negative diplococci is sufficient to support a tentative diagnosis of meningococcal disease. For confirmatory identification, other species of *Neisseria*, *Kingella* and *Moraxella* have to be taken into account (Table 168.4). Differentiation characteristics are the production of acid from glucose

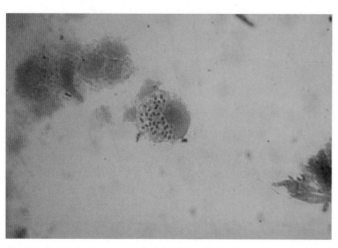

Fig. 168.8 Gram stain of a urethral discharge from a male who has gonorrhea. Note the intracellular Gram-negative diplococci with neutrophils.

Table 168.3 Specimens and culture media for the isolation of *N. gonorrhoeae* and *N. meningitidis*

Species	Disease	Specimen/site	Media for cultivation
N. gonorrhoeae	Cervicitis	Endocervix, urethra (Bartholin's glands, rectum, pharynx)	Selective
	Pelvic inflammatory disease (PID)	Endocervix, endometrium, fallopian tubes	Selective, nonselective
	Disseminated infection (DGI)	Endocervix, urethra, skin lesions Joint fluid Blood	Selective, nonselective Nonselective, selective Blood culture medium
	Ophthalmia	Conjunctiva	Nonselective, selective
N. meningitidis	Meningitis/septicemia	Cerebrospinal fluid Blood Nasopharynx Skin lesions	Nonselective, blood culture medium Blood culture medium Selective, nonselective Nonselective

Table 168.4 Characteristics of the most common human *Neisseria* spp.

Species	Colony morphology on chocolate agar	ACID FROM		Lactose	Sucrose	Fructose	Reduction of nitrate
		Glucose	Maltose				
N. gonorrhoeae	Gray-brown, translucent, smooth (0.5–1 mm diameter)	+	–	–	–	–	–
N. meningitidis	Gray-brown, translucent, smooth (1–3 mm diameter)	+	+	–	–	–	–
N. lactamica	Gray-brown, translucent, smooth (1–2 mm diameter)	+	+	+	–	–	–

and maltose. Gonococci acidify only glucose and *N. lactamica* produces acid from glucose, maltose and lactose, although a number of commensal *Neisseria* spp. may be misidentified as *N. meningitidis* on the basis of carbohydrate oxidation. Enzyme tests may further differentiate these species.[1] Isolation of *N. meningitidis* can also be finally confirmed by NAATs/PCR, DNA sequence or MALDI/TOF analysis.

Infections caused by other Neisseriaceae

The so-called nonpathogenic *Neisseria* spp. colonize the human nasopharynx and oropharynx. They comprise eight species (*N. lactamica, N. cinerea, N. polysaccharea, N. sicca, N. subflava, N. flavescens, N. mucosa* and *N. elongata*). These species do not grow on the enriched antibiotic-containing media used for the isolation of gonococci and meningococci.[1]

Strains of *N. lactamica, N. subflava, N. cinerea* and *N. polysaccharea* can be isolated from the selective media and differentiated by their patterns of acid production (see Table 168.4).[1] Without additional tests, including chromogenic enzyme substrate tests and serologic tests, the eight species may be misidentified as meningococci or gonococci.

Neisseria lactamica produces acid from lactose and can thus be differentiated from meningococci. This and other nonpathogenic neisserial species are only occasionally associated with disease, although *N. lactamica* has been isolated from cases of meningitis or sepsis in both adults and children (Table 168.5).

Neisseria animalis, N. denitrificans, N. canis, N. dentiae, N. macacae and *N. iguanae* are present in the oropharynx of guinea pigs, cats, cows, monkeys and iguanas, respectively, and have not been associated with human disease.[1]

In general, the nonpathogenic *Neisseria* spp. are susceptible to penicillin, ampicillin and tetracyclines. Only *N. mucosa* is penicillin resistant and sensitive to chloramphenicol. Some strains of *N. lactamica* have an altered penicillin-binding protein 2 as found in relatively penicillin-resistant *N. meningitidis*. Rare strains of *N. sicca, N. flavescens* and *N. subflava* are penicillin resistant because of production of β-lactamase. Such strains are a potential source of β-lactamase genes that are transferable to meningococci and gonococci.[1]

THERAPY AND MANAGEMENT

Gonorrhea

Without treatment male urethral infection subsides after 2–3 months. Repeated infection, if untreated, leads to stricture of the urethra. Such sequelae are now rare, because the signs of urethritis bring most men to diagnosis and treatment. In 10–20% of women, gonorrhea results in ascending genital infection and PID, manifested by endometritis, salpingitis, tubo-ovarian abscess and pelvic peritonitis. Infertility due to fallopian tube obstruction is the most common and serious sequela of PID and occurs in 15–20% of women after a single episode and in 50–80% of women after three or more episodes.[62] In addition, disseminated gonococcal infections may occur. In the pre-antibiotic era, *N. gonorrhoeae* was a frequent cause of endocarditis and meningitis. Patients with gonorrhea may have concurrent sexually transmitted disease (STD) infections. *Chlamydia trachomatis* can be recovered from 15–30% of men who have gonococcal urethritis and from 35–50% of women who have endocervical gonorrhea.[63]

After the emergence of sulfonamide-resistant strains, penicillin was introduced as treatment for gonorrhea. Since 1976, gonococcal isolates with a decreased sensitivity for penicillin (minimum inhibitory concentration (MIC) >0.1 mg/1) have been recovered. This chromosomally encoded penicillin insensitivity results from mutations at the *pen* A, *pen* B, *env* and *mtr* genes, which can be spread by

Table 168.5 Nonpathogenic neisserial species rarely isolated from clinical disease in humans

Neisserial species	Clinical disease observed when isolated
N. lactamica	Meningitis or sepsis in adults and children
N. cinerea, N. polysaccharea, N. sicca, N. subflava	Native and prosthetic endocarditis, often in patients with heart abnormalities or intravenous drug use
N. sicca	Native and prosthetic valve endocarditis Meningitis cases Rarely pneumonia and osteomyelitis
N. subflava	Rarely endocarditis, meningitis and sepsis
N. flavescens	Once in an outbreak of meningitis Occasionally in sepsis resembling chronic meningococcemia
N. mucosa	Occasional endocarditis, meningitis, ocular infections, cellulitis, pneumonia and empyema.
N. cinerea	Conjunctivitis in newborns (ophthalmia neonatorum) Proctitis and lymphadenitis Meningitis in patients with facial trauma Pneumonia in immunodeficient patients
N. elongata	Endocarditis or sepsis Wound infections, osteomyelitis after oral surgery
N. weaveri	Human wounds due to dog bites

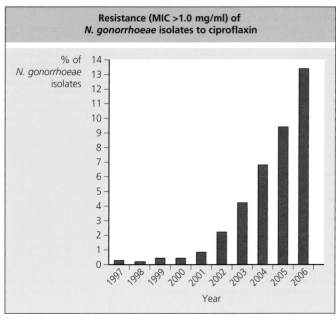

Resistance (MIC >1.0 mg/ml) of *N. gonorrhoeae* isolates to ciproflaxin

Fig. 168.9 Resistance (MIC >1.0 mg/ml) of *N. gonorrhoeae* isolates to ciprofloxacin, United States, 1997–June 2006. Redrawn from Centers for Disease Control and Prevention.[40]

natural transformation. Mutations in the *pen* genes alter penicillin-binding proteins, reducing their affinity to penicillin. The *mtr* locus encodes an efflux pump. Mutations of *mtr* and *env* alter the permeability of the gonococcal membrane. These strains represent 10–16% of all gonococci in the Western world. In 1976, strains of gonococci that were totally resistant to penicillin due to β-lactamase production were also recovered. These isolates contain a plasmid (Pc^r) that carries the genes for a TEM-1 type β-lactamase. Even though the prevalence of penicillinase-producing *N. gonorrhoeae* (PPNG) remains stable at about 5–10% in Western Europe and the USA, it is no longer common practice to treat gonococcal infections with penicillin. One reason is that therapy failure has implications for the infected patient as well as for public health.[64] Antibiotic regimens for gonorrhea require high patient compliance and an efficacy of 100%. Fluoroquinolones (i.e. ciprofloxacin, ofloxacin or levofloxacin) are also no longer recommended for treatment of gonococcal infections[40] due to the sharp increases in antibiotic resistance[65] (Fig. 168.9). The high-level quinolone resistance (MIC >0.1–16 mg/l) is chromosomally mediated, mainly due to mutations in *gyrA* (the gene encoding DNA gyrase) and *parC* (topoisomerase IV). Tetracycline is not recommended as primary treatment of uncomplicated gonococcal infections due to the high-level of tetracycline resistance caused by a conjugative plasmid into which the *tetM* transposon has inserted.

Present recommendations for treatment of uncomplicated gonorrhea are based on regimens that provide high efficacy, that have potential effect against concurrent STDs (particularly *C. trachomatis*) and that can be administered as a single dose to obtain maximal

patient compliance.[40] Typical regimens are ceftriaxone (one intramuscular dose) or a single oral dose of cefixime. Each of the therapies also includes a single oral dose of azithromycin (or doxycycline for 1 week) for the treatment of co-infecting *C. trachomatis*. One oral dose of azithromycin is most often active against both gonococci and *C. trachomatis*. Doxycycline is contraindicated during pregnancy. Pregnant women who have gonococcal infection are treated with ceftriaxone followed by 7–10 days of erythromycin.[40]

Treatment of PID has been performed with a large number of antibiotic combinations. The important role of both gonococci and *C. trachomatis* in producing PID has been elucidated and, although the role of various anaerobes in PID has not yet been ascertained, many studies have shown that anaerobic cover is essential for treatment of PID patients. The recommended regimens now include intravenous cefotetan or cefoxitin plus doxycycline and/or metronidazole.[40] The recommended regimen for treatment of outpatients is a 2-week combination of oral ofloxacin and clindamycin or metronidazole. Amoxicillin–clavulanic acid together with doxycycline also covers the major pathogens responsible for PID. Azithromycin in combination with amoxicillin–clavulanic acid may also give excellent activity against *N. gonorrhoeae*, anaerobes and *C. trachomatis*.

Complicated gonococcal infection in males (acute epididymitis) is treated with a single dose of ceftriaxone plus doxycycline for 10 days. Treatment of disseminated gonorrhea always starts with ceftriaxone. Children who have gonococcal infection are treated with ceftriaxone. The latest USA recommended treatment regimens are available at http://www.cdc.gov/std/treatment.

Meningococcal disease

The mainstay of treatment for patients who have meningococcal disease is benzylpenicillin or a third-generation cephalosporin (e.g. ceftriaxone).[11] For most cases of uncomplicated meningococcal meningitis, 7-day treatment is adequate. When the etiology is not known at admission, ceftriaxone or cefotaxime is used for the first 24–48 hours to cover the possibility of other bacterial pathogens.[11] β-Lactamase-producing strains have occasionally been recovered. These strains harbor the same plasmid as many PPNG. In addition, there are

N. meningitidis strains that are not β-lactamase positive but have decreased sensitivity to penicillin due to reduced affinity of penicillin to penicillin-binding proteins 2 and 3, resulting from an altered *penA* gene. Although the frequency of relatively penicillin-resistant meningococci is low, continued surveillance is necessary. Cefotaxime or ceftriaxone is used when relatively penicillin-resistant strains are isolated. Treatment of meningococcal septic shock with plasmapheresis or inhibitors of inflammatory mediators is still in the experimental phase.

PREVENTION

Gonococcal infection

Condoms provide a high degree of protection from acquisition of gonorrhea, as well as other STDs. Other preventative measures are early diagnosis and treatment, partner notification and screening, and case finding. A new approach is the use of topical microbicides for intravaginal or intrarectal use.

Attempts to develop a gonococcal vaccine have been hampered by the high degree of antigenic variability in pili, outer membrane proteins and LOS during the natural course of infection. There are currently no suitable animal models for testing gonococcal vaccine efficacy. Transfected animals expressing human proteins involved in *Neisseria* infection such as transferrin receptors, CR3, CD46, CEACAMs and Toll-like receptors may aid vaccine development.

Meningococcal disease

Prevention of meningococcal disease is based on chemoprophylaxis and vaccination.[47]

Chemoprophylaxis

The aim of chemoprophylaxis is to reduce secondary cases of meningococcal disease and to arrest outbreaks. The risk of a secondary case among close contacts in the household setting is 150–1000 times higher than that in the general population. Children are at greatest risk, but secondary disease can occur at all ages. Risk is maximal in the week following recognition of the index case but extends for several weeks.

Many antibiotics used for therapy do not effectively eradicate or prevent carriage of meningococci because of inadequate levels in oropharyngeal secretions. Rifampin (rifampicin), ceftriaxone, azithromycin and the quinolones are effective against meningococci in the naso- and oropharynx.[11] However, rifampin resistance can develop rapidly and quinolone resistance in meningococci has recently been reported. Ceftriaxone as a single intramuscular dose is 97% effective in household contacts 1–2 weeks after infection. The advantage of ceftriaxone is that it can be used in pregnancy and in small children.

Chemoprophylaxis is recommended only for close household contacts of cases and other intimate contacts. Patients who have meningococcal disease should receive chemoprophylaxis before discharge from the hospital, because parenteral antibiotic treatment of meningococcal disease (except ceftriaxone) is unreliable in eliminating meningococci from the nasopharynx.

Polysaccharide vaccines

Polysaccharide vaccines reduce the incidence of infection among military recruits, reduce the progress of epidemics of serogroup A disease and protect susceptible complement factor-deficient individuals.[11] Capsule polysaccharide vaccines are available for the pathogenic meningococcal serogroups A, C, Y and W135. These vaccines are safe, with mild local adverse events, and have good efficacy (>85%) in older children and adults. However, due to lack of a T-helper response, the vaccines are poorly immunogenic below 2 years of age, fail to induce immunologic memory and provide protection for only 3–5 years. Polysaccharide vaccines are used by travelers visiting countries with a high incidence of meningococcal disease. A polysaccharide vaccine against serogroup B meningococci is not available due to carbohydrate mimicry and poor immunogenicity.

The immunogenicity of polysaccharide vaccines is greatly improved by chemical conjugation to a protein carrier. The resulting polysaccharide conjugate vaccines are safe, immunogenic in young infants and induce long-term memory. Polysaccharide conjugate vaccines against serogroups A, C, W135 and Y are now available. These vaccines are so far safe and immunogenic, are anticipated to provide long-term protection (as they induce a T-cell-dependent response) and are effective in young children.[66] Introduction of the C conjugate meningococcal vaccines in 2000 markedly reduced the incidence of serogroup C disease in the UK with estimated vaccine efficacies of 88% in young children and 95% in young adolescents. Immunization also decreased nasopharyngeal carriage by 66% and transmission of the pathogen (herd immunity).[67] However, widespread use of monovalent serogroup conjugate vaccines may become ineffective when the capsule types switch due to genetic exchange or strains arise that show reduced capsule expression.

Outer membrane protein vaccines

Complement-mediated killing of encapsulated strains is also achieved with cross-reactive antibodies directed against outer membrane components. Developed outer membrane vesicle (OMV) vaccines with a low LOS composition show efficacies of 50–80% in clinical trials, but do not protect young children and are in general too strain specific, i.e. the vaccines can be used against clonal disease outbreaks, but not for prevention of sporadic disease caused by diverse strains. Multivalent vaccine strains based on common variants of PorA (a major inducer and target of bactericidal antibodies) may provide protection against multiple subtypes of *N. meningitidis*. Recently, novel conserved candidate vaccine antigens have been identified using a 'reverse vaccinology' approach.[68] Currently, the lipoproteins GNA1870 and GNA2132, the conserved surface proteins OMP85, NspA and NadA, as well as PorA, pilin and LOS conjugates, are being evaluated for their vaccine potential.

REFERENCES

References for this chapter can be found online at http://www.expertconsult.com

Luce Landraud
Sylvain Brisse

Chapter |**169**|

Enterobacteriaceae

INTRODUCTION

As a whole, the family Enterobacteriaceae can be considered ubiquitous as members are found in various ecologic sources such as soil, water, vegetation and animals.[1-3] Some species are important pathogens of plants,[4] while many species are part of the normal flora of many animals including humans. Because many Enterobacteriaceae species are believed to be natural inhabitants of the gut, the terms 'enteric bacteria' or 'enterics' are sometimes used to refer to the taxonomic family Enterobacteriaceae. However, this practice is not advised, since these terms can cover all species of the gut (including Enterobacteriaceae) and some Enterobacteriaceae members (e.g. the epiphytes or plant pathogens) do not have the gut as a natural habitat.

Some Enterobacteriaceae species are more frequently associated with infection in animals and humans.[2] Some of the most important pathogens in human history, such as the agent of plague *Yersinia pestis*, belong to Enterobacteriaceae, and members of the family represent a huge public health concern (e.g. *Salmonella enterica* serotype Typhi, *Shigella*, *Escherichia coli*). Two main types of infectious disease are associated with Enterobacteriaceae: intestinal diseases and extraintestinal diseases. The transmission route of intestinal infection is classically orofecal with exogenous ingestion of specific pathogens, either by person-to-person transmission or, more often, by environmental (water and food) contamination. An endogenous pathway of infection is also possible (e.g. bacterial translocation from the gut to blood), as is more often observed in immunocompromised hosts or persons with underlying conditions such as cirrhosis or chemotherapy.

This chapter focuses on aspects of taxonomy, pathogenesis, clinical diagnosis and management of human Enterobacteriaceae infections. Other aspects have been covered elsewhere.[1-3,5]

TAXONOMY, PHYLOGENY AND CLONAL RELATIONSHIPS

In the prokaryotic taxonomy, Enterobacteriaceae represent the only family within the Order Enterobacteriales, itself one of 15 Orders within class Gammaproteobacteria, which belongs to phylum Proteobacteria (sometimes still referred as 'purple bacteria and their relatives'). Based on 16S rRNA gene sequences, the closest phylogenetic relatives of Enterobacteriaceae appear to be the Pasteurellaceae, the Vibrionaceae, and members of the Orders Aeromonadales and Alteromonadales (Fig. 169.1).

The family Enterobacteriaceae currently includes (as of mid-2009) more than 210 species and 50 genera, and these numbers will doubtless continue to increase rapidly. Release 7.7 of the Taxonomic Outline of Bacteria and Archaea includes 43 Enterobacteriaceae genera

(http://www.taxonomicoutline.org). A history of taxonomic changes and synonyms of species is maintained at http://www.bacterio.cict.fr. Recent taxonomic changes for taxa of medical relevance include:

* the proposal of *Escherichia albertii* for *eae*-positive diarrhea-causing strains that are closely related to *Shigella boydii* serotype 13 and were previously attributed to *Hafnia alvei*;

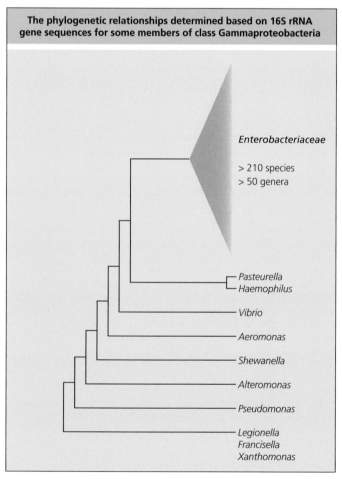

Fig. 169.1 A schematic representation of the phylogenetic relationships determined based on 16S rRNA gene sequences for some members of class Gammaproteobacteria. Based on currently available data, the bacterial groups that are most closely related to Enterobacteriaceae are families Pasteurellaceae and Vibrionaceae, Order Aeromonadales, genus *Shewanella* and Order Alteromonadales. Data from the Ribosomal Database Project, http://rdp.cme.msu.edu.

- the demonstration that *Plesiomonas shigelloides*, which is associated with water-borne diarrhea, belongs to Enterobacteriaceae even if it is oxidase positive;
- the creation of genus *Cronobacter* that includes several former *Enterobacter* species, including *C. sakazakii*;
- the realization that most '*E. cloacae*' nosocomial isolates actually belong to *E. hormaechei*; and
- the transfer of *Calymmatobacterium granulomatis*, the agent of granuloma inguinale (donovanosis), to genus *Klebsiella*, as it is closely related to *K. pneumoniae*.

Further, one should note that since its proposal, the validity of genus *Raoultella* has been questioned by several authors.[3] The recent review by Janda[3] provides detailed information on some of the newest Enterobacteriaceae taxa, including a review of the evidence for their medical significance.

A precise phylogeny of Enterobacteriaceae genera and species would be useful for taxonomic purposes and would allow understanding of the evolution of characteristics such as biochemical capabilities, host range, ecology and virulence. Unfortunately, the 16S rRNA molecule is poorly informative within this family,[6] and sequencing of other genes will be needed to establish a robust phylogeny of Enterobacteriaceae species.

All *Salmonella* strains are currently classified into two species: *S. enterica* and *S. bongori*. The type strain of a proposed third species, *Salmonella subterranea*, does not appear to belong to the genus *Salmonella* based on gene sequences, and the taxonomic position of this species within *Salmonella* should be reconsidered. *Salmonella enterica* itself is subdivided into six subspecies: *enterica, arizonae, diarizonae, houtenae, indica* and *salamae*. *Salmonella enterica* subsp. *enterica* is by far the most important from a medical standpoint, representing 99% of clinical infections. For details of *Salmonella* nomenclature, including serovar naming, see Figure 169.2.

The genus *Escherichia* currently includes the species *E. coli, E. fergusonii, E. albertii, E. hermanii, E. vulneris* and *E. blattae*. Clinically, *E. coli* is by far the most important species. Sequence comparisons indicate that *E. fergusonii* and *E. albertii* are closely related to *E. coli*, while the three remaining species may be evolutionarily more distant.

The clonal diversity of *E. coli* strains was initially disclosed based on multilocus enzyme electrophoresis (MLEE), but is currently best described by large-scale multilocus sequence typing (MLST) approaches.[7,8] Genome-wide sequence data of multiple strains are now being produced.[9] As shown earlier, based on DNA–DNA hybridization[10] and MLEE studies,[11] the genomic species that includes *E. coli* strains also includes *Shigella* strains, with the exception of *Shigella boydii* serotype 13 (Fig. 169.3). Hence, *Shigella* species were distinguished historically based on clinical and biochemical characteristics, but *Shigella* strains are phylogenetically more closely related to some *E. coli* strains than are some *E. coli* strains between themselves. In addition, the three taxonomic *Shigella* species *S. flexneri, S. dysenteriae* and *S. boydii* do not correspond to three phylogenetic clusters within the *E. coli* species.[12] Rather, the major *Shigella* clusters may comprise strains from two or more *Shigella* 'species'. In contrast, both *S. sonnei* and *S. dysenteriae* group 1 form unique and genetically homogeneous clusters.

Other pathotypes of *E. coli*, such as enteropathogenic *E. coli* (EPEC), enterotoxigenic *E. coli* (ETEC) or enterohemorrhagic *E. coli* (EHEC), also show multiple independent origins and parallel evolution (see Fig. 169.3).[8,12,14] There are currently several MLST schemes in use and efforts are ongoing to harmonize the set of genes used to identify *E. coli* strains. In the near future, nearly complete genome sequences of multiple *E. coli/Shigella* strains will be available (see, e.g., http://xbase.bham.ac.uk).

DIAGNOSTIC MICROBIOLOGY

All Enterobacteriaceae are Gram-negative, nonspore-forming bacilli. They are either motile by peritrichous flagella (except *Tatumella ptyseos*) or nonmotile. With a few exceptions (e.g. *Klebsiella granulomatis*), they grow rapidly on ordinary laboratory media, under either aerobic or anaerobic conditions. Growth is generally optimal at 99°F (37°C). Some specific properties are common: all species utilize glucose fermentatively (often with gas production), are oxidase negative (with the exception of *Plesiomonas shigelloides*) and catalase positive, and reduce

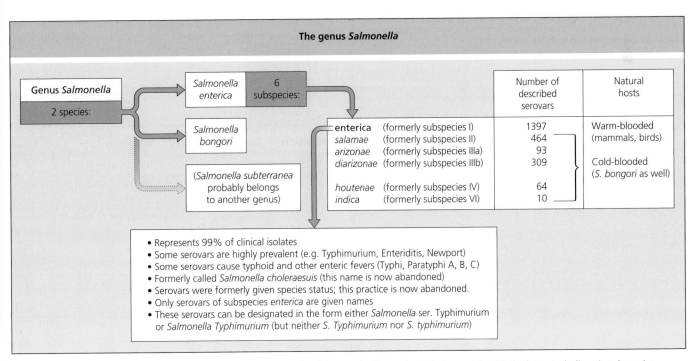

Fig. 169.2 The genus *Salmonella* includes two species, *S. bongori* and *S. enterica* (formerly *S. choleraesuis*), with the latter including six subspecies. Nomenclature has evolved from a system where all serovars (the combination of O antigen and the two phases of the H antigen) were considered as species (e.g. *Salmonella typhi*) into the current system, which gives names to serovars of subspecies *S. enterica* subsp. *enterica* (e.g. *S. enterica* subsp. *enterica* serotype Enteritidis), but designates the serovars of other subspecies and of *S. bongori* simply by their antigenic formula. More details can be found at http://www.bacterio.cict.fr/s/salmonella.html.

The polyphyletic origin of *Shigella* and *Escherichia coli* pathotypes

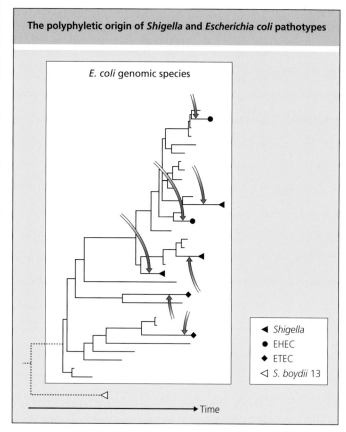

Fig. 169.3 Schematic representation of the polyphyletic origin of *Shigella* and *Escherichia coli* pathotypes, which are each found on several branches that are nested inside the diversity of *E. coli*. *Shigella* (black triangles), enterotoxigenic *E. coli* (ETEC; black diamonds) and enterohemorrhagic *E. coli* (EHEC; black circles) pathotypes have several independent origins from ancestral strains that have incorporated virulence genes by horizontal transfer (grey arrows). Among the *Shigella*, only *Shigella boydii* serotype 13 (open triangle) represents a lineage distinct from the phylogenetic cluster corresponding to the *E. coli* species.

nitrates to nitrites (excepted *Photorhabdus* and *Xenorhabdus*). Some useful features for identification of Enterobacteriaceae species that are common in clinical samples are given in Table 169.1; more details on identification methods can be found in other reference texts.[5]

In classic nonselective media, colonies are circular and convex, with a smooth surface and a diameter of 1–3 mm after 24 hours. Selective media are used to recover Enterobacteriaceae from fecal samples or other specimens containing complex flora. These media enhance the growth of particular Enterobacteriaceae species, while inhibiting non-desired species. Classically, these media (e.g. MacConkey lactose- or sorbitol-containing media) contain substrate(s) selectively used by one or a few species and facilitate distinction between colonies. More precise distinction of genera and species is obtained by differences in biochemical activity (enzyme profiles, carbon source utilization, pH-based reactions). Several miniaturized tests are available commercially (e.g. Api 20E or Biotype-100 strips from BioMerieux). Typically, isolates are identified by comparison of their biochemical profile with a reference database that contains the percentages of positive results for each substrate/species pair. More automated identification systems based on the same approach are classically used in larger microbiology laboratories.[15] One limitation of this approach is that isolates that are biochemically atypical or correspond to rare or novel species (thus not incorporated in the reference databases) cannot be identified or can even be misidentified. Typically, Enterobacteriaceae species that are common pathogens are easily identified but identification of environmental species can be problematic. Automated methods can also test antimicrobial susceptibility, which is important in regard to the increase of resistant strains isolated in human infections.

In some species, serotyping remains the predominant means by which routine identification is performed beyond the species level, given the high epidemiologic and medical relevance of serotype characterization. This is the case, for example, for *Salmonella* strains. In fact, biochemical profiling is not sufficient for diagnosis of the serotypes causing typhoid or typhoid-like fevers (Typhi, Paratyphi A, B and C). Serotyping of Enterobacteriaceae is based on antigenic variation of the O (somatic, corresponding to the polysaccharide side chain of the lipopolysaccharide), H (flagellar) and K (capsular) surface antigens. In some species, most or all strains do not have a capsule (*E. coli*, *Salmonella*), whereas the capsule is the predominant and most discriminatory antigen of *Klebsiella*. Serotyping is typically performed

Table 169.1 Major properties used to identify the most common Enterobacteriaceae implicated in human infections

Species	BIOCHEMICAL TESTS					Remarks
	TDA	VP	ONPG	Indole production	Citrate (Simmons)	
Escherichia coli	(–)	(–)	(+)	(+)	(–)	Utilization of inositol (–)
Citrobacter spp.	(–)	(–)	(+)	Variable	(+)	Urease variable, H$_2$S (–) except *C. freundii*
Shigella spp.	(–)	(–)	(–) except *S. sonnei*	(+)*	(–)	Utilization of xylose (–)
Salmonella enterica	(–)	(–)	(–) except *S. arizonae*	(–)	(+) except Typhi and Paratyphi A	H$_2$S (+)
Yersinia spp.	(–)	(–)	Variable	Variable	(–)	H$_2$S (–), urease (+) except *Y. pestis*
Enterobacter spp.	(–)	(+)	(+)	(–)	(+)	LDC (–) except *E. aerogenes* and *E. gergoviae*, ODC (+)
Klebsiella spp.	(–)	(+)[†,‡]	(+)[†]	(–) except *K. oxytoca*	(+)[†]	ODC (–) except *K. ornithinolytica*
Serratia spp.	(–)	(+)	(+)	(–)	(+)	Gelatin hydrolysis (+) except *S. fonticola*

(Continued)

Table 169.1 Major properties used to identify the most common Enterobacteriaceae implicated in human infections—cont'd

Species	TDA	VP	ONPG	Indole production	Citrate (Simmons)	Remarks
				BIOCHEMICAL TESTS		
Proteus spp.	(+)	(−)	(−)	(−) except *P. vulgaris*	Variable	H_2S (+), urease (+)
Morganella morganii	(+)	(−)	(−)	(+)	(−)	H_2S (−), urease (+)
Providencia spp.	(+)	(−)	(−)	(+)	(+)	H_2S (−)

*30–70% positive reaction for *S. dysenteriae* or *S. flexneri*, and negative for *S. Sonnei*
†Except *K. pneumoniae* subsp. *rhinoscleromatis*.
‡Except *K. pneumoniae* subsp. *ozaenae*.
(−), 70–100% negative reaction; (+), 70–100% positive reaction; variable, different reactions between different species or <70% positive/negative reaction for strains of the species. H_2S, hydrogen sulfide production; LDC, lysine decarboxylase; ODC, ornithine decarboxylase; ONPG, O-nitrophenyl-β-D-galactopyranoside; TDA, phenylalanine deaminase; VP, Voges–Proskauer.

by slide agglutination using sets of O, H and K antisera, and the resulting combination of antigens defines the serotype (also called serovar). The most familiar serotyping scheme is the Kauffman–White scheme used for *Salmonella*, which distinguishes more than 2540 serotypes.[16] In *E. coli*, serotyping is important for identification of particular pathovars such as the EHEC strains or for identification of *E. coli* strains that possess the K1 capsular type and are implicated in neonatal infections. Serotyping is also used for *Shigella* identification. In *Klebsiella*, K typing can confirm identification of *K. pneumoniae* subspecies *rhinoscleromatis* and *ozaenae*, as the former has capsular type K3 (although rare *K. pneumoniae* subsp. *pneumoniae* are K3) and the latter is most often K4 (and sometimes K5).

Finally, knowledge of specific virulence factors and the pathogenesis of infection allowed the development of molecular diagnostic methods. For example, virulence factors of pathogenic strains include specific adhesins which confer the ability to colonize the intestinal mucosal surface, and specific factors which interfere with the normal physiology of epithelial cells. These genotypic methods are very important in particular situations, for example to make the distinction between diarrheagenic *E. coli* and commensal strains, or to detect toxin-producing *E. coli* strains causing the hemolytic–uremic syndrome. Advances in genomic characterization of virulence factors will continue to allow the development of new diagnostic methods based for example on nucleic acid-based probes, polymerase chain reaction (PCR) methods or DNA arrays.[17]

GENERAL PATHOPHYSIOLOGIC CONSIDERATIONS

Enterobacteriaceae are associated with both intestinal and extraintestinal infections, among which, ordered by frequency, are urinary tract infection, bacteremia, pneumonia, abdominal or pelvic infection, surgical site infections, meningitis and various abscesses including wound infections (Fig. 169.4). Despite the fact that many Enterobacteriaceae are part of the normal facultative flora of the gastrointestinal tract of mammals, this family represents a major contributor to human infections, ranking among the most frequent groups of pathogens in many clinical sources.

The balance between host defenses and virulence factors of Enterobacteriaceae members is a key factor that determines commensalism or disease (Fig. 169.5). Commensal bacteria themselves represent an important barrier against infection, as colonization of the gut by harmless commensals protects the host from intruding pathogens. Recognition by the host of the commensal flora occurs through the tolerance phenomenon.[18,19] The tolerogenic process that maintains homeostasis is based on various specific interactions between

microbes and the digestive mucosa. The physical barrier of the mucus together with antibacterial molecules creates a distance that maintains commensal bacteria separate from the epithelial surface. Specific features of commensal species, such as inhibition of nuclear factor kappa B (NF-κB) by *Lactobacillus casei*, or particular characteristics of epithelial cells, such as the reduced expression of Toll-like receptor 4 (TLR4) at the gut surface epithelium, reduce the effects of bacterial stimuli, thus avoiding inflammation that would be detrimental for the host.[20] Enteric bacteria modulate inflammation leading to host responses that are compatible with their survival and restrain other intestinal resident flora members.[19,21] The specific digestive Enterobacteriaceae pathogens *E. coli*, *S. enterica*, *Shigella* spp. and *Yersinia*, as well as examples of mechanisms by which they breach the intestinal barrier, are described in more detail below.

Extraintestinal infections by Enterobacteriaceae occur through microbial colonization of normally sterile sites. Each anatomic site presents specific molecular structures and defenses against infection, and bacteria must therefore express specific colonization factors to adhere to these structures and specific virulence factors to counter these defenses.

Many pathogenicity factors have been described in Enterobacteriaceae. These factors are often clustered in chromosomal regions called pathogenicity islands (PAIs), which were first described in uropathogenic and diarrheagenic *E. coli*.[22,23] Most pathogenic Enterobacteriaceae are characterized by specific sets of PAIs (Table 169.2) whereas these PAIs are absent in nonpathogenic strains. PAIs are acquired by horizontal transfer and are typically associated with tRNA genes, flanked by repeated sequences, and may differ from the core genome in guanine and cytosine (G+C) content and in codon usage.

CLINICAL MANIFESTATIONS

Intestinal infections

The most important enteric pathogens are *S. enterica*, some strains of *E. coli*, *Shigella* and *Y. enterocolitica*. Although other Enterobacteriaceae are occasionally implicated in gastrointestinal infections, clinical significance is sometimes controversial (e.g. for *Plesiomonas shigelloides* or diarrhea-associated *K. pneumoniae*). Indeed, Enterobacteriaceae isolated from stool specimens during acute diarrhea could reflect the drastic change in stool flora, rather than being the cause of the symptoms.

Escherichia coli

Six distinct pathotypes of diarrheagenic *E. coli* are classically distinguished: enterotoxigenic, enteropathogenic, enterohemorrhagic, enteroinvasive, enteroaggregative and diffusely adherent *E. coli*. Identification

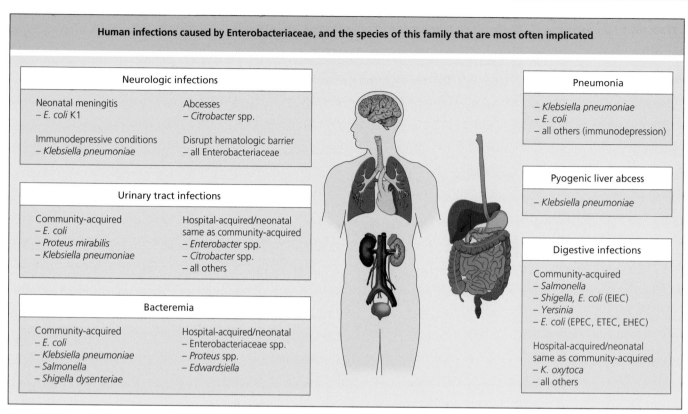

Human infections caused by Enterobacteriaceae, and the species of this family that are most often implicated

Neurologic infections

Neonatal meningitis – *E. coli* K1	Abcesses – *Citrobacter* spp.
Immunodepressive conditions – *Klebsiella pneumoniae*	Disrupt hematologic barrier – all Enterobacteriaceae

Urinary tract infections

Community-acquired – *E. coli* – *Proteus mirabilis* – *Klebsiella pneumoniae*	Hospital-acquired/neonatal same as community-acquired – *Enterobacter* spp. – *Citrobacter* spp. – all others

Bacteremia

Community-acquired – *E. coli* – *Klebsiella pneumoniae* – *Salmonella* – *Shigella dysenteriae*	Hospital-acquired/neonatal – Enterobacteriaceae spp. – *Proteus* spp. – *Edwardsiella*

Pneumonia

– *Klebsiella pneumoniae*
– *E. coli*
– all others (immunodepression)

Pyogenic liver abcess

– *Klebsiella pneumoniae*

Digestive infections

Community-acquired
– *Salmonella*
– *Shigella, E. coli* (EIEC)
– *Yersinia*
– *E. coli* (EPEC, ETEC, EHEC)

Hospital-acquired/neonatal
same as community-acquired
– *K. oxytoca*
– all others

Fig. 169.4 Human infections caused by Enterobacteriaceae and the species of this family that are most often implicated.

of diarrheagenic *E. coli* strains requires their distinction from commensal *E. coli* strains, which is rendered possible by their specific sets of virulence factors, sometimes in combination with serotyping. Table 169.3 summarizes clinical, epidemiologic and biologic features of the distinct pathotypes.

Enterotoxigenic Escherichia coli (ETEC)

First described in Calcutta in 1956, ETEC is a major etiologic agent of diarrhea in infants younger than 2 years of age in developing countries, with an estimated 1.5 million deaths per year.[24] The illness caused by ETEC is abrupt with a short incubation period. Diarrhea is watery, similar to *Vibrio cholerae* infection, and fever is often absent. Two clinical syndromes are distinguished: weaning diarrhea, mostly observed among children in the developing world, and travelers' diarrhea. Immunologic protective response could explain the decrease in incidence after 5 years of age. Co-infection with ETEC and other enteric pathogens is common, rising to 40% of cases in endemic areas. ETEC is endemic all year round in numerous countries from Africa, Asia and Latin America. However, the infection is more common in warm and wet months. ETEC may be the cause of 20–40% of travelers' diarrhea and represents the most frequent cause of diarrhea for North American and European travelers visiting developing countries.[24]

Two classes of enterotoxins contribute to the pathogenesis of ETEC:

- the LT-I and LT-II heat-labile oligomeric toxins, which are closely related to cholera enterotoxin; and
- STa and STb heat-stable monomeric toxins.

A large number of ETEC fimbrial antigens have been characterized constituting multiple Colonization FActors (CFAs; more than 22 CFAs are known). The initial nomenclature that designated them as 'colonization factor' (CFA/I to IV) was replaced in the mid-1990s by a uniform designation composed of the initials 'CS' for 'coli surface antigen' and number (e.g. CS2), except for CFA/I.[24]

Unfortunately, ETEC is still difficult to recognize in minimally equipped laboratories. Serotyping was rapidly abandoned because ETEC isolates may belong to a large number of serotypes that change over time. Several immunoassays (including radioimmunoassay and enzyme linked immunosorbent assays) were widely used in ETEC diagnosis until the use of PCR to detect LT- and ST-producing *E. coli*, either in isolated colonies or directly from stools. DNA probes and PCR methods were also developed to detect ETEC colonization factors.

Enteropathogenic Escherichia coli (EPEC)

EPEC infections cause diarrhea in infants younger than 2 years except for rare cases in adults attributed to ingestion of large inocula. Outbreaks are common in developed countries, where EPEC is a major cause of infant diarrhea, with high mortality rates. Clinical manifestations include profuse watery diarrhea, vomiting and fever, all of which contribute to severe dehydration.

EPEC pathogenesis consists of bacterium-to-bacterium localized adherence pattern (LA phenotype), signal transduction and intimate adherence of the bacteria to the enterocyte membrane with disruption of the apical cytoskeleton.[25] Infection by EPEC induces attaching and effacing (A/E) lesions characterized by effacement of microvilli and intimate adherence to the epithelial cell membrane, with formation of pedestal-like structures. Two specific genetic elements are implicated: the EPEC adherence factor (EAF) plasmid encoding a cluster of 14 genes coding for the expression and assembly of the bundle-forming pilus (BFP) and a 35 kb chromosomal pathogenicity island called the locus of enterocyte effacement (LEE).[25] This locus encodes a type III secretion system (T3SS) and multiple EPEC-secreted protein (Esp) effectors. One of these, the translocated intimin receptor (Tir), acts as a receptor for intimin (Eae), a 97 kDa bacterial outer membrane protein. Adherence of EPECs to epithelial cells induces increases in the intracellular calcium levels, host cell protein phosphorylation with activation of kinases that leads to changes in intestinal water and electrolyte secretions. The formation of A/E lesions reduces the

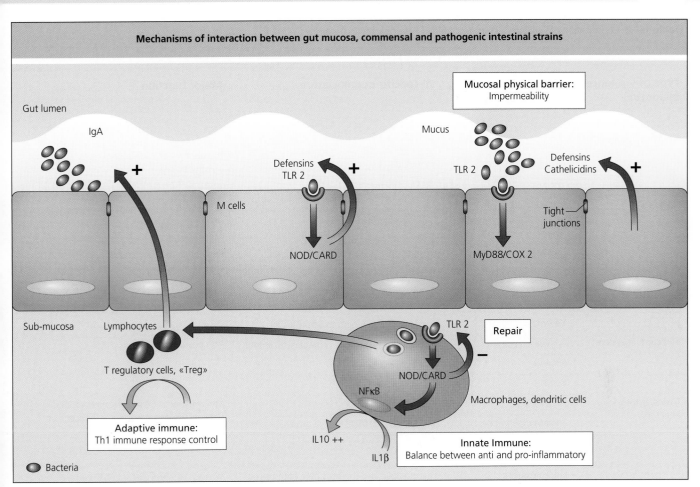

Fig. 169.5 Interplay between intestinal bacteria and the host. At the proximity of the intestinal mucosa, physical barriers exclude bacteria by the impermeability of the epithelium with tight junctions, and by production of factors excreted by epithelial cells themselves such as defensins or cathelicidins. The mucus is composed of mucin glycoproteins that interplay with bacteria, which are trapped and maintained at a distance from the epithelium. When the intestinal mucosa is exposed to bacteria (pathogens or commensal in hosts with underlying conditions), an effective immune activation is essentially based on three major regulated events. (1) Activation of TLR2/MyD88-dependent signaling is essential for effective intestinal repair in response to epithelial damage in the presence of commensal bacteria. (2) Innate immune mechanisms with activation of macrophages, dendritic cells or neutrophils are central in the control of local inflammation (NOD2/CARD15 pathway). A central role of the NOD/CARD system implicated in the controlled production of NF-κB is demonstrated. (3) Induction of regulatory T cells by commensal bacteria, with low induction of Th1 differentiation, is observed and explains at least in part the associated tolerance.

Table 169.2 Classification of virulence factors described in Enterobacteriaceae species

| Type of virulence factor (VF) | Bacterial source | DESCRIPTION | |
		VF-specific nomenclature	Major function
Colonization factors, adhesins	*Escherichia coli*	P-fimbriae: type 1 common pili; sfa fimbriae: CFA/I to IV in ETEC; bundle-forming pilus (BFP) and Tir in EPEC; AAF/I and AAF/II in EAEC; Afa adhesins in DAEC	Adherence to target epithelial cells via specific receptors
	Shigella	–	
	Salmonella	Curli	
	Yersinia	Invasin	
	Proteus	MR/P fimbriae; PMF (*P. mirabilis* fimbriae), ATF (ambient temperature fimbriae), NAF (nonagglutinating fimbriae)	
	Klebsiella	Type 1 common fimbriae, type 3 fimbriae, type 6 fimbriae	

Table 169.2 Classification of virulence factors described in Enterobacteriaceae species—cont'd

Type of virulence factor (VF)	Bacterial source	VF-specific nomenclature	Major function
Component of secretion system	*Escherichia coli*	T3SS *sep/esp* locus in EPEC and EHEC	Molecular needle that permits export of secreted bacterial proteins across bacterial membranes and injection directly into target eukaryotic cells
	Salmonella	T3SS *inv/spa* locus	
	Shigella	T3SS *mxi/spa* locus (also described in EIEC)	
	Yersinia	T3SS *ysc* locus	
Flagella	Many members of Enterobacteriaceae except *Shigella*	–	Mobility, proinflammatory activity
Capsular polysaccharide	*Escherichia coli*	K1 antigen	Resistance to antimicrobial complement activity and prevention of antibacterial serum resistance
	Salmonella serotype Typhi	Vi antigen	
	Klebsiella	K capsular antigens: K1, K2, K4 and K57 emergent capsule	
	Yersinia	YadA, AIL (attachment invasion locus)	
Iron capture system	*Escherichia coli*	Aerobactin, chu protein, yersiniabactin in EAEC	Iron acquisition
	Shigella	*foc, fet, iuc* and *iut* loci	
	Yersinia	Yersiniabactin	
Toxins, cytotoxic effectors	*Shigella* spp.	Pic serine protease	Mucolytic activity; modification of 28S ribosomal subunit leading to apoptosis of target cells
	Shigella dysenteriae	Shiga-toxin (Stx) (ADP ribosyltransferase toxins)	
	Enterohemorrhagic *Escherichia coli*	Shiga-like toxin (Stx)	
	Enterotoxigenic *Escherichia coli*	Thermolabile and thermostable enterotoxins (LT, ST)	Increase of intracellular cAMP causes modification of apical ion channel activity in target cells
	Enteroaggregative *Escherichia coli*	EAST-1, antiaggregative toxin, plasmid-encoded toxin, Pic protease	Unknown
	Uropathogenic *Escherichia coli*	Hemolysin alpha (RTX toxins), CNF1	Proinflammatory activity; modification of Rho GTPase (for CNF1)

T3SS effectors

Effectors targeting or mimicking Rho GTPase family members	*Salmonella*	SopE2, SopE, SptP	Modification of cytoskeletal actin and macropinocytosis
	Shigella	IpaA, IpaC, IpgB1, IpgB2	
	Yersinia	YopT, YopE, YpkA/YopO	
Effectors targeting innate immune signaling pathways	*Salmonella*	SipB (SspB), AvrA, SspH1, SpvC	Apoptosis in macrophages and dendritic cells; inhibition of NF-κB signaling and IL-8 production
	Shigella	OspG, OspF, IpaB	
	Yersinia	YopJ	
Effectors targeting actin polymerization directly	Enteropathogenic *Escherichia coli*	Tir	Actin nucleation and pedestal formation
	Salmonella	SipA (SspA), SipC (SspC)	Induction of actin polymerization
	Shigella	IcsA (VirG), IcsP, VirA	Actin nucleation
	Yersinia	YopH	Antiphagocytic activity targeting a major focal adhesin
Effectors promoting intracellular survival	*Salmonella*	SseF, SseG, SseJ, SopD2, SifA, PipB2, SspH2, SptP	Contribution of Sif formation and microtubule formation
	Shigella	IcsB	Host cell survival and prevention of autophagic recognition of IcsA/VirG

cAMP, cyclic adenosine monophosphate; DAEC, diffusely adherent *E. coli*; EAEC, enteroaggregative *E. coli*; EHEC, enterohemorrhagic *E. coli*; EIEC, enteroinvasive *E. coli*; EPEC, enteropathogenic *E. coli*; ETEC, enterotoxigenic *E. coli*; IL, interleukin; NF-κB, nuclear factor kappa B.

Table 169.3 *Escherichia coli* and intestinal infections

Pathotype of *E. coli*	Clinical manifestations	Histologic effects	Specific virulence factors	Diagnostic methods	References
Enterotoxigenic *E. coli* (ETEC)	Watery diarrhea; travelers' diarrhea; endemic cholera-like illness in children; developing countries	LT-B subunit binding GM1 and LT-A subunit increase cyclic AMP production, leading to chloride and neutral sodium chloride secretion	LT (enterotoxin, heat labile) and ST (enterotoxin, heat stable); various colonization factors (CFs) including CS1 at CS7, CFA/I and CFA/II	Immunologic detection of LT (ELISA, passive latex agglutination); specific cytopathic effects on CHO cells; detection of LT or ST gene (*stx*) (PCR)	Qadri et al.[24] Nataro & Kaper[25]
Enteropathogenic *E. coli* (EPEC)	Watery diarrhea with vomiting and fever; children <2 years; developing countries	A/E adhesion; actin-rich pedestal	Outer membrane intimin adhesin (*eae* gene); LEE pathogen (T3SS, *esc* genes, Esp effectors); EAF plasmid (bundle-forming pilus); intimin receptor Hp90 or Tir; EAST-1 (*astA* gene)	A/E adhesion effect on Hep-2 cytotoxic assay; detection of *eae* gene and/or EAF probe DNA (typical strain) (PCR or hybridization); O:H serotyping (O55, O86, O111, O119, etc.)	Nataro & Kaper[25] Franckel & Phillips[26]
Enterohemorrhagic *E. coli* (EHEC)	Late bloody diarrhea, hemolytic–uremic syndrome triad (thrombocytopenia, hemolytic anemia, renal failure); children and young adults; industrialized countries	A/E adhesion; actin-rich pedestal (identical to EPEC)	Outer membrane intimin adhesin (*eae* gene); LEE pathogen (T3SS, *esc* genes, Esp effectors); pO157 plasmid with notably enterohemolysin gene (in O157:H7 strains); *stx* genes ++ (specific virulence); EAST-1 (*astA* gene)	Detection of *stx* (PCR or hybridization), accessory detection of *eae* gene; O:H serotyping (O157:H7 ++, O26, O103, O111, etc.)	Nataro & Kaper[25]
Enteroinvasive *E. coli* (EIEC)	Classic watery diarrhea; minority dysentery syndrome	*Shigella*-like invasion of epithelium	Large virulence plasmid (220 kb, 100 genes); TTSA type secretion (*mxi/spa* locus); Ipa, Ipg and Osp effectors; Vir regulators; IcsA/VirG	Guinea pig keratoconjunctivity or Sereny test; DNA probe hybridization (17 kb pMR17-*Eco*RI fragment or 2.5 kb *Hind*III fragment pInv-ial); detection of *ial* gene (PCR)	Nataro & Kaper[25] Parsot[27]
Enteroaggregative *E. coli* (EAEC)	Watery diarrhea; travelers' diarrhea; children and adults; HIV patients; developing and industrialized countries	Adherence to epithelial cells with typical 'stacked-brick' pattern; mucoid biofilm formation; toxic effects	Large plasmid (typical strains); EAST-1; transcriptional activator gene; *she* patho-island; HPI *Yersinia* island; 18.30 kDa outer membrane adhesin; AAF/I, AAF/II, AFA/III factors	Adherence with specific pattern in HEp-2 cell assays; detection of CVD432 (PCR)	Jenkins et al.[28] Huang et al.[29] Weintraub[30]
Diffusely adherent *E. coli* (DAEC)	Watery diarrhea persistent in young children; developing and industrialized countries	—	Afa, dra operon; others?	DA pattern in HEp-2 adherence assays; detection of *daaC* gene (PCR or hybridization)	Le Bouguenec & Servin[31]

A/E adhesion, 'attaching and effacing' adhesion; ELISA, enzyme linked immunosorbent assay; PCR, polymerase chain reaction.

absorptive capacity of the intestinal epithelium and could also explain diarrhea. Moreover, the two EPEC effectors EspF and Map (mitochondrial-associated protein) act to disrupt tight junction integrity and to induce apoptotic cell death, respectively, disrupting intestinal barrier function.[32]

Diagnosis of EPEC has long been determined by serotyping, as EPEC corresponds to only a few serotypes. In fact, the hallmark of EPEC infection is the ability to induce the A/E histopathologic effect, which can be reproduced in cell culture. A diagnostic method that relies on the fluorescent actin staining (FAS) test is very specific when associated with negative Shiga toxin production (see EHEC section). However, this phenotypic test is not easy to perform. Genotypic tests were developed for the detection of the three major characteristics of EPEC: the *eae* gene responsible for the A/E phenotype, an EAF probe (not constant, with atypical strains) and absence of *stx* genes coding for Shiga toxins.

Enterohemorrhagic Escherichia coli (EHEC)

First reported in 1983, EHEC strains are responsible for gastrointestinal illnesses including severe abdominal pain and grossly bloody diarrhea that can be accompanied by the hemolytic–uremic syndrome (HUS) several days after the onset of diarrhea (sometimes 10–15 days later). HUS is specifically associated with thrombocytopenia and hemolytic anemia, as well as acute renal failure which often requires dialysis treatment. EHEC constitutes the most common etiologic agent of infectious HUS in children and appears as an emergent diarrheic agent in industrialized countries.[33] Contamination by food, particularly of bovine origin, caused the first outbreaks reported in the USA, but water-borne and person-to-person transmission were also reported.[34]

Also named STEC for *stx*-producing *E. coli*, EHEC infection is recognized based on the association of the LEE pathogenicity island (containing an *eae* gene as in EPEC), which confers an A/E histopathology effect, and the production of a cytotoxin of the Stx family including a prototype Stx1, identical to Stx1 of *S. dysenteriae* type 1 and Stx2 variants.[34] The presence of Stx toxins diffusing in the circulation appears to be a determinant in the development of HUS, leading to vascular damage in the colon and kidneys, specifically by induction of apoptosis.[35] Other toxins have been described in EHEC, such as EAST-1 (also present in the enteroaggregative *E. coli* (EAEC) pathotype) and hemolysin.

Bacteriologic diagnosis is not easy and depends on early investigation, as HUS is often observed several days after the onset of diarrhea, when patients no longer have STEC in their stools. The recommended diagnostic method consists of detecting DNA encoding *stx* and *eae* factors directly in the fecal flora. Initially restricted to the O157:H7 serotype, which does not ferment D-sorbitol (as opposed to other *E. coli* strains), EHEC were detected by sorbitol nonfermenting colonies in specific agar. At present, the increase in incidence of *stx*-producing *E. coli* of other serotypes (e.g. O26, O103, O111 and O145), which do not have specific biochemical characteristics, complicates the detection of STEC in stools.[25]

Enteroinvasive Escherichia coli (EIEC)

First described in 1971 as being capable of causing diarrhea in volunteers, EIEC is closely similar to *Shigella* biochemically as well as for its genetic and pathogenic characteristics (see Phylogeny section). EIEC infections are mostly described in developing countries, appearing in the form of outbreaks. Although person-to-person transmission can occur, as also described for shigellosis, diarrhea is usually food- or water-borne.

The major virulence factor is a 220 kb plasmid, named the virulence plasmid (VP). The pathogenic mechanism of EIEC is virtually identical to that of *Shigella* (see below). Although EIEC can be responsible for a dysenteric syndrome with blood, mucus and leukocytes in stools, this clinical presentation is less frequent than upon infection with *Shigella*. Watery diarrhea is common and indistinguishable from ETEC infections.

For bacteriologic diagnosis, specific polynucleotide probes have been defined based on virulence factor sequences, which are detected by a multiplex PCR system or hybridization.[17,36]

Enteroaggregative Escherichia coli (EAEC)

This pathotype was first described in 1991 as 'enteroadherent *E. coli*' for non-EPEC adherent strains associated with diarrhea.[37] Nataro and colleagues[25] later recognized two phenotypes, diffuse (see below) and aggregative adherence (AA), characterized by a stacked-brick formation of bacterial cells attached to HEp-2 cells, consisting of the first description of EAEC. EAEC is an important emerging agent in developing countries, mostly in children younger than 2 years of age.[30] This pathogen is also an important cause of diarrhea in HIV-infected patients and travelers. The typical illness is a watery, mucoid, secretory diarrhea with low-grade fever. Vomiting is classically absent. Although the exact mechanism of pathogenesis is not fully understood, a model in three stages was proposed:[25]

- adherence to intestinal mucosa by aggregative fimbriae (AAF/I and AAF/II);
- stimulation of mucus production and mucoid biofilm production; and
- elaboration of EAEC cytotoxins responsible for damage to intestinal cells.

A 108 kDa plasmid encodes a toxin that elicits destructive lesions in the rat ileal loop and could constitute a putative enteroaggregative virulence factor. Another EAEC heat-stable enterotoxin encoded by the *astA* gene is a 4.1 kDa homologue of the ST protein (EAST-1); however, although this may play a role, it is detected in only 40% of cases of EAEC. The diagnosis of EAEC diarrhea is difficult and is performed in only a few laboratories. The gold standard method for the identification of EAEC is the HEp-2 adherence assay with the characteristic aggregative or 'stacked-brick' adherence pattern. EAEC strains are highly heterogeneous and many strains are auto-agglutinable, which excludes serotyping as a bacteriologic diagnostic method. DNA probe CVD432, corresponding to an anti-aggregative protein transporter gene *aat* encoded on a plasmid, was proposed as a good candidate (89% sensitive and 99% specific compared to the HEp-2 adherence test). More recently, multiplex PCR was proposed to identify EAEC.[28] However, as EAEC strains could lack some virulence markers, the HEp-2 adherence assay remains the preferred diagnostic test.

Diffusely adherent Escherichia coli (DAEC)

Diffusely adherent *E. coli* constitutes a heterogeneous group of isolates which are associated with watery diarrhea in children older than 1 year of age. All DAEC strains are defined by a diffuse adherence (DA) pattern to HEp-2 or HeLa culture cells. This adherence phenotype is due to the production of adhesins encoded by a family of operons related to *afa/dra/daa* genes.[31,38] These adhesive structures are both afimbrial (such as Afa) or fimbrial (such as F1845 encoded by daaC or Dr) and have been demonstrated to recognize the Cromer blood group antigen Dr(a) on the human decay-accelerating factor. Afa/Dr DAEC was reported initially in extraintestinal *E. coli* infection by a uropathogenic strain[39] and does not appear specific to strains associated with diarrheal diseases (DAEC). Moreover, these structures were also described among commensal *E. coli* from normal digestive flora. Although the interaction between Afa/Dr adhesins and receptors leads to cell signaling resulting in actin modification, the implication of Afa/Dr DAEC strains in diarrhea remains controversial.[38]

Shigella

Symptoms of shigellosis are mild watery diarrhea or more severe inflammatory bacillary dysentery, characterized by fever, abdominal cramps, and blood and mucus in stools. A large proportion of all diarrheal episodes worldwide are attributed to *Shigella*, with 1.1 million fatal cases annually; approximately 99% of cases occur in developing countries.[40]

The four *Shigella* species, a genus first described by K. Shiga, are now known to be part of the genomic species *E. coli*, with the exception of *S. boydii* serotype 13, which is closely related to *E. albertii*.[41] The genus *Shigella* includes *S. dysenteriae*, *S. flexneri*, *S. sonnei* and *S. boydii*, each being subdivided into several serotypes based on O antigen variation. *Shigella dysenteriae* is responsible for the most severe form and the majority of fatal shigellosis cases; *S. flexneri* and *S. sonnei* are found predominantly in developing and industrialized countries, respectively.[42]

Shigella are facultative intracellular pathogens derived from *E. coli* by parallel acquisition of virulence factors, including chromosomal PAIs and the pINV virulence plasmid (see above, Taxonomy and EIEC sections). Evolution of *Shigella* has also involved substantial loss of gene functions, such as flagella and fimbriae. Various PAIs have been described, including sequences encoding several iron acquisition systems (e.g. *iuc* or *fec* locus) or specific toxins (enterotoxin ShET1 encoded by setA1 and set1B). The prominent virulence determinant of *Shigella* is the large virulence plasmid (pINV) which encodes approximately 100 genes including the T3SS machinery, regulators VirB and MxiE, and several protein effectors and chaperones that stabilize the T3SS substrates. The *mxi/spa* locus encodes the components of the T3SS machinery, deriving from flagellar architecture consisting of a needle protruding from the basal body to the bacterial surface.[43] This essential machinery is required for the translocation of approximately 25 effector proteins from the bacterial cytoplasm into epithelial cells, leading to bacterial invasion and intracellular survival[42] (Fig. 169.6).

Shigella's effectors modulate the immune response, favoring bacterial invasion and intracellular survival.[40,42] Severe tissue damage during *Shigella* infection results from an adaptive inflammatory response with caspase-1 dependent macrophage killing. Tissue destruction and secretion by *Shigella* of enterotoxins 1 and 2 (shET1, shET2) which induce fluid secretion into the intestine explain diarrhea. In addition,

S. dysenteriae serotype 1 secretes the Shiga toxin, responsible not only for vascular lesions in the colon but also in the central nervous system (CNS) and kidney, thus being associated with life-threatening complications.

Salmonella

The genus *Salmonella* includes the two species *S. bongori* and *S. enterica*, the latter being subdivided into six subspecies (see Fig. 169.2). *Salmonella enterica* subsp. *enterica* is responsible for 99.9% of human infections. To date, more than 2540 serovars of *S. enterica* have been described, with 1400 of these within the subspecies *enterica*. Two major forms of salmonellosis are distinguished: enterocolitis (gastroenteritis) and typhoid (enteric) fever. *Salmonella enterica* serovars Typhi and Paratyphi A, B and C and Sendai are responsible for typhoid and typhoid-like fevers and are only known to infect humans. Typhoid fever is characterized by a systemic infection where bacteria colonize the liver, spleen and bone marrow, associated with discrete gastrointestinal symptoms. This systemic illness leads to an estimated 20 million cases and 200 000 deaths worldwide each year. The population structure of the genetically monomorphic serotype Typhi has recently been disclosed,[44] indicating that most genotypic variants that diversified from the ancestor of Typhi approximately 50 000 years ago still survive in the present human population. This observation is best explained by the superposition of two epidemiologic patterns, with outbreaks of acute infection leading to a proportion (approximately 5%) of asymptomatic carriers that allow the survival and transmission of most Typhi genotypes over long periods of time.

Gastroenteritis can be caused by a large number of serovars including Typhimurium and Enteritidis, the most frequent ones in many countries. Infection is localized to the intestine, without systemic

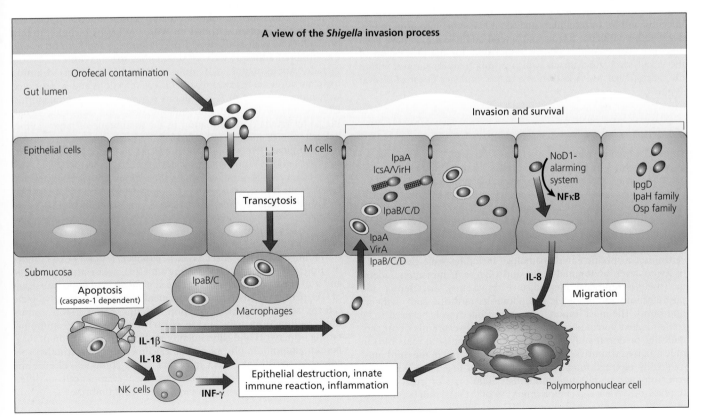

Fig. 169.6 A view of the *Shigella* invasion process. *Shigella* transmitted by the fecal–oral route reach the large intestine, transcytose across the epithelial layer through M cells, and encounter resident macrophages. *Shigella flexneri* is capable of survival in macrophages, inducing apoptosis and release of proinflammatory cytokines such as IL-1β or IL-8. IL-8 induces a massive infiltration of neutrophils, which destroy the integrity of the epithelial layer. Once released from macrophages, bacteria invade the epithelial cells from the basolateral side, escape to phagosomal vesicles, and move in the intracellular cytoplasm by polymerization of actin, ultimately invading neighboring cells. Adapted from Schroeder & Hilbi.[40]

diffusion in most cases. Some serovars cause disease in both humans and animals and have large host ranges, whereas others are more host restricted.

Typically acquired by contaminated foods or water, *Salmonella* colonize the intestine and can translocate across the intestinal epithelium by multiple mechanisms including invasion of M cells, via solitary intestinal lymphoid tissue[45] or a subset of dendritic cells,[46] or by disruption of tight junctions.[47] Translocation of *Salmonella* allows interaction with intestinal epithelial cells through their basolateral surface and leads to the production of proinflammatory cytokines and chemokines. Interaction between TLR5 and the major subunit of bacterial flagella, encoded by *fliC*, has been highlighted.[48] Although downregulation of *fliC* expression in *Salmonella* helps to explain how bacteria could evade the host immune defense in mesenteric lymph nodes, TRL5-dependent detection of flagellin seems to facilitate dissemination to these lymphoid tissues.[46,48]

Similar to *Shigella*, *Salmonella* injects effectors directly into the cytoplasm of epithelial cells. Manipulation of the host cytoskeleton leads to macropinocytosis and active invasion of enterocytes.[49] Specific targets of *Salmonella* effectors are a Ras subfamily of GTPases, the Rho GTPases. These proteins are essential targets for bacterial virulence factors. The active form is associated with GTP interacting with effectors at the eukaryotic membrane cell, while the inactive form associated with GDP is sequestered in the cytosol by GDP dissociation inhibitor (GDI)-Rho protein. The switch between activation and inactivation of Rho GTPases constitutes a specific balance implicated in the regulation of the organization of the actin cytoskeleton and in various essential physiologic events. Different *Salmonella* effectors targeting Rho GTPases alter the function and lead to internalization of the bacteria in nonphagocytic cells. After internalization, *Salmonella* are enclosed in a spacious phagosome, the SCV (for *Salmonella* containing vacuole), derived from membrane ruffles.

Two major *Salmonella* pathogenicity islands (SPIs), SPI-1 and SPI-2, are required for invasion of the epithelial cells in the early steps of infection and for intracellular survival and systemic infection, respectively. Other virulence factors and several additional SPIs have been described. For example, SPI-7 is responsible for the production of the Vi polysaccharide capsule, which is important for survival within the macrophage and is known as a major virulence factor of serovar Typhi.[50]

Yersinia

Three taxonomic species of the genus *Yersinia* – *Y. enterocolitica*, *Y. pseudotuberculosis* and *Y. pestis* – cause human infections. *Yersinia pestis*, the agent of plague, has species status in the nomenclature for obvious clinical and historic reasons, even if *Y. pestis* actually corresponds to a recently emerged pathogenic clone of *Y. pseudotuberculosis*.[51] As plague is discussed in Chapter 120, and a recent review is available,[52] it will not be developed further in this chapter.

Yersinia enterocolitica is the most common species causing enteric yersiniosis, a specific enteric pathology including acute gastroenteritis (with fever, abdominal pains and diarrhea), mesenteric adenitis (pseudo-chirurgical appendicular symptoms), bacteremia and postinfectious immunologic complications (arthritis and erythema nodosum). The most important source of infection is believed to be contaminated porcine products. Most cases of yersiniosis occur sporadically, predominantly affecting young children (<10 years old) in industrialized countries. This infection could represent the third most frequently reported food-borne gastroenteritis in Europe.[53] A recent epidemiologic study found more than 5000 cases of gastroenteritis implicating *Yersinia* spp., representing 5% of the total number of intestinal infections observed between 1997 and 2004.[53]

Pathogenic *Yersinia* invade Peyer's patches and disseminate to lymphoid tissues, including liver and spleen, where they suppress and reorient the immune system. The bacteria contain a plasmid that encodes a T3SS, which is essential for virulence expression of *Yersinia*.[54] The virulence plasmid also encodes many effectors (named

Yop for '*Yersinia* outer proteins'), which translocate via the T3SS directly into eukaryotic cells and prevent proinflammatory warning signals by hijacking the host's intracellular machinery.[55] YopH constitutes a potent tyrosine phosphatase targeting a focal adhesion protein that is essential for phagocytosis.[55] Other effectors modulate the activities of Rho GTP binding proteins. YopE is a GTPase activating protein, YopT a cysteine protease and YpkA/YopO a multifunctional protein with both serine–threonine kinase activity and GDI activity. The latter protein prevents phagocytosis by macrophages and modifies cytoskeletal dynamics.[55–57] YopP/YopJ is able to interfere with inflammatory pathways, inhibiting the phosphorylation and degradation of IκB, the inhibitor of NF-κB.[58]

Extraintestinal infections

Urinary tract infections

Urinary tract infections (UTIs) are among the most common bacterial infections in humans and account for significant morbidity and high medical costs (see Chapters 53, 55 and 56).

The uroepithelium is a specialized stratified transitional epithelium composed of three cell layers, which prevent the entry of pathogens. The apical membrane of umbrella cells exhibits extended horizontal compact structures called 'plaques' and 'hinges'. These structures cover the totality of the bladder uroepithelium and are required for its impermeability.[59,60] Nevertheless, both plaques and hinges are highly detergent-insoluble lipid domains, thus assimilated to lipid rafts, and it has been reported that uropathogenic *E. coli* (UPEC) may penetrate the bladder uroepithelium through lipid rafts.[61] Moreover, plaques and hinges contain integral membrane proteins called uroplakins (UPIa, UPIb, UPII and UPIIIa/b) and UPIa is the receptor for one important adhesive appendage of UPEC, the type 1 pili.[60]

UPEC differs from commensal *E. coli* by the presence of specific virulence factors such as adhesins, toxins, capsule and iron uptake systems, which are often encoded by PAIs.[22] Adhesins include the fimbrial adhesins such as the type 1 pili, P-fimbriae and S-fimbriae, and the afimbrial adhesins such as AfaE. Other specific virulence factors include various toxins. α-Hemolysin (Hlyα) is the most common toxin encountered in extraintestinal *E. coli* infections and is associated with more than half of *E. coli* strains responsible for pyelonephritis. Hlyα seems to interfere with inflammatory and apoptotic signaling pathways via pore formation in the membrane of target epithelial cells, which modifies the intracellular calcium concentration.[62,63] A co-regulated Hlyα toxin, CNF1, is found in one-third of all UPEC strains[64,65] and in some K1 *E. coli* strains.[66] These specific UPEC virulence factors act together to bypass the various host defense mechanisms of the urinary tract.

Other common Enterobacteriaceae associated with UTIs are *Klebsiella pneumoniae* and *Proteus mirabilis*.[67,68] These species infect specific groups of patients such as those with diabetes mellitus or neuropathic bladders and urinary catheters. A common pathogen in both community and hospitalized UTIs, *K. pneumoniae* possesses a number of virulence determinants, including adhesins, urease activity, capsule and iron-scavenging systems.[69–71] *Proteus mirabilis* is an important agent of UTI, particularly in hospitalized patients and notably those who are catheterized. A hallmark of infection with this species is stone formation, resulting from active urease which hydrolyzes urea to ammonia, raising urinary pH and subsequently leading to precipitation of magnesium ammonium phosphate and calcium phosphate. Another specific characteristic of *Proteus* infections is the ability to colonize the surfaces of catheters, linked to the capacity of swarmer cells to differentiate between and to express large numbers of fimbriae.[67,72]

Respiratory tract infections

Enterobacteriaceae may cause community-acquired pneumonia in the elderly and are implicated in inhalational pneumonia.[73] In particular, *K. pneumoniae* and *E. cloacae* are among the most frequent bacteria responsible for ventilation-associated pneumonia, after *Staphylococcus aureus* and *Pseudomonas aeruginosa*. *Klebsiella pneumoniae* was originally described as the agent of Friedländer's pneumonia, a severe lobar pneumonia, and remains an important cause of hospital- and community-acquired pneumonia, even though the incidence of community-acquired pneumonia has decreased in North America and Europe[74] (see 'Other infections and rare or emerging Enterobacteriaceae pathogens' below, and Chapter 28).

Meningitis and neurologic infections

Two clinically distinct situations can be described for neurologic infections by Enterobacteriaceae: primary infection associated with bacteremia, especially observed in neonates, and direct inoculation after traumatic or surgical disruption of the CNS (e.g. during neuroperitoneal dialysis).

The *E. coli* pathotype neonatal meningitis *E. coli* (NMEC) is the most common cause of Gram-negative neonatal meningitis, the incidence of which seems to be increasing. Eighty percent of strains express the K1 capsular type and belong to a limited number of serogroups (O1, O45, O18, O7, O16, O83).[34,75] Levels of bacteremia correlate with the development of meningitis.[34] As well as its classic antiphagocytic function, the K1 capsular polysaccharide also shows structural similarities with human tissue components, leading to an immune tolerance and resistance to antibacterial serum activity, thus possibly contributing to the high virulence by high resistance to antibacterial serum activity.[76] Some other virulence factors leading to invasion of the blood–brain barrier have been described for the NMEC pathotype, such as the outer membrane protein A, Ibe membrane proteins and the cytotoxic necrotizing factor.[77]

Citrobacter koseri is another classic bacterium described in neonatal neurologic infections, in particular as a cause of devastating neonatal meningitis characterized by the formation of multiple brain abscesses. The ability of *C. koseri* to survive phagolysosome fusion and replicate within macrophages, which could be dependent on *fliP* expression, may contribute to the establishment of a chronic CNS infection.[78]

One possible clinical complication of *K. pneumoniae* liver abscess is meningitis (see 'Other infections and rare or emerging Enterobacteriaceae pathogens', below).

Bacteremia

Bacteremia is a major complication of infection by Enterobacteriaceae as it can lead to severe sepsis with acute organ failure and septic shock (see Chapter 44).

The primary source of bacteremia is urinary tract infections. Other classic sources of blood infections include the digestive tract, implicating both specific intestinal pathogens and opportunistic enteric bacteria, which can translocate from the intestinal lumen to blood in hosts with underlying conditions (e.g. digestive solid tumor, cholecystitis or immunosuppressive treatment). *Salmonella* serovars that cause typhoid fever and, more rarely, nontyphoidal *Salmonella* can cause sepsis.[79]

Other infections and rare or emerging Enterobacteriaceae pathogens

Many if not most Enterobacteriaceae can cause infection, even if rarely, and those species that are considered medically most important are described in Table 169.4. *Klebsiella* spp., principally *K. pneumoniae* and to a lesser extent *K. oxytoca*, are responsible for frequent hospital-acquired infections and can occur in the form of outbreaks, in particular in immunocompromised persons and neonatal intensive care units (ICUs).[70] *Klebsiella pneumoniae* ranks second in frequency to *E. coli* among nosocomial Gram-negative bacteremia isolates.

However, *K. pneumoniae* cannot be viewed only as an opportunist pathogen, as it causes a number of distinctive infections in previously healthy persons in the community.[69] An update on the virulence and clinical characteristics of *Klebsiella* infections has recently been published.[74] *Klebsiella pneumoniae* owes its name to Friedländer's pneumonia, a severe

form of lobar pneumonia that used to devastate chronic alcoholics. In addition, two chronic and somewhat neglected diseases of the upper respiratory airways, rhinoscleroma and ozena, are also associated with strains related to *K. pneumoniae*, which were given subspecific status based on clinical criteria: *K. pneumoniae* subsp. *rhinoscleromatis* and *K. pneumoniae* subsp. *ozaenae*, respectively. Note that the etiologic role of *K. pneumoniae* subsp. *ozaenae* in ozena is still not well established. Finally, renewed interest in *K. pneumoniae* is now emerging due to the increasing prevalence of pyogenic liver abscesses, especially – but not exclusively – in Asian countries. Pyogenic liver abscesses are generally community acquired and often without underlying hepatobiliary diseases. Moreover, *K. pneumoniae* liver abscesses can be associated with metastatic complications including meningitis and endophthalmitis. Most reports implicate hypermucoviscous strains of the capsular serotype K1.[90] A recent population study by MLST[91] has defined a number of virulent clones of *K. pneumoniae*, one of which is associated with pyogenic liver abscess and two of which correspond to *K. pneumoniae* subsp. *rhinoscleromatis* and *K. pneumoniae* subsp. *ozaenae*, respectively. These two subspecies should therefore be regarded as clones of *K. pneumoniae* that have evolved particular characteristics.[91]

Klebsiella planticola and *K. terrigena* are often misidentified as *K. pneumoniae* or *K. oxytoca*; as a result, knowledge of their clinical importance remains poor (note that the validity of genus *Raoultella*, which was proposed for the two former species, has been questioned). Cytotoxin-producing *K. oxytoca* were recently shown to be a cause of antibiotic-associated hemorrhagic colitis.[92]

Klebsiella (*Calymmatobacterium*) *granulomatis* is the causative agent of donovanosis (granuloma inguinale), a chronic genital ulceration (see Chapter 60). This species was shown to have a very close phylogenetic relationship to *Klebsiella* members and it has been proposed that it should be reclassified as *Klebsiella granulomatis*.[83,93] Specific diagnosis is possible by detection of typical intracellular Donovan bodies in biopsy samples and amplification of DNA sequences of the *phoE* gene *in situ*.[93] In fact, comparison of *phoE* sequences of *K. granulomatis* and *K. pneumoniae* suggests that the former may represent particular strains of *K. pneumoniae*.[91]

Serious infections by *Cronobacter* (formerly *Enterobacter*) *sakazakii* with fatal outcome have been described, in particular in children. This species has been associated with small outbreaks or sporadic cases of sepsis, meningitis and necrotizing enterocolitis reported in infants younger than 1 month, especially in premature babies and neonatal ICUs. High morbidity and mortality were associated with neurologic forms of this infection. Powdered infant formulae were incriminated as a source of *C. sakazakii* infections.[94]

Other species such as *Enterobacter cloacae* (itself a complex of several species), *Citrobacter freundii*, *Citrobacter koseri*, *Proteus mirabilis*, *Hafnia alvei*, *Morganella morganii*, *Serratia marcescens* and others can cause disease in humans. These are generally considered as opportunistic pathogens, as they ordinarily occur as commensals in the gastrointestinal tract. The clinical significance of most unusual Enterobacteriaceae species remains unclear, given limited data, and specific virulence factors remain unknown in most.

Rare pathogenic species are more difficult to identify with classic methods than more frequent pathogens. Molecular methods, such as the sequencing of 16S rRNA or *rpoB* genes, are especially helpful in these cases and may also lead to the discovery of novel species. For example, some strains that were misidentified as *Hafnia alvei* expressing the *eae* gene have now been reclassified as *Escherichia albertii*, leading to reconsideration of the implication of *H. alvei* in gastrointestinal disease.[95]

PREVENTION, MANAGEMENT AND CONTROL OF INFECTIONS

Symptomatic treatment

Rapid oral rehydration using intravenous fluids is the first recommended therapy in digestive Enterobacteriaceae infections, specifically during EPEC infection affecting very young children or ETEC-related

Table 169.4 Unusual, emerging or recently reclassified Enterobacteriaceae species causing human infections

Species	Human infections	Properties	Risk factors	Recent references
Escherichia albertii	Diarrhea	*Eae*-positive strains, previously misidentified as *Hafnia alvei*; closely related to *Shigella boydii* serotype 13	–	Hyma et al.[41]
Enterobacter (Cronobacter) sakazakii	Bacteremia, meningitis and cerebrolysis, necrotizing enterocolitis	Described in 1980, phenotypically close to *E. cloacae* but sorbitol negative, specific yellow pigment, α-glucosidase activity detected in specific agar medium	Neonatality, low birth weight	Drudy et al.[80] Bowen & Braden[81]
Klebsiella pneumoniae subsp. *rhinoscleromatis*	Rhinoscleroma, a chronic granulomatous disease of upper airways	Related to *K. pneumoniae* but ONPG negative; no acid production with lactose; urease, LDC and citrate negative; K3 capsular type	Nutritional deficiency, tropical and subtropical areas	Botelho-Nevers et al.[82] Brisse et al.[91]
Klebsiella pneumoniae subsp. *ozaenae*	Ozena, a chronic rhinitis with atrophic nasal mucosa	Closely related to *K. pneumoniae* but always urease negative; K4 or rarely K5	Developing countries	Botelho-Nevers et al.[82] Brisse et al.[91]
Klebsiella granulomatis	Donovanosis (granuloma inguinale)	Previously named *Calymmatobacterium granulomatis*; uncultured in defined medium	Southern Africa or Asia, Papua New Guinea, northern and central Australia	Carter et al.[83]
Enterobacter hormaechei	Intra-abdominal abscesses, urinary tract infections, bacteremia	Often misidentified as *E. cloacae*; a frequent cause of nosocomial infections	–	Hoffmann et al.[84]
Edwarsiella tarda	Gastrointestinal disease (controversial), bacteremia, wound infections with abscesses following trauma in aquatic environment	Described in 1965, resides in intestine of cold-blooded animals and water. LDC, ODC, H_2S and indole reaction positive; absence of fermentation of most sugars except glucose and maltose	Immunocompromised	Slaven et al.[85]
Hafnia alvei	Bacteremia, respiratory tract infections associated with abscesses, gastroenteritis (controversial)	Voges–Proskauer reaction positive, indole production negative, absence of fermentation of lactose, motility at 22°C positive	Immunocompromised	Janda[3]
Kluyvera ascorbata	Urinary tract infections, soft tissue infections, intra-abdominal abscesses	Described in 1936, including four species (*ascorbata, cryocrescens, cochleae, georgiana*) closely related to *E. coli* but esculin negative, citrate and malonate positive, growth in KCN	Neutropenia, underlying malignancy	Cheruvattath et al.[86]
Leclercia adecarboxylata	Bacteremia, wound infections, pneumonia	Described in 1962, closely related to *E. coli* but lysine decarboxylase negative, malonate positive; acid production from arabitol and cellobiose but not from adonitol and sorbitol	Immunocompromised status, neutropenia, cirrhosis	Temesgen et al.[87]
Pantoea agglomerans	Bacteremia associated with venous catheter, bone or joint infections, soft tissue infections with abscesses	Includes strains originally named *Enterobacter agglomerans* or *Erwinia herbicola*; presents a characteristic LDC-, ADH- and ODC-negative profile	Blood products, intravenous fluids; wounds from thorns or knives	Cruz et al.[88]
Plesiomonas shigelloides	Water-borne gastrointestinal infections	Oxidase positive	Consumption of seafood or untreated water; biliary tract diseases or acute cholangitis	Salerno et al.[89]

ADH, antidiuretic hormone; H_2S, hydrogen sulfide production; LDC, lysine decarboxylase; ODC, ornithine decarboxylase.

diarrhea and shigellosis.[24] Symptomatic treatment of EHEC infections is critical for management of HUS, which requires dialysis in more than half of cases[33] (see Chapters 34 and 35 for a discussion on the management of these conditions).

Antimicrobial resistance and emergence of multidrug resistance

Resistance mechanisms to antimicrobial agents can be intrinsic and acquired. The latter mechanisms result from mutational events (especially for quinolone resistance) or, more often, acquisition of various mobile genetic elements such as transposons and plasmids.

Recent changes have been witnessed regarding the epidemiology of resistance of Enterobacteriaceae. In particular, strains producing extended-spectrum β-lactamases (ESBLs) and expressing multidrug resistance to different antibiotic families are spreading rapidly. ESBLs can hydrolyze a wide range of β-lactam substrates including cephalosporins. First observed in the early 1980s in Germany and France, these enzymes evolved by mutation of common penicillinases and were initially widespread in *Klebsiella*,[96] especially for β-lactamases of the SHV family since this species harbors a chromosomal gene that is the progenitor of the plasmid-harbored SHV ESBLs.[97] During the 1990s, most outbreaks were reported in ICUs, involving unrelated strains of the same species and dissemination to different species. During this period, most ESBL-positive Enterobacteriaceae strains belonged to *K. pneumoniae, P. mirabilis, E. coli* and *E. aerogenes*, and were especially isolated in hospital infections. A significant increase in fecal carriage of ESBL-producing Enterobacteriaceae was also noted.[98] Risk factors for infection by ESBL-producing Enterobacteriaceae included, as is common for other nosocomial infections, increased length of hospital stay, admission to the ICU or pre-existing co-morbidities. A more specific factor for ESBL-producing Enterobacteriaceae infection is prior use of third-generation cephalosporins.[96] Note that family Enterobacteriaceae is the evolutionary source of several important β-lactamases which have diversified in the chromosome of Enterobacteriaceae members before being mobilized and evolving into ESBL enzymes. This is the case, for example, for CTX-M in *Kluyvera*,[13] SHV and LEN in *K. pneumoniae*,[97] or TEM in a yet-undiscovered ancestral Enterobacteriaceae species (as deduced from its close sequence relatedness to SHV).

The past few years have witnessed the emergence of ESBLs of the CTX-M family, first described in Japan in 1986. CTX-M enzymes hydrolyze cefotaxime in preference to ceftazidime and are prevalent among community-acquired infections. In *E. coli*, one predominant CTX-M15 clone represented two-thirds of all EBSLs isolated in 2004 in the UK.[99,100] CTX-M is also a common ESBL identified in Enterobacteriaceae isolated in fecal flora.

Carbapenems (the most widely used is imipenem, followed by meropenem and ertapenem) constitute classic antibiotic molecules used in infections by ESBL-producing strains. Three distinct mechanisms have been described for carbapenem resistance:

- outer membrane protein mutation causing decreased permeability;
- production of carbapenemases (four classes encoded either on chromosomes or plasmids are known; classes A and B are mostly identified in Enterobacteriaceae); and
- altered affinity of the penicillin-binding proteins for carbapenems.[101]

Some carbapenemases such as IMI-1, the first acquired carbapenemase identified in *Serratia marcescens* (isolated in Japan in 1991), or KPC-1, reported from a *K. pneumoniae* isolate from the USA in 2001, are β-lactamase enzymes that hydrolyze most β-lactams, conferring a high level of resistance even to carbapenems and thus compromising treatment. Their dissemination has significantly increased over the last decade among various Enterobacteriaceae, as the corresponding genes are often located on transferable plasmids.[102]

Vaccination and prevention

Prevention of digestive infections depends on adequate treatment of drinking water and food contamination control, which remains very difficult in many places in the world.

Vaccination constitutes a major perspective and challenge for the control of frequent Enterobacteriaceae infections specifically against digestive illnesses which affect several million people in developed countries.[24,103–105] In addition, the emergence and rapid dissemination of multidrug resistance and the challenges faced by the development of novel agents should encourage vaccine development. Multiple vaccination programs are currently being developed, such as:

- the rCTB-CF ETEC vaccine consisting of a combination of recombinant cholera toxin B subunit and formalin-inactive ETEC bacteria;[24,106]
- a clinical trial to obtain *Shigella* protective vaccines (http://clinicaltrials.gov/ct2/home); and
- enterohemorrhagic *E. coli* vaccines to prevent human disease as well as carriage of STEC in animals.[33]

REFERENCES

📖 References for this chapter can be found online at http://www.expertconsult.com

Pseudomonas spp., *Acinetobacter* spp. and miscellaneous Gram-negative bacilli

INTRODUCTION

Strictly aerobic Gram-negative bacilli have become increasingly important as human pathogens over the past 20 years.[1,2] Molecular methods for identification have led not only to a number of changes in taxonomy, but also contributed important insights into the clinical significance and epidemiology of these organisms. While *Pseudomonas aeruginosa*[1] remains the clinically most prevalent species among the nonfermenting Gram-negative bacilli, other species, mainly *Acinetobacter baumannii*, have emerged as important nosocomial pathogens contributing significantly to morbidity and mortality.[2] *Stenotrophomonas maltophilia* and *Burkholderia cepacia* are commonly isolated from patients in the setting of the intensive care unit (ICU) and patients with cystic fibrosis (CF).[3] Species of *Acidovorax, Alcaligenes, Brevundimonas, Comamonas, Chryseobacterium (Flavobacterium), Pandoraea* and *Ralstonia* groups have increasingly been recognized as potential pathogens since the late 1980s.[3]

EPIDEMIOLOGY

Most of the nonfermenting Gram-negative bacilli can survive or even replicate under adverse environmental conditions. *Pseudomonas* spp. and other nonfermenting aerobic Gram-negative bacilli, in particular *Acinetobacter* spp., may survive for extended time periods in dry, cold or warm environments, and have been isolated from a variety of surfaces as well as from medical products and foods such as dairy products, poultry and frozen foods. Most species are saprophytic organisms and can also be recovered from water, soil, plants, vegetables, insects and various other sources due to their ability to use a wide variety of substrates as sole carbon and energy sources and to grow in environments providing only limited nutrients.[1-3] Even though several of these species have been isolated from clinical specimens, the clinical significance of many of them remains to be determined. However, combining intrinsic resistance to antimicrobial agents, resistance to the protective conditions of the skin (such as dryness, low pH, the resident normal flora and toxic lipids) and the mucous membranes (such as the presence of mucus, lactoferrin and lactoperoxidase), and high resistance to environmental conditions, these organisms may pose an important problem in the susceptible host and in health-care facilities.

PATHOGENIC ROLE

Aerobic nonfermenting Gram-negative bacilli can be isolated as part of the transient physiologic flora. Although most species are considered low-virulent, saprophytic organisms, others such as *P. aeruginosa* and

A. baumannii are recognized as important human pathogens worldwide and can be responsible for severe nosocomial, health-care-associated and (less frequently) community-acquired infections contributing significantly to morbidity and mortality.[1,2]

ANTIBIOTIC THERAPY

Most nonfermenting aerobic Gram-negative bacilli have a high intrinsic resistance which makes them frequently multiresistant to the major classes of antimicrobial agents, often leaving few therapeutic options.[1-3] Antimicrobial therapy should be guided by *in-vitro* susceptibility testing results; when possible, minimal inhibitory concentrations (MICs) of the respective antimicrobials should be determined, in particular in cases of severe infection. Various mechanisms of both intrinsic and acquired resistance have been identified, their type and frequency varying widely among different species.

This chapter deals with *P. aeruginosa, A. baumannii* and other potentially pathogenic nonfermenting aerobic Gram-negative bacilli.

Pseudomonas aeruginosa and Other *Pseudomonas* spp.

NATURE AND TAXONOMY

The taxonomic classification of *Pseudomonas* spp. has undergone significant changes since the proposition of the genus in 1894 and at times more than 800 different species have been included in the genus *Pseudomonas*. Historically, phenotypic characterization and subsequent classification were attempted on the basis of utilization of various organic compounds as sole energy sources.[4] Based on rRNA–DNA hybridization, five different groups have been identified that were previously included in *Pseudomonas* spp.:[1]

- I: *Pseudomonas* spp.;
- II: *Burkholderia* spp. and *Ralstonia* spp.;
- III: *Comamonas* spp.;
- IV *Brevundimonas* spp.; and
- V: *Xanthomonas* spp. and *Stenotrophomonas* spp.

One example of these nomenclature changes is *Stenotrophomonas maltophilia* which was formerly designated *Pseudomonas maltophilia* in 1961 and then *Xanthomonas maltophilia* in 1983 (Table 170.1).

The taxonomic status of *Pseudomonas* spp. other than *P. aeruginosa* has evolved significantly (see Table 170.1). Some species, such as *P. fluorescens* and *P. putida*, are heterogeneous and several biovars have been recognized: five biovars in *P. fluorescens* (I–V) and two biovars in *P. putida* (A and B), which differ in a few metabolic properties.[1]

Table 170.1 Current nomenclature of nonfermenting Gram-negative bacilli*

Genus	Current name	Previous name(s)
Achromobacter	*Achromobacter denitrificans*	*Alcaligenes xylosoxidans* subsp. *denitrificans*, *Alcaligenes denitrificans* CDC group VD-3
	Achromobacter piechaudii	*Alcaligenes piechaudii*
	Achromobacter ruhlandii	*Alcaligenes ruhlandii*
	Achromobacter xylosoxidans	*Alcaligenes xylosoxidans* subsp. *xylosoxidans*, *Alcaligenes denitrificans* subsp. *xylosoxidans*, *Achromobacter xylosoxidans* CDC groups IIIa, IIIb
Acidovorax	*Acidovorax delafieldii*	*Pseudomonas delafieldii*
	Acidovorax facilis	*Pseudomonas facilis*
	Acidovorax temperans	*Pseudomonas temperans*
Acinetobacter	*Acinetobacter baumannii*	*Acinetobacter anitratus*, *A. calcoaceticus*, *Diplococcus mucosus*, *Micrococcus calcoaceticus*, *Alcaligenes haemolysans*, *Mima polymorpha*, *Herellea vaginicola*, *Bacterium anitratum*, *Moraxella lwoffi* var. *glucidolytica*, *Neisseria winogradskyi*, *Achromobacter anitratus*, *Achromobacter mucosus*
	Acinetobacter baylyi	
	Acinetobacter bouvetii	
	Acinetobacter calcoaceticus	*Acinetobacter anitratus*, *Acinetobacter calcoaceticus* subsp. *anitratus*
	Acinetobacter gerneri	
	Acinetobacter grimontii	
	Acinetobacter haemolyticus	*Acinetobacter anitratus*
	Acinetobacter johnsonii	
	Acinetobacter junii	
	Acinetobacter lwoffii	*Acinetobacter anitratus*, *Moraxella lwoffi*, *Acinetobacter calcoaceticus* subsp. *lwoffi*
	Acinetobacter parvus	
	Acinetobacter radioresistens	
	Acinetobacter schindleri	
	Acinetobacter tandoii	
	Acinetobacter tjernbergiae	
	Acinetobacter towneri	
	Acinetobacter ursingii	
	Acinetobacter venetianus	
Agrobacterium	*Agrobacterium tumefaciens*	
Alcaligenes	*Alcaligenes faecalis*	*Alcaligenes odorans*, *Pseudomonas odorans*
Bergeyella	*Bergeyella zoohelcum*	*Weeksella zoohelcum*
Brevundimonas	*Brevundimonas aurantiaca*	*Caulobacter henricii* subsp. *aurantiacus*
	Brevundimonas diminuta	*Pseudomonas diminuta*
	Brevundimonas intermedia	*Caulobacter intermedius*
	Brevundimonas subvibrioides	*Caulobacter subvibrioides*
	Brevundimonas variabilis	*Caulobacter variabilis*
	Brevundimonas vesicularis	*Pseudomonas vesicularis*
Burkholderia	*Burkholderia ambifaria*	
	Burkholderia anthina	
	Burkholderia arboris sp. nov.	
	Burkholderia cenocepacia	
	Burkholderia cepacia	*Pseudomonas cepacia*, *Pseudomonas multivorans*, *Pseudomonas kingae* CDC group EO-1
	Burkholderia diffusa sp. nov.	
	Burkholderia gladioli	*Pseudomonas gladioli*, *Pseudomonas marginata*
	Burkholderia latens sp. nov.	
	Burkholderia mallei	*Pseudomonas mallei*, *Actinobacillus mallei*
	Burkholderia metallica sp. nov.	
	Burkholderia multivorans	
	Burkholderia pseudomallei	*Pseudomonas pseudomallei*
	Burkholderia pyrocinia	
	Burkholderia seminalis sp. nov.	
	Burkholderia stabilis	
	Burkholderia vietnamensis	
Chryseobacterium	*Chryseobacterium gleum*	*Flavobacterium gleum* CDC group IIb
	Chryseobacterium indologenes	*Flavobacterium indologenes* CDC group IIb
	Chryseomonas luteola	*Pseudomonas luteola* CDC group Ve-1

(Continued)

Table 170.1 Current nomenclature of nonfermenting Gram-negative bacilli*—cont'd

Genus	Current name	Previous name(s)
Comamonas	Comamonas aquatica Comamonas kerstersii Comamonas terrigena Comamonas testosteroni	 Pseudomonas terrigena Pseudomonas testosteroni CDC group EF-19
Cupriavidus	Cupriavidus necator	Wautersia eutropha, Ralstonia eutropha, Pseudomonas/Alcaligenes eutrophus
Delftia	Delftia acidovorans	Comamonas acidovorans, Pseudomonas acidovorans
Elizabethkingia	Elizabethkingia meningoseptica	Chryseobacterium meningosepticum, Flavobacterium meningosepticum CDC group IIa, Flavobacterium meningosepticum
Myroides	Myroides odoratus	Chryseobacterium odoratum, Flavobacterium odoratum CDC group M-4f
Ochrobactrum	Ochrobactrum anthropi Ochrobactrum intermedium	Achromobacter Vd Ochrobactrum sp. nov.
Oligella	Oligella ureolytica Oligella urethralis	CDC group IVe Moraxella urethralis, CDC group M-4
Pandoraea	Pandoraea spp.	Burkholderia spp.
Pedobacter	Pedobacter heparinum Pedobacter piscium	Sphingobacterium heparinum Sphingobacterium piscium
Pseudomonas	Pseudomonas aeruginosa Pseudomonas alcaligenes Pseudomonas chlororaphis Pseudomonas delafieldii Pseudomonas fluorescens Pseudomonas kingii Pseudomonas mendocina Pseudomonas oryzihabitans Pseudomonas pertucinogena Pseudomonas pseudoalcaligenes Pseudomonas putida Pseudomonas sp. group 1 Pseudomonas stutzeri Pseudomonas stutzeri-like Pseudomonas-like group 2	 Pseudomonas aureofaciens CDC group Vb-2 Bordetella pertussis rough phase IV Pseudomonas alcaligenes biotype B Pseudomonas denitrificans CDC group Vb-1 CDC group Vb-3 CDC group IV-d
Ralstonia	Ralstonia pickettii	Burkholderia pickettii, Pseudomonas pickettii, CDC groups Va-1, Va-2, Pseudomonas thomasii
Rhizobium	Rhizobium radiobacter Rhizobium rhizogenes Rhizobium rubi Rhizobium vitis	Agrobacterium radiobacter, Agrobacterium tumefaciens, Agrobacterium radiobacter CDC group Vd-3 Agrobacterium rhizogenes Agrobacterium rubi Agrobacterium vitis
Shewanella	Shewanella algae Shewanella hanedai Shewanella putrefaciens	 Alteromonas hanedai Pseudomonas/Alteromonas putrefaciens, CDC group Ib, Achromobacter putrefaciens
Sphingobacterium	Sphingobacterium antarcticum Sphingobacterium faecium Sphingobacterium mizutaii Sphingobacterium multivorum Sphingobacterium spiritivorum Sphingobacterium thalpophilum Sphingobacterium yabuuchiae	 Flavobacterium mizutaii Flavobacterium multivorum CDC group IIk-2 Flavobacterium spiritivorum, Sphingobacterium versatilis CDC group IIk-3 Flavobacterium thalpophilum Flavobacterium yabuuchiae
Sphingomonas	Sphingomonas paucimobilis	Pseudomonas paucimobilis CDC group IIk-11
Stenotrophomonas	Stenotrophomonas maltophilia	Xanthomonas maltophilia, Pseudomonas maltophilia
Weeksella	Weeksella virosa	Flavobacterium genitale CDC group II-f

*The list is limited to those potentially involved in human infections.[1,6,7]

EPIDEMIOLOGY

Currently, there are 160 *Pseudomonas* spp.,[1] most of which are ubiquitous organisms and are widely distributed in nature.[5] To date, a total of 12 *Pseudomonas* spp., including *P. aeruginosa, P. fluorescens, P. luteola, P. putida* and *P. stutzeri*,[6] have been implicated in human infections. The increasing importance of *Pseudomonas* spp. can be attributed in part to the increasing usage of broad-spectrum antimicrobial agents and the resulting selective pressure in favor of these inherently resistant Gram-negative organisms. Also, the increasing number of immunocompromised and intensive care patients as well as the increase in invasive procedures may have contributed to the emergence of mainly saprophytic organisms as important nosocomial pathogens. *P. aeruginosa* remains the most prevalent aerobic nonfermenting Gram-negative organism identified as the causative pathogen in a large variety of nosocomial infections.

Recent studies have shown the ability of individual *P. aeruginosa* strains to acquire or discard genomic segments, giving rise to strains with customized genomic repertoires that can survive in a wide range of environmental habitats that can serve as reservoirs for the infecting organisms.[7] Studies have identified a variety of environmental reservoirs in hospitals and nursing homes. For example, *P. aeruginosa* has been isolated from surgical instruments, disinfectants (quaternary ammonium compounds) and contact lens cleaning solutions, as well as in ventilatory equipment in ICUs and surgical equipment such as an ultrasonic aspirator used in neurosurgical procedures.[5,8] Surveys using molecular typing methods (exotoxin A typing) also linked *P. aeruginosa* isolates from sinks, wash basins and toilets to those isolated from the hands of staff and the urinary tracts of paraplegic patients, and transmission over a 6-month period in an ICU for newborns has been related to a source implicating air valves in the ventilator tubes.[9] *Pseudomonas* spp. are not part of the normal flora and colonization of healthy individuals with *Pseudomonas* spp., particularly *P. aeruginosa*, is rare.[10] While *P. aeruginosa* has been isolated from many different sites, including the respiratory tract, genitourinary tract and skin, recovery of these bacteria, especially mucoid variants, should prompt the search for infections.[1] In contrast, intestinal colonization reaches 18% in hospitalized patients and figures up to 73% have been reported in patients recovering from gastrointestinal surgery. In neutropenic patients intestinal colonization has been identified as the source of subsequent *P. aeruginosa* bloodstream infection.

Several *Pseudomonas* spp. other than *P. aeruginosa*, particularly *P. fluorescens, P. stutzeri* and *Sphingomonas paucimobilis* (*P. paucimobilis*), are more frequently isolated from clinical specimens than other *P. non-aeruginosa* and have been implicated in a variety of infections in adult and pediatric patients. There have also been individual reports of common source outbreaks due to these organisms.

EPIDEMIOLOGIC MARKERS

A variety of typing methods using both phenotypic and molecular techniques have been assessed for epidemiologic and clinical purposes. A selection of conventional and molecular methods is summarized in Table 170.2.

Conventional phenotypic methods

Conventional methods such as biochemical profiles, antibiotic susceptibility patterns, bacteriophage and bacteriocin susceptibilities, as well as outer membrane protein profiles and multilocus enzyme electrophoresis, are based on unstable properties of the organisms and phenotypic characters may change during the course of an outbreak or during a prolonged period of occurrence of endemic cases with apparently identical pathogens. To date, molecular methods have largely replaced conventional typing methods. Various different methodologies are used.

Restriction fragment length polymorphism (RFLP)

DNA probes specific for genes coding for exotoxin A (*exoA*), alginate (*algD*), elastase (*lasB*) or pilin (*PAK*), can be used for differentiating isolates from different patients, provided that at least two DNA probes are used (5% of *P. aeruginosa* strains are deficient in the *exoA* gene).

Pulsed-field gel electrophoresis (PFGE)

Advantages of this method include a very high discriminatory power, making it uniquely suitable for outbreak investigation. On the downside, PFGE is a labor-intensive method and time to result ranges between 48 and 96 hours.

Random amplified polymorphic DNA (RAPD) polymerase chain reaction (PCR)

RAPD-PCR has been shown to be a useful tool for typing of *P. aeruginosa*. RAPD-PCR has only a moderate discriminatory power that is lower than that of PFGE, but can be improved by combining RAPD with an RFLP analysis of the fragments. Although allowing for a quick estimate in a defined epidemiologic outbreak setting, this method is not suitable for large-scale epidemiologic studies.

Multilocus sequence typing (MLST)

MLST is a sequence-based, highly discriminative typing method that was developed in the late 1990s and has been applied to a variety of bacterial pathogens including *Neisseria meningitidis, Streptococcus pneumoniae, Staphylococcus aureus, S. epidermidis, A. baumannii*[11] and *P. aeruginosa*.[12] For MLST of *P. aeruginosa*, sequences of the conserved regions of the housekeeping genes *acsA, aroE, guaA, mutL, noD, ppsA* and *trpE* are used.[13] Compared to PFGE, MLST showed a higher sensitivity for the detection of genetic relatedness in recent studies, while the discriminator power of PFGE was higher than that of MLST in *P. aeruginosa*.[12]

DIAGNOSTIC MICROBIOLOGY

Bacteriology of *Pseudomonas* spp.

Pseudomonas spp. are thin, rod-shaped, nonspore-forming Gram-negative bacilli with a guanine/cytosine content of 57–68 mol%. *Pseudomonas* spp. are motile due to one (e.g. *P. aeruginosa, P. stutzeri, P. oryzihabitans*; Fig. 170.1) or more polar flagella (e.g. *P. fluorescens, P. putida, P. luteola*).[1,5] *Pseudomonas* spp. including *P. aeruginosa* can be recovered from clinical and environmental specimens using standard collection, transport and storage techniques, and can be cultured using standard broth or solid media including all nonselective (e.g. Columbia or tryptic-soy agar) as well as a number of selective media including MacConkey agar. While selective media containing inhibitors such as acetamide, nitrofurantoin or cetrimide may be helpful for the isolation of *Pseudomonas* spp., inhibition of some strains of *P. aeruginosa* (isolated from specimens from CF patients) by cetrimide and nalidixic acid has been reported.

Pseudomonas spp. grow at temperatures between 82°F and 108°F (28–42°C) and visible growth is usually achieved within 24–48 hours. Colonies of *P. aeruginosa* on solid media are usually flat (Fig. 170.2), but a variety of culture variants including small colony variants (SCV)[14] and mucoid forms have been described. Mucoid forms are particularly observed in patients suffering from CF and can pose problems for identification and susceptibility testing. Pyoverdin (fluorescein, yellow) is produced by all fluorescent *Pseudomonas* spp.; *P. aeruginosa* may also produce pyocyanin (blue), pyorubin (red) or pyomelanin (black). The distinct green color of *P. aeruginosa* colonies usually results from a combination of pyoverdin and pyocyanin. *P. aeruginosa* can be separated from the other fluorescent *Pseudomonas* spp. (e.g. *P. fluorescens, P. putida*) by its ability to grow at 108°F (42°C).

Table 170.2 Epidemiologic markers for *Acinetobacter baumanii* and *Pseudomonas aeruginosa* typing

Epidemiologic markers		Species	Principles and characteristics	Advantages	Drawbacks
Phenotypic	Biotyping	*A. baumannii*	Utilization of substrates, production of enzymes, biotyping schemes for identification, commonly carbon-source utilization test using levulinate, citraconate, L-phenylalanine, phenylacetate, 4-hydroxybenzoate and L-tartrate	Rapid, easy to perform, inexpensive, also useful for identification to species level	Unstable, variability of metabolic characters, limited discriminatory power
		P. aeruginosa	Utilization of substrates, production of enzymes, biotyping schemes for identification	Rapid, easy to perform, API 20NE panel or automated identification systems (Vitek, MicroScan, Phoenix), inexpensive	Unstable, variability of metabolic characters, poorly discriminating
	Resistance phenotype	*A. baumannii*, *P. aeruginosa*	Antimicrobial susceptibility pattern always obtained, multiple resistance markers	Rapid, easy to perform, standardized (national/international guidelines), automated systems (Vitek, MicroScan, Phoenix) can be used, early and often useful during outbreak	Unstable profiles, plasmid acquisition or loss during an outbreak, derepression of inducible enzymes, mutations, poorly discriminating, unreliable
	Serotyping	*A. baumannii*	O-antigenic polysaccharide of the lipopolysaccharide, 34 O-antisera	No advantages for *A. baumannii*	Not all strains typeable, low discriminatory power
		P. aeruginosa	Based on somatic O-specific antigen (LPS), polyclonal/monoclonal antibodies, 20 serotypes, 17 antisera (IATS)	Rapid, early results, easy to perform, inexpensive	50–70% of CF strains nontypeable, polyagglutination of some CF strains, reproducibility of anti-LPS monoclonal antibodies is 75%, only available in specialized laboratories
	Phage typing	*A. baumannii*	Two systems (21 and 14 phages, respectively)	Limited requirements, inexpensive	Lack of reproducibility, low discriminatory power, approx. 20% of strains nontypeable, only available in specialized laboratories
		P. aeruginosa	Colindale set of 21 phages, cell surface receptors (OM, LPS, slime)	Limited requirements, inexpensive	Lack of reproducibility, low discrimination, insensitivity of CF- and LPS-defective strains, only available in specialized laboratories
	Pyocin typing	*P. aeruginosa*	R, F, S pyocins, specific lytic activity, 105 types, 26 subtypes	Limited requirements, inexpensive	Poor discrimination, complexity of the system, time-consuming technique, only available in specialized laboratories
Genotypic	Plasmidotyping	*A. baumannii*	Plasmids present in many *A. baumannii* strains	No advantage for *A. baumannii* typing	Plasmids are easily transferable and may be gained or lost, cumbersome technique
		P. aeruginosa	Relatively rare plasmid in *P. aeruginosa*, plasmids of 1.2–60 MDa in 15% of strains	No advantage for *P. aeruginosa* typing	Low frequency, acquisition or loss during epidemics
	Genomic DNA, total DNA	*P. aeruginosa*	Polymorphism of DNA, REA endonucleases (EcoR1, HindII, SmaI), conventional agarose gel electrophoresis	Good discriminatory power	Large number of fragments making resolution of bands difficult to interpret

Method	Species	Principle	Advantages	Disadvantages
DNA RFLP	*P. aeruginosa*	Detection of genes coding for exotoxin A (*exoA*), elastase (*lasB*), alginate (*algD*), two probes necessary	Good discriminatory power, good correlation with ribotyping	Laborious techniques, small numbers of isolates can be compared
Ribotyping (ribosomal DNA)	*A. baumannii*	*Hind*III, *Hinc*II, *Eco*R1, *Cla*I	Results comparable to AFLP, automated systems available	Limited discriminatory power, labor intensive, PFGE and others provide more accurate results for *A. baumannii*
	P. aeruginosa	Three genes coding for rRNA, probes for 16S and 23S RNA, restriction enzymes (*Eco*R1, *Cla*I, *Sal*I)	Universal, excellent reproducibility, stable ribotype patterns within outbreaks	Laborious techniques, sensitivity and specificity not established for *P. aeruginosa*
Pulsotyping (PFGE)	*A. baumannii*	*Apa*I and/or *Sma*I	Gold standard for *A. baumannii*, highest discriminatory power, interlaboratory reproducibility possible with standardized protocols	Labor intensive
	P. aeruginosa	DNA fingerprinting, restriction enzymes *Dra*I, *Spe*I	The most specific discriminatory technique	Interpretation somewhat delicate, heavy workload
RAPD-PCR	*A. baumannii*	Amplification of random DNA sequences	Fast, easy and low cost, relatively high discriminatory power	Inter- and intralaboratory reproducibility difficult to achieve, not suited for large-scale epidemiologic studies, discriminatory power inferior to PFGE
	P. aeruginosa	Amplification of random DNA sequences	Fast, easy and low cost, relatively high discriminatory power	Inter- and intralaboratory reproducibility difficult to achieve
Repetitive extragenic palindromic (REP)-PCR	*A. baumannii*	PCR-based typing method, amplification of highly-conserved REP sequences using specific primers	Simple, rapid	Inter- and intralaboratory reproducibility remains to be determined, expensive
AFLP	*A. baumannii*	PCR-based typing method, amplification of restriction fragments (*Hind*III and *Taq*I) using specific primers	Can be used for typing and species identification, relatively robust method, high discriminatory power	*Acinetobacter* only, requires a high level of standardization and extensive experience, cumbersome and expensive, restricted to reference laboratories, not suited for routine epidemiologic analyses, data are not readily transportable
MLST	*A. baumannii*, *Acinetobacter* genomic species 13TU, *P. aeruginosa*	Amplification and sequencing of several specific loci in different housekeeping genes: *A. baumannii* and *Acinetobacter* genomic species 13TU: *gltA*, *gyrB*, *gdhB*, *recA*, *cpn60*, *gpi*, *rpoD*; *P. aeruginosa*: *acsA*, *aroE*, *guaA*, *mutL*, *nuoD*, *ppsA*, *trpE*	Highly portable, highly reproducible	Time-consuming, very expensive
PCR/ESI-MS)	*A. baumannii*	Amplification of specific sequences of six housekeeping genes (*efp*, *trpE*, *adk*, *mutY*, *fumC*, *ppa*), detection by ESI-MS	Results similar to MLST, easy, high throughput, fastest method to date	Novel method, not suited for routine laboratories, expensive equipment, detailed evaluation warranted

AFLP, amplified fragment length polymorphism; CF, cystic fibrosis; ESI-MS, electrospray ionization mass spectrometry; IATS, International Antigenic Typing Scheme; LPS, lipopolysaccharide; MLST, multilocus sequence typing; OM, outer membrane; PCR, polymerase chain reaction; PFGE, pulsed-field gel electrophoresis; RAPD, random amplified polymorphic DNA; REA, restriction endonuclease analysis; RFLP, restriction fragment length polymorphism.

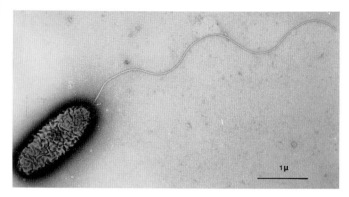

Fig. 170.1 *Pseudomonas aeruginosa* monotrichous polar flagellum seen on electron microscopy. Courtesy of Professor A Marty.

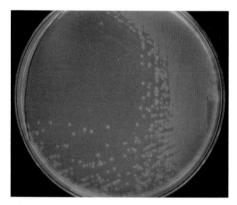

Fig. 170.2 *Pseudomonas aeruginosa* colonies on agar medium. Courtesy of Professor E Bingen.

Characteristics differentiating *Pseudomonas* spp. are shown in Table 170.2. This simplified scheme for identification of these bacteria is mainly based on morphologic features (flagella), pigment production and the main metabolic characteristics. Automated systems can usually identify *P. aeruginosa* from clinical specimens; however, additional testing is often required for identification of *Pseudomonas* spp. including mucoid or other forms of *P. aeruginosa* from CF patients.

Other methods to identify *Pseudomonas* spp. include conventional and real-time PCR, probes directed at or sequencing of species-specific 16S rRNA,[15] fluorescence in situ hybridization (FISH) and matrix-assisted laser desorption/ionization-time of flight (MALDI-TOF) mass spectrometry.[16]

PATHOGENICITY AND PATHOGENESIS

Pseudomonas aeruginosa expresses a variety of virulence factors. While host-related factors also play an important role in the course of *P. aeruginosa* infection, some specific bacterial factors have been characterized in recent years (Table 170.3).

Host-related factors

As with other opportunistic infections, host-related factors such as anatomic and physiologic barriers play an important role in the pathogenesis of *P. aeruginosa* infections. Several of the more severe and more frequent *P. aeruginosa* infections such as burn wound infections, as well as colonization of the upper respiratory or gastrointestinal tract, largely depend on the impairment of the natural barriers provided by intact skin or mucous membranes. Animal studies showed that *P. aeruginosa* can cause lethal infections originating from as little as 10 colony forming

units (cfu) inoculated into burned skin, while similar infections of the intact skin require five to six logs more organisms.

As in skin infections, disruption of the integrity of the corneal mucosa has been identified as the major factor in severe *P. aeruginosa* infections of the eye. Mucosal surfaces provide protection against *P. aeruginosa* colonization and infection by a variety of mechanisms such as mucus-containing antimicrobial factors including lysozyme, lactoferrin and defensins, the presence of physiologic flora, and muco-ciliary clearance. However, if impaired by underlying diseases such as CF or therapeutic interventions such as antimicrobial or anti-cancer chemotherapy, *P. aeruginosa* has a high propensity for colonization and infection of the respective site.

A variety of soluble factors involved in the pathogenesis of *P. aeruginosa* infections, such as complement, collectins, cytokines, chemokines and immunoglobulins, as well as cellular mediators, have been characterized. A detailed summary of their function can be found elsewhere.[1,17]

Bacterial factors

Virtually all major classes of bacterial virulence systems (see Table 170.3) have been reported in *P. aeruginosa* such as endo- and exotoxins, pili, flagella, proteases, lipases, iron-binding proteins and exopolysaccharides. Adherence of *P. aeruginosa* to host tissue is in part promoted by pili (encoded by the *pilA* gene, regulated by *rpoN*, *pilS* and *pilR*), flagella (*fliC* (flagellin) and *fliD* (protein caps)) and other appendage-like structures that have recently been identified in multidrug-resistant strains of *P. aeruginosa*. In addition, lipopolysaccharide may bind to the cystic fibrosis transmembrane conductance regulator (CFTR). Defective expression (ΔF508 allele) of the CFTR has been identified as one of the factors contributing to the hypersusceptibility of CF patients to chronic *P. aeruginosa* infection. Recent studies have identified numerous CFTR-dependent factors that are recruited to the epithelial plasma membrane in response to infection and that are needed for bacterial clearance. Several factors mediating resistance to host defenses have been identified in *P. aeruginosa*, including lipopolysaccharide O (LPS O) preventing lysis by complement and a variety of proteases (e.g. protease IV, elastolytic proteases and alkaline protease) that are involved in the evasion of innate immunity, degradation of cells and host proteins, and syndecan 1.

Manifestation of infection largely depends on the expression of a variety of toxins or other substances that damage host cells such as ferripyochelin that has been shown to destroy endothelial cells alone or in combination with hydrogen peroxide. Toxins that may be produced by *P. aeruginosa* include exotoxin A (an inhibitor of protein biosynthesis by means of inactivating elongation factor 2), leukocidin, plcHR (a hemolytic phospholipase C), pyocyanin and rhamnolipids. Most of the toxins and hydrolytic enzymes that are involved in virulence are regulated by a complex system, many components of which are influenced by environmental factors. In *P. aeruginosa* three major quorum-sensing systems have been identified to date, termed las, rhl and PQS. These interacting quorum-sensing systems seem to play an important role in the regulation of biofilm formation and expression of virulence factors. Degradation of acyl-homoserine lactones, the signaling molecules of the quorum-sensing system, has even been discussed as a treatment option. In addition, the GacS/GacA two-component system positively controls the transcription of two sRNAs (RsmY, RsmZ) that are crucial for the expression of virulence genes and which regulate the response to oxidative stress in *P. fluorescens*. The spread of *P. aeruginosa* and invasion of the bloodstream requires a smooth LPS substituted with O side chains and is likely enhanced by bacterial factors stimulating the release of tumor necrosis factor (TNF) and quorum-sensing molecules.

Mucoid *Pseudomonas aeruginosa*

In the early 1960s the importance of mucoid variants of *P. aeruginosa* was recognized. Mucoid strains are morphologic and functional variants of *P. aeruginosa* characterized by the ability to produce copious

Table 170.3 *Acinetobacter baumanii* and *Pseudomonas aeruginosa* virulence-associated factors

Category	Pathogen	Classes of virulence factors (examples)	Effects in humans
Enzyme	A. baumannii	Antibiotic-inactivating enzymes (β-lactamases) Proteases Protein S	Inactivation of antimicrobial agents Tissue damage Interference with phagocytosis
	P. aeruginosa	Adhesins (exoenzyme S) Antibiotic-inactivating enzymes (β-lactamases) Elastolytic activity (two enzymes Las A, Las B) Glycolipid-rhamnolipid (heat-stable) Hemolysins (phospholipase C) Neuraminidase Cytoplasmic lectins, *P. aeruginosa* lectin I (PA I), PA II Proteases (alkaline and neutral metalloproteinase)	Binding specificity for glycolipids (glycosphingolipid) Inactivation of antimicrobial agents Break down elastin of blood vessels, hemorrhages Disruption of phospholipids of cell membranes, hydrolysis of lung surfactant and ciliostatic action Enhances pilin-mediated adherence PA I specific for D-galactose, PA II specific for D-mannose Tissue damage (active on elastin, collagen, fibrin), digestion of protecting host defense proteins
Structural	A. baumannii	Aerobactin Fimbriae Iron-repressible outer membrane receptor proteins Iron-uptake components Lipopolysaccharide Lipopolysaccharide (hydrophobic sugars in the O side chain) Outer membrane proteins Pili Polysaccharide capsule	Increased virulence (mechanism to be determined) Adhesion to epithelial cells Increased virulence (mechanism to be determined) Survival in the bloodstream Proinflammatory response Adhesion to host cells Interference with cell permeability Adhesion to epithelial cells Interference with phagocytosis, survival in dry environment
	P. aeruginosa	Lipopolysaccharide Mucopolysaccharide capsule (alginate) Pili (fimbriae) Siderophores (pyochelin and pyoverdin)	Cascade of inflammatory events Adhesion to epithelial cells, barrier to antibiotics, increased viscosity of bronchial secretions (cystic fibrosis) Adhesion to epithelial cells Help growth in iron-limited condition, generation of toxic oxygen-free radicals
Toxin	A. baumannii	Lipid A Outer membrane protein A (Omp 38)	Toxicity, pyrogenicity Cytotoxicity, apoptosis, cell death
	P. aeruginosa	Cytotoxins (leucocidin) Endotoxins Exotoxin A Phenazine pigment (pyocyanin)	Cytopathic effects on leukocytes and alteration of phospholipids of cell membrane Septic shock Tissue damage, inhibition of phagocytes, inhibition of protein synthesis Ciliary disruption

amounts of alginate, an acetylated polymer of D-mannuronic and L-glucuronic acids regulated by ClpXP proteases, AlgB, Alg8 and Alg44[18] (Figs 170.3, 170.4). Alginate has been implicated in the pathogenesis of respiratory tract infections due to *P. aeruginosa* in CF patients as well as in chronic oropharyngeal colonization.

In vivo, in areas with impaired local defenses, such as in the airways of CF patients, the organism grows in microcolonies surrounded by a thick polysaccharide matrix. In autopsied lungs of CF patients there are microcolonies adherent to the walls of larger airways and in the alveoli. Mucoid *P. aeruginosa* is present in abundance in foci of active inflammation in small bronchioles but not in destroyed parenchymal areas. This observation is consistent with the simultaneous role of bacterial growth in the active inflammatory process and of toxins produced by *P. aeruginosa* diffusing away from microcolonies. Several studies have addressed the role of antibodies against alginate and their failure to confer protection against infection in CF patients, showing that the bio-

film-like growth may interfere with the opsonizing capabilities of the alginate antibodies. An exopolysaccharide–alginate conjugate vaccine has been discussed as a therapeutic approach.

CLINICAL MANIFESTATIONS

Bacteremia/bloodstream infection

Assessment of the incidence of *P. aeruginosa* bloodstream infection (BSI) is difficult. While in older series *P. aeruginosa* accounted for 20–35% of all BSI isolates, this figure has been considerably lower in recent series, where 4.4% were due to *P. aeruginosa*. In another recent study analyzing 24 179 nosocomial BSIs from 52 hospitals in the USA over a 7-year period, *P. aeruginosa* accounted for 3.8% of all BSI isolates from non-ICU wards and 4.7% from ICUs, making it the

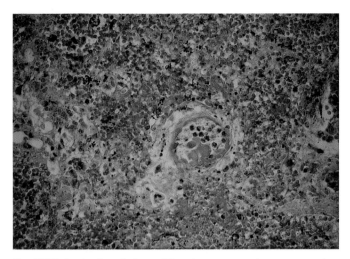

Fig. 170.3 Anatomic pathology of *Pseudomonas aeruginosa* pneumonia showing acute inflammatory exudate, necrosis of alveolar membranes and fibrinous thrombosis in a venula. Hematoxylin–eosin stain. Courtesy of Professor Groussard.

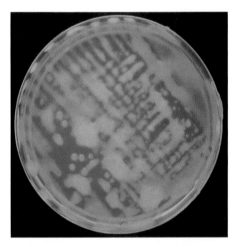

Fig. 170.4 Mucoid colonies of a strain of *Pseudomonas aeruginosa* isolated from a patient with cystic fibrosis. Courtesy of Professor E Bingen.

Table 170.4 Predominant sites and incidences of nosocomial infections due to *Acinetobacter baumanii*, *Burkholderia cepacia*, *Pseudomonas aeruginosa* and *Stenotrophomonas maltophilia*

Organism	Clinical presentation	Incidence (% of patients)
Pseudomonas aeruginosa	Bloodstream infection Pneumonia (VAP) Urinary tract infection Wound infection Cystic fibrosis respiratory infection Burn wound infection	3–5 21–24 11–15 8–10 70–90 1–10
Stenotrophomonas maltophilia	Bloodstream infection Pneumonia (VAP) Urinary tract infection Wound infection Cystic fibrosis respiratory infection Burn wound infection	<1 to 6 2 3–9 8–17 – –
Burkholderia cepacia	Bloodstream infection Pneumonia (VAP) Urinary tract infection Wound infection Cystic fibrosis respiratory infection Burn wound infection	<1 <1 4 – 80 –
*Acinetobacter baumannii**	Bloodstream infection Pneumonia (VAP) Urinary tract infection Wound infection Cystic fibrosis respiratory infection Burn wound infection	<1 to 14 5–10 10–30 2–32 – –

–, no data available; VAP, ventilator-associated pneumonia.
*Includes *Acinetobacter* genomic species 2, 3 and 13TU.

seventh and fifth most commonly isolated pathogen, respectively. In this series *P. aeruginosa* BSI had an incidence of 2.1 per 10 000 hospital admissions.[19] Historically, crude mortality rates of 50–70% have been reported in patients with *P. aeruginosa* BSI, while more recent studies found crude mortality rates of 28% in non-ICU and 48% in ICU patients, respectively,[19] as well as an attributable mortality ranging from 15% to 44%.

Secondary *P. aeruginosa* BSI most often originates from the respiratory tract (Table 170.4) while other sources such as the urinary tract or burn wounds are less common. Colonization of the gastrointestinal tract, which may develop in the presence of a variety of risk factors such as hospitalization in an ICU, the presence of neutropenia or treatment with cytotoxic chemotherapy, has also been discussed as a source of *P. aeruginosa* BSI, particularly in neutropenic patients receiving chemotherapy. Approximately 50% of these patients develop intestinal carriage, compared to only 5–15% of the general population, and translocation of *P. aeruginosa* has been implicated as the potential mechanism for invasion and metastatic infection. In addition, contaminated medical equipment used for endoscopic retrograde cholangiopancreatography (ERCP), placement of left ventricular assist devices and other invasive procedures have been reported as sources of *P. aeruginosa* BSI.[20]

The clinical presentation of *P. aeruginosa* BSI may range from benign transient bacteremia to fulminant septic shock with high mortality. The usual presentation does not differ from sepsis due to other Gram-negative pathogens. In neutropenic patients, typical skin lesions (e.g. ecthyma gangrenosum; see Chapter 12) may present and point to *P. aeruginosa* as the causative pathogen. Even though these lesions may on rare occasions present in non-neutropenic patients or be associated with other pathogens such as *Aspergillus* spp. or *Mucor* spp., the presence of ecthyma gangrenosum in a septic patient should prompt antimicrobial chemotherapy active against *P. aeruginosa*.[1]

Endocarditis

Pseudomonas aeruginosa is the second most common cause of endocarditis due to non-HACEK Gram-negative bacilli (after *Escherichia coli*), accounting for 22% (n=11) of all cases caused by non-HACEK Gram-negative bacilli in a recent observational study from the International Collaboration on Endocarditis-Prospective Cohort Study (ICE-PCS) database, including 2761 cases of definite endocarditis from 61 hospitals in 28 countries.[21] In contrast to older studies that reported endocarditis due to *P. aeruginosa* predominantly in intravenous drug users,[20] the ICE-PCS study found that 57% of patients with non-HACEK Gram-negative endocarditis had a health-care-associated infection, whereas intravenous drug use was observed in only 4% of patients. Implanted endovascular devices and prosthetic heart valves were frequent risk factors.[21] The in-hospital mortality of patients with endocarditis due to *P. aeruginosa* reached 21% in recent studies despite high rates of cardiac surgery (55%).[21]

Lower respiratory tract infections (see also Chapter 28)

Pseudomonas aeruginosa is a leading cause of nosocomial infections and is responsible for 10% of all hospital-acquired infections. It is the most common Gram-negative pathogen causing ventilator-associated pneumonia (VAP) and is consistently associated with a measurable attributable mortality.[22,23]

Since *P. aeruginosa* is also a frequent colonizer of endotracheal tubes and the nasopharynx of patients with mechanical ventilation receiving antimicrobial chemotherapy, the significance of a culture from the upper respiratory tract yielding *P. aeruginosa* in the absence of clinical and/or radiologic signs of pneumonia is less clear. The delay in eradication of *P. aeruginosa* in patients with VAP may be explained by an increased apoptosis in neutrophils.[22]

Typical pathologic features include necrosis of alveolar septa (see Fig. 170.3) and arterial walls, with areas of focal hemorrhage and, in intact areas, infiltration with macrophages, mononuclear cells and polymorphonuclear leukocytes. A different lung pathology has been described in bacteremic pneumonia, which is rarely seen and mainly affects patients with severe underlying conditions. Risk factors are listed in Table 170.5.

The clinical course is characterized by a rapid progression with a diffuse and often bilateral infiltration, usually in combination with pleural effusion. On cross-section, the lesions are nodular, hemorrhagic with necrotic foci or umbilicated nodules surrounded by dark hemorrhage. Intra-alveolar hemorrhage with patchy alveolar septal necrosis is seen on microscopy. The lesions contain many bacteria but lack infiltration with macrophages, mononuclear cells and polymorphonuclear leukocytes. Similar to fulminant pneumonia caused by Panton–Valentine leukocidin (PVL)-positive *S. aureus*, pulmonary edema and necrotizing bronchopneumonia are associated with a poor prognosis. This form of pneumonia is generally complicated by bloodstream invasion that often spreads metastatically to distant sites of infection. The case fatality rate in patients with fulminant bacteremic pneumonia due to *P. aeruginosa* is extremely high (up to 80–100% of cases).

Historically, community-acquired pneumonia due to *P. aeruginosa* was mainly seen in immunocompromised patients, such as HIV/AIDS patients with low CD4 counts or patients suffering from CF, but it has also been reported in previously healthy patients with no underlying immunosuppression.

Inappropriate antibiotic therapy, mainly due to lack of coverage against *P. aeruginosa*, has been identified as a significant risk factor for adverse outcome.[24]

Skin and soft tissue infections

Commonly seen skin and soft tissue infections in otherwise healthy patients are dermatitis or superinfections of predisposing skin lesions. Folliculitis due to *P. aeruginosa* has been repeatedly described and outbreaks have been linked to swimming pools, whirlpools, hot tubs and, recently, contamination of an industrial closed loop water recycling system in a cardboard factory.[25]

Burn wound sepsis

Pseudomonas aeruginosa is the most common cause of burn wound sepsis, which is the predominant form of skin and soft tissue infection complicating severe thermal injury. The mortality rate is high (50–78%) despite improvements in management and antibiotic therapy.[20] The incidence of *P. aeruginosa* BSI, however, has declined considerably from 10% of burn patients in older reports to about 1% in more recent studies.[26]

Colonization of the burned skin surface by *P. aeruginosa* may result from the patient's own flora or from environmental sources. The bacteria penetrate into the subcutaneous tissues via hair follicles and breaks in the burned skin, and may enter the bloodstream with the

Table 170.5 Sources, means of transmission and risk factors for nosocomial infections due to aerobic Gram-negative bacilli

Organisms and reference	Settings*	Sources/means of transmission	Risk factor/comments
Achromobacter (Alcaligenes) xylosoxidans	ICU, hemodialysis units	Contaminated chlorhexidine solution, dialysis fluid, aerosols, respirators	Aqueous source, hemodialysis, severe underlying disease
Acinetobacter baumannii	ICU	Contaminated ventilators, intravascular catheters	Severely ill patients, cross-contamination, outbreaks
Burkholderia cepacia	ICU	Airborne transmission, contaminated skin preparations, ventilator, thermometer, antiseptic solutions	Cystic fibrosis patients, hand carriage, immunocompromised patients
Elizabethkingia (Chryseobacterium) meningosepticum	NICU	Contaminated water, ice, disinfectants, humidifiers	Wounds, mechanical ventilation
Pseudomonas aeruginosa	ICU, burns units	Contaminated equipment, solutions, antiseptics, endogenous	Cross-contamination, exposure to broad-spectrum antibiotics, severely ill patients, outbreaks in burn patients
Pseudomonas putida, Pseudomonas fluorescens	ICU	Contaminated blood and blood by-products, antiseptics	Large (burn) wounds, intravascular devices
Stenotrophomonas maltophilia	ICU, hematology/ oncology units	Contaminated devices, disinfectants, catheters	Dialysis fluids, exploratory procedures, neutropenia, respiratory devices, tracheostomized patients, backflow from nonsterile tubes

*Most frequently reported occurrence. ICU, intensive care unit; NICU, neonatal intensive care unit.

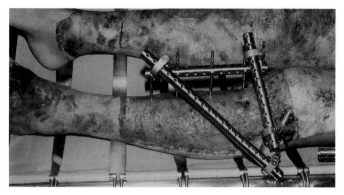

Fig. 170.5 Burned leg superinfected with *Pseudomonas aeruginosa*. Courtesy of Professor H Carsin.

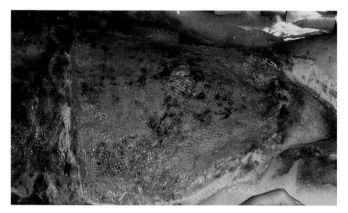

Fig. 170.6 Burned abdominal wall superinfected with *Pseudomonas aeruginosa*. Courtesy of Professor H Carsin.

help of the proteolytic enzymes they produce. Other virulence factors (see Table 170.3) contribute significantly to the severity of the burn infection, which can be the source of bloodstream invasion. Recently Gr-1⁺/CD11b⁺ cells have been identified as an accelerator of sepsis stemming from *P. aeruginosa* wound infection in thermally injured mice. Sepsis requires specific management in burn centers (Figs 170.5, 170.6). Recent studies comparing BSI in burn patients due to *P. aeruginosa*, *A. baumannii*, *Klebsiella pneumoniae* and *S. aureus* showed that *K. pneumoniae* had the greatest impact on mortality relative to all other pathogens.

Ecthyma gangrenosum

This focal skin lesion constitutes a rare manifestation of *P. aeruginosa* BSI. The lesion is characterized by an erythema surrounded by hemorrhage, necrosis of skin tissues and bacterial invasion. These extensive and destructive lesions of the skin are particularly seen in neutropenic patients, but have also been reported in non-neutropenic pediatric and adult patients.

Eye infections

Pseudomonas aeruginosa is the most common Gram-negative pathogen causing infections of the eye, despite not forming part of the normal ocular flora. Infections most commonly originate from an exogenous source and are related to (superficial) injuries. Ocular infections vary from mild (conjunctivitis) to extremely severe (orbital cellulitis).

Keratitis

Keratitis is the most frequent eye infection. Keratitis due to *P. aeruginosa* has only been reported secondary to an injury of the corneal

surface. Recent studies support this observation, stating that *P. aeruginosa* does not cause keratitis in animals with an intact cornea. The predominant predisposing factors in *P. aeruginosa* keratitis are wearing of contact lenses, congenital abnormalities, burns or trauma, altered host defenses (in particular patients with HIV infection) and prematurity. Contact lens-associated keratitis due to *P. aeruginosa* has mainly been observed in association with extended-wear contact lenses, inappropriate disinfecting regimens and poor hygiene. The bacteria may adhere to the lens, resulting in the development of a thick coat of mucopolysaccharides forming a biofilm similar to that seen on other prosthetic devices. Viral keratitis (herpes simplex) may also be associated with secondary bacterial infection.

Exocellular products of *P. aeruginosa* and strong adhesion to the exposed basement membrane of the epithelium increase the corneal damage; exotoxins, proteases and phospholipases degrade the corneal stroma, resulting in extensive loss of collagen fibers from the stroma. Keratitis due to *P. aeruginosa* may progress rapidly, leading to endophthalmitis and loss of eyesight.

Endophthalmitis

Endophthalmitis most often results from an endogenous origin, occurring by hematogenous spread from other infected sites. It may also occur after intraocular inoculation of *P. aeruginosa* by trauma, burns or ocular surgery, or following keratitis. Endophthalmitis may present as an acute fulminant disease with severe pain, chemosis and decreased acuity, and can progress rapidly to panophthalmitis. The prognosis is poor without appropriate local and systemic management.

Urinary tract infections

Urinary tract infections due to *P. aeruginosa* are usually health-care associated. Common risk factors include the presence of a foreign body (e.g. long-term catheter or stent), surgery or any cause of obstruction of the urinary flow or persistent infection (e.g. chronic prostatitis). While *P. aeruginosa* urinary tract infections usually affect patients with prolonged hospitalization, patients receiving antimicrobial therapy over a prolonged period of time and/or patients with the above-mentioned risk factors, infections in otherwise healthy children with no known risk factors have also been reported.

P. aeruginosa urinary tract infections have no specific clinical presentation but tend to evolve with frequent recurrences, treatment failures and chronic evolution. A characteristic picture of ulcerative or necrotic lesions and multiple renal abscesses is seen in patients who have metastatic bacteremia with urinary tract invasion.[20]

Ear infections

Pseudomonas aeruginosa is frequently isolated from the external auditory canal, particularly in infants. Infections may range from benign transient colonization to severe infections with a prolonged clinical course that may be associated with permanent neurologic sequelae and adverse outcome. *P. aeruginosa* has been identified as the cause of a mild superficial infection of the external ear canal (e.g. swimmer's ear). Although this benign infection usually resolves without sequelae, it may proceed to invasion of the epithelium between cartilage and bone in the lateral portion of the auditory canal, penetrating soft tissue, cartilage and bone.

Malignant (necrotizing) otitis externa

Malignant otitis externa or necrotizing otitis externa is a severe invasive ear infection, clinically characterized by decreased hearing, otalgia, otorrhea, early facial nerve paralysis and a swollen erythematous external auditory canal. Adjacent soft tissue is often involved and the infection may progress to the middle ear, mastoid, temporal bone and cranial nerves. Clinical presentation may include visible extension with cellulitis and bone erosions, and purulent discharge from the inner ear if the tympanic membrane is perforated.[20] *P. aeruginosa* may be isolated from superficial swabs of the external auditory canal and from surgical specimens. Most cases occur in elderly people with diabetes mellitus, but cases have also been reported from patients suffering from AIDS, elderly patients without immunosuppression or infants with severe underlying diseases.

Management of this severe and extensive ear infection requires prolonged antibiotic therapy, surgical debridement and drainage. The fatality rate is high (about 15–20%). Relapses are frequent and malignant external otitis requires prolonged follow-up.

Miscellaneous

Central nervous system infections

Infections of the central nervous system (CNS) are rarely due to *P. aeruginosa*. Meningitis, epidural or subdural empyema and brain abscesses have been reported in adults and children, usually as a result of either direct inoculation (head trauma, surgery) or a contiguous infection (sinus, mastoid), or following bloodstream infection.

Bone and joint infections

Bone and joint infections are infrequently caused by *P. aeruginosa*. As in CNS infections, direct inoculation (trauma, surgery), contiguous infection from surrounding tissue or resulting from hematogenous seeding following BSI are the most common routes of infection. Recent studies in war casualties found that *P. aeruginosa* was more frequently seen in primary osteomyelitis, whereas Gram-positive pathogens were more likely to be isolated from recurrent episodes.

Infections predominantly occur in patients with predisposing factors such as diabetes mellitus, intravenous drug use and chronic debilitation. More frequently reported associations include:

- vertebral osteomyelitis and arthritis involving the sternoclavicular or sternochondral joints in intravenous drug users;
- vertebral osteomyelitis in elderly patients following genitourinary instrumentation or surgery; and
- osteochondritis of the foot in children following puncture wounds or in patients with diabetic foot ulcers.

While *P. aeruginosa* seems to have a particular affinity for cartilaginous joints of the axial skeleton, infections at a distant site such as

pneumonia rarely spread to the vertebral column or the axial skeleton. Following pelvic surgery or femoral catheterization, osteomyelitis of the pubic symphysis has also been reported as well as rare cases of pelvic osteomyelitis in children.

The clinical presentation may be discrete, and pain, swelling, fever and other systemic signs are variable.[20] The diagnosis of these infections may be difficult as blood cultures are frequently negative and imaging studies may also be normal in the earlier stages.

PATHOGENICITY AND CLINICAL MANIFESTATIONS OF *PSEUDOMONAS* SPP. OTHER THAN *P. AERUGINOSA*

Some of the non-*aeruginosa Pseudomonas* spp. have been isolated from human clinical specimens (blood, urine, stools) and occasional cases of opportunistic infection as a result of transfusions, contamination of indwelling catheters, antiseptics or dialysis fluid, and various other mechanisms of transmission have been reported. For example, *P. fluorescens*, a psychrophilic organism, may grow at 39°F (4°C), which favors its presence in blood products and infusates such as heparin. Outbreaks of bacteremia, respiratory infections in adult and pediatric CF and non-CF patients, wound infections and rare cases of community-acquired pneumonia have been reported. These *Pseudomonas* spp., particularly *P. fluorescens*, *P. stutzeri* and *Sphingomonas paucimobilis* (*P. paucimobilis*), have also been implicated in rare cases of brain abscess, arthritis, endophthalmitis and keratitis. Most cases occur in patients with severely impaired host defenses such as immunocompromised patients in the ICU setting (Table 170.6).[20]

ANTIMICROBIAL RESISTANCE AND THERAPY

Although *P. aeruginosa* is most frequently involved in nosocomial infections, it is not the most resistant organism in the group of aerobic nonfermenting Gram-negative bacilli. Although these organisms are intrinsically resistant to many antimicrobials, several antimicrobial agents from different classes remain potentially active against *P. aeruginosa* and other *Pseudomonas* spp. (Tables 170.7, 170.8). However, the percentage of multi- or pandrug-resistant clinical

Table 170.6 Epidemiology and pathogenicity of *Acinetobacter* spp. and *Pseudomonas* spp.

Species	Habitat and epidemiology	Clinical significance
Acinetobacter non-*baumannii*, i.e. *A. johnsonii, A. junii, A. lwoffii, A. radioresistens, A. ursingii*	Ubiquitous, soil, water, sewage water, hospital environment, antiseptics, injectable solutions, more susceptible to antibiotics than other species	Outbreaks of pseudobacteremia involved in catheter-related bloodstream infection, isolation from wounds, urine, blood, cerebrospinal fluid
A. baumannii (*Acinetobacter* genomic species 2, 3, 13TU)	Hospital environment, colonized patients, health-care personnel	Opportunistic pathogen, severe infections mostly in immunocompromised patients
Pseudomonas alcaligenes, P. pseudoalcaligenes	Environment, water, plants, hospital environment, rare opportunistic pathogens	Occasional bacteremia (contaminated blood products, solutions)
P. putida, P. fluorescens, P. aeruginosa	Soil, water, plants, hospital sinks, floor, food spoilage (eggs, meat, fish, milk), opportunistic pathogens	Rarely isolated from clinical specimens, rare cases of colonization in patients with cystic fibrosis, bacteremia, urinary tract infection, wounds
P. stutzeri	Ubiquitous, soil, water, sewage water, hospital environment, antiseptics, injectable solutions, relatively more frequent than other non-*aeruginosa Pseudomonas* spp., opportunist, more susceptible to antibiotics than other species	Outbreaks of pseudobacteremia, isolation from pus, urine, blood, cerebrospinal fluid, contamination of bone marrow transplant
P. aeruginosa, P. fluorescens	Hospital environment, patients, health-care personnel	Opportunistic pathogen, severe infections mostly in immunocompromised patients

Table 170.7 Resistance mechanisms in *Acinetobacter baumannii* and *Pseudomonas aeruginosa*

Antibiotic class	Antibiotics	Organism	Mechanisms	Genetic basis (examples)
Aminoglycosides	Aminoglycosides	A. baumannii	Aminoglycoside-modifying enzymes	aph(3')-VIa and aac(6')-I
	Aminoglycosides	A. baumannii	Ribosomal (16s rRNA) methylation	
	Aminoglycosides	A. baumannii	Efflux	AdeABC, AdeM
	Aminoglycosides	P. aeruginosa	Enzymatic inactivation	aph(3')-IIb
	Aminoglycosides	P. aeruginosa	Reduced permeability	PprA, PprB
Fosfomycin	Fosfomycin	P. aeruginosa	Altered transport system	Chromosomal mutation (GlpT), plasmid-mediated (fosA, fosB)
Quinolones	Quinolones	A. baumannii	Modification of target binding site	gyrA, parC
	Quinolones	A. baumannii	Efflux	AdeABC, AdeM
	Quinolones	P. aeruginosa	Altered DNA gyrase target	gyrA, parC
	Quinolones	P. aeruginosa	Efflux	mexCD-oprJ, mexAB-oprM
Rifampin (rifampicin)	Rifampin	P. aeruginosa	Altered DNA polymerase target	arr-2
Tetracyclines and glycylcyclines	Tetracyclines and glycylcyclines	A. baumannii	Tetracycline-specific efflux	Tet(A), tet(B)
	Tetracyclines and glycylcyclines	A. baumannii	Ribosomal protection	tet(M)
	Tetracyclines and glycylcyclines	A. baumannii	Multidrug efflux	AdeABC
β-Lactams	Carbapenems	A. baumannii	Multidrug efflux	AdeABC
	Carbapenems	A. baumannii	Carbapenemases	OXA, IMP
	Carbapenems	P. aeruginosa	Altered protein porin D2	Chromosomal, orpD
	Carbapenems	P. aeruginosa	Imipenemase	VIM, IMP
	Cephalosporins	P. aeruginosa	Reduced permeability	Chromosomal
	Cephalosporins	P. aeruginosa	β-Lactamase inactivation (83%)	AmpC, PSE-1, PSE-3, PSE-4, OXA-10 (=PSE-2), IMP-1, TEM-1, TEM-2, OXA-1
	Monobactams	P. aeruginosa	β-Lactamase inactivation	AmpC, PSE-1, PSE-3, PSE-4, OXA-10 (=PSE-2), IMP-1, TEM-1, TEM-2, OXA-1
	Penicillins	A. baumannii	Altered penicillin binding proteins (PBPs)	Chromosomal (altered PBP-4)
	Penicillins	P. aeruginosa	Altered PBP targets	Chromosomal (altered PBP-4)
	β-Lactams	A. baumannii	β-Lactamases	TEM, SHV, ADCs, VEB, PER, CTX-M, OXA, IMP, VIM, SIM
	β-Lactams	A. baumannii	Outer membrane proteins	CarO (29-kDa), 22-, 33-, 36-, 43-, 44-, 47-kDa, HMP-AB, OmpW
	β-Lactams	A. baumannii	Efflux	AdeABC

Table 170.8 Antibiotic susceptibility of *Acinetobacter baumannii* and *Pseudomonas aeruginosa*

Antibiotics		A. BAUMANNII		P. AERUGINOSA	
		MIC$_{50}$ (mg/l)	MIC$_{90}$ (mg/l)	MIC$_{50}$ (mg/l)	MIC$_{90}$ (mg/l)
β-Lactams	Ampicillin	64	>256	64	>256
	Ampicillin–sulbactam	1	16	32	256
	Amoxicillin	32	256	32	>256
	Amoxicillin–clavulanic acid	2	256	32	256
	Mezlocillin	16	512	16	128
	Piperacillin	8	512	8	512
	Piperacillin–tazobactam	4	128	4	128
	Ticarcillin	64	512	32	512
	Ticarcillin–clavulanic acid	32	256	16	512
	Cefazolin	256	512	128	512
	Cefuroxime	32	128	32	256
	Ceftriaxone	8	128	8	128
	Cefotaxime	16	128	16	64
	Ceftazidime	4	128	4	32
	Cefepime	4	16	4	16
	Imipenem	0.06	0.25	1	2
	Meropenem	0.25	1	0.5	2
	Aztreonam	16	64	4	16
Aminoglycosides	Amikacin	2	8	0.5	2
	Gentamicin	1	32	0.5	8
	Tobramycin	0.5	8	0.125	4
Quinolones	Ofloxacin	0.5	16	2	4
	Ciprofloxacin	0.5	64	0.06	0.25
	Levofloxacin	0.25	8	1	32
	Moxifloxacin	0.12	16	4	32
Miscellaneous	Trimethoprim–sulfamethoxazole	2	256	128	≥128

From Zhanel *et al.*[27]

P. aeruginosa strains has increased considerably in the past decade and often leaves few therapeutic options. Antimicrobial agents with potential antipseudomonal activity include semisynthetic penicillins such as carboxypenicillins (ticarcillin), ureidopenicillins (piperacillin), some third- (group IIIb) and fourth-generation cephalosporins (ceftazidime, cefpirome, cefepime), carbapenems (imipenem, meropenem), monobactams (aztreonam), aminoglycosides (gentamicin, tobramycin, amikacin), fluoroquinolones (ciprofloxacin, levofloxacin) and polymyxins (polymyxin B, polymyxin E). Novel agents that display *in-vitro* activity against *P. aeruginosa* belong to well-known classes and include doripenem, ceftobiprole and ceftaroline. There is an urgent need for antimicrobials active against multidrug-resistant Gram-negative bacilli, and new antimicrobial classes active against *Pseudomonas* spp. need to be developed. A summary of antipseudomonal treatment options in various indications is given in Table 170.9.

P. aeruginosa displays a wide array of resistance determinants, most of which are chromosomally located. The incidence of plasmids in *P. aeruginosa* is relatively low. Mechanisms of resistance include altered outer membrane permeability (altered protein porins or lack of protein porin OprD), production of chromosomally and plasmid-mediated β-lactamases, aminoglycoside-inactivating enzymes and an efflux mechanism actively pumping out different antibiotic classes from the bacterial cell.

β-Lactamases, as well as IMP, GES and VIM metallocarbapenemases, may be augmented by a number of efflux systems and decreased OprD expression which together confer multidrug resistance to β-lactam antibiotics. In clinical settings these are often encountered in combination with other mechanisms conferring resistance to fluoroquinolones and aminoglycosides, thus considerably limiting the remaining therapeutic options.

Recent multicenter studies report rates of multidrug-resistant (i.e. resistance to three or more antimicrobial classes) *P. aeruginosa* ranging from 3% to 50%, with considerable variation between countries.

The therapy of serious *Pseudomonas* infections should be based on the results of adequately performed antimicrobial susceptibility testing, including determination of minimal inhibitory concentrations (MICs). Of note, in mucoid strains of *P. aeruginosa* determination of MICs and susceptibility testing using commercial systems may not be accurate, and the addition of agar dilution or gradient diffusion techniques (such as E-test) may be warranted. Data shown in Table 170.8 indicate current susceptibility rates, but due to considerable geographic variation empiric therapy should be based on local susceptibility data.

Pseudomonas spp. other than *P. aeruginosa* are generally more susceptible to currently used antimicrobial agents including trimethoprim–sulfamethoxazole. Based on *in-vitro* susceptibilities, carbapenems and fluoroquinolones remain the drugs of choice, while aminoglycosides have considerably less activity, especially in *P. putida* and *P. fluorescens* which are also resistant to trimethoprim–sulfamethoxazole. While *P. stutzeri* is usually susceptible to all antipseudomonal agents, higher rates of resistance to aztreonam and β-lactam antibiotics have been reported in *P. putida*, *P. fluorescens* and *P. oryzihabitans*.

Treatment of infections due to *P. aeruginosa* with a single agent is possible using third-generation cephalosporins such as ceftazidime or cefpirome, carbapenems such as imipenem or meropenem, or fluoroquinolones such as ciprofloxacin if the strain is susceptible.[28] A meta-analysis of controlled clinical trials has also shown that monotherapy (β-lactam) provided similar survival compared to combination therapy (β-lactam and aminoglycoside) in patients with cancer and neutropenic fever.[29] However, especially with fluoroquinolones and carbapenems, resistance may develop quickly during therapy and close microbiologic

Table 170.9 Empiric antibiotic therapy for *Acinetobacter baumannii* and *Pseudomonas aeruginosa* infections

Choices	Organism	Drugs	Indications
Monotherapy	*P. aeruginosa*	Antipseudomonal penicillins: ticarcillin, piperacillin, azlocillin; Cephalosporins: ceftazidime, cefoperazone, cefpirome; Carbapenems: imipenem, meropenem; Fluoroquinolones: ciprofloxacin	Limited to nongranulocytopenic patients, non-life-threatening infections
	A. baumannii	Carbapenems: imipenem, meropenem; Fluoroquinolones: ciprofloxacin, levofloxacin; Polymyxins: colistin (in carbapenem-resistant strains); Glycylcycline: tigecyclin (in multidrug-resistant strains)	Due to high and increasing resistance therapy must be based on susceptibility testing results
Conventional combinations	*P. aeruginosa*	Azteonam, ticarcillin or ceftazidime plus tobramycin, imipenem plus amikacin, ciprofloxacin plus ceftazidime, ciprofloxacin plus fosfomycin	Severe *P. aeruginosa* infections – pneumonia, bacteremia, burns (plus topical), malignant external otitis media (plus surgery), central nervous system infection (plus intrathecal), cystic fibrosis (plus topical, colistin or tobramycin inhalative)
	A. baumannii	Combination of two *in vivo* active compounds such as imipenem plus ciprofloxacin or amikacin, combination of any monotherapy drug with sulbactam or polymyxin	Critically ill patients with severe infections; data on sulbactam and polymyxin therapy are from *in vitro* and animal models and from rare case studies in humans
Alternatives	*P. aeruginosa*	Antipseudomonal penicillin plus fluoroquinolone, aztreonam plus aminoglycoside, aminoglycoside plus fluoroquinolone	
	A. baumannii	Various combinations of β-lactams and amikacin, imipenem plus rifampin (rifampicin)	Salvage therapy, combinations of antibacterial agents that are resistant by *in-vitro* testing should be used with great caution or avoided

monitoring is advised including repeated determination of susceptibility. In addition to systemic antimicrobial therapy, other interventions such as surgical debridement or local antimicrobial therapy have been shown to be useful in specific infections due to *P. aeruginosa*.

Central nervous system infections due to *P. aeruginosa* require bactericidal antibiotics that reach high concentrations in cerebrospinal fluid (CSF). Patients with meningitis require a combination of ceftazidime, which is highly concentrated in CSF when the meninges are inflamed, and an aminoglycoside. If there is obstruction of the subarachnoid space the aminoglycoside may be instilled directly into the ventricular system. *P. aeruginosa* brain abscesses may require surgical intervention in addition to prolonged antibiotic therapy.[20]

Malignant external otitis, which may present as an extremely severe infection, usually requires a combination of local surgical debridement and drainage together with antimicrobial therapy consisting of a (local) aminoglycoside or quinolone preparation and a parenteral antipseudomonal β-lactam.

In burn wound sepsis frequent emergence of resistance due to high bacterial counts and limited access of antibiotic to burn sites has been reported. Local procedures with topical agents and surgical debridement of necrotic tissue are always applied in addition to systemic antibiotics.[20]

Strategies for the treatment of pneumonia due to *P. aeruginosa* have emphasized the importance of early initiation of appropriate empiric therapy because the majority of fatal cases occur within the first 48–72 hours. For treatment of severe infections such as pneumonia or bacteremia, combination therapy is generally recommended (antipseudomonal β-lactam and an aminoglycoside), but there is a poor correlation between clinical response and the *in-vitro* synergistic effects of antibiotics.[20] In CF patients, eradication of *Pseudomonas* spp. as well as other pathogens such as *Burkholderia cepacia* or *Stenotrophomonas maltophilia* from the airways occurs temporarily only, whatever strategy is used. Proper management of acute exacerbations of *Pseudomonas* lung infection in these patients usually requires combination therapy and higher dosing. Fluoroquinolones have been used successfully both in adult and pediatric CF patients, and a combination of ciprofloxacin with fosfomycin has demonstrated *in-vitro* synergy. Repeated courses of aggressive antibiotic therapy every 3 months in combination with other measures such as mucolytics, antiproteases, topical (inhalative) antibiotic therapy and physiotherapy have increased the long-term survival of patients with CF. Current treatment options have been extensively reviewed elsewhere.[30] Administration of antibiotics directly into the tracheobronchial tree has been shown to increase local antibiotic concentrations. Inhalation therapy utilizing aminoglycosides and colistin is generally well tolerated, although some reduction of the maximum expired volume per second has occasionally been observed. Currently, tobramycin and polymyxin B are being used successfully in prevention and therapy of respiratory tract infections due to *P. aeruginosa* as well as *B. cepacia* in patients with CF.

PREVENTION

Prevention plays a major role in controlling *Pseudomonas* infections. Preventative measures can be based on the identification of sources and interruption of ways of transmission (see Table 170.2) and a variety of guidelines have been established in the USA and in European countries, implementing isolation policies, administrative and regulatory measures and hospital epidemiology surveillance. Attempts to reduce the risk of colonization and subsequent infection in high-risk patients have included:

* elimination of endogenous nosocomial *P. aeruginosa* and reduction of oropharyngeal, intestinal and skin colonization in ICU patients;
* prevention of cross-contamination and monitoring of various sources of *P. aeruginosa*; and
* prevention of contamination in burns patients, in surgical wounds and in the oropharyngeal area in ventilated patients.

Active vaccination has been discussed for high-risk patients and a variety of antigenic determinants are being evaluated as potential vaccine targets including outer membrane proteins, flagella and pili. In addition, vaccination with live attenuated strains has been shown to be efficacious in animal models. Current approaches to vaccines and immunotherapy against *P. aeruginosa* have recently been reviewed in detail.[31]

Acinetobacter Species

NATURE AND TAXONOMY

The genus *Acinetobacter* has undergone significant taxonomic modification over the last 30 years. To date, the genus *Acinetobacter* consists of 32 different species, 17 of which have been assigned names (see Table 170.1). While most *Acinetobacter* spp. are considered to be of minor clinical importance, *A. baumannii* and unnamed *Acinetobacter* genomic species 3 and 13TU have emerged as important clinical pathogens, contributing significantly to morbidity and mortality. Due to their phenotypic similarity, these three species have been grouped together with the environmental organism *A. calcoaceticus* in the so-called *A. calcoaceticus–A. baumannii* (Acb) complex. Overall, *A. baumannii* has emerged as one of the most significant nosocomial pathogens over the past decades, especially in patients with impaired host defenses in the ICU and has been implicated in a variety of infections including BSI, pneumonia and meningitis.

In severe nosocomial infections, mortality rates as high as 64% have been reported. Similar to methicillin-resistant *Staph. aureus* (MRSA), major epidemiologic features of these organisms include their propensity for clonal spread and their involvement in hospital outbreaks, as well as the ability to express or acquire resistance determinants, making it one of the most resistant organisms known to date.

EPIDEMIOLOGY

Acinetobacter spp. are widely distributed in nature and can be isolated from virtually 100% of soil and freshwater samples when appropriate enrichment and culture techniques are used. Nevertheless, current studies indicate that not all *Acinetobacter* spp. are found naturally in the environment (some such as *A. schindleri* and *A. ursingii* have until now only been recovered from human specimens) and that the clinically important species in particular (e.g. *A. baumannii*) are in fact not ubiquitous.[3] A variety of *Acinetobacter* spp. recovered from the axilla, groin and toe webs, the oral cavity, the respiratory tract and normal intestine have also been identified as part of the commensal human flora. In contrast, some *Acinetobacter* spp., such as *A. baylyi*, *A. bouvetii*, *A. grimontii*, *A. tandoii*, *A. tjernbergiae* and *A. towneri*, that were isolated from activated sludge have as yet never been observed in human specimens. Studies investigating the colonization of human skin and mucous membranes found *Acinetobacter* spp. in up to 44% of nonhospitalized individuals and in up to 75% of patients hospitalized on a regular ward. The most frequently isolated species were *A. lwoffii* (58–61%), *A. johnsonii* (20%), *Acinetobacter* genomic species 15BJ (12%), *A. junii* (10%), *A. radioresistens* (8%) and *Acinetobacter* genomic species 3 (5%), whereas *A. baumannii* was found only rarely on human skin (0.5–3%) and in human feces (0.8%), and was not found at all in *Acinetobacter* genomic species 13TU.[32] Recent studies investigating potential skin contamination in healthy US soldiers did not report any *Acinetobacter* spp., but the lack of enrichment techniques and long transport time may have contributed to this finding. In addition, seasonal and geographic variations in skin colonization with *Acinetobacter* spp. have been reported from different geographic locations where *Acinetobacter* genomic species 3 (36%), *Acinetobacter* genomic species 13TU (15%), *Acinetobacter* genomic species 15TU (6%) and *A. baumannii* (4%) were the most frequently recovered species, whereas *A. lwoffii*, *A. johnsonii* and *A. junii* were only rarely found.[33,34]

Molecular epidemiology

Only after 1986, when the taxonomy of the genus *Acinetobacter* was revised and molecular methods provided the necessary tools to identify *Acinetobacter* at the species level, did detailed studies of the epidemiology of the different members of this genus became possible. Commonly used methods include ribotyping, pulsed-field gel electrophoresis, random amplified polymorphic DNA analysis, amplified fragment length polymorphism (AFLP) and, most recently, multilocus sequence typing (MLST)[11]Bartual, 2005 and polymerase chain reaction/electrospray ionization mass spectrometry (PCR/ESI-MS).[35]

Acinetobacter outbreaks published between 1977 and 2004 (http://www.outbreak-database.com) have recently been extensively reviewed in two studies.[36,37] Recent studies increasingly report outbreaks involving multidrug-resistant *A. baumannii*. The persistence of endemic strains of *A. baumannii* over an extended period of time and the spread of single clones within a medical center have been documented in several institutions worldwide, with some studies linking individual outbreaks to a common source such as computer keyboards, blood pressure cuffs, enteral nutrition or dust in the interior of a mechanical ventilator and inside continuous venovenous hemofiltration (CVVH) dialysis machines, while others failed to identify a common source despite extensive environmental surveillance.

Several large studies failed to detect major interinstitutional spread of *A. baumannii* while other recent studies from New York, London and Johannesburg reported involvement of several different medical centers within a city, or even of health-care facilities in several cities within one country. Following reports of the so-called European clones I, II and III,[38] some authors suggested that a few epidemic strains may be involved in outbreaks across countries; however, in contrast to the aforementioned multisite outbreaks, no epidemiologic link in time or space could be established.

DIAGNOSTIC MICROBIOLOGY

Acinetobacter spp. are nonfermenting, nonmotile, oxidase-negative, aerobic Gram-negative coccobacilli usually found in diploid formation or in chains of variable length (Fig. 170.7) and may be mistaken for Gram-negative (or even Gram-positive) cocci. Strictly aerobic, *Acinetobacter* spp. grow well on most routinely used solid media at temperatures of 68–111°F (20–44°C). *Acinetobacter* spp. isolated from human specimens grow readily at 99°F (37°C). In contrast to the species of the *Acinetobacter calcoaceticus–baumannii* complex, several other *Acinetobacter* spp. do not grow on MacConkey agar or may show hemolysis on sheep blood agar (*A. haemolyticus*, *Acinetobacter* genomic species 6, 13BJ, 14BK, 15BJ, 16 and 17).

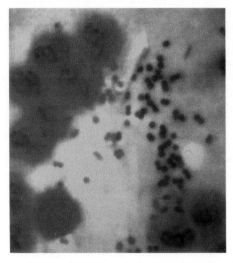

Fig. 170.7 Morphology of *Acinetobacter baumannii* on Gram stain. Preparation from a lung infection in mice. Courtesy of Dr ML Joly-Guillou.

While presumptive identification at the genus level is possible using the above-mentioned criteria, unambiguous identification of *Acinetobacter* spp. to the genus level is possible by transformation of the naturally transformable tryptophan auxotroph *A. baylyi* ADP1 by crude DNA of any *Acinetobacter* to wild-type phenotype.[39] There are several methods that can be used for the identification of *Acinetobacter* spp., unfortunately none of which is readily available in the routine laboratory. Phenotypic identification of 11 of the 12 initially described genomic species (but not of the novel species) is possible using a scheme proposed by Bouvet and Grimont.[40] Molecular methods include amplified 16S ribosomal DNA restriction analysis (ARDRA), high-resolution fingerprint analysis by AFLP, ribotyping, tRNA spacer fingerprinting, restriction analysis of the 16S–23S rRNA intergenic spacer sequences, sequence analysis of the 16S–23S rRNA gene spacer region, sequencing of the *rpoB* (RNA polymerase β-subunit) gene and its flanking spacers, PCR/ESI-MS and MALDI-TOF mass spectrometry,[41] as well as methods to identify *A. baumannii* by detection of the bla_{OXA-51}-like carbapenemase gene or using differences in the *gyrB* genes to differentiate between *A. baumannii* and *Acinetobacter* genomic species 13TU by means of a conventional PCR amplifying a specific region of the *gyrB* gene. While most of these methods are not suitable for the routine laboratory, some of the novel methods such as MALDI-TOF mass spectrometry may be an interesting option in the future, but require further evaluation.

Species identification using currently available commercial systems such as API 20NE, Vitek 2, Phoenix and MicroScan WalkAway remains problematic, especially since *A. baumannii*, *Acinetobacter* genomic species 3 and *Acinetobacter* genomic species 13TU are uniformly identified as *A. baumannii* by the most widely used identification systems.

PATHOGENICITY AND PATHOGENESIS

Several factors may be responsible for the virulence of *Acinetobacter* spp., including the presence of a polysaccharide capsule formed of L-rhamnose, L-glucose, D-glucuronic acid and D-mannose that makes the surface of strains more hydrophilic, factors facilitating adhesion to human epithelial cells in the presence of fimbriae and/or mediated by the capsular polysaccharide; enzymes such as butyrate esterase, caprylate esterase and leucine arylamidase potentially involved in damaging tissue lipids; and the LPS component of the cell wall and the presence of lipid A, which are likely to participate in the pathogenicity of *Acinetobacter* spp.

Recent studies using whole genome sequencing identified a large number of antibiotic drug resistance determinants as well as several pathogenicity islands,[42] a significant number of which likely originated in other bacterial species including *Pseudomonas* spp., *Salmonella* spp. and *E. coli*.[42] Relevant genes included those encoding the cell envelope, pilus biogenesis, iron uptake and metabolism, as well as sensor kinases that are important for the regulation of virulence determinants in other Gram-negative organisms such as *P. aeruginosa*. Several studies in *A. baumannii* have described siderophore-mediated iron acquisition systems, biofilm formation, adherence and outer membrane protein function and a specific lipopolysaccharide.

Important elements of the host response may include Toll-like receptor signaling and the stimulation of proinflammatory cytokines; the LPS of *Acinetobacter* seems to be equally potent to *E. coli* LPS at similar concentrations. Humoral immune responses include antibodies targeted toward iron-repressible outer membrane proteins and the O-polysaccharide component of LPS that have bactericidal and opsonizing *in-vitro* activity. While several potential host response mechanisms have been described in recent studies, the role of the host responses in the pathogenesis of *A. baumannii* infections remains to be determined.

CLINICAL MANIFESTATIONS

Acinetobacter spp. (mainly *A. baumannii*) have been implicated as the causative pathogen in nearly all types of nosocomial infection, including BSI, pneumonia, urinary tract infection, wound infection and meningitis. Crude mortality in patients with *A. baumannii* BSI ranges from 32% to 52%[43] but mortality rates as high as 64% have been reported in patients with meningitis due to *A. baumannii*.

Pneumonia

Acinetobacter baumannii accounts for 5–10% of cases of ICU-acquired pneumonia in the USA and is usually observed in patients with a prolonged ICU stay. The proportion of nosocomial pneumonia due to *A. baumannii* in institutions where this organism is endemic may be much higher. Predisposing factors include endotracheal intubation, surgery, prior antibiotic therapy and underlying pulmonary disease. The clinical presentation may include multilobular involvement, pleural effusion and formation of a bronchopulmonary fistula. Mortality rates of up to 70% have been reported, but as with other severe *A. baumannii* infections this may reflect the patients' underlying condition rather than the virulence of the organism. Community-acquired pneumonia due to *A. baumannii* has mainly been reported from tropical regions of Australia and Asia, and affects patients with impaired host defenses such as those with diabetes, renal failure, chronic alcohol abuse or underlying pulmonary disease. Similar to infections with community-acquired MRSA, it is characterized by a fulminant clinical course, secondary BSI and a high mortality of 40–60%.

Bloodstream infection

In a recent series analyzing almost 25 000 cases of nosocomial BSI, *A. baumannii* was the tenth most common pathogen, accounting for 1.3% of all monomicrobial BSIs (0.6 BSIs per 10 000 admissions).[19] *Acinetobacter baumannii* BSI tends to occur late during hospitalization, a mean of 26 days after hospital admission.[19] Sources include intravascular catheters, pneumonia, urinary tract infection and wound infection. Crude mortality in patients with *A. baumannii* BSI ranged from 16.3% to 43.4% and was exceeded only by the crude mortality in patients with BSI due to *P. aeruginosa* and *Candida* spp. Even though a significantly higher mortality was seen in *A. baumannii* BSI compared to BSIs due to other Gram-negative pathogens and in patients with colonization or infection due to multidrug-resistant *A. baumannii*, none of the studies formally adjusted for severity of illness or comorbidities. *Acinetobacter* spp. other than *A. baumannii* – in particular *A. johnsonii*, *A. lwoffii* and *Acinetobacter* genomic species 3, as well as *A. haemolyticus*, *A. junii*, *A. radioresistens* and *Acinetobacter* genomic species 10, *A. ursingii* and *A. schindleri* – have been mainly associated with catheter-related BSIs.

Wound infection

Acinetobacter baumannii has been implicated in 2.1% of ICU-acquired skin/soft tissue infections, but has recently been isolated from up to 32.5% of wound infections in combat casualties sustained in Iraq or Afghanistan. Colonization and infection of burn wounds with *A. baumannii* has also been reported. Even though colonization is one of the major risk factors for BSI in these patients, the impact of *A. baumannii* infection on the outcome of burn patients or combat casualties remains to be determined.

Miscellaneous

Acinetobacter baumannii is responsible for 1.6% of ICU-acquired urinary tract infections. Most cases of pyelonephritis and other UTIs have been associated with a urinary catheter or nephrolithiasis. Nosocomial, post-neurosurgical *A. baumannii* meningitis has increasingly been reported. Risk factors include neurosurgery and external ventricular drainage, and crude mortality rates up to 70% have been reported. Other infections include endocarditis (commonly associated with prosthetic valves), endophthalmitis or keratitis, as well as osteomyelitis and arthritis.

MANAGEMENT AND RESISTANCE

Antibiotic resistance

Prior to the 1970s it was possible to treat *Acinetobacter* infections with a range of antibiotics, including aminoglycosides, β-lactams and tetracyclines. However, since 1980 successive surveys have shown increasing resistance in clinical isolates of *Acinetobacter* spp. High proportions of strains are now resistant to most commonly used antibacterial drugs including aminopenicillins, ureidopenicillins, cephalosporins of the first (cephalothin) and second generation (cefamandole), cephamycins such as cefoxitin, chloramphenicol and tetracyclines, and resistance to all known antibiotics (i.e. pandrug resistance) has now emerged in *A. baumannii*. Therapy of serious *A. baumannii* infections should be based on the results of adequately performed antimicrobial susceptibility testing, and empiric therapy should consider recent institutional level susceptibility data.[2] To date, carbapenems remain the agents of choice for serious *A. baumannii* infections, but increasing resistance has been reported from several countries including Portugal, Spain, France and the USA. In the case of multi- or pandrug-resistant strains, combination therapy or the use of agents such as rolistin may be considered. A detailed review of the currently available antimicrobial agents and their potential use in the therapy of *A. baumannii* infections has recently been published.[19] Newer compounds with anti-Gram-negative activity such as tigecycline (with reported MIC_{90}s between 2 and 32 µg/ml)[44] or doripenem will most likely not have better activity against *A. baumannii* than the currently existing antimicrobials.

Burkholderia Species

NATURE AND TAXONOMY

Burkholderia spp. (as well as *Ralstonia* spp.) were transferred from rRNA group II of the former genus *Pseudomonas*. The genus *Burkholderia* currently consists of more than 35 species, most of which have been assigned species names. Some of the novel *Burkholderia* spp. have recently been reclassified as *Pandoraea* spp. All *Burkholderia* spp. are genetically related on the basis of DNA–DNA homologies, 16S rRNA sequences and phenotypic characters. They are ubiquitous organisms, being widespread in water, soil and plants, and are present in the human environment.

The *B. cepacia* complex currently harbors nine genovars:

- I: *B. cepacia*;
- II: *B. multivorans*, *B. gladioli*;
- III: genovar III, *B. cenocepacia*;
- IV: *B. stabilis*;
- V: *B. vietnamensis*;
- VI: genovar VI;
- VII: *B. ambifaria*;
- VIII: *B. anthina*; and
- IX: *B. pyrrocinia*

and represents the most frequently isolated clinical pathogen among the *Burkholderia* spp., followed by *B. mallei* and *B. pseudomallei*. It has recently been proposed that five other species be added to the novel species within the *B. cepacia* complex: *Burkholderia latens* sp. nov., *Burkholderia diffusa* sp. nov., *Burkholderia arboris* sp. nov., *Burkholderia seminalis* sp. nov. and *Burkholderia metallica* sp. nov.[16]

EPIDEMIOLOGY

Similar to *P. aeruginosa* or *Stenotrophomonas maltophilia*, *Burkholderia* spp. can be isolated from a variety of environmental sources. *Burkholderia cepacia* is an environmental organism that has no specific nutritional requirements and may survive for months in water, sinks, antiseptic solutions (chlorhexidine, quaternary ammoniums, povidone–iodine), pharmaceutical products, dialysis fluid and various injectable solutions. It may also survive on environmental surfaces[5] and has been found in nebulizers, ventilatory equipment and many other medical and dental devices (see Table 170.5).

Person-to-person transmission has been reported for strains of the *B. cepacia* complex, but so far there are no reports of person-to-person transmission of *B. mallei* and *B. gladioli*. Overall, about 3% of pediatric and 7% of adult CF patients are colonized or infected with strains of the *B. cepacia* complex, with a considerable geographic variation of species. *Ralstonia pickettii* (*B. pickettii*) and *B. gladioli* are ubiquitous organisms that can be found in water and soil and may play a role as nosocomial pathogens. Rare outbreaks of infection have been described and emergence of multidrug resistance is a potential problem.[5] *Burkholderia mallei* and *B. pseudomallei* are predominantly found in Asia, Africa and South America. *Burkholderia pseudomallei*, the causative agent of melioidosis, can be isolated from environmental samples such as soil and water.

Transmission to humans usually occurs by percutaneous inoculation, ingestion or inhalation from the environment; however, person-to-person transmission, zoonotic disease and laboratory-acquired infections have been reported. While cases of human melioidosis have been detected worldwide, the highest incidence has been reported from north-east Thailand and the Northern Territory of Australia where *B. pseudomallei* accounts for up to 36% of cases of fatal community-acquired pneumonia and is the most common cause of this infection. *Burkholderia mallei* is the causative agent of glanders, a disease primarily affecting horses and donkeys. In contrast to *B. pseudomallei*, *B. mallei* does not survive in the environment, although laboratory infections have been reported.[45]

DIAGNOSTIC MICROBIOLOGY

Identification tests for *Burkholderia* spp. are summarized in Table 170.10. While commercial test systems such as API 20NE, Phoenix, MicroScan and Vitek 2 can identify bacteria of the *B. cepacia* complex, misidentification is frequent and differentiation of species within the complex, as well as differentiation from other nonfermenting Gram-negative rods such as *Achromobacter* spp. or *Ralstonia* spp., may require additional testing. Of note, *B. gladioli* is often misidentified as *B. cepacia* complex by commercial test systems. *Burkholderia pseudomallei* may be falsely identified as *B. cepacia*, *B. mallei*, *P. stutzeri* or other *Pseudomonas* spp. *Burkholderia pseudomallei* and *B. mallei* cannot be distinguished by morphology or serologic tests, and molecular methods such as 16S rRNA gene sequencing may be required for species identification.

PATHOGENICITY AND PATHOGENESIS

Although only weakly virulent with a limited invasive capacity in the normal host, *B. cepacia* has become an important nosocomial pathogen. *Burkholderia cepacia* has been isolated from a variety of nosocomial infections including BSI, urinary tract infection, arthritis, peritonitis, endophthalmitis and pneumonia,[20] most commonly in patients with impaired host defenses such as CF patients or patients in the ICU. The predominant site of infection is the respiratory tract (Table 170.11).

Table 170.10 Diagnostic microbiology of *Burkholderia* species

Characteristics	*Burkholderia cepacia*	*Burkholderia mallei*	*Burkholderia pseudomallei*
Call length (µm)	1.6–3.2	1.4–4.0	1.5
Flagella number	>1	0	>1
Pigment (diffusible)	+		+
Oxidase	+	+	+
Poly-β-hydroxybutyrate accummulation	+	+	+
Gelatin	V	+	+
Lipase (Tween 80 hydrolysis)	+	V	
Denitrification		+	+
Arginine dihydrolase		+	+
Growth at 105.8°F	V	+	+
Guanine + cytosine content in DNA (%)	67.4	69.0	69.5

Main characteristics differentiating species.[1,11] Red indicates a positive result, white a negative result. V, variable.

Table 170.11 Infections due to *Acinetobacter baumanii* and *Pseudomonas aeruginosa*

Infection		Associated factors
Respiratory tract infections	*A. baumannii* pneumonia, nosocomial, 60% mortality with BSI	Mechanical ventilation Endotracheal or tracheostomy tube Neurologic disease
	P. aeruginosa pneumonia (30–60% mortality rate)	Nasogastric tube Prolonged stay in intensive care unit Broad-spectrum antibiotics
	P. aeruginosa pneumonia, nosocomial, with BSI (80–100% mortality rate)	Neutropenia Underlying malignant neoplasm Cytotoxic chemotherapy Chronic bronchiectasis (terminal state) Diabetes mellitus Severe immunodepression Severe burns
	A. baumannii pneumonia (community acquired, 60% mortality in bacteremic pneumonia)	Chronic obstructive pulmonary disease Smoking Alcoholism
	P. aeruginosa respiratory tract infection in people with cystic fibrosis (ultimately fatal unless a pulmonary transplant is carried out)	Presence of the lethal genetic disease cystic fibrosis Chronic colonization with *P. aeruginosa* Progressive lung deterioration Altered immune response to *P. aeruginosa*
Bloodstream infection (BSI)	*A. baumannii*	Prolonged stay in intensive care unit, mechanical ventilation, underlying immunosuppression, intravenous devices Leukemia, lymphoma Colonization with *A. baumannii* Various endoscopic instrumentation procedures
	P. aeruginosa	Prolonged stay in intensive care unit, broad-spectrum antibiotics, invasive procedures, underlying immunosuppression, intravenous devices Leukemia, lymphoma Mechanical ventilation, Intravenous drug use Trauma Prematurity Ulceration of the gastrointestinal tract Solid organ or bone marrow transplant Various endoscopic instrumentation procedures

Table 170.11 Infections due to *Acinetobacter baumanii* and *Pseudomonas aeruginosa*—cont'd

Infection		Associated factors
Skin and soft tissue infections	*P. aeruginosa*	Burn wound sepsis Wound infection Ecthyma gangrenosum Invasive procedures, surgery Dermatitis, pyoderma
Urinary tract infections	*A. baumannii*	Invasive procedures, urinary catheters
	P. aeruginosa	Acute (rare) Chronic (obstruction)
Endocarditis	*P. aeruginosa*	Intravenous drug use Prosthetic heart valves
Miscellaneous	*A. baumannii*	Meningitis (secondary)
	P. aeruginosa	Brain abscesses, meningitis (secondary, following neurosurgical procedures) Bone and joint infections (chronic osteomyelitis) Ear infections (otitis externa, malignant external otitis) Eye infections (keratitis, endophthalmitis, contact lens keratitis)

Virulence factors of *B. cepacia* include exoproducts (proteases, lipases, exopolysaccharides) that act in addition to the LPS forming part of O-antigen and which are responsible for severe pneumonia and sepsis in CF patients. Cellular virulence factors have recently been reviewed in detail.[46]

Attachment to epithelial cells is mediated by pili, followed by penetration, biofilm formation and invasion, which is in part aided by flagella and LPS. In addition, intracellular survival of clinical *B. cepacia* has been demonstrated. As in *Pseudomonas* spp., quorum-sensing system(s) may be responsible for the regulation of virulence factors in *B. cepacia*.

In *B. pseudomallei*, host-related factors such as diabetes, chronic renal disease or alcoholism seem to play a major role in the acquisition and clinical course of disease. Production of LPS and the ability of *B. pseudomallei* to survive intracellularly have been identified as important factors in the pathogenesis of melioidosis. The latter is conferred by the production of a capsular polysaccharide and the ability to form small colony variants or mucoid variants.

CLINICAL MANIFESTATIONS

While several *Burkholderia* spp. such as *B. gladioli* or *B. thailandiensis* have been isolated only occasionally from clinical specimens, the *B. cepacia* complex (including *B. cepacia*, *B. multivorans*, *B. cenocepacia*), *B. mallei* and *B. pseudomallei* are classified as human pathogens. *Burkholderia gladioli* has been reported to cause disease in patients with CF or chronic granulomatous disease and other immunocompromising conditions.

Respiratory tract infection and pneumonia are the most frequent manifestations of infection due to bacteria of the *B. cepacia* complex, most commonly *B. cepacia*. In patients with CF, increased mortality and a higher rate of fatal complications following lung transplantation has been associated with *B. cepacia* colonization. While chronic colonization of the respiratory tract with little or no clinical symptoms is frequent, cases of fulminant necrotizing pneumonia and sepsis with a rapidly fatal outcome have been reported. In addition, *B. cepacia* has been associated with catheter-related BSI, ventilator-associated pneumonia, skin and soft tissue infections following burns, surgery or invasive diagnostic procedures.

Although *Burkholderia mallei* is normally found in infections of horses and *B. pseudomallei* is present in soil and water, these organisms can also cause glanders and melioidosis in humans. Clinical manifestations of melioidosis (*B. pseudomallei*) in humans include pneumonia, genitourinary manifestations, osteomyelitis and skin or soft tissue abscesses, commonly associated with BSI and sepsis (see Chapter 119). Clinical presentation of BSI may range from transient bacteremia to fulminant septic shock with mortality rates of up to 87%.

MANAGEMENT AND RESISTANCE

In-vitro efficacy against *B. cepacia* has been demonstrated for ureido-penicillins, third-generation cephalosporins, carbapenems, fluoro-quinolones, trimethoprim–sulfamethoxazole, chloramphenicol and minocycline.[47] Among the novel antimicrobials, tigecycline has shown less activity compared to minocycline. However, resistance to several classes of antimicrobial agents is often observed, especially in patients receiving multiple courses of antibiotics over a prolonged period of time, such as CF patients. Therapy of *B. cepacia* infections should be based on the results of antimicrobial susceptibility testing. In cases of multi- or pandrug-resistant strains, combination therapy is recommended and the use of agents such as polymyxins may be considered. In addition, inhalation therapy in combination with intravenously administered antimicrobials can control pulmonary exacerbation by *B. cepacia* infection.[48] Management of *B. mallei* and *B. pseudomallei* infections are discussed elsewhere in this book (see Chapter 119).

Stenotrophomonas maltophilia

NATURE AND TAXONOMY

Stenotrophomonas maltophilia is an opportunistic pathogen that was transferred from the genus *Pseudomonas* via the *Xanthomonas* group to the newly defined genus *Stenotrophomonas*. *Stenotrophomonas maltophilia* is a ubiquitous environmental bacterium that has also emerged as an important nosocomial pathogen contributing substantially to morbidity and mortality of immunocompromised patients, particularly in the ICU setting.[49]

EPIDEMIOLOGY

Stenotrophomonas maltophilia can be readily isolated from soil, plants, water and raw milk, and can also be recovered from the hospital environment where it has been isolated from ventilatory equipment and from respirometers, as well as from dialysis fluids and antiseptic solutions (see Table 170.5). There is a high incidence of infections due to *S. maltophilia* in immunocompromised patients such as those with solid malignancies, leukemia or lymphoma.[49] In addition, *S. maltophilia* is increasingly implicated in pulmonary infections in CF patients (see Table 170.4). Recent surveys report a point prevalence of 11% of CF patients with transient colonization with *S. maltophilia*, thus affecting approximately 30% of these patients during a 6-month period, even though the importance of *S. maltophilia* in patients with CF remains to be determined.

DIAGNOSTIC MICROBIOLOGY

Stenotrophomonas maltophilia grows readily on most routinely used media. These bacteria are characterized by the presence of a single or a small number of polar flagella (motile bacteria), frequently pigmented colonies (yellow or yellowish orange) and a negative oxidase reaction. *Stenotrophomonas maltophilia* acidifies sugars (except for rhamnose and mannitol) and is generally proteolytic.

PATHOGENICITY AND PATHOGENESIS

Stenotrophomonas maltophilia produces proteolytic enzymes and other pathogenic extracellular enzymes such as DNAse, RNAse, elastase, lipase, hyaluronidase, mucinase and hemolysin, which may contribute to the severity of *S. maltophilia* infection in immunocompromised patients.

CLINICAL MANIFESTATIONS

Stenotrophomonas maltophilia, particularly in immunocompromised patients, has been implicated as the causative pathogen in respiratory tract infections, endocarditis, bacteremia, meningitis and urinary tract infections. In addition, it is also known to cause severe cutaneous infections (ecthyma gangrenosum similar to that due to *P. aeruginosa*), cellulitis and abscesses, and has been identified as one of the most common causes of infection in wounds resulting from agricultural machinery.

MANAGEMENT AND RESISTANCE

Stenotrophomonas maltophilia displays intrinsic resistance to most classes of antimicrobial agents as a result of chromosomally mediated mechanisms, poor permeability of the outer membrane and naturally produced inactivating enzymes. Mechanisms of resistance include production of several β-lactamases, rendering it susceptible only to latamoxef and combinations of ticarcillin plus clavulanic acid or piperacillin plus tazobactam, as well as carbapenemase production conferring resistance to carbapenems.[50] Few strains are susceptible to gentamicin, neomycin and kanamycin, and susceptibility to doxycycline is reported in less than 50% of strains. Resistance to tetracyclines is associated with alteration of outer membrane proteins.

Currently, trimethoprim–sulfamethoxazole remains the drug of choice for treatment of infections due to *S. maltophilia* although *in-vitro* studies indicate that ticarcillin–clavulanic acid, minocycline, some of the new fluoroquinolones and tigecycline may be useful alternative agents in case of resistance or allergy.[50] Due to increasing rates of resistance, therapy should always be guided by susceptibility testing. Of note, susceptibility testing results may not correctly predict clinical treatment response. In addition, novel fluoroquinolones such as moxifloxacin have displayed reasonable *in-vitro* activity. Severe infections may require combination therapy including ticarcillin plus clavulanic acid or piperacillin plus tazobactam, quinolones, and trimethoprim–sulfamethoxazole.

Miscellaneous Aerobic Nonfermenting Gram-Negative Bacteria

Many other nonfermenting Gram-negative bacilli have been identified from clinical specimens. Some are increasingly involved in human infection.[3,5,51] These genera and species have undergone many taxonomic changes; some have been identified recently and the wide use of analysis of ribosomal 16S RNA gene sequences has allowed a clearer taxonomic position to be established for most of these organisms. The following section includes a short description of the pathogenic role of nonfermenting Gram-negative bacteria involved in human infections and of the management of these infections. For easy reading, the generic groups are described in alphabetical order.

ACHROMOBACTER SPP.

See *Alcaligenes* spp. and *Ochrobacterium* spp.

AGROBACTERIUM SPP.

See *Rhizobium* spp.

ALCALIGENES SPP. (INCLUDING ACHROMOBACTER SPP.)

The genera *Alcaligenes*, *Achromobacter* and *Ochrobacterium* have undergone confusing taxonomic changes in the past decade (see Table 170.1). Currently *Alcaligenes faecalis* remains the only *Alcaligenes* spp. of clinical importance, after several other *Alcaligenes* spp. have been transferred to the genus *Achromobacter*, including *A. denitrificans*, *A. xylosoxidans*, *A. ruhlandii* and *A. piechaudii*.

Epidemiology

The natural habitat of *Alcaligenes* spp. is the same as that of *Pseudomonas* spp. In the hospital environment, *A. faecalis* and *A. xylosoxidans* have been isolated from various environmental sources such as respirators, hemodialysis systems, intravenous solutions and disinfectants.[1]

Diagnostic microbiology

Achromobacter spp. and *Alcaligines* spp. are Gram-negative nonfermenting rods, strictly aerobic and motile, with one to eight peritrichous flagella, usually described as degenerated. They are oxidase-positive, catalase-positive and indole-negative. In contrast to *A. xylosoxidans*, the species *A. faecalis*, *A. piechaudii* and *A. denitrificans* are not saccharolytic. Not all *Alcaligenes* spp. or *Achromobacter* spp. possess specific physiologic or biochemical characteristics allowing a biochemical identification to species level.

Pathogenesis and clinical manifestations

Alcaligenes spp. and *Achromobacter* spp. have been isolated from various clinical sources such as blood, feces, sputum, urine, cerebrospinal fluid, wounds, burns and swabs taken from throat, eyes and ear discharges. *Alcaligenes* strains do not seem to possess any specific virulence determinants. They are infrequent causes of hospital-acquired infections in patients who often have severe underlying disease. Rare cases of peritonitis, pneumonia, bacteremia, meningitis and urinary tract infections have been reported in the literature.[52] In many instances the organism is considered to be a colonizer.[52] Nosocomial outbreaks of infection are usually associated with an aqueous source of contamination. *Alcaligenes* spp. are predominantly isolated from respiratory tract specimens and recovery of these organisms from the sputum of CF patients has been associated with an exacerbation of pulmonary symptoms.

Alcaligenes xylosoxidans has been implicated in BSI (mostly catheter related), pneumonia, endocarditis, meningitis, osteomyelitis, peritonitis and urinary tract infection, often in patients with underlying malignancy, HIV and CF.

Management

As with other nonfermenting Gram-negative bacteria, available susceptibility data for *Alcaligenes* spp. and *Achromobacter* spp. are based on a limited number of isolates, and antimicrobial therapy should be guided by appropriate susceptibility testing. *Alcaligenes faecalis* is generally resistant to aminoglycosides, chloramphenicol and tetracyclines and usually susceptible to trimethoprim–sulfamethoxazole and β-lactam antibiotics such as ureidopenicillins, ticarcillin–clavulanic acid, cephalosporins and carbapenems. *Alcaligenes xylosoxidans* has been shown to be usually susceptible to ureidopenicillins, imipenem and polymyxins and variably resistant to fluoroquinolones. In contrast to *A. faecalis*, *Achromobacter* spp. are often resistant to cephalosporins. There have been several reports of resistance to broad-spectrum penicillins in *A. xylosoxidans* due to constitutive β-lactamase production; three different types of cephalosporinase and the presence of other β-lactamases have been demonstrated.

BERGEYELLA SPP.

See *Weeksella* spp.

CHROMOBACTERIUM SPP.

The genus *Chromobacterium* contains only one species, *C. violaceum*. On agar plates these bacteria usually form violet colonies (violacein). The bacterium has some fermentative activities on sugars and is proteolytic. Nonpigmented strains may be misidentified as *Aeromonas* spp.

Found in soil and water in tropical climates, *C. violaceum* has been implicated in skin, soft tissue and bloodstream infections, mainly in patients with neutrophil dysfunction.[53] In immunocompromised patients, bacteremia may be associated with a high mortality.[53] Empiric treatment can be attempted using imipenem, fluoroquinolones, gentamicin, tetracycline or trimethoprim–sulfamethoxazole.

CHRYSEOBACTERIUM SPP., ELIZABETHKINGIA SPP., FLAVOBACTERIUM SPP. AND MYROIDES SPP.

The clinically important *Chryseobacterium* spp. (*C. meningosepticum* and *C. indologenes*) have been reclassified from the genus *Flavobacterium* (see Table 170.1), while other *Flavobacterium* spp. such as *F. multivorum*

and *F. spiritivorum* have been moved to the genus *Sphingobacterium*. In addition, *F. odoratum* has been reclassified as *Myroides odoratus* and *M. odoratimimus*.

Chryseobacterium meningosepticum has recently been reclassified as *Elizabethkingia meningoseptica*.[54] *Chryseobacterium* spp. and *Elizabethkingia* spp. are ubiquitous organisms that can be found not only in soil and water but have also been recovered from foods and from the hospital environment. Epidemiologic studies have traced the bacterial source to contaminated water, ice machines and humidifiers. Phenotypic markers used for the delineation of outbreaks of *E. meningoseptica* infections were serology based on the O-antigenic type; nine O-serovars have been identified (A–H and K).

Microbiology

Chryseobacterium spp. usually grow between 41°F and 86°F (5–30°C), but strains isolated from human specimens including *E. meningoseptica* readily grow at 99°F (37°C). On nutrient agar they produce colonies 1–2 mm in diameter, which are frequently pigmented light yellow or yellowish orange (nondiffusible pigment, Fig. 170.8). The metabolism is strictly aerobic and sugars are metabolized by the oxidative pathway, except for *Myroides odoratus* (*C. odoratum*) and *Sphingobacterium multivorum* (*F. multivorum*) which do not acidify glucose. Indole-positive species (i.e. *E. meningoseptica*, *C. gleum*) are usually strongly proteolytic; esculin, citrate and urease tests are variably positive.

Clinical manifestations

Elizabethkingia meningoseptica and *C. indologenes* have been isolated from patients with sepsis, osteomyelitis, meningitis and endocarditis.[55] Meningitis due to *E. meningoseptica* has often been observed in neonates but has been reported infrequently in immunocompromised adult patients. Bloodstream infections due to *E. meningoseptica* and *C. indologenes* have been associated with intravascular catheters or contaminated infusates and often present as benign transient bacteremia. In otherwise healthy individuals *E. meningiseptica* has also been implicated in cellulitis, arthritis and community-acquired pneumonia.[55]

Management

Elizabethkingia meningoseptica and *Chryseobacterium* spp. are intrinsically resistant to many commonly used antimicrobial agents including aminoglycosides, third-generation cephalosporins, penicillins (mezlocillin, piperacillin, ticarcillin), aztreonam, imipenem and tetracycline.

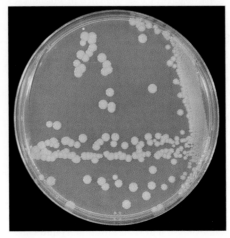

Fig. 170.8 Colonies of *Flavobacterium–Chryseobacterium* group grown on Mueller–Hinton agar. Courtesy of Professor H Monteil.

However, most of these species, including *E. meningoseptica*, are generally susceptible to agents that are usually active against Gram-positive bacteria such as rifampin (rifampicin), clindamycin, erythromycin and vancomycin. Cases of neonatal sepsis have been treated with clindamycin combined with piperacillin. Recent studies have reported the highest *in-vitro* activities in minocycline, rifampin, trimethoprim–sulfamethoxazole and levofloxacin. *Chryseobacterium indologenes* is uniformly resistant to aztreonam, third-generation cephalosporins, aminoglycosides, erythromycin, clindamycin, vancomycin and teicoplanin. Therapy should be guided by antimicrobial susceptibility testing using MICs, since disk-diffusion results are unreliable in predicting susceptibility of *Chryseobacterium* spp. Interpretation of MICs, however, is complicated by the lack of Clinical and Laboratory Standards Institute (CLSI) clinical breakpoints.[51]

COMAMONAS SPP., DELFTIA SPP. AND ACIDOVORAX SPP

Previously designated as *Pseudomonas* rRNA homology group III, the family Comamonadaceae now includes the genera *Comamonas*, *Delftia* and *Acidovorax*. The genus *Comamonas* consists of four named species – *C. aquatica*, *C. kerstersii*, *C. terrigena* and *C. testosteroni* – that have been isolated from human specimens, as well as several other species that so far have been recovered from environmental samples only. The genus *Delftia* consists of *D. acidovorans*, formerly designated *Comamonas acidovorans*. Three clinically relevant species – *Acidovorax facilis*, *A. delafieldii* and *A. temperans* – currently belong to the genus *Acidovorax* in addition to several environmental species that have recently been identified or reclassified from the genus *Pseudomonas*.

Members of these genera are aerobic, Gram-negative, oxidase-positive rods that are commonly found in soil, water and on plants, but are seldom implicated in human infections. Rare cases of catheter-related bacteremia (*C. testosteroni*, *D. acidovorans*, *Acidovorax* spp.), meningitis (*C. testosteroni*), endocarditis (*C. testosteroni*, *D. acidovorans*), conjunctivitis (*C. testosteroni*) and otitis media (*D. acidovorans*) have been reported.[56]

OCHROBACTRUM SPP.

Derived from the genus *Achromobacter*, two species have been recognized as clinical pathogens: *Ochrobactrum anthropi* and *O. intermedium*. These nonfastidious bacteria grow readily on most conventional media and can be identified to genus level by classic biochemical tests; however, no biochemical reaction can separate the two species.

Ochrobactrum spp. are environmental organisms and are considered opportunistic pathogens of low virulence in humans. *Ochrobactrum anthropi* has been associated with catheter-related bloodstream infections, and individual cases of meningitis, endocarditis and other infections have been published. In contrast, *O. intermedium* has only been implicated in one case of pyogenic liver infection; however, due to the biochemical indistinguishability, these data should be interpreted with caution.

Ochrobactrum spp. are usually resistant to most β-lactam antibiotics except carbapenems. Aminoglycosides (except tobramycin in *O. intermedium*), fluoroquinolones, tetracycline and trimethoprim–sulfamethoxazole are usually active. In addition, *O. intermedium* is resistant to polymyxins.[51]

OLIGELLA SPP.

This genus was created in 1987 and includes *Oligella urethralis* (derived from *Moraxella urethralis* and CDC group M-4) and *Oligella ureolytica* (derived from CDC group IVe). These small rods, often occurring in pairs, grow slowly on blood agar and exhibit only limited metabolic activity. They are oxidase- and catalase-positive. *O. ureolytica* is motile, while *O. urethralis* is not. Both species have been implicated in bacteremia, arthritis and genitourinary infections including urosepsis, although the causative role could not be established in all cases.[57]

Both species are usually susceptible to most antimicrobial agents, with *O. ureolytica* being the more resistant species. Therapy should be guided by the results of antimicrobial susceptibility testing.

RALSTONIA SPP.

Ralstonia spp. were reclassified from *Pseudomonas* rRNA group II and originally consisted of *R. pickettii* (formerly *Burkholderia pickettii* or *Pseudomonas pickettii*) and *R. eutropha* (formerly *Alcaligenes eutrophus*). More recently, *R. eutropha* has been reclassified as *Cupriavidus necator*, after intermittently being named *Wautersia eutropha*.[58] Both are emerging pathogens isolated from infections in immunocompromised patients or from respiratory tract infections in CF patients.[59]

RHIZOBIUM SPP.

The genus *Rhizobium* currently consists of four species – *R. radiobacter*, *R. rhizogenes*, *R. rubi* and *R. vitis* – all of which were transferred from the genus *Agrobacterium* (see Table 170.1). *Rhizobium* spp. are phytopathogenic organisms, present in water, soil and environmental plants; they are strictly aerobic coccobacilli, motile with peritrichous flagella (one to six). They grow easily on conventional media, produce oxidase and catalase, and can be identified by most commercially available systems.

Thus far, only *R. radiobacter* has been implicated in infections in humans, mostly device related. Individual cases of endocarditis, catheter-related BSI, peritonitis and urinary tract infections have been published.[60]

Rhizobium spp. are generally susceptible to cephalosporins (second- and third-generation), ticarcillin, imipenem, tetracyclines, colistin, trimethoprim–sulfamethoxazole and fluoroquinolones. In device-related infections, removal of the device may be necessary.[60]

SHEWANELLA SPP.

Shewanella putrefaciens, formerly designated CDC group Ib, *Alteromonas*, *Pseudomonas* and *Achromobacter putrefaciens*, currently belongs to the genus *Shewanella*, which also includes *Shewanella algae*. *Shewanella* spp. grow in media used for Enterobacteriaceae and produce H_2S, which may result in misidentification as *Salmonella* spp. or *Proteus* spp., even though *Shewanella* spp. are nonfermenting. *Shewanella putrefaciens* is present in the environment and has occasionally been isolated from meningitis, otitis media, keratitis, intra-abdominal infections and bacteremia, most cases occurring in immunocompromised patients.[61] In contrast, *Shewanella algae* accounts for the majority of clinical isolates and has been associated with a broad range of diseases, including BSI, peritonitis, osteomyelitis, skin and soft tissue infections, and otitis media.[61]

Shewanella spp. are generally resistant to penicillins but susceptible to third-generation cephalosporins, imipenem, ciprofloxacin, aminoglycosides, trimethoprim–sulfamethoxazole and tetracyclines.[61]

SPHINGOBACTERIUM SPP.

Two species of the genus *Sphingobacterium*, *S. multivorum* and *S. spiritivorum*, are derived from several *Flavobacterium* spp. and CDC groups IIk-2 and -3 (see Table 170.1). In addition, the genus also harbors *S. antarcticum*, *S. faecium*, *S. thalpophilum* and *Sphingobacterium* genospecies 1 and 2. *Sphingobacterium mizutaii* has been transferred to the genus *Flavobacterium*. Other species formerly included in the genus,

S. heparinum and *S. piscium*, have been reclassified as *Pedobacter* spp., none of which has been implicated in clinical manifestations in humans. *Sphingobacterium* spp. are characterized by colonies that develop a yellow pigment after a few days at room temperature. *Sphingobacterium multivorum*, *S. spiritivorum* and *S. thalpophilum* have been isolated from a variety of infections including bloodstream infections, peritonitis, wound infections, urinary tract infections and abscesses.[62]

Sphingobacterium spp. *in vitro* are usually resistant to aminoglycosides and polymyxin B and susceptible to fluoroquinolones and trimethoprim–sulfamethoxazole.

WEEKSELLA SPP. AND *BERGEYELLA* SPP.

Weeksella virosa (see Table 170.1) and *Bergeyella zoohelcum* have both been implicated in infections in humans. While *W. virosa* has been recovered from urine and vaginal swabs, *B. zoohelcum* has been implicated in wound infections following animal bites but individual cases of BSI and meningitis have also been reported.[63] Both grow as pigmented colonies (brown or yellow) and can be distinguished by urease (positive in *B. zoohelcum*) and susceptibility to polymyxin B (*B. zoohelcum* is resistant). Both organisms are usually susceptible to most antimicrobial agents, but susceptibility testing is nevertheless warranted in all cases.

REFERENCES

References for this chapter can be found online at http://www.expertconsult.com

Chapter | **171** | *Francis Mégraud*
Philippe Lehours
Steven FT Thijsen

Curved and spiral bacilli

INTRODUCTION

The curved and spiral bacilli are a heterogeneous group of bacteria that share little morphology.

Helicobacter pylori was previously called *Campylobacter pylori*[1] and in the first part of the 20th century *Campylobacter* was called *Vibrio*. *Campylobacter*, *Helicobacter* and *Vibrio* spp. all produce infections of the gastrointestinal tract. Moreover, they are all Gram-negative organisms and have a similar, curved shape. Using nucleic acid sequence determination of 16S rRNA, the genera *Campylobacter* and *Helicobacter* have been classified (together with *Arcobacter*, *Sulfurospirillum* and *Wolinella*) as members of the superfamily VI of Gram-negative bacilli now called Epsilonproteobacteria (Table 171.1).[2] Only Epsilonproteobacteria that are involved in human infections are discussed in this chapter.

Treponema, *Borrelia* and *Leptospira* are all members of Spirochaetales. These spirochetes are thin, helical, Gram-negative bacteria.

Campylobacter spp., *Helicobacter pylori* and *Vibrio cholerae*

CAMPYLOBACTER SPP.

Nature

Campylobacter spp. are microaerophilic, Gram-negative, curved rods which obtain their energy by using fatty acids and amino acids rather than carbohydrates, and are adapted to life in mucus of the digestive tract. With the genera *Arcobacter* and *Sulfurospirillum*, they form the family Campylobacteraceae. At least 16 species and six subspecies have been differentiated.[2] Not all, however, cause disease in humans.[3] *Campylobacter jejuni* and *Campylobacter coli* are responsible for enteric infections and are the most common Campylobacters found in humans. *Campylobacter fetus* is the third most frequently isolated, but is mostly involved in systemic diseases. The other species (e.g. *Campylobacter lari*, *Campylobacter upsaliensis*) occur only anecdotally. They also lead to enteric infections. Clinical aspects of *Campylobacter* diarrhea are discussed in more detail in Chapter 35.

Epidemiology

Campylobacter spp. infections can be considered as zoonoses, because the primary reservoir for *Campylobacter* spp. is animals. These bacteria are essentially present in the digestive tract of animals, especially birds, where they do not cause disease. Only *C. fetus* spp. *venerealis* causes

septic abortion in cattle. Humans can become infected by ingesting contaminated food or water or through contact with infected animals, including pets. The majority of *Campylobacter* spp. infections are sporadic, although outbreaks mostly of limited size do occur. Large outbreaks involving water as a vehicle have also been described. *Campylobacter* enteritis is more common than *Salmonella* and *Shigella* enteritis and is a major cause of travelers' diarrhea. Infections can be caused by the ingestion of undercooked, contaminated poultry or contaminated milk as well as by cross-contamination of foods which will

Table 171.1 Epsilonproteobacteria of potential clinical interest[2]

FAMILY CAMPYLOBACTERACEAE		FAMILY HELICOBACTERACEAE
Genus Campylobacter	**Genus Arcobacter**	**Genus Helicobacter**
Campylobacter jejuni	*Arcobacter butzleri*	*Helicobacter pylori*
Campylobacter coli	*Arcobacter cryaerophilus*	*Helicobacter acinonychis*
Campylobacter concisus	*Arcobacter nitrofigilis*	*Helicobacter aurati*
Campylobacter curvus	*Arcobacter skirrowii*	*Helicobacter bilis*
Campylobacter fetus		*Helicobacter bizzozeronii*
Campylobacter gracilis		*Helicobacter canadensis*
Campylobacter helveticus		*Helicobacter canis*
Campylobacter hominis		*Helicobacter chrolecystus*
Campylobacter hyointestinalis		*Helicobacter cinaedi*
Campylobacter lanienae		*Helicobacter felis*
Campylobacter lari		*Helicobacter fennelliae*
Campylobacter mucosalis		*Helicobacter ganmani*
Campylobacter rectus		*Helicobacter hepaticus*
Campylobacter showae		*Helicobacter mesocricetorum*
Campylobacter sputorum		*Helicobacter muridarum*
Campylobacter upsaliensis		*Helicobacter mustelae*
Related species:		*Helicobacter nemestrinae*
Bacteroides ureolyticus		*Helicobacter pametensis*
		Helicobacter pullorum
		Helicobacter rodentium
		Helicobacter salomonis
		Helicobacter trogontum
		Helicobacter typhlonius
		Candidatus H. bovis
		Candidatus H. suis
		Related species:
		'H. winghamensis'
		'H. muricola'
		CLO-3
		'Gastrospillum hominis'

be consumed raw.[4] This is an important consideration since the simple preventive measure of cleaning cutting boards, cutlery and hands with soap and hot water may not be often applied in kitchens.[5] Eating undercooked beef was also identified as a risk factor in a case control study in France.[6] As for other enteric infections, taking acid suppressing drugs, especially proton pump inhibitors, is a risk factor for *Campylobacter* infection.[7]

It has been estimated that there are 1.4 million cases annually in the USA.[8] Transmission of the disease from human to human has also been described but seldom occurs. In temperate countries there is a peak incidence in summer and early autumn, although infections occur throughout the year.[9] The highest incidence is found in young children, with a second peak in young adulthood. Infants can also be infected but the risk factors appear to be different.[10] The incidence in developing countries, with less hygienic living conditions, is even higher than in developed countries and direct transmission from poultry to humans seems to occur.

Pathogenesis

Campylobacter bacilli are acid sensitive. Because of the relative barrier imposed by the gastric acid environment, infection is more likely to occur when large numbers of bacteria are ingested. Histologic examination of gut biopsies obtained from patients who have *Campylobacter* enteritis reveals inflammation and edema of the mucosa, with infiltration of neutrophils in the lamina propria. *Campylobacter* colonizes the small bowel but lesions are mainly restricted to the ileum and colon.

In vitro co-culture of epithelial cells with *C. jejuni* has shown that these bacteria can adhere and penetrate into the cells. *C. jejuni* can adhere to epithelial cells via a number of different adhesins: a surface exposed lipoprotein (JlpA) which binds to Hsp90α,[11] a fibronectin-binding protein (CadF),[12] an ABC binding protein (Peb1)[13] and a putative autotransporter (CapA).[14] *C. jejuni* is able to circumvent the induction of innate immunity, Toll-like receptors 5 and 9 not being efficiently stimulated. *C. jejuni* is also able to synthesize proteins which may play a role in internalization and cytoskeletal rearrangement.[15] Cia proteins (for *Campylobacter* invasion antigens) are secreted through the flagella filament upon contact with a eukaryotic cell and appear to contribute to the invasion.[16] *C. jejuni*'s translocation may occur by a transcellular as well as a paracellular route. The disruption of tight junctions of epithelial cells leads to proinflammatory cytokine response[17] and allows the bacterium to move to the basolateral side and reinvade epithelial cells or be taken up by macrophages.

During this process the transcription factors nuclear factor kappa B (NF-κB) and MAP kinases are activated,[18] contributing to both inflammatory diarrhea and clearance of the infection. In addition, *C. jejuni* produces a cytolethal distending toxin (CDT) acting on the cell cycle and leading to apoptosis.[19] Nevertheless, despite the numerous pathogenicity studies performed, the role of CDT in diarrheal disease caused by *C. jejuni* remains unclear.

The molecular mimicry of human ganglioside with the lipo-oligosaccharide (LOS) molecules present in strains of *C. jejuni* expressing the O:19 antigen has been implicated in the association of *C. jejuni* infection with the Guillain–Barré syndrome.[20]

Immune persons in endemic areas, where infections are frequent, can become asymptomatic carriers. Infection can have a protracted course in the case of immune deficiencies, such as in patients suffering from hypogammaglobulinemia. In AIDS patients, opportunistic infections with *C. jejuni* and atypical *Campylobacter* spp. also suggest a role for cellular immunity.

The presence of *Campylobacter*-specific secretory IgA and serum IgA in breast milk correlates with protection against diarrhea. IgG also plays an important role against disease.[21]

An interesting mechanism to avoid elimination by the immune system has been developed by *C. fetus*. Almost all *C. fetus* strains express a surface protein that abrogates complement C3b binding. This prevents opsonization, thereby conferring resistance to killing by phagocytes and adding to the pathogenicity of the species.[22]

In summary, pathogenesis remains poorly understood, in part because of the lack of an animal model that mimics human diarrheal disease, but also because of the genetic variability within the organism resulting from genomic reorganization and phase variation that has made it difficult to identify genomic correlates of virulence.[23]

Prevention

Preventive measures for *Campylobacter* spp. infections include adequate heating of contaminated food and reinforcement of hygiene in the kitchen in order to avoid cross-contamination as well as adequate disinfection of drinking water supplies. Eradication of the animal reservoir is extremely difficult and costly but adequate measures taken in poultry farms and abattoirs can at least decrease the level of contamination.

Development of vaccines is an alternative but no vaccine against campylobacteriosis is currently available.[24] However, several approaches are being followed – for example, the development of:

- live attenuated vaccines;
- vaccines based on heat-killed/formalin-killed bacteria with or without mucosal adjuvants;
- subunit vaccines delivered together with adjuvants; and
- live attenuated *Salmonella* strains expressing *Campylobacter* proteins.[21]

While the link between *Campylobacter* infection and Guillain–Barré syndrome may stimulate the development of a vaccine, whole-cell vaccines cannot be used until we know more about the determinants of this disease.

Diagnostic microbiology

The curved motile rods can be observed in a fecal sample using Gram staining or darkfield microscopy. Culturing *Campylobacter* spp. necessitates special conditions, sometimes difficult to implement.[25] Cultures are commonly performed with an atmosphere comprising 5% oxygen, 10% carbon dioxide and 85% nitrogen. Some species, such as *Campylobacter rectus* and *Campylobacter hyointestinalis*, also require hydrogen in the atmosphere for growth. Selective culture media contain antibiotics such as cefoperazone to suppress the growth of normal Gram-negative intestinal bacteria, vancomycin to suppress the growth of Gram-positive bacteria, and an antifungal compound, as well as blood or charcoal, to neutralize inhibiting factors such as oxygen-free radicals. Commonly used media are Skirrow's, Butzler's, Karmali's agar and cefoperazone charcoal deoxycholate agar. An important disadvantage of selective media is that some *Campylobacter* spp. such as *C. hyointestinalis*, *C. fetus* and *C. upsaliensis*, which are sensitive to antibiotics used in these selective media, can be missed. To circumvent this problem, membrane filtration of feces can be performed to eliminate contaminants followed by culturing on nonselective media. However, this filtration technique is less sensitive than direct plating.

Although the most important species (i.e. *C. jejuni* and *C. coli*) grow at 107.6°F (42°C), some species (e.g. *C. fetus*) grow best at 98.6°F (37°C) and will be missed when cultures are only incubated at 107.6°F (42°C). Typically, *C. jejuni* and *C. coli* colonies with a gray color and growing flat and confluently are visible after 2–3 days of culture. Definite identification of suspect colonies is performed using standard biochemical tests showing positive oxidase and catalase tests.

Campylobacter jejuni is the only *Campylobacter* spp. that is capable of hydrolyzing hippurate, which is essential for its differentiation from other Campylobacters, especially *C. coli*; however, some *C. jejuni* strains may appear hippurate negative. Growth at 77°F (25°C) is essential for diagnosing *C. fetus*. Given the high level of resistance of Campylobacters to quinolones, the nalidixic acid susceptibility test is no longer a key test in *Campylobacter* identification. Molecular identification – polymerase chain reaction (PCR), sequencing – is now being performed more frequently in this group of bacteria. A comparison of seven PCRs, mostly multiplex PCRs, to differentiate well-characterized strains showed a perfect sensitivity and specificity for *C. coli* but not for *C. jejuni*.[26] Real-time PCR has also been used successfully.[27]

Campylobacter spp. can also be detected using PCR directly on feces. The sensitivity is much higher than detection by culture.[28] However, the specificity cannot be proven given the lack of a reference method. Typing of isolates is important for epidemiologic studies. More than 60 serotypes of *C. jejuni* and *C. coli* have been identified with the Penner O typing system but molecular typing methods are now commonly used, including polymerase chain reaction restriction fragment length polymorphism (PCR-RFLP) of the *fla* gene, macrorestriction of the genomes, amplified fragment length polymorphism and multilocus sequence typing.[29] Serology can also be helpful in diagnosing a *Campylobacter* spp. infection because serum IgG and IgM levels start to rise in response to infection 5 days after infection and reach a peak 2–4 weeks later. This is a key investigation in the diagnosis of *C. jejuni*-associated Guillain–Barré syndrome.

Clinical features

Most *Campylobacter* spp. infections manifest as acute enteritis.[30] The ensuing diarrhea can vary from modest to voluminous stools that may be watery or bloody. The infection can also run a subclinical course, especially in hyperexposed populations. Disease will develop 1–3 days after ingestion of the bacilli and symptoms usually disappear after a week. Stool samples typically remain positive for *Campylobacter* spp. for several weeks. In most cases, *Campylobacter* enteritis is a self-limiting disease and it tends to be more severe in patients at the extremes of life. Fever, malaise and abdominal pain may precede diarrhea or may be the most predominant signs. Infection with *Campylobacter* spp. gives rise to inflammation of the gut mucosa. The accompanying pain and fever may also lead to symptoms resembling inflammatory bowel disease. When pain is the major feature of the infection, differentiation from appendicitis may be difficult. *Campylobacter jejuni* can grow in bile and can occasionally cause acute cholecystitis and pancreatitis.[31]

Only a few patients who have a *C. jejuni* infection develop systemic disease. Bacteremia can occur, but generally in patients who have an underlying disease.[32]

A postinfectious reactive arthritis may occur[33] which is very similar to the complication seen after enteritis caused by *Salmonella* spp., *Shigella* spp. or *Yersinia* spp. and appears to be associated with the presence of the HLA-B27 antigen. It also appears that *C. jejuni* is the major cause of postinfectious irritable bowel syndrome.[34]

C. jejuni has also been associated with a rare form of mucosaassociated lymphoid tissue (MALT) lymphoma called immunoproliferative small intestinal disease (IPSID).[35]

Another important complication of *Campylobacter* enteritis is the Guillain–Barré syndrome.[20] A variant, Miller Fisher syndrome, can also occur. *Campylobacter jejuni* enteritis is the infection most frequently observed before Guillain–Barré syndrome and occurs in 20–40% of cases. The risk of developing Guillain–Barré syndrome after *Campylobacter* spp. infection is estimated at 1 per 2000 infections. Major neurologic sequelae exist in 20% of the cases.

Campylobacter coli infections are very similar to infections with *C. jejuni*, but they tend to follow a less severe course.

Infections with *C. fetus* tend to disseminate from the intestine, especially in patients who have conditions that cause impaired immunity, such as chronic alcoholism, diabetes mellitus, malignancies and HIV infection, and in the elderly. Systemic *C. fetus* infections can lead to endocarditis, thrombophlebitis, mycotic aneurysm, meningitis, bone and joint infections and septic abortion.

Campylobacter upsaliensis, C. lari and *C. hyointestinalis* can also cause enteritis. *Campylobacter consisus, C. gracilis, C. curvus, C. mucosalis, C. rectus, C. showae, C. sputorum* and *Bacteroides ureolyticus* can be associated with periodontal infections.

HELICOBACTER PYLORI

Helicobacter pylori was cultured for the first time in 1982, from the stomach which was previously thought to be sterile.[36] Currently this bacterium is considered to be the most important bacterium responsible for chronic infections. It is also the first bacterium known to be involved in a cancer in humans. Clinical aspects of *Helicobacter* infection are discussed in more detail in Chapter 33.

Nature

Helicobacter spp. are spiral-shaped, flagellate Gram-negative bacilli. They are microaerophilic and use amino acids and fatty acids rather than carbohydrates to obtain their energy. At present, about 23 species of *Helicobacter* and two candidate species have been identified, only eight of which cause disease in humans (see Table 171.1).[2] *Helicobacter pylori* is the third bacterium for which the entire genome has been sequenced[37] and the first for which the genome of two strains has been sequenced.[38]

Diagnostic microbiology

Invasive methods for diagnosing *H. pylori* infection depend on endoscopy to obtain biopsies. These biopsies can then be processed for histologic examination and stained with hematoxylin–eosin, Giemsa stain or silver stain. *H. pylori* is usually abundant and its typical morphology and the presence of polymorphs make diagnosis easy. However, previous treatment with proton pump inhibitors may render histologic diagnosis more difficult. The use of immunoperoxidase staining can be considered when atypical bacilli are detected. The examination of a smear can be performed in the endoscopic ward using either darkfield examination of a wet smear or Gram staining.

Because *H. pylori* is a fragile organism, transport conditions are extremely important for culture. Biopsies can be transported in saline for 3–4 hours, but (commercially) available transport medium must be used if preservation for up to 24 hours is necessary. The biopsies must be maintained at a low temperature (39°F/4°C) before being ground with a homogenizer and plated on media enriched with 5–10% blood and supplemented with antibiotics to inhibit growth of contaminant bacteria. The plates must then be incubated for up to 12 days in a microaerobic atmosphere. Growth usually occurs within 3–4 days. *Helicobacter pylori* colonies are easily identified by their morphology and their urease, catalase and oxidase activities. These tests are sufficient when the bacteria are grown from the stomach; molecular tests must be added when they are grown from other specimens.

The urease test is specific for *H. pylori*. A color change is observed if *H. pylori* urease is present when the biopsy is introduced into a medium containing urea and a pH indicator. Tests using semisolid agars show an optimal sensitivity after 24 hours. In contrast, strip tests show a high sensitivity after just 2 hours.

Polymerase chain reaction for diagnosing *H. pylori* infection does not require specific transport conditions and can be performed with a urease test kit sent by mail. Several genes can be targeted: urease, 16S rRNA, 23S rRNA, 29 kDa antigen, *cag*A gene or *vac*A gene. A real-time PCR has been developed which allows detection of both *H. pylori* and its resistance to macrolides. Primers target the 23S rRNA gene and the dissociation curve of the amplicons indicates the mutation present.[39]

Less invasive methods for obtaining material are aspiration of gastric juice or a capsulated string. Diagnosis can also be made using noninvasive tests. The urea breath test measures urease production by *H. pylori*. Samples of breath air are collected by having the patient blow into a tube before and 30 minutes after ingestion of ^{13}C-labeled urea. The tubes can be maintained for months and sent by mail to a laboratory that has a mass spectrometer in order to measure the [13]C:[12]C ratio.

Another method is based on the detection of *H. pylori* antigens in stools using enzyme-linked immunosorbent assay (ELISA). Polyclonal antibodies were first used as a reagent. A second generation of tests employs monoclonal antibodies and gives excellent results.

Antibodies are mainly detected by ELISA. There are numerous kits commercially available with different sensitivities and specificities. Immunoblot methods can also be used. Detection of specific antibodies has also been proposed but shows a lower sensitivity than in blood.

Rapid one-step immunoassays have been developed for detection either of *H. pylori* antigens in stools or *H. pylori*-specific antibodies in blood or urine, but they do not reach a sufficient level of sensitivity.

Since none of the tests is perfect in terms of sensitivity, a combination of tests is recommended.[40] All tests have a comparable sensitivity except for the smear examination, the agar-based urease and rapid serology tests which are inferior. The urea breath test is ideal for follow-up 4–6 weeks after eradication therapy. Serology cannot be used for this purpose because the antibody titer may be high for months after the disappearance of *H. pylori*.[41]

VIBRIO CHOLERAE

Nature

Vibrio cholerae is a Gram-negative, comma-shaped rod belonging to the family Vibrionaceae. Its natural habitat consists of fresh-water and salt-water environments. Based on differences in the composition of the major cell wall antigen (O), 139 serotypes have been differentiated. *V. cholerae*, which belongs to either serogroup O1 or serogroup O139, has been associated with epidemic cholera. *V. cholerae* serogroup O1 can be subdivided into El Tor and classic biotypes as well as the Ogawa, Inaba and Hikojima serotypes. Other serogroups of *V. cholerae*, in addition to nontoxigenic *V. cholerae* O1 or O139, do not cause epidemic cholera; they may, however, cause individual cases of diarrhea.

Epidemiology

Cholera has raged in seven pandemics since 1817. It is possible that an eighth is superimposed on the seventh. The fifth and sixth pandemics were caused by the classic biotype and originated in the Indian subcontinent. The seventh and current one was caused by the El Tor strain and began in 1961 in Indonesia. It has gradually affected most of Asia and Africa and is found incidentally in parts of Europe. In 1991, this pandemic reached South America and has since spread throughout Latin America (Fig. 171.1).[42] Persons who have blood group O are at higher risk of El Tor cholera than those with blood group A, B or AB.[43] This is particularly important for Latin America, where 73% of the population carries the blood type O. An episode of classic cholera protects nearly entirely against recurrent cholera of either biotype, but an episode of El Tor cholera does not protect against future attacks.

In 1992, a novel *V. cholerae* variant O139 (synonym Bengal), which has the same origin as the El Tor strain, emerged in southern Asia. This 1992 epidemic was the first one caused by a serogroup other than O1, and it occurred in populations assumed to be largely immune to *V. cholerae* O1. The impact of a *V. cholerae* O139 infection on the risk of a subsequent *V. cholerae* infection, either O1 or non-O1, has not yet been determined. The Bengal strain has the potential to spread pandemically. It has now affected areas throughout the Indian subcontinent, neighboring states and other parts of Asia. Cases occurring as far away as the USA and Western Europe have also been described.

The distribution and subdistribution of 632 reported outbreaks have been reviewed from the Program for Monitoring Emerging Diseases (ProMED) from 1995 to 2005.[44] Of the reported outbreaks, 66% occurred in sub-Saharan Africa followed by South East Asia. In West and Southern Africa, the most commonly cited risk factor was heavy rainfall and flooding. The lack of infrastructure and economic development, and especially poor sanitation and the lack of clean water have made many parts of Africa susceptible to cholera.[45] The largest identified risk factor for cholera outbreaks is a contaminated water source. In more developed regions, the risk factor is more likely to be related to seafood or vegetables that have not been properly washed or cooked.

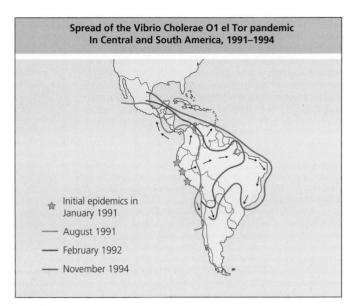

Fig. 171.1 Spread of the *Vibrio cholerae* O1 El Tor pandemic in Central and South America, 1991–94. Adapted from Tauxe *et al.*[43]

Vibrio cholerae, including serogroups O1 and O139, exist as natural inhabitants of aquatic ecosystems and are therefore facultative human pathogens. Within the marine environment they attach to zooplankton and are able to form biofilm, facilitating environmental persistence. *V. cholerae* O1 and O139 are endemic in freshwater zooplankton[46] and indeed an important role of the environment was supported by the correlation between cholera incidence and elevated sea surface temperature. Following events related to El Niño, it was shown that the detection of *V. cholerae* followed ambient temperature increases and coincided with or preceded annual outbreaks of cholera in the summer.[47] The extreme weather conditions of higher temperature, increased rainfall and consequent flooding may explain the global increase in the number of reported outbreaks from 1997 to 1999.[48] Finally, it should be noted that underreporting of cholera is a notorious problem, and the estimation of between 3 and 5 million cases and 120 000–200 000 deaths per year due to cholera could represent a small proportion, perhaps only 10–20% of all cases.[49,50]

Pathogenesis

The infectious dose is high due to the acid sensitivity of the bacteria. Persons who have impaired gastric acidity or who take acid-suppressing medication have an increased risk of infection. In addition, *H. pylori* gastritis is also associated with an increased risk of cholera.[51] The surviving bacteria adhere to and colonize the small intestine epithelial cells, producing the cholera toxin and causing acute watery diarrhea. In the intestine *V. cholerae* is faced with growth inhibitory substances (e.g. bile salts) and defense factors (e.g. complement and defensins), against which it has developed survival strategies. The powerful enterotoxin then released is a 68 kDa protein consisting of an active (A) subunit and five binding (B) subunits (Fig. 171.2). The cholera toxin is released from *V. cholerae* via an extracellular protein secretion machinery which excretes more than 90% of the toxin.[53]

The genes encoding the cholera toxin are part of a single-stranded DNA filamentous bacteriophage CTXΦ.[54] More precisely, the cholera toxin is composed of two types of subunit, a single toxic-active A subunit (CTA) and a circular B subunit heptamer (CTB) responsible for toxin binding to cells. CTA is synthesized as a single polypeptide chain, which is post-translationally modified via the action of a *V. cholerae* protease which generates two fragments, CTA1 and CTA2. CTA1 possesses an ADP-ribosylating activity whereas CTA2 inserts CTA into CTB.[55] The CTB subunits attach to the GM1 ganglioside receptor in

Fig. 171.2 Mechanism of action of *Vibrio cholerae* toxin. The toxin binds to the GM1 ganglioside receptor on the intestinal mucosal cell membrane via the binding (B) subunits (a). The active portion of the A subunit enters the cell and activates adenyl cyclase (b), which results in the accumulation of cyclic adenosine monophosphate (cAMP), derived from adenosine triphosphate (ATP), along the cell membrane (c). The cAMP causes active secretion of sodium (Na$^+$), chloride (Cl$^-$), potassium (K$^+$), bicarbonate (HCO$_3^-$) and water (H$_2$O) out of the cell into the lumen of the intestine (d). Adapted from Murray *et al.*[52]

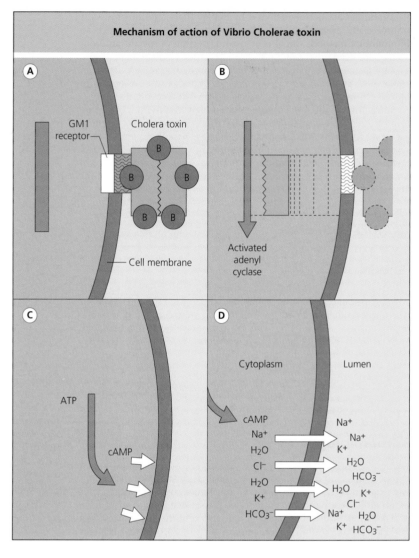

the lining of the mucosal cells; the cholera toxin is then endocytosed by the cell either through caveoli-coated vesicles or clathrin-coated vesicles and travels to the endoplasmic endothelium reticulum, probably in association with the actin cytoskeleton via lipid drafts.[56,57] The A subunit triggers a cascade of reactions involving cyclic adenosine monophosphate, prostaglandins, 5-hydroxytryptamine and calmodulin.[58] This results in an increased level of intracellular cAMP leading to an increase in intestinal chloride secretion and a decrease in sodium chloride absorption. The outcome is a passive watery excretion that leads to diarrhea. The volume typically exceeds 1 liter per hour in adults and 10 ml/kg per hour in children. Since cholera results from a locally acting enterotoxin, it is not accompanied by systemic manifestations caused by a cytokine-induced acute-phase reaction.

The complete genome sequences of the two chromosomes of *V. cholerae* O1 El Tor, now available, helped to unveil the mechanisms of cholera pathogenesis. The bacteria contain two chromosomes, one of which is approximately 3 Mb and codes for virulence factors such as the cholera toxin.[59] A toxin co-regulated pilus (TCP) was identified as the most important colonization factor. The bacterium first colonizes the intestinal surface utilizing TCP and then may receive a signal that induces full cholera toxin and TCP expression and the onset of disease. The genes required for TCP synthesis (*tcp* operon) are located on a pathogenicity island (PI) named Vibrio PI (VPI). VPI contains a G+C content lower than the rest of the genome (35.6% vs 47.7%) suggesting an external origin.[60–62] VPI also encodes a regulator (ToxT) which has been demonstrated to coordinate the expression of TCP and cholera toxin. ToxT is under the control of several regulatory systems that are known

to respond to various environmental conditions (osmolarity, pH and nutriment composition) and to bacterial cell density.[63–65]

Motility, surface antigens (capsule, lipopolysaccharide, outer membrane proteins) and hemagglutination protease are additional important virulence factors. Finally, the role of extracellular capsular polysaccharides in intestinal adherence, virulence and biofilm formation has also been characterized.

In *V. cholerae*, quorum-sensing regulation is considered as the key mechanism coordinating virulence gene expression with that of cell population density. *V. cholerae* contains two well-characterized quorum-sensing systems, CqsA/S and LuxS/PQ.[66] It has been proposed that biofilm formation increases acid resistance of *V. cholerae* and is critical for entry into the host as it passes the stomach milieu. Once in the intestinal environment, quorum-sensing signals within the biofilm repress virulence factor gene expression, such as genes encoding for the cholera toxin and TCP.[67,68] The bacterium then detaches from the biofilm and colonizes the intestines where quorum-sensing signals are low and cholera toxin and TCP are expressed.

Prevention

Cholera is difficult to eradicate from water and is likely to remain a serious threat to public health for some time. Measures to prevent cholera include separating sewage and drinking water systems, disinfection of drinking water and food, hygiene measures (e.g. hand washing with soap), active case finding and effective case management with the use of oral rehydration. Breast-feeding provides important protection to infants, not because of transmission of maternal antibodies but because of the lower exposure to contaminated food and water. During epidemics, the bodies of persons who died of cholera should be disinfected and buried rapidly, and the consumption of food at gatherings, including funerals, should be discouraged.

The currently licensed, parenteral, killed cholera vaccine is no longer recommended by the World Health Organization (WHO) because of its limited protective efficacy. To induce mucosal immunity, oral vaccines, both inactivated (whole cell/cholera toxin B-subunit or WC-BS) and live (CVD103-HgR), have been developed.[69] WC-BS is currently recommended by the WHO (Dukoral; licensed by SBL Vaccine, Sweden) and consists of four batches of heat- or formalin-killed whole-cell *V. cholerae* O1, representing both serotypes (Inaba and Ogawa) and both biotypes (classic and El Tor), supplemented with purified recombinant cholera toxin B-subunit.

Mass vaccination campaigns of populations considered to be at high risk of cholera outbreaks have been performed in several countries. When the WC-BS vaccine was studied in Bangladesh, a short-term protection of 6 months was found in 85% of adults and children over 6 years of age; the protection was as good after two doses as after three. However, the duration of protection dramatically decreased after 1 year. Similar protection rates were obtained in other studies in Peru (86% protection efficacy), Mozambique (60.5% protection efficacy), Uganda and Darfour after two or three doses.[70–72] Vaccines that include the B-subunit of the toxin provide cross-protection against heat-labile enterotoxigenic *Escherichia coli*, a result of the close relationship between the two toxins.[73,74] A variant of the Dukoral killed whole cell vaccine containing no recombinant CTB-subunit has been produced and tested in Vietnam. It is administered in two doses 1 week apart and an efficacy of 66% against *V. cholerae* El Tor was obtained after 8 months in all age groups tested.[75]

CVD103-HgR consists of a live attenuated, genetically modified *V. cholerae* O1 Inaba strain which has been engineered to produce CTB but not the A subunit of CT, and produces higher resistance to the homologous classic strain than to the El Tor strain. Attenuation of El Tor has led to several new candidate vaccines that have proven safe and highly effective against El Tor cholera.[76] The vaccine (Orochol; licensed by Berna Biotech, Switzerland) is given orally along with buffer to neutralize stomach acidity. The vaccine is available in two formulations, either a low-dose formulation for nonendemic countries or a 10-fold higher dose formulation for cholera-endemic developing countries. The vaccine is currently licensed in several industrialized countries. The safety and immunogenicity of a single dose of Orochol has been demonstrated.[77–79]

Because immunity against the O1 type is not protective against O139, *V. cholerae* O139 type vaccines have been developed. New attenuated strains of serogroup O139 for use as oral vaccines (CVD112 and Bengal 15), as well as new candidate vaccines, have been developed.[80–82] A bivalent O1 and O139 whole-cell oral vaccine without CTB was also recently developed in Vietnam and shown to be safe and immunogenic in both adults and children, generating 90% anti-O1 and 68% anti-O139 vibriocidal responses after administration of a two-dose regimen. It elicits a robust immune response and can be produced at a low cost.[83,84] Similar results were obtained during a randomized placebo-controlled trial in adults and children in a cholera-endemic area in Kolkata, India.[85]

Diagnostic microbiology

For rapid diagnosis, darkfield examination of a fresh, unstained stool specimen is highly sensitive and specific; a characteristic finding is the 'shooting star' phenomenon caused by the motility of the single polar flagellum of the organism. The diagnosis of cholera is confirmed when *V. cholerae* is identified in a stool culture on thiosulfate-citrate-bile salts-sucrose (TCBS) agar directly or after enrichment in alkaline peptone water, taking advantage of *V. cholerae*'s tolerance to alkaline conditions. Sucrose-positive, smooth, yellow colonies grown on TCBS agar are submitted to an oxidase test and the identification of *V. cholerae* is completed by biochemical and serologic tests.

Once identified at the species level, additional tests include serotyping for O antigens and the three antigen variants recognized, as well as biotyping to differentiate classic and El Tor biotypes. A rapid, colorimetric immunodiagnostic method is available for the detection of *V. cholerae* O1. The immunochromatographic strip test may be the simplest, most rapid and most sensitive and specific test for the detection of *V. cholerae*. Two rapid immunodiagnostic test kits based on the use of monoclonal antibodies have been developed for the direct detection of *V. cholerae* O139: a co-agglutination test and Bengal DFA (a direct fluorescent-antibody test). In epidemic settings in developing countries, a bacteriologic diagnosis is not indicated in all suspected cases because the management of dehydrating diarrhea is guided by the extent of fluid loss rather than by the nature of the infecting organism. In contrast, the diagnosis should be confirmed in individual cases of suspected cholera in the developed world.

Such classical methods can be time-consuming. Thus molecular methods, when available, are more suitable for *Vibrio* spp. detection directly from environmental water samples, since they can detect dead bacteria and viable but nonculturable (VNC) bacteria. Several molecular techniques based on DNA amplification have been developed and could be useful in the detection of *V. cholerae* O1 directly from environmental water in cholera endemic areas and in complementing the identification of toxigenic strains isolated by culture.[86–88]

Clinical features

Cholera is an acute diarrheal disease in which the fluid loss is responsible for all other clinical manifestations of the disease. Most cases are so mild that they may escape detection, but a small percentage are so serious that death can occur within a few hours of the onset of symptoms. *V. cholerae* needs to be considered among the possible diarrheal causes in children living in endemic areas.[50,89] In Latin America, well-established case management has kept fatality rates low (at about 1%). In contrast, cholera in Africa has been sporadic and as a result less well recognized. The fatality rates there also tend to be higher (about 10%).[90] Children are more likely to have only subclinical infection or mild diarrhea, whereas adults tend to develop more severe disease and require hospitalization.

Cholera is in principle a self-limiting disease if dehydration is sufficiently corrected. Cholera gravis is a voluminous painless watery diarrhea that can lead to dehydration and even death within a few hours. The case fatality rate for untreated cholera gravis is 50%. Symptoms include nausea, vomiting (especially early in the illness) and muscle cramps, followed by signs of hypovolemic shock. With adequate treatment, mortality is reduced to 1% or less in all age groups. After an incubation period of between 18 hours and 5 days, symptoms are generally abrupt and include watery diarrhea and vomiting. The most distinctive feature of cholera is the painless purging rice-water stools with a fishy odor. The vomitus is generally a clear, watery, alkaline fluid. The rate of diarrhea may reach 500–1000 ml/h in severe cases, leading to severe dehydration. Most patients have no urine output until the dehydration is corrected. Because *V. cholerae* does not invade the epithelial lining of the intestine, there is little inflammatory response and hence the stool contains few if any leukocytes and patients are afebrile. Metabolic abnormalities may also occur, including hypokalemia as the result of potassium loss, acidosis from both bicarbonate loss and increased lactate production resulting from anaerobic glycolysis, and hypoglycemia due to deficient gluconeogenesis resulting in seizures and other neurologic abnormalities. Hyperventilation (Kussmaul breathing) may occur as a result of the metabolic acidosis. Shock from cholera can precipitate abortion in pregnant women, although this is less likely to occur if rehydration is prompt.

Complications include acute renal failure, low blood glucose concentrations and electrolyte imbalance, especially hypokalemia, but these are generally from improper treatment. Severe muscle cramps of arms and legs are common. They are probably due to the electrolyte imbalance, although the exact explanation is not known. They subside within a few hours of treatment.[50]

Management

The management of cholera patients consists of two components:
- rehydration, which is critical; and
- antimicrobial therapy, which is optional and intended to shorten the duration of the illness and prevent spread of the disease.

Effective fluid replacement can be expected to reduce mortality to less than 1% of the severely affected individuals. If fluids are given promptly, nearly all deaths are avoided. However, as effective treatment is not always available in remote areas where cholera occurs, cholera deaths are still common. Mild and moderately dehydrated patients can be treated using oral rehydration solution (ORS), which has three basic components: sugars, salts and water. Physiologically, the sugar acts as the vehicle whereby salts can be absorbed by the mucosal cell; water follows passively.[91] Patients on ORS should remain on ORS until the diarrhea stops. Severely dehydrated patients should be treated intravenously. When intravenous solutions and equipment are not available, severely dehydrated patients may be treated through a nasogastric tube.

Antibiotic treatment serves to shorten the illness and save rehydration fluids. Incomplete courses have contributed to antibiotic resistance. Options are guided by local sensitivity patterns. These are tetracycline (250 mg q12h for 7–10 days) or amoxicillin (250 mg q6h for 5 days). Tetracyclines and quinolones are not recommended during pregnancy. During epidemics, prophylactic antibiotics should be used for the immediate family only and should be limited to single-dose therapy. Reports from several cholera-endemic countries of strains resistant to antibiotics, including tetracycline, ampicillin, kanamycin, streptomycin, sulphonamides and fluoroquinolones, have emerged with a trend of spatial and temporal fluctuations. On a molecular basis, conjugative plasmids, transposons, integrons, mutations and proton-motive-force-dependent efflux have been associated with this antibioresistance.[92,93]

Apart from fluid replacement, novel and potentially useful strategies to reduce diarrhea in cholera have been developed. First, the inhibition of toxin binding is a particularly attractive approach because binding inhibitors can be administered prophylactically in high-risk areas or as therapy after the infection has begun, as well as administrated orally.[94] Second, enkephalin inhibitors such as racecadotril can be effective in *V. cholerae* and *E. coli*-related pediatric diarrhea.[95] Third, small-molecule thiazolidinone inhibitors of CFTR Cl⁻ conductance have been shown to be effective in preventing Cl⁻ and fluid secretion in human intestinal cells and rodents.[96] In conclusion, all of these new agents could be promising compounds for cholera treatment, but further studies must be carried out to prove their antidiarrheal efficacy *in vivo*.

Other pathogenic *Vibrio* spp.

Vibrio parahaemolyticus is a halophilic, or salt-requiring, *Vibrio* sp. that has been related to food poisoning and ingestion of raw or inadequately cooked seafood. The epidemiology results from the ubiquitous presence of the organism in coastal waters. The median incubation time is estimated at 23 hours (range, 5–92 hours); secondary cases are rare. Preventive measures include the use of boiled water for cooking food. It is not known whether clinical disease confers immunity. There is no effective vaccine available. Stool culture on selective TCBS agar demonstrates distinct opaque green colonies; final identification is made using standard biochemical tests. The clinical picture ranges from mild, watery diarrhea with low-grade fever to frank dysentery. Specific treatment is not required in most cases because the illness is self-limiting and no benefit has been established from antimicrobial agents.

Other less common halophilic *Vibrio* spp. include *Vibrio vulnificus*, *Vibrio alginolyticus*, *Vibrio fluvialis*, *Vibrio hollisae* and *Vibrio damselae*. Molecular methods, especially PCR, can be used for identification or detection of these species, including in the environment. In contrast to the *Vibrio* spp. discussed so far, *V. vulnificus* and *V. alginolyticus* are associated more frequently with soft tissue wound infection and sepsis than with diarrhea.[97] *V. vulnificus* may be considered an emerging pathogen and its virulence is the strongest among the noncholera *Vibrio* spp. Pathogenicity is generally reserved for the immunocompromised host and is related to disease states that exhibit high serum iron levels, including liver disease. Prevention involves avoidance of contaminated salt water. Immunocompromised patients should be warned against the ingestion of raw oysters and shellfish. At higher latitudes, severe *V. vulnificus* infections have been reported in association with very hot weather conditions and sea water temperatures above 68°F (20°C).

A *Vibrio* polysaccharide conjugate vaccine may be useful in the management of *V. vulnificus* infections. Antibodies that react with the capsular polysaccharide of the organism are detectable in infected patients and in persons without known exposure to the organism, suggesting that cross-reacting antibodies are present in the general population.

V. vulnificus infections are the cause of two main clinical syndromes:
- primary sepsis secondary to ingestion of raw oysters; and
- localized infection from wound exposure to salt water in which the organism lives.

Both syndromes demonstrate characteristic skin lesions of the trunk and extremities. They are characterized by hemorrhagic bullae which progress to necrotic ulceration. Necrotizing fasciitis of the foot associated with *V. vulnificus* can cause death within 48 h and has an overall mortality rate of 50%, even with appropriate antibiotic and surgical treatment.[98] Besides these two syndromes, *V. vulnificus* may also cause acute diarrhea in those on antacid therapy. Early suspicion is critical, because *V. vulnificus* is not always susceptible to aminoglycosides, and tetracycline is the first-choice treatment.

V. alginolyticus may cause bacteremia and death in immunocompromised hosts. Among immunocompetent hosts, it may cause cellulitis and otitis media in swimmers and fishermen.

Vibrio mimicus, a nonhalophilic *Vibrio*, produces a clinical spectrum that is indistinguishable from that of *V. parahaemolyticus*. The epidemiology of *V. mimicus* reflects a global distribution; outbreaks have been associated with heavy contamination of water sources. Prevention involves adequate purification of water sources and proper cooking practices. The diagnosis is confirmed by identifying the agent on TCBS agar and subsequent specific antiserum testing. Treatment is limited to fluid and electrolyte replacement.

V. alginolyticus represents a diagnostic obstacle, because it is often outnumbered by other *Vibrio* spp. in environmental and seafood samples. As *V. parahaemolyticus* is the species responsible for most seafood-borne outbreaks worldwide,[99] the differentiation of this species from other *Vibrio* spp. is of great importance. For this purpose Bauer *et al.* have recently developed a novel multiplex PCR for the identification of *V. parahaemolyticus*, *V. cholerae* and *V. vulnificus* which could be very useful for clinical laboratories.[100]

Treponema spp., *Borrelia* spp. and *Leptospira* spp.

The order of the Spirochaetales is divided into the families Spirochaetaceae and Leptospiraceae. These families include, among others, the genera *Treponema*, *Borrelia* and *Leptospira* (Table 171.2). Syphilis and endemic treponematoses are discussed in Chapters 57 and 104, respectively. Infection caused by *Borrelia burgdorferi* (Lyme disease) is covered in Chapter 43. The remainder of this chapter deals with *B. recurrentis*, leptospirosis and *Spirillum* infections.

Table 171.2 Order Spirochaetales

Spirochaetaceae		Etiologic agent	Human disease
Family Spirochaetaceae	Genus *Cristispira*		None
	Genus *Serpulina*		None
	Genus *Spirochaeta*		None
	Genus *Treponema*	*Treponema pallidum* subsp. *pallidum*	Syphilis
		Treponema pallidum subsp. *endemicum*	Bejel
		Treponema pallidum subsp. *pertenue*	Yaws
		Treponema carateum	Pinta
	Genus *Borrelia*	*Borrelia recurrentis*	Epidemic relapsing fever
		Many *Borrelia* spp.	Endemic relapsing fever
		Borrelia burgdorferi, Borrelia garinii, Borrelia afzelii	Lyme borreliosis
Family Leptospiraceae	Genus *Leptonema*		None
	Genus *Leptospira*	*Leptospira interrogans*	Leptospirosis

The genera *Treponema*, *Borrelia* and *Leptospira* contain pathogens associated with human infections. The genera *Cristispira*, *Serpulina*, *Spirochaeta* and *Leptonema* are not known to cause disease in humans.

BORRELIA RECURRENTIS

Nature and epidemiology

The louse-borne epidemic relapsing fever, caused by *Borrelia recurrentis*, is transmitted by the human body louse and is associated with unhygienic living circumstances. The tick-borne endemic relapsing fever is caused by different *Borrelia* spp. and is transmitted by the *Ornithodorus* tick.

Pathogenesis and prevention

When lice are crushed, *B. recurrentis* is released and penetrates the skin or mucous membranes. Organisms can be detected in the blood when the patient has a fever. They sequester in internal organs in the afebrile periods. Mutational changes in the antigenic properties of the organism and consequent antibody production account for the relapses, which end when sufficient borrelicidal antibody has been developed.

Preventive measures are similar to those recommended for Lyme disease and involve the elimination or avoidance of the spirochete vector. A vaccine is not yet available for public health purposes.

Diagnostic microbiology

Diagnosis is based on the clinical presentation and detection of the bacteria in the blood. Spirochetes are found in the majority of wet or stained blood smears. They have also been detected in the CSF of patients who have signs of central nervous system involvement. Up to 10% show positive serologic tests for syphilis.

An early clinical diagnosis of louse-borne relapsing fever is not difficult during epidemics. In contrast, the initial differential diagnosis in an isolated case includes many different diseases such as malaria, typhoid fever, leptospirosis and dengue fever.[101]

Clinical features

Epidemic louse-borne relapsing fever and endemic tick-borne relapsing fever have very similar clinical manifestations; heterogeneity reflects differences in, for example, spirochete strains and the condition of the patient. Louse-borne relapsing fever and tick-borne relapsing fever both have a very acute onset of high fever with chills and muscle and joint aches. Headache and lethargy may be accompanied by neurologic findings, including meningitis and seizures leading to coma. Photophobia and iridocyclitis may develop, causing permanent damage to the sight. Coughing may result from bronchitis or pneumonia. A 2-day truncal rash may occur at the end of the first febrile period. Abdominal tenderness with enlargement of liver and spleen may be associated with jaundice, lymphadenopathy and hemorrhagic diathesis.

The first bout of fever usually lasts 3–6 days, sometimes with fatal complications including myocarditis, cerebral hemorrhage and hepatic failure. The fever may suddenly reappear after a 7–10-day interval. Louse-borne disease typically has a longer incubation period and a more elongated cycle of febrile and afebrile periods, and is associated with a single relapse. Tick-borne disease manifests with multiple relapses that taper off in duration and intensity.

Management

First-choice antibiotic is doxycycline 100 mg q12h for 5–10 days. One 500 mg dose of erythromycin is the second-choice option. Antibiotic treatment may be accompanied by a Jarisch–Herxheimer reaction that cannot be prevented by prior corticosteroid therapy[102] and that reflects clearance of the spirochetemia. It may be advisable to give the first dose of antibiotics at a lower dose (e.g. erythromycin 250 mg) to limit the severity of the Jarisch–Herxheimer reaction (see Chapter 125 for further management guidelines).

LEPTOSPIRA INTERROGANS SPP.

Nature

Leptospira interrogans spp. are thin, motile, coiled bacilli. The serotypes of the *Leptospira interrogans* sp. group include *icterohaemorrhagiae, canicola, pomona, autumnalis, grippotyphosa, hebdomadis, ballum* and *australis*.[103] Each of these has a different natural habitat. For example, *L. interrogans* serotype *icterohaemorrhagiae* is most commonly found in rats, *L. interrogans* serotype *canicola* in dogs and *L. interrogans* serotype *pomona* in pigs.

Epidemiology

Leptospirosis is a zoonosis that occurs worldwide (see Chapter 124). In the USA, rats are the most common vector for human infection, followed by dogs, livestock, rodents, wild mammals and cats. Humans are dead-end hosts because person-to-person transmission is very rare. The peak incidence is during the summer and early autumn; young adult men often become infected, for example, after recreational exposure to contaminated water. Leptospirosis has long been considered an occupational disease affecting farmers, veterinary surgeons and abattoir workers through indirect contact with infected animals via urine-contaminated water or soil.[104]

Pathogenesis

Leptospira spp. penetrate the intact mucous membranes or abraded skin, enter the bloodstream and spread to all parts of the body, including the cerebrospinal fluid (CSF) and eyes. Liver damage is subcellular and may lead to jaundice. Renal failure may result from a direct toxic effect of the leptospires on the tubules. Meningeal irritation may occur when the leptospires enter the CSF. They are abundant during the early stage of the meningeal disease and disappear when serum antibodies develop. A chronic or recurrent uveitis may result from leptospires persisting in the corpus vitrium of the eye. Myalgia, particularly of the calves, may be an early sign, and pathologic changes such as polymorphonuclear infiltration of the muscle occur late.[105]

Prevention

Effective control of leptospirosis is difficult because leptospires can establish a symbiotic relationship with many hosts, even if they have been vaccinated, and persist in the renal tubules (with excretion in the urine) without causing illness or pathologic changes in the kidneys. In addition, wild animals represent a reservoir from which domestic animals are continually infected. Widespread vaccination of livestock and pets in the USA has reduced the incidence of infection in some species, although adequately vaccinated dogs can still infect humans.[106] Immunization of rice fieldworkers in China with polyvalent vaccines has been practiced. In France a vaccine against serovar *icterohaemorrhagiae* is available for human use.[107] Prohibition of recreational activities in contaminated waters and measures to reduce the number of rats have been successful in reducing the incidence of disease. Prevention can be considered using 200 mg doxycycline once a week for heavily exposed individuals such as soldiers who train in the jungle.[108]

Diagnostic microbiology

Isolating the organism from patient material or the detection of seroconversion confirms the clinical suspicion of leptospirosis. Leptospires can be isolated from blood or CSF during the first 10 days of illness. During the second week, they appear in the urine and can be detected in biopsies from various organs. Tween 80-albumin is viewed as the best available medium.[109] Cultures should be maintained in the dark for up to 6 weeks at 82–86°F (28–30°C). Leptospires grow in semisolid media in a ring 0.5–1 cm below the surface, appearing 6–14 days after inoculation. They remain viable in heparinized blood for more than 1 week and can be mailed to a reference laboratory for identification.

The laboratory technique most commonly used to diagnose leptospirosis is a two-step serologic procedure, although antibiotic treatment may interfere with antibody development and account for false-negative results.

Macroscopic slide agglutination is used for screening purposes, followed by a microscopic agglutination test (MAT) with live antigens for determining antibody titers and identifying serotypes. Both tests use pools of antigens representative of most serogroups. Nevertheless, cross-reactions often occur and serologic tests cannot accurately identify the serotype responsible for infection. Currently, the sensitivity and specificity necessary for reliable clinical diagnosis is best achieved using a battery of 23 antigens. The presumptive diagnosis may be based on a microscopic agglutination titer of 1:100 or greater or on a positive slide agglutination test. Agglutinins appear after 1 week of illness and decline after the third or fourth week. For areas in the world where laboratory resources are limited a dipstick assay using a broadly reactive leptospiral antigen on a solid support for the detection of IgM antibodies was demonstrated to have satisfactory specificity and sensitivity.[110]

Other techniques to identify leptospires include darkfield examination and silver staining. Polymerase chain reaction has proven valuable as a rapid, sensitive and specific means of diagnosing leptospiral infection, especially during the first 10 days of illness when the clinical expression of the disease may be confusing.[111]

Clinical manifestations

Leptospirosis may evolve subclinically or clinically. It has an incubation period of approximately 7–12 days; clinical illness typically follows a biphasic course. During the initial phase of 4–7 days, patients present with sudden onset of fever, severe general malaise, muscular pain (especially in the calves) and conjunctival congestion; leptospires can be isolated from most tissues. Two days without fever follow. During the second phase of up to 30 days, leptospires are still detectable in the urine, kidney and vitreous body. Circulating antibodies emerge and meningeal inflammation, uveitis and rash develop.[112]

Icteric leptospirosis, or Weil's disease, occurs in 10% of the clinically ill patients; 90% remain anicteric. Icteric leptospirosis can be caused by any type of leptospire including *L. interrogans* subtype *icterohaemorrhagiae*. Prominent features are renal and liver malfunction, hemorrhage and impaired consciousness; the mortality rate is 5%.[113] The combination of a direct serum bilirubin level of less than 20 mg/100 ml (342 mmol/l), a marked elevation in serum creatine phosphokinase and an elevation in transaminase (SGOT and SGPT) of less than 200 units is suggestive of the diagnosis.[114] Hepatocellular necrosis rarely occurs and no residual hepatic dysfunction ensues. Hepatomegaly is found in 25% of cases. The severity of the illness probably reflects the degree of the vasculitis.

Anicteric leptospirosis is a more common and less severe form of leptospirosis. It has a sudden onset and is accompanied by remittent fever and chills, persistent headache, severe myalgia, malaise, prostration and abdominal pain with nausea and vomiting lasting up to 7 days. During the following so-called immune stage, the fever virtually subsides. Delirium and meningism, however, may develop. Several organ systems can be affected, including the lungs, which may show pulmonary infiltrates, and the eyes.[115] A rash may develop as well. Distinct erythematous pretibial lesions can be found in the Fort Bragg fever syndrome, which is caused by *L. interrogans* serotype *autumnalis*.

MANAGEMENT

Severely ill patients should be treated with intravenous penicillin or amoxicillin for 7 days (Table 171.3).[116,117] Less severely ill patients should receive oral doxycycline for 7 days.[118] Severe disease is not limited to adults but may also affect children, who benefit from antibiotics even late during the illness.[119] Careful monitoring and supportive therapy are important in order to prevent possible complications, including renal failure, hypotension and major hemorrhage.

Table 171.3 Treatment options for leptospirosis

| Bacteria | ANTIBIOTIC | |
	First choice	Second choice
Leptospira icterohaemorrhagiae, copenhagi (Weil's disease) *Leptospira hardjo* (milker's disease) *Leptospira grippotyphosa*	Penicillin G 1 MU q4–6h iv for 7 days Alternative: Amoxicillin 500 mg q6h for 7 days	Doxycycline 100 mg q12h po for 7 days

Adapted from Speelman *et al.*[117]

SPIRILLUM MINUS

Rat-bite fever can be caused by either *Streptobacillus moniliformis* or *Spirillum minus*. The first description of the spirillum dates back to 1888 when Carter reported a spiral organism which he called *Spirillum minor* in the blood of wild rats. Later the organism was named *Spirocheta morsus muris* and in 1924 the organism was renamed *Spirillum minus*.[120]

Nature

The literature on *Spirillum minus* is very puzzling since largely conflicting properties of the organism have been reported. The basic problem lies in the fact that the description of the organism is purely morphologic.[121] No biochemical properties or nucleotide sequence data are available. *Spirillum minus* is a Gram-negative spiral micro-organism. It measures 0.2–0.5 mm in width and 3–5 mm in length. It possesses two to three windings and is actively motile by means of bipolar tufts of flagella.

Epidemiology and pathogenesis

Spirillum minus can be detected in the oropharynx of rats and small rodents. Infections occur throughout the world. Data on incidence are lacking so the widely held belief that infections with *S. minus* are more often seen in the Pacific region cannot be substantiated. Transmission from human to human has not been documented.

Prevention

No studies have been reported on the use of prophylactic antibiotics after a rat bite.

Diagnostic microbiology

The spiral bacteria can be made visible using darkfield microscopy or Giemsa staining of blood smears, smears from eschars or lymph node aspirates. *Bergey's Manual of Determinative Microbiology* states that the organism cannot be cultured on artificial media but can be detected in the blood of mice or guinea-pigs 3 weeks after intraperitoneal injection of clinical samples.[121] A practical problem concerning this approach is the fact that these animals are the natural reservoir of these spirilla.

Animal inoculation studies should include control animals and pre-inoculaton evaluation for spirilla.[122] Most reports in the literature do not describe if such controls were performed.

Diagnosis of *S. minus* infection in the literature is based on clinical presentation,[123] direct visualization of the organism[124] or animal inoculation.[122] These spirilla could not be cultured on artificial media. Other reports indicate an easily cultivable *S. minus* as an etiologic agent for endocarditis[125,126] and recurrent fever.[127] These spirilla could be cultured on simple media such as blood agar and an antibiogram could be established. Further characterization of the spirilla is warranted to determine if we are dealing with one or multiple species or even genera.[128] No specific serologic test can be used; however, the VDRL is positive in 50% of cases.

Clinical features

Spirillum minus rat-bite fever is also called sodoku: 'so' means rat and 'doku' means poison in Japanese.[120] The initial lesion of the rat bite usually heals promptly. One to 36 days after the exposure the patient becomes ill and develops fever. At the site of the bite, the wound reactivates and an eschar develops. Regional lymphadenitis is present in the majority of cases. A violaceous maculopapular rash on palms and soles, very similar to the one seen in syphilis, is a common feature. If untreated, relapsing fever will develop. As compared to the rat-bite fever caused by *Streptobacillus moniliformis*, sodoku has a longer incubation period and arthritis is not a frequent event.

Management

Penicillin is the treatment of choice although no clear-cut guidelines can be presented about dose and duration. A Jarisch–Herxheimer reaction can occur after initiation of antibiotic therapy. Tetracycline can be used for patients with an allergy for penicillin.

REFERENCES

 References for this chapter can be found online at http://www.expertconsult.com

Gram-negative coccobacilli

INTRODUCTION

The Gram-negative coccobacilli that are important human pathogens including *Bordetella*, *Brucella*, *Francisella*, *Haemophilus*, *Legionella*, *Pasteurella* and *Yersinia* spp. *Actinobacillus*, *Aggregatibacter*, *Cardiobacterium*, *Eikenella*, *Kingella* and *Moraxella* spp. occasionally cause human disease. All of these genera except *Yersinia* are fastidious, requiring special nutrients and growth factors for isolation. Like other members of the Enterobacteriaceae, *Yersinia* spp. are not exacting in their growth requirements.

The genera *Brucella*, *Francisella*, *Pasteurella* and *Yersinia* cause zoonotic infections in humans. *Legionella* infections are acquired through exposure to environmental contamination. *Haemophilus* and most *Bordetella* infections arise through person-to-person transmission. Rarely *Bordetella bronchiseptica*, an animal pathogen, produces opportunistic human infections.

Bordetella Species

NATURE

Bordetella spp. are minute Gram-negative coccobacilli. They often demonstrate bipolar staining. They may be nonmotile or motile by means of peritrichous flagella. *Bordetella pertussis* and *Bordetella parapertussis* are nonmotile. *Bordetella* spp. are strictly aerobic (except for *B. petrii*) and the optimum temperature for growth is 95–98.6°F (35–37°C). No acid is produced from carbohydrates. There are eight species in the genus (a further putative species, *Bordetella ansorpii*, is awaiting confirmation of its validity); these differ in their fastidiousness and growth requirements. *Bordetella pertussis* is the most exacting and requires special media for isolation; *Bordetella parapertussis* is slightly less exacting; *Bordetella bronchiseptica* grows on ordinary laboratory media. Multilocus enzyme electrophoresis, insertion sequence polymorphisms and sequencing data derived from 16S rDNA sequence analysis and microarray-based comparative genome hybridization have confirmed the close genetic relatedness of all known *Bordetella* species.[1] *Bordetella pertussis* and *B. parapertussis* are probably human adapted subspecies of *B. bronchiseptica*. The genomes of *B. pertussis*, *B. parapertussis*, *B. bronchiseptica*[2] and *B. avium*[3] have all been sequenced.

Bordetella pertussis and *B. parapertussis* are human pathogens of the respiratory tract causing pertussis or whooping cough. *B. bronchiseptica* and *B. avium* are primary respiratory tract pathogens of birds and mammals. *B. bronchiseptica*, *B. hinzii*, *B. holmesii*, *B. trematum*, *B. petrii*, *B. ansorpii* and *B. avium* may infrequently cause infection in humans, particularly in the immunocompromised host.

EPIDEMIOLOGY

Pertussis is highly contagious, being transmitted via aerosolized droplets of respiratory secretions, and in the prevaccine era nearly all children became infected between the ages of 1 and 5 years. Attack rates range from 50% for school contacts to 80–90% for close family contacts. Patients disseminate organisms for weeks or months and are highly infectious in the nonspecific catarrhal and early paroxysmal stages of the infection. It is therefore easy for the infection to spread to susceptible individuals before the possibility of whooping cough is considered. There is little evidence of asymptomatic carriage.

Whooping cough is still a major disease worldwide and an important cause of death in malnourished children. It is estimated that there are over 51 000 000 cases each year worldwide and 300 000 deaths.[4] In most populations the disease is endemic, with epidemics occurring every 4 years in late winter and spring. There is no animal reservoir.

With the use of whole-cell pertussis vaccine the incidence of pertussis in children aged 1–5 years declines sharply but there is an increase in the incidence of the disease in children younger than 1 year. Unfortunately, these young infants are those at greatest risk of morbidity and mortality from pertussis. Females are more likely to be infected than males. Immunized contacts may become transiently colonized. Adolescents and adults with waning vaccine-induced immunity are increasingly suffering from pertussis, which often goes undiagnosed because the infection may be atypical, and these older patients act as a source of transmission to young children. It has been suggested that up to 20% of adults with a prolonged cough may be suffering from pertussis.[4] There are three serotypes of *B. pertussis* pathogenic for humans, which contain agglutinins 1,2; 1,2,3; and 1,3. Strains may switch serotype both *in vitro* and *in vivo*. For this reason, a genotypic method of classification, based on techniques such as restriction fragment length polymorphism (RFLP) or pulsed-field gel electrophoresis (PFGE) is preferable.

PATHOGENICITY

Bordetella pertussis, *B. parapertussis* and *B. bronchiseptica* all possess a virulence control system regulated by the BvgAS operon.[1] BvgAS is a two-component phospho-relay system that responds to environmental conditions by switching between three phenotypic phases. The Bvg⁺ phase occurs with respiratory tract colonization and is associated with the expression of a number of virulence factors. The Bvgⁱ phase is associated with respiratory transmission and Bvg⁻ is an avirulent phase that enables *B. bronchiseptica* to survive in the environment.[1] Some Bvg-regulated genes are expressed in all three subspecies. Others, although they are present in all three subspecies, are differently expressed. Importantly the *ptx-ptl* operon which encodes pertussis toxin (PT) is present in *B. pertussis*, *B. parapertussis* and *B. bronchiseptica* but only expressed in the Bvg⁺ phase of *B. pertussis*.

Table 172.1 Virulence factors of *Bordetella pertussis**

Toxin	Synonyms	Composition	Actions	Comments
Filamentous hemagglutinin	FHA	Protein	Adhesin	Highly immunogenic component of acellular pertussis vaccines
Pertactin	PRN	Outer membrane protein	Adhesin	Enhances protective immunity
Pertussis toxin	PT	Protein	Attachment to ciliated respiratory epithelium Activation of cAMP, HSF, LPF, IAP Impairs leukocyte function Haemolytic	Adjuvant component of acellular pertussis vaccines
Adenylate cyclase toxin	ACT	Protein	Activation of cAMP Antiphagocytic Anti-inflammatory Haemolytic	Calmodulin-activated RTX toxin
Dermonecrotic toxin	DNT	Polypeptide	Vascular smooth muscle contraction Dermal necrosis	
Tracheal cytotoxin	TCT	Glycopeptide	Ciliostasis Inhibits DNA synthesis	
Lipopolysaccharide	LPS	Lipopolysaccharide	Endotoxin	
Fimbriae	FIM	Protein	Facilitates persistent tracheal colonization	Component of some acellular pertussis vaccines

cAMP, cyclic adenosine monophosphate; HSF, histamine sensitizing factor; IAP, islet-activating protein; LPF, lymphocytosis promoting factor; RTX, repeats in toxin.
*With the exception of pertussis toxin, similar toxins are expressed in *B. parapertussis* and *B. bronchiseptica.*

Bordetella pertussis produces a number of adhesins and toxins, which are important in pathogenesis[1] (Table 172.1).

Filamentous hemagglutinin (FHA), pertactin (PRN) and fimbriae (FIM) are adhesins that play a role in colonizing the ciliated respiratory tract epithelium. Pertussis toxin (PT) is a four-polypeptide toxin with many biologic activities: a histamine-sensitizing factor, a lymphocytosis-promoting factor, an enhancer of insulin secretion and a potent adjuvant. It is composed of two subunits, A and B. Subunit B mediates toxin binding and subunit A carries out the toxin's biologic activities. Pertussis toxin activates adenyl cyclase, resulting in increased cyclic adenosine monophosphate (cAMP) in the host cell. Adenylate cyclase toxin (ACT) is an extracytoplasmic protein that can enter leukocytes. Once inside the cells, ACT is activated by calmodulin to catalyze the production of cAMP from adenosine triphosphate (ATP). The increased cAMP interferes with leukocyte function. Dermonecrotic toxin (DNT) is a heat-labile toxin that can cause vascular smooth muscle contraction resulting in focal ischemic necrosis. Tracheal cytotoxin (TCT) is a peptide derived from bacterial peptidoglycan. It causes ciliostasis, inhibits DNA synthesis and kills ciliated epithelial cells, which are then sloughed off. The endotoxin lipo-oligosaccharide (LOS) of *B. pertussis* probably also plays a part in pathogenicity.[1]

Following inhalation, *B. pertussis* adheres to ciliated epithelium in the trachea and bronchi. Adhesion is mediated by filamentous hemagglutinin, pertactin and possibly pertussis toxin. The bacilli then begin to multiply, producing pertussis toxin, which disrupts cell function; tracheal cytotoxin, which inhibits ciliary motion; and adenylate cyclase toxin, which interferes with phagocytosis. The dermonecrotic toxin causes local necrosis. The organisms remain localized on the respiratory epithelium. They do not invade.

PREVENTION

Prevention of pertussis depends on immunization. Whole-cell pertussis vaccines consist of killed suspensions of whole bacterial cells adsorbed with the adjuvant aluminum hydroxide. To be effective the vaccine must contain all three agglutinogens, 1, 2 and 3. Pertussis vaccine was introduced into the UK during the 1950s and resulted in a steady decline in the size of pertussis epidemics until the mid-1970s.

Many concerns have been voiced about the safety of whole-cell vaccines and fears of possible neurologic sequelae. In the UK these fears resulted in a dramatic fall in the rate of vaccine uptake and three large epidemics of pertussis occurred in the late 1970s (Fig. 172.1). Since that time, parental confidence in the vaccine has gradually been restored and the number of cases has again declined. There is no strong evidence that whole-cell pertussis vaccine does produce long-term adverse effects but it may trigger the appearance of pre-existing neurologic problems. A severe adverse reaction to a previous dose of vaccine is a contraindication for further doses. Vaccination should be delayed in children who are unwell.

A number of acellular pertussis vaccines, containing up to five *B. pertussis* antigens, including pertussis toxin, filamentous hemagglutinin, pertactin and fimbrial antigens FIM2 and FIM3, have been developed and have replaced whole-cell pertussis vaccine in the routine infant immunization program in many developed countries, including the UK.[5] They are generally less reactogenic than whole-cell preparations and may be used for booster immunization in older children and adults.

As the incidence of pertussis in older children and adults is increasing there may be a case for using acellular pertussis vaccine to boost waning vaccine-induced immunity in older age groups. Whole cell pertussis vaccine should be avoided for adolescents and adults because of significant degrees of reactogenicity.

DIAGNOSTIC MICROBIOLOGY

With careful sampling and culture techniques *B. pertussis* can be recovered for up to 3 months after the onset of the illness. Nasopharyngeal aspirates, pernasal swabs or nasopharyngeal swabs are the specimens of choice. Dacron TM or rayon pernasal swabs should be used to increase recovery of *B. pertussis* as this organism has a greater affinity for Dacron than for cotton wool. Samples collected using Dacron swabs

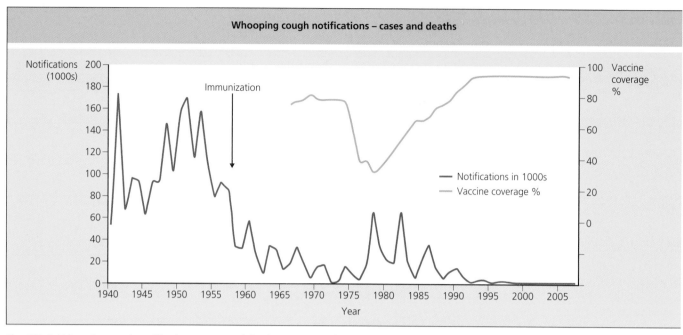

Whooping cough notifications – cases and deaths

Fig. 172.1 Whooping cough notifications – cases and deaths. Figures are for England and Wales 1940–2007. Data supplied by the Health Protection Agency Centre for Infections.

are preferable for polymerase chain reaction (PCR) testing. These samples are far superior to 'cough plates'. Material collected for bacterial culture should be plated immediately on a suitable medium. If this is not possible it should be placed in a charcoal transport medium.[1] The traditional Bordet–Gengou agar, a potato infusion agar containing 10% glycerol and 20% sheep blood, has the disadvantage of a short shelf life. Better growth is obtained on charcoal blood agar, which can be made selective by the addition of cephalexin.

Cultures should be incubated in a moist aerobic atmosphere at 98.6°F (37°F) for at least 7 days. After 3–5 days of incubation, typical 'bisected pearl' colonies appear (Fig. 172.2). Suspect colonies should be checked by Gram staining and identified using slide agglutination with type-specific antisera. *B. pertussis* and *B. parapertussis* can be differentiated by a series of simple tests; *B. bronchiseptica* can be identified using a commercial galley test kit such as API 20NE.

Bordetella pertussis has three major surface agglutinogens (1, 2 and 3) which form the basis of a serotyping scheme. There are three serotypes responsible for infections: 1,2; 1,3 and 1,2,3. The serotype of an isolate can be determined by slide agglutination using cross-absorbed antisera. Type 1,3 is the most common serotype, accounting for 90% of isolates.

Direct immunofluorescence may be applied to respiratory secretions to give a rapid diagnosis, but this method lacks sensitivity and specificity[1] and has been largely superseded by PCR-based detection. Real-time PCR methods are more sensitive than culture, especially for specimens collected more than 3–4 weeks into the illness and following antibiotic treatment. A number of different primers have been used, including *IS481* which detects *B. pertussis* (and *B. holmesii*); *IS1001*, which detects *B. parapertussis* and *B. holmesii*; and *ptxA* which is specific for *B. pertussis*.[6]

Serologic diagnosis of *B. pertussis* is based on ELISA assay of IgG and IgA antibodies to pertussis toxin. A rise in titer of IgG or IgA (twofold or greater) to pertussis toxin in acute and convalescent phase samples taken at least 2 weeks apart is considered significant. In adolescents and adults a single high titer of antipertussis toxin IgG has a good predictive value of acute pertussis infection, with reported sensitivity of 76% and specificity of 99%.[5] Serology is unreliable in young infants.

CLINICAL MANIFESTATIONS

Bordetella pertussis is the cause of pertussis, or whooping cough. In a typical case, following an incubation period of 7–14 days, the patient develops red eyes, a runny nose, mild cough and sneezing ('catarrhal stage'), clinically indistinguishable from many viral upper respiratory tract infections. After about 1 week the cough becomes more severe and the patient experiences paroxysmal bouts of a severe, hacking cough. A paroxysm consists of repeated coughing followed by an inspiratory gasp as the patient finally inspires. This is the characteristic 'whoop'. Paroxysms may be triggered by a variety of stimuli, including cold air and loud noises. A child may become cyanosed during a paroxysm and can suffer fatal hypoxia. Often the child vomits at the end of a paroxysm and is left exhausted. The 'paroxysmal stage' may last for 1–4 weeks. This is followed by a lengthy 'convalescent stage' as the paroxysms decline and the patient slowly recovers. Many cases, but not all, develop a lymphocytosis.

Common complications include pneumonia (which may be primary or secondary to a supervening infection with another pathogen) and otitis media. The child may suffer cerebral hypoxia during a paroxysm which can lead to encephalopathy or fitting. Other possible complications include intraventricular hemorrhage, subconjunctival hemorrhages, umbilical or inguinal herniae, fractured ribs, ruptured diaphragm and rectal prolapse. Pertussis is most severe in very young

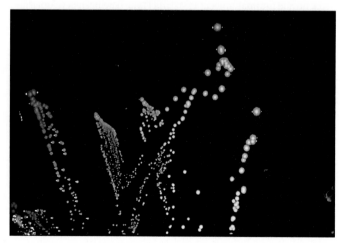

Fig. 172.2 Colonies of *Bordetella pertussis* on charcoal blood agar.

infants and in this age group the presentation may be atypical with no characteristic paroxysmal whooping. Similarly, partially immunized children and adults may have an atypical form of pertussis.[1]

Bordetella parapertussis is a cause of acute bronchitis or pertussis-like infections in children.[1] *Bordetella bronchiseptica* may rarely cause pneumonia, meningitis or whooping cough in highly immunocompromised patients.[1]

MANAGEMENT

Antimicrobial therapy for pertussis, when administered early in the course, can decrease transmission to susceptible contacts and possibly ameliorate symptoms. Macrolides are the antibiotics of choice and appear to reduce the severity and duration of the disease. Trimethoprim–sulfamethoxazole (co-trimoxazole) or fluoroquinolones are alternatives for older patients who are unable to tolerate erythromycin. Corticosteroids may be indicated in infants who have life-threatening disease. Secondary bacterial infections should be treated with appropriate antibiotics.

Brucella Species

NATURE

Brucella spp. are small, nonmotile, nonsporing, noncapsulate Gram-negative coccobacilli. They are aerobic, but some strains require 5–10% carbon dioxide for primary isolation. Growth on culture media is improved by the addition of serum or blood. Growth *in vitro* is slow and primary isolation may require up to 4 weeks' incubation. *Brucella* spp. are catalase-positive and usually oxidase-positive, but urease activity and hydrogen sulfide production are variable. *Brucella* is a monospecific genus, *Brucella melitensis*, with multiple biovars. In practice it is more useful to refer to separate species, which have differing host specificities. There are six species of *Brucella* (and two provisional species, *B. pinnipediae* and *B. cetaceae*, awaiting full validation), four of which can infect humans (Table 172.2). *B. melitensis* is the most virulent and is responsible for the majority of human infections. Both *Brucella abortus* and *Brucella suis* cause considerable morbidity in countries where brucellosis persists in domestic animals. The genomes of *B. melitensis*,[7] *B. abortus*[8] and *B. suis*[9] have been sequenced.

EPIDEMIOLOGY

Brucella spp. can infect a wide variety of domestic and wild animals. Brucellosis is a true zoonosis because humans acquire the infection directly or indirectly from infected animals. About 500 000 cases of human brucellosis are reported annually worldwide but this almost certainly is a gross underestimate of the true incidence.

Brucellosis is prevalent in Mediterranean countries, the Middle East, the Indian subcontinent, Mongolia and Central and South America.[10] Some countries have eradicated brucellosis, including the UK, much of northern Europe, Australia, New Zealand and Canada.

In their natural hosts, *Brucella* spp. cause chronic infections that are mild or asymptomatic. The bacteria localize in the reproductive tissues of ruminants, which are rich in mesoerythritol. Erythritol stimulates the multiplication of *Brucella* spp. This accounts for the main symptoms of brucellosis in animals – sterility or abortion. Erythritol is not present in human tissue. *Brucella* organisms are shed in large numbers in the products of conception, in urine and in milk, and when the animals are slaughtered. Humans are infected either by direct contact with infected animals or animal products or indirectly by ingesting infected milk or dairy produce.

In endemic areas the majority of cases occur in dairymen, herdsmen, abattoir workers, butchers and veterinary surgeons. Children may become infected in rural areas of developing countries if they live in close proximity with domestic animals. The general public generally acquires the infection through the ingestion of unpasteurized milk and milk products such as fresh soft cheese. Case-to-case transmission in humans is very rare. Self-inoculation with live *Brucella* vaccine is a recognized risk among veterinary surgeons. Laboratory workers are at risk of acquiring brucellosis through the inhalation of aerosols.[11] This may occur when staff handle as yet unidentified Gram-negative coccobacilli without adequate safety precautions. Brucellosis is considered a potential biologic weapon via airborne transmission.

Brucella melitensis is responsible for the majority of human infections and is primarily food-borne. The primary hosts for *B. melitensis* are sheep and goats. *Brucella abortus* and *B. suis* infections are generally sporadic and occur in people who work with cattle or pigs, respectively. *Brucella canis* infections are the least common in humans and are generally laboratory acquired.[12]

PATHOGENESIS

Brucella spp. are facultative intracellular parasites, surviving and multiplying within cells of the reticuloendothelial system. The organisms enter the body by inhalation, ingestion or after penetration of intact skin, abrasions or the conjunctival mucosa. The lipopolysaccharide (endotoxin) of smooth strains (S-LPS) is a major virulence determinant. S-LPS is antiphagocytic, facilitates cell entry, inhibits the fusion of *Brucella*-containing vacuoles (BCV) with lysosomes and inhibits host cell apoptosis. A two-component regulatory system, BvrR/BvrS is important for invasion and intracellular survival, and acts by regulating the expression of outer membrane proteins, Omp 3a (Omp25) and Omp 3b (Omp22).[13] The altered expression of surface proteins permits Brucellae to bind to and penetrate host cells.

Table 172.2 *Brucella* species pathogenic to humans

Species	Primary host	Humans as secondary host
Brucella abortus (biovars 1–6, 9)	Cattle, camels, yaks, buffalo	++
Brucella melitensis (biovars 1–3)	Goats, sheep, camels	++++
Brucella suis biovars 1–3 biovar 2 biovar 4 biovar 5	 Pigs Hares Reindeer Small rodents	 + + + +
Brucella canis	Dog, fox, coyote	+
Brucella pinnipediae, B. cetaceae	Minke whales, dolphins, porpoises, seals	+

The type IV secretion system (VirB) of *Brucella*, encoded by *virB* operon, is also important for adherence, cell entry and bacterial survival and replication within macrophages.[13]

After ingestion by phagocytic cells, the organisms proliferate in the local lymph nodes. The infection spreads hematogenously to tissues rich in elements of the reticuloendothelial system, including the liver, bone marrow, lymph nodes and spleen. Organisms may also localize in other tissues, including joints, central nervous system, heart and kidneys.

Endotoxin and hypersensitivity to *Brucella* antigens may cause some of the symptoms of brucellosis, including fever and weight loss. Antibodies against the *Brucella* LPS appear within a few days of the onset of the acute phase of the disease and are important in preventing re-infection. However, cell-mediated immunity, particularly the production of activated mononuclear phagocytes, is more important in promoting recovery.

PREVENTION

The ideal method of prevention of human brucellosis is to eliminate the disease from domestic livestock. This has been achieved in several countries. There are effective vaccines for cattle (S19) and goats (Rev-1).

Where eradication has not been achieved, people who are occupationally exposed should minimize the risk of infection by wearing protective clothing, gloves, goggles and masks. These measures are particularly important when handling animals that have recently given birth or aborted.

In the past, live, attenuated animal vaccines have been given to workers at high risk of contracting brucellosis. However, these vaccines may produce infection in humans and are far from ideal. Candidate vaccines, including an LPS–protein conjugate vaccine and a live attenuated strain are under development.[14] *Brucella* spp. are killed by heating at 140°F (60°C) for 10 minutes. Boiling or pasteurizing milk will therefore eliminate the risk of transmission via dairy products.

DIAGNOSTIC MICROBIOLOGY

Clinicians should inform laboratory staff when brucellosis is suspected so that they can handle samples and cultures in a containment level 3 laboratory and in a biologic safety cabinet to avoid laboratory-acquired infections. A definitive diagnosis depends on the isolation of *Brucella* spp. from cultures of blood, bone marrow or tissue taken early in the disease. Bone marrow cultures are reported to give a slightly higher yield than peripheral blood cultures but, since modern blood culture methods can produce positive results in up to 80% of cases, bone marrow cultures are not generally required or advocated. Biphasic Castaneda bottles were traditionally recommended to reduce the risk of contamination during subculturing. Cultures should be incubated at 98.6°F (37°F) for at least 6 weeks before they are discarded. Modern semiautomated blood culture techniques (e.g. Bactec®, Bact-Alert®) are suitable for the isolation of *Brucella* spp. The lysis centrifugation method also gives good results. These commercial systems may give positive results in a matter of days rather than weeks, depending on the initial inoculum of organisms in the sample. In developing countries where automated blood culture systems are not available, blood clot culture is more sensitive than whole blood culture.

Positive cultures should be subcultured onto serum dextrose agar or a similar medium. Selective culture media are not necessary for human blood cultures but may be required for contaminated material. *Brucella* spp. produce small, smooth, translucent colonies after 48 hours of incubation at 98.6°F (37°C) in air plus 5–10% carbon dioxide. Commercial galley-test identification systems may

misidentify *Brucella* spp. as *Moraxella phenylpyruvica*,[11] and isolates should be sent to a reference laboratory for further tests to confirm the identity and to determine the biovar of the strain. This classification is based on the production of hydrogen sulfide, urease activity, the tolerance of the organism to the bacteriostatic dyes basic fuchsin and thionin and agglutination with monospecific antisera. Tbilisi (Tb) phage typing is also used to define *Brucella* spp. A real-time multiplex PCR assay has been described which can also be used to confirm the identity and species of *Brucella* isolates.[15] A number of PCR assays for diagnosing brucellosis in clinical samples have been described and can provide a rapid diagnosis of acute brucellosis and also an early detection of relapses. Antigen detection is another potential diagnostic tool.

Many serologic tests have been described for brucellosis. Interpretation of results is often difficult since both IgG and IgM antibodies can persist for a long time. A sample of serum should be collected as early as possible in the course of the disease. The serum agglutination test (SAT) using *B. abortus* strain 119 is widely used. False-negative results can occur if serum samples are not diluted beyond 1:320, owing to a prozone phenomenon. False-positive reactions may occur due to cross-reactivity with strains of *Escherichia coli*, *Vibrio cholerae*, *Yersinia enterocolitica* and *Francisella tularensis*. The SAT measures both IgM and IgG. To measure the quantity of specific IgG, serum is first treated with 2-mercaptoethanol to inactivate IgM. IgG and IgA antibodies seem to be the best indicators of acute infection. A rise in antibody titer is observed in more than 97% of patients who have acute brucellosis and positive blood cultures. An initial IgM antibody response is followed after 1–2 weeks by a rise in IgG. During recovery the IgG antibody titers slowly decline over a period of months but IgM antibodies may persist at a low level in the serum for several years. Sustained IgG antibody titers or a second rise in IgG antibody levels are seen in chronic infection or relapse. The SAT test cannot be used to diagnose *B. canis* infection.

Commercial ELISA tests based on antibodies to S-LPS are highly sensitive but appear to be less specific than the SAT. Rapid point-of-care tests, including fluorescent polarization immunoassay (FPA) and immunochromatographic *Brucella* IgM/IgG lateral flow assay (LFA) are highly sensitive and specific and have been used successfully to diagnose brucellosis in endemic areas.

CLINICAL MANIFESTATIONS (SEE ALSO CHAPTER 123)

Brucellosis is a systemic infection that can affect any tissue of the body. The protean, vague clinical symptoms are generally not specific for brucellosis. The possibility of brucellosis should be considered in any fever of unknown origin, especially in patients who have occupational exposure or have recently traveled in endemic areas.

MANAGEMENT

Before the introduction of antibiotics, brucellosis was a chronic, relapsing illness. A number of antimicrobial agents are active against *Brucella* spp. *in vitro* but they are not always clinically effective. *Brucella* spp. are sequestered intracellularly, so agents that achieve adequate intracellular concentrations should be used. It is also necessary to give a prolonged course of treatment to reduce the rate of relapsing infection. The World Health Organization (WHO) recommendations for treating brucellosis are either an oral regimen of doxycycline plus rifampin (rifampicin) daily for at least 6 weeks or oral doxycycline for 6 weeks supplemented by parenteral streptomycin daily for the first 2–3 weeks.[12] Gentamicin may be a suitable alternative to streptomycin (see also Chapter 123).

Franciscella Species

NATURE

Francisella spp. are very small, faintly staining, pleomorphic Gram-negative, nonmotile and nonspore-forming coccobacilli. They are strictly aerobic, oxidase-negative and weakly catalase-positive. The organisms are surrounded by a thin, lipid-rich capsule. They attack carbohydrates slowly, producing acid but no gas. *Francisella tularensis* requires cysteine or cystine for growth and grows slowly at 98.6°F (37°C) on suitably enriched media.

Francisella tularensis causes tularemia in animals and humans. Within the species *F. tularensis* there are four subspecies, which differ in their virulence and their epidemiology (Table 172.3). *F. tularensis* subsp. *tularensis* (type A) is the most virulent and is found primarily in North America. There are two distinct genetic clades of *F. tularensis* subsp. *tularensis*; clade A1 is found in the central United States and has a high case-fatality rate; clade A2 occurs in the western USA and has a lower case-fatality rate. *Francisella tularensis* subsp. *holarctica* (type B) is more widely distributed than *F. tularensis* subsp. *tularensis* and is less virulent. The genomes of strains of both clades of *F. tularensis* subsp. *tularensis* have been sequenced.[16]

EPIDEMIOLOGY

The majority of human infections with *F. tularensis* occur in the northern hemisphere between latitudes 30° and 71°. It is well recognized in North America, Scandinavia and Russia, but has not been described in the UK.[17] The organism is found in many species of wild and domestic animals, birds, fish and blood-sucking arthropods. *Francisella tularensis* may persist in water, possibly in association with free-living amebae.

In the USA the most important reservoirs of *F. tularensis* are rabbits, hares, muskrats and ticks. In Scandinavia and Russia, rodents (such as voles and mice) and mosquitoes are important reservoirs. The modes of transmission to humans include tick or mosquito bites, contact with infected animal tissues, inhalation of an infectious aerosol or ingestion of contaminated meat or water. There is an increased risk of tularemia in occupations that bring people into contact with infected material.

There are approximately 200 cases each year reported in the USA, with over 60% occurring in the southern and southern-central states of Missouri, Oklahoma, Arkansas, Texas and Kansas. Most infections occur in males. Infections usually occur in summer following insect bites or winter when animals are hunted and trapped.

PATHOGENICITY

The infectious dose in humans depends on the subspecies and the route of entry. Inhalation of fewer than 10 organisms of *F. tularensis* subsp. *tularensis* can result in infection and up to 30% of untreated infections can be lethal.[17] The infecting dose rises to 10^8 when the organisms are ingested. Laboratory workers are at high risk through handling infected laboratory animals or cultures of the organism. *Francisella tularensis* is a hazard group 3 pathogen. *Francisella tularensis* subsp. *tularensis* (type A) is more virulent to animals and humans than the other subspecies. The low infecting dose, aerosol transmission, high virulence and high mortality of consequent infection with *F. tularensis* subsp. *tularensis* mean that this organism is a potential bioweapon.

It does not produce an exotoxin. Virulence determinants of *F. tularensis* include the lipopolysaccharide (LPS), capsule and type IV pili. The *Francisella* pathogenicity island (FPI) contains 19 genes that are necessary for intracellular growth and virulence. Genes within the FPI are regulated by the Mg1A protein.[18] The application of new molecular methods should further elucidate the molecular basis of *F. tularensis* pathogenicity, which is still poorly understood.

After entry into the body, the organisms spread to the regional lymph nodes, from where they may disseminate via the lymphatic system or bloodstream to involve multiple organs. There is probably a transient bacteremia at this early stage. *Francisella tularensis* is a facultative intracellular parasite and can multiply and survive for prolonged periods within macrophages, hepatocytes and endothelial cells. Intracellular survival is associated with a failure of phagosome–lysosome fusion and the bacteria replicate in the cell cytosol. The bacilli are protected from humoral antibodies, which are directed against carbohydrate antigens. Recovery from tularemia depends on cell-mediated immunity, which is directed against the protein antigens of the organism.

PREVENTION

Prevention of tularemia is best achieved by avoiding exposure to the organism. Gloves, masks and goggles should be worn when skinning or eviscerating animals. Animals that look sick should be left intact. Game meat should be thoroughly cooked and fresh water that is possibly contaminated should not be drunk. Ticks should be promptly removed and chemical insect repellants may be used.

A live attenuated vaccine (LVS) was used to immunize laboratory staff working with *F. tularensis* in the USA until recently. It provided good protection against an aerosol challenge of 10 organisms of a virulent strain

Table 172.3 *Francisella tularensis* subspecies and biovars

Subspecies	Geographical distribution	Virulence in humans	Virulence in rabbits	Main animal hosts
Tularensis (type A) Clade 1*	Central United States	+++	+++	Rabbits, hares, ground squirrels
Clade 2†	Western United States			
Holartica (type B) Biovar I	North America, Europe, Siberia, Far East, Kazakhstan	++	+	Rodents, beavers, muskrats
Biovar II	Eurasia			
Biovar japonica	Japan			
Mediasiatica	Central Asia	+	+	Rodents, rabbits
Novocida‡	North America	+	?	Muskrats

*Clade 1 is associated with distribution of Lone Star tick and American dog tick; it has a high case-fatality rate.
†Clade 2 is associated with distribution of Rocky Mountain wood tick and deer fly; it has a low case-fatality rate.
‡Low virulence and usually infections only occur in immunocompromised hosts.

of *F. tularensis* subsp *tularensis* but the degree of protection declined as the infecting dose increased. Problems with LVS, including reversion to virulence and variable immunogenicity, have led to its withdrawal. New novel epitope-based and subunit tularemia vaccines are being developed.[19]

DIAGNOSTIC MICROBIOLOGY

Isolation of *F. tularensis* from clinical material is potentially hazardous and it is imperative that the laboratory is notified if tularemia is suspected so that appropriate containment precautions can be taken. *Francisella tularensis* is a category 3 pathogen and should only be knowingly handled at containment level 3 in a biologic safety cabinet by trained and experienced staff.

The detection of *F. tularensis* in a Gram-stained smear of aspirates or other samples is rarely successful. PCR methods have been described that can be applied to clinical samples and to identify the subspecies of an isolate.

The organism requires cysteine or cystine for growth. Specialized media such as cysteine–glucose–blood agar have been devised, but *F. tularensis* will grow on some media that are routinely used for other organisms. Chocolate blood agar is often supplemented with cysteine (e.g. IsoVitaleX) and will then support the growth of *F. tularensis*. Similarly, *F. tularensis* will grow on buffered charcoal yeast extract agar (BCYE), which is normally used to isolate *Legionella* spp.

Cultures should be incubated at 98.6°F (37°F) with additional carbon dioxide in the atmosphere of incubation. *Francisella tularensis* grows slowly, taking 2–4 days to produce visible colonies, and cultures should be incubated for 3 weeks before being discarded as negative. The addition of penicillin to the medium will suppress the overgrowth of contaminants.

Colonies of *F. tularensis* are blue-gray, round, smooth and somewhat mucoid. They are β-hemolytic on blood-containing media. The identity of the organism can be confirmed by slide agglutination or fluorescent antibody staining. Alternatively, PCR targeting the *fopA* or *tul4* gene may be used.[20] Biochemical tests are of little value. Some commercial identification tests may misidentify *F. tularensis* as *Aggregatibacter actinomycetemcomitans*. Further subspeciation should only be undertaken in a reference laboratory.

Real-time PCR tests for the diagnosis of tularemia have been described. Many cases of tularemia are diagnosed serologically. An agglutination test using killed *F. tularensis* antigen or an ELISA is generally used. A fourfold rise in antibody titer or a single titer of more than 1:160 is considered diagnostic. IgG and IgM antibodies can persist for months or years and it may be difficult to distinguish past from current infection. Infections with *Brucella* spp. can give rise to antibodies that cross-react with *F. tularensis*. A commercial latex agglutination test is also available.

CLINICAL MANIFESTATIONS (SEE ALSO CHAPTER 121)

The clinical manifestations of *F. tularensis* infection depend on the portal of entry, the virulence of the infecting organism and the immune status of the individual host.

MANAGEMENT

Streptomycin remains the drug of first choice for treating all forms of tularemia. Gentamicin is an acceptable alternative. Ciprofloxacin and other quinolones have been used successfully to treat tularemia. Tetracycline and chloramphenicol have been used to treat infections but both are bacteriostatic for *F. tularensis* and there is a high rate of relapse when these agents are used. *Francisella tularensis* produces a β-lactamase, and β-lactamase-stable β-lactams, such as cefotaxime, ceftriaxone and imipenem, may be of use, although they have not been fully evaluated. For postexposure prophylaxis oral doxycycline or ciprofloxacin for 14 days is recommended.[21]

Haemophilus Species

NATURE

Haemophilus spp. are small, pleomorphic, nonmotile, nonsporing Gram-negative rods or coccobacilli. They are aerobic and facultatively anaerobic. Growth is often enhanced by the addition of 5–10% carbon dioxide to the incubation atmosphere. The oxidase and catalase reactions vary among the species. *Haemophilus* spp. require one or both of two accessory growth factors (X and V). X factor can be provided by hemin, protoporphyrin IX or other iron-containing porphyrins. X-dependent *Haemophilus* spp. cannot synthesize protoporphyrin from δ-aminolevulinic acid, a process involving several enzyme-mediated steps, some or all of which may be defective. V factor is nicotinamide adenine dinucleotide (NAD) or NAD phosphate or certain unidentified precursors of these compounds. It is essential for oxidation–reduction processes.

The differential requirements for X and V factors are important criteria for defining *Haemophilus* spp., which are obligate parasites of humans and animals. The species of *Haemophilus* associated with infections in humans are shown in Table 172.4. *Haemophilus influenzae* is the major human pathogen in the group. Some strains of *H. influenzae* have a polysaccharide capsule, of which there are six distinct antigenic types, designated a–f. The most important is type b, which has a capsule consisting of polyribosyl ribitol phosphate (PRP). *Haemophilus influenzae* type b (Hib) strains are associated with the majority of invasive infections.

Haemophilus influenzae biogroup *aegyptius* (formerly *Haemophilus aegyptius*) is a cause of epidemic conjunctivitis and Brazilian purpuric fever.[22] *Haemophilus ducreyi* is the causative agent of chancroid. *Haemophilus aphrophilus*, *H. paraphrophilus* and *H. parainfluenzae* are occasionally implicated in infective endocarditis and in brain and liver abscesses. *Haemophilus pittmaniae*[23] is part of the normal oropharyngeal flora that has been isolated from various sites of infection, including blood and bile. *Haemophilus haemolyticus* is a pharyngeal commensal that has classically been differentiated from *H. influenzae* by the demonstration of β-hemolysis on blood agar. However a significant number of *H. haemolyticus* strains are nonhemolytic and may be erroneously identified as *H. influenzae*.[24] Neither hemolytic nor nonhemolytic strains of *H. haemolyticus* have ever been implicated as the cause of infection.

The two species *H. aphrophilus* and *H. paraphrophilus* have recently been combined as a single species and reassigned to the genus *Aggregatibacter* as *Aggregatibacter aphrophilus* sp. nov. comb.[25] Similarly, *Haemophilus segnis* has been reassigned as *Aggregatibacter segnis*. The name *H. quentini* has been proposed for a group of *Haemophilus* strains isolated from neonatal and female genital tract infections which were previously termed a cryptic genospecies of *Haemophilus* but this name has not to date been validly published.

The genome of *Haemophilus influenzae* strain Rd was the first bacterial genome to be fully sequenced.[26]

EPIDEMIOLOGY

Haemophilus influenzae is an obligate parasite of human mucous membranes; it is not found in any other animal species. It colonizes the throat and nasopharynx, and to a lesser extent the conjunctivae and genital tract. The respiratory tract is colonized by *Haemophilus* spp. – mainly *H. parainfluenzae* and noncapsulate strains of *H. influenzae* (ncHi) – in 25–84% of healthy people. The carriage rates for Hib are much lower (3–5%).

Table 172.4 Species of *Haemophilus* associated with infection of humans

Species	REQUIREMENT FOR			Hemolysis	ACID FROM			
	X factor	**V factor**	**CO$_2$**		**Glucose**	**Sucrose**	**Lactose**	**Mannose**
H. influenzae	+	+	–	–	+	–	–	–
H. influenzae biogroup *aegyptius*	+	+	–	–	+	–	–	–
H. haemolyticus	+	+	–	+‡	+	–	–	–
H. parainfluenzae	–	+	–	–	+	+	–	+
H. pittmaniae	–	+	–	+	+	+	–	+
H. parahaemolyticus	–	+	–	+	+	+	–	–
*H. aphrophilus**	h	–	+	–	+	+	+	+
*H. paraphrophilus**	–	+	+	–	+	+	+	+
H. segnis†	–	+	–	–	w	w	–	–
H. ducreyi	+	–	–	–	–	–	–	–

h, requires hemin for primary isolation; w, weak reaction.
H. aphrophilus and *H. paraphrophilus* have been reassigned to the genus *Aggregatibacter* as *Aggregatibacter aphrophilus* sp. nov. comb.
†*H. segnis* has been reassigned to the genus *Aggregatibacter* as *Aggregatibacter segnis*.
‡*H. haemolyticus* strains can be nonhemolytic.

Table 172.5 Spectrum of infections caused by *Haemophilus influenzae*

Infection	Age group affected	Strains
1. Invasive infections: 　Meningitis 　Epiglottitis 　Pneumonia 　Septic arthritis 　Osteomyelitis 　Cellulitis 　Bacteremia	90% children <4 years old* 10% older children and adults	90% type b (Hib) 10% ncHi 1% types e and f
2. Neonatal and maternal sepsis	Neonates Parturient mothers	>90% ncHi
3. Noninvasive respiratory infections: 　Otitis media 　Sinusitis 　Conjunctivitis 　Acute exacerbations of chronic bronchitis	Children and adults	>90% ncHi2

ncHi, noncapsulated *Haemophilus influenzae*.
*Figures reflect prevaccine incidence and age distribution.

Haemophilus influenzae is associated with two types of infection, invasive infections and noninvasive infections which have distinctive epidemiologic profiles (Table 172.5).

Haemophilus influenzae type b meningitis principally affects children aged 2 months to 2 years. Epiglottitis occurs in slightly older children, with the peak incidence being in children aged 2–3 years. Risk factors for invasive disease are mainly socioeconomic and include overcrowding, attendance at day-care centers, chronic illness and lack of access to good health care facilities.

Invasive Hib infections are distributed worldwide but the incidence varies from country to country with very high incidence rates being found in certain racial groups, for example Apache and Navajo Native Americans, Alaskan Inuit and Australian Aborigines (Table 172.6). In these racial groups the peak incidence of infection occurs at a younger age. By contrast, a very low incidence rate has been reported in Hong Kong Chinese. There is seasonal variation, with most cases occurring in the winter months.

The introduction of vaccines effective against Hib in infants has dramatically reduced the incidence of invasive disease in children in countries using this vaccine, and consequently the epidemiology is changing.

The noninvasive infections of the respiratory tract associated with *H. influenzae* include otitis media, sinusitis, acute exacerbations of chronic bronchitis and conjunctivitis. The majority of these infections are caused by noncapsulate strains and many occur in adults. There is often an underlying physiologic or anatomic abnormality. These infections have a worldwide distribution and all of them are more common in the winter months.

Haemophilus influenzae biogroup *aegyptius* is associated with an acute pediatric condition of seasonal conjunctivitis and septicemia (Brazilian purpuric fever).

Table 172.6 Annual incidence of *Haemophilus influenzae* type b meningitis

Country	Incidence*
England	25
Finland	26
USA (Texas, North Carolina, Maryland, California)	19–69
Australia (New South Wales, Victoria)	20–25
Hong Kong Chinese	2.7
Gambia	60
Alaskan Inuit	282
Apache Native Americans	254
Australian Aborigines	454

*Figures for incidence per 100 000 children under the age of 5 years and are from various countries and ethnic groups prior to the introduction of routine immunization with Hib conjugate vaccine.

PATHOGENICITY

Haemophilus influenzae is transmitted by aerosols of respiratory secretions or by direct contact with contaminated material. The primary event is colonization of the nasopharynx. Prior infection with respiratory viruses (e.g. influenza) promotes colonization and subsequent infection by *Haemophilus* spp. Noninvasive infections of the respiratory tract result from contiguous spread of organisms colonizing the respiratory tract. Acute sinusitis, otitis media and acute exacerbations of chronic bronchitis usually follow a viral infection. This predisposes to secondary infection with potentially pathogenic components of the local resident bacterial flora by mechanisms including obstruction to the outflow of respiratory secretions, depression of local immunity and suppression of mucociliary clearance. The majority of these infections are caused by noncapsulate strains.

There are a number of microbial factors that promote colonization, including fimbriae and other adhesins, lipo-oligosaccharide (LOS) and IgA1 protease.[27] LOS consists of two covalently linked moieties, lipid A and core oligosaccharide. LOS is a ciliotoxin and is important for colonization, persistence and survival of the bacteria in the human host. The lipid A moiety mediates the endotoxic effects that are associated with severe infection.

IgA1 protease inactivates secretory IgA, facilitating bacterial access to the mucosal surface. Fimbriae and the autotransporter proteins, Hap, HMW1/HMW2 and Hia/Hsf are associated with binding to respiratory tract epithelium. Hap is found in both noncapsulate and capsulate strains and promotes the entry of bacteria into epithelial cells. HMW1/HMW2 proteins are expressed by the majority of noncapsulate *H. influenzae* but are not found in capsulate strains. Hia is found in nearly all noncapsulate strains. Its analogue, Hif, is expressed in almost all capsulate strains. Possession of the outer membrane protein P2 is another important virulence factor for noncapsulate *H. influenzae*. Lipoprotein D (LPD) is a highly conserved 42 kDa surface lipoprotein found in all *H. influenzae*, which impairs respiratory ciliary function.

Invasive infections, notably meningitis and epiglottitis, are mainly caused by Hib and result from invasion of the bloodstream. The pathogenesis of these infections has been elegantly elucidated using an infant rat model.[28] The capsule of type b *H. influenzae* is the single most important virulence determinant for invasion because it protects the organism from phagocytosis and complement-mediated lysis. The rarity of infections in the first 2 months of life correlates with the presence of maternal antibodies to PRP and the occurrence of infection in early infancy with the absence of antibodies having such specificity. As the mean level of PRP antibodies in the population rises, so Hib infections become less common. It is unclear whether natural antibody production is stimulated by exposure to Hib or to some other organism (e.g. *Escherichia coli* K100) that possesses cross-reacting antigens.

Brazilian purpuric fever is caused by a single clone of *H. influenzae* biogroup *aegyptius*.[29] The LOS phenotype is a critical determinant of virulence for *H. influenzae* biogroup *aegyptius*.

PREVENTION

Vaccination

Haemophilus influenzae type b conjugate vaccines have now been developed in which the PRP is covalently linked to a protein carrier. Several different protein carriers have been used, including tetanus toxoid, diphtheria toxoid, a non-toxic mutant diphtheria and an outer membrane protein complex from *Neisseria meningitidis* group B. These vaccines produce a lasting anamnestic response, which is not age related. They can be given effectively to infants as young as 2 months of age and are also effective in high-risk groups of patients who have a poor response to polysaccharide vaccines. The Hib vaccine can be given concurrently with diphtheria–tetanus–pertussis immunization. In the UK Hib vaccine is administered at 2, 3 and 4 months as a component of a pentavalent vaccine (diphtheria, tetanus, acellular pertussis, Hib and inactivated polio vaccine), with a booster dose (Hib combined with meningococcus C vaccine) being given at 12 months of age. Countries where Hib vaccine is routinely offered have witnessed a dramatic decline in the occurrence of Hib infections (Fig. 172.3; see also Chapter 3).

Immunization of infants with conjugate Hib vaccine results in a reduction in the rate of nasopharyngeal colonization by Hib and a marked herd immunity effect.

Haemophilus influenzae type b vaccine is recommended after splenectomy, or for patients who have functional asplenia, together with pneumococcal vaccine and meningococcal vaccine.

There is currently considerable interest in developing vaccines for nontypeable *H. influenzae*. A 10-valent pneumococcal conjugate vaccine, using *H. influenzae*-derived protein D as a carrier protein for the pneumococcal polysaccharide, showed protection against both pneumococcal and noncapsulate *H. influenzae* otitis media.[30] Several candidate antigens are being investigated (Table 172.7).[31]

Chemoprophylaxis

Oral rifampin for 4 days is recommended for eradicating carriage of *H. influenzae* type b and has been used to prevent secondary infection in household and nursery contacts. Its efficacy is unproven. Widespread use of the vaccine may soon render chemoprophylaxis unnecessary.

DIAGNOSTIC MICROBIOLOGY

Gram-stained smears of cerebrospinal fluid, pus, sputum or aspirates from joints, middle ear or sinuses may provide a rapid diagnosis. *Haemophilus influenzae* tends to stain poorly and dilute carbol fuchsin is a better counterstain than neutral red or safranin.

Rapid tests for Hib capsular antigens, such as latex agglutination or a PCR-based method, can be applied to clinical material. False-positive latex agglutination results have been reported in cerebrospinal fluid samples collected from children who had recently received Hib vaccine.

Specimens should be plated on appropriate culture media as soon as possible. Chocolate agar is the most commonly used medium for culturing *Haemophilus* spp. It can be used without further

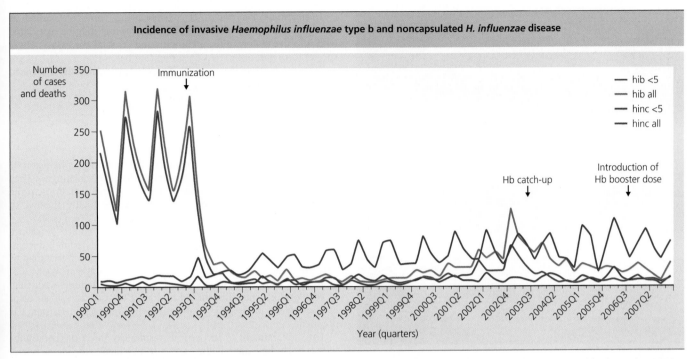

Fig. 172.3 Incidence of invasive *Haemophilus influenzae* type b and noncapsulated *H. influenzae* disease. Figures are for the period from October 1990 to June 2008 in England and Wales. Data supplied by the Health Protection Agency Centre for Infections.

Table 172.7 Candidate vaccine antigens of noncapsulate *Haemophilus influenzae* (ncHi)

Antigen	Protective in animal model	Comments
Lipo-oligosaccharide (LOS)	+	Common epitopes among ncHi strains
P6	+	Highly conserved lipoprotein
OMP26	+	Highly conserved
OMP P5	+	Highly conserved
Lipoprotein D (LPD)	+	Recombinant deacylated form (protein D) used as carrier protein for pneumococcal conjugate vaccine
OMP P2		>50% of total OMP of ncHi Heterogeneous and conserved regions
HtrA	±	
HMW1/HMW2	+	Found in >75% ncHi strains
P4 lipoprotein	+	Highly conserved

supplementation for specimens from normally sterile sites. The addition of bacitracin to chocolate agar will assist the recovery of *H. influenzae* from respiratory samples because it will suppress the growth of other respiratory organisms. Good growth can also be obtained on certain transparent media that contain blood extracts (e.g. Levinthal's agar or Fildes peptic digest agar).

The cultures should be incubated at 98.6°F (37°C) in an aerobic atmosphere enriched with 5–10% carbon dioxide. After 24 hours of incubation, colonies of noncapsulate *H. influenzae* are small, circular, smooth and pale gray. Capsulated strains produce somewhat larger, mucoid colonies, which have a characteristic seminal odor. On clear media, such as Levinthal's agar, colonies of capsulated strains exhibit iridescence when viewed obliquely with transmitted light. Type b capsulated strains can also be detected by the presence of precipitin haloes on transparent media containing hyperimmune Hib antiserum.

Confirmation of the identity of colonies depends on demonstrating a requirement for X factor, V factor, or both. This is usually performed as a disk test. The culture is plated onto a nutrient agar that is deficient in both X and V factors, and paper disks containing X factor alone, V factor alone, and both X and V factors are placed on the surface of the agar. After overnight incubation, growth is observed around the disks supplying the required growth factors (Fig. 172.4). An alternative method of demonstrating X-factor requirement is the porphyrin test.[32]

Haemophilus influenzae strains should be typed to determine their capsular serotype. This is normally carried out by slide agglutination using type-specific antisera. This method is prone to misinterpretation, with problems of autoagglutination, cross-reacting antisera and observer error. The definitive method of typing *H. influenzae* is capsular genotyping using a PCR-based method.[33]

CLINICAL MANIFESTATIONS

Haemophilus influenzae is associated with two distinct types of infection: invasive and noninvasive infections.

Invasive infections

Haemophilus influenzae type b (Hib) meningitis is the commonest and most serious manifestation of systemic infection with *H. influenzae*. Prior to the use of Hib conjugate vaccine, Hib meningitis principally occurred in young children between the ages of 2 months and 2 years. In countries that have introduced routine infant immunization with Hib conjugate vaccine the incidence

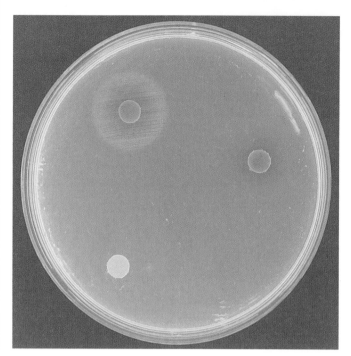

Fig. 172.4 Growth factor requirement of *Haemophilus influenzae*. Strain of *H. influenzae* sown on Columbia agar plate. Filter paper disks containing X factor, V factor, and both X and V factors have been placed on the surface of inoculated plate, but colonies of *H. influenzae* grow only around the disk with both X and V factors.

Haemophilus aphrophilus, *H. paraphrophilus* (now reclassified as *Aggregatibacter aphrophilus*) and *H. parainfluenzae* may be associated with infective endocarditis, meningitis and cerebral abscesses.[34] These species form part of the HACEK group (see below).

Haemophilus segnis (*Aggregatibacter segnis*) is occasionally associated with acute appendicitis.

MANAGEMENT

Cefotaxime, ceftriaxone and related third-generation cephalosporins are the antibiotics of choice for treating *Haemophilus* meningitis. They are bactericidal for *H. influenzae*, achieve high concentrations in the meninges and cerebral tissues, and have proved highly effective in clinical practice.

Chloramphenicol was formerly the treatment of choice. Resistance may be encountered but in most parts of the world this remains uncommon. Ampicillin is also effective but resistance due to a β-lactamase is now encountered in an unacceptably high percentage of strains. For example, 13% of Hib strains in the UK are β-lactamase-producing. In view of this, ampicillin should no longer be used as a single agent in *Haemophilus* meningitis in countries where ampicillin resistance is prevalent.

For the treatment of less serious respiratory infections, oral antibiotics including amoxicillin, amoxicillin–clavulanate, tetracycline, erythromycin or newer macrolides such as clarithromycin or azithromycin are all effective. β-Lactamase-mediated amoxicillin resistance may again be a problem. In the UK, 19% of noncapsulate isolates are β-lactamase producers. Occasional strains are resistant to ampicillin by an intrinsic mechanism.

of invasive *H. influenzae* infections has dramatically declined. *Haemophilus* meningitis can also occur in neonates, in whom the causative organism is almost invariably noncapsulate and the presentation can resemble group B streptococcal sepsis. Meningitis caused by either type b or noncapsulated strains can occur in older children and adults.

Epiglottitis is a life-threatening infection that is almost always caused by Hib. It occurs in children, aged 2–5 years, with a peak incidence in those aged 2–3 years. Examination of the larynx is potentially hazardous because it may provoke respiratory obstruction. The diagnosis should be based on the clinical findings confirmed by blood culture results (see also Chapter 24).

Other less common invasive *H. influenzae* infections include pneumonia, periorbital cellulitis, osteomyelitis, septic arthritis and a bacteremia with no obvious focus of infection. *Haemophilus influenzae* pneumonia is a major cause of mortality in young children in the developing world.

Noninvasive infections

A variety of local infections, principally in the respiratory tract, may be seen. These include otitis media, sinusitis, conjunctivitis and acute exacerbations of chronic bronchitis (see Chapter 26). Most of these infections are caused by noncapsulated strains of *H. influenzae*. *Haemophilus influenzae* is an important cause of purulent conjunctivitis. This may be sporadic but can occur in outbreaks. Severe conjunctivitis associated with severe sepsis and a high mortality was first described in 1984 in Brazilian children aged 1–4 years. The causative organism is a clone of *H. influenzae* biogroup *aegyptius*, which is indistinguishable in routine laboratory tests from noncapsulate *H. influenzae*.

Rarely *H. influenzae* may be associated with other infections, including endocarditis, urinary tract infections, cholecystitis, salpingitis and epididymo-orchitis. Many of these unusual infections are associated with pre-existing damage, including the presence of urinary stones or gallstones.

Haemophilus ducreyi

EPIDEMIOLOGY

Haemophilus ducreyi (see Chapter 60) is the causative agent of the sexually transmitted disease chancroid, or soft sore. Chancroid is endemic in tropical areas, particularly central and southern Africa, South East Asia, India and the Caribbean where it is responsible for 25–50% of genital ulcers.[35] It occurs sporadically in other parts of the world and recently there have been major outbreaks in Canada and the USA. It is more common in nonwhite, uncircumcised males and in low socioeconomic groups living in poor hygienic conditions. Infection may be asymptomatic or inapparent in females. Genital ulcers, including chancroid, are associated with increased transmission of HIV. Co-infection with *Treponema pallidum* or herpes simplex virus (HSV) is common. The incidence of *H. ducreyi* has been decreasing over recent years, whilst the incidence of HSV type 2 genital ulcers has increased. The reason for this declining incidence is unclear.

PATHOGENICITY

Haemophilus ducreyi has not been isolated from nonhuman sources and is sexually transmitted. The organisms gain access via a break in the epithelium and establish infection in a focal area of mucosa or skin in the genital tract. An inoculum of 10^4 organisms is required to initiate infection. The pathogenesis of chancroid is poorly understood. Hemolysin is important in epithelial cell invasion and ulcer formation. Superoxide dismutase enzymes contribute to survival of the bacteria within the host. Potential virulence factors include fimbriae, LPS, cytotoxins and outer membrane proteins (OMP).[35]

PREVENTION

The use of condoms dramatically reduces the transmission of *H. ducreyi*. All sexual partners should be identified by contact tracing and treated. Education is vitally important. *Haemophilus ducreyi* hemolysin is a possible candidate for vaccine development.

DIAGNOSTIC MICROBIOLOGY

Gram-stained examination of material from ulcers or buboes reveals pleomorphic coccobacilli or short rods. The organisms are more commonly extracellular but may be intracellular. Characteristically they resemble 'shoals of fish'. However, ulcer material is generally contaminated with other bacteria and direct Gram staining identifies only about 10% of culture-positive cases and microscopy is not recommended as a diagnostic test.[36] Specimens collected from the base and margins of ulcers using a saline-moistened swab or by aspirating a bubo should be plated directly onto culture plates which should be incubated in a humid atmosphere with 5% carbon dioxide at 91.4°F (33°C) for 2–3 days.[36]

Haemophilus ducreyi is a fastidious organism that grows slowly on chocolate agar. In general a suitable medium contains a growth supplement such as IsoVitaleX and is made selective by the addition of vancomycin. The sensitivity of culture is low but can be increased somewhat by using more than one medium.

The appearance of colonies of *H. ducreyi* varies with the medium used. Typically, after 24 hours' incubation the colonies are pinpoint, yellow-gray and translucent or semiopaque. Cultures often appear mixed, with a variety of colonial forms. The colonies are very cohesive and can be pushed across the agar surface with an inoculating loop.

Haemophilus ducreyi requires X factor but not V factor for growth. It can be identified using a number of rapid test systems, including API-ZYM and RapIDNH.

PCR is the most sensitive diagnostic technique and has been shown to be 95% sensitive compared to culture.[36] Multiplex PCR tests that also amplify *Treponema pallidum* and HSV have been developed.[37]

CLINICAL MANIFESTATIONS

These are described in Chapter 60.

MANAGEMENT

The susceptibility of *H. ducreyi* to antimicrobial agents varies from one geographic area to another. Many strains are β-lactamase producers and resistance to tetracycline and trimethoprim–sulfamethoxazole is common. Azithromycin and ceftriaxone exhibit excellent *in-vitro* activity against *H. ducreyi* and have the advantage that they can be used as single-dose therapy.[38] Ciprofloxacin and erythromycin are alternative agents, but strains with intermediate resistance to both of these agents have been reported.

Buboes should be drained to prevent sinus formation.

HACEK Group

NATURE

The HACEK group of organisms includes *H. parainfluenzae*, *H. aphrophilus*, *H. paraphophilus*, *Actinobacillus actinomycetemcomitans*, *Cardiobacterium hominis*, *Eikenella corrodens* and *Kingella kingae*. *Haemophilus aphrophilus* and *Haemophilus paraphrophilus* have now been reassigned to the genus *Aggregatibacter* and combined as a single species, *Aggregatibacter aphrophilus* sp. nov. comb. Similarly, *Actinobacillus actinomycetemcomitans* has been renamed *Aggregatibacter actinomycetemcomitans* sp. nov.[23] It was previously thought that the genus *Cardiobacterium* consisted of a single species, *C. hominis*. However a second species, *C. valvarum*, has now been described[39] which has also been associated with infective endocarditis. All of the HACEK group are small, fastidious, pleomorphic Gram-negative bacilli that form part of the normal commensal flora of the oropharynx and are infrequent causes of human infections. They are slow growing, their growth being enhanced by the use of enriched culture media and an increased carbon dioxide tension.

Cardiobacterium hominis and *Eikenella corrodens* usually require hemin (X factor) and carbon dioxide on primary isolation and may be misidentified as *Haemophilus* spp.; these requirements are lost on subculture. The colonies of *E. corrodens* have a characteristic 'bleach-like' odor and often 'pit' the surface of the agar. Colonies of *K. kingae* produce slight β-hemolysis on blood agar.

CLINICAL MANIFESTATIONS

Collectively, the HACEK group of organisms causes 3% of all cases of infective endocarditis[40] and is responsible for a variety of other infections (see Chapter 47).

Aggregatibacter actinomycetemcomitans was originally thought to be a secondary pathogen in actinomycotic infections caused by *Actinomyces israelii*. It is now recognized as a cause of periodontal infections, brain and other soft tissue abscesses, osteomyelitis and infective endocarditis.[41]

Cardiobacterium hominis and *C. valvarum* have been implicated in cases of natural and prosthetic valve endocarditis[42] but rarely cause other types of infection.

Eikenella corrodens tends to cause indolent infections, often in association with other organisms. Infections associated with *E. corrodens* include periodontitis, human bite wounds, sinusitis, meningitis, brain abscess, pulmonary infections, pelvic infections, endocarditis, osteomyelitis and septic arthritis.[43] Clenched fist injuries are the most serious human bite wounds and are sustained when the knuckles of the assailant's hand strike the teeth of the adversary.

Kingella spp. (*K. kingae* and *K. denitrificans*) are associated with endocarditis and osteoarticular infections. Since the introduction of routine Hib immunization in the USA, and consequent decline in Hib septic arthritis, *K. kingae* has emerged as a major cause of septic arthritis in children less than 2 years of age.[44] *K. kingae* expresses an RTX toxin which is cytotoxic to respiratory epithelium, synovial cells and macrophage-like cells.[45]

Haemophilus parainfluenzae and *Aggregatibacter aphrophilus* (formerly *H. aphrophilus* and *H. paraphophilus*) may cause endocarditis. *Haemophilus parainfluenzae* has been reported as a rare cause of the spectrum of infections associated with *H. influenzae*: meningitis, epiglottitis, septic arthritis, osteomyelitis, pneumonia and bacteremia. *Aggregatibacter aphrophilus* has been implicated in cases of brain abscesses, septic arthritis, osteomyelitis, epiglottitis and meningitis.

PREVENTION

Approximately 60% of cases of endocarditis caused by HACEK organisms are associated with poor oral hygiene, bad dentition or recent dental work.[40] Prevention of endocarditis should therefore be based on good dental and oral hygiene in patients at risk of endocarditis.

MANAGEMENT

The treatment of endocarditis caused by HACEK organisms should be based on antimicrobial susceptibility tests, including tests for β-lactamase activity. Since many of these organisms are slow growing, such tests can be problematic. Currently, third-generation cephalosporins, including cefotaxime or ceftriaxone, are the drugs of choice for treating endocarditis caused by the HACEK organisms.

Eikenella corrodens is generally susceptible to penicillin, but consideration should be given to the possibility of β-lactamase-producing aerobic and anaerobic organisms when treating mixed infections, such as human bites.

Legionella Species

NATURE

Legionella spp. are slender, aerobic, noncapsulated, non-spore-forming pleomorphic Gram-negative coccobacilli. In clinical material they often appear as coccobacilli but they tend to form elongated filamentous forms on some culture media. They are motile with a single polar flagellum. *Legionella* spp. stain poorly with Gram stain. Basic fuchsin is a better counterstain for these organisms. They do not attack carbohydrates, and nitrate is not reduced. The cell wall contains branched-chain fatty acids with high concentrations of ubiquinones, which give characteristic profiles by gas–liquid chromatographic analysis. The genome sequences of several *L. pneumophila* strains (Philadelphia, Paris, Lens and Corby) have been established.[46]

Legionella spp. are nutritionally fastidious and will not grow on ordinary culture media. A suitable medium for their isolation is buffered charcoal yeast extract (BCYE) supplemented with L-cysteine, α-ketoglutarate and ferric ions. The pH of the medium should be adjusted to pH 6.[9] *Legionella* can grow in the temperature range 68–107.6°F (20–42°C). There are more than 50 species of *Legionella* and human infections have been documented for 19 of these species

Table 172.8 *Legionella* species associated with disease	
Species	**Number of serogroups**
Legionella pneumophila	15
Legionella anisa	1
Legionella bozemanii	2
Legionella cincinnatensis	1
Legionella dumoffii	1
Legionella feeleii	2
Legionella gormanii	1
Legionella hackeliae	2
Legionella jordanis	1
Legionella longbeachae	2
Legionella lansingensis	1
*Legionella lytica**	1
Legionella maceachernii	1
Legionella micdadei	1
Legionella oakridgensis	1
Legionella parisiensis	1
Legionella sainthelensi	2
Legionella tucsonensis	1
Legionella wadsworthii	1

*Formerly called *Legionella*-like amebal pathogens (LLAP).

(Table 172.8). Infections due to species other than *L. pneumophila* are rare and usually occur in immunocompromised hosts. The exception is *Legionella longbeachae* serogroup 1 which is a major cause of community-acquired pneumonia in Australia.[47] More than 90% of human infections are caused by *Legionella pneumophila* serogroup 1.

Some *Legionella* grow very poorly on BCYE but can be isolated by co-cultivation with amebae. Originally called *Legionella*-like amebal pathogens (LLAPs), they have been renamed as *L. lytica*, *L. drozanskii*, *L. falloni* and *L. rowbothamii*.[48]

EPIDEMIOLOGY

Legionella spp. are distributed worldwide. They are found in fresh water streams, rivers, ponds and lakes and in moist soil and mud. The organisms are able to survive in moist environments for long periods of time and can withstand temperatures of 32–154°F (0–68°C) and a pH range of 5.0–8.5. They can survive chlorination and can proliferate in air-conditioning cooling towers, hot water systems, shower heads, taps, whirlpool spas and respiratory ventilators. The organisms are located in biofilms on the surfaces of these systems, where they are far less susceptible to the effects of biocides and chlorine. The growth of *Legionella* spp. is aided by coexisting bacteria and algae, which provide nutrients, and protozoa, in which the *Legionella* spp. can live and multiply.

The exact incidence of *Legionella* infections is difficult to determine. There is no doubt that exposure to *Legionella* spp. is a fairly frequent event and serologic surveys suggest that asymptomatic infection and seroconversion are common. Large-scale surveys of pneumonia suggest that *Legionella* spp. cause 2–5% of community-acquired pneumonia and up to 30% of nosocomial pneumonia.

Cases may be sporadic or occur as part of an outbreak. The original description of Legionnaires' disease was of an outbreak of a febrile respiratory illness in delegates at an American Legion convention in Philadelphia in 1976. A total of 221 people developed pneumonia and 34 died.[49] Retrospective studies have revealed that the first proven case occurred in 1947 and the first known epidemic was in 1965 in Washington, DC.

Sporadic cases are reported throughout the year, but most cases of epidemic infection occur in the summer and autumn, presumably because warmer weather encourages proliferation of the bacteria in water. The disease tends to occur in the middle-aged and elderly, especially in people who have impaired respiratory and cardiac function, who are heavy smokers or who are immunocompromised. Cases have been documented in children. Person-to-person spread has not been demonstrated. Surgery is a major predisposition in nosocomial infection, with transplant patients at the greatest risk.

Legionella is a good example of an organism that has been present in the environment for a long time but has been brought into close contact with humans as a result of technical developments. Organisms are disseminated via contaminated water droplets from nebulizers and humidifiers and in aerosols from cooling towers, whirlpools and evaporative condensers. Infection arises from inhalation of contaminated aerosols, direct instillation during surgery or possibly by ingestion of contaminated water. Hospital equipment that has been rinsed in tap water prior to use may be a source of infection.

There are more than 50 species and 64 subgroups in the genus *Legionella*. *L. pneumophila* contains 15 different serogroups. *L. pneumophila* serogroup 1 can be subdivided into subtypes, on the basis of monoclonal antibody typing or genotyping. Identifying the subtype of a strain is of importance in defining outbreaks where an environmental isolate can be matched to isolates from human cases of legionellosis. Several different methods have been used to genotype strains of *L. pneumophila*, including pulsed-field gel electrophoresis (PFGE), restriction fragment length polymorphism (RFLP) analysis, multilocus sequence typing (MLST), amplified fragment length polymorphism (AFLP) and sequence-based typing (SBT).

PATHOGENICITY

Legionella spp. residing in water are transmitted to humans via aerosols. Droplet nuclei of less than 5 µm will reach the alveoli, where the organisms are ingested by alveolar macrophages. *Legionella* is a facultative intracellular parasite and multiplies freely within the macrophages. The bacteria bind to the alveolar macrophages via complement receptors and are engulfed in phagosomes. Phagolysosome fusion is inhibited by an unknown mechanism that prevents intracellular killing. The bacteria multiply within the phagosomes. When the supply of nutrients is depleted the bacteria respond by expressing virulence proteins which lead to lysis of the host cell and release of bacteria, which are then taken up by other macrophages and the infection cycle is repeated.[50] This process produces chemotactic substances that attract polymorphonuclear leukocytes and monocytes. The inflammatory response results in a destructive pneumonia.

There are two phases in the life cycle of *Legionella pneumophila* – an intracellular replicative phase (RP) and an infectious nonreplicating transmissive phase (TP) which promotes transmission to a new host. Bacilli in the RP are avirulent, not flagellated and sodium resistant, whereas those in the TP are virulent, flagellated and motile. Complex regulatory systems govern the differentiation between these two phases.[51] In the TP the bacteria express genes concerned with transmission and host cell attack including substrates of the dot/Icm secretion system type IV pilus and more than 90 proteins; RP bacteria express components of aerobic metabolism. Switch is linked not only to expression of virulence trait but also to motility.

The virulence factors of *L. pneumophila* have not been fully determined. A 24 kDa protein, macrophage infectivity potentiator (mip), appears to be required for virulence. The major outer membrane protein may be important in the uptake of *Legionella* spp. by macrophages. A variety of extracellular enzymes are produced by *Legionella* spp., including proteases, esterases and hemolysins, but these have not been shown to be important virulence factors. The virulence of *L. pneumophila* may be enhanced by multiplication in amebae.

PREVENTION

Prevention of legionellosis depends upon identification of the environmental source and reduction of *Legionella* colonization. The most commonly used method of decontamination is periodic superheating and flushing of water supplies. This method is particularly useful for urgent disinfection during an outbreak. Hyperchlorination is no longer recommended because chlorine decomposes in hot water and *Legionella* spp. are relatively chlorine tolerant. Biocides are relatively ineffective. The most effective method appears to be copper–silver ionization units, which generate metallic ions that disrupt and kill bacterial cells.[52] Despite these costly measures it is often impossible to eliminate *Legionella* spp. from water supplies.

New water systems should be designed to minimize the risk of heavy colonization with *Legionella* spp., avoiding 'dead spaces', stagnation, materials that support the growth of *Legionella* spp. and the build-up of sediment. Regular monitoring for *Legionella* spp. is also advisable, particularly in high-risk areas.

Several putative vaccines have been developed that induce cell-mediated immunity in guinea pigs. These may be an option in the future for highly susceptible patients.

DIAGNOSTIC MICROBIOLOGY

Definitive diagnosis of legionellosis depends on culturing *Legionella* organisms, detecting *Legionella* antigens or DNA in body fluids or demonstrating a serologic response to the infection.

Legionella spp. can be cultured from sputum, endotracheal aspirates, bronchoalveolar lavages, lung biopsies and pleural fluid. Sputum samples should not be diluted in saline, because this can prove inhibitory to some

Legionella spp., but in distilled water. Gram-stained smears of the sample will reveal poorly staining Gram-negative rods or coccobacilli, which are suggestive of legionellosis. Direct immunofluorescence of the smear using a monoclonal antibody to a major outer membrane protein common to all the serogroups of *L. pneumophila* can give a rapid provisional diagnosis but this test is not as sensitive as culture and will only detect *L. pneumophila*.

Cultures should therefore also be carried out. The sample should be cultured on a specific medium such as BCYE. *Legionella* spp. do not grow on blood agar. It is possible to render BCYE semiselective by the inclusion of antibiotics, but this may prove inhibitory to some strains of *Legionella* spp. It is therefore prudent to culture samples on both BCYE and BCYE supplemented with antibiotics. Contaminated material, such as sputum, can be heated at 122°F (50°C) for 30 minutes to suppress the growth of other less heat-stable organisms prior to inoculating the culture plates. Cultures should be incubated at 98.6°F (37°C) in 2–5% carbon dioxide for up to 14 days. *Legionella* spp. are slow growing, and on primary isolation it may take 3–5 days for colonies to appear. Cultures should not be regarded as negative until they have been cultured for at least 10 days. Colonies of *Legionella* spp. have a ground-glass appearance, which may be white, gray, pale blue or purple-tinged (Fig. 172.5). Often the colonies will fluoresce under ultraviolet light.

Colonies that grow on BCYE but not blood agar, that are catalase-positive, oxidase-negative and have a characteristic Gram-stain morphology should be regarded as presumptive *Legionella* spp. *Legionella pneumophila* hydrolyzes hippurate, starch and gelatin but in general biochemical tests are not of great help in identifying *Legionella* spp. Serologic typing using direct or indirect fluorescent antibody tests with polyclonal or monoclonal antibodies will confirm the identity of clinical isolates. Sequence analysis of the *mip* gene can be used to differentiate most *Legionella* spp.[53] Other schemes based on the 5S rRNA gene and partial 16S rRNA gene sequencing have also been described, but are less discriminatory than *mip* gene sequencing. Real-time PCR based on the *mip* gene can also be used to provide a rapid diagnosis.

Legionella lytica (and other LLAPs) can be isolated on BCYE if the cultures are incubated at 86°F (30°C).

Urine samples can be examined for *Legionella* soluble antigen using either an enzyme immunoassay or a radioimmunoassay kit. These tests are specific for *L. pneumophila* serogroup 1 (which causes 70–80% of human infections) and can give a rapid diagnosis. However, they will not detect infections caused by other *Legionella* spp. Rapid immunochromatographic tests for urinary antigen are also commercially available, including the Binax NOW urinary antigen test. The antigen persists in the urine for 1–2 weeks but some patients continue to excrete antigen for months.

Serologic tests can be used to make a diagnosis of legionellosis. The most commonly used technique is an indirect fluorescent antibody test (IFAT), but other techniques, such as ELISA or a rapid microagglu-

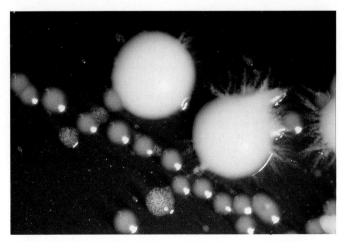

Fig. 172.5 Colonies of *Legionella pneumophila* on BCYE agar, showing the typical ground-glass appearance. With permission from Harrison TG, Taylor AG (eds). A laboratory manual for *Legionella*. Chichester: Wiley; 1998.

tination test, are also available. A fourfold or greater rise in antibody titer in a patient who has had clinical pneumonia indicates *Legionella* infection. It may take weeks or even months for the antibody titer to rise, and antibodies can persist for years, so serology is less useful than culture or antigen detection in the diagnosis of acute cases. Serology is much more useful in epidemiologic studies. The only validated serologic test is for *L. pneumophila* serogroup 1. Cross-reacting antibodies may be found in patients who have *Campylobacter* spp. infection.

CLINICAL MANIFESTATIONS

Asymptomatic *Legionella* infections are relatively common, as demonstrated by seroepidemiologic surveys. Symptomatic *Legionella* infection can present in two distinct ways: a severe pneumonia (Legionnaires' disease) and an acute influenza-like illness known as Pontiac fever. Clinical aspects are discussed in detail in Chapter 27.

MANAGEMENT

Macrolides or quinolones are the treatments of choice. In the patient who is acutely ill with Legionnaires' disease, a macrolide (e.g. azithromycin or clarithromycin) or a quinolone (e.g. levofloxacin or moxifloxacin) should be administered. The co-administration of rifampin does not appear to give any additional benefit.

Cases of Pontiac fever resolve spontaneously without the need for antibiotic therapy.

Moraxella Species

NATURE

Moraxella spp. are Gram-negative diplococci that morphologically and phenotypically resemble *Neisseria* spp. They are strictly aerobic, oxidase-positive, catalase-positive, DNAse-positive and asaccharolytic. *Moraxella catarrhalis* is now recognized as an important cause of upper and lower respiratory tract infections in children and adults.

Moraxella lacunata is associated with conjunctivitis. *Moraxella nonliquefaciens* is a commensal in the upper respiratory tract and may be a secondary invader in respiratory infections. *Moraxella osloensis* is a common commensal in the genital tract and may be misidentified as *Neisseria gonorrhoeae*. Unlike *N. gonorrhoeae*, *M. osloensis* grows well on blood agar. *M. osloensis* has been reported in cases of septic arthritis, osteomyelitis and bacteremia. These three organisms will not be further discussed.

EPIDEMIOLOGY

Moraxella catarrhalis is exclusively found in humans. The nasopharyngeal carriage rate of *M. catarrhalis* is 1–5% in healthy adults, but up to 75% of infants and young children are colonized with this organism.[54] This marked disparity may reflect the age-dependent development of secretory IgA antibodies. Nasopharyngeal carriage rates are significantly higher in the autumn and winter months. It also appears that the carriage rate is higher in adults who have chronic lung disease than in healthy adults.

PATHOGENICITY

M. catarrhalis is a mucosal pathogen, causing infections of the upper respiratory tract in young children and the lower respiratory tract in chronic obstructive airways disease (COPD). A number of potential virulence factors have been identified among the outer membrane proteins of *Moraxella catarrhalis*. These include the adhesins UspA1/A2, MID/Hag, CD and McaP, and the nutrient uptake proteins LbpA, LpbB, TbpA, TbpB and CopB. UspA1 and UspA2 are thought to have a role in infections in COPD patients since they bind to fibronectin which is produced in abundance in the chronically damaged airways. Lipo-oligosaccharide (LOS) is another highly conserved surface component that has been implicated as a possible virulence factor.[31]

PREVENTION

Currently there is considerable interest in the development of a vaccine to prevent *M. catarrhalis* infections. UspA1, UspA2 proteins and MID/Hag are the most immunogenic of these proteins but they exhibit considerable heterogeneity between strains. The functional adhesive domains of these proteins are more conserved and it may be possible to combine these with more conserved proteins[55] (Table 172.9).

DIAGNOSTIC MICROBIOLOGY

Moraxella catarrhalis grows well on blood agar and chocolate agar, producing small, nonhemolytic, grayish-white colonies that slide across the agar surface, like a hockey puck, when pushed with a bacteriologic loop. It may be difficult to distinguish *M. catarrhalis* from commensal *Neisseria* spp. in respiratory tract specimens, and the use of selective media may be necessary. Gram-stained films reveal Gram-negative diplococci but *M. catarrhalis* often resists destaining and thus may appear to be Gram-positive (Fig. 172.6). *M. catarrhalis* is DNAse positive, reduces nitrate and hydrolyses tributyrin, tests that differentiate it from the majority of *Neisseria* spp.

PCR tests can be applied to clinical material without the need for bacterial culture. A multiplex PCR for the detection of *Haemophilus influenzae*, *Moraxella catarrhalis* and *Streptococcus pneumoniae* has been successfully used to identify the bacterial etiology of middle ear infections.[56]

CLINICAL MANIFESTATIONS (SEE ALSO CHAPTER 25)

Moraxella catarrhalis is an important cause of otitis media and sinusitis in children, being the third most common cause of these conditions after *S. pneumoniae* and *H. influenzae*.[54]

In adults *M. catarrhalis* is associated with acute exacerbations of chronic bronchitis, being the third most common isolate after *H. influenzae* and *S. pneumoniae*. *Moraxella catarrhalis* may cause pneumonia, especially in the elderly and is associated with a poor prognosis. There have been several reports of nosocomial outbreaks of

Table 172.9 Candidate vaccine antigens of *Moraxella catarrhalis*

Antigen	Action	Comments
UspA1	Adhesin	Highly immunogenic Contains both conserved and variable regions
UspA2	Induces serum resistance	Highly immunogenic Contains both conserved and variable regions
MID/Hag	IgD binding Adhesin Hemagglutinin	Highly immunogenic Contains both conserved and variable regions
OMP CD	Porin	Highly conserved
McaP	Adhesin	Highly conserved

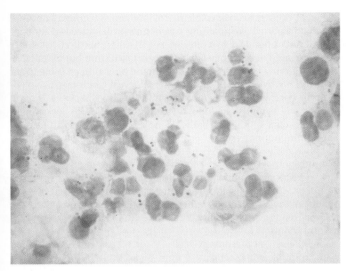

Fig. 172.6 Gram-stained smear of sputum containing *Moraxella catarrhalis*. Sample from a patient suffering an acute exacerbation of chronic bronchitis showing Gram-negative diplococci and leukocytes (*Moraxella catarrhalis*).

lower respiratory tract infections due to *M. catarrhalis* in respiratory units. *Moraxella catarrhalis* may occasionally cause invasive infections, including bacteremia, meningitis and endocarditis.

MANAGEMENT

Before 1977 no β-lactamase-positive isolates of *M. catarrhalis* had been reported. By 1980, 75% of *M. catarrhalis* isolates in the USA were β-lactamase-positive and now virtually all strains of *M. catarrhalis* are β-lactamase-positive. Among isolates collected in a European study from 1997 to 1999, more than 90% of *M. catarrhalis* carried BRO-1 β-lactamase.[57] There are two *M. catarrhalis* β-lactamases, BRO-1 and BRO-2, which are unique to this genus. There is some evidence that, in mixed infections, *M. catarrhalis* β-lactamases can protect other respiratory pathogens such as *S. pneumoniae* and *H. influenzae* from the action of β-lactam antibiotics. The β-lactamases of *M. catarrhalis* are chromosomal and inducible; therefore ampicillin therapy should be avoided.

Many infections due to *M. catarrhalis* can be treated with oral antibiotics, including amoxicillin–clavulanate, trimethoprim–sulfamethoxazole, tetracyclines (contraindicated in children aged under 7 years), cefaclor, clarithromycin, azithromycin and ciprofloxacin.

Pasteurella Species

NATURE

Pasteurella spp. are very small, nonmotile, nonspore-forming Gram-negative bacteria that are coccoid, oval or rod-shaped. They often exhibit bipolar staining. They are aerobic and facultatively anaerobic. Most species are catalase-positive and oxidase-positive. They attack carbohydrates readily, forming acid but no gas. Nitrates are reduced to nitrite. *Pasteurella* spp. will grow on ordinary laboratory media at 98.6°F (37°C). There are 15–20 species included in the genus *Pasteurella*, but it is probable that not all of these are true members of the genus. The type species is *Pasteurella multocida*. *Pasteurella multocida* is subdivided into four subspecies – *multocida*, *septica*, *gallicida* and *tigris*.

EPIDEMIOLOGY

Pasteurella spp. are distributed worldwide. They are commensals or parasitic organisms in the upper respiratory tract and gastrointestinal tracts of many domestic and wild animals and birds.

Pasteurella multocida is found in the oropharynx of 50–90% of domestic cats, 50–70% of dogs and 50% of pigs. It is the cause of hemorrhagic septicemia and bronchopneumonia in cattle and water buffalo, pneumonia in pigs and sheep, swine atrophic rhinitis, snuffles in rabbits and fowl, and fowl cholera in chickens, ducks and turkeys. It is generally carried asymptomatically by cats and dogs but may infect bites inflicted on these animals by feline or canine assailants. Humans become infected through contact with infected animals.

Pasteurella multocida can remain viable in soil and water for up to 4 weeks and may survive in animal carcasses for up to 3 months. Most human infections are caused by *P. multocida* subsp. *multocida* and *P. multocida* subsp. *septica*, though other species are sometimes implicated (Table 172.10).

PATHOGENICITY

Pasteurella multocida is transmitted to humans by contact with infected animals. The most common source of infection is bites, scratches, or licks from cats or dogs (see Chapter 68). Respiratory tract infections in those handling animals may result from airborne transmission. In a few patients it is not possible to document an animal source of the infection.

Virulence in *P. multocida* is associated with the degree of encapsulation. Strains with large capsules are more resistant to phagocytosis *in vivo*. There are five serogroups based on capsular antigens – A, B, D, E and F – and 16 serotypes (1–16) based on lipopolysaccharide (LPS) antigens. Capsular types A and D produce an exotoxin (PMT), encoded by the *toxA* gene. The role of this toxin in human infections is not known. *Pasteurella multocida* lipopolysaccharide is an important virulence factor. Fimbriae are probably important adhesins. Other putative virulence factors include neuraminidases, iron-sequestering proteins, surface adhesins and metabolic enzymes.[58]

PREVENTION

The only way of effectively preventing *Pasteurella* infections is to avoid contact with domestic or wild animals. Animal bites should be cleaned promptly and devitalized tissue should be debrided. Prophylactic antibiotics may be indicated after cat and dog bites, particularly if the patient is immunocompromised or diabetic or the wound affects the hands or face.

DIAGNOSTIC MICROBIOLOGY

A clinical history of animal bites will, in most instances, alert the laboratory to the possibility of *Pasteurella* spp. Samples should be cultured on blood agar plates at 98.6°F (37°C) for 24 hours. *Pasteurella multocida*

Table 172.10 Species of *Pasteurella* most commonly associated with infections in humans

- *Pasteurella multocida* subsp. *multocida*
- *Pasteurella multocida* subsp. *septica*
- *Pasteurella canis*
- *Pasteurella dagmatis*
- *Pasteurella stomatis*

grows as small, gray, nonhemolytic colonies, with a strong odor of indole. Gram-stained films reveal small Gram-negative coccobacilli. The organisms often show bipolar staining in methylene blue preparations. The identity of the organism can be confirmed by a series of biochemical and serologic tests and serology.

CLINICAL MANIFESTATIONS

Pasteurella infections in humans usually present as destructive soft tissue infections of acute onset following a bite or scratch from a domestic or wild animal. Open wounds may be infected by animal licks. Some *Pasteurella* infections present as respiratory infections, which may be chronic. In other cases the patient presents with a bacteremic infection. Approximately one-third of patients who have bacteremia have underlying cirrhosis.

MANAGEMENT

Animal bites should be carefully cleaned, irrigated and debrided. Penicillin is the treatment of choice for *Pasteurella* infections. Other agents with good activity include ampicillin, amoxicillin–clavulanate, cefuroxime and ciprofloxacin. Many infected animal bites have a polymicrobial etiology and it is prudent to use a regimen that provides good cover against both anaerobes and streptococci, such as amoxicillin–clavulanate. A strain of *P. multocida* that produced ROB-1 β-lactamase has been reported.

Yersinia Species

NATURE

Yersinia spp. are members of the Enterobacteriaceae. They are short, pleomorphic Gram-negative rods or coccobacilli, which often exhibit bipolar staining. *Yersinia pestis* is nonmotile. Other species are nonmotile at 98.6°F (37°C) but motile at temperatures less than 86°F (30°C) by means of peritrichous flagella. They are aerobic and facultatively anaerobic, oxidase-negative and catalase-positive. They are nonlactose fermenters. *Yersinia pestis* is urease-negative, and *Yersinia enterocolitica* and *Yersinia pseudotuberculosis* are both urease-positive. *Yersinia* spp. grow on simple laboratory media and are tolerant of bile salts. The optimal temperature for growth is 82–86°F (27.8–30°C). They do not form spores or capsules, but *Y. pestis* produces a capsule-like envelope. They share antigens with other members of the Enterobacteriaceae.

Multilocus sequence typing suggests that *Y. pestis* is a clone derived from *Y. pseudotuberculosis*.[59] The genome of five strains of *Y. pestis* and one strain of *Y. pseudotuberculosis* have been sequenced.[60]

The genus *Yersinia* contains three important human pathogens associated with zoonotic infections – *Y. pestis* causes plague, and *Y. pseudotuberculosis* and *Y. enterocolitica* give rise to infections known as yersiniosis.

Because these two diseases are very different they are described separately.

PLAGUE

The clinical features, pathogenesis, epidemiology and treatment of plague are discussed in detail in Chapter 120.

Diagnostic microbiology

Plague should be suspected in febrile patients exposed to flea bites or rodents in endemic parts of the world. It is important to notify the laboratory if plague is suspected so that appropriate precautions can be taken. There is a considerable risk of laboratory-acquired infection. Material suspected of containing *Y. pestis* must be handled in a containment level 3 laboratory in a category I or III exhaust protective cabinet by experienced, trained personnel. Smears taken from bubo aspirates, blood, sputum or cerebrospinal fluid should be examined using Gram stain and methylene blue. Gram stain will reveal Gram-negative pleomorphic coccobacilli with rounded ends. Wright–Giemsa or Wayson staining will demonstrate bipolar staining. *Yersinia pestis* appear light blue with dark blue polar bodies. Smears can also be examined by direct immunofluorescence.

Material can be cultured on blood agar or MacConkey agar or in broth cultures. Cultures should be incubated at 80°F (26.7°C). Tiny, translucent, nonhemolytic colonies appear on blood agar after 24 hours. After further incubation the colonies enlarge and become opaque. *Yersinia pestis* grows rather poorly on MacConkey agar and the colonies tend to autolyse after 2–3 days. In fluid culture *Y. pestis* tends to form chains.

The identity of presumptive colonies of *Y. pestis* can be confirmed using cultural and biochemical tests. Typically, *Y. pestis* is oxidase-negative, catalase-positive, urea-negative, indole-negative and lactose-negative. However strains may be misidentified as *Y. pseudotuberculosis* or other members of the Enterobacteriaceae. Alternatively, definitive identification can be made by detection of F1 antigen by immunofluorescence of the organisms. A bacteriophage that lyses *Y. pestis* but not *Y. pseudotuberculosis* can be used as a rapid identification in reference laboratories. A real-time PCR assay for *Y. pestis pla* gene has been developed.[61] A serologic diagnosis can be made using a passive hemagglutination test using tanned sheep red cells to which F1 antigen has been adsorbed, or a complement fixation test. A fourfold or greater rise in titer or a single titer over 1:16 in convalescent serum indicates plague infection. For large-scale seroepidemiologic surveys an ELISA test for antibodies to F1 antigen can be used.

YERSINIOSIS

Yersiniosis encompasses a wide spectrum of infections caused by *Y. enterocolitica* and *Y. pseudotuberculosis*. The clinical features range from gastroenteritis, enterocolitis or mesenteric adenitis to sepsis.

Epidemiology

Yersinia enterocolitica is harbored in the gastrointestinal tract of a wide range of mammals, including rodents, cattle, sheep, pigs, cats and dogs. Infected animals tend to become chronic carriers and excrete large numbers of bacilli, which can contaminate water and dairy products. Humans are infected by eating inadequately cooked meat (especially pork) or other food contaminated with *Yersinia* spp. Infection may also arise following contact with an infected domestic animal. In the USA, outbreaks associated with dairy products, chocolate and milk have been reported. Rarely, water is the source of the infection. The ability of *Y. enterocolitica* to grow at 39°F (4°C) means that refrigerated meat and meat products can become a potent source of infection. Infections are more common in children than in adults. Most cases occur in the autumn and winter. *Yersinia enterocolitica* sepsis has been reported following the transfusion of blood that has been stored for more than 3 weeks at 39°F (4°C).

Yersinia enterocolitica is a well-recognized cause of abdominal pain and diarrhea in Scandinavia and northern Europe. It is less commonly seen in the USA. Cases have been reported from other parts of the world. In Europe, infections are generally sporadic and the predominant serotypes are 03 and 09. In the USA, sporadic infections are less common but food-borne outbreaks caused by serotypes 03 and 09 have been described.[62]

Yersinia pseudotuberculosis infection is less commonly seen. The organism is harbored in the gastrointestinal tract of rodents, farm animals and birds. Human infections have been reported from all parts of the world but, as with *Y. enterocolitica*, it is more common in northern Europe than elsewhere. Infection is generally seen in children and affects males more frequently than females. The majority of infections occur in the winter.

Pathogenicity

Yersinia enterocolitica generally gains entry to the body via the gastrointestinal tract. The infecting dose is 10^8–10^9 organisms/ml. Within the ileum the organisms invade the mucosa via specialized follicle-associated epithelial cells (M cells) that are involved in antigen uptake. Adherence and invasion of epithelial cells requires two chromosomal genes, *inv* and *ail*.[63] Following invasion the bacteria enter Peyer's patches and macrophages, where they can survive intracellularly and multiply. This results in a severe gastroenteritis. The bacteria may also spread to the mesenteric lymph nodes causing mesenteric adenitis, which may mimic acute appendicitis.

The organisms may disseminate through the body, producing sepsis and splenic and hepatic abscesses. A reactive polyarthritis can occur, particularly in HLA-B27-positive patients.

Yersinia pseudotuberculosis usually gives rise to mesenteric adenitis. Both species produce V-W and YOPs antigens, which are essential for virulence, and an outer membrane protein, invasin, which is involved in adherence to and invasion of cells (Table 172.11). A clone of *Y. pseudotuberculosis* has been identified as the cause of a toxic-shock syndrome associated with a desquamating, erythematous rash called Far East scarlet-like fever.

Prevention

Prevention of yersiniosis depends on good animal husbandry and careful slaughtering techniques to minimize contamination of meat with orofecal material. Meat should not be consumed raw and should not be stored at 39°F (4°C) for prolonged periods before consumption. There is no effective vaccine.

Diagnostic microbiology

Material for culture will include stool specimens, blood, lymph nodes and food samples. Specimens should be cultured on blood agar and MacConkey agar at 80°F (26.7°C) for 24 hours. Heavily contaminated

Table 172.11 Virulence factors of *Yersinia* species

Virulence factor	Gene	Location	*Y. pestis*	*Y. entero-colitica*	*Y. pseudotuberculosis*	Action
Pigment	*hms*	Chromosomal	+	+	+	Promotes biofilm formation and blocks proventriculus in flea vector for *Y. pestis*
Phospholipase D	*ymt*	pFra plasmid	+	−	−	Promotes survival of *Y. pestis* in flea vector
F1 antigen	*caf1*	pFra plasmid	+	−	−	Fibrillar capsule inhibits macrophage activity
Plasminogen activator	*pla*	pPst plasmid	+	−	−	Activates mammalian plasminogen and anticomplementary Promotes dissemination from subcutaneous inoculation of *Y. pestis*
Lipopolysaccharide	*rfb*	Chromosomal	+	+	+	Endotoxin
Yersiniabactin	*irp2*	Chromosomal	+	+	+	Siderpophore-essential for full virulence of *Y. pestis* by subcutaneous inoculation
V antigen, low calcium response plasmid, *Yersinia* outer proteins (YOPs)	*yopH, yopM, yopE, ypkA/yopO, yopJ/ yopP, yadA, lcrV*	pLCR/pYV plasmid	+	+*	+	YOPs production essential for virulence of *Y. pestis* YOPs deregulate signaling pathways in host Type III secretion system, adhesin
pH 6 antigen	*psaA*	Chromosomal	+	+	+	Fibrillar surface protein Binds host lipoprotein Antiphagocytic
Invasin	*inv*	Chromosomal	−	+	+	Invasion of epithelial cells
Ail protein	*ail*	Chromosomal	−	+	+	Host cell attachment and serum resistance

* Yop T exclusive to *Y. enterocolitica*.

samples such as feces can be subjected to a cold enrichment technique whereby the sample is inoculated into phosphate-buffered saline and incubated at 39°F (4°C) for 3 weeks or more. The broth is subcultured at weekly intervals on to MacConkey agar or a special selective medium, CIN (cefsulodin, irgasan, novobiocin) agar. A chromogenic medium for detecting *Y. enterocolitica* has been described.[64] *Yersinia pseudotuberculosis* is rarely isolated from feces.

Presumptive colonies of *Yersinia* spp. are identified using a range of physical and biochemical tests. The serotype can be determined using slide agglutination tests.

A serologic diagnosis depends on demonstrating a significant rise of serotype-specific antibodies.

Clinical manifestations

A variety of clinical presentations have been documented in yersiniosis. The commonest form is acute gastroenteritis due to *Y. enterocolitica*. This is often indistinguishable from *Salmonella* or *Campylobacter* gastroenteritis. The commonest presentation of *Y. pseudotuberculosis* infection is mesenteric adenitis, which can mimic acute appendicitis.

Management

Yersinia enteritis and mesenteric adenitis do not generally require antimicrobial chemotherapy. Sepsis, extraintestinal foci of infection and enteritis in immunocompromised patients should be treated with antimicrobials. *Yersinia enterocolitica* is generally resistant to penicillin, ampicillin and first-generation cephalosporins. Aminoglycosides, quinolones, tetracyclines and third-generation cephalosporins have all been used successfully to treat *Y. enterocolitica* infections. *Yersinia pseudotuberculosis* is usually sensitive to benzylpenicillin and ampicillin.

REFERENCES

References for this chapter can be found online at http://www.expertconsult.com

Anaerobic bacteria

INTRODUCTION

Infections caused by anaerobic bacteria are common, and may be serious and life-threatening. Anaerobes are the predominant components of the bacterial flora of normal human skin and mucous membranes,[1] and are therefore a common cause of bacterial infections of endogenous origin. Because of their fastidious nature, these organisms are difficult to isolate from infectious sites and are often overlooked. Delay in appropriate therapy against these organisms often leads to clinical failures. Their isolation requires appropriate methods of collection, transportation and cultivation of specimens.[2–4] Treatment of anaerobic bacterial infection is complicated by the slow growth of these organisms, which makes diagnosis in the laboratory only possible after several days, by the often polymicrobial nature of the infection and by the growing resistance of anaerobic bacteria to antimicrobial agents.

NATURE

Anaerobic bacteria do not grow on solid media in the presence of room air (10% carbon dioxide and 18% oxygen), whereas facultative anaerobic bacteria grow both in the presence and in the absence of air. Microaerophilic bacteria grow poorly or not at all aerobically, but grow better under 10% carbon dioxide or anaerobically. Anaerobes can be divided into strict anaerobes that are unable to grow in the presence of more than 0.5% oxygen and moderate anaerobes that are capable of growing at between 2% and 8% oxygen.[4] Anaerobes generally do not possess catalase, but some clinical isolates produce superoxide dismutase that can protect them from oxygen.

The clinically important anaerobic bacteria in decreasing frequency are:

- six genera of Gram-negative rods (*Bacteroides, Prevotella, Porphyromonas, Fusobacterium, Bilophila* and *Sutterella* spp.);
- Gram-positive cocci (primarily *Peptostreptococcus* spp.);
- Gram-positive spore-forming (*Clostridium* spp.) and nonspore-forming bacilli (*Actinomyces, Propionibacterium, Eubacterium, Lactobacillus* and *Bifidobacterium* spp.); and
- Gram-negative cocci (mainly *Veillonella* spp.) (Table 173.1).[4–6]

The frequency of recovery of anaerobic bacterial strains differs in various infectious sites (Table 173.2). Mixed infections caused by numerous aerobic and anaerobic organisms are observed commonly in clinical situations (Fig. 173.1).[2,3]

Approximately 95% of the anaerobes isolated from clinical infections are members of these genera. The remaining isolates belong to species not yet described, but these usually can be assigned to the appropriate genus on the basis of morphologic characteristics and fermentation products. The frequency of recovery of anaerobic strains differs in various infectious sites.

The taxonomy of anaerobic bacteria has changed in recent years because of improved characterization methods using genetic studies.[4,6] The ability to differentiate between similar strains enables better characterization of type of infection and predicted antimicrobial susceptibility.[4]

EPIDEMIOLOGY

Most infections are caused by anaerobes that belong to the normal flora. Anaerobic infection generally occurs when members of the normal flora contaminate a previously sterile body site or gain access to the body from an external source of normal flora such as a bite. They also occur when the local defenses are decreased in capacity. Some anaerobic infections are caused by contamination of wounds by soil containing anaerobes. Such is the case with some *Clostridium* infections. *Clostridium difficile* enterocolitis can lead to epidemics in the hospital. In geriatric wards and nurseries in particular these bacteria are transmitted by hands from one patient to another. *Clostridium botulinum* causes food poisoning due to the presence of the toxin produced by *C. botulinum* in food.[7]

Gram-positive spore-forming bacilli

Anaerobic spore-forming bacilli belong to the genus *Clostridium*. Morphologically, the clostridia are highly pleomorphic, ranging from short, thick bacilli to long filamentous forms, and are either ramrod straight or slightly curved. The clostridia found most frequently in clinical infections are *Clostridium perfringens* (Fig. 173.2), *Clostridium septicum, Clostridium ramosum, Clostridium novyi, Clostridium sordellii, Clostridium histolyticum, Clostridium fallax, Clostridium bifermentans* and *Clostridium innocuum*.

Clostridium perfringens, the most commonly recovered *Clostridium* isolate, is an inhabitant of soil and of intestines of humans and animals, and is the most frequently encountered histotoxic *Clostridium* species. This micro-organism, which elaborates a number of necrotizing extracellular toxins,[8] is easily isolated and identified in the clinical laboratory. It can be characterized in direct smears of a purulent exudate by the presence of stout gram-variable rods of varying length, frequently surrounded by a capsule. *Clostridium perfringens* can cause a devastating illness with a high mortality rate. Bacteremia caused by *Clostridium* spp. is associated with extensive tissue necrosis, hemolytic anemia and renal failure.

Clostridium septicum has often been found to be associated with malignancy. The intestinal tract is thought to be the source of the organism, and most of the isolates are recovered from blood and subcutaneous tissue.[9] *Clostridium sordellii* infections have been reported in women undergoing therapeutic abortion, during natural childbirth, and in injection drug users.[10]

Table 173.1 Predominant anaerobic bacteria

Gram-positive cocci	*Peptostreptococcus* spp.: *P. magnus, P. asaccharolyticus, P. prevotii, P. intermedius, P. anaerobius, P. micros* Microaerophilic streptococci (not true anaerobes)
Gram-positive nonspore-forming bacilli	*Propionibacterium* spp.: *P. acnes, P. propionicum, P. granulosum Eubacterium tentum Bifidobacterium* spp.: *B. eriksonii, B. dentium Actinomyces* spp.: *A. israelii, A. naestundii, A. viscosus, A. odontolyticus, A. meyerii*
Gram-positive spore-forming bacilli	*Clostridium* spp.: *C. perfringens, C. ramosum, C. septicum, C. novyi, C. histolytica, C. sporogenes, C. difficile, C. bifermentans, C. butyricum, C. innocuum, C. sordellii, C. botulinum, C. tetani*
Gram-negative bacilli	*Bacteroides fragilis* group: *B. fragilis, B. thetaiotaomicron, B. distasonis, B. vulgatus, B. ovatus, B. uniformis* Other *Bacteroides* spp.: *B. gracilis, B. ureolyticus Bilophila wadsworthia, Sutterella* spp. Pigmented *Prevotella* spp.: *P. melaninogenica, P. intermedia, P. denticola, P. loescheii, P. corporis, P. nigrescens* Other *Prevotella* spp.: *P. oris, P. buccae, P. oralis* group (*P. oralis, P. buccalis, P. veroralis*), *P. bivia, P. disiens Porphyromonas* spp.: *P. asaccharolytica, P. gingivalis, P. endodontalis Fusobacterium* spp.: *F. nucleatum, F. necrophorum, F. gonidiaformans, F. naviforme, F. mortiferum, F. varium*

Table 173.2 Anaerobic bacteria most frequently encountered in specific infection sites

Organism		Infection site
Gram-positive cocci	*Peptostreptococcus* spp. Microaerophilic streptococci (not obligate anaerobes)	Respiratory tract, intra-abdominal and soft-tissue infections Sinusitis, brain abscesses
Gram-positive bacilli	Nonspore-forming: *Actinomyces* spp.	Intracranial abscesses, chronic mastoiditis, aspiration pneumonia, head and neck infections
	Propionibacterium acnes	Shunt infections (cardiac, intracranial), infections associated with foreign body
	Bifidobacterium spp.	Chronic otitis media, cervical lymphadenitis, abdominal infections
	Spore-forming: *Clostridium perfringens*	Soft-tissue infection, sepsis, food poisoning
	Clostridium septicum	Sepsis, neutropenic enterocolitis
	Clostridium difficile	Colitis, antibiotic-associated diarrheal disease
	Clostridium botulinum	Botulism
	Clostridium tetani	Tetanus
	Clostridium ramosum	Soft-tissue infections
Gram-negative bacilli	*Bacteroides fragilis* group	Intra-abdominal and female genital tract infections, sepsis, neonatal infections
	Pigmented *Prevotella* and *Porphyromonas* spp.	Orofacial infections, aspiration pneumonia, periodontitis
	Prevotella oralis	Orofacial infections
	Prevotella oris-buccae	Orofacial infections, intra-abdominal infections
	Prevotella bivia, Prevotella disiens	Female genital tract infections
	Fusobacterium nucleatum	Orofacial and respiratory tract infections, brain abscesses, bacteremia
	Fusobacterium necrophorum	Aspiration pneumonia, bacteremia

Although *C. botulinum* is usually associated with food poisoning, wound infections caused by this organism are being recognized with increasing frequency. Proteolytic strains of types A and B have been reported from food poisoning and wound infections. Infant botulism occurs with types A, B and F.[7] Disease caused by *C. botulinum* is usually an intoxication produced by ingestion of contaminated food (uncooked meat, poorly processed fish, improperly canned vegetables) containing a highly potent neurotoxin.[8] The polypeptide neurotoxin is relatively heat labile, and food containing this toxin may be rendered innocuous by exposure to 212°F (100°C) for 10 minutes. Infection of a wound with *C. botulinum* occurs rarely and can produce botulism.

Clostridium difficile has been incriminated as the causative agent of antibiotic-associated and spontaneous diarrhea and colitis.[11] *Clostridium tetani* is found in soil and is rarely isolated from human feces. Infections caused by this bacillus are a result of contamination of wounds with soil containing *C. tetani* spores.[8] The spores will germinate in devitalized tissue and produce the neurotoxin that is responsible for the clinical findings.

Laboratory diagnosis of *C. difficile*

Most laboratories use direct stool toxin assays (as opposed to organism detection assays) given their relatively rapid turnaround time. This practice has made investigation of the changing epidemiology of *C. difficile* more challenging, since isolation of a pathogen from culture is needed for epidemiologic surveillance.[12]

Direct stool toxin assays

Cytotoxicity assay Cytotoxicity assay (also known as tissue culture assay) is the gold standard for the diagnosis of *C. difficile*.[13] The test is

performed by adding a prepared stool sample (diluted, buffered and filtered) to a monolayer of cultured cells. If *C. difficile* toxins (A and/or B) are present, they exert a cytopathic effect characterized by rounding of fibroblasts in tissue culture (see Fig. 173.1).

Because only a few toxin molecules per cell are sufficient to cause rounding, the cytotoxicity assay can detect as little as 10 pg of toxin B, making it the most sensitive *C. difficile* test (94–100%).[14,15] In addition, the sample is preincubated with neutralizing antibody against the toxins, allowing for high specificity (99%). However, most clinical laboratories do not perform this assay routinely given its relatively high cost and long turnaround time (48 hours).

Enzyme immunoassay Enzyme immunoassay (EIA) allows direct detection of *C. difficile* toxin.[16] Commercially available reagents can detect toxin A alone or both toxins A and B. EIA for both toxins is

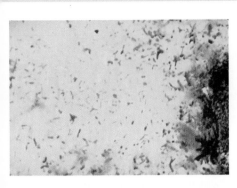

Fig. 173.1 Gram stain of a perirectal abscess caused by polymicrobial aerobic and anaerobic flora.

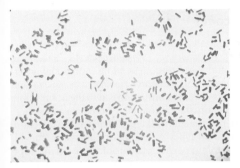

Fig. 173.2 Gram stain of *Clostridium perfringens*.

preferred because clinical cases may involve strains with a mutation in toxin A (rendering the EIA for toxin A ineffective) or strains that produce only toxin B.[17–20] In one study of 276 stool samples positive for *C. difficile* by EIA, for example, 19% were positive for toxin A alone, 48% for toxin B alone, and 33% for both toxins.[21]

EIA is the preferred diagnostic assay in most clinical laboratories because the technique is relatively simple and results are available within 24 hours. Despite good specificity (up to 99%), EIA is reported to have only moderate and variable sensitivity (60–95%).[12] There is a relatively high false-negative rate since 100–1000 pg of toxin must be present for the test to be positive.[22] Up to three serial EIA tests may increase the diagnostic yield by as much as 10% if the initial test is negative, although this incurs excessive cost without substantially enhancing diagnosis.[23] Supplementing negative EIA stool tests with tissue culture assay may also be useful.

Organism detection assays

An inherent problem with detection of the organism rather than the toxin is that up to 30% of hospitalized patients are colonized without disease.[3] Some laboratories use one of these methods to screen stool samples, with subsequent cytotoxin testing for positive samples.[24]

Anaerobic culture

Anaerobic culture is used less frequently for diagnosis of *C. difficile*. Although the test is extremely sensitive, anaerobic culture requires about 3 days. In addition, the assay cannot distinguish toxin-producing strains from nontoxin-producing strains.[15] To address this limitation, some laboratories perform an EIA on anaerobic culture isolates to determine whether they are toxin-producing strains; this approach appears to be more sensitive than assays that use stool specimens directly[25] (see 'Direct stool toxin assays' above).

Anaerobic culture is not a routinely used diagnostic tool in most clinical laboratories since it is relatively slow and labor intensive. However, it remains an important tool for epidemiologic surveillance.[12]

Polymerase chain reaction

Real-time polymerase chain reaction (PCR) using primers targeting a region of the toxin B gene could be a useful tool for diagnosis of *C. difficile* infection.[26] In a study evaluating 618 stool samples comparing PCR and EIA techniques with anaerobic culture (the 'gold standard'), sensitivity and specificity were better for PCR than EIA (67% vs 94% and 92% vs 97%, respectively).

Common antigen testing

Common antigen testing detects glutamate dehydrogenase (GDH) antigen, an essential enzyme produced constitutively by all *C. difficile* isolates. Some laboratories use this method to screen stool samples, with subsequent cytotoxin testing for positive samples.[24,27]

Endoscopy

Endoscopy can be a useful adjunctive tool for the diagnosis of *C. difficile* in the following settings:

- high clinical suspicion for *C. difficile* with negative laboratory assay(s);
- prompt *C. difficile* diagnosis needed before laboratory results can be obtained;
- failure of *C. difficile* infection to respond to antibiotic therapy; and
- atypical presentation with ileus or minimal diarrhea.[10,28]

Endoscopy is not warranted in patients with classic clinical findings and a positive stool toxin assay. In the setting of fulminant colitis, care should be taken to introduce minimal amounts of air given the risk of perforation. Gross and histologic findings obtained by endoscopic evaluation are discussed in detail above.

Gram-positive, nonspore-forming bacilli

Anaerobic, Gram-positive, nonspore-forming rods comprise part of the microflora of the gingival crevices, the gastrointestinal tract, the vagina and the skin. Several distinct genera are recognized: *Actinomyces*, *Arcanobacterium*, *Atopobium*, *Bifidobacterium*, *Eubacterium*, *Lactobacillus*, *Mobiluncus*, *Propionibacterium* and *Pseudoramibacter*. The most frequently recovered species are *Propionibacterium*, *Eubacterium*, *Bifidobacterium* and *Lactobacillus*.

The *Actinomyces*, *Arcanobacterium* and *Bifidobacterium* spp. are Gram-positive, pleomorphic, anaerobic to microaerophilic bacilli.

Actinomyces israelii, *Actinomyces naeslundii* and *Propionibacterium propionicum* are normal inhabitants of the human mouth and throat and are the most frequent cause of actinomycosis. The organisms have been recovered from intracranial abscesses, chronic mastoiditis, aspiration pneumonia and peritonitis.[3,5] The lesions of actinomycosis occur most commonly in the tissues of the face, neck, lungs, pleura and female and male genital and urinary tracts. Bone, pericardial and anorectal lesions are less common, but virtually any tissue may be invaded; even disseminated infection with bacteremia has been described.[29]

Most organisms of the genus *Eubacterium* and anaerobic lactobacilli seem to be nonpathogenic. They are almost invariably isolated as part of mixed flora in the oral, vaginal and gastrointestinal areas. These organisms have been recovered most commonly in infections associated with predisposing or underlying conditions that include malignancy, previous surgery, immunodeficiency, diabetes mellitus, the presence of a foreign body, dental extraction and broad-spectrum antibiotic therapy.[30]

Propionibacterium spp. ordinarily are not pathogens, but can be found in association with implanted cardiac prostheses or central nervous system (CNS) shunts or as a cause of endocarditis on previously damaged valves. They have been recovered from parotid and dental infections, brain abscesses, conjunctivitis associated with contact lens, peritonitis and foreign body and pulmonary infections. The most common species, *Propionibacterium acnes*, may be isolated from blood cultures but is associated only rarely with bacteremia or endocarditis. Because these organisms are part of the normal skin flora, they are common laboratory contaminants or may grow in blood cultures from skin contamination if the skin surface has been improperly decontaminated before the blood sample is drawn. *Propionibacterium acnes* can cause bacteremia, especially in association with shunt and infections,[31,32] and is believed to play a role in the pathogenesis of acne vulgaris.[33]

Gram-negative bacilli

Bacteroides fragilis group are the most frequently recovered species of Bacteroidaceae in clinical specimens (Fig. 173.3). *Bacteroides fragilis* group are resistant to penicillins, mostly through the production of β-lactamase. They include several members – the most commonly isolated ones are *B. fragilis* (the most commonly recovered member), *Bacteroides thetaiotaomicron*, *Bacteroides distasonis*, *Bacteroides ovatus* and *Bacteroides vulgatus*. These organisms are part of the normal gastrointestinal flora[1] and predominate in intra-abdominal infections and other infections that originate from the gut flora (i.e. perirectal abscesses, decubitus ulcers).[3,5] *Bilophila wadsworthia* and *Centipeda periodontii* are new genera and species found in abdominal and endodontal infection, respectively.[34]

Pigmented *Prevotella* spp. (*Prevotella melaninogenica*, *Prevotella intermedia*), *Porphyromonas* spp. (*Porphyromonas asaccharolytica*) and non-pigmented *Prevotella* spp. (*Prevotella oralis*, *Prevotella oris*) are part of the normal oral and vaginal flora and are the predominant Gram-negative anaerobic species isolated from respiratory infections and their complications, aspiration pneumonia, lung abscess, chronic otitis media, chronic sinusitis, abscesses around the oral cavity, human bites, paronychia, brain abscesses and osteomyelitis.[35] *Prevotella bivia* and *Prevotella disiens* are important isolates from obstetric and gynecologic infections.

Fusobacterium species

Fusobacterium spp. are moderately long and thin organisms with tapered ends, and have typical fusiform morphology (Fig. 173.4). The species of *Fusobacterium* seen most often in clinical infections are *Fusobacterium nucleatum*, *Fusobacterium necrophorum*, *Fusobacterium mortiferum* and *Fusobacterium varium*. *Fusobacterium nucleatum* is the predominant *Fusobacterium* sp. from clinical specimens, and is often associated with oral, pulmonary and intracranial infections.[36] *Fusobacterium* spp. are frequently isolated from abscesses, obstetric and gynecologic infections, blood and wounds.

A growing resistance of Gram-negative anaerobic bacilli to penicillins has been noted in the past decade.[37] These include the pigmented *Prevotella* and *Porphyromonas*, *Prev. oralis*, *Prev. disiens*, *Prev. bivia* and *Fusobacterium* spp. The main mechanism of resistance is through the production of the enzyme β-lactamase. Testing for antimicrobial susceptibility and the ability to produce β-lactamase of all Gram-negative anaerobic bacilli can assist in the selection of appropriate antimicrobials.

The recovery rates of the different anaerobic Gram-negative bacilli in infected sites are similar to their distributions in the normal flora.[3,5] The *B. fragilis* group were more often isolates in sites proximal to the gastrointestinal tract (abdomen, bile), pigmented *Prevotella* spp. were more prevalent in infections proximal to the oral cavity (bones, sinuses, chest), and *Prev. bivia* and *Prev. disiens* were more often isolates in obstetric and gynecologic infections (see Table 173.2). Knowledge of this common mode of distribution allows for logical choice of antimicrobials that are adequate for the therapy of infections in these sites.

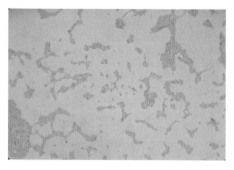

Fig. 173.3 Gram stain of *Bacteroides fragilis*. Courtesy of Mike Cox.

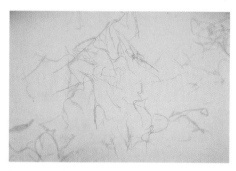

Fig. 173.4 Gram stain of *Fusobacterium nucleatum*. Courtesy of Mike Cox.

Gram-positive cocci

The species most commonly isolated are *Peptostreptococcus magnus*, *Peptostreptococcus asaccharolyticus*, *Peptostreptococcus anaerobius*, *Peptostreptococcus prevotii* and *Peptostreptococcus micros*. Additional anaerobic cocci include *Coprococcus*, *Peptococcus*, *Ruminococcus sarcina* and *Staphylococcus saccharolyticus*. These organisms are part of the normal flora of the mouth, upper respiratory tract, intestinal tract, vagina and skin.

These organisms can be isolated in all types of anaerobic infection. They also predominate in all types of respiratory infection (including chronic sinusitis, mastoiditis, acute and chronic otitis media, aspiration pneumonia and lung abscess), and necrotizing, subcutaneous and soft-tissue infections.[38] They are generally recovered mixed with other aerobic or anaerobic organisms, but in many cases they are the only pathogens recovered. This may be of particular significance in cases of bacteremia. Microaerophilic streptococci are not true anaerobes as they can also become aerotolerant after subculture; however, they grow better anaerobically and are often grouped under anaerobes in many studies. These organisms include the *Streptococcus anginosus* group (previously called *Streptococcus milleri* group, which includes *Streptococcus constellatus* and *Streptococcus intermedius*) and *Gemella morbillorum* (previously called *Streptococcus morbillorum*). Microaerophilic streptococci are of particular importance in chronic sinusitis and brain abscesses. They are also recovered from obstetric and gynecologic infections and abscesses.[39]

Gram-negative cocci

There are three genera described as anaerobic Gram-negative cocci: *Veillonella*, *Acidaminococcus* and *Megasphaera* spp. There are two described species of *Veillonella* and only one each of the other two genera. *Veillonella* is the most frequently involved of the three genera and *Veillonella* spp. are part of the normal flora of the mouth, vagina and the small intestine of some persons. Although they are rarely isolated from clinical infections, these organisms have been recovered occasionally from almost every type of anaerobic infection.[40]

PATHOGENICITY

Anaerobes as part of the normal flora (Table 173.3)

The human body mucosal and epithelial surfaces are colonized with aerobic and anaerobic micro-organisms.[1] Differences in the environment, such as oxygen tension, pH and variations in the ability of bacteria to adhere to these surfaces, account for changing patterns of colonization. Microflora also vary in different sites within the body system, as in the oral cavity; for example, the micro-organisms present in the buccal folds vary in their concentration and types of strain from those isolated from the tongue or gingival sulci. However, the organisms that prevail in one body system tend to belong to certain major bacterial species, and their presence in that system is predictable. The relative and total counts of organisms can be affected by various factors, such as age, diet, anatomic variations, illness, hospitalization and antimicrobial therapy. However, these sets of bacterial flora, with predictable pattern, remain stable through life, despite their subjection to perturbing factors. Anaerobes outnumber aerobic bacteria on all mucosal surfaces, and certain organisms predominate in the different sites (see Table 173.3).

Knowledge of the composition of the flora at certain sites is useful for predicting which organisms may be involved in an infection adjacent to that site and can assist in the selection of a logical antimicrobial therapy, even before the exact microbial etiology of the infection is known. Recognition of the normal flora can also help the clinical microbiology laboratory to identify appropriate culture media that will be selective in inhibiting organisms that may interfere with the growth of certain anaerobic bacteria.

The anaerobic microflora of the skin is largely made up of the genus *Propionibacterium*[34] (mostly *Propionibacterium acnes*) and, to a lesser extent, *Peptostreptococcus* spp. The perineum and lower extremity may harbor members of the colonic and vaginal flora.

The microflora of the upper airways, including oral cavity, nasopharynx and oropharynx, is complex and contains many types of obligate anaerobes. The distribution of bacteria within the mouth seems to be a function of their ability to adhere to the oral surfaces. The differences in numbers of the anaerobic microflora probably occur because of considerable variations in the oxygen concentration in parts of the oral cavity. The ratio of anaerobic bacteria to aerobic bacteria in saliva is approximately 10:1. The total count of anaerobic bacteria in the saliva and elsewhere in the oral cavity reach 10^7–10^8 bacteria/ml. The predominant anaerobic bacteria in the upper airways include *Fusobacterium* spp. (especially *F. nucleatum*), pigmented *Prevotella* and *Porphyromonas* spp., *Prev. oralis* and *Peptostreptococcus* spp. These organisms also predominate in oropharyngeal, otolaryngologic and pulmonary infections.

The gastrointestinal flora varies in bacterial concentration at different levels. The stomach acidity reduces the number of organisms swallowed from the oropharynx. The stomach, duodenum, jejunum and proximal ileum normally contain relatively few bacteria. However, the flora becomes more complex, and the number of different bacterial species increase in the distal portion of the gastrointestinal tract. Interruption in intestinal motility may result in an increase in the number of anaerobic and aerobic bacteria. The bacterial counts in the small intestine are relatively low, with total counts of 10^2–10^5 organisms/ml. The organisms that predominate up to the ileocecal valve are Gram-positive facultative, whereas below that structure *Bacteroides*, *Peptostreptococcus* and *Clostridium* spp. and coliform bacteria are the major isolates.[2] The mean number of bacteria in the colon exceeds 10^{11} bacteria/g fecal material. Approximately 99.9% of these bacteria are anaerobic (ratio of aerobes to anaerobes is 1:1000–10 000). In the colon 300–400 different species or types of bacteria can be found, many of which are not yet identified.

The female genital flora is composed of mixed aerobic and anaerobic flora. However, the concentration and type of bacteria is less stable than that of the gastrointestinal flora and can be influenced by antimicrobial therapy, pregnancy and gynecologic surgery. A concentration of 10^8 organisms/ml is found during the reproductive years. Changes occur in the number of organisms at the various stages of the menstrual cycle.[41] The predominant aerobic organisms are aerobic lactobacilli, and the predominant anaerobic bacteria are anaerobic *Lactobacillus*, *Peptostreptococcus*, *Prevotella* and *Bacteroides* and *Clostridium* spp. Other anaerobic isolates include *Porphyromonas*, *Fusobacterium*, *Bilophilia*, *Bifidobacterium*, *Actinomyces*, *Eubacterium* and *Propionibacterium* spp. Enterobacteriaceae can be found in postmenopausal flora. Bacterial vaginosis is associated with an increase in the number of anaerobic flora and a decrease in the concentration of lactobacilli.[42]

Most infections caused by anaerobic bacteria originate from the endogenous mucosal membrane and skin flora. An exception is *C. difficile*, the major cause of antibiotic-associated colitis. Anaerobes belonging to the indigenous flora of the oral cavity can be recovered from various infections adjacent to that area, such as cervical lymphadenitis, subcutaneous abscesses and burns in proximity to the oral cavity, human and animal bites, paronychia, tonsillar and retropharyngeal abscesses, chronic sinusitis, chronic otitis media, periodontal abscess, thyroiditis, aspiration pneumonia and bacteremia associated with one of the above infections.[3,5] The predominant anaerobes recovered in these infections are *Prevotella*, *Porphyromonas*, *Fusobacterium* and *Peptostreptococcus* spp., which are all part of the normal flora of the mucous surfaces of the oropharynx (Fig. 173.5).

A similar correlation exists in infections associated with the gastrointestinal tract. Such infections include peritonitis after rupture of a viscus, liver and spleen abscess, abscess and wounds near the anus, intra-abdominal abscess, and bacteremia associated with any of these

Table 173.3 Normal flora

Site	NO. OF ORGANISMS/g FECAL MATERIAL			Predominant anaerobic bacteria
	Aerobes	Anaerobes	Anaerobe/aerobe ratio	
Skin	–	–	–	*Propionibacterium acnes* *Peptostreptococcus* spp.
Mouth/upper respiratory tract	10^8–10^9	10^9–10^{11}	Nasal washings 3–5:1 Saliva 1:1 Tooth surface 1:1 Gingival crevice 1000:1	Pigmented *Prevotella* and *Porphyromonas* spp. *Fusobacterium* spp. *Peptostreptococcus* spp. *Actinomyces* spp.

Gastrointestinal tract:
  Upper
  Lower
	10^2–10^5
	10^5–10^9
		10^3–10^7
		10^{10}–10^{12}
			Stomach 1:1
			Small bowel 1:1
			Ileum 1:1
			Colon 1000:1
				Bacteroides fragilis group
				Clostridium spp.
				Peptostreptococcus spp.
				Bifidobacterium spp.
				Eubacterium spp.

Female genital tract	10^8	10^9	Endocervix 1–5:1 Vagina 1–5:1	*Peptostreptococcus* spp. *Prevotella bivia* *Prevotella disiens*

For predominant anaerobic bacteria in the gastrointestinal tract, all organisms can be found in both the upper and lower gastrointestinal tracts.

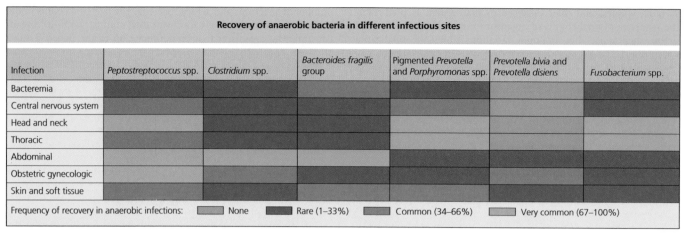

Fig. 173.5 Recovery of anaerobic bacteria in different infectious sites.

infections.[3,5] The anaerobes that predominate in these infections are *B. fragilis* group, *Clostridium* spp. (including *C. perfringens*) and *Peptostreptococcus* spp.

Another site where a correlation exists between the normal flora and the anaerobic bacteria recovered from infected sites is the genito-urinary tract. The infections involved are amnionitis, septic abortion and other pelvic inflammations.[3,5] The anaerobes usually recovered from these sites are species of anaerobic Gram-negative bacteria and *Peptostreptococcus* spp. Organisms belonging to the vaginal–cervical flora are also important pathogens of neonatal infections. They can be acquired by the newborn before delivery in the presence of amnionitis or during passage through the birth canal.

Conditions predisposing to anaerobic infection

The clinical situations that predispose to anaerobic infections include exposure of the sterile body sites to a high inoculum of indigenous mucous membrane flora. Poor blood supply and tissue necrosis lower the oxidation and reduction potential and favor the growth of anaerobic bacteria. Any condition that lowers the blood supply to an affected area of the body can predispose to anaerobic infection. Therefore, trauma, foreign body, malignancy, surgery, edema, shock, colitis and vascular disease may predispose to anaerobic infection. Other predisposing conditions include diabetes mellitus, splenectomy, immunosuppression, hypogammaglobinemia, neutropenia, leukemia, collagen vascular disease and cytotoxic drugs. Previous infection with aerobic or facultative organisms may make the local tissue conditions more favorable for the growth of anaerobic bacteria. The human defense mechanisms may also be impaired by anaerobic conditions and anaerobic bacteria. The noted effects include impairments in phagocytosis and intracellular killing (often caused by encapsulated anaerobes[43] and by succinic acid produced by *Bacteroides* spp.), inhibition of chemotaxis (by *Fusobacterium*, *Prevotella* and *Porphyromonas* spp.), degradation of serum proteins by proteases (by *Bacteroides* spp.) and production of leukotoxins (by *Fusobacterium* spp.).[44]

Suppuration, abscess formation, thrombophlebitis and gangrenous destruction of tissue associated with gas formation are the hallmarks of anaerobic infection (Table 173.4). Anaerobes are especially common in chronic infections, and they are commonly seen after failure of therapy with antimicrobials that are effective against them, such as aminoglycosides, trimethoprim–sulfamethoxazole (co-trimoxazole) and earlier quinolones.

Certain infections are very likely to involve anaerobes as important pathogens, and their presence should always be assumed. Such

Table 173.4 Clinical signs of anaerobic infection

Infection adjacent to a mucosal surface

Foul-smelling discharge

Necrotic gangrenous tissue and abscess formation

Free gas in tissue

Bacteremia or endocarditis with no growth on aerobic blood cultures

Infection related to the use of antibiotics effective against aerobes only

Infection related to tumors or other destructive processes

Infected thrombophlebitis

Infection after bites

Black discoloration of exudates containing *Bacteroides melaninogenicus*, which may fluoresce under ultraviolet light

'Sulfur granules' in discharges caused by actinomycosis

Clinical presentation of gas gangrene

Clinical condition predisposing to anaerobic infection (after maternal amnionitis, perforation of bowel, etc.)

infections include brain abscess, oral or dental infections, human or animal bites, aspiration pneumonia and lung abscesses, peritonitis after perforation of viscus, amnionitis, endometritis, septic abortions, tubo-ovarian abscess, abscesses in and around the oral and rectal areas, pus-forming necrotizing infections of soft tissue or muscle and postsurgical infections following procedures on the oral or gastrointestinal tract or female pelvic area.[5] Certain solid malignant tumors, such as colon, uterine and bronchogenic carcinomas, and necrotic tumors of the head and neck, have the tendency to become infected with anaerobic bacteria.[45] The anoxic conditions in the tumor and exposure to the endogenous adjacent mucous flora may predispose to these infections.

Virulence factors

Anaerobic bacteria contain a number of components that have been defined as virulence factors in facultative bacteria including toxins, polysaccharide capsules, and lipopolysaccharides. Most of these also have been shown to be virulence factors in anaerobic species. The capacity to survive and grow under anaerobic conditions has also led to the identification of other properties of anaerobes which may play a role in virulence.

Toxins

The most clearly identified virulence factors for anaerobic bacteria are the exotoxins produced by clostridial species including botulinum toxins, tetanus toxin, *C. difficile* toxin A and B, and five toxins produced by *C. perfringens* (as well as many other clostridial species); these are among the most virulent bacterial toxins in mouse lethality assays. Alpha toxin is the major toxin produced by *C. perfringens*, but studies have shown a complex interaction between alpha and theta toxin in the production of experimental gas gangrene.[1,2] Both toxins appear to be involved in upregulation of intercellular adhesion molecule (ICAM)-1 and platelet aggregating factor (PAF), which contributes to vascular leukostasis and absence of a polymorphonuclear leukocyte (PMN) response to the infection.[3]

Clinical expression of these histotoxic clostridial syndromes depends upon the site of toxin production and the physiologic effects of the toxin (see 'Epidemiology, microbiology, and pathophysiology of *Clostridium difficile* infection', 'Clostridial myonecrosis' and 'Botulism').

An enterotoxin has also been identified in *Bacteroides fragilis*, which is a metalloprotease.[4] Strains producing the toxin have been recovered from patients with diarrhea and from healthy controls but seem to be more common in those with diarrhea.[5]

Capsular polysaccharides

In the same way that *Clostridium* spp. serve as the prototypes for toxins produced by anaerobes, *B. fragilis* has been studied as a unique virulent anaerobe. The organism constitutes 0.5% of normal colonic flora and yet is the most common anaerobe isolated from intra-abdominal infections and is the most frequent anaerobic bacteremic isolate.[6] This explains why investigators have chosen to examine *B. fragilis* virulence factors in more detail.

Based upon the rat model of intra-abdominal sepsis, it became apparent that *B. fragilis* alone among the anaerobes studied was capable of provoking abscesses without a synergistic facultative organism and that heat-killed *B. fragilis* retained this capacity.[7] Following extraction and purification of the polysaccharide capsule of a prototype strain, this complex sugar was also able to provoke abscesses in the model system. Further study of the capsular polysaccharide has led to an appreciation that it is actually a complex of polysaccharides with zwitterionic properties (containing alternating oppositely charged sugars).[8,9] Adherence of the capsular polysaccharide complex to mesothelial cells *in vitro* stimulates ICAM-1 and tumor necrosis factor (TNF); pretreatment of mice with antibodies to ICAM-1 or TNF results in failure of the animals to develop intraperitoneal abscesses in a mouse model of intra-abdominal sepsis.[10]

Lipopolysaccharides

Anaerobic Gram-negative bacteria, like all Gram-negative bacteria, contain lipopolysaccharide (LPS) that can be extracted from the envelope, but the biologic activity of this endotoxin (mouse lethality assays, the chick embryo death test, and the Shwartzman reaction) is 100–1000 times less than that of LPS from Enterobacteriaceae.[11] The LPS of *B. fragilis* contains a lipid A moiety (the endotoxin portion of LPS), but there are structural and chemical composition differences which render this LPS less potent than the LPS of *Escherichia coli*.[11]

Other anaerobic Gram-negative bacteria, such as fusobacteria, are thought to contain endotoxin with substantial biologic activity. One study of extracted LPS from a strain of *Fusobacterium nucleatum* found biologic activity equal to the LPS of Enterobacteriaceae and correlated this with inhibition of gingival fibroblasts.[29] Thus, LPS of fusobacteria may play a pathogenic role in periodontal disease and presumably accounts for the severity of illness with Lemierre disease[30,31] (see 'Anaerobic bacterial infections').

Volatile fatty acids

Another virulence factor of anaerobes is the production of short chain volatile fatty acids. Production of these fatty acids is a characteristic feature of the metabolic system of anaerobes that is used to identify these microbes in the microbiology laboratory and may be responsible for the characteristic putrid drainage. These volatile fatty acids have been shown to inhibit phagocytic killing of bacteria.[32,33]

Ability to tolerate oxygen

A number of anaerobic bacteria, including *B. fragilis*, can tolerate exposure to oxygen. These organisms contain varying concentrations of superoxide dismutase, an enzyme present in aerobic bacteria which protects against the toxic effects of oxygen.[34] The ability to survive exposure to oxygen is a different type of factor which facilitates the survival and thus pathogenicity of the organism.

Formation of and host defense to abscesses

As noted above, an abscess is a unique biologic phenomenon, representing at one and the same time a pathologic process and host defense to contain infection. Within the fibrous capsule of a well-formed abscess, bacteria and PMN coexist; these same neutrophils *in vitro* will kill the bacteria.

Anaerobes contribute to the severity of infection through their synergy with their aerobic counterparts and with each other.[22] Anaerobic bacteria generally take longer than aerobic bacteria to become virulent. This is because some of the major virulence factors of certain anaerobic bacteria (i.e. the production of a capsule) are expressed only after the infection has become chronic.[43]

Anaerobic bacteria possess several virulence factors that assist them to adhere to and invade epithelial surfaces. These factors include the presence of surface structures (such as capsule polysaccharide or lipopolysaccharide), production of superoxide dismutase and catalase, immunoglobulin proteases, coagulation promoting, spreading factors (such as hyaluronidase, collagenase and fibrinolysin), adherence factors and the production of toxins.[44] Other factors that enhance the virulence of anaerobes include mucosal damage, oxidation–reduction potential drop and the presence of hemoglobin or blood in an infected site.

An indirect pathogenic role of some anaerobes is their ability to produce the enzyme β-lactamase. Several anaerobic bacteria can produce β-lactamase (Table 173.5). β-Lactamase-producing bacteria (BLPB) can protect not only themselves but also other penicillin-susceptible organisms from the activity of penicillins. This can occur when the enzyme β-lactamase is secreted into the infected tissue or abscess fluid in sufficient quantities to degrade the β-lactam ring of penicillin before it can kill the susceptible bacteria.[46]

In-vitro and *in-vivo* studies have demonstrated protection of penicillin-susceptible bacteria from penicillin by aerobic and anaerobic BLPB (i.e. protection of group A streptococci by *Staphylococcus aureus* or *Bacteroides* spp.).[46] The predominant anaerobic BLPB are pigmented *Prevotella* and *Porphyromonas*, *Bacteroides* and *Fusobacterium* spp.

Table 173.5 Principal β-lactamase-producing anaerobes

Fusobacterium spp.: *F. nucleatum*, *F mortiferum*, *F. varium*

Pigmented *Prevotella* and *Porphyromonas* spp., *Prevotella oralis* group

Other *Prevotella* spp.: *P. oris*, *P. buccae*, *P. bivia*, *P. disiens*

Bacteroides fragilis group, *Bacteroides splanchnicus*

Bilophila wadsworthia

Clostridium spp.: *C. ramosum*, *C. clostridioforme* and *C. butyricum*

PREVENTION

Proper therapy of acute infections can prevent the occurrence of chronic infections where anaerobes predominate. In settings where anaerobic infections are expected to occur, such as intra-abdominal and wound infections after surgery, proper antimicrobial prophylaxis reduces the chance of such infections.

Prevention and early therapy of conditions that may lead to anaerobic infection can reduce their rate. Preventing oral flora aspiration by improving the neurologic status of the patient, repeated suctioning of oral secretions, improving oral hygiene and maintaining lower stomach pH can reduce the risk of aspiration pneumonia and its complications. Skin and soft-tissue infections can be prevented by irrigation and debridement of wounds and necrotic tissue, drainage of pus and improvement of blood supply.

Prophylactic therapy before surgery is generally administered when the operative field is expected to be contaminated by the normal flora of the mucous membrane at the operated site. Cefazolin is effective in surgical prophylaxis in sites distant from the oral or rectal areas, when anaerobic cover is not required. Cefoxitin, cefotetan or ertapenem are used in procedures that involve the oral, rectal or vulvovaginal surfaces because their spectrum includes the anaerobic flora likely to be encountered.

COLLECTION, TRANSPORT AND DIAGNOSTIC MICROBIOLOGY

Collection of specimens for anaerobic bacteria

The proper management of anaerobic infection depends on appropriate documentation of the bacteria causing the infection. Without such an approach, the patient may be exposed to inappropriate, costly and undesirable antimicrobial agents with adverse side-effects. Some laboratories may fail to recover certain or all of the anaerobes present in a specimen. This situation can occur particularly when the specimen is not promptly placed under anaerobic conditions for transport to the laboratory. If care is not taken to avoid specimen contamination with normal flora, anaerobes may not be recovered.

Appropriate cultures for anaerobes are especially important in polymicrobial infections.[4] Techniques or media that are inadequate for isolation of anaerobes because of a lack of an anaerobic environment, or because of an overgrowth of aerobic organisms, can be misleading. This may cause the clinician to direct therapy toward only the isolated aerobic organism(s).

The most acceptable documentation of an anaerobe is through recovery of anaerobic organisms from the infected site. Three essential elements require the physician's cooperation with the microbiology laboratory for appropriate documentation of anaerobic infection: collection of appropriate specimens, their expeditious transportation and careful laboratory processing.

Specimens must be obtained free of contamination so that saprophytic organisms or normal flora are excluded and culture results can be interpreted correctly. Because indigenous anaerobes are often present on the surfaces of skin and mucous membranes in large numbers, even minimal contamination of a specimen with normal flora can give misleading results. On this basis, specimens can be designated according to their acceptability for anaerobic culture to the acceptable or the unacceptable category. Materials that are appropriate for anaerobic cultures should be obtained using a technique that bypasses the normal flora (Table 173.6). Unacceptable or inappropriate specimens can yield normal flora also and therefore have no diagnostic value.

Acceptable specimens (Table 173.7) include blood specimens, aspirates of body fluids (pleural, pericardial, cerebrospinal, peritoneal

Table 173.6 Methods for collection of specimens for anaerobic bacteria

Infection site	Methods
Abscess or body cavity	Aspiration by syringe and needle Incised abscesses: syringe or swab (less desirable); specimen obtained during surgery after cleansing the skin
Tissue or bone	Surgical specimen using tissue biopsy or curette
Sinuses or mucus surface abscesses	Aspiration after decontamination or surgical specimen
Ear	Aspiration after decontamination of ear canal and membrane; in perforation, cleanse ear canal and aspirate through perforation
Pulmonary	Transtracheal aspiration, lung puncture, bronchoscopic aspirate (using double lumen catheter and quantitative culture)
Pleural	Thoracentesis
Urinary tract	Suprapubic bladder aspiration
Female genital tract	Culdocentesis after decontamination, surgical specimen Transabdominal needle aspirate of uterus Intrauterine brush (using double lumen catheter and quantitative culture)

Table 173.7 Appropriate and inappropriate specimens for anaerobic culture

Appropriate	Inappropriate
Feces or rectal swabs Throat or nasopharyngeal swabs Sputum or bronchoscopic specimens Routine or catheterized urine Vaginal or cervical swabs Material from superficial wound or abscesses not collected properly to exclude surface contaminations Material from abdominal wounds obviously contaminated with feces (e.g. an open fistula)	All normally sterile body fluids other than urine (e.g. blood, pleural and joint fluids) Urine obtained by suprapubic bladder aspiration Percutaneous transtracheal aspiration or direct lung puncture Culdocentesis fluid obtained after decontamination of the vagina Material obtained from closed abscesses Material obtained from sinus tracts or draining wounds

and joint fluids), urine collected by percutaneous suprapubic bladder aspiration, abscess contents, deep aspirates of wounds and specimens collected by special techniques, such as transtracheal aspirates or direct lung puncture. Specimens of the lower respiratory tract are difficult to obtain without contamination with indigenous flora. Double-lumen catheter bronchial brushing and bronchoalveolar lavage, cultured quantitatively, can be useful. Direct needle aspiration is probably the best method of obtaining a culture, and the use of swabs is much less desirable. Specimens obtained from sites that are normally sterile may be collected after thorough skin decontamination, as is the case for the collection of blood, or spinal, joint or peritoneal fluids.

Transportation of specimens

Prompt delivery of specimens to the laboratory to allow for microbiologic processing is essential. Various transport devices are available that generate an oxygen-free environment. These systems generally contain an oxygen-free environment provided by mixture of carbon dioxide, hydrogen and nitrogen, plus an indicator that illustrates aerobic conditions. The specimens should be placed into an anaerobic transporter as soon as possible after collection. Aspirates of liquid specimen or tissue are always preferred to swabs, although systems for the collection of all culture forms are commercially available.

Liquid specimens may be inoculated into a commercially available anaerobic transport vial. A plastic or glass syringe without a needle may also be used for transport. After the specimen is collected and all air bubbles are expelled, the syringe is capped. Because air gradually diffuses into the plastic syringe, no more than 30 minutes should elapse before the specimen is processed. This inexpensive transport device for liquid specimens is especially useful in the hospital where it can be rapidly transported to the microbiology laboratory.

Swabs may be placed in the sterilized tubes containing carbon dioxide or prereduced, anaerobically sterile Carey and Blair semisolid media. Tissue specimens or swabs can be transported in an anaerobic jar or in a Petri dish inside a sealed plastic bag that can be rendered anaerobic by use of a catalyzer.

Laboratory diagnosis

For the laboratory diagnosis of *Clostridium difficile*, see above.

Certain findings are suggestive of anaerobic infection (Table 173.8). However, laboratory diagnosis of anaerobic infections begins with the examination of a Gram-stained smear of the specimen (see Fig. 173.1). The appearance of the Gram-stained organisms will give important preliminary information regarding the types of organism present, suggest appropriate initial therapy and serve as a quality control on the final culture analysis. The laboratory should be able to recover all of the morphologic types in the approximate ratio in which they are seen.

The techniques for cultivation of anaerobes should provide optimal anaerobic conditions throughout processing. Detailed procedures of these methods can be found in microbiology manuals.[4] Briefly, these methods could be the prereduced tube method, the anaerobic glove-box technique (Fig. 173.6), which provides an anaerobic environment throughout processing, or the anaerobic jar or bag systems, which are more simplified.

As a minimum requirement for the recovery of anaerobes, specimens should be inoculated onto enriched blood agar medium (containing vitamin K1 and hemin) and a selective medium (for *Bacteroides* spp.), such as laked sheep blood agar with kanamycin and vancomycin, should be used. The use of a selective medium along with a nonselective one increases the recovery rate and can shorten the time to identification of organisms.

Although prereduced vitamin K1-enriched thioglycolate broth is generally used as a back-up culture, this medium alone should never be used as a substitute for a solid medium. The major limitation of liquid media is the possibility of overgrowth of slow-growing strict anaerobes by rapid-growing aerobic and facultative organisms. Selective media can supplement nonselective media in increasing the bacterial yield and facilitating recovery.

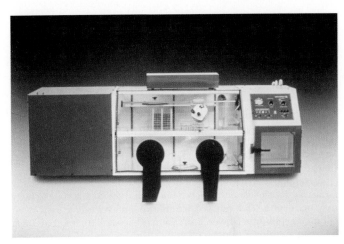

Fig. 173.6 Anaerobic glove-box used in the microbiology laboratory for processing of specimens and identifying anaerobic bacteria. Courtesy of Mike Cox.

Cultures should be placed immediately under anaerobic conditions and incubated for 48 hours or longer. Plates should then be examined for approximate number and types of colonies present. Each colony type should be isolated, tested for aerotolerance and identified.

An additional period of 36–48 hours is generally required to identify completely the anaerobic bacteria to a species or genus level using biochemical tests. Kits containing these biochemical tests are commercially available. These are good with fast-growing anaerobes (i.e. *B. fragilis* and *C. perfringens*). Rapid enzymatic tests have recently been introduced. This panel test enables identification of the anaerobes after only 4 hours of aerobic incubation and seems to be as good as the biochemical tests. Other rapid tests that have potential use and can also be used directly on clinical isolates are direct fluorescent microscopy and direct gas–liquid chromatography. Direct fluorescent microscopy can identify *Actinomyces* spp. and *Propionibacterium propionicus*. This method is inaccurate in identification of *B. fragilis* group, pigmented *Prevotella* and *Porphyromonas* spp. Gas–liquid chromatography of metabolites can be employed to assist in the identification of anaerobes. Direct cellular fatty acid analysis using gas–liquid chromatography with capillary column can also be useful. Nucleic acid probes and PCR methods are also being developed for rapid identification of anaerobic bacteria.

Most clinical microbiology laboratories are able to identify the major anaerobic bacteria. Peptostreptococci are generally not speciated because they are usually susceptible to commonly used antimicrobials. *Clostridium* spp. can be identified by the presence of spores and their ability to survive 30 minutes exposure to ethanol or heating to 176°F (80°C) for 10 minutes. Speciation requires biochemical testing. Nonspore-forming Gram-positive bacilli can be speciated by gas–liquid chromatography and biochemical tests. *Propionibacterium* spp., which are often a contaminant, can be separated from other nonspore-forming Gram-positive bacilli by using a catalyze test and indole reaction. *Bacteroides fragilis* group organisms grow on 20% bile and are generally catalase positive. Pigmented *Prevotella* and *Porphyromonas* spp. produce black or brown pigment within a week when growing on rabbit blood agar medium. *Fusobacterium* spp. have a distinct morphology on Gram stain and, in contrast to *Bacteroides* spp., are susceptible to kanamycin.

Identification of an anaerobe to a species level is often cumbersome, expensive and time-consuming, taking up to 72 hours. Identification is most helpful in selecting an antibiotic against a species that has predictable antibiotic susceptibility. The level of speciation adequate for identifying an anaerobe is often controversial.

Occasionally, species identification of an organism will provide the diagnosis, as with *C. difficile* in patients who have colitis or *C. botulinum* in infants with botulism. However, because most anaerobes are endogenous, there are rarely epidemiologic reasons to perform complete

---

Table 173.8 Bacteriologic findings suggestive of anaerobic infection

Organisms seen on Gram stain that cannot be grown in aerobic cultures

Typical morphology for anaerobes on Gram stain

Anaerobic growth on proper media containing antibiotic-suppressing aerobes

Growth in anaerobic zone of fluid or agar media

Gas, foul-smelling odor in specimen or bacterial culture

Characteristic colonies on anaerobic plates

Colonies of pigmented *Prevotella* or *Porphyromonus* spp. may fluoresce red under ultraviolet light, and older colonies produce a typical dark pigment

identification. Identifying *B. fragilis* group, which often cause bacteremia and septic complications, has significant prognostic value.

Antimicrobial susceptibility testing

The antimicrobial susceptibility of anaerobes has become less predictable. Resistance to several antimicrobials, especially by anaerobic Gram-negative bacilli and *Fusobacterium* spp., has increased over the past decade.[38] It is important, therefore, to perform susceptibility testing for anaerobes recovered from sterile body sites, those with particular epidemiologic or prognostic significance (e.g. *C. difficile*), or those that are clinically important and have variable susceptibilities.

Screening of anaerobic Gram-negative bacilli isolates (particularly *Prevotella*, *Bacteroides* and *Fusobacterium* spp.) for β-lactamase activity may be helpful. This can provide information regarding their penicillin susceptibility. However, occasional bacterial strains may resist β-lactam antibiotics through other mechanisms.

Routine susceptibility testing of all anaerobic isolates is extremely time-consuming and in many cases unnecessary. Susceptibility testing should be limited to anaerobes isolated from blood cultures, bone, CNS and serious infections, as well as to those isolated in pure culture from properly collected specimens. Antibiotics tested should include penicillin, a broad-spectrum penicillin, a penicillin plus a β-lactamase inhibitor, clindamycin, a second-generation cephalosporin (e.g. cefoxitin), an extended-spectrum fluoroquinolone, tigecycline, metronidazole and a carbapenem (e.g. imipenem).

The method recommended by the Clinical and Laboratory Standards Institute (CLSI), formerly the National Committee for Clinical Laboratory Standards (NCCLS), includes agar dilution testing, microbroth and macrobroth dilution.[47] Newer methods include the E-test and the spiral gradient end-point system.

CLINICAL MANIFESTATIONS

Anaerobic bacteria have been recovered in infections at all anatomic locations. However, their frequency of isolation and the types of bacterial isolate depend on the microbial flora at their source or at the adjacent mucocutaneous sites.

Central nervous system infections

Anaerobic bacteria can cause a variety of intracranial infections. These organisms induce brain abscess, subdural empyema and infrequently cause epidural abscess and meningitis. The main source of brain abscess is an adjacent, generally chronic infection in the ears, mastoids, sinuses, oropharynx, teeth or lungs.[48] Ear or mastoid infection tends to spread to the temporal lobe or cerebellum, whereas facial sinusitis often causes abscess of the frontal lobe. Hematogenous spread often occurs after dental, oropharyngeal or pulmonary infection. Rarely bacteremia of another origin or endocarditis can lead to such infection.

Meningitis caused by anaerobes is rare and can follow respiratory infection or develop as a complication of a cerebrospinal fluid shunt. Shunt infections are generally caused by skin flora such as *Prop. acnes*,[11] or in instances of ventriculoperitoneal shunts that perforate the gut, by anaerobes of enteric origin (i.e. *B. fragilis*).[49] *Clostridium perfringens* has been reported as a cause of brain abscesses and meningitis after head injuries or after intracranial surgery.[2]

The anaerobic bacteria generally recovered from brain abscesses that complicate respiratory and dental infections include *Prevotella*, *Porphyromonas*, *Bacteroides*, *Fusobacterium* and *Peptostreptococcus* spp. Microaerophilic and other streptococci are also often isolated. Actinomyces are less frequently encountered.

At the stage of encephalitis, antimicrobial therapy accompanied by measures to control the increase in intracranial pressure can prevent abscess formation. Once an abscess has formed, surgical excision or drainage may be needed, combined with a long course of

antibiotics (4–8 weeks). Some neurosurgeons advocate complete evacuation of the abscess, whereas others advocate repeated aspirations.[50] In patients who have multiple abscesses or in those who have abscesses in essential brain areas, repeated aspirations are preferable. High-dose antibiotics for an extended period may represent an alternative approach in this group of patients and have often replaced surgical drainage.[50]

Because of the difficulty involved in the penetration of various antimicrobial agents through the blood–brain barrier, the choice of antibiotics is restricted. The antimicrobials advocated for these infections are metronidazole, penicillins, meropenem and chloramphenicol. However, the choice may vary according to the specific isolates and their susceptibilities. A significant improvement in the mortality rate has been associated with the introduction of computed tomography (CT) and use of metronidazole therapy.

Head and neck and upper respiratory tract infections

Anaerobic bacteria can be recovered from a variety of head and neck and upper respiratory tract infections and predominate more in their chronic forms (Table 173.9). These include chronic otitis media, sinusitis and mastoiditis, tonsillar, peritonsillar and retropharyngeal abscesses, all deep neck space infections, parotitis, sialadenitis, thyroiditis, odontogenic infections, and postsurgical and nonsurgical head and neck wounds and abscesses. The predominant organisms are of oropharyngeal flora origin and include *Prevotella*, *Porphyromonas*, *Bacteroides*, *Fusobacterium* and *Peptostreptococcus* spp.

Most dental infections involve anaerobes. These include endodontal pulpitis and periodontal (gingivitis and periodontitis) infections, periapical and dental abscesses, and perimandibular space infection.[28,51] Pulpitis may progress to an abscess and eventually involve the mandible and other neck spaces. In addition to the organisms mentioned above, microaerophilic streptococci and *Streptococcus salivarius* can also be involved.

Vincent's angina (or trench mouth) is a distinct form of ulcerative gingivitis; the causative organisms include *Fusobacterium* spp. and anaerobic spirochetes.[2]

Deep neck infections after oral, dental and pharyngeal infections are usually polymicrobial. These include mediastinitis after perforation of the esophagus, extension of retropharyngeal abscess or cellulitis, and dental abscess.[52]

Otitis media

Anaerobes were isolated in 5–15% of patients who had acute otitis media[52a] and 42% of culture-positive aspirates of patients who had serous otitis media.[52b] The predominant isolates in acute otitis media were *Peptostreptococcus* spp. and *Peptostreptococcus acnes*. These organisms, as well as Gram-negative anaerobic bacilli, were recovered in serous otitis media.

Several studies reported the recovery of anaerobes in about 50% of the patients who have chronic suppurative otitis media.[3,5,52c,d] The infection is often polymicrobial and the predominant anaerobes were Gram-negative bacilli and peptostreptococci, and the common aerobes were *Pseudomonas aeruginosa* and *Staph. aureus*. Many of these organisms can produce β-lactamase and might have contributed to the high failure rate of β-lactam antibiotics in the therapy of this infection. Anaerobes were isolated from 23 out of 24 (96%) specimens of chronic mastoiditis[52e] and from most patients who have intracranial abscesses that complicate chronic suppurative otitis media.[3,5,48]

Anaerobes were recovered from infected cholesteatomas.[52f,g] The production of organic acids by anaerobic bacteria may promote the process of bone destruction in cholesteatoma.[52g] Because infected cholesteatoma contains bacteria similar to those recovered from chronically infected ears, it may serve as a nidus for chronic infection.

Table 173.9 Aerobic and anaerobic bacteria isolated in head and neck and upper respiratory tract infections

Type of infection	Aerobic and facultative organisms	Anaerobic organism
Otitis media and mastoiditis: acute chronic	*Streptococcus pneumoniae* *Haemophilus influenzae** *Moraxella catarrhalis** *Staphylococcus aureus** *Escherichia coli** *Klebsiella pneumoniae** *Pseudomonas aeruginosa**	*Peptostreptococcus* spp. Pigmented *Prevotella* and *Porphyromonas* spp.* *Bacteroides* spp.* *Fusobacterium* spp.* *Peptostreptococcus* spp.
Peritonsillar and retropharyngeal abscess	*Streptococcus pyogenes* *Staphylococcus aureus**	*Fusobacterium* spp.* Pigmented *Prevotella* and *Porphyromonas* spp.*
Recurrent tonsillitis	*Streptococcus pyogenes* *Haemophilus influenzae** *Staphylococcus aureus**	*Fusobacterium* spp.*
Suppurative thyroiditis	*Streptococcus pyogenes* *Staphylococcus aureus**	Pigmented *Prevotella* and *Porphyromonas* spp.* *Peptostreptococcus* spp.
Sinusitis: acute chronic	*Haemophilus influenzae** *Streptococcus pneumoniae* *Moraxella catarrhalis** *Staphylococcus aureus** *Streptococcus pneumoniae* *Haemophilus influenzae**	*Peptostreptococcus* spp. Pigmented *Prevotella* and *Porphyromonas* spp.* *Fusobacterium* spp.* *Bacteroides fragilis* group*
Cervical lymphadenitis	*Staphylococcus aureus** *Mycobacterium* spp.	Pigmented *Prevotella* and *Porphyromonas* spp.* *Peptostreptococcus* spp.
Postoperative infection disrupting oral mucosa	*Staphylococcus* spp.* Enterobacteriaceae* *Streptococcus pyogenes*	*Fusobacterium* spp.* *Bacteroides* spp.* Pigmented *Prevotella* and *Porphyromonas* spp.* *Peptostreptococcus* spp.
Deep neck abscesses and parotitis	*Streptococcus* spp. *Staphylococcus* spp.*	*Bacteroides* spp.* *Fusobacterium* spp.* *Peptostreptococcus* spp.*
Odontogenic complications	*Streptococcus* spp. *Staphylococcus* spp.*	Pigmented *Prevotella* and *Porphyromonas* spp.* *Peptostreptococcus* spp.
Oropharyngeal: Vincent's angina and necrotizing	*Streptococcus* spp. *Staphylococcus* spp.*	*Fusobacterium necrophorum**

* Organisms that have the potential of producing β-lactamase.

Sinusitis

Sinus disease may develop when allergy, viral infection, or anatomic obstruction occurs, preventing normal drainage. In the first stages of infection, the most common pathogens are similar to those recovered in acute otitis media: *Streptococcus pneumoniae, Haemophilus influenzae* and *Moraxella catarrhalis*. Anaerobic organisms become involved as the infection becomes chronic and the levels of tissue oxygen decline.[52h] The transition in the bacterial flora from aerobic to anaerobic flora has been demonstrated.[52i] An elevated serum antibody level to *Prevotella* and *Fusbacterium* spp. was demonstrated in patients with chronic sinusitis.[52j] Although anaerobes are generally isolated from only about 7% of patients who have acute sinusitis (generally in maxillary sinusitis secondary to periodontal infection), they can be isolated from up to 67% of patients who have chronic infection.[3,5,52k] An average of three anaerobes per aspirate were recovered in patients who had chronic sinusitis.[52l]

Sinus infection may spread via anastomosing veins or contiguously to the CNS. Complications include orbital cellulitis,[52m] meningitis, cavernous sinus thrombosis, and epidural, subdural and brain abscesses.[3,5]

Parotitis

Viral parotitis can be caused by paramyxovirus (mumps), Epstein–Barr virus, coxsackievirus, HIV, and influenza A and parainfluenza virus. Acute suppurative parotitis is generally caused by *Staph. aureus*, streptococci and, rarely, aerobic Gram-negative bacteria. Anaerobes, mostly *Peptostreptococcus, Bacteroides*, and pigmented *Prevotella* and *Porphyromonas* spp., have also been recognized as an important cause of this infection.[52n] Empiric antibiotic therapy should be directed against both aerobic and anaerobic bacteria. Surgical drainage may be indicated when pus has formed.

Cervical lymphadenitis

The anterior cervical, the submandibular or the posterior cervical nodes are the most prevalent sites of infection. The most common causes in children are viruses. The organisms causing acute unilateral infection associated with facial trauma or impetigo are *Staph. aureus* and *Streptococcus pyogenes*. *Bartonella henselae* and mycobacterial infections are important in chronic infections. Anaerobes (mostly *Fusobacterium* and *Peptostreptococcus* spp.) were isolated in about 25%

of the infections, often in pure culture.[27] Their recovery was associated with a primary dental, periodontal or tonsillar infection.

Infection after head and neck surgery

Infections after head and neck surgery are caused by the exposure of the surgical site to the oropharyngeal flora, by the decreased blood supply and by the presence of necrotic tissue. They are common after surgery for malignant tumors. The wounds are generally infected by polymicrobial aerobic and anaerobic flora; the average number of isolates varies from one to nine (average six).[53] The most common isolates are peptostreptococci, *Staph. aureus*, anaerobic Gram-negative bacilli (i.e. *Bacteroides* spp.), *Fusobacterium* spp. and Enterobacteriaceae. The presence of this flora warrants the use of antimicrobial agents that are effective against these organisms in the prophylaxis and therapy of this infection.[54]

Tonsillitis

Indirect evidence is mounting that anaerobes are involved in both acute and chronic tonsillitis. The evidence is mainly derived from studies of complications of anaerobic tonsillitis (i.e. bacteremia, abscesses) where anaerobes play a major role. The organisms associated with the infection are *Fusobacterium* spp., peptostreptococci and Gram-negative anaerobic bacilli. Polymicrobial flora predominate in peritonsillar and retropharyngeal abscesses, where the number of isolates is between one and 12 (average five anaerobes and two aerobes).[3,5,55] Anaerobes have also been isolated from the cores of tonsils of children with recurrent group A β-hemolytic streptococci (GABHS) infection[23,46,56] and non-GABHS tonsillitis.[56] These organisms can be isolated from 25% of suppurative cervical lymph nodes and are mostly associated with the presence of dental or tonsillar infections.[27] Anaerobic organisms were associated with thrombophlebitis of the internal jugular veins, which often causes postanginal sepsis.[3,5]

The pathogenic role of anaerobes in the acute inflammatory process in the tonsils is also supported by several clinical observations:

- their recovery in tonsillar or retropharyngeal abscesses, often without any aerobic bacteria;[55]
- their isolation from tonsils in Vincent's angina;[5]
- the recovery of encapsulated pigmented *Prevotella* and *Porphyromonas* spp. in acutely inflamed tonsils;
- the isolation of anaerobes from the core of recurrently inflamed non-GABHS tonsils;[56] and
- the response to antibiotics in patients who have non-GABHS tonsillitis.[57,58]

Furthermore, immune response against *Prev. intermedia* can be detected in patients who have non-GABHS tonsillitis[59] and against *Prev. intermedia* and *F. nucleatum* in patients who recovered from peritonsillar cellulitis or abscesses[60] and infectious mononucleosis.[61]

Metronidazole therapy alleviated the symptoms of tonsillar hypertrophy and shortened the duration of fever in patients who had infectious mononucleosis.[57] Because metronidazole has no antiviral or aerobic antibacterial efficacy, suppression of the oral anaerobic flora may contribute to diminishing the inflammation induced by the Epstein–Barr virus. This is supported by the increased recovery of *Prev. intermedia* and *F. nucleatum* during the acute phases of mononucleosis.[62]

Recurrent pharyngotonsillitis and failure to eradicate the GABHS with penicillin can be a serious clinical problem. One explanation for penicillin failure is that repeated administrations result in selection of BLPB.[46] β-Lactamase-producing strains of pigmented *Prevotella* and *Porphyromonas* spp., *B. fragilis*, *Fusobacterium* spp., *Haemophilus influenzae* and *Staph. aureus* were isolated from the tonsils of more than 75% of children with recurrent GABHS tonsillitis[23,46,63,64] and from 40% of children with non-GABHS tonsillitis.[56] Similar organisms were recovered from patients who had adenoiditis and adenoid hypertrophy.[65]

The recovery of these bacteria in more than three-quarters of the patients who had recurrent GABHS tonsillitis,[46,63,64] the ability to measure β-lactamase activity in the core of these tonsils[66] and the response of patients to antimicrobials effective against BLPB (i.e. clindamycin

or amoxicillin plus clavulanic acid)[46,67,68] support the role of these aerobic as well as anaerobic organisms in the inability of penicillin to eradicate GABHS tonsillitis.

Pleuropulmonary infections

Aspiration of oropharyngeal secretions or gastric contents, and severe periodontal or gingival disease are the most prevalent risk factors for developing anaerobic pleuropulmonary secretion. The infection can progress from pneumonitis into necrotizing pneumonia and pulmonary abscess, with or without empyema.[69] The lesions tend to develop in the dependent pulmonary segments, in either of the superior segments of the lower lobes and in the posterior segments of the upper lobes. The infection is generally polymicrobial where the causative organisms of community-acquired infection (in 60–80% of cases) are aerobic and anaerobic members of oropharyngeal flora. The anaerobes isolated are *Prevotella*, *Porphyromonas*, *Fusobacterium* and *Peptostreptococcus* spp., and the aerobes are β-hemolytic streptococci and microaerophilic streptococci (Table 173.10).[70] Anaerobes can also be recovered in about one-third of patients who have nosocomial-acquired aspiration pneumonia and pneumonia associated with tracheostomy with and without mechanical ventilation,[71] where they are generally recovered mixed with Enterobacteriaceae, *Pseudomonas* spp. and *Staph. aureus*. Specimens for culture should be obtained in a manner that will avoid their contamination by the oral flora. They can be obtained using bronchoalveolar lavage, bronchoscopy via bronchial brush protected in a double-lumen plugged catheter (using quantitative cultures in the last two methods), percutaneous transtracheal aspiration, lung biopsy and thoracentesis (of empyema fluid). Management of these infections includes drainage of the pleural space in the presence of empyema, and antimicrobials effective against the anaerobic and aerobic bacteria (see Chapter 29).

Intra-abdominal infections

Secondary peritonitis and intra-abdominal abscesses generally occur because of the entry of enteric micro-organisms into the peritoneal cavity through a defect in the wall of the intestine or other viscus as a result of obstruction, infarction or direct trauma. Perforated appendicitis, inflammatory bowel disease with perforation and gastrointestinal surgery are often associated with polymicrobial infections caused by aerobic and anaerobic bacteria, where the number of isolates can average 12 (two-thirds are generally anaerobes). Diverticulitis and its complications is also associated with such an infection.[72]

The initial infection that follows perforation is peritonitis. This is a synergistic infection in which more than one organism is involved. Characteristically, the more types of bacteria that can be isolated, the graver the morbidity. The specific micro-organisms involved in peritonitis are generally those of the gastrointestinal tract flora where anaerobes outnumber aerobes in the ratio 1:1000–10 000.[1] Of the more than 400 bacterial species that constitute the gut flora, only the virulent ones survive in the peritoneum to cause the infection. The more distal the perforation in the gastrointestinal tract, the more numerous are the types and number of organisms that spill into the peritoneal cavity. An average of 11.6 organisms per specimen (8.5 anaerobes and 3.1 nonanaerobes) was recovered in a study of 71 patients with gangrenous and perforated appendicitis.[73] The predominant aerobic and facultatives are *E. coli* and *Streptococcus* spp. (including *Enterococcus* spp.), and the most frequently encountered anaerobes are the *B. fragilis* group, and *Peptostreptococcus*, *Clostridium*, *Fusobacterium* and *Eubacterium* spp. (see Table 173.10).[3,5]

Intra-abdominal infections are characteristically biphasic: in the initial stages a generalized peritonitis occurs, which is primarily associated with *E. coli* sepsis, and in the later stages, in which the infection is contained and intra-abdominal abscesses emerge, *B. fragilis* can be recovered.[74]

The clinical manifestations of secondary peritonitis are a reflection of the underlying disease process. Fever, diffuse abdominal pain, nausea and vomiting are characteristic. Physical examination reveals signs of peritoneal inflammation, including rebound tenderness, abdominal wall rigidity and decrease in bowel sounds. These early findings may be followed by signs and symptoms of shock.

Table 173.10 Aerobic and anaerobic bacteria isolated in various types of infection

Type of infection	Aerobic and facultative organisms	Anaerobic organism
Pleuropulmonary	*Staphylococcus aureus** viridans streptococci *Pseudomonas aeruginosa** Enterobacteriaceae*	Pigmented *Prevotella* spp. (*P. denticola, P. melaninogenica,* *P. intermedia, P. nigrescens, P. loescheii*) Nonpigmented *Prevotella* spp. (*P. oris, P. buccae, P. oralis*) *Fusobacterium nucleatum* *Peptostreptococcus* spp. (*P. micros, P. anaerobius, P. magnus*) *Bacteroides fragilis* group Nonspore-forming Gram-positive rods (*Actinomyces, Eubacterium,* *Lactobacillus* spp.)
Intra-abdominal	*Escherichia coli* *Enterococcus* spp. *Pseudomonas aeruginosa**	*Bacteroides fragilis* group *Bilophila wadsworthia* *Peptostreptococcus* spp. (especially *P. micros*) *Clostridium* spp.
Female genital tract	*Streptococcus* (groups A, B, others) *Escherichia coli* *Klebsiella pneumoniae* *Neisseria gonorrhoeae* (in sexually active patients) *Chlamydia* spp. (in sexually active patients) *Mycoplasma hominis* (in postpartum patients)	*Peptostreptococcus* spp. *Prevotella* spp. (especially *P. bivia, P. disiens*) *Bacteroides fragilis* group *Clostridium* spp. (especially *C. perfringens*) *Actinomyces, Eubacterium* spp. (in intrauterine contraceptive device-associated infections)
Skin and soft tissue	*Staphylococcus aureus* *Streptococcus* (*Strep. milleri group*, groups A and B, viridans group) *Enterococcus* spp.[‡] Enterobacteriaceae[‡] *Pseudomonas aeruginosa**	*Peptostreptococcus* spp. (*P. magnus, P. micros, P. asaccharolyticus*) Pigmented *Prevotella* spp.[†] *Actinomyces* spp. *Fusobacterium nucleatum*[†] *Bacteroides fragilis* group[‡] *Clostridium* spp.[‡]

* Recovered in hospital-acquired infection.
[†] After exposure to oral flora.
[‡] After exposure to colonic flora.

The manifestations of shock from a ruptured viscus merge with those of peritonitis and may be followed by toxemia, restlessness and irritability, a higher temperature, an increase in pulse rate, chills and convulsions. Biliary tract infection is caused by *E. coli, Klebsiella* and *Enterococcus* spp. Anaerobes (mostly *B. fragilis* group and rarely *C. perfringens*) can be recovered in complicated infections associated with carcinoma, recurrent infection, obstruction, bile tract surgery or manipulation.[75]

Laboratory studies reveal an elevated blood leukocyte count in excess of $12\,000/mm^3$ with a predominance of polymorphonuclear forms. Radiographs of the abdomen may reveal free air in the peritoneal cavity, evidence of ileus or obstruction and obliteration of the psoas shadow. Diagnostic ultrasound, gallium and CT scanning[76] may be useful in detecting appendiceal or other intra-abdominal abscesses. Postoperative wound infections can occur after appendectomy.

Appropriate management of mixed aerobic and anaerobic intra-abdominal infections requires the administration of antimicrobials that are effective against both aerobic and anaerobic components of the infection[2,5] as well as surgical correction and drainage of pus.[77] Single and easily accessible abscesses can be drained percutaneously, thus avoiding a surgical procedure. The outcome of the infection depends on a variety of factors that include the general condition of the patient (as measured by the Apache score[78]), the site of perforation, the bacteriology of the infection and the antimicrobial chosen for therapy. The principle of using antimicrobial coverage effective against both the aerobic and anaerobic offenders has become the cornerstone of practice and its efficacy has been confirmed by numerous studies.[77]

The choice of therapy should cover Enterobacteriaceae and anaerobes (mainly *B. fragilis* group), and can be achieved by combination or single-agent therapy. Single-agent therapy provides the advantage of avoiding the ototoxicity and nephrotoxicity of aminoglycosides and may be less expensive. However, a single agent may not be effective against hospital-acquired resistant bacterial strains, and the use of a single agent is devoid of antibacterial synergy, which may be important

in immunocompromised hosts. However, for otherwise healthy persons, when therapy is initiated without a long delay, single agents provide adequate therapy. An anti-Enterobacteriaceae agent, such as an aminoglycoside, a quinolone or a third-generation cephalosporin, plus an anti-anaerobic agent, such as clindamycin, metronidazole or cefoxitin, is used as combination therapy. Single-agent therapy includes a carbapenem (e.g. imipenem, meropenem, ertapenem), tigecycline, or a penicillin plus a β-lactamase inhibitor (i.e. ticarcillin–clavulanate).[77] The need to add therapy directed at *Enterococcus* spp. is controversial and some authorities advocate adding such a drug (i.e. amoxicillin or vancomycin). However, these organisms are isolated in only 10–20% of cases and rarely in pure culture (see also Chapter 37).

Antimicrobial prophylaxis before colonic surgery includes either an oral preparation such as erythromycin plus neomycin or a parenteral antimicrobial such as cefoxitin. Use of prophylaxis has reduced the rate of postsurgical wound infection (see also Chapter 132).[79]

Female genital tract infection

Female genital tract infections involving anaerobes are polymicrobial and include the following: bacterial vaginosis; soft-tissue perineal, vulvar and Bartholin gland abscesses; endometritis; pyometra; salpingitis; tubo-ovarian abscesses; adnexal abscess; pelvic inflammatory disease, which may include pelvic cellulitis and abscess; amnionitis; septic pelvic thrombophlebitis; intrauterine contraceptive device-associated infection; septic abortion; and postsurgical obstetric and gynecologic infections.[3,5,80,81] Obtaining proper cultures is often difficult, and avoiding their contamination by the normal genital flora can be achieved by use of culdocentesis, laparoscopy or quantitative endometrial cultures of transcervical samples obtained with a telescoping catheter.

The predominant anaerobes include *Prev. bivia, Prev. disiens* and *Peptostreptococcus, Porphyromonas* and *Clostridium* spp. *Bacteroides fragilis* group is less often isolated in these infections than in intra-abdominal infection.[81] *Actinomyces* spp. and *Eubacterium nodatum* are commonly isolated in infections associated with intrauterine devices. *Mobiluncus* spp. may be involved with bacterial vaginosis.[3,5,80] The aerobic organisms also isolated mixed with these anaerobes include Enterobacteriaceae, *Streptococcus* spp. (including groups A and B), *Neisseria gonnorhoeae* and *Chlamydia* spp. (in sexually active females) and *Mycoplasma hominis* (see Table 173.10).

Clinical findings associated with the presence of anaerobes include gas in the tissues, abscess formation and foul-smelling discharge. Management of polymicrobial pelvic infection includes the use of anti-microbials effective against all potential aerobic and anaerobic pathogens. Additionally, coverage against sexually transmissible pathogens should be provided. The therapeutic regimens include doxycycline, levofloxacin or gentamicin in combination with cefoxitin, cefotetan, ampicillin–sulbactam, clindamycin or metronidazole.[82]

Skin and soft-tissue infections

Skin and soft-tissue infections that generally involve anaerobes include superficial infections, such as infected cutaneous ulcers, cellulitis, pyoderma, paronychia, hidradenitis suppurativa and a variety of secondary infected sites. These include secondary infected diaper rash, gastrostomy or tracheostomy site wounds, infected subcutaneous sebaceous or inclusion cysts, eczema, psoriasis, poison ivy, atopic dermatitis, eczema herpeticum, scabies or kerion infections, and post-surgical wound infection.[3,5,83–86]

Subcutaneous tissue infections that may also include skin involvement include cutaneous and subcutaneous abscesses, breast abscess, decubitus ulcers, infected diabetic (vascular or trophic) ulcers (Fig. 173.7), bite wound (Fig. 173.8), anaerobic cellulitis (Fig. 173.9) and gas gangrene, bacterial synergistic gangrene, infected pilonidal cyst or sinus, Meleney's ulcer and burn wound infection.[84,86] Anaerobic soft-tissue infections that occur deeper are necrotizing fasciitis (see Fig. 10.5), necrotizing synergistic cellulitis, gas gangrene and crepitus cellulitis.[87] These infections can involve the fascia and the muscle surrounded by the fascia, and can induce myositis (Fig. 173.10) and myonecrosis.

The organisms recovered from soft-tissue infections vary according to the type of infection. However, the location and the circumstances leading to the infection can influence the type of organism involved in the infection. Cultures from lesions involving anaerobes frequently contain bacterial species that are members of the 'normal flora' of the region of the infection (Fig. 173.11).

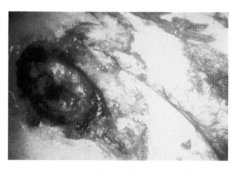

Fig. 173.9 Polymicrobial necrotizing cellulitis. The initial lesion is a reddish-brown bleb and is accompanied by local tenderness.

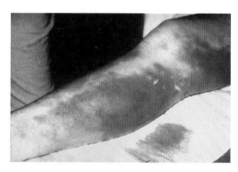

Fig. 173.10 Anaerobic streptococcal myositis involving muscle and fascial planes.

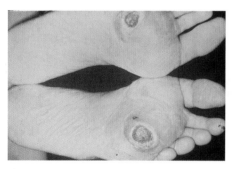

Fig. 173.7 Infected diabetic ulcer.

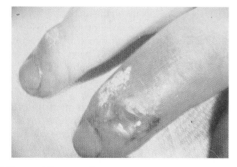

Fig. 173.8 Human bite wound.

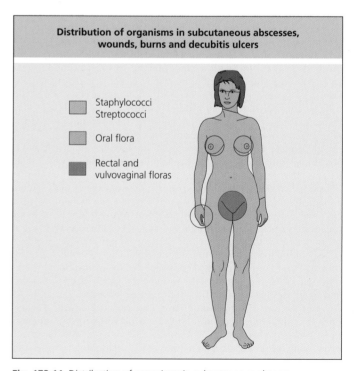

Distribution of organisms in subcutaneous abscesses, wounds, burns and decubitis ulcers

- Staphylococci Streptococci
- Oral flora
- Rectal and vulvovaginal floras

Fig. 173.11 Distribution of organisms in subcutaneous abscesses, wounds, burns and decubitis ulcers.

Aspirates from wounds and subcutaneous tissue infections and abscesses of the rectal area (decubitus ulcer, perirectal abscess) or those that originate from the gut flora (i.e. diabetic foot infection) tend to yield organisms found in the colonic flora.[3,5,84–87] These include *B. fragilis* group, *Clostridium* spp., Enterobacteriaceae and *Enterococcus* spp. In contrast, infections in and around the oropharynx, or those that originate from that site, generally contain members of the oral flora (i.e. paronychia, bites, breast abscess). These include pigmented *Prevotella* and *Porphyromonas*, *Fusobacterium* and *Peptostreptococcus* spp. Skin flora organisms such as *Staph. aureus* and *Streptococcus* spp. or nosocomially acquired organisms can be isolated at all body sites (see Table 173.10). In addition to oral flora, human bite infections often contain *Eikenella* spp. and animal bites harbor *Pasteurella multocida*.[88]

Infections involving anaerobes are generally polymicrobial, and in some (i.e. decubitus ulcers, diabetic foot ulcer) they are often complicated by osteomyelitis or bacteremia.[89] Deep tissue infections such as necrotizing cellulitis, fasciitis and myositis often involve *Clostridium* spp., *Strep. pyogenes* or a polymicrobial combination of aerobic and anaerobic bacteria. They often contain gas in the tissues and putrid-like pus with a gray thin quality, and are associated with a high rate of bacteremia and mortality.[87,90]

Management of deep-seated soft-tissue infection includes surgical debridement, drainage and vigorous surgical management. Improvement of oxygenation of the involved tissues through enhancement of blood supply and administration of hyperbaric oxygen, especially in clostridial infection, may be helpful, although there is no formal evidence demonstrating the benefit of hyperbaric oxygen.

Osteomyelitis and septic arthritis

Osteomyelitis caused by anaerobic bacteria is often indistinguishable from infection caused by aerobic bacteria. Anaerobes are especially notable in osteomyelitis of the long bones after trauma and fracture, osteomyelitis related to peripheral vascular disease, and decubitus ulcers and osteomyelitis of cranial and facial bones.[89,91] Most of these infections are polymicrobial.

Anaerobic osteomyelitis of cranial and facial bones is generally caused by spread from a contiguous soft-tissue source or from sinus, ear or dental infection. The high number of anaerobes within the oral flora accounts for their importance in cranial osteomyelitis. The predominance of intestinal anaerobes in pelvic osteomyelitis has been related to their spread from decubitus ulcers.[5] The anaerobes in osteomyelitis associated with peripheral vascular disease access the involved bone from adjacent soft-tissue ulcers. Osteomyelitis of long bones is generally caused by hematogenic spread, trauma or the presence of a prosthetic device.

Anaerobic streptococci and *Bacteroides* spp. are the most common organisms at all sites, including osteomyelitis associated with bites and cranial infection. Pigmented *Prevotella* and *Porphyromonas* spp. are especially prevalent in skull and bite infections, whereas members of the *B. fragilis* group are associated with vascular disease or neuropathy. Fusobacteria, which are members of the oral flora, are most frequently isolated from bites and from cranial and facial infections. Clostridia are most often found in long bones, especially in association with environmental wound contamination after trauma. Because clostridia colonize the lower gastrointestinal tract, they may contaminate compound fractures of the lower extremities.

Septic arthritis caused by anaerobic bacteria is uncommon, and is often associated with hematogenous and contiguous spread of infection, trauma and prosthetic joints.[79,82] Most cases of septic arthritis caused by anaerobes are monomicrobial. The predominant isolated anaerobes are peptostreptococci and *Prop. acnes* (often in prosthetic joint infection), *B. fragilis* and fusobacteria (often in infections of hematogenic origin), and clostridia (associated with trauma).

Bacteremia

The incidence of anaerobes in bacteremia is 5–15%.[90] However, in the 1990s the incidence was lowered to approximately 4% (0.5–12%) of all cases of bacteremia, with variation by geographic location, hospital patient demographics and especially patient age.[92] Recent studies, however, documented a resurgence in bacteremia due to anaerobic bacteria.[93] This increase is explained by the higher incidence of anaerobic bacteremia in immunosuppressed patients and patients with complex underlying disease.[93] The most prevalent blood culture isolates are *B. fragilis* group (over 75% of anaerobic isolates). Other common isolates include *Clostridium* spp. (10–20%), *Peptostreptococcus* spp. (10–15%), *Fusobacterium* spp. (10–15%) and *Prop. acnes* (2–5%).

The specific organisms involved in bacteremia largely depend on the portal of entry and underlying disease. Recovery of *B. fragilis* group and clostridia is mostly associated with a gastrointestinal source, pigmented *Prevotella* and *Porphyromonas* spp. and fusobacteria with oropharynx and pulmonary sources, fusobacteria with the female genital tract, *Prop. acnes* with foreign body, and peptostreptococci with all sources, but especially with oropharyngeal, pulmonary and female genital tract sources. The predominance of these isolates in conjunction with the specific sources is related to the origin of the primary infection and the endogenous flora at the infection site.

The predisposing factors to anaerobic bacterial bacteremia include malignant neoplasms; hematologic disorders; organ transplant; recent gastrointestinal, obstetric, or gynecologic surgery; intestinal obstruction; decubitus ulcers; dental extraction; the newborn; sickle cell disease; diabetes mellitus; postsplenectomy; and the use of cytotoxic agents or corticosteroids.[3,5]

The clinical presentation of anaerobic bacteremia is similar to that seen with aerobic infection, except for the signs of infection at the portal of entry of infection. It commonly includes fever, chills, hypotension, leukocytosis, shock, disseminated intravascular coagulation and anemia. Features typical of anaerobic infection include metastatic lesions, hyperbilirubinemia and suppurative thrombophlebitis. Mortality rate varies between 15% and 30% and is improved with early and appropriate antimicrobial therapy and resolution, when present, of the primary infection.

MANAGEMENT

The recovery from an anaerobic infection depends on prompt and proper management. The principles of managing anaerobic infections include neutralizing toxins produced by anaerobes, preventing their local proliferation by changing the environment and hampering their spread into healthy tissues.

Toxin neutralization by specific antitoxins may be employed, especially in infections caused by *Clostridium* spp. (tetanus and botulism). Controlling the environment is achieved by debriding of necrotic tissue, draining the pus, improving circulation, alleviating the obstruction and increasing the tissue oxygenation. Certain types of adjunct therapy such as hyperbaric oxygen (HBO) may also be useful. The primary role of antimicrobials is in limiting the local and systemic spread of the organism.

Hyperbaric oxygen

There is controversy regarding whether HBO should be used in infection of spore-forming Gram-positive anaerobic rods. There are several uncontrolled reports that demonstrated efficacy in individual cases.[3,5,94] However, because no well-controlled studies are available, the efficacy of HBO is unproved. Using HBO in conjunction with other therapeutic measures is not contraindicated, except when it may delay the execution of other essential procedures. Topical application of oxygen-releasing compounds may be useful as an adjunct to other procedures.

Surgical therapy

In many cases surgical therapy is the most important and sometimes the only form of treatment required, whereas in others surgical therapy is an important adjunct to a pharmacologic approach. Surgery is important in draining abscesses, debriding necrotic tissues, decompressing closed space infections and relieving obstructions. When surgical drainage is not used, the infection may persist and serious complications can develop.

Antimicrobial therapy

Appropriate management of mixed aerobic and anaerobic infections requires the administration of antimicrobial drugs effective against both the aerobic and the anaerobic components. A number of factors should be considered when choosing appropriate antimicrobial agents. They should have efficacy against all target organisms, induce little or no resistance, achieve sufficient levels in the infected site, and have minimal toxicity and maximum stability.

Antimicrobials often fail to cure the infection. Among the reasons for this are the development of bacterial resistance, achievement of insufficient tissue levels, incompatible drug interaction and the development of an abscess. The environment of an abscess is detrimental to many antibiotics. The abscess capsule interferes with the penetration of drugs, and the low pH and the presence of binding proteins or inactivating enzymes (i.e. β-lactamase) may impair their activity. The low pH and the anaerobic environment within the abscess are especially unfavorable for the aminoglycosides and quinolones. However, an acidic pH, high osmolarity and an anaerobic environment can also develop in the absence of an abscess.

When choosing antimicrobials (see Table 173.13) for the therapy of mixed infections, their aerobic and anaerobic antibacterial spectrum (Fig. 173.12) and their availability in oral or parenteral form should be considered (Table 173.11). Some antimicrobials have a limited range of activity. For example, metronidazole is active only against anaerobes and therefore cannot be administered as a single agent for the therapy of mixed infections. Others (i.e. carbapenems) have wide spectra of activity against Enterobacteriaceae and anaerobes.

The selection of antimicrobial agents is simplified when reliable culture results are available. However, this may be difficult to achieve in anaerobic infections because of the problems in obtaining appropriate specimens. For this reason, many patients are treated empirically on the basis of suspected, rather than established, pathogens. Fortunately, the types of organism involved in many anaerobic infections and their antimicrobial susceptibility patterns tend to be predictable. However, the pattern of resistance to antimicrobials may vary in a particular hospital and resistance to antimicrobial agents may emerge while a patient is receiving therapy.

The susceptibility of the B. fragilis group to the frequently used antimicrobial drugs has been studied systemically over the past two decades. These surveys have failed to reveal strains resistant to chloramphenicol or metronidazole and minimal resistance (<1%) to

imipenem or the combinations of a penicillin and β-lactamase inhibitors, but resistance to other agents varies. The rate differs among various medical centers and generally increases with extensive use of some antimicrobial agents (penicillins, cephalosporins and clindamycin).[95]

Aside from susceptibility patterns, other factors influencing the choice of antimicrobial therapy include the pharmacologic characteristics of the various drugs, their toxicity, their effect on the normal flora and bactericidal activity. Although identification of the infecting organisms and their antimicrobial susceptibility may be needed for selection of optimal therapy, the clinical setting and Gram-stain preparation of the specimen may indicate the types of anaerobe present in the infection as well as the nature of the infectious process.

Antimicrobial agents

Some classes of agent have poor activity against anaerobic bacteria. These include the aminoglycosides, the monobactams and the currently available quinolones. Antimicrobial agents suitable for use in controlling aerobic infections are discussed in more detail below.[96,97]

Penicillins

Penicillin G (benzylpenicillin) is still the drug of choice against most non-BLPB. These include anaerobic streptococci, Clostridium spp. and nonsporulating anaerobic bacilli, and most non-β-lactamase-producing Gram-negative anaerobic rods (i.e. Bacteroides, Fusobacterium, Prevotella and Porphyromonas spp.).[96] However, in addition to the B. fragilis group, which is known to resist the drug, many other anaerobic Gram-negative rods are showing increased resistance. These include Fusobacterium spp., pigmented Prevotella and Porphyromonas spp. (prevalent in orofacial infections), Prev. bivia and Prev. disiens (common in obstetric and gynecologic infections), and Bilophila wadsworthia and Bacteroides splanchinus. Resistance to penicillin of some Clostridium spp. through production of β-lactamase has also been noted. These included C. ramosum, C. clostridioforme and C. butyricum.

The increase in the number of penicillin-resistant bacterial strains has important implications for antimicrobial therapy. Many penicillin-resistant bacteria can produce enzymes that degrade penicillins or cephalosporins by releasing the enzyme in the area of the infection. Therefore, these organisms may protect not only themselves but also penicillin-sensitive pathogens. Penicillin therapy directed against a susceptible pathogen might therefore be rendered ineffective by the presence of BLPB.[46]

The use of combinations of β-lactamase inhibitors (such as clavulanic acid, sulbactam or tazobactam) plus a β-lactam antibiotic (ampicillin, amoxicillin, ticarcillin or piperacillin) can overcome this phenomenon in organisms that produce a β-lactamase that can be

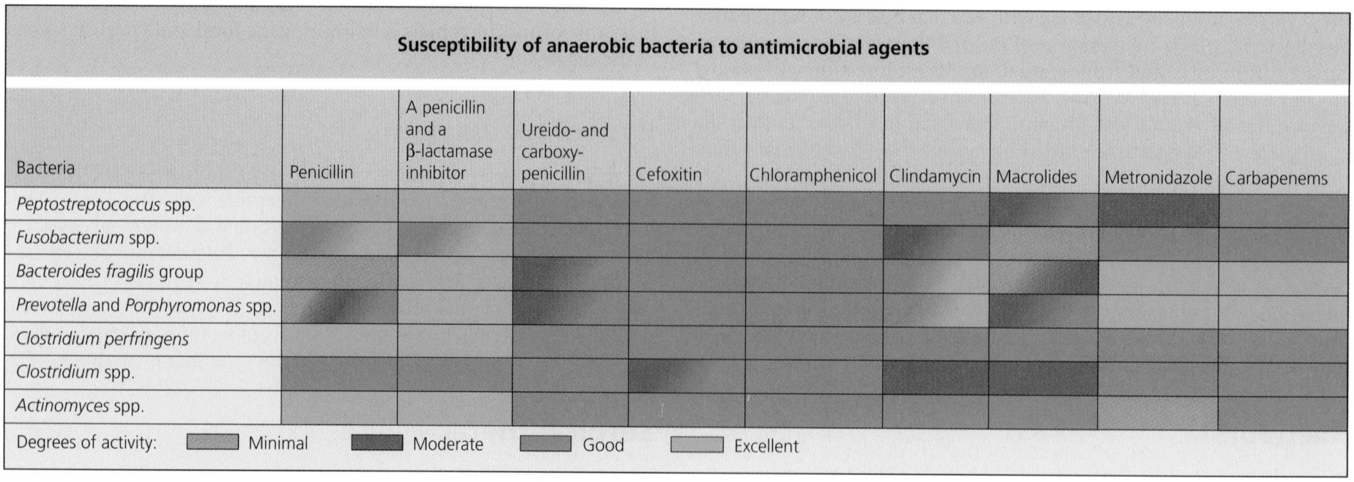

Susceptibility of anaerobic bacteria to antimicrobial agents									
Bacteria	Penicillin	A penicillin and a β-lactamase inhibitor	Ureido- and carboxy-penicillin	Cefoxitin	Chloramphenicol	Clindamycin	Macrolides	Metronidazole	Carbapenems
Peptostreptococcus spp.									
Fusobacterium spp.									
Bacteroides fragilis group									
Prevotella and Porphyromonas spp.									
Clostridium perfringens									
Clostridium spp.									
Actinomyces spp.									

Degrees of activity: ▭ Minimal   ▭ Moderate   ▭ Good   ▭ Excellent

Fig. 173.12 Susceptibility of anaerobic bacteria to antimicrobial agents.

Table 173.11 Antimicrobial drugs recommended for the therapy* of site-specific anaerobic infections

	Surgical prophylaxis	Parenteral	Oral
Intracranial	1. Penicillin 2. Vancomycin	1. Metronidazole[4] 2. Chloramphenicol	1. Metronidazole[4] 2. Chloramphenicol
Dental	1. Penicillin 2. Erythromycin	1. Clindamycin 2. Metronidazole[4], chloramphenicol	1. Clindamycin, amoxicillin + CA 2. Metronidazole[4]
Upper respiratory tract	1. Cefoxitin 2. Clindamycin	1. Clindamycin 2. Chloramphenicol, metronidazole[4]	1. Clindamycin, amoxicillin + CA 2. Metronidazole[5]
Pulmonary	NA	1. Clindamycin[5] 2. Ticarcillin + CA, ampicillin + SU[6], imipenem or meropenem	1. Clindamycin[8] 2. Metronidazole[5], amoxicillin + CA
Abdominal	1. Cefoxitin 2. Clindamycin[3]	1. Clindamycin[3], cefoxitin[3], metronidazole[3] 2. Imipenem or meropenem ertapenem, piperacillin-tazobactam, tigecycline	1. Clindamycin[8], metronidazole[8] 2. Amoxicillin + CA
Pelvic	1. Cefoxitin 2. Doxycycline	1. Cefoxitin[6], clindamycin[3] 2. Piperacillin–tazobactam[6], ampicillin + SU[6], metronidazole[6]	1. Clindamycin[6] 2. Amoxicillin + CA[6], metronidazole[6]
Skin and soft tissue	1. Cefazolin[7] 2. Vancomycin	1. Clindamycin, cefoxitin 2. Metronidazole + vancomycin 3. Tigecycline	1. Clindamycin, amoxicillin + CA 2. Metronidazole + linezolid
Bone and joint	1. Cefazolin[7] 2. Vancomycin	1. Clindamycin, imipenem or meropenem 2. Metronidazole + vancomycin, piperacillin–tazobactam	1. Clindamycin 2. Metronidazole + linezolid
Bacteremia with BLPB	NA	1. Imipenem or meropenem, metronidazole 2. Cefoxitin, ticarcillin + CA	1. Clindamycin, metronidazole 2. Chloramphenicol, amoxicillin + CA
Bacteremia with non-BLPB	NA	1. Penicillin 2. Clindamycin, metronidazole, cefoxitin	1. Penicillin 2. Metronidazole, chloramphenicol, clindamycin

* Therapies are given as drug(s) of choice (alternative drugs). BLPB, β-lactamase-producing bacteria; CA, clavulanic acid; NA, not applicable; SU, sulbactam.
1, drug(s) of choice; 2, alternative drugs; 3, plus aminoglycoside; 4, plus a penicillin; 5, plus a macrolide (i.e. erythromycin); 6, plus doxycycline; 7, in location proximal to the rectal and oral areas use cefoxitin; 8, plus a quinolone (only in adults).

bound by the inhibitor. However, if other mechanisms of resistance emerge, blockage of the enzyme β-lactamase will not prevent resistance. Other mechanisms of resistance include alteration in the porin canal through which the antimicrobial penetrates into the bacteria and changes in the penicillin-binding protein that inhibit binding of the drug into the bacterial cell wall.

The semisynthetic penicillins, carbenicillin, ticarcillin, piperacillin and mezlocillin are generally administered in large quantities to achieve high serum concentrations. These drugs have good activity against Enterobacteriaceae and most anaerobes in these concentrations. However, they are not absolutely resistant to β-lactamase produced by Gram-negative anaerobic bacilli.

Cephalosporins

The efficacy of cephalosporins varies against *Bacteroides* spp.[96,97] The activity of the first-generation cephalosporins against anaerobes is similar to that of penicillin G, although on a weight basis they are less active. Most strains of the *B. fragilis* group and many *Prevotella* and *Porphyromonas* spp. are resistant by virtue of cephalosporinase production. The second-generation cephalosporin cefoxitin is relatively resistant to this enzyme and is therefore the most effective cephalosporin against the *B. fragilis* group. However, 5–15% of *B. fragilis* group may be resistant, reflecting hospital use pattern. Because of its wide antibacterial coverage, it is often used for the therapy and prophylaxis of mixed infections. Cefoxitin is relatively inactive against most species of *Clostridium* (including *C. difficile*); *C. perfringens* is an exception.

Other second-generation cephalosporins, such as cefotetan and cefmetazole, have a longer half-life than cefoxitin. These two agents are as effective as cefoxitin against *B. fragilis*, but have poor efficacy against other members of the *B. fragilis* group (i.e. *B. thetaiotaomicron*). Third-generation cephalosporins have activity against *Bacteroides* spp. that is inferior to that of second-generation cephalosporins.

Carbapenems (imipenem, meropenem, ertapenem)

The β-lactam carbapenems imipenem and meropenem have excellent activity against a broad spectrum of aerobic and anaerobic bacteria, including β-lactamase-producing *Bacteroides* spp. and Enterobacteriaceae and *Pseudomonas* spp.[97] Resistance of *B. fragilis* group is very rare (<1%). Ertapenem has similar efficacy but is not active against *Pseudomonas* spp. and *Acinetobacter* spp.[98]

Chloramphenicol

Chloramphenicol shows excellent *in-vitro* activity against most anaerobic bacteria, and resistance is rare. The drug is also effective against many Enterobacteriaceae and Gram-positive cocci. However, the experience of using this drug in intra-abdominal sepsis was disappointing. The toxicity of chloramphenicol, the rare but fatal aplastic anemia and the dose-dependent leukopenia, limit its use, especially in neutropenic patients.

Clindamycin and lincomycin

Clindamycin and lincomycin are effective against anaerobes and have good activity against aerobic Gram-positive cocci.[96] Clindamycin has broader coverage against anaerobes, including β-lactamase-producing *Bacteroides* spp. Resistance of *B. fragilis* group is 5–10%, and some *Clostridium* spp. other than *C. perfringens* are resistant. Antibiotic-associated colitis caused by *C. difficile* was first described after clindamycin therapy. However, colitis has been associated with many other antimicrobial agents, including penicillins and cephalosporins.

Metronidazole

Metronidazole has excellent activity against anaerobes. However, its antibacterial efficacy is limited to anaerobic bacteria. Microaerophilic streptococci, *Prop. acnes* and *Actinomyces* spp. are often resistant. Concern was raised about the carcinogenic and mutagenic effects of this drug; however, these effects were shown only in one species of mice and were never substantiated in other animals or humans.[3,5]

Macrolides (erythromycin, azithromycin, clarithromycin)

The macrolides erythromycin, azithromycin and clarithromycin have moderate-to-good *in-vitro* activity against anaerobic bacteria other than *B. fragilis* group and fusobacteria. They are active against *Prevotella* and *Porphyromonas* spp., microaerophilic and anaerobic streptococci, Gram-positive nonspore-forming anaerobic bacilli and certain clostridia. They show relatively good activity against *C. perfringens* and poor or inconsistent activity against Gram-negative anaerobic bacilli.[99]

Glycopeptides (vancomycin, teicoplanin)

The glycopeptides are effective against all Gram-positive anaerobes (including *C. difficile*), but are inactive against Gram-negative bacilli.

Tetracyclines

Tetracycline is of limited use because of the development of resistance by all types of anaerobe, including *B. fragilis* group. The newer tetracycline analogues doxycycline and minocycline are more active than the parent compound. Because there is significant resistance to these drugs, they can be used if the organisms are susceptible or in less severe infections in which a therapeutic trial is feasible.

Tygecycline

Tygecycline, a glycylcycline, is a direct analogue of minocycline with a 9-glycylamide moiety. It has activity against both Gram-negative and Gram-positive bacteria, anaerobes and certain drug-resistant pathogens including methicillin-resistant *Staph. aureus*.[100] It is active against *Streptococcus anginosus* group (which includes *Strep. anginosus*, *Strep. intermedius* and *Strep. constellatus*), *Bacteroides fragilis*, *Bacteroides thetaiotaomicron*, *Bacteroides uniformis*, *Bacteroides vulgatus*, *Clostridium perfringens* and *Peptostreptococcus micros*.[101]

Quinolones

The first generation of fluoroquinolones such as ciprofloxacin and ofloxacin are inactive against most anaerobic bacteria. However, some broad-spectrum quinolones, which have recently become clinically available or are under active development, have significant anti-anaerobic activity. Quinolones with low activity against anaerobes include ciprofloxacin, ofloxacin, levofloxacin, fleroxacin, pefloxacin, enoxacin and lomefloxacin. Compounds with intermediate anti-anaerobic activity include sparfloxacin and grepafloxacin. Trovafloxacin, gatifloxacin and moxifloxacin yield low minimum inhibitory concentrations (MICs) against most groups of anaerobes. Quinolones with the greatest *in-vitro* activity against anaerobes include clinafloxacin and sitafloxacin.[102] The use of the quinolones is restricted in growing children and during pregnancy because of their possible adverse effects on cartilage.

Table 173.12 Antimicrobial drugs of choice for anaerobic bacteria

	Drug of choice	Alternative drugs
Peptostreptococcus spp.	Penicillin	Clindamycin, chloramphenicol, cephalosporins
Clostridium spp.	Penicillin	Metronidazole, chloramphenicol, cefoxitin, clindamycin
Clostridium difficile	Vancomycin	Metronidazole, bacitracin
Fusobacterium spp.	Penicillin	Metronidazole, clindamycin, chloramphenicol
Bacteroides (BL–)	Penicillin	Metronidazole, clindamycin, chloramphenicol
Bacteroides (BL+)	Metronidazole, a carbapenem, a penicillin and β-lactamase inhibitor, clindamycin	Cefoxitin, chloramphenicol, piperacillin, tigecycline

Gram-negative bacilli include *Bacteroides fragilis* group and *Prevotella*, *Porphyromonas* and *Fusobacterium* spp.
BL, β-lactamase.

Other agents

Bacitracin is active against pigmented *Prevotella* and *Porphyromonas* spp. but is inactive against *B. fragilis* and *Fusobacterium nucleatum*.[2] Quinupristin–dalfopristin shows antibacterial activity against anaerobic organisms tested, including *C. perfringens* and *Lactobacillus* and *Peptostreptococcus* spp.[103] Linezolid is active against *F. nucleatum*, other fusobacteria and *Porphyromonas*, *Prevotella* and *Peptostreptococcus* spp.[104] Little clinical experience has, however, been gained in the treatment of anaerobic bacteria using these agents.

Choice of antimicrobial agents

The parenteral antimicrobials that can be used in most infectious sites (Tables 173.11, Table 173.12) are clindamycin, metronidazole, chloramphenicol, cefoxitin, a penicillin (e.g. ticarcillin, ampicillin, piperacillin) and a β-lactamase inhibitor (e.g. clavulanic acid, sulbactam, tazobactam), tigecycline, and a carbapenem (e.g. imipenem, meropenem, ertapenem).

An agent effective against Gram-negative enteric bacilli (e.g. aminoglycoside, a fluoroquinolone) or an antipseudomonal cephalosporin (e.g. cefepime) are generally added to clindamycin, metronidazole and, occasionally, cefoxitin when treating intra-abdominal infections to provide coverage for these bacteria. As failure of therapy in intra-abdominal infections has been noted more often with chloramphenicol, this drug is not recommended.

Penicillin can be added to metronidazole in the therapy of intracranial, pulmonary and dental infections to cover for microaerophilic streptococci, *Actinomyces* spp. and *Arachnia* spp. A macrolide (i.e. erythromycin) is added to metronidazole in upper respiratory infections to treat *Staph. aureus* and aerobic streptococci. Penicillin is added to clindamycin to supplement its coverage against *Peptostreptococcus* spp. and other Gram-positive anaerobic organisms.

Table 173.13 Activity of antimicrobial agents against anaerobes

Agent	Comments
Nearly always active	
Metronidazole	Inactive versus microaerophilic streptococci (e.g. *Streptococcus milleri*), *Propionibacterium* and *Actinomyces* spp.; bactericidal versus most Gram-negative anaerobic strains
Carbapenems	Resistant to most *Bacteroides* β-lactamases, although a novel β-lactamase that cleaves carbapenems was found in rare *B. fragilis* strains*
β-Lactam plus β-lactamase inhibitors	The addition of a β-lactamase inhibitor to a β-lactam dramatically increases activity against anaerobes that produce a β-lactamase
Chloramphenicol	Good activity versus virtually all clinically significant anaerobes†
Usually active	
Clindamycin	*B. fragilis* group: 10–20% of strains resistant; some clostridia other than *C. perfringens* are resistant
Cefamycins	*B. fragilis* group: 5–15% of strains resistant with considerable institutional variation at least partly reflecting use patterns; poor activity versus clostridia
Antipseudomonal	Relatively resistant to β-lactamases of *Bacteroides* spp; penicillins large doses usually employed
Variable activity	
Penicillin	Inactive versus some or most penicillinase-producing anaerobes, including most of the *B. fragilis* group and many strains of *Prevotella melaninogenica*, *P. intermedia*, *P. bivia*, *P. disiens* and some clostridia
Cephalosporins	Less activity *in vitro* than penicillin G versus most anaerobes and limited other than cefamycins published clinical experience to document efficacy
Tetracycline	Inactive versus many anaerobes and most strains of *B. fragilis*; doxycycline and minocycline are somewhat more active than tetracycline
Vancomycin	Active against Gram-positive anaerobes; inactive versus Gram-negative anaerobes
Macrolides	Inactive versus many *Fusobacterium* spp. and some *B. fragilis* spp.; ketolides also show reduced activity versus fusobacteria
Fluoroquinolones	'Third-generation' (gatifloxacin, moxifloxacin and gemifloxacin) show good *in-vitro* activity; limited published data
Tigecycline	Active against nearly all anaerobes including strains of *B. fragilis* that are resistant to β-lactams, clindamycin and quinolones. Minimum inhibitory concentrations are somewhat higher for clostridia‡
Penicillin	Inactive versus some or most penicillinase-producing anaerobes, including most of the *B. fragilis* group and many strains of *Prevotella melaninogenica*, *P. intermedia*, *P. bivia*, *P. disiens* and some clostridia
Cephalosporins	Less activity *in vitro* than penicillin G versus most anaerobes and limited other than cefamycins published clinical experience to document efficacy
Tetracycline	Inactive versus many anaerobes and most strains of *B. fragilis*; doxycycline and minocycline are somewhat more active than tetracycline
Vancomycin	Active against Gram-positive anaerobes; inactive versus Gram-negative anaerobes
Poor activity	
Aminoglycosides	
Trimethoprim–sulfamethoxazole	
Monobactams (aztreonam)	

*Edwards R, *et al*. J Antimicrob Chemother 1999;43:273–6.
†While *in-vitro* activity is excellent, clinical failures with chloramphenicol have been documented, rendering this drug less preferable than other active agents for the treatment of anaerobic infections.
‡Snydman DR, *et al*. J Antimicrob Chemother 2005;55:1024–8.

Doxycycline is added to most regimens in the treatment of pelvic infections to provide therapy for *Chlamydia* and *Mycoplasma*. Penicillin is still the drug of choice for bacteremia caused by non-BLPB. However, other agents should be used for the therapy of bacteremia caused by BLPB.

Because the duration of therapy for anaerobic infections, which are often chronic, is generally longer than for infections caused by aerobic and facultative anaerobes, oral therapy is often substituted for parenteral therapy. The agents available for oral therapy are limited and include clindamycin, amoxicillin plus clavulanic acid, chloramphenicol and metronidazole.

Clinical judgment, personal experience, safety and patient compliance should direct the physician in the choice of the appropriate antimicrobial agents. The duration of therapy generally ranges between 2 and 4 weeks, but should be individualized depending on the response. In some cases, such as lung abscesses, treatment may be required for as long as 6–8 weeks, but can often be shortened with proper surgical drainage.

REFERENCES

 References for this chapter can be found online at http://www.expertconsult.com

Mycobacteria

INTRODUCTION

Cardinal Richelieu (1585–1642), Nicolai Paganini (1782–1840), Heinrich Heine (1797–1856), Anton Chekhov (1860–1904), Franz Kafka (1883–1924), Eleanor Roosevelt (1884–1962) and George Orwell (1903–1950) all shared a common fate. Each of these famous people died of tuberculosis. In some cases their disease was not understood, while in other cases management of the disease was inadequate, mostly because of a lack of effective therapeutic agents.

Clearly, the presence of a concurrent disease (especially AIDS) as well as the overall state of person's health and host defense mechanisms are critical determinants of the morbidity and mortality rates of tuberculosis. However, even more complex factors strongly influence the incidence of tuberculosis including poverty, ignorance and indifference about the disease, and the lack of access to adequate health care. In the World Health Organization (WHO) report on global tuberculosis control,[1] 22 countries were identified as having a 'high burden' of tuberculosis. Based on surveillance and survey data, it is estimated that there were 8.8 million new cases of tuberculosis in 2005 (136 per 100 000), including 3.9 million (60 per 100 000) new smear-positive, and thus, highly infectious cases. The goals of the WHO global tuberculosis control program are to detect 70% of tuberculosis cases in the high-burden countries and to successfully treat 85% of the identified cases.

In addition to *Mycobacterium tuberculosis*, the two most important key players in global mycobacterial disease are *M. leprae* and *M. ulcerans*. During the past years notably *M. avium* complex and the rapidly growing mycobacteria have been the subject of extensive investigations as well, largely because of the increasing incidence of human disease and awareness of disease caused by nontuberculous mycobacteria (NTM).[2–5] As a consequence, accurate laboratory diagnosis of all mycobacterial species, a major focus of this chapter, is an important element for effective treatment and control of any mycobacterial disease.

GENERAL CHARACTERISTICS OF MYCOBACTERIAL ORGANISMS

Lehmann and Neumann first introduced the genus *Mycobacterium* into the scientific literature in 1896. The subsequent history of the genus has been profoundly influenced by the fact that only very few of the more than over 100 currently recognized species have been a devastating cause of human disease and suffering, above all *M. tuberculosis*. Thus, studies of microbial physiology, structure, genetics and diagnostic tools have mainly focused on *M. tuberculosis* and secondarily on *Mycobacterium leprae*.

The genus *Mycobacterium* is the only genus in the family of the Mycobacteriaceae[6] and is related to other mycolic acid-containing genera. All mycobacteria are aerobic (though some species are able to grow under a reduced oxygen atmosphere), nonspore-forming, nonmotile, slightly curved or straight rods. The most prominent feature of mycobacteria that is uniformly present and distinctive to the genus is the lipid-rich cell envelope.[7,8] Indeed, it is the complex cell envelope of mycobacteria that confers upon these bacteria the property of 'acid-fastness' (i.e. resistance to decolorization when stained with carbolfuchsin and decolorized with dilute hydrochloric acid). Uniformly, they do not stain well with Gram stain. Mycobacteria possess a cell wall polysaccharide that resembles that of Gram-positive bacteria; however, the mycobacterial peptidoglycan contains lipids in place of proteins and polysaccharides.[9] Furthermore, the mycobacterial envelope contains a plasma membrane that is quite similar in structure and function to the plasma membrane of other bacteria, except for the presence of lipoarabinomannan (LAM), lipomannan and phosphatidylinositol mannosides (Fig. 174.1). As a whole, the cell wall component of the

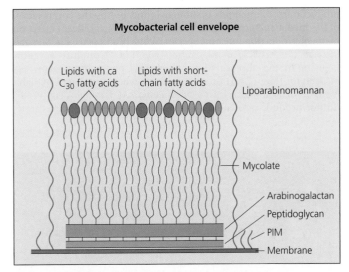

Fig. 174.1 Mycobacterial cell envelope. This model displays the asymmetric array of the structural elements extending from the plasma membrane that surrounds the cytoplasm of the mycobacterial cell. The arabinogalactan is covalently linked to the peptidoglycan, which along with the lipoarabinomannan (LAM) and phosphatidylinositol mannosides (PIM) are associated with the plasma membrane. The cell wall lipids are shown in a possible arrangement with the mycolates linked to the arabinogalactan. Two classes of polar lipids with medium and short chain fatty acids complement the varying hydrocarbon chains of the mycolates to create an even cell envelope. There is evidence for a small number of porins within the hydrophobic bilayer. Adapted from Brennan & Draper.[10]

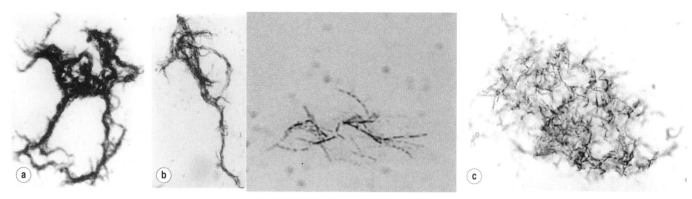

Fig. 174.2 Microscopic clusters of three different species of mycobacteria. (a) Serpentine cording of *M. tuberculosis*. (b) Cross-banding of *M. kansasii*. (c) Loose clusters of *M. avium* complex. Photomicrographs taken from Attorri *et al*.[11]

envelope confers size, shape, protection against osmotic pressure, and probably protects the plasma membrane from deleterious molecules in the environment of the cell. In summary, the peptidoglycan confers cell shape while the next layer of the envelope, arabinogalactan esterified to the mycolic acids, provides for a hydrophobic permeability barrier. Other important fatty acids are waxes, phospholipids and mycoserosic and phthienoic acids, and tuberculostearic acid (10-R-methyl-octadecanoic) acid is a unique cell component within the Actinomycetales, including the mycobacteria.[8]

In 1947, Middlebrook first described growth of tubercle bacilli in the shape of serpentine cords ('cording'). For many years cording was correlated with virulence and considered a distinctive feature of *M. tuberculosis* (Fig. 174.2). However, it is now known that several mycobacterial species display cording and the correlation with virulence, if any, is unclear. Cord factor appears to be a mixture of mycolate-containing molecules including the original cord factor associated with *M. tuberculosis*, trehalose 6,6'-dimycolate.

Many species of mycobacteria are capable of producing carotenoids (carotene and xanthophylls) and this feature can be an important aid in the presumptive identification of a mycobacterial organism. The production of carotenoids is strongly influenced by the composition of the media and growth conditions. Light has a significant effect on pigment production for some species. Scotochromogens, e.g. *M. scrofulaceum* (Fig. 174.3) or *M. szulgai* (Fig. 174.4) produce a yellow pigment in the absence of light, whereas photochromogens, e.g. *M. kansasii* (Fig. 174.5) produce pigment when stimulated by light. Nonphotochromogens, e.g. *M. tuberculosis* or *M. fortuitum* (Fig. 174.6) do not produce carotenoids. The function of mycobacterial carote-

noids is largely unknown, but some evidence suggests that carotenoids provide protection against phototoxic effects.

The genome of mycobacteria displays a typical bacterial chromosomal structure, i.e. a single large circular DNA molecule with a G+C content of 60–70 mol% (except *M. leprae*; <57%). The complete

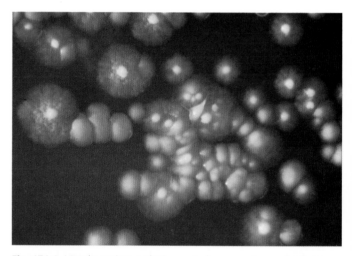

Fig. 174.4 *Mycobacterium szulgai*, a scotochromogenic mycobacterium, grown on Middlebrook 7H10 agar.

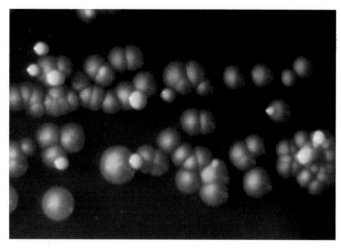

Fig. 174.3 *Mycobacterium scrofulaceum*, a scotochromogenic mycobacterium, grown on Middlebrook 7H10 agar.

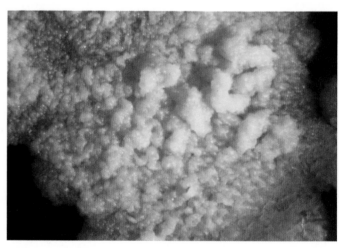

Fig. 174.5 *Mycobacterium kansasii*, a photochromogenic mycobacterium, grown on Middlebrook 7H10 agar, after exposure to light.

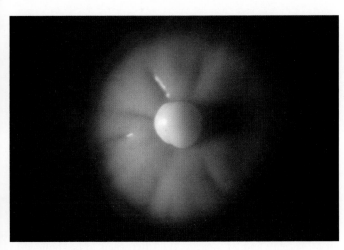

Fig. 174.6 *Mycobacterium fortuitum*, a nonchromogenic rapid grower, grown on Middlebrook 7H10 agar.

genome sequence of *M. tuberculosis* H37Rv (4.41 Mb) has recently been deciphered.[12] Most of the NTM, in particular *M. avium* complex, *M. scrofulaceum* and the rapid growers, contain plasmids. The size and number of plasmids vary; their function is largely unknown. There has been considerable speculation that plasmids in mycobacteria include DNA sequences that encode a variety of virulence factors.

However, plasmids would appear to have no role in antibiotic resistance or virulence in *M. tuberculosis*, since the organism does not contain plasmids.

Overall, the analysis of genetic relatedness confirms the classic classification scheme based on pigmentation and growth rate. Genome sequence information has also revealed interesting information about differences within the *M. tuberculosis* complex. For example, comparisons of *M. tuberculosis* H37Rv (a human isolate that is also virulent in mice) with bacille Calmette–Guérin (BCG) Pasteur showed that 18 variable sequence regions are missing in BCG Pasteur. Perhaps even more intriguing is the presence of two large tandem duplications in BCG Pasteur, whereas other BCG strains lack one of these duplications and neither of the duplications is seen in *M. tuberculosis* H37Rv. Furthermore, the genome size of *M. bovis* is significantly smaller than that of *M. tuberculosis* which seems at odds with the fact that *M. bovis* has a significantly wider host range than *M. tuberculosis*.[13,14]

Very recently, sequence information has placed in doubt the longheld belief that *M. tuberculosis* evolved from an animal pathogen (i.e. *M. bovis*). Rather, it indicates that all members of the *M. tuberculosis* complex, i.e. *M. tuberculosis*, *M. bovis*, *M. bovis* BCG, *M. caprae*, *M. africanum*, *M. microti*, '*M. canettii*' and *M. pinnipedii* (Table 174.1), gradually evolved from a common ancestor and '*M. canettii*' segregated some 2.4–2.8 million years ago. *M. tuberculosis*, in its present form, is estimated to be only some 35 000 years old and was always a human pathogen.[18,19] Sequence analysis of the paralogous genes in a large set of *M. tuberculosis* strains collected worldwide confirmed the very ancient origin of '*M. canettii*'.[20,21]

Table 174.1 Major characteristics of the *Mycobacterium tuberculosis* complex

Species	Geographic distribution	Remarks	Identifying features
M. tuberculosis	Widespread, humans are the definite host; disease also in elephants and other mammals	Based on genetic analyses present day *M. tuberculosis* is relatively young (~35 000 years old)	Usually PZA susceptible, nitrate reductase activity positive, niacin positive, aerobic
M. bovis	Widespread, broad host range including nonhuman primates, cattle, goats, cats, dogs, buffalo, badgers, possums, deer and bison. Humans are viewed as a 'spillover' host	Mainly extrapulmonary manifestation in humans	PZA resistant, nitrate reductase activity negative, niacin negative, microaerophilic
M. bovis BCG	Nonvirulent vaccine strain	First reported in 1908 as a nonvirulent strain of *M. tuberculosis*; appears to be a regulatory mutant of *M. bovis*	PZA resistant, nitrate reductase activity negative, niacin negative, aerobic
M. caprae	Mainly in goats, few infections in humans		PZA susceptible, nitrate reductase activity negative, niacin negative, microaerophilic
M. africanum		Type I and type II	Mostly PZA susceptible, predominantly nitrate reductase activity negative, niacin variable, microaerophilic
M. microti	Initially considered strictly an animal pathogen (e.g. voles, llamas, cats), several human cases were reported in 1998[15]		'Croissant-like' cell morphology; does not grow well in culture; identification via molecular methods
'*M. canettii*'	East Africa, occurrence appears to be limited to the African continent	Based on genetic studies ancestor of all members of the *M. tuberculosis* complex, ~2.4–2.8 million years old; 'living fossil'	Smooth colonies, distinct patterns upon DNA typing
M. pinnipedii	Pinnipeds as major hosts		

Adapted and modified from van Soolingen et al.,[15] Vincent & Gutierrez[16] and Grange.[17]
PZA, pyrazinamide.

EPIDEMIOLOGY AND CLINICAL MANIFESTATIONS OF THE MOST IMPORTANT MYCOBACTERIAL PATHOGENS

Tuberculosis

Tuberculosis is the second most common infectious cause of adult mortality, and is ranked tenth of all causes of loss of healthy life worldwide. Of the estimated 8.8 million cases in 2005, 7.4 million were found in Asia and sub-Saharan Africa (Fig. 174.7).[1] Of these, a total of 1.6 million died of tuberculosis, including 195 000 patients infected with HIV. Before the development of effective chemotherapy, the mortality rate for tuberculosis was 50–60%. Following the discovery of isoniazid (INH) and rifampin (rifampicin; RMP), the majority of pulmonary and extrapulmonary tuberculosis became treatable. Nevertheless, treatment of tuberculosis remains problematic in many areas because of the lack of/or intermittent access to therapy, poor adherence to therapy, poor drug quality, and above all, the worldwide emergence of resistance.[22]

Multidrug-resistant *M. tuberculosis* strains (i.e. resistant to INH and RMP at least) are responsible for more than 4% of all newly and previously treated tuberculosis cases. A 'virtually untreatable form of tuberculosis' (BBC News, September 2006) has emerged recently, XDR-TB (extensively drug-resistant tuberculosis). Occurring worldwide, including highly industrialized countries such as the USA, such XDR strains are resistant against INH and RMP as well as against the two most important second-line drug classes, a fluoroquinolone (e.g. ciprofloxacin) and an injectable drug (e.g. amikacin).[23]

Tuberculosis in the most common form is a chronic pulmonary disease classified as either primary or post-primary disease.[24] Post-primary disease can be a consequence of either reactivation (endogenous infection) or re-infection (exogenous infection). By far the most common (95%) route of infection is inhalation of infectious droplet nuclei, but exposure to *M. tuberculosis* bacilli neither always leads to infection nor are all patients with disease infectious. The risk of infection is directly related to the number and distribution of tubercle bacilli in the inhaled and respired air, emphasizing the importance of infectious droplet nuclei to airborne transmission. Unless a patient receives prophylaxis, symptomatic disease eventually occurs in 5–10% of infected patients. The appearance and extent of disease varies with only one-half of infected patients developing disease within the first 2 years. Hematogenous spread of tubercle bacilli from the lung probably invariably occurs, but the bacteremia is usually occult and does not produce symptoms or disease. Nevertheless, hematogenous dissemination accounts for the occurrence of extrapulmonary involvement of lymph nodes, kidneys, reproductive organs, bones, and gastrointestinal tract (see Chapter 30).

Compared to the global incidence of tuberculosis there is a small proportion of human disease caused by other members of the *M. tuberculosis* complex such as *M. bovis* and *M. africanum*. Human infections with *M. caprae*[25] appear to be very infrequent; the same holds for *M. microti*[15] and '*M. canettii*'. The latter seems to be confined to the African continent only,[20,26] and *M. pinnipedii* appears to affect seals only.[27]

Leprosy

Leprosy (Hansen's disease) is a chronic disease of the skin, nerves and mucous membranes. The immunologic response (e.g. hypersensitivity) becomes an important component of the pathogenesis of the disease. The clinical manifestations of leprosy have been separated into six categories (Ridley–Jopling classification scheme).[28] The system is both a clinical classification based on the nature and severity of symptoms and a histopathologic classification. The classification groups are: (1) polar tuberculoid; (2) borderline tuberculoid; (3) borderline; (4) borderline lepromatous; (5) lepromatous (subpolar); and (6) lepromatous polar.

Lepromatous leprosy is the most severe form of the disease with numerous skin lesions involving face and nose. Acid-fast bacilli (AFB) are numerous and present in immature macrophages which contrasts

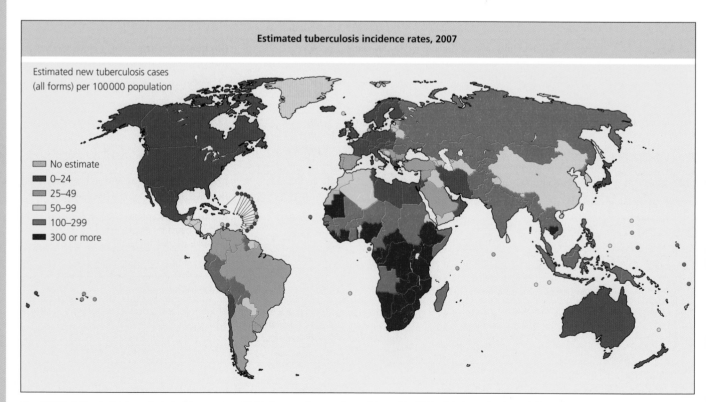

Estimated tuberculosis incidence rates, 2007

Estimated new tuberculosis cases (all forms) per 100 000 population

- No estimate
- 0–24
- 25–49
- 50–99
- 100–299
- 300 or more

Fig. 174.7 Estimated tuberculosis incidence rates, 2007. Data and map adapted from World Health Organization. Global tuberculosis control: surveillance, planning, financing. WHO Report 2008, Geneva: WHO/HTM/TB/2008.393.

to tuberculoid leprosy, where macrophages have matured into epithelioid cells (see also Chapter 103), and AFB are hard to detect.

Epidemiology of leprosy is difficult to assess because of the lack of a diagnostic skin test, inability to cultivate the organism *in vitro* and the nature of the geographic distribution of endemic disease. Even though the disease is of great antiquity, the source for *M. leprae*, the mode of transmission and the portal of entry are not clear to date. Human-to-human transmission through nasal secretions has been accepted for a long time. However, there is evidence that the disease may also be airborne, vector-borne or vehicle-borne. The worldwide implementation of the standardized multidrug therapy has dramatically decreased the number of registered leprosy patients from 10–12 million cases in the mid 1980s to 1.15 million cases in the late 1990s.[29] Nevertheless, the annual confirmed new cases (500 000–700 000) suggest that therapy largely fails to avoid transmission.[30] The vast majority of patients are in the developing world, predominantly South East Asia and mostly in India.

Care and treatment of leprosy have two equally difficult components. The first is treatment of active disease, especially in patients with physical deformities or at risk of developing deformities. The second is care of effectively treated patients, but with disabling or debilitating deformities due to the pathology associated with the various manifestations of leprosy.

Buruli ulcer/Bairnsdale ulcer

Mycobacterium ulcerans is the etiologic agent of Buruli ulcer in Africa and Bairnsdale ulcer in Australia,[4] an emerging disease involving chronic and necrotizing skin ulcers. Occurring mostly in rural tropical regions it is the third most common mycobacterial disease in immunocompetent humans after tuberculosis and leprosy (Fig. 174.8). Disease typically begins as a lump under the skin, followed by a shallow ulcer at the site of the lump. *M. ulcerans* produces a toxin that causes necrosis. The type of disease ranges from a localized nodule or ulcer to widespread ulcerative or nonulcerative disease including, for instance, osteomyelitis.

Treatment with antimicrobial agents has widely been unsuccessful. Surgical removal of the affected tissue, often followed by skin grafting, is the method of choice. If untreated, *M. ulcerans* disease may even lead to severe sequelae such as blindness or loss of limbs. Disease control in endemic regions is limited to early case detection with surgical treatment.

Adequate surveillance data are missing for most of the endemic aereas, therefore the incidence and prevalence of Buruli ulcer are not precisely defined. Ghana, an exception, has reported an overall national prevalence rate of active lesions of 20.7 per 100 000, but the rate was

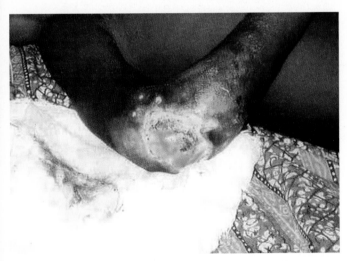

Fig. 174.8 Buruli ulcer on the elbow of an African girl caused by *M. ulcerans*. Courtesy of F Portaels.

as high as 150.8 per 100 000 in districts where the disease was more endemic.[31] There is growing evidence that *M. ulcerans* also produces disease in reptiles and mammals. *M. ulcerans* is a heat-sensitive, fastidious organism and has an unusually long generation time. Promising molecular tests have been developed which may help to accelerate diagnosis.[32]

Nontuberculous mycobacterial diseases

Diagnostic criteria, clinical presentation and treatment of diseases caused by more than 20 NTM have been meticulously reviewed.[3–5] The official ATS/IDSA statement covers other important aspects such as taxonomy, epidemiology, pathogenesis and laboratory aspects. In addition, the clinical significance and laboratory diagnostic aspects of NTM have been reviewed.[33–35] Therefore, the following discussion only focusses on the most prominent NTM species causing disease in humans (Table 174.2).

Mycobacterium avium complex

Mycobacterium avium complex (MAC) is common not only in soil, water and animals, but also in certain food (e.g. hard cheese). It also colonizes pools and hot water tubs. Portals of infection are probably both gastrointestinal and pulmonary by ingestion of contaminated water and food and inhalation of aerosols.

Mycobacterium avium complex causes disseminated disease usually (but not exclusively) in people with HIV infection, but may also be responsible for pulmonary disease in immunocompetent patients and cervical lymphadenitis in normal hosts, mostly children.[4,36]

Disseminated MAC disease was rarely reported before the advent of the HIV epidemics. Based on complete follow-up information, disseminated MAC disease occurred in 20–35% per year of people with HIV infection.[37] However, this dates back 10 years and MAC prophylaxis (rifabutin, azithromycin or clarithromycin) and the use of highly active antiretroviral therapy (HAART) have significantly decreased the incidence of MAC disease in people with HIV infection.

Disseminated MAC disease in people with HIV infection is a progressive illness characterized by intermittent fever, sweats, weakness, anorexia and weight loss. Patients may have nausea, diarrhea and vomiting along with abdominal pain. The microbiologic hallmark of MAC disease is a positive blood or bone marrow culture; however, duodenal, rectal, spleen or liver biopsies may be diagnostic as well (Fig. 174.9). The level of the bacteremia ranges from intermittently culture positive to 10^6 cfu/ml. The level of infection of bone marrow may be orders of magnitude higher than in blood.[38] Disseminated MAC infection in people with HIV infection clearly decreases survival. Treatment with a macrolide and another agent improves survival and the quality of life. MAC disease in people with HIV infection may also be focal, including pulmonary infection, peripheral lymphadenitis and cutaneous infection (see Chapter 91).

The majority (≥90%) of disseminated MAC disease is caused by *M. avium*. Overall, *M. intracellulare* is isolated about as frequently as *M. avium*, but the isolation of *M. avium* has been associated with a poorer prognosis. Other species should be considered for symptomatic patients as well, such as *M. triplex*, *M. genavense*, and *M. conspicuum* or, for patients with cutaneous infections, *M. haemophilum* (see Table 174.2). Disseminated MAC disease in HIV-negative patients is usually associated with congenital immunodeficiency, immunosuppression, malignancy or a specific immunodeficiency such as a deficiency in interferon gamma (IFN-γ) production or IFN-γ receptors. In children without HIV infection disseminated MAC disease with visceral involvement has been associated with a high mortality rate (82%).

Mycobacterium avium complex pulmonary disease is seen worldwide with an overall incidence of about 1/100 000 persons. The incidence of pulmonary disease appears to be increasing, but this may be due in part to increased surveillance and awareness by the medical community. MAC pulmonary disease may be associated with a history of chronic lung infection including cystic fibrosis. However, the

Table 174.2 Nontuberculous mycobacteria

Clinical disease/specimen/site	Occurrence	Species	Growth rate	Recovered from environment	Geographic distribution	Risk factors, additional remarks	Microbiologic and diagnostic features
Cutaneous, wound	Common	M. chelonae	Rapid	Yes	Widespread	Contact lenses, ocular surgery (LASIK-associated), implants, catheters	
Cutaneous, wound	Common	M. fortuitum	Rapid	Yes	Widespread	Central catheters, postsurgical wounds, mammoplasty, nail salon furunculosis	
Cutaneous, wound	Common	M. haemophilum	Very slow	Yes?	Australia, Europe, North America	AIDS, organ transplant recipients, lymphoma, children; infections at the cooler sites of the body including the extremities	Fastidious, requires hemin or ferric ammonium citrate, growth at 30–32°C, growth stimulated by CO_2, may be missed by the laboratory
Cutaneous, wound, bone	Common	M. marinum	Rapid/slow	Yes	Widespread	Skin abrasion or trauma; in immunocompetent and immunocompromised patients; 'fish tank granuloma', 'swimming pool granuloma'	Photochromogen, optimum growth (32°C)
Cutaneous, wound	Unknown	M. mucogenicum	Rapid	?	Unknown	Catheters	
Cutaneous, ulcers, bones	Common (tropics)	M. ulcerans	Very slow	Yes	Ghana, Uganda, South East Asia, Central and South America, Australia	Normal host, third most prevalent Mycobacterium isolated from human specimens and continuing to emerge; Buruli ulcer (Africa), Bairnsdale ulcer (Australia)	Fastidious, vulnerable upon pretreatment, very slow growth at 30°C, microaerophilic
Cutaneous, wound	Uncommon	M. abscessus	Rapid	Yes	Widespread		
Cutaneous, wound	Uncommon	M. avium complex	Slow	Yes	Widespread		
Cutaneous	Uncommon	M. kansasii	Slow	Yes	Widespread		Photochromogenic
Cutaneous	Uncommon	M. smegmatis	Rapid	Yes	Unknown		
Cutaneous, wound	Unknown	M. conspicuum	Slow	No	Unknown		
Cutaneous, urine, fluids (BAL, joint), blood	Unknown	M. immunogenicum	Rapid	Yes	Unknown	Respiratory pseudo-outbreaks (contaminated bronchoscopy equipment), catheters	Culture at 25–30°C, M. abscessus-chelonae-like
Cutaneous, tenosynovitis	Unknown	M. malmoense	Slow			AIDS is not a predisposing factor	Microaerophilic
Cutaneous	Unknown	M. novocastrense	Rapid	Yes	Unknown	Potential human pathogen	Scotochromogenic M. marinum-like
Disseminated	Common	M. xenopi	Slow	Yes	Worldwide	Hot water systems	Thermophilic

Disease	Frequency	Species	Growth rate		Distribution	Clinical/epidemiology	Characteristics
Disseminated	Common	*M. avium complex*	Slow	Yes	Widespread	AIDS, hairy cell leukemia, congenital immunodeficiencies	Usually nonpigmented, pigmented colonies occur, three colony variants
Disseminated	Common	*M. chelonae*	Rapid	Yes	Widespread		
Disseminated, blood or bone marrow, joint fluid	Common	*M. haemophilum*	Very slow		Australia, Europe, North America	Common and continuing to emerge	
Disseminated	Common	*M. kansasii*	Slow	Yes	Europe, USA		Photochromogenic
Disseminated	Uncommon	*M. abscessus*	Rapid	Yes			
Disseminated, blood, bone marrow, liver, spleen	Uncommon	*M. genavense*	Slow	Yes	Widespread, isolated from pet birds	Disease in humans established, especially in AIDS patients and malnourished patients	Grows very slowly if at all, prefers slightly acidic medium (pH 6.0)
Disseminated	Uncommon	*M. malmoense*	Very slow	Yes		AIDS	
Disseminated	Unknown	*M. celatum*	Slow	No	Europe, USA	Disease in humans established	Two copies of 16S rRNA gene
Disseminated Osteomyelitis, cellulitis		*M. smegmatis*	Rapid			Catheters	
Disseminated, blood	Unknown	*M. conspicuum*	Slow	No			
Disseminated Spinal osteomyelitis Lymphadenitis	Unknown	*M. lentiflavum*	Slow	No		Disease in humans established, especially HIV and AIDS patients	
Disseminated		*M. simiae*	Slow			Infections in immunocompromised patients	
Disseminated, lymph node, spinal fluid, pericardial and peritoneal fluid	Unknown	*M. triplex*	Slow	No	Unknown	Disease in humans established	*M. simiae-avium*-like
Intestinal		*M. paratuberculosis*	Slow	Yes			Fastidious, cause of Johne's disease in cattle; association with *M. paratuberculosis* and Crohn's disease in humans (?)
Lymphadenitis	Common	*M. avium complex*	Slow	Yes	Widespread	Childhood	
Lymphadenitis	Common	*M. malmoense*	Very slow	Yes	UK, Northern Europe	Childhood	Slow growth
Lymphadenitis	Common before 1980	*M. scrofulaceum*	Slow	Yes	Widespread	Childhood	
Lymphadenitis	Uncommon	*M. abscessus*	Rapid	Yes			
Lymphadenitis	Uncommon	*M. chelonae*	Rapid	Yes			
Lymphadenitis	Uncommon	*M. fortuitum*	Rapid	Yes			

(Continued)

Table 174.2 Nontuberculous mycobacteria—cont'd

Clinical disease/specimen/site	Occurrence	Species	Growth rate	Recovered from environment	Geographic distribution	Risk factors, additional remarks	Microbiologic and diagnostic features
Lymphadenitis	Uncommon	*M. haemophilum*	Slow	Yes?		Also in immunocompetent children	
Lymphadenitis, soft tissue	Unknown	*M. bohemicum*	Slow	Yes	Unknown	Potential pathogen	
Lymphadenitis	Unknown	*M. heidelbergense*	Slow	No	Germany	Resembles *M. malmoense*	
Lymphadenitis, pulmonary	Unknown	*M. tusciae*	Slow	Yes	Tuscany	Potential pathogen	
Lymphadenitis, disseminated	Unknown	*M. interjectum*	Slow/rapid	No		Disease in humans established	
Lymphadenitis	Unknown	*M. szulgai*	Slow				
Pulmonary	Common	*M. abscessus*	Rapid	Yes	Widespread, predominantly USA	Symptoms and radiographic presentation similar to *M. fortuitum*. Also in patients with gastroesophageal disorders with chronic vomiting	
Pulmonary	Common	*M. avium complex*	Slow	Yes	Widespread	Chronic lung disease, cystic fibrosis	
Pulmonary		*M. heidelbergense*	Slow	Yes	?	Lung tumor	
Pulmonary	Common	*M. kansasii*	Slow	Yes	Localized USA, UK, Europe, South Africa	Alcoholism, malignancy, AIDS, chronic lung diseases (COPD, pneumoconiosis); seen in gold miners	Photochromogen, intensely pigmented, large, beaded, acid-fast, elongated bacilli
Pulmonary	Common	*M. malmoense*	Very slow	Yes	Localized UK, Northern Europe	Pneumoconiosis, silicosis, industrial dust disease; common and continuing to emerge	
Pulmonary		*M. smegmatis*	Rapid	Yes		Rare, associated with lipoid pneumonia	
Pulmonary	Common	*M. xenopi*	Slow	Yes	Localized UK, Europe, Canada, infrequently in the USA	Underlying lung disease; common and continuing to emerge; associated with hospital water systems	Pigmented, optimum growth at 45°C
Pulmonary	Uncommon	*M. asiaticum*	Slow	Yes	Localized Australia, USA		
Pulmonary	Uncommon	*M. fortuitum*	Rapid	Yes		Similar to lung disease with *M. abscessus*; gastroesophageal disorders with chronic vomiting	

Site	Frequency	Species	Growth		Distribution	Pathogenicity	Remarks
Pulmonary	Uncommon	*M. gordonae*	Slow	Yes	Widespread	Frequent contaminant and debatable cause of disease	'Tap-water' scotochromogen
Pulmonary	Uncommon	*M. haemophilum*	Slow		Unknown, seems localized		
Pulmonary	Uncommon	*M. immunogenum*	Rapid				
Pulmonary	Uncommon	*M. shimoidei*	Slow		Australia, Japan		
Pulmonary		*M. scrofulaceum*	Slow		South Africa	AIDS but also HIV-negative patients; seen in gold miners	Produces niacin
Pulmonary	Uncommon	*M. simiae*	Slow	Yes	Israel, Thailand, France, USA, Australia	Underlying lung disease, pneumonia; often environmental contaminant	
Pulmonary	Uncommon	*M. szulgai*	Slow	Yes?	Europe, Japan, USA	Clinical picture often indistinguishable from tuberculosis; underlying disease (COPD, history of tuberculosis), alcoholism, smoking	Scotochromogen, slow growth at 25–37°C, no growth at 42°C
Pulmonary	Uncommon	*M. terrae*	Slow				
Pulmonary, sputum	Unknown	*M. alvei*	Rapid	Yes	Unknown, first isolated and described in Spain	Potential human pathogen	
Pulmonary	Unknown	*M. branderi*	Slow	No	Scandinavia	Potential pathogen	
Pulmonary	Unknown	*M. brumae*	Rapid	Yes	Unknown	Potential human pathogen	
Pulmonary	Unknown	*M. celatum*	Slow	No	Europe, USA		Contains two copies of 16S rDNA
Pulmonary, sputum	Unknown	*M. confluentis*	Rapid	No	Unknown	Potential human pathogen	Brown pigment
Pulmonary	Unknown	*M. conspicuum*	Slow	No	Europe	Disease in humans established	
Pulmonary	Unknown	*M. heckeshornense*	Slow	No	Unknown	Potential pathogen	*M. xenopi*-like organism
Pulmonary	Unknown	*M. interjectum*	Slow/rapid	No		Disease in humans established	
Pulmonary	Unknown	*M. intermedium*	Slow/rapid	No	Unknown	Disease in humans established	Photochromogen
Pulmonary	Unknown	*M. kubicae*	Slow		Unknown	Potential human pathogen	
Pulmonary, sputum?	Unknown	*M. mageritense*	Rapid	No	Spain, unknown	Potential human pathogen	
Pulmonary, wound	Unknown	*M. mucogenicum*	Rapid	Yes	Unknown	Disease in humans established	
Pulmonary	Unknown	*M. triplex*	Slow	No	Unknown	Disease in humans established	*M. avium* complex-like
Urine	Unknown	*M. hassiacum*	Rapid	Yes	Unknown	Nonpathogen?	Scotochromogen
Wound	Unknown	*M. branderi*	Slow	No	Unknown	Disease in humans established	

(Continued)

Table 174.2 Nontuberculous mycobacteria—cont'd

Clinical disease/ specimen/site	Occurrence	Species	Growth rate	Recovered from environment	Geographic distribution	Risk factors, additional remarks	Microbiologic and diagnostic features
Wound, soft tissue, blood	Unknown	M. fortuitum (3rd biovariant)	Rapid	Yes	Unknown		
Wound, pulmonary	Unknown	M. gondii	Rapid	No	Unknown	Nosocomial?	Pigmented, M. smegmatis-like
Wound Osteomyelitis	Unknown	M. wolinskyi	Rapid	No	Unknown	Post-traumatic and postsurgical. wounds	M. smegmatis-like
Wound Tenosynovitis (hand)		M. terrae	Slow				
Bone	Uncommon	M. chelonae	Rapid	Yes	Widespread		
Bone	Uncommon	M. fortuitum	Rapid	Yes	Widespread		

Information compiled and adapted from a variety of sources including Falkinham,[2] Tortoli,[3] American Thoracic Society,[4] Khan,[5] Vincent & Gutierrez,[16] Grange,[17] Pfyffer & Vincent,[33] Pfyffer,[34] Brown-Elliott & Wallace.[35]
BAL, bronchoalveolar lavage.

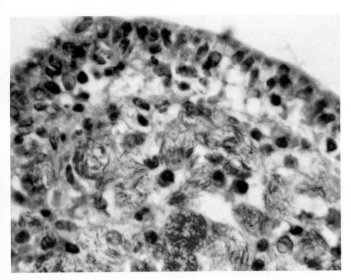

Fig. 174.9 Acid-fast stain of a section of small intestine from a patient with HIV infection and disseminated *M. avium* disease. The photomicrograph shows many acid-fast bacilli within a villus tip of the intestinal tract biopsy. The cuboidal cells at the periphery of the tip are in disarray and appear abnormal with cell nuclei not evenly distributed at the base of the cells. There is no evidence of granuloma, but the overwhelming number of mycobacteria may be partially obscuring the host's cellular response. The histopathology is consistent with the symptoms of patients with MAC gastrointestinal tract infections, including abdominal pain, diarrhea and wasting. Courtesy of LS Young.

traditionally recognized presentation of MAC pulmonary disease has been an apical fibrocavitary lung disease, sometimes showing large cavities, in males in their late forties and early fifties who have a history of smoking and, sometimes, alcohol abuse.[4] In postmenopausal, nonsmoking, white females, MAC pulmonary disease also presents with nodular and interstitial nodular infiltrates, frequently involving the right middle lobe or lingula ('Lady Windermere Syndrome').[4] In patients without underlying HIV infection, symptoms may vary and be nonspecific, including chronic productive cough, dyspnea, sweats, malaise and fatigue (see Chapter 30).

Mycobacterium avium complex cervical lymphadenitis is mostly a pediatric disease and primarily seen in children under 5 years of age. Lymphadenitis in immunocompetent children usually presents as an insidious, painless, unilateral process involving one or more lymph nodes. Mycobacteria isolated from infected lymph nodes are mostly (60–80%) MAC with the remainder being *M. scrofulaceum* and *M. tuberculosis* (see Chapter 30). *Mycobacterium avium* complex lymph node infection of children over 12 years of age is rarely simple lymphadenitis and may indicate disseminated disease and immunodeficiency.

Thus, MAC disease is frequently seen as disease in persons with and without underlying HIV infection. Although there are some similarities in the manifestation of MAC disease in both groups, the mortality rate, extent and pathologic manifestations of disease are frequently dissimilar.[36] Also, distinction between true infection with MAC and transient colonization may be difficult.

Mycobacterium kansasii

It appears that tap water is the major reservoir of *M. kansasii*. While being the second most common cause of NTM disease in the USA,[4] it is also seen in other parts of the world, i.e. in Europe (UK) and among mine workers in South Africa.[34] After MAC *M. kansasii* is the second most common NTM that causes disseminated disease in patients with AIDS.[4] Generally, the organism primarily affects middle-aged men. Risk factors are chronic obstructive pulmonary disease, pneumoconiosis, malignancy, previous mycobacterial disease and alcoholism. *Mycobacterium*

kansasii pulmonary disease parallels in many ways the clinical course of tuberculosis in terms of clinical symptoms and chest X-ray.

Rapid growers

Although the number of newly discovered rapidly growing mycobacteria is increasing constantly and the pathogenic potential of many of them is well recognized,[35] the vast majority (>90%) of disease in humans is caused by three species: *M. fortuitum* (see Fig. 174.6), *M. chelonae* and *M. abscessus*. These species are important causes of cutaneous, pulmonary and postsurgical wound infections (skin, soft tissue, bone), especially following catheter placement, augmentation mammaplasty and cardiac bypass surgery. Disseminated disease is rare and almost invariably occurs in immunocompromised patients, but disease is not common in people with HIV infection.

The distribution of rapidly growing mycobacteria appears to be worldwide. The three species associated with human disease have been isolated from drinking water, natural waters, ice machines, as well as in waste water and soil. The ubiquitous nature of these microorganisms, their resistance to many disinfectants and their ability to grow on unusual substrates such as polyhalogenated phenols account for the fact that rapidly growing mycobacteria are found as contaminants of medical equipment, prosthetic valves and disinfectants.

The incidence of pulmonary disease caused by rapidly growing mycobacteria is unclear (80% by *M. abscessus*), but an increased awareness of these species as human pathogens is leading to greater insight into the true incidence of disease. Nevertheless, the isolation of rapidly growing mycobacteria from respiratory tract specimens must be interpreted with great caution because contamination and colonization are common. True infection is usually associated with chronic pulmonary disease such as cystic fibrosis, previous mycobacterial lung disease and bronchiectasis due to previous respiratory infection. Rapidly growing mycobacteria are intrinsically resistant to antituberculous agents including INH, RMP and pyrazinamide (PZA).

PATHOGENICITY

The pathogenicity of mycobacterial infections in the immunocompetent host has as much to do with the immune response of the host as with destructive virulence properties of the mycobacterial pathogen. Thus, the principal virulence factor of mycobacteria is the ability to invade and persist or replicate within macrophages. Tubercle bacilli are believed to attach to macrophages by binding to the mannose receptor on the macrophage via the mycobacterial cell envelope LAM. Alternatively, tubercle bacilli can indirectly bind via CR1/CR3 complement receptors or Fc receptors.

The bacilli enter the macrophage by phagocytosis and once internalized the bacilli are surrounded by a membrane-bound vacuole to form a nascent phagosome. With the maturation of the phagolysosome, bacilli are exposed to a variety of antimicrobial factors including reactive oxygen intermediates, hydrolytic activities and a highly acidic pH. Cytokine-activated macrophages may also produce reactive nitrogen intermediates, although this has been conclusively shown only in murine macrophages. Virulent mycobacteria obstruct the maturation of phagosomes, inhibiting acidification, and can escape from the phagolysosome into the cytoplasm. Other bacilli appear able to adapt to life within the phagolysosome.

Recent evidence indicates that the maturation of the phagolysosome varies depending on the bacterial pathogen and even between intracellular pathogens.[39,40] The composition of the phagosome membrane is determined in part by the infecting mycobacteria; for example, phagosomes containing *M. avium* do not contain the vacuolar H+-ATPase that is needed for acidification of the phagosome. Phagosomes containing either *M. tuberculosis* or *M. avium* bacilli are frequently incompetent for fusion with endocytic organelles, suggesting a mechanism for the block in phagolysosome fusion. Inhibition of acidification can occur as a consequence of the exclusion of a proton pump (as with *M. avium*) or fusion with a lysosome that does not contain a pump or perhaps by the release of an ammonia metabolizing enzyme such as glutamine synthetase. Once mycobacteria have modified or adapted to the intracellular environment the bacilli may proliferate, but the mechanism of intracellular replication of mycobacteria is poorly understood.

The immunopathogenesis of mycobacterial infections primarily involves a cell-mediated immune response. This response includes the activation of macrophages to identify and inhibit or kill mycobacteria and the detection and lysis of phagocytes in which mycobacteria are in a state of growth and replication (Fig. 174.10).

Mycobacterial antigens are presented by antigen-presenting cells (monocyte/macrophage lineage) resulting in secretion of interleukin (IL)-2 and clonal proliferation of CD4+ and CD8+ lymphocytes (α/β T cells).[42] Mycobacterial antigens arising from the phagosome are presented by major histocompatibility complex (MHC) class II molecules while antigens arising from the cytoplasm are presented by MHC class I molecules.[39] This difference determines, in part, the fate

of the antigen-presenting cell, stimulation or destruction, because the presentation of antigen arising from the cytoplasm indicates that the cell has failed to control the mycobacteria. The release of IFN-γ by the clonally expanded CD4 cells, but also to a lesser extent by CD8 cells, natural killer (NK) cells and γδ cells, activates macrophages. This initiates a cascade of events including the hydrolysis of vitamin D that leads to further activation of macrophages and the release of tumor necrosis factor (TNF) by the activated macrophages. The sequence of cellular responses at the site of mycobacterial infection appears to be polymorphonuclear granulocytes (PMNs), NK cells, γδ cells and then α/β T cells; however, with time the α/β T cells become predominant in the cellular response. The sequence of recruitment is probably determined by the proximity of the cells to the site of infection; for example, γδ cells are likely to be one of the first cells recruited to the site of *M. tuberculosis* infection in the lung. The PMNs produce highly proteolytic enzymes that cause tissue liquefaction while each of the T-cell types possesses cytotoxic activity. Activated macrophages have an increased capacity for seeking out, engulfing and destroying mycobacteria, but the production of TNF by macrophages contributes to tissue necrosis and, therefore, to the immunopathology of the disease.

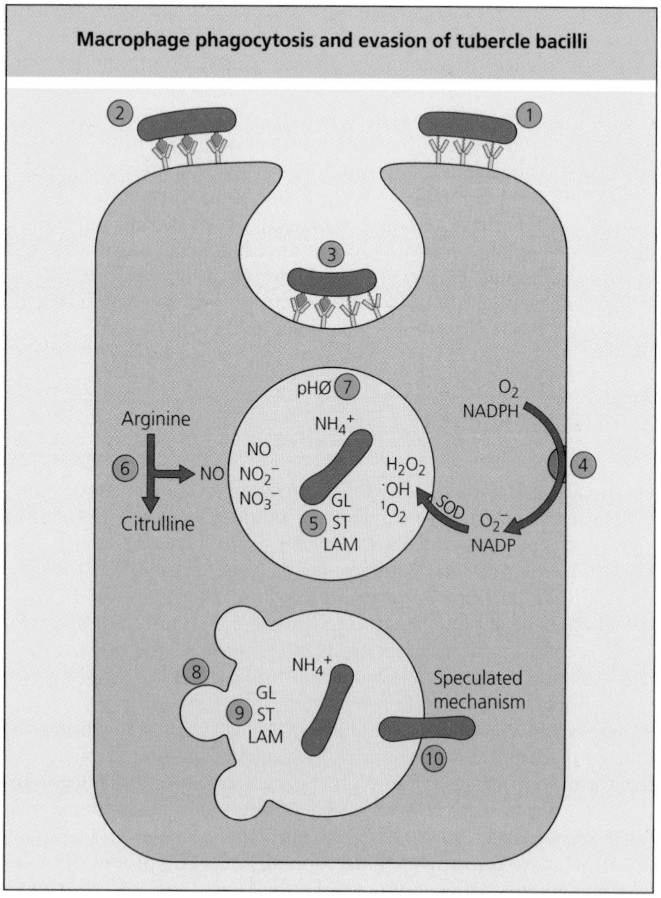

On the other hand, mycobacteria are equipped to resist oxidative killing by phagocytic cells. This resistance is controlled by the *katG* promoter in the mycobacterial genome. The *katG* gene encodes an enzyme with catalase, peroxidase and peroxynitritase activities.[43]

Granulomas develop as a mycobacterial infection becomes more chronic. Granulomas are aggregates of activated macrophages that take on epithelial cell-like morphology (epithelioid cells), and typically, lymphocytes are found at the periphery of the granuloma. Although the formation of a granuloma effectively contains the mycobacteria where they can be killed, bacilli can persist within giant cells (fused epithelioid cells) and the granuloma may never sterilize. With time a fibrotic wall (collagen) will encapsulate the granuloma and the center of the granuloma may become necrotic with a cheese-like appearance, which is the source of the descriptive word caseation. Hippocrates termed granulomas 'tubercles' because they were similar in morphology to the tubers of plants, hence the name tuberculosis.[17]

Host–pathogen interactions involving phagocytic uptake, intracellular survival, host immune responses and antigenic variation are highly complex and have been extensively reviewed.[41,42,44]

Macrophage phagocytosis and evasion of tubercle bacilli

Fig. 174.10 Macrophage phagocytosis and evasion of tubercle bacilli. The tubercle bacilli bind via lipoarabinomannan (LAM) (1) or complement receptors (2); phagocytosis occurs (3) with the activation of an oxidative burst (4); glycolipids (GL), sulfatides (ST) and LAM can downregulate the oxidative burst (5); reactive nitrogen intermediates may play a role in antimycobacterial activity (6), as does the acidic pH of the phagolysosome (7). Finally, the production of ammonia by tubercle bacilli may diminish the effect of reactive nitrogen intermediates (8) and contribute to the failure to form a phagolysosome fusion (9). Tubercule bacilli may evade the antimycobacterial activities of the phagolysosome by producing a hemolysin that releases the bacilli into the cytoplasm (10). NADP, nicotinamide adenine dinucleotide phosphate; NADPH, nicotinamide adenine dinucleotide phosphate, reduced form; SOD, superoxide dismutase. Adapted from Chan & Kaufmann.[41]

LABORATORY DIAGNOSIS OF MYCOBACTERIA

General remarks

The detection and identification of mycobacteria in clinical specimens requires profound expertise and is associated with a considerable safety risk when specimens are handled improperly. Given the low infectious dose of *M. tuberculosis* for humans (50% infective dose, <10 AFB), specimens from known or suspected cases of tuberculosis must be considered potentially infectious and handled with appropriate precautions.[45] Aerosol-generating manipulations should be conducted in a biosafety cabinet class II. Level 3 facilities are required for laboratories associated with higher risk (processing specimens for culture, identification and susceptibility testing; extraction of DNA from culture). Only in complying with the generally accepted biohazard precautions will safety for both laboratory personnel and the environment be assured.

The technologies available to assist in the laboratory diagnosis of mycobacterial infections have improved remarkably.[16,34,46,47] Major achievements are:

- fully automated, nonradiometric culture systems for culture and drug susceptibility testing;
- nucleic acid amplification assays for the direct detection of *M. tuberculosis* complex in clinical specimens;

- identification at the species level by nucleic acid probes, line probe assays and gene sequencing;
- molecular assays for the rapid detection of antimicrobial resistance; and
- DNA typing methods for answering questions relating to transmission routes, to reactivation versus re-infection of disease or to the genetic diversity of strain populations.

In discussing diagnostic mycobacteriology it is important to emphasize two general principles of laboratory medicine. First, the quality of any clinical test is highly dependent on the quality of the specimen, including the time of collection in the course of the disease, the appropriateness and sufficiency of the specimen, and the prompt and proper transport of the specimen to the laboratory. Second, the intended purpose of the test must be understood by the physician who orders the test. Was the test designed to screen for disease, to provide a definitive diagnosis based on a clinical index of suspicion, to confirm another test, to monitor therapy (test of cure), or to provide epidemiologic information? Use of a test for a purpose for which it was not designed and evaluated could be misleading. For example, nucleic acid amplification assays for the direct detection of M. tuberculosis complex in clinical specimens were evaluated as diagnostic assays for the very first detection of disease and explicitly not for monitoring response to therapy or cure.

The Centers for Disease Control and Prevention and other expert institutions recommend that AFB smear results be available and positive results be reported within 24 hours of specimen receipt.[48] The time required for identification and susceptibility testing of M. tuberculosis should average 14–21 days and 15–30 days, respectively.[48,49] With the new molecular tests available this goal will easily be achieved and partial results be available to the clinician even more rapidly.

Collection of specimens

The most critical step in the laboratory diagnosis of any infectious disease often occurs before the specimen arrives at the laboratory.[34,46,50] The quality, quantity, timing, transport and appropriateness of the specimen have a greater impact on the outcome of a laboratory test than almost any other factor (Table 174.3). It is important that physicians notify the laboratory if they suspect an uncommon or fastidious mycobacterial infection (such as M. ulcerans, M. genavense or M. haemophilum) because these and other species of mycobacteria have

Table 174.3 Specimen types and requirements for the diagnosis of mycobacterial infections

Specimen type	Requirements	Collection	Note
Abscess fluid	10 ml*	Collect with syringe, submit in sterile container	Dry swab or swab submitted in transport medium unacceptable
Blood	5–10 ml (adult) 1–5 ml (child)	SPS tube, tube with heparin or citrate, Isolator tube	EDTA tube and coagulated blood unacceptable Do not refrigerate
Fluids (pleural, pericardial, peritoneal, synovial, etc.)	10–15 ml*	Collect with syringe, submit in sterile container	Swabs unacceptable
Bone	Bone chip	Sterile container, no fixative	Formalin-fixed unacceptable
Bone marrow	100 mg* or 1–3 ml aspirate	SPS tube, heparin or citrate tube, isolator tube	Aspirate volumes >5 ml may be primarily peripheral blood Do not refrigerate
Bronchoalveolar lavage or bronchial washing	≥5 ml	Sterile container	Avoid contamination of bronchoscope with tap water (possible false-positive results)
Cerebrospinal fluid	5–10 ml*	Sterile tube	
Gastric lavage	5–10 ml	Sterile container, collecting in morning before arising and eating	Neutralize with 10% sodium carbonate if delayed processing
Lymph node	Whole node or part*, caseous part	Sterile container	Formalin-fixed unacceptable
Skin biopsy	Sterile container, aspirate	Biopsy at periphery or aspirate from under margin of lesion	Note if suspicion of M. ulcerans, M. haemophilum or M. marinum (need special culture conditions or extended incubation)
Sputum	5–10 ml	Early morning sputum in sterile plastic container	Use sterile hypertonic saline for induced sputum, avoid exposure to tap water Do not pool sputum specimens
Stool	≥1 g	Sterile plastic container, no transport medium	Refrigerate, but do *not* freeze
Tissue biopsy	1 g*	Sterile container	Caseous portion, formalin-fixed unacceptable
Urine	50 ml*	First morning specimen, catheter urine in sterile container	24-hour urine and pooled urine specimens unacceptable Refrigerate

SPS, sodium polyanetholsulfonate.
*As much as possible (up to or in excess of the weight/volume shown).
Adapted and modified from Pfyffer,[34] CLSI,[46] Kent & Kubica[50] and Della Latta.[51]

growth requirements that are significantly different from the majority of other species of mycobacteria isolated from clinical specimens.

Respiratory specimens

Sputum is the best specimen for the diagnosis of pulmonary tuberculosis. Expectorated sputum specimen should be collected early in the morning on three occasions. The wide-mouthed, sterile, plastic container (wax free) with a tight fitting cap containing the sputum specimen should be immediately transported to the laboratory or held at 39.2°F (4°C) until processed. Prompt processing of sputum is required to minimize overgrowth of mycobacteria by the normal respiratory tract microflora. Alternative respiratory tract specimens are induced sputum, endotracheal aspiration, bronchial washings or aspirates taken during bronchoscopy, and gastric lavage. Bronchoscopes must be carefully cleaned and decontaminated after collecting specimens from patients.

Gastric lavage

Gastric lavage (for swallowed sputum) is useful for collecting specimens from patients who, for a variety of reasons, are unable to produce sputum by other means. Gastric lavage is the specimen of choice from infants and children (up to 12 years) suspected of having pulmonary tuberculosis. *M. gordonae* is frequently found in many hospital water supplies and especially in ice machines, and use of such contaminated water during the collection of a gastric aspirate may result in a false-positive smear or culture. A gastric lavage must be promptly sent to the laboratory because it must be processed as soon as possible or neutralized with 10% sodium carbonate to avoid loss of mycobacteria due to gastric acidity. As with expectorated sputum specimens, gastric lavage specimens should be collected early in the morning, before eating, and on three separate occasions.

Urine

Three early morning midstream urine specimens should be collected into a sterile plastic container with a leak-proof cap. Large volumes of urine can be concentrated by filtration, but 24-hour urine should not be used because of contamination and dilution of any mycobacteria present.

Blood and bone marrow

Blood, bone marrow aspirates or cores are ideal specimens for the diagnosis of disseminated mycobacterial infections, in particular of MAC infections. If blood has to be transported before inoculation of the medium, sodium polyanethol sulfonate (SPS), heparin or citrate may be used as an anticoagulant. Blood collected in EDTA and coagulated blood are not acceptable for culture, neither is direct inoculation of blood onto a solid medium. If blood cannot immediately be processed by the laboratory, it should be stored at room temperature.

Other fluids

Pleural, pericardial, synovial and ascitic fluids as well as pus and cerebrospinal fluid (CSF) may also be submitted for diagnostic analyses. *Mycobacterium tuberculosis* meningitis is a medical emergency and CSF specimens should be collected, transported and processed in a manner that reflects the urgent nature of such a diagnosis.

Tissues

Tissue should be submitted for both histology and mycobacteriology. As tissue is preferred over necrotic material or pus for culture, it is therefore important to have fresh tissue and not swabs submitted to the microbiology laboratory. Formalin-preserved tissue should be submitted for histologic studies. Although not suitable for culture, formalin-preserved and paraffin-embedded tissue may be submitted for polymerase chain reaction (PCR) analysis, especially if AFB are observed on microscopic examination of the tissue sections.

Feces

Feces are not a particularly useful specimen for the diagnosis of tuberculosis or other mycobacterial infections, with the exception of suspected gastrointestinal tract infection with MAC in HIV-positive patients. However, the recovery of MAC from feces is poor (low sensitivity) even in HIV-positive patients. If *M. avium* is isolated from the feces the positive predictive value of the culture is high, meaning that the patient is likely to develop disseminated disease.[52] To avoid overgrowth of normal gastrointestinal tract microflora, feces must be rather harshly decontaminated, but this is likely to also decrease the yield of mycobacteria.[53]

Processing

Contaminated specimens

Most respiratory tract specimens are expected to be contaminated with normal respiratory tract microflora. In addition, the mucin matrix both protects and traps micro-organisms and makes the specimens difficult to process. Therefore such specimens have to be decontaminated (to reduce or eliminate other micro-organisms that would be likely to overgrow the mycobacteria that might be present in the specimen) and liquefied. The most common agents used to pretreat respiratory specimens are N-acetyl-L-cysteine (NALC) and dithiothreitol (DTT or sputolysin). Both NALC and DTT are unstable in air and must be prepared fresh. A combination of NALC and sodium hydroxide is most commonly used for digesting and decontaminating sputum. Other agents used for digestion and decontamination are zephiran (benzalkonium chloride)-trisodium phosphate, oxalic acid, cetylpyridinium chloride (CPC)-sodium chloride, and sulfuric acid.[34,46,50,51] Finally, the pretreated specimen is centrifuged to increase sensitivity of microscopy and the recovery of mycobacteria from culture.

There is no ideal method for digesting and decontaminating respiratory tract specimens. Invariably, mycobacteria are lost during decontamination. Detailed descriptions of the various procedures for digesting and decontaminating sputum and other contaminated specimens have been well described elsewhere.[34,46,50,51]

Uncontaminated specimens

The primary concern about specimens from sterile body sites is the quantity of specimen submitted for smear and culture. Swabs usually contain insufficient material for culture, and 1 g of tissue or 10 ml of fluid are ideal. To improve recovery of mycobacteria, centrifugation should be used to concentrate large volumes of fluids. Aseptically collected tissues and fluids from normally sterile body sites usually do not require processing. These specimens can initially be inoculated on a chocolate agar plate to check for purity. If sterile, specimens are concentrated and inoculated into a liquid growth medium as well as on solid media without decontamination.

Acid-fast stain and smear microscopy

An acid-fast stain remains the most rapid and least expensive method for directly detecting mycobacteria in clinical specimens, and is highly specific. Nevertheless, the laboratory must be aware that there are organisms other than mycobacteria with various degrees of acid-fastness such as *Rhodococcus* spp., *Nocardia* spp. and *Legionella micdadei*, as well as cysts from *Cryptosporidium*, *Isospora*, *Cyclospora* and *Microsporidium* spores. The presence of AFB in a specimen from a patient with signs and symptoms of tuberculosis or another mycobacterial infection is an important guide to effective treatment and the initiation of public health measures. Furthermore, an acid-fast stain can quickly assess patient infectiousness, and is also used to confirm that a culture is acid fast. The detection limit of an acid-fast stain has been estimated to be 5000–10 000 bacilli/ml of sputum; overall sensitivity is between 22% and 78%.[55] The importance of the acid-fast stain and the need for a prompt turnaround time cannot be overemphasized. In laboratories that do not perform cultures, an acid-fast stain can be performed using a specimen treated for a short time with 5% sodium hypochlorite. Above all, the predictive value of a positive smear for *M. tuberculosis* in expectorated sputum is very high (~90%).

The three stains that are commonly used to detect AFB are Ziehl–Neelsen, Kinyoun and auramine–rhodamine fluorochrome stains.[51] With each of these procedures, acid-fastness is defined as resistance to decolorizing with acid–alcohol (e.g. 3% hydrochloric acid in 95% ethanol). When mycobacteria are stained with Gram's crystal violet and safranin they often appear as beaded Gram-positive bacilli or fail to stain at all. It is important to note, however, that culture media, incubation conditions and the age of the culture influence the acid fastness of mycobacteria. The critical role of the mycobacterial cell wall in acid fastness is underscored by the observation that INH causes a loss of 'acid fastness' in susceptible strains of *M. tuberculosis*.

The preparation of the smear is the critical first step in performing an acid-fast stain. Using a glass slide cleaned with ethanol, make a smear of approximately 1 × 2 cm of a single specimen or isolate. For CSF specimens previously concentrated by centrifugation, three drops of the concentrate are placed on a clean glass slide, one drop at a time. The drop is allowed to air dry before the next drop is added. The slide is air dried or alternatively dried at 176°F (80°C) for 15 minutes in a biosafety cabinet class II – it is important to note that heat fixing may not kill all the mycobacteria on the slide. Mycobacteria appear brightly fluorescent against a dark background in the auramine–rhodamine stain and the increased sensitivity of the fluorescence stain compared with the other stains is used to rapidly screen slides at a lower (250–450×) magnification. However, fluorescent objects must be examined at 800–1000× magnification to confirm morphology. Positive fluorescent smears should be confirmed with either the Ziehl–Neelsen or Kinyoun stains. The Ziehl–Neelsen stain requires that the carbolfuchsin stain be heated for the stain to penetrate the mycobacterial cell. In contrast, heating is unnecessary with the Kinyoun stain because the concentration of basic fuchsin and phenol have been increased to ensure that the basic fuchsin penetrates the mycobacterial cell wall. Using a 100× oil immersion lens, 100–300 fields of a properly prepared smear and stain should be examined. It should be remembered that in examining even 100–300 fields, only 1–4% of a 1 × 2 cm smear would be examined. Mycobacteria usually appear as pink, slender rod-shaped bacilli; however, pleomorphic shapes are common and range from coccoid to long rods with curves or bends (Fig. 174.11).

Culture

In detecting approximately 10^2 viable organisms/ml of specimen, culture is more sensitive than smear microscopy. Also, it is the only reliable means to monitor effectiveness of therapy in tuberculosis patients.[55] A variety of solid (e.g. Löwenstein–Jensen, Ogawa, Middlebrook agar) and liquid media (see below) are available for the culture of mycobacteria from clinical specimens. It is highly recommended to use a combination of solid and liquid media to ensure good recovery for subsequent species identification and susceptibility testing. The macroscopic and microscopic characteristics, together with the rate of growth and pigmentation, are valuable in making a presumptive identification (see Fig. 174.2).

Manual culture systems used for the detection of mycobacteria are the Septi-Chek Acid-Fast Bacillus Biphasic System (Becton Dickinson Microbiology Systems, Sparks, MD), the MB Redox Tube System (Heipha Diagnostika, Eppelheim, Germany), and the Mycobacteria Growth Indicator Tube (MGIT; Becton Dickinson). The Septi-Chek AFB system consists of Middlebrook 7H9 broth and a plastic paddle with modified Löwenstein–Jensen medium, Middlebrook 7H11 agar and chocolate agar. Comparison studies with conventional culture

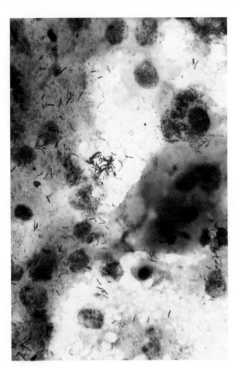

Fig. 174.11 Ziehl–Neelsen acid-fast stain of sputum containing 4+ tubercle bacilli. Courtesy of S Froman and A Gaytan.

and the BACTEC 460 TB System indicated that the Septi-Chek AFB Biphasic System is reliable and practical.[56] MB Redox tubes contain modified Kirchner medium enriched with growth supplements, antibiotic compounds and a redox indicator (tetrazolium salt) which is reduced to a pink-, red- and violet-colored formazan by mycobacteria. The accumulation of reduced dye on the surface of the bacilli results in the appearance of visible microcolonies.[57] The MGIT contains a highly enriched Middlebrook 7H9 broth in conjunction with a fluorescence quenching-based oxygen sensor (silicon rubber impregnated with a ruthenium pentahydrate). Growth is detected by exposing an inoculated MGIT to ultraviolet light and examining for fluorescence, which is an indication of growth and oxygen consumption. The performance of these manual systems in combination with conventional solid media is satisfactory.[56–59]

The radiometric, semiautomated BACTEC 460 TB System, commercially developed in the early 1980s by Becton Dickinson, became a 'gold standard' for the rapid detection of mycobacteria (Table 174.4). In the BACTEC 460 TB System growth of mycobacteria is detected by measuring the release of $^{14}CO_2$ from ^{14}C-labeled palmitate, which is the primary carbon source in the BACTEC 460 TB 12B culture medium. This technology has significantly improved recovery rates and detection time (for references, see[34]). However, as with all liquid media, neither colony morphology nor mixed cultured can be recognized. Other limitations of the BACTEC 460 TB System are the costs, the problem of radioactive waste disposal, labor intensity and the potential for needle punctures among technicians. Due to these disadvantages the BACTEC 460 TB System is gradually vanishing from clinical mycobacteriology laboratories.

The studies published to date on the nonradiometric automated systems – BACTEC MGIT 960 (Becton Dickinson), ESP Culture System II (Trek Diagnostic Systems, Cleveland, OH) and MB/BacT (bioMerieux, Marcy-L'Etoile, France) – indicate similar performance in terms of recovery rates and time to detection in comparison with conventional culture and the radiometric BACTEC.[60–62] Though costly, these new systems are convenient, labor-saving, do not require the use of radioisotope, offer continuous monitoring of the cultures and electronic data management, and address safety more appropriately.

Table 174.4 Semiautomated and fully automated systems for the detection of *Mycobacterium tuberculosis* complex and other mycobacteria in clinical specimens

Instrument/medium	Manufacturer	Detection system	SIRE/PZA/second line drugs susceptibility testing
BACTEC 460 • BACTEC 12B medium (modified 7H9 broth) • No medium available for blood and bone marrow	Becton Dickinson Microbiology Systems, Sparks, MD, USA	Detection of radioactively labeled CO_2 released during the catabolism of 14C-labeled palmitic acid in the growth medium	Yes/Yes/Yes
BACTEC 9000MB • MYCO/F medium + supplements (modified 7H9 broth) • MYCO F/LYTIC medium for blood and bone marrow	Becton Dickinson Microbiology Systems, Sparks, MD, USA	Detects changes in O_2 concentration in the growth medium using an O_2 sensor based on fluorescence quenching	No/No/No
BACTEC MGIT 960 • MGIT (modified 7H9 broth) • No medium available for blood and bone marrow	Becton Dickinson Microbiology Systems, Sparks, MD, USA	O_2 sensor based on fluorescence quenching	Yes/Yes/Yes
BACTEC 9050 • BACTEC MYCO F/LYTIC (medium for blood and bone marrow)	Becton Dickinson Microbiology Systems, Sparks, MD, USA	Fluorogenic system	No/No/No
ESP Culture System II • ESP Myco (modified 7H9 broth)	Trek Diagnostic Systems, Cleveland, OH, USA	Detects production on consumption of gas by measuring changes in partial pressure of gas phase of culture medium	Yes/No/No
MB/BacT/ALERT 3D • Bact/ALERT MP (modified 7H9 broth) • Bact/Alert ML Mycobacteria lytic (medium for blood)	BioMérieux, Marcy-L'Etoile, France	Detects changes in CO_2 concentration in gas phase of the growth medium using a colorimetric sensor and reflected light	No/No/No

PZA, pyrazinamide; SIRE, streptomycin, isoniazid, rifampin and ethambutol.

For many years the Isolator System (Wampole, Cranbury, NJ) and the radiometric BACTEC 13A blood culture medium (Becton Dickinson) were the only reliable systems for mycobacterial blood cultures. Since the Isolator Sytem is associated with a not negligible safety risk and the BACTEC 13A medium is no longer commercially available, blood and bone marrow specimens are increasingly cultivated in MYCO/F LYTIC bottles (Becton Dickinson) or the MB/BacT ALERT blood medium (bioMérieux). These two culture systems were as sensitive as and faster for the detection of MAC bacteremia than the older standard systems, Isolator and the radiometric BACTEC 13A medium.[63] Also, BacT/ALERT FA blood cultures and BACTEC MYCO/F LYTIC vials equally supported ample growth of *M. tuberculosis*.[64]

Identification

Traditional methods (Runyon groups, morphologic features and growth aspects)

In 1958, Ernest Runyon proposed that by dividing mycobacteria into four groups based on the rate of growth and pigmentation one could make a preliminary identification. Rapid growers were separated from slowly growing mycobacteria according to the time required to produce clearly visible colonies (≤7 days for rapid growers; the most accurate measure of growth is made with subcultures). Slowly growing mycobacteria were separated based on pigment production: scotochromogenic (see Figs 174.3, 174.4), photochromogenic (see Fig. 174.5) and nonphotochromogenic (see Fig. 174.6). Fifty years later, the Runyon groups remain a valuable guide for a presumptive identification of mycobacteria isolated by solid culture, and the logic of this classification has been corroborated by 16S rRNA sequence analysis.

Even with biochemical identification only, the correlation between an initial classification into a Runyon group and the final identification ranges from 87% (nonphotochromogens) to 97% (rapid growers).[50]

The first challenge for the clinical mycobacteriology laboratory is to distinguish between members of the *M. tuberculosis* complex (see Table 174.1) and NTM, a taxonomically imprecise, but clinically useful distinction.

Growth of *M. tuberculosis* on Middlebrook 7H10 or 7H11 agar at 95°F (35°C) is usually detected in 2–3 weeks. The colonies are beige colored, rough, dry, corded, flat and with irregular borders (Fig. 174.12). On egg media such as Löwenstein–Jensen or Ogawa media the colonies are frequently warty and granular and with time heap into a cauliflower shape (Fig. 174.13). Although the growth of *M. tuberculosis* is quite distinct and it is not unreasonable for an experienced mycobacteriologist to make a presumptive report of *M. tuberculosis* based on the rate and appearance of growth, identification must always be confirmed by standard procedures.

Three clinically significant species of mycobacteria have lower optimal growth (86°F/30°C): *M. ulcerans*, *M. marinum* and *M. haemophilum*. In addition, *M. haemophilum* requires hemin for growth and, therefore, specimens suspected to harbor this species should be inoculated onto chocolate agar, Middlebrook 7H10 agar with hemolyzed blood or 7H10 agar with a hemin-containing paper strip.

Mycobacterium avium complex organisms isolated from blood or sputum appear as either glossy, whitish colonies or smaller, translucent colonies on Middlebrook 7H10 or 7H11 agar after 10–14 days (Fig. 174.14). A third, less frequently encountered morphology resembles the dry and flat colonies of *M. tuberculosis*. In older cultures colonies may even become verrucose and develop pigment. However, these colony variant types are not observed on egg-based

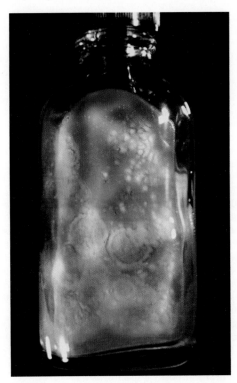

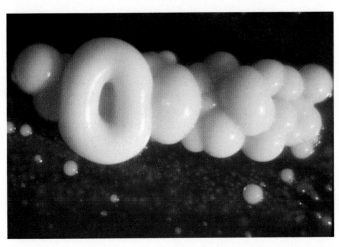

Fig. 174.14 *M. avium* grown on Middlebrook 7H10 agar. The two most frequent morphologies are shown (beige opaque colonies and smaller translucent colonies).

Fig. 174.12 Primary isolate of *M. tuberculosis* grown from sputum on Löwenstein–Jensen medium displaying characteristic beige, rough and dry-appearing growth. Courtesy of S Froman and A Gaytan.

media. The initial distinction between colony types is important because the transparent variants tend to be more resistant to antimicrobial agents.

Conventional biochemical tests

For many decades the salient biochemical features of mycobacteria represented the 'gold standard' for identification at the species level. Details about the many biochemical tests used in the conventional identification of mycobacteria are described in a variety of sources. Wayne and Sramek[65] and Kent & Kubica[50] described strategies for the use of these tests. Their value in today's clinical mycobacteriology laboratory has, however, become limited.

For more than 10 years mycolic acids have been extracted by saponification and derivatives prepared with either a phenyl ester or a fluorescent compound, for detection by high performance liquid chromatography (HPLC). The HPLC pattern of an unknown species is then compared with a library of known patterns usually facilitated by a decision analysis system.[66] The equipment cost and the expertise required to perform HPLC analyses has restricted use of this technology mostly to large hospital, and reference and public health laboratories.[46] Alternatively, whole cell fatty acid analysis can be performed by commercially available instrumentation and software (e.g. Microbial Identification Systems, Newark, DL).

Nevertheless, with the increasing number of new mycobacterial species it is well accepted today that biochemical tests are in many instances insufficient for accurate identification. Therefore, the ultimate identification scheme of mycobacteria mainly relies on molecular methods, along with some phenotypic tests.

Molecular methods

For some time nucleic acid probes (AccuProbe; Gen-Probe, San Diego, CA) have been commercially available for the identification of *M. tuberculosis* complex, *M. intracellulare*, MAC, *M. gordonae* and *M. kansasii* from culture. The AccuProbe culture confirmation test is based on the use of acridinium ester labeled DNA probes that are complementary to species-specific rRNA which is released from the mycobacteria using a combination of a lysing reagent, sonication and heat. If a stable RNA–DNA duplex forms, the acridinium label is protected within the helix from a selection reagent while free acridinium label is inactivated. Stable duplexes are detected by the addition of an alkaline hydrogen peroxide solution, which in combination with the bound acridinium ester generates chemiluminesence. The amount of light produced is measured in a luminometer as relative light units (RLUs).

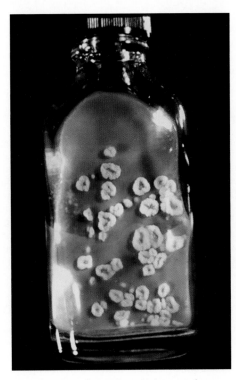

Fig. 174.13 Primary isolate of *M. tuberculosis* grown from sputum on Löwenstein–Jensen medium displaying 'cauliflower' or verrucose colonies. These are also characteristic of other mycobacteria including MAC and rapid growers, especially as a culture ages. Courtesy of S Froman and A Gaytan.

The AccuProbe test cannot be used for direct detection of mycobacteria in clinical specimens. In general, the AccuProbe tests are highly reliable and simple to perform. They are very specific and sensitive for *M. tuberculosis* complex and *M. gordonae* (100%); for the other species sensitivity is less (range 85–100%).

A more recent development is the line probe assay. In the INNO-LiPA multiplex probe assay (INNO-LiPA MYCOBACTERIA; Innogenetics, Ghent, Belgium), probes consist of the ~280 bp internal transcribed spacer (ITS) region in between the 16S and the 23S rDNAs. With this assay both *M. tuberculosis* complex as well as a number of NTM can easily be identified.[67] The GenoType kits of Hain Lifescience (Nehren, Germany) are based on similar technology and are able to identify 23 (GenoType CM) and 14 (GenoType AS) additional species, respectively. Concordant results have been obtained for 92.6% of previously sequenced mycobacterial strains with the CM Assay and 89.9% with the AS Assay.[68] Non-*Mycobacterium* species were also identified. Most attractively, the GenoType technology is able to separate most species within the *M. tuberculosis* complex.

Another way to identify mycobacteria at the species level is via PCR and PCR-restriction enzyme analysis (PRA). Telenti *et al.*[69] established a method based on the *hsp65* gene encoding for the 65 kDa heat shock protein and developed an algorithm of species identification based on the restriction profiles generated by Hae*III* and Bst*EII*. Although the method is widely used the major drawbacks of the technique are the facts that ambiguous profiles may occur and the database is very complex (http://app.chuv.ch/prasite/index.html).

Today, it is generally accepted that gene sequencing for identification purposes remains the 'gold standard' for identification. Identification of species-specific signatures within variable regions of highly conserved genes such as the 16S rDNA gene or *hsp65* gene generated PCR protocols using genus-specific primers followed by direct sequencing of the PCR products.[16,47] In addition to these genes, other targets such as the gene encoding the 32 kDa protein, the *sod* gene, the *gyrB* gene coding for the gyrase subunit B, the *rpoB* gene coding for the RNA polymerase, the *dnaJ* gene, or the ITS 16S–23S sequence may be used (for refs., see[16]). Even with the possibilities of gene sequencing the user has to be aware that each protocol has its limitations. For example, on 16S rDNA sequencing, *M. kansasii* is indistinguishable from *M. gastri*, *M. abscessus* from *M. chelonae*, and *M. ulcerans* from *M. marinum*.

Direct detection of *M. tuberculosis* complex by nucleic acid amplification

A vast number of studies have concentrated on the four commercially available nucleic acid amplification (NAA)-based kits designed to detect *M. tuberculosis* complex directly from clinical specimens:

- the Amplicor *M. tuberculosis* Test (Roche Molecular Systems, Inc., Branchburg, NJ);
- the Amplified *M. tuberculosis* Direct Test (MTD; GenProbe);
- the BDProbeTec Strand Displacement Amplification (SDA; Becton Dickinson); and
- GenoType Mycobacteria Direct (Hain Lifescience).

The Amplicor *M. tuberculosis* PCR assay is based on amplification of a 584 bp region of the 16S rRNA gene sequence. Incorporation of dUTP instead of dTTP prevents carry-over in the amplification reaction. Experience has shown that the specificity for smear-positive specimens ranges from 90% to 100% for respiratory specimens and from 87.5% to 100% for extrapulmonary specimens. Sensitivity appears to be significantly lower for smear-negative specimens, from 50% to 95% for respiratory specimens and from 17% to 70% for extrapulmonary specimens.

The amplified *M. tuberculosis* direct (MTD) test uses transcription-mediated amplification and a hybridization protection assay to qualitatively detect the *M. tuberculosis* complex. Mycobacterial rRNA is released by sonication from bacilli present in a clinical specimen, denatured with heat and transcribed into cDNA with a reverse transcriptase.

One part of the oligonucleotide used in the reverse transcription step includes a promoter region for a high efficiency RNA polymerase (e.g. phage T7 polymerase); the other part of the oligonucleotide includes a 16S rRNA target-specific sequence. As a result of cycles of denaturation, reverse transcription and RNA synthesis, the mycobacterial rRNA is amplified under isothermal conditions (108°F/42°C). *Mycobacterium tuberculosis* complex-specific amplicons are detected using the GenProbe hybridization protection assay (see above). Based on published reports, overall specificity of the MTD ranges from 92% to 100%. For respiratory specimens the sensitivity is between 91% and 100% for smear-positive specimens and between 65% and 92% for smear-negative specimens. For nonrespiratory specimens, the sensitivity is between 88% and 100% for smear-positive specimens and between 63% and 100% for smear-negative specimens.

The BDProbeTec SDA is an isothermal enzymatic process that co-amplifies sequences of the IS*6110* (specific to *M. tuberculosis* complex) and the 16S rRNA gene (common to most mycobacterial species). By nicking the recognition sequence in double-stranded DNA by a restriction endonuclease and extension of that site with a polymerase that synthesizes a new strand of DNA while displacing the existing one, the assay has similarly a high specificity. Sensitivity for smear-positive specimens was between 98.5% and 100% and between 33% and 85% for smear-negative specimens.

In a large retrospective study that included 824 respiratory species, AFB smear, Cobas Amplicor MTB and BDProbeTec revealed similar specificity (99.7%, 99.9% and 99.9%, respectively), whereas overall sensitivity of the three tests was 61.5%, 78% and 86.2%, respectively (proportion of smear-positive specimens was <61%).[70]

The GenoType Mycobacteria Direct is based on the nucleic acid sequence-based amplification (NASBA) and DNA strip techniques, allowing the 23S rRNA amplification-based detection of *M. tuberculosis* complex, *M. avium*, *M. intracellulare*, *M. kansasii* and *M. malmoense* directly from specimens. Although data are still very limited, this method may turn out to be promising.[71]

From the numerous studies including both respiratory and extrapulmonary specimens it is obvious that NAA-based diagnostic tests are:

- appropriate, if there is a clinical suspicion of tuberculosis;
- always performed in conjunction with culture; and
- not to be requested to monitor therapeutic success.[46,47]

Most importantly, laboratories perfoming such assays should be part of external quality control schemes.[72]

DNA fingerprinting

Molecular typing helps to differentiate relapses from exogenous re-infections in patients and to demonstrate false-positive cases due to contaminated bronchoscopes or laboratory cross-contamination of clinical specimens during workup. It also allows the definition of prevalent families of strains and elucidates the intraspecies genetic micro-evolution. Most importantly, it helps to identify transmission chains. Lastly, DNA typing methods are also useful in identifying members within the *M. tuberculosis* complex such as *M. microti*, *M. caprae* or *M. canettii*. For *M. tuberculosis* in particular, a number of methods have been developed to carry out DNA typing rapidly. The most important ones are as follows.[16]

IS*6110* restriction fragment length polymorphism

The IS*6110*-based analysis of *M. tuberculosis* centers on differences in fragment length and copy number of this insertion element. There are 0–20 copies of the 1355 bp IS*6110* in most strains of *M. tuberculosis*. If strains of *M. tuberculosis* contain a small number of IS*6110* only, the resulting patterns often do not discriminate between strains. The distribution of IS*6110* within the genome appears to be stable over several months to years. IS*6110*-based restriction fragment length polymorphism (RFLP) is conceptually straightforward[73] and standardized to facilitate interlaboratory comparability of patterns.[74] Basically, the method involves extraction of genomic DNA, restriction of the DNA with an appropriate enzyme (e.g. PvuII) and electrophoretic separation of the restriction fragments (RFLP analysis). The IS6110 pattern is revealed by Southern hybridization using a labeled fragment of the IS6110 sequence. A computer-based method of analysis of the IS6110 patterns was described by Heersma et al and software is commercially available.[75] A drawback of this method is the large amount (about 2 μg) that is required for analysis. Therefore, other PCR-based typing methods were developed that have comparable discrimination and reproducibility to RFLP analysis.

Spacer oligonucleotide typing ('spoligotyping')

This method uses PCR primers to amplify the 36 bp direct repeats (DRs) in the genomic direct-repeat region of M. tuberculosis complex DNA.[76] The resulting PCR products are hybridized to 43 different oligonucleotides fixed to a membrane. The 43 oligonucleotides were derived from the sequences of the spacer DNA between the DRs. This method is able to discriminate the members of the M. tuberculosis complex.[16] Spoligotyping also allows the identification of prevalent groups of strains, e.g. the Beijing strain, a genotype frequently encountered in China, in other regions of Asia and the former Soviet Union, or the 'W' strain, an evolutionary branch of the Beijing family which caused a large outbreak in the USA.

PCR assays targeting loci other than IS6110

Genotyping based on a variable number of tandem repeats (VNTRs) of different classes of interspersed genetic elements, the mycobacterial interspersed repetitive units (MIRUs), is an elegant alternative to the labor-intense classic IS6110-based DNA typing. It relies on:

- PCR amplification of multiple loci using primers specific for the flanking regions of each repeat locus; and
- the determination of the sites of the amplicpons which reflect the numbers of the targeted MIRU-VNTR copies.

A standardization of the method has recently been proposed.[77]

ANTIMICROBIAL RESISTANCE AND SUSCEPTIBILITY TESTING

Resistance

During bacterial multiplication resistance to antimycobacterial drugs develops spontaneously and with a defined frequency. Genetic mutations resulting in resistance of M. tuberculosis to RMP lead to an estimated prevalence of 1 in 10^8 bacilli in drug free environments. Antimicrobial resistance in mycobacteria is fundamentally a reflection of the large populations of mycobacteria present in infected tissues and fluids and the frequencies of individual gene mutations that result in a resistant phenotype. In pulmonary tuberculosis there are 10^7–10^9 bacilli in lung cavities, but only 10^2–10^4 bacilli in caseous lesions. The likelihood of spontaneous mutations leading to an INH- and RMP-resistant phenotype of M. tuberculosis (MDR-TB) is very low, i.e. in 10^{-14} ($10^{-6} \times 10^{-8}$) AFB. Therefore, the worldwide emergence of resistant strains cannot be explained by the phenomenon of natural mutations only. More important is the man-made impact leading to the high rate of acquired resistance,[22] mainly because of the patients' nonadherence to therapy (see above).

Antimicrobial resistance in M. tuberculosis is classically defined as a significant difference in the activity of an antimycobacterial drug between a wild-type strain and another strain. A wild-type strain is defined as a strain isolated from a patient before treatment and less than 1% of a population of that strain is resistant to any antimycobacterial agent. Resistance emerges as a consequence of individual mutations in mycobacterial genes that lead to a structural or functional change such that an antimycobacterial agent is no longer active against that strain. In the recent past, several resistance mechanisms

at the molecular level have been elucidated (for references, see[78]). For example, there is compelling evidence that resistance to INH results from a mutation or a combination of mutations in the katG, ahpC, inhA, ndh or the kasA genes of M. tuberculosis (Table 174.5). In M. tuberculosis, resistance to RMP is a result of a mutation within an 81 bp (27 amino acid) sequence of the core region of the rpoB gene (RNA polymerase β subunit); streptomycin resistance has been attributed to mutations in either the rrs gene (16S rRNA gene) or the rpsL gene (ribosomal protein S12). Quinolone resistance has been ascribed to mutations in the gyrA genes and pyrazinamide resistance to mutations in the pncA gene that encodes pyrazinamidase/nicotinamidase activity. The targets for the major classes or types of antimycobacterial agent are shown in Figure 174.15. Antibiotic resistance does not appear to transfer between strains of mycobacteria by either plasmid exchange or resistance transfer factors. The M. tuberculosis MDR as well as the XDR phenotypes appear to be entirely the result of a stepwise accumulation of individual mutations.

Intrinsic resistance to antimicrobial agents is also common in both slowly and rapidly growing NTM. In most instances, this form of resistance appears to be the result of the impermeability of the mycobacterial cell envelope. For example, most MAC isolates are resistant to RMP despite the fact that the isolate has a wild-type rpoB gene. However, M. avium resistance to INH may reflect the lack of an effective antimicrobial activity rather than or in addition to a lack of permeability.[82] Both M. chelonae and M. abscessus are intrinsically resistant to quinolones, while M. fortuitum is susceptible.

Antimicrobial agents

There are a variety of antimicrobial agents available for the treatment of mycobacterial infections; however, until recently almost all clinical studies of these agents were focused on M. tuberculosis and to a lesser extent M. leprae. The emergence of MAC as an important opportunistic infection associated with HIV infection and increased recognition that rapidly growing mycobacteria are a significant cause of human disease led to an expansion in our knowledge about the activity of certain agents against these and other mycobacteria. Although MAC is resistant to INH and only variably susceptible to RMP, MAC infections can be successfully treated with a macrolide and other agents such as ethambutol (EMB) plus rifabutin. Infections caused by rapidly growing mycobacteria must be treated with antimicrobial agents other than the primary antituberculous agents INH, RMP, EMB and PZA. For most other species there is often only limited information about the effectiveness and efficacy of antimycobacterial agents, perhaps with the exception of M. kansasii and M. marinum. The antimicrobial agents recommended for the treatment of various mycobacterial infections are shown in Table 174.6; however, it is not always appropriate to perform susceptibility tests on all of the agents because of a lack of standardized procedures and well-established interpretive criteria[83] (see also Chapter 143).

Susceptibility testing

The susceptibility testing of mycobacteria and the definition of antimicrobial resistance have been influenced by decades of focus on M. tuberculosis. Thus, there is more information about antimicrobial agents and the susceptibility testing of M. tuberculosis than for all other species of mycobacteria. Indeed, susceptibility testing of many NTM has been largely extrapolated from experience with M. tuberculosis, including adoption of the same interpretive criteria. In some instances this extrapolation has proven to provide useful and reliable information, but in other situations this practice can be misleading. Therefore, with the exception of testing of M. tuberculosis isolates against the first-line antimycobacterial agents, susceptibility testing of mycobacteria should be performed in laboratories with extensive experience. Although the laboratory can provide valuable but limited guidance in the interpretation of results, the application of those results to the treatment of a patient with an uncommon mycobacterial infection is

Table 174.5 Mycobacterial genes with mutations associated with antimicrobial resistance

Antimicrobial agent	Species	Gene(s) involved	Proportion of resistance (%)	Gene function	Mechanisms of action
Rifampin (rifampicin)	M. tuberculosis M. africanum M. leprae M. avium	rpoB	>96	β-subunit of RNA polymerase	Inhibition of transcription
Isoniazid	M. tuberculosis M. tuberculosis M. tuberculosis M. tuberculosis M. leprae M. tuberculosis	katG inhA locus ndh ahpC acpM (kasA)	20–80 15–43 10 10–15	Catalase-peroxidase Enoyl ACP reductase NADH dehydrogenase II Alkyl hydroperoxidase β-ketoacyl ACP synthase	Inhibition of mycolic acid biosynthesis and multiple effects on DNA, lipids, carbohydrates, NAD metabolism
Ethambutol	M. tuberculosis	embCAB	47–65	Arabinosyltransferase	Inhibition of arabinogalactan synthesis
Streptomycin	M. tuberculosis M. smegmatis M. tuberculosis	rpsL rrs	52–59 8–21	S12 Ribosomal protein 16S rRNA	Inhibition of protein synthesis
Pyrazinamide	M. tuberculosis	pncA	72–97	Nicotinamidase/prazinamidase	Acidification of cytoplasm and de-energized membrane
Fluoroquinolones	M. tuberculosis M. smegmatis	gyrA gyr B	75–94 In vitro	DNA gyrase subunit A and subunit B	Inhibition of DNA gyrases
Azithromycin–clarithromycin	M. avium M intracellulare M. chelonae M. abscessus	V domain 23S rRNA	95	23S rRNA	
Amikacin–kanamycin	M. tuberculosis	rrs	>6	16S rDNA	Inhibition of protein synthesis
Ethionamide	M. tuberculosis	etaA/ethA inhA	37 56	Flavin mono-oxygenase	Inhibition of mycolic acid biosynthesis

Proportion of resistance represents the estimated percentage of resistance that can be accounted for by mutations in the respective genes. Mutations in katG, ahpC, inhA and/or kasA collectively probably account for 90% of isoniazid resistance.
Adapted from Zhang et al.[78] Percentage figures taken in part from Zhang & Telenti.[79]

likely to require the involvement of a physician with experience in the management of such infections.

Drug susceptibility testing is mandatory on initial isolates of *M. tuberculosis* and related species from all patients. If culture remains positive over an extended period of time, susceptibility testing should be repeated to monitor a possible development of drug resistance. The current guidelines of the Clinical Laboratory Standards Institute (CLSI) recommend repeating susceptibility testing at least every 3 months.[83]

There are three accepted methods for drug susceptibility testing of *M. tuberculosis*: the absolute concentration method, the resistance ratio method and the agar proportion method, the latter being used most widely on the Western hemisphere.

Agar proportion method

This method is based on the concept of 'critical concentrations' of antituberculosis agents and the percentage of resistant tubercle bacilli within a test population ('critical proportion'). Critical concentrations for antituberculosis agents were established on an empiric clinical basis. Therapeutic success was unlikely if the proportion of drug-resistant mutants within a population of *M. tuberculosis* isolated from a patient exceeded a threshold of 1% at a concentration of the antituberculosis agent that was known to be therapeutically effective against a 'wild-type' or fully susceptible strain. The critical concentration may not be the same as the peak serum concentration of a drug and there might be an interest in applying the use of the minimum inhibitory

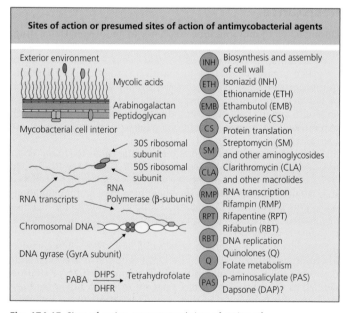

Fig. 174.15 Sites of action or presumed sites of action of antimycobacterial agents. DHFR, dihydrofolate reductase; DHPS, dihydropteroate synthase; PABA, p-aminobenzoic acid; PAS, p-aminosalicylic acid. Figure adapted from Parsons et al.[80] and Young.[81]

Table 174.6 Antimycobacterial agents ranked by clinical use

Species	Primary or first choice	Secondary or second choice	Notes
M. tuberculosis	INH, RMP, PZA, EMB	SM, amikacin, ciprofloxacin, linezolid	Treatment plan varies depending on incidence of INH resistance in community, if MDR or XDR, patient adherence, clinical manifestation, other factors
M. bovis	INH, RMP, EMB		Uniformly PZA resistant, usually 9–12 months' therapy recommended
M. leprae	Dapsone, RMP, clofazimine, clarithromycin	Ethionamide, prothionamide, minocycline	Treatment plan varies depending on paucibacillary or multibacillary disease
M. avium *M. intracellulare*	Azithromycin or clarithromycin, ethambutol, rifabutin Surgical excision (lymphadenitis/children)	Amikacin, streptomycin, moxifloxacin	PZA resistant, INH resistance is usual; drugs and doses vary depending on immunocompetency, disseminated or pulmonary or other, and treatment vs prophylaxis
M. chelonae *M. fortuitum* *M. abscessus*	Amikacin, cefoxitin, ciprofloxacin, clarithromycin, doxycycline or minocycline, sulfonamides	Imipenem, levofloxacin, tobramycin (*M. chelonae* only), linezolid	All resistant to INH, PZA, RMP, SM, EMB and clofazimine. *M. chelonae* uniformly resistant to cefoxitin. EMB may be useful for treating *M. smegmatis*. Contamination with these species is common, confirm clinical significance
M. kansasii	RMP, INH, EMB	Pyridoxine, clarithromycin, rifabutin, sulfamethoxazole	PZA resistance is uniform. Only test RMP; testing of INH and EMB can be misleading. Clarithromycin resistance occurs. Treatment for 12 or more months
M. scrofulaceum	Surgical excision without chemotherapy (lymphadenitis)	Azithromycin, clarithromycin	INH and PZA resistant
M. ulcerans	Surgical excision, RMP, amikacin	EMB, trimethoprim–sulfamethoxazole, SM, ciprofloxacin, sparfloxacin	Chemotherapy rarely effective
M. marinum	Clarithromycin, minocycline, doxycycline, RMB, rifabutin, EMB, trimethoprim–sulfamethoxazole		INH and PZA resistant
M. haemophilum	Clarithromycin, rifabutin, ciprofloxacin Surgical debridement		Limited clinical experience
M. simiae	Treat like *M. avium* complex		INH, RMP, EMB and PZA resistant
M. xenopi	Azithromycin, clarithromycin, RMP	Rifabutin, SM	
M. celatum	Clarithromycin		RMP and PZA resistant
M. genavense	EMB, RMP, rifabutin, clarithromycin	Amikacin, clofazimine	PZA resistant

First-choice agents are expected to be active against wild-type isolates (i.e. from untreated patients); second-choice agents are less preferred, usually due to toxicity, expense or unclear efficacy.
EMB, ethambutol; INH, isoniazid; MDR, multidrug resistance; PZA, pyrazinamide; RMP, rifampin; SM, streptomycin; XDR, extensive drug resistance.
Adapted from American Thoracic Society[4] and Clinical Laboratory Standards Institute;[83] see also Chapter 143.

concentration (MIC) in the future. However, there are no standardized methods for MIC testing of mycobacteria and the testing of *M. tuberculosis* continues to follow the conventions of critical concentrations and the 1% growth inhibition threshold.

The proportion method can be applied as either a direct or an indirect test.[83] Inoculating several dilutions of a standardized suspension of mycobacteria onto Middlebrook 7H10 agar plates is the basis of the agar proportion method. The number of colony forming units (cfu) that grow on the drug-containing plates or quadrants are compared with the number of cfu on a drug-free plate or quadrant. If the number of cfu that grow on drug-containing medium exceeds 1% of the total number of cfu on the drug-free medium, then the isolate is con-

sidered 'resistant' to that drug at that concentration. The agar proportion method is standardized[83] against which all newer developments of culture-based drug susceptibility testing have to be validated (see below).

Modified proportion method by the BACTEC 460 TB System

The radiometric proportion method is simply an adaptation of the agar proportion method to the BACTEC 460 TB 12B medium and radiometric measurement of growth inhibition. As a consequence of this particular technique, drug susceptibility results become available more rapidly, i.e. between 5 and 10 days. Critical concentrations have been established for both first- and second-line antituberculous drugs.[83,84] The isolate is inoculated into BACTEC 460 TB 12B medium with or without the addition of test drug. The concentration of mycobacteria inoculated into medium without drug is 100-fold less than the concentration inoculated into BACTEC 460 TB media with drug.

In some clinical situations the BACTEC 460 method might be best considered a screening test because the method does not allow an estimate of the percentage of resistant bacilli and is vulnerable to major errors (false susceptibility or resistance) due to mixed populations of mycobacterial species. Indeed, when an MDR isolate of *M. tuberculosis* is detected for the first time using the BACTEC 460 TB method, the identity of the isolate should be verified and the presence of a contaminant or mixed culture be ruled out before proceeding with testing secondary agents. Although the importance of promptly reporting an MDR isolate of *M. tuberculosis* cannot be overstated, the consequences of a false report of multidrug resistance must be recognized as well.

Drug testing by nonradiometric growth-based methods

Some of the new, nonradiometric methods such as the BACTEC MGIT 960 and the ESP Culture System II show excellent agreement with the agar proportion method and the BACTEC 460 TB System for drug susceptibility testing.[85–87] However, to date, only the BACTEC MGIT 960 System offers PZA testing.[88] Likewise, critical concentrations for second-line drugs for this system have been established in a large multicenter study.[89] For INH and RMP, the BACTEC MGIT 960 was also in 99–100% agreement with the resistance ratio method, and showed a concordance for EMB and PZA of 85% and 92%, respectively. Good correlation was also found for second-line drugs.[90]

Mycobacterium avium complex, *Mycobacterium kansasii* and other slowly growing NTM

In-vitro susceptibility testing of MAC and most of the other NTM, using the methods and interpretive criteria described for *M. tuberculosis*, has little value as a guide to antimicrobial treatment. One important exception is *M. kansasii*, for which *in-vitro* results based on the interpretive criteria used with *M. tuberculosis* correlate well with clinical efficacy. For many uncommon NTM (e.g. *M. simiae* and *M. szulgai*) there are few clinical cases to form a basis for interpretive criteria. As pointed out above, it is often difficult to distinguish between contamination, colonization, infection and disease with many of the NTM, especially the rapidly growing mycobacteria.

In general, the *in-vitro* susceptibility testing of MAC has limited value primarily because of the lack of a correlation with clinical response and, therefore, the lack of interpretive criteria.[83] The important exceptions are for azithromycin and clarithromycin because these macrolides have proven clinical and microbiologic efficacy in the prophylaxis and treatment of MAC disease, with interpretive criteria based, at least in part, on monotherapy trials in humans. Although wild-type MAC is uniformly susceptible to macrolides, macrolide resistance develops quickly with monotherapy. An analysis of these resistant isolates showed that over 95% of clinically significant macrolide resistance in MAC is a consequence of mutations in the V domain of the 23S rRNA gene.[82] Therefore, clinically significant macrolide resistance can be defined as an MIC for clarithromycin and azithromycin at pH 6.8 of $\geq 64\,\mu g/ml$ and $\geq 512\,\mu g/ml$, respectively.[83]

Mycobacterium avium complex isolates from patients with breakthrough azithromycin or clarithromycin prophylaxis can be tested against one macrolide. Testing one drug is sufficient, since all evidence indicates that resistance crosses between these macrolides. If a patient has not received macrolide prophylaxis, it is unnecessary to perform a susceptibility test on initial MAC isolates from blood or tissue to guide treatment. However, establishing baseline MIC values for a MAC isolate may prove valuable in interpreting susceptibility test results for a subsequent isolate from the same patient weeks or months later. Susceptibility testing is also warranted if a patient relapses, if the infection is intractable or if the clinical situation is desperate. Testing may assist in deciding to add drugs; however, macrolide treatment should probably be continued even in the face of resistance.

The interpretation of *in-vitro* test results for EMB should not be attempted at this time. Ethambutol is commonly used as a 'second' agent in the treatment of MAC to prevent macrolide resistance, but EMB has little or no therapeutic activity alone against MAC.[91] The drug does, however, increase the activity of other agents, including macrolides, and this may influence the mutation frequency.[92] The CLSI now recommends that MAC be tested by establishing MICs via the BACTEC 460 TB System or via the microtiter method.[83]

Mycobacterium marinum is predictably susceptible to RMP and EMB; alternative agents are amikacin and kanamycin as well as tetracyclines, ciprofloxacin, clarithromycin and trimethoprim–sulfamethoxazole (co-trimoxazole). Susceptibility testing of *M. marinum* isolates using methods and interpretive criteria described for *M. tuberculosis* appears to be inappropriate.[83] Wild-type isolates of *M. haemophilum* are susceptible to quinolones, rifamycins, clarithromycin and azithromycin, and are likely to be resistant to INH, streptomycin, EMB and PZA.[93] *Mycobacterium simiae* is highly resistant to antimycobacterial agents; however, there are exceedingly few cases of disease on which to base any firm conclusions about susceptibility and clinical usefulness. Clarithromycin in combination with EMB and perhaps a quinolone such as ofloxacin appears to be effective.[4,94]

Rapid growers

Although four methods have been described for measuring the *in-vitro* susceptibility of rapidly growing mycobacteria, the CLSI now recommends only the broth microdilution method.[83] Broth microdilution provides a quantitative result and better supports the growth of *M. chelonae*. The broth microdilution method is essentially a modification of a standard method for nonmycobacteria that grow aerobically. Commercially prepared broth microdilution panels can be used if the appropriate drugs are available at the necessary concentrations. Alternatively, broth microdilution panels can be prepared in-house. The agents that should be tested are listed in Table 174.6. Testing rapidly growing mycobacteria should be restricted to laboratories with more extensive experience.

Practical value of molecular detection of resistance

Apart from the growth-based strategies and the numerous alternative ways to test drug susceptibility (e.g. colorimetry, flow cytometry, bioluminescence or quantitation of mycobacterial antigens) there are protocols available which detect the gene mutations involved in resistance of *M. tuberculosis* against antimicrobial agents. Although they are capable of providing the clinician with susceptibility results within 1–2 days, most of these protocols are not yet ready for the routine clinical mycobacteriology laboratory, mainly because, very often, more than a single mutation is responsible for drug resistance, making the whole issue very complex (e.g. mutations at least on four different genes are involved in INH resistance). However, since over 97% of all RMP-resistant strains carry a mutation in a specific short core region of the *rpoB* gene, molecular detection of point mutations in this case is a straightforward approach. Detection of these mutations is reliably achieved by gene sequencing or, more simply, by the use of the commercially available line probe assays.

In analyzing 360 smear-positive respiratory specimens, sensitivity and specificity of the INNO-LiPA Rif. TB test (Innogenetics) were 100% and 96.6%, respectively.[95] Hillemann *et al.*[96] studied over 140 strains of *M. tuberculosis*, among them 103 MDR-TB strains, and reported 100% concordance between the GenoType MTBDR Assay

(Hain) and gene sequencing. Using the same assay, in 95.1% of RMP-resistant strains the mutations in the *rpoB* gene and in 73% of the INH-resistant strains mutations in the *katG* gene could be detected.[97] Brossier *et al.*[98] recommended the MTBDR test as a rapid method to detect RMP-resistant (concordance 100% with DNA sequencing) and high-level INH-resistant (concordance 89%) strains, but not for low-level INH-resistant strains of *M. tuberculosis* (concordance 17%). The MTBDR test has recently been modified (MTBDRplus Assay; Hain) to detect a broader variety of mutations in the *rpoB* and *inhA* genes.[99] A very promising development appears to be a line probe-based assay designed to detect mutations in the *pncA* gene by Sekiguchi *et al.*:[100] in testing some 250 strains of *M. tuberculosis*, sensitivity and specificity of the assay were both 100% compared to conventional PZA susceptibility testing.

IMMUNODIAGNOSTIC TESTS FOR TUBERCULOSIS

Historically, the first immunodiagnostic test was the tuberculin skin test (TST). Shortcomings of this test include the inability to distinguish active disease from patient sensitization, unknown predictive values and cross-reaction with NTM. None of the numerous serologic tests has found wide clinical use, mainly because of the lack of sensitivity and specificity.

In contrast, the recently developed and commercially available whole-blood IFN-γ assays are promising candidates to improve the current level of diagnostic accuracy for tuberculosis infection, particularly if skin testing remains equivocal. The two test systems – the QuantiFERON-TB Gold In-Tube (QFNG-IT; Cellestis, Victoria, Australia) and the T-SPOT.TB (Oxford Immunotec, Oxford, UK) – are not affected by BCG vaccination, do not cross-react with the majority of NTM and are less prone to variability and subjectivity associated with placing and reading of the TST (Table 174.7).

Although both tests measure T-cell INF-γ responses to similar *M. tuberculosis*-specific antigens over a 16- to 24-hour incubation period, they are based on different technologies. The T-SPOT.TB assay is based on ELISPOT methodology and requires the isolation and incubation of peripheral blood mononuclear cells (PBMC) and the standardization of 250 000 PBMC in each of its test wells. The T-SPOT.TB assay requires, overall, two working days, and may be more laborious than the QFNG-IT. Nevertheless, the use of a standardized number of washed PBMC might contribute to the greater sensitivity reported in the literature. In contrast, the QFNG-IT has technical advantages over the T-SPOT.TB assay, since the stimulation of T-cell IFN-γ response in whole blood is performed in tubes precoated with the *M. tuberculosis* antigens. Also, the enzyme-linked immunosorbent assay (ELISA) is simple and rapid to perform. Since background noise may occur, a 'Nil' control is required to adjust for this background, as well as for heterophile antibody effects and nonspecific IFN-γ in blood samples.

It is important to stress that neither of these new tests distinguishes between latent and active infection. To date, there are a large number of publications available which focus on the performance characteristics of each test; however, there are only few published head-to-head comparisons of the QFNG-IT and the T-SPOT.TB assays specifying their feasibility in different patient cohorts. In a recent systematic review of the literature Pai *et al.*[102] concluded that QFNG-IT has a specificity of 99% (T-SPOT.TB 96%) among non-BCG-vaccinated participants and a specificity of 96% (T-SPOT.TB 93%) among BCG-vaccinated participants, while the T-SPOT.TB appears to be more sensitive than QFNG-IT and TST. Diel *et al.*[103] compared both IFN-γ release assays in TST-positive persons recently exposed to pulmonary tuberculosis cases. In this study, factors independently influencing the risk of *M. tuberculosis* infection and their interactions with each other were evaluated by multivariate analysis. There were five variables which significantly predicted a positive IFN-γ release assay result, i.e. age, AFB-positivity of the source case, cough, cumulative exposure time and foreign origin of the patient. There was excellent agreement between the two assays (93.9%, kappa = 0.85), with QFNG-IT finding 30.2% of

Table 174.7 Characteristics of the commercially available tests for the diagnosis of tuberculosis infection

Variable	Tuberculin skin test	QuantiFERON-TB Gold/ QuantiFERON-TB Gold In-Tube	ELISPOT T-SPOT.TB
Administration	*In vivo* (intradermal)	*Ex vivo*, ELISA-based	*Ex vivo*, ELISPOT-based
Antigens	PPDS or RT-23	ESAT-6, CFP-10 and TB7.7	ESAT-6 and CFP-10
Standardized	Mostly	Yes	Yes
Reading prone to subjectivity	Yes	No	No
Units of measurement	Millimeters of induration	Units of IFN-γ	IFN-γ spot-forming cells
Definition of positive test results	5, 10 and 15 mm	Patient's IFN-γ ≥0.35 U/ml (after subtracting IFN-γ response in nil control)	≥6 spot-forming cells in the antigen wells, with 250 000 cells/well, and at least double-negative well
Indeterminate	If anergy (rarely tested)	Poor response to mitogen (<0.5 U/ml in positive control) or high background response (>8.0 U/ml in nil well)	Poor respone to mitogen (<20 spot-forming cells in positive control well) or high background (>10 spot-forming cells in negative well)
Time to result	48–72 h	Same day (but longer if run in batches)	16–24 h (but longer if run in batches)
Consultation(s)	2	1	1
Cost per test (US dollars) Materials Labor/other Total cost	11.58	17.29 20.02 37.31	57.33 20.02 77.35

Adapted from Menzies *et al.*[101]

contacts positive and T-SPOT.TB finding 28.7% of them. Overall, the IFN-γ release assays were more accurate indicators of the presence of latent tuberculosis than TST.

In HIV-positive asymptomatic individuals (n=286) both QFNG-IT and T-SPOT.TB assay were more sensitive than TST (20.0% and 25.2%, respectively, compared with 12.8% [TST]), but seemed, as a whole, to be less sensitive than in immunocompetent patients.[104]

The performance of IFN-γ release assays in children is less understood. Without the inconvenience and complications associated with TST they are acceptable substitutes for TST, however, the sensitivity and specificity of IFN-γ release assays compares well with the TST.[105] In latent tuberculosis the agreement between QFNG-IT and T-SPOT. TB assay was very good (92%) in children, with moderate agreement betweeen TST and QFNG-IT (77%) and TST and T-SPOT.TB (75%), respectively.[106] For culture-confirmed active tuberculosis, however, the same authors stated that the sensitivity of the TST was 83%, compared to 80% for the QFNG-IT and 58% for the T-SPOT.TB.

Basically, the problem of indeterminate results occurs with both IFN-γ release assays. In HIV-infected individuals, T-SPOT.TB provided more indeterminate results than the QFNG-IT (8 vs 1/256, $p < 0.01$),[104] similar to that confirmed by others (14% versus 1.8%).[107] Indeterminate results appear to be dependent on the number of CD4 cells inasmuch as patients with a CD4 count ≤200 cells/ml were significantly more likely to have an indeterminate result.[104,107] In children less than 4 years of age indeterminate results were more often seen using the QFNG-IT than the T-SPOT.TB.[108] In applying the T-SPOT.TB assay after indeterminate results have been obtained from the QFNG-IT test 65% of the 40 patients yielded a valid result.[109]

Since the experience with IFN-γ release assays is still limited, longitudinal studies are needed to define their predictive values, especially in children and high-risk populations.[110] A large meta-analysis has pointed out very clearly areas of uncertainty and recommendations for research.[101] Other problems concern the phenomena of conversions, reversions and nonspecific variations in serial testing[111] and altered performance characteristics of the assays in conjunction with ethnicity (e.g. Malay and Indian race versus Chinese race).[112]

From the present state of knowledge it is obvious that application of IFN-γ release assays for tuberculosis infection should be tailored to different high-risk groups. In addition, caution should be exercised in their current use in immunosuppressed patients.

REFERENCES

References for this chapter can be found online at http://www.expertconsult.com

Mycoplasma and Ureaplasma

INTRODUCTION

Mycoplasma and *Ureaplasma* belong taxonomically to the order Mycoplasmatales in the class Mollicutes ('soft skin'). Apart from being human pathogens, some organisms of the order Mollicutes are economically important plant and animal pathogens. The initial divisions of mycoplasmas into different species were based on inhibition of growth of the organisms on agar media containing homologous antibodies. In later studies, sequencing of the genome of mycoplasmas has confirmed the relevance of the initial classification method.

Over 120 named *Mycoplasma* species exist; 13 *Mycoplasma* species, two *Acholeplasma* species and one *Ureaplasma* species have been isolated from humans. However, only four are well-established human pathogens:

- *Mycoplasma pneumoniae;*
- *Mycoplasma hominis;*
- *Mycoplasma genitalium;* and
- *Ureaplasma urealyticum.*

Apart from the species mentioned above, several other species of *Mycoplasma* occur in the human endogenous flora of the mouth and the genital tract (*M. buccale, M. faucium, M. orale* and *M. salivarum*).

NATURE

Mycoplasma and *Ureaplasma* are the smallest organisms so far identified as being capable of reproducing in broth and on agar media; on the latter they form barely visible colonies.[1] They also have the smallest known genome of any 'free living' organism. They differ from eubacteria by lacking peptidoglycan. The absence of peptidoglycan and β-lactam receptors explains the resistance to β-lactam antibiotics.

Mycoplasma pneumoniae Infection

EPIDEMIOLOGY

Mycoplasma pneumoniae is one of the most common causes of atypical pneumonia.[2,3] It is transmitted from person to person by infected respiratory droplets during close contact and particularly affects young adults. The incubation period after exposure is, on average, 2–3 weeks.[4] Infection is more frequent during the fall and winter, but can develop year round.[5] The cumulative attack rate in families approaches 90% and immunity is short.[6]

Outbreaks of *Mycoplasma* infection have been described in military recruits,[7] institutions for developmentally disabled individuals[8] and hospitals.[9]

PATHOGENESIS

Mycoplasma pneumoniae grows under both aerobic and anaerobic conditions. The organism most commonly exists in a filamentous form (Fig. 175.1) and has adherence proteins that attach to epithelial membranes with particular affinity for respiratory tract epithelium.[10–13]

Once attached, *M. pneumoniae* produces hydrogen peroxide, causing injury to epithelial cells and their associated cilia (Fig. 175.2). However, many of the pathogenic features of infection with *M. pneumoniae* are believed to be immune mediated rather than induced directly by the bacteria.[13,14]

The organism may persist in the respiratory tract for several months after initial infection and sometimes for years in hypogammaglobulinemic patients, possibly because the organism attaches strongly and invades epithelial cells.

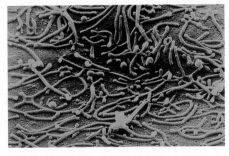

Fig. 175.1 Electron micrograph of a *Mycoplasma* organism producing filamentous structures in a broth culture. This gives the organism the appearance of a fungal mycelium. ('Myco' in mycoplasma refers to this feature.)

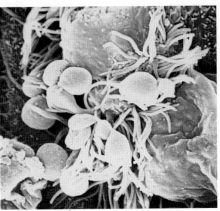

Fig. 175.2 Swelling ('ballooning') of cilia in tissue cell cultures experimentally infected by *Mycoplasma hominis.* Courtesy of Per-Anders Mårdh.

CLINICAL MANIFESTATIONS (SEE TABLE 175.1)

Atypical pneumonia

Mycoplasma pneumoniae is one of the most common causes of atypical pneumonia (Fig. 175.3) and together with *Chlamydia pneumoniae* and *Legionella* spp. represents 7–20% of cases of community-acquired pneumonia (CAP) for which a pathogen can be identified.[15,16] However, the incidence may be higher in patients with milder disease. The incidence of CAP due to *M. pneumoniae* varies depending on the techniques used for diagnosis, the age of the patients and whether the series include outpatients, hospitalized patients, or both. Several prospective studies showed that the incidence of *M. pneumoniae* is between 5% and 22.8%.[17] Pneumonia can be present without any findings on chest auscultation.

Asthma[18]

Mycoplasma pneumoniae has been linked to asthma. An infection with *M. pneumoniae* may precede the onset of asthma or exacerbate asthma symptoms. Chronic infection with *M. pneumoniae* has been suspected to play a part in some patients with asthma. A role for immunoglobulin E-related hypersensitivity and induction of T-helper type 2 immune response leading to inflammatory response in *M. pneumoniae*-infected patients with asthma has also been proposed. As macrolides are both antimicrobials and anti-inflammatory drugs, their therapeutic role in reducing asthma symptoms needs further clinical studies.

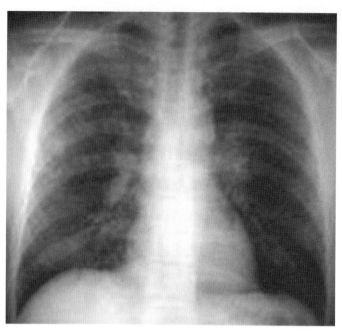

Fig. 175.3 Posteroanterior chest radiograph shows poorly defined reticulonodular pattern and ground-glass opacities in the right lung and poorly defined small nodular opacities in the left lung. The patient was a 37-year-old man with *Mycoplasma pneumoniae*. Source: Image Consult, 2008.

Table 175.1 Clinical manifestations of infection due to *Mycoplasma* and *Ureaplasma*

	M. pneumoniae	M. hominis	M. genitalium	Ureaplasma urealyticum
Atypical pneumonia	+++	–	–	–
Asthma	+++	–	–	–
Upper respiratory tract infection	+++	+	–	+
Hemolysis	+++	–	–	–
Skin disease	+++	–	–	–
CNS involvement	+	+	–	+
Hepatitis	+	–	–	–
Arthralgia	+	++	–	–
Arthritis	+	++	–	–
Sexually transmitted disease	–	+++	+++	++
Urinary tract infection	–	+++	–	–
Postpartum	–	+++	–	–
Fever	+	+++	–	–
Pelvic inflammatory disease	–	+++	+++	+++
Chorioamnionitis	–	+++	–	–
Endocarditis	–	+	–	–
Wound infection	–	+	–	–
Preterm delivery	–	–	–	++
Chronic lung disease	–	–	–	++

Mycoplasma pneumoniae infection may worsen asthma symptoms and can produce wheezing in children who do not have asthma. On the other hand, the role of *M. pneumoniae* in patients with chronic obstructive pulmonary disease and its exacerbations has not been established.[19]

Upper respiratory tract diseases

Most patients with respiratory infections due to *M. pneumoniae* do not develop pneumonia, but can have intractable, nonproductive cough, wheezing, dyspnea and signs of upper respiratory tract infection such as pharyngitis (6–59%), rhinorrhea (2–40%) and bullous myringitis (2–35%).[14,20]

Extrapulmonary diseases[17,19]

Extrapulmonary complications of *M. pneumoniae* infections may include hemolytic anemia, mucocutaneous lesions, meningoencephalitis and other CNS manifestations, and arthritis.

An autoimmune response is thought to play a role in these manifestations; however, the bacterium can be isolated from most extrapulmonary sites.[21]

Hemolytic anemia

Antibodies (IgM) to the 'I' antigen on erythrocyte membranes appear during the course of infection and produce a cold agglutinin response in about 60% of patients. Note, however, that cold agglutinins can also occur in other respiratory infections and they are not a surrogate diagnostic marker of *Mycoplasma* infection. Although hemolysis may be severe, it is usually not clinically significant.[5]

Mucocutaneous lesions

Dermatologic manifestation may range from a mild erythema multiforme (Fig. 175.4) to Stevens–Johnson syndrome.[22–25] Antibiotics may intensify the dermatosensitive potential of *M. pneumoniae*.[25]

Meningoencephalitis and other central nervous system manifestations

Central nervous system (CNS) manifestations occur in approximately 0.1% of the patients with *M. pneumoniae* infection and in up to 7% requiring hospitalization.[21] CNS involvement occurs most frequently in children and presents with encephalitis.[26] Other manifestations

include aseptic meningitis, peripheral neuropathy, transverse myelitis, cranial nerve palsies (Bell's palsy) and cerebellar ataxia.[27,28]

Although uncommon, CNS involvement is associated with 8% mortality and 23% of severe sequelae.[21]

Other

Nonspecific gastrointestinal symptoms such as hepatitis and rarely pancreatitis can occur.[29,30] Arthralgia is common, arthritis is rare.[31] Cardiac or renal involvement and uveitis are unusual.[14,32,33]

Although the isolation of *M. pneumoniae* on SP-4 medium is possible, culture requires 2–3 weeks (Fig. 175.5). As such, clinical laboratories do not attempt to culture *M. pneumoniae* and the specific diagnosis of *M. pneumoniae* infection relies upon nonculture techniques.

Cold agglutinins

Cold agglutinins develop in approximately 50–75% of all patients 1–2 weeks after infection.[34–36] However, other bacterial, rickettsial and viral infections can also produce cold agglutinins. Since it is neither sensitive nor specific, the test is not helpful.

Serology

Antibody titers rise 7–9 days after infection (Fig. 175.6). In the past, the most widely used approach for serodiagnosis was the complement fixation (CF) test, which measured predominantly 'early' IgM and IgG antibody. More recently, enzyme immunoassay (EIA) techniques have been used with a sensitivity of 97.8% and a specificity of 99.7%. EIAs are more sensitive for detecting acute infection and can be comparable in sensitivity to polymerase chain reaction (PCR).[37]

Polymerase chain reaction

Direct PCR detects genomic DNA and may be highly sensitive and specific in patients with respiratory tract infections. Real-time PCR may be superior.[38] PCR can also be used on respiratory secretions, cerebrospinal fluid (CSF) and other tissue samples.

TREATMENT

Empiric therapy of atypical pneumonia

Indolent onset, extrapulmonary involvement and normal white blood cell count are findings that favor the presence of atypical pneumonia. Macrolides (azithromycin, clarithromycin and erythromycin) are considered as first-line treatment.[35] Azithromycin 500 mg orally once

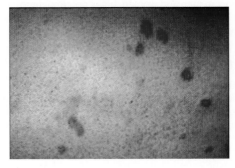

Fig. 175.4 The red spots on this person's back appear where blisters (bullae) caused by erythema multiforme have ruptured and the overlying skin removed (denuded). The resulting lesions are yellow-crusted ulcers (erosions). Erythema multiforme may be associated with herpes simplex infection, *Mycoplasma* pneumonia or other medical conditions such as streptococcal infection or tuberculosis, or may result from exposure to chemicals or medications.

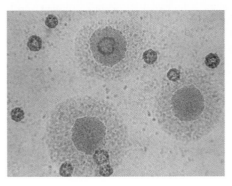

Fig. 175.5 Colonies of *Mycoplasma hominis* on PPLO agar with 'fried egg' appearance. Courtesy of Per-Anders Mårdh.

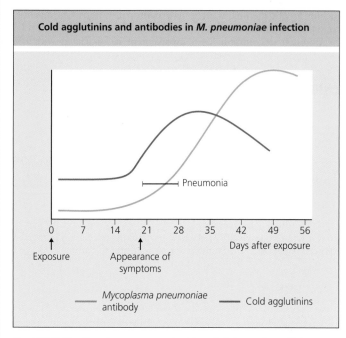

Fig. 175.6 Kinetics of appearance of cold agglutinins and specific antibodies to *Mycoplasma pneumoniae* related to time after being taken ill with *M. pneumoniae* pneumonia.

daily, followed by 250 mg orally for 4 days (or 500 mg for 3 days), is the most common regimen used. Erythromycin is less expensive but is commonly associated with gastrointestinal side-effects. Other antibiotics, such as tetracyclines (doxycycline 100 mg orally twice daily) and fluoroquinolones (levofloxacin and moxifloxacin), may be used. Although the duration of treatment for atypical pneumonia has not been firmly established, it is usual to treat for 10–14 days.[5] No studies have been performed which evaluate the treatment of patients with extrapulmonary findings of *M. pneumoniae* infection. For hemolytic anemia, some patients responded to steroids or plasmapheresis.[13]

Mycoplasma hominis

This organism has been isolated from the fallopian tubes of women with acute salpingitis.[39] The bacteria can be part of the normal genital flora for sexually experienced men and women.[40] The organism spreads through the cervical canal via the uterus and by the lymphatic vessels of the parametrium to the tubes. The percentage of women with vaginal colonization of *M. hominis* increases after puberty in direct proportion to sexual experience. In a study by McCormack[40] genital colonization with *M. hominis* was found in 1 of 91 women without a prior history of sexual activity, but in 15 of 97 sexually active women with multiple lifetime partners.[40] The rate of colonization is higher in sexually active women than in men,[41] probably because women are more susceptible to colonization.[41] Newborns are likely to become colonized during passage through the birth canal. This colonization is transient and the proportion of infants colonized decreases proportionally with age. Infants more than 3 months of age are rarely if ever colonized.[42] *Mycoplasma hominis* is common in women who lack a lactobacilli-dominated vaginal flora and have a mixture of bacterial species in the vagina. Many of these species are strictly anaerobic. Up to 75% of all women with bacterial vaginosis are carriers of *M. hominis*.[43]

IDENTIFICATION

Mycoplasma hominis is the smallest free-living bacterium. It can be detected in cultures within a few days. *Mycoplasma hominis* will escape detection using automated blood culture detection systems such as

BacT/ALERT,[44] unless cultures are routinely incubated for 3–5 days using special media.[45]

To improve recovery of *M. hominis*, clinical specimens should be immediately inoculated onto culture media and not allowed to dry. After plating, cultures should be promptly incubated or kept at 39°F (4°C). The best laboratory culture medium is beef heart infusion broth (PPLO), supplemented with fresh yeast extract and horse serum. *Mycoplasma hominis* grows suboptimally *in vitro* under atmospheric conditions. Colonies develop best on agar when incubated at 95% nitrogen and 5% CO_2 atmosphere.[41]

SUSCEPTIBILITY

Susceptibility testing has not been standardized for *Mycoplasma* and there is no proven correlation between laboratory findings and clinical outcome.

Mycoplasma hominis is susceptible *in vitro* to tetracyclines and clindamycin, and is moderately susceptible to rifampin (rifampicin) and chloramphenicol. It is resistant to aminoglycosides, erythromycin and trimethoprim.[46] Fluoroquinolones are active *in vitro* but resistance may develop during treatment.[47] *Mycoplasma hominis* is susceptible to linezolid and quinupristin–dalfopristin but clinical data are not available.[48]

CLINICAL FEATURES

Mycoplasma hominis has been associated with genitourinary tract and nongenital infections. Genitourinary tract infections that have been linked to *M. hominis* include:

- pyelonephritis;
- pelvic inflammatory disease;
- chorioamnionitis; and
- postpartum and postabortal fever.

Nongenitourinary infections that have been linked to *M. hominis* include:

- septicemia;
- wound infections;
- central nervous infections;
- joint infections;
- lower respiratory tract infections; and
- endocarditis.

Urinary tract infections

Mycoplasma hominis can frequently be recovered from the lower genitourinary tract in men and women, but is not thought to cause cystitis, epididymitis or prostatitis. However, it can cause acute pyelonephritis, especially after instrumentation or if obstruction is present.[49,50]

Postpartum and postabortal fever

Ten percent of cases of postpartum and postabortal fever are related to the presence of *M. hominis*.[51] *Mycoplasma hominis* was also found in 8% of blood cultures of women with fever after abortion[51] but not in women without fever. More evidence of the pathogenicity of *M. hominis* is the fourfold rise in antibody titers in approximately 50% of women who had postabortal fever, as compared to only 2 of 53 controls who experienced abortion without fever.

Pelvic inflammatory disease

The role of *M. hominis* as a cause of pelvic inflammatory disease (PID) remains controversial.[49] *Mycoplasma hominis* has been isolated from the fallopian tubes of women with salpingitis and in whom an antibody response could be established.[39,52] *Mycoplasma hominis* is rarely present in patients with salpingitis who do not also have evidence of concurrent chlamydial or gonococcal vaginitis or bacterial vaginosis.[53] Therefore, its role as a primary pathogen in salpingitis is still uncertain. *Mycoplasma hominis* may also increase the risk for tubal occlusion and infertility.

Chorioamnionitis

Mycoplasma hominis has been isolated from women with premature labor and chorioamnionitis and from 30% of children with birth weight below 2500 g who were born by Caesarian section with intact membranes.[54] However, the exact role of *M. hominis* in chorioamnionitis is still to be defined.

Nongenitourinary tract infections

Central nervous system disease

Infection in the CNS of neonates is probably acquired in utero or via passage through the birth canal.[55] The CNS infections related to *M. hominis* are brain abscess complicating a subdural hematoma,[56] meningitis[57] and meningoencephalitis.[55]

Arthritis

Mycoplasma hominis arthritis is characterized by the presence of fever, leukocytosis and purulent joint effusion with a negative Gram stain. A study reported 16 cases of septic arthritis due to *M. hominis*, where half of them had undergone manipulation of the urinary tract before the onset of infection.[58] *Mycoplasma hominis* arthritis was also described in patients with immune defects,[59] immunosuppression or following joint replacement or trauma.[58]

Wound infections

Mycoplasma hominis has been associated with infected pelvic hematoma[60] and infected Caesarian wounds, and is also occasionally found in other surgical wounds. Since the signs and symptoms of *M. hominis* wound infection are not specific, it can only be suspected when there are abnormal findings such as polymorphonuclear leukocytes with a negative Gram stain, negative routine cultures and a poor response to β-lactam or aminoglycoside therapy.[46,61,62]

Bacteremia

Positive blood cultures can be found after recent trauma[60] or a urologic surgical procedure. *Mycoplasma hominis* can also cause transient bacteremia after delivery, usually with no fever.[63]

Endocarditis

Mycoplasma hominis is a rare cause of native and prosthetic valve endocarditis.[64]

Respiratory tract

Mycoplasma hominis has been isolated from respiratory secretions in 1–3% of healthy persons, 8% of patients with chronic respiratory complaints and 14% of persons engaging in orogenital sex.[65] A few cases of empyema have been reported[66] but in general *M. hominis* is rarely capable of causing lower respiratory tract infections.

Prosthetic joint infection

A few cases of prosthetic joint infection have been described. Some were successfully managed with debridement followed by long courses of therapy with oral doxycycline or clindamycin.[58]

Mycoplasma genitalium

Mycoplasma genitalium (Fig. 175.7) is an emerging sexually transmitted infection.[67] Studies support a higher prevalence than gonococcus but lower prevalences than *C. trachomatis*. A role for this pathogen has also been suggested in chronic cases of nongonococcal urethritis.[68] Likewise, *M. genitalium* has been recovered from the urethra of HIV-infected men[69] and can be found in urethral cultures from men with and without discharge. In a recent study in women in the second and third trimester of pregnancy, *M. genitalium* was recovered from vaginal lavage samples in 1.6% of women who had reached the second trimester. This percentage increased in those who returned for repeat examination in the third trimester. *Mycoplasma genitalium* is a cause of cervicitis and endometritis.[70] Carriage of *M. genitalium* was associated with mucopurulent discharge, frequent vaginal douching, smoking and a history of miscarriage.[71] *Mycoplasma genitalium* was not associated with bacterial vaginosis (BV).

DIAGNOSIS

The organism is difficult to culture and most studies used PCR for identification. Antibodies were detected in 40% of women with PID with a microimmunofluorescence test.[72] Since such antibodies were detected by immunoblotting in approximately half of the women with proven tubal factor infertility, a definite diagnosis is difficult to make.

Mycoplasma genitalium has an antibiotic susceptibility pattern similar to *M. pneumoniae* and it appears to be sensitive to macrolides, especially azithromycin and tetracycline.

Ureaplasma urealyticum

Ureaplasma urealyticum (Fig. 175.8) derives its name from the fact that it possesses the enzyme urease. This organism was previously called T-strain *Mycoplasma* as it produced tiny (T) colonies in comparison to those of *Mycoplasma*. *Ureaplasma urealyticum* remains the single species in the genus *Ureaplasma*, although there have been some proposals for a differentiation based, for example, on biochemical and serology characteristics. Fourteen different serotypes of *U. urealyticum* were described.[73] One biovar of human *Ureaplasma* (biovar no. 1) has been called *Ureaplasma parvum*.[74]

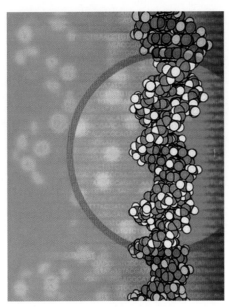

Fig. 175.7 Genome of *Mycoplasma genitalium*. With permission from *Nature*.

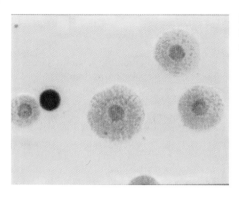

Fig. 175.8
Ureaplasma urealyticum.

CLINICAL MANIFESTATIONS

The presence of *U. urealyticum* in the genital tract is associated with sexual activity.[75] A large number of studies questioned the role of *U. urealyticum* in the pathogenesis of nongonococcal nonchlamydial urethritis.[73] Those studies were not consistent and are therefore difficult to interpret. Large randomized studies are needed in order to establish if *U. urealyticum* is a urethral colonizer or has a role in the sexual transmission of disease.[76,77] *Ureaplasma urealyticum* is found in the lower genital tract in up to 75% of women of reproductive age and can ascend to the fallopian tubes.[39] Treatment of infertile couples with tetracycline has provided inconclusive support to the role of *U. urealyticum* as a cause for infertility. A higher rate of recovery of *U. urealyticum* from babies with low weight and a statistical correlation of carriage of *U. urealyticum* with preterm birth has also been established. In addition, the colonization of *U. urealyticum* in the respiratory tract of premature neonates (<34 weeks) was associated with the development of chronic lung disease.[30,78] Despite high rates of colonization of the respiratory tract of newborns with *U. urealyticum* and the need for assisted ventilation, including several cases of respiratory insufficiency and death,

until now there have been no studies proving the etiologic role of *U. urealyticum* in chronic lung disease in preterm births.[73] However, *U. urealyticum* can cause meningoencephalitis in newborns.

Ureaplasma urealyticum splits urea and therefore is capable of producing stones in the urinary tract.

DIAGNOSIS

Ureaplasma species can be detected in culture within 48 hours. Growth in a broth medium containing urea and an indicator causing a color change has been used to diagnose ureaplasmas.[1] Tests of the urea-splitting capability of *U. urealyticum* can also be carried out on agar media where the colonies turn dark brown after adding the test substrate. However, the use of molecular-based techniques, such as 16S rRNA gene-based PCR tests, detects *U. urealyticum* with much higher sensitivity rates than culture.[79–81] *Ureaplasma urealyticum* is known to have a similar susceptibility pattern to *Mycoplasma* spp.

THERAPY

Ureaplasma species are typically susceptible to antibiotics such as tetracyclines, macrolides and the newer fluoroquinolones.

REFERENCES

References for this chapter can be found online at http://www.expertconsult.com

Patrick Kelly
Emmanouil Angelakis
Didier Raoult

Chapter | **176**

Rickettsia and rickettsia-like organisms

INTRODUCTION

Rickettsia and rickettsia-like organisms are fastidious, obligate intracellular, coccobacilli that are transmitted to vertebrate hosts by arthropods. Traditional methods to classify bacteria are not useful for strict intracellular organisms as they have few phenotypes. The advent of molecular methods has enabled very accurate determinations of phylogenetic relationships between intracellular bacteria, and the order Rickettsiales has been reclassified to contain the genera *Anaplasma, Ehrlichia, Neorickettsia, Orientia, Rickettsia* and *Wolbachia*.[1] Phylogenetic studies have shown that several bacteria previously classified in the order Rickettsiales did not belong to the α subgroup of the Proteobacteria phylum;[1] the genus *Bartonella* was moved to the α_2 subgroup and the genus *Coxiella* to the γ subgroup (see Fig. 176.1).

Molecular studies have also greatly facilitated the detection and description of new organisms and the *Rickettsia* genus now contains 24 recognized species classified into three groups based on their genomic, antigenic, morphologic and ecologic patterns: the spotted fever group (SFG), the typhus group and the *R. bellii* group.[1] Similarly, the number of *Bartonella* spp. and the clinical syndromes caused by these organisms have increased rapidly. While infections with *Anaplasma* and *Ehrlichia* spp. were previously considered only of veterinary importance, studies over the past two decades have revealed several new species or strains that are pathogenic in both people and animals. In this chapter we describe the infections caused by rickettsiae and rickettsia-like organisms.

Spotted Fever Group Rickettsiae

NATURE

The SFG rickettsiae are obligate, intracellular, Gram-negative, coccobacilli (1.0–2.0 × 0.3–0.7 μm) that can infect vertebrate (endothelium, vascular smooth muscle and macrophages) and invertebrate cells (hemocytes and salivary gland epithelium). The SFG rickettsiae have a high content of lipopolysaccharides which are highly immunogenic and are responsible for the considerable serologic cross-reactivity between the different species within the group. There are, however, also species-specific antigens and these include the rickettsial outer membrane proteins A and B, rOmpA and rOmpB, respectively.[2] Until recently it appeared that there was a single pathogenic *Rickettsia* on each continent. However, between 1984 and 2004, nine more species or subspecies of tick-borne SFG rickettsiae were identified as emerging pathogens.

Rickettsia felis is also a newly described pathogenic SFG rickettsia and has pili which are probably involved in cell attachment and conjugation.[3]

The structure and the genome of *R. akari* is similar to that of other *Rickettsia* species.[4]

EPIDEMIOLOGY

Most SFG rickettsiae are found in only one or a limited number of species of ticks and hence the distribution of the various tick species determines the risk areas for SFG rickettsioses.[5] People are not considered good reservoirs for SFG rickettsiae as they are seldom infested with ticks for long periods and rickettsemia is normally of only short duration, especially with antibiotic intervention.

The reservoir and vector of *R. felis* is the cat flea (*Ctenocephalides felis*) which transmits the organism transovarially. It appears that *R. felis* is transmitted to people by flea bites.[6]

Rickettsia akari is found in the mouse mite (*Liponyssoides sanguineus*) which is the vector and reservoir of infection. Transmission might also occur with the use of contaminated needles in intravenous drug users.[6]

PATHOGENICITY

Ticks inject virulent SFG rickettsiae in their saliva while feeding and these adhere to endothelial cells, the most important target cells. Adherence is receptor mediated and results in changes to the actin cytoskeletal structure and phagocytosis of organisms into the cell.[7] The resultant phagosome lyses very rapidly and organisms are released into the cytoplasm. Some organisms escape from infected endothelial cells at the tick attachment site and spread via lymphatics to regional lymph nodes causing lymphadenomegaly. They also enter the bloodstream and infect endothelial cells throughout the body.

PREVENTION

There are no vaccines against the SFG rickettsiae and prevention depends on reducing exposure to vectors by avoiding infested areas and controlling ticks and fleas on domestic animals. People living in endemic areas and travelers to these areas should use effective tick repellants on their clothing such as DEET (*N*,*N*-diethyl-m-toluamide) or permethrins. Wearing light-colored clothes facilitates early tick detection and removal before they can attach. Prevention of rickettsialpox depends on rodent and mite control.

DIAGNOSTIC MICROBIOLOGY

The typical clinical picture of the SFG rickettsioses is high fever (103–104°F/39.5–40°C), headache and characteristic rash. Common nonspecific laboratory abnormalities include mild leukopenia, anemia and thrombocytopenia.[8]

Direct diagnosis

Rickettsia spp. can be isolated from blood or tissue samples in cell cultures (Vero, L929, HEL, XTC-2 or MRC5 cells) in biosafety level 3 laboratories.[8] Direct immunofluorescence techniques on tissues have moderate sensitivity (53–75%) but are nearly 100% specific.[9] Greater sensitivity may be achieved with polymerase chain reaction (PCR) assays amplifying sequences of several genes including 16S rDNA, *rOmpA*, *rOmpB*, *gltA* (citrate synthase) and gene D.[8]

Indirect diagnosis

Currently, the indirect microimmunofluorescence assay (IFA) is the most commonly used technique for the diagnosis of SFG rickettsioses.[10] Infection with the various SFG rickettsiae cannot always be differentiated by comparing IFA titers against the different members of the group. If differences in IFA assay titers between SFG rickettsiae are less than two serum dilutions, Western blot assays targeting two high-molecular-weight proteins (*rOmpA* and *rOmpB*)[11] and cross-absorption studies are needed to determine the SFG rickettsiae causing infection.[8]

CLINICAL MANIFESTATIONS

Currently, there are 14 SFG rickettsiae that are pathogenic in people (Table 176.1).

Rickettsia africae is the etiologic agent of African tick bite fever (ATBF) which is probably the most prevalent SFG rickettsiosis in the

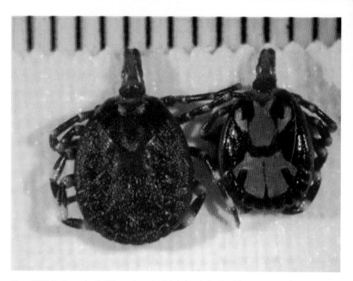

Fig. 176.1 Female (left) and male (right) adult *Amblyomma variegatum*, vector and reservoir of *Rickettsia africae*.

world. It is transmitted by *Amblyomma hebraeum* and probably also by *A. variegatum* (Fig. 176.1), with the majority of these ticks being infected and hence vectors of *R. africae* in sub-Saharan Africa. Fever is common (88%) and accompanying clinical signs are generally mild and include regional lymphadenomegaly (57%). A rash is seen in 49% of the patient and may be vesicular. To date no deaths or severe manifestations have been reported in patients with ATBF.[8]

Rickettsia rickettsii is the agent of Rocky Mountain spotted fever (RMSF) which is the most severe of the SFG rickettsioses. In the USA the major vectors are *Dermacentor andersonii* (wood tick) and *D. variabilis* (American dog tick) while in Central and South America the major vector is *Amblyomma cajennense* (Cayenne tick). The incubation period of RMSF is 2–14 days and initial signs include high fever (>102°F/39°C) and headache. Although a macular rash, which appears first on the wrists and ankles before generalizing, is a characteristic

Table 176.1 Prevalence of signs and prognoses for the more common spotted fever group rickettsioses

Spotted fever group	Fever	Rash	Eschar	Regional lymphadenopathy	Fatality rate without treatment
African tick bite fever	88%	49%	53–98%	49–57%	None
Rocky Mountain spotted fever	Yes	90%	Rare	None	20–25%
Mediterranean spotted fever	100%	87%	53%	Rare	1–2.5%
Israeli spotted fever	Yes	100%	90%	None	0–3.5%
Astrakhan fever	Yes	94%	23%	Rare	None
Japanese spotted fever	Yes	100%	91%	None	None
Queensland tick typhus	Yes	100%	65%	70%	Two fatal cases
Flinders Island spotted fever	Yes	100%	25–55%	55%	None
Siberian tick typhus	Yes	Common	62–77%	Uncommon	None
Lymphangitis-associated rickettsiosis	Yes	Common	75%	100%	None
TIBOLA-DEBONEL	45%	Uncommon	100%	100%	None
Far Eastern spotted fever	Yes	Common but often faint	Yes	20%	None
Flea-borne spotted fever	Common	Common	None	Yes	None
Rickettsialpox	Common	Common	Common	None	None

feature of RMSF it occurs in fewer than 50% of patients in the first 3 days of illness. In untreated patients, signs progress with the development of the vasculitis.

Rickettsia conorii has recently been shown to comprise three subspecies.[8]

- *Rickettsia conorii* subsp. *conorii* is the agent of Mediterranean spotted fever (MSF). After an incubation period of about 6 days, there is an abrupt onset of high fever (>102°F/39°C) and flu-like symptoms.[12] Typically, an eschar or tache noire (black spot) develops at the site of tick attachment. After about 4 days, a generalized maculopapular rash develops that also involves the palms and soles but spares the face (Fig. 176.2). Most patients will recover over 10 days without treatment but the rash may still be visible for 10–20 days after remission of clinical symptoms. Severe forms of MSF are seen in 5–6% of patients and the mortality rate is around 2%.

- *Rickettsia conorii* subsp. *israelensis* is transmitted by *R. sanguineus* and causes Israeli spotted fever.[8] This disease has similar clinical features to MSF. Although Israeli spotted fever is typically milder and of shorter duration than classic MSF, several fatal cases and severe forms have been described.

- *Rickettsia conorii* subsp. *caspia* causes Astrakhan fever in the Caspian Sea area in Russia and Chad.[8] The disease is similar to MSF but eschars are seen in relatively few patients (23%).

Rickettsia japonica causes Japanese or Oriental spotted fever which occurs particularly along the coast of south-western and central Japan. The rash is usually found on the palms of the hands and the soles of the feet and may become petechial after a few days before it disappears over about 2 weeks. Up to 20% of patients may have severe disease, with encephalitis, disseminated intravascular coagulopathy, multiorgan failure and acute respiratory distress syndrome having been reported.[8]

Rickettsia australis is the agent of Queensland tick typhus and is transmitted principally by *Ixodes holocyclus* in Australia.[8] An eschar at the site of tick attachment and lymphadenopathy are found in 65% and 70% of cases, respectively.

Rickettsia honei causes Flinders Island spotted fever. The organism might be the most widely distributed of the SFG rickettsiae as it has recently been identified in Thailand and Texas.[8] Patients with Flinders Island spotted fever have a sudden onset of fever, headache, myalgia, joint swelling and pain, and a slight cough in some patients.

Rickettsia sibirica subsp. *sibirica* is the agent of Siberian or North Asian tick typhus which occurs in Asiatic Russia and is transmitted by *Dermacentor* spp.[8] The disease is usually mild and there are seldom severe complications.

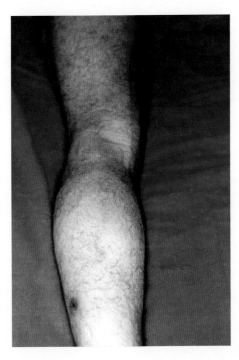

Fig. 176.3 Lymphangitis expanding from the inoculation eschar on the left leg to an enlarged, painful lymph node in the left groin of a patient with *Rickettsia mongolotimonae* infection. From Fournier, *et al.*[14]

Rickettsia sibirica subsp *mongolotimonae* infections have now been described in 11 patients.[13] Infections cause a 'lymphangitis-associated rickettsiosis' with signs including fever, maculopapular rash, eschar, enlarged regional lymph nodes and rope-like lymphangitis (Fig. 176.3).

Rickettsia massiliae was recently isolated from a patient with a maculopapular rash, eschar and slight hepatomegaly. The organism is transmitted by *Rhipicephalus* spp. in Europe and Central Africa.[15]

Rickettsia slovaca is transmitted by *Dermacentor marginatus* and *D. reticulatus*. Long considered nonpathogenic, *R. slovaca* has recently been found to be the agent of 'TIBOLA' (tick-borne lymphadenopathy) and 'DEBONEL' (*Dermacentor*-borne necrosis-erythema-lymphadenopathy) in Spain.[8]

Rickettsia heilongjiangensis is the agent of Far Eastern spotted fever and is found in *D. silvarum* in China and *Haemaphysalis* spp. from Siberia and the Russian Far East.[16] Infections result in fever, headache, rash, eschar, regional lymphadenopathy and conjunctivitis (Fig. 176.4).

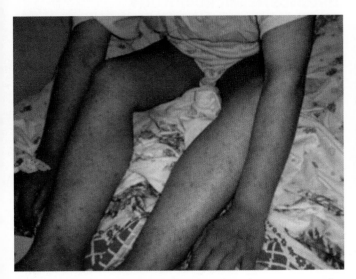

Fig. 176.2 Maculopapular rash in a patient with Mediterranean spotted fever from Algeria. Courtesy Dr Nadjet Mouffok.

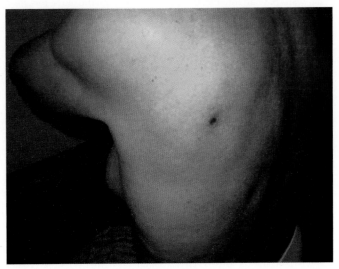

Fig. 176.4 Eschar and faint macular rash in a patient with *Rickettsia heilongjiangensis* infection. From Mediannikov, *et al.*[17]

Rickettsia aeschlimannii occurs in *Hyalomma* spp. in Africa and Europe. Two patients have been described with *R. aeschlimannii* infections but there is evidence that these may be more widespread in southern Europe.[8]

Rickettsia parkeri occurs in *Amblyomma maculatum* in the southern United States. Although the organism has been known for over 60 years, it has only recently been recognized as a pathogen in two patients.[18]

Rickettsia felis, previously known as the ELB agent, is the recently described agent of 'flea-borne spotted fever'.[19] Clinical signs are nonspecific, most commonly including fever, headache and rash. Other signs that have been reported are marked fatigue, myalgia, photophobia, conjunctivitis, abdominal pain, vomiting and diarrhea, and solitary black crusted skin lesions surrounded by a livid halo.

Rickettsia akari causes rickettsialpox which is transmitted by the mouse mite and has been reported in the USA, Ukraine, Slovenia and Korea. The incubation period is about 10 days and clinical signs include fever, headache and myalgia. There is usually an inoculation eschar and regional lymphadenopathy. About 4 days after the first clinical signs, a rash appears which has macular then papular and then vesicular lesions. The disease is usually mild and self-limiting.

MANAGEMENT

In practice, doxycycline (200 mg/day) is the drug of choice and may be used for 3–14 days, depending on the severity of the infection. It should be given for at least 3 days after clinical defervescence and resolution of signs.[8] When doxycycline cannot be used, chloramphenicol (50–75 mg/kg) can be effective but there are treatment failures and side-effects. Josamycin has been used successfully in pregnant women and children,[10] but children treated with azithromycin or clarithromycin required shorter courses of therapy and defervescence occurred in under 7 days.

Typhus Group Rickettsiae

NATURE

Both *R. prowazekii* and *R. typhi* are Gram-negative, obligate intracellular bacilli and, as with other members of the genus *Rickettsia*, their outer walls have an inner leaflet that is thicker than the outer. *Rickettsia prowazekii* is a category B bioterrorism agent and has a genome of 1.1 Mb with a single circular chromosome and a high proportion of noncoding DNA (24%).[20] The genome of *R. typhi* is nearly identical to that of *R. conorii* and other SFG rickettsiae.

EPIDEMIOLOGY

The human body louse, which lives in clothing, is the only established vector of *R. prowazekii* (Fig. 176.5). People are usually infected when feces from infected lice contaminate skin that has been scarified due to pruritus caused by the lice. Infections may also occur when conjunctivae or mucous membranes are exposed to the crushed bodies or feces of infected lice. Further, transmission might occur with inhalation of infected feces and through aerosols of feces-infected dust.

Murine typhus is one of the most prevalent rickettsial diseases throughout the world. The principal vectors are the rat flea (*Xenopsylla cheopis*) and the rat louse (*Polyplax spinulosa*). Other possible vectors are the cat flea (*Ctenocephalides felis*) and the mouse flea (*Leptopsyllia segnis*).[21]

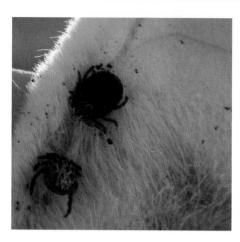

Fig. 176.5 The human body louse (*Pediculus humanus humanus*), the vector of *Rickettsia prowazekii*, feeding on a rabbit.

PATHOGENICITY

After local infection by *R. prowazekii* at the site of the louse bite, the organism infects the endothelial cells of capillaries and small blood vessels, producing a vasculitis. Tissue biopsies reveal perivascular infiltration with lymphocytes, plasma cells, polymorphonuclear leukocytes and histiocytes, with or without necrosis of the vessel.[22] Unlike SFG rickettsiae, *R. prowazekii* multiplies to large numbers within cells but does not cause significant injury to cells before they lyse. Infection of endothelial cells and the resultant vascular inflammation and hemostatic alterations are the principal pathogenic features of *R. typhi*.[22]

PREVENTION

Preventing epidemic typhus depends on eliminating human body lice with insecticides such as permethrin powder (1%) at doses of 30–50 g for an adult and 15–25 g for a child. Doxycycline can be used for chemoprophylaxis in visitors to high-risk areas. Vaccines using crude antigen and/or inactivated rickettsiae are partially protective against epidemic typhus but have undesirable toxic reactions and are difficult to standardize.[6]

Control of murine typhus depends on elimination of flea vectors and their mammalian reservoirs.

DIAGNOSTIC MICROBIOLOGY

Epidemic typhus should be considered in patients with body lice and in poor people living in unhygienic conditions. Murine typhus should be considered in patients who are exposed to rodents and their fleas and who have prolonged fever and rash with or without lymphadenopathy.

Direct diagnosis

Rickettsia typhi can be isolated in shell vials containing Vero or L929 cells,[9] while *R. prowazekii* can be isolated in shell vials with human embryonic lung (HEL) fibroblasts in a biosafety level 3 containment laboratory. Direct immunodetection of organisms in tissues enables diagnosis before seroconversion and facilitates early and appropriate treatment. PCR and sequencing methods are useful, sensitive and rapid tools to detect and identify typhus group rickettsiae in blood and skin biopsies. Recently a 'suicide' PCR has been reported.[23]

Indirect diagnosis

The indirect immunofluorescence antibody assay is the reference method for diagnosing typhus group rickettsioses,[9] although an immunoperoxidase assay has been developed as an alternative for *R. typhi*.[9] Cross-adsorption followed by IFA and Western blotting can differentiate antibodies to the organisms, but the expense of the technique limits its use.

CLINICAL MANIFESTATIONS

Epidemic typhus occurs in two clinical forms: the primary febrile illness and the recrudescence of infection (Brill–Zinsser disease). After an incubation period of 10–14 days, patients may develop malaise and vague symptoms before the abrupt onset of fever (100%), headache (100%) and myalgia (70–100%). A rash is seen in 20–60% of patients[6] and typically begins in the axillary folds and upper trunk on about the fifth day of illness. In uncomplicated epidemic typhus, fever usually resolves after 2 weeks of illness if untreated, but recovery of strength usually takes 2–3 months. Without treatment, the disease is fatal in 13–30% of patients.[10] People who survive epidemic typhus remain infected with *R. prowazekii* for life. When stressed, they may experience a recrudescence, known as Brill–Zinsser disease, and they may become the source of a new epidemic if they become infested with body lice.[10]

Murine typhus is usually mild and many cases may be overlooked. When present, signs in untreated patients last for 7–14 days, when there is usually a rapid return to health. The fatality rate may reach 4%.[10]

MANAGEMENT

Doxycycline (200 mg/day) is the recommended treatment and a single oral dose of doxycycline (200 mg) usually leads to defervescence within 48–72 hours. Treatment, however, is recommended for 7–15 days, or for at least 2 days after fever resolves. Chloramphenicol (2 g/day) can be given to patients who cannot be given tetracyclines and is the drug of choice in pregnancy, except near parturition when gray syndrome may develop.[21]

Scrub Typhus

NATURE

Orientia tsutsugamushi, the causative agent of scrub typhus, is an obligate, intracellular, Gram-negative bacterium (0.5 × 1.2–3.0 µm) that has a different cell wall structure and genetic makeup to other rickettsiae.[24] Although the species is genetically stable, there is enormous genetic and antigenic variability between strains of *O. tsutsugamushi*. There are three antigenically distinct prototype strains: Karp, Kato and Gilliam originally isolated from New Guinea, Japan and Burma, respectively.[25]

EPIDEMIOLOGY

Orientia tsutsugamushi causes scrub typhus in the 'tsutsugamushi triangle' because of its vector which is bounded to the north by Siberia and the Kamchatka Peninsula, to the south by Australia, to the east by Japan and to the west by Afghanistan and India[25] (Fig. 176.6). The disease is transmitted by the bites of larval trombiculid mites (chiggers) of the genus *Leptotrombidium*. *Leptotrombidium deliense* is the most important vector species in South East Asia and southern China, whereas *L. akamushi*, *L. scutellare* and *L. pallidum* are the main vectors in Korea and Japan, and *L. chiangraiensis* is the likely vector in Thailand.[24]

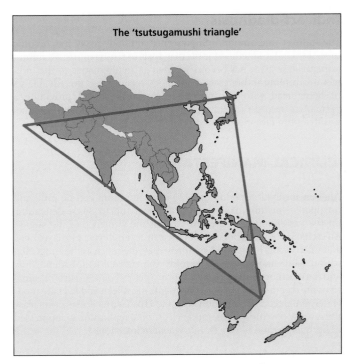

The 'tsutsugamushi triangle'

Fig. 176.6 The 'tsutsugamushi triangle'.

PATHOGENICITY

Target cells of the bacteria are mainly endothelial cells but macrophages and polymorphonuclear leukocytes are also infected. The bacteria can induce apoptosis in a variety of host cells by retarding the release of intracellular calcium.[26] In murine macrophages, *O. tsutsugamushi* produces inflammatory cytokines such as tumor necrosis factor (TNF) and interleukin (IL)-6. Tumor necrosis factor production appears to be inhibited by the production of IL-10.[24]

PREVENTION

Weekly doses of 200 mg doxycycline can prevent scrub typhus, but the efficacy of the daily 100 mg doxycycline dose regimen commonly used for malaria chemoprophylaxis has not been evaluated. Topical DEET applied to exposed skin and to the tops of boots and socks will prevent chiggers from feeding.

DIAGNOSTIC MICROBIOLOGY

The eschar is the single most useful diagnostic clue. Concurrent leptospirosis and scrub typhus should be considered in patients who are at risk and who have atypical clinical features of either disease.

Direct diagnosis

Orientia tsutsugamushi can be isolated from blood or tissues injected into white mice, chicken embryos and various cell lines such as HeLa, Vero, BHK, McCoy and L929.[27] Detection of organisms by PCR of peripheral blood and skin biopsy is a sensitive test but should be performed before antibiotic treatment or seroconversion.[24] Recently, a real-time PCR assay was described that can be used to diagnose scrub typhus by detecting major outer membrane antigen genes.[28]

Indirect diagnosis

The indirect microimmunofluorescence antibody assay has become the gold standard method for the diagnosis of scrub typhus. An immunoperoxidase assay has been developed as an alternative to the indirect microimmunofluorescence antibody assay; it has the advantages of being read with a conventional microscope and providing a permanent record of results.[9] Western blot assays differentiate true-positive from false-positive reactions with cross-reacting antibodies.

CLINICAL MANIFESTATIONS

After an incubation period of 5–20 days, infections can be mild and unapparent or fulminant and rapidly fatal (up to 30%) depending on the susceptibility of the host and/or the virulence of the strain.[6] An eschar is common but may not be seen as the chigger bite is painless and often occurs in areas not routinely examined such as the anogenital region, axilla and between skin folds. Generalized lymphadenopathy and the maculopapular rash may appear after 2–3 days. Gastrointestinal signs are common and in 30% of patients the spleen and liver are moderately enlarged.[6] Co-infection with the HIV-1 virus does not increase the severity of scrub typhus, rather HIV-1 viral replication is suppressed in both in-vivo and in-vitro O. tsutsugamushi infections.[6]

MANAGEMENT

Chloramphenicol (2 g/day) was the first recommended treatment of scrub typhus as it is a cheaper alternative to the tetracyclines. Currently, however, a 1-week course of oral doxycycline (200 mg/daily) is the treatment of choice for uncomplicated cases. Chloramphenicol- and doxycycline-resistant strains of O. tsutsugamushi have been reported in Thailand and azithromycin has been shown to be an alternative antimicrobial treatment in areas where doxycycline-resistant scrub typhus is prevalent.[29] Recently, a patient with leptospirosis and scrub typhus was successfully treated by early plasma exchange and a 7-day course of moxifloxacin therapy.[30]

Ehrlichioses

NATURE

Ehrlichia are obligate, intracellular, Gram-negative bacteria that survive in phagosomal vacuoles within the host cell. With Romanowsky stains they appear as mulberry-like structures, known as morulae, in monocytes or neutrophils. Two forms can be differentiated by electron microscopy, dense-cored cells and reticulate cells, both of which are capable of binary fission.[31]

EPIDEMIOLOGY

Ehrlichia chaffeensis is the agent of human monocytic ehrlichiosis while E. ewingii causes human granulocytic ehrlichiosis. The principal vector of both organisms is Amblyomma americanum, the Lone Star tick. Organisms are transmitted transtadially (larva to nymph to adult) but not transovarially (adult to larva). To date white-tailed deer (Odocoileus virginianus) appear to be the major reservoir of both E. chaffeensis and E. ewingii.[8]

PATHOGENICITY

Ehrlichia chaffeensis preferentially infects mononuclear leukocytes while E. ewingii infects neutrophils. Within the cell the organisms remain in the phagosome and inhibit its fusion with lysosomes. Ehrlichiae spread from the site of tick attachment via the lymphatics and bloodstream and infect cells around the body.[32]

PREVENTION

Avoidance of tick-infested areas is the first line of defense in preventing cases of human ehrlichiosis. If the use of protective clothing is not practical, insect repellents containing DEET can be used.

DIAGNOSTIC MICROBIOLOGY

In endemic areas, the disease should be suspected in all patients presenting with fever, headache, elevated liver transaminases, thrombocytopenia and leucopenia, even if there is no history of tick attachment.

Direct diagnosis

Occasionally, diagnoses can be made when morulae are seen in monocytes in Romanowsky stained peripheral blood smears, buffy coat preparations or cerebrospinal fluid (CSF). Various cell lines have been used for isolation, including a canine hysticytic line (DH82), a human monocytic leukemia line (THP-1), HEL-22 cells (fibroblast-like cells), Vero cells and a human promyelocytic leukemia cell line (HL-60).[31] Detection of ehrlichial DNA/RNA in peripheral blood is probably the best method to diagnose human monocytic ehrlichiosis (HME) in the acute phase. Most often this is with primers that amplify a section of the 16S rRNA gene.[31]

Indirect diagnosis

Most diagnoses are made using the indirect microimmunofluorescence antibody assay. Many diagnoses are made retrospectively with convalescent phase sera as relatively few patients (30%) seen in the acute phase of HME have reactive antibodies.[33] Immunoblotting procedures have higher specificity than the indirect microimmunofluorescence antibody assay but are generally only available in research laboratories.

CLINICAL MANIFESTATIONS

The main clinical signs reported are fever (98%), malaise (30–80%), headache (77%), myalgias (65%), vomiting (36%), cough (25%) and neurologic signs with changes in mental status (20%).[32] A skin rash that involves the trunk and extremities, and less commonly the face, occurs in 12–36% of patients and is more common in children (67%). Although age (>60 years) is an independent risk factor for severe or fatal HME in some studies, many severe or fatal cases have been described in apparently healthy children or young adults. These also occur in immunocompromised patients.[32]

Human infections with E. ewingii were first reported in 1999. This organism appears to be less virulent than E. chaffeensis and most of the reported patients have been immunosuppressed.[34]

MANAGEMENT

Doxycycline (4 mg/kg q12h; maximum 100 mg/dose) has become the antimicrobial agent of choice, even in children.[31] In patients allergic to doxycycline, tetracycline (25 mg/kg q6h; maximum 500 mg/dose) or rifampin (rifampicin; 20 mg/kg q12h; maximum 600 mg) are acceptable alternatives.[31] Antimicrobial therapy should be continued for at least 3 days after the patient becomes afebrile with the minimum course being between 5 and 10 days.

Anaplasmosis

NATURE

Anaplasma spp. are small, often pleomorphic or coccoid, Gram-negative, nonmotile cells ranging from 0.3 to 0.4 μm in diameter. Lipopolysaccharides and lipo-oligosaccharides have not been detected in the cell wall of *Anaplasma* and it is unknown if they contain peptidoglycan.[35]

EPIDEMIOLOGY

Anaplasma phagocytophilum is the agent of human granulocytic anaplasmosis which is transmitted by *Ixodes* spp.: *I. scapularis* is the most important vector in North America, *I. ricinus* in Europe and *I. persulatus* in Eastern Europe and Asia.[35] Human granulocytic anaplasmosis is seasonal, with most cases occurring between May and October when tick vectors are most active, particularly the nymphs which are difficult to detect because of their small size.[34]

PATHOGENICITY

The bacteria presumably infect neutrophils migrating to the site of tick attachment and disseminate as these cells migrate further. Infections might also spread if the organisms replicate locally in macrophages or endothelial cells and drain to local lymph nodes and the systemic bloodstream.[36]

PREVENTION

Vaccines against *A. phagocytophilum* are not currently available. People at risk should be informed of measures to prevent exposure to vectors including the use of insect repellants such as DEET or permethrin on clothes and shoes.

DIAGNOSTIC MICROBIOLOGY

Clinical signs are not specific, as are laboratory abnormalities which can include leukopenia, a left shift, thrombocytopenia and elevated hepatic transaminases.

Direct diagnosis

The diagnosis can be confirmed by using Romanowsky stains to identify typical clusters of organisms.[37] *Anaplasma phagocytophilum* can be isolated in tissue cultures of a promyelocytic leukemia (HL-60) cell line or primary bone marrow cells. Several primer sets have been used to amplify different target sequences of *A. phagocytophilum* in clinical samples as well as in ticks.[38]

Indirect diagnosis

The indirect microimmunofluorescence antibody assay has been used most frequently. There is serologic cross-reactivity in indirect microimmunofluorescence antibody assays between *E. chaffeensis* and *A. phagocytophilum* as these organisms are related and have common antigens such as the heat shock proteins. Enzyme immunoassays have also been used to detect antibodies to *A. phagocytophilum*.[39]

CLINICAL MANIFESTATIONS

The incubation period after tick attachment is 7–10 days and, although the majority of patients recall tick attachment or exposure, other routes of transmission such as exposure to deer blood, blood transfusion or perinatal infection have been reported.[36] Clinical signs include high fever, rigors, generalized myalgias, severe headache, arthralgia, nausea and a nonproductive cough. Rash is rare (<11%) and patients may present with atypical pneumonitis and Sweet's syndrome.[36] Fatal cases have been reported in the USA and the case fatality rate is estimated to be about 1%.[40]

MANAGEMENT

The recommended therapy for adults is oral doxycycline (200 mg/day).[37] Children older than 8 years should also be treated with doxycycline given in divided doses with dosage adjusted to the patient's weight (4.4 mg/kg q24h; maximum 100 mg/dose).[37] Rifamycin has excellent activity and can be used in cases of tetracycline allergy or pregnancy.[37]

Q Fever

NATURE

Morphologically, *Coxiella burnetii* is a Gram-negative, strictly intracellular, pleomorphic coccobacillus 0.2–1.0 μm in diameter. The organism may occur as either a small-cell or large-cell variant.[41] The small-cell variant is a compact, small rod with a very electron-dense center of condensed nucleoid filaments. The large-cell variant is larger and less electron dense and is the metabolically active intracellular form of the *C. burnetii*.

Antigenic variation or phase variation is an important characteristic of *C. burnetii* and is associated with changes in the lipopolysaccharide of the outer membrane. Organisms isolated from acutely infected animals express the phase I antigen and are very infectious. After serial passage in eggs or tissue culture, the lipopolysaccharide is modified and there is an antigenic shift to phase II organisms which are minimally infectious. Phase II organisms revert to phase I following passage in a vertebrate host. There are no distinct morphologic changes associated with this phase variation.

EPIDEMIOLOGY

Coxiella burnetii has been found worldwide, with the notable exception of New Zealand. A wide variety of ticks, rodents, birds, and wild and domestic mammals can be infected, but domestic ruminants are the major reservoirs for *C. burnetii* infections in humans. Although cattle, sheep and goats may remain chronically infected for weeks to years, the majority of infections are subclinical. Infected animals can shed large numbers of organisms in birth products (>10^9/g), feces and urine, and a major risk factor for people developing Q fever is contact with infected domestic livestock. Most human cases occur sporadically but outbreaks occur with high-risk occupations (farmers, hunters, workers in meat, milk or hide and fleece processing plants, slaughterhouses, veterinary schools, etc.).[41]

Infections occur principally by inhalation of infected aerosols with just a single organism being sufficient to cause infection. This has led to *C. burnetii* being designated a Category B biothreat agent by the US Centers for Disease Control and Prevention. The organisms may remain infective in aerosols for up to 2 weeks and in the soil for as long as 5 months. In some outbreaks, however, there is no direct contact with infected farms or animals and their products. In these outbreaks the source has been ascribed to windborne spread of *C. burnetii* from infected areas in the vicinity.[41]

PATHOGENICITY

The target cells of *C. burnetii* are monocytes and macrophages. Most infections occur via the respiratory route and involve the alveolar macrophages.[41] The Kupffer cells of the liver are involved in infections that take place via the digestive tract. Attachment to the host cell is followed by passive entry into the phagolysosome, where production of a potent acid phosphatase protects the organism from enzyme attack. Disturbance of cytokine regulatory processes, allowing survival and replication of *C. burnetii* within host cells, is also important in establishing infection. Subsequently, there is a bacteremia which, in overt clinical cases in humans, coincides with fever.

PREVENTION

Appropriate tick control strategies and good hygiene practices can decrease environmental contamination. Infected fetal fluids and membranes, aborted fetuses and contaminated bedding should be incinerated or buried. Vaccination of people in high-risk occupations should be considered. In Australia, a formalin-inactivated, whole cell *C. burnetii* (Henzerling strain, Phase I) vaccine (Q-Vax, CSL) has proven highly effective in reducing Q fever in abattoir workers.[42]

DIAGNOSTIC MICROBIOLOGY

While Q fever should be considered in patients who have close contact with domestic ruminants and cats, exposure to animals may not be reported as organisms persist in the environment for many years.

Direct diagnosis

Although *C. burnetii* does not grow on artificial media, it may be isolated in embryonated eggs, laboratory animals such as guinea pigs and mice, and in a number of tissue culture cell lines.[41] The shell vial assay may improve recovery of organisms from patients with endocarditis. A number of PCR assays have been described which detect various DNA sequences in *C. burnetii* and these have been shown to detect organisms in around 65% of patients with acute and chronic Q fever.[43]

Indirect diagnosis

The indirect microimmunofluorescence antibody assay has become the reference technique. Immunoglobulin M antibodies reactive with phase II *C. burnetii* appear rapidly, reach high titers within 14 days and persist for 10–12 weeks. Immunoglobulin M antibodies reactive with phase I antigens are usually at a much lower titer during acute infection. Immunoglobulin G antibodies reactive with phase II antigens reach peak titers about 8 weeks after the onset of symptoms, while those reactive with phase I antigens develop only very slowly and remain at lower titers than antibodies to phase II antigens, even after a year. In chronic Q fever, where there is persistence of organisms, the IgG titers to phase I and phase II antigens may both be high, and the presence of IgA antibody to phase I antigen is usually, although not exclusively, associated with chronic infection.

CLINICAL MANIFESTATIONS

The incubation period depends on the route of exposure, the inoculum dose and the age of the patient, but is usually about 3–4 weeks. Around 38% develop a mild, flu-like, self-limiting illness with low fever, headache, chills, sweating, cough, nausea and bradycardia relative to body temperature.[41] There is an inverse relationship between severity of disease and age, and infections in children may go unnoticed. Other frequently occurring signs include pneumonia which is found in almost 40% of patients and may be the only sign in 17%.

Women infected before they are pregnant do not have increased risks of abortion or premature delivery. When infections occur during pregnancy, however, fetal death or premature delivery is seen in almost every patient.[44] Chronic infections of the uterus develop in about 50% of patients and this may lead to abortions in subsequent pregnancies.

Chronic Q fever is seen in around 0.5% of patients and occurs months to years after infection. Endocarditis is the major clinical presentation of chronic Q fever and particularly involves the mitral and aortic valves. In other patients with chronic Q fever there may be osteoarticular infections, chronic hepatitis, chronic pulmonary infections and a chronic fatigue syndrome.

MANAGEMENT

Prompt treatment of acute Q fever with oral doxycycline, 100 mg twice a day for 14 to 21 days, is the treatment of choice. Co-trimoxazole for the duration of pregnancy is recommended for pregnant women as it might decrease the possibility of abortion and premature delivery. In patients with endocarditis, treatment with hydroxychloroquine (600 mg/day initial dose and titration to achieve a plasma level of 1 mg/ml) and doxycycline (200 mg/day) for 18 months to 3 years is required before serology shows cure.

Bartonellosis

NATURE

The *Bartonella* are Gram-negative bacilli or coccobacilli that belong in the α_2 subgroup of the class Proteobacteria.[45] The principal human pathogens are *B. bacilliformis*, *B. quintana* and *B. henselae*, but eight other species have been implicated in human disease: *B. elizabethae*, *B. koehlerae*, *B. alsatica* and *B. vinsonii* subsp. *berkhoffii* in endocarditis, *B. vinsonii* subsp. *arupensis* in bacteremia and heart valve disease, *B. grahamii* in neuroretinitis, *B. clarridgeiae* in cat-scratch disease and *B. washoensis* in myocarditis (Table 176.2).

EPIDEMIOLOGY

Each *Bartonella* species is adapted to a mammalian reservoir host where organisms occur within erythrocytes and endothelial cells and cause a long-lasting bacteremia. They are transmitted between hosts by arthropod vectors, mainly sandflies, body lice, fleas and ticks.

Bartonella bacilliformis occurs only in remote Andean valleys of Peru, Ecuador and Columbia and humans are the main reservoir of infection. The sandfly *Lutzomyia verrucarum* is the most important vector.[46]

Humans are the only known reservoir of *B. quintana* and the body louse (*Pediculus humanis corporis*) is recognized as its major vector. Recent studies have implicated *Ctenocephalides felis* in the transmission of *B. quintana*.[47]

The major vector of *B. henselae* is the cat flea (*Felis domesticus*) and large numbers of viable organisms can be found in flea feces. Contaminated cats' claws and teeth enable transmission of organisms by bites or scratches or when cats lick open wounds.[48]

Table 176.2 *Bartonella* species reported to date: epidemiologic and clinical data

Bartonella spp.	Reservoir host	Vector-detection in arthropods	Disease in humans	First cultivation
B. bacilliformis	Human	Sandfly (*Lutzomia* spp.)	CD, END	1919
B. talpae	Mole	Unknown	Unknown	1911
B. peromysci	Unknown	Unknown	Unknown	1942
B. vinsonii subsp. *vinsonii*	Rodents	Unknown	Unknown	1946
B. quintana	Human, cats	Human body lice/fleas	TF, BA, BAC, END	1961
B. henselae	Cats, rats, dogs	Fleas (*Ctenocephalides felis*)	CSD, BA, BAC, LMF, END, PH, RET	1990
B. elizabethae	Rodents, dogs	Fleas	END (1 case)	1993
B. grahamii	Voles, rodents	Fleas?	RET (1 case)	1995
B. taylorii	Rats	Fleas?	Unknown	1995
B. doshiae	Voles	Fleas?	Unknown	1995
B. clarridgeiae	Cats, dogs	*Ctenocephalides felis*	Unknown	1995
B. vinsonii subsp. *berkhoffii*	Dogs, coyotes, gray foxes	Fleas and ticks	END	1995
B. vinsonii subsp. *arupensis*	Rodents, cattle	Deer ticks	BAC (1 case)	1999
B. tribocorum	Rats	Unknown	Unknown	1998
B. koehlerae	Cats	Fleas	END (1 case)	1999
B. alsatica	Rabbit	Fleas or ticks	END (1 case)	1999
B. bovis (*weissii*)	Cows, cats	Unknown	Unknown	1999
B. washoensis	Rodents, dogs	Unknown	MYOC (1 case)	2000
B. birtlesii	Rats	Unknown	Unknown	2000
B. schoenbuchensis	Wild roe deer	Unknown	Unknown	2001
B. capreoli	Wild roe deer	Unknown	Unknown	2002
B. chomelii	Cows	Unknown	Unknown	2004
B. rattimasilliensis	Rats	Unknown	Unknown	2004
B. phoceensis	Rats	Unknown	Unknown	2004

BA, bacillary angiomatosis; BAC, bacteremia; CSD, cat-scratch disease; END, endocarditis; LMF, lymphadenopathy; MYOC, myocarditis; PH, peliosis hepatitis; RET, retinitis; TF, trench fever

PATHOGENICITY

Bartonella are rapidly cleared from the blood into a primary niche, most likely endothelial cells.[49] At about 5-day intervals, further waves of erythrocyte infection occur from the primary niche, perhaps reflecting the duration of the infection cycle in these cells. *Bartonella* in erythrocytes do not cause clinical signs in most reservoir hosts; the exception is *B. bacilliformis* which is associated with severe hemolytic anemia and Oroya fever.

In endothelial cells, *B. bacilliformis*, *B. quintana* and *B. henselae* have the unique ability to cause vasculoproliferative lesions (verruga peruana, bacillary angiomatosis and bacillary peliosis) by stimulating angiogenesis and the formation of new capillaries from old ones.

PREVENTION

Control of the arthropod vectors is most important. Cat fleas live on both cats and dogs and are best controlled by fumigating areas where cats and dogs live. People infested with body lice should bathe and use a pediculicide such as permethrin lotion, shampoo or powder on the hair-covered areas of the body. Sandflies can be controlled by spraying the environment with long-acting insecticides. Individual protection depends on avoiding exposed biotopes at night and the use of insect repellents (DEET) or mosquito nets treated with permethrin/deltamethrin.

DIAGNOSTIC MICROBIOLOGY

There are no pathognomonic clinical features in patients with bartonelloses and definitive diagnoses can only be made using laboratory testing.

Direct diagnosis

Bartonella grow on most blood-enriched media when incubated at 99°F (37°C) in an atmosphere containing 5% carbon dioxide. *Bartonella* can also be isolated in various cell lines in tissue culture with a shell-vial culture technique increasing the recovery rate.[50] Recently, pre-enrichment culture in *Bartonella* α Proteobacteria growth medium before subinoculation of agar plates has been reported to improve the isolation of *Bartonella* from clinical specimens.[51] Isolates are best identified using PCR-based methods which have also been shown to be more sensitive than culture in detecting organisms in tissues and blood.[45]

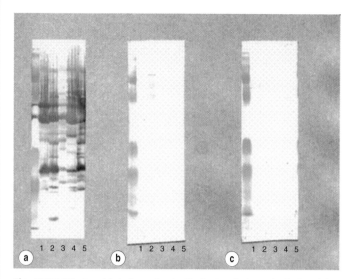

Fig. 176.7 Western blot of a patient with *Bartonella henselae* before (a) and after cross-adsorption with (b) *B. quintana* or (c) *B. henselae*. Line 1: *B. quintana*; Line 2: *B. henselae*; Line 3: *B. elizabethae*; Line 4: *B. vinsonii* subsp. *berkhoffii*; Line 5: *B. alsatica*.

Indirect diagnosis

The most commonly used technique is the indirect microimmuno-fluorescence antibody assay although enzyme-linked immunosorbent assays have also been described. Care should be taken in interpreting serology results from immunocompromised patients who might not mount significant antibody responses. Also, serology should be interpreted with caution in endocarditis patients as there are significant cross-reactions with other agents causing 'culture-negative' endocarditis such as *C. burnetii* and *Chlamydia* spp. Western blot analysis after cross-adsorption study has been shown to be a powerful tool for the identification of *Bartonella* at the species level in endocarditis (Fig. 176.7).

CLINICAL MANIFESTATIONS

A number of different clinical conditions have been associated with *Bartonella* infections.

Carrion's disease

Carrion's disease is caused by *B. bacilliformis*. Clinical signs are seen mostly in children and teenagers and include fever, malaise, hyporexia, nausea and vomiting, hepatomegaly, lymphadenopathy, pallor and a systolic murmur. Mortality rates can be high in untreated patients, reaching 90%, especially if infections are complicated with other diseases such as salmonellosis.[45]

Trench fever

The etiologic agent is *B. quintana*. After an incubation period of 2–3 weeks, there is a sudden onset of fever, retro-orbital headache and intense pain in the long bones of the legs, in particular the tibias.[45] While fatal cases have not been reported, the disease may persist for 4–6 weeks and result in prolonged disability.

Cat-scratch disease

Bartonella henselae is the major etiologic agent of cat-scratch disease which is now generally recognized to be the most common cause of chronic benign lymphadenopathy. In 75% of patients the adenopathy might be accompanied by mild systemic signs including fever, malaise, fatigue, headache, anorexia, weight loss and emesis that usually resolve within 2 weeks. Most cases are self-limiting, with the adenopathy resolving spontaneously in 2 weeks to 4 months.[45]

Atypical manifestations of cat-scratch disease occur in about 15% of patients. The most common is Parinaud's oculoglandular syndrome where there is unilateral conjunctivitis with preauricular lymphadenopathy that probably results from inoculation into the conjunctiva rather than the skin.

Bacillary angiomatosis

Bacillary angiomatosis is a vascular proliferative disease caused by *B. henselae* or *B. quintana*.[45] It was first described in HIV-infected patients but also occurs in organ transplant recipients and in immunocompetent patients. Lesions most often involve the skin but can occur at other sites including bone marrow, spleen, liver and lymph nodes.

Bacillary peliosis

This rare condition is caused by *B. henselae* infections of the parenchymal vasculature which results in the development of cystic, blood-filled spaces, particularly in the liver (peliosis hepatic) but also in the spleen, bone marrow or lymph nodes.[45]

Bacteremia

Persistent bacteremia is now one of the most frequently reported manifestations of re-emergent *B. quintana* infections among homeless people and alcoholics.[45] Prolonged bacteremia can also occur with *B. henselae* in HIV-infected patients. These infections may be asymptomatic or associated with an insidiously developing, prolonged symptom complex of malaise, fatigue, weight loss and recurring high-grade fevers.

Endocarditis

Bartonella endocarditis in immunocompetent and immunocompromised patients and infections with these organisms should be suspected in all patients with endocarditis that is 'culture-negative' by routine blood culture techniques.[45]

MANAGEMENT

In patients with Oroya fever, ciprofloxacin (patients <7 years, 10 mg/kg q12h; patients 7–14 years, 250 mg q12h; patients >14 years, 500 mg q12h; all for 10 days) or chloramphenicol (50 mg/kg q6h for 3 days, then 25 mg/kg/day for a further 11 days) are the drugs of choice and significantly reduce mortality.[52] The current recommendation is that *B. quintana* bacteremia be treated with intravenous gentamicin (3 mg/kg/day for 14 days) and doxycycline (200 mg/day for 28 days). While *B. henselae* is susceptible to most antibiotics *in vitro*, most typical cases of cat-scratch disease respond very poorly to antimicrobial therapy. In immunosuppressed patients the use of antibiotics is associated with rapid clinical improvement. In patients with suppurative lymph nodes, needle aspiration is an appropriate treatment.[52]

REFERENCES

References for this chapter can be found online at http://www.expertconsult.com

Chlamydia

INTRODUCTION

The chlamydial diseases seldom occur abruptly and they are not easily recognized; rather, chlamydial infections may run an insidious, chronic course, causing severe damage only after years of infection.[1] Their possible role in chronic diseases with an inflammatory component has led to renewed interest in these organisms. Their obligatory intracellular growth makes normal bacteriologic analysis difficult.[2] The sequencing of whole genomes of several chlamydial species[3] has provided new possibilities for studying these organisms and our concepts of the nature of chlamydiae are changing accordingly. Their small genomes as well as the wide variety of associated clinical syndromes make *Chlamydia* promising in future studies of disease pathogenesis in general.

NATURE

The current classification of chlamydial species is rapidly evolving and there are proposals to name new species and even new genera.[4] The suggested genus *Chlamydophila* has been criticized on the basis of intracellular evolution which is different from extracellular bacterial evolution in general, and the name *Chlamydia* should be conserved. *Chlamydia trachomatis* is a human pathogen with its closest relatives found in the mouse (*C. muridarum*) and pig (*C. suis*). *Chlamydia pneumoniae* is a human pathogen with strains reported in the horse, marsupials and amphibians. *Chlamydia psittaci* is a pathogen of birds, *C. abortus* and *C. pecorum* are pathogens of ruminants, *C. felis* is a pathogen of cats and *C. caviae* is found in guinea pigs. All except the last species also cause diseases in humans. Numerous *Chlamydia*-like or *Chlamydia*-related bacteria have been isolated recently, but their pathogenic potential and distribution require further studies.[5] Like *Legionella*, these new agents are able to multiply in amebae and have been called environmental *Chlamydia*-like agents.

Chlamydiae are small, Gram-negative bacteria that are obligatory intracellular parasites, the general properties of which are outlined in Table 177.1. They are not cultivable on synthetic media. They exist in nature in two forms: a nonreplicating, infectious dense particle called the elementary body (EB); and a loose, larger, intracellular form, the reticulate body (RB), which is able to multiply by binary fission but is noninfectious (Fig. 177.1).[6] The EB is a spherical particle about 300 nm in diameter; it can be stored at –94 °F (–70 °C) in sucrose-containing buffers and cultured in cell cultures.

Chlamydiae have a double layer membrane of Gram-negative bacteria with a periplasmic space. They are usually devoid of peptidoglycan, but seem to use it when dividing.[7] The circular genomes of *C. pneumoniae* and *C. trachomatis* contain 1 230 000 and 1 039 000 base pairs, respectively, with just over 1000 potential genes.[3] Species-specific plasmid is present in 10 copies in *C. trachomatis*,[8] but is not found in the human type of *C. pneumoniae*. The major outer membrane protein (MOMP) forms the outer membrane of the particle with some minor proteins, of which two are rich in cysteine. *Chlamydia trachomatis* has nine and *C. pneumoniae* 21 genes for putative membrane proteins (PMPs). Cysteine-rich proteins apparently have replaced the peptidoglycan with their S–S bridges in maintaining the rigidity of the chlamydial membrane. On electron microscopy, the surface can be seen to consist of a hexagonal pattern with substructures made up of a few rosettes with short spikes (Fig. 177.2).[9]

The MOMP of *C. trachomatis* contains four variable regions, which divide it into about 20 immunotypes denoted alphabetically.[10] The MOMP of *C. pneumoniae* is more homogeneous and the surface structure differs from that of *C. trachomatis*. Chlamydial lipopolysaccharide (LPS) is of rough type, weakly endotoxic, and situated in the outer membrane. It contains three KDO-residues, in which the α-2-8 bond is specific for *Chlamydia*. It is 10 times less toxic than typical LPS but induces production of interleukin (IL)-8 via Toll-like receptor 4 (TLR-4) in the presence of CD14.[11]

Table 177.1 General properties of *Chlamydia*

- Obligatory intracellular Gram-negative parasites
- Elementary body–reticulate body cycle
- Lack of peptidoglycan
- Common group antigen (lipopolysaccharide)
- Tendency to persistent infections
- Host immune defense participates in the development of lesions

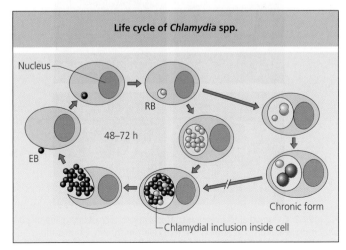

Life cycle of *Chlamydia* spp.

Nucleus

RB

48–72 h

EB

Chronic form

Chlamydial inclusion inside cell

Fig. 177.1 Life cycle of *Chlamydia* spp.

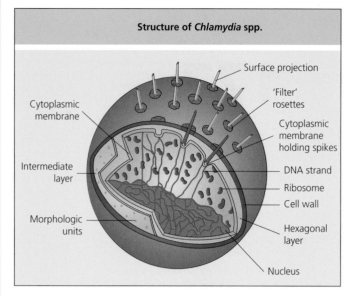

Structure of *Chlamydia* spp.

Surface projection

'Filter' rosettes

Cytoplasmic membrane holding spikes

DNA strand

Ribosome

Cell wall

Hexagonal layer

Nucleus

Cytoplasmic membrane

Intermediate layer

Morphologic units

Fig. 177.2 Structure of *Chlamydia* spp. Courtesy of Dr A Matsumoto.

In the multiplication cycle, the EBs attach to the surface of susceptible cells and are passively engulfed by activity of the cell. *Chlamydia trachomatis* lymphogranuloma venereum (LGV) biotype is wrapped by heparan sulfate that is taken from the cell by the chlamydial organism, which can then use heparin receptors on the cell surfaces; *C. pneumoniae* and *C. psittaci* may also use glycosaminoglycans in the attachment but there apparently are other receptors, too.[12]

The chlamydial surface can prevent the fusion of the endocytic vacuole with lysosomes, and travels on microtubules joining to the exocytic pathway. The EB envelope changes, transforming the metabolically inactive inert EB into the metabolically active RB, which is 0.8–1 μm in diameter. In the process, the disulfide bridges are reduced and MOMP acts as a porin. DNA, RNA and proteins are synthesized within the RB, which divides successively by binary fission. The endosomal walls intercept nearby trans-Golgi vesicles that incorporate sphingomyelin and glycerophospholipids into the swelling chlamydial inclusion (Figs 177.3, 177.4). Metabolically active RBs acquire nutrients and metabolic building blocks, including nucleotides and ATP ('energy' parasites) from host cells.[13] Chlamydial LPS is present in RBs and also seems to attach to host cell membranes.

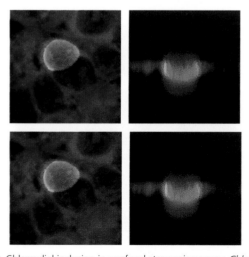

Fig. 177.3 Chlamydial inclusion in confocal stereomicroscopy. *Chlamydia pneumoniae* cultured in human line (HL) cells are shown. Fluorescein isothiocyanate (FITC)-labeled anti-LPS monoclonal antibody stain. Courtesy of Dr A Laurila.

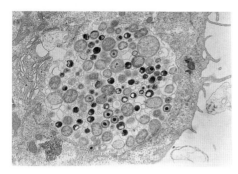

Fig. 177.4 Electron microscopy of chlamydial inclusion. Reticulate bodies and transition stages to dense elementary bodies are shown. *Chlamydia pneumoniae* cultured in HL cells. Courtesy of Dr CH von Bonsdorff.

Chlamydiae use their type III secretion system (TTSS) to gain control over the host cell and interfering cellular immune defense mechanisms by proteolytic proteins. Apoptosis is prevented during the growth period but induced in nearby inflammatory cells.[14] A chlamydial cytotoxin and proteolytic enzymes secreted through the TTSS have been demonstrated.[15] Eventually, the inclusion body may contain several thousand chlamydial RBs. At the end of the replication cycle, chlamydiae start to condense into EBs, and apoptosis and proteolysis are promoted in order to liberate the new infectious particles. Sometimes the mature inclusion is expelled intact but usually the inclusion bursts open, releasing infective chlamydial particles and the cell dies. The whole cycle takes 2–3 days. Depletion of tryptophan or iron or the presence of penicillin or interferon gamma (IFN-γ) in subinhibitory concentrations induces an aberrant, slowly metabolizing form of RB, which can persist for long periods. In chronic infections this may be the dominant form of *Chlamydia*.[13] The microscopic appearance of chlamydial inclusion varies with different strains, and the inclusions of *C. trachomatis* contain glycogen.

EPIDEMIOLOGY

Chlamydia trachomatis is transmitted by direct contact and via vectors such as flies and contaminated towels in poor sanitary conditions in trachoma-endemic areas. Newborn infants contract the infection from their mother, sometimes before birth, and can infect their siblings via excretions. In industrialized countries, *C. trachomatis* is by far the most common bacterial sexually transmitted disease (STD). The incidence is greatest in young sexually active people and varies widely among different areas, from very low levels in Scandinavian countries to 15–40% in some urban areas of other developed countries.

Chlamydia pneumoniae is a common respiratory pathogen worldwide. In tropical countries, infections are common during the first years of life, especially in urban slums. In industrialized countries, children begin to seroconvert at school age at the rate of 10% each year. The rate seems to depend on population density, but at the age of 15 years 25–50% of populations have demonstrable antibodies against the agent. The antibody prevalence continues to rise; nearly all elderly people have measurable antibodies. Because antibodies are lost by a few years after an acute infection, this steady increase points to repeated infections during life and to possible chronic infections. Spread via droplets has been proposed. Asymptomatic carriers are found but their number is disputed and there is a possibility that only some people are effective transmitters of the agent. In sparsely inhabited areas in high latitudes, *C. pneumoniae* has caused epidemics at intervals of 5–7 years. In lower latitudes, the interval between epidemics is shorter and an endemic situation can be found near the equator. In military garrisons with susceptible recruits, the slow epidemics are prolonged and can last 6 months.

Avian *C. psittaci* is contagious in dried droppings of diseased birds for several days and is typically transmitted by the inhalation of dust. Patients are usually turkey or duck farmers, plant processors or persons who have contact with diseased caged or wild birds. Person-to-person transmission occasionally occurs. Infections caused by *C. psittaci* strains from mammals are less well known. Ovine abortion strains are known to cause septic abortions in pregnant women who are in contact with affected farm cattle. Pet cats can be a source of *C. felis* infections. *Chlamydia*, like *Legionella*, are able to multiply in amebae[5] but the significance of this property in epidemiology is so far not known.

PATHOGENICITY

Owing to their unique life cycle, in which they parasitize only living, metabolically active cells, chlamydiae are not harmless commensals.[3] It is not known whether the pathogen stays dormant inside cells, protected from antibodies, for prolonged periods only to be activated later by some signal, or whether there is a special form of chronically infecting *Chlamydia* spp. In chronic persistent infections *in vitro*, it is possible that chlamydiae respond with morphologically abnormal forms, in which internal proteins such as heat shock proteins (hsps) are produced and antigens of mature EBs are diminished.[16]

Chlamydiae are potent inducers of cytokines, such as IFN-γ and IL-1, which prevent the multiplication of the agent *in vitro*.[13] In chronic infections such as trachoma, there are findings that point to diminished cell-mediated immunity and increased humoral immunity.[17] Chlamydial immunity is relatively short-lived, immunotype specific and re-infections are common. Active therapy of episodes in the community can lead to 'arrested immunity', in which re-infections are common, but chronic infections fortunately rare.[18]

In repeated chlamydial infections[19] there is a hypersensitivity component, apparently caused by common internal cross-reactive proteins. Chlamydial hsp60, a protein produced in chronic infections, has been blamed for the hypersensitivity reactions seen.[20] Moreover, it is related to the host's hsp60 and may initiate autoimmune reactions.

In chronic chlamydial infections, chlamydia can persist in noncultivable form and damage results partly from persistent inflammation. Blinding trachoma was thus named after *C. trachomatis* and long-term sequelae of lymphogranuloma venereum – rectal strictures, elephantiasis and esthiomena (genital elephantiasis) – have been known for some time, but infertility and ectopic pregnancies caused by tubal occlusion have only recently been associated with chronic *C. trachomatis* infection.

Chlamydia pneumoniae is able to disseminate inside white blood cells from lungs in the circulation[21] and thus may disseminate widely. This is obviously one reason why it has been associated with a wide variety of diseases. Most important is the association of *C. pneumoniae* with atherosclerosis.[22] Over 70 seroepidemiologic surveys have repeatedly demonstrated that the presence of elevated antibodies against *C. pneumoniae* is associated with an increased risk of having a cardiac event. The antibody findings are further supported by the presence of circulating immune complexes containing *C. pneumoniae* antibodies and antigens, pointing to an access of chlamydial components into the circulation. Human hsp60 and chlamydial hsp60 co-localize in atherosclerotic plaques and coronary angioblasty releases chlamydial components from the lesions. Final demonstration of the common presence of the agent in the atherosclerotic lesion has been obtained by immunoelectron microscopy, immunohistochemistry, nucleic acid demonstration by polymerase chain reaction (PCR), *in-situ* hybridization and even isolation of the agent from lesions.[23]

The important question is, does this presence have an effect on the atherosclerotic process? *C. pneumoniae* may simply be an innocent bystander in atherosclerotic lesions carried there in blood. However, it is an intracellular pathogen, able to multiply in macrophages, endothelial cells and smooth muscle cells. This multiplication is accompanied by induction of cytokines, adhesion molecules, growth factors and proteases. Oxidative substances appear as the host defense mechanisms against chlamydial infection. Chlamydial LPS induces foam cell formation in macrophages, the characteristic pathologic feature of the atherosclerotic plaque. Several well-known risk factors for coronary heart disease are also associated with a chronic *C. pneumoniae* infection, such as smoking, elevated cholesterol levels, lowered levels of high-density cholesterol and elevated blood pressure.[24] Animal experiments point to the possibility that it could even initiate the process[25] and that this could be prevented with antibiotics. Recently it was found that children as young as 11 years with signs of persistent *C. pneumoniae* infection show early signs of atherosclerosis including intimal thickening of their aortas.[26] *Chlamydia* can also be found in the vessel walls at the age of 14 years, decades before the complications of atherosclerosis, myocardial and cerebral infarctions start to appear.

Preliminary small-scale intervention trials with positive results encouraged pharmaceutical companies to begin intervention trials with antibiotics known to be effective in acute chlamydial infections, although animal and cell culture trials had shown them to be ineffective in chronic infections.[27,28] All the patients had advanced atherosclerosis and in this phase antibiotic treatment had no effect on the lesions formed.[29] The results mean that in advanced atherosclerosis usual antichlamydial antibiotics are ineffective and treatment of chronic infections demands further studies.[30]

The association of *C. pneumoniae* with childhood and adult asthma seems to be accepted[31] but its association with chronic neurologic diseases is debated.[32] There are reports of the association of *Chlamydia* with some forms of cancer (*C. trachomatis* with cervical cancer, *C. pneumoniae* with lung cancer, *C. psittaci* with ocular adnexal MALT lymphoma).[33] These diseases have remained mostly unstudied, although some animal models and successful intervention trials have been reported.

PREVENTION

Vaccines against *Chlamydia* spp. have been under development for 40 years without evident success. *Chlamydia trachomatis* has several immunotypes making development of a vaccine complicated, and the protective antigens of *C. pneumoniae* are not known. Knowledge of the complete genome and progress in immunology may alter this situation in the future.[34]

In 1998 the World Health Organization (WHO) started a project to eradicate trachoma. It is based on SAFE strategy (lid Surgery, Antibiotic mass treatment, Facial cleanliness and Environmental hygiene). Mass medication campaigns, washing the face every second day with clear water and wiping it with a towel that is not shared with other people is effective. Latrine hygiene is effective in controlling flies that spread trachoma. Evidence supports the effectiveness of this approach and there is a possibility that trachoma will be eradicated before 2020.[35]

The advent of nucleic acid amplification tests (NAATs) has led some countries to introduce screening in order to eradicate *C. trachomatis* from the population.

DIAGNOSTIC MICROBIOLOGY

The clinical features of chlamydial infections, such as their slow onset, the low numbers of infectious agents present and the cross-reactions seen in serology and some nucleic acid amplification tests, make usual diagnostic methods difficult.[36,37]

Chlamydia trachomatis infections

Culture

Culture was originally the gold standard in *C. trachomatis* diagnosis but due to its low sensitivity it is unsatisfactory. Although it is recommended in legal cases and in order to test antibiotic sensitivity, laboratories performing *Chlamydia* culture are nowadays rare.

Samples for culture should contain live cells from the diseased area and this can be problematic if the pathogen has invaded deeper tissues.

The sample is collected in a medium that contains sucrose, aminoglycosides, vancomycin and antifungal agents. McCoy cell lines and green monkey kidney cell lines are commonly used. Centrifugation onto cells and the addition of cytostat (usually cycloheximide) into the growth medium are needed for optimal growth. Multiwell plates are suitable for mass isolation attempts, but vials are better protected from cross-contamination. *Chlamydia trachomatis* can be stained by Lugol's iodine; immunofluorescence staining using LPS-specific monoclonal antibody gives a more clear-cut result but it stains all *Chlamydia* spp. The culture result is available in 2–3 days, but blind passage can improve the outcome.

Antigen detection

All enzyme immunoassay (EIA) kits for the diagnosis of *C. trachomatis* measure the common LPS group antigen that is present in all chlamydiae and produced in large amounts during the growth cycle. However, they lack sensitivity seen in NAATs and their use has diminished lately.

Direct fluorescent antibody (DFA) staining has been successfully used in *C. trachomatis* diagnosis. This test seems to be marginally more sensitive than EIA; moreover, the quality of the sample can be controlled in the stained smear. However, the interpretation demands expertise and is tiring to the reader, and therefore the test is often used only in the confirmation of EIA test results.

Serology

In individual *C. trachomatis* infections serologic tests are often of questionable value, although serology has been important in epidemiologic and disease association studies. The infection is often superficial without detectable seroconversion. Proper antibiotic therapy can also prevent antibody formation. The use of the complement fixation (CF) test in *C. trachomatis* infections is limited to lymphogranuloma venereum. Microimmunofluorescence (MIF) testing, if properly done, can differentiate between species and even immunotypes. It is, however, demanding and can be performed in relatively few laboratories. *Chlamydia trachomatis* antibodies start to appear at the sexually active age and peak at about 30 years of age. They are more often found in females than in males; the opposite is seen with *C. pneumoniae* antibodies, where males predominate. In *C. trachomatis* infections, MIF testing is usable in lymphogranuloma venereum, perihepatitis and infant pneumonitis, it can also give a clue to the triggering agent in reactive arthritis.

Enzyme immunoassay tests based on chlamydial EBs or chlamydial LPS (group antigen) are commercially available but have not gained wide popularity. Species-specific EIA kits based on peptides are also available. Their use in infertility studies can reveal tubal occlusions.

Nucleic acid amplification tests

The use of NAATs has altered the former concept of culture as the 'gold standard' of *C. trachomatis* diagnosis and has replaced other diagnostic methods. Several methods are commercially available. A great advantage is the possibility of using mailed morning void urine, tampons and self-collected samples for detection. To avoid leakage of urine during mailing, even self-collected dry swabs have been tried.

Nucleic acid (NA) tests are not without problems and some of the early ones have been removed from the market. In the case of *C. trachomatis* NA detection tests are usually based on its plasmids, but also on 16S RNA or chromosomal DNA. There have been reports on plasmid-free variants and, in 2006, a new plasmid variant was found to cause an epidemic in Southern Sweden, where 25% of the cases were caused by it and it was not detectable with most commonly used NAATs. The problem is now well known and diagnostic firms seem to have solved the problem.

There is no consensus as to whether a positive result should be confirmed with another test method, if the success of therapy should be monitored, and whether young females should be retested after 3–12 months. All these have been recommended but are not in general use. Cost is a major reason for this. In screening general populations, pooling of urine samples can save expense.

Chlamydia pneumoniae infections

Culture

The same principles as in *C. trachomatis* culture are used for *C. pneumoniae*, with the exception that HEp-2 or HL cells are used. *Chlamydia trachomatis* can be found in samples in amounts toxic for cells but *C. pneumoniae* cultures in primary isolation usually contain only a few inclusions. The consensus is that serology in acute infections is more sensitive than culture.[37]

Antigen detection

Direct fluorescent antibody staining from respiratory samples is still more difficult when compared to genital swabs and is used only occasionally. Since EIA detection tests are based on common chlamydial LPS they can be used in respiratory samples to obtain a presumptive diagnosis of chlamydial respiratory infection. This possibility has been used in only a few studies.

Nucleic acid amplification tests

In theory, NAATs should be as good for *C. pneumoniae* as for *C. trachomatis*. So far, most studies have been done with in-house kits and commercial kits have been slow to appear on the market. In acute infections NAATs are more sensitive than culture. One difficulty is to get representative samples from the pneumonic area because upper respiratory tract specimens can remain negative. In positive cases, a possible carriage status must be remembered.

Serology

Serology has been the method most commonly used for *C. psittaci* and *C. pneumoniae*. The need for paired samples considerably lessens the value of serology in acute situations.

Microimmunofluorescence testing seems, for the moment, to be the most convenient test for the serologic diagnosis of an acute *C. pneumoniae* infection.[37] In primary infections, the diagnosis can be obtained from the first sample that contains IgM antibodies specific for *C. pneumoniae*. The possibility of a false-positive reaction due to IgM rheumatoid factor should always be kept in mind, especially in elderly patients. In elderly patients undergoing re-infections, the rapid response can be missed if the first serum sample is not collected early enough after the onset of disease. Apart from the situation in which strong group reaction interferes with the result, an experienced reader can interpret the reaction to differentiate the species. In MIF testing, strains of *C. pneumoniae* react much more uniformly than do those of *C. trachomatis*.

The time-honored CF test has traditionally been used for the diagnosis of chlamydial respiratory tract infections. The CF test in *C. pneumoniae* infections is sensitive only in primary infections of young adults.

Enzyme immunoassay tests for species-specific serology are currently replacing MIF due to their easy laboratory performance. They seem to be more sensitive, especially in acute infections of children.

Other *Chlamydia* and *Chlamydia*-like organisms

Serology by CF test has been used traditionally in diagnosis of psittacosis. The number of different species makes MIF cumbersome and there are few studies on the definite causative agent in chlamydioses of humans. Isolation in cell cultures can be attempted and the ability of *C. psittaci* to cause laboratory infections should be kept in mind. NAATs are not currently commercially available. Wide spectrum pan-*Chlamydia* probes which detect numerous species have been tried. Several *Chlamydia*-like agents have been associated with human diseases by isolation, serology and lately by NAATs. Environmental *Chlamydia*-like agents can be isolated in cultures of amebae. They can interfere as laboratory contaminants in *Chlamydia* NAATs.

Diagnosis of chronic chlamydial infections

Diagnosing chronic chlamydial infections is problematic. The number of infective organisms can be small and the site of infection can be difficult to reach. Culture often remains negative, especially if the sample is from a peripheral site. Antibody responses can be quite variable or even lacking. However, persistently elevated titers, especially of IgA type, have been suggested as a marker of chronic infection but their value in individual diagnosis is doubtful, especially if a single sample is collected. Enzyme immunoassay tests have been inferior when compared to the MIF test in chronic infections. Measurements of local antibodies in asthma patients and antibodies to chlamydial hsp60, with or without combination with inflammation markers such as C-reactive protein (CRP), have been used in some studies.

Antigen detection by immunohistochemistry is sensitive and diagnostic but, like nucleic acid-based methods (e.g. NAATs, *in-situ* hybridization), it is currently used in research laboratories only. The value of demonstrating circulating immune complexes that contain chlamydial antigens in blood samples has been proposed, but the technique is quite demanding. Detection of nucleic acid in circulating white blood cells is nowadays frequently used. The lack of international standards is reflected in the fact that in comparative study populations, the positivity can vary between 0% and 80%. A newly described method is to measure the presence of chlamydial LPS in the circulation, but none of these approaches indicates the site of the infection.

All these markers can also be found in otherwise healthy persons, suggesting common prevalence of chronic chlamydial infections.[21] All markers are affected by age and season so for.

CLINICAL MANIFESTATIONS

The diseases associated with chlamydial infection are listed in Table 177.2 and discussed in relevant chapters. *Chlamydia pneumoniae* has been associated with a wide variety of diseases, but in most cases these associations are highly speculative so far.

Table 177.2 Diseases associated with *Chlamydia* spp., or in which a possible association has been proposed

Species	Infection	Distribution	Disease	Incidence
Chlamydia trachomatis	Acute	Females	Cervicitis	About 30%
			Endometritis	Common
			PID	10–70%
			Perihepatitis, splenitis, appendicitis	Isolated case reports
			Bartholinitis	Rare
		Males	Urethritis	10–30%
			Epididymitis	Rare
		Both sexes	Conjunctivitis	Uncommon
			Reactive arthritis	Common cause
		Neonates	Conjunctivitis	10%
			Infant pneumonitis	By definition
	Chronic	Female	Chronic PID	Common
		Both sexes	Trachoma	By definition
Chlamydia pneumoniae	Acute	Both sexes	Pneumonia, endemic	10%
			Pneumonia, epidemic	Up to 50%
			Acute bronchitis	5%
			Sinusitis	5%
			Otitis media	Case reports
			Common cold, subclinical	10% of school children annually
			Carditis	Case reports
			Reactive arthritis	Case reports
	Chronic	Both sexes	COPD, asthma	10–50% (?)
			Atherosclerosis	50–80 % (?)
			Alzheimer's disease	?
			Multiple sclerosis	?
Chlamydia psittaci	Acute	Both sexes	Psittacosis–ornithosis	By definition
Chlamydia abortus	Acute	Female	Infectious abortion	Rare
Chlamydia felis	Acute	Both sexes	Conjunctivitis	Rare

MANAGEMENT (SEE CHAPTERS 15 AND 27)

Chlamydiae are sensitive to tetracyclines, macrolides, azalides and newer fluoroquinolones. An antimicrobial effect is also seen with rifampin (rifampicin), clindamycin and chloramphenicol. Chlamydiae are resistant to aminoglycosides, vancomycin and cephalosporins.

Chronic forms seem to be very resistant to treatment and in intervention trials even 1-year courses of monotherapy have shown no evidence of eradication.[29] Novel drugs effective against chronic chlamydial forms are currently sought.

REFERENCES

References for this chapter can be found online at http://www.expertconsult.com

Opportunistic and systemic fungi

Opportunistic Fungi

INTRODUCTION

Fungal infections have become increasingly important clinically because of the rising incidence of immunocompromised patients as a result of infection, malignancy (especially leukemia), chemotherapy and immunosuppressive therapy, especially in transplantation medicine and in critical care. Moreover, the use of current antimicrobial prophylactic strategies has likely contributed to the changing epidemiology of invasive mycoses. Table 178.1 gives a list of medically important fungi that can cause disseminated infection in humans. Table 178.2 shows the variables that likely account for the current trends in the epidemiology of opportunistic fungal infections.

Candidiasis

NATURE

Candida spp. are yeast-like fungi that can form true hyphae as well as pseudohyphae. They are ubiquitous in soil and food and can be found as normal commensals on skin and mucosal membranes of the human gastrointestinal, genitourethral and respiratory tracts.

Candida spp. that under certain conditions are clinically important are *C. albicans, C. guilliermondii, C. krusei, C. parapsilosis, C. tropicalis, C. kefyr, C. lusitaniae, C. rugosa, C. dubliniensis* and *C. glabrata*. The fungal origin of these lesions was first proposed in 1839.[2]

EPIDEMIOLOGY

Since the introduction of antibiotics in the 1940s, there has been a sharp increase in the incidence of candidal infections. In a survey of 180 hospitals from 1980 to 1990, *Candida* spp. were the sixth most commonly isolated nosocomial pathogens, most frequently cultured from the urinary tract (46%).[3] *Candida* spp. were the fourth most common cause of bloodstream infection (8%) in US hospitals and were associated with a mortality of 29% (compared to 17% for bloodstream infections caused by nonfungal pathogens).[3,4]

Approximately 50% of invasive *Candida* infections are caused by non-*albicans Candida* spp., which appears to be stable distribution.[4] A surveillance program of bloodstream infections (BSIs) in the USA, Canada, Latin America and Europe from 1997 through 1999 detected 1184 episodes of candidemia in 71 medical centers (32 in the USA,

23 in Europe, 9 in Latin America and 7 in Canada). Overall, 55% of the yeast BSIs were due to *C. albicans*, followed by *C. glabrata* (20%), *C. parapsilosis* (15%), *C. tropicalis* (9%) and miscellaneous *Candida* spp. (6%).[5]

Changes in the frequency of invasive candidiasis are most notable in the following subgroups of patients: those hospitalized in critical care units, patients with hematologic malignancies, hematopoietic stem cell transplant (HSCT) recipients and organ transplant recipients.[1] In a review of 74 published studies,[6,7] the most important risk

Table 178.1 Fungi causing disseminated infection in humans

Fungi	Medically important species
Penicillium	*Penicillium marneffei*
Candida	*C. albicans, C. guilliermondii, C. krusei, C. lusitaniae, C. parapsilosis, C. pseudotropicalis, C. rugosa, C. stellatoidea, C. tropicalis, Torulopsis (or Candida) glabrata*
Cryptococcus	*C. neoformans var. neoformans, C. neoformans var. gattii*
Aspergillus	*A. fumigatus, A. flavus, A. niger, A. terreus, A. nidulans*
Mucorales	*Rhizopus oryzae, R. arrhizus, R. rhizopodiformis, Rhizomucor pusillus, Absidia oryzae, A. corymbifera, A. ramosa, Mucor circinelloides*
Histoplasma	*H. capsulatum*
Coccidioides	*C. immitis*
Blastomyces	*B. dermatitidis*
Sporothrix	*S. schenckii*
Fusarium	*F. solani, F. oxysporum, F. moniliforme, F. dimerum, F. chlamydosporum, F. anthophilum*
Trichosporon	*T. beigelii, T. capitatum*
Geotrichum	*G. candidum*
Rhodotorula	*R. rubra*
Dematiaceous molds (pheohyphomycetes)	*Pseudallescheria boydii (Scedosporium apiospermum), Bipolaris, Alternaria, Scedosporium prolificans*

Table 178.2 Variables that likely account for the current trends in the epidemiology of opportunistic fungal infections[1]

- Increasing number of susceptible hosts
- Greater laboratory expertise in the detection and identification of fungi
- Use of new transplantation modalities for hematopoietic stem cell transplantation (e.g. CD34+ selected autografts and peripheral blood stem cell transplantation)
- Evolution in organ transplantation practices
- Advances in surgical technology
- Use of corticosteroid-sparing regimens and an overall conservative approach to immunosuppression
- Use of novel immunosuppressive agents
- Use of antimicrobial prophylactic practices (e.g. use of fluconazole for antifungal prophylaxis, ganciclovir for cytomegalovirus prophylaxis, quinolones for Gram-negative bacterial prophylaxis)

factors for nosocomial colonization and infection with *Candida* spp. were underlying diseases (hematologic cancer (OR 1.7–45); renal failure (OR 1.4–22); hepatic failure (OR 7–42)); invasive procedure or devices (central venous or arterial catheter (OR 5.8–26); urinary catheter (OR 13)); interhospital transfer of a patient (OR 21), prolonged use of multiple antibiotics (OR 1.7–25) and especially the usage of vancomycin (OR 275).[6] In mice and humans, vancomycin has been shown to enhance gastrointestinal colonization with *C. albicans*.[3]

Among HSCT recipients, an overall decrease has been documented in the frequency of candidal infections, as well as a shift toward isolation of non-*albicans* species of *Candida*.[8,9] It has been proposed that use of fluconazole as antifungal prophylaxis largely accounts for these trends.[8] Antifungal prophylaxis with fluconazole during neutropenia and acute graft-versus-host disease (until day 75 after transplantation) was associated with a significant reduction in the incidence of invasive candidiasis and improved survival rates.[9] However, although *C. albicans* was the most common colonizing isolate before transplantation, fluconazole-resistant species such as *C. krusei* and *C. glabrata* were isolated after transplantation and exposure to fluconazole.[9] In another study, fluconazole prophylaxis was the most important determinant for the relative increase in isolation of *C. krusei* (OR 27.07) and *C. glabrata* (OR 5).[8]

A meta-analysis of 16 randomized controlled trials, however, showed that fluconazole prophylaxis in neutropenic non-bone marrow transplant patients did not decrease fungus-related mortality or systemic fungal infections.[10] Moreover the mortality due to invasive candidiasis was significantly higher than that due to invasive aspergillosis in adult HSCT-recipients (48.9% vs 35.5%, respectively).[11]

Among organ transplant recipients, invasive *Candida* infections are most relevant for liver and pancreas transplant recipients. An overall decline in the incidence of invasive candidiasis has been noted in liver transplant recipients, even in the absence of systemic antifungal prophylaxis: many centers now report incidences of less than 10%.

Molecular typing has shown that in the majority of cases, candidemia arises from an endogenous origin after previous colonization. This holds true for *C. albicans* and most non-*albicans Candida* spp. except for infections with *C. parapsilosis*, which are thought to arise mainly from infected biomaterials, intravenous fluids or the hands of health-care workers. Also, human-to-human transmission (patient-to-patient, nurse-to-patient and between sexual partners) has become increasingly important.

Recurrence of oropharyngeal candidiasis in patients who have AIDS has been shown to be mostly due to recurrence of the same strain (relapse), although infection with a new strain also occurs.

PATHOGENICITY

Intact barrier function is an essential feature of host defense against candidiasis. The virulence of the *Candida* spp. has been shown to correlate with its ability to adhere to epithelial cells (especially *C. albicans*) or plastic polymers such as intravascular or urethral catheters (*C. tropicalis*). The fungus is capable of secreting proteinases and lipases that can assist invasion, although the clinical importance of these enzymes is not clear.[12]

After candidal invasion of the dermis or bloodstream, neutrophils constitute the first line of defense, followed by monocytes and eosinophils, which can kill *Candida* spp. via oxidative and nonoxidative pathways. Patients who have neutropenia are particularly at risk of developing candidiasis, which underscores the importance of neutrophils in host defense against this fungus. The clinical outcome of infection is primarily determined by the host defense status. Clinical and experimental data suggest that:

- an impairment of acquired cellular immunity (e.g. in HIV infection) predisposes mainly to mucocutaneous candidiasis (gastrointestinal and vaginal); and
- impaired innate immunity, especially neutrophil function, with or without impaired T-lymphocyte function, is the major risk factor for the development of systemic candidiasis.

In the rare chronic mucocutaneous candidiasis syndrome, various combinations of defect in T-lymphocyte response to *Candida* spp. have been described[13,13a,13b] (see Chapter 72).

The role of humoral acquired immunity in the body's defense against candidal infection remains to be determined,[12] although evidence is increasing that the innate immunity is an important part of the host defense against *Candida*.[14]

DIAGNOSTIC MICROBIOLOGY

In general, a diagnosis of candidiasis faces the dual problem of:

- differentiating between colonization and infection; and
- underdetection of deep-seated infection.

In culture, *Candida* spp. grow rapidly at 77–98.6°F (25–37°C) on simple media. On special culture media, hyphae or elongating pseudohyphae are formed. *Candida* spp. grow in routine ventilated blood culture flasks and on agar plates as smooth creamy white colonies. A differential culture medium (CHROMagar Candida) can distinguish between *C. albicans* and certain non-*albicans Candida* spp.

The yield from blood cultures in disseminated disease using commercial blood culture systems is approximately 80%, but low for certain *Candida* spp., such as *C. glabrata*. However, improved culture techniques such as biphasic cultures and lysis–centrifugation may greatly improve the diagnostic yield (Table 178.3).[15]

Specimens for microscopic evaluation give a better diagnostic yield after treatment with 10% potassium hydroxide, which lyses epithelial cells. The demonstration of blastoconidia (budding yeast), hyphae and pseudohyphae is highly suggestive but not diagnostic for tissue invasion. Staining with optical brighteners such as calcofluor white or Blankophor P is a sensitive method for the detection of fungi, but requires a fluorescent microscope. Although in the routine clinical microbiology laboratory the Gram stain is commonly used to detect yeast in blood culture slides (yeasts commonly stain Gram-positive), morphologic details are more difficult to detect compared to staining with an optical brightener. Spores from molds in blood culture, which might be present in invasive fusariosis or scedosporiosis, might then be misinterpreted as yeast infection. *Candida* species identification can be achieved by the germ tube test, which enables identification of *C. albicans* and *C. dubliniensis* (but not most non-*albicans Candida* spp.) by showing the formation of hyphal elements within 90 minutes. Alternatively, rapid species identification can be achieved directly on positive blood culture bottles using peptide nucleic acid fluorescent *in situ* hybridization (PNA-FISH).[16]

Table 178.3 Detection of fungal infections

Diagnostic technique	Major features	Useful	Not useful
Microscopy/histopathology	Rapid Relies on distinctive appearance of organism	Histopathologic identification of: *Cryptococcus* *Blastomyces* *Histoplasma* *Coccidioides*	Cannot give a specific species classification for: *Aspergillus* *Candida*
Culture-based methods • Traditional culture • Automated blood culture methods	Inexpensive Early detection of growth Capital expense	*Cryptococcus* grows rapidly *Aspergillus* – tissue sample *Candida* and bloodstream infections *Cryptococcus* and *Histoplasma*	Slow growth for most endemics Poor sensitivity for *Candida* and *Aspergillus* blood samples No value for *Aspergillus*
Nonculture methods • Antigen • Antibody • PCR	Sensitive and specific Moderately sensitive and specific Still experimental	*Cryptococcus* and *Histoplasma* *Aspergillus*–galactomannan may be useful Endemic mycoses Potential use for *Candida* and *Aspergillus*	No reliable tests for other mycoses No reliable tests for opportunistic fungi

Early initiation of adequate antifungal therapy was shown to have significant impact on hospital mortality, with those patients receiving very early antifungal therapy showing a significant survival benefit.[17,18] However, as the time to detection for commercial blood culture systems is too long for blood culture to be used as an early marker to initiate antifungal therapy,[15] there is a need for biologic markers that help to identify patients who require early antifungal therapy in order to benefit from this window of opportunity and to reduce hospital mortality. Biologic markers that detect *Candida* spp. and are available commercially include cell wall components such as mannan and antimannan antibody and (1,3)-β-D glucan (BG).

The diagnostic sensitivity and specificity of detection of mannan and antimannan reported in patients with candidemia was encouraging, but only if the detection of antigen and antibody was combined.[19] The cell wall component BG is present in many fungi, including *Candida* spp., and may circulate in patients with invasive candidiasis.[20] This antigen may be a useful tool for identifying patients who require antifungal therapy in the intensive care unit (ICU) setting. However, serum BG levels are not specific for fungal infection and may also be positive in bacteremic patients.[21,22]

Recent studies indicate that the performance of these biomarkers in patients with hematologic malignancy depends on the phase of the treatment of the underlying condition.[23] Circulating antibodies could be detected in patients who developed candidemia after their first episode of neutropenia and before blood cultures yielded yeast, indicating that *Candida* infection may occur long before clinical manifestation of the disease.[24] Molecular diagnosis by polymerase chain reaction (PCR) appears very promising since fungal DNA can be detected in the blood of infected patients before conventional methods. Furthermore, a broad range of yeasts and molds can be identified to species level. Automation of sample preparation and use of real-time PCR systems will help standardize the procedure and reduce false-positive results due to contamination, but commercial and clinically validated formats are not yet available.

Susceptibility testing and interpretative breakpoints

Intensive efforts in the USA and Europe to develop standardized, reproducible and clinically relevant susceptibility testing methods for the fungi have resulted in reference documents from the Clinical Standards Laboratory Institute (CLSI/NCCLS M27-A3) and from the European Committee on Antimicrobial Susceptibility Testing (EUCAST Definitive Document E.DEF 7.1).[25,26]

An important requirement for an *in-vitro* susceptibility test is that a reproducible result is obtained and that the assay is capable of separating wild-type isolates from non-wild-type isolates, i.e. those isolates that harbor a resistance mechanism. It has been shown with *Candida* that even subtle methodologic factors can individually or collectively impact on the chosen endpoint and the minimum inhibitory concentration (MIC) result.[27] Both CLSI and EUCAST methods allow reading after 24 hours of incubation which provides clinicians with useful susceptibility information sooner.

Breakpoints have been established for many antifungal agents although different approaches were followed by the CLSI and EUCAST. For breakpoint determination the EUCAST Antifungal Susceptibility Testing Subcommittee has taken into account pharmacokinetic (PK)–pharmacodynamic (PD) data of the specific drug, dosing regimens, toxicology, resistance mechanisms, wild-type MIC distributions and clinical outcome data.[28] The validation of the EUCAST method for fluconazole was performed using clinical data sets from patients with oropharyngeal candidiasis and candidemia. Using the EUCAST method the response for those infected with a strain with a MIC of 4 mg/l was 66% but reached 100% when the dose was greater than 100 mg/day, whereas the response for those infected with strains with MICs >8 mg/l was only 12%. Hence, an MIC of 2 mg/l or 4 mg/l was able to predict successful treatment.[28] Others have also shown that the fluconazole MIC of the isolate has a major impact on the response of the patient as well as on hospital mortality.[29]

Reliable and convincing interpretive breakpoints are not yet available for amphotericin B. The reference methods do not reliably identify amphotericin B-resistant isolates. However, amphotericin B resistance appears to be uncommon among isolates of *C. albicans*, *C. tropicalis* and *C. parapsilosis*.

Antifungal resistance

Resistance is relatively uncommon in patients with invasive candidiasis and the level of resistance has been stable below 3% of bloodstream isolates for many years. Resistance to fluconazole was common in oropharyngeal candidiasis in the period prior to the introduction of highly active antiretroviral therapy (HAART) and multiple underlying resistance mechanisms were identified. In fungi, acquired resistance appears to develop primarily when a large number of micro-organisms are exposed for a relatively long period to a fungistatic drug. With the use of HAART and the greater number of alternative drugs with a different mode of action, resistance can be managed more successfully.

Elevated MIC values of echinocandins with occasional treatment failure have been reported for strains of Candida, and resistance was associated with amino acid substitutions in two 'hot-spot' regions of Fks1, the major subunit of glucan synthase.[30] The Fks1-mediated resistance mechanism is conserved in a wide variety of Candida spp. and can account for intrinsic reduced susceptibility of certain species. Fks1 mutations confer resistance in both yeasts and molds, and sporadic Aspergillus fumigatus isolates resistant to echinocandins have been found.

CLINICAL MANIFESTATIONS

The clinical manifestations of Candida infection can be divided into mucocutaneous infections and deep-seated infections. Mucocutaneous infections include thrush, candidal esophagitis, nonesophageal gastrointestinal candidiasis, candidal vaginitis and cutaneous candidiasis syndromes. Deep-seated infections include chronic disseminated candidiasis (hepatosplenic candidiasis), candidemia and candidiasis of various organ systems.

Mucocutaneous candidiasis

The most common clinical manifestation of candidal infection is oral thrush (acute pseudomembranous candidiasis), which presents as curd-like plaques on examination. It is diagnosed by the demonstration of yeast hyphae and pseudohyphae in a Gram-stained direct smear, 10% potassium hydroxide preparation, calcofluor preparation or culture of scrapings. Oral thrush should alert the physician to the possibility of an underlying disease.

Candidal esophagitis is frequently associated with AIDS, lymphoma or leukemia, although it can occur in people who are not immunocompromised. In up to 30% of cases of esophagitis there are no oral lesions on examination. Seventy-five percent of women with vulvovaginal candidiasis have no risk factors. Diagnosis is made on the basis of the combination of clinical symptoms, microscopy with 10% potassium hydroxide (include a wet preparation as well to exclude Trichomonas vaginalis and clue cells) and/or culture. The vaginal pH in candidiasis should be in the normal range (4.0–4.5); a pH higher than 4.7 indicates bacterial vaginosis, trichomoniasis or a mixed infection.

Chronic mucocutaneous candidiasis is a relatively rare disease characterized by protracted and persistent infections with Candida spp. of skin, mucosal membranes, hair and nails, and is frequently associated with endocrinopathies or autoimmune disorders. Severe disease may prove fatal, usually due to bacterial sepsis. Disseminated candidiasis is a rare complication.[13]

Deep organ infection

Disseminated candidiasis and candidemia constitute major clinical and diagnostic problems. Overall, the recovery of blood cultures depends on the Candida spp., with the commercial blood culture systems being positive in less than 40% of candidemia cases due to C. glabrata, although increased blood volume, ventilation of culture flasks and Isolator lysis–centrifugation cultivation have improved the diagnostic yield to 82%. The value of surveillance cultures is controversial, although absence of C. albicans in surveillance cultures has a high predictive value for the absence of disseminated candidiasis in patients who have leukemia or lymphoma or in bone marrow transplant patients.[3] However, isolation of C. tropicalis in surveillance

cultures is highly suggestive of disseminated infection because more than 50% of these patients will develop candidemia. Skin and eye lesions are present in only 10% of cases of disseminated candidiasis.

Virtually every organ can be infected by Candida spp. Candidal meningitis and encephalitis usually occur as a complication of disseminated candidiasis. In disseminated candidiasis, 62% of cases developed candidal myocarditis, with electrocardiographic changes mimicking infarction and supraventricular tachycardias. Candida spp. are the major cause of fungal endocarditis, with up to 41% of cases caused by non-albicans spp. In most cases, blood cultures are positive. Candida pneumonia is usually associated with disseminated candidiasis. Primary candidal pneumonia is rare. Diagnosis is based on transbronchial biopsy.

In abdominal surgery, heavy growth of Candida spp. in the first culture (intraoperative or from abdominal drain) or an increasing fungal load in serial cultures has been shown to be highly predictive of the development of candidiasis.

Infection of the urinary tract with Candida spp. is difficult to discriminate from colonization or from disseminated candidiasis. Microscopic urine analysis does not discriminate, unless renal casts containing yeasts are found, and quantitation of candiduria (such as is used for bacterial urinary infections) is not a reliable indicator of deep infection. Any patient who has persistent candiduria without a recent history of urinary tract instrumentation should be evaluated for diabetes mellitus, renal insufficiency or genitourinary tract abnormalities.[31]

'Candida hypersensitivity syndrome'

For many years, C. albicans has been mentioned as the cause of a chronic syndrome called Candida hypersensitivity syndrome, also known as chronic candidiasis, Candida-related complex and 'the yeast connection'.[32] Symptoms include general malaise, fatigue and nonspecific gastrointestinal, genitourinary and neuropsychiatric complaints.

The syndrome is said to be caused by intestinal and vaginal fungal overgrowth, inflammation, production of fungal toxins and invasion of mucous membranes. Therapy usually consists of a rigorous 'yeast elimination' diet and long-term antifungal treatment. In an effort to characterize the disease, 100 individuals who had chronic fatigue syndrome were evaluated, including eight who had been given a diagnosis of 'yeast connection'. No differences in laboratory or physical findings, including candidal skin testing, could be detected between patients and control subjects.[33] A prospective randomized clinical trial comparing nystatin treatment with placebo failed to show an improvement in the systemic complaints[34] and analysis of the diet demonstrated nutritional imbalances that could lead to the development of nutritional deficiencies if the diet were followed over a prolonged period of time. The American Academy of Allergy and Immunology reviewed the literature and concluded that the Candida hypersensitivity syndrome is 'speculative and unproven'.[35]

MANAGEMENT

Recently the mycoses study group of the Infectious Diseases Society of America (IDSA) has published practice guidelines for the treatment of invasive candidiasis.[36] These will be followed throughout this part of the chapter. The current drugs approved for treatment of systemic fungal diseases in the USA are listed in Table 178.4. Their mechanism of action is shown in Figure 178.1.

Mucocutaneous candidiasis
Oropharyngeal candidiasis

Initial mild disease can be treated with clotrimazole troches (one 10 mg troche five times daily) or nystatin (available as a suspension of 100 000 U/ml (46 ml q6h) or as flavored 200 000 U pastilles, one

Table 178.4 Drugs approved for treatment of systemic fungal diseases

Class	Generic name	Brand name	Available formulation(s)	Year initially approved
Polyene	Amphotericin B	Fungizone (Apothecon Products, Princeton, NJ)	Intravenous, oral solution	1958
Polyene	Amphotericin B lipid complex	Abelcet (Liposome, Princeton, NJ)	Intravenous	1995
Polyene	Amphotericin B cholesteryl sulfate	Amphotec (SEQUUS Pharmaceuticals, Menlo Park, CA)	Intravenous	1996
Polyene	Amphotericin B liposomal	AmBisome (Fujisawa Healthcare, Deerfield, IL)	Intravenous	1997
Pyrimidine	Flucytosine	Ancoban (ICN Pharmaceuticals, Costa Mesa, CA)	Oral tablet, intravenous	1972
Azole	Ketoconazole	Nizoral (Janssen Pharmaceutica, Titusville, NJ)	Oral tablet	1981
Azole	Fluconazole	Diflucan (Pfizer, New York, NY)	Intravenous, oral tablet, oral suspension	1990
Azole	Itraconazole	Sporanox (Janssen Pharmaceutica, Titusvilie, NJ)	Intravenous, oral capsule, oral solution	1992
Azole	Voriconazole	Vfend (Pfizer, New York, NY)	Intravenous, oral tablet	2002
Echinocandin	Caspofungin	Cancidas (MSD, Whitehouse Station, NJ)	Intravenous	2001

or two 4–5 times daily, for 7–14 days). Oral fluconazole (100–200 mg/day for 7–14 days orally) is recommended for moderate-to-severe disease. Recently it was shown that a single dose of fluconazole of 750 mg was as efficacious as a full 2-week course of 150 mg daily for the treatment of oropharyngeal candidiasis.[37] Recommended therapy for refractory disease includes itraconazole solution (200 mg/day for 7–14 days orally); voriconazole (200 mg/day orally); posaconazole (400 mg/day orally) or amphotericin B oral suspension.[36] Intravenous echinocandin or amphotericin B deoxycholate at 0.3 mg/kg per day were also shown to be effective and may be used as last-resort therapy in patients with refractory disease.

Although suppressive therapy is effective for the prevention of recurrent infections, to reduce the likelihood of development of antifungal resistance it should be used only if the recurrences are frequent or disabling. Denture-related disease may require thorough disinfection of the denture for definitive cure.

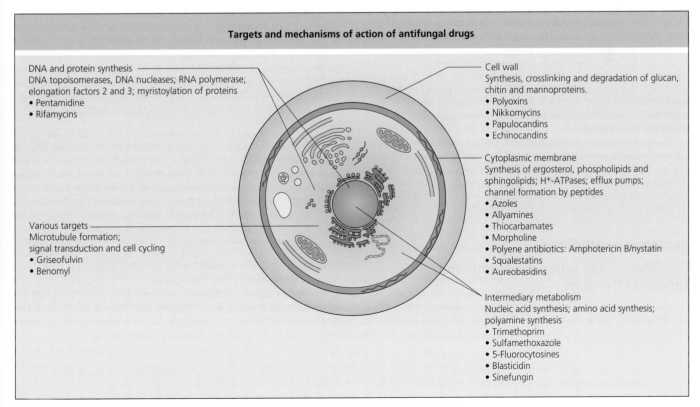

Targets and mechanisms of action of antifungal drugs

DNA and protein synthesis
DNA topoisomerases, DNA nucleases; RNA polymerase; elongation factors 2 and 3; myristoylation of proteins
• Pentamidine
• Rifamycins

Various targets
Microtubule formation;
signal transduction and cell cycling
• Griseofulvin
• Benomyl

Cell wall
Synthesis, crosslinking and degradation of glucan, chitin and mannoproteins.
• Polyoxins
• Nikkomycins
• Papulocandins
• Echinocandins

Cytoplasmic membrane
Synthesis of ergosterol, phospholipids and sphingolipids; H+-ATPases; efflux pumps; channel formation by peptides
• Azoles
• Allyamines
• Thiocarbamates
• Morpholine
• Polyene antibiotics: Amphotericin B/nystatin
• Squalestatins
• Aureobasidins

Intermediary metabolism
Nucleic acid synthesis; amino acid synthesis; polyamine synthesis
• Trimethoprim
• Sulfamethoxazole
• 5-Fluorocytosines
• Blasticidin
• Sinefungin

Fig. 178.1 Targets and mechanisms of action of antifungal drugs.

Esophageal candidiasis

Systemic therapy is required for effective treatment of esophageal candidiasis. Although symptoms of esophageal candidiasis may be mimicked by other pathogens, a diagnostic trial of antifungal therapy is often appropriate before endoscopy to search for other causes of esophagitis. A 14- to 21-day course of fluconazole (200–400 mg/day orally) is preferred. For patients who are unable to tolerate an oral agent, fluconazole may be administered intravenously or an echinocandin or amphotericin B deoxycholate at a dose of 0.3–0.7 mg/kg daily is considered appropriate. Suppressive therapy should be used occasionally in patients with disabling recurrent infections. Patients with refractory esophageal candidiasis should be treated with itraconazole oral solution (200 mg/day) or posaconazole 400 mg twice daily or voriconazole 200 mg twice daily. Intravenous amphotericin B (0.3–0.7 mg/kg per day as needed to produce a response) or an echinocandin may be used in patients with otherwise refractory disease.[36]

For *Candida*-associated denture stomatitis, the treatment of choice is fluconazole (50 mg/day for 2 weeks) combined with chlorhexidine.

Vulvovaginal candidiasis

This may be classified into complicated (severe, resistant species, impaired host defenses) and uncomplicated forms. Uncomplicated vaginitis is seen in 90% of patients and responds readily to short-course oral or topical treatment with any of the therapies listed above, including a single dose of fluconazole. In contrast, the recurrent complicated vaginitis seen in 10% of patients is defined as severe or recurrent disease, infection due to *Candida* spp. other than *C. albicans* and/or vulvovaginal candidiasis in an abnormal host. Complicated vulvovaginal candidiasis requires topical therapy administered intravaginally daily for 7 days or multiple doses of fluconazole (150 mg every 72 hours for three doses).[36] *Candida glabrata* may fail to respond to azole therapy, including voriconazole, and may respond to topical boric acid 600 mg/day for 14 days, topical 17% flucytosine cream alone or in combination with 3% amphotericin B cream, administered daily for 14 days. Azole-resistant *C. albicans* infections are rare.

Recurrent vaginitis is defined as four or more episodes of symptomatic vulvovaginal candidiasis within 1 year and is usually due to azole-susceptible *C. albicans*. After control of causal factors (e.g. uncontrolled diabetes), induction therapy with 2 weeks of a topical or oral azole should be followed by a maintenance regimen for 6 months. Recurrent vulvovaginal candidiasis is managed with fluconazole (150 mg orally every week). If fluconazole therapy is not feasible, topical clotrimazole (200 mg twice daily), clotrimazole (500 mg vaginal suppository once weekly) or other intermittent topical azole treatments are recommended.[36]

The persistent immunologic defect of chronic mucocutaneous candidiasis requires a long-term approach.[13] Systemic therapy is needed and all of the azole antifungal agents have been used successfully. The dosages required are similar to those used for other forms of mucocutaneous candidiasis. As with HIV-infected patients, development of resistance to these agents has also been described.

Systemic candidiasis

Candidemia and intravenous catheter-related candidal infections

Candida bloodstream infections are frequently associated with clinical evidence of the sepsis syndrome and high associated attributable mortality. In addition, hematogenous seeding may compromise the function of one or more organs.

All patients with a positive blood culture should be treated, even if the sample is drawn from a catheter. Additionally, indwelling intravascular catheters should be removed or changed, preferably without using a wire for replacement.[36] The evidence for this recommendation is strongest in the non-neutropenic patient population. In neutropenic patients, the role of the gut as a source for disseminated candidiasis is evident from autopsy studies, but in an individual patient it is difficult to determine the relative contribution of gut versus catheter as the primary source of fungemia. An exception is made for fungemia due to *C. parapsilosis*, which is very frequently associated with catheters.

The standard treatment for candidemia is fluconazole (loading dose of 12 mg/kg (800 mg), daily maintenance dose of 6 mg/kg (400 mg)) or an echinocandin (caspofungin: loading dose of 70 mg, then 50 mg/day; micafungin: 100 mg/day; anidulafungin: loading dose of 200 mg, then 100 mg/day). An echinocandin is favored for patients with moderately severe to severe illness or for patients with recent exposure to azoles.[36] Transition to fluconazole may be considered if isolates are susceptible to fluconazole, for infection due to *C. parapsilosis*, and in clinically stable patients. For infection with *C. glabrata*, an echinocandin is preferred. Voriconazole is effective for candidemia, but offers little advantage over fluconazole. The drug is recommended as step-down oral therapy for selected cases such as candidemia due to *C. krusei*. Polyenes, such as lipid-formulations of amphotericin B or amphotericin B deoxycholate, are alternatives if there is intolerance or in resource-limited situations.[36]

An echinocandin is recommended for most neutropenic patients. Fluconazole is an option in less critically ill patients and voriconazole if mold coverage is also warranted.

Antifungal treatment should be continued for at least 2 weeks after the last positive blood culture or after the clinical symptoms have subsided, and patients should be followed for 3–6 months to detect long-term sequelae due to hematogenous seeding.

Timely initiation of adequate antifungal therapy is important to improve clinical outcome[17,18] and empiric therapy should be considered in critically ill patients with risk factors for invasive candidiasis but with no known cause for the fever. For suspected candidiasis in non-neutropenic patients empiric therapy is similar to proven candidiasis with either fluconazole or an echinocandin as initial therapy. In neutropenic patients lipid-formulations of amphotericin B, echinocandins or voriconazole are recommended.

Recommended treatment of central nervous system (CNS) candidiasis is lipid formulation of amphotericin B (3–5 mg/kg) with or without flucytosine. The flucytosine dose should be adjusted to produce serum levels of 40–60 μg/ml. Fluconazole can be used as step-down therapy at a dose of 400–800 mg/day (6–12 mg/kg).

Treatment should be continued until all signs and symptoms, cerebrospinal fluid (CSF) abnormalities and radiologic abnormalities have resolved. Intraventricular devices should be removed. The occurrence of a brain abscess worsens the prognosis considerably. The indication for surgery remains to be determined but surgical drainage, if feasible, is probably advisable.[36]

Native valve *Candida* endocarditis should be treated with combined antifungal treatment (lipid formulation of amphotericin B with or without 5-fluorocytosine (5-FC)) and early valve replacement. An echinocandin may be considered as an alternative therapy. Without surgical intervention, the mortality is high (90%); with combined surgical and medical treatment, the mortality has dropped to 45%. Fluconazole therapy (400–800 mg/day) can be considered as step-down therapy in patients with susceptible isolates, who are clinically stable and who have clearance of *Candida* from the bloodstream. Treatment should continue for at least 6 weeks after valve replacement, but a longer duration is recommended in patients with perivalvular abscesses and other complications.

Because recurrences have occurred years later patients should be followed up for at least 2 years. Primary therapy with fluconazole has been successfully used on occasion, but fluconazole is more often employed as part of a long-term suppressive regimen.

In *Candida* urinary tract infection, the clinical circumstances dictate the management because candiduria can represent colonization, cystitis, pyelonephritis, disseminated candidemia or a fungus ball.

Treatment is not recommended for asymptomatic candiduria unless the patient belongs to a group at high risk of dissemination: neutropenic patients, low birth weight infants and patients who will undergo urologic manipulations. Neutropenic patients and neonates with *Candida* urinary tract infection should be managed as described for invasive candidiasis, while those undergoing urologic procedures should receive fluconazole at a dosage of 200–400 mg/day or amphotericin B deoxycholate at a dosage of 0.3–0.6 mg/kg per day for several days before and after the procedure.[36]

For cystitis oral fluconazole at a dosage of 200 mg/day (3 mg/kg) for 2 weeks is recommended if the infection is due to a fluconazole-susceptible *Candida* spp. For fluconazole-resistant isolates amphotericin B deoxycholate (0.3–0.6 mg/kg per day) for 1–7 days or oral flucytosine (25 mg/kg four times daily) for 7–10 days is recommended. There is no role for echinocandins, voriconazole or posaconazole as these drugs do not achieve clinically useful levels in the urine. Bladder irrigation with amphotericin B (50 g/ml in sterile water or 5% glucose administered continuously over a three-way Foley catheter for 5–7 days) is not recommended but may be useful in fluconazole-resistant infection, most notably *C. glabrata*. If there is a fungus ball in the urinary tract, the treatment is surgical.

Peritonitis is usually classified based on the cause of the inflammatory process and is further differentiated into primary, secondary and tertiary peritonitis. In primary peritonitis, no breach in the gastrointestinal tract is present. Secondary peritonitis is the most frequent form of peritonitis and is the result of a local infectious process within the abdominal cavity, with or without a hollow viscous perforation, and can lead to diffuse peritonitis. Tertiary peritonitis is an ill-defined entity and is generally referred to as a persistent or recurrent peritonitis after initial adequate treatment for secondary peritonitis.[38] *Candida* is more frequently isolated in nosocomial peritonitis, especially in immunocompromised patients and those receiving broad-spectrum antibacterial agents. Upper gastrointestinal tract perforations are also commonly associated with *Candida* infection.[38]

In critically ill patients with secondary or tertiary peritonitis, the significance of the recovery of *Candida* spp. remains controversial. Therefore, the diagnosis should be based on specimens that are collected perioperatively and processing should include microscopic examination. As mortality rates of *Candida* peritonitis in critically ill patients are high, typically 50–75%, immediate antifungal therapy is recommended, preferably in combination with surgical intervention.[38] Drugs of choice include fluconazole for susceptible *Candida* isolates, and voriconazole or the echinocandins for unknown or less-susceptible species. Antifungal therapy should last for 2–3 weeks. Surgical patients with recurrent gastrointestinal perforation are at increased risk for *Candida* peritonitis and may benefit from prophylactic antifungal therapy.

Chronic disseminated candidiasis (hepatosplenic candidiasis) is difficult to treat; this syndrome is not acutely life-threatening but does require prolonged therapy to produce a cure. Fluconazole at 6 mg/kg per day is generally preferred in clinically stable patients. Lipid formulations of amphotericin B at a dosage of 3–5 mg/kg per day or amphotericin B deoxycholate at 0.5–0.7 mg/kg per day may be used in acutely ill patients or patients with refractory disease. Some but not all experts recommend an initial 1–2 week course of amphotericin B for all patients, followed by a prolonged course of fluconazole. The echinocandins are alternatives for initial therapy.[36] Therapy should be continued until calcification or resolution of lesions, particularly in patients receiving continued chemotherapy or immunosuppression. Premature discontinuation of antifungal therapy may lead to recurrent infection.

Prophylaxis

Antifungal prophylaxis is highly controversial because the relationship between candidal colonization and dissemination is often not clear and azole prophylaxis may select for *Candida* spp. that are resistant to azoles.

Postoperative prophylaxis is recommended for high-risk liver, pancreas and small bowel transplant recipients with fluconazole at a dosage of 200–400 mg (3–6 mg/kg per day) or with liposomal amphotericin B at a dosage of 1–2 mg/kg per day. For ICU patients fluconazole prophylaxis has only been shown to be beneficial in adult units with high-risk patients and a high incidence of invasive candidiasis.[39] In hematology patients with chemotherapy-induced neutropenia, fluconazole at a dosage of 400 mg (6 mg/kg) daily, posaconazole at a dosage of 200 mg three times daily or caspofungin at a dose of 50 mg daily have been shown to prevent invasive fungal infection when administered for the duration of the neutropenia.[36] Itraconazole oral solution at a dosage of 200 mg/day is considered an alternative but is commonly less well tolerated. For HSCT recipients with neutropenia fluconazole at a dosage of 400 mg (6 mg/kg) daily, posaconazole at a dosage of 200 mg three times daily or micafungin at a dosage of 50 mg daily is recommended during the period of risk of neutropenia.[36] Besides pharmacologic prophylaxis, simple measures such as hand disinfection by medical personnel are of paramount importance, especially in preventing the spread of *C. parapsilosis*.[4]

Aspergillosis

NATURE

Aspergillus spp. can cause disease in humans by:
- colonization and subsequent allergic reactions;
- colonization of pre-existing cavities (fungus ball or aspergilloma); or
- tissue invasion.

Aspergilli are found ubiquitously in organic debris such as hay, decaying vegetation (compost piles), soil, potted plants, in pepper and spices and in construction sites. The genus *Aspergillus* contains over 250 species, although only a few are associated with disease. Recently the use of polyphasic taxonomy, which combines phenotypic features of the fungi with molecular sequence analysis, has significantly changed the classification of aspergilli. New cryptogenic species have been identified that cannot be differentiated from conventional species by microscopic morphologic features. For instance, within *Aspergillus* section *Fumigati* 30 new species have been described.[40] The clinical implications of the new species are unknown, although *in vitro* several new species are less susceptible to licensed antifungal agents compared to the conventional species.

EPIDEMIOLOGY

Worldwide, aspergillosis is the most common invasive mold infection.[41]

In a large cohort of 11 802 patients with hematologic malignancies it was shown that the overall incidence of invasive fungal infection was 4.6% with 69% of cases occurring in patients with acute myeloid leukemia.[42] Mold infection was observed in 2.9% of patients, with *Aspergillus* spp. being responsible for almost 90% of cases. Autopsy studies indicate that approximately 15% of patients have a mixed fungal infection which is not diagnosed during life in the majority of patients. In hematology patients with invasive aspergillosis the survival at 12 weeks was 52.2%.[43] Receipt of an allogeneic HSCT or solid-organ transplant, progression of underlying disease, prior respiratory disease, receipt of corticosteroid therapy, renal impairment, low monocyte counts, disseminated aspergillosis, diffuse pulmonary lesions, pleural effusion, and proven or probable (as opposed to possible) aspergillosis were predictors of increased overall mortality.[43] In most centers *Aspergillus fumigatus* is the most prevalent species and the lungs and the brain are the most common sites of infection.

The reported prevalence of allergic bronchopulmonary aspergillosis (ABPA) in patients who have asthma varies from 6% to 28%. In cystic fibrosis, 6–25% of patients are reported to have ABPA.[44]

PATHOGENICITY

The main route of infection in aspergillosis is airborne, via inhalation of the 2.5–3.0 μm conidia (spores), which settle in lungs, nose or paranasal sinuses. However, most studies suffer from a lack of correlation between air spore counts and the rate of infection. Hospital water supply has also been recognized as a source of infection, but transmission via water appears to play a modest role compared to the airborne route.[45] Other routes of infection are traumatized skin, especially due to burns, insertion openings of indwelling intravenous catheters and intravenous drug use. Patient-to-patient transmission is very uncommon, but has been reported via transplantation of an infected organ and through a patient with skin aspergillosis.

The main risk factors for invasive aspergillosis include prolonged profound granulocytopenia ($<0.5 \times 10^9/l$), especially in allogeneic HSCT recipients, high-dose corticosteroid therapy, chronic granulomatous disease, AIDS with a CD4+ lymphocyte count below 50/l, and treatment with cytotoxic drugs such as ciclosporin. Less commonly encountered risk factors are diabetes mellitus, alcohol excess, influenza, prematurity and exposure to aspergilli in large quantities.[46]

In chronic granulomatous disease, phagocytes are unable to generate the respiratory burst to kill micro-organisms. The fact that these patients and patients who have neutropenia are at risk of developing invasive aspergillosis underscores the importance of phagocytes in host defense. Alveolar macrophages and neutrophils play a major role in the defense against aspergilli.[47] Alveolar macrophages form the first line of defense by ingesting and killing conidia, even in the absence of opsonins. When conidia escape and germinate to form hyphae, granulocytes will adhere to and kill the fungus. The conidia that have not been cleared may germinate in the alveolar spaces and hyphal forms invade the pulmonary tissue and vasculature, leading to hematogenous dissemination to other organs (brain). However, blood cultures are rarely positive, except for *A. terreus*. Conidia that stay in the dormant state can survive for many days in the reticuloendothelial system. Killing of aspergilli by phagocytes is impaired by corticosteroids.

The role of humoral immunity is double edged. In ABPA, aspergilli elicit an anti-*Aspergillus* IgE antibody response, which evokes a type I immediate hypersensitivity reaction. Anti-*Aspergillus* IgG antibodies have been demonstrated in ABPA, aspergilloma and in the convalescence phase of invasive aspergillosis. These antibodies do not seem to play a significant role in host defense.

The fungus secretes various metabolic products (gliotoxin) and enzymes, such as phospholipases, hemolysin and elastase, which may play a role in virulence.[46] However, the biologic significance of these agents is not clear, since molecular studies in which gene-deletion mutants have been constructed do not show diminished virulence.

DIAGNOSTIC MICROBIOLOGY

Aspergillus is a mold that grows in tissue with dichotomously branching and regular septate hyphae (Fig. 178.2). Optical brighteners, such as Blankophor P, can be used to detect fungal elements directly

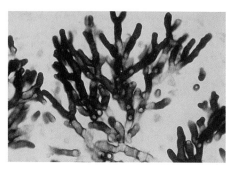

Fig. 178.2 *Aspergillus* hyphae.

in clinical specimens. However, the microscopic characteristics are not specific for *Aspergillus* spp., as other molds such as *Fusarium* or *Scedosporium* have similar microscopic morphology. At best the *Aspergillus*-like microscopic morphology can be differentiated from zygomycetes, which present as nonseptate, irregular hyphae that commonly branch at 90°. Therefore, identification to the species level can be achieved only by culture or molecular tests. *Aspergillus* spp. readily grow on standard bacteriologic media, although mycologic media will give a higher yield and are therefore recommended. Identification to the species level should always be performed with clinically relevant isolates, as *Aspergillus* spp. differ in their susceptibility to antifungal agents.

Aspergilli can be isolated from the sputum of 1–6% of healthy individuals. Also, *Aspergillus* colonization is found in patients who have chronic lung disease, cigarette smokers and those who have HIV infection. In these patient groups a positive culture is often not associated with invasive disease.[48] However, for high-risk patients, such as allogeneic bone marrow transplant recipients (60%), persons with hematologic cancer (50%), and those with signs of neutropenia (60%) or malnutrition (30%), a positive culture result is associated with invasive disease.[48]

In the high-risk patients the diagnostic yield of cultures is low and a negative culture does not rule out the presence of invasive disease. Therefore, other tests and procedures, such as nonculture-based methods and high-resolution CT scan, are used to diagnose invasive aspergillosis. The detection of circulating galactomannan (GM) by Enzyme Immuno Assay (Platelia Aspergillus, BioRad Laboratories, France) has become an important tool in the management of neutropenic patients with hematologic malignancy, although significant heterogeneity has been reported between centers using this assay.[49] Often GM is detected in serial serum samples although the antigen can also be detected in bronchoalveolar lavage (BAL) fluid or CSF.[50] Serum reactivity has been reported in patients treated with certain antibiotics such as piperacillin–tazobactam and the diagnostic sensitivity is significantly reduced in patients receiving mold-active antifungal agents.[51]

Other nonculture-based methods include (1,3)-β-D glucan (BG) antigen which is released by a variety of fungi and circulates in patients with invasive fungal infection. BG is released by *Candida*, *Aspergillus* and *Fusarium*, but infections due to zygomycetes and *Cryptococcus* will not be detected. In addition, extensive research has been performed to investigate the utility of PCR for the diagnosis of invasive aspergillosis. Although numerous studies have shown that circulating *Aspergillus* DNA can be detected early in high-risk patients, a clinically validated commercial assay is currently not available.[52]

To facilitate the validation of diagnostic tools and the performance of clinical trials, consensus definitions have been proposed. These definitions are based on host factors, clinical features (including radiology) and mycology and were recently revised.[53] In addition to culture, GM and BG are accepted as mycologic evidence for invasive aspergillosis, but not PCR.

CLINICAL MANIFESTATIONS

Aspergillosis can manifest as either fungal colonization, which can cause allergic disease and saprophytic disease (aspergilloma), or invasive disease.

The spectrum of disease caused by *Aspergillus* spp. includes:
- noninvasive aspergillosis – sinotracheobronchial colonization, allergic (bronchopulmonary) aspergillosis, aspergilloma (i.e. secondary saprophytic colonization of pre-existing cavities) and obstructing bronchial aspergillosis (mainly in patients who have AIDS); and
- invasive aspergillosis with pulmonary involvement such as acute bronchopneumonia, cavitation or slowly progressive bronchopneumonia, or extrapulmonary involvement of paranasal sinuses, CNS, skin, bone and heart.

Allergic bronchopulmonary aspergillosis

Allergic aspergillosis can either manifest as an extrinsic allergic alveolitis, causing a hypersensitivity pneumonitis in nonatopic patients, or it can cause ABPA in atopic individuals.

The major criteria for the diagnosis of ABPA are:[44]

* asthma;
* immediate cutaneous reaction to *A. fumigatus*;
* total serum IgE concentration (>1000 ng/ml);
* elevated *A. fumigatus*-specific serum IgE levels;
* precipitating antibodies to *A. fumigatus* in the serum;
* peripheral blood eosinophilia (not essential for diagnosis);
* chest roentgenographic infiltrates (not essential for diagnosis); and
* central bronchiectasis.

Eight criteria for ABPA diagnosis were initially identified, but only some of them are essential. The nonessential criteria (e.g. pulmonary infiltrates or blood eosinophilia) may be present only at the time of exacerbation or during the acute phase of the disease. The presence of bronchiectases in ABPA signifies more permanent lung damage.[44]

Aspergilloma

Aspergillomas are fungus balls that colonize pre-existing cavities in the lungs and occasionally in the sinuses and the nose. They can cause massive hemoptysis, which is fatal in 10% of cases.[46] Other symptoms can include fever, malaise and weight loss. A pulmonary CT scan may show a cavitary mass surrounded by air. Microscopic and cultural identification of *Aspergillus* spp. in a sputum smear and high antibody titers to *Aspergillus* support the diagnosis. Over 95% of patients have detectable IgG antibodies to *Aspergillus*, and antibody levels usually decrease after successful surgical removal of the aspergilloma.

Aspergillomas have been subdivided into simple and complex according to the radiologic appearance. Other chronic forms of *Aspergillus* infection of the lung that have systemic symptoms have been described. These entities include chronic necrotizing pulmonary aspergillosis (CNPA), semi-invasive aspergillosis, chronic invasive pulmonary aspergillosis, symptomatic pulmonary aspergilloma and *Aspergillus* pseudotuberculosis.[54] Diagnostic criteria for chronic pulmonary aspergillosis with response parameters have been proposed.[54]

Invasive aspergillosis

Invasive aspergillosis is a life-threatening aggressive disease that affects immunocompromised patients. High-resolution CT has proved to be a more sensitive and specific tool than conventional chest X-ray in neutropenic patients to diagnosis invasive aspergillosis. Lesions associated with invasive aspergillosis include nodular infiltrates, the halo sign and the air crescent sign, but these may be due to other micro-organisms such as other molds or bacteria.[55] In the absence of specific clinical symptoms and sensitive diagnostic tools, high-risk patients commonly received antifungal therapy empirically if their fever persisted for more than 3–5 days despite broad-spectrum antibacterial therapy. However, the availability of GM and high-resolution CT has enabled an alternative approach in which antifungal therapy is started pre-emptively if circulating antigen is detected and CT lesions consistent with fungal disease are observed.[56] Prospective studies that compare the benefits of management strategies, i.e. empiric versus pre-emptive treatment strategies, are underway.

Although HSCT recipients and other patients with hematologic malignancy are at highest risk for invasive aspergillosis, the disease is increasingly reported in critically ill patients.[57] The diagnosis of invasive aspergillosis in this patient group is challenging as circulating GM is detected in only 42% of patients. Culture and GM detection in BAL fluid appeared to be most useful, with a sensitivity of 88% for GM detection.[57]

Invasive aspergillosis is classified according to the revised consensus definitions in the categories proven, probable or possible disease.[53] For definite proof of invasive aspergillosis, a biopsy is required which shows tissue invasion by hyphae in combination with identification of an *Aspergillus* species. CT-guided lung biopsy might be a feasible tool, even in thrombocytopenic patients, with a promising diagnostic yield.[58]

Although *in-vitro* susceptibility testing is not routinely performed in invasive aspergillosis, the emergence of azole-resistant aspergillosis was recently described.[59] The *A. fumigatus* isolates were cross-resistant against azoles and the presence of resistance was associated with treatment failure.[59] In patients failing azole therapy it seems appropriate to determine the *in-vitro* activity of antifungal agents to help guide the treatment.

Extrapulmonary aspergillosis

Extrapulmonary dissemination of pulmonary aspergillosis, especially to the brain, is a well-known complication in the immunocompromised host. Meningitis due to *Aspergillus* spp. can occur, but is rare. A multivariate discriminant analysis of autopsy-proven fungal infections of the CNS demonstrated that a combination of pulmonary infiltrates and focal neurologic disease in an immunocompromised patient is more likely to be caused by *Aspergillus* spp. than by either *Candida* spp. or *Cryptococcus neoformans*. Definitive diagnosis is made by biopsy,[53] although the detection of GM in CSF is also highly indicative of CNS aspergillosis.

Virtually any organ can be infected by *Aspergillus* spp. The fungus may cause local infection in the ear or eye (endophthalmitis, keratomycosis). Direct bony invasion or hematogenous spread can occur, causing osteomyelitis. In the gastrointestinal tract, aspergillosis can lead to fatal perforation. Black necrotizing skin lesions can be a sign of disseminated aspergillosis. As in candidiasis, aspergilli can form fungal balls in the urinary tract, which present as renal colic.

Fungal sinusitis

Fungal sinusitis should be considered in all patients who have chronic sinusitis.[60] Clinical features and predisposing conditions are listed in Table 178.5. It is important to distinguish between noninvasive and invasive sinusitis because the latter can progress through invasion into soft tissue, cartilage and bone into the palate and nose or it can invade cerebral blood vessels, resulting in ischemic infarction and direct infection of the brain.

Chronic indolent invasive sinonasal infections occur in immunocompetent hosts in regions with high levels of environmental spores, such as the Sudan, Saudi Arabia and other tropical or desert areas, and occasionally in patients with diabetes in other locales. *Aspergillus flavus* is the most common causative agent of these infections, in contrast to the frequent isolation of *A. fumigatus* from sites of infection in immunocompromised hosts. These infections have a progressive clinical course over months to years, with invasion of the surrounding tissues: the ethmoid sinuses, orbit and subsequent cranial bone osteomyelitis and intracranial extension.

Radiologic findings associated with fungal sinusitis are calcifications and loss of bony sinus margins, as well as features that are common in bacterial sinusitis, such as air–fluid levels of more than 8 mm of mucoperiosteal thickening.

To distinguish between invasive and noninvasive fungal sinusitis, adequate tissue biopsies as described in Table 178.5 are necessary. The presence of hyphae excludes chronic bacterial sinusitis. In superficial fungal disease, hyphae are found only in mucopurulent material within the sinus. In invasive fungal infection, hyphae penetrate into the sinus submucosa, blood vessels or bone. The main differential diagnosis is zygomycosis.

Aspergillosis and AIDS

Aspergillosis and AIDS is discussed in Chapter 91.

Table 178.5 Key clinical points in the diagnosis and treatment of fungal sinusitis

Type	Clinical clues	Most common causes	Diagnosis	Initial management
Noninvasive fungal sinusitis	Immunocompetent patient; intractable symptoms despite adequate treatment for bacterial sinusitis; allergic rhinitis, asthma, nasal polyps. Calcifications in sinus on CT; proptosis in children	Hyaline molds; *Aspergillus* spp.; *Fusarium* spp.; dematiaceous molds; *Bipolaris* spp.; *Curvularia lunata*; *Pseudallescheria boydii*	Aspiration of sinus contents should be followed by silver impregnation staining and culture of aspirate; sinus contents often have the consistency of peanut butter or cottage cheese; in patients who have diabetes mellitus or other conditions involving immunocompromise, biopsy of healthy and diseased mucosa and bone should be considered to rule out tissue invasion	Surgery is necessary to establish drainage and to remove impacted mucus, polyps or fungus ball
Invasive fungal sinusitis	Fever, headache, epistaxis and cough in an immunocompromised patient; diabetes mellitus; hemochromatosis; protein-calorie malnutrition; leukemia; neutropenia. Nasal mucosal ulcer or eschar; calcifications in sinus on CT; orbital apex syndrome; proptosis in adults	Hyaline molds, zygomycetes; *Rhizopus oryzae*; *Cunninghamella bertholetiae*; *Aspergillus* spp.; *Fusarium* spp.; dematiaceous molds; *P. boydii*	Early endoscopic evaluation should be followed by biopsy of healthy and diseased mucosa and bone; sinus contents should be followed by silver impregnation staining culture of aspirate; if the results of endoscopic evaluation are negative, open biopsy should be performed immediately	Emergency surgery is necessary to remove necrotic and devitalized tissue; treatment with amphotericin B should be initiated on demonstration of tissue invasion and before culture results become available; immunosuppression should be reversed including discontinuation of corticosteroids and treatment of iatrogenic neutropenia

Adapted from DeShazo et al.[60]

MANAGEMENT[61]

In ABPA, the treatment of choice is a combination of systemic corticosteroids and itraconazole. Two double-blind, randomized, placebo-controlled trials have shown a benefit of adding itraconazole to corticosteroid therapy, which is the mainstay of therapy for ABPA. The mechanism of this effect is to eradicate *Aspergillus* species from the lung and diminish the antigenic stimulus for bronchial inflammation. The trials demonstrated that adding itraconazole had a significant ability to ameliorate disease, as assessed by the reduction in corticosteroid dose, increased interval between corticosteroid courses, eosinophilic inflammatory parameters and IgE concentration, as well as improvement in exercise tolerance and pulmonary function.[44,62] Itraconazole may be useful as a corticosteroid-sparing agent. Detailed therapeutic guidelines are provided by Walsh et al.[61]

For aspergillomas, the natural history is variable and therapy must be individualized. A conservative approach is prudent. Surgical resection (or where available, selective radiologic embolization of the feeding vessels) is indicated for hemoptysis. Spontaneous resolution of pulmonary aspergillomas has been reported. In patients treated with azoles resistance can emerge, which is commonly directed against multiple compounds of the azole class depending on the underlying resistance mechanism.[63]

The medical treatment options for invasive pulmonary aspergillosis are listed in Table 178.6. For neutropenic patients, the isolation of *Aspergillus* spp. from any sterile site or from respiratory specimens warrants immediate diagnostic work-up. Early initiation of antifungal therapy in patients with strongly suspected invasive aspergillosis is warranted while a diagnostic evaluation is conducted. The same is true for any sudden intracranial event in this group, especially in the presence of pulmonary infiltrates, with or without fever.[65]

Although significant experience exists with amphotericin B deoxycholate, because of significantly better survival and improved responses of initial therapy with voriconazole, primary therapy with amphotericin B deoxycholate is not recommended. At week 12, there were successful outcomes in 52.8% of the patients treated with voriconazole compared to 31.6% of those receiving amphotericin B.[66] Two issues with voriconazole must be taken into account: the occurrence of transient visual disturbances in about 30% of patients, and the considerable number of drugs showing important interactions with voriconazole, most notably drugs that are metabolized by the cytochrome p450 enzymes such as ciclosporin A. Another problem remains the intravenous administration of voriconazole in patients with renal insufficiency. As the cyclodextrin is known to accumulate in patients with kidney failure, the dose should be reduced which also reduces the exposure of the active drug. Especially in the ICU setting this restricts the use of voriconazole. In addition, evidence is accumulating that therapeutic drug monitoring is necessary to guide adequate drug exposure in the patient.

Based on the results of a randomized trial comparing two initial doses of liposomal amphotericin B (3 mg/kg per day and 10 mg/kg per day) which showed comparable efficacy with voriconazole, liposomal amphotericin B may be considered an alternative for primary therapy. The echinocandin caspofungin was investigated in a phase II trial for primary therapy of invasive aspergillosis in patients with hematologic malignancy, but the response rate was only 31%, thereby providing insufficient evidence for a recommendation for first-line therapy. Caspofungin, micafungin, liposomal amphotericin B, itraconazole and posaconazole are recommended for salvage therapy. In that setting the diagnosis should be confirmed and a change of class appears appropriate.

There is insufficient evidence to support the use of a combination of antifungal agents for primary therapy of invasive aspergillosis. A study compared the efficacy of voriconazole (31 patients) to voriconazole

Table 178.6 First- and second-line therapy for invasive aspergillosis

Generic (trade) name	Dosage	Comments
Amphotericin B deoxycholate	0.8–1.25 mg/kg iv q24h	High doses in neutropenia; significant interaction with ciclosporin
Itraconazole	Intravenous form, recently available 200 mg iv q24h; 200 mg q8h for 4 days, then 200 mg po q12h (for cerebral disease 400 mg q12h)	If patient can eat and does not take hepatic cytochrome P450-inducing co-medication; significant interaction with ciclosporin; measure itraconazole serum levels; new itraconazole cyclodextrin oral solution has better bioavailability; limited data on iv use >14 days
Voriconazole	Loading 6 mg/kg q12h, thereafter 3 mg/kg q12h or 200 mg po q12h	At least as effective as liposomal amphotericin B for empiric antifungal therapy in febrile neutropenia[64] More effective than D-AmB for invasive aspergillosis[64]
Caspofungin	70 mg iv on day 1, 50 mg iv thereafter	FDA approved for refractory aspergillosis
Lipid-formulations of amphotericin (all iv)		
Liposomal amphotericin (AmBisome)	1–5 mg/kg q24h	Less toxic than amphotericin B deoxycholate, but higher dosage needed to be equally effective
Amphotericin B colloidal dispersion (ABCD, Amphotec)	4–6 mg/kg q24h	Less toxic than amphotericin B deoxycholate, but higher dosage needed to be equally effective; expensive
Amphotericin B lipid complex (ABLC, Abelcet)	5 mg/kg q24h	Less toxic than amphotericin B but higher dosage needed to be equally effective; expensive

Adapted from Denning.[41]

and caspofungin (16 patients) in patients with invasive aspergillosis who had failed to amphotericin B therapy. Salvage therapy with the combination of voriconazole and caspofungin was associated with reduced mortality compared with therapy with voriconazole, independent of other prognostic variables.[67] However, the patients who had received voriconazole alone had been treated between 1997 and 2001, while those who received the combination had been treated between 2001 and 2004, which might bias the results due to other improvements in supportive care that could have had a positive impact on the survival of patients.

Another issue that remains unresolved is the choice of antifungal in patients who have breakthrough infection during mold-active prophylaxis. Azoles, especially posaconazole, are increasingly used to prevent invasive fungal infection in high-risk patients. There are no studies that address the optimal choice of antifungal drug although it seems appropriate to change to another drug class.

The optimal duration of therapy is unknown and dependent on the extent of invasive aspergillosis, the response to therapy and the patient's underlying disease(s) or immune status. A reasonable course would be to continue therapy to treat microfoci, after clinical and radiographic abnormalities are resolving, cultures (if they can be readily obtained) are negative, and reversible underlying predispositions have abated. Duration of therapy should be guided by clinical response and radiologic follow-up. Continuation of antifungal therapy through re-induction cancer chemotherapy, or resumption of antifungal therapy in patients with apparently resolved fungal infection who are about to receive re-induction chemotherapy, is worthy of consideration. The ultimate response of these patients to antifungal therapy is largely related to host factors, such as the resolution of neutropenia and the return of neutrophil function, lessening immunosuppression and the return of graft function from a bone marrow or organ transplant, as well as the extent of aspergillosis when diagnosed.

The administration of antifungal agents is one of the three cornerstones of treating invasive fungal infections. The other two, surgical interventions in order to reduce the fungal burden, and resolution or reduction of the immune suppression, should be considered in every patient with invasive aspergillosis.

PREVENTION

If untreated, the mortality of invasive aspergillosis reaches 100%.[41]

Preventive measures include reduction of environmental exposure of patients from sources of infection and antifungal prophylaxis. Specialized air-handling systems capable of excluding *Aspergillus* spores, such as high-efficiency particulate air (HEPA) filtration with or without laminar air flow ventilation, have proven to be very effective in reducing spore counts. However, there is evidence that 50–70% of patients acquire *Aspergillus* infection in the community and go on to develop clinical disease during admission. In those patients air-handling measures will not be effective. The alternative approach is targeted antifungal prophylaxis for hematologic patients who are at high risk for developing invasive fungal infections.

Two recent randomized studies in neutropenic patients and patients with graft-versus-host disease have shown that prophylaxis with posaconazole was more effective than fluconazole or itraconazole in preventing invasive fungal infection.[68,69] Significantly fewer patients with neutropenia in the posaconazole treatment group developed invasive aspergillosis (1% vs 7%, *p* <0.001) and survival was significantly longer among recipients of posaconazole than among recipients of fluconazole or itraconazole (*p*=0.04). In these high-risk populations prophylaxis might be a useful management strategy.

Cryptococcosis

NATURE

Cryptococcosis is a systemic infection caused by the encapsulated yeast-like fungus *Cryptococcus neoformans*. As early as 1894, Otto Busse described 'corpuscular' tumor-like lesions caused by 'coccidia species'. Since then *C. neoformans* has been known by a variety of names, including *Saccharomyces neoformans* and *Torula histolytica*.

Table 178.7 Names in current and former use in the *C. neoformans/C. gattii* species complex and with reference to the different typing nomenclatures in current use

Cryptococcus neoformans, type strain CBS 132 (teleomorph *Filobasidiella neoformans*)

Cryptococcus neoformans var. *neoformans* (serotype D). Synonyms: *Saccharomyces neoformans* and *Torula nasalis*

Cryptococcus neoformans var. *grubii* (serotype A). Synonyms: *Candida psicrophylicus* and *Saccharomyces hominis*

Intervarietal *grubii* × *neoformans* hybrids

Serotype AD hybrids. CBS 132, the type strain of *C. neoformans* var. *neoformans* is a serotype AD hybrid

Cryptococcus gattii (teleomorph *Filobasidiella bacillispora*)

No infraspecific taxa are described, but four different genotypes do occur:

- AFLP genotype 4 = serotype B (or C). Synonyms: *Cryptococcus neoformans* var. *gattii*, *Candida hondurianus*, *Torulopsis neoformans* var. *sheppei*, *Cryptococcus neoformans* var. *shanghaiensis* and *Saccharomyces subcutaneous tumefaciens*
- AFLP genotype 5 = serotype B or C. Synonym: *Cryptococcus bacillisporus*
- AFLP genotype 6 = serotype B (or C)
- AFLP genotype 7 = serotype B or C

Interspecific *gattii* × *neoformans* hybrids

Serotype BD hybrid = AFLP genotype 8
Serotype AB hybrid = AFLP genotype 9

Adapted from Bovers et al.[70]

An overview of names in current and former use in the *C. neoformans/C. gattii* species complex and the different typing nomenclatures was given by Bovers et al.[70] (Table 178.7).

Cryptococcus neoformans or *C. gattii* commonly cause pulmonary infection, which most likely starts with inhalation of infectious basidiospores, although this transmission route is not yet fully understood. Inhaled basidiospores may cause infection in mice and are more effective than yeast cells in causing cryptococcosis. Humans probably come into contact with *C. neoformans* frequently as the majority of children have been exposed to *C. neoformans* before they reach the age of 5 years,[71] and antibodies are present in adults without a history of disease. In immunocompetent individuals *C. neoformans* infection is either cleared or remains dormant. In immunocompromised individuals, however, *C. neoformans* can disseminate, most notably to the CNS causing meningoencephalitis. *Cryptococcus gattii* primarily infects otherwise healthy individuals, with exception of serotype C isolates of *C. gattii* that were found to be implicated in HIV-associated infections.[70]

EPIDEMIOLOGY

Cryptococcus neoformans var. *grubii* occurs throughout the world and causes 99% of the cryptococcal infections in persons with HIV. *Cryptococcus neoformans* var. *neoformans* also occurs worldwide, but appears to be a more common cause of infection in Europe.[70] *Cryptococcus gattii* infections have been geographically restricted to tropical and subtropical climates. However, recently an outbreak was detected in Vancouver Island (British Columbia, Canada), which has a temperate climate, with an incidence of *C. gattii* infection between 8.5 and 37 cases per million residents per year between 1999 and 2003.[72] This incidence is significantly higher than areas where *C. gattii*

is typically observed such as Australia.[72] The peak incidence of disease coincides with the flowering season of the eucalyptus tree, namely November through February.

Cryptococcal meningitis is the most common life-threatening fungal infection in people who have HIV infection. Recently the global burden of disease was estimated using published studies.[73] The incidence ranged from 0.04% to 12% per year among persons with HIV. Sub-Saharan Africa had the highest yearly burden estimate, with a median incidence of 3.2% which is equivalent to 720 000 cases (range: 144 000–1.3 million). The median incidence was lowest in Western and Central Europe and Oceania (approximately 0.1% each). Globally, approximately 957 900 cases (range: 371 700–1 544 000) of cryptococcal meningitis occur each year, resulting in 624 700 deaths by 3 months after infection.[73]

The use of novel immunosuppressive agents may also have a role in the changing frequency, spectrum and clinical presentation of opportunistic mycoses. With the declining incidence of *C. neoformans* infection in HIV-infected patients treated with HAART, organ transplant recipients have re-emerged as one of the leading groups of immunocompromised patients at risk for cryptococcal infections.[74] Cryptococcosis is the third most commonly occurring invasive fungal infection in solid-organ transplant (SOT) recipients, representing approximately 8% of invasive fungal infections.[74]

PATHOGENICITY

Cryptococcus neoformans is a facultative intracellular organism. Its pathogenicity depends upon the immune status of the host, virulence factors of the *C. neoformans* strain and the size of the inoculum.

Risk factors for cryptococcosis include (in decreasing order of frequency):
- HIV infection (especially with a low CD4$^+$ lymphocyte count);
- corticosteroid treatment;
- organ transplantation;
- chronic leukemia;
- lymphoma; and
- sarcoid, even without corticosteroid treatment.

The main fungal virulence factors consist of its:
- ability to grow at body temperature;
- polysaccharide capsule;
- production of melanin and mannitol;
- alpha mating type; and
- mannoprotein-4.[75]

The polysaccharide capsule is known to interfere with phagocytosis, antigen presentation and leukocyte migration, and it can activate immunosuppressive T lymphocytes.[76] Most clinical cryptococcal strains develop large capsules during infection.[76] The cryptococcal metabolic products melanin and mannitol can function as antioxidants that can protect the yeast against oxidative attacks of phagocytes.

The first line of host defense consists of alveolar macrophages, followed by infiltration of neutrophils and later T lymphocytes, natural killer lymphocytes and monocytes. Neutrophils can kill opsonized cryptococci *in vitro*. There is evidence that the capsular polysaccharide of *C. neoformans* plays an active role in interfering with neutrophil migration into the subarachnoid space during inflammation,[77] despite the presence of the neutrophil attractant interleukin (IL)-8 in the CSF.

However, the role of neutrophils in host defense against *C. neoformans* is not clear because patients who have severe neutropenia are not at risk of developing cryptococcosis. Experimental data have shown that functional T lymphocytes are essential in restricting cryptococcal spread. With intact T-lymphocyte function, confinement of yeasts and granuloma formation has been observed. Occasionally, *C. neoformans* can be found in granulomatous pulmonary lesions and reactivates upon decreasing host resistance and appears analogous to the primary complex in tuberculosis.

DIAGNOSTIC MICROBIOLOGY

Cryptococcus neoformans grows on routine laboratory media such as Sabouraud's agar, producing white-to-cream colored mucoid colonies, which develop within 36–72 hours. Unlike nonpathogenic cryptococci, *C. neoformans* replicates at 98.6°F (37°C). For blood cultures, the lysis–centrifugation (Isolator) method has been recommended. Because *C. neoformans* is susceptible to cycloheximide, media containing cycloheximide should not be used. A rapid test to identify *C. neoformans* is the urease test because cryptococci produce large amounts of urease in the presence of urea (as do all basidiomycetous yeasts). To distinguish *C. gattii* from *C. neoformans* var. *neoformans*, glycine-L-canavanine-bromothymol blue agar can be used.

Microscopically, *C. neoformans* can be distinguished from other yeasts by its capsule, which is visualized by an India ink preparation (Fig. 178.3). The preparation is made by mixing equal volumes of sample fluid and ink, and ideally one should be barely able to read a newspaper through the preparation. The preparation typically shows budding yeast with a double refractive wall, distinctly outlined capsule and refractive inclusions in the cytoplasm. Occasionally, short hyphal yeast forms can be seen.

The laboratory diagnosis of cryptococcosis is rather straightforward compared with that of other fungal infections (see Table 178.3).

Latex agglutination tests (or enzyme-linked immunosorbent assay, ELISA) for cryptococcal antigen in body fluids are sensitive and specific and detect all serotypes. Due to differences between various commercial kits, absolute titer values are not interchangeable. In general, however, a positive test at a dilution of greater than 1:4 is highly suggestive of cryptococcal infection. False-positive results can be caused by rheumatoid factor or (rarely) through cross-reaction with other micro-organisms such as *Trichosporon beigelii* and the bacterium *Capnocytophaga canimorsus* or contamination of the specimen with agar or agarose in the laboratory. In CSF, false-negative results can be caused by either low or high antigen titers (prozone effect, especially in patients who have AIDS) or because of immune complex formation. Pronase pre-treatment of the sample reduces both prozone reactions and rheumatoid factor interactions. Antigen testing in CSF is more sensitive than India ink preparation or culture. In patients who have pulmonary cryptococcosis without dissemination, serum samples may test negative for cryptococcal antigen. However, in these cases, *C. neoformans* antigen is likely to be positive in BAL fluid. Cryptococci are occasionally isolated from the sputum. In patients who are not immunocompromised it is safe to keep the patient under close observation

without starting treatment. In all other cases, a careful search for infection of other sites should be made (including CSF examination) and there should be a low threshold for initiating therapy.

Antibodies to *C. neoformans* have no diagnostic value and are found in healthy people as well as in those with cryptococcosis. Presumably, antibodies have a favorable prognostic value when they become positive during convalescence in patients who do not have AIDS. In pulmonary cryptococcosis, antibodies may interfere with antigen testing due to the formation of complexes, necessitating pronase pre-treatment of the samples.

CLINICAL MANIFESTATIONS

Although *C. neoformans* usually enters the body through the lungs, the main site of infection is the CNS. However, any other organ can be involved, mainly skin, bone, prostate and eye. The clinical picture of cryptococcosis in patients who have AIDS resembles that in severely immunocompromised patients who do not have HIV infection. In SOT recipients the use of calcineurin inhibitors, which is the mainstay of immunosuppression in this patient group, may affect the clinical presentation of cryptococcal disease, but appears to have no influence on the incidence.[74]

In the immunocompetent host, disease is usually more focal, with cryptococcoma formation (especially with *C. gattii*), and disease is more often confined to the lungs.[78] Although survival is higher for infection with *C. gattii*, it causes more neurologic complications, residual disease and relapses than *C. neoformans* var. *neoformans* and *grubii*.[78]

Pulmonary involvement

The clinical picture of pulmonary cryptococcosis depends upon the immune status of the host. In the immunocompetent host, one-third of patients are asymptomatic and in some cases isolation of *C. neoformans* may represent colonization. The majority of patients present with pulmonary symptoms such as cough (54%), chest pain (46%) and sputum production (32%). If the cryptococcosis is confined to the lungs, cultures and antigen titers in CSF, blood and urine can be negative.

Compared with the immunocompetent host, cryptococcosis in the immunocompromised patient who does not have HIV infection has a more rapid course with early dissemination. In SOT recipients 54% of patients had pulmonary disease. Patients receiving a calcineurin inhibitor-based regimen were less likely to have disseminated disease and more likely to have cryptococcosis limited to the lungs.[79] This is thought to be due to the anticryptococcal activity of these compounds.[79] In SOT recipients pulmonary cryptococcosis may be detected in asymptomatic patients, but may also present as acute respiratory failure, which is associated with a grave prognosis.[74]

Patients who have HIV infection and pulmonary cryptococcosis are almost invariably symptomatic, presenting with fever (84%), cough (63%), dyspnea (50%), weight loss (47%) and headache (41%). They have disseminated disease, as shown by positive cultures and antigen testing in CSF, blood and urine. Most patients have low CD4+ lymphocyte counts, often less than 100 000/ml.

Pulmonary cryptococcosis is diagnosed through antigen detection or culture of expectorated sputum, BAL, transbronchial lung biopsy (Fig. 178.4) or needle aspiration. In all cases, serum and CSF analysis for antigen and cryptococcal culture should be performed to assess dissemination.

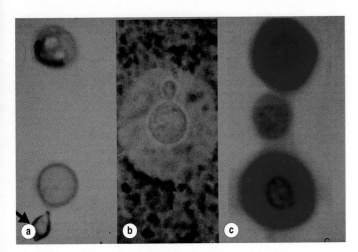

Fig. 178.3 *Cryptococcus neoformans.* (a) Cytologic preparation of CSF, (b) India ink preparation, (c) Mayer's mucicarmine stain. With permission from Jaster and Malecha. Cryptococcal meningitis, New England Journal of Medicine, Dec 1996. Copyright 1996 Massachusetts Medical Society. All rights reserved.

Central nervous system involvement

If the CNS is involved in cryptococcosis, both the brain and the meninges are usually diffusely affected. In the immunocompromised patient, cryptococcomas and focal signs of disease are rare. Approximately

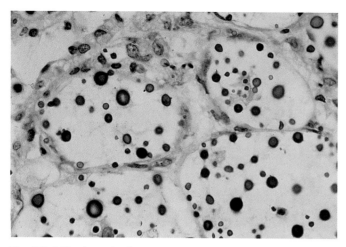

Fig. 178.4 Histology of pulmonary cryptococcosis.

70–90% of patients present with signs of subacute meningitis or meningoencephalitis: headache, fever, irritability, dizziness, memory loss, personality change, somnolence, confusion or obtundation.

Classic signs of meningitis such as nuchal rigidity are often absent. Papilledema is seen in one-third and cranial nerve palsies in one-fifth of cases. Symptoms may wax and wane over weeks to months and are often nonspecific.

Cryptococcal meningoencephalitis in immunocompromised patients who do not have HIV infection resembles the clinical picture in patients who do have HIV infection, with three exceptions:

- the duration of symptoms is usually shorter in patients who have AIDS, due to paucity of the inflammatory response and high fungal burden;
- patients who have AIDS present more often earlier in the disease with a second site of infection such as lungs, skin or blood; and
- concomitant illness such as infections (e.g. due to *Toxoplasma gondii*) or neoplasms is more likely.

Because focal neurologic symptoms due to cryptococcosis occur in only 10% of patients who have HIV infection, these symptoms should alert the physician to concomitant pathology. Patients who are successfully treated for cryptococcosis but who present with insidious mental impairment, ataxia or other neurologic signs should be evaluated for hydrocephalus by CT. Shunting is indicated for hydrocephalus.

Analysis of CSF in cryptococcal meningitis will typically yield the following findings:

- high opening pressure (reflecting raised intracranial pressure);
- CSF glucose level that may be either low or normal; and
- elevated or normal protein levels.

Usually, the CSF contains remarkably few cells with mononuclear predominance, especially in patients who have AIDS. Cryptococci can be cultured or identified directly through staining with India ink (see Diagnostic microbiology, above); cryptococcal antigen levels in CSF and serum are almost always positive. Semiquantitative CSF cultures showed baseline CSF colony-forming units to be an important prognostic factor, with a high burden associated with high mortality.[80]

Cerebral CT findings can be normal in 50% of patients who have cryptococcal meningitis, regardless of whether they have HIV infection. In patients who do not have AIDS, the CT may reveal hydrocephalus, gyral enhancement and/or multiple focal nodules with or without contrast enhancement. In patients who have AIDS, diffuse cortical atrophy is more common. Cerebral MRI appears to be more sensitive than CT in cryptococcal meningoencephalitis. The finding of pseudocysts and choroidal ependymal granulomas (cryptococcomas) is thought to be relatively specific for cryptococcosis. Lesions due to *C. neoformans* var. *gattii* tend to be fewer in number, bigger in size and

surrounded by edema as compared to those caused by *C. neoformans* var. *neoformans* and *grubii*.

Other sites of infection

About 10–15% of patients will develop skin manifestations, which can present in many forms, including papular, nodular or ulcerative lesions, or as cellulitis. In patients who do not have AIDS, skin lesions can be the sole site of infection; however, in patients who have AIDS, cryptococcal skin lesions are almost always a sign of disseminated disease. A diagnosis of cryptococcal skin disease is confirmed by biopsy.

The eye is a frequent site of infection and any part of the eye may be involved. Visual loss is a distinct threat, especially in cases of endophthalmitis, although some patients have visual loss without signs of endophthalmitis, possibly due to optic neuritis or elevated intracranial pressure. Early diagnosis and rapid treatment are essential to preserve sight.

From 5% to 10% of patients have bone lesions, which are mostly osteolytic and have to be distinguished from cold abscesses (e.g. due to tuberculosis) or neoplasms.

Many other body sites can be affected by *C. neoformans*. In men, the prostate gland is thought to serve as an extraneural reservoir and source of relapse.

MANAGEMENT[81]

In isolated pulmonary cryptococcosis and other non-CNS disease in patients who do not have HIV infection, patients can be treated according to their risk and disease severity. In the immunocompetent asymptomatic patient who has minor lesions on the chest radiograph and no extrapulmonary dissemination, careful observation or fluconazole monotherapy (200–400 mg/day for 3–6 months) is justified because many undergo spontaneous regression. Every patient who has symptomatic or disseminated disease or a compromised immune system should be treated with antifungal medication. In all cases, lumbar puncture should be performed to exclude meningeal involvement.

There is no consensus about the treatment schedule for pulmonary cryptococcosis and other non-CNS disease. For patients who have extensive lobar consolidation or mass lesions (more frequent with *C. gattii*), surgical resection of the lesions can be warranted.

All patients who have cryptococcal meningitis should be treated, regardless of their immune status, because 10–20% will either die or develop serious neurologic sequelae. For patients who have cryptococcal meningitis and AIDS, the antifungal regimen of choice is amphotericin B (0.7 mg/kg/day) plus 5-FC (100 mg/kg/day) for 2 weeks, followed by consolidation therapy with fluconazole 400 mg/day for 8–10 weeks, and subsequent lifelong maintenance therapy at 200 mg/day. This regimen has been shown to reduce the mortality from about 15% to 6% in the first 2 weeks in a double-blind, randomized, multicenter trial.[82] Combination therapy of amphotericin B and flucytosine will sterilize CSF within 2 weeks of treatment in 60–90% of patients. The addition of flucytosine to amphotericin B was independently associated with earlier CSF sterilization,[80] and 5-FC is thought to be important in preventing early relapse. In patients treated with amphotericin B and 5-FC, factors independently associated with mycologic failure at 2 weeks were high serum antigen titer and abnormal brain imaging at baseline.[83] Hematologic malignancy, abnormal neurology at baseline and prescription of 5-FC for less than 14 days were independently associated with treatment failure at 3 months.[83] Recently a randomized, open-label, phase II trial showed that amphotericin B combined with fluconazole at a dosage of 400 mg/day or 800 mg/day was safe and effective.[84] There was a trend towards better outcomes in the combination therapy arms at days 42 and 70.[84]

For consolidation therapy, it is unlikely that there is any added benefit to routine substitution of fluconazole with extended-spectrum azoles, such as itraconazole, voriconazole or posaconazole.

Itraconazole (400 mg/day) was inferior to fluconazole during the consolidation and clearance phases.

It has been shown that maintenance therapy can be safely discontinued if the CD4 cell count is ≥200 for 3 months.[85]

For patients who have cryptococcal meningitis (Table 178.8), but who do not have AIDS, the regimen of choice is less well defined. In SOT recipients the use of the lipid formulations of amphotericin B (liposomal amphotericin B at a dosage of 3–4 mg/kg/day or amphotericin B lipid complex at a dosage of 5 mg/kg/day) is favored over amphotericin B deoxycholate, because many transplant recipients receiving calcineurin inhibitors have renal function impairment and any further worsening of organ dysfunction should be avoided.[74] A total treatment duration of 4–6 weeks has been successful, but the relapse rate may be lower with longer treatment courses or azole consolidation therapy.

It is advisable to follow patients closely over the first 6–12 months because most relapses occur in the first year after treatment. In male patients who do not have AIDS, positive urine culture after prostatic massage can predict a high risk for recurrence and prolonged oral treatment is advisable in these cases.

For patients with elevated baseline opening pressure, lumbar drainage should remove enough CSF to reduce the opening pressure by 50%. Patients should initially undergo daily lumbar punctures to maintain CSF opening pressure in the normal range. When the CSF pressure is normal for several days, the procedure can be suspended. Occasionally patients who present with extremely high opening pressures (≥400 mmH$_2$O) may require a lumbar drain, especially when frequent lumbar punctures are required to or fail to control symptoms of elevated intracranial pressure. In cases where repeated lumbar punctures or use of a lumbar drain fail to control elevated pressure symptoms, or when persistent or progressive neurologic deficits are present, a ventriculoperitoneal shunt is indicated. There are no data to support the routine use of direct intraventricular therapy (e.g. via an Ommaya reservoir).

Despite wide use of triazole (and other antifungal) drugs, drug resistance has not yet been a serious concern in cryptococcal infections.

PROGNOSIS

For patients who do not have AIDS or cancer, the mortality rate due to cryptococcal infections is about 25–30%. After initial curative treatment, 20–25% of patients who do not have AIDS relapse. Among cured patients, 40% have significant neurologic deficits such as visual loss, cranial nerve palsy, motor dysfunction, personality change and decreased mental function due to chronic increased intracranial pressure or hydrocephalus. Mortality in patients after SOT is 33–49%.[74]

For patients who have AIDS, the mortality rate during initial therapy has been 10–25%, and 30–60% of patients die within 12 months. The relapse rate without maintenance treatment is 50–60%. Currently, the prognosis is mainly determined by the response to HAART. The prognosis for patients who have a malignancy is worse than for patients who have AIDS, but this probably reflects the course of the underlying disease rather than the cryptococcosis.

Adverse prognostic clinical features in patients who do not have HIV infection are listed in Table 178.9.

Immune reconstitution inflammatory syndrome

Immune reconstitution inflammatory syndrome (IRIS) has emerged as a major complication in patients with AIDS receiving HAART, with an estimated incidence of 4–16 cases per 100 person-years in AIDS-associated cryptococcosis.[86] IRIS has also been reported in SOT-related cryptococcosis, with a prevalence of 4.8%. IRIS comprises a constellation of clinical manifestations due to an inflammatory tissue response in patients experiencing improvement in cellular immunity after reduction or cessation of immunosuppressive therapy. Fungemia, an extremely low CD4 cell count, cryptococcosis as an AIDS-defining illness, lack of CSF sterilization at week 2, introduction of HAART within 1–2 months after the diagnosis of cryptococcosis, and a rapid decrease in HIV load after HAART have been recognized as risk factors for IRIS in HIV patients.[87]

There is no evidence-based treatment for IRIS but anti-inflammatory drugs may be considered for major complications related to inflammation in the CNS and other severe manifestations. It is important to distinguish IRIS from worsening of the cryptococcosis.

Table 178.8 Preferred treatment options for cryptococcal disease in HIV-negative patients

Pulmonary and other non-CNS disease

Mild-to-moderate symptoms or culture-positive specimen from this site
- Fluconazole, 200–400 mg q24h for 6–12 months
- Itraconazole, 200–400 mg q24h for 6–12 months
- Amphotericin B, 0.5–1 mg/kg q24h (total 1000–2000 mg)

Severe symptoms and immunocompromised hosts

Treat like CNS disease

CNS

Induction/consolidation: amphotericin B 0.7–1 mg/kg q24h plus flucytosine 100 mg/kg q24h for 2 weeks, then fluconazole 400 mg q24h for a minimum of 10 weeks

Amphotericin B 0.7–1 mg/kg q24h plus flucytosine 100 mg/kg q24h for 6–10 weeks

Amphotericin B 0.7–1 mg/kg q24h for 6–10 weeks

Lipid formulation of amphotericin B 3–6 mg/kg q24h for 6–10 weeks

The clinician must determine whether to follow lung therapeutic regimen or CNS (disseminated) regimen for treatment of infection in other body sites (e.g. skin). When other disseminated sites of infection are noted or the patient is at risk for disseminated infection it is important to rule out CNS disease. Duration of therapy is based on resolution of disease.
Adapted from Saag et al.[81]

Table 178.9 Adverse prognostic clinical features in cryptococcal meningitis in patients who do not have HIV infection

- Initial positive India ink examination of CSF
- High CSF opening pressure
- Low CSF glucose
- Low CSF leukocyte count (<20/µl)
- Cryptococci isolated from extraneural sites
- Initial CSF (or serum) antigen titer >32
- Corticosteroid treatment or lymphoreticular malignancy

Recurrent cryptococcal disease
- Abnormal CSF glucose concentration after ≥4 weeks of therapy
- Absence of anticryptococcal antibodies
- Post-treatment CSF (or serum) cryptococcal antigen titer of ≥8
- No decrease in antigen titers during therapy
- Daily corticosteroid treatment ≥20 mg prednisone after completion of antifungal therapy

A retrospective study of patients who had AIDS demonstrated only a prognostic value of antigen levels in the CSF, not in serum. There is substantial variability in titers with the different antigen detection kits used.

Mucormycosis and Infections by Other Zygomycetes

NATURE

Mucormycosis refers to disease caused by fungi belonging to the order Mucorales. Other names for the disease include phycomycosis and zygomycosis, the latter including diseases caused by Entomophthorales. Both Mucorales and Entomophthorales belong to the class Zygomycetes.

The major forms of zygomycosis include rhinocerebral, pulmonary, cutaneous, gastrointestinal and disseminated diseases. *Rhizopus*, *Mucor*, *Rhizomucor* and *Absidia* are the most common organisms that cause zygomycosis in humans. The taxonomy of the genus *Absidia* has recently been revised and the thermotolerant *Absidia* species have been renamed *Mycocladus* species.[88]

EPIDEMIOLOGY

Although these organisms are ubiquitous and grow in decaying organic material, mucormycosis is an uncommon disease and occurs almost exclusively in patients who have an underlying disease, with the exception of *Apophysomyces elegans*, which has been reported as a causative agent of zygomycosis, especially in immunocompetent patients. Some investigators report an increase in the prevalence of zygomycosis, which might be associated with the increased use of voriconazole that has no activity against zygomycetes.[89] A comprehensive review of 926 cases of zygomycosis, however, indicated that the increase in cases occurred before the clinical use of voriconazole, especially in bone marrow transplant recipients.[90]

Risk factors for mucormycosis are listed in Table 178.10. Diabetes mellitus and neutropenia are the most commonly encountered risk factors.

PATHOGENICITY

Infection with Mucorales usually occurs through inhalation of spores or deposition of spores in the nasal turbinates. Cutaneous mucormycosis is the primary presentation in immunocompetent patients, and results from direct inoculation of abraded skin.[93]

After pulmonary infection, the first line of defense is provided by alveolar macrophages. In animal studies, alveolar macrophages from healthy mice have been shown to inhibit germination of *Rhizopus oryzae* spores. In contrast, alveolar macrophages from corticosteroid-treated mice or diabetic mice fail to inhibit spore germination and the mice are rapidly killed by pulmonary and disseminated disease.

Table 178.10 Risk factors for mucormycosis

- Diabetes mellitus, especially with ketoacidosis
- Immunosuppression, especially corticosteroid treatment
- Iron overload with or without deferoxamine treatment (e.g. hemodialysis, hemochromatosis)
- Hematologic disease, especially neutropenia
- Intravenous drug use (CNS mucormycosis)
- Sustained skin trauma (cutaneous mucormycosis)
- Kwashiorkor (gastrointestinal mucormycosis)

From Sugar[91] and Yohai et al.[92]

Neutrophils play an important role in the second line of host defense. It is not known how diabetes mellitus or corticosteroids interfere with elimination of the fungi. Normal human serum can inhibit the growth of *Rhizopus* spp., unlike serum from patients who have diabetic ketoacidosis, which enhances fungal growth. The presence of elevated available serum iron predisposes the host to mucormycosis, and treatment with the iron chelator deferasirox (desferrioxamine) was shown to be as effective as liposomal amphotericin B in an experimental model of invasive zygomycosis.[94] Deferasirox treatment also enhanced the host inflammatory response to mucormycosis and showed synergistic interaction with liposomal amphotericin B for improving survival and reducing tissue fungal burden.[94] This opens new perspectives for the treatment of invasive zygomycosis, but the experience with deferasirox in a limited number of clinical cases is variable.

As in aspergillosis, a hallmark of mucormycosis is angioinvasion, resulting in thrombosis and tissue necrosis. The fungus has a predilection for veins over arteries.

DIAGNOSTIC MICROBIOLOGY

Mucorales grow at temperatures of 77–131°F (25–55°C) with an optimal temperature of 82.4–86°F (30°C). Clinical isolates will grow at 98.6°F (37°C) in the laboratory 2–5 days after incubation under aerobic conditions.[93] Cycloheximide inhibits their growth, so culture media containing cycloheximide should not be used. The recovery of zygomycetes in culture of clinical specimens is reduced by refrigeration of the sample, vigorous homogenization of the specimen and exposure to antifungal drugs.

On light microscopy, Mucorales have irregularly shaped, nonseptate broad (10–20 mm in diameter) hyphae with right-angle branching, visualized with hematoxylin and eosin staining, periodic acid–Schiff (PAS) reaction or Grocott–Gomori methenamine silver nitrate stains.

There are currently no biologic markers that can be detected in patients with invasive zygomycosis. Zygomycete antigens are not detected with the galactomannan and $(1,3)$-β-D-glucan assay.

CLINICAL MANIFESTATIONS

The clinical manifestations of mucormycosis can be divided into seven syndromes:

- rhinocerebral;
- pulmonary;
- cutaneous;
- gastrointestinal;
- CNS;
- disseminated; and
- miscellaneous (e.g. bones, kidney, heart or mediastinum).

The clinical manifestations depend upon the underlying disease. In patients who have diabetic ketoacidosis, rhinocerebral disease is the most common manifestation. Leukemic patients who have neutropenia are susceptible to rhinocerebral, pulmonary and disseminated disease. Children who have kwashiorkor (protein–calorie malnutrition) are especially at risk of developing gastrointestinal mucormycosis. Patients treated with deferoxamine because of iron or aluminum overload mainly present with disseminated mucormycosis.

In general, clues to the diagnosis of mucormycosis are signs of vasculitis with tissue necrosis, such as a black discharge or eschar on the skin, palate or nasal mucosa. Also, any radiographic imaging that reveals a lesion that surrounds vessels without a mass effect in an immunocompromised patient is suggestive of mucormycosis.

A biopsy with culture and microscopic evaluation is needed in order to discriminate between mucormycosis, other invasive fungal infections including aspergillosis and infection caused by Gram-negative bacteria such as *Pseudomonas* spp.

About 60% of rhinocerebral mucormycosis cases occur in diabetic patients. It is a rapidly fulminant disease, presenting with fever, nasal mucosal ulceration or necrosis, sinusitis (in 26% as an early sign), headache and facial pain or orbital involvement.

Typically, when a ketoacidotic diabetic patient who has decreased consciousness does not wake up within 24–48 hours after correction of serum glucose and electrolytes, (rhino)cerebral mucormycosis should be considered and the palate should be inspected for a black necrotic eschar resulting from extension of the disease towards the oropharynx. In rare cases, rhinocerebral disease may follow a chronic course.

The pulmonary form of mucormycosis occurs especially in severely neutropenic hematologic patients or those who have diabetes mellitus. It presents with cough, fever, chest pain and dyspnea and progresses rapidly. The diagnosis of pulmonary zygomycosis is difficult to make as the clinical presentation is very similar to that of invasive aspergillosis in patients with cancer. However, concomitant sinusitis and voriconazole prophylaxis were significantly associated with zygomycosis.[95] CT images such as masses, halo sign, air crescent sign and cavities did not discriminate between aspergillosis and zygomycosis. Only the presence of 10 or more nodules and pleural effusion on the initial CT were associated with zygomycosis.[95]

Cutaneous mucormycosis usually occurs in people who have sustained trauma (including indwelling postoperative catheters) or who have an underlying illness such as diabetes mellitus. Occasionally, cutaneous mucormycosis is a manifestation of systemic disease. Gastrointestinal mucormycosis is primarily found in patients who have extreme malnutrition. All segments of the gastrointestinal tract can be involved. The clinical symptomatology mimics an intra-abdominal abscess.

Central nervous system mucormycosis is rare and occurs most frequently as a direct extension from the nose or paranasal sinuses, or is associated with intravenous drug use. Cerebral lesions appear on CT scanning as low-density masses with variable peripheral enhancement. Gadolinium-contrast MRI can suggest cavernous sinus thrombosis and thrombosis of other vessels as indirect signs of infection, or ocular muscle involvement may be demonstrated.

MANAGEMENT

Mucormycosis is a rapidly progressive disease that warrants immediate aggressive combined surgical and medical treatment. All devitalized tissue should be removed, if necessary repeatedly, followed by reconstructive surgery in a later phase. Optimal treatment of the underlying disease is vital, including rapid correction of diabetic ketoacidosis. Intravenous lipid formulation of amphotericin B in high (initial) doses of 5 mg/kg per day is the treatment of choice. Recently, in a case series of 41 patients, it was shown that the combination of a polyene with caspofungin was more effective than amphotericin B alone for the treatment of invasive zygomycosis.[96] Patients treated with polyene–caspofungin therapy (six evaluable patients) had superior success (100% vs 45%, $p=0.02$) and Kaplan–Meier survival time ($p=0.02$), compared with patients treated with polyene monotherapy. Patients treated with amphotericin B lipid complex had inferior success (37% vs 72%, $p=0.03$) and a higher clinical failure rate (45% vs 21%, $p=0.04$), compared with patients who received other polyenes.[96]

PROGNOSIS

The prognosis of mucormycosis depends largely upon the underlying disease and in general the prognosis is better for those who have diabetes mellitus. In the review of 929 cases of invasive zygomycosis, analysis of survival by decade revealed that overall mortality improved from 84% in the 1950s to 47% in the 1990s.[90] However, mortality due to zygomycosis has remained essentially unchanged since the 1960s, when amphotericin B deoxycholate was widely introduced.

Survival was 3% for cases that were not treated, 61% for cases treated with amphotericin B deoxycholate, 57% for cases treated with surgery alone and 70% for cases treated with antifungal therapy and surgery. By multivariate analysis, infection due to *Cunninghamella* species and disseminated disease were independently associated with increased rates of death.[90] Adverse prognostic factors in rhinocerebral disease include hemiparesis or hemiplegia, bilateral infections, nondiabetic co-morbidity and extensive facial necrosis.

Gastrointestinal mucormycosis has a high mortality and is usually diagnosed at autopsy.

Penicilliosis

NATURE

Penicilliosis is caused by the fungus *Penicillium marneffei*, a dimorphic mold with yeast-like growth in tissue.

The fungus is endemic in South East Asia and was originally isolated from the bamboo rat *Rhizomys sinensis*. It causes deep-seated infections in humans and rodents.

EPIDEMIOLOGY

Before the AIDS era, most patients in endemic regions (tropical Asia, especially Thailand, north-eastern India, China, Hong Kong, Vietnam and Taiwan) affected with penicilliosis had no known underlying disease. Now, the infection mainly affects patients who have HIV infection and is recognized as an AIDS-defining opportunistic infection. In Thailand's Chiang Mai province it is the third most common HIV-related opportunistic infection (after tuberculosis and cryptococcosis).[97]

PATHOGENICITY

Penicillium marneffei is a facultative intracellular organism that can survive and replicate in macrophages. It was also shown that deficiency of CD4+ T-cell-dependent immunity contributes to the development of fatal disseminated penicilliosis in AIDS patients. Whether infection occurs as a consequence of zoonotic (animal) or sapronotic (environmental) transmission remains unknown to date.[98] The fungus can be cultured from the internal organs of four species of rodents but has also been recovered from soil specimens.

Penicillium marneffei evokes three patterns of tissue response:
- in the immunocompetent host, granuloma formation with central necrosis;
- suppurative abscesses are found in various organs; and
- in the immunocompromised host, an anergic necrotizing reaction in lung, liver and skin is seen, with diffuse infiltration of macrophages in tissues with proliferating yeast.

Antibody-mediated immunity does not seem to play a major role in host defense, although the host–fungus interaction is poorly understood.[98]

Penicilliosis affects all ages and both sexes, although 90% of the cases reported in the English literature are male.[99]

DIAGNOSTIC MICROBIOLOGY

In culture, *P. marneffei* is the only known *Penicillium* spp. that exhibits temperature-dependent dimorphic growth. The fungus grows as a mold at 77°F (25°C) and looks grayish and downy. It produces a distinctive red diffusible pigment, which is visible on agar media. At 98.6°F (37°C) it grows as a yeast on Sabouraud's glucose agar with cerebriform colonies that do not produce the red pigment.

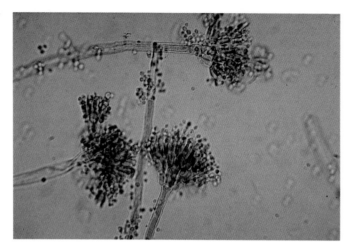

Fig. 178.5 Lactophenol cotton blue preparation of *Penicillium brevi compactum*.

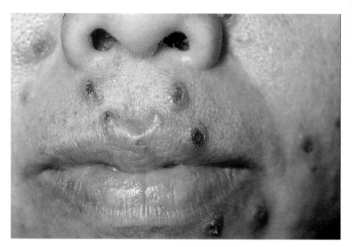

Fig. 178.6 HIV-infected patient with *Penicillium marneffei* infection with molluscum contagiosum-like lesions.

On microscopic examination (Fig. 178.5) *Penicillium* spp. appear as short, septate, branching hyphae as well as sausage-shaped cells that divide by fission instead of budding, and may show a central septum, which distinguishes it from *Histoplasma capsulatum*. *Penicillium* spp. can be identified both inside macrophages and extracellularly when tissue preparations are stained with PAS, Wright or Giemsa stain. Clinical specimens that are commonly used for microscopy and culture include bone marrow aspirate, blood, lymph node biopsies, skin biopsies, skin scrapings, sputum, BAL pellet, pleural fluid, liver biopsies, CSF, pharyngeal ulcer scrapings, palatal papule scrapings, urine, stool samples, and kidney, pericardium, stomach or intestine specimens.[98] Several nonculture-based methods have been developed and evaluated for rapid diagnosis of penicilliosis using the detection of circulating fungal antigens and fungal DNA.[98] Assays that detect *Aspergillus* galactomannan cross-react with *P. marneffei* antigen.

CLINICAL MANIFESTATIONS

In patients who are not immunocompromised, the clinical picture may strongly resemble that of tuberculosis or histoplasmosis (e.g. generalized lymphadenopathy, fever, weight loss, anemia and a nonproductive cough). In patients who have HIV infection, the disease is usually disseminated, affecting skin, reticuloendothelial system, lung and gut. Other tissues that may be involved are liver and spleen, kidney, bone, joints and pericardium. In contrast to histoplasmosis and tuberculosis, adrenal involvement and CNS infections are rare. The molluscum contagiosum-like lesions of skin and mucosa indicate disseminated disease (Fig. 178.6)[99] Most patients acquire skin lesions on the face and neck.

Chest radiographs show patchy infiltration and sometimes abscess formation. Abdominal CT scanning often demonstrates hepatomegaly or hepatosplenomegaly, but the diffuse microabscesses that cause the hepatomegaly are usually indistinguishable.

The diagnosis is made by culturing *P. marneffei* from blood, bone marrow, skin scrapings or liver biopsy specimen or by identifying the organism microscopically in a touch smear of a skin biopsy or bone marrow aspirate.

MANAGEMENT

In-vitro susceptibility testing shows that the fungus is highly susceptible to miconazole, itraconazole, ketoconazole and flucytosine, moderately susceptible to amphotericin B and the least susceptible to fluconazole.[98] Recommended treatment of penicilliosis is amphotericin B (0.5–1.0 mg/kg/day for 2 weeks), followed by itraconazole 200–400 mg/day for

6 weeks for people who do not have HIV infection, and indefinitely for patients who have HIV infection.[100] If treated appropriately, the reported response rate ranges between 59%[69] and 75%.[100]

Prevention with itraconazole in advanced HIV disease is successful, but does not provide survival benefit.

Fusariosis

Fusarium spp. are found in soil with a worldwide distribution and are important plant pathogens. Infections with *Fusarium* spp. are uncommon and are most frequently caused by *Fusarium solani* (50%) followed by *F. oxysporum* (approximately 20% of cases). In humans *Fusarium* spp. may cause a wide range of infections, including superficial (keratitis and onychomycosis), locally invasive and disseminated infections. *Fusarium* spp. may also cause allergic diseases (sinusitis) in immunocompetent individuals and mycotoxicosis in humans and animals following ingestion of food contaminated by toxin-producing *Fusarium* spp.[101] Immunocompromised patients at high risk for fusariosis are those with prolonged and profound neutropenia and/or severe T-cell immunodeficiency. Infections in these patient groups are characterized by rapid dissemination. Fusariosis may be acquired through inhalation of airborne conidia, but skin breakdown (trauma, burns, onychomycosis or cellulitis at toes and fingers) has also been shown to lead to disseminated infection. *Fusarium* spp. may also be recovered from hospital water, and water-related activities and showering appear to be a mechanism for transmission to the immunocompromised host.[102] Most patients have prolonged and severe (<100 neutrophils/ml) neutropenia. The disease mimics aspergillosis and presents with an abrupt onset of fever, often combined with sinusitis, painful ecthyma gangrenosum-like skin lesions, pulmonary involvement and myalgia.

Histopathologic tissue examination with PAS or Gomori methenamine silver staining reveals vascular invasion by hyphae with infarction and necrosis. Contrary to aspergillosis, 50–70% of cases with disseminated fusariosis have positive blood cultures.[101] This may be due to the formation of yeast-like structures during invasive infection, which might be misinterpreted as yeast infection on microscopic examination of positive blood cultures.

Fusarium spp. grow rapidly on agar media but growth is inhibited by cycloheximide. Localized infection is likely to benefit from surgical debridement, while systemic antifungal agents are required in disseminated disease. Different species may exhibit different susceptibility to antifungal agents, with *F. solani* commonly being resistant to azoles and with high MICs of amphotericin B, and *F. oxysporum* showing susceptibility to voriconazole and posaconazole.[101] High-dose amphotericin B is therefore recommended for *F. solani* and *F. verticilloides*, and high-dose amphotericin B or voriconazole for other species. Performing *in-vitro* susceptibility testing may help to guide antifungal therapy. Response rates are below 50% and depend on the underlying condition of the patient and the possibility of immune reconstitution. Successfully treated disseminated fusariosis tends to recur with repeated bone marrow suppression.

Systemic Fungi

Infections with systemic fungi are acquired by inhaling the airborne conidia (asexual spores) of dimorphic, exogenous fungi. In the lungs, these fungi convert to tissue forms that may disseminate to other internal organs as well as the skin. The etiologic agents, and consequently the prevalence and geographic distribution of their respective mycoses, tend to be restricted to certain geographic areas. The classification as systemic or endemic mycoses is not exclusive, as many opportunistic and subcutaneous mycoses often exhibit systemic clinical manifestations as well as discrete areas of endemicity.

This section will focus on four common systemic and endemic mycoses: blastomycosis, coccidioidomycosis, histoplasmosis and paracoccidioidomycosis. All are caused by dimorphic fungi. The fungi that cause coccidioidomycosis and histoplasmosis exist in nature, where they are associated with dry soil or soil mixed with guano. The agents of blastomycosis and paracoccidioidomycosis undoubtedly exist in nature, but their habitats have not been clearly defined. Inhalation of conidia of any of these fungi can lead to pulmonary infection, which may or may not be symptomatic. If symptoms are not transient, self-resolving or otherwise immediately manifested, the organism may have become dormant and entered a latent phase with the potential to produce active disease in the future. Alternatively, progressive pulmonary disease may develop with possible dissemination to other parts of the body. Except for a few extremely rare cases, these infections are not contagious, and there is scant evidence of transmission among humans or animals. Table 178.11 compares some of the epidemiologic features of these systemic mycoses.

Although most symptomatic cases of blastomycosis, coccidioidomycosis, histoplasmosis and paracoccidioidomycosis occur in patients without significant pre-existing and predisposing disease, individuals with defects of cell-mediated immunity have long been recognized to be at risk for these mycoses if they are exposed by residence or travel in the appropriate endemic areas. In recent years, these infections have increasingly emerged as opportunistic mycoses in patients with HIV/AIDS, either due to new exposure or reactivation of previously latent infections. As described earlier in this chapter, the AIDS pandemic has revealed another endemic and systemic, dimorphic, opportunistic pathogen, *Penicillium marneffei*, which is prevalent in South East Asia.

Blastomycosis, coccidioidomycosis, histoplasmosis and paracoccidioidomycosis are caused respectively by the following dimorphic fungi: *Blastomyces dermatitidis*, *Coccidioides immitis* or *Coccidioides posadasii*, *Histoplasma capsulatum* and *Paracoccidioides brasiliensis*. Each species grows as a mold in nature or the laboratory at temperatures below 98.6°F (37°C). On routine fungal culture media at 77–86°F (25–30°C), they produce mycelial colonies that vary in texture, pigment and growth rate, but may be indistinguishable from each other or many saprophytic molds. The ecology and geographic distribution of these fungi are summarized in Table 178.12. Microscopically, the hyphae are uniform in width, hyaline (not pigmented), branched, septate and similar in appearance except for the production of asexual spores or conidia, which are helpful aids to their identification. In the host, or under the appropriate growth conditions *in vitro*, they convert to a distinctive form of growth that is found in tissue: *B. dermatitidis*, *H. capsulatum* and *P. brasiliensis* produce characteristic budding yeast cells, and *C. immitis* and *C. posadasii* produce spherules.

Genetic and molecular research on these fungi in recent years has identified specific genes and signal transduction pathways that trigger host recognition and morphogenetic conversion, which are essential for their pathogenicity.[104] Molecular phylogenetic studies have determined that these pathogenic fungi are closely related and classified within the same family of the Phylum Ascomycota. All four of these infections begin in the lungs and Chapter 31 provides detailed descriptions of pulmonary blastomycosis, coccidioidomycosis, histoplasmosis and paracoccidioidomycosis.

Table 178.11 Epidemiologic features of fungal infections

Feature	Blastomycosis	Coccidioidomycosis	Histoplasmosis	Paracoccidioidomycosis
Geographic areas of high endemicity	Yes	Yes	Yes	Yes
Saprophytic form (<95°F): hyaline, septate hyphae	Yes	Yes	Yes	Yes
Predominant tissue forms	Yeasts	Spherules	Yeasts	Yeasts
High infection rate in endemic areas	?	Yes	Yes	Yes
At least 90% of infections are initiated by inhalation	Yes	Yes	Yes	Yes
Approximate percentage of infections that are asymptomatic	?	≥60	>95	>95
At least 90% of infections are self-limited	?	Yes	Yes	Yes
Approximate percentage of immunocompetent patients	>90	>90	>90	>90
Approximate percentage of males among patients with disease	50–90	75–90	80–90	95
Relative frequency of disease among AIDS patients in the endemic areas	Rare	Common	Common	Infrequent

From Larone et al.[103]

Table 178.12 Summary of systemic mycoses

Mycosis	Etiology	Ecology	Geographic distribution	Mycelial form*	Tissue form
Blastomycosis	*Blastomyces dermatitidis*	Unknown (riverbanks?)	Endemic along Mississippi, Ohio and St Lawrence River valleys and south-eastern USA	Slow to moderate growth rate. Colonies are white to tan, flat, velvety or cottony. Hyaline septate hyphae and short conidiophores bearing single globose to pyriform conidia, 2–10 μm	Thick-walled yeasts with broad-based, usually single, buds, 8–15 μm
Coccidioidomycosis	*Coccidioides immitis* and *C. posadasii*	Soil	Semiarid regions of south-western USA, Mexico, Central and South America	Moderate to rapid growth rate. Colonies are white to brown, flat to wooly. Hyaline septate hyphae and arthroconidia, 3 × 6 μm	Spherules, 10–80 μm or larger, containing endospores, 2–4 μm
Histoplasmosis	*Histoplasma capsulatum* var. *capsulatum* and *H. capsulatum* var. *duboisii*	Bat and avian habitats (guano); alkaline soil	Global; endemic in Ohio, Missouri and Mississippi River valleys, central Africa (var. *duboisii*)	Slow growth rate. Colonies are white to brown, flat to wooly. Hyaline septate hyphae and arthroconidia, 3 × 6 μm	Oval yeasts, 2 × 4 μm, intracellular in macrophages
Paracoccidioidomycosis	*Paracoccidioides brasiliensis*	Unknown (soil?)	Central and South America	Slow growth rate. Colonies are flat to velvety, white to brown. Hyaline septate hyphae and rare globose conidia and chlamydospores	Large, multiple budding yeasts, 15–30 μm or larger

*Colony descriptions are for typical isolates grown at 77°F (25°C) on Sabouraud's glucose agar.

Blastomycosis

Blastomycosis is a chronic infection characterized by granulomatous and suppurative lesions, but the clinical manifestations may be protean. Following inhalation of airborne conidia, dissemination may occur to any organ, but preferentially to the skin and bones. Although the prevalence of blastomycosis is greatest on the North American continent, autochthonous cases have been documented in Africa, South America and Asia. It is endemic for humans and dogs in the eastern United States and south-eastern Canada. Early histopathologic evidence confirmed that both cutaneous and systemic manifestations originated in the lung; however, the respiratory episode may be completely asymptomatic.

MYCOLOGY

At temperatures below 95°F (35°C), *B. dermatitidis* grows as a mold, producing a colony of uniform, hyaline, septate hyphae and conidia. Isolates vary in their rate of growth, colony appearance, and degree and type of conidiation. Many strains produce a white, cottony mycelium that becomes tan to brown with age (Table 178.13). On enriched media at 98.6°F (37°C), *B. dermatitidis* converts to growth in the yeast form and produces colonies that are folded, pasty and moist.

The mycelia produce abundant conidia from short lateral conidiophores on the aerial hyphae. The conidia are spherical, ovoid or pyriform in shape, smooth walled and up to 10 μm in diameter. Because the colony and conidia of *B. dermatitidis* may be confused with many other fungi, identification must be confirmed by conversion to the characteristic yeast form. This conversion can be accomplished by *in-vitro* cultivation on rich medium (e.g. brain–heart infusion, chocolate agar or Kelly's medium) at 98.6°F (37°C). Under these conditions

Table 178.13 Species-specific exoantigens* for the identification of systemic dimorphic fungal pathogens

Fungus	Exoantigens
Coccidioides immitis	HS, F, HL
Histoplasma capsulatum	h, m
Blastomyces dermatitidis	A
Paracoccidioides brasiliensis	1, 2, 3

*Exoantigens are detected by precipitin lines of identity in immunodiffusion tests of concentrated culture supernatant fluids versus reference antigens and antisera.

or in tissue, *B. dermatitidis* grows as a thick-walled spherical yeast that usually produces single buds (Fig. 178.7). The bud and parent yeast have a characteristically wide base of attachment and the bud often enlarges to a size equal to that of the parent cell before they separate. Yeast cells are multinucleated and normally range in size from 8 μm to 15 μm, although some cells reach a diameter of 30 μm.

The sexual or teleomorphic form is *Ajellomyces dermatitidis*. Sexual reproduction may be stimulated *in vitro* with appropriate tester mating strains, but patients are only infected with haploid strains of one mating type, which reproduce asexually.

ECOLOGY AND EPIDEMIOLOGY

The natural habitat of *B. dermatitidis* has not been resolved. Over the years, *B. dermatitidis* has been isolated, but never repeatedly, from soil samples collected in rural environments, including a chicken house, a

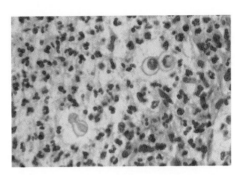

Fig. 178.7 *Blastomyces dermatitidis*, yeast form in hematoxylin- and eosin-stained section of microabscess from a cutaneous lesion. This shows large spherical yeasts characterized by thick, highly refractile cell walls, single budding and a broad attachment between the parent yeast cell and bud.

cattle crossing and several river banks. Positive samples were collected in Wisconsin from a beaver dam associated with a large outbreak of blastomycosis and from a fishing site involved in another outbreak. Several clusters of cases, with or without recovery of *B. dermatitidis* from environmental samples, have implicated river banks, fresh water and soil.[105]

Dogs are commonly infected and there are numerous reports of isolated cases in other animal species, but there is no evidence that an animal reservoir perpetuates *B. dermatitidis*. It probably resides in nature in a protected and dormant condition during most of the year, until it is stimulated by a suitable climatic or other specific but transient event to propagate and produce conidia that become airborne and infectious.

Because *B. dermatitidis* is not readily recoverable from nature and an adequate skin test antigen is not available for conducting population surveys of exposure, the geographic distribution of blastomycosis has been estimated from reports of human and canine cases. The endemic area extends broadly eastward from states that border the Mississippi River. Blastomycosis is endemic in southern Canada east of Manitoba and, in the USA, in Illinois, Wisconsin, Minnesota, Ohio, the Atlantic Coastal states, and the south-eastern states with the exception of Florida. Blastomycosis is rare in the New England and western states. The highest incidence occurs in Arkansas, Kentucky, Illinois, Louisiana, Mississippi, North Carolina, Tennessee and Wisconsin. Within these areas, local pockets of high endemicity have been identified. Canine cases exhibit the same endemic pattern as those of humans. Indeed, blastomycosis may occur more frequently in dogs than in humans. Clinical reports have also documented autochthonous cases in both northern and southern Africa, as well as India, Israel, Mexico and Venezuela. Reports of the infection occurring elsewhere are dubious because the diagnosis was questionable or the patients had a history of travel to an endemic area.

The data from large clinical reviews indicate that blastomycosis occurs more frequently during middle age and in males. Although the disease can occur at any age, 60% of patients were between the ages of 30 and 60 years. Among the hundreds of cases compiled in several reviews, less than 4% of the patients were under 20 years of age and blastomycosis was rarely reported in children. However, in more recent studies, especially involving outbreaks, blastomycosis occurred equally in both sexes and two-thirds of the patients associated with outbreaks have been children (<16 years old).[105]

The male to female ratios reported in several surveys involving hundreds of patients vary from 6:1 to 15:1, but lower ratios have been reported in smaller studies and the overall sex ratio of outbreak cases is approximately 1. Perhaps both sexes are equally susceptible to acute blastomycosis, but males are more inclined to develop chronic or disseminated disease. The other systemic mycoses also occur more often in males (Table 178.14), and male animals are more suscep-

tible (or less resistant) than females to challenge with *B. dermatitidis*. Blastomycosis may be similar to histoplasmosis in that children are equally susceptible to infection and disease, but the sex-related differences are manifested after puberty.

Genetic or racial differences in prevalence have not been confirmed. Socioeconomic and occupational data have associated blastomycosis with poverty, malnutrition, manual labor, agriculture, construction work and exposure to dust and wood. The incidence of blastomycosis among immunocompromised patients, including patients with AIDS, is comparatively lower than that observed with other systemic mycoses.

PATHOGENICITY

Evidence has linked experimental virulence of strains of *B. dermatitidis* with the amount of α-1,3-glucan in the cell walls. This polysaccharide has been shown to vary in strains of *H. capsulatum* and *P. brasiliensis* that differ in virulence.[109] However, the best characterized virulence factor is BAD1, a cell wall adhesin and immunodominant antigen. This protein contains multiple copies of a 25-amino acid tandem repeat, which binds to CR3 complement receptors and elicits both antibodies and cell-mediated immune responses.[110,111] Compared with less virulent mutants, the wild type contains less surface-bound BAD1. Although the mechanisms whereby BAD1, as well as α-1,3-glucan, contribute to virulence have not been fully elucidated, Klein and associates have postulated that shedding of BAD1 by virulent strains may neutralize macrophage defenses by occupying receptors, diminishing their ability to bind yeast cells.[111] In the alveoli, *B. dermatitidis* induces an inflammatory response characterized by the infiltration of both macrophages and neutrophils and leading to the subsequent formation of granulomata. Both conidia and yeast cells are susceptible to the killing mechanisms of neutrophils and macrophages.[110,111]

If the pathogenesis of blastomycosis resembles that of histoplasmosis and coccidioidomycosis, most infections may be subclinical and resolve spontaneously. However, because specific and sensitive skin test antigens are lacking, the extent of exposure to *B. dermatitidis* in the general population has not been determined. In addition, calcification is uncommon and there is little radiologic or histopathologic evidence of residual blastomycotic lesions. The best evidence for the existence of subclinical blastomycosis derives from the reported outbreaks, where specific serologic and skin test reactions documented exposure to *B. dermatitidis* in the absence of symptoms.[105]

PREVENTION

There are no clear guidelines for the prevention of blastomycosis. However, the BAD1 antigen may be an excellent vaccine candidate for future study.[112]

DIAGNOSTIC MICROBIOLOGY

Microscopic examination

Blastomycosis is best diagnosed by direct examination or positive culture of sputa, skin lesions or other specimens. In calcofluor white or KOH preparations of pus, exudate, sputum, BAL fluid or other specimens, a diagnosis can be established detecting the characteristic yeast cells of *B. dermatitidis* (see Table 178.12 and description above). In tissue stained with hematoxylin and eosin, the yeast cytoplasm stains darkly and the cell wall appears colorless (Fig. 178.7). The multinucleated yeast cells are often abundant in cutaneous lesions. If the yeasts are sparse, fungal cell wall stains, such as PAS or methenamine silver, are helpful.

Table 178.14 Summary of serologic tests for antibodies to systemic dimorphic fungal pathogens in patients without AIDS

Mycosis	Test	Antigen	Diagnosis	Prognosis	Limitation/specificity
			SENSITIVITY AND VALUE		
Blastomycosis	CF	By	Less than 50% of cases positive; reaction to homologous antigen only is diagnostic	Fourfold change in titer	Highly cross-reactive
	ID	Bcf	Up to 80% of cases positive, i.e. A band	Loss of A band	More specific than CF test
	EIA	A	Up to 90% of cases positive (titer ≥1:16)	Change in titer	92% specificity
Coccidioidomycosis	TP	C	Early primary infection; 90% cases positive	None	None
	CF	C	Titer ≥1:32 5 secondary disease	Titer reflects severity (except in meningeal disease)	Rarely cross-reactive with H
	ID	C	More than 90% cases positive, i.e. F and/or HL band		More specific than CF test
Histoplasmosis	CF	H	Up to 83% of cases positive (titer ≥1:8)	Fourfold change in titer	Cross-reactions in patients with blastomycosis, coccidioidomycosis, cryptococcosis, aspergillosis; titer may be boosted by skin test with H
		Y	Up to 94% of cases positive (titer ≥1:8)	Fourfold change in titer	Less cross-reactivity than with H
	ID	H(10X)	Up to 85% of cases positive, i.e. m or m and h bands	Loss of h	Skin test with H may boost m band; more specific than CF test
Paracoccidioidomycosis	CF	P	80–95% of cases positive (titer ≥1:8)	Fourfold change in titer	Some cross-reactions at low titer with aspergillosis and candidiasis sera
	ID	P	98% of cases positive (bands 1, 2 and/or 3)	Loss of bands	Band 3 and band m (to H) are identical

A, antigen A of *B. dermatitidis*; Bcf, culture filtrate of *B. dermatitidis* yeast phase; By, yeast phase of *B. dermatitidis*; C, coccidioidin; CF, complement fixation; EIA, enzyme immunoassay; H, histoplasmin; ID, immunodiffusion; P, culture filtrate of *P. brasiliensis* yeast phase; TP, tube precipitin; Y, yeast phase of *H. capsulatum*.[106–108]

Culture

On most routine culture media, *B. dermatitidis* produces a mold with variable macroscopic features and conidia. Cultures should be incubated at 86°F (30°C) or room temperature for at least 4 weeks. Their identification is confirmed by growth on a rich medium at 98.6°F (37°C) and conversion to the characteristic yeast form. Alternatively, the identity of a culture may be established by an immunodiffusion test to detect a *B. dermatitidis*-specific antigen (antigen A). As indicated in Table 178.13, the technique has also been expanded to identify other dimorphic pathogens. In addition, DNA probes are commercially available to identify cultures of *B. dermatitidis*, as well as other agents of systemic mycoses.[113]

Serology

Since the tests for complement fixing antibodies and delayed-type skin reactivity lack specificity and sensitivity, they are not helpful unless the patient is negative to heterologous fungal antigens; even then, positive, monospecific serologic tests to *B. dermatitidis* may not indicate active infection. Serologic tests for antibodies to the specific antigen

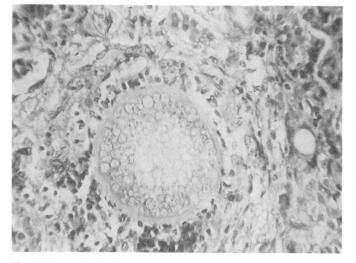

Fig. 178.8 *Coccidioides immitis*, spherule in hematoxylin- and eosin-stained section of lung lesion. This shows refractile cell wall and internal endospores.

A, which can be detected by the immunodiffusion test or an enzyme immunoassay (EIA), are more suggestive of infection, but negative tests do not exclude blastomycosis. Table 178.14 summarizes the conventional serologic tests for antibodies to *B. dermatitidis* and other systemic fungi. The most useful serologic procedure is an EIA for antibodies to antigen A, and EIA titers reflected the severity of disease (see Table 178.14). False-positive results may occur with sera from patients with histoplasmosis

CLINICAL MANIFESTATIONS

Two classic forms of blastomycosis are recognized: pulmonary, often with dissemination, and chronic cutaneous blastomycosis. A wide variety of symptoms, pathology and radiographic appearances may be observed in blastomycosis. The most common symptoms include cough, weight loss, chest pain, skin lesions, fever, hemoptysis and localized swelling. After the lung, the most frequently involved organs are the skin, bones and genitourinary tract, followed by the central nervous system, liver or spleen.

Primary pulmonary blastomycosis may be asymptomatic or present as acute or subacute pneumonia, ranging from mild to severe (see Chapter 31 for a detailed clinical description). In chronic cutaneous blastomycosis, lesions initially occur as one or more subcutaneous nodules that eventually ulcerate. Lesions are more common on exposed skin surfaces, such as the face or extremities. Spread may occur by extension to contiguous areas and require weeks or months for the ulcerative process to evolve. If untreated, elevated granulomatous lesions with advancing borders will develop. The yeast cells can be observed in microabscesses near the dermis. Extensive, often verrucous, epithelial hyperplasia overlying the abscesses may develop and resemble carcinoma. These extensive cutaneous lesions are characteristically discolored and crusty, and tend to heal and scar in the central, older areas. The active microabscesses found at the leading edge of the lesion can be aspirated or biopsied, and the typical yeast cells of *B. dermatitidis* can be observed on direct microscopic examination.

Dissemination may be widespread and unpredictable in blastomycosis and include the genitourinary tract, CNS and spleen, as well as the skin and bones. Less frequently, the liver, lymph nodes, heart and other viscera are infected. The progressive systemic form of blastomycosis develops in patients with unresolving pulmonary infection, but the degree of pulmonary involvement is not related to the extent of dissemination. This infection may be chronic, with few organisms present, or multiple pulmonary foci may be demonstrable at the time generalized systemic disease develops.

In fulminant cases, the dermal lesions may be more severe than those of chronic cutaneous blastomycosis and are seen in about 75% of cases. Overall, skeletal involvement occurs in approximately a third of patients. Osteomyelitis and, in some cases, draining sinuses to the skin develop, and should be examined for the presence of characteristic yeast cells. Because of the frequency of bone involvement and because almost any bone can be affected, whenever blastomycosis is diagnosed a complete radiographic examination is advisable. Arthritis may develop by extension from infected bone or by direct dissemination from the lung without bone infection. In up to 22% of patients the urogenital tract is involved, especially the prostate, male genitalia, kidney and adrenals. Metastasis to the CNS, resulting in meningitis or brain abscess, occurs in up to 10% of patients.

Primary cutaneous blastomycosis is initiated by traumatic autoinoculation or contamination of an open wound with infectious material. The lymphatics and regional lymph nodes are involved, but the infection remains localized and often resolves without treatment. The natural history and pathology are similar to subcutaneous mycoses (see Chapter 179) and systemic dissemination is rare in the immunocompetent host.

There are well-documented series of patients with HIV/AIDS and blastomycosis. However, the incidence of blastomycosis in HIV-positive patients is not as high as co-infection with other endemic

mycoses. Because of the presumed rural reservoir of *B. dermatitidis* or its low census in nature, patients with AIDS may be exposed less often than similar patients in the endemic areas for coccidioidomycosis or histoplasmosis. Alternatively, the host defenses against *B. dermatitidis* may be less dependent upon cell-mediated immunity. Cases of blastomycosis and AIDS have presented with acute miliary pneumonia and a relatively higher frequency of CNS disease. The management of blastomycosis in immunocompromised patients is more difficult and the prognosis is worse.

MANAGEMENT

As demonstrated by several outbreak cases, primary blastomycosis in immunocompetent individuals may not require therapy (see Chapter 31). Patients with protracted, severe or progressive primary infection, chronic pulmonary or disseminated blastomycosis require treatment. Depending on the manifestations of disease and the integrity of the underlying host defenses, chemotherapeutic success rates with amphotericin B, ketoconazole or itraconazole currently vary between 70% and 95%. Mortality is higher in patients with AIDS and other immunocompromising conditions. Recent guidelines recommend itraconazole for mild to moderate disease, and a lipid formulation of amphotericin B (AMB) followed by itraconazole for more severe forms.[114]

Fluconazole can be an effective alternative for the treatment of non-life-threatening cases of blastomycosis, especially in patients who may not have responded to another drug. Its only advantage over itraconazole may be in patients with involvement of the CNS, which is penetrated well by fluconazole.

Blastomyces dermatitidis is quite susceptible to amphotericin B, which is the recommended treatment for patients with life-threatening or severe disease (e.g. involvement of multiple organs), those with meningitis, or blastomycosis in immunocompromised patients, as well as patients who do not respond to an azole.[114]

The protocol for administration of conventional amphotericin B or a lipid formulation and monitoring renal function are the same as its application for other mycoses. Most patients experience adverse side-effects, including renal dysfunction, fever, anorexia, phlebitis, hypokalemia, nausea, chills, headache and anemia.

Lipid emulsions of amphotericin B have the advantage of delivering higher doses with diminished toxicity. Adult respiratory distress syndrome due to overwhelming pulmonary blastomycosis requires aggressive treatment. Blastomycosis in patients with AIDS may require suppressive therapy following the initial course of treatment with amphotericin B, similar to the management of cryptococcosis and histoplasmosis in patients with AIDS. Suppressive treatment in AIDS patients would be daily itraconazole or possibly fluconazole for CNS disease.[114]

In addition, voriconazole appears to be effective. In a retrospective review of 24 patients with endemic mycoses who were treated with voriconazole (often as salvage cases), 20 patients showed improvement or stabilization of their disease after 2 months and at subsequent follow-up.[115]

Corrective surgery may be necessary as an adjunct to antibiotic treatment. Because of the occurrence of relapse or reactivation blastomycosis, patients should be observed for years after treatment and resolution of disease.

Coccidioidomycosis

Coccidioidomycosis is caused by either of two phenotypically indistinguishable species, *Coccidioides immitis* or *Coccidioides posadasii*, dimorphic fungi that normally live in well-defined geographic areas. Both the agents and coccidioidomycosis are almost entirely limited to these endemic regions. It was recognized quite early that coccidioidomycosis is confined to the south-western USA, contiguous regions of northern Mexico and specific areas of Central and South America. The natural reservoir was established by isolating *Coccidioides* species from soil samples collected throughout the endemic areas, and the environmental conditions under which the fungus was propagated have been described. From mycelial culture filtrates, the skin test antigen coccidioidin was developed to detect exposure to *C. immitis* or *C. posadasii* and used to conduct population surveys of skin reactivity. The more common primary form is a mild respiratory ailment, also called valley fever or San Joaquin Valley fever.

MYCOLOGY

Coccidioides posadasii was described by Fisher *et al.*[116] They compared the genotypes of isolates of '*C. immitis*' from different geographic regions and, based on their phylogenetic analyses of these populations, determined that the majority of isolates outside California belong to a different species, which they named *C. posadasii* to honor Dr Posadas who described the first case. Although the two species differ in their geographic distribution and genotype, differences in their phenotypes or pathogenicity have yet to be delineated. Because they cannot be distinguished by simple laboratory tests, the more familiar name, *C. immitis*, will be used here.

The life cycle of *C. immitis* (or *C. posadasii*) encompasses several distinct morphologic structures that are produced under different conditions. In nature and in the laboratory, either species grows as a mold, producing hyaline, branching, septate hyphae. As the culture ages, characteristic arthroconidia are formed, usually, but not invariably, in alternate hyphal cells. With time, the arthroconidial chains fragment to release the unicellular, barrel-shaped arthroconidia, which are approximately 3 μm × 6 μm in size, easily airborne and small enough to be inhaled into the alveoli. They are highly resistant to desiccation, temperature extremes and deprivation of nutrients, and may remain viable for years. Under appropriate growth conditions the arthroconidia will germinate to recycle the saprophytic mycelial form.

Following their inhalation, the arthroconidia become spherical. In the infected host, *C. immitis* exists as spherules (spherical thick-walled structures, 15–80 μm in diameter) that are filled with a few to several hundred endospores (see Fig. 178.8). As a spherule enlarges, the nuclei undergo mitosis, the cytoplasm condenses around these nuclei and a cell wall forms around each developing endospore. At maturation, the spherule ruptures to release its endospores (2–5 μm in size), which may enlarge to form mature spherules. Hyphae as well as spherules may be observed in the tissues and sputum of patients with coccidioidal cavities of the lungs.

On routine mycologic media, such as inhibitory mold or Sabouraud's agar, at the usual incubation temperature of 77–86°F (25–30°C), different isolates of *C. immitis* produce a wide variety of colony types. Because numerous infectious arthroconidia are produced in culture and can be readily aerosolized in the dry state, cultures should be examined only under a safety cabinet that protects both the laboratory worker and the environment. Spherules can be produced in the laboratory on a complex medium at 104°F (40°C) under 20% CO_2.

ECOLOGY AND EPIDEMIOLOGY

In the USA, the geographic areas endemic for coccidioidomycosis and from which *C. immitis* can be isolated from the environment correspond to the Lower Sonoran life zone. These areas are characterized by a semiarid climate, alkaline soil and characteristic indigenous desert plants and rodents. The endemic foci in Mexico, Argentina and other areas of Central and South America are associated with ecologically similar environments. The mycelia, which can be found several inches beneath the soil surface, can be recovered at the surface after the spring rains. As the weather becomes hot and dry, the mycelia convert to infectious arthroconidia, accounting for the peak infection rate during the summer. In the endemic areas, natural infections also occur among indigenous fauna, such as desert rodents, dogs and cattle.

Inhalation of the arthroconidia of *C. immitis* leads to infection and acquisition of a positive delayed-type hypersensitivity response to coccidioidin. More than half of these infections are benign and most of the others are symptomatic but self-limited (see Table 178.11). Approximately 1% of these cases will develop progressive pulmonary disease, dissemination, or both. Some individuals have an increased risk of developing disseminated disease following primary infection (Table 178.15). These include persons in certain ethnic groups: Filipinos, African-Americans, Latin Americans and Native Americans. This ethnic predilection for severe disease clearly indicates the importance of the genetic background of the host in mounting an effective immune response to infection.

In addition to ethnicity, males, women in the third trimester of pregnancy, persons with a cellular immunodeficiency (including AIDS) and individuals at the extremes of age are more susceptible to severe disease (Table 178.15). In addition, risks for severe pulmonary disease include diabetes, cigarette smoking, low income and old age.

The areas of endemicity defined by case reports and by isolation of *C. immitis* from soil have been confirmed by skin test surveys with coccidioidin. Within the endemic areas, which include portions of the south-western USA (California, Arizona, New Mexico, Nevada, Utah and Texas) and north-western Mexico, the percent reactivity varies; some of the highest rates are found in Phoenix and Tucson, Arizona, and Kern County, California. Isolated cases of coccidioidomycosis occurring outside the established areas of endemicity have been attributed to fomite transmission of the arthroconidia or to patient travel through the endemic area.

Numerous outbreaks of primary infection have been reported among individuals simultaneously exposed to a heavy aerosol of arthroconidia. Coccidioidomycosis is therefore an occupational hazard for construction workers, archeology students and others who disrupt the soil in the endemic areas.

PATHOGENICITY

In vivo, potent cell wall antigens are released when the arthroconidia develop into spherules. Although arthroconidia and endospores are readily engulfed by alveolar macrophages, killing is enhanced by activation of macrophages with the appropriate T cells or cytokines.[117] When stimulated by spherules, leukocytes from both patients and skin test-positive subjects secrete potentially protective cytokines, such as interferon gamma (IFN-γ) and IL-12.

Table 178.15 Risk factors for disseminated coccidioidomycosis

Age	Infants and elderly
Sex	Male
Genetics	Filipino > African-American > Native American > Hispanic > Asian
Serum CF antibody titer	>1:32
Pregnancy	Late pregnancy and postpartum
Delayed-type hypersensitivity skin test	Negative
Depressed cell-mediated immunity	Malignancy, chemotherapy, steroid treatment, HIV infection

Investigators have identified several potential virulence factors. For example, *C. immitis* produces a serine proteinase with broad specificity for host substrates, such as elastin, collagen, IgG and IgA. Other proteinases have also been detected and are thought to contribute to the development of spherules and release of endospores.[117]

Many of the patients who develop disseminated coccidioidomycosis have depressed cell-mediated immunity. There is a marked inverse relationship between the antibody titer (see below) and specific cell-mediated immunity, as measured by skin test and, *in vitro*, by the numbers of CD4[+] and CD8[+] T lymphocytes, the responsiveness of T cells to mitogens or antigens, and the production of cytokines. In severe coccidioidomycosis, patients have elevated antibody titers, circulating immune complexes and depressed cellular immunity. This condition has been related to increased antigen burden, populations of suppressor cells, immune complexes and impaired lymphocyte circulation. Immune complexes are detected in serum of patients with coccidioidomycosis and correlate with the severity of disease.

In the mouse model of experimental coccidioidomycosis, specific anergy is correlated with the amount of coccidioidal antigen present. Recovery often leads to restoration of immune functions. However, the impaired cellular immune responses are likely governed by whether T-helper 1 (Th1) or Th2 responses predominate early in infection.[117] In strains of mice that differ in susceptibility to *C. immitis*, protective responses are correlated with the secretion of IFN-γ, which is a Th1-associated cytokine and potent activator of macrophages. Conversely, much of the immunopathology may be attributable to excess production of tumor necrosis factor (TNF). Perhaps the genetic predisposition to disseminated coccidioidomycosis (see Table 178.15) is related to genetic control of the T-cell response to *C. immitis*.

PREVENTION

Coccidioides immitis cannot be eliminated from the soil, but public health efforts to reduce the dust associated with dispersion of the arthroconidia are helpful in areas of high endemicity. Another approach has focused on the development of a vaccine for persons at risk. In mice and humans, cell-mediated immunity to *C. immitis* confers excellent protection against disease. Spherule-derived vaccines in the past were not successful, but several new approaches to identify specific candidate epitopes are currently under investigation.[117]

DIAGNOSTIC MICROBIOLOGY

Microscopic examination

A definitive diagnosis of coccidioidomycosis requires the finding of spherules of *C. immitis* in sputum, draining sinuses or tissue specimens (see Fig. 178.8). Clinical exudates should be examined directly in 10% or 20% KOH, with or without calcofluor white, and tissue obtained from biopsy can be stained with hematoxylin and eosin or special fungal stains, such as Gomori methenamine silver or the PAS stain, which stain fungal cell walls black or reddish, respectively. Direct microscopic examination of cutaneous or deep tissue specimens, either in calcofluor/KOH preparations or histologic sections, yields positive results in approximately 85% of proved cases. However, sputum specimens are positive by direct examination or culture in less than half of the cases.

Culture

Clinical specimens are cultured on inhibitory mold, Sabouraud's agar or other routine fungal medium. Colonies of *C. immitis* develop within 1 or 2 weeks and are examined for the production of characteristic arthroconidia. Microscopic preparations of mycelia should always be prepared under a biosafety hood. The identification of *C. immitis* can be readily confirmed by demonstrating the production of exoantigen F (see Table 178.13). Alternatively, DNA-based identification is available with commercial kits.

With the exception of tissue scrapings, biopsies and surgical specimens, cultures are more often positive than microscopic examinations of clinical material. However, use of both procedures will optimize the opportunity to establish a diagnosis. Between 25% and 50% of sputa, bronchial washes, spinal fluids and urine specimens yield positive cultures. Positive blood cultures are infrequent but significantly associated with acute, disseminated coccidioidomycosis and a poor prognosis.

Skin tests

As noted above, coccidioidin, a standardized toluene extract of mycelial culture filtrate, is used for skin testing, and a positive test for delayed-type hypersensitivity is denoted by induration exceeding 5 mm in diameter. Another *C. immitis* antigen, prepared from cultured spherules and termed spherulin, is more sensitive but less specific than coccidioidin. Skin testing with either antigen does not induce or boost an immune response. The skin test becomes positive within 2 weeks after the onset of symptoms and before the appearance of antibodies and often remains positive indefinitely. A positive reaction has no diagnostic significance without a history of conversion, but a negative test can be used to exclude coccidioidomycosis, except in patients with severe disseminated coccidioidomycosis who may have become anergic. Indeed, a negative skin test in confirmed cases is associated with a grave prognosis. Conversely, a positive skin test in healthy subjects implies immunity to symptomatic reinfection.

Serology

As indicated in Table 178.14, tube precipitins or latex agglutinins measure specific IgM antibodies. They assist in the diagnosis of primary infections because these antibodies are detected in 90% of patients within 2 weeks after the appearance of symptoms and disappear in most cases by 4 months.

The CF test, which measures IgG antibodies to coccidioidin, is a useful diagnostic and prognostic tool. The CF titer correlates with the severity of disease. Most patients with secondary coccidioidomycosis develop a titer of 1:16 or higher, whereas in nondisseminated cases the titer is almost invariably lower. Therefore, a critical titer of 1:32 or higher reflects active, disseminated disease. However, a lower titer does not exclude disseminated disease, because many patients, such as those with single extrapulmonary lesions, notably coccidioidal meningitis, do not develop high titers. Multiple serum specimens are helpful because a change in the CF titer reflects the prognosis. The CF titer declines with recovery and eventually disappears, while a rising titer indicates active, uncontrolled infection and a poor prognosis.

The immunodiffusion (ID) method can be used to detect both TP and CF antibodies by using reference antisera and heated (TP only) and unheated antigen. Antibodies to two specific heat-labile antigens, termed F (or CF) and HL, may be detected.

CLINICAL MANIFESTATIONS

Following inhalation of arthroconidia, the primary infection in most individuals is asymptomatic. Others may develop flu-like symptoms: fever, chest pain, cough or weight loss. Radiographic examination often reveals discrete nodules in the lower lobes. Primary pulmonary coccidioidomycosis is detailed in Chapter 31.

Only about 1% of primary cases progress to secondary or disseminated coccidioidomycosis. The numerous manifestations of secondary coccidioidomycosis include chronic and progressive pulmonary disease, single or multiple extrapulmonary dissemination or generalized systemic infection. Chronic pulmonary coccidioidomycosis usually involves a single, thin-walled cavity, but patients may develop enlarging or multiplying nodules or cavities. Dissemination may be fulminant or chronic, with periods of remission and exacerbation.

Extrapulmonary lesions most frequently involve the meninges, skin or bone. Chronic cutaneous coccidioidomycosis develops from initial lesions that usually appear on the face or neck and that, over a period of years, evolve into thick, raised, verrucous lesions with extensive epithelial hyperplasia. Bone involvement may accompany generalized systemic disease. Both osteomyelitis of long bones, vertebrae and other bones and arthritis may occur. Draining sinus tracts may evolve from subcutaneous and osseous lesions.

Coccidioidomycosis is the AIDS-defining illness for many patients, who commonly present with fever and chills, weight loss and night sweats. After pulmonary disease, coccidioidal meningitis is a frequent complication. Serologies are often negative in AIDS patients and the mortality rate is high. Diffuse pulmonary disease and a low CD4+ lymphocyte count (<50/µl) carry a poor prognosis.

MANAGEMENT

Symptomatic treatment is usually adequate for the patient with primary coccidioidomycosis, although ketoconazole may reduce the symptoms. However, if the primary infection is persistent or severe, or if there is evidence of dissemination, fluconazole or itraconazole should be administered for 2–6 months.

The chronicity of the disseminated disease usually requires prolonged therapy. Successful treatment may require continuous administration for more than a year. Chronic coccidioidal meningitis is often treated with fluconazole, which has excellent penetration across the blood–brain barrier. Some cases may require the intrathecal administration of chemotherapy. Grave disease is treated with amphotericin B in the usual formulation or as a lipid preparation to provide a higher dosage with reduced toxicity. For patients with AIDS, the total dose of amphotericin B should be at least 1.0 g, after which a maintenance regimen of itraconazole or fluconazole may be started. Patients treated with amphotericin B or azoles are more likely to relapse if the delayed skin test becomes negative and the CF antibody titers equal or exceed 1:256.

Histoplasmosis

Histoplasmosis is caused by the thermally dimorphic fungus, *Histoplasma capsulatum*. The infection occurs worldwide and is initiated by inhalation of microconidia produced by the mold form (see Table 178.12). The incidence varies considerably, being negligible in many parts of the world but significant in local regions of endemicity where most of the native population has been infected. Ninety-five percent of these infections are unapparent and detected only by the manifestation of residual lung calcification(s), a delayed hypersensitivity skin test reaction to histoplasmin, or both. The skin test antigen, histoplasmin, is a standardized culture extract similar to coccidioidin.

MYCOLOGY

There are three varieties of *H. capsulatum*, but most human cases are caused by *H. capsulatum* var. *capsulatum*, while *H. capsulatum* var. *duboisii* is found in Africa (see below), and *H. capsulatum* var. *farciminosum* causes infection in horses. Although *H. capsulatum* can undergo sexual reproduction with a compatible mating strain, clinical isolates reproduce asexually, being haploid and clonal. *Histoplasma capsulatum* and *B. dermatitidis* are closely related ascomycetous fungi and members of the same teleomorphic or sexual genus, *Ajellomyces*.

Histoplasma capsulatum is a thermally dimorphic fungus. At temperatures below 95°F (35°C) it grows as a mold, often white or brown in color, and at 98.6°F (37°C) it grows as a yeast with small, heaped and pasty colonies. *Histoplasma capsulatum* characteristically grows

slowly. Under optimal conditions, the mold colony develops after 1 or 2 weeks and conidia are produced shortly thereafter. However, cultures of clinical specimens sometimes require incubation periods of 8–12 weeks before there is detectable growth. Primary isolates are often brown and become white with prolonged cultivation.[113]

Microconidia and macroconidia are produced directly by the aerial hyphae at temperatures below 95°F (35°C). The microconidia are globose and 1–5 µm in diameter. Upon dehydration, they are easily dislodged by the wind and become airborne. Their small size enables the microconidia to be inhaled into the alveoli. The macroconidia are larger and more distinctive. At 98.6°F (37°C) the mold converts to growth as a small, budding yeast. Conversion is often difficult to effect *in vitro* but is enhanced by a rich, complex medium, such as brain–heart infusion agar. The yeast cells are small, ellipsoidal, approximately 1–3 µm × 3–5 µm in size, and virtually identical to the yeasts observed *in vivo* within phagocytes (see Table 178.12 and Fig. 178.9).

ECOLOGY AND EPIDEMIOLOGY

In nature, *H. capsulatum* lives in soil with a high nitrogen content and is associated with bat and avian habitats. *Histoplasma capsulatum* has been isolated many times from bird roosts, chicken houses, bat caves and similar environments. Conidia, when dry, are easily airborne and spread by wind currents, as well as by birds and bats. *Histoplasma capsulatum* is most prevalent in the environment where the infection is most endemic, namely in the Ohio–Mississippi Valley: in Missouri, Kentucky, Tennessee, Indiana, Ohio and southern Illinois. This region also has the highest population of starlings, which tend to congregate in large numbers. The excrement from these birds provides an ideal medium for the enrichment of *H. capsulatum*. In South America, the chief reservoir appears to be chicken coops and bat caves.

In cases of histoplasmosis from Africa, both *H. capsulatum* var. *capsulatum* and *H. capsulatum* var. *duboisii* have been isolated. Infections elsewhere are due to the global variety, *H. capsulatum* var. *capsulatum*. *Histoplasma capsulatum* var. *duboisii* causes African histoplasmosis, which is distinguished from the usual infection by:

- a greater frequency of skin and bone lesions;
- diminished pulmonary involvement;
- pronounced giant cell formation; and
- larger, thick-walled yeast cells in tissue.

Although these clinical features are characteristic and reproducible, *H. capsulatum* var. *duboisii* cannot be reliably differentiated *in vitro* from the type species on the basis of morphology, physiology and antigenic composition.

Much of the knowledge concerning the prevalence of histoplasmosis has been derived from global skin test surveys with histoplasmin. The region with the highest level of reactivity is the central USA, along the river valleys of Ohio, Mississippi, St Lawrence and Rio Grande,

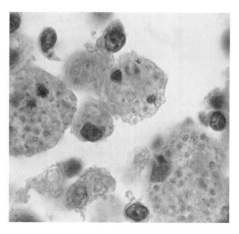

Fig. 178.9 *Histoplasma capsulatum*. Small yeast cells packed inside macrophages in a Giemsa-stained smear of bone marrow aspirate.

where in some locales 80–90% of the population may be skin test positive by the age of 20 years. Foci of high reactivity exist elsewhere in the world, such as southern Mexico, Indonesia, the Philippines and Turkey. In the USA alone, projections based on skin test surveys have led to estimations that more than 40 million people have been exposed with 500 000 new infections every year. Of these, perhaps 55 000–200 000 cases will be symptomatic, 1500–4000 will require hospitalization annually and 25–100 deaths will occur. These projections were made prior to 1980 and do not reflect the increasing incidence of opportunistic histoplasmosis in patients with AIDS.

Outbreaks or epidemics of acute respiratory histoplasmosis result from the simultaneous exposure of a large number of people. These epidemics are not caused by direct spread among humans or animals. Rather, the sudden release leads to multiple exposure of a heavy inoculum that has accumulated in a dormant environment. Silos, air-conditioning units contaminated with bird droppings, and accumulations of guano in caves, attics or parks have all been implicated as reservoirs for *H. capsulatum* in outbreaks of this type.

Males develop symptomatic histoplasmosis more often than females and approximately 75% of cases occur in males. Before puberty, the attack rate for males and females is identical and the percentage of positive skin test reactors is the same for both sexes at all ages. These epidemiologic data suggest that either adult males are inherently more susceptible to the disease or females are more resistant. Severity of disease and mortality are greater at the age extremes, in infancy and after the age of 50.

In addition to humans, many wild and domestic animals are susceptible to histoplasmosis. Some animals, including the bat, may act as vectors to disseminate the organism in nature.

PATHOGENICITY

All clinical forms are believed to evolve from the same natural history. Microconidia are inhaled from an exogenous source and penetrate to the alveoli, where they convert to small, budding yeast cells. The conversion of *H. capsulatum* to the yeast form at 98.6°F (37°C) is essential for pathogenicity, and expression of yeast-specific genes has been correlated with virulence and thermal tolerance.[118] The yeast cells are readily phagocytized by alveolar macrophages. At this stage, the yeast-laden macrophages may be cleared through the upper respiratory tract. They may also disseminate through the circulation, spreading the yeasts to other reticuloendothelial organs, and/or they may invoke a tissue response *in situ*. The tissue reaction may involve an early influx of neutrophils and lymphocytes, but the pyogenic inflammatory response gives way to epithelioid cell tubercle formation. In the course of these various possible reactions, the intracellular yeasts may or may not be inactivated by the phagocytes, depending upon the immune status of the host.

The phagocytized yeast cells of *H. capsulatum* are able to survive intracellularly by a calcium-dependent process, block acidification within the phagolysosome and multiply within macrophages.[119] However, macrophages from immunized animals, as well as normal macrophages activated by immune lymphocytes or cytokines, restrict the growth of intracellular yeasts. In experimental, self-limited murine histoplasmosis, various parameters of cell-mediated immunity are depressed during the height of antigen (yeast) burden, suppressor T cells and macrophage-like suppressor cells are detected, and production of IL-1 and IL-2 is impaired. Concomitant with resolution of the infection, the number of suppressor cells in the spleen diminishes and T helper cells increase.[110] These correlations of competent cell-mediated immune responses with resistance to infection are supported by the clinical data. Similar to coccidioidomycosis, there is an inverse relationship between the magnitude of the cell-mediated immune response, as measured by delayed-type hypersensitivity or *in-vitro* lymphoblastogenesis and high levels of specific antibody, which correlate with the severity of the disease. Additional evidence suggests that TNF may be crucial in the induction of protective T-cell responses.[110]

DIAGNOSTIC MICROBIOLOGY

Microscopic examination

Histoplasmosis can be diagnosed on finding the yeast cells in clinical material. Suitable specimens include sputa, tissue from biopsy or surgical specimens, spinal fluid and blood. The buffy coat of a blood specimen may reveal yeast-filled macrophages. Bone marrow obtained when patients are febrile may contain yeast cells. Smears of infected sputum, blood, marrow or tissue that have been fixed with methanol and stained with the Wright or Giemsa stain will reveal the characteristically small, ellipsoidal yeast cells (approximately 2 × 4 μm) inside macrophages. With either stain, the larger end of the yeast cell contains an eccentric, red-staining mass (see Fig. 178.9).

Culture

Sputum specimens should be collected early in the morning and purulent or sanguineous portions should be selected for culture. A bronchial wash is even more likely to be positive. Because *H. capsulatum* may grow very slowly, cultures should be incubated for up to 12 weeks, if possible, before discarding as negative. If a sporulating mold develops, *H. capsulatum* can be identified by the presence of its characteristic macroconidia (see Table 178.12) and by conversion to the yeast form by growth on an enriched medium at 98.6°F (37°C), by the detection of *H. capsulatum*-specific exoantigens (see Table 178.13) or by using a specific DNA probe.

Lysis-centrifugation is the most sensitive and rapid method to recover dimorphic fungi from blood, especially *H. capsulatum*.[113]

Skin test

The antigen, histoplasmin, is a standardized culture filtrate preparation and 0.1 ml is injected intradermally. A positive reaction is indicated by induration of >5 mm diameter after 48 hours. As with coccidioidin, a positive test, if specific, denotes previous sensitization to *H. capsulatum*. Without a history of prior negativity, the positive test has no diagnostic significance. Histoplasmin is a polyvalent mixture of antigens, only some of which are specific for *H. capsulatum*. Because some antigenic determinants are shared by other pathogenic fungi, cross-reactions can occur. For example, some individuals sensitive to *B. dermatitidis* or *C. immitis* will give a false-positive reaction to histoplasmin. Therefore, along with histoplasmin, it is routine to administer coccidioidin in the USA or coccidioidin and paracoccidioidin in South America. A reaction to a single antigen is generally considered specific. Reactions to two antigens may be caused by sensitization to one or both, although the larger reaction is often considered more specific.

Serology

Specific antibodies to *H. capsulatum* antigens can be detected during infection. Two serologic tests are now widely accepted because of their convenience, availability and utility: the measurement of antibodies by complement fixation (CF) and the immunodiffusion (ID) test for precipitins. Both tests may be helpful in the diagnosis and prognosis of histoplasmosis, provided the results are properly interpreted (see Table 178.14).

CF tests detect antibodies to two antigens of *H. capsulatum*: histoplasmin and a standardized suspension of killed yeast cells. Because of the possibility of cross-reactivity, patient sera are tested concomitantly against other fungal antigens, such as coccidioidin, spherulin, *B. dermatitidis* or *Paracoccidioides brasiliensis*. Serum antibodies specific for *H. capsulatum* antigens can be detected by the CF test 2–4 weeks following exposure. Most laboratories perform the CF test on twofold dilutions of patient serum, beginning with a dilution of 1:8. With resolution of the infection, the antibody titer gradually declines and disappears (i.e. titer <1:8), in most cases by 9 months. The CF test with either *H. capsulatum* yeast or mycelial (histoplasmin) antigen is very sensitive and 90% of patients are positive (i.e. titer >1:8). A titer of 1:32 that persists or rises over the course of several weeks indicates active disease in patients with an established diagnosis of histoplasmosis. Unfortunately, in sensitive patients, the skin test antigen may boost the CF antibody titer to histoplasmin and the elevated titer may remain for as long as 3 months. If a patient's serum is reactive to more than one antigen or if it is anticomplementary, the ID test should be conducted.

Precipitins can be detected by immunodiffusion (ID) of serum and antigen in agarose. The ID test becomes positive in up to 80% of patients with histoplasmosis by the third or fourth week of infection. This test, while less sensitive and requiring a longer time to become positive, is more specific than the CF test. There are two specific precipitin bands, m and h (see Table 178.13). The m line, which is observed more frequently, appears soon after infection and may persist in the serum up to 3 years following recovery. The h band is more transient. Because it disappears soon after the disease, the presence of serum antibodies to the h antigen is better correlated with active infection. As with the CF titer, the m band may be boosted by the administration of the histoplasmin skin test.

An excellent radioimmunoassay (RIA) test for antigenemia and antigenuria has been developed by MiraVista Diagnostics (Indianapolis, IN, USA).[120] Tests for polysaccharide antigen in the serum have been detected in 79% of patients with disseminated histoplasmosis and 97% had a positive test for antigen in the urine. After treatment with amphotericin B, serum titers dropped in all the patients and urine titers dropped in 91% of patients. Testing either serum or urine had prognostic value, detecting relapses in AIDS patients. The antigen can also be measured in CSF or BAL fluid specimens. However, the test lacks optimal specificity because patients with other systemic mycoses have been shown to yield positive tests for the antigen.

PREVENTION

Several approaches are currently underway to develop an effective vaccine for histoplasmosis.[112]

CLINICAL MANIFESTATIONS

The manifestations of infection with *H. capsulatum* are numerous. The initial pulmonary episode may be acute or chronic, or dissemination may occur by hematogenous or lymphatic spread from the lungs to other organs. Most normal individuals are able to contain the infection. The granulomata that form may undergo fibrosis and residual scars may remain in the lungs or spleen. Resolution appears to confer some immunity to re-infection. This process occurs without symptoms in 95% of all persons with acute, primary histoplasmosis, whether disseminated or confined to the lung. For a description of the pneumonic forms of histoplasmosis, see Chapter 31.

The gamut of clinical forms and pathology observed in pulmonary histoplasmosis can also occur in any other part of the body. The yeast cells are probably disseminated throughout the body while inside macrophages. The most common sites of involvement, after the lung, are the reticuloendothelial tissues of the spleen, liver, lymph nodes and bone marrow. However, lesions have been documented in almost every organ. Dissemination may be completely benign and unapparent except for the presence of calcified lesions, usually in organs of the reticuloendothelial system.

Alternatively, disseminated histoplasmosis may be acute and progressive. In such cases, the pulmonary symptoms are insignificant and patients may have splenomegaly and hepatomegaly, weight loss, anemia and leukopenia. Granulomatous lesions and macrophages packed with yeast cells can be observed throughout the liver, spleen, marrow and, quite often, the adrenals. Acute progressive histoplasmosis is often fulminant and rapidly fatal; ultimately every organ can become diseased. This form of histoplasmosis is an opportunistic disease associated with compromised cell-mediated immunity, such as patients with AIDS or those receiving immunosuppressive drugs and those with underlying lymphomatous neoplasia. In most cases, the compromising condition served to reactivate a quiescent lesion that was originally acquired years earlier. Within the endemic area, infants with histiocytosis may develop disseminated histoplasmosis that is characteristically fulminant. Chronic disseminated histoplasmosis may evolve from protraction of the acute disease. This form is progressive, with eventual involvement of every organ, especially the mucocutaneous areas around the eye, tongue and anus.

Within the vast endemic regions, histoplasmosis is often the initial AIDS-defining condition among HIV-infected patients. The survival time for patients with AIDS is significantly shorter for those with disseminated histoplasmosis. Important risk factors for the development of histoplasmosis in AIDS patients include environmental exposure to likely sources of *H. capsulatum* (chicken coops), positive CF antibodies to histoplasmin, chronic medical condition(s), herpes simplex infection and a CD4+ lymphocyte count of <150 000/ml.[121]

MANAGEMENT

Most primary pulmonary infections with *H. capsulatum* go undetected and require no treatment. Symptomatic cases in immunocompetent persons are treated with itraconazole. This recommendation applies to patients with progressive pulmonary or disseminated disease, as well as mild to moderate or stable disease.[120] Severe cases of any form are treated initially with amphotericin B followed by itraconazole. The regimen of amphotericin B is similar to that applied to other systemic mycoses. Recovery following treatment with amphotericin B is generally faster and fewer relapses occur than are experienced with blastomycosis and coccidioidomycosis. Arrested pulmonary lesions are often removed surgically. Less severe cases in non-immunocompromised patients may be treated with itraconazole. AIDS patients with histoplasmosis may be treated initially with a lipid formulation of AMB and then placed on maintenance therapy with itraconazole. Cases of meningitis due to *H. capsulatum* are treated with an amphotericin B preparation followed by fluconazole. As noted earlier, voriconazole has been used successfully in a limited number of patients with endemic mycoses.[115]

Paracoccidioidomycosis

Paracoccidioidomycosis (South American blastomycosis) is caused by the thermally dimorphic fungus, *Paracoccidioides brasiliensis*. The infection is restricted to endemic areas of Central and South America. It is a chronic, granulomatous disease that begins with a primary, pulmonary, usually inapparent infection that disseminates to produce ulcerative granulomata in the mucosal surfaces of the nose, mouth and gastrointestinal tract. In addition to the skin and lymph nodes, the infection may spread to the internal organs.

MYCOLOGY

Colonies of *P. brasiliensis* grow very slowly and the macroscopic features of the mold colony are variable and nonspecific. Various asexual reproductive structures are produced by *P. brasiliensis*, including chlamydospores, arthroconidia and singly borne conidia. In the absence of conidia, which may not be produced for 10 weeks in culture, the mycelia and colony may be indistinguishable from *B. dermatitidis* or many saprophytic molds. The yeast cells, which can be induced by cultivation on a rich medium at 95–98.6°F (35–37°C), are readily identified by their unique appearance. As shown in Figure 178.10, the yeasts produce multiple buds, each attached to the parent yeast by a narrow base. The yeast cells are large, up to 30 μm in diameter, and

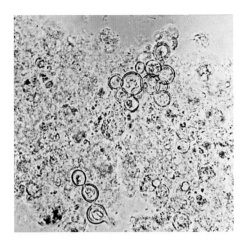

Fig. 178.10 *Paracoccidioides brasiliensis.* Large multiply budding yeast cells in a potassium hydroxide preparation of a scraping of cutaneous paracoccidioidomycosis.

have thinner walls than the yeasts of *B. dermatitidis*. These forms have been described as 'pilot wheels'.

ECOLOGY AND EPIDEMIOLOGY

The natural habitat of *P. brasiliensis* has not been proven, but is presumed to be soil. The organism has been recovered only sporadically and not repeatedly from soil in Venezuela and Argentina. Like *B. dermatitidis*, its environmental niche and life cycle in nature are unknown. There is no evidence of an animal vector or transmission of the infection. Human infections are presumed to follow exposure to the organisms from an exogenous source. Most patients are males (>90%), agricultural workers, often malnourished, and usually 30–60 years of age.

Thousands of cases of paracoccidioidomycosis have been reported from Brazil, Venezuela and Colombia, and fewer cases from Argentina, Ecuador and other South and Central American countries, with the exception of Chile and the Caribbean nations. Discrete endemic foci exist within this broad area of geographic distribution. However, all cases are isolated and outbreaks have not been observed. The endemic zones are associated with moderate temperatures (57–86°F/14–30°C) and rainfall, elevation of 500–6500 feet, subtropical forests and river valleys, but not all areas fitting this description have paracoccidioidomycosis.

Skin test surveys have been conducted with various antigens derived from *P. brasiliensis*. These paracoccidioidins exhibit cross-reactivity with histoplasmin and it is difficult to interpret double reactions of equal size in the same individual. As with the skin test antigens of the other dimorphic, systemic pathogens, paracoccidioidin elicits a delayed, indurative reaction that indicates previous exposure. The percentage of reactivity in the endemic areas varies up to 75% and occurs equally in both men and women. Significant risk factors for infection (i.e. positive skin test) include agricultural occupations, association with certain aquatic environments and contact with bats. Many patients with paracoccidioidomycosis are malnourished and exhibit depressed cell-mediated immune responses.

PATHOGENICITY

Paracoccidioides brasiliensis, like the other systemic fungi, causes disease in males more frequently than females (see Table 178.11), although skin test surveys have revealed comparable reactivity between the sexes, implying equal exposure. Sex-linked differences may be associated with the generally more potent cellular immunity of females. Limited studies indicate that physiologic concentrations of sex hor-

mones do not directly inhibit these fungi. However, a protein from the mycelial cytosol of *P. brasiliensis* has been shown to bind estrogen but not testosterone or other hormones. Binding blocks conversion of the mycelium to yeast at 98.6°F (37°C) and may explain the resistance of females to paracoccidioidomycosis.[122] Once yeast cells of *P. brasiliensis* have developed in the lung, yeast cell wall polysaccharides, such as α-glucan, are associated with virulence and the ability to stimulate granulomata.

DIAGNOSTIC MICROBIOLOGY

Sputum, tissue or scrapings of mucocutaneous lesions may reveal the multiply budding yeast cells that are pathognomonic for *P. brasiliensis* (see Fig. 178.10). Specimens should be cultured at 77–86°F (25–30°C) on mycologic media. The yeast form often grows better at 95°F (35°C) or 96.8°F (36°C) than 98.6°F (37°C).

The ID test is extremely useful. As indicated in Table 178.14, nearly all patients have at least one of three specific precipitin lines, which are detected by identity with reference serum. The ID test also has prognostic value, as the bands disappear with clearing of the infection, and the number of bands is somewhat correlated with the severity of the disease. The CF test is quantitative and useful for assessing prognosis, but cross-reactions occur with other fungi.

CLINICAL MANIFESTATIONS

The initial contact with *P. brasiliensis* occurs by inhalation. This episode is unapparent and the organism becomes quiescent for an indefinite period or the lesion may resolve. This asymptomatic infection results in the acquisition of a positive delayed skin test reaction to paracoccidioidin. The eventual development of symptomatic disease depends upon the host–fungal interaction, i.e. the integrity of the cell-mediated immune responses of the individual, environmental conditions (e.g. temperature, nutrients), host conditions (e.g. age, sex, state of nutrition) and the virulence of the strain of *P. brasiliensis*.

Acute or subacute disease

Patients under 30 years of age may develop an acute, progressive infection characterized by lymphonodular lesions in the lung. This 'juvenile' form is rare. The yeasts may disseminate to the reticuloendothelial tissue, lymph nodes, liver, spleen, skin, bone, joints or other organs. The severity and duration of the illness depend upon the extent of organ involvement and it may be fatal within a period of several weeks or months.

Chronic disease

More than 90% of cases are the chronic 'adult' type and develop from activation of latent cells, usually after several years. Lesions may be localized in the lung or metastasis may occur from the lung to other organs, particularly the skin and mucocutaneous tissue, lymph nodes, spleen, liver, adrenals and combinations thereof. Mucocutaneous, often petechial, lesions frequently develop on the corners of the mouth, lips, gingiva or tongue. Pulmonary lesions are granulomatous nodules that may cavitate but rarely calcify.

MANAGEMENT

Patients should be assessed for malnourishment, alcoholism and extensive tobacco use, all of which exacerbate the disease. Since many of the antifungal drugs are effective against *P. brasiliensis*, the initial treatment choice may reflect the expense and local availability of antifungal agents. Sulfonamide derivatives are among the earliest but less effective drugs. Trimethoprim–sulfamethoxazole (TMP–SMZ) is the currently recommended formulation of this type. The azoles are much more effective. Itraconazole is currently the drug of choice and a clinical cure rate approaching 100% is achievable with a daily dose of 100 mg for 6 months. Relapses are rare. Fluconazole is also effective, producing cures in about 90% of patients who received 200–400 mg/day for 6 months. Although amphotericin B is highly effective against paracoccidioidomycosis, it should be reserved for patients who fail to respond or cannot tolerate one of the azoles. After initiating therapy, serologies are checked every few months to monitor the effectiveness of treatment. Some clinicians recommend a maintenance regimen of TMP–SMZ or itraconazole for up to 1 year after serologic tests become negative or indefinitely for patients with AIDS.

REFERENCES

 References for this chapter can be found online at http://www.expertconsult.com

Malcolm D Richardson
Caroline B Moore
Richard C Summerbell
Aditya K Gupta

Chapter | **179** |

Superficial and subcutaneous fungal pathogens

Superficial Fungal Pathogens

The majority of superficial fungal infections are caused by three groups of fungi: dermatophytes, *Candida albicans* and *Malassezia* spp.[1-3]

NATURE

Candida albicans is the principal agent of candidiasis. *Malassezia* spp. are lipophilic (lipid-requiring) yeasts found on the body surface as commensals and are agents of the skin disease tinea versicolor (pityriasis versicolor). In addition, they may be causal in the allergically mediated condition seborrheic dermatitis.

Other fungi cause less common types of superficial disease. Yeasts in the genus *Trichosporon* may cause white piedra, superficial colonizations of the scalp, and axillary and pubic hair shafts. The melanized yeast-like organism *Hortaea werneckii* (also known by several older names all ending in 'werneckii') causes the dark skin lesions of tinea nigra. The rare hair shaft colonization black piedra is caused by *Piedraia hortae*. Finally, approximately 35 nondermatophytic filamentous fungi and a few yeasts have been authenticated as causing onychomycosis (i.e. fungal nail disease). Most prominent among these are members of the genera *Scytalidium*, *Aspergillus*, *Scopulariopsis*, *Fusarium* and *Onychocola*.

EPIDEMIOLOGY

Dermatophytosis is among the most common of all communicable diseases. Because many cases are never brought to medical attention, fully reliable incidence figures do not exist. Onychomycosis, in which the great majority of cases are dermatophytic, may account for 10–30% of all superficial mycoses. In the USA Medicare insurance for seniors (≥65 years old) in 1 year paid for consultations involving 662 000 patients, or 2.7% of the senior population, at a cost of over US$43 000 000. Less than 10% of those aged under 30 years and more than 20% of those aged over 75 years had tinea unguium (dermatophytic onychomycosis; Table 179.1) in population studies.[4] Tinea capitis in children is common in some areas. In an urban center in the USA up to 4% of children presenting with nondermatologic complaints at a clinic were infected by *Trichophyton tonsurans*, whereas up to 30% of asymptomatic adults accompanying infected children were carriers.[5] A study of 224 children in a Philadelphia school reported 3% symptomatic and 14% asymptomatic, infected children.[6] Tinea pedis has been found to affect 1.5% of pediatric patients, 5.9% of 11–15 year olds[5] and up to 45% of adult marathon runners.[7] There is a significant age-dependent association between sporting activities and pedal

dermatophytosis.[8] Many of the most prevalent dermatophytes are cosmopolitan, but certain species, especially agents of tinea capitis, have defined endemic regions (see Table 179.1).

Cutaneous candidiasis is particularly common in infants, at least 10% of whom have candidal skin colonizations. Fifty per cent of this colonized group go on to become symptomatic, usually with candidal diaper dermatitis. Many adults harbor an indigenous strain of *C. albicans*; up to 30% of healthy women, for example, are culture positive for this species in vaginal swab samples, at least when pregnant or taking oral contraceptives. The lower gut may serve as a reservoir when other body sites are free of *C. albicans*. Normal skin only rarely yields *C. albicans* but the yeast may rapidly colonize chronically moist or damaged skin, including moist dermatophyte lesions.

Malassezia spp. have been found as skin commensals in over 90% of humans surveyed.[1,2] In the temperate zone they only occasionally proliferate to the point of causing the finely scaly maculae of tinea versicolor, but in the tropics the prevalence may reach 50% of the population. *Malassezia* spp. in patients who have HIV and other immunocompromised patients may cause pustular hair follicle inflammations referred to as *Malassezia* folliculitis, and may be associated with an increased prevalence of seborrheic dermatitis.[9] In atopic individuals, *Malassezia* spp. growing commensally on skin may serve as a triggering allergen in atopic dermatitis.[9] A possible association between *Malassezia* and neonatal acne or cephalic pustulosis is under investigation.

White piedra is found worldwide, but is now uncommon because of modern hygiene. Black piedra is native to South East Asia, the Pacific and South America, and affects other primates in addition to humans. It is uncommon when discouraged but is cultivated in some cultures. Tinea nigra is of tropical or subtropical origin; about 150 indigenous US cases were reported between 1950 and 1988, in addition to many more cases acquired by travelers, mostly in the Caribbean. *Scytalidium* infections of nails, soles or palms are usually acquired in the tropics. *Scytalidium dimidiatum*, the most common infectious species, has rapidly growing pantropical forms as well as a distinctive slow-growing Indian subcontinent form that may be transmitted among family members in the Indian Diaspora. Most other agents of nondermatophytic onychomycosis are cosmopolitan saprobic molds and, despite their opportunistic potential, are more frequently seen as insignificant contaminants of body surfaces than as etiologic agents.[10]

PATHOGENICITY

Dermatophytes normally infect only the keratinized stratum corneum of the epithelial skin layers. They degrade keratin and other skin proteins. They are restricted to the stratum corneum by cellular immune components, and by the iron limitation and other effects mediated by transferrin. A twofold higher prevalence in males than females may reflect

Table 179.1 Definition and distribution of dermatophytoses

Area of infection	Disease name	Prevalent agents	Geographic area
Scalp	Tinea capitis	*Trichophyton tonsurans*	Cosmopolitan, especially urban Americas, Latin America
		Microsporum canis	Cosmopolitan; predominant dermatophyte in parts of south and east Europe
		Trichophyton violaceum	Endemic to Middle East, North Africa
		Trichophyton soudanense	Endemic to sub-Saharan Africa
Beard area	Tinea barbae	*Trichophyton rubrum*, *Trichophyton verrucosum*	Cosmopolitan
Glabrous skin (trunk, limbs, face)	Tinea corporis	*Trichophyton rubrum*, *Trichophyton mentagrophytes* complex, *Microsporum canis*, *Epidermophyton floccosum*	Cosmopolitan
		Trichophyton megninii	Endemic to Portugal, Sardinia
Scalp, glabrous skin	Favus	*Trichophyton schoenleinii*	Relict in rural Africa, central Asia; formerly widespread
Palms	Tinea manuum	*Trichophyton rubrum*, *Trichophyton mentagrophytes* complex	Cosmopolitan
Groin	Tinea cruris	*Trichophyton rubrum*, *Trichophyton mentagrophytes* complex, *Epidermophyton floccosum*	Cosmopolitan
Soles, toe webs	Tinea pedis	*Trichophyton rubrum*, *Trichophyton mentagrophytes* complex, *Epidermophyton floccosum*	Cosmopolitan
Nails	Tinea unguium (dermatophytic onychomycosis)	*Trichophyton rubrum*, *Trichophyton mentagrophytes* complex	Cosmopolitan

inhibition by progesterone. Involvement of an autosomal dominant susceptibility allele has been proposed in the common chronic form of *Trichophyton rubrum* infection.[11] An indication of the relative importance of lymphocytes in host defense is seen in HIV infection, in which helper T-cell counts below 100 cells/ml correlate with a marked increase in onychomycosis,[12] including the unusual 'proximal white' form.

Dermatophytes differ in their host interactions. Anthropophilic dermatophytes (Table 179.2), specific to human disease, are distinguished from zoophilic dermatophytes, which have specific animal associations but may be transmitted to humans, and from geophilic dermatophytes, which are occasionally pathogenic to humans or animals but primarily grow on decaying keratinous material. The *Trichophyton mentagrophytes* complex, containing four sibling species distinguishable by molecular study, has both anthropophilic and zoophilic variants. Infection of humans by zoophilic dermatophytes usually elicits a pronounced inflammatory response.[14] Such inflamed lesions may resolve spontaneously, unlike the often chronic lesions of anthropophilic dermatophytoses.

The common anthropophilic dermatophytes include lower body dermatophytes associated with sites other than the scalp, and dermatophytes strongly adapted for tinea capitis, less commonly causing other tineas. *Trichophyton rubrum*, *T. mentagrophytes* complex and *Epidermophyton floccosum* are the common lower body species. Tinea capitis dermatophytes consist of two major groups distinguished by their colonization of hair (see Table 179.2). In the 'ectothrix' group, hair shafts are externally ensheathed with masses of arthroconidia (spores). In the 'endothrix' group, the hair shafts are heavily invested internally by arthroconidia. An anomalous scalp infection, favus,

caused by the now rare *Trichophyton schoenleinii*, is distinguished by the presence of follicles transformed into scutula, that is, pits lined with fungal mycelium.

Tinea capitis agents primarily cause new infections in children, and may cause dramatic outbreaks. *Microsporum audouinii* infections spontaneously resolve at 15–19 years of age, but most endothrix agents cause lifelong asymptomatic infections in some adult carriers[6] and occasionally cause new tinea corporis or other infections in adults. New anthropophilic tinea capitis infections are usually acquired via shared headgear, bedding or grooming and haircutting instruments. Adults who acquire new infections caused by endothrix species usually have intimate contact with infected children. Anthropophilic lower body dermatophytoses are often acquired via the feet, either from family members or in communal aquatic or exercise facilities. After infecting the feet, these fungi may go on to infect other body sites.

Zoophilic dermatophytes (see Table 179.2) usually cause tinea corporis or tinea capitis in humans. They may be transmitted directly from infected animals or from fomites, such as fence posts in cattle yards. *Microsporum canis* may cause limited outbreaks among humans before virulence is attenuated.[15]

Candida albicans is often acquired in the birth canal or in infancy from caregivers. Generally, an individual harbors only one or two strains. Cutaneous candidiasis is predisposed to by warm, moist conditions with abrasion, especially in the diaper rash of infancy but also in adult occupations that involve wet hands. In the latter cases, paronychia or interdigital erosion frequently results. Intertriginous candidiasis occurs in moist body folds and is exacerbated by diabetes mellitus or obesity. Chronic mucocutaneous candidiasis (CMC), in which skin

Table 179.2 Common and formerly common dermatophytes and their infectivity

Anthropophiles (type of scalp infection if characteristic)	Zoophiles (type of human scalp infection) [principal hosts]	Geophiles (type of human scalp infection)
Epidermophyton floccosum	*Microsporum canis* (ectothrix) [cat, dog]	*Microsporum gypseum* (ectothrix)
Microsporum audouinii (ectothrix)	*Microsporum gallinae* [fowl]	*Microsporum praecox*
Microsporum ferrugineum (ectothrix)	*Microsporum nanum* [swine]	*Microsporum racemosum*
Trichophyton concentricum	*Microsporum persicolor* [vole]	*Microsporum vanbreuseghemii*
Trichophyton megninii (ectothrix)	*Trichophyton equinum* [horse]	The listing of geophiles does not include species that have not been well substantiated to cause human disease. These species are not properly considered dermatophytes according to Ajello[13]
Trichophyton mentagrophytes complex (phylogenetic species *Trichophyton interdigitale*)	*Trichophyton mentagrophytes* complex (phylogenetic species *Trichophyton interdigitale*, *Trichophyton mentagrophytes*, *Trichophyton erinacei*) [rodents, rabbits, hedgehogs]	
Trichophyton rubrum	*Trichophyton simii* [monkey]	
Trichophyton schoenleinii (favus)	*Trichophyton verrucosum* [cattle]	
Trichophyton soudanense (endothrix)		
Trichophyton tonsurans (endothrix)		
Trichophyton violaceum (endothrix)		

and mucosa are extensively colonized by *C. albicans*, results from inherited defects in cellular immunity.[16] Particular associated conditions include congenital thymus dysplasias, polyendocrine deficiencies and leukocyte dysfunctions such as chronic granulomatous disease. In this latter disease, the impaired production of toxic oxygen species prevents killing of *Candida* spp. within phagocytes.

Malassezia spp. are also generally acquired as commensal surface flora in early infancy. They primarily use fatty acids secreted by the skin. Corticosteroid use, Cushing's disease, malnutrition and immunosuppression may contribute to an increased frequency of tinea versicolor; HIV infection and miscellaneous immunosuppressions predispose to folliculitis.

Nondermatophytic onychomycosis caused by genera other than *Scytalidium* is strongly predisposed to by advanced age.

Details regarding the prevention of infection caused by agents of superficial fungal infection, diagnosis, clinical manifestations and management can be found in Chapter 13.

DIAGNOSTIC MICROBIOLOGY

Superficial mycotic infections are best tested by the combination of direct microscopy for fungal elements in hydroxide (KOH, NaOH) slides, and fungal culture. Direct microscopy may be facilitated by the use of fluorescent fungal cell wall dyes such as calcofluor or Congo red. Histopathology performed with fungal stains has been suggested as an alternative to 'KOH and culture' for onychomycosis, but the ability of this technique to distinguish dermatophyte from nondermatophyte infections has received only preliminary investigation.

Dermatophytes in direct microscopy show cylindrical fungal filaments that may include chains of rounded arthroconidia. At times filaments may be converted entirely into arthroconidia, such as within or around hair shafts in tinea capitis. In superficial white onychomycosis caused by *T. mentagrophytes* complex members, microscopy may show 'frondose branching', an appressed, palmate spreading of fungal hyphae between keratin lamellae. In nails, soles and palms, all morphologies of dermatophyte filaments overlap with those of other potentially infectious fungi, especially *Scytalidium* spp.

Generally, dermatophyte filaments from the growing fronts of infection, such as the peripheral 'ring' in classic ringworm and adjacent to the nailbed in tinea unguium, will be alive and will stain with vital stains such as neutral red.[17] Those from prior growth fronts, such as centers of ringworm lesions or extruded, distal nail, tend to be senescent and will not yield a culture. For this reason, sampling tinea at its extending margin, and subungual onychomycosis at the juncture of nail and nailbed, is recommended. Tinea corporis is sampled by using a scalpel to remove skin scale from the advancing lesion margin after light disinfection with an ethanol swab. In subungual onychomycosis, heavily contaminated debris is scraped from the undersurface of the nail and discarded; then, after swabbing with ethanol, friable material is scraped from the nail undersurface as close as possible to the nailbed. Clippings may also be taken. In superficial white onychomycosis, white, opaque areas on the upper nail surface are scraped. As with subungual onychomycosis, superficial debris is scraped and discarded before sample collection. In tinea pedis of the sole and tinea manuum, in which growth fronts may not be apparent, the affected area should be scraped broadly so that the whole is represented in the sample.

Even with expert sampling approximately 10–25% of nail samples positive for fungal filaments in direct microscopy fail to yield a culture.[17] That such a finding accurately reflects the active infection can be confirmed by vital staining,[18] and should not be mistaken for a technical 'false-negative' culture result. Also, approximately 45–50% of toenails and 60% of fingernails clinically suggestive of onychomycosis fail to yield any evidence of fungal infection.[19] Dermatophyte colonization in very degraded nails may be partially supplanted by secondary invaders such as *Pseudomonas* bacteria and *Scopulariopsis* mold (the latter may also appear as a sole agent of onychomycosis or as a contaminant), and the original etiologic agent may be difficult to trace.

Hair from tinea capitis or barbae is plucked so that the hair root, the best source of inoculum, is included. In 'black dot' tinea capitis, in which hairs are fragile, a few hair roots may be extracted with the tip of a scalpel and included along with surface scrapings of the lesion. *Microsporum* scalp lesions typically show strong yellow–green fluorescence under a Wood's light and can be presumptively diagnosed in this manner. In zoophilic tinea corporis and other lesions with vesicles or bullae, the apices of these may be clipped and included in the sample. Moist, suppurating lesions may be sampled with a swab. Swab samples may make direct microscopy difficult and are best evaluated by culturing.

For culture, scrapings or fragments from clippings are usually planted on Sabouraud's agar supplemented with antibacterials and the selective antifungal cycloheximide. Common commercial equivalents include Mycosel, Dermasel and Mycobiotic. Dermatophytes and *C. albicans* are among the small minority of fungi able to grow well on these media. Potato glucose or potato flake agar with cycloheximide is preferred by some laboratories because the distinctive pigmentation of some species is enhanced. A cycloheximide-free medium is generally used for nails, and also recommended for soles and palms because nondermatophytic etiologic agents such as *Scytalidium* and *Fusarium* spp. must also be isolated from at least some of these sites. The most common of such media are plain Sabouraud's agar supplemented with antibacterials only, and two restrictive media: Littman oxgall agar and inhibitory mold agar. These media, unlike plain Sabouraud's agar, inhibit fast-growing contaminant molds from overgrowing the slower growing etiologic agents.

The characteristics and criteria used in identifying dermatophytes have been summarized.[20–22] Since most dermatophyte species are susceptible to similar therapies (duration of therapy may vary, e.g. between *Microsporum* spp. and the more rapidly inhibited endothrix *Trichophyton* spp. in tinea capitis), species identification is salient primarily to recognize situations in which animal hosts or familial or institutional carriers constitute potential sources of re-infection and continuation of outbreaks. Zoophilic dermatophyte species and the endothrix tinea capitis agents are most notorious in these situations, but unusual outbreaks of anthropophilic lower body dermatophytoses may also be detected and controlled through species identification.

Candidiasis in skin and nails is recognized in direct microscopy by the presence of budding yeast cells and candidal-type filaments; the yeast cells bud through a narrow constriction, unlike *Malassezia* yeasts, and the filaments give rise to budding cells on side branches, unlike dermatophyte filaments. Although filaments indicate an invasive condition in cutaneous candidiasis, and are usually found in any genuine case of infection, masses of budding cells alone may be seen in some nail specimens. In fingernails, this often indicates nearby paronychia that was not sampled directly. In some cases, however, especially with toenails, yeast cells merely indicate harmless growth of *Candida* spp. (other than *C. albicans*) of the normal skin flora in crevices in onychomycotic or traumatized nails. *Candida albicans* should normally be identified when isolated from skin; there are a number of inexpensive, specific, rapid tests for this species such as rice-tween, cornmeal-tween or oxgall medium tests for formation of chlamydospores under a cover slip. *Candida* spp. other than *C. albicans* need not be identified to species level from superficial sites except in rare cases in which they are isolated from material with conclusive evidence of invasive yeast infection (e.g. formation of filaments with lateral budding cells) in direct microscopy. Because *C. albicans* commonly contaminates moist dermatophyte lesions without significantly exacerbating symptoms, and because normal flora yeasts may proliferate harmlessly in nail crevices, the laboratory gold standard for any diagnosis of cutaneous yeast infection is the specific presence of yeast-type filamentous elements within cutaneous tissue in direct microscopy.

Tinea versicolor is recognized in direct microscopy by the rounded yeast cells and short hyphal fragments ('spaghetti and meat balls') of *Malassezia* spp. Culture is normally unnecessary and may be problematic when attempted. Although there is considerable research interest in quantitative cultural analysis of *Malassezia* spp. in seborrheic dermatitis, clinical diagnosis based on symptoms remains the gold standard.

Other purely microscopic diagnoses not requiring culture include black and white piedra. Tinea nigra evinces distinctive dark filaments in direct microscopy, but is also readily cultured to yield the etiologic agent, *H. werneckii*. No other organism shows melanized, two-celled

yeasts budding from annellidic apertures heavily fringed with collarette remnants. Mycology laboratories must also recognize the microscopically distinctive corynebacterial and actinomycetous elements found in erythrasma, trichomycosis axillaris and pitted keratolysis.[1] All intertriginous skin samples should be stained with methylene blue preparations to detect erythrasma. In specimens from this infection, methylene blue deeply stains delicate branching filaments less than 1 mm in diameter, often seen breaking up into smaller bacillary or coccoid forms. The poorly understood 'dermatophilus-like' agent of pitted keratolysis[1] also stains in methylene blue, and shows a mixture of coccoid cells and short filaments, at least some of which appear tapered and, in broader regions, subdivide to give rise to a second or third longitudinal series of cells. In trichomycosis axillaris, hair is heavily ensheathed in corynebacterial cells (gram-positive rod and coccus forms less than 1 mm in diameter). These may be readily distinguished in crushed preparation in hydroxide from the over 2 mm in diameter arthroconidia and yeast cells seen in the macroscopically similar white piedra.

The correct diagnosis of onychomycosis caused by nondermatophyte molds can be especially challenging. These nondermatophyte filamentous fungi can easily be ascertained as causing onychomycosis if distinctive morphologic elements such as conidiophores are seen in addition to filaments in direct microscopy of nail specimen, or if a fungus from warm latitudes, such as a *Scytalidium*, is isolated in an area in which only such fungi occur in infected patients. Most cases are more ambiguous. A fungal species such as *Aspergillus sydowii* may be isolated either as a contaminant or as an etiologic agent, and filaments seen in direct microscopy may be either nonviable dermatophyte elements or genuine nondermatophyte elements. Therefore, even exclusive and heavy isolation of such a nondermatophyte from a specimen positive for fungal filaments does not guarantee that the nail is infected by the same nondermatophyte.[10] The current gold standard, which may not be easy to attain in practice, is:

- first to demonstrate fungal elements in direct microscopy compatible with the suspected agent; and
- second, in culture, to show, through correlating the results of two nail samples collected at least 1 week apart, that the nondermatophyte in question consistently grows from the diseased nail.

True mixed infection by a dermatophyte and a nondermatophyte may occur, but again can only be demonstrated scientifically by showing a consistent presence of the latter in more than one serial sample.

Subcutaneous Fungal Pathogens

Although subcutaneous fungal infections exhibit extraordinary heterogeneity, they have certain features in common – infection is usually acquired from nature and not from infected humans or animals, and the endemic areas are delineated by an ecosystem that consists of altitude, temperature, rainfall, type of soil and type of vegetation. Most patients belong to low socioeconomic groups or live in rural areas. Subcutaneous mycoses arise from inoculation of soil or vegetation into the skin by minor trauma, and most patients have an occupation connected either with agriculture or an outdoor activity and do not use appropriate footwear.

The group of fungi that cause the majority of subcutaneous infections in humans are termed black molds.[2,23–25] Black molds are a heterogeneous group of darkly pigmented (dematiaceous) fungi, widely distributed in the environment, that occasionally cause infection in humans. The taxonomy and terminology of dematiaceous fungal infections is baffling. The term chromoblastomycosis was introduced in 1922 and was later modified in 1935 to a broader term 'chromomycosis'. More recently, the term 'phaeohyphomycosis' was proposed to cover 'all infections of cutaneous, subcutaneous and systemic nature caused by hyphomycetous fungi that develop in the host tissues in the form of dark walled dematiaceous septate mycelial elements'. In 1981, the term was further expanded to include deuteromycota and ascomycota whose tissue forms are filamentous and dematiaceous. This certainly excludes infections by fungi that produce thick-walled 'sclerotic bodies' in the tissues and are classically labeled as chromoblastomycosis. The line of demarcation is, however, only histopathologic and very thin because some of the fungi (e.g. *Exophiala dermatidis*), in addition to mycelial forms, produce rounded structures closely resembling sclerotic bodies. Thus, there has been plenty of overlap in the nomenclature of these cases, especially during the 1970s and 1980s.

The clinical spectrum of infection includes mycetomas, chromoblastomycosis, sinusitis and superficial, cutaneous, subcutaneous and systemic phaeohyphomycosis. During the past few years, there have been reports of infections caused by black molds in previously healthy individuals and in immunocompromised patients. Molecular studies have contributed to our understanding of the epidemiology of these infections. In addition, data on antifungal susceptibility tests have become available. Surgical excision and antifungal therapy (usually itraconazole) remain the standard treatment for these infections.

There are many extensive reviews of all the infections described here.[1–3,18,26,27] Specific references are cited here where new information, particularly concerning diagnosis and therapy, supersedes that found in the general texts. A special issue of *Medical Mycology* entitled: 'The dark world of black fungi – a major area of concern' reviews many topics outlined here.

NATURE

Chromoblastomycosis

Chromoblastomycosis (also known as chromomycosis, Carrión mycosis, Lane–Pedroso mycosis, verucoid dermatitis and black blastomycosis) is a term that describes a group of chronic localized infections of the skin and subcutaneous tissue, most often involving the limbs.[19,29,30] It is characterized by raised crusted lesions. It is most often caused by several species of brown-pigmented (dematiaceous) fungi.

Entomophthoramycosis

Rhinofacial conidiobolomycosis is a chronic mycosis affecting the subcutaneous tissues. It originates in the nasal sinuses and spreads to the adjacent subcutaneous tissue of the face, causing disfigurement. Basidiobolomycosis is a chronic subcutaneous infection of the trunk and limbs. For an exhaustive review of entomophthoramycosis, refer to Ribes *et al.*[20]

Lobomycosis

Lobomycosis, also known as keloidal blastomycosis or Lobo disease, is an uncommon and chronic subcutaneous mycosis. It is characterized by slowly developing, variably sized cutaneous nodules after a traumatic event. The dermal nodules manifest as smooth, verrucose or ulcerated surfaces that can attain the size of a small cauliflower-like keloid. The onset of the disease is generally insidious. The increase in size or number of lesions is a slow process, progressing over a period of 40–50 years. The lesions are composed of granulomatous inflammatory tissue containing numerous globose or subglobose to lemon-shaped, yeast-like fungal cells singly or in simple and branched chains.

Lobomycosis is a chronic dermal infection that presents a wide spectrum of clinical–dermatologic manifestations, mainly characterized by the development of keloid lesions as well as nodular, verrucoid and sometimes ulcerous forms. The etiologic agent at an international level, according to the consensus nomenclature, has been called *Loboa loboi*, even though recently it has been accommodated as *Lacazia loboi*.

Mycetoma

Mycetoma is a chronic suppurative infection of the skin, subcutaneous tissue and bone.[21] It usually affects the hand or foot and may be caused by various fungi (eumycetoma) or actinomycetes (actinomycetoma). The micro-organisms are inoculated into subcutaneous tissue by minor trauma. A characteristic feature of mycetoma is the production of grains in the infected tissue; these grains are compact masses of fungal or actinomycete elements and they discharge to the outside through sinus tracts.

Phaeohyphomycosis

Phaeohyphomycosis is a rare infection caused by dematiaceous fungi, involving the skin and subcutis, paranasal sinuses or central nervous system (CNS).[22] Phaeohyphomycosis refers to subcutaneous and deep-seated infections caused by brown-pigmented (dematiaceous) molds that adopt a septate mycelial form in tissue. This term was also created to separate various clinical infections caused by dematiaceous molds from the distinct subcutaneous infection known as chromoblastomycosis. Unlike mycetoma and chromoblastomycosis, phaeohyphomycosis is not limited to the skin or subcutaneous tissues, and elicits a wider variety of inflammatory responses.

Phaeohyphomycosis is characterized by a nodule, cyst or pyogranuloma. Histopathologically, the lesions show brown-walled hyphae in the dermis, subcutis or sometimes in the epidermis.

Rhinosporidiosis

Rhinosporidiosis is a chronic granulomatous infection of the mucous membranes caused by *Rhinosporidium seeberi*. The disease is characterized by the chronic and benign evolution of polyps that primarily affect the mucous membranes, especially the nostrils and ocular conjunctiva; visceral dissemination is rare.

Sporotrichosis

Sporotrichosis is a subacute or chronic infection caused by the dimorphic fungus *Sporothrix schenckii*. After implantation, this organism can cause cutaneous or subcutaneous infection, which commonly shows lymphatic spread. Occasionally, widespread disseminated infection also occurs.

EPIDEMIOLOGY

Chromoblastomycosis

Chromoblastomycosis is encountered mainly in arid parts of tropical and subtropical regions. Most cases occur in Central and South America, but chromoblastomycosis has also been reported in South Africa, Asia and Australia. Another major focus appears to be Madagascar.[17,29] Although common in rural areas, the disease lacks epidemic potential.

Chromoblastomycosis is caused by various dematiaceous fungi, to which a number of names have been given. There is therefore a great deal of confusion in the nomenclature used by various authors. The most frequently involved etiologic agents, beginning with the most common, are *Phialophora verrucosa*, *Fonsecaea pedrosoi*, *Fonsecaea compacta*, *Cladosporium carrionii* and *Rhinocladiella aquaspersa* (*Ramichloridium cerophilum*). Sporadic cases of chromoblastomycosis can also be caused by other dematiaceous molds. These organisms form characteristic thick-walled, dark brown muriform sclerotic cells in tissue.

The etiologic agents of chromoblastomycosis are widespread in the environment, being found in soil, wood and decomposing plant matter. Human infection usually follows the traumatic inoculation of the fungus into the skin. Minor trauma, such as cuts or wounds due to thorns or wood splinters, is often sufficient. The disease is most prevalent in rural parts of warmer climates where people go barefoot. There is no human-to-human transmission.

Chromoblastomycosis is unusual in children and adolescents. Except in Japan, men contract the disease much more frequently than women, reflecting the importance of occupational exposure. Men have a greater opportunity for soil contact and predisposition to injury while working in the fields. The majority are aged 30–50 years. The rarity of the disease in children exposed to the same environmental conditions as adults suggests a long period of latency.

Entomophthoramycosis

Entomophthoramycosis occurs mainly in the tropical rain forests of East and West Africa, South and Central America, and South East Asia.

Conidiobolus coronatus (*Entomophthora coronata*), the causative organism of rhinofacial conidiobolomycosis, lives as a saprophyte in soil and on decomposing plant matter in moist, warm climates. It can also parasitize certain insects.

A few cases of conidiobolomycosis have been caused by *Conidiobolus incongruus* which has been reported to affect the lower extremities.[30] This species rarely produces infections in humans but reported cases have involved deep structures such as lung, mediastinum, heart, liver and gastrointestinal tract.[30]

The most widely held view is that *Basidiobolus ranarum* is the sole agent causing basidiobolomycosis, and that *B. meristosporus* and *B. haptosporus* are synonyms of the former; not all authors are of this opinion, however. *Basidiobolus ranarum* has been recovered from soil and decaying vegetation; it has also been isolated from the gut of frogs, toads and lizards that had apparently swallowed infected insects. It is still uncertain how the disease is acquired and what is the length of incubation. Inoculation through a thorn prick or an insect bite has been suggested, as has contamination of a wound or other abrasion. The infection is most common in children. More detailed aspects of entomophthoramycosis caused by *B. ranarum* can be found in the review by Gugnani.[31]

For an exhaustive review of the epidemiology of entophthoramycosis, refer to Ribes *et al.*[20]

Lobomycosis

In lobomycosis, the onset of the disease is generally insidious and difficult to document. The increase in size and number of lesions is a slow process; it can take 40–50 years. This latency period often makes it important to note the patient's history of travel or stay in areas of endemicity to arrive at a proper diagnosis. The history often reveals the cause being a trauma, for example an arthropod sting, a snake bite, a cut from an instrument, or a wound acquired while cutting vegetation. The causal agent of lobomycosis appears to be saprobic in aquatic environments, which probably plays an extremely significant part in its life cycle. Recent reports have substantiated the Amazon basin as an endemic area for the disease.[32]

The human disease is endemic in the tropical zone of the New World. There have been isolated cases reported in Holland and a doubtful case in Bangladesh. Identification of the disease in dolphins widened the geographic distribution of the disease. Seven cases of lobomycosis involving two species of dolphins, namely marine dolphins (*Tursiops truncatus*) and marine freshwater dolphins (*Sotalia fluviatilis*), have been reported in Florida, the Texas coast, the Spanish–French coast, the South Brazilian coast and the Surinam River estuary. Although lobomycosis in dolphins has been reported in the USA, only one human case has been reported from the USA.[33] Although identification of the disease in dolphins has widened its known geographic distribution, the source of the organism is still unknown

All attempts to isolate the fungus from lesions of infected people have failed. In the dermis it appears as spheric or elliptic budding cells. Although it is accepted that the infection is exogenous in origin, the natural habitat of the causal fungus remains unknown.

The organism gains entry through the skin; it develops *in situ* for an unspecified period (several years) and then reaches the subcutaneous tissue. The disease is most prevalent in men aged 30–40 years; it is much less common in women and children.

Mycetoma

Mycetomas are most common in arid tropical and subtropical regions of Africa and Central America, particularly those areas bordering the great deserts.[2] However, sporadic cases have been reported from many parts of the world. The countries surrounding the Saharan and Arabian deserts form the most important endemic area, not only because of the number of new cases occurring each year, but also because of the diversity of causal organisms. Mycetoma is also endemic in certain regions of India and in Central and South America.

Mycetomas are caused by various actinomycetes and fungi that occur as saprophytes in the soil or on vegetation. Individual species of fungi or actinomycetes are often associated with particular geographic areas. About six species of fungi are common causes of eumycetoma and five aerobic actinomycetes are common etiologic agents of actinomycetoma. The geographic distribution of these environmental organisms is influenced by climate.

In the arid regions of the tropics and subtropics, the most frequent etiologic agents are *Madurella mycetomatis*, *Actinomadura madurae*, *Actinomadura pelletieri* and *Streptomyces somaliensis*. These organisms are encountered in the great deserts of Africa and Asia and on their fringes, as well as in south-eastern Europe. In the relatively humid mountain regions of Latin America, *Nocardia brasiliensis* is the predominant organism while *Madurella grisea* is a less prominent cause of infection.

In the occasional cases of mycetoma that occur in temperate regions, the principal isolates have been *Pseudallescheria boydii*, *A. madurae* and *M. mycetomatis*. Mycetomas occur more frequently in men than in women. Adults aged between 20 and 50 years are the most commonly affected, although cases in children have also been reported. Most patients come from rural districts in the tropics and subtropics, but cases often occur in some countries with a temperate climate, such as Romania.

Trauma is a critical factor in acquisition of the infection. The organisms may be implanted at the time of injury, or later as a result of secondary contamination of the wound. Traumas are often due to vegetable matter (grasses, wisps of straw, hay). In the tropics and subtropics thorny trees such as the acacia are abundant and are often used for fuel. Wounds caused by the thorns may facilitate the entry of soil organisms, or the causative agents may grow on the thorns and be implanted directly into the subcutaneous tissue. It is not surprising, therefore, that mycetomas affect mainly the feet of country-dwellers who walk barefoot.

The vast majority of organisms causing mycetomas are saprophytes of the external environment: *Nocardia* spp. exist in the soil; other species are encountered not only in the soil, but also on living and dead plants. However, little is known about their behavior outside the human host.

Phaeohyphomycosis

Black molds are widely encountered in soil and wood. In addition, some organisms can produce yeast-like synanamorphs that adapt to aqueous environments. Typically, the infection is acquired by the inoculation of the fungus through a penetrating injury. In addition, other possible portals of entry have been suggested, including the inhalation of spores with lung or sinus invasion, the ingestion of contaminated food or water with subsequent penetration through the gastrointestinal tract, contamination of the skin at the insertion of a vascular catheter, and contamination of the catheter itself. Some cases of systemic infection have no apparent portal of entry.

Phaeohyphomycosis has a worldwide distribution, but subcutaneous infection is most often seen in the rural population of tropical parts of Central and South America. Most cases of cerebral or paranasal sinus infection have been reported from the USA. There is little information on the incidence of phaeohyphomycosis. The number of organisms implicated as etiologic agents of phaeohyphomycosis is increasing. More than 80 different molds, classified in 40 different genera, have been incriminated. These fungi have often been given different names at different times, and there is therefore a great deal of confusion in the nomenclature used in different reports.

Among the more important etiologic agents, *Alternaria*, *Bipolaris*, *Curvularia*, *Exophiala*, *Exserohilum* and *Phialophora* spp. and *Xylohypha bantiana* can be included. Many of these organisms are found in soil or decomposing plant debris; others are plant pathogens.[34] The most important predisposing factor for cutaneous and subcutaneous infection is exposure to contaminated material present in the environment (decaying wood, plants).

Human infection follows inhalation or traumatic implantation of the fungus. In addition to these agents of phaeohyphomycosis, others are being reported. For example, *Colletotrichum* spp., which are common plant pathogens, have been reported as a cause of subcutaneous phaeohyphomycosis in patients undergoing chemotherapy for hematologic malignancies and may cause life-threatening phaeohyphomycosis in immunosuppressed patients.[35]

Rhinosporidiosis

Rhinosporidiosis is endemic in India[36] and Sri Lanka, where the incidence is estimated at 1.4% of the pediatric population, as well as in South America and Africa. Occasional cases have been reported from the USA, South East Asia and other parts of the world. Some arid countries of the Middle East also show a high incidence of the disease. The etiologic agent is an endosporulating organism, *Rhinosporidium seeberi*. So far, all attempts to isolate this fungus from lesions have failed. The life cycle of the parasite is complicated. In tissue, large, thick-walled sporangia (spherules) are formed. Large numbers of spores are produced within the sporangia and, when the spores are mature, they are released through a pore in the wall. Each spore may develop to form a new sporangium. Little is known about the natural habitat of *R. seeberi*, but it is believed that stagnant pools of water may be the source of human infection. The most prevalent location of the disease is the nasal cavity

The disease is most prevalent in rural districts, particularly among people working or bathing in stagnant water (such as rice fields). Men are more commonly affected than women. In arid countries most infections are ocular and dust is postulated to be a vector.

The disease affects mostly males (70–90%) and the incidence is greater in those aged between 20 and 40 years. Ocular infection is more prevalent in women, while nasal and nasopharyngeal infection preferentially affects males.

Sporotrichosis

Sporotrichosis is worldwide in distribution, but occurs most frequently in temperate humid climatic regions.[37] At present, the largest number of reported cases comes from the North American continent.[38] Other regions where the infection is endemic include South America,[38] South Africa and South East Asia.

The causative agent is a dimorphic fungus, *Sporothrix schenckii*, which is found in the soil and on plants and sphagnum moss. It grows in nature as a mycelium, but in tissue it forms small, budding cells.

It is not clear whether the infection is more common among men than women. Incidence in the different age groups is also variously assessed, but children are less often affected than adults.

Sporotrichosis caused by the dimorphic fungus *Sporothrix schenckii* is widely distributed throughout the world, especially in tropical and subtropical regions. Classically, infection is caused by traumatic inoculation of soil, plants and organic matter contaminated with the fungus, occasionally by inhalation. Some leisure and occupational activities such as agriculture and floriculture have been associated with transmission of the disease. To date, the largest epidemic of sporotrichosis occurred in Witwatersrand, South Africa, in the 1940s when about 3000 miners were infected from wood timbers in the mines. However, the literature about epidemics is scant and usually related to a common source of infection.[37,38]

Since 1998, the Infectious Diseases and Zoonosis Services of the Evandro Chagas Clinical Research Institute (IPEC), Oswaldo Cruz Foundation (Fiocruz), Brazil, have been diagnosing a growing number of cases of human and feline sporotrichosis emanating from the city of Rio de Janeiro and its surroundings.

Although the main clinical characteristics of human and feline sporotrichosis have been described elsewhere,[39] many questions related to the mechanism of zoonotic transmission and to the context in which this transmission occurs remain unanswered.

Recently, the role of felines in the transmission of sporotrichosis to humans has gained importance.[38] In Rio de Janeiro from 1998 to 2004, 759 humans, 64 dogs and 1503 cats were diagnosed with sporotrichosis. Of them, 85% of dogs and 83.4% of patients were reported to have had contact with cats with sporotrichosis, and 55.8% of the latter reported cat bites or scratches. Unusual manifestations were diagnosed in humans. Canine sporotrichosis presented as a self-limited mycosis. Feline sporotrichosis varied from subclinical infection to severe systemic disease with hematogenous dissemination of *Sporothrix schenckii*. The zoonotic potential of cats was demonstrated by the isolation of *S. schenckii* from skin lesion fragments and from material collected from their nasal and oral cavities. An accompanying editorial commentary on this report has been published by Hay & Morris-Jones.[37]

PATHOGENICITY

Chromoblastomycosis

The causative fungi require implantation through the skin into subcutaneous tissue. The lesion appears at the site of skin trauma or puncture wound. However, the inoculation may have occurred so long before that no history of injury can be elicited. In general, the disease remains localized to the area surrounding the initial infection. In rare cases, hematogenous spread to the brain, lymph nodes, liver, lungs and other organs is observed.

Entomophthoramycosis

Pathogenicity of the causal organisms is a reflection of inoculum size and frequency of exposure in endemic areas. For an exhaustive review of the pathogenicity of the agents causing entomophthoramycosis, refer to Ribes *et al.*[20]

Lobomycosis

Lobomycosis develops following trauma to the skin, but in most clinical histories the event is so minimal that it is not remembered. The disease runs an extremely slow course and years may elapse before the patient seeks medical advice. The organism has been transmitted successfully to an armadillo and to tortoises. In addition, the infection has been maintained through nine generations in the footpads of mice. Most of our knowledge of the etiologic agent of lobomycosis is derived from histopathologic and electron microscopy studies.[27]

The fungus is abundant in lobomycotic skin lesions. It is a remarkably homogenous, spherical intracellular yeast, 5–12 μm in diameter. *L. loboi* is predominantly an intracellular pathogen. Organisms, singly or in chains, reside predominantly in macrophage vacuoles. They probably reproduce by budding; linear or radiating chains of as many as 20 organisms linked by tubules have been observed.[27]

Mycetoma and phaeohyphomycosis

The organisms causing these conditions are not regarded as being pathogenic. Typically, the infection is acquired by the inoculation of the fungus through a penetrating injury

Rhinosporidiosis

Studies on the virulence of *R. seeberi* have not been carried out. Nothing is known about the mode of infection. It is most likely that trauma is an essential factor in the initiation of disease. Spores of *R. seeberi* are not able to penetrate intact epithelium. Because the nose and eyes are the most common sites of the disease it is suggested that the organisms are transmitted in dust and water.

Sporotrichosis

Sporothrix schenckii usually enters the body through traumatic implantation, but occasionally the fungus is introduced through inhalation of the conidia. Because the infection can also be hematogenously disseminated, it may be that the yeast cells are able to resist phagocytosis and intracellular killing by host effector cells, although *in-vitro* data suggest that the yeast cells are readily killed in the presence of human serum. Host defense mechanisms in response to *S. schenckii* have not been extensively studied.

For many years it has been known that the epidemiology of *S. schenckii* may change with time. The observation has also been made that the human population is now more resistant through better nutrition and living standards or reduced contact with environmental spores. There is also some evidence that phenotypic changes may occur that could affect the ability of *Sporothrix* to infect. Findlay & Vismer[40] showed that when natural isolates of *Sporothrix* were grown in culture media containing a wood source, the fungus became a much more prolific producer of conidia. It has been suggested that wood may enhance the invasive potential of *Sporothrix*. An additional view is that the production of melanin by *Sporothrix* may enhance the ability of the fungus to scavenge free oxidative radicals from host phagocytic cells.[41] *Sporothrix schenckii* conidia and yeast forms can synthesize melanin in the external environment.[41]

PREVENTION

Avoidance of skin penetration is the best means of preventing chromoblastomycosis, entomophthoramycosis and phaeohyphomycosis. Suitable footwear will help to prevent chromoblastomycosis.

Very little is known about the ecology of *Loboa loboi*. However, the agent is probably introduced directly into the dermis through a penetrating injury, such as a thorn prick or an insect bite, or close, abrasive contact with a dolphin. In areas where infections have been reported it would be advisable to avoid penetrating injuries.

The causative agents of mycetoma normally live as saprophytes in the soil. Because the most common site for mycetoma is the foot it is reasonable to assume that the wearing of appropriate footwear would prevent infection. Avoidance of trauma to the hands and other areas is difficult to encourage because most infections seem to be related to outdoor activities.

Rhinosporidiosis can be prevented by avoiding eye and nose contact with contaminated dust and water.

Occupations that predispose persons to sporotrichosis include gardening, farming, masonry, floral work, outdoor labor and other activities involving exposure to contaminated soil or vegetation such as sphagnum moss or roses. Wearing gloves and protective clothing while carrying out these activities may therefore prevent traumatic implantation of the fungus through the skin.

DIAGNOSTIC MICROBIOLOGY

Chromoblastomycosis

Microscopic examination of wet preparations of pus, scrapings or crusts from lesions can permit the diagnosis of chromoblastomycosis if clusters of the characteristic small, round, thick-walled, brown-pigmented

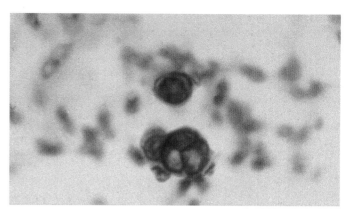

Fig. 179.1 Chromoblastomycosis. Thick-walled, septate, dematiaceous muriform cells. With permission from Richardson MD, *et al*. Slide atlas of fungal infection: subcutaneous and unusual fungal infections, Oxford: Blackwell, 1995.

sclerotic cells are seen (Fig. 179.1). These cells are often divided by longitudinal and transverse septa.

The definitive diagnosis of chromoblastomycosis depends on the isolation of the etiologic agent in culture. Identification of the individual etiologic agents is difficult.

Entomophthoramycosis

Microscopic examination of smears or tissue from the nasal mucosa will reveal broad, nonseptate, thin-walled mycelial filaments.

The culture of causal organisms of entomophthoramycosis is difficult. To optimize the recovery of fungus from clinical material, specimens must be inoculated on the largest possible number of media.

For an exhaustive review of the diagnosis of entomophthoramycosis, refer to Ribes *et al.*[20]

Lobomycosis

The etiologic agent of lobomycosis is an obligate pathogen of humans and lower mammals that has yet to be isolated and grown *in vitro*; therefore, nothing is known of its basic cultural characteristics and growth. Diagnosis is based on demonstrating the presence of globose, thick-walled, yeast-like cells ranging from 5 to 12 μm in diameter in lesion exudate or tissue sections. The organism multiplies by budding and thus mother cells with single buds are often observed. However, characteristic sequential budding leads to the production of chains of cells that are linked to each other by a tubular connection, or isthmus. Budding may occur at more than one point on a cell, giving rise to branched or radiating chains of cells. These thick-walled, hyaline, spherical cells with chains of cells interconnected by tubular connections are the basis on which a diagnosis of lobomycosis rests. The thick-walled, budding hyaline cells with catenate chains of conidia can be readily observed in tissue smears or exudates mounted in 10% potassium hydroxide or in calcofluor white preparations. Tissue sections can be stained with the use of periodic acid–Schiff digest, Grocott–Gomori methenamine-silver nitrate or Gram stains.

Microscopic examination of specimens of pathologic material will reveal numerous hyaline, round or ovoid cells with an average diameter of 9 μm (Fig. 179.2). These cells closely resemble the yeast forms of *Paracoccidioides brasiliensis* or *Histoplasma duboisii*. The cells are enclosed in a double-contoured membrane and are capable of budding. They often form chains and appear to be joined together by bridge-like structures within the chain. If the individual elements show multiple budding, the chains are divided into branches.

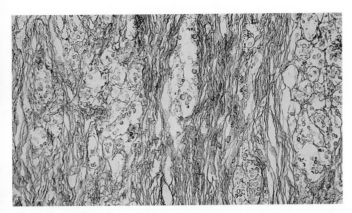

Fig. 179.2 Lobomycosis. Yeast cells are attached to each other in short chains. Nonbudding and single-budding cells are also present.

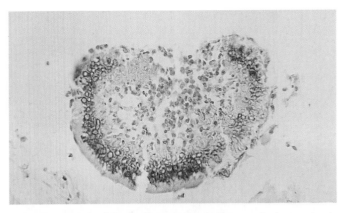

Fig. 179.3 Granule of *Madurella mycetomatis*. The granules have a deeply pigmented periphery of compact hyphae. Randomly oriented, poorly pigmented fungal elements in the interior of the granule are less compact.

Loboa loboi has never been successfully cultured. This distinguishes it from *P. brasiliensis*, which it closely resembles morphologically. The globose and subglobose budding cells of *L. loboi* resemble budding cells of *P. brasiliensis* in tissue. However, the central mother cells of *P. brasiliensis* become large and thick-walled compared to the daughter cells, which remain smaller. In contrast, yeast cells of *L. loboi* remain consistent in diameter, giving rise to branching chains of blastoconidia. In addition, the cell wall of *L. loboi* contains constitutive melanin,[42] which can be detected by the use of the Fontana–Masson histologic stain. The walls of cells of *P. brasiliensis* are not known to contain melanin. *Loboa loboi* has never been cultured *in vitro*. On the other hand, *P. brasiliensis* can be grown in artificial culture and is known to be a dimorphic pathogen.

Serologic tests have high sensitivity but lack specificity because of antigenic cross-reactivity with fungi from the genus *Paracoccidioides*.[27]

Molecular methods have been used in an attempt to characterize the causative agent of lobomycosis.[42,43] Fungal-specific primers targeted for highly conserved genomic nucleic acid sequences were used in a polymerase chain reaction (PCR) to amplify DNA from lobomycosis lesions in a bottlenose dolphin. Sequence alignments of this DNA possessed high homology to fungal ribosomal DNA sequences found in the genus *Cladosporium*. When used for *in-situ* hybridization, the riboprobe transcribed from a cloned PCR-generated fragment bound to *L. loboi* cells. These results support the hypothesis that *L. loboi* in dolphin tissue is a fungus.

A new monotypic genus, *Lacazia*, with *Lacazia loboi* as the type species, was recently proposed[42,43] to accommodate the obligate etiologic agent of lobomycosis in mammals. The continued placement of *L. loboi* in the genus *Paracoccidioides* as *Paracoccidioides loboi* O.M. Fonseca et Lacaz was found to be taxonomically inappropriate. The older name *Loboa loboi* Ciferri *et al.* was considered to be a synonym of *P. brasiliensis*.

Mycetoma

The diagnosis of mycetoma depends on the identification of grains. These should, if possible, be obtained by puncture from a softened, but not ulcerated, nodule with a syringe. Failing this, grains can be obtained with a dissecting needle or by aspiration from the secretion flowing from a sinus.[44] If there is no pus flowing from the lesion, small fragments of tissue should be removed. If possible, between 20 and 30 grains should be obtained; these should be rinsed in sterile saline before being cultured.

Gross examination of the grains may give a clue to the etiologic diagnosis. Black grains suggest a fungal infection, minute white grains often indicate a *Nocardia* infection, and larger white grains the size of a pinhead may be of either fungal or actinomycotic origin. Small, red grains are specific to *Actinomadura pelletieri*, but yellowish-white grains may be actinomycotic or fungal in origin. Their shape, consistency and structure must be carefully determined.

Direct microscopic examination will confirm the diagnosis of mycetoma and will also reveal whether the causative organism is a fungus or an actinomycete.[44] Actinomycotic grains contain very fine filaments (<1 μm diameter), whereas fungal grains contain short hyphae (2–4 μm diameter), which are sometimes swollen. This can be seen by direct microscopic examination of crushed grains in potassium hydroxide, but it is much more readily observed in stained histologic sections (Fig. 179.3).

Although the identification of the causal agents of mycetoma can often be deduced from the morphologic characteristics of the grains, it is also important to isolate the organism in culture. Agar plates should be inoculated with several grains (or with secretion or tissue fragments). Cultures should be retained for up to 6 weeks before being discarded. The actinomycetes grow much more slowly than the fungi.

Madurella mycetomatis is the commonest cause of eumycetoma in Sudan and other countries in tropical Africa. Currently, the early diagnosis of mycetoma is difficult. In attempting to improve the identification of *M. mycetomatis* and, consequently, the diagnosis of mycetoma, a specific oligonucleotide primer based on the sequence of the internal transcribed spacer (ITS) regions spacing the genes encoding the fungal ribosomal RNAs has been described.[45] More recently, the molecular identification of black-grain mycetomas has been reported.[46]

Phaeohyphomycosis

One common factor among these fungi is their melanin formation in the cell wall in culture and, in most cases, in human tissue. Microscopic examination of stained histopathologic sections or wet preparations of clinical material, such as pus or skin scrapings, can permit the diagnosis of phaeohyphomycosis if brown-pigmented septate mycelium with occasional branching is seen (Fig. 179.4).

Identification of the etiologic agent is essential for correct management, and this depends on its isolation in culture.[34] No serologic tests are available.

Rhinosporidiosis

Microscopy of clinical material reveals round or ovoid organisms that, depending on age, vary in diameter with a prominent wall.[47-49] These mature forms are known as sporangia. Sporangia measure up to 350 mm in diameter and have a cell wall measuring about 5 mm. The sporangia may be filled with up to 12 000 endospores, 7–15 μm in diameter (Fig. 179.5). The immature forms of the organism are known as trophocytes; they are smaller than sporangia, have a relatively thinner wall and do not contain endospores. Trophocytes mature into sporangia. Endospores develop within sporangia. Endospores are released

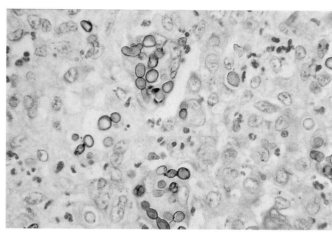

Fig. 179.4 Subcutaneous phaeohyphomycosis caused by *Bipolaris spicifera*. The fungal elements are stained with Fontana–Masson, which accentuates and confirms the presence of melanin or melanin-like pigment in the fungal cell walls.

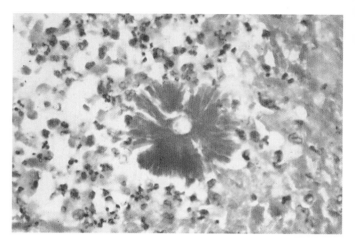

Fig. 179.6 Asteroid body in cutaneous sporotrichosis. A yeast-like cell of *Sporothrix schenckii* with faintly basophilic, retracted cytoplasm is intimately surrounded by elongated spicules of Splendore–Hoeppli material.

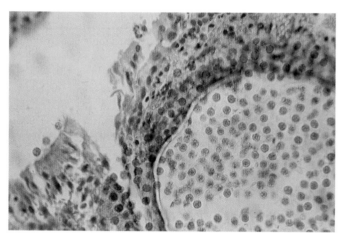

Fig. 179.5 Rhinosporidiosis.

upon maturity and thereafter develop into trophocytes. The organisms are abundant and appear in various sizes and stages of development. It is not necessary to perform special staining because of the size of the agent.

Rhinosporidium seeberi has traditionally been classified as a fungus on the basis of morphologic and histochemical characteristics. Recent molecular studies have generated conflicting results.[27,50] The organism may be either a cyanobacterium or a protist. Using consensus PCR, a portion of the *R. seeberi* 18S rRNA gene directly from infected tissue has been amplified.[51] Analysis of the aligned sequence and inference of phylogenetic relationships showed that *R. seeberi* is a protist from a novel clade of parasites that infect fish and amphibians. Fluorescent *in-situ* hybridization and *R. seeberi*-specific PCR showed that this unique 18S rRNA sequence is also present in other tissues infected with *R. seeberi*. These data support the *R. seeberi* phylogeny recently suggested by others. *Rhinosporidium seeberi* is not a classic fungus, but rather the first known human pathogen on the basis of a previously aligned dataset of the DRIPs clade (named after the organisms *Dermocystidium*, the rosette agent, *Ichthyophonus* and *Psorospermium*), a novel clade of aquatic protistan parasites (*Ichthyosporea*).

Immunologic methods have been used to identify the causal agent of rhinosporidiosis *in situ* where the immunolocalization of *R. seeberi* antigens using sera from individuals infected with *R. seeberi* and tissue from Sri Lankan patients with rhinosporidiosis was determined by electron microscopy.[52] This study found that the expression of this antigen occurs only in the final developmental stages of *R. seeberi* mature sporangia. The data may explain why circulating antibodies to

R. seeberi were not detected previously in studies that used endospores as antigen in immunoassays. This appears to be the first report in which an antigenic material with a potential role in the immunology of rhinosporidiosis has been described.

Sporotrichosis

Direct examination of clinical material, such as pus or tissue, is often disappointing because the organism is seldom abundant. However, it can be of value if conducted with painstaking care. The detection of typical ovoid or cigar-shaped cells or asteroid bodies of *S. schenckii* will confirm the diagnosis (Fig. 179.6).

The definitive diagnosis of sporotrichosis depends on the isolation of the etiologic agent in culture. Identifiable mycelial colonies will appear in 2–5 days. The color usually changes from cream or light brown to dark brown or black with age. Confirmation of the identification depends on the morphologic characteristics of the mycelial form and its conversion to the yeast form.

CLINICAL MANIFESTATIONS

Chromoblastomycosis

The lesions of chromoblastomycosis are usually unilateral and occur mainly on the exposed parts of the body, particularly the feet and lower legs.[17,29,53] Other less common sites include the hands, arms, shoulders and neck. The initial lesion is a painless papule or nodule on an erythematous and occasionally verrucous base. The condition may also present as an abscess surrounded by infiltration or as a psoriasiform lesion with erythema and scaling. As the disease develops, the affected limb becomes enlarged. Small satellite nodules may occur at the edge of the original lesion. Itching often occurs and may be severe.

The primary lesion develops very slowly, its diameter increasing by only 1–2 mm per year. It is firm and elastic in consistency and colored red or violet verging on gray. There is a warty, papillomatous margin surrounding a center that may be flat, smooth or scaly, with areas of scarring.

Later in the disease, the lesion may become pedunculated or ulcerated (if bacterial superinfection occurs). However, the lesions usually retain a warty, dry character.

Secondary lesions may appear, especially along the lymphatics draining the site of infection; here again, development is slow and symptoms are few. The lymph nodes are only involved if there is superimposed bacterial infection.

In endemic areas the unilateral development of vegetative, atrophic and scarred lesions on a lower limb is suggestive of chromoblastomycosis. The condition must be distinguished from a number of other fungal infections including blastomycosis, lobomycosis, paracoccidioidomycosis, phaeohyphomycosis, rhinosporidiosis and sporotrichosis. It must also be differentiated from prototh ecosis, leishmaniasis, verrucous tuberculosis, certain leprous lesions and syphilis. On the upper limbs the erythematosquamous lesions can be confused with psoriasis or subacute or discoid lupus erythematosus. Mycologic and histologic investigations are indispensable for confirmation of the diagnosis.

Entomophthoramycosis

Entomophthoramycosis is a chronic subcutaneous infection of the trunk and limbs. The subcutaneous swelling that characterizes this disease is usually localized to the buttock and thighs, but may also be found on the arm, leg or shoulder.

The initial swelling may be rapid or slow in onset and is hard and painless. The spread is slow but relentless, and a large mass is formed that is attached to the skin but not to the underlying tissue (unlike *Conidiobolus* infection). This is a disfiguring infection, but the skin covering the lesions does not ulcerate. Lymphatic obstruction may occur and can result in massive lymphedema. There is no functional impairment as long as the joints are not blocked by the volume of the swellings. The underlying bone and joints are not affected by the disease.

The disease is most common among adult males, particularly those living or working in tropical rain forests. Infection is acquired through inhalation of spores or their introduction into the nasal cavities by soiled hands.

Very rarely, *B. ranarum* can cause gastrointestinal basidiobolomycosis.[31]

Conidiobolus infection generally begins with unilateral involvement of the nasal mucosa. The most common nasal symptom is obstruction, but frequent nose bleeding can occur and is evidence of the development of a nasal polyp in the anterior region of the inferior turbinate. Subcutaneous nodules then develop in the nasal and perinasal regions and may be associated with epidermal lesions.

The spread of the infection is slow but relentless. It is usually confined to the face, and the development of gross facial swelling involving the forehead, periorbital region and upper lip is very distinctive. As a rule, the lesions are firmly attached to the underlying tissue, although the bone is spared. The skin remains intact. Spread to the lymph nodes has been reported. Even if, in advanced cases, the diagnosis is obvious from the appearance, mycologic and histologic examinations are essential for its confirmation.

The disease can be diagnosed with confidence on the basis of appearance and the results of the mycologic and (in particular) the histologic examination. Specimens must be taken from the subcutaneous tissue where the infection develops.

For an exhaustive review of the clinical manifestations of entomophthoramycosis, refer to Ribes *et al.*[20]

Lobomycosis

Lobomycosis is an indolent infection that first manifests as a papule or small nodule of normal pink skin color or with a grayish tinge. The nodule then proliferates and, by partial or total coalescence, may form extensive multilobar lesions. The disease spreads by peripheral extension or autoinoculation from scratching, or it may follow the draining lymphatics, especially in elderly people. Because of the slow growth of lobomycosis lesions, patients do not present themselves for treatment until many years have passed and usually after the lesions have become large.

The lesions are located in the dermis and subcutis and may form massive tumors, which are firm and resistant to pressure at the outset, but which later become hard and fibrous and resemble a keloid. The typical keloid-like skin lesions appear only after several months. If there is ulceration, depressed scars may remain; their surface is smooth and shiny in places, owing to atrophy of the underlying epidermis, and wrinkled and fissured elsewhere.

The disease may be symptomless or cause itching and burning, and trauma to the affected area may be especially painful. The most common sites of infection are the coolest parts of the body – the limbs, face, ears and buttocks. Differentiation of keloidiform lesions on the ears from lepromatous leprosy is difficult, but in lobomycosis the presentation is unilateral. The lesions may cover a whole limb. If the head is involved, the patient may be so grossly disfigured as to be completely excluded from social life. With a few exceptions there are no adenopathies. No deaths from lobomycosis have been reported.

Lesions may be keloid scars or irregular fibrous changes of the skin without secretion. Leprosy, leishmaniasis and chromoblastomycosis can produce similar lesions. Mycologic and histologic examination will confirm the diagnosis.

Mycetoma

Mycetoma is a chronic, suppurative infection of the subcutaneous tissue and contiguous bones. The lesion appears to begin at a site of minor trauma and continues to spread locally over the ensuing months and years.

The clinical features of the disease are fairly uniform, regardless of the type of organism causing it. Eumycetoma follows a slower and generally less destructive course than actinomycetoma. Spread to the internal organs and involvement of the regional lymph nodes is rare, occurring in no more than 2–5% of cases.

The feet are by far the most common site of involvement and account for two-thirds or more of cases. Other sites include the lower legs, hands, head, neck, chest, shoulder, arms and abdomen.

In most cases, the first sign of the disease is a small, hard, usually painless, subcutaneous nodule that is not attached to the underlying tissue. It is covered by taut thinned skin, which is reddish-violet in color. A number of small nodules may coalesce to form a larger and frequently multilobar nodule.

Over the ensuing months the nodule begins to soften on the surface, caves in, ulcerates and partly empties, discharging a viscous, purulent fluid containing grains. If there is little fluid, the grains may not escape. The lesion then broadens out at the surface and also spreads inward to infect muscles and bones. The lesions, which are covered with depigmented and scarred skin, present as swellings, which are often covered with a crust. Later, the lesions develop sinus tracts that discharge pus and blood containing the characteristic grains.

The infection slowly spreads to adjacent tissue, including bone; this often causes considerable deformity. Mycetomas of the feet make the arches convex, thus preventing the toes from touching the ground. However, the general health of the patient is not affected. Pain, burning and pruritus may occur but are usually mild. Depending on the location and size of the lesion, and also on whether there is any bone involvement, limb function may be impaired.

Radiologic examination is useful in determining the extent of bone destruction. Abnormalities include periosteal reactions, sclerosis, endosteal reactions, cortical erosions and joint destruction. CT scanning is also helpful in delineating the extent of lesions.

Bacterial superinfection is not uncommon and is largely responsible for adenopathies and impairment of the general health. Visceral and especially cerebral metastases are the most serious complications; they cause cachexia and are often fatal. Fortunately, they are rare.

In most cases, the diagnosis of mycetoma of the feet presents no problems, but it may be difficult if other body sites are involved, particularly in regions where the disease is not endemic and if no grains have been discharged at the time of examination.

The characteristic feature of mycetoma is the presence in a fistulated swelling of grains that are found to contain actinomycotic or fungal filaments. This finding distinguishes mycetoma from chromoblastomycosis, cutaneous tuberculosis, certain syphilitic or leprous lesions, botryomycosis and other conditions.

Phaeohyphomycosis

Phaeohyphomycosis can be divided into a number of distinct clinical forms, including cutaneous and subcutaneous infection, paranasal sinus infection, cerebral infection and invasive and systemic disease.[54] The disease spectrum of noncutaneous phaeohyphomycosis includes sinusitis, pulmonary disease, CNS infection, ocular disease, arthritis, osteomyelitis, fungemia, endocarditis, peritonitis and gastrointestinal disease.

Subcutaneous phaeohyphomycosis

Subcutaneous phaeohyphomycosis usually follows the traumatic implantation of the fungus into the subcutaneous tissue. Minor trauma, such as cuts or wounds from thorns or wood splinters, is often sufficient. The principal etiologic agents include *E. jeanselmei*, *Exophiala spinifera*, *Exophiala dermatitidis* (*Wangiella dermatitidis*), *Phialophora richardsiae* and *Phialophora parasitica*.[54]

The lesions occur mainly on the arms and legs. Other less common sites include the buttocks, neck and face. The initial lesion is a firm, sometimes tender, subcutaneous nodule that may enlarge slowly to form a painless cystic abscess. Lesions are attached to the skin but not to the underlying tissue or bone. Unless the cyst ruptures, the overlying skin remains unaffected. In immunosuppressed patients with subcutaneous phaeohyphomycosis, the lesions are more likely to drain through sinuses.

Phaeohyphomycosis in transplant recipients

Infection of subcutaneous tissue by black fungi has only been reported in six transplant patients, all of whom were solid organ recipients.[55] These patients presented with indolent, localized infections at least 1 year after transplant, while on maintenance immunosuppressive regimens. They were cured by surgical resection, either alone or in conjunction with antifungal agents. A further case report illustrates the features of subcutaneous phaeohyphomycosis occurring in a bone marrow transplant recipient receiving high doses of immunosuppressive agents, in whom widespread subcutaneous infection due to *E. jeanselmei* was not eradicated by repeated resections and therapy with amphotericin B and flucytosine.[56] The infection was eventually cured after the addition of itraconazole to the therapeutic regimen. Results of *in-vitro* testing of the isolate for susceptibility to a combination of amphotericin B, flucytosine and itraconazole confirmed the potential role of combination antifungal therapy in the setting of refractory infection.

Local recurrence of subcutaneous phaeohyphomycosis in transplant recipients after medication or surgical treatment is also seen.

Paranasal sinus infection

This form of phaeohyphomycosis is becoming more common. The principal etiologic agents include *Alternaria* spp., *Bipolaris spicifera*, *Bipolaris hawaiiensis*, *Curvularia lunata* and *Exserohilum rostratum*.

It is a slowly progressive condition that may remain confined to the sinuses or spread to contiguous structures. Affected people usually complain of longstanding symptoms of allergic rhinitis, nasal polyps or intermittent sinus pain. Patients present with nasal obstruction and facial pain, with or without proptosis. The sinuses are filled with a thick, dark, tenacious, inspissated mucus.

CT scanning is the best method for evaluating the extent of the infection. The typical finding is a large mass filling one or more of the sinuses.

Alternaria and *Curvularia* spp. occasionally cause necrotic lesions of the nasal septum in patients with leukemia or AIDS.

Cerebral phaeohyphomycosis

This form of phaeohyphomycosis may follow hematogenous dissemination of infection from the lungs, or it may result from direct spread from the nasal sinuses. Involvement of the CNS carries a poor prognosis. The routes of infection have not been clearly established, but the most likely port of entry seems to be the respiratory tract, although direct inoculation into the brain and extension from the sinuses, ear and pulmonary infections have also been reported. Most cases are due to *X. bantiana* (*Cladosporium trichoides*). Other etiologic agents include *Bipolaris* spp. and *E. dermatitidis*. Many cases of cerebral infection with *X. bantiana* have occurred in people with no obvious predisposing factors.

The symptoms of cerebral phaeohyphomycosis are gradual in onset. Persistent headache is the most common presenting symptom. The most frequent clinical findings include focal neurologic signs, hemiparesis and fits. Fever is minimal or absent. Chest radiographs are normal.

CT scans of the head will often reveal a unilateral, well-circumscribed lesion, with the frontal lobes of the brain being the most common location. Cerebrospinal fluid (CSF) findings are varied. The opening pressure may be raised, the protein concentration may be increased, the glucose concentration may be reduced, and pleocytosis may be present. It is most unusual to recover the fungus from the CSF. The diagnosis is seldom established until neurologic resection is performed.

Cutaneous infection

Alternaria spp. and *Exophiala spinifera* have been seen in and isolated from crusted, ulcerated or scaling skin lesions.[54] Many of these infections have followed traumatic implantation and a substantial proportion have occurred in leukemic patients or transplant recipients. The arms and legs are the more common sites of infection.

Other forms of phaeohyphomycosis

Dematiaceous molds have caused endocarditis after valve insertion or replacement, and peritonitis in patients on continuous peritoneal dialysis.[2] Fungemia due to black fungi is unusual.[22] Fever without a clear source of infection is the most frequent presentation. In a series of 23 cases occurring in a tertiary hospital, fever was the most frequent clinical manifestation, and only one patient developed signs of deep-seated infection, with a clinical picture of necrotizing pneumonia similar to that caused by *Aspergillus* spp.[22]

The lesions of subcutaneous phaeohyphomycosis can be confused with the small initial lesions of chromoblastomycosis, sporotrichosis, blastomycosis, coccidioidomycosis and paracoccidioidomycosis, as well as with cutaneous leishmaniasis. Lymphangitic spread of sporotrichosis and the development of verrucous lesions in the other conditions makes the distinction easier.

In people who are not immunosuppressed, the clinical presentation of phaeohyphomycosis of the paranasal sinuses cannot be distinguished from that of *Aspergillus* infection. In immunosuppressed patients, *Aspergillus* sinusitis is a fulminant and often lethal condition, unlike phaeohyphomycotic sinusitis. However, both groups of organisms can cause black necrotic lesions of the nasal septum.

Bacterial brain abscess is the most common initial diagnosis in patients with cerebral phaeohyphomycosis. In occasional patients, the diagnosis of cryptococcosis, histoplasmosis, coccidioidomycosis or sporotrichosis must be excluded.

Rhinosporidiosis

Rhinosporidium seeberi causes the production of large polyps or wart-like lesions that occur predominantly on the mucous membranes. The nasal mucosa is affected in more than 70% of cases. The onset of the disease in the nose is insidious and the patient remains unaware of its presence until symptoms of obstruction develop. In some cases, the patient complains of itching and unilateral coryza. Rhinoscopic examination will reveal papular or nodular smooth-surfaced lesions that gradually become pedunculated and acquire a papillomatous or proliferative appearance. They are pink, red or violet in color. The polyps may obstruct the nasal passages, particularly in the event of even slight trauma. If located low in the nostril, they may protrude and hang onto the upper lips. If they are sited in the posterior part of the fossa, they may partially obstruct the pharynx or larynx and cause dysphagia or dysphonia and dyspnea.

In some cases the eyes are affected, the lesions being located on the conjunctiva. Initially these are small, flat granulations that may grow to form multilobed polyps of a pale pink color. At the same time there is diffuse vascular dilatation, photophobia and lacrimation, which is often due to involvement of the lacrimal sac and duct.

The ears may also become involved; depending on their size and location, these polyps may impair hearing.

Lesions may also develop on the male genital organs (the penis and, in exceptional cases, the urethra) and on the vulva and vagina in women. They may resemble flat or acuminate condylomas; lesions in the anus present as polyps and may sometimes be mistaken for hemorrhoids.

Cutaneous rhinosporidiosis, which is very rare, is generally due to spread from a neighboring mucosal lesion. It presents initially as minute papillomas; these gradually become larger and pedunculated. The surface is irregular, verrucous and polypous.

Cutaneous lesions are usually asymptomatic, but depending on their location (especially if they are on the sole of the foot) or their size they may cause pain. The surface of ulcerated rhinosporidiosis lesions is dotted with white spots, which are more readily discerned when depressed with a glass spatula; on microscopy these are seen to be sporangia.

Dissemination to the internal organs or bones is rare. In most cases the general health of the patient is unimpaired.

The appearance of pedunculated or unpedunculated polyps or nodules covered with white dots on the nasal mucosa or the conjunctiva should suggest the diagnosis of rhinosporidiosis. The condition must be distinguished from cryptococcosis, cutaneous tuberculosis, leprous lesions, leishmaniasis, treponematoses, and myospherulosis, an iatrogenic condition related to the application of nasal substances.

Sporotrichosis

The clinical manifestations of sporotrichosis are rather variable, which helps to explain the large number of different classification schemes that have been proposed.[57] The most common clinical presentation is a localized cutaneous or subcutaneous lesion. Lymphatic spread may then lead to the development of further cutaneous lesions. Much less commonly, the fungus may cause infection of the lungs, joints, bones, eyes and meninges. Widespread disseminated infection has been reported in patients with diabetes, alcoholics, drug abusers and patients with AIDS.

Cutaneous sporotrichosis

Cutaneous sporotrichosis tends to affect exposed sites, mainly the limbs and especially the hands and fingers. The right hand is affected more frequently than the left. The initial lesion develops at the site of implantation of the fungus. It is a painless nodule that is movable at first but that later becomes attached to the neighboring tissue. The skin turns red then violaceous, and the nodule breaks down to form an ulcer, which discharges a serous or purulent fluid. The edge of the ulcer is often irregular and it may become edematous, vegetative and crusted.

After a period of a few days to several weeks, the primary lesion may become surrounded by satellite lesions, or further nodules along the course of the draining lymphatics may develop. These soon become palpable and ulcerate through to the skin. In most cases, however, the lymphangitis heals or remains static for a long time without ulcers forming. In most cases the regional lymph nodes are not involved. However, this is not an invariable rule. Any involvement of these lymph nodes is evidence of a superimposed bacterial infection and they may ulcerate in turn.

Apart from these very typical lesions, sporotrichosis may present a different clinical picture. Extension over large areas of skin, often described as the disseminated cutaneous form, may occur. Flat, infiltrated or papulopustular or nodulopustular lesions may develop. Whether oozing, proliferative, papillomatous or verrucous, the lesions of sporotrichosis are generally painless but often pruritic. Several ulcers may be interconnected by subcutaneous fistular passages. Confluent lesions may form a purulent and warty plaque with a continually expanding margin, whereas the center becomes atrophied, smooth and shiny.

Primary cutaneous lesions may heal spontaneously, leaving behind unsightly and even disfiguring scars, which may be a functional impediment. However, secondary lesions may persist for several years.

Extracutaneous sporotrichosis

Pulmonary sporotrichosis is a rare but well-recognized condition. It may be primary, following the inhalation of spores, and may be accompanied by enlargement of the hilar or tracheobronchial lymph nodes. It may, however, also be of a secondary character, caused by hematogenous dissemination. The symptoms are nonspecific and include a productive cough, fever and weight loss. Hemoptysis may occur and can be massive and fatal. The course may be chronic. The typical radiologic finding is a single, nodular upper lobe lesion, which may or may not cavitate. The natural course of the lung lesion is gradual progression to death.

Most patients with osteoarticular sporotrichosis also have preceding cutaneous lesions. This condition presents as stiffness and pain in a large joint. The onset is indolent. In almost all cases of arthritis, the knee, elbow, ankle or wrist is involved. Osteomyelitis seldom occurs without arthritis; the lesions are usually confined to the long bones nearby affected joints.

Endophthalmitis, although very rare, may result in blindness; chorioretinitis has also been reported. Cases of meningitis have also been seen.

The development of a cutaneous lesion on the limbs following trauma is suggestive of sporotrichosis, particularly if the patient is resident in an endemic region. The development of multiple ulcers along lymphatics is also suspicious. At a later stage of development sporotrichosis must be distinguished from mycoses such as blastomycosis, chromoblastomycosis and paracoccidioidomycosis, and from leishmaniasis, verrucous tuberculosis and tertiary syphilis. The diagnosis ultimately depends on mycologic and histologic examination.

MANAGEMENT

There are no trials comparing different strategies for the treatment of infection caused by black fungi. Treatment depends on the clinical form of the disease and is reviewed by Silveira & Nucci.[23] Cutaneous and subcutaneous phaeohyphomycosis are usually treated with complete surgical excision of the lesion, resulting in complete cure in the majority of cases. In addition, various antifungal agents have been used. Itraconazole is considered the drug of choice, and the dose has ranged from 200 to 600 mg daily. The duration of treatment is not established. Although unusual, progression or recurrence of disease, even with adequate itraconazole serum levels, has been observed. Whenever possible, surgical resection is also recommended for lesions in other organs, in association with an antifungal agent.

A number of reviews expanding many of the guidelines given here have been published.[24,58]

Chromoblastomycosis

Chromoblastomycosis is a difficult condition to treat.[17,29] Surgical excision should be reserved for small lesions; it carries a high risk of local dissemination and should only be attempted in conjunction with antifungal treatment.

There is no ideal antifungal treatment for chromoblastomycosis.[19] The most commonly used drug is flucytosine (150–200 mg/kg per day given as four divided doses), but resistance is a frequent problem during long-term treatment. Amphotericin B is not effective as monotherapy but appears to be effective in combination with 5-fluorocytosine (5-FC). Ketoconazole is effective in combination with 5-FC. Fluconazole is reported to be successful.

Much better results have been obtained when 5-FC (4 g/day given as four divided doses) is combined with oral thiabendazole (1 g/day given as two divided doses). Treatment should be continued for at least 1 month after clinical cure is obtained. Itraconazole (400 mg/day) has given promising results in a few patients. Itraconazole is particularly effective when combined with liquid nitrogen cryotherapy.[19] Recent trials have shown terbinafine (50 mg/day) to be effective, even in chronic cases.[19] The local application of heat to the lesions may be beneficial.

Entomophthoramycosis

Conidiobolomycosis

There is no standard treatment for all forms of this disease. Treatment has so far been disappointing. Surgical resection of infected tissue is seldom successful and may hasten the spread of infection. The condition can be treated with saturated potassium iodide solution (up to 10 ml q8h as tolerated) or amphotericin B. Long-term results are poor.

Patients with rhinofacial conidiobolomycosis treated with fluconazole (200 mg/day for 4 months) have been completely cured or have exhibited considerable improvement. Some patients have responded to combination treatment with amphotericin B and terbinafine,[59] or a combination of itraconazole and fluconazole.[60]

Trimethoprim–sulfamethoxazole, amphotericin B and fluconazole are useful in the treatment of C. incongruus infection[61] but clinical failure has been reported during treatment with amphotericin B and flucytosine.

Basidiobolomycosis

The therapy of choice still appears to be saturated potassium iodide solution (30 mg/kg per day) which should be given for 6–12 months. Oral ketoconazole (400 mg/day) has sometimes been successful, but amphotericin B has seldom been helpful. Surgical resection is not curative.

Ribes et al.[20] provides an exhaustive review of the treatment of entomophthoramycosis.

Lobomycosis

Antifungal drugs are ineffective. Amphotericin B, griseofulvin, sulfonamides and ketoconazole have been employed without adequate clinical responses.

Cure can only be achieved by surgical excision, the extent of the lesions permitting. Care must be taken during surgery of lobomycosis to avoid contaminating healthy tissue. Cryosurgery has also been used. Unfortunately, however, recurrence after excision is common. In advanced cases, the extensive excision required to remove the lesion may not be justified if the infection is not life-threatening. In cases involving larger areas of infection, treatment with clofazimine (300 mg/day) is recommended. The drug must be used, after initial clinical improvement, for at least 2 years at 100 mg/day. At present, the disease does not have a satisfactory medical treatment. The course of the disease is slow and chronic and the prognosis is poor. Lobomycosis never heals spontaneously and is never fatal, but it may be a very serious impediment.

Mycetoma

Early actinomycetomas (and some late and advanced cases) respond well to treatment.[62,63] The drug of choice is streptomycin sulfate (1000 mg/day intramuscularly). This should be combined with trimethoprim–sulfamethoxazole (co-trimoxazole) 960 mg q12h in cases caused by S. somaliensis, A. pelletieri or N. brasiliensis. Other regimens include trimethoprim–sulfamethoxazole and amikacin, and streptomycin combined with either dapsone or trimethoprim–sulfamethoxazole. If no response is seen after 3 weeks of treatment, other regimens can be substituted. These include streptomycin and rifampin (rifampicin), or streptomycin and sulfadoxine plus pyrimethamine. Therapy must be continued for months or even years. In favorable cases, edema and tenderness regress, discharge of secretion and grains diminishes, and sinuses dry up and close.

Even after symptoms and clinical signs have disappeared, the disease has become clinically silent and laboratory tests have become normal, it is recommended that treatment be continued for the same period of time as was required to achieve these results.

The response of eumycetoma to antifungal treatment is disappointing.[62,63] Madurella mycetomatis and P. boydii infections have been known to respond to ketoconazole (400 mg/day), but it is essential to test liver function before starting and during treatment with this drug. Long-term treatment with itraconazole has resulted in improvement in M. grisea mycetoma. The fungal agents causing mycetoma are resistant to amphotericin B and 5-FC. Terbinafine has been successful in the treatment of maduromycetoma.

Mycetoma due to Acremonium spp. and P. boydii appears to respond to fluconazole (200 mg daily for 10–12 weeks).

Surgical excision is the method of choice if the eumycotic lesions are small enough for total removal to be possible. Amputation is often required in advanced cases with bone involvement, particularly when there is no response to drug treatment. Prostheses and rehabilitation are indispensable in every case of mutilating surgery.

Phaeohyphomycosis

Subcutaneous phaeohyphomycosis

Incision and drainage of subcutaneous lesions is seldom successful. Surgical resection is required. Treatment with amphotericin B has cured or improved unresectable lesions, but later relapse has been common. Itraconazole and terbinafine have been successful in the treatment of phaeohyphomycosis.

Paranasal sinus infection

Complete surgical debridement combined with amphotericin B treatment is essential to halt the progression of this form of phaeohyphomycosis. Even so, it is not uncommon for the condition to recur. The need for repeated debridement is most evident in patients with disabling symptoms or erosion of the bone separating the paranasal sinus from the brain.

Oral treatment with itraconazole (100–400 mg/day) appears promising, although the optimum dosage and duration of treatment have not been defined.

Necrotic nasal septum lesions due to Alternaria spp. or Curvularia spp. have been cured after surgical excision.

Cerebral phaeohyphomycosis

In no case has a patient survived without surgical resection of the lesion. Treatment with amphotericin B on its own is ineffective. Lesions that have not been completely removed have usually proved fatal. A single case of cerebral phaeohyphomycosis due to Cladosporium spp. responded partially to fluconazole (300 mg/day for 5 weeks).

Cutaneous infection

Surgical debridement of cutaneous lesions combined with parenteral amphotericin B is the most effective method of treatment. Topical antifungal treatment is seldom helpful.

Other forms of phaeohyphomycosis

Too few patients have been treated for firm recommendations to be possible. However, the response to amphotericin B has been partial at best. Surgical resection of lesions or oral treatment with itraconazole should be considered.

In *in-vitro* tests the new azole antifungals, including voriconazole, appear to be as active as itraconazole against a number of agents of phaeohyphomycosis.

Rhinosporidiosis

The treatment of choice is surgical excision. No drug treatment has proved effective. If left untreated, the polyps will continue to enlarge slowly. Local injection of amphotericin B may be used as an adjunct treatment to prevent reinfection and spread of the disease.[27] In very rare cases, widely disseminated or deep-seated visceral lesions may develop. Spontaneous remission is unusual.

Sporotrichosis

Saturated potassium iodide solution remains the treatment of choice for patients in developing countries who contract cutaneous sporotrichosis, owing to its ease of administration and low cost.[64] However, new drugs are needed, especially for disseminated sporotrichosis.[64] The starting dose is 1 ml q8h, and this is increased to 4–6 ml q8h. Treatment should be continued for at least 1 month after clinical cure is obtained, which may take 2–4 months. Intolerance (iodism) is frequent and consequently therapy is often stopped.

If the patient cannot tolerate potassium iodide, oral itraconazole (100–200 mg/day) can be used.[65] Treatment should be continued for up to 6 months. The most appropriate therapeutic regimen appears to be 200 mg/day during the entire treatment period, or 200 mg/day at the beginning of treatment, reduced to 100 mg/day after improvement. Many cases treated in this way are cured relatively quickly. Cutaneous sporotrichosis has also been successfully treated with terbinafine (125 mg/day).[66]

Local heat, on its own or in combination with drug treatment, has been shown to improve cutaneous lesions. Besides thermotherapy, the simple warming of diseased limbs in winter months has proved helpful.

Amphotericin B has cured some patients with extracutaneous forms of sporotrichosis, but failures are common. In cases of arthritis or osteomyelitis, better results have been obtained when the drug has been combined with surgical debridement.

Itraconazole (400 mg/day) has given good results in patients with extracutaneous infection, especially in those who have not responded to fluconazole.[66] The Mycoses Study Group of the Infectious Diseases Society of America has published detailed practice guidelines for sporotrichosis.[67] Their recommendations were derived primarily from multicenter, nonrandomized treatment trials, small retrospective series and case reports. The treatment of choice for fixed cutaneous or lymphocutaneous sporotrichosis is itraconazole 100–200 mg/day for 3–6 months.

REFERENCES

References for this chapter can be found online at http://www.expertconsult.com

Protozoa: intestinal and urogenital amebae, flagellates and ciliates

This chapter discusses the amebae, flagellates and ciliates that parasitize the intestinal and urogenital systems of humans (Table 180.1). With the exception of *Trichomonas vaginalis*, all of the organisms live in the intestinal tract. Intestinal protozoa vary in pathogenicity and prevalence, but, with rare exceptions, all have a worldwide distribution.

NATURE

Amebae, flagellates and ciliates are single-celled eukaryotic organisms belonging to the subkingdom or phylum Protozoa. In general, the organisms related to human infection change their form and function from the active, feeding trophozoites to the resting cyst form. All protozoa contain a nucleus, often with a karyosome near its center. The cytoplasm is composed of the endoplasm (which immediately surrounds the nucleus) and the ectoplasm (which functions as the locomotion apparatus). Reproduction is relatively simple and is accomplished through repeated asexual multiplication by binary fission. Although not completely clear, *Blastocystis hominis* is currently classified with the protozoa and will be discussed in this chapter.

EPIDEMIOLOGY

Intestinal amebae, flagellates and ciliates are transmitted through fecally contaminated food, water or other materials. Prevalence is correlated with socioeconomic conditions, and higher infection rates occur in people who have poor personal hygiene, who live in areas with poor sanitation, or men who have sex with men.[1] Contaminated water supplies are a particular problem because the usual levels of chlorination may not kill cysts.[2] Filtration is required. Endemic and epidemic disease has been traced to water supplies that use surface water which either is not filtered or has been improperly filtered.

These organisms generally have a cystic stage that develops when conditions in the environment are unfavorable for continued multiplication. The cyst wall is thicker than the trophozoite membrane and thus provides protection. Once these cysts have been transferred to a new host, usually by fecal–oral contamination from person to person, the organisms excyst. Excystation factors include osmotic changes in the environment, enzymatic action of the enclosed organism on the inner surface of the cyst wall and, among the parasitic protozoa, favorable pH and enzymatic action of the host tissues. Transmission of those protozoa with no identified cyst stage has not been totally explained.

Entamoeba histolytica

Infections with *E. histolytica* are seen worldwide and are more prevalent in the tropics. In 2003, over 500 million people were estimated to be infected with *E. histolytica*, 50 million had extensive symptoms, including colitis or extraintestinal abscesses, and there were 110 000 deaths.[3] For every case of invasive disease diagnosed, there are at least 10–20 asymptomatic individuals excreting infective cysts. Population groups with a higher incidence of amebiasis include people from the developing world or recent immigrants from there to the developed nations.

Social changes seen in the late 1960s – open expression of homosexuality, increased sexual contacts, increased frequency of sexual activities and anonymity of sexual partners – contributed to dramatic increases in sexually transmitted organisms, including *E. histolytica*. Clinical presentations within the homosexual community often differ from those seen in the heterosexual population and almost 50% of all homosexual men found to be infected with *E. histolytica* are asymptomatic.[4] However, it is an accepted fact that the ameba

Table 180.1 Amebae, flagellates and ciliate that parasitize the intestinal and urogenital systems of humans

Type	Species	Pathogenicity*
Amebae	*Entamoeba histolytica*	1
	Entamoeba dispar	2
	Entamoeba hartmanni	2
	Entamoeba coli	2
	Entamoeba polecki	2
	Entamoeba moshkovskii	1
	Entamoeba gingivalis[†]	2
	Endolimax nana	2
	Iodamoeba bütschlii	2
	Blastocystis hominis	6
Flagellates	*Dientamoeba fragilis*	1
	Giardia lamblia	1
	Trichomonas vaginalis[‡]	1
	Pentatrichomonas (Trichomonas) hominis	2
	Trichomonas tenax[†]	2
	Chilomastix mesnili	2
	Enteromonas hominis	2
	Retortamonas intestinalis	2
Ciliate	*Balantidium coli*	1

*Pathogenic = 1; nonpathogenic = 2; pathogenicity controversial = 6.
[†]Body site: mouth.
[‡]Body site: urogenital system.

morphologically identified as *E. histolytica* is actually two separate and distinct species. *E. histolytica* is the pathogenic species and is considered the etiologic agent of amebic colitis and extraintestinal amebiasis, while *E. dispar* is the nonpathogenic species and does not invade tissue or cause intestinal symptoms. Therefore, in epidemiologic studies prior to the development of specific reagents for the identification of true *E. histolytica*, those organisms identified as *E. histolytica* were actually in the *E. histolytica/E. dispar* group.

Entamoeba moshkovskii, which is morphologically identical to *E. histolytica* and *E. dispar* but biochemically and genetically different, has been considered until recently to be primarily a free-living (nonpathogenic) ameba. However, human isolates have now been detected in North America, Italy, South Africa, Bangladesh, India, Iran and Australia.[1] Recent studies suggest that infection with this species can cause diarrhea and other intestinal disorders.[1] Since *E. moshkovskii* is indistinguishable in its cyst and trophozoite forms from *E. histolytica* and *E. dispar*, it is not possible to differentiate the three species on the basis of traditional microscopic examination. Therefore, past studies on the prevalence of *E. histolytica* may be flawed if the possible presence of *E. dispar* and *E. moshkovskii* was not considered.

Epidemiologic evidence of sexual transmission of *E. histolytica* has grown significantly since the early 1970s, particularly in New York City and San Francisco. In San Francisco, the incidence of reported symptomatic intestinal amebiasis increased by over 1000% from 1978 to 1988 among homosexual men between 20 and 39 years of age.[4] Direct oral–anal contact (anilingus) leads to fecal exposure and oral contact with a variety of intestinal pathogens. Transmission can also occur during oral–genital sex after anal intercourse has occurred. Active heterosexuals can acquire infection with *E. histolytica* through sexual activities that provide an opportunity for fecal–oral contamination. The key factor is not necessarily homosexuality, but the frequency of sexual activity and potential for fecal–oral contact. In a study from Japan, symptomatic amebiasis in the east-southeast area of Tokyo is a disease that predominantly afflicts males, and the high rates of patients who engaged in male homosexual or bisexual practices suggest that amebiasis is likely to be a sexually transmitted disease in homosexual or bisexual men. These infections were confirmed to be true *E. histolytica*, primarily zymodeme II.[5]

With the advent of AIDS, and the subsequent modifications in sexual practices within homosexual communities, the incidence of *E. histolytica* infection has decreased. In recent years, the increased incidence of disease caused by coccidian parasites, *Cystoisospora belli* and *Cryptosporidium* spp. and the microsporidia, *Enterocytozoon bieneusi* and *Encephalitozoon intestinalis* has become much more of a problem in patients who have AIDS.

In certain urban areas (Mexico City, Mexico; Medellin, Colombia; and Durban, South Africa), the incidence of invasive disease is considerably higher than in the rest of the world. Contributing factors may include poor nutrition, tropical climate, decreased immunologic competence of the host, stress, altered bacterial flora in the colon, traumatic injuries to the colonic mucosa, alcoholism and genetic factors.

The human is the reservoir host for *E. histolytica/E. dispar* and can transmit the infection to other humans, primates, dogs, cats and possibly pigs. The cyst stages are very resistant to environmental conditions and remain viable in the soil for days. The asymptomatic cyst passer who is a food handler is thought to play the most important role in transmission.

It has been postulated that a colonization–blocking vaccine could eliminate *E. histolytica* as a cause of human disease, particularly as humans serve as the only significant reservoir host, and a number of potential protective antigens are being investigated.[6]

Blastocystis hominis

Blastocystis hominis is transmitted via the fecal–oral route through contaminated food or water; the cysts survive in water for up to 19 days at normal temperatures.[2,7,8] Although other modes of transmission are not defined, the incidence and apparent worldwide distribution suggest the traditional route of infection. When genotypic results from animal isolates were compared with the diversity of genotypes of 102 human *Blastocystis hominis* isolates, 67.4 % (62/92) of isolates from mammals and birds were identical to human *B. hominis* genotypes. Thus, the possibility of zoonotic transmission appears to be very likely.[9] Prevention would involve improved personal hygiene and sanitary conditions.

Giardia lamblia (intestinalis, duodenalis)

Various peer-reviewed journal publications through 2007 use different terms for the species of *Giardia* that infect humans; however, we have decided to maintain *G. lamblia* for this chapter. Transmission is by ingestion of viable cysts, and contaminated food and drink are the usual sources. These zoonotic protozoa are responsible for disease in a broad range of hosts, including humans, have a low infectious dose enhancing the possibility of transmission, have transmission stages that are small and environmentally resistant, and are insensitive to the disinfectants commonly used in the water industry.[10] This infection is found in children or in groups that live in close quarters.[11,12] Also there may be outbreaks caused by poor sanitation facilities or breakdowns; travelers and campers often experience such outbreaks.[13,14] There is also an increase in the prevalence of giardiasis in the male homosexual population, probably as a result of anal and/or oral sexual practices.[15]

Decreased gastric acid production may predispose people to infection with *G. lamblia*. Normal gastric acidity may act as a barrier to infection; patients who have had a gastrectomy are prone to infection with *G. lamblia*. Reduction in gastric acid also occurs as a result of malnutrition and both factors may, as a group, increase susceptibility to infection with this organism. Impairment of the host's immune system may also play a role.

Lower incidence of giardiasis in infants up to 6 months of age may be associated with breast-feeding and some protection against infection via secretory IgA; however, lower incidence may also be related to a decreased exposure to *G. lamblia* in breast-fed infants.

Giardiasis is one of the common causes of travelers' diarrhea and is worldwide in distribution. Visitors in areas endemic for *Giardia* spp. are more likely to become symptomatic than the inhabitants of that area; this is probably because the latter have developed immunity from previous, and possibly continued, exposure to the organism. A number of outbreaks in the USA have been attributed to resort or municipal water supplies, such as Oregon, Colorado, Utah, Washington, New Hampshire and New York.[16–18] High infection rates were also reported from hikers and campers who drank stream water. Because some of these areas were remote from human habitation, infected wild animals, especially the beaver, were suspected of being the source.[13,17,19–21] Surveys show human infection rates of 2–15% in various parts of the world.

Because of potential wild animal reservoirs and possibly domestic animal reservoir hosts, measures in additional to personal hygiene and improved sanitation have to be considered.[22,23] Iodine is recommended as an effective disinfectant for drinking water, but it must be used according to directions.[24,25] Filtration systems have also been recommended, although they have certain drawbacks, such as clogging.

Isoenzyme studies, used for parasite identification and classification, have provided information related to organism pathogenicity, possible implication in water-borne outbreaks, and the potential cause of human disease. The examination of isoenzyme patterns of *G. duodenalis* (*G. lamblia*) obtained from humans and animals showed no obvious correlation between clinical symptoms and isoenzyme patterns. These studies also demonstrated significant differences between isolates from within a single region and those from other distant geographic locations.[26,27]

Dientamoeba fragilis

Dientamoeba fragilis infection is commonly associated with enterobiasis, and it has been suggested that *D. fragilis* may infect *Enterobius* spp. eggs and thus bypass gastric acidity. Although clinical infections with

D. fragilis occur, they are not often reported. This is probably because the infection is self-limiting, stool examination is not requested and laboratory identification is difficult. However, there exists a growing body of case reports from numerous countries around the world that have linked this protozoal parasite to clinical manifestations such as diarrhea, abdominal pain, flatulence and anorexia. A number of studies have even incriminated *D. fragilis* as a cause of irritable bowel syndrome, allergic colitis, and diarrhea in human immunodeficiency virus patients.[28–30] The incubation period for clinical disease is not clearly defined.

Trichomonas vaginalis

Infection with *T. vaginalis* is acquired primarily through sexual intercourse; asymptomatic men therefore need to be diagnosed and treated. The organism can survive for some time in a moist environment such as damp towels and underclothes; however, this mode of transmission is thought to be very rare.

Balantidium coli

Domestic pigs are probably the most important reservoir host for human infection with *B. coli*. In areas in which pigs are the main domestic animal, the incidence of human infection can be quite high (e.g. New Guinea). Human infection is fairly rare in temperate areas; however, once the infection is established, it can develop into an epidemic, particularly when environmental sanitation and personal hygiene are poor. This situation has been seen in mental hospitals in the USA. Preventive measures involve increased attention to personal hygiene and sanitation, as the mode of transmission is ingestion of infective cysts through contaminated food or water.

PREVENTION

Transmission of the majority of the intestinal protozoa occurs through ingestion of infective cysts, which can be acquired from food, water and person to person by the fecal–oral route. These infections tend to be found more frequently in groups that live in close quarters or in certain population groups. There may be outbreaks due to poor sanitation facilities or breakdowns as evidenced by infections in travelers and campers; certainly this has been found for giardiasis. Although amebiasis is usually associated with poor sanitation and underdeveloped areas of the world, sexual transmission has also been documented, mainly among urban homosexual men. Prevention in this group is directly related to limiting sexual practices that provide an opportunity for fecal–oral contamination. The single most effective practice that prevents the spread of infections with intestinal protozoa, particularly in the childcare setting, is thorough hand washing by the children, staff and visitors. In the case of *D. fragilis*, it has been suggested that the trophozoites may infect *Enterobius* spp. eggs, thus allowing protection from gastric acidity; however, under most circumstances, total prevention of enterobiasis and/or infection with *D. fragilis* is neither realistic nor possible. *T. vaginalis* is acquired primarily though sexual intercourse, hence the need to diagnose and treat asymptomatic males. The organism can also survive for some time in a moist environment such as damp towels and underclothes; however, this manner of transmission is considered rare.

Although incomplete epidemiologic investigation and reporting make it difficult to determine the significance of the water-borne transmission of giardiasis accurately, the water-borne route seems to be more important for this protozoan than for other more commonly recognized water-borne pathogens, with the possible exception of *Cryptosporidium* spp. Iodine has been recommended as an effective disinfectant for drinking water, but it must be used according to directions. Because of the potential for wild animal and possibly domestic animal reservoir hosts related to *Giardia* spp., measures in addition

to personal hygiene and improved sanitary measures have to be considered and implemented. If appropriate procedures are followed, conventional water filtration should trap most protozoan parasites, including *Giardia*. One should avoid swallowing water when in lakes, rivers, pools or hot tubs; also do not drink directly from lakes, rivers, streams, or springs. Filtration devices for hikers and campers are also available; however, one should look for 'reverse osmosis', 'absolute 1 micron', 'Standard 53' and the words 'cyst reduction' or 'cyst removal'. Boiling water, at a rolling boil, for 1 minute is sufficient to kill organisms, including *Giardia* spp. and *Cryptosporidium* spp. It is also important to thoroughly wash all fruits and vegetables if eating uncooked, use safe water for washing food, peel fruit, and avoid unpasteurized milk or dairy products.

PATHOGENICITY

Some of the intestinal protozoa are nonpathogenic and produce no disease; however, microscopists must be able to distinguish pathogenic from nonpathogenic species. The presence of nonpathogenic species indicates that the person has been exposed to fecal contamination. Several species can cause mild to severe gastrointestinal symptoms, and *E. histolytica* may produce extraintestinal lesions. However, pathogenic or potentially pathogenic protozoa do not always produce symptoms or they may remain after symptoms have resolved. Asymptomatic individuals may serve as reservoirs for the infection. Detection of a potentially pathogenic protozoan does not necessarily prove that the organism is causing the illness. Patients may have diarrhea caused by other organisms such as *Salmonella* spp., *Shigella* spp., *Escherichia coli* or rotavirus. Current intestinal protozoan pathogens included in this chapter are: *Entamoeba histolytica*, *Blastocystis hominis*, *Giardia lamblia*, *Dientamoeba fragilis* and *Balantidium coli*. *Trichomonas vaginalis*, a urogenital flagellate, is also considered pathogenic, and may cause mild to severe vaginitis and other urogenital problems.

Entamoeba histolytica

Although many people worldwide are infected with *E. histolytica*, only a small percentage develops clinical symptoms. Morbidity and mortality caused by *E. histolytica* vary, depending on geographic area, organism species (*E. histolytica* vs *E. dispar*) and the immune status of the patient.

During the 1980s and 1990s several publications reviewed the issues regarding pathogenic *E. histolytica* vs nonpathogenic *E. dispar*. On the basis of current knowledge, pathogenic *E. histolytica* is considered to be the etiologic agent of amebic colitis and extraintestinal disease, whereas nonpathogenic *E. dispar* produces no intestinal symptoms and is not invasive in humans.[31–33] (See also Chapter 110.) Diamond & Clark[34] redescribed the two species as *E. histolytica* (Schaudinn 1903), which is the invasive human pathogen, and *E. dispar* (Brumpt 1925), which is noninvasive and which does not cause disease. During the past several years, extensive work has been published related to the pathogenesis of *E. histolytica*.[35,36]

Blastocystis hominis

The true role of this organism in terms of colonization or disease and the relevance of organism numbers require additional clarification. In studies of patients with irritable bowel syndrome, there are patients in whom the presence of *B. hominis* did not appear to be incidental.[37,38] The first report of a possible relationship between intestinal obstruction and a concomitant *B. hominis* infection has also been published.[39] In patients with other underlying conditions, the symptoms may be more pronounced.[40] There is evidence to indicate there are several ribodeme types, and there may be a relationship between ribodeme type and pathogenicity, only some of which will be responsible for increased intestinal permeability and symptoms.[41,42]

Giardia lamblia

The majority of individuals infected with *G. lamblia* are asymptomatic. Preliminary studies indicate that there may be two different strains of *G. lamblia*, Group A and Group B, associated with different degrees of virulence. Group A appears to be more pathogenic and is associated with symptomatic infection. Isoenzyme and molecular studies also support the differences between these two groups.[43–47]

Dientamoeba fragilis

During the past several years, the pathogenicity of *D. fragilis* has been associated with a wide range of symptoms.[28–30] However, it appears that there may be both pathogenic and nonpathogenic variants. Evidence for two genetically distinct forms has been obtained using polymerase chain reaction-restriction fragment length polymorphism (PCR-RFLP) analysis of ribosomal genes.[48,49]

Trichomonas vaginalis

Trichomonas vaginalis is site specific and usually cannot survive outside the urogenital system. After introduction, proliferation begins, with resulting inflammation and large numbers of trophozoites in the tissues and the secretions. Nutrient acquisition and cytoadherence, immune system evasion and regulation of virulence genes are virulence factors associated with pathogenesis.[50] It appears that interference with trichomonads, mucin receptors and proteinases may form a strategy to prevent colonization with this pathogenic flagellate.[51]

Balantidium coli

Some infections with *B. coli* produce no symptoms, while others cause symptoms with severe dysentery similar to that seen in patients with amebiasis. Symptoms usually include diarrhea or dysentery, tenesmus, nausea, vomiting, anorexia and headache. Insomnia, muscular weakness and weight loss have also been reported. Diarrhea may persist for weeks to months prior to the onset of dysentery. There may be tremendous fluid loss, with a type of diarrhea similar to that seen in cholera or in some coccidial or microsporidial infections.

On contact with the mucosa, *B. coli* may penetrate the mucosa with cellular infiltration in the area of the developing ulcer, which may extend to the muscular layer. The ulcers may vary in shape, and the ulcer bed may be full of pus and necrotic debris. Although the number of cases is small, extraintestinal disease has been reported (peritonitis, urinary tract infection, inflammatory vaginitis).[52]

DIAGNOSTIC MICROBIOLOGY

Because intestinal symptoms are nonspecific, diagnosis requires laboratory identification of the organisms present. Immunodiagnostic methods for antibody detection are useful for the diagnosis of extraintestinal amebiasis, but their utility is limited for intestinal disease.

Organism morphology varies and species characteristics often overlap. For reliable identification, microscopists must be able to differentiate all species regardless of their potential for causing disease. Special attention will be given to the clinically significant intestinal pathogens, especially *E. histolytica*, *B. hominis*, *G. lamblia*, *D. fragilis* and *B. coli*.

Identification of amebae in fecal specimens

Trophozoites and cysts are diagnostic stages of the amebae, and either or both stages can be detected in feces. Microscopists must be able to distinguish trophozoites and cysts from epithelial cells, polymorphonuclear leukocytes and macrophages, as well as from pus cells, yeasts, pollen, molds, and vegetable and crystalline artifacts.

Trophozoite motility in physiologic saline mounts of fresh material and cytoplasmic inclusions, such as erythrocytes in trophozoites and chromatoid bodies in cysts, can be observed. Iodine solutions are used for temporary cyst stains of fresh or fixed specimens. Cyst characteristics are less variable than those of trophozoites, and species of cysts can often be identified in iodine-stained wet mounts. However, examination of permanent stained smears using oil immersion (×1000) is recommended for definitive identification of trophozoites and cysts. Size is not a reliable feature for species differentiation of either trophozoites or cysts except when separating the *E. histolytica/E. dispar* group from the nonpathogen *Entamoeba hartmanni*.

The microscopist must observe the cytoplasmic and the nuclear characteristics of several organisms before making a final identification. Although cysts are more easily identified than trophozoites, several cysts (particularly if they are immature) should be observed to ensure that the identification is reliable. If two species are identified, there should be distinct populations of each.

Sometimes, although amebic organisms are seen, species cannot be identified. In these instances, the laboratory should report 'unidentified ameba trophozoites (or cysts)'; if the genus can be determined but the species cannot, 'unidentified *Entamoeba* trophozoites or cysts' should be reported, and another specimen should be requested.

Entamoeba histolytica

Intestinal infection is usually diagnosed by the microscopic identification of organisms in feces or in sigmoidoscopic material from ulcerations (Fig. 180.1). Nonpathogenic amebae can be confused with pathogens (Figs 180.2–180.5). Only trophozoites are found in tissue lesions, but both trophozoites and cysts may be found in the intestinal lumen. Some patients who have invasive disease may have only trophozoites in fecal specimens, and examination of permanent stained smears may be required to establish the diagnosis.

Suspected amebic abscesses are often diagnosed by positive serologic tests. Aspirates of abscesses or intestinal lesions may contain amebic trophozoites, sometimes with ingested erythrocytes seen in direct wet mounts or in permanent stains such as trichrome or iron-hematoxylin stains.[52,53] Other species of intestinal amebae are not pathogenic but must be differentiated from *E. histolytica*. *Entamoeba polecki* is seen occasionally in refugees from South East Asia and may be confused with *E. histolytica*, as can *E. moshkovskii*.[52] *Entamoeba gingivalis* is a common inhabitant of the oral cavity, particularly in patients who have poor oral hygiene. It resembles *E. histolytica* but has no known cyst stage. As a result, trophozoites of *E. gingivalis* may lead to the misdiagnosis of amebic lung abscess by morphologic examination of pulmonary material, especially sputum.

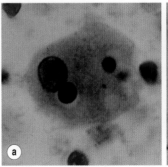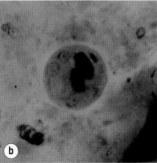

Fig. 180.1 (a) *Entamoeba histolytica*, trophozoite containing ingested red blood cells (the presence of red blood cells confirms the organism is the true pathogen, *E. histolytica*). (b) *Entamoeba histolytica/E. dispar*, cyst containing four nuclei and chromatoidal bars with smooth, rounded edges (trichrome stain). Note: from the cyst morphology, it is not possible to differentiate pathogenic *E. histolytica* from nonpathogenic *E. dispar*.

Fig. 180.2 *Entamoeba hartmanni.*
(a) Trophozoite. (b) Cyst containing up to four nuclei and chromatoidal bars with smooth, rounded edges (trichrome stain). Note: *E. hartmanni* measures smaller than *E. histolytica/E. dispar*; the trophozoite is <12 μm and the cyst is <10 μm.

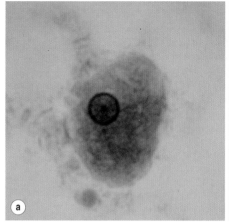
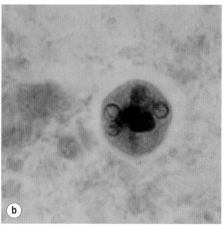

Fig. 180.3 *Entamoeba coli.* (a) Trophozoite containing a single nucleus in which the karyosome is eccentric (tends to be centrally located in *E. histolytica/E. dispar*). (b) Cyst contains more than five nuclei (d'Antoni's iodine).

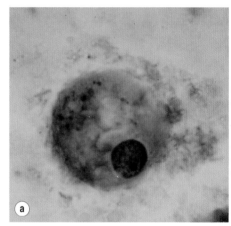
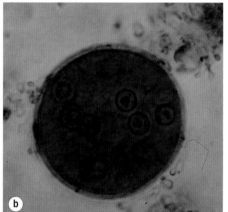

Fig. 180.4 *Endolimax nana.* (a) Trophozoite containing a single nucleus with no peripheral chromatin (large karyosome only) and vacuolated cytoplasm. (b) Cyst containing four nuclei (three easily visible) (trichrome stain).

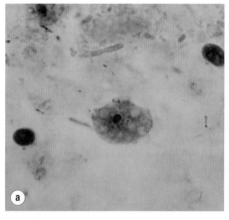
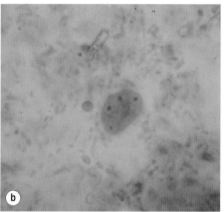

Currently, there are several immunoassays that can be used to identify organisms in the genus *Entamoeba* (*E. histolytica/E. dispar* group) and other reagents that can differentiate pathogenic *E. histolytica* from nonpathogenic *E. dispar*. The antigen detection enzyme-linked immunosorbent assay (ELISA) kits are based on specific amebic adhesin molecules found in the feces of people infected by either *E. histolytica* or *E. dispar*. The second ELISA reagent is able to detect the adhesin produced by *E. histolytica* in feces. Another immunoassay product is available for the detection of *E. histolytica* and *E. dispar* in fecal specimens; however, this kit does not differentiate between the two organisms, but is specific for the *E. histolytica/E. dispar* group.[54] These procedures are simple, sensitive and specific. It is important to remember that these kits require fresh stool specimens; specimens preserved in any of the routine stool collection fixatives are not acceptable. Polymerase chain reaction methods are also being developed for the differentiation of *E. histolytica* from *E. dispar*.[55]

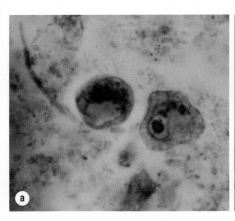 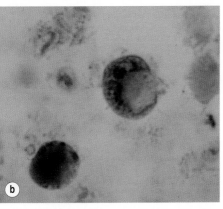

Fig. 180.5 *Iodamoeba bütschlii.* (a) Trophozoite containing a single nucleus with a large karyosome and cyst containing a single nucleus and a large glycogen vacuole. (b) Cyst containing a single nucleus and a large glycogen vacuole – note the size of the karyosome (trichrome stain). There is also a *Blastocystis hominis* central body form present at the lower left of the image.

Serologic testing for intestinal disease is not recommended unless the patient has true dysentery; even in these patients, the titer (e.g. indirect hemagglutination) may be low and difficult to interpret. The definitive diagnosis of intestinal amebiasis should not be made without demonstrating the organisms. When extraintestinal disease is suspected, serologic tests are much more relevant. Indirect hemagglutination and indirect fluorescent antibody tests (FAs) have been reported positive with titers of ≥1:256 and ≥1:200, respectively, in almost 100% of cases of amebic liver abscess.[52] Positive serologic results, in addition to clinical findings, make the diagnosis highly probable. In the absence of rapid serologic tests for amebiasis (tests with very rapid turnaround times for results), the decision as to causative agent often must be made on clinical grounds and on results of other diagnostic tests such as scans.

Histologic diagnosis of amebiasis can be made when trophozoites within the tissue are identified and differentiated from host cells, particularly histiocytes and ganglion cells. Periodic acid–Schiff staining is often used; the organisms will appear bright pink with a green–blue background (depending on the counterstain used). Hematoxylin and eosin staining will also allow typical morphology to be seen. As a result of sectioning, some organisms will exhibit the evenly arranged nuclear chromatin with the central karyosome, and some will no longer contain the nucleus.

Blastocystis hominis

The characteristic form of *B. hominis* that is usually seen in human fecal specimens varies in size from 6 to 40 μm and contains a large central body resembling a vacuole, which may be involved with carbohydrate and lipid storage. The amebic form can occasionally be seen in diarrheal fluid but may be difficult to recognize.[56] Generally, *B. hominis*

will be identified on the basis of the typical round form containing the central body.[52] Routine stool examinations are very effective in recovering and identifying *B. hominis* (Fig. 180.6), although the permanent stained smear is the procedure of choice because the examination of wet preparations may not easily reveal the organism. The organisms should be quantitated on the report form, that is, as rare, few, moderate, or many. It is also important to remember that other possible pathogens may be present and should be ruled out before a patient is treated for *B. hominis*.

Identification of flagellates in fecal specimens

The flagellates are a more diverse group than the amebae. The type of motility, shape, number of nuclei and other characteristics, such as an undulating membrane, sucking disk, cytostome, spiral groove, and the number and location of flagellae, are important characteristics used to identify flagellate trophozoites. The organism shape and size, number and position of nuclei, and absence or arrangement of fibrils are used to identify flagellate cysts.

In some cases, species can be determined by the examination of either direct or concentrated wet mounts. Species of cysts may be identified in iodine-stained mounts. However, permanent stains are always recommended for every stool specimen submitted; organisms identified in wet preparations may not represent all types of organism present.

Giardia lamblia

Diagnosis is usually established by the demonstration of cysts or, occasionally, trophozoites in feces (Fig. 180.7). Nonpathogenic

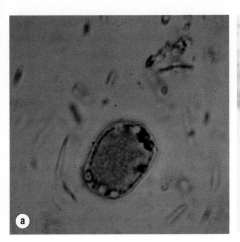 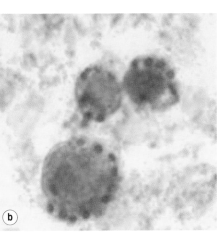

Fig. 180.6 *Blastocystis hominis.* (a) Central body form with large 'empty' area (appears like a vacuole) with multiple nuclei around the edges (d'Antoni's iodine). (b) Three central body forms with the large empty area surrounded by nuclei (trichrome stain).

flagellates can be seen in Figure 180.8. Because of the variable shedding of organisms, several stool specimens should be examined before the infection is ruled out. In some cases, a series of stools can be examined and be negative, and yet the patient still has giardiasis. It is important for the laboratory and the clinician to recognize this fact. Permanent stains are recommended for the definitive diagnosis of this infection.

When *G. lamblia* organisms are not found in stool specimens, duodenal aspirates, string test mucus or biopsied mucosal tissue can be examined. The string test[52] is used to collect mucus from the duodenal area and its use may be less traumatic for the patient than other methods. Materials obtained by drainage, aspiration or the string test can be examined by simple, direct wet mounts. Biopsy tissue may be processed and stained by the usual histopathologic methods; however, before preservation, a fresh imprint smear of the mucosal surface on a slide can be made and stained with trichrome or Giemsa stain.

Immunoassay methods (enzyme immunoassay, FA, immunochromatographic assay) are available and may be appropriate in test ordering situations. Education of the medical staff will be mandatory to ensure that tests are appropriately ordered and that there is complete understanding of the limits of the information generated (test results limited to absence or presence of *G. lamblia*). Recently, industrial companies and municipalities have shown a great deal of interest in these reagents. This is particularly relevant when the water sources are used for drinking and/or recreational purposes.[52]

Dientamoeba fragilis

Permanent stains are required to diagnose this infection, and multiple specimens may be required because shedding varies from day to day. The delicately staining trophozoites are usually binucleate, although the nuclei may be in different planes of focus (Fig. 180.9). The nuclei tend to be fragmented and can often be seen in a 'tetrad' formation. They must be differentiated from the trophozoites of *Endolimax nana*, *Iodamoeba bütschlii* and *Entamoeba hartmanni*. Nuclear characteristics, the presence of binucleate forms, tremendous size variation and the absence of cysts will aid in identification of this organism.

A permanent stained smear should be examined for every stool specimen submitted to the laboratory for an ova and parasite examination.[52,53] If this approach is not used, then many infections with this organism can be missed. If a laboratory periodically finds and identifies *G. lamblia*, but never sees *D. fragilis*, then collection and diagnostic methods should be reviewed.

Fig. 180.7 *Giardia lamblia.* (a) Trophozoites in mucus – note the sucking disk area, linear axonemes, curved median bodies and two nuclei (trichrome stain). (b) Cysts containing multiple nuclei, linear axonemes and curved median bodies (iron-hematoxylin stain).

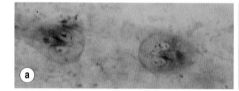
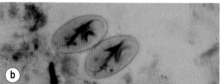

Fig. 180.8 *Chilomastix mesnili.* (a) Trophozoite with single nucleus and clear feeding groove/cytostome. (b) Cyst containing single nucleus and curved fibril called the 'shepherd's crook' (trichrome stain).

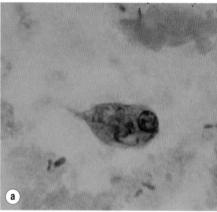
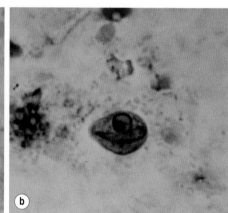

Fig. 180.9 *Dientamoeba fragilis.* (a) Trophozoite with single nucleus fragmented into a 'tetrad' configuration. (b) Trophozoite containing two nuclei, each showing fragmented chromatin (trichrome stain). There is no known cyst form for this organism.

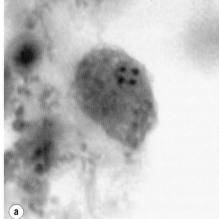
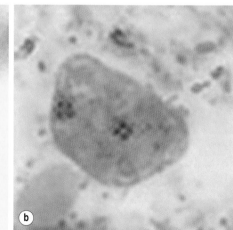

Identification of flagellates in urogenital specimens

Trichomonas vaginalis

Infections with *T. vaginalis* are usually detected by finding the motile trophozoites in wet mounts of vaginal fluid, prostatic fluid or sediments of freshly passed urine. In wet mounts, the trophozoites move with a nervous, jerky motion and possess an undulating membrane, which extends only one-half the length of the organism (Fig. 180.10). In old urine specimens, the organisms may be dead or badly distorted and thus cannot be identified or may be confused with host cells.

Specimens include vaginal fluid, scrapings or washings. They may be examined in a saline wet mount or as a stained smear, or the material can be cultured. Although some consider that wet-mount examinations are as efficient as cultures in revealing infections, current evidence suggests that cultivation methods are superior.[57,58] Immunofluorescent and ELISA methods have also been described. Organisms may be difficult to recognize in permanent stains; however, if a dry smear is submitted to the laboratory, Giemsa or Papanicolaou stain can be used. Chronic *T. vaginalis* infections may cause atypical cellular changes that can be misinterpreted, particularly on the Papanicolaou smear. Organisms are routinely missed on Gram stains. The number of false-positive and false-negative results reported on the basis of stained smears strongly suggests that identification should be confirmed by observation of motile organisms, either from the direct wet mount or from appropriate culture media.

For culture, it is mandatory that the specimen be collected correctly, immediately inoculated into the proper medium and properly incubated. Excellent methods are available using plastic envelopes containing appropriate media. This envelope approach allows both immediate examination and culture in one self-contained envelope. These systems are commercially available and serve as the specimen transport container, the growth chamber during incubation and the 'slide' during microscopy.[52,59]

Monoclonal antibodies and DNA probe procedures for the detection of *T. vaginalis* have been reported as being very effective.[60,61] An enzyme immunoassay has been developed for the detection of the *T. vaginalis* antigen from vaginal swabs.[62,63] The predictive value of a positive test was 82% and that of a negative test was 99.3%. Commercial products based on these methodologies should be very helpful in diagnosing this infection. Serologic tests have been tried; however, none is commercially available.

Identification of ciliates in fecal specimens

Balantidium coli

In human feces, *B. coli* trophozoites are readily recognized by their large size, their shape and their rapid, rotating motion. Cysts are less easily identified, but they usually cause few diagnostic problems. The morphology of trophozoites and cysts is seen in Figure 180.11.

Examination of direct saline mounts is the most practical method of detecting these protozoa. Cysts can be recovered by concentration, but in human infections trophozoites are usually more numerous than cysts. Iodine-stained mounts and permanent stains are of little value because the organisms tend to overstain and may resemble helminth eggs and/or debris.[52]

CLINICAL MANIFESTATIONS AND MANAGEMENT

The clinical manifestations and management of infections caused by these organisms is discussed in Chapters 49, 108 and 110.

REFERENCES

References for this chapter can be found online at http://www.expertconsult.com

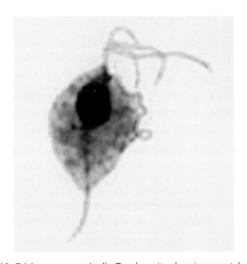

Fig. 180.10 *Trichomonas vaginalis.* Trophozoite showing axostyle, flagella, and part of the undulating membrane (Giemsa stain). There is no known cyst form for this organism.

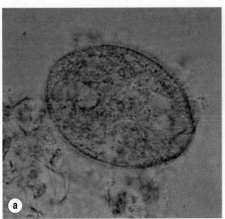
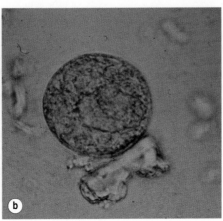

Fig. 180.11 *Balantidium coli.* (a) Trophozoite – note the cilia around the edges ('fuzzy football'). (b) Cyst – note the cilia are difficult to see within the cyst wall (d'Antoni's iodine – light preparation, pale color).

Protozoa: intestinal coccidia and microsporidia

Intestinal coccidia and microsporidia have primarily gained attention as etiologic agents of HIV-associated diarrhea and intestinal disease among persons with other cellular immunodeficiency, including organ transplant recipients or patients undergoing chemotherapy. These organisms, however, are not only opportunistic pathogens, but are also the cause of common, worldwide intestinal infections in immunocompetent children and adults. Also, newly described microsporidia are recognized as causing a wide range of organ or systemic infections in immunocompromised patients.

NATURE

Intestinal coccidia

The intestinal coccidia are obligate intracellular protozoa that belong to the phylum Apicomplexa, subphylum Sporozoa, and infect small intestinal enterocytes. Species of four genera (*Cryptosporidium, Cyclospora, Isospora, Sarcocystis*) are pathogenic in humans.[1-3]

The most frequent agents of human cryptosporidiosis are the bovine *Cryptosporidium* species, *C. parvum*, and *C. hominis*, of which humans and rarely domestic animals are the natural reservoir.[1,4,5] Also, other zoonotic cryptosporidia, including *C. meleagridis, C. felis, C. canis, C. muris* and *C. suis*, have been identified in stools of patients with HIV infection and in HIV-seronegative children living in resource-poor countries.[5-7] *Isospora belli* has been identified as the only accepted cause of human isosporiasis.[3] Intestinal organisms that were previously termed blue-green algae, cyanobacterium-like bodies or coccidia-like bodies were characterized as belonging to the coccidians, and are named *Cyclospora cayetanensis*.[2]

Microsporidia

The term 'microsporidia' is a nontaxonomic designation commonly used to describe a group of obligate intracellular protist-like parasites belonging to the phylum Microsporidia. The nomenclatural status of Microsporidia is ambiguous at present.[8] Microsporidia are considered specialized parasites that evolutionarily seem to be derived from an endoparasitic chytrid ancestor on the earliest diverging branch of the fungal phylogenetic tree,[9] but their exact relationship to the fungi remains to be determined.[10] Approximately 1200 species have been identified that are parasitic in every major animal group, and 14 or these can infect humans (see Table 181.1). To date, seven genera (*Enterocytozoon, Encephalitozoon, Anncaliia, Nosema, Pleistophora, Trachipleistophora* and *Vittaforma*) and unclassified microsporidia (referred to collectively as *Microsporidium*) have been implicated in human infections.[11,12]

EPIDEMIOLOGY

Cryptosporidium species

Cryptosporidial infections have been detected on all continents. Cumulative prevalence rates are between 1% and 3% in industrialized nations and between 5% and 10% in developing countries.[13] Children, particularly those less than 2 years of age, have a higher prevalence of infection than adults. Seroepidemiologic studies indicate that cryptosporidiosis may be more common than is estimated based upon surveys of fecal oocyst shedding. Seroprevalence rates in developed countries range between 25% and 35%, and in developing countries they are up to 65%. In severely immunodeficient patients with HIV infection, cryptosporidiosis is among the most important causes of chronic diarrhea, accounting for 10-20% of diarrheal episodes.[14]

Sources of infectious cryptosporidial oocysts are humans and animals. Oocysts are transmitted by the fecal-oral route and infection may be acquired from contaminated surfaces, ground and recreational water, pets and farm animals (particularly cattle and sheep), contaminated foods and person-to-person contact, including transmission between household members, sexual partners, children in day-care centers and nosocomial infections involving both medical care staff and patients. An increasing number of outbreaks of cryptosporidial infections attributed to drinking water have been reported, including an outbreak in Milwaukee, USA in 1993 that affected over 400 000 persons.[15] Ingestion of as few as 10 oocysts may cause diarrhea.

Cyclospora species

Cyclospora spp. have been identified worldwide in stool specimens of immunocompromised and immunocompetent patients, including travelers, but the source of infection appears to be restricted to tropical and subtropical areas. The parasite is transmitted by the fecal-oral route and infection is most probably acquired from contaminated water or food (particularly raspberries and green leafy vegetables) from tropical or subtropical countries.[16] It is not known whether animals can be infected and serve as sources for human infection. Direct person-to-person transmission is unlikely because excreted oocysts require days to weeks to become infectious. Warm temperatures and high humidity facilitate sporulation.[17]

Isospora species

Isospora belli is endemic in many parts of Africa, Asia and South America, and is particularly common in patients from developing countries who have AIDS and chronic diarrhea; for example, it occurs in 10-20% of such patients in Haiti or Africa. Modes of transmission are not known but it is assumed that they comprise water and/or food that contains oocysts.

Microsporidia

Reported human infections are globally dispersed. Although microsporidiosis appears to occur most frequently in persons infected with HIV, it is emerging as an infection in otherwise immunocompromised hosts, such as organ transplant recipients or patients undergoing chemotherapy, and in immunocompetent individuals, including travelers, the elderly and children.[10,11]

The sources of microsporidia infecting humans and modes of transmission are uncertain. Because microsporidial spores are released into the environment via stool, urine and respiratory secretions, possible sources of infection may be persons or animals infected with microsporidia as well as contaminated water and food.[10,12] Ingestion of microsporidial spores is the most probable mode of transmission. Transmission by the aerosol route has also been considered because spores have been found in respiratory specimens of patients who have *Encephalitozoon* spp. infection.[18] Epidemiologic and experimental studies in mammals suggest that *Encephalitozoon* spp. can be transmitted transplacentally from mother to offspring, but no congenitally acquired human infections have been reported.

PATHOGENICITY

Cryptosporidium species

Cryptosporidium spp. develop intracellularly at the microvillous border of enterocytes (Fig. 181.1). Infected cells lack microvilli at the site of parasite attachment and the mucosal surface appears disrupted. In immunocompetent individuals, infection is usually limited to the intestine. In immunocompromised patients, organisms are found throughout the entire gastrointestinal tract and within epithelial cells of the biliary tree, the pancreatic ducts and the airways. In the intestines, cryptosporidial infection induces atrophy, blunting or loss of villi, crypt hyperplasia, and infiltration of lymphocytes, neutrophils, plasma cells and macrophages into the lamina propria. Cryptosporidial infection has been associated with marked reduction in the brush border enzyme activities, including sucrase, lactase and maltase deficiency, with impaired absorption of vitamin B12 and D-xylose, and with increased permeability of the intestinal epithelium to organic molecules. Malabsorption and intestinal injury appear to correlate with the number of organisms infecting the intestine. No specific virulence determinants of the parasite have been clearly linked to direct or indirect damage of intestinal host tissues. Putative virulence factors include molecules that are involved in parasite attachment to host cells and host cell membrane disruption.

The immune responses to cryptosporidial infection involves both innate and adaptive immune responses. CD4+ lymphocytes and interferon gamma (IFN-γ) play key roles in the memory response.[19] Severe or persistent cryptosporidiosis has primarily been observed in HIV-infected patients with marked CD4+ cell immunodeficiency,[14] and rarely in persons with IFN-γ deficiency[20] or with X-linked hyper-IgM syndrome which leads to secondary hypogammaglobulinemia and impaired cellular immune function.[21]

Isospora species

Isospora belli develops within parasitophorous vacuoles deep in the cytoplasm of the enterocyte. Histologic abnormalities associated with isosporiasis range from minimal changes of the small intestinal architecture to marked villous atrophy, crypt hyperplasia and inflammatory infiltrates in the lamina propria consisting of eosinophils, neutrophils, lymphocytes and plasma cells. The mechanisms by which these changes occur are unknown. As a result of the intestinal injury, malabsorption and steatorrhea have been documented.[3,17]

Cyclospora species

Cyclosporiasis is associated with villous atrophy, crypt hyperplasia and inflammatory infiltrates. The mechanisms that lead to the clinical features are unknown.

Microsporidia

Microsporidiosis has been associated with abnormalities in structure and function of infected organs but how the different microsporidial species cause disease is not sufficiently understood.[10,11]

Enterocytozoon bieneusi infection generally appears to be limited to intestinal enterocytes (Fig. 181.2) and biliary epithelium. Patients who have severe cellular immunodeficiency appear at highest risk of developing microsporidial disease but little is known about immunity to *E. bieneusi* infection due to the lack of tissue culture or small animal models.[10] It is not understood whether microsporidial infection in these patients is primarily a reactivation of latent infection acquired before the state of suppressed immunity or whether microsporidial disease is caused by recently acquired infection.

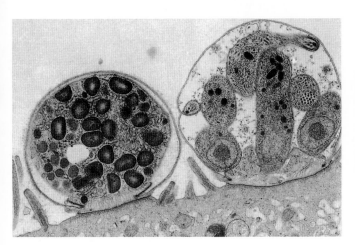

Fig. 181.1 Intestinal cryptosporidial infection. Transmission electron micrograph of duodenal tissue of a patient with HIV infection showing two different developmental stages of *Cryptosporidium* spp. on the brush border of the mucosal surface: mature schizont with merozoites (right), undifferentiated zygote (left). *Cryptosporidium* spp. develop intracellularly just under the plasma membrane of the host cell. Courtesy of MA Spycher.

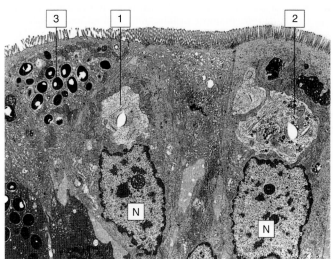

Fig. 181.2 Intestinal *Enterocytozoon bieneusi* infection. Transmission electron micrograph showing duodenal epithelium of a patient with HIV infection who has *Enterocytozoon bieneusi* infection. The different developmental stages between the enterocyte nuclei (N) and the microvillous border include: (1) a proliferative plasmodium; (2) late sporogonial plasmodia; and (3) mature spores. Courtesy of MA Spycher.

Encephalitozoon cuniculi and *E. hellem* infect a variety of cells including epithelial and endothelial cells, fibroblasts, kidney tubule cells, macrophages and possibly other cell types in numerous mammalian hosts, for example rabbits, rodents, carnivores, monkeys and humans.[12,22] In mammals, they usually cause latent asymptomatic or chronic mildly symptomatic infection, but interstitial nephritis and severe neurologic disease caused by central nervous system vasculitis and granulomatous encephalitis may occur. The parasites are able to persist in their animal hosts despite an active immune response. Microsporidial infection activates antibody production, although antibodies alone do not appear to yield protection. The role of a competent cellular immune response in suppressing microsporidial multiplication is suggested by epidemiologic studies in humans, and has been established experimentally.[23] *In-vitro* studies demonstrated the importance of IFN-γ and tumor necrosis factor in resistance to *Encephalitozoon* spp.[23,24] The pathogenesis of human *Encephalitozoon* infection has yet to be defined. Rare histologic and clinical investigations in immunodeficient patients have indicated that *E. cuniculi* and *E. hellem* usually cause disseminated infection in this patient group.[11,12,18,22]

PREVENTION

Cryptosporidiosis

Cryptosporidial oocysts are remarkably resistant to many common disinfectants, including chlorine-based compounds.[25] Therefore, the water industry studied alternative methods to inactivate water-borne oocysts, including a water disinfection device delivering germicidal ultraviolet (UV) light which yielded promising results.[26] However, control of surface-water contamination and adequate filter systems are required to guarantee the complete removal of cryptosporidia from water supplies.

Cyclosporiasis, isosporiasis

Avoiding food or water that may be contaminated with feces may prevent cyclosporiasis and isosporiasis, but details of the sources of infection and the modes of transmission are unknown.

Microsporidiosis

Laboratory experiments indicate that the thick-walled spores may survive in the environment for months or years depending on the temperature and humidity. Exposure to recommended working concentrations of most disinfectants, boiling and autoclaving seem to kill *Encephalitozoon* spp. spores but no data are available for *Enterocytozoon* spp. Recent studies demonstrated successful disinfection of *Encephalitozoon* spp. in water using chlorine and ozone disinfection.[10,27]

DIAGNOSTIC MICROBIOLOGY

Stool examination by light microscopy is the most important test to diagnose intestinal coccidia and intestinal microsporidia. In many laboratories, tests for *Cryptosporidium* spp., *Isospora* spp., *Cyclospora* spp. and microsporidia must be specifically requested because the general request of 'stool for O & P' (ova and parasites) often does not mean that the specific methods to detect these organisms are applied. Microsporidial species that cause systemic infection are best detected in urine sediments.

Cryptosporidium species

Examination of stool specimens by light microscopy

To visualize the *Cryptosporidium* spp. oocysts in fecal smears, acid-fast staining (e.g. modified cold Kinyoun technique; Fig. 181.3) and the immunofluorescence (IF) technique are among the most sensitive, specific and widely used methods. The IF detection procedure is more sensitive than the acid-fast staining but the difference in sensitivity may not be of clinical relevance when watery stools of patients with HIV infection are examined. These patients usually excrete an amount of oocysts that can easily be detected using acid-fast staining. The oocysts should be measured in order to distinguish *Cryptosporidium* spp. (4–6μm in diameter) from *Cyclospora* spp. (8–10μm). Enhanced sensitivity of stool examination can be obtained by concentrating oocysts, preferably with the formalin-ethyl acetate (FEA) technique.

The exact sensitivity of the coprodiagnostic techniques is not known but some data raise questions about the widely held belief that these techniques are sufficient to meet the needs of clinicians and epidemiologists.[28] The minimum number of oocysts in human stool specimens that can be detected by the FEA stool concentration technique and the IF staining procedure was found to be unexpectedly high: 5000–10 000 oocysts per gram of stool in watery stool specimens and 10 000–50 000 oocysts per gram of stool in formed stool. Examination of multiple specimens may be necessary, because clinical studies have shown that examination of single stool specimens may have an insufficient diagnostic yield. Furthermore, in a prospective analysis of jejunal biopsies in patients who have AIDS, *Cryptosporidium* spp. were present in more than 10% of patients whose stool examinations were negative. These results, however, were in contrast to another study that only identified organisms on biopsy in one-third of patients shedding *Cryptosporidium* spp. in their feces.

Stool antigen detection techniques have been developed but the sensitivity of currently available tests is not better than microscopic techniques.[29] Molecular diagnostic methods have improved diagnostic yields but currently are not ready to use in routine laboratories.[30]

Cytologic diagnosis

Aspiration of duodenal fluid or small intestinal brushing can be used for diagnosis when upper endoscopy is performed. Examination of centrifuged duodenal aspirates under the microscope may be the most sensitive diagnostic procedure.

Histologic examinations

Cryptosporidium spp. appear basophilic by examination under the light microscope of small intestinal tissue sections stained with hematoxylin and eosin. The intracellular organisms seem to project into the intestinal lumen because of their apical extracytoplasmic localization. Under electron microscopy the unique ultrastructural features of different developmental stages of the parasite can be seen (see Fig. 181.1), but this is rarely necessary for diagnostic purposes.

Serology

Specific IgM or IgG antibodies to *Cryptosporidium* spp. can be detected within 2 weeks of onset of symptoms in most patients. In the majority of patients IgG titers may persist for long periods. Serologic testing is mainly used as an epidemiologic tool and has no diagnostic application, particularly because antibody persistence limits its use in the diagnosis of acute infection.

Cyclospora species

Diagnosis of *Cyclospora* spp. is dependent on detection by light microscopy of the refractile oocysts, 8–10μm in diameter, in wet mounts of fresh stool specimens or in acid-fast stained smears prepared from stool concentrated by the FEA sedimentation.[17,31] Acid-fast stained oocysts vary in appearance from faint pink to deep red, and many organisms remain as unstained spheres (see Fig. 181.3). The sensitivity of the coprodiagnostic techniques is unknown. In many patients' specimens, however, the number of oocysts detected per slide is low, indicating that not all symptomatic patients excrete a large enough number of oocysts for laboratory detection to be assured. Examination of small intestinal tissue of patients who have *Cyclospora* infection

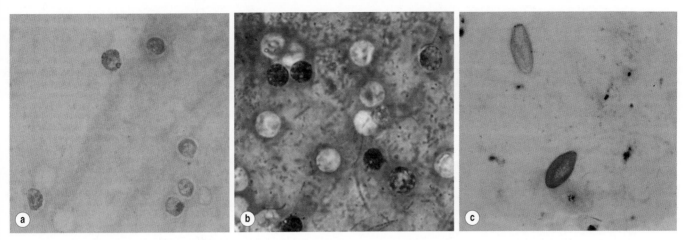

Fig. 181.3 Acid-fast stained smears of fecal specimens showing intestinal coccidia. (a) *Cryptosporidium* spp., round, 4–6 μm diameter. (b) *Cyclospora* spp., round, 8–10 μm diameter. Courtesy of EG Long. (c) *Isospora belli*, elliptical, 23–33 μm long and 10–19 μm wide. Modified Kinyoun stain.

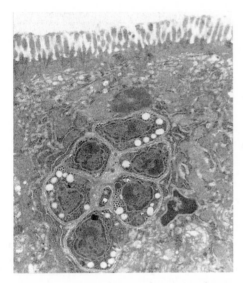

Fig. 181.4 Intestinal *Cyclospora* infection. Transmission electron micrograph of duodenal epithelium obtained from a patient with HIV infection who has *Cyclospora cayetanensis* infection. A mature schizont filled with numerous merozoites is shown. Courtesy of AM Deloul and FP Chatelet.

often did not reveal any parasites. The presence of intracellular parasites has rarely been documented in aspirated duodenal or jejunal fluid and on duodenal and jejunal biopsy (Fig. 181.4).

Isospora species

Diagnosis of *I. belli* is usually achieved by detection under the light microscope of the parasite oocysts in wet preparations or acid-fast stained smears of concentrated stool specimens (see Fig. 181.3). Repetitive stool examinations may be necessary because the parasite may be excreted intermittently or in low numbers. Histologic examination of small intestinal tissue sections may reveal the parasite within enterocytes.

Microsporidia

Diagnosis of microsporidial infection is dependent on morphologic demonstration of the organisms themselves. This can be difficult because of the organisms' small size and staining properties hamper visualization of the spores and developing stages using routine staining techniques. The spores, the stages by which microsporidia are usually identified, are small, ranging in size from 1 to 3.5 μm in diameter.

Evaluation of patients who have suspected microsporidiosis should begin with examination of body fluids by light microscopy using special staining techniques. Definitive species identification of microsporidia is made using electron microscopy, antigenic analysis, and molecular analysis. Collection of fresh material (without fixative) may be useful for cell culture and for future molecular analysis.[11]

Examination of stool specimens

In patients who have suspected enteric microsporidiosis, examination of stool specimens by light microscopy is the first step. It is at least as sensitive as examination of biopsy specimens. Detection of microsporidial spores requires adequate illumination and magnification [i.e. ×630 or ×1000 magnification (oil immersion)], and special staining methods. The two most commonly used stains are the chromotrope stain, which appears to be the most specific (Fig. 181.5),[32] and chemofluorescent agents, which might be more sensitive but may produce false-positive results.[33] An epidemiologic comparison of these techniques resulted in the recommendation to screen specimens with chemofluorescent agents and to confirm the results with the chromotrope stain.

Fig. 181.5 Detection of microsporidia in stool samples. Smear of a formalin-fixed, unconcentrated stool specimen of a patient who has AIDS and chronic diarrhea, showing pinkish-red-stained spores of *Enterocytozoon bieneusi*. Chromotrope staining (oil immersion).

The differences in spore size between *Enterocytozoon* (1–1.5 μm in diameter) and *Encephalitozoon* spp. (2–3 μm in diameter) often permit a tentative diagnosis of the genus from examination of stool under the light microscope. The microsporidian should be identified to the level of genus by electron microscopy or molecular analysis because *Encephalitozoon* spp. have a propensity for dissemination, and have a different drug sensitivity pattern compared with *Enterocytozoon bieneusi*.

Immunofluorescent procedures for diagnosis of *Encephalitozoon*-like microsporidial spores are promising but not widely available. Diagnostic application of polyclonal antibodies in fecal samples has been hampered by background staining, cross-reactions with yeast and bacteria, and low sensitivity. Monoclonal antibodies against *Encephalitozoon* spp.[34] and against spores of *Enterocytozoon bieneusi* have been generated.[35]

Histologic examination

Among patients with HIV infection who suffered from chronic diarrhea, stool examinations proved as sensitive as endoscopic evaluation for all pathogens except cytomegalovirus and *Leishmania*.[14] Examination of duodenal and terminal ileal tissue has resulted in detection of microsporidia but the parasites are rarely found in colonic tissue sections.

Only highly experienced pathologists have reliably and consistently identified microsporidia in tissue sections using routine techniques such as hematoxylin and eosin stain. Ultra-thin plastic sections stained with methylene blue-azure II–basic fuchsin or with toluidine blue may facilitate detection but these techniques are not routinely used. In our experience, tissue Gram stains such as Brown–Brenn or Brown–Hopps have proved to be the most useful for the rapid and reliable identification of HIV-associated microsporidia in routine paraffin-embedded tissue sections (Fig. 181.6). Others prefer a silver stain (Warthin–Starry stain) or the chromotrope-based staining technique.

Cytologic diagnosis

Microsporidial spores have been detected in sediments of duodenal aspirate, bile or biliary aspirates, urine (Fig. 181.7), bronchoalveolar lavage fluid, cerebrospinal fluid (CSF) and in smears of conjunctival swabs, sputum and nasal discharge.[11] Microscopic examination of centrifuged duodenal aspirate obtained during endoscopy appears to be the most sensitive technique for diagnosis of intestinal microsporidiosis. Because microsporidial infection often involves multiple organs, detection of microsporidia in virtually any tissue or bodily fluid should prompt a thorough search of other sites. In particular, urine specimens of patients suspected of having disseminated microsporidiosis should be examined.

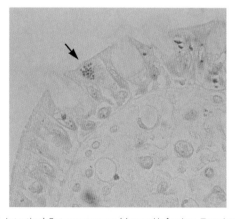

Fig. 181.6 Intestinal *Enterocytozoon bieneusi* infection. Terminal ileal tissue obtained by ileocolonoscopy in a patient who has AIDS and chronic diarrhea caused by *Enterocytozoon bieneusi* infection. Gram-positive or Gram-labile microsporidial spores (arrow) are found in supranuclear location within small intestinal enterocytes. Brown–Brenn stain.

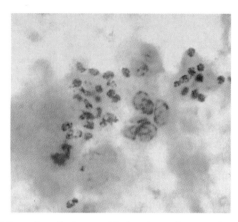

Fig. 181.7 Detection of microsporidia in urine sediment. Urine sediment from a patient who has AIDS and disseminated *Encephalitozoon hellem* infection, showing Gram-labile intracellular and extracellular microsporidial spores. Gram stain (oil immersion).

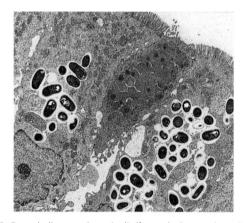

Fig. 181.8 *Encephalitozoon intestinalis* (formerly *Septata intestinalis*): developing spores within enterocytes separated by a fibrillar matrix. *Encephalitozoon intestinalis* develop within parasitophorous vacuoles, unlike *E. bieneusi*, which develop in direct contact with enterocyte cytoplasm. Courtesy of MA Spycher.

Electron microscopy

Microsporidial ultrastructure is unique and pathognomonic for the phylum and, with rare exceptions, ultrastructural features can distinguish between most genera of microsporidia (Fig. 181.8; see Fig. 181.2).[36,37]

Serology

Serologic assays (including carbon immunoassay, indirect IF test, enzyme-linked immunosorbent assay and Western blot immuno-detection) have been useful in detecting antibodies to *E. cuniculi* in several species of animals, but reliable serologic tests for diagnosis of human microsporidiosis are lacking. This lack of availability is partly because *Enterocytozoon* spp. have not been continuously propagated in cell culture or laboratory animals.

Cell culture

Encephalitozoon spp., *Trachipleistophora* spp., *Vittaforma corneae* and *Anncaliia algerae* have been isolated using cell culture systems, but these tests are fastidious and costly, and the most common human species, *E. bieneusi*, has not been continuously propagated.

Molecular techniques

Universal panmicrosporidian and species-specific primer pairs that amplify the short regions of the small subunit rRNA gene have been developed,[22,38] but, at present, these techniques are confined to research laboratories. Recently, simultaneous detection of four human pathogenic microsporidia from patients' specimens by oligonucleotide microarray has been described.[39] Diagnosis and identification of *Enterocytozoon bieneusi* and the different *Encephalitozoon* spp. have been successfully performed with fresh stool specimens, formalin-fixed stool specimens, intestinal tissue obtained by endoscopic biopsy, urine specimens and other body fluids.[10] *In-situ* hybridization to visualize *E. bieneusi* in tissue sections has been developed.

CLINICAL MANIFESTATIONS

Cryptosporidiosis

For cryptosporidiosis the mean incubation period between infection and onset of symptoms is approximately 7–14 days (range 5–28 days). The severity and duration of illness vary depending on the immune status of the hosts. Children, the elderly and individuals with nutritional deficiencies may suffer from a more severe and prolonged disease, as is observed in immunodeficient patients. Whether cryptosporidiosis in immunocompromised patients is mainly a reactivation of latent infection or whether clinical illness is caused by recently acquired infection is not known.

Immunocompetent patients

In immunocompetent patients, cryptosporidia cause a self-limiting, usually watery, diarrhea lasting 10–14 days (range 2–28 days), but the clinical presentation varies from asymptomatic shedding of oocysts to severe disease that may last up to 3 months.[15,40] Patients often complain of abdominal pain, flatulence, loss of appetite, nausea and vomiting, and may suffer from low-grade fever, anorexia, malaise, weakness, fatigue, myalgias and headaches. The diarrhea and abdominal pain are often made worse by eating. Cough appears significantly more frequent in children with cryptosporidiosis than in children with diarrhea of another etiology, but the parasite has rarely been documented in the airways of immunocompetent individuals. Single case reports of pancreatitis associated with cryptosporidiosis and reactive arthritis have been described. Poorly understood lasting adverse effects of infection in children may include deficits of linear growth and cognitive sequelae, even if cryptosporidial infection is otherwise symptomless.[41,42]

Immunocompromised patients

In immunocompromised patients, particularly individuals with HIV infection, cryptosporidiosis is a more severe, often chronic and incurable illness that can be life-threatening. The main clinical presentation is watery diarrhea that can lead to severe dehydration, electrolyte depletion, malnutrition and weight loss. In addition, infection of the biliary tract and the gallbladder, resulting in acalculous cholecystitis, sclerosing cholangitis ('AIDS cholangiopathy') and stenosis of the papilla of Vater, frequently occurs. Infection of the epithelial cells of the respiratory tract, including sinuses, is increasingly described, but it is not clear whether this finding is of clinical relevance because most of these patients have a concomitant respiratory infection. Systemic cryptosporidiosis has not been described.

The clinical course of HIV-associated cryptosporidiosis is highly variable. Four clinical patterns of disease have been identified:

- asymptomatic shedding of oocysts;
- transient diarrhea with transient or chronic shedding of oocysts;
- chronic diarrhea; and
- fulminant disease that leads to cachexia and death within months.

Most patients who have severe illness have CD4+ lymphocyte counts below 50 cells/µl. Spontaneous clinical recovery may occur and is mainly correlated with higher CD4+ lymphocyte counts, but a benign course of the diarrhea may also occur in severely immunodeficient patients. Clinical observations suggest that cryptosporidial disease is more severe if co-infections caused by other enteropathogens are present. Concurrent dual or multiple intestinal infection is found in up to 50% of patients who have HIV-associated cryptosporidiosis.

Cyclosporiasis

The spectrum of *Cyclospora*-associated illness is not yet fully defined but it may range from asymptomatic carriage of the organism to severe and prolonged diarrhea in immunocompetent and immunocompromised patients. Patients who have AIDS tend to have a more prolonged and severe illness, and *Cyclospora*-associated cholangiopathy has been described in this group.[16,17]

The incubation period between infection and onset of symptoms ranges between 2 and 11 days and is usually about 7 days. In symptomatic infections the main clinical manifestation is mild to severe watery diarrhea, accompanied by abdominal cramps, bloating, increased flatus, nausea, anorexia, substantial weight loss and fatigue. Vomiting is less common and about 25% of the patients report fever and myalgias.

If not treated, diarrhea is self-limiting but may last for several weeks (range 2–107 days), and remissions and relapses may occur during gradual resolution of the illness. *Cyclospora* infection does not appear to provide lasting immunity.

Isosporiasis

In immunocompetent persons, *I. belli* infection causes self-limited watery diarrhea accompanied by malaise, anorexia, cramping abdominal pain, weight loss and, less frequently, low-grade fever. In immunocompromised patients, the illness is more severe and prolonged, or chronic if untreated. Also, acalculous cholecystitis and two single cases of disseminated extraintestinal isosporiasis in patients with AIDS have been reported.

Microsporidiosis in immunocompromised patients

The spectrum of clinically manifest microsporidial infection is diverse and includes intestinal, ocular, muscular, cerebral, respiratory and urinary tract disease (Table 181.1).[10,11] The most prevalent microsporidial disease is HIV-associated chronic diarrhea.[14] Disseminated microsporidial infections are being increasingly recognized in patients who have AIDS.

Diarrhea, cholangitis, acalculous cholecystitis

Two microsporidial species – *Enterocytozoon bieneusi* and *Encephalitozoon intestinalis* – cause chronic diarrhea and wasting, cholangiopathy and acalculous cholecystitis in patients who have HIV infection or who are otherwise immunodeficient, particularly when CD4+ lymphocyte counts drop below 50–100/µl.

Enterocytozoon bieneusi is estimated to be one of the most important HIV-associated intestinal pathogens, present in 5–30% of those with otherwise unexplained diarrhea. The main symptoms are chronic nonbloody diarrhea, anorexia, weight loss and bloating. Some patients experience intermittent diarrhea and a few excrete microsporidial spores without having diarrhea. The stool is watery or soft, and diarrhea seems to be worsened by most foods. Some of the patients report abdominal pain or nausea and vomiting. Laboratory evidence for intestinal malabsorption is common. *E. bieneusi* itself is not immediately life-threatening, but diarrhea is debilitating, and weight loss may lead to cachexia, which is a significant cause or cofactor in the deaths of many patients. Up to one-third of patients who have intestinal microsporidiosis have

Table 181.1 Microsporidial species pathogenic in humans, and clinical manifestations

Microsporidial species	Clinical manifestations
Enterocytozoon bieneusi	Diarrhea, wasting syndrome Cholangiopathy, cholangitis, acalculous cholecystitis Sinusitis, bronchitis, pneumonitis
Encephalitozoon intestinalis (formerly *Septata intestinalis*)	Diarrhea Cholangiopathy, cholangitis, acalculous cholecystitis Sinusitis, bronchitis, pneumonitis Urinary tract infection, nephritis Bone lesions; nodular cutaneous lesions
Encephalitozoon cuniculi	Systemic infection Keratoconjunctivitis Sinusitis, pneumonitis Urinary tract infection, nephritis Hepatitis Peritonitis Symptomatic and asymptomatic intestinal infections Seizures, encephalitis
Encephalitozoon hellem	Systemic infection Keratoconjunctivitis Sinusitis, bronchitis, pneumonia Nephritis, ureteritis, cystitis, prostatitis, urethritis
Anncaliia connori (formerly *Brachiola connori* and *Nosema connori*)	Systemic infection
Trachipleistophora anthropophthera	Systemic infection including brain, heart, kidney, eye
Pleistophora ronneafiei	Myositis
Trachipleistophora hominis	Myositis, keratoconjunctivitis, sinusitis
Anncaliia vesicularum (formerly *Brachiola vesicularum*)	Myositis
Anncaliia algerae (formerly *Brachiola algerae* and *Nosema algerae*)	Keratitis, myositis
Vittaforma corneae (formerly *Nosema corneum*)	Keratitis Urinary tract infection
Nosema ocularum	Keratitis
Microsporidium ceylonensis	Corneal ulcer
Microsporidium africanum	Corneal ulcer

dual or multiple co-infection with other intestinal pathogens. The parasite has also been detected in the biliary tree and/or gallbladder of patients who have cholangitis and acalculous cholecystitis. Imaging procedures often reveal dilatation of both intrahepatic and common bile ducts, irregularities of the bile duct wall and gallbladder abnormalities such as wall thickening, distention or the presence of sludge.[11,14]

Encephalitozoon intestinalis primarily causes diarrhea, and the parasite may also spread into the biliary tract and gallbladder, causing cholangitis and cholecystitis. In contrast to *Enterocytozoon bieneusi*, systemic dissemination to kidneys and other sites may occur.[43]

Systemic microsporidiosis

There are three microsporidial genera, *Encephalitozoon* spp., *Trachipleistophora* spp. and *Vittaforma corneae*, which have been found to disseminate in severely immunodeficient patients who have HIV infection.[22,44–46] Disseminated infection caused by *Anncaliia* (formerly *Brachiola connori* or *Nosema connori*) was found at autopsy in a 4-month-old athymic boy reported in 1973.

Encephalitozoon spp. were initially identified in patients who had AIDS and keratoconjunctivitis.[47] Subsequently the spectrum of recognized *Encephalitozoon*-associated disease has expanded to include keratoconjunctivitis, bronchiolitis, sinusitis, pneumonitis, nephritis, ureteritis, cystitis, prostatitis, hepatitis, peritonitis, diarrhea and encephalitis.[18,22] Clinical manifestations may vary substantially, ranging from an asymptomatic carrier state to organ failure.

Trachipleistophora anthropophthera was identified at autopsy in cerebral, cardiac, renal, pancreatic, thyroid, hepatic, splenic, lymphoid and bone marrow tissue of two patients who had AIDS and initially presented with seizures.[45]

Urinary tract infection

Predominant genitourinary signs and symptoms caused by *Encephalitozoon* infections have been observed. Clinical manifestations included asymptomatic microhematuria, urethritis, prostatitis, acute cystitis and interstitial nephritis associated with dysuria, gross hematuria and progressive renal insufficiency.[18]

Respiratory tract infection

In most patients who have respiratory tract microsporidial infection, including bronchiolitis, pneumonia and progressive respiratory failure, intestinal or systemic microsporidiosis was also present. Single cases of patients have been reported in whom sinusitis causing nasal obstruction and persistent mucopurulent nasal discharge caused by *E. bieneusi* or *Encephalitozoon* spp. was a predominant manifestation of systemic microsporidiosis.

Keratoconjunctivitis

HIV-associated ocular microsporidiosis caused by *Encephalitozoon* spp. is restricted to the superficial epithelium of the cornea and conjunctiva. Most patients exhibit bilateral coarse punctate epithelial keratopathy (Fig. 181.9), conjunctival inflammation resulting in redness and foreign body sensation, decreased visual acuity and photophobia. In patients who initially present with symptomatic keratoconjunctival microsporidiosis, dissemination of the parasite may be common, but clinical manifestations other than keratoconjunctivitis may be mild or absent.[48]

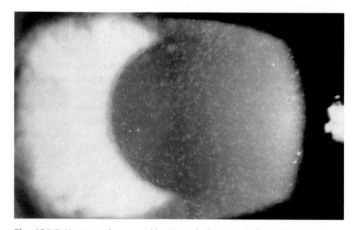

Fig. 181.9 Keratopathy caused by *Encephalitozoon hellem*. Slit-lamp demonstration of punctate epithelial keratopathy in a patient who has AIDS and keratoconjunctivitis caused by *Encephalitozoon hellem*. Ocular microsporidiosis can often be diagnosed by examination under the light microscope of a smear obtained by a nontraumatic conjunctival swab. Courtesy of M Diesenhouse and DA Schwartz.

Cerebral microsporidiosis

Microsporidia was first accepted as the etiologic agent of a neurologic disorder in two children, reported in 1959 and 1984. Both presented with seizures and might have had impaired immune responses. *Encephalitozoon cuniculi* and *Trachipleistophora anthropophthera* were detected in CSF or brain tissue of patients with HIV infection who presented with fever and somnolence or seizures and mental decline. MRI disclosed multiple small, contrast-enhancing, mostly ring-like lesions localized to the hippocampus, mesencephalon and cerebral cortex (Fig. 181.10).[45,49]

Myositis

Myositis caused by *Pleistophora* spp. has been described in an HIV-seronegative patient and in a patient with HIV infection, both of whom had severe cellular immunodeficiency. Newly characterized microsporidia, *Trachipleistophora hominis* and *Anncaliia* (formerly *Brachiola vesicularum*), were detected in muscle biopsies of patients who had AIDS and presented with myositis.[44,50]

Microsporidiosis in immunocompetent persons

Enterocytozoon bieneusi and *Encephalitozoon* spp. are associated with self-limiting watery diarrhea in immunocompetent adults as well as in children, particularly among persons who reside or have traveled in tropical countries.[51] An unexpectedly high prevalence (17%) of intestinal microsporidiosis due to *Enterocytozoon bieneusi* was found in HIV-seronegative elderly patients in Spain.[52]

Deep stromal infections of the cornea caused by different microsporidial species have been described in otherwise seemingly healthy persons who presented with severe keratitis or a corneal ulcer or who were contact lens wearers (see Table 181.1).

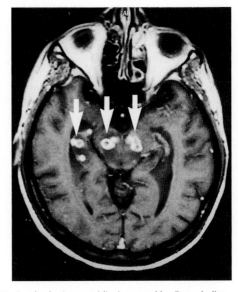

Fig. 181.10 Cerebral microsporidiosis caused by *Encephalitozoon cuniculi* in a patient with HIV infection. The MRI shows multiple small contrast-enhancing, mostly ring-like, partly micronodular, lesions in hippocampal, mesencephal and intracortical regions (arrows), partly accompanied by slight edema, and congestion of the right ethmoid sinus. *Encephalitozoon cuniculi* was isolated from CSF. From Weber *et al.*,[49] with permission from Massachusetts Medical Society.

MANAGEMENT

Cryptosporidiosis

The efficacy of antiparasitic therapy of cryptosporidiosis remains controversial.[53] Among immunocompetent patients, diarrhea due to cryptosporidial infection is usually self-limiting but chronic infection may cause malnutrition in children in developing countries. Nitazoxanide may be useful in immunocompetent individuals with cryptosporidiosis. In a randomized, placebo-controlled trial in apparently immunocompetent children and adults in Egypt, nitazoxanide (500 mg q12h for 3 days in adults, 100–200 mg q12h in children) decreased the duration of diarrhea and cryptosporidial oocyst shedding.[54]

In contrast, in patients who have AIDS no agent has proven effective in the absence of treatment of HIV infection.[53] A randomized trial in HIV-infected persons with cryptosporidiosis in Mexico suggested a shorter duration of diarrhea and oocyst clearance with nitazoxanide treatment among patients with CD4+ lymphocyte counts above 50/μl but no effect was found among patients with CD4+ cell counts below 50/μl.[55] Because the latter group of patients is mainly in need of effective antiparasitic therapy, and because diarrhea in HIV-infected persons with CD4+ cell counts above 50/μl frequently improves due to improved immune function, the usefulness of nitazoxanide in patients with AIDS is doubtful. Case series and a randomized, controlled trial suggested that treatment with oral paromomycin (500 mg q6h for at least 4 weeks) may result in decreased oocyst shedding and improved intestinal function and morphology,[56] but other investigators have not found any clinical benefit.[57] *In-vitro* studies have indicated that nitazoxanide activity may be enhanced by the co-administration of azithromycin or rifabutin,[58] but clinical experience of such combinations is lacking. Hyperimmune bovine colostrum has been found in *in-vitro* experiments in animal studies and in single patients to reduce or eradicate cryptosporidia, but these results could not be reproduced in larger human studies.

Symptomatic treatment of diarrhea may include drugs that affect gut motility such as loperamide, diphenoxylate, opiates, somatostatin and octreotide. Immune reconstitution following initiation of potent antiretroviral therapy of patients who have HIV infection results in cessation of oocyst shedding and diarrhea, but cryptosporidial infection is controlled rather than cured because failure of antiretroviral therapy often results in relapse of cryptosporidiosis.[59]

Cyclosporiasis

A placebo-controlled trial showed that trimethoprim–sulfamethoxazole (TMP–SMX [co-trimoxazole]; double-strength TMP 160 mg/SMX 800 mg q12h for 7 days) was clinically successful and shortened oocyst shedding in immunocompetent patients who have cyclosporiasis.[60] In this study, 3 days of treatment with TMP–SMX was not sufficient to eradicate *Cyclospora*. Trimethoprim 160 mg/SMX 800 mg q6h for 10 days cured HIV-associated cyclosporiasis but the relapse rate was high (43%). Maintenance therapy with double-strength TMP–SMX three times per week did prevent relapses in these patients. For patients who cannot tolerate sulfonamides, a 1-week course of ciprofloxacin (500 mg q12h) may be an alternative although it was not as effective as TMP–SMX in a randomized trial.[61]

Isosporiasis

Immunocompetent and immunocompromised patients respond promptly to therapy with TMP–SMX (double-strength TMP 160 mg/SMX 800 mg q6h for 10 days).[62] In patients with sulfonamide allergies, pyrimethamine 75 mg/day plus folinic acid 10 mg/day may be successful. To prevent the high rate of relapses in patients who have AIDS, maintenance therapy with double-strength TMP–SMX, three times per week, or pyrimethamine 25 mg/day plus folinic acid 5 mg/day, is recommended. In case of sulfonamide intolerance, a 1-week course of ciprofloxacin (500 mg q12h) may be an alternative although it was not as effective as TMP–SMX in a randomized trial among HIV-infected Haitians.[61]

Microsporidiosis

Albendazole, fumagillin, its analog TNP-470, and nikkomycin Z have been found to inhibit completely or partially the replication or spore germination of *Encephalitozoon* spp. and *Vittaforma corneae* propagated in cell cultures, but did not destroy mature microsporidial spores, so that these may sustain infection.[63–65] Numerous other anti-protozoal drugs and antibiotics have been tested *in vitro*, with negative findings. *In-vitro* systems to investigate *Enterocytozoon bieneusi* are not available.

Among HIV-infected persons with access to antiretroviral therapy and immune reconstitution, the occurrence of microsporidiosis has been substantially reduced.[59] Little information on clinical experience in the therapy of human microsporidiosis is available, and only two controlled treatment trials have been conducted,[64,65] confirming previ-ous case observations which indicated that albendazole can result in clinical cure of HIV-associated encephalitozoonosis in parallel with the cessation of spore excretion. In contrast, albendazole is not effective for the treatment of *Enterocytozoon bieneusi* infection and does not reduce the parasite load although previous observations had suggested that clinical improvement may occur in some patients. Oral purified fumagillin was used in a pilot study and subsequently in a small randomized trial to treat HIV-associated diarrhea due to *E. bieneusi*. Fumagillin appeared to eradicate the parasite transiently in many patients but serious adverse events and parasitic relapse were observed.[65,66]

REFERENCES

References for this chapter can be found online at http://www.expertconsult.com

Govinda S Visvesvara
Augusto Julio Martinez
(deceased)

Chapter | **182**

Protozoa: free-living amebae

NATURE

The concept that small free-living amebae, particularly *Acanthamoeba* spp. have the potential to cause disease in humans was developed by CG Culbertson of the Indiana University School of Medicine and the Eli Lilly Laboratories in 1958. The basis of this observation was a chance discovery of an ameba growing in a batch of monkey kidney cell cultures that were to be used for growing polio virus for the development of polio vaccine. This ameba, described as *Acanthamoeba* sp. (Lilly A-1), was found to produce, on intracerebral, intraspinal and intranasal inoculations, meningoencephalitis in cortisone-treated monkeys and mice.[1–3] This isolate is now called *Acanthamoeba culbertsoni*.

The first case of amebic meningoencephalitis in humans, attributed initially to *Acanthamoeba* although later the causative organism was identified as a species of *Naegleria*, was described in Australia in 1962. It is now known that besides *Acanthamoeba* spp., two other free-living amebae, *Naegleria fowleri* and *Balamuthia mandrillaris*, also cause central nervous system (CNS) disease in humans and other animals.[1–4] Recently, however, *Sappinia diploidea*, now reidentified as *Sappinia pedata*, a saprophytic ameba that has been previously isolated from the fecal specimens of lizards, elks and bisons, was identified in a brain biopsy specimen of a previously healthy 38-year-old man who developed visual disturbances, headache and a seizure.[5-6] This suggests that there are cases of human infections caused by free-living amebae other than *Acanthamoeba*, *Balamuthia* and *Naegleria* spp. that may have been either misdiagnosed or unrecognized.

Taxonomy

The free-living amebae, according to the classic taxonomic system, were classified under the subphylum Sarcodina and superclass Rhizopodea.[3] The International Society of Protistologists abandoned the older hierarchical system and recently replaced it with a new classification system emphasizing modern morphologic approaches, biochemical pathways and molecular phylogenetics. According to this new schema the Eukaryotes have been classified into six clusters or 'Super Groups', namely Amoebozoa, Opisthokonta, Rhizaria, Archaeplastida, Chromalveolata and Excavata. *Acanthamoeba* and *Balamuthia* are included under Super Group Amoebozoa (Acanthamoebidae), along with *Sappinia* (Flabellinea: Thecamoebidae), and *Naegleria fowleri* under Super Group Excavata (Heterolobosia: Vahlkampfiidae).[7]

The free-living amebae (*Acanthamoeba*, *Naegleria*, *Balamuthia*, *Hartmannella* and *Vahlkampfia* spp.) and the parasitic amebae (e.g. *Entamoeba histolytica*) move by producing cytoplasmic bulges, the lobopodia, from the surface of the body. In contrast to *E. histolytica*, which is a mitochondria-lacking ameba that causes gastrointestinal disease, *Naegleria*, *Acanthamoeba* and *Balamuthia* are mitochondria-bearing amebae that cause diseases of the CNS of humans and animals, which almost always lead to death. The term amphizoic amebae indicates the ability of these amebae to exist as free-living in nature and as parasites within host tissue; this differentiates them from the truly parasitic *E. histolytica*.[8]

Although several species of *Naegleria* have been described, so far only one species, *N. fowleri* (*Naegleria aerobia* and *Naegleria invadens* are non-valid synonyms), is known to infect the human CNS. Several of the more than 20 species of *Acanthamoeba* that have been described so far cause not only a chronic granulomatous CNS disease in humans and other animals, but also infect the cornea (*Acanthamoeba* keratitis), the skin, the nasal sinuses and pulmonary tissues. The disease caused by *Acanthamoeba* spp. has been described as granulomatous amebic encephalitis (GAE). *Balamuthia mandrillaris*, the only known species of *Balamuthia*, causes GAE and skin infections in humans and other animals.[1–3]

Naegleria fowleri

Naegleria fowleri is also described as an ameboflagellate because it has a transient flagellate stage in its life cycle in addition to a feeding and dividing form, the trophozoite, and a resistant cyst stage (Fig. 182.1). The trophozoite, measuring 10–25 μm, normally feeds on bacteria and multiplies by binary fission. However, it is able to differentiate into a pear-shaped biflagellate stage in response to sudden changes in the ionic concentration of its environment. When the conditions become unfavorable the trophozoite differentiates into a resistant cyst stage. The trophozoite is usually uninucleate; the nucleus is spherical and contains a large, centrally placed, dense nucleolus. Additionally, numerous dumbbell-shaped mitochondria, vacuoles, lysosomes and ribosomes are present within the cytoplasm. Cysts are round and contain a single nucleus with a central dense nucleolus; the dense cyst walls are plugged with one or more flat pores. The cysts are 7–14 μm in diameter, with a mean of 10 μm.[3,8]

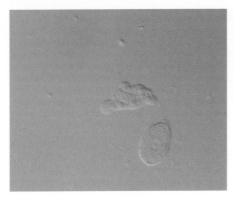

Fig. 182.1 *Naegleria fowleri*. The trophozoite can be differentiated from the cyst by its characteristic lobopodial locomotion; both are taken from culture. Differential interference contrast.

Acanthamoeba spp.

In 1930 Aldo Castellani isolated an ameba from a yeast culture; it was later named as *Acanthamoeba castellanii*.[1-3] Currently, more than 24 species have been identifed in the genus *Acanthamoeba* based on morphologic criteria such as size of the trophozoites and cysts as well as differences in the cyst wall configuration. The various species are included in three different groups:

- Group I comprises those species that have large trophozoites with cysts that range in size from 16 to 30 μm (e.g. *A. astronyxis*, *A. comandoni*, *A. tubiashi*);
- Group II includes by far the largest number of species with cysts measuring around 18 μm or less (e.g. *A. castellanii*, *A. polyphaga*, *A. rhysodes*, *A. hatchetti*); and
- Group III consists of species with subtle differences in cyst morphology, also measuring 18 μm or less (e.g. *A. culbertsoni*, *A. royreba*, *A. lenticulata*).

Currently, identification of species based on morphologic criteria such as size are considered unreliable and hence sequencing of the 18S rDNA is being used not only to differentiate isolates but also to understand the phylogeny of *Acanthamoeba*. Based on sequence differences, 15 genotypes (T1–T15) of *Acanthamoeba* have been established.[1-4] The acanthamebae are also called opportunistic amebae because they produce disease principally in immunodeficient individuals.

The life cycle of *Acanthamoeba* spp. consists of two stages: a feeding and reproducing trophozoite stage and a resistant cyst stage (Fig. 182.2). The trophozoites feed on bacteria and detritus present in the milieu and multiply by binary fission. They are uninucleate and are 15–45 μm in size. The nucleus has a centrally placed, large, densely staining nucleolus. The cytoplasm is finely granular and contains numerous mitochondria, ribosomes and lysosomes. Cysts are 10–25 μm in size and are double walled: the outer wall (the ectocyst) is wrinkled and contains protein; the inner wall (the endocyst) is usually stellate, polygonal, oval or spherical and contains cellulose. Pores covered by opercula are present at the point of contact between the ectocyst and the endocyst. Cysts are uninucleate.

Balamuthia mandrillaris

Balamuthia mandrillaris, previously called leptomyxid ameba, is the only species included under the genus *Balamuthia*. Based on molecular analysis, all isolates studied so far appear to be homogeneous and belong to one genotype. *Balamuthia mandrillaris* has two stages in its life cycle (Fig. 182.3). The trophozoite is irregular in shape and measures from 12 to 60 μm with a mean size of about 30 μm. Although usually uninucleate, binucleate forms are occasionally seen. The nucleus contains a large centrally placed nucleolus. Occasionally, in infected human tissues, trophic stages containing a large nucleus with two or three nucleolar bodies have been observed. Cysts are also uninucleate, more or less spherical, and range in size from 12 to 30 μm with a mean of 15 μm. Cysts appear to be double walled with a wavy

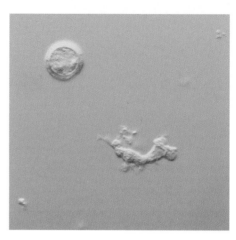

Fig. 182.3 *Balamuthia mandrillaris*. The trophozoite is irregularly shaped whereas the cyst is spherical; both are taken from culture. Differential interference contrast.

ectocyst and a spherical endocyst when viewed under the light microscope. However, ultrastructurally the cysts are tripartite with an outer thin and irregular ectocyst, an inner thick endocyst and a middle amorphous fibrillar mesocyst.[1,2]

Cultivation

Acanthamoeba spp. and *N. fowleri*, but not *B. mandrillaris*, can be cultivated on non-nutrient agar plates coated with suitable Gram-negative bacteria such as *Escherichia coli* or *Enterobacter aerogenes*. The amebae will feed on the bacteria, multiply and differentiate into cysts within a few days. They can be easily subcultured by transplanting a small piece of agar containing trophozoites and/or cysts onto a fresh agar plate coated with bacteria as before. *Naegleria fowleri* and *Acanthamoeba* spp. can also be grown successfully on mammalian cell cultures. *Balamuthia mandrillaris* will not grow on bacteria-coated agar plates. However, it can be isolated from infected human or animal tissue by inoculating monkey kidney or human lung fibroblasts with the triturated tissue and from which a continuous culture can be established by periodic transfers.

Naegleria fowleri and *Acanthamoeba* spp. can be grown axenically (bacteria free) in a complex chemical medium. Although several different formulations are available, in our laboratory we use a modified version of Nelson's medium that contains a 0.5% solution of liver digest, 0.5% glucose and a low osmolarity buffered salt solution supplemented with 3–5% fetal bovine serum. *Acanthamoeba* spp. can also be easily grown in a medium composed of 2% proteose peptone, 0.5% yeast extract and 0.1% glucose made up in a low osmotic buffered salt solution with or without serum. Additionally, *N. fowleri* and several species of *Acanthamoeba* have also been grown in a chemically defined medium consisting of several different amino acids, vitamins, hemin and salts. *Balamuthia mandrillaris* has also been grown in an axenic medium, thus facilitating the screening of various pharmaceutical agents.[9]

EPIDEMIOLOGY

Naegleria fowleri is widely distributed throughout the world and has been isolated from fresh water, thermal discharges of power plants, heated swimming pools, hot springs, aquariums, soil, dust in air, sewage and even from nasal passages of children. *Naegleria fowleri* is thermophilic and grows well, even at temperatures of up to 113°F (45°C). It is therefore not surprising that primary amebic meningoencephalitis (PAM) cases have occurred in the hot summer months when many people engage in aquatic activities in lakes, ponds and swimming pools that may harbor these amebae in large numbers.

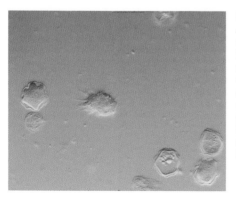

Fig. 182.2 *Acanthamoeba castellanii*. The trophozoite has spiny acanthopodia whereas the cyst has an outer wrinkled ectocyst and a stellate endocyst; both are taken from culture. Differential interference contrast.

In colder climates these amebae will probably encyst and remain dormant in the sediments of fresh water lakes, ponds, rivers and swimming pools.[1–3,10]

Acanthamoeba spp. have been isolated from soil, sewage, fresh, brackish and sea water, bottled mineral water, cooling towers of electric and nuclear power plants, physiotherapy pools, jacuzzis, heating and ventilating and air conditioning units, eye wash stations, dialysis machines, dust in the air, bacterial, fungal and mammalian cell cultures, contact lens paraphernalia, the nose and throat of patients who have respiratory complaints and healthy individuals, and biopsy or autopsy specimens of cornea, lungs, nasal sinuses, skin and CNS tissue of humans and animals. Acanthamoebae have generated considerable interest in recent years because they act, under laboratory conditions, as hosts for pathogenic bacteria such as *Legionella* spp, *Mycobacterium avium*, *Listeria monocytogenes*, *Burkholderia pseudomallei*, *Vibrio cholerae*, *Escherichia coli* serotype O157, *Francisella tularensis*, *Helicobacter pylori* and *Afipia felis*. Recently, *Mycobacterium massiliense* has been isolated from human clinical specimens such as sputum, liver, lung abscesses and even human feces. Additionally, a virus (mimivirus) about the size of a small bacterium with a 1.2 megabase genome has been discovered in *A. polyphaga*. Acanthamoeba is therefore of great public health importance.[1–3]

Cases of GAE may occur at any time of the year and therefore transmission has no relation to climatologic changes.

Balamuthia mandrillaris has only recently been isolated from soil and it may probably occur in water also. It is, therefore, believed to have the same habitat as *Acanthamoeba* spp. and *N. fowleri*. *Balamuthia mandrillaris* has also been isolated from biopsy and autopsy specimens of humans and other animals.[1,3]

PATHOGENICITY

Naegleria fowleri

Primary amebic meningoencephalitis occurs in active healthy children and young adults with no known history of immune disorder. Most patients who have PAM have a history of swimming, diving or playing under water; the ameba enters through the nasal passages and the nasal mucosa is the initial site of the primary lesions. The route of invasion into the brain is through the fila olfactoria of the olfactory nerves. The trophozoites cross the cribriform plate and reach the subarachnoid space, which is richly vascularized and bathed in the cerebrospinal fluid (CSF), thus constituting an ideal medium for their proliferation and subsequent dissemination into the brain parenchyma and other areas of the CNS.[1–3]

Naegleria fowleri is a highly pathogenic and virulent ameba. However, the minimum number of amebae required to cause infection and death in humans is not known. Experiments with infection have shown that mice, when just a few amebae are instilled intranasally, die of PAM in a similar fashion to humans. However, different isolates of *N. fowleri* vary in their degree of virulence: some are highly virulent whereas other isolates are only moderately virulent. Furthermore, any isolate can become avirulent on prolonged cultivation in an axenic medium. It is believed that the probability of infection in nature may depend upon the number and virulence of the amebae.[3,11]

The trophozoite of *N. fowleri* is highly phagocytic and induces necrosis of the CNS tissue. It is believed to ingest human tissue directly by producing a food cup or amebostome and by producing lysosomal hydrolases and phospholipases that degrade myelin. It has also been shown experimentally that the amebae exert a contact-dependent cytolysis mediated possibly by a multicomponent system that consists of a heat-stable hemolytic protein, heat-labile cytolysin and/or phospholipase A enzyme.[1–3,11,12]

The incubation period of PAM varies from 2 to 15 days depending on the size of the inoculum and the virulence of the amebae. In experimental infections with a mildly virulent *N. fowleri*, the incubation period has been as long as 3–4 weeks.[1–3]

Acanthamoeba spp.

Granulomatous amebic encephalitis, caused by *Acanthamoeba* spp., usually occurs in chronically ill, debilitated individuals, in immunosuppressed patients including those who have AIDS, or in those who have received broad-spectrum antibiotics or chemotherapeutic medications.[1–3] *Balamuthia mandrillaris* causes infection in both immunodeficient and immunocompetent individuals. The pathogenesis of GAE is complex and poorly understood. It is believed that the immunity is predominantly T-cell mediated and therefore depletion of CD4+ and T-helper lymphocytes permits the growth and development of the amebae. The incubation period is unknown and several weeks or months may elapse before the disease becomes apparent. The respiratory tract or the skin may act as the portal of entry. One hypothesis is that ulceration of the skin may enable the amebae to enter.[1] The route of invasion to the brain must be via the bloodstream because there are no lymphatic channels within the brain.[1,13] Furthermore, trophozoites and cysts are often seen around blood vessels and within necrotic CNS tissue. The acanthamoebae are known to secrete enzymes such as lysosomal hydrolases, aminopeptidases and phospholipases, which may contribute to CNS damage.[1,2]

According to more recent studies the initial process of invasion, in case of *Acanthamoeba*, occurs when a 136-kDa mannose-binding protein (MBP), a lectin, expressed on the surface of the ameba, adheres to mannose glycoproteins on the surface of the epithelial cells and causes destruction of the epithelial cells. *Acanthamoeba* may also produce food cups on its surface and ingests the epithelial cells.[14] *Balamuthia*, like *Acanthamoeba*, probably invades human tissue by interacting with the host connective tissue and ingesting bits and pieces of host tissue as well as by producing enzymes that will degrade the tissue, thus helping *Balamuthia* to ingest.[15]

Acanthamoeba keratitis

Acanthamoeba keratitis (AK) is inflammation of the cornea caused by ocular trauma or by contact lens wear and the use of nonsterile homemade saline solution that has been contaminated with bacteria and fungi, which support the growth and multiplication of *Acanthamoeba* spp. The latter may adhere to the corneal epithelial cells as well as secrete proteolytic and collagenolytic enzymes that may damage the corneal epithelium and thus contribute to the pathogenesis of AK. If proper treatment is not provided, AK may lead to a vascularized scar within a thin cornea, causing impaired vision or perforation of the cornea and loss of the eye.[1–4,16]

PREVENTION

Primary amebic meningoencephalitis

The trophic and the cyst forms of *N. fowleri* are susceptible to chlorine and are killed at 1 mg/l, provided the water temperature is 78.8 °F (26 °C) or below. If, however, the water temperature is above 78.8 °F the chlorine concentration may need to be increased to 2 mg/l. It is therefore important for swimming pools to be maintained properly with adequate chlorination at all times. As it is not possible to disinfect natural bodies of waters such as lakes and ponds in which *N. fowleri* may be found, appropriate warnings should be posted, particularly during the hot summer months.[1,2]

Granulomatous amebic encephalitis

New and creative preventive measures need to be formulated because GAE produced by *Acanthamoeba* spp. and *B. mandrillaris* occurs principally in immunocompromised individuals. As *Acanthamoeba* spp. can grow and colonize hot water tanks, jacuzzis, filters used in heating, ventilating and air conditioning units, and in-line filters used for purifying portable water supplies and eye wash stations, periodic inspection of these systems is recommended.[1–3]

Acanthamoeba keratitis

It is recommended that eye care professionals educate patients about the proper care and use of contact lenses. Contact lenses and contact lens paraphernalia, particularly the solutions, should be kept meticulously clean. Contact lens wearers should follow the directions and recommendations of the manufacturers and eye care professionals. Additionally, contact lenses should not be used during swimming or other water sports.[16]

DIAGNOSTIC MICROBIOLOGY

Primary amebic meningoencephalitis

In individuals who have PAM, the CSF is characterized by pleocytosis, with a predominance of polymorphonuclear leukocytes but without bacteria. The CSF pressure is elevated (100–600 mmHg). Glucose concentration may be slightly reduced or normal, but the protein content is elevated, ranging from 100 mg/100 ml to 1000 mg/100 ml. CT scans show obliteration of the cisterns around the midbrain and the subarachnoid space over the cerebral hemispheres. Differential diagnosis of PAM from acute pyogenic or bacterial meningoencephalitis is dependent upon the detection of the ameba in the CSF *in situ* under a microscope. Smears of CSF should also be stained with Giemsa or trichrome stains for the delineation of the characteristic nuclear morphology. Gram stain is not useful. Care must be taken to differentiate amebic trophozoites from macrophages. Many cases have been diagnosed retrospectively based on examination of hematoxylin and eosin-stained sections or immunohistochemical tests.[1–3]

Recently, a real time multiplex polymerase chain reaction (PCR) assay has been developed which identifies *N. fowleri* DNA in the CSF within 5 hours of receipt of the specimen, thus greatly facilitating a quick diagnosis so that anti-*N. fowleri* therapy can be initiated promptly.[17] Serologic tests are of no value in the diagnosis of PAM because most patients die too early (within 3–7 days) in the disease process to mount a detectable immune response.[1–3]

Granulomatous amebic encephalitis

Examination of the CSF in patients who have GAE reveals lymphocytic pleocytosis with mild elevation of proteins and normal levels of glucose. Visual detection of *Acanthamoeba* spp. trophozoites in the CSF has rarely been reported. However, *Acanthamoeba* spp. have been identified in brain biopsies from several patients. Molecular techniques such as PCR and real-time PCR have also been used recently to identify *Acanthameba* in the CSF, brain and corneal tissue as well as in tear fluid.[1–3,18] CT scans and MRI are nonspecific and of limited value in the diagnosis. Single or multiple heterogeneous, hypodense, non-enhancing, space-occupying lesions that involve the basal ganglia, cerebral cortex, subcortical white matter, cerebellum and pons may be encountered, suggesting a brain abscess, brain tumor or intracerebral hematoma.

Brain and skin biopsies are important diagnostic procedures. *Acanthamoeba* spp. can be easily cultured from the brain, skin, lung and corneal tissue by placing a portion of the tissue that has been minced on non-nutrient agar plates coated with a layer of Gram-negative bacteria. Specimens for culture should be processed as quickly as possible. The incubation temperature depends upon the source of the samples. The agar plate should be incubated at 86°F (30°C) if the specimens originate from cornea or skin, but at 98.6°F (37°C) if the specimens are from the brain, the lung or any other internal organ. Amebae, if present in the samples, will feed on bacteria and multiply by binary fission. If the plates are examined under the light microscope, distinctive track marks with an ameba at the end of each track may be seen. The amebae will differentiate into cysts after a few days of incubation. Amebae can be identified to the level of genus on the basis of the characteristic morphology of trophozoites and

cysts. Additionally, *Naegleria* spp. can be identified if flagellates appear within 2–4 hours of a loopful of amebae from the agar plate being suspended in distilled water. Identification to the species level, however, is difficult on the basis of morphology alone; nonmorphologic methods such as serology, isoenzyme analysis or DNA profiles therefore need to be used.[1–3,18]

Balamuthia mandrillaris will not grow on bacteria-coated agar plates. However, *B. mandrillaris* can be isolated from the CNS by inoculating monkey kidney cell culture with brain extract and subsequently growing the amebae in an axenic medium.[9]

Acanthamoeba keratitis

For the diagnosis of AK, deep corneal scraping and biopsy is recommended. Unfixed specimens should be processed for culture. Smears should also be prepared and fixed with methanol, Schaudinn's fixative or a spray-on fixative, and stained with Giemsa–Wright or Hemacolor, or with Wheatly's or Masson's trichrome stain. Hemacolor staining is quick and stains the distinctive cyst wall pinkish-red. The trichrome stains the nucleolus of the trophozoite reddish-pink and the cytoplasm greenish-purple and is therefore useful in differentiating trophozoites of *Acanthamoeba* spp. from the host cells.[1–3] Confocal microscopy has also been used recently to diagnose AK.[19]

CLINICAL MANIFESTATIONS

Primary amebic meningoencephalitis

The first case of PAM was reported in 1962.[1–3] Although at that time the case was thought to be caused by *Acanthamoeba* sp., it is now considered to be caused by *N. fowleri*. It is believed that more than 200 cases of PAM have occurred worldwide as of March 2008. Further, as many as 121 cases have been reported in the USA alone. Primary amebic meningoencephalitis has also been described in a South American tapir and cattle.[1]

Primary amebic meningoencephalitis is an acute, fulminating and usually fatal CNS disease that occurs mainly in healthy young adults and children with a recent history of watersport activities. Primary amebic meningoencephalitis has a rapid onset and a short incubation period that lasts from 3 to 7 days. It is characterized by the sudden onset of bifrontal or bitemporal headaches, fever, nausea, vomiting and stiff neck. Nuchal rigidity usually occurs with positive Kernig's and Brudzinski's signs. Abnormalities in taste or smell and cerebellar ataxia may be seen early but photophobia occurs late in the clinical course. An increase in intracranial pressure has been reported in most patients. Generalized seizures leading to lethargy, confusion, coma and death within 48–72 hours have been reported in a number of patients.[1] Focal myocardial necrosis has also been reported.

Pathologic features

At autopsy the cerebral hemispheres are swollen and edematous. The olfactory bulbs and the orbitofrontal cortices are necrotic and hemorrhagic. Because of increased intracranial pressure, uncal and cerebellar tonsillar herniations are usually seen. The arachnoid membrane is severely congested with scant purulent exudate. Amebic trophozoites are usually seen within the Virchow–Robin spaces with minimal or no inflammatory reaction (Fig. 182.4). Cysts are not seen within the CNS lesions. Necrotizing angiitis may occasionally be seen.[1,2]

Granulomatous amebic encephalitis produced by *Acanthamoeba* spp. and *Balamuthia mandrillaris*

Granulomatous amebic encephalitis caused by *Acanthamoeba* spp. occurs principally in individuals who are immunosuppressed (either iatrogenically or because of AIDS) and GAE caused by *B. mandrillaris*

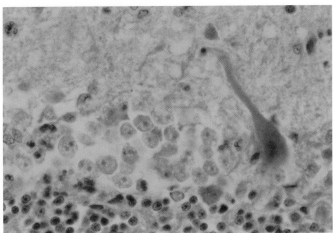

Fig. 182.4 CNS section demonstrating numerous trophozoites of *Naegleria fowleri*. Note the absence of cysts. (H & E.)

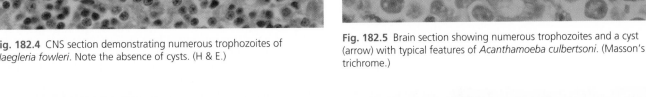

Fig. 182.5 Brain section showing numerous trophozoites and a cyst (arrow) with typical features of *Acanthamoeba culbertsoni*. (Masson's trichrome.)

occurs in either the very young or very old and in individuals who have AIDS. In the USA as many as 120 cases attributable to *Acanthamoeba* spp. (70 in people with AIDS) and 101 attributable to *B. mandrillaris* have occurred. Additionally, several cases of GAE caused by *Acanthamoeba* spp. and *B. mandrillaris* have been described in gorillas, a baboon, monkeys, dogs, sheep and cows.[1,3,20]

The clinical manifestations and pathologic features of GAE are similar regardless of which of these two organisms is the cause. It is an insidious disease and has a long and protracted clinical course. Clinical signs include personality changes, headache, low-grade fever, nausea, vomiting, lethargy, hemiparesis, seizures, depressed levels of consciousness and coma. Third and sixth cranial nerve palsies may be seen in some patients. Clinically, GAE may mimic bacterial leptomeningitis, tuberculous or viral meningitis, or single or multiple space-occupying lesions. Cerebellar ataxia and diplopia have been described in some patients. Pneumonitis with the presence of trophozoites and cysts within pulmonary alveoli has also been described.[1] In most cases of GAE, however, final diagnosis is made at autopsy.

Pathologic features

The cerebral hemispheres are edematous. Encephalomalacia with multifocal areas of cortical softening and hemorrhagic necrosis may be seen. Multifocal necrotic lesions may also be seen in the posterior fossa structures, midbrain, thalamus, brain stem and cerebellum. Trophozoites and cysts of the infecting organisms are seen, most often in the necrotic lesions in basal ganglia, midbrain, brain stem and cerebral hemispheres (Fig. 182.5). Microglial nodules may be seen within the necrotic tissues. Occasionally, angiitis may be seen with perivascular cuffing by inflammatory cells, chiefly lymphocytes, a few plasma cells and macrophages. In patients who have advanced AIDS there is very little inflammation. Trophozoites and cysts can easily be identified by light microscopic examination of the tissue sections. Also in patients who have AIDS, multiple ulcerations of the skin with acute and chronic inflammation may be seen and the ulcers may contain trophozoites and cysts of the infecting ameba (Fig. 182.6). The kidneys, prostate gland, adrenal glands, lungs and liver may also be involved, suggesting hematogenous dissemination. The ulcerated skin may serve as a portal of entry for the amebae in some patients. Several cases of skin and nasal infection without dissemination into the CNS have also been reported.[1,21–24]

In general, the trophic and cyst stages of *Acanthamoeba* spp. and *B. mandrillaris* look similar in formalin-fixed and hematoxylin and eosin-stained sections under the light microscope. In some patients, however, differential identification of *B. mandrillaris* can be made if the nuclei of the amebae in the sections possess two or three nucleolar

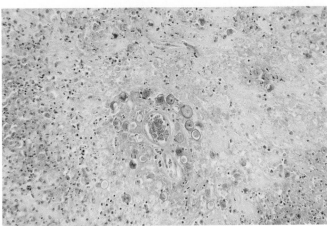

Fig. 182.6 Trophozoites and cysts of *Acanthamoeba* sp. surrounding a blood vessel in a skin biopsy of a patient who has AIDS. A diffuse but modest inflammatory reaction is seen.

elements because these are not seen in *Acanthamoeba* spp. (Fig. 182.7). A definitive identification may be arrived at by carrying out immunohistochemical analysis of the tissue sections using rabbit anti-*Acanthamoeba* spp. or anti-*B. mandrillaris* sera. The cyst wall of *B. mandrillaris* is characteristically tripartite and hence can be identified definitively by electron microscopy analysis of brain sections.[1–3]

Acanthamoeba keratitis

Acanthamoeba keratitis is a sight-threatening chronic inflammation of the cornea. It is associated with contact lens wear and the use of homemade nonsterile saline solution, corneal abrasion or trauma. Although the first case of AK in the USA was reported in a farmer from south Texas with ocular trauma of the right eye, wearing contact lenses and using nonsterile homemade saline was found to be a risk factor for AK in 1985 because most of the 24 patients reported in the previous 2 years were contact lens wearers.[1–3,16] By December 1996, more than 700 cases of AK were estimated to have occurred worldwide. Recently, an increase in the AK cases in the Chicago (Illinois) area was reported during May 1, 2003 and September 15, 2006.[25] An in depth epidemiologic survey conducted by CDC because of a multistate outbreak of *Acanthamoeba* keratitis revealed that the national increase in the number of *Acanthamoeba* keratitis cases was associated

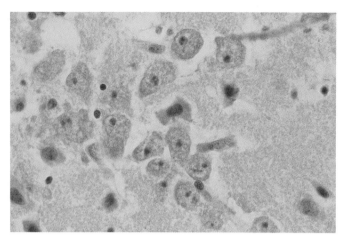

Fig. 182.7 CNS section showing many trophozoites of *Balamuthia mandrillaris*. More than one nucleoli can be seen within the nuclei of the trophozoite.

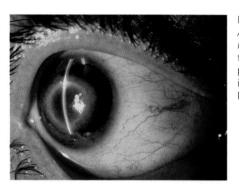

Fig. 182.8
Acanthamoeba keratitis. Note the typical central or paracentral ring infiltrate. Courtesy of Dr Theodore.

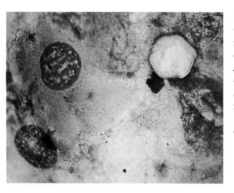

Fig. 182.9
Characteristic star-shaped morphology of the cyst of *Acanthamoeba* sp. demonstrated by a corneal scraping stained with Hemacolor. Courtesy of Dr Theodore.

with the use of Advanced Medical Optics Complete® MoisturePlus™ multipurpose contact lens solution leading to an international recall by the manufacturer.[26] Additionally, another study revealed that most contact lens solutions marketed in the US do not have sufficient disinfection activity against *Acanthamoeba* spp.[27]

The hallmark of AK is severe ocular pain, photophobia, a central or paracentral 360° stromal ring infiltrate (Fig. 182.8), recurrent breakdown of corneal epithelium with a waxing and waning clinical course and a corneal lesion refractory to the usual antibacterial, antiviral and antimycotic medications.[1-3]

When examined under the light microscope, corneal scrapings and/or sections of biopsied corneal tissue reveal trophozoites and cysts of *Acanthamoeba* spp. infiltrated between the lamellae of the cornea (Fig. 182.9). Polymorphonuclear leukocytes, eosinophils, lymphocytes, macrophages and plasma cells have also been seen occasionally. Ulceration, descemetocele formation and perforation are often seen in the later stages of AK.[1-3]

MANAGEMENT

Primary amebic meningoencephalitis

Primary amebic meningoencephalitis has almost always resulted in death. A few patients, however, have survived, probably because of early diagnosis and aggressive treatment with amphotericin B, miconazole (not available in the USA) and rifampin (rifampicin).[28] Amphotericin B and miconazole can be administered intrathecally or intravenously, alone or in combination, and rifampin can be given orally. A 9-year-old girl from California, one of the patients who survived this disease in the USA, was treated as follows:

- intravenous amphotericin B 1.5 mg/kg body weight per day in two divided doses for 3 days and then 1 mg/kg for 3 days;
- intrathecal amphotericin B 1.5 mg/day for 2 days followed by 1 mg/day for 8 days;
- intravenous miconazole 350 mg/m² body surface area per day in three divided doses for 9 days;
- intrathecal miconazole 10 mg/day for 1 day followed by 10 mg every other day for 8 days; and
- oral rifampin 10 mg/kg per day in three divided doses for 9 days.

The patient was also given sulfisoxazole (sulphafurazole) q6h for 3 days, but this was discontinued once *N. fowleri* was identified as the cause of the disease. Dexamethasone and phenytoin were given to lower the intracranial pressure and seizure activity, respectively. Amebae disappeared from the CSF after 3 days of treatment. Although cell counts and biochemistry of the CSF were abnormal for several months afterwards, the patient recovered completely without any neurologic sequelae.[28] It has also been reported that a boy from Texas, USA, recovered from PAM after intravenous amphotericin B and treatment in a hyperbaric chamber.[29]

Granulomatous amebic encephalitis

Although it is known from *in-vitro* experiments that several drugs, including pentamidine, propamidine, dibromopropamidine, miconazole, paromomycin, neomycin, ketoconazole and 5-fluorocytosine, have inhibitory effects on several isolates of *Acanthamoeba*, there is as yet no effective treatment for GAE and therefore the prognosis is poor.[1-3] This is partly due to the difficulty in the diagnosis of GAE because of a lack of clear-cut symptoms, lack of a reliable noninvasive diagnostic test and lack of knowledge of the care givers; diagnosis is often made at the time of postmortem. The disease has been identified in only a very few patients before death. Several patients who were diagnosed premortem, however, have reportedly recovered from this disease. *Acanthamoeba rhysodes* was isolated from the CSF of a Nigerian patient with neurologic disease who showed clinical improvement after treatment with sulfamethazine. He was discharged from the hospital but was lost to follow-up.[1-3]

Acanthamoeba culbertsoni was isolated from the CSF of an Indian patient with CNS impairment who recovered after treatment with chloramphenicol.[2,3] A 7-year-old girl from Barbados with a 'brain tumor' recovered without any neurologic sequelae after surgical excision. *Acanthamoeba healyi* was isolated from the 'tumor' and also demonstrated in the hematoxylin and eosin-stained, formalin-fixed sections. The patient also received oral ketoconazole treatment for 8 months postoperatively.[30,31] Prognosis of patients who have disseminated skin infections without CNS involvement is, however, good. In an immunocompromised (without HIV/AIDS) patient with *A. rhysodes* skin infection, skin ulcers healed after the following treatment regimen: cleansing of skin ulcers twice daily with chlorhexidine gluconate solution followed by the application of 2% ketoconazole cream. The patient was also given 4 mg/kg intravenous pentamidine isethionate for 1 day. Because of pentamidine toxicity the dosage was cut to 2700 mg and given over a 4-week period. Thereafter, he was given itraconazole orally at a dose of 200 mg daily for 8 months, resulting in the total healing of the skin lesions.[21] However, several patients with GAE caused by *Acanthamoeba* spp., as well as *Acanthamoeba* cutaneous infections without CNS involvement, have been successfully treated with a combination of pharmaceuticals including pentamidine isethionate, sulfadiazine, flucytosine, and itraconazole.[21–24,29] Another drug, miltefosine, a hexadecylphosphocholine, has also been shown to have amebicidal potential and miltefosine has been successfully used to treat GAE patients in Austria.[33,34] For *Acanthamoeba* cutaneous infection without CNS involvement, topical applications of chlorhexidine gluconate and ketoconazole cream in addition to the above have resulted in therapeutic success.[1–3]

Recently, voriconazole, a triazole compound, was used to clear cutaneous infection in a patient recovering from lung transplantation.[24] Another recent case with a cadaveric liver transplant was initially treated empirically with a combination of drugs including sulfadiazine, pyrimethamine, cefotaxime, chloramphenicol, gentamicin, isoniazid, rifampin and pyrazinamide to cover *Toxoplasma*, bacterial and tuberculous infections. Since the patient did not show any improvement a lobectomy was performed and *Acanthamoeba* was identified in the tissue sections. Pyrimethamine was stopped and rifampin was continued at 600 mg q8h and co-trimoxazole at 960 mg q8h was added to the regimen. The patient improved and is alive 11 years after *Acanthamoeba* infection was diagnosed.[35]

Although the majority of patients with *Balamuthia* GAE have died, a few patients have survived the infection. For example, two patients, a 60-year-old man and a 6-year-old girl from California, and a 70-year-old woman from New York have survived balamuthiasis after treatment with a combination of pentamidine isethionate, sulfadiazine, macrolide antibiotics (azithromycin–clarithromycin), fluconazole an d flucytosine (5-fluorocytosine).[36,37] Two Peruvian patients with cutaneous lesions became well after prolonged therapy with albendazole and itraconazole. One of the Peruvian patients had a large lesion on the chest wall that was surgically removed. Surgical excision of the lesion may have reduced the parasite load, thus helping in the recovery process.[38]

Acanthamoeba keratitis

Treatment of AK with topical application of polyhexamethylene biguanide or chlorhexidine gluconate in combination with propamidine isethionate appears to be the treatment of choice, as several patients have been treated successfully in this way.[1–3] Many patients have also been treated with topical application of propamidine isethionate 0.1% and dibromopropamidine, in conjunction with neosporin. Ketoconazole and clotrimazole appear to be effective *in vitro* and *in vivo*. Other reports of successful treatment with 0.1% hexamidine di-isethionate eye drops have been reported. Some patients have also been treated successfully with combinations of topical propamidine and miconazole and systemic ketoconazole, or topical clotrimazole or oral itraconazole with topical miconazole.[39] Medical cure has been achieved with the administration topically of polyhexamethylene biguanide[40] or chlorhexidine with or without propamidine.[41,42] Debridement of the cornea, penetrating keratoplasty and corneal grafting have also been performed with good results in some patients. Recurrence of AK has been reported after corneal transplantation, probably caused by cysts of *Acanthamoeba* spp. still present in the corneal stroma.

Disclaimer

The findings and conclusions in this report are those of the authors and do not necessarily represent the views of the Centers for Disease Control and Prevention.

REFERENCES

 References for this chapter can be found online at http://www.expertconsult.com

Blood and tissue protozoa

Organisms of the genera *Plasmodium, Babesia, Toxoplasma, Leishmania* and *Trypanosoma* are the most prevalent protozoa able to invade blood and human tissues. They cause diseases of immense socioeconomic impact, most of them having a limited (although extensive) geographic distribution.

Malaria is considered separately in Chapter 111.

Babesiosis

Human babesiosis is an uncommon tick-borne parasitic zoonotic disease that was first described by Babes in Rumanian cattle in 1888. It was not reported as a human disease until 1957.

NATURE

The genus *Babesia* belongs to the family Piroplasmida, closely related to *Plasmodium* and *Theileria* genus, and comprises over 70 species that parasitize mammals and birds. Infection in cattle is widespread and it is an economically important disease. Most human cases in Europe are caused by *Babesia divergens* and by *Babesia microti* in the USA. A number of *Babesia*-like piroplasms are being increasingly found infecting humans. Among them, former *Babesia* WA1 and CA5, endemic of western North American states, have been recently renamed *Babesia duncani*.[1]

EPIDEMIOLOGY AND PATHOGENICITY

Babesiosis in humans occurs predominantly in the USA. It is highly endemic in the coastal areas of Massachusetts, Connecticut and New York State, where seroprevalence rates reach 4–6%, indicating that subclinical infections are common. In these areas rodents are the main reservoir and humans are usually infected by the bite of an infected nymph of *Ixodes scapularis* tick. Transfusions of blood or blood products have caused a few cases. Subclinical infections are common in endemic areas. Serosurveys in the USA have found 3–8% of samples positive for *B. microti* and up to 16% for *B. duncani*.

In Europe *B. divergens* is the main causative agent of bovine babesiosis. The seroprevalence for this species in exposure-selected human populations reaches 1.5–11.5% but only a few clinical cases have been reported, with splenectomized patients being at highest risk.[2–4]

Suspected or confirmed cases of babesiosis have also been reported from Colombia, Mexico, India, China, Taiwan, Japan, Egypt and South Africa.

PREVENTION

General recommendations include avoidance of known endemic areas, especially in the warm months of the year. Clothes should be sprayed with tick repellents before going on outdoor activities and on return the skin should be thoroughly examined for the presence of ticks.

DIAGNOSTIC MICROBIOLOGY

Babesia spp. are intraerythrocytic parasites that may resemble plasmodium trophozoites, but the hemozoin pigment present in the late stages of malarial trophozoite development is never present in babesiosis. Schizonts and gametocytes are not formed. Multiple erythrocyte parasitization is common and organisms are occasionally arranged in a characteristic Maltese cross shape (Fig. 183.1).

Parasitemia usually persists, demonstrable by light microscopy, for 3–12 weeks.

Serologic diagnosis can be made using indirect immunofluorescent antibody (IFA) assay. A serum titer of at least 1/256 is diagnostic of recent *B. microti* infection. Within a few weeks, most patients who have active infection have serum titers equal to or higher than 1/1024, falling over a few months to levels under 1/256. Due to the lack of cross-reactivity,

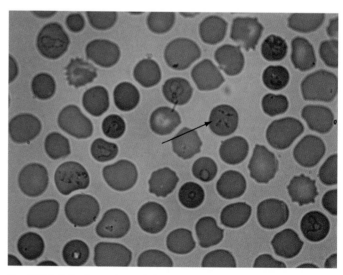

Fig. 183.1 *Babesia* spp. heavy infection. Single and multiple intraerythrocytic parasites can be seen. The arrow marks a typical Maltese cross arrangement.

individuals exposed to the infection on the west coast of the USA should also be tested for antibodies to the *Babesia* WA1 species.[5] *B. microti*, WA1 and *B. divergens* have limited serologic cross-reactivity.

CLINICAL MANIFESTATIONS

The clinical forms of babesiosis vary widely depending upon the immune status of the host and the species of *Babesia* involved.

In the American Northwest, the symptoms of *B. microti* infection (Nantucket fever) range from a nonspecific flu-like self-limited febrile illness to severe haemolytic anemia. It is most severe in those who are older or asplenic. The usual incubation period is 1–3 weeks. The onset is gradual with nonspecific symptoms such as malaise, fatigue, anorexia, headache, emotional lability, myalgias and arthralgias. Blood leukocytes are not elevated and platelets are usually decreased. There may be a haemolytic anemia. The mortality is less than 10% of symptomatic cases.

The European clinical cases diagnosed occur mainly in asplenic patients who present with a high fever and severe haemolytic anemia, and the infection is usually fatal.

MANAGEMENT

Early treatment is recommended for all diagnosed cases to prevent long-term sequelae and potential transmission through blood donation.

The standard treatment is clindamycin, 1200–2400 mg/day q6–8h plus 650 mg of quinine q6–8h; both drugs are given for 5–10 days. Combination of atovaquone (750 mg q12h) and azithromycin (500 mg on day 1 and 250 mg per day thereafter) for 7 days is also effective and is associated with fewer adverse reactions.[6] Chloroquine is not recommended. Blood transfusion and general supportive treatment may be needed for severe disease. Exchange transfusion has been used in an attempt to decrease parasite load, but its usefulness has not been demonstrated. It is recommended to rule out co-infection by *Borrelia burgdorferi* and other tick-transmitted micro-organisms.

Toxoplasmosis

Toxoplasmosis is a widespread zoonosis, caused by the coccidian parasite *Toxoplasma gondii*, first recognized in 1908. *Toxoplasma* (from the Greek, meaning 'shaped as a bow') is a one-species genus.

Humans are usually infected orally, developing few, if any, symptoms of infection. The infection persists for life without signs of disease. However, during immunosuppression quiescent parasites multiply, resulting in neurologic disease or, more rarely, other organ manifestations. Congenital transmission is a cause of major concern as it is frequently associated with severe disease in the newborn and retinochoroiditis later in life.

NATURE

Toxoplasma gondii is a parasite of many species of mammals and birds. The main forms of the parasite lifecycle are oocysts, tachyzoites and bradyzoites.

The oocysts result from the sexual multiplication that takes place exclusively in the intestinal epithelium of cats and other felines. They are present in feline feces, and after maturing in the environment become the source of infection for noncarnivorous animals.

In the secondary host (all hosts but felines) *T. gondii* cells have two forms:

- rapidly multiplying tachyzoites (*tachy*, rapid); and
- 'dormant' bradyzoites (*brady*, slow).

When the host is infected by oocysts, tachyzoites or bradyzoites, a disseminated infection by tachyzoite forms takes place. Tachyzoites multiply inside the host cells, which rupture when 8–32 tachyzoites are produced. The tachyzoites released infect new cells. When the immune response controls the infection, some surviving parasites persist for many years in tissue cysts, which are sacs containing hundreds or thousands of *T. gondii* bradyzoites. They represent the parasite reservoir present in secondary hosts. Tissue cysts can be found in any tissue, but are most common in muscle and brain.

Cats become infected from eating birds, small rodents or other sources of raw meat. Humans and other animals become infected from either oocysts in soil and contaminated food or tissue cysts in raw meat. When acute infection occurs during pregnancy, tachyzoites are able to infect the placenta and, in a second step, the fetus. The parasite can also be acquired by organ transplantation or blood transfusion.

EPIDEMIOLOGY

Seroprevalence to *Toxoplasma gondii* in sheep and cattle varies widely but has been frequently found above 25%; however, it is lower in pigs and poultry and is declining in intensive reared animals. The prevalence of oocyst-shedding cats in Europe has been found to be less than 0.3%.[7]

Infection rates in humans are very variable and depend upon eating habits and environmental factors. It has been estimated that one-third of mankind is infected.[8,9]

Patients with schizophrenia and other psychiatric disorders have been found to have higher seroprevalence of *T. gondii* than matched controls but an etiologic link has not been proved.[10]

Human disease caused by *T. gondii* is much more restricted than the infection itself, and is generally a consequence of either intrauterine acquisition or immunocompromise.

PATHOGENICITY AND IMMUNITY

Toxoplasma gondii tachyzoites invade cells from nearly every organ, where they survive inside parasitophorous vacuoles. Resistance to the infection has been found to be enhanced by interferon gamma (IFN-γ) and diminished by IL-6. Extracellular tachyzoites are lysed by complement combined to specific antibody, and CD4+ and CD8+ T lymphocytes, lymphokine-activated killer and natural killer cells play a major role in infection control.

PREVENTION

Toxoplasmosis can be prevented at three different levels:

- prevention of primary infection;
- prevention of vertical transmission and congenital disease; and
- prevention of disease in infected immunocompromised individuals.

To prevent primary infection, the exposure to parasite can be reduced by health education (Table 183.1). No vaccine is presently available. Maternal immunity due to toxoplasmosis passed before conception protects the fetus from the infection. Immunodeficient patients receiving trimethoprim–sulfamethoxazole (co-trimoxazole) as prophylaxis for *Pneumocystis* infection are substantially protected from toxoplasmosis.

Toxoplasma gondii IgG serology should be included in the initial workup of pre-transplant patients and transplantation of a solid organ from a seropositive donor to a seronegative recipient should be avoided if possible. If such a transplant is performed, then the recipient should have anti-*T. gondii* treatment for at least 2 months.

Individuals who have HIV infection and are seronegative for *T. gondii* should avoid being exposed to the parasite. For those patients who have HIV infection and are seropositive for *T. gondii*, further serologic tests do not provide useful information.

Table 183.1 Toxoplasmosis primary preventive measures

- Do not eat undercooked or raw red meat or eggs. Cook meat until it is no longer pink in the center
- While handling raw meat avoid touching your mouth or contaminating other food. Normal hygienic washing of hands and utensils will suffice
- Cured or smoked meat is generally considered safe from *Toxoplasma*. Freeze it at −4°F (−20°C) for at least 24 hours as an additional precaution
- Consume only pasteurized or ultra-heat-treated (UHT) sterilized milk and dairy products
- Wash or peel all fruits and vegetables to be eaten uncooked
- Control insect pests and their access to foodstuffs
- Avoid living with cats or kittens. If unfeasible take special care: change the cat litter box daily and rinse it with nearly boiling water. Wear gloves and wash your hands well with soap and water immediately after. Prevent your cat from hunting birds and rodents or eating raw meat
- Use gloves and wash your hands well after gardening and other outdoor activities with soil contact.

Routine serologic screening during pregnancy remains controversial. It is aimed at detecting acute maternal infections. It is, however, sometimes difficult to establish an early and reliable diagnosis of acute maternal infection. When acute infection is diagnosed in a pregnant woman, anti-*T. gondii* treatment, further assessment of fetal infection and abortion may be offered.

DIAGNOSTIC MICROBIOLOGY

The diagnosis of *T. gondii* past infection is usually made by reactive IgG testing. The suspicion of acute or recent infection may rely on a single serum sample but a reliable serologic diagnosis requires paired sera. A typical acute infection would have rising titers of positive IgM with the IgG negative or positive with low avidity. Nevertheless, in some cases, reactive IgM may be undetectable or may persist for more than 12 months.[11,12] The functional affinity of specific IgG antibodies (avidity) is initially low, and usually increases during the subsequent 3–6 months, although in some cases it may take much longer periods.[13]

Congenital infection in the newborn by IgM or IgA testing detects only one half of infected infants.[14]

Parasite demonstration by polymerase chain reaction (PCR) of tissue or body fluids is the most efficient diagnostic tool for active infection. Examination of stained tissue or fluid smears, growth in tissue cultures and experimental animal inoculation may be used.[15,16] The most sensitive method for chorioretinitis is PCR plus relative concentration measures of antitoxoplasma antibodies in serum and aqueous humor.[17]

CLINICAL MANIFESTATIONS

There are three different forms of toxoplasmosis: congenital infection, acute extrauterine infection and toxoplasmosis of the immunocompromised host.

Congenital toxoplasmosis

Toxoplasmosis acquired in utero can be asymptomatic or may produce signs of disease that can be present at birth or later in life.

The risk of congenital toxoplasmosis depends upon the time of acquisition of acute maternal infection.[18] Vertical transmission of *T. gondii* increases with gestation age (15–25% in the first trimester of pregnancy, 30–54% in the second and 60–65% in the third). Conversely, the severity of congenital disease is increased when infection occurs in early pregnancy.

Signs of infection at delivery are present in 21–28% of those infected in the second trimester and ≤11% of those infected in the third trimester. Overall, 10% are born with severe disease.

Clinical manifestations of congenital toxoplasmosis include strabismus, chorioretinitis, encephalitis, microcephaly, hydrocephalus, psychomotor retardation and convulsions, as well as nonspecific manifestations such as anemia, jaundice, hypothermia, thrombocytopenia, diarrhea and pneumonitis. The characteristic triad of hydrocephalus, cerebral calcifications and chorioretinitis resulting in mental retardation, epilepsy and impaired vision is the most severe and extreme form of the disease. Cerebral lesions may calcify, providing retrospective evidence of congenital toxoplasmosis.

Toxoplasma gondii chorioretinitis in immunocompetent patients is frequently secondary to congenitally acquired infection (Fig. 183.2). The proportion of congenitally infected asymptomatic individuals who develop chorioretinitis later in life (usually in the first four decades) is unknown, but may well be over two-thirds. Up to 30% of patients relapse after treatment.

Acquired toxoplasmosis

In 90% of cases, no clinical symptoms are apparent during acute infection. Most symptomatic patients present with enlarged lymph nodes that are located mainly in the head or neck area. Malaise and low-grade fever are present in less than 50% of symptomatic cases. Although *T. gondii* organisms are not usually seen, the histologic picture of acute *T. gondii* lymphadenopathy is usually diagnostic. Occasionally the lymph node histopathology can be mistaken for that of cat-scratch disease, lymphoma and other infections.[19]

Rare manifestations of acute infection include chorioretinitis, myositis and heart, lung, liver or central nervous system (CNS) symptomatic involvement.

Toxoplasmosis in the immunocompromised host

Toxoplasmosis is a serious disease in patients who have profound immunosuppression such as those who have had a transplant or who have AIDS.

In transplant patients, the incidence and severity of the disease depends upon previous exposure to the parasite of donor and recipient, the type of organ transplanted and the degree of immunosuppression induced. The disease can be due to reactivation of a chronic silent infection or an acute primary infection acquired from the transplanted organ. The risk of developing toxoplasmosis for seronegative recipients of an organ from a seropositive donor is 57% for heart, 20% for kidney and minimal for liver transplants, reflecting the tropism of tissue cysts for striated muscle.[20] Incidence in bone marrow transplants is usually under 5%.[21] The disease manifests as a systemic disease with diverse

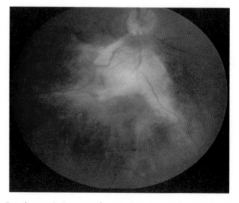

Fig. 183.2 Fundoscopic image of toxoplasmic chorioretinitis. Most cases presenting in adults represent a late manifestation of congenitally acquired toxoplasmosis.

degrees of multiorgan involvement including pneumonitis, carditis, hepatitis, myositis and encephalitis.

In patients who have AIDS, the clinical manifestations are usually related to CNS dysfunction or ocular lesions. Myocarditis is frequently found at autopsy, but is rarely clinically apparent. Infections of lung and other organs have also been reported.

Patients who become infected with *T. gondii* risk developing toxoplasmosis when their CD4⁺ T-lymphocyte count is less than 100 000/ml. The onset of *T. gondii* encephalitis is usually subacute. Fever and malaise usually precede the first neurologic symptoms. Headache, confusion, neuropsychiatric manifestations, seizures or other focal signs strongly suggest the diagnosis. Diagnosis is based upon clinical data, neuroradiology (an MRI scan is the procedure of choice) and response to therapy. *T. gondii* encephalitis in patients who have AIDS usually presents as multiple abscesses in the basal ganglia or the grey–white matter junction with a contrast-enhanced ring (Fig. 183.3). Diffuse *T. gondii* encephalitis is an uncommon rapidly fatal form.

In immunocompromised patients there is no good serologic marker of active toxoplasmosis. The presence of anti-*T. gondii* antibody means previous exposure and therefore present infection, but not necessarily disease. The absence of specific antibodies makes toxoplasmosis unlikely.

MANAGEMENT

Congenital toxoplasmosis

In gestational toxoplasmosis, the drug therapy may be intended to treat the mother, the fetus or the newborn (Fig. 183.4). Spiramycin is a macrolide antibiotic that concentrates in the placenta, and is used early after maternal infection aiming to decrease vertical transmission. Spiramycin 3 g/day q8h is given to pregnant women who have an acute infection from diagnosis to delivery unless fetal infection is proved.

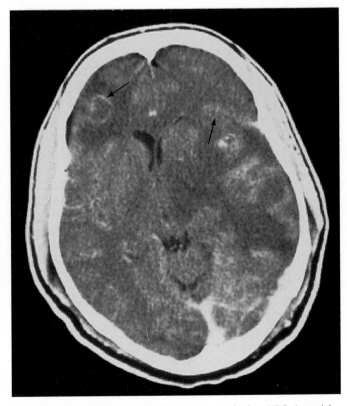

Fig. 183.3 Toxoplasmic encephalitis in a person who has AIDS. A cranial CT scan shows bilateral contrast-enhanced ring lesions with peripheral edema and mass effect.

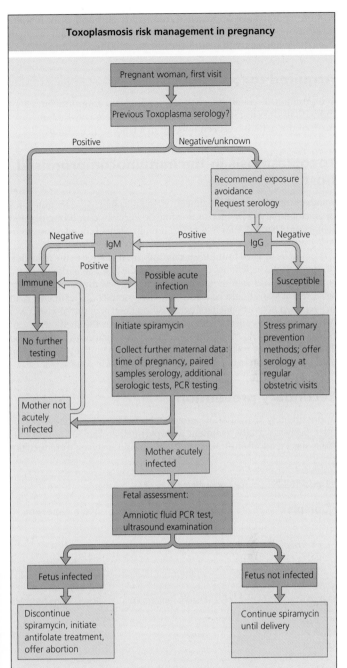

Fig. 183.4 Toxoplasmosis risk management in pregnancy.

In such a case, the maternal regimen is switched to sulfadiazine 4 g plus pyrimethamine 25 mg and folinic acid 15 mg a day until delivery, although no study has proved the benefit of such treatment.[22,23] All infected newborns should have anti-*T. gondii* treatment (sulfadiazine 50 mg/kg q12h plus pyrimethamine 1 mg/kg/day and folinic acid 5 mg/kg/day for at least 6 months). No treatment regimen seems to decrease the rate of chorioretinitis.[24]

To confirm fetal infection, ultrasound fetal examination and sampling the amniotic fluid for *T. gondii* PCR and culture are recommended. Fetal blood sampling obtained by cordocentesis has been commonly used to detect fetal antibodies and for *T. gondii* culture. Cordocentesis had an inherent risk of fetal loss of 2–3% and has been replaced by amniotic fluid PCR testing.

Termination of pregnancy is commonly offered to women who seroconvert in the first 8 weeks of pregnancy and to those infected in the first 22 weeks of pregnancy when fetal infection is confirmed.

A more conservative approach recommends abortion only if there is ultrasonographic evidence of hydrocephalus, although a small percentage of cases with neurologic disease will then be born.[25]

Acquired toxoplasmosis

Symptomatic *T. gondii* infection in nonpregnant immunocompetent individuals does not need to be treated unless there is visceral involvement or the patient has been infected in a laboratory accident.

Toxoplasmosis in the immunocompromised host

Standard anti-*T. gondii* treatment is sulfadiazine 4g/day q6h plus pyrimethamine as a first 100mg loading dose followed by 50mg/day and folinic acid 15mg/day for 6–8 weeks. If brain edema is of relevance corticosteroids should be given, but the clinical response to anti-*T. gondii* therapy would be masked by the unspecific improvement due to the reduction of edema. If the patient has not improved in the first 2 weeks of therapy a control CT or MRI scan should be repeated to review the empiric diagnosis. A repeat scan should be carried out after completing treatment. With this regimen 80% of patients survive, although 50% of the survivors will have neurologic sequelae. Serious adverse effects to the medication can be expected in 40% of patients. In cases of intolerance to sulfadiazine, 75–100mg/day of pyrimethamine alone or with clindamycin has been used. Azithromycin has been used as a reserve agent in some cases.

Secondary prevention

Approximately 80% of AIDS patients relapse after an initial episode of toxoplasmosis. Daily treatment with pyrimethamine 50mg plus sulfadiazine 1g and folinic acid 10–15mg should be given to reduce the relapse rate to 5–10%. Preventive treatment can be safely discontinued if immune system function is restored.[26]

Leishmaniasis

Leishmaniasis is the term used to describe a group of chronic parasitic diseases caused by a number of species of the genus *Leishmania*. The infection can be localized in the skin or mucous membranes or disseminated in the reticuloendothelial system. It is usually a zoonosis transmitted by *Phlebotominae* sandflies, which are endemic in areas of Southern Europe, Asia, Africa and the Americas.

NATURE

The genus *Leishmania*, along with the genus *Trypanosoma*, belongs to the order Kinetoplastida, which comprises flagellated protozoa that possess a characteristic extranuclear DNA mass called the kinetoplast.

Leishmania parasites are classified into two broad groups:
- New World *Leishmania* spp.; and
- Old World *Leishmania* spp.

Closely related species are grouped into complexes (Table 183.2). Members of *Leishmania braziliensis* complex have been renamed *Leishmania* subgenus *viannia*.

Sandflies are small (3–4mm), hairy mosquito-like insects, which transmit the disease. Old World sandflies belong to the genus *Phlebotomus*; New World species belong to the genera *Lutzomyia* and *Psychodopygus*.

Sandflies become infected when taking a blood meal containing infected macrophages, which are present in blood or skin. *Leishmania* live in the digestive tract of the insect as flagellated parasites (the

Table 183.2 Summary of epidemiology of leishmaniasis

Complex	Main pathogenic species	Main reservoir	Geographic distribution (maps)	Clinical disease (rarely)
Leishmania donovani	L. donovani	Humans	India, Bangladesh, Burma	VL, PKDL, CL
		Canids	Sudan, Kenya, Somalia	VL (PKDL, CL)
	L. infantum	Dogs; also found in rats	Extending from the Mediterranean to China	VL, CL
	L. chagasi (infantum)	Foxes, dogs, opossums	South of Mexico to northern South America	VL, CL
Not included in a complex	L. major	Gerbils, girds and other rodents	Arid areas north of the Sahara, Arabia and central Asia	CL (LR)
		Rodents	Sub-Saharan savannah	CL
	L. tropica	Humans	Towns in East Mediterranean countries, Middle East and central Asia	CL (LR)
	L. aethiopica	Hyraxes	Highlands of Ethiopia and Kenya	CL, DCL (MCL)
	Leishmania sp.	Hyraxes?	Namibia	CL
Leishmania mexicana	L. mexicana	Forest rodents	Tropical forests of southern Mexico, Belize and Guatemala	CL
	L. amazonensis	Forest rodents	Tropical forests of South America	CL, DCL
	L. venezuelensis, L. garnhami, L. pifanoi	Undetermined	Venezuela	CL
Leishmania braziliensis	L. braziliensis	Forest rodents, peridomestic animals	Tropical forests of South and Central America	CL, MCL (VL)
	L. guyanensis	Sloths, arboreal ant-eaters	Guyana, Surinam, areas of Brazil.	CL, MCL
	L. panamensis	Sloths	Panama, Costa Rica, Colombia	CL MCL
	L. peruviana	Dogs	Areas of Peru and Argentina	CL

CL, cutaneous leishmaniasis; DCL, diffuse cutaneous leishmaniasis; LR, leishmaniasis recidivans (chronic lupoid leishmaniasis); MCL, mucocutaneous leishmaniasis; PKDL, post-kala-azar dermal leishmaniasis; VL, visceral leishmaniasis. Common names are in parentheses.

promastigote form). The parasites divide in the midgut of the insect except for the *viannia* group, which multiply in the hindgut. The highly motile promastigotes migrate to the buccal cavity of the insect, which regurgitates them on biting, thereby infecting a vertebrate host. Promastigotes rapidly penetrate macrophages and transform into an aflagellated oval body measuring 2–3.5 mm across and called an amastigote (literally, without whip). Amastigotes live as obligate intracellular parasites inside the macrophages where they multiply and are phagocytosed by other mononuclear cells when the host cell ruptures. The infection may disseminate to internal organs, spread locally to mucous membranes or persist as a chronic skin lesion.

EPIDEMIOLOGY

Leishmaniasis is endemic in 88 countries (see Chapter 117, Fig. 117.1). The world prevalence and annual incidence have been estimated to be 12 and 1.5–2 million people, respectively. The incidence of all forms of the disease is steadily increasing.[27] Some individuals may be asymptomatic Leishmania carriers.[28]

The vast majority of patients are infected by sandflies, but rare cases in which infection is transmitted by blood transfusion have been reported. Transmission by sharing needles among intravenous drug abusers may occur.

PATHOGENICITY

The internalization of *Leishmania* in the macrophage results from the interaction of complement CR3 and fucose–mannose receptors with the parasite major surface protein (Gp63) cysteine proteases and membrane lipophosphoglycan. Parasite survival inside the parasitophorous vacuole is facilitated by iron superoxide dismutase and acidic phosphatase secreted by the parasite. In animal models, susceptibility to infection is mediated by two subsets of CD4+ T lymphocytes, named T-helper Th1 and Th2.

The CD8+ T lymphocytes also play a major protective role. The host's immune system, parasite species and strain-dependent factors interact to create the full spectrum of clinical disease.

DIAGNOSTIC MICROBIOLOGY

The laboratory diagnosis can be made by demonstrating *Leishmania* by microscopy or culture, detecting parasite DNA by PCR techniques or demonstrating immune response by serology or leishmanin cutaneous tests.

To study skin lesion, smears can be prepared from the tissue juice of the raised edge of an ulcer. The sample can be aspirated with a needle or scraped with a blade. Parasites can be detected by microscopy or culture in only 30% of cases of leishmaniasis recidivans, 50% of cases of mucocutaneous leishmaniasis (MCL) and 70% of cases of cutaneous leishmaniasis (CL).

In cases of visceral leishmaniasis (VL) sternal bone marrow aspirate is the sample of choice for parasitologic diagnosis (62–100% sensitivity). Splenic fluid aspirate has a higher diagnostic rate (95–100%), but splenic rupture may complicate the procedure. Other samples such as blood, lymph nodes or liver tissue may be of value. To increase positive yield of microscopic examination, samples should be routinely cultivated in special media. The use of a microcapillary culture method has been found more sensitive and rapid than traditional tube cultures.[29,30] Most PCR-based tests show higher sensitivity than standard parasitologic methods and, in some cases, species identification can be accomplished by PCR testing. Post-treatment-positive PCR on bone marrow is associated with a higher risk of relapse.[31,32]

Serologic testing is useful in the diagnosis of VL and can be of value in cutaneous forms of leishmaniasis. The sensitivities and specificities of the tests vary depending on the manufacturer, the area of acquisition, proportion of HIV co-infected patients and controls used. Indirect fluorescent antibody test (IFAT) is sensitive and group specific, and its sensitivity is 80–100% in VL patients who do not have HIV infection and 77–89% in MCL. In CL, low titers can occasionally be found. Cross-reactivity has been found in the sera of patients who have leprosy, tuberculosis, Chagas disease, African trypanosomiasis, malaria and schistosomiasis. Newer direct agglutination test and tests based on the detection of antibodies against recombinant kinesin protein of 39 kDa (rK39) are more specific with similar sensitivity. An rK39 based dip-strip test is suitable for field conditions. A proportion of individuals who have HIV infection and VL have persistently negative serology; rK39 dip tests in co-infected European patients had a sensitivity of 20–22% while in Sudan sensitivities of 98–95% have been reported.[33–36]

CLINICAL MANIFESTATIONS

Most cases of leishmanial infection are probably subclinical. The disease produced can be classified in two groups: VL (also called kala-azar) and cutaneous leishmaniasis. Cutaneous disease can be divided into Old World cutaneous leishmaniasis, New World cutaneous leishmaniasis and MCL. Less frequent forms include diffuse cutaneous leishmaniasis (DCL), cutaneous recidivans leishmaniasis and post-kala-azar dermal leishmaniasis (PKDL).

Visceral leishmaniasis

The population at higher risk includes children under 5 years of age, immunocompromised patients and those who are malnourished. The incubation period is usually 2–8 months. Most patients do not recall having a suggestive skin lesion during the previous months. The onset is usually as an insidious febrile illness, but can be sudden with a high fever and chills. An enlarged spleen and moderately enlarged liver and lymph nodes can be detected on physical examination. As the disease progresses, signs of anemia, ecchymoses and abdominal discomfort become apparent. Anemia is due to splenic sequestration, hemodilution, bone marrow infiltration, hemolysis and bleeding. Thrombocytopenia and leukopenia are also common. In advanced disease, massive spleen enlargement, emaciation, ascites, subcutaneous edema, diarrhea, bleeding and severe anemia develop.

The mortality of untreated disease is 85–95%. Intercurrent infections are the cause of death in most cases.

Visceral leishmaniasis in immunocompromised patients

Patients who have HIV infection and immunosuppressed transplant recipients have an increased risk of developing the disease.[37] In Southern Europe, the prevalence of leishmaniasis among AIDS patients is 2–9%. This represents 10 000 times the rate in the general population. Several years may elapse from exposure to development of the disease. Immunodepressed patients may develop VL when infected with strains that in immunocompetent individuals cause only cutaneous disease. Atypical manifestations of VL encountered in these patients include localized lesions on bony prominences (Fig. 183.5), tongue, larynx, intestinal tract and lung, and Kaposi's sarcoma. Most of these atypical manifestations have also been recognized in non-AIDS patients who have advanced disease. In immunocompromised patients the disease almost invariably relapses after treatment.[38] Some patients may develop manifestations in atypical locations or localized visceral leishmaniasis mostly in areas where parasitized leukocytes were gathered by an inflammatory response.

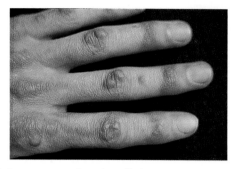

Fig. 183.5 Cutaneous manifestation of kala-azar in AIDS.

Old World cutaneous leishmaniasis

There are four cutaneous forms of leishmaniasis with distinctive clinical and immunologic features.

Oriental sore or localized CL appears on the site of the sandfly bite after approximately 2–4 weeks. The lesion begins as an asymptomatic papule, which enlarges and forms a well-circumscribed ulcer with a raised violaceous border. The lesion spontaneously resolves over a period of months, leaving a depressed scar.

Leishmaniasis recidivans presents as a chronic skin lesion that appears on the skin areas where an oriental sore has been. It has also been called 'chronic relapsing CL' and 'chronic lupoid leishmaniasis' because it closely resembles lupus vulgaris both clinically and histologically.[39]

Diffuse cutaneous leishmaniasis is a rare form of diffuse skin infection characterized by heavy parasitization of skin macrophages and absence of an effective cellular response. The lesions do not ulcerate and spread locally and at distant sites.

Post-kala-azar dermal leishmaniasis consists of symmetric macules or nodules on the face and sometimes on the trunk and extremities of patients, months to years after having VL.[40]

New World cutaneous leishmaniasis

Cutaneous leishmaniasis and MCL in the Americas take several clinical forms. The most notorious are chiclero ulcer, uta, cutaneous diseases caused by *Leishmania (Viannia) braziliensis* and MCL.

Chiclero ulcer caused by *Leishmania mexicana* was originally seen in latex (chicle) collectors who entered the forest. The lesion appears as a destructive ulcer of the pinna of the ear or the face and progresses over months (Fig. 183.6).

In uta, a disease of young children caused by *Leishmania peruviana*, the skin ulcer heals in 3–6 months leaving a disfiguring scar, usually on the face.

The cutaneous diseases caused by *Leishmania (Viannia) braziliensis* complex consist usually of multiple shallow ulcers that have a tendency to metastasize along the lymphatic vessels. They evolve to MCL in 5% of cases. Untreated, such diseases persist for years. Relapses after treatment are common.

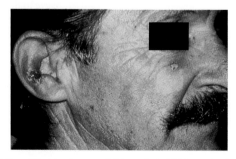

Fig. 183.6 New World cutaneous leishmaniasis (chiclero ulcer).

Mucocutaneous leishmaniasis, a markedly disfiguring, life-threatening disease, is typically caused by *L. braziliensis* and appears during the first 10 years after resolution of cutaneous disease. It consists of a pseudotumoral destructive lesion. It usually starts in the nasal mucosa and spreads to oronasopharyngeal mucosa, larynx and skin of the lips and nose. Death may be due to pneumonia, laryngeal obstruction, secondary sepsis or starvation. Spontaneous cure is rare and response to therapy is poor. Differential diagnoses include carcinoma, syphilis, yaws, rhinoscleroma and rhinosporidiasis.

MANAGEMENT

Treatment schemes can be divided in two groups – those applied to localized CL and those for extensive disease (VL, MCL and DCL).

Most cutaneous sores will slowly resolve spontaneously providing lifelong immunity. Indications for treatment are imported disease infection by *L. braziliensis* complex and sores in potentially disabling sites. Surgical excision and cryotherapy are suitable for small lesions. For larger lesions infiltration of the sore with antimonials is used: 0.5–1.5 ml of parenteral solution is carefully injected into the edges and base of the ulcer and three doses are given 3 days apart. Systemic treatment is recommended for all forms of *L. v. braziliensis* complex infections.

Alternative treatments include topical aminosidine (paromomycin) ointment (once daily for 1 month), and oral allopurinol (5 mg/kg q6h) plus probenecid (500 mg q6h) for 1 month and oral miltefosine (2.5 mg/kg/day for 28 days).

For VL, amphotericin B, antimonials, aminosidine or miltefosine may be used.

The membrane of *Leishmania* amastigotes contains ergosterol. For this reason, antifungals that interfere with the ergosterol pathway can be used in leishmaniasis. New lipid-associated amphotericin compounds are theoretically targeted against *Leishmania* because the amphotericin B–lipid complexes are cleared from blood by the monocellular/macrophagic system where the parasite persists. Liposomal amphotericin at total doses of up to 21 mg/kg are used following different dosage regimens. In Europe is common to use 3 mg/kg during the firsts 5 days followed by one or two more doses at day 10 or at days 14 and 21.

Antimonials, either meglumine antimoniate or stibogluconate sodium, are given at an antimony dose of 20 mg/kg/day. The duration of treatment is 1 month for VL and 2–3 months for DCL and PKDL. If the patient is not thrombocytopenic, intramuscular administration is recommended. Intravenous drug should be infused over 2 hours to prevent cardiac arrhythmia. Other common side-effects are pancreatitis, arthralgia, myalgia, exfoliative rash and abdominal cramps. In areas of India were antimonial resistance is widespread, parenteral administration of aminosidine (11 mg/kg/day intramuscularly for 3 weeks), an aminoglycoside with parasiticidal activity has been used successfully.[41]

Miltephosin is an orally administered drug that given at 2.5 mg/kg/day for 28 days cured 94% of Indian VL cases.[42]

Continuous suppressive treatment with one dose of antimonials every 2–4 weeks is indicated for patients who have HIV infection and leishmaniasis after a full course of treatment. Amphotericin every 2–4 weeks is also being used. Pentamidine might prevent relapses when used as prophylaxis against *Pneumocystis jirovecii* infection. When suppressive therapy was discontinued after successful antiretroviral therapy, relapses were observed only in patients with CD4 counts under 350.[43]

Trypanosomiasis

Trypanosomes produce two clinically and epidemiologically different diseases that are presented separately:

- American trypanosomiasis or Chagas disease; and
- African trypanosomiasis or sleeping sickness.

Table 183.3 Features of human trypanosomes

Species	T. brucei gambiense T. brucei rhodesiense	T. cruzi
Geographic distribution	Sub-Saharan Africa	Central and South America
Name of disease produced	Sleeping sickness	Chagas disease
Main affected organ	Brain	Heart, colon, esophagus
Vector (common name)	*Glossina* (tsetse fly)	*Reduvidae* (kissing bugs)
Mode of transmission	Bite (insect saliva)	Insect feces
Multiplying form in man	Trypomastigote	Amastigote

When a human host is infected, the organisms multiply in the inoculation area, then pass into the blood; in a third phase they localize in some internal organs causing chronic disease.

Trypanosomes pass through the morphologic stages of amastigote and trypomastigote. The differences between the main species that can be found in humans are summarized in Table 183.3.

CHAGAS DISEASE (AMERICAN TRYPANOSOMIASIS)

Chagas disease is named after Carlos Chagas, who discovered *Trypanosoma cruzi* and described its lifecycle and the clinical features of the disease.

The disease starts as an acute febrile illness followed by a long asymptomatic period and a chronic symptomatic stage characterized by distention and abnormal function of the heart and gastrointestinal tract.

Epidemiology

Chagas disease is endemic in most Latin American countries. Low income families of rural areas are most frequently affected and up to 30% of the population have the infection in the most affected regions. The World Health Organization estimates that there are 7 694 500 infected persons.

Hemipterous insects of the Reduviidae family (kissing bugs) are responsible for an estimated 41 200 new cases annually. The parasite has a sylvatic cycle maintained by reduviids that feed on wild animals, and which occasionally bite humans. It may also persist in a domestic cycle maintained by reduviids that live in the cracks of mud huts, feeding on humans, house rodents and domestic animals. In some areas, these two cycles overlap. As asymptomatic individuals may harbour a low number of parasites in their blood for many years, transmission by blood product transfusion, especially platelets, is a major cause for concern.

Vertical transmission occurs in approximately 1–10% of infected mothers, causing more than 14 000 new cases per year. Oral transmission through contaminated food is a less common route of infection.

Pathogenicity

Triatomid bugs infect when taking a blood meal from a host infected by *T. cruzi*. The parasite develops in the gut of the insect and infective trypomastigotes are released with insect feces. *Triatoma* spp. bite humans at night and defecate soon after they are engorged, contaminating the skin with trypomastigotes that penetrate through skin erosions or mucosal surfaces (typically the conjunctiva). The parasite multiplies inside cells as amastigotes. Some amastigotes differentiate into trypomastigotes, which disseminate through the circulation and may eventually be eaten by a reduviid bug.

Although the histopathology of Chagas disease is characteristic, the pathophysiologic mechanism that leads to these changes is not clearly understood. As a result of an inflammatory process (and perhaps a neurotoxin) the conducting system of the heart and the myenteric plexus are damaged. The mononuclear cell response gradually controls the infection, but does not usually eradicate it. In the late stages of the disease, only small numbers of parasites are found in cardiac muscle and the gastrointestinal tract. Neuronal depletion of the myenteric plexus leads to asynchronous peristaltic movement and, in the most severe cases, the esophagus, colon or other internal ducts dilate to enormous size.

Prevention

General improvement in housing standards or at least the use of non-cracking plaster and the regular use of residual insecticides is recommended to eliminate domestic vectors. Organ or blood donors at risk should be serologically screened for trypanosome infection. Maternal screening is aimed to detect newborns at risk.

Diagnostic microbiology

Direct parasitologic diagnosis can be obtained by visualizing the parasite in blood or tissue. Serology is especially useful for screening and for patients who have undetectable parasitemia. Xenodiagnosis is a sensitive method but is slow and cumbersome.

Parasitemia is usually detectable in the acute phase of disease by staining the buffy coat. Needle aspiration or slit-skin smear of inoculation lesions may be positive.

Serology is a reliable sensitive method of diagnosis. It usually becomes positive 1 month after infection and, in untreated individuals, frequently remains positive for life. Cross-reactivity exists with leishmaniasis, malaria, toxoplasmosis, pemphigus foliaceus, infectious mononucleosis, *Trypanosoma rangeli* and mycobacterial infections.

PCR techniques may be especially useful in early detection of infection in newborns, and in assessing suspected cross-reacting serology or combined infections. The potential of PCR in defining a parasitologic cure is a subject of current research.

Clinical manifestations

The disease evolves through three different clinical stages: acute infection, asymptomatic period and chronic disease.

Acute infection is symptomatic in only one-third of those infected. The severity and intensity of signs are greatest in younger patients, but the prevalence of infection increases with age. Symptomatic patients may develop an inflammatory lesion at the site of inoculation and an enlarged satellite lymph node. Manifestations of acute disease are fever, generalized lymphadenopathy, moderate hepatosplenomegaly, erythematous rash and myocarditis. Most patients survive the acute stage and gradually become asymptomatic within a few months. Congenitally infected newborns may be asymptomatic or present with enlarged liver and spleen. Most severe cases develop myocarditis or meningoencephalitis.

The indeterminate form is the asymptomatic period during which the infection can only be detected by serology or PCR, although some degree of esophageal dysfunction or cardiac disease may be found when appropriate diagnostic methods are used.

The chronic symptomatic stage develops in one-third of those infected, usually 5–15 years after infection (Figs 183.7, 183.8). Chronic cardiomyopathy is eventually present in 27%, digestive manifestations in 6% and neurologic disorders in 3% of infected individuals.

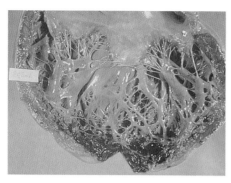

Fig. 183.7 A dilated heart from a fatal case of chagasic cardiomyopathy. Chronic heart disease is the commonest cause of death in Chagas disease. Courtesy of Dr J Cohen, Cordoba, Argentina.

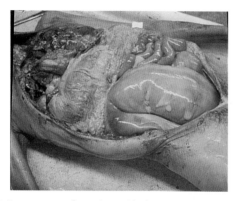

Fig. 183.8 Post-mortem of a patient with chagasic megacolon. Grossly enlarged colon as shown here or other duct dilation is characteristic of chronic Chagas disease. Courtesy of Dr J Cohen, Cordoba, Argentina.

Congestive heart failure, arrhythmias and embolic disease characterize chagasic cardiomyopathy, which is the most common cause of death in Chagas disease.[44] The presence of right bundle branch block or any of these conditions with suggestive epidemiologic data strongly suggest *T. cruzi* infection.

Esophageal disorders include achalasia, cardiospasm and enlargement. Megacolon results in constipation and abdominal pain. Associated complications include esophagitis, esophageal hemorrhage, esophageal cancer, volvulus and obstructive intestinal disease.

Latent disease reactivates in immunocompromised patients. In one series of AIDS patients who had Chagas disease, 87% developed encephalitis and 21% acute myocarditis.

Management

Antiparasitic therapy is recommended at least for the acute and recently acquired forms and parasitemic immunocompromised patients. Recent data suggest that it may also be beneficial in later stages.[45,46] Nifurtimox and benznidazole are the only two parasiticidal drugs routinely being used against *T. cruzi*.

Nifurtimox treatment is seldom available. Benznidazole (5–7 mg/kg/day in two divided doses for 2 months) seems slightly more active and better tolerated.

Pre-emptive benznidazole therapy is recommended for chagasic patients undergoing bone marrow or organ transplantation.[47] Cardiac complications may need a pacemaker or anticoagulation.

Esophageal disease is treated with cardiac dilatation in early cases. Surgery is reserved for severe esophageal or colonic dilatation.

AFRICAN TRYPANOSOMIASIS

Two African trypanosomes of the *brucei* complex infect humans:
- *Trypanosoma brucei gambiense*, which usually produces chronic infections; and
- *Trypanosoma brucei rhodesiense*, which tends to produce a more acute disease.

After an initial stage of parasitization restricted to the bloodstream, some individuals develop encephalitis. One of its most striking symptoms is a somnolence/insomnia disorder after which the disease was named 'sleeping sickness'.

Epidemiology

The vector of *T. brucei* subspecies is a fly of the genus *Glossina* (tsetse fly), which is geographically confined to tropical Africa; 80% of cases occur in Congo. It is estimated that at least 300 000 people are presently infected and 45 000 new cases occur annually.

Several *Trypanosoma* spp. infect wild and domestic animals and the infection is an important economic problem.

Trypanosoma b. rhodesiense is transmitted by *Glossina morsitans*. This fly lives in the dry savannas of East Africa, feeding mainly on the wild ungulates, which represent the main reservoir. *Trypanosoma b. gambiense* is endemic in West Africa. Humans are considered to be the main reservoir. Transmission usually occurs in the shaded riverine areas where *Glossina palpalis* and *Glossina tachinoides* live and breed.

Nature

The vector fly is infected when taking a blood meal containing trypanosomes. The ingested parasites transform and multiply in the insect midgut and migrate to the salivary glands from where new hosts are infected by biting. In the human host the parasite multiplies asexually in the interstitial space and spreads through the lymphatic vessels to the lymph nodes and blood (Fig. 183.9).

Pathogenicity

The parasite can produce hundreds of antigenically different surface glycoproteins serially. This process enables it to elude the host immune

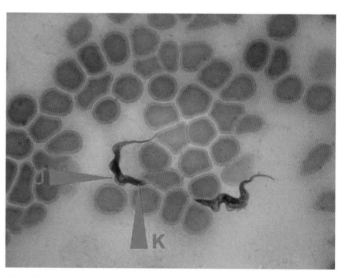

Fig. 183.9 *Trypanosoma brucei* in a Giemsa-stained blood smear. Note the central nucleus on an undulating (U) membrane and a clump of mitochondrial DNA called a kinetoplast (K).

response, resulting in a characteristic fluctuating parasitemia pattern throughout the course of infection. After a variable period, the parasite reaches the CNS, causing meningitis and choroid plexus breakdown. Large amounts of IgM are produced in the serum and cerebrospinal fluid (CSF). Characteristic plasmacytic morular cells can be seen in tissues, blood, bone marrow and CSF. Autoimmune phenomena, circulating immune complex deposition and increased vessel permeability play an important role in pathogenesis.

Prevention

Massive clearance of *Glossina* spp. habitats, insecticide spraying, destruction of wild game, periodic mass treatment and enforced relocation of entire populations were successfully used in the past. A more recent development for control is the use of *Glossina* spp.-attracting traps. Active surveillance is recommended periodically in areas of *T. b. gambiense* and during epidemics in *T. b. rhodesiense* areas. Travelers visiting endemic areas should be warned of the types of activity that may increase the chances of being bitten by tsetse flies and report any possible exposure. Mosquito repellents may be useful.

Diagnostic microbiology

The diagnosis of the disease essentially depends upon the careful repeated microscopic examination of blood or CSF samples. Increased intrathecal synthesis of IgM is a sensitive marker of CNS involvement.[48] Lymph node and bone marrow aspiration may be positive in cases with a low parasitemia. *In-vitro* culture and a miniature anion exchange column test are also feasible. Serologic screening can be carried out with the card agglutination test for trypanosomiasis (CATT) but confirmatory tests are needed.[49] PCR testing is available in some reference laboratories.

Clinical manifestations

In African trypanosomiasis, the disease develops in two stages:
- a hemolymphatic stage that spares the nervous system; and
- a second stage defined by CNS involvement.

The disease produced by *T. b. gambiense* usually develops chronically whereas in *T. b. rhodesiense* infection the disease tend to be more acute, without a clear distinction between stages.

An infective bite by a *Glossina* spp. fly may produce an inoculation chancre. Within days or weeks, the parasite disseminates to the blood. In the Gambian form of the disease, an enlarged neck lymph node may be present (Winterbottom's sign) and the patient may remain asymptomatic for years. In the hemolymphatic stage, the symptoms may be few and nonspecific: undulant fever, headache, malaise, weight loss, anemia, edema, arthralgia, diarrhea and pruritus.

On physical examination there may be erythematous circinate papules on the trunk, disproportionate pain to soft tissue pressure (Kerandel's sign) and discrete enlargement of lymph nodes, liver and spleen. Pancarditis is common in the more acute forms, when it constitutes a major cause of death. Some degree of anemia, thrombocytopenia, leukocytosis, hypogonadism, renal disease and thymus atrophy may be seen.

The CNS manifestation that gave the disease its name is the disappearance of the circadian distribution of sleep and wakefulness, which are therefore fragmented throughout the day and night. Other CNS manifestations include altered reflexes, paresthesiae, pareses, dyskinesia, choreoathetosis, epilepsy, slurred speech, mood changes, lethargy, delirium and psychosis. Without treatment, nearly all patients will develop neural involvement and die.

Management

The choice of the antiparasitic drug will depend upon whether the CNS is infected. Pentamidine or suramin can be used when the CNS is spared from infection. Melarsoprol and eflornithine are effective for both hemolymphatic and neural stages. Suramin dosage is 20 mg/kg/day (maximum 1500 mg), one intravenous injection every 5 days for 25 days. Pentamidine dosage is 4 mg/kg/day, one dose every second day for 20 days. *Trypanosoma b. rhodesiense* and some strains of *T. b. gambiense* do not respond to pentamidine.

Melarsoprol, a toxic trivalent arsenical derivative, has been the treatment of choice for patients who have had CNS involvement for five decades. Relapse after treatment occurs in up to 6% of cases and is reduced by nifurtimox combination therapy.[50] Frequently fatal arsenic-related encephalopathy occurs in 10% of cases and prednisolone treatment may reduce its incidence.

Being much less toxic, intravenous eflornithine (400 mg/kg/day in two divided doses for 7 days) plus nifurtimox (15 mg/kg/day given orally q8h for 10 days) appears to be a promising first-line therapy for second-stage sleeping sickness.[51]

General supportive treatment, anticonvulsant preventive therapy and early recognition and treatment of associated parasitic and bacterial infections are essential.

INFECTION BY OTHER *TRYPANOSOMA* SPECIES

Trypanosoma rangeli is an American parasite transmitted by triatomids. In some areas of Central America, human parasitization by *T. rangeli* is more frequent than that by *T. cruzi*. Although regarded as nonpathogenic to humans, it is medically important as a source of misdiagnosis of Chagas disease.

Animal pathogenic trypanosomes are lysed by apolipoprotein L-I, a component of human high-density lipoprotein (HDL). Patients with very low levels of high-density lipoproteins (such as those with Tangier's disease) may be susceptible to those trypanosomes. Two human cases by *Trypanosoma evansi* in India and *Trypanosoma lewisi* from Thailand have been recently reported.

REFERENCES

 References for this chapter can be found online at http://www.expertconsult.com

HD Alan Lindquist
John H Cross

Chapter | **184**

Helminths

Helminths are the most common parasites infecting humans. The world population is over six billion and there are probably a similar number of helminthic infections occurring in humans. They are transmitted to humans by food, water, soil and arthropod and molluscan vectors. Once established, they can be found in all organs, particularly intestines but also in liver, lungs, blood and occasionally in brain and other organs. This chapter describes some of these worms, their biology, epidemiology, pathogenicity, clinical aspects, diagnosis and prevention.

NATURE

The word helminth comes from the Greek meaning worm and refers to all types of worm, both free-living and parasitic. The major parasitic worms are found primarily in two major phyla:

* the Nematoda or roundworms; and
* the Platyhelminthes or flatworms, which are divided into the Trematoda or flukes and the Cestoda or tapeworms (Table 184.1). Structurally the helminths have an outer covering called a cuticle or tegument. It may be tough or delicate and essentially protects the organism, especially from digestion, while in the host intestinal tract. This structure may also possess spines, hooks, cutting plates and stylets used for attachment or to aid in penetration. There are also suckers or acetabula used by the flatworms for attachment. Some species have lytic glands near the mouth and the secretions digest host tissue for food or lyse tissues during migration.

The helminths have digestive systems of various types, excretory systems and massive reproductive systems. Most of the trematodes are hermaphroditic, one worm possessing both male and female reproductive organs; the schistosomes, on the other hand, have separate sexes. Each segment of a tapeworm has both male and female sex organs, whereas the nematodes have separate sexes. Some worms produce larvae, but most produce eggs, which pass in the host's excrement. Worms in the circulatory system produce larvae, which are carried in the blood, are ingested by blood-sucking arthropods and are then transmitted to the next host via the bite. The life cycles of the parasites are highly variable, from simple direct egg transmission to complex cycles involving one or more intermediate hosts (Figs 184.1–184.4).

EPIDEMIOLOGY

Helminthic infections are the most common parasites of humans. The highest prevalence occurs in tropical countries with poor or inadequate food supplies, and where insect, molluscan and other invertebrate vectors abound and sanitary conditions are poor.

Nematodes

Intestinal nematodes

Over one billion people, primarily children, are infected with *Ascaris lumbricoides*. In some areas of Indonesia infection rates are as high as 90%.[1] Nearly one billion people are infected with hookworm, *Necator americanus*, *Ancylostoma duodenale* or both. The former has a worldwide distribution, whereas the latter is found in certain parts of Africa, China, India and Japan. Hookworm prevalences are highly variable, being 35% in the Philippines and 90% in Indonesia, with infection rates highest in adult males.[1] Up to 800 million people are infected with *Trichuris trichiura*; both sexes and all age groups are infected, and in the Cameroons 3.1–97.3% of 22 000 children were found to be infected.[2]

Strongyloides stercoralis, like other soil-transmitted helminths, is endemic in areas with high humidity, warm temperatures and poor sanitation. The prevalence of this parasite varies from 10% to 20% in areas of Africa, South America and Asia. In surveys conducted in Indonesia and the Philippines using the Harada–Mori filter paper test-tube technique on single-stool specimens the prevalence rates were usually less than 1%.[1,3] There are reports, however, of rates as high as 25% in areas with concomitant high prevalence of human T-lymphocyte leukemia/lymphoma virus-1 virus infections.[4]

Pinworm or *Enterobius vermicularis* is a common nematode in temperate regions with an estimated 200 million infections worldwide. It is a parasite that most individuals acquire in childhood, but it is not uncommon in adults in a family with infected children. It is a common nematode infection in the USA. A high prevalence of pinworm is also reported in male homosexuals.[5]

Tissue nematodes

Larva migrans is a syndrome caused primarily by nematode parasites of lower animals. Larvae of dog hookworms such as *Ancylostoma braziliensis* and *A. caninum* penetrate human skin and migrate through this tissue causing a creeping eruption or cutaneous larva migrans. This occurs worldwide, but mostly in areas with warm, moist climates. *Ancylostoma caninum* can also cause an enteritis in humans, especially in Australia.[6] The larvae of dog and cat ascarids or *Toxocara* spp. cause visceral larva migrans in children when embryonated eggs are ingested. The larvae provoke granuloma formation, often in the central nervous system (CNS) and eye. Seroprevalence rates for *Toxocara* antibodies are high in England and France.

Although there are now seven recognized species of *Trichinella*, the only species that is important to humans is *T. spiralis*. This species has a worldwide distribution in the temperate regions,[7] whereas the other species are reported from animals in Africa (*T. nelsoni*), Arctic regions (*T. nativa*) and Palearctic and Nearctic regions (*T. pseudospiralis, T. britovi, T. murrelli*) and the Australian region (*T. papuae*). *Trichinella* spp.

Table 184.1 The major parasitic worms

Nematodes (roundworms)	Intestinal *Ascaris lumbricoides* *Enterobius vermicularis* *Ancylostoma duodenale*	*Necator americanus* *Strongyloides stercoralis* *Trichostrongylus* spp.	*Trichuris trichiura* *Capillaria philippinensis*
	Tissue *Trichinella spiralis* Visceral larva migrans (*Toxocara canis* or *Toxocara cati*) Ocular larva migrans (*Toxocara canis* or *Toxocara cati*) Cutaneous larva migrans (*Ancylostoma braziliensis* or *Ancylostoma caninum*) *Dracunculus medinensis*	*Angiostrongylus cantonensis* *Angiostrongylus costaricensis* *Gnathostoma spinigerum* *Anisakis* spp. (larvae from saltwater fish)	*Phocanema* spp. (larvae from saltwater fish) *Contracaecum* spp. (larvae from saltwater fish) *Capillaria hepatica* *Thelazia* spp.
	Blood and tissues (filarial worms) *Wuchereria bancrofti* *Brugia malayi* *Brugia timori* *Loa loa*	*Onchocerca volvulus* *Mansonella ozzardi* *Mansonella streptocerca* *Mansonella perstans*	*Dirofilaria immitis* (usually lung lesion; in dogs, heartworm) *Dirofilaria* spp. (may be found in subcutaneous nodules)
Platyhelminthes (flatworms) Cestodes (tapeworms)	Intestinal *Diphyllobothrium latum* *Dipylidium caninum*	*Hymenolepis nana* *Hymenolepis diminuta*	*Taenia solium* *Taenia saginata*
	Tissue (larval forms) *Taenia solium* *Echinococcus granulosus*	*Echinococcus multilocularis* *Multiceps multiceps*	*Spirometra mansonoides* *Diphyllobothrium* spp.
Trematodes (flukes)	Intestinal *Fasciolopsis buski* *Echinostoma ilocanum*	*Heterophyes heterophyes* *Metagonimus yokogawai*	
	Liver/lung *Clonorchis (opisthorchis) sinensis* *Opisthorchis viverrini* *Fasciola hepatica*	*Paragonimus westermani* *Paragonimus mexicanus* *Paragonimus heterotremus*	*Paragonimus skrjabini* *Paragonimus* spp.
	Blood *Schistosoma mansoni* *Schistosoma haematobium*	*Schistosoma japonicum* *Schistosoma intercalatum*	*Schistosoma mekongi*

Adapted from Garcia LS. Classification of human parasites. Clin Infect Dis 1997;25:21–3.

are ubiquitous and found in a wide variety of animal life. Transmission occurs among animals by the ingestion of *Trichinella*-infected meat. All types of carnivous mammals and birds are susceptible to infections. Most human infections are obtained by eating infected pigs and wild animals. Reports of trichinosis are sporadic, usually among groups who have participated in a communal meal. An epidemic in France reported several thousand with some deaths after the consumption of 'steak tartare' prepared from imported horse meat.[8]

The 'firey serpent of Medina' or *Dracunculus medinensis* (also known as the guinea worm) is reported from 17 African countries, Yemen, Saudi Arabia, India and Pakistan. Ten million people may be infected, and in some areas 50% of a population may have the infection every year. Sex prevalences are variable, but most infection occurs in those aged 15–40 years. Transmission is seasonal and closely related to rainfall, when the population of the major copepod vectors (*Cyclops* spp.) are abundant. Education programs are underway to eradicate the parasite.[9]

Angiostrongyliasis, or parastrongyliasis, is caused by the molluscan-borne nematodes *Angiostrongylus cantonensis*, the rat lung worm and *A. costaricensis*. The former is endemic in rats (*Rattus* spp.) in Asia, the Pacific Islands, Australia, India, Africa, the Caribbean and Louisiana and Florida in the USA. *Angiostrongylus costaricensis* is reported in Latin America and Texas, but most human infections are reported from Costa Rica. Human infection with *A. cantonensis* is reported primarily from Taiwan and Thailand, with infection acquired from eating the snails *Achatina fulica* in Taiwan and *Pila ampullacae* in Thailand. In

Taiwan most infections are in children of both sexes while in Thailand the parasitosis is seen mostly in adult males. Two human infections have been reported in Louisiana.[10–12] *Angiostrongylus costaricensis* is usually seen in children who accidently ingest the slug *Vaginulus plebeius* on vegetation. Rats (*Rattus* spp.), cotton rats (*Sigmodon* spp.) and rice rats (*Oryzomys* spp.) are natural hosts for *A. costaricensis*.

Anisakiasis is caused by third-stage larvae of *Anisakis simplex* and *Pseudoterranova decipiens*, which are acquired by eating species of raw marine fish and squid. The adult worms, related to *Ascaris*, are found in marine mammals worldwide, but most infections in humans have occurred in Japan and other countries where people eat uncooked marine fish and squid.

Gnathostoma spp. larvae can invade human tissue and most infections are reported from Thailand and Japan, and occasionally Mexico. *Gnathostoma spinigerum* is the most common species reported. *Gnathostoma hispidium* has also been found in humans. Dogs and cats are the natural hosts for adult worms. Copepods serve as the first intermediate host, and fish, frogs, snakes and chicken are the second intermediate hosts. Infections are more common in adults of both sexes.

Blood and tissue nematodes (see Chapter 115)

The filarids are a group of nematodes located in the lymphatics, subcutaneous and cutaneous tissues. There are seven major filarids of humans transmitted by arthropods in tropical and subtropical parts of the world.

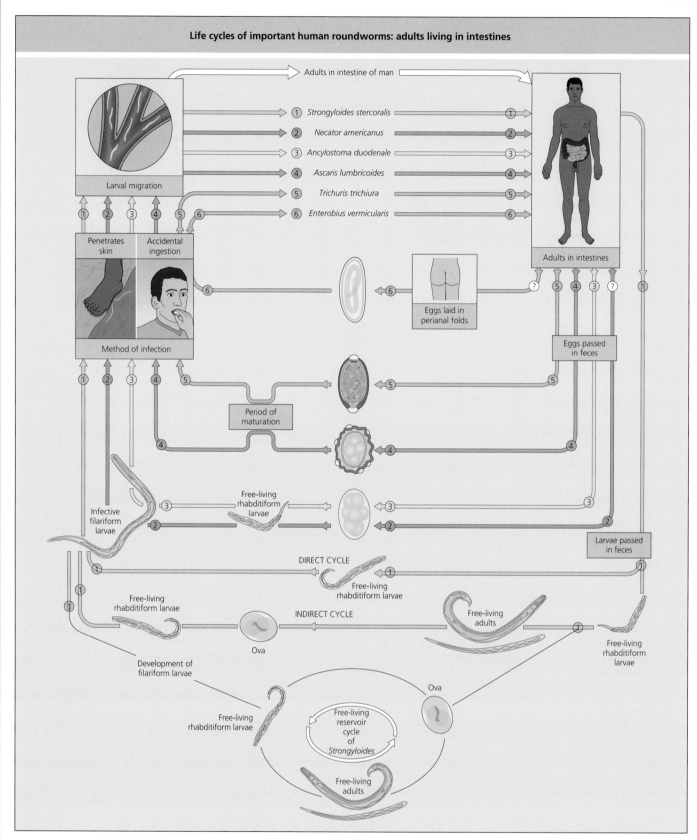

Fig. 184.1 Life cycles of important human roundworms: adults living in the intestines.

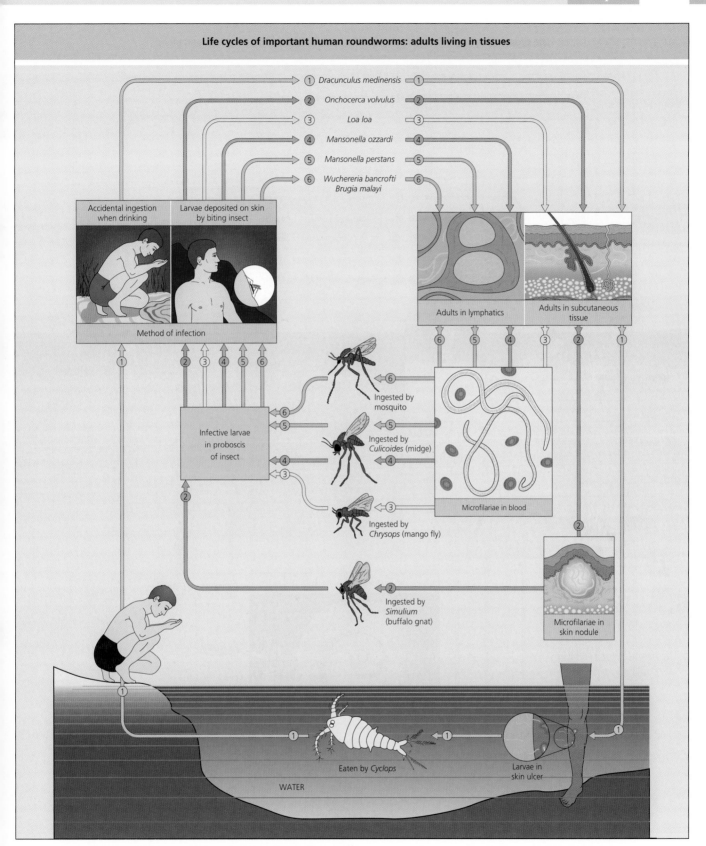

Fig. 184.2 Life cycles of important human roundworms: adults living in tissues.

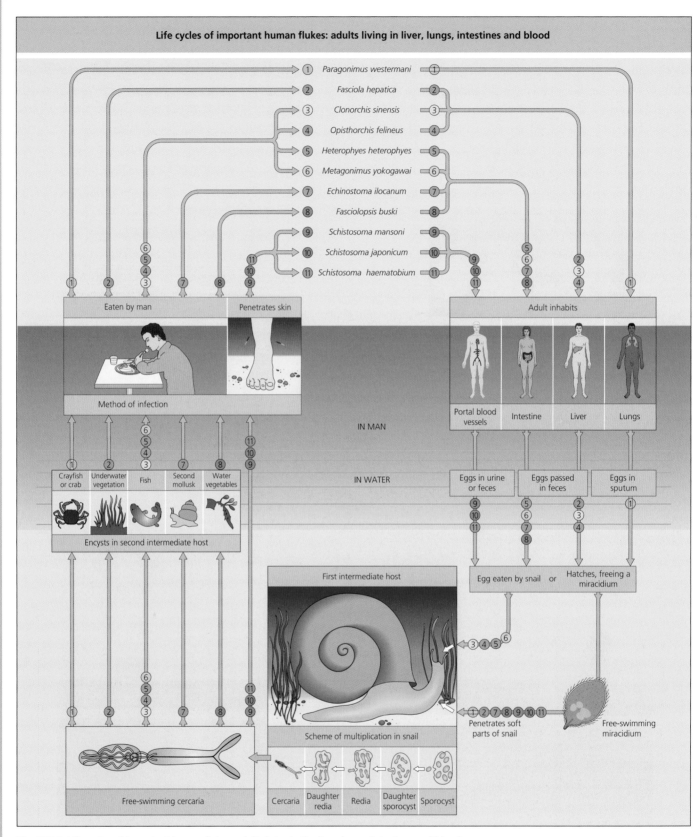

Fig. 184.3 Life cycles of important human flukes: adults living in the liver, lungs, intestines and blood.

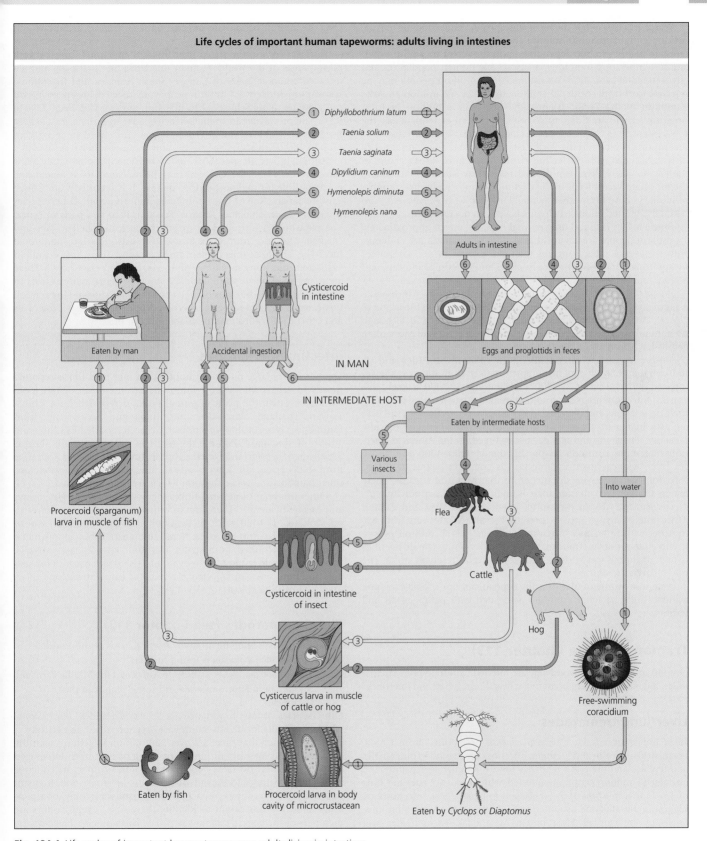

Fig. 184.4 Life cycles of important human tapeworms: adults living in intestines.

Wuchereria bancrofti is the most widespread, being endemic in Asia, Africa, Central and South America and the Pacific Islands. Prevalence rates are highly variable depending upon the vector mosquito population, temperature, humidity, a susceptible human population and environmental sanitation. An estimated 115 million people may be infected worldwide, with 50 million in Africa, 62 million in Asia, 2 million in the Pacific Islands and less than 1 million in Latin America.[13] There are different vectors in different endemic areas; the most extensive is *Culex quinquefasciatus*, whereas *Aedes polynesiensis* is the important vector in the Pacific Islands. There is a nocturnal periodicity associated with the feeding habits of the mosquitoes, except in the Pacific where there is a diurnal periodicity of microfilariae and the mosquito vector feeds in the daytime. Although a limited number of monkeys have been experimentally infected with *W. bancrofti*,[14] no naturally infected animal reservoirs have been documented.

Brugia malayi is found only in rural Asia and infects approximately 13 million people.[13] Many of the islands of Indonesia are endemic, with prevalence rates from less than 1% to over 30%.[15] The major mosquito vectors are *Mansonia*, *Anopheles* and *Aedes* spp. and cats, and *Macaca* and *Presbytis* spp. monkeys are known reservoir hosts.

Brugia timori is found only in the Lesser Sunda Islands of Indonesia. A prevalence rate of 25% was reported in a population on the island of Flores.[16] *Anopheles barbirostris* is a major mosquito vector and, although no naturally infected reservoirs have been found, cats and Mongolian gerbils have been experimentally infected.[17]

Onchocerca volvulus is endemic in 26 countries in Africa and six in Central and South America. Approximately 18 million people are infected and as a result 270 000 are blind and 500 000 severely disabled.[18] Infections are more common in males than females, reflecting male occupations and their higher exposure to vector flies. Prevalences are also higher in areas close to running water where the blackfly *Simulium damnosum* and related species breed. In the Americas infections are more common in the highlands 1000–4000 feet above sea level, whereas in Africa infection is common below 1000 feet. Infections decrease with distance from the rivers and streams. There are no animal reservoirs and there is no microfilarial periodicity.

Loa loa, the African eye worm, is endemic in West and Central Africa where *Chrysops* spp. are present. Prevalence rates vary from 8% to 40%, with infections increasing with age; 20–30 million people live in endemic areas. Transmission by the day-biting female deerflies is highest during wet seasons. Monkeys serve as reservoir hosts. The microfilariae are diurnal.

A unique feature of filarids is the dependency upon *Wolbacter* spp., a intracellular bacterial symbiont associated with pathogenesis and fertility.[19,20]

Trematodes (see Chapter 113)

Over 40 million people worldwide are infected with food-borne trematodes; the most important occur in the liver, lungs, blood and intestines.

Liver/lung trematodes

The Chinese liver fluke, *Clonorchis sinensis*, is reported from China, Japan, Korea, Taiwan and Vietnam. Infections are highest in older males and females and there is a tendency toward familial aggregations. An estimated 7 million people are infected, with prevalence rates in China of 15–24.6%, in Korea 11.7–30.8% and in Japan 2.9%. Infections are highest in the snail and fish intermediate hosts in the warmer months. Snails in the families Hydrobiidae, Melaniidae, Assimineidae and Thiaridae are first intermediate hosts, and fish, primarily of the family Cyprinidae, are second intermediate hosts. *Opisthorchis viverrini* is endemic in Thailand, Laos and Vietnam. The infection is found in an estimated 10 million people in all age groups, increasing from childhood to adulthood, and in both sexes. Prevalences vary from 7.3% to 53.2% in Thailand. *Bithynia* spp. are important snail hosts and *Cyclocheilichthys* spp. freshwater fish are important second intermediate hosts. Dogs, cats and other fish-eating mammals are reservoir hosts.

Over 10 million people are infected with *O. felineus* in Europe and Siberia.[21]

Fasciola hepatica, the sheep liver fluke, is endemic in most sheep-raising areas of the world. Human infections are increasing and are most common in parts of Europe, South America and the Middle East. Approximately 2.4 million people are infected. Sheep, goats and cattle are the natural hosts, with infection rates varying from 25% to 92%. The prevalence in humans reaches 65% in Bolivia, 24–53% in Ecuador, 10% in Peru and 2–17% in Egypt.[21] Infections are more common in adults who acquire infection from eating watercress salads.

Although over 40 species of *Paragonimus* are described, only a few infect humans and the Oriental lung fluke, *Paragonimus westermani*, is responsible for the most serious disease. It is reported from China, Taiwan, Japan, Korea, the Philippines and Thailand. Other species occur in China, Thailand, Mexico, Ecuador, Peru and parts of Africa. The parasitosis is acquired by eating metacercariae-laden crabs and crayfish. The juice from crabs is used for seasoning and traditional medicine. The juice may contain metacercariae. There are 20 million suspected infections in China, and over 600 000 elsewhere.[21] There are many snail hosts, with *Semisulcospira* spp. being major vectors in China and Korea. The crabs *Eriocheir* and *Potamon* spp. and the crayfish *Cambaroides* spp. are important second intermediate hosts. Dogs, cats and other carnivorous mammals are reservoir hosts.

Intestinal trematodes

There is a very large number (about 70) of intestinal flukes reported mostly in Asians who acquire infections because of eating raw food. *Fasciolopsis buski*, the giant intestinal fluke, is reported from China, Taiwan, Thailand, Bangladesh and India and occasionally from Indonesia. Over 200 000 infections have been reported in China and 10 000 in Thailand.[21] Pigs are the reservoir host, and snails such as *Segmentina*, *Hippeutis* and *Gyraulus* spp. are important vectors. Cercariae from snails encyst on water plants such as water caltrop, watercress, water bamboo and water chestnut which are eaten uncooked.

Other important intestinal flukes include *Echinostoma*, *Heterophyes* and *Metagonimus* spp. There are an estimated 150 000 cases of echinostomiasis, 240 000 cases of heterophyiasis and 650 000 cases of metagonimiasis, most in China, Korea and Japan. Echinostome metacercariae are acquired from snails, fish and other aquatic animals, whereas *Heterophyes* and *Metagonimus* infective stages occur in fish. All ages and both sexes are infected as a result of eating the second intermediate hosts uncooked.

Blood trematodes (see Chapter 112)

Schistosomiasis is endemic to many tropical areas of the world:
- *Schistosoma japonicum* is found in Asia;
- *S. haematobium* and *S. mansoni* in Africa and the Middle East; and
- *S. mansoni* in South America and some islands in the Caribbean.

Other species of less importance are *S. mekongi* and *S. intercalatum*, which are focally located in South East Asia and Africa, respectively.

It is estimated that there are over 200 million infections, with the prevalence and intensity of infections being highest in children aged 5–15 years. Infection rates depend upon water contact in endemic areas. Despite the widespread distribution of snails and frequent opportunities for water contact, high transmission only occurs at a few sites. It is important to identify these sites.[22] Snail vectors are members of the genera *Bulinus* spp. for *S. haematobium*, *Biomphalaria* spp. for *S. mansoni* and *Oncomelania* spp. for *S. japonicum*. *Bulinus* and *Biomphalaria* spp. are strictly aquatic whereas the *Oncomelania* are amphibious snails. There are some animal hosts for *S. mansoni*, but humans are the most important source of infection. Humans are also the most important host for *S. haematobium*, whereas many domestic and wild animals are a reservoir host for *S. japonicum*. Although *S. japonicum* is endemic on Taiwan, the strain of parasite on the island will not infect humans. It is considered to be a zoophilic strain.[23]

Cestodes (see Chapter 113)

Cestode or tapeworm infections are acquired by ingestion of intermediate hosts containing the infective larval stages:

- the beef tapeworm *Taenia saginata* and pork tapeworm *T. solium* are acquired by ingesting the cysticercus stage in beef or pork;
- the fish tapeworm *Diphyllobothrium latum* is acquired by eating raw fish infected with the plerocercoid or sparganum stage; and
- *Hymenolepis nana* and *H. diminuta* are rodent tapeworms that use fleas and beetles as intermediate hosts.

Taenia saginata is reported worldwide, with high infection rates in Africa and Asia. Most infections occur in adults. The cysticercus is found only in bovids; however, in parts of Asia, especially in Taiwan, pigs are a recognized source of infection for a strain of the parasite, namely *T. saginata* (*asiatica*).[24]

Taenia solium is found sporadically in pigs worldwide, with many human cases reported from Mexico and Central and South America, South West Asia and Africa. Human cysticercosis is also present in these areas. Certain areas of Irian Jaya in Indonesia report many cases of cysticercosis because of the habit of eating uncooked pork.

Hymenolepis nana is the most common tapeworm in North America and is particularly reported in children worldwide. *Hymenolepis diminuta* is not common but reported occasionally in South East Asia.

There is a high prevalence of *D. latum* in humans in Scandinavia, Finland, Alaska, Canada and Northern USA. Other species of *Diphyllobothrium* are reported from Japan and South America.

Sparganosis or infections with the larval stage of *Spirometra* spp. is reported occasionally from many parts of the world. Infection is acquired by ingesting copepods or second intermediate host (frogs, toads or other aquatic animals). Infections in southern Asia are attributed to the use of fresh animal tissues as poultices.

Echinococcus granulosus and *E. multilocularis* are associated with human hydatid disease, whereas *E. vogeli* and *E. oligarthrus* rarely cause disease in humans. *Echinococcus granulosus* is the most important and found primarily in sheep-raising areas. Strains of the parasite are also found in goats, swine, cattle, horses and camels.

The parasitoses are found worldwide, with canines serving as the definitive host and animals such as sheep as intermediate hosts. Humans acquire infection by ingesting eggs from dogs, whereas dogs acquire the infection by eating sheep liver and other organs containing cysts with large numbers of scolices. Infections usually occur in the young and the cysts develop over a period of years.

Echinococcus multilocularis has a limited distribution in dogs, foxes, wolves and cats as the reservoir hosts and larval stages in wild rodents, especially voles. The parasite, however, is reported to be moving southward in the USA. Rare human infections are acquired by the ingestion of eggs passed by the canines. Infection with any of the *Echinococcus* spp., however, is related to poor sanitary conditions in populations with a low level of education and in people closely associated with canine reservoir hosts.

PATHOGENICITY

Helminths seem to live in peaceful coexistence with their hosts and usually cause few problems. However, if there are many worms, there may be severe disease. The parasites, especially in the intestines, can cause obstruction and possibly perforation. The worms also secrete or excrete toxic substances, which affect the tissues. Lytic substances, such as those secreted by hookworms to obtain blood, can induce inflammation and there may be changes due to malabsorption and competition for nutrients. Larval stages may be more pathogenic, secreting antigenic substances that cause hypersensitivity, while the antigens promote antibody production and cellular immune responses. Worms in the wrong place can be highly pathogenic.

Helminths have intricate life cycles and disease is usually associated with the larval migratory pathways and the final habitat of adult worms in the host. The amount of pathology and disease varies with the parasitosis.

Nematodes living in the intestine (see Chapter 108)

Enterobius vermicularis

The life cycle of *Enterobius vermicularis* is presented in Figure 184.1. Pinworm resides in the large bowel, where mating occurs. Gravid females migrate out of the anus and deposit eggs on the perianal skin. Eggs under the fingernails in children lead to re-infection when the fingers are placed in the mouth. Eggs can be released onto the bedsheets and become disseminated throughout the household when the sheets are shaken. The eggs will survive for 2 weeks in a humid and cool environment. When eggs are ingested they hatch in the intestine and the larvae migrate to the large intestine to mature in 6 weeks.

Ascaris lumbricoides

Infection with *Ascaris lumbricoides* can occasionally be highly pathogenic. The life cycle is presented in Figure 184.1. The adult male worm may measure 15–31 cm by 2–4 mm and the female 20–35 cm by 3–6 mm. The female can live for a year or more and produce 240 000 eggs/day. The eggs pass in the feces and embryonate in the soil in 10–14 days. Upon ingestion the egg hatches in the intestine and the liberated larva penetrates the mucosa and passes to the liver via the portal vessels and then to the lungs. After a few weeks the larva penetrates the alveolar air sac, passes up the pulmonary tree, is coughed up and swallowed and becomes sexually mature in the small intestines in 60–75 days.

Trichuris trichiuria

Trichuris trichiuria has a direct life cycle (see Fig. 184.1). Adult females in the large intestine deposit eggs in the fecal stream and after a few weeks in the soil they become embryonated. When eggs are swallowed they hatch in the intestine and the larva moves down the bowel to the colon. The worms bury their narrow anterior end into the mucosa with the wider posterior end extended freely into the lumen of the colon. The females lay eggs after 3 months and produce 3000–10 000/day. The females measure 35–55 mm and the males 30–45 mm.

Hookworms

A number of hookworm species can enter the human body, but most are natural parasites of animals other than humans (i.e. zoonotic parasites). The species from lower animals usually cause a creeping eruption or cutaneous larva migrans. Only two hookworms are considered to be important human species:

- *Necator americanus*; and
- *Ancylostoma duodenale*.

Both species measure about 10–13 mm for females and 6–11 mm for males and can be 0.4–0.6 mm in width. The anterior mouths have cutting plates or teeth and the males have bell-shaped bursal rays at the posterior end that are used for holding females during copulation. The vulva is mid-central and eggs pass from the females into the fecal stream and out with host feces onto the soil. Female worms pass 5000–10 000 (*N. americanus*) and 10 000–20 000 (*A. duodenale*) eggs/day. In warm, moist climates the eggs embryonate in the soil and rhabditiform larvae are released. Within a few days the larvae molt and develop into filariform larvae or the infective stage. The larvae climb to the top of the soil or grass, cling together and wait for a human host to come by. They usually penetrate the skin between the toes or other body surfaces. Some *A. duodenale* larvae may be ingested in water and enter the oral mucosa. The larvae are carried by the blood to the heart and then the lungs where they remain for a period, break out into the alveoli, pass up the pulmonary tree and are swallowed. The parasite matures in the small intestine, copulates and produces eggs in about 5 weeks (see Fig. 184.1).

The infections can remain active for as long as 13 years. The attachment of adult worms can cause small erosive lesions, hemorrhage, tissue cytolysis and neutrophilic infiltration. The worms change attachment sites regularly, leaving old sites oozing blood and plasma. Iron deficiency anemia and blood loss result from long-term infection with a large number of worms.

Pathologic changes occur in the bone marrow due to blood loss. Liver function may change as a result of anemia, as well as reduced capacity for albumen synthesis. Hookworm disease with iron deficiency anemia, hypoproteinemia and hepatosplenomegaly may contribute to thousands of deaths each year.

Strongyloides stercoralis

Strongyloides stercoralis is a unique nematode having a parasitic life cycle and a free-living cycle, with males and females present in the free-living cycle (see Fig. 184.1) and only females present in the parasitic life cycle. The parasitic females measure 1.5–2.5 mm and have a long cylindric esophagus. The vulva is in the posterior third of the body and the paired uteri contain thin-shelled eggs.

The eggs are deposited in the small intestinal epithelium and hatch soon after release. The first-stage or rhabditiform larva passes in the feces and develops into a second-stage and then a third or infective-stage filariform larva after a few days. The third-stage larvae penetrate the skin and migrate through the body and via the blood to the lungs; after several days they migrate up the respiratory tree and are swallowed. The larvae enter the intestinal mucosa and mature, and the female worms produce eggs parthenogenetically. Some larvae transform into infective forms in the bowel, penetrate the mucosa, migrate and develop into adults. This is internal autoinfection and can lead to hyperinfection in the immunocompromised host. Some rhabditiform larvae transform into rhabditoid free-living male and female adults in the soil and reproduce. The eggs hatch, releasing rhabditiform larvae, which develop into filariform larvae that can enter the skin of a host.

Cellular immunity is responsible for keeping infections under control, but when immunity is affected by disease or immunosuppression, the parasite multiplies unabated and this leads to hyperinfection and dissemination.

Capillaria philippinensis

Intestinal capillariasis is a disease in which the parasite can multiply in the digestive tract. *Capillaria philippinensis* is a tiny worm; females measure 2.5–5.3 mm and males 1.3–3.9 mm. The anterior body is narrow and the posterior is slightly wider and contains reproductive organs and digestive tract. The females deposit eggs, which must reach water where they embryonate. When these are eaten by small freshwater fish the eggs hatch and the larvae develop into infective stages in 3 weeks. When humans eat the fish the larvae mature in 2 weeks. After mating the females first produce larvae that will mature in the gut, whereas the second-generation worms produce thick-shelled eggs, which pass out in the feces. The parasites can multiply rapidly, producing thousands of progeny.[25] If the patient is not treated the disease can be fatal. Over 200 000 worms were recovered from 1 liter of bowel fluid at one autopsy. The worms enter the crypts and cause atrophy, the villi are flattened and denuded, the mucosal glands are denuded and the lamina propria is infiltrated with inflammatory cells. Other organs are also affected by malnutrition and hypokalemia. Most of the pathology is in the jejunum.[26]

Nematodes living in tissues

Trichinella spiralis

Trichinella spiralis is related to other trichiurids in having a slender anterior and a wider posterior end. Female worms measure 2–4 mm and males 1–1.5 mm. Infections are acquired by eating uncooked muscle containing encysted larvae from infected animals, usually pigs.

The larvae are digested from the cyst, pass to the small intestines and burrow beneath the epithelium where they develop into adults, re-enter the gut lumen and reproduce. The larvae produced enter the gut wall, are picked up by the blood and carried throughout the body to striated muscle where they become encysted. The larvae entering the muscle cell cause alterations in morphology, which results in the characteristic 'nurse cell'. Morphologic and molecular changes occur in the cell until it eventually becomes calcified. The larvae can remain alive for many years in the cell. Chronic inflammatory cells may surround the parasitized muscle cell.

Filarial nematodes

The filarial nematodes are long and slender and are found in the lymphatics, tissues and body cavities. The life cycles of some of the filarids are presented in Figure 184.2. Microfilariae are produced by female worms and arthropods are the vectors (see Chapter 115).

Wuchereria bancrofti, Brugia malayi *and* Brugia timori

The lymphatic filarids *W. bancrofti*, *B. malayi* and *B. timori* produce microfilariae that usually appear in the blood between 2200 and 0200 hours (nocturnal periodicity). *Wuchereria bancrofti*, found in some of the Pacific Islands, produces microfilariae that appear in the blood in the daytime (diurnal periodicity). Mosquitoes obtain blood at night and the larvae develop into the infective stage in 10–14 days. At the next feeding the infective larvae migrate from the thoracic muscles of the mosquito to the proboscis and crawl into the hole made by the bite. The larvae migrate in the host until they reach the definitive habitat and develop into adults. The worms copulate and the females produce microfilariae; the life cycle of *W. bancrofti* is a few months longer than that of *B. malayi*. Infections may persist for several years.

The pathogenesis of lymphatic filariasis has been a matter of debate and a model integrating various aspects of the parasitosis has been proposed.[27] It has also been suggested that *Wolbachia*, an endosymbiont of filarids, may be associated with the pathogenesis.[19,20] On the other hand, the pathology of lymphatic filariasis may be associated with immunologic responsiveness. Some people who have the infection are microfilaremic but without antibodies or disease, whereas other are amicrofilaremic and have antibodies. There is an inflammatory stage with lymph channel irritation. Adult worms can be found in the lymph vessels, primarily the axillary, epitrochlear, inguinal and pelvic nodes as well as those in the testis, epididymis and spermatic cord.

Onchocerca volvulus

Onchocerca volvulus adults are coiled in fibrous tissue nodules in the subcutaneous tissue. The females may reach 50 cm in length and 0.5 mm in diameter and the microfilariae produced are released into the interstitium of the skin. Males are smaller, being 5 cm in length. Microfilariae are picked up by biting flies or black flies of the genus *Simulium* and after developing to the infective stage the larvae are introduced into a host at the next feeding. The larvae migrate through the tissue and after many months settle down, usually in pairs, and become encapsulated (see Fig. 184.2).

The microfilariae leave the nodule and migrate through the dermis, provoking a dermatitis and blindness.

Loa loa

The African eye worm *Loa loa* actually moves through subcutaneous tissue and often traverses the conjunctiva. The males are 3–4 cm and the females 4–7 cm in length and 3–5 mm wide. Microfilariae have a diurnal periodicity and are ingested by species of *Chrysops* at the time of a blood meal. The larvae develop to the infective stage in 10–13 days and enter the host through the hole made by the bite at the next feeding (see Fig. 184.2). The adult worms cause little damage as they migrate quickly through the tissue.

Dracunculus medinensis

Dracunculus medinensis is similar to the filarids. The females measure up to 120 cm long and 2 mm wide and the males 2 cm. The worms mature in the connective tissue; gravid females then migrate to the subcutaneous tissue where they cause ulcers through which larvae are released when the lesion is immersed in water. The larvae are ingested by copepods and develop into infective larvae in 2 weeks. When the copepods are ingested in drinking water the larvae are liberated, penetrate the digestive tract and develop into adults in the connective tissue in a year (see Fig. 184.2).

Angiostrongylus cantonensis

Angiostrongylus cantonensis is found naturally in the lungs of rats. The larvae produced by the females move up the pulmonary tree, are swallowed and pass out in the rat feces. Mollusks (snails and slugs) serve as intermediate hosts and, when eaten by rats, the larvae are digested out of the snail tissue, migrate from the gut to the brain, and after 3 weeks migrate to the lungs. Larvae are produced by adult females a few weeks later. Humans who ingest snails or slugs acquire the infective larvae, which migrate to the CNS and cause eosinophilic meningitis. The females reach 2–3 cm and the males 1–2 cm in length and 0.2–0.3 mm in width. In most human infections the larvae die in the brain and cord and elicit an inflammatory reaction in the meninges. Eosinophils, monocytes and foreign body giant cells infiltrate around the dead worms. Tissue necrosis is also evident. Larvae are reported in the eye, and are often recovered from cerebrospinal fluid (CSF). Adult worms have been found on a few occasions in the pulmonary artery.[10]

Anisakis simplex and *Pseudoterronova decipiens*

Anisakis simplex larvae measure 2–3 cm by 0.3–0.6 mm and *Pseudoterranova decipiens* 2–3 cm by 0.3–1.2 mm. They are found in the muscle and body cavity of marine fish and squid. When eaten by marine mammals (e.g. whales, seals, porpoises) the worms mature in the stomach and the females deposit eggs in the feces. In the ocean, a larva hatches from the egg and is eaten by a small marine crustacean. When the crustacean with a third-stage larva is eaten by fish, the freed larva migrates to the abdominal cavity. When infected fish are eaten raw by humans the liberated larvae penetrate the stomach or small intestine and provoke a foreign body reaction around the worm.

Gnathostoma spinigerum

Gnathostoma spinigerum is a robust nematode with a large globose head surrounded by rows of spines. The females measure 1–1.5 cm by 1–2.5 mm and the males 1–2.5 cm by 1–2 mm. The adults are coiled in the wall of the digestive tract of dogs and cats. Eggs pass in the feces, embryonate in fresh water and are ingested by copepods. The larvae hatch and develop into the second larval stage. When the copepod is eaten by a second intermediate host, the third-stage larva develops, and when this is eaten by a dog or cat the worm penetrates the gut wall and matures. Humans who eat infected fish, frogs or other aquatic food, raw or fermented, acquire the infection and the larvae migrate through the tissue in a fashion similar to that of cutaneous larva migrans. The CNS may be invaded, resulting in an eosinophilic myeloencephalitis with eosinophilic pleocytosis and bloody and xanthochromic CSF. The eye may also be invaded, causing palpebral edema, exophthalmos and subconjunctival hemorrhage.

Larva migrans

Cutaneous larva migrans is caused by dog or cat hookworm larvae that enter the skin and are unable to complete the life cycle. They either migrate through subcutaneous tissue or encyst in the tissue and the larvae may cause serpiginous erythematous tracts. The tracts eventually become dry and encrusted.

Visceral larva migrans is caused by the dog and cat ascarid larvae (*Toxocara* spp.) that escape from eggs that are accidentally swallowed. The larvae migrate through the tissue and encyst as second-stage larvae. The migrating larvae produce tracts with hemorrhagic necrosis.

Trematodes living in liver, lungs, intestines and blood

Although many trematodes infect humans, only a few are considered to be important pathogens. These flat worms are found in all organs, especially the intestines, and a few are found in the liver, lungs and blood. The life cycles of the important trematodes are presented in Figure 184.3.

The opisthorchid liver flukes

Clonorchis sinensis, *Opisthorchis viverrini* and *Opisthorchis felineus* are found in the bile ducts. The worms are hermaphroditic and about 1.5 cm long and tapered at both ends. Eggs produced pass down the bile ducts to the intestine and out with the feces. In water, snails of a number of species (*Parafossarulus*, *Thiara* and *Bithynia*) serve as the first intermediate host; they ingest the egg and the miracidium is released from the egg. After reproducing by polyembryony, cercariae are produced that leave the snail and encyst as metacecariae in freshwater fish (cyprinids or carp). When the fish is eaten raw or improperly cooked the metacercariae are digested out of the fish and migrate down the bowel and then into the bile passages. Cholangiocarcinoma is a possible complication and DNA carcinogens may be associated with infection. There may also be an association with nitrosamines, which are commonly found in Asian foods.[28]

Fasciolopsis buski

Fasciolopsis buski is the largest intestinal trematode of humans, measuring 5–7 cm by 8–20 mm by 1–3 mm. It has an oral and ventral sucker, two large ceca, two branched testes and a central and coiled uterus. Eggs pass in the feces into water and the hatched miracidium enters a specific planorbid snail. Cercariae released from the snail attach to aquatic vegetation and form into metacercariae. When eaten the metacercariae excyst and attach to the mucosa of the small intestine.

Fasciolia hepatica

Fasciolia hepatica is acquired by eating aquatic vegetation on which the metacercariae are attached. Upon ingestion the metacercariae are released and penetrate the gut wall, traverse the peritoneal cavity, pass through the liver capsule into the liver parenchyma and into the bile duct. Worms may also re-enter the liver parenchyma. The worms are large, 4 cm in length and 1.5 cm wide, with a large cephalic cone at the anterior end. The egg passes down the bile duct to the intestines and out with the feces. It hatches in the water and the miracidium enters into snails of the genus *Lymnea*. Cercariae are released and encyst on all varieties of aquatic vegetations.

Paragonimus westermani

Paragonimus westermani usually resides in pairs in the lung. They are reddish brown, plump bodied and shaped like coffee beans, and measure about 1.2 cm long, 0.6 cm wide and 0.4 cm thick. They have two large branching testes in the posterior half of the body. Eggs enter the alveoli, are coughed up and swallowed, and pass out in the feces or in sputum. The egg hatches in water, enters a specific snail and multiplies; released cercariae enter crabs and crayfish where the metacercariae encyst. When the infected crustacean is eaten the metacercariae are released from the cyst, penetrate the gut wall and enter into the peritoneum, diaphragm and lung.

Young migrating worms produce local hemorrhage and cellular infiltration. These worms may settle in ectopic locations and evoke a pronounced tissue reaction. In the lung and other locations a leukocytic infiltration develops around the worm and fibrous tissue infiltrates to form a cyst wall. Eggs may migrate into pulmonary tissue and other locations and evoke granulomatous reactions. Cerebral paragonimiasis often develops, with hemorrhage, eosinophils, a yellowish exudate and Charcot–Leyden crystals. Some lesions may eventually calcify.

Other species of *Paragonimus* can also infect humans and invade subcutaneous tissue and the abdominal cavity.

Other intestinal fluke infections

Most intestinal fluke infections are innocuous unless there is a large number of worms. The eggs of the heterophyids are tiny and may be carried by the lymphatics and venules to ectopic locations such as the heart and evoke granulomas. Eggs of the intestinal flukes pass in the feces and hatch in water and the miracidia enter snails. Cercariae emerging from the snails enter fish and other aquatic animal life; when these animals are eaten the metacercariae excyst and develop into adults in the small intestine.

Human schistosomes

Human schistosomes are found in the venous bloodstream. Eggs are passed into water and the miracidia released search out specific snails in which to continue the life cycle. Cercariae released from the snails penetrate the skin and the larval schistosomulae migrate to the lungs and then to the mesenteric and vesical veins. Eggs carried back through the mesenteric veins to the liver are responsible for granuloma formation.

The schistosomes are the only trematodes with separate sexes. They have oral and ventral suckers. The females are 1.5–2.5 cm in length and 0.2–0.3 mm in diameter. The male is 0.5–2.0 cm and, although flat, usually curls up to form the gynecophoral canal in which the female lies. The female leaves the male, crawls to the small venules close to the lumen of the gut or urinary bladder and deposits eggs. The miracidium releases enzymes to work with the spines on the *S. mansoni* and *S. haematobium* eggs to digest the tissue and enter the lumen of the intestine and bladder. Some eggs are carried back via the venules and veins to the liver. Infections are known to persist for many years.[29] The life cycles of the human schistosomes are presented in Figure 184.3.

Cestodes living in the intestines and tissues

Adult tapeworms residing in the intestines do not cause serious disease, but larval stages of two species are highly pathogenic. The adults in the intestines pass eggs, which are taken up by an intermediate host (see Fig. 184.4).

Eggs of *T. saginata* and *T. solium* are ingested by bovids and swine and the larval or cysticercus stages develop in muscles. When the meat is eaten insufficiently cooked the cysticerci are released and develop into adults in the small intestine.

The life cycles of the fish tapeworm *D. latum* and related species involves two intermediate hosts. The egg hatches in water and the corricidium is taken in by a copepod and develops into a procercoid larva. When eaten by a fish the larva develops into a pleroceroid larva and when the fish is eaten the larva becomes an adult in the intestine.

Hymenolepid cestodes often require an insect (beetles and fleas) as an intermediate host. *Hymenolepis nana* can also be acquired by ingestion of the egg. Some strains of *H. nana* are also capable of internal autoinfection.

Morphologically, all tapeworms have a scolex and neck, and immature, mature and gravid proglottids. The scolex of *D. latum* has a sucking groove as a hold-fast organ, whereas the other tapeworms have a scolex with four suckers, and *T. solium* and *H. nana* have a rostellum on the scolex with rows of hooklets. Each mature proglottid is hermaphroditic with both male and female sex organs. The length and width of each species varies with the longest being *D. latum* (2–15 m), followed by the taeniids (1–4 m), *H. nana* (1.5–4 cm) and *H. diminuta* (1–6 cm).

Larval stages of tapeworms also infect humans (Fig. 184.5). Infection with the plerocercoid larva of diphyllobothriid species such as *Spirometra* is the cause of sparganosis. The larvae acquired from eating aquatic animals or drinking copepods in water penetrate the gut

wall and migrate through the tissue. Animal poultices used in Asia are another source of infection. The larvae cause painful inflammatory swellings or transient lesions. The parasite may invade the eye causing periorbital edema.

Humans who become infected with the eggs of *T. solium* may develop cysticercosis. The larvae invade the muscles, brain, eye and skin. Although the cyst may remain intact and dormant for years, it may eventually break and the released fluids cause granulomas and calcification.

Echinococcosis or hyatid disease develops in humans who accidentally ingest the eggs of the dog tapeworms *E. granulosus* or *E. multilocularis*. The egg hatches in the duodenum and the oncosphere penetrates the gut and becomes established in the liver and other organs. A cyst develops brood capsules and protoscolices proliferate from the inner germinal epithelium of the brood capsule. An outer laminated acellular limited membrane forms and the cyst develops over many years. Unilocular cysts develop with *E. granulosus* and multilocular alveolar cysts with *E. multilocularis*. Cysts develop in many organs. The adult worms are parasites of canines and the intermediate host can be any animal, but most often are sheep for *E. granulosus* and rodents for *E. multilocularis*.

PREVENTION

Most parasitic infections can be prevented if good sanitary practices are followed. The soil-transmitted nematodes can be controlled and possibly eradicated with proper disposal of feces. This is true for most intestinal parasites, even those that require an intermediate host. The disposal of fecal matter into water bodies containing molluscan intermediate hosts perpetuates trematode infections. The construction and use of sanitary privies will go a long way toward preventing infections of all types, but in most endemic areas these practices are usually not followed and indiscriminate defecation is the trend. Infection with skin-penetrating helminths such as hookworm and *Strongyloides* spp. can be prevented by wearing shoes and protective clothing.

Arthropod-borne helminthiasis, such as filariasis, can be prevented by the use of insecticides in houses. Breeding areas of the vectors can also be treated with insecticides. The use of repellents will also help, as will sleeping under insecticide-impregnated bed nets.

The avoidance of water known to harbor snail vectors will prevent schistosome infections. The destruction of snail breeding areas and the use of molluscicides will help to control infections.

The ingestion of raw foods should be restricted in endemic areas. The eating of raw fish is a practice in many countries, and if this is discouraged certain trematode and cestode infections could be prevented. The cooking of marine fish would prevent anisakiasis. Similarly the cooking of aquatic vegetation would prevent trematode infection such as fascioliasis and fasciolopsiasis. Undercooked beef and pork are responsible for trichinosis and tapeworm infections and thorough cooking will destroy the parasites. Freezing foods will kill most parasites and in the future irradiation of foods will make food safe.[30] Microwave treatment, however, is not considered adequate for destroying parasites.

The use of anthelmintics can be used to eliminate helminthic infections. Mebendazole, albendazole and praziquantel have been used in mass treatment campaigns for some nematode and trematode infections. Antifilarial drugs have been used in mass treatment programs and have even been included in table salt distributed to a population group. Reduction of infections in a population will be of significant benefit and will augment control and eventual eradication programs (see Chapter 115). These methods along with education programs would be a definite adjunct to prevention and control.

DIAGNOSIS

The diagnosis of helminthic infections depends upon the location of the parasite in the body. The majority of worms are in the digestive tract and the diagnosis is made by stool examination. Blood is examined for

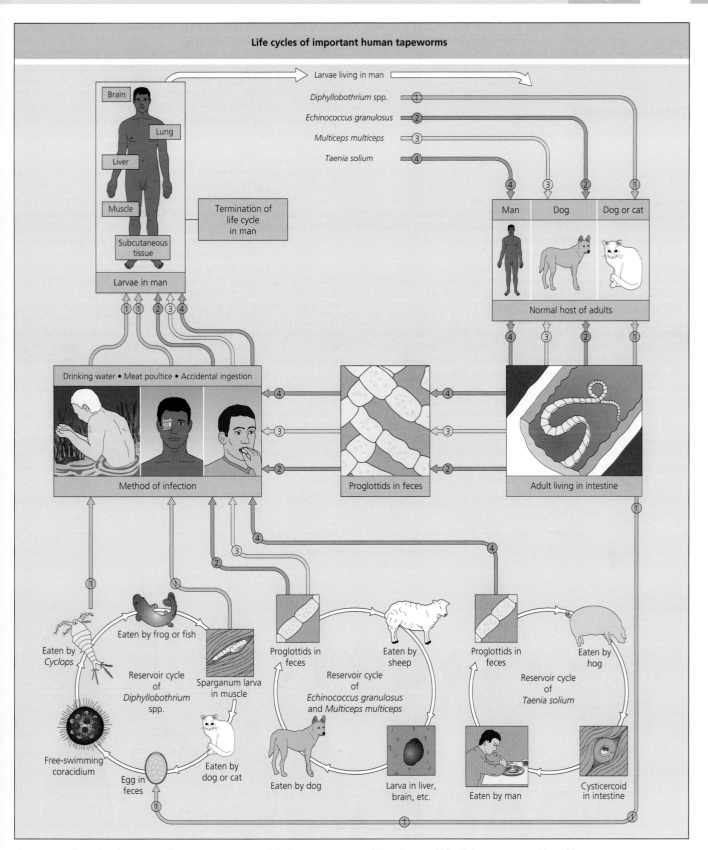

Fig. 184.5 Life cycles of important human tapeworms; adults living in tissues and intestines and blood: humans are accidental hosts.

parasites in the circulatory system, and urine and sputum are examined for worms in the genitourinary systems and respiratory passages. Tissue parasites are diagnosed by biopsies and by immunologic methods. Many techniques have been developed to aid in the diagnosis and most of these have been presented in detail.[31]

Stool specimens

Intestinal parasites are detected by microscopic examination of one or preferably more than one stool specimen.[32] The stools should be collected in a clean dry container and examined as soon as possible after being passed. A direct examination is made by making wet films on a clean microscope slide. A small portion of feces is mixed with a drop of saline on the slide and examined under low-power (3100) and high-power (3450) magnification, if needed. The preparation should not be too thick; it should be thin enough to read newsprint through. Iodine stain preparations can also be used, especially for protozoan infections, but do not add a great deal to the observation of helminth eggs and larvae. If a stool specimen cannot be examined within a few hours after passage it should be placed into 10% formalin or another preservative. The examination can then be done when it is more convenient.

Concentration techniques are also available. The simplest is sedimentation of feces in a tube or sedimentation flask and the sediment is then examined microscopically. The formalin–ethyl acetate technique, in which the stools are mixed with saline and passed through gauze or a screen, is widely used. The material collected is centrifuged several times in saline and finally formalin. Ethyl acetate is added and the preparation is centrifuged slowly. The detritus layer and supernatant are poured off and the sediment examined microscopically. The zinc sulfate flotation method is another simple technique in which small samples of feces are mixed thoroughly with zinc sulfate (1.18 sp gr or 1.2 sp gr for formalized stools). This may be centrifuged or permitted to stand for a period and the surface fluids examined for eggs. This method is unsatisfactory for operculated eggs, however. Eggs from various helminths as well as larvae of hookworm and *Strongyloides* are depicted in Figures 184.6 and 184.7.

The Kato method to examine stools has been modified into the Kato–Katz technique for estimating the number of eggs in the feces. Screened feces are placed into a small hole in a template, which delivers 41.7 mg feces onto a microscope slide. A Cellophane square soaked in a glycerine–malachite green is placed onto the feces and the preparation is permitted to stand for 30–60 minutes. The glycerine clears the fecal material and eggs can be seen against a green background. This technique is especially good for thick-shelled eggs such as those of *A. lumbricoides*, *T. trichiura* and *S. mansoni*. The preparation should be examined within 30 minutes for thin-shelled eggs such as hookworm, which may dissolve if they stand for too long. The number of eggs observed is multiplied by 24 to obtain the number of eggs/g of feces. The Kato method uses only the glycerine-soaked Cellophane and is not quantitative.

Fecal cultures can be used to recover nematode larvae, especially of the hookworms and *Strongyloides* spp. The feces are mixed with charcoal with a small amount of water and placed into a Petri dish with moist filter paper lining the bottom of the dish. This is kept at room temperature for several days and the larvae will migrate to the surface of the charcoal. The culture is placed into a Baermann apparatus consisting of a funnel with rubber tubing attached to the stem and a pinch-clamp closing the tube. A sieve is placed into the top of the funnel and lined with gauze. The funnel is filled with warm water and the culture placed onto the gauze. The apparatus stands at room temperature for 10–12 hours and the fluid is drawn off through the tubing into a glass flask. Larvae can be collected from the flask and examined microscopically to determine the species.

The Harada–Mori technique is also used to culture feces and recover larvae. Filter paper strips are coated on one side with feces and placed into a tube containing a small amount of water. The tube is kept upright so that the filter paper is kept moist by capillary action. After 4–10 days the filter paper is removed and the water examined for larvae.

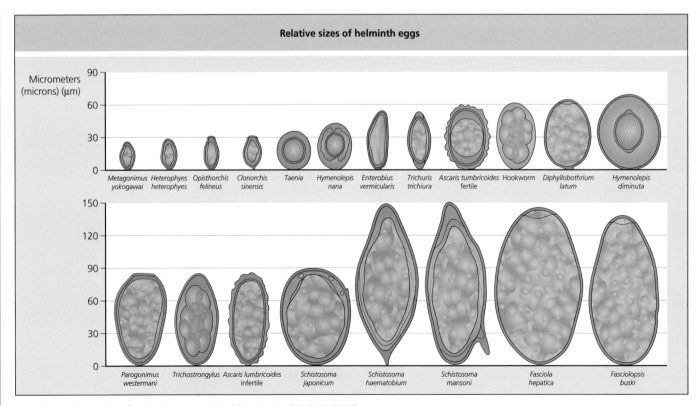

Fig. 184.6 Relative size of helminth eggs. HHS Publication No. (CDC 89–8116)

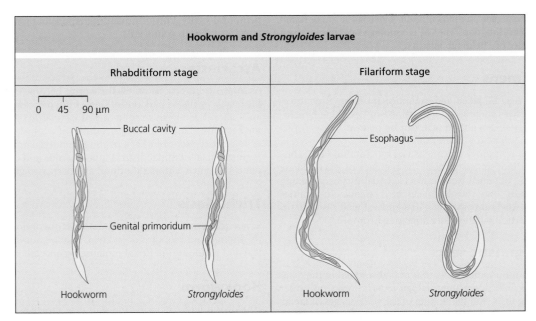

Fig. 184.7 Hookworm and *Strongyloides* larvae. HHS Publication No. (CDC 89–8116)

An agar plate culture for *Strongyloides* spp. has been developed.[33] A few grams of feces are placed into the center of the agar and the plate is incubated at room temperature for 48 hours. Tracks are made by the parasite in the agar and the larvae can be recovered by a Pasteur pipette and placed onto a microscope slide for identification.

Eggs of some parasites can be picked up on perianal swabs. Swabs such as scotch tape or paddle swabs are placed on the perianal area and then placed under a microscope for examination. Pinworm, tapeworm and *A. lumbricoides* eggs can be recovered.

Eggs of *Schistosoma* spp. can be found in feces using some of the above-mentioned examinations. An egg-hatching technique can also be used in which feces are placed into a sidearm flask and water added until it reaches a level just below the sidearm. When the suspension settles more water is added until the level is above the sidearm. A dark cloth or bag is placed over the flask without covering the sidearm. The sidearm is then placed into the light and hatching miracidia from the schistosome eggs will be attracted to the light. They can be examined microscopically.

Specimens can be collected directly from the duodenum and examined for helminthic infections. Material collected by duodenal aspiration can be examined microscopically for *Strongyloides* and *Ascaris* spp. and flukes.

The Entero-Test or string capsule is also available for examining duodenal specimens. A gelatin capsule containing a string is swallowed and the end of the string taped to the cheek. The string in the capsule contains a small weight that carries the string down the duodenum after the capsule dissolves. After 4 hours the string is pulled up and the mucus adhering to the string is placed onto a microscope slide and examined.

Tapeworm proglottids are at times found in stool specimens. These segments should be washed in water and placed between two microscope slides. The slides are than tied together with string and the specimens placed into a fixative – alcohol, formalin, acetic acid (AFA). After fixation the worms can be stained and examined for specific identification. If the proglottids have rosette-shaped uterine branches the worm can be identified as a diphyllobothriid. The number of uterine branches of *Taenia* spp. can be counted and the specimen identified as *T. solium* (6–11) or *T. saginata* (15–20). India ink can be injected into the uterine pore and the branches are then more easily counted.

Adult trematodes found in feces should be washed and placed between two microscope slides that are then tied together with string. The specimens are than placed into a fixative such as AFA. After fixation the worms can be stained and examined for speciation.

Sputum specimens

Sputum to be examined for eggs or larvae should be mixed with 3% sodium hydroxide, centrifuged and the sediment examined.

Urine specimens

Urine specimens will sometimes help in the diagnosis of *S. haematobium* eggs or microfilariae of *W. bancrofti* and *O. volvulus*. The urine specimen is centrifuged and the sediment examined.

Blood samples

Several of the filarial infections can be diagnosed by the examination of drops of blood from finger or ear lobe pricks. The blood is placed onto a microscope slide and covered with a coverglass and examined under low power for thrashing microfilariae. For specific identification thick blood smears are made with several drops of blood, the smear is permitted to dry for several hours and then stained with Giemsa stain. Identifications are based upon, for example, microfilarial sizes, cephalic space and tail nuclei. Microfilariae of *W. bancrofti*, *B. malayi*, *B. timori* and *L. loa* are present in the blood. *Onchocerca volvulus* microfilariae are found in skin snips.

Blood should be obtained at night for most lymphatic filariae and in the daytime for *L. loa*. Microfilariae can also be recovered from blood by membrane filtration. In some cases of lymphatic filariasis adult worms may be seen by ultrasound and the worms can be seen 'dancing' in the lymph channels.[34]

Cerebrospinal fluid

Cerebrospinal fluid is examined for evidence of helminthic infections. Eosinophilic pleocytosis is suggestive of angiostrongyliasis, paragonimiasis, cysticercosis, gnathostomiasis and schistosomiasis. Larvae of *A. cantonensis* are reported in CSF, especially in children, and *T. spiralis* larvae can be found in the CSF in very heavy infections. The CSF is centrifuged and the sediment examined for evidence of a helminth infection.

Tissue specimens

Tissue specimens may be taken and examined for helminthic infections. Muscle biopsies can be sectioned, stained and examined microscopically for *T. spiralis*, or the muscle can be pressed between two glass slides and examined for trichina larvae.

Rectal and bladder biopsy specimens can be examined for schistosome eggs. Skin biopsies may reveal the presence of microfilariae of *O. volvulus*. Fluid obtained from suspected hydatid cysts, although dangerous to obtain, may reveal scolices of *E. granulosus*. Biopsies can also be made when anticipating a diagnosis of gnathostomiasis, sparganosis or infection with another migrating helminth.

Immunodiagnostic tests

There are myriad immunodiagnostic tests available to aid in the diagnosis of helminthic infections. Immunologic tests, however, only offer a presumptive diagnosis, and the finding of the worms, eggs or larvae provides the definitive diagnosis. Immunologic tests are useful when the parasite is not demonstrated such as in cases of toxocariasis and in some cases of cysticercosis and echinococcosis. Immunodiagnostic tests have been developed for most parasitic diseases to detect antibodies as well as antigens. Techniques in molecular biology have also been emerging and may eventually become valuable tools in detecting helminthic infections.[35]

Detailed information on immunologic and molecular methods in the diagnosis of parasitic diseases has been presented elsewhere.[36] Older tests such as complement fixation are still of value in the diagnosis of cysticercosis, paragonimiasis and schistosomiasis, especially for indicating active infections. Gel diffusion has been used in fascioliasis and the circumoval precipitation test (COPT) is used to detect antibodies in cases of schistosomiasis. In the latter, eggs of schistosomes develop precipitates around the shell in the presence of antibody-positive sera.

The enzyme-linked immunosorbent assay (ELISA) is currently one of the most widely used tests for many parasitoses. Indirect fluorescent antibody is also used, especially on tissue and parasite sections, to detect antigenic material. The indirect hemagglutination test along with EIA (enzyme immunoassay) is used for hydatid disease and EIA for cysticercosis. An EIA test is now recommended for strongyloidiasis, toxocariasis and other larval migrans. It is also of value in the diagnosis of paragonimiasis, schistosomiasis, trichinosis, angiostrongyliasis, gnathostomiasis and filariasis. *Taenia*-specific antigens can be detected in human feces by ELISA.[37]

The immunoblot or Western blot is being applied to the diagnosis of most helminthiases, especially fascioliasis, schistosomiasis, paragonimiasis and cysticercosis. Molecular diagnostics have been reported for most species of parasites, and mostly applied to research laboratories; the detection of DNA by the polymerase chain reaction (PCR) is reported for the most important human helminths. For example, a PCR assay has been developed to detect *W. bancrofti* DNA in blood[38] and a PCR to determine the presence of *W. bancrofti* DNA in vector mosquitoes.[39]

CLINICAL MANIFESTATIONS

An intestinal helminthiasis is usually unnoticed unless a large worm is found by the patient in the feces.

Pinworms

Pinworms generally cause little disease, but in children infections lead to perianal itching, eczema, nose-picking, pica and loss of sleep. Worms may migrate into the vagina, uterus and fallopian tubes and peritoneal cavity. Pinworms can be responsible for recurrent urinary tract infections in young girls.

Ascariasis

Ascariasis is innocuous unless the worms become erratic and migrate into vital organs or pass out of one of the orifices – nose, mouth or anus. Erratic ascariasis may be caused by anesthesia, trauma or some medications. A bolus of a large number of worms can cause volvulus or intussusception, blockage of the bile ducts, cholangitis, intestinal perforation, abdominal distress, pneumonitis and cough. Infection is often associated with malnutrition and decreased growth.

Trichuriasis

Severe trichuriasis can lead to abdominal discomfort, dysentery, colitis, anemia and bloody stools. There may be nutritional loss, weight loss and malnutrition. Rectal prolapse occurs with some infections.

Hookworm

Hookworm larvae entering the skin may provoke a ground itch and secondary bacterial infections. Migrating larvae can cause pneumonitis and eosinophilia, and worms in the intestine can cause abdominal pain, nausea, vomiting and diarrhea. Large numbers of worms sucking blood cause iron deficiency anemia, hypoproteinemia and hepatosplenomegaly, and children will have impaired mental, physical and sexual development. Severe malnutrition develops, especially with concomitant infections with *A. lumbricoides* and *T. trichiura*.

Toxocariasis

Toxocariasis (visceral larva migrans) causes hypereosinophilia, hepatomegaly and symptoms of chronic pulmonary inflammation with cough. There may also be visual difficulties due to retinochoroiditis or peripheral retinitis.

Strongyloides stercoralis

Early infections with *S. stercoralis* are similar to hookworm infections, causing ground itch and pneumonitis. Worms in the intestines cause inflammation, irritation, diarrhea, intestinal bleeding and melena. Sprue-like symptoms may also develop, along with malabsorption, weight loss and eosinophilia. Dermal lesions may occur with urticarial eruptions on the buttocks, termed larval currens. Immunocompromised people, especially those with human T-cell leukemia virus 1 (HTLV-1) associated lymphoma, are at risk of developing disseminated strongyloidiasis and present with severe enteritis, a protein-losing enteropathy, bronchitis, pneumonia, pleural effusion, cough and a blood-tinged sputum with rhabditiform larvae; this is often referred to as the 'hyperinfection syndrome'. Eosinophilia is usually absent in these cases. Death may result. Disseminated strongyloidiasis may also present as Gram-negative pneumonia or meningitis, or as a polymicrobial bacteremia, with bacteria being spread by worms migrating from the bowel.

Capillariasis philippinensis

Capillariasis philippinensis leads to a protein-losing enteropathy, malabsorption, electrolyte imbalance, weight loss, wasting and death. Patients initially present with abdominal pain, borborygmi and diarrhea. Untreated infections usually lead to death.[25]

Trichinosis

Trichinosis is asymptomatic except when a large number of trichina larvae are ingested. Adult worms in the small intestines cause symptoms of gastroenteritis, nausea, abdominal pain, anorexia, diarrhea, fever and weight loss. During the migratory phase, muscle and joint pain develop, followed by periorbital edema and eosinophilia. Larvae can cause cell destruction, acute inflammatory changes and interstitial myocarditis. The infection can also cause neurologic and pulmonary complications.

Lymphatic filariasis (see Chapter 115)

Symptoms associated with lymphatic filariasis are associated with the host's immune status; little immunity is associated with more severe disease. Early symptoms are fever, lymphangitis, lymphedema and lymphadenitis, which may be transitory and occur periodically. Scrotal involvement leads to orchitis, hydrocele and chyluria. Worms may block the lymph flow leading to lymphatic varicoses and eventual skin fibrosis, thickening and elephantiasis. Renal lesions may also occur, with microfilariae in the urine and chyluria. There may be enlargement of the legs, arms, scrotum, mammary glands and vulva. Tropical pulmonary eosinophilia with fever, splenomegaly, pulmonary infiltrates and hypereosinophilia is associated with *W. bancrofti* and *B. malayi* infections. Microfilariae are absent and are probably destroyed by host immune mechanisms in chronic infections.

Subcutaneous migration of *L. loa* may cause transient swelling known as Calabar swellings, which are a local reaction to the worm and its products. It is characterized by fever, eosinophilia and the urticarial swellings, which are more common in Caucasians. Migrating adult worms may pass over the bridge of the nose or through the conjunctiva across the eyeball. Migration of the worms in abnormal locations can cause symptoms in the scrotum, bowel, kidney and heart, but not usually in natives living in the African endemic areas. Visitors suffer more than indigenous populations.

Oncocercomas due to *O. volvulus* develop over bony prominences. Some nodules develop in deeper tissue and are unnoticeable. Dermatitis and blindness are caused by the microfilariae. Recent investigations suggest that the inflammatory response in the eye is induced by the endosymbiotic *Wolbachia* bacteria released by dead microfilariae.[20] Lymph nodes in the groin may show lymphocyte depletion and fibrosis, followed by 'hanging groin', especially in Africans. In the Americas nodules commonly develop on the upper part of the body, whereas in Africa the nodules develop on lower parts of the body.

Guinea worm

Guinea worm in the subcutaneous tissue elicits allergic manifestations such as itching. When the female worms get close to the skin there is a localized erythema followed by pruritus, nausea, vomiting, diarrhea or asthmatic symptoms. The worm will secrete a toxic substance that causes a blister, which breaks when the area comes in contact with water, and the female releases larvae when the lesion opens up. The area becomes painful. The worm will eventually die and is resorbed or becomes calcified.

Angiostrongylus cantonensis and *Angiostrongylus costaricensis*

Migrating third-stage larvae of *A. cantonensis* may cause vague symptoms of gastroenteritis, vomiting, headache and fever. Once the worms reach the CNS they cause headache, nausea, vomiting, stiff neck, myalgia, pain and paresthesia. Coma may be a feature of heavy infections. Worms have been seen in the eyes of some patients. There may be paralysis of eye muscles. Frequent signs are abnormal tendon reflexes including abnormal Achilles' reflex, a positive Kernig's sign and impaired sensorium and vision. Infections with a large number of worms may be fatal.[10]

Abdominal angiostrongyliasis due to *A. costaricensis* resembles acute appendicitis. A tumor-like mass is palpable in the right lower quadrant. There may be fever, diarrhea or vomiting, along with eosinophilia.[40]

Gnathastome and anisakid larvae

Shortly after ingestion of gnathostome larvae there are symptoms of nausea, vomiting, pruritus and urticaria, and at times upper abdominal pain. Larval invasion into the liver will cause right upper quadrant tenderness and changes in liver function. In the lung there is a pulmonary infiltration and pneumothorax in patients with pleural infusion. Larvae migrating through the subcutaneous tissue and skin cause a rash along with red pruritic painless swellings. Invasion of the CNS often leads to death.

Anisakid larvae in the throat may lead to a 'tickle-throat', causing cough, but when they invade the mucosa of the intestinal tract they provoke eosinophilic granuloma formation, severe abdominal pain, nausea, vomiting and diarrhea. Usually, only a single worm is involved and the symptoms disappear when it is removed.

Trematodes

The trematodes, like the nematodes, cause little disease unless a large number of worms are involved. The liver flukes (*C. sinensis, O. viverrini, O. felineus*) in the bile ducts may cause symptoms early in the infection such as hepatomegaly, jaundice, diarrhea, anorexia, epigastric pain and fever. Repeated infection over a period of years may lead to ductal fibrosis, obstruction, cholangitis, cholecystitis and cirrhosis, and in some patients cholangiocarcinoma.

The sheep liver fluke *F. hepatica*, because of its large size, may block the bile ducts and cause cholangitis. Toxic secretions cause fever, chills, jaundice, an enlarged tender liver, cough, vomiting, abdominal symptoms and eosinophilia. Young worms may attack the pharyngeal mucosa, causing bleeding and edema. This occurs after eating raw sheep liver containing the parasite. The condition has been called halzoun.

The large intestinal fluke *F. buski* may cause intestinal blockage and toxemia when there is a large number of worms. Eosinophilia is common and ulcers may develop, which often hemorrhage. It causes abdominal distention, hunger pains and increased appetite, diarrhea and a foul-smelling yellowish stool. Allergic manifestations, nausea, vomiting, ascites and cachexia develop as a result of toxins secreted by the worms. Other intestinal flukes cause little disease, but tiny eggs of the heterophyids may enter the mucosa and are carried to ectopic locations such as the brain and heart, provoking granuloma formation. Echinostomes may produce inflammation and ulceration with diarrhea and abdominal pain.

The young lung fluke of *P. westermani* produces little disease during migration, but once established in the lung may cause fever, dyspnea, cough, chest pain and the production of a rusty sputum. At first the disease is often thought to be tuberculosis. The worms may enter the cranial cavity and invade the brain causing fever, headache, nausea, vomiting and visual disturbances, convulsions and meningeal signs.

Schistosome infections (see Chapter 112)

There may be petechial hemorrhages at the site of penetration where schistosome cercariae enter the skin. There will be localized edema and pruritus. After a few weeks there are toxic or allergic reactions and symptoms include fever, nausea, abdominal pain, rigor, urticarial rashes and eosinophilia. This acute stage is known as Katayama syndrome. In the chronic stage granulomas have formed around the eggs in tissue and hepatomegaly develops and the spleen becomes enlarged. This is followed by esophageal varices and finally ascites. Intestinal disease, usually with *S. mansoni* and *S. japonicum*, may involve the entire intestine or more often the large bowel. There may be abdominal cramps, tenderness and bloody mucoid stools. A protein-losing enteropathy, weight loss and anemia may also develop.

Features of *S. haematobium* infection are dysuria, urinary frequency and hematuria. Eosinophils in the urine are not uncommon. Heavy infections, with the deposition of many eggs in the bladder tissue, can lead to squamous cell carcinoma.

Pulmonary involvement can be a feature of all schistosome infections, and causes cor pulmonale with dyspnea, cough and hemoptysis.

Cerebral manifestations are common in oriental schistosomiasis, with symptoms of lethargy and confusion followed by speech difficulties and optical field defects. *Schistosoma mansoni* occasionally causes the spinal cord symptoms of a transverse myelitis, usually in the lumbar region. Flaccid paralysis of the lower limbs is also reported.

Tapeworm (see Chapter 113)

Tapeworm, even the larger ones, in the small intestines provoke few symptoms. Patients usually become aware of being infected only when worm segments are passed in the feces. If *D. latum* attaches to the proximal portion of the jejunum vitamin B12 deficiency results, with the development of pernicious anemia. This was seen in Finland but is now very rare. Sparganosis associated with other diphyllobothriid species causes painful inflammatory swellings, which may be transient. Spargana in the eyes cause intense reactions and periorbital edema.

Taenia spp. in the intestine are asymptomatic in most patients, but some have hunger pains, abdominal discomfort and indigestion. Patients usually become symptomatic when proglottids are found in the feces or passing from the anus. Eosinophilia is not uncommon. Cysticercosis or infection with larvae of *T. solium* is a serious disease, especially if there are cysticerci in the CNS. Cysticerci in the muscle are asymptomatic, but can give rise to myositis, fever and eosinophilia. The cysticerci usually die and become calcified. Cysticerci in the eye cause visual symptoms such as a decrease in visual acuity, retinal edema and hemorrhage. Neurocysticercosis results in arachnoiditis with CSF pleocytosis and an increase in CSF pressure. Obstructive hydrocephalus, cerebral infarction, epilepsy, papilledema, vomiting, headache, a toxic gait and intellectual deterioration may also develop. Dead or dying parasites may exacerbate symptoms, and location of the parasite in the CNS is responsible for a variety of CNS symptoms.

Hyperinfections with *H. nana* may cause diarrhea, loss of appetite, abdominal pain, headache, weakness, and at times epileptoid convulsion, dizziness and eosinophilia. *Hymenolepis diminuta* may cause diarrhea.

Hydatid disease (see Chapter 114)

There are usually no symptoms with hydatid disease until the cysts are large and in vital organs. Many years are usually required for a cyst to reach a significant size. Cysts in the liver may put pressure on the bile ducts and blood vessels. Large cysts in the lung can cause cough, shortness of breath and chest pains. Involvement of the CNS results in different symptoms depending upon the location of the cyst. Leaks of hydatid fluid sensitize the patient and can cause anaphylactic shock. A cyst in the eye causes proptosis.

MANAGEMENT (SEE CHAPTERS 113, 115 AND 150)

Management of helminthic infection is variable and depends upon the specific parasite, the location in the host and the number of worms involved.

REFERENCES

References for this chapter can be found online at http://www.expertconsult.com

Index

Note: Page numbers in **bold** refer to major discussions. Page numbers suffixed by (i) refer to illustrations and page number suffixed by (t) refer to tables. Page numbers suffixed by (PP) refer to Practice Points.

Index

Index